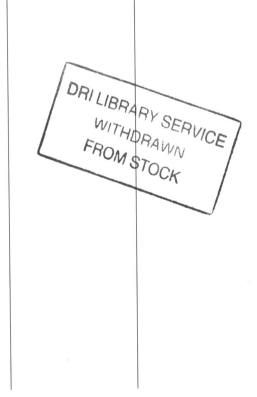

PEDIATRIC ENDOCRINOLOGY AND INBORN ERRORS OF METABOLISM

PEDIATRIC ENDOCRINOLOGY AND INBORN ERRORS OF METABOLISM

Editor

Kyriakie Sarafoglou, MD

Director, Leo Fung Center for Congenital Adrenal Hyperplasia
& Disorders of Sex Development
Division of Pediatric Endocrinology
Division of Genetics & Metabolism
University of Minnesota Medical School
University of Minnesota Children's Hospital-Fairview
Minneapolis, Minnesota, USA

Associate Editors

Georg F. Hoffmann, MD
Univ.-Prof. Dr. med., Prof. h.c. (RCH)

Geschäftsführender Direktor
Universitäts-Kinderklinik
Direktor Abteilung I (Schwerpunkte: Allgemeine Kinderheilkunde,
Stoffwechsel, Gastroenterologie, Nephrologie)
Heidelberg, Baden-Württemberg, Germany

Karl S. Roth, MD

Professor & Chair
Department of Pediatrics
Creighton University School of Medicine
Omaha, Nebraska, USA

Consulting Editor
Howard Courtney, M.Phil.

New York   Chicago   San Francisco   Lisbon   London   Madrid   Mexico City
Milan   New Delhi   San Juan   Seoul   Singapore   Sydney   Toronto

The McGraw·Hill Companies

1 2 3 4 5 6 7 8 9 0   CTP/CTP   12 11 10 9 8

ISBN 978-0-07-143915-2
MHID 0-07-143915-3

This book was set in *Electra LH* by Aptara®, Inc.
The editor was Jim Shanahan.
The production supervisor was Catherine Saggese.
The cover designer was Janice Bielawa.
The text designer was Alan Barnett.
The indexer was Ann Blum.
Project Management was provided by Sandhya Joshi, Aptara®, Inc.
China Translation & Printing Services Ltd. was printer and binder.

This book is printed on acid-free paper.

Library of Congress Cataloging-in-Publication Data

Sarafoglou, Kyriakie.
    Pediatric endocrinology and inborn errors of metabolism/Kyriakie
Sarafoglou; associate editors, Georg Hoffmann, Karl Roth; consulting
editor, Howard Courtney.
       p.; cm.
    Includes bibliographical references and index.
    ISBN-13: 978-0-07-143915-2 (alk. paper)
    ISBN-10: 0-07-143915-3 (alk. paper)
  1. Pediatric endocrinology. 2. Metabolism, Inborn errors of. I.
Hoffman, Georg. II. Title.
    [DNLM: 1. Endocrine System Diseases. 2. Child. 3. Metabolism, Inborn
Errors. WS 330 S243p 2008]
RJ418.S37 2008
618.92'4—dc22
                                   2007045992

DEDICATION

To the memory of Robert Gorlin and Thomas Moshang

CONTENTS

CONTRIBUTORS

Brage S. Andresen, PhD
Associate Professor of Human Genetics
Institute of Human Genetics
Research Unit for Molecular Medicine
Århus University Hospital, Skejby
Århus, Denmark

Stephen Ball, PhD, FRCP
Senior Lecturer in Endocrinology
School of Clinical Medical Sciences
University of Newcastle Medical School
Newcastle Upon Tyne, United Kingdom

Manisha Balwani, MD, MS
Assistant Professor
Department of Genetics and Genomic Sciences
   and Medicine
Mount Sinai School of Medicine
New York, New York, USA

Andrew J. Bauer, MD
Associate Professor of Pediatrics
Fellowship Program Director in Pediatric Endocrinology
   Uniformed Services University, Bethesda, MD
Chief, Pediatric Endocrinology
Walter Reed Army Medical Center,
Washington, DC, USA

Melena Bellin, MD
Fellow, Pediatric Endocrinology
University of Minnesota Medical School
University of Minnesota Children's Hospital, Fairview
Minneapolis, Minnesota, USA

Michael J. Bennett PhD, FRCPath, FACB
Professor of Pathology and Laboratory Medicine
University of Pennsylvania School of Medicine
Holder, Evelyn Willing Bromley Endowed Chair
   in Clinical Labortories and Pathology
Director, Metabolic Disease Laboratory
Children's Hospital of Philadelphia
Philadelphia, Pennsylvania, USA

Susan A. Berry, MD
Professor of Pediatrics, Ophthalmology, and Genetics,
   Cell Biology & Development
Director, Division of Genetics and Metabolism
Institute of Human Genetics
University of Minnesota Medical School
University of Minnesota Children's Hospital, Fairview
Minneapolis, Minnesota, USA

Bala Bhagavath, MD
Assistant Professor
Warren Alpert Medical School of Brown University
Division of Reproductive Endocrinology and Infertility
Women and Infants Hospital
Providence, Rhode Island, USA

Nenad Blau, PhD
Professor of Clinical Biochemistry
Division of Clinical Chemistry and Biochemistry
University Children's Hospital Zurich
Zurich, Switzerland

Walter O. Bockting, PhD
Associate Professor
Department of Family Medicine and Community Health
Coordinator of Transgender Health Services, Program in
   Human Sexuality
Behavior Specialist, Leo Fung Center for Congenital Adrenal
   Hyperplasia and Disorders of Sex Development
University of Minnesota Medical School
Minneapolis, Minnesota, USA

Peter Burgard, PD Dr. phil
Pädiatrische Psychologie
Zentrum für Kinder- und Jugendmedizin der Universität Heidelberg
Klinik I (Schwerpunkte: Allgemeine Kinderheilkunde,
   Stoffwechsel, Gastroenterologie, Nephrologie)
Heidelberg, Germany

Bruce R. Carr, MD
Holder, Paul C. MacDonald Distinguished Chair in
   Obstetrics and Gynecology
Professor of Obstrtrics and Gynecology
Director, Division of Reproductive Endocrinology and Infertility
University of Texas Southwestern Medical Center
Dallas, Texas, USA

Marcelle I. Cedars, MD
Professor, Department of Obstetrics, Gynecology, and
   Reproductive Sciences
Vice Chair for Clinical Programs
Director, Division of Reproductive Endocrinology
Director of Reproductive Laboratories
University of California-San Francisco
UCSF Medical Center
San Francisco, California, USA

James C. M. Chan, MD
Professor of Pediatrics
University of Vermont
Director of Research
The Barbara Bush Children's Hospital
Maine Medical Center
Portland, Maine, USA

Tim Cheetham, MD
Senior Lecturer in Pediatric Endocrinology
School of Clinical Medical Sciences (Child Health)
Sir James Spence Institute of Child Health
Royal Victoria Infirmary
Newcastle Upon Tyne, United Kingdom

George P. Chrousos, MD, FAAP, MACP, MACE, FRCP
Professor and Chairman
First Department of Pediatrics
Athens University Medical School
Aghia Sophia Children's Hospital
Athens, Greece

Tina M. Cowan, PhD, FACMG
Associate Professor of Pathology and Pediatrics
Director, Stanford Biochemical Genetics Laboratory
Stanford University Medical Center
Stanford, California, USA

Gregory M. Enns, MB, ChB
Director, Biochemical Genetics Program
Division of Medical Genetics
Stanford University Medical School
Stanford, California, USA

Brian Fowler, PhD
Professor in Clinical Chemistry
Head of Laboratories, Metabolic Unit
University Children's Hospital
Basel, Switzerland

J. Paul Frindik, MD
Associate Professor of Pediatrics
Division of Pediatric Endocrinology
University of Arkansas for Medical Sciences
Arkansas Children's Hospital
Little Rock, Arkansas, USA

Brigitte I. Frohnert, MD, PhD, FAAP
Fellow, Pediatric Endocrinology
University of Minnesota Medical School
University of Minnesota Children's Hospital-Fairview
Minneapolis, Minnesota, USA

K. Michael Gibson, PhD, FACMG
Professor of Pediatrics and Pathology
University of Pittsburgh School of Medicine
Director, Biochemical Genetics/Nutrition Laboratory
Division of Medical Genetics
Children's Hospital of Pittsburgh
Pittsburgh, Pennsylvania, USA

Dorothea Haas, MD
University Hospital
Center for Pediatric and Adolescent Medicine
Division of Inborn Metabolic Diseases
Heidelberg, Germany

Kathryn D. Harrington, MD
Pediatric Resident
University of Minnesota Medical School
University of Minnesota Children's Hospital, Fairview
Minneapolis, Minnesota, USA

Georg F. Hoffmann, MD, Univ.-Prof. Dr. med., Prof. h.c. (RCH)
Geschäftsführender Direktor
Universitäts-Kinderklinik
Direktor Abteilung I (Schwerpunkte: Allgemeine Kinderheilkunde,
   Stoffwechsel, Gastroenterologie, Nephrologie)
Heidelberg, Baden-Württemberg, Germany

Irene Hong-McAtee, MD, FAAP, MSCR
Assistant Professor of Pediatrics
Division of Pediatric Endocrinology and Diabetes
University of Kentucky School of Medicine
Lexington, Kentucky, USA

Christopher P. Houk, MD, FAAP
Associate Professor of Pediatrics
Division of Pediatric Endocrinology
Medical College of Georgia
Backus Children's Hospital at
   Memorial Health University Medical Center
Savannah, Georgia, USA

Keith Hyland, PhD
Director, Department of Neurochemistry
Vice President, Medical Neurogenetics
Atlanta, Georgia, USA

Andrea Kelly, MD
Assistant Professor of Pediatrics
University of Pennsylvania School of Medicine
Fellowship Director, Division of Endocrinology/Diabetes
The Children's Hospital of Philadelphia
Philadelphia, Pennsylvania, USA

Richard I. Kelley, MD, PhD
Professor of Pediatrics
Johns Hopkins University School of Medicine
Director, Clinical Mass Spectrometry Laboratory
Kennedy Krieger Institute
Baltimore, Maryland, USA

Stephen F. Kemp, MD, PhD
Professor of Pediatrics and Medical Humanities
Division of Pediatric Endocrinology
University of Arkansas for Medical Sciences
Arkansas Children's Hospital
Little Rock, Arkansas, USA

Douglas S. Kerr, MD, PhD
Professor, Pediatrics, Biochemistry, and Nutrition
Case Western Reserve University School of Medicine
Director, Center for Inherited Disorders of Energy Metabolism
Pediatric Endocrinology and Metabolism
Rainbow Babies and Childrens Hospital
University Hospitals Case Medical Center
Cleveland, Oklahoma, USA

David M. Koeller, MD
Associate Professor of Pediatrics
Chief, Division of Metabolism
Director, Metabolic Clinic
Oregon Health & Science University
Portland, Oregon, USA

Prof. Dr. Christian Körner, PhD
Universitätskinderklinik / Universitätsklinik für Kinder- und
   Jugendmedizin
Heidelberg, Germany

Peter A. Lee, MD, PhD
Professor of Pediatrics
Penn State College of Medicine
The Milton S Hershey Medical Center
Hershey, Pennsylvania, USA

James V Leonard PhD, FRCP, FRCPCH
Professor Emeritus
Clinical and Molecular Genetics Unit
Institute of Child Health
University College London and Former Consultant Paediatrician,
Great Ormond Street Hospital for Children
London, United Kingdom

Xiaoping Luo, MD
Professor of Pediatrics
Chairman, Department of Pediatrics
Tongji Hospital
Director, Center for the Diagnosis of Genetic Metabolic Diseases
Tongji Medical College Huazhong University of Science
    and Technology
Wuhan, Hubei, China

Maria Alexandra Magiakou, MD
Assistant Professor of Pediatric Endocrinology
First Department of Pediatrics
Athens University "Agia Sofia" Children's Hospital
Athens, Greece

Dietrich Matern, MD, FACMG
Associate Professor of Laboratory Medicine
Head, Biochemical Genetics Laboratory
Mayo Clinic College of Medicine
Rochester, Minnesota, USA

Ertan Mayatepek, MD
Professor and Chairman
Department of General Pediatrics
University Children's Hospital
Dusseldorf, Germany

Bradley S. Miller, MD, PhD, FAAP
Assistant Professor
Director of Growth Programs
Division of Endocrinology
Department of Pediatrics
University of Minnesota Medical School
University of Minnesota Children's Hospital-Fairview
Minneapolis, Minnesota, USA

Chantal F. Morel, MD, FRCPC, FCCMG
Clinical and Metabolic Geneticist
Assistant Professor, Department of Medicine
University of Toronto
University Health Network and Mount Sinai Hospital
Toronto, Ontario, Canada

Andrew A. M. Morris, PhD, FRCPCH
Consultant and Honorary Senior Lecturer in
    Paediatric Metabolic Medicine
Willink Unit,
Royal Manchester Children's Hospital
Manchester, United Kingdom

Thomas Moshang, Jr., MD
Professor of Pediatrics (CHOP), Emeritus
University of Pennsylvania School of Medicine
Children's Hospital of Philadelphia
Philadelphia, Pennsylvania, USA

Sogol Mostoufi-Moab, MD
Instructor
University of Pennsylvania School of Medicine
Children's Hospital of Philadelphia
Philadelphia, Pennsylvania, USA

Brandon Nathan, MD
Assistant Professor of Pediatrics
Associate Director, Pediatric Endocrinology Fellowship Program
University of Minnesota Medical School
University of Minnesota Children's Hospital-Fairview
Minneapolis, Minnesota, USA

William L. Nyhan MD, PhD
Professor of Pediatrics
Director Biochemical Genetics Laboratory
University of California San Diego Medical Center
La Jolla, California, USA

Karel Pacak, MD, PhD, DSc
Chief, Clinical Neuroendocrinology Unit
Section on Medical Neuroendocrinology
Reproductive Biology and Medicine Branch
National Institute of Child Health and Human Development
National Institutes of Health
Bethesda, Maryland, USA

Darius A. Paduch, MD, PhD
Assistant Professor of Urology and Reproductive Medicine
Director, Male Infertility-Genetics Laboratory
Center for Male Reproductive Medicine and Microsurgery
Weill Medical College of Cornell University
New York, New York, USA

Sherly Pardo-Reoyo, MD
Fellow Department of Genetics and
    Genomic Sciences and Medicine
Mount Sinai School of Medicine
New York, New York, USA

Anna Petryk, MD
Assistant Professor
Department of Pediatrics, and Genetics, Cell Biology
    and Development
University of Minnesota Medical School
University of Minnesota Children's Hospital, Fairview
Minneapolis, Minnesota, USA

Jordan Pinsker, MD
Assistant Professor of Pediatrics
F. Edward Hébert School of Medicine
Uniformed Services University of the Health Sciences
Tripler Army Medical Center
Honolulu, HI
Honolulu, Hawaii

Michel Polak, MD, PhD
Professeur des Universités/Praticien Hospitalier
Service d'Endocrinologie Pédiatrique and
Institut National de la Santé et de la Recherche Médicale
Hôpital Necker Enfants Malades
Paris, France

Lynda E. Polgreen, MD
Assistant Professor of Pediatrics
Division of Pediatric Endocrinology
University of Minnesota Medical School
University of Minnesota Children's Hospital
Minneapolis, Minnesota, USA

Constantin Polychronakos, MD
Professor, Pediatrics and Human Genetics
Director, Pediatric Endocrinology and Diabetes
McGill University Faculty of Medicine
McGill University Health Center
Montreal Quebec, Canada

Zubin Punthakee, MD
Assistant Professor, Pediatrics and Medicine
Division of Endocrinology and Metabolism
McGill University Faculty of Medicine
McGill University Health Center
Montreal Quebec, Canada

Sandeep Raha, PhD
Assistant Professor of Pediatrics
McMaster University Faculty of Medicine
McMaster University Medical Center
Hamilton, Ontario, Canada

Mitchell P. Rosen, MD
Assistant Professor
Department of Obstetrics, Gynecology and Reproductive Sciences
University of California-San Francisco
UCSF Medical Center
San Francisco, California, USA

Betsey Schwartz, MD
Division of Pediatric Endocrinology
Park Nicollet Methodist Hospital
St. Louis Park, Minnesota, USA

David S, Rosenblatt MDCM, FCCMG, FRCPC, FCAHS
Professor and Chairman, Department of Human Genetics
Professor, Departments of Medicine and Pediatrics
Director, Division of Medical Genetics, Department of Medicine
McGill University
Montreal, Quebec, Canada

Karl S. Roth, MD
Professor & Chair
Department of Pediatrics
Creighton University School of Medicine
Omaha, Nebraska, USA

Kumud Sane, MD
Assistant Professor
Division of Pediatric Endocrinology
University of Minnesota Medical School
Minneapolis, Minnesota, USA

Shashikant M. Sane, MD
Professor and Chairman,
Pediatric Radiology
Childrens Hospitals and Clinics of Minnesota
Minneapolis, Minnesota, USA

Claude Sansaricq MD, PhD
Professorial Lecturer
Ex Associate Professor
Department of Genetics and Genomic Sciences and Pediatrics
Ex Director IEM Facilities

Mount Sinai School of Medicine
New York, USA

Kyriakie Sarafoglou, MD
Director, Leo Fung Center for CAH & Disorders of
    Sex Development
Division of Pediatric Endocrinology
Division of Genetics & Metabolism
University of Minnesota Medical School
University of Minnesota Children's Hospital, Fairview
Minneapolis, Minnesota, USA

Juergen R. Schäfer, PD
Department of Internal Medicine
Cardiology, Angiology and CAD Prevention
University Hospital Giessen and Philipps University Marburg
Marburg, Germany

Andreas Schulze, MD, FRCPC
Associate Professor of Paediatrics & Biochemistry
Medical Director, Newborn Screening Program
Department of Pediatrics
Division of Clinical and Metabolic Genetics
The Research Institute Genetics and Genome Biology Program
University of Toronto
The Hospital for Sick Children, Toronto
Ontario, Canada

Peter N. Schlegel, MD
Professor in Urology and Reproductive Medicine
Chairman, Department of Urology
Weill Medical College of Cornell University
New York, New York, USA

Radhakant Sharma, PhD
Department of Neurochemistry
Horizon Molecular Medicine
Atlanta, Georgia, USA

Hilary Smith, MD
Pediatric Resident
Children's Hospital of Pittsburgh
University of Pittsburgh School of Medicine
Pittsburgh, Pennsylvania, USA

Stephen B. Sondike, MD
Section Head, Adolescent Medicine
Charleston Area Medical Center
Associate Professor of Pediatrics
West Virginia School of Medicine
Charleston, West Virginia, USA

Muhidien Soufi, MD
Department of Internal Medicine
Cardiology, Angiology and CAD Prevention
University Hospital Giessen and Philipps University Marburg
Marburg, Germany

Charles A. Stanley, MD
Professor of Pediatrics
University of Pennsylvania School of Medicine
Director, Hyperinsulinism Center
Division of Endocrinology and Diabetes
The Children's Hospital of Philadelphia
Philadelphia, Pennsylvania, USA

Julia Steinberger, MD, MS
Associate Professor in Pediatric Cardiology
Director, Pediatric Lipid Clinic

Medical Director, Pediatric Echocardiography Laboratory
University of Minnesota Medical School
University of Minnesota Children's Hospital, Fairview
Minneapolis, Minnesota, USA

Robert D. Steiner, MD
Professor of Pediatrics and Molecular and Medical Genetics
Vice Chair for Research in Pediatrics
Deputy Director, Oregon Clinical and Translational Research Institute
Oregon Health & Science University
Portland, Oregon, USA

Constantine A. Stratakis MD, D(Med)Sci
Director and Chief
Section on Endocrinology and Genetics
DEB & Heritable Disorders Branch
National Institute of Child Health and Human Development
National Institutes of Health
Bethesda, Maryland, USA

Arnold W. Strauss, MD
BK Rachford Professor and Chair
Department of Pediatrics
University of Cincinnati College of Medicine
Director, Cincinnati Children's Research Foundation
Chief Medical Officer, Cincinnati Children's Hospital Medical Center
Cincinnati, Ohio, USA

Marshall L. Summar, MD
Associate Professor of Pediatrics and Molecular Physiology & Biophysics
Center for Human Genetic Research and Division of Medical Genetics
Vanderbilt University Medical Center
Nashville, Tennessee, USA

Mark A. Tarnopolsky, MD, PHD, FRCPC
Professor of Pediatrics and Medicine,
Hamilton Hospitals Assessment Centre Endowed Chair in
    Neuromuscular Disorders
Director of Neuromuscular and Neurometabolic Clinic
McMaster University Medical Center
Hamilton, Ontario, Canada

Christian Thiel, PhD
Universitätskinderklinik / Universitätsklinik für
    Kinder- und Jugendmedizin
Heidelberg Abteilung
Heidelberg, Germany

Beat Thöny, PhD
Division of Clinical Chemistry and Biochemistry
University Children's Hospital Zurich
Zurich, Switzerland

Johan L.K. van Hove, PhD, MBA
Associate Professor of Pediatrics
Section Head, Clinical Genetics and Metabolism
Department of Pediatrics
University of Colorado, Denver
Denver, Colorado, USA

Guy Van Vliet, MD
Professor of Pediatrics
University of Montreal
Chief, Endocrinology Service
Sainte-Justine Mother and Child University Hospital Center
Montreal Quebec, Canada

Eric Vilain, MD, PhD
Professor of Human Genetics, Pediatrics and Urology
Chief, Medical Genetics
Director, Laboratory of Sexual Medicine, Department of Urology
David Geffen School of Medicine at UCLA
Los Angeles, California, USA

Costa Voulgaropoulos, MD
Pediatric Endocrinologist
Department of Pediatric Endocrinology and Diabetes
Childrens Hospitals and Clinics of Minnesota
St. Paul, Minnesota, USA

Ronald J.A. Wanders, PhD
Professor of Pediatrics and Clinical Chemistry
Director, Laboratory of Genetic Metabolic Disease.
Emma Children's Hospital Academic Medical Center
University of Amsterdam
Amsterdam, The Netherlands

Robert J. Ward, MD
Assistant Professor of Radiology
Boston University School of Medicine
Boston, Massachusetts, USA

David A. Weinstein, MD, MMSc
Associate Professor of Pediatrics
Director, Glycogen Storage Disease Program
Division of Pediatric Endocrinology
University of Florida College of Medicine
Gainesville, Florida, USA

Joseph I. Wolfsdorf, MB, BCh
Professor of Pediatrics
Harvard Medical School
Clinical Director and Associate Chief,
Division of Endocrinology,
Director, Diabetes Program
Children's Hospital-Boston
Boston, Massachusetts, USA

Nadir Yehya, MD
Resident, Department of Pediatrics
Childrens Hospital Los Angeles
University of Southern California
Los Angeles, California, USA

Chunli Yu, MD, FACMG
Assistant Professor
Director, Biochemical Genetics Laboratory
Department of Human Genetics and Pediatrics
Emory University
Decatur, Georgia, USA

Arthur B. Zinn, MD, PhD
Associate Professor of Genetics and Pediatrics
Department of Genetics
Case Western Reserve University School of Medicine
Rainbow Babies and Children's Hospital
Cleveland, Ohio, USA

Johannes Zschocke, Prof. Dr. med., PhD
Professor of Human Genetics
Medical University Innsbruck
Innsbruck, Austria

PREFACE

From its initial conception, *Pediatric Endocrinology and Inborn Errors of Metabolism* (PE-IEM) was created with a dual purpose in mind: to be both a comprehensive, *clinically-focused* medical reference for specialists encompassing the full range of endocrine and metabolic disorders; and to be an information bridge providing inroads into the fundamental concepts of the two interrelated disciplines. The contributors and editorial team strove to make the chapters on inborn errors approachable by endocrinologists and the endocrine chapters approachable by metabolic specialists through what became the underlying precept of the textbook—explanation not simplification. Following this paradigm, chapters first elucidate the mechanisms underlying a disorder and how they relate to the corresponding phenotypes through clinically relevant discussions of genetics and pathophysiology, thus framing the basis of disease; and, second, provide complete and detailed discussions of clinical features, laboratory evaluations, treatment modalities and follow-up management. Rather than simply listing signs and symptoms under the assumption that their occurrence within a disorder is always self-explanatory, *PE-IEM* explains through the pathophysiology why and how these manifestations occur. Many years ago, one of my mentors in medical school told me, "If you know the pathway, you know the disorder." As a result of this step-wise approach, we hope that medical professionals at any level involved in caring for endocrine and metabolic patients will find this textbook a useful resource.

Many single specialty textbooks are similar in size to *PE-IEM*. However, by carefully defining our focus we have provided even more detailed and clinically relevant information concerning presentation, diagnosis and treatment, yet expanded to encompass two specialties all within a single volume. To achieve this goal, we had to address the question: *What is the most pertinent information needed for the practicing physician to fully understand the etiology and pathophysiology of a disease in order to make informed decisions concerning the diagnosis and management of a patient?* To remain a single volume, we focused on describing disease pathogenesis, and, where relevant, the most frequently recurring mutations in relation to phenotype, rather than on lengthy discussions of a disorder's historical background and itemized accounts of the discovery of each mutation, both of which can be found in many textbooks and on established internet databases, such as:

- Online Mendelian Inheritance in Man—http://www.ncbi.nlm.nih.gov/sites/entrez?db=OMIM)

- Gene Tests—http://www.genetests.org

- The Metabolic and Molecular Bases of Inherited Disease—http://www.ommbid.com

However, what is not easily found in other textbooks or on the internet is a single organized source that provides detailed information for the practicing physician concerning the pathophysiology, diagnosis and management of both inborn errors of metabolism and endocrine disorders. By combining the two disciplines, a physician contemplating the differential diagnosis of a patient with hypoglycemia, for example, will need only one textbook to find full coverage of the potential underlying disorders (i.e., hyperinsulinism, glycogen storage diseases, organic acidurias, fatty acid oxidation disorders, adrenal insufficiency and disorders of growth).

An important feature of this textbook, and one that further aids in the differential diagnosis, is that many sub-types of disorders—even rare ones—covered within a chapter are individually discussed following a specific format. Disease-oriented chapters begin with a full description of the etiology/pathophysiology of the overall disorder. Then, in most cases, each individual sub-type of a disorder is structured in the following format: *Etiology/Pathophysiology; Presentation; Diagnosis; Treatment.* Thus, with *PE-IEM*, the reader can readily and consistently find the information (s)he seeks. The structured format also has the added benefit of addressing the heterogeneity of contributors and writing styles created by any multi-author textbook.

Other unique features of *PE-IEM* include the *At-A-Glance* page that begins every disease-oriented chapter which serves as a quick reference summary for easy access to the biochemical profile, presentation, occurrence rate, locus, etc., of a disease in order to find the information needed to differentiate between sub-types of a disorder. To address the subtle but significant differences among the sub-types of a disease, many contributors went the extra step by using multiple graphics to show how the different enzymatic defects affect a pathway rather than a single graphic with a multitude of defect markers. The other purpose behind multiple, individualized graphics is to assist readers outside the specialty by visualizing which precursors and metabolites are affected in the sub-types of a disease. Finally, to create a medical reference that presents a more balanced world-view of current modes of diagnosing and treating pediatric patients with inborn errors of metabolism and endocrine disorders, the editors invited scientific leaders from a wide range of countries to contribute and collaborate on the 50 chapters that encompass *PE-IEM*.

Many individuals contributed their time and expertise to create this textbook. The opportunity of working with and learning from so many esteemed colleagues was, without question, the highlight of editing a textbook. During the collaborative process of putting together the textbook certain individuals went above and beyond the call of duty and it is appropriate that their efforts be recognized. Georg Hoffmann, James Shanahan, Howard Courtney and Karl Roth—without their dedication and support, this textbook would not have been possible. Similarly, I must mention Brad Miller and Tina Cowan—both of whom made invaluable contributions, often in times of need, for which I am eternally grateful. I would also like to give special thanks to Toni Moran; and to Noelle Gray for her editorial assistance.

Kyriakie Sarafoglou, MD

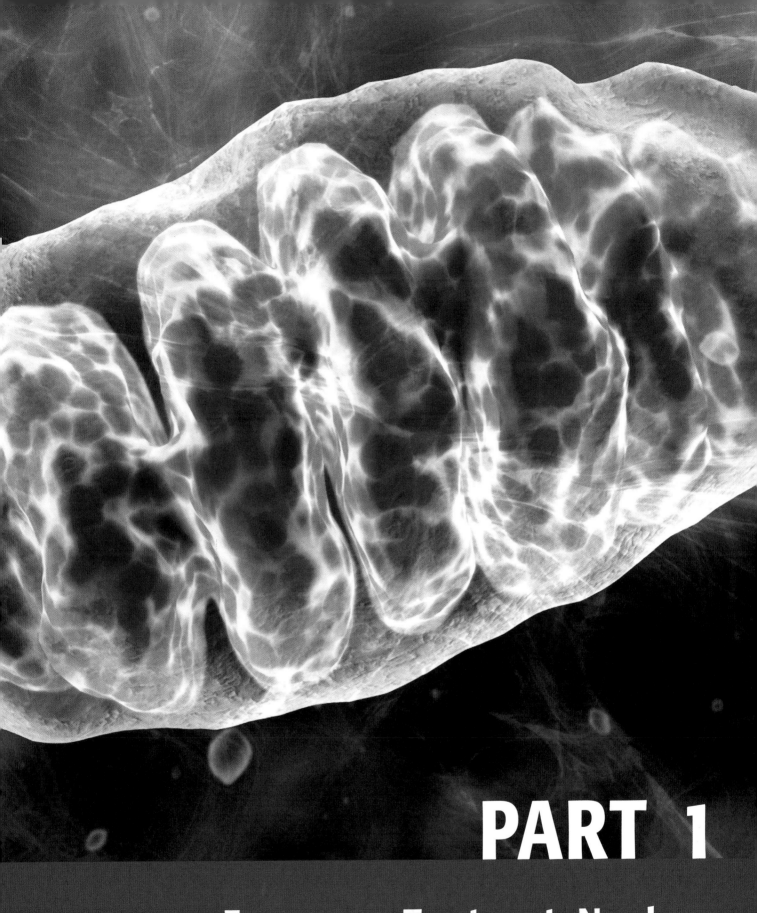

PART 1

Emergency Treatment, Newborn Screening, and Molecular Testing

IN THIS PART

Previous page: Mitochondria

CHAPTER

1

Emergency Assessment and Management of Suspected Inborn Errors of Metabolism and Endocrine Disorders

Susan A Berry, MD, Brandon Nathan, MD, Georg F. Hoffmann, MD, Kyriakie Sarafoglou, MD

In the acute phase, endocrine and metabolic emergencies can be life-threatening disorders. In some cases, patients will present without a diagnosis because the underlying disorder remains dormant until the metabolic stress of an acute disorder (e.g. fever, trauma, etc.) exceeds the body's threshold for compensation and thus exacerbates the disease.

The driving force in the early recognition and treatment of these emergencies is maintaining a suspicion that an endocrine or metabolic disease may be the underlying cause. This suspicion guides the next steps in the emergency care of these patients, namely, in laying the groundwork for ordering appropriate tests (for diagnostic purposes, it is important that critical samples are retrieved during an acute phase prior to treatment), gathering a focused family history that may offer clues to the diagnosis, and ensuring that the correct emergency treatment is initiated.

Overall, the emergency physician and pediatrician most likely will be confronted with more endocrine-related emergencies than metabolic. While most individual metabolic disorders are rare, in the aggregate, inborn errors occur with the same frequency as juvenile diabetes. However, it is also likely that physicians will start seeing more metabolic patients in emergency situations, with the mandatory implementation and expansion of newborn screening programs (in the United States, several European and Arabic countries). The resulting earlier diagnosis extends life expectancy in patients with inborn errors of metabolism that were once catastrophic in the first years of life. Physicians should take immediate steps to evaluate and treat the infant, and have access to a regional metabolic disorder subspecialty center, to either refer the patient or seek advice. It should also be noted that those inborn errors discussed below do not comprise an exhaustive list of all the known disorders of metabolism, many of which do not present as acutely decompensated states.

EMERGENCY ASSESSMENT AND MANAGEMENT OF INBORN ERRORS OF METABOLISM

The emergency assessment and management of patients with rare inborn errors of metabolism (IBEM) can seem a complex and formidable task if the managing physician focuses on the relative rarity and unique characteristics of each individual disorder. However, by categorizing disorders into general subgroups, a more focused emergency management approach can be undertaken. *The most important observation to facilitate management is the simple one that the patient might have an IBEM.* Continuing to include this group of disorders in the differential diagnosis of acute catastrophic illness is essential to planning an effective strategy for emergency treatment. It should be noted that there are no organized clinical studies that have formally applied the strategies describe here. This information is based on cumulative clinical experience and review of the literature. As the practice of IBEM management evolves, protocols such as these may become more established, and evidence-based conclusions should emerge.

Newborn Blood-Spot Screening and Emergency Management

With the advent of expanded newborn blood-spot screening, increasingly children have the diagnosis of their IBEM established soon after birth. In locations providing such screening, typically by use of tandem mass spectrometry, emergency treatment that is specific to a given disorder can be expedited. The availability of expanded newborn blood-spot screening can be very helpful if a newborn suddenly deteriorates, even if the results of the expanded newborn screening are not yet available, but the sample has been taken and sent. In such instances, contact with the newborn screening laboratory may provide an immediate specific diagnosis or rule out relevant metabolic disorders, respectively. For facile management of patients with

known diagnoses, it is highly recommended that the treating metabolic physician prepare an emergency management plan that is provided to the patient or family in a written form (ideally a laminated card). The information should include a prominent announcement of medical intensity, the patient's name, diagnosis, a brief summary of the nature of the patient's condition, recommended initial steps for management, and complete contact information (so that the emergency physician can communicate with the treating metabolic physician). Prompt initiation of treatment, combined with timely consultation, will provide the highest likelihood of successful and effective intervention. Action sheets prepared by an expert panel of the American College of Medical Genetics are an important new resource for initiation of treatment for IBEM; they can be found at www.acmg.net/resources/policies/ACT/condition-analyte-links.htm. Figure 1-1 shows an example of such an emergency letter, in this case for a child with medium-chain acyl-CoA dehydrogenase (MCAD) deficiency.

Acute Presentation of IBEM: History and Clinical Findings

In the absence of a known diagnosis, the treating physician will need to rely on history and a keen sense that the presentation of the patient is atypical, prompting consideration of a diagnosis of an IBEM. A more extended history that includes establishing an ongoing pattern of illness, abnormal neurological status, or family history of early death (e.g., sudden infant death syndrome [SIDS]) may yield details suggestive of an inborn error of metabolism. Of note, most inborn errors of metabolism are autosomal recessive conditions, so family history may not be definitive in determining whether a patient has such a condition. However, the observation of consanguinity is a strongly suggestive factor, and a known diagnosis in a sibling should prompt the assumption that the newly presenting patient has the same disorder.

UNIVERSITY OF YOURSTATE
METABOLIC DISEASES CARE TEAM

MEDICAL ALERT
Medium chain acyl Co-A dehydrogenase (MCAD) deficiency

Re: Affected Patient
        Date of Birth mo/dy/yr

To whom it may concern:

This patient has a genetic biochemical disorder due to an inability to generate ketones from fat in a normal fashion (beta-oxidation defect). Patients with this condition are susceptible to severe and sudden hypoglycemia (low blood sugar) upon fasting. When liver glycogen stores are depleted by fasting, she cannot make ketones to serve as fuel. Because of the metabolic block, low blood sugar and acidosis ensue with vomiting, lethargy and eventual coma or death if treatment is not begun. It is essential that these guidelines be followed if one is to anticipate and prevent a serious complication:

1. During any illness, it is essential that sugar-containing clear liquids in increased amounts should be administered.

2. If she vomits and/or is unable to drink during such an illness, she should be admitted to the hospital and receive intravenous fluids containing glucose and electrolytes. Glucose should be administered at a concentration of D10 at 1.5 x maintenance levels. Blood glucose, electrolyte, liver function and ammonia levels should be monitored.

3. **In case of an emergency please call us: (612) 273-xxxx and ask for the doctor on call for pediatric metabolism at the University of YourState**. A physician is on call for this service 24 h a day. Affected's regular metabolic provider is Reallya Expert, MD. Her dietician is Mrs. Special Diet, RD. They can be reached for non-emergent questions at 612-625-xxxx.

FIGURE 1-1. Example emergency letter for a child with MCAD deficiency.

A careful history that documents the recurrence of similar episodes is significant in assisting the consideration of an IBEM as a potential etiology for metabolic decompensation. If such a history is ascertained, the suspicion of an IBEM should be markedly heightened, and treatment should be initiated. Older age at presentation (e.g., childhood or adolescence) should not preclude the potential diagnosis of an IBEM. Milder forms of almost all IBEMs have been described, and affected patients can suffer decompensation later in life at times of notable physical stress (e.g., childbirth, trauma, steroid therapy, etc.) (1–7). A history of abnormal neurological status is also an important feature. If developmental delay, seizures, or hypotonia are known preceding health issues, the suspicion for an IBEM in an acutely presenting patient should be increased. In one series, most patients presenting with previously unknown IBEMs had one of these findings (8).

A partial list of clinical findings that may accompany acute presentations of IBEMs is provided in Table 1-1. Unfortunately, these findings are rather nonspecific, so the diagnosing physician will need to maintain a high index of suspicion to consider IBEMs

in their differential diagnosis. A potential clue to heighten this suspicion may be that the patient may seem sicker or have more extreme laboratory values than might be anticipated given his or her antecedent history. Calvo and colleagues (8) analyzed the most frequent presenting symptoms in a series of patients with IBEMs presenting to an emergency department. Their findings concluded neurological signs or history (i.e., hypotonia, developmental delay, feeding disturbance, and altered sensorium) to be the most frequent symptom class, present in 85%

of patients, followed by digestive symptoms (typically vomiting), seen in 58.5%. Perhaps most important, their study pointed out that neurological and digestive symptoms were associated in 51% of patients, emphasizing the observation that IBEM patients are likely to have multiple symptoms when presenting acutely (8). The researchers also noted that typically the presenting symptoms of these patients require immediate intervention that precedes definitive diagnosis.

It is important to remember that beyond these findings in the patient's history, some queries or observations that suggest an IBEM will not be made unless specifically sought. A clinical history of specific food refusal may be suggestive of an IBEM. Examples include protein refusal in urea cycle disorders or aminoacidopathies or aversion to sweets and fruits in disorders of fructose metabolism. A history of maternal liver disease in pregnancy is a suggestive clue for disorders of fatty acid oxidation (9). The observation of an unusual odor such as "sweaty feet" odor can be found in patients with isovaleric acidemia and glutaric acidemia type II, or the presence of a sweetish, fruity smell in urine or earwax can be discerned in patients with maple syrup urine disease (10).

Initial Laboratory Assessment in Acute Presentation of an IBEM

Table 1-2 lists laboratory studies that should be undertaken for the paired goals of diagnosis and ongoing management of an IBEM. Although results of some testing will not be available during the immediate management phase, for some IBEMs, the only time that significant diagnostic metabolites can be detected is during an acute episode of decompensation. Thus testing during the presenting illness may be the only time at which the physician has the opportunity to gather information yielding a diagnosis for the patient. Achieving accurate measures of ammonia and lactate requires special attention to sample collection and handling. Both

TABLE 1-1 Presenting Findings in Acute Decompensation of IBEM	
• Hypoglycemia	• Symptoms of cardiac decompensation
• Acidosis	• Evidence of muscle dysfunction
• Respiratory distress, particularly tachypnea	Pain
• Vomiting	Rhabdomyolysis
• Evidence of hepatic dysfunction	Weakness
Coagulopathy/bleeding	• Symptoms of infection
Hepatomegaly	• Seizures
Jaundice	• Abnormal neurological exam
	• Altered sensorium

TABLE 1-2   Laboratory Studies for Management of Suspected Acute Decompensation of IBEM

- Complete blood count (WBC differential and platelet count)
- Electrolytes
- Blood glucose
- BUN and creatinine
- ALT, AST, bilirubin
- Coagulation studies (INR, PTT)
- Venous blood gases
- Uric acid

- Plasma ammonia
- Plasma lactate and pyruvate
- Creatine kinase
- Urinalysis, especially urine ketones
- Screening diagnostic studies
    - Plasma amino acids
    - Urine organic acids
    - Plasma acylcarnitine profile
    - Plasma carnitine
    - Urine acylglycine panel

require free-flowing samples that should be placed on ice and transported immediately to the laboratory for processing. If the diagnosis of an IBEM is already established, some of these studies can be deferred. However, the diagnostic studies noted in Table 1-2 are also important for later management of the inter-current illness.

Anion Gap, Ammonia, Creatine Kinase, and Ketones Four laboratory values carry special significance in the diagnosis and early management of a possible IBEM. Observation of abnormalities in these laboratory studies makes the diagnosis of an IBEM more likely, but they are highlighted here because they may not be among common studies done in emergency situations. Recognition of their utility may prompt their ascertainment in a setting where these laboratory tests would not be among the first tests otherwise selected. These tests, along with hypoglycemia, are critical observations that may direct significant changes in management and additional diagnostic considerations and testing.

1. *Anion gap (>16). The most specific laboratory finding suggestive of an IBEM is a remarkably elevated anion gap,* where the gap is calculated as [Na]−{[Cl] + [bicarbonate]} because the number of clinical conditions that can cause an anion gap of this degree is limited. Although an anion gap of this magnitude can be due to shock with consequent lactic acidosis, to diabetic ketoacidosis, or to significant renal failure and/or cardiomyopathy, the clinical history and findings, along with initial standard laboratory testing, should reveal these etiologies, leaving only unexplained anions from inborn errors of metabolism and significant poisonings in the differential diagnosis (11). An elevated anion gap indicates that there are additional organic compounds circulating; in the context of IBEMs, these are unconjugated organic acids, including lactic acid. Persistent lactic acidosis even after correction of the hypoxic state and/or poor circulation is suspicious for an IBEM and often is the predominant finding in disorders of pyruvate metabolism, such as pyruvate dehydrogenase complex and pyruvate carboxylase (PC) deficiencies. Other metabolic disorders associated with lactic acidosis are multiple carboxylase deficiencies due to either biotinidase deficiency or holocarboxylase synthase deficiency, organic acidopathies (e.g., methylmalonic, propionic, isovaleric, and glutaric type I acidemias), glycogen storage disease type I, gluconeogenesis defects, fatty acid oxidation defects, and mitochondrial disorders, including glutaric acidemia type II.

2. *Ketones.* Urinary ketone or serum ketone values can be highly significant, particularly in the neonate. In a clinical setting where ketosis is more extreme than anticipated (e.g., significant ketones with less than 12 hours of fasting) and where glucose elevation is not evident, an IBEM should be considered. Ketoacidosis can be a prominent secondary phenomenon in IBEM, as in the previously mentioned organic acidopathies, maple syrup urine disease (MSUD), holocarboxylase synthase deficiency, glycogen storage diseases, including type III and type IV, and glycogen synthase, and disorders of gluconeogenesis (e.g., phosphoenolpyruvate carboxykinase [PC] deficiency and fructose-1,6-diphosphatase deficiency). Other disorders presenting with elevated urinary and serum ketones include idiopathic ketotic hypoglycemia, a poorly characterized disorder of unknown cause, and rare disorders of ketone use such as β-ketothiolase and succinyl-CoA-3-ketoacid CoA transferase (SCOT) deficiencies. Conversely, the absence of ketones after significant fasting suggests a possible disorder of fatty acid oxidation, hyperinsulinism, or a rare defect in ketone synthesis. Measurement of plasma free fatty acids at the same time as ketone bodies will assist in distinguishing between these disorders. Free fatty acids will be low in a hyperinsulinemic state and elevated in disorders of fatty acid oxidation or defects in ketone synthesis.

3. *Elevated ammonia.* The observation of markedly elevated ammonia levels, especially without other signs of acute hepatic dysfunction, is also highly significant. The normal range for ammonia is age-dependent, with values up to 150 µM/L normal in a premature infant in a premature infant, but values greater that 50 µM/L are abnormal in older infants and children. In cases of hepatic failure of any etiology, the underlying etiology for hyperammonemia is often revealed through the general history and additional laboratory findings. While there are inborn errors of metabolism that have evidence of acute hepatic failure as a primary presenting finding, the observation of marked hyperammonemia with otherwise minimal or no hepatic dysfunction suggests an IBEM, most often either a urea cycle defect or organic acidemia, particularly propionic acidemia and methylmalonic acidemia. Elevated ammonia also can be seen as a presenting finding in disorders of fatty acid oxidation in the setting of the generalized hepatic dysfunction that can accompany their acute presentation, so the presence of abnormal liver function tests does not reduce the suspicion of an IBEM.

4. *Elevated creatine kinase.* Observation of significant elevations in creatine kinase in a child or young adult in the absence of evidence of a previously existing muscular dystrophy is unusual and suggests an IBEM with myopathy or cardiomyopathy or both (e.g., defects in β-oxidation of long- and very-long-chain fatty acids, disorders of the carnitine cycle and transport, disorders of the electron transport chain, and some forms of glycogen storage disease, particularly types III and V). When noted, caution should be exercised because IBEMs with this finding also may have associated rhabdomyolysis and/or hypoglycemia as complicating factors of which this elevation may be a harbinger.

Beyond these four values, significant metabolic acidosis is a less specific but extremely common manifestation of "toxic" metabolites. Overall, the observation of laboratory values that seem atypical for the history preceding the presentation, as well as "atypical" clinical findings should prompt the treating physician to expand the differential diagnosis to include IBEMs. For example, hepatomegaly and cardiomyopathy, when associated with hypoglycemia and metabolic acidosis, can be the presenting manifestations of defects in β-oxidation of long- and very-long-chain fatty acids, including disorders of the carnitine cycle and transport, whereas cardiomyopathy and/or skeletal myopathy are the presenting manifestations of mitochondrial diseases or glycogen storage disease type II (Pompe).

Acute Management of IBEMs

With the consideration that an ill patient may have an IBEM, a strategy that combines diagnostic studies with immediate intervention is ideal. The features of IBEMs that may cause acute decompensation revolve around conditions affecting the metabolism of small molecules, yielding failures in fuel use, generation of toxic metabolites, or both. As a general rule, intervention should strive to reverse the catabolic process that was the likely precipitant of decompensation. A mandatory first step is to interrupt intake of potentially toxic dietary precursors by stopping all oral intake. With the extremely rare exception of pyruvate dehydrogenase complex deficiency, the most effective strategy to achieve the combined goal of fuel repletion and reduction of toxic metabolites is immediate infusion of intravenous glucose at a rate of 8–10 mg/kg/min. In the treatment of acute decompensation of metabolic disease, this infusion rate should be maintained even if elevated blood glucose levels ensue. Blood glucose levels should be monitored, and if they become abnormal, an insulin drip (0.05 U/kg/h) should be used to maintain normal blood glucose levels while maintaining the glucose infusion (11). If renal function is adequate, fluid volumes should be administered at a rate 1.5 times maintenance levels because high fluid volume facilitates the excretion of toxic metabolites. If the patient is febrile, this represents an additional physiological stress, so medication to reduce fever should be administered and fluid volumes increased to reflect increased insensible loss. Acetaminophen can be used in almost all circumstances unless there is evidence of marked acute hepatic failure. Antibiotic therapy is recommended in every patient because sepsis is an important consideration in differential diagnosis and may be present concomitantly leading to further catabolism.

The initial phase of treatment facilitates the reduction of offending precursor load and provides a caloric source to reduce catabolism. Careful monitoring of vital signs and intake and output and ongoing measurement of acute laboratory values are essential to the successful initial management of a patient with an IBEM. Beyond the desired achievement of acid–base and fluid–electrolyte balance, additional interventions may be appropriate based on the most likely diagnosis that can be deduced from laboratory values. The initial basic laboratory tests obtained should be available soon after beginning treatment and should yield diagnostic clues if the diagnosis is unknown. The results of the special metabolic investigations relevant to the diagnosis of potentially treatable metabolic disorders should be available within 24 hours or, at the latest, within 48 hours.

Subsequent management can be based on presumptive diagnosis after initial laboratory values are received. The general management strategy after acute measures have been applied centers around a general classification of the IBEM symptoms being related to the accumulation of toxic metabolites, abnormalities in energy supply, or both. After initial laboratory values are available, this classification can be applied more readily. Prietsch and colleagues (12) outlined a therapeutic classification of metabolic disorders, describing disorders of intoxication type (group 1), disorders with reduced fasting tolerance (group 2), disorders with disturbed mitochondrial energy metabolism (group 3), disorders of neurotransmission (group 4), and disorders with no specific emergency treatment available (group 5) (12). For this summary of acute interventions, the first two groups assume the highest profile for acute management. Table 1-3 summarizes this classification scheme, focusing on disorders that are best suited to management using the following suggested strategies (groups 1 and 2), but it also includes information about the latter three groups for reference.

Early-Phase Management of an IBEM with Toxic Metabolites

Through initiation of the management strategy just described, the most essential therapeutic intervention is that of limiting the exogenous and endogenous burden of the offending precursor (primarily protein for aminoacidopathies, urea cycle abnormalities, and organic acidemias; dietary restriction and reversal of catabolism for long-chain fatty acid disorders; and cessation of dietary intake of sugars for disorders where the enzyme block causes accumulation of toxic metabolites, e.g., fructose for hereditary fructose intolerance or galactose for classical galactosemia). In many of these conditions, reversal of catabolism is also essential. The use of a glucose infusion and fluid volume will suffice for initial care for many of these conditions, but for the next phase of care, additional nutritional support and detoxification agents, if appropriate, should be provided because glucose alone will not be sufficient to reverse endogenous catabolism and maintain anabolism.

If the patient has a known or strongly suspected disorder of protein metabolism, additional caloric supplementation can be provided by beginning infusion of intralipids at a dose of 1 g/kg/day and increasing to reach a total caloric intake of 100–120 kcal/kg/day. It is imperative that this latter therapy not be initiated unless the diagnosis is known and/or a fatty acid oxidation disorder has been ruled out. Although protein intake should be stopped initially in disorders where amino acids or their metabolites are toxic, the duration of withdrawal should not exceed 24–48 hours, at which time protein intake should be resumed gradually, with the route determined by the clinical situation of the patient.

If the patient has a known or suspected organic acidemia, L-carnitine can be administered at a dose of 75–200 mg/kg/day. This is most efficient if administered intravenously because the bioavailability is higher by this route (13). If ammonia is a toxic metabolite, then specific addition of intravenous scavenger agents (14) such as Ammonul (sodium benzoate–sodium phenylacetate) at a dose of 250 mg/kg (5.5 g/m²) as a loading dose over 1–2 hours, followed by the same dose over 24 hours, is warranted. L-Arginine also should be provided (0.2 g/kg = 2 mL/kg of 10% arginine HCl).

A central line should be used for administration of these medications. If the initial ammonia level is >500 micromol/l or this regimen is not effective over the course of 6–8 hours, then dialysis may be required to reduce ammonia levels. As specific laboratory information is available, the regimen should be tailored specifically to optimize treatment for that condition (i.e., addition of specific cofactors or vitamins or addition of disease-specific drugs such as 2-(2-nitro-4-trifluoromethylbenzoyl)-cyclohexane-1,3-dione [NTBC] for hereditary tyrosinemia (15).

Early-Phase Management of an IBEM with Fuel Depletion

The preliminary management strategy of supplying glucose at 8–10 mg/kg/minute typically will result in correction of signs of acute metabolic decompensation in disorders where fasting is the primary precipitating factor in clinical presentation. This infusion rate provides sufficient glucose to yield euglycemia in nocturnal treatment of glycogen storage disease (16). Use of this strategy should be effective in disorders of glucose synthesis or release (i.e., disorders of gluconeogenesis or glycogen storage) or fatty acid oxidation disorders, where the inability to generate ketones from fat may be the limiting resource as liver glycogen stores become exhausted.

TABLE 1-3 Classification of IBEM Based on Emergency Intervention Strategy (Selected Examples)

Disorders with Toxic Metabolites	Emergency Therapy Strategy
Urea cycle disorders	Discontinue intake of offending precursors
Ornithine carbamyl transferase deficiency	
Carbamyl phosphate synthase deficiency	Reverse endogenous catabolism
Argininosuccinic aciduria	Glucose D_{10} at 1.5 × maintenance
Citrullinemia	Consider Intralipid at 1 g/kg/day (*only* if not FAO)
Aminoacidopathies	
Hepatorenal tyrosinemia	Provide detoxification measures if available:
Maple syrup urine disease	*UCDs*
Organic acidemias	Na-Benzoate and Na-phenylbutyrate (Ammonul)
Propionic acidemia	N-Carbamylglutamate (for NAGS deficiency)
Methylmalonic acidemia	Dialysis
Isovaleric acidemia	*Organic acidemias*
Glutaric acidemia, type 1	Carnitine
3-Methylcrotonyl-CoA carboxylase deficiency	Dialysis
Long-chain fatty acid oxidation disorders	*Tyrosinemia*
VLCAD deficiency	Nitrosone (TBC)
Trifunctional protein deficiency	*MSUD*
LCHAD deficiency	Rarely dialysis
Carbohydrate disorders	
Galactosemia	
Hereditary fructose intolerance	
Fructose-1,6-diphosphatase deficiency	

Disorders of Energy Utilization/Reduced Fasting Tolerance	**Emergency Therapy Strategy**
Glycogen storage diseases (types I, III, and IX)	Give IV glucose at 8–10 mg/kg/min
Fatty acid oxidation disorders	
MCAD deficiency	
SCAD deficiency	
Carnitine transporter deficiency	
Disorders of ketogenesis/ketolysis	
Hyperinsulinism	

Disorders with Abnormal Mitochondrial Energy Metabolism	**Emergency Therapy Strategy**
Pyruvate dehydrogenase complex deficiency	*Avoid* high glucose in PDHC, consider intralipids at 1 g/kg/day
Mitochondrial respiratory chain defects	Correct (lactic) acidosis

Disorders of Neurotransmission	**Emergency Therapy Strategy**
Pyridoxine-responsive seizures	Trial infusion of pyridoxine and folinic acid
Pyridoxale phosphate–responsive seizures	Oral pyridoxale phosphate
Folinic acid–responsive seizures	

Disorders without Specific Emergency Treatments	**Emergency Therapy Strategy**
Nonketotic hyperglycinemia	No disease-specific treatment: treat symptoms noted
Sulfite oxidase deficiency and related disorders	Monitor coagulation in CDG
Congenital disorders of glycosylation	

Ammonul = sodium benzoate–sodium phenylacetate; FAO = fatty acid oxidation disorder.
Source: after Prietsch et al. (12).

TABLE 1-4   Peri- and Postmortem Samples

Plasma

Heparinized plasma (~5 mL) kept deep
rozen (−80°C).

Blood spots

Blood should be dropped on filter paper
(Guthrie cards) for analysis of acylcarnitines
and amino acids

Blood

Whole blood (10–15 mL) anticoagulated
with EDTA should be deep frozen
for later extraction of DNA
for studies of molecular biology.

Urine

All urine available should be collected and,
if in enough quantity, filled in
different tubes and deep frozen.

CSF

CSF (in 1-mL portions) should be collected
in a tube and deep frozen (−80°C).

Skin biopsy

Skin for fibroblast culture must be taken with
sterile precautions into medium and the cell
culture established. Fibroblasts are preferably
cultured premortem; however, a skin biopsy
may be obtained up to 24 hours postmortem
(or even later) and stored 1–2 days at ambient
temperature in culture medium or 0.9%
NaCl–do *not* freeze!
Needle biopsies should be considered before
death because histological and enzymatic
mitochondrial studies in postmortem tissues are
almost uninterpretable (if necessary, muscle
biopsies may be obtained up to 1
hour postmortem). The acquisition of open
organ biopsies is only indicated in exceptional
cases. It should be discussed with the
laboratory/metabolic specialist (samples
are partly frozen immediately at −70°C
or in liquid nitrogen, partly to be stored
in glutaraldehyde for electron microscopy).

Liver biopsy

Three or more samples of 1 cm^3 each should be
snap frozen in liquid nitrogen and stored on
dry ice at −80°C or in liquid nitrogen
for histochemistry and enzymology.

**Muscle (skeletal or heart) and
other tissue biopsy**

As indicated for liver tissue. Specific investigations
of these samples depend on the history,
clinical symptoms, and routine laboratory data.
The spectrum of specific analysis to be done on
postmortem samples is rather broad and to
be discussed with a metabolic specialist. It most
often includes analysis of amino acids, organic
acids, carnitine, and the profile of acylcarnitines.
These studies may lead to specific enzymology
and molecular studies, or clinical and laboratory
data may suggest these studies directly.

The treatment of pyruvate dehydrogenase complex deficiency is the one major exception to the empirical use of higher-rate glucose infusions as an initial therapy. Children with this rare disorder present with significant lactic (and pyruvic) acidemia, and infusion of high-dose glucose exacerbates their clinical course. If glucose infusion results in rapid progression of weakness in the face of increasing lactic acidosis, this specific diagnosis should be considered, and intralipid infusion with normal saline should be substituted for reduced glucose infusion. The use of L-carnitine as an acute empirical measure is controversial because some speculate that this may exacerbate cardiomyopathy in long-chain fatty acid disorders, but for management of short- or medium-chain fatty acid oxidation disorders, carnitine should be administered at 75–125 mg/kg/day by mouth or intravenously. Conversely, if the patient has a known disorder of long-chain fatty acid oxidation, administration of medium chain triglycerides (MCT) oil provides critical energy substrate.

The ultimate goal of therapy is not simply to reverse the metabolic emergency but to prevent irreversible damage to the patient's brain. The diseases leading to acute intoxication, such as maple syrup urine disease, the classical organic acidurias, and the urea cycle defects, carry the greatest risk of major sequelae. Additional supportive therapeutic measures are used informally in some centers to enhance this goal. These may include mannitol for the treatment of cerebral edema, which also may enhance detoxification through increased diuresis. Increased intracranial pressure may be monitored neurosurgically. Overall supportive care is critical in patients in intensive-care units, with especial vigilance for the detection and prompt treatment of infection.

Postmortem Investigations

In the event of death when metabolic disease is suspected, it is important to store adequate amounts of biological fluids and available tissues for further diagnostic procedures. Without diagnosis, genetic counseling of the parents, reliable risk assessment, and early specific intervention in case of recurrence in future children are not possible. The use of these samples should be planned carefully in accordance with advice from specialists in inborn errors of metabolism.

In the case of SIDS, it is important to recognize that defects of fatty acid oxidation may be responsible, particularly long-chain fatty acid oxidation defects, which can lead to respiratory arrest and heart block or arrhythmias. In most cases, autopsy reveals an excess of fat droplets in the liver or heart, but even in the absence of steatosis, blood spots always should be collected on a filter paper for analysis of acylcarnitines by electrospray tandem mass spectrometry and for the common MCAD mutation. Most amino acids also will be analyzed from this sample. With the exception of the mitochondrial fatty acid oxidation defects, most inborn errors of metabolism, such as urea cycle defects, organic acidemias, congenital lactic acidosis, and carbohydrate disorders, do not cause SIDS but rather acute illness with obvious clinical symptoms that precedes death by hours or days, as well as preceding chronic symptomatology.

Table 1-4 highlights the representative peri- and postmortem samples that are recommended to be taken for investigations if a child dies (suddenly) of an unknown, possible metabolic disease. It must be remembered that autolysis during the process of dying causes the intracellular fluid to mix with extracellular fluid. Misleading changes of plasma metabolites may be encountered. Plasma and/or serum samples from the last days of life that still may be available at a clinical laboratory therefore are especially valuable and should be retrieved.

EMERGENCY ASSESSMENT AND MANAGEMENT OF SELECT ENDOCRINE DISORDERS

Hypoglycemia

Hypoglycemia is the most common metabolic problem in neonates and results from an imbalance between total-body glucose use and hepatic glucose production. Even with the frequency of hypoglycemia, controversy still exists as to the definitive blood glucose cutoff level that universally is considered safe (i.e., no risk of long-term sequelae). With no conclusive evidence or consensus, a safe approach is to use a blood glucose concentration of less than 50 mg/dL (2.75 mmol/L) for all ages. Since hypoglycemia is a symptom and not a diagnosis, it is important for the clinician to remain on the alert for clinical signs and conditions that might lead to severe hypoglycemia. At the same time, there must be a low threshold for investigating and diagnosing hypoglycemia with frequent blood glucose measurements and treating hypoglycemia promptly in order to maintain blood glucose levels in the normal range.

The body's ability to maintain an appropriate concentration of blood glucose reflects the dynamic balance between intake, tissue use (i.e., glycolysis and glycogen synthesis), and endogenous production (i.e., glycogenolysis and gluconeogenesis) of glucose. Glucose homeostasis is regulated primarily by the anabolic hormone insulin (which accelerates the uptake/removal of glucose and gluconeogenic substrates from blood into tissues, promotes intracellular glucose metabolism, and initiates glycogen synthesis) and several catabolic counterregulatory hormones (i.e., glucagon, cortisol, growth hormone, epinephrine, and norepinephrine) that stimulate the production and release of glucose.

Elevated blood glucose levels activate the release of insulin, which acts on three main target tissues (muscle, liver, and adipose tissue) through the following processes: 1) increases glucose transport and metabolism, 2) stimulates glycolysis and glycogen synthesis in the liver, 3) suppresses lipolysis, 4) promotes the synthesis of long-chain fatty acids, 5) stimulates triglyceride synthesis from glycerol and fatty acids in adipose tissue, 6) increases cellular uptake of amino acids and stimulates protein synthesis, and 7) promotes the storage of carbohydrate and lipids.

Decreased blood glucose levels decrease insulin levels and activate the release of counterregulatory hormones, which result in mobilization of fuel reserves and an increase in the endogenous production of glucose by 1) inhibiting glucose-using pathways and the storage of metabolic fuels, 2) stimulating glycogenolysis, 3) inhibiting glycogen synthesis, glycolysis, and lipogenesis, and 4) activating gluconeogenesis, lipolysis and ketogenesis.

Brain tissue is highly dependent on glucose and is one of the primary determinants of the body's rate of glucose use. As such, glucose use rates are highest in infants (8 mg/kg/minute), where the brain accounts for a larger percentage of total body weight, and decrease with age as total body mass increases (children: 6–8 mg/kg/minute; adolescents: 4–6 mg/kg/minute; adults: 2–4

mg/kg/minute). In infants, glycogen reserves are smaller (depleted in less than 12 hours), and at the same time, infants have higher glucose requirements. In addition, delayed maturation of glyconeogenic enzymes, impaired ketogenesis from free fatty acids, and delayed glycogenolytic response to glucagon predispose infants to hypoglycemia.

The symptoms of hypoglycemia are not specific, particularly in the newborn. Subtle symptoms such as poor feeding, weakness, headache, confusion, irritability, and hunger may be the only manifestations, and they may not be associated with the classical adrenergic effects such as tachycardia, anxiety, and diaphoresis. Seizures and coma are the usual presentations of severe hypoglycemia.

The spectrum of diseases presenting with hypoglycemia is broad but can be narrowed significantly by the age at presentation, how long before or after a feeding the hypoglycemia occurred, maternal history during pregnancy and delivery, and history of intrauterine stress or increased risk for septicemia.

Infants of mothers with gestational diabetes are at risk for transient hypoglycemia at birth because of development of islet cell hyperplasia stimulated by the maternal elevated glucose concentrations. When infants of mothers with severe preeclampsia or acute fatty liver disease (AFLP) or hemolysis, elevated liver enzymes, and low platelets (HELLP) syndrome develop hypoglycemia, it may be due to a fatty oxidation disorder (17).

Intrauterine growth restricted (IUGR) and small-for-gestational age (SGA) babies also may experience transient hypoglycemia the first couple of months after birth, most likely due to decreased glycogen and protein stores, immaturity of the enzymes involved in glucose homeostasis, and elevated insulin secretion. Infants with persistent hypoglycemia and increased requirements of intravenous glucose to maintain normoglycemia (>10–12 mg/kg/minute) have hyperinsulinism (see Chapter 4), the most common cause of intractable hypoglycemia in infants up to 6 months of age. Micropenis and hypoglycemia in a male infant suggest hypoglycemia due to congenital hypopituitarism. Other inherited causes of hypoglycemia include hypopituitarism, organic acidemias, glycogen storage diseases (except for glycogen type II disease, Pompe disease), disorders of gluconeogenesis, galactosemia, and fructose intolerance (presenting after introduction of sucrose or fructose in the diet). In a toddler or an older child, hypoglycemia can be caused by accidental ingestion of sulfonylureas, salicylates, and acetaminophen. Munchhausen by proxy, where a caregiver injects insulin into a child causing hypoglycemia, also should be kept in mind as a possibility in

cases of unexplained hypoglycemia with elevated insulin levels and low C-peptide levels. The circulating elevated serum C-peptide results from the conversion of proinsulin to insulin and is not part of the insulin preparations used to treat diabetes.

Children with gastroesophageal reflux and Nissan fundoplication are at risk for dumping syndrome, which is characterized by postprandial hypoglycemia caused by an excessive insulin secretion after a sharp rise in plasma glucose.

Laboratory Evaluation At the time of hypoglycemia, a critical blood sample should be obtained before glucose administration in order to elucidate the defect in glucose homeostasis. Measurement of insulin, free fatty acids, serum ketones, growth hormone (GH), cortisol, acylcarnitine profile, lactate/pyruvate, and ammonia should be the first lab tests requested. If there is enough blood, additional studies can include plasma amino acids, carnitine levels, and C- peptide. The first voided urine after the hypoglycemic episode also should be saved and sent for determinations of ketones, urinary organic acids, and urinary reducing substances and a toxicology screen. Measurement of serum/urinary ketones and free fatty acids can provide valuable information. When free fatty acids (FFAs) are decreased, ketones also will be low due to the decreased availability of FFAs to undergo β-oxidation in the mitochondrion. Low FFAs and ketones in the presence of elevated GH and cortisol levels suggests hyperinsulinism, even if insulin levels are low. Decreased FFAs and ketones differentiate the hypoglycemia due to hyperinsulinism from fatty oxidation defects, where FFAs are elevated and ketones, although present, are low for the degree of hypoglycemia.

When both GH and cortisol levels are low during the time of hypoglycemia, it is suggestive of hypopituitarism. When either GH or cortisol is low, it suggests isolated GH deficiency or cortisol deficiency due to primary or secondary adrenal insufficiency. Hypoglycemia associated with metabolic acidosis, ketoacidosis, lactic acidosis, and elevated ammonia levels suggests an organic acidemia.

Hypoglycemia associated with hepatomegaly and lactic acidosis suggests either glycogen type I disease or a defect in glyconeogenesis such as fructose-1,6-biphosphatase deficiency or phosphoenolpruyvate carboxykinase deficiency (PEPCK). Hypoglycemia with hepatomegaly, renal tubular acidosis, acute liver failure, and urine positive for reducing substances suggests fructose intolerance or galactosemia.

Treatment The immediate goal in treatment of hypoglycemia in the emergency setting is normalization of blood glucose levels and involves intravenous administration of a bolus of 25% dextrose at 1 mL/kg and initiation of intravenous fluids providing 10% dextrose at one-half maintenance or at a glucose rate of 6–8 mg/kg/minute. The plasma glucose should be monitored frequently until stabilization at a level above 70 mg/dL. When hypoglycemia is refractory to high rates of intravenous glucose administration, hyperinsulinism should be suspected (see Chapter 4). The coexistence of hyperkalemia, hyponatremia, and/or hyperpigmentation and/or ambiguous genitalia in a female should initiate a workup for adrenal insufficiency and hydrocortisone therapy (see Chapter 29). If critical lab tests were not obtained at the time of hypoglycemia and provocative testing is planned to obtain critical values, the fasting should be initiated only after a defect of β-oxidation has been ruled out.

Thyrotoxic Crisis/Thyroid Storm

Thyrotoxic crisis or thyroid storm is extremely rare in the pediatric population but remains a life-threatening endocrine emergency that requires prompt recognition and therapy. Thyroid storm results from the release of preformed thyroid hormone from degenerating thyroid follicles. Symptoms of thyroid storm most often mimic those of a hypermetabolic rate and include fever as high as 106°F, hyperhydrosis, cutaneous flushing, altered mental status, hypertension, widened pulse pressure, and supraventricular tachycardias. Extreme agitation and restlessness may be present and progress to delirium or overt psychosis. Congestive heart failure with pulmonary edema can occur, which eventually may progress to cardiovascular insufficiency and shock. Other manifestations include diarrhea, hepatobilliary inflammation with jaundice, and profound apathy progressing to stupor or coma as the disease progresses.

Most cases of thyroid storm occur in individuals with Graves disease, the most common etiology for hyperthyroidism in the pediatric population, but thyroid storm also may be encountered in patients with Hashimoto thyroiditis (hashitoxicosis), a toxic solitary nodule or toxic multinodular goiter, TSH-secreting tumors, or from exogenous thyroid hormone administration (18,19). Even with marked elevations of free thyroxine and/or triiodothyronine levels in these patients, the vast majority of these patients do not experience thyroid storm. Therefore, it is likely that other precipitating factors cause progression of the hyperthyroidism to a thyrotoxic crisis. Thyroid storm is encountered most commonly in patients with long-standing hyperthyroidism and poor nutritional status. Other factors that may precipitate

a thyroid storm include treatment with ^{131}I, thyroidectomy, withdrawl of antithyroid medication, anesthesia, surgery, infection, trauma, and stress. Severe thyrotoxic states also may be masked or lessened by concurrent endocrine disease such as diabetic ketoacidosis (20).

Early recognition and initiation of therapy for the hyperthyroid neonate or child with thyroid storm are crucial to prevent cardiovascular collapse and possible death. When thyrotoxic crisis is suspected, a several-tiered approach should be directed at the following areas:

1. *Cardiovascular stabilization.* Appropriate support of intravascular volume for signs of shock should be initiated first. Once cardiovascular status is stabilized, β-blockade using propranolol, esmolol, metoprolol, atenolol, or labetolol should be used unless evidence for congestive heart failure is present. Nonspecific β-blockade with propanolol at 10 μg/kg by slow intravenous push every 10–20 minutes to a maximum of 5 mg will control sympathetic hyperactivity and decrease conversion of T_4 to T_3. Maintenance therapy with propanolol at 2 mg/kg/day in three to four divided doses or atenolol at 1–2 mg/kg/day once a day would control tachycardia. Propanol is contraindicated in patients with asthma.

2. *Reduction of thyroid hormone levels.* Propylthiouracil (6–10 mg/kg/day divided every 6–8 hours, maximum 1200 mg/day) is used most commonly because of its ability to both limit new synthesis of thyroid hormone by blocking an organification step and to inhibit conversion of T_4 to T_3. Alternatively, methimazole (0.5–1 mg/kg/dose every 8 hours) may be used. In the setting of thyrotoxicosis, large doses of iodine in the form of Lugol solution and a saturated solution of potassium iodide complement the effects of antithyroid medications by blocking the release of prestored hormone and decreasing iodide transport and oxidation in follicular cells. The decrease of organification due to increased doses of iodide is known as the *Wolf–Chaikoff effect.* However, the thyroid gland escapes the inhibition if high doses of iodide beyond the acute phase because the iodide transport system adapts to the higher concentrations of iodide (usually within 48 hours). Of note, iodine therapy should be given 1 hour after initiation of the antithyroid medication in order to avoid stimulation of new thyroid hormone synthesis before the blockade of iodine organification takes effect. The dosing during thyrotoxicosis is 3–5 drops every 8 hours of Lugol iodide (or SSKI) or 10% sodium iodide 125–250 mg/day intravenously over 24 hours. Angioedema and laryngeal edema are life-threatening reactions to iodide that occur rarely. Contrast agents

such as iopanoic acid 100–200 mg /day or 500 mg every third day can be used as a second line of therapy. Corticosteroids (methylprednisone 1 mg/kg intravenously every 12 hours or dexamethasone 0.1 mg/kg/dose also may be beneficial in limiting the inflammatory response and may have an added benefit of inhibiting peripheral conversion of thyroxine to triiodothyronine as well.

3. *Supportive care.* Management of fever using acetaminophen (15 mg/kg orally or rectally every 4 hours) and cooling blankets.

4. *Treatment of coexisting pathology.* Since sepsis has been associated with thyroid storm, an infectious workup should be considered and broad-spectrum antibiotic coverage initiated if indicated clinically.

5. *Evaluation and therapy for other autoimmune endocrine disorders.* Adrenal insufficiency occurs rarely with thyroid storm but should be suspected in a nonresponsive patient with thyrotoxic crisis. In this situation, a low threshold for administration of "stress dose" hydorocortisone (50–100 mg/m^2) should be considered. Other endocrine diseases such as diabetic ketoacidosis also should considered because hyperglycemia arbitrarily can reduce the level of T_3 in these situations (21,22).

Acute Adrenal Insufficiency

Adrenal insufficiency (AI) always should be considered in the differential of a nonresponsive patient with signs of hypotension, hypoglycemia, hyponatremia, and hyperkalemia. The most common cause in infants is the salt-wasting form of congenital adrenal hyperplasia (CAH) due to 21-hydroxylase deficiency. Other causes of AI include acute infection (particularly meningococcemia), hemorrhage into the adrenal gland, and rapid tapering of steroids in children with a suppressed hypothalamic–pituitary–adrenal (HPA) axis due to prolonged use of oral or inhaled steroids (>10–14 days). In older boys and men X-linked adrenoleukodystrophy may present with isolated AI. Since the HPA axis suppression may last for several months after discontinuation of the steroid therapy, these children can be at risk of adrenal crisis during this period in the presence of stress.

Similarly, patients with known disorders of the adrenal gland (e.g., congenital adrenal hyperplasia, autoimmune adrenalitis [Addison disease], and adrenoleukodystrophy) are at risk of adrenal crisis during acute illness or stress if "stress doses" of hydrocortisone are not given. The signs and symptoms of AI vary depending on whether cortisol secretion, aldosterone secretion, or both are affected

---

TABLE 1-5   Signs and Symptoms of Severe Adrenal Crisis

- Persistent vomiting without diarrhea
- Mental status changes
- Cardiovascular instability, including hypotension, tachycardia, and other signs of shock only minimally responsive to crystalloid or colloid fluid boluses
- Electrolyte abnormalities, including hyponatremia, hyperkalemia, hypoglycemia, normal anion gap, metabolic acidosis
- Eosinophilia

(see Table 1-5). Patients with cortisol deficiency may present with hypoglycemia, weakness, fatigue, anorexia, nausea, vomiting, dizzy spells, and orthostatic hypotension (cortisol deficiency reduces cardiac output). Signs of aldosterone deficiency include hyponatremia, salt cravings, hyperkalemia, elevated renin, and hypotension due to intravascular volume depletion. Metabolic acidosis may be present due to poor tissue perfusion.

Hyperpigmentation of mucosal surfaces, skin lines, or previous scars results from increased production of ACTH in primary adrenal insufficiency.

Treatment Initial therapy for adrenal crisis is directed at support of the cardiovascular system. Isotonic fluids (0.9% normal saline or lactated Ringer's solution 20 mL/kg) should be administered to support intravascular volume. Additional boluses of isotonic solutions should be repeated as necessary for ongoing hypotension. Dextrose can be administered as boluses of 10% glucose per 2–4 mL/kg as needed for hypoglycemia. Dextrose also should be added to ongoing intravenous fluids, administered at 1.5 to 2 times maintenance.

The other mainstay of initial therapy is glucocorticoid administration. Before starting intravenous glucocorticoids, a sample should be obtained for a cortisol and ACTH determination. Hydrocortisone sodium succinate should be given as an intravenous bolus at an initial dose of 25 mg for an infant or toddler, 50 mg for a younger child, and 100 mg for an adolescent or young adult. Following the initial bolus, hydrocortisone sodium succinate is administered intravenously at 100 mg/m^2 in four divided doses during the first 24 hours. The patient's response is monitored by evaluating arterial blood pressure, heart rate, peripheral perfusion, and urine output. Once the patient is stable, the dose of hydrocortisone can be weaned by approximately 50% per day until a physiological replacement dose of 6–8 mg/m^2/day is reached (8–12 mg/m^2/day in patients with CAH).

In the presence of hyperkalemia, if the serum concentration is 5.5–7 mEq/L and the electrocardiogram (ECG) shows only peaked T waves, infusion of intravenous fluids without potassium and close monitoring are recommended. However, patients with higher concentrations of potassium and ECG abnormalities require immediate treatment. Some of the interventions include 1) calcium gluconate 10% given at a dose of 0.5 mL/kg to antagonize enhanced membrane excitability, 2) intravenous bicarbonate 7.5% 2–3 mL/kg given over 30–60 minutes to correct metabolic acidosis or a combination of glucose and insulin infusion (1 unit of insulin for evey 5–6 g of carbohydrate given), both the preceding measures promote potassium transport into the cells; and 3) agents such as K$^+$-binding resins (Kayexalate) can also be used at a dose of 1 g/kg to increase the elimination of potassium from the body.

Sometimes patients with aldosterone deficiency or resistance (pseudohypoaldosteronism) may present with hyponatremia and hyperkalemia and in shock secondary to salt wasting. In these instances, hydrocortisone therapy can be initiated along with fluid rescusitation, while awaiting the diagnostic testing to rule out cortisol deficiency.

In some cases of CAH such as 11-hydroxylase or 17-hydroxylase/lyase deficiency, adrenal crisis is not associated with salt wasting; instead, hypokalemia and/or hypertension may be present. Symptomatic hypokalemia can be treated with 0.5–1 mEq/kg/hour of potassium and continuous cardiac monitoring.

A proposed diagnostic and treatment protocol is outlined in Table 1-6.

TABLE 1-6   Initial Diagnostic Evaluation and Therapeutic Intervention in Suspected Adrenal Crisis

- *Administer intravenous fluids*
  - Normal saline (0.9 NaCl) or lactated Ringer's solution 20 mL/kg bolus over 20–30 minutes as needed to support intravascular volume
  - D$_{10}$W 2–4 mL/kg* as necessary to correct hypoglycemia
- *Diagnostic evaluation*
  - In patients without a previous history of adrenal disorders, the following laboratory tests should be obtained prior to initiation of hydrocortisone therapy (if possible):
    - ACTH
    - Cortisol
    - 17-Hydroxyprogesterone (if CAH suspected) and a karyotype in an infant with ambiguous genitalia
    - Plasma renin activity and aldosterone in the presence of hyponatremia and hyperkalemia
- Therapeutic intervention
  - Hydrocortisone sodium succinate 50–100 mg/m^2 intravenous bolus or intramuscularly if patient is symptomatic and IV access is not easily accessible
- Maintenance fluids
  - Patient should be placed on D$_5$ NS** (no potassium) at 1.5 to 2 times maintenance rate
- Maintenance glucocorticoids
  - After initial intravenous bolus, hydrocortisone sodium succinate should be continued at a dose of 50–100 mg/m^2/day divided every 6 hours for 24 hours and then decreased by 50% each day as long as the patient is stable
  - Mineralcorticoids (Fludrocortisone, Florinef)
  - No mineralcorticoids need be given (hydrocortisone at preceding stress doses has strong mineralcorticoid activity)
  - Once hydrocortisone is decreased from stress doses, Florinef 0.1 mg qd should be considered in children as well as sodium chloride in infants if salt wasting is present

* = 10% glucose; ** = 5% glucose, normal saline.

Diabetic Ketoacidosis

Diabetic ketoacidosis (DKA) remains the leading cause of morbidity and mortality in pediatric diabetes patients. The metabolic consequences of DKA are life-threatening, and great care must be taken to address each one of these disturbances during the course of therapy for the pediatric patient. Specific to the pediatric population is the risk of cerebral edema during DKA therapy, which occurs at a rate as high as 1% of all such patients. Evidence-based guidelines have been published recently that outline current standards of care for the treatment of DKA in children (23).

Therapy for DKA is aimed primarily at supporting intravascular volume, reversing metabolic disturbances, and preventing complications, notably cerebral edema. The potential complications resulting from DKA are listed in Table 1-7. The etiology for each complication and guidelines for therapy are described in detail below:

1. *Shock secondary to intravascular volume depletion.* Patients presenting in DKA have a significant degree of dehydration (usually 10% to 15% of total body weight) and universally will require initial isotonic fluid rehydration. Dehydration is caused both by osmotic diuresis due to hyperglycemia and by vomiting related to ketoacidosis. Most patients should receive a rapid bolus of 10–15 ml/kg of 0.9% NaCl followed by a combination of maintenance fluids plus replacement of the total fluid deficit over the next 36–48 hours. The composition of these fluids at a minimum should be 0.45% NaCl though initial rehydration with 3/4 normal saline (two-bag system), or even 0.9% NaCl is also acceptable. Patients who are hypotensive or show evidence for cardiovascular instability should receive additional boluses of isotonic fluids.

2. *Metabolic acidosis.* The acidosis observed in DKA is an anion gap metabolic acidosis resulting primarily from the increased release of ketone bodies from the liver. β-Hydroxybutyrate and, to a lesser degree, acetoacetate are the primary ketone bodies observed. A smaller degree of the overall metabolic acidosis stems from increased levels of lactate from poor tissue perfusion and/or infection in selected patients. Insulin administration causes an eventual inhibition of gluconeogenesis and lipolysis, slowing the rate of ketone body formation and acidosis. After the initial fluid bolus, regular insulin should be given intravenously at a rate of 0.1 or 0.05 U/kg/hour for children younger than age 3 years. Alternatively, frequent (every 2 hours) sub-

TABLE 1-7	Potential Complications Associated with DKA

- Shock
- Metabolic acidosis
- Hypokalemia/hyperkalemia
- Hypolgycemia
- Cerebral edema

cutaneous doses of lispro insulin at a dose of 0.1 U/kg can be given subcutaneously if intravenous therapy is not feasible. Insulin therapy should continue at this rate or may be decreased (0.05 U/kg/hour) if intravenous fluid dextrose concentrations exceed 10%. Due to the potential increased risk of cerebral edema (see below), bicarbonate therapy should be reserved for cases of decreased cardiac contractility, persistent hyperkalemia, or cardiopulmonary arrest. Other theoretical concerns regarding bicarbonate therapy can be worsening tissue hypoxia by potential left shift of the oxygen–hemoglobin dissociation curve. Persistent acidosis in the absence of measurable ketone bodies should prompt an evaluation for other etiologies. Non–anion gap hyperchloremic metabolic acidosis commonly occurs in situations where excess chloride was given during the course of therapy.

3. *Hypokalemia or hyperkalemia.* DKA results in depletion of total-body stores of potassium, particularly from the intracellular space. As acidosis progresses, an extracellular shift of potassium from the intracellular space occurs in exchange for hydrogen ions to minimize the ongoing acidosis. In addition, high obligate urinary losses of potassium occur secondary to the ongoing osmotic diuresis and from activation of the renin–angiotensin–aldosterone system to assist with restoration of intravascular volume. Initial potassium levels therefore may be low, normal, or high in DKA. Hyperkalemia may occur in severely dehydrated patients with very poor renal perfusion. Most commonly, potassium levels are normal, but they will drop precipitously after intravenous fluid administration and insulin therapy due to the following factors: 1) an increase in the shift of potassium and glucose to the intracellular space during the insulin-mediated restoration of carbohydrate metabolism, 2) an increase in potassium and hydrogen ions entering the cell during the correction of metabolic acidosis, and 3) dilution of the extracellular potassium concentrations due to expansion of extracellular volume during correction of dehydration. Therefore, it is

crucial to add moderate to high concentrations of potassium in the intravenous fluids concurrent with insulin administration unless hyperkalemia is noted. Either potassium chloride or a combination of other potassium salts (e.g., potassium acetate or phosphate) at a concentration of 40 mEq/L should be added to the intravenous fluids. Concentrates as high as 60–80 mEq/L may be required to maintain normal potassium levels during therapy.

4. *Hypoglycemia.* It is imperative to monitor blood glucose levels closely once intravenous fluids and insulin therapy are initiated. Despite the high levels most patients present with, blood glucose levels tend to fall rather precipitously following an initial intravenous fluid bolus. This occurs because of the increase in renal perfusion, glomerular filtration, and subsequent glucosuria following restoration of intravascular volume. Once intravascular volume is supported sufficiently, the care provider should aim to lower blood glucose levels by approximately 100 mg/dL/hour to avoid rapid shifts in blood osmolality. As glucose levels continue to fall during therapy, changes to the intravenous fluid composition should be made to avoid hypoglycemic events and to allow for continued correction of ketoacidosis. Therefore, once blood glucose reaches 250 mg/dL or less, either dextrose should be added or the concentration should be increased in the intravenous fluids before lowering the insulin infusion rate.

5. *Cerebral edema.* Identifying high-risk patients, maintaining vigilant observation for signs of cerebral edema, and instituting therapy quickly when clinical signs are present help in the prevention of morbidity and mortality from cerebral edema. Almost all patients with severe DKA have some degree of cerebral swelling. The mechanism of cerebral edema is not known. An association between the rapid fall in blood glucose, the decrease in serum sodium, the rapid administration of intravenous fluids with or without changes in serum sodium, the rapid correction with alkali therapy, and hypophosphatemia is suggested as potential mechanisms of cerebral edema. Young age (<5 years), severe acidosis, high levels of blood urea nitrogen (BUN), and a falling sodium trend during therapy increase the risk for the development of cerebral edema. Vigilant monitoring, including hourly neurological checks, should be performed in all patients with DKA, especially in high-risk patients. If clinical suspicion of cerebral edema is high, therapy should be given immediately, prior to any imaging

TABLE 1-8   Protocol for DKA Management

Ongoing Laboratory Evaluation

- *Initial:* Electrolytes, pH venous, phosphorus, serum osmolality, serum betahydroxybutyrate, CBC (if clinically indicated)
- *Hourly:* Bedside glucose level—until serum glucose is less than 500 mg/dL and paired samples are within 10% of each other
- *Every 2 hours:* Electrolytes, pH venous—until insulin drip is discontinued

Therapy

- Insulin
  - *Insulin regular drip*
    - Age < 3 years, start at 0.05 U/kg/h
    - Age ≥ 3 years, start at 0.1 U/kg/h
- Intravenous fluids
  - *Initial bolus*
  - Sodium chloride 0.9% (NS) (20 mL/kg) over 1 hour
  - Repeat 10 mL/kg NS bolus as needed for hypotension
  - *Maintenance + deficit intravenous fluids*
  - Rate of fluid
    - Intravenous rate is approximately twice maintenance
      - 100 mL/kg/day for 1–10 kg
      - 50 mL/kg/day for next 10 kg (11–20 kg)
      - 20 mL/kg/day for every kilogram thereafter), *or* 3000 mL/m^2
  - Type of fluid
    - After NS bolus, if plasma glucose > 300 mg/dL *and*
      - If serum K+ <3.5 mEq/L: D$_5$W* 0.45% NaCl + 60 mEq/L KCl
      - If serum K+ 3.5–6 mEq/L: D$_5$W 0.45% NaCl + 40 mEq/L KCl
      - If serum K+ >6 mEq/L: D$_5$W 0.45% NaCl
    - After NS bolus, if plasma glucose < 300 mg/dL *and*
      - If serum K+ <3.5 mEq/L: D$_{10}$W** 0.45% NaCl + 60 mEq KCl
      - If serum K+ 3.5–6 mEq/L: D$_{10}$W 0.45% NaCl + 40 mEq KCl
      - If serum K+ >6 mEq/L: D$_{10}$W 0.45% NaCl

* = 5% glucose; ** = 10% glucose, NS = normal saline (0.9% NaCl).

study. Mannitol 0.25–1 g intravenously over 20 minutes is the most commonly used therapy, although 3% hypertonic saline (5–10 mL/kg) intravenously over 20–30 minutes is an acceptable alternative.

6. *Other considerations.* Although infrequent, some cases of DKA may be associated with severe infections, including invasive fungal disease. Body phosphate stores also may be depleted and can be restored by substituting potassium phosphate for KCl during therapy (Table 1-8).

Hypercalcemia

Hypercalcemia can result in the precipitation of calcium salts in soft tissues, particularly in the renal interstitium, making it by definition, a "dangerous" endocrine emergency. Signs and symptoms are subtle and often nonspecific, making it an easy diagnosis to overlook.

Children with mild hypercalcemia (<13 mg/dL) may be asymptomatic. Common complaints associated with long-standing or more severe hypercalcemia include nausea, vomiting, constipation, muscle weakness, polyuria, polydipsia, and depression. In the patient with longer-standing hypercalcemia, flank or abdominal pain secondary to nephrolithiasis also may be a presenting sign. Extreme hypercalcemia (>15 mg/dL) can result in central nervous system (CNS) effects such as irritability, seizures, and coma.

The initial diagnostic evaluation should be aimed at establishing whether the hypercalcemia is parathyroid hormone (PTH)–dependent or independent (Table 1-9). Therapy ultimately should be aimed at the underlying etiology (see Chapter 39 for a full discussion), but a number of temporizing measures can be employed to stabilize the patient with hypercalcemia.

Immediate treatment for hypercalcemia should include generous intravenous fluid administration, along with a loop diuretic to promote calciuresis. A typical regimen would include an initial fluid bolus using isotonic fluids (0.9% NaCl) of 20 mL/kg over 1 hour, followed by D$_5$ normal saline with a minimum of 20 mEq/L of potassium chloride at twice maintenance. Furosemide (Lasix) should be given at a dose of 1 mg/kg intravenously every 6 hours, or bumetamide (Bumex) can be substituted at a dose of 0.05–0.1 mg/kg intravenously every 12–24 hours (maximum 10 mg/day). Careful attention must be paid to potassium levels during this period because hypokalemia may result from the frequent loop diuretic administration. This therapy should result in initial restoration of intravascular volume, increased renal perfusion, and calciuria. Therapy should be continued until serum calcium levels fall below 12 mg/dL. In cases associated with hypervitaminosis D, a low-calcium diet and oral glucocorticoids (prednisone 1–2 mg/kg/day [maximum dose 60 mg/day] up to 3–5 days) can be used as an adjunctive therapy to inhibit vitamin D–mediated absorption of calcium from the gastrointestinal tract.

In the rare situation where calcium levels are significantly elevated (>14 mg/dL) and intravenous fluids and/or diuretics cannot be

TABLE 1-9   Diagnostic Evaluation of Hypercalcemia

- Ca, Mg, PO$_4$
- Ionized Ca
- PTH
- 25-(OH)$_1$-vitamin D$_3$
- 1,25-(OH)$_2$-vitamin D$_3$
- Urine Ca:Cr ratio
- BUN/creatinine
- PTH-related peptide (if oncologic diagnosis suspected)
- Renal ultrasound
- TSH, free T$_4$ (in cases of suspected hyperthyroidism)
- Morning cortisol or ACTH stimulation test (in cases of suspected adrenal insufficiency)

used or are ineffective, bisphosphanates (Pamidronate 1 mg/kg intravenously over 4 hours) or calcitonin (4–8 IU/kg subcutaneously every 12 hours) can be used as temporary stabilizing measures to acutely drop serum calcium levels. Bisphosphanates cause decreased bone resorption by inhibiting osteoclast activity and recruitment. Bisphosphanates have been employed successfully in several pediatric hypercalcemic cases and may be particularly useful in children with hypercalcemia secondary to immobilization or from cancer therapy. Calcitonin causes a transient inhibition of osteoclast activity, as well as decreased calcium absorption from the gastrointestinal tract. The most commonly available calcitonin is derived from salmon (although a recombinant human form is also available) and may cause an allergic reaction in susceptible individuals. Skin testing prior to administration should be entertained if a potential reaction is suspected. If these measures are not effective, peritoneal or hemodialysis should be considered.

Hypocalcemia

Hypocalcemia commonly presents with neuromuscular symptoms, including muscle cramps, paresthesias, muscle spasms and seizures. Interruptions to normal cardiac function also may occur, resulting in arrythmias, myocardial depression, and hypotension and making hypocalcemia a life-threatening endocrine disturbance. In infants or younger children, symptoms may be much more nonspecific and can include lethargy, poor feeding, irritability, and apnea. Physical examination findings in moderate to severe hypocalcemia are highlighted by the Chvostek (facial muscle twitching after tapping on facial nerve) and Trousseau (carpopedal spasm after inflating a sphygmomanometer to a pressure above resting blood pressure) signs. Hypocalcemia may result from disturbances in any of the normal mediators of calcium regulation, including PTH activity, vitamin D levels, acid–base balance, and renal function. Table 1-10 describes the initial diagnostic evaluation of the patient with acute hypocalcemia.

In severe cases of hypocalcemia, initial therapy first should include intravenous administration of calcium gluconate (100–200 mg/kg or 1–2 mL/kg of the standard 10% calcium gluconate preparation). Rapid infusion of calcium is likely to result in only a transient rise in calcium levels but, more important, may cause dangerous bradycardia. Therefore, calcium boluses should be given over approximately 30 minutes. Care also must be taken to ensure adequate, safe vascular access because extravasation of calcium salts can lead to significant tissue necrosis. For patients with a persistent calcium requirement demanding intravenous

TABLE 1-10	Diagnostic Evaluation of Hypocalcemia

- Total Ca
- Mg
- Phosphorus
- Alkaline phosphatase
- Ionized calcium
- Urine calcium:creatinine ratio
- PTH
- 25-hydroxyvitamin D
- 1,25-dihydroxyvitamin D
- Blood urea nitrogen
- Creatinine

boluses every 4–8 hours, a continuous drip at a rate of 1–2 mg of elemental calcium per kilogram per hour should be initiated. Oral calcium salts should be started as soon as possible, in particular when hyperphosphatemia is present. A safe starting dose is 50 mg/kg/day of oral elemental calcium, but 200 mg/kg/day may be required in severe cases.

Once calcium levels have stabilized, therapy should be tailored toward correction of the underlying etiology (e.g., hypoparathyroidism, vitamin D deficiency, or familial hypocalcemic hypercalciuria). This may include initiation of vitamin D_2 (ergocalciferol) or vitamin D_3 (cholecalciferol) and 1,25-dihdroxyvitamin D_3 (calcitriol). In cases of vitamin D deficiency, a starting dose of 1000–2000 IU/day can be given for 2 months or longer depending on the degree of deficiency and whether or not rachitic signs are present. Calcitriol, administered at a dose of 20–60 ng/kg/day, should be given to patients with hypoparathyroidism or other forms of disease causing decreased PTH activity or secretion (e.g., pseudohypoparathyroidism or autosomal dominant hypocalcemia). Care must be given not to push calcium levels into the normal or high range in disorders where hypercalciuria is likely to occur (e.g., hypoparathyroidism). This may result in additional precipitation products and nephrocalcinosis. Other considerations include correction of alkalotic states that promote decreases in ionized calcium, correction of hypomagnesemia that can impair the secretion of PTH, and lowering of serum phosphate levels because this can result in soft tissue calcium salt deposits once calcium therapy has begun.

Hyponatremia

Hyponatremia is defined as a serum sodium concentration of less then 130 mEq/L. Some of the causes of hyponatremia include gastrointestinal (GI) illness; water intoxication due to improper dilution of the formula,

psychogenic polydipsia, or the syndrome of inappropriate secretion of antidiuretic hormone (SIADH); increased renal sodium loss secondary to kidney disease or aldosterone deficiency (either isolated or as part of adrenal insufficiency); pseudohypoaldosteronism; and edema-forming states such as congestive heart failure, nephrotic syndrome, and cirrhosis. Hyponatremia associated with hyperkalemia is caused by aldosterone deficiency states, including salt-wasting CAH due to 21-hydroxylation deficiency, 3β-dehydrogenase deficiency, and lipoid adrenal hyperplasia.

Symptoms usually do not develop until the serum sodium concentration is less than 125 mEq/L, and their development is more indicative of the rate of serum sodium decline than the serum sodium absolute value. Symptoms associated with hyponatremia range from anorexia, headache, nausea, vomiting, and irritability to disorientation, seizures, and coma.

Laboratory Evaluation Initial evaluation of hyponatremia includes serum electrolytes, with BUN/creatinine and glucose, serum and urine osmolalities, urinalysis, and urine electrolytes. Hyponatremia in the presence of normal creatinine and low or normal BUN suggests water intoxication due to psychogenic polydipsia, dilute formula, or SIADH. A urine osmolality greater than the serum osmolality suggests SIADH and differentiates from water intoxication due to polydipsia or dilute formula, where both urine and serum osmolality would be low. Adrenal insufficiency and hypothyroidism occasionally can present with an SIADH picture caused by increased free water gain and negligible sodium loss.

A high urinary sodium concentration (>20 mEq/L) reflects sodium and water loss from the kidney due to sodium-wasting nephropathy, hypoaldosteronism, and adrenal disorders associated with aldosterone deficiency. A low urinary sodium concentration (<20 mEq/L) suggests extrarenal sodium and water losses as the kidney appropriately increases sodium reabsorption, as seen in GI disorders and severe burns.

If hyponatremia is associated with hyperkalemia and hypoglycemia, causes of adrenal insufficiency should be investigated by measuring ACTH, cortisol, aldosterone, renin, 17-hydroxyprogesterone, 17-hydroxypregnenolone, and DHEAS levels. Elevated aldosterone and renin levels in presence of hyponatremia and hyperkalemia suggest pseudohypoaldosteronism, whereas a low aldosterone level and elevated renin level suggest aldosterone deficiency.

Elevated 17-hydroxyprogesterone, ACTH, and DHEAS levels and a low cortisol level in addition to low aldosterone and elevated renin suggest salt-wasting CAH due to 21-hydroxylase deficiency, whereas an elevated 17-hydroxypregnenolone level instead of 17-hydroxyprogesterone suggests CAH due to 3β-dehydrogenase deficiency. Elevated renin and ACTH levels with low adrenal steroids suggest primary adrenal insufficiency.

Treatment When treating hyponatremia and deciding the rate of fluid administration and serum sodium correction, the risks of hyponatremia-induced cerebral edema must be weighed against the risk of developing osmotic demyelination syndrome (ODS) (24). Cerebral edema results from the osmotic movement of the water in brain cells in the setting of hypo-osmolarity, whereas ODS, previously termed *central pontine myelinolysis*, occurs when water moves too rapidly out of brain cells during administration of hypertonic saline solutions. Patients with ODS present with mental status changes, spastic quadriparesis, and pseudobulbar palsies after a period of improvement with fluid administration.

Patients with hyponatremia who develop seizures, severe lethargy, or coma should be treated with hypertonic saline 3%, with a target rate of correction of 1.5–2 mEq/L per hour for the first 3–4 hours or more briefly if the symptoms improve (1 mEqL/kg of 3% saline would correct the serum sodium by 1 mEq/L/hour). The maximum rise in serum sodium concentration should not exceed 10 mEq/L during the first 24 hours. In these patients, the high likelihood of cerebral edema outweighs the risk of possible ODS. Patients with acute (<48 hours duration) hyponatremia tolerate aggressive sodium therapy better than patients with symptomatic chronic hyponatremia because the adaptive mechanism of the brain to hyponatremia (mobilization of organic osmolytes by brain cells to preserve cell volume) has not taken full effect. For seizure control, phenytoin at 5–10 mg/kg should be given intravenously. Close monitoring of fluid balance, serum sodium, and serum and urine osmolality is essential. The remission of symptomatic hyponatremia in patients with SIADH or other causes of water intoxication is followed by fluid restriction rates of normal saline to below insensible losses or complete fluid restriction if sodium is less than 125 Meq/L (25). The fluid restriction can be lessened slowly as soon as the serum sodium rises. A formula to calculate the change in serum sodium concentration in pediatric patients when 1 L of intravenous fluids (IVFs) is used is the following (26):

$$\text{Serum Na change (mEq/L) with 1 L of IVFS} = [\text{Na content in IVFs (mEq/L)} - \text{measured Na (mEq/L)}]/[0.6 \times \text{Wt (kg)} + 1]$$

In hyponatremic patients with mild symptoms, the risk of ODS outweighs the risk of cerebral edema. Slow sodium correction at 0.5 mEq/L/hour with a maximum sodium increase of 10–12 mEq/L prevents the development of ODS.

Hypovolemic hyponatremia should be treated with normal saline fluid administration, and if adrenal insufficiency is suspected, cortisol administration at 100 mg/m²/day divided in four intravenous doses should be added to the regimen.

Hypernatremia

Hypernatremia is a serum sodium concentration greater than 145 mEq/L, more often caused by water deficiency (i.e., inadequate water intake, increased renal or GI fluid loss, profuse sweating, burns, and skin disease) than by sodium excess (i.e., unduly high sodium bicarbonate or hypertonic saline intravenously). Patients with excessive mineralocorticoid secretion or action, as in hyperaldosteronism, apparent mineralocorticoid excess (AME), Liddle syndrome, dexamethasone-suppressible hyperaldosteronism (DSH), Cushing syndrome, and CAH due to 11-hydroxylase deficiency or 17,20-hydroxylase/lyase deficiency, have modest hypernatremia (<150 mEq/L) because of sodium's osmotic activity that drives water into the extracellular fluid space. Hypernatremia in disorders of mineralocorticoid excess usually is associated with low renin and hypokalemic alkalosis.

Inadequate water intake results from either an impaired thirst mechanism or lack of access to water (i.e., physically or mentally impaired, inadequate breast-feeding, etc.). Causes of increased renal fluid loss include diuretics and osmotic glucosuria seen in patients in DKA, whereas causes of increased renal water loss include central diabetes insipidus (CDI) or nephrogenic diabetes insipidus (NDI).

Infants may present with muscle weakness, tachypnea, irritability, lethargy, and high-pitched cry. Polyuria and polydipsia may be present in patients with hypernatremia due to CDI or NDI. Shock rarely develops in infants because extracellular fluid and plasma volumes remain preserved until severe dehydration (>10% loss of body weight). In severe dehydration, skin turgor is reduced, and abdominal skin may feel like dough.

Laboratory Evaluation Initial evaluation of hypernatremia includes serum electrolytes, with BUN/creatinine and glucose, serum and urine osmolalities, urinalysis, and urine electrolytes. Patients with hypernatremia due to pure sodium overload would have increased urinary sodium excretion (>100 mEq/L). Patients with hypernatremia due to nephrogenic diabetes insipidus (NDI) or

central diabetes insipidus (CDI) have low urine osmolality, increased serum osmolality, and decreased sodium excretion in the urine (<20 mEq/L).

Patients with extrarenal fluid losses (i.e., GI, burns, etc.) have decreased sodium excretion in the urine, as in NDI or CDI, but decreased serum osmolality and appropriately elevated urine osmolality (>700 mOsm/kg). Urinary sodium excretion is elevated (>20 mEq/L) in severe osmotic diuresis or with diuretic use.

If hypernatremia is associated with hypokalemia and/or hypertension, the laboratory evaluation should include aldosterone, renin, adrenal profile including deoxycorticosterone, corticosterone, 17-hydroxyprogesterone, cortisol, and adrenal androgens. Hypernatremia, hypokalemia, and/or hypertension, when associated with elevated levels of deoxycorticosterone and corticosterone and low 17-hydroxyprogesterone, cortisol, aldosterone, renin, and androgen levels, suggest CAH due to 17,20-hydroxylase deficiency, whereas when associated with elevated deoxycorticosterone, androgens, and 17-hydroxyprogesterone with low aldosterone, renin, and cortisol, they suggest CAH due to 11β-hydroxylase deficiency. The 24-hour urine for free cortisol should be tested if Cushing syndrome is suspected. If the only hormonal abnormalities are low aldosterone and renin, evaluation to rule out apparent mineralocorticoid excess (AME), Dexamethasone-suppressible hyperaldosteronism (DSH), or Liddle syndrome should follow. Hyperaldosteronism should be suspected in cases where aldosterone is high with low renin.

Treatment Determination of the patient's volume status is the first step in the treatment of hypernatremia. A hypovolemic patient is treated initially with normal saline (0.9%) until the patient is hemodynamically stable, and then fluids should be changed to a hypotonic solution (0.45%).

Patients with hypernatremia due to diabetes insipidus require water replacement with intravenous hypotonic saline or free water along with DDAVP in CDI and hydrochlorothiazide in NDI (for details of treatment, see Chapter 41).

Because of the risk of cerebral edema, correction of hypernatremia in normovolemic patients should target lowering the serum sodium by 0.5–1 mEq/L/hour, with a maximum decrease of 10 mEq/24 hours. No more than half the deficit should be replaced within the first 24 hours, with the remainder corrected over the next 1–2 days.

The same formula described under hyponatremia for calculation of the sodium concentration per hour using 1 L of IVFs is applicable in hypernatremia.

REFERENCES

1. Feinstein JA, O'Brien K. Acute metabolic decompensation in an adult patient with isovaleric acidemia. *South Med J.* 2003;96:500–503.

2. Finkelstein JE, Hauser ER, Leonard CO, et al. Late-onset ornithine transcarbamylase deficiency in male patients. *J Pediatr.* 1990;117:897–902.

3. Heringlake S, Boker K, Manns M. Fatal clinical course of ornithine transcarbamylase deficiency in an adult heterozygous female patient. *Digestion.* 1997;58:83–86.

4. Lucke T, Perez-Cerda C, Baumgartner M, et al. Propionic acidemia: Unusual course with late onset and fatal outcome. *Metabolism.* 2004;53:809–810.

5. Shaw PJ, Dale G, Bates D. Familial lysinuric protein intolerance presenting as coma in two adult siblings. *J Neurol Neurosurg Psychiatry.* 1989;52:648–651.

6. von Wendt L, Simila S, Ruokonen A, et al. Argininosuccinic aciduria in a Finnish woman presenting with psychosis and mental retardation. *Ann Clin Res.* 1982;14:145–147.

7. Yorifuji T, Kawai M, Muroi J, et al. Unexpectedly high prevalence of the mild form of propionic acidemia in Japan: Presence of a common mutation and possible clinical implications. *Hum Genet.* 2002;111:161–165.

8. Calvo M, Artuch R, Macia E, et al. Diagnostic approach to inborn errors of metabolism in an emergency unit. *Pediatr Emerg Care.* 2000;16:405–408.

9. Browning MF, Levy HL, Wilkins-Haug LE, et al. Fetal fatty acid oxidation defects and maternal liver disease in pregnancy. *Obstet Gynecol* 2006;107:115–120.

10. Burton BK. Inborn errors of metabolism in infancy: A guide to diagnosis. *Pediatrics.* 1998;102:E69.

11. Claudius I, Fluharty C, Boles R. The emergency department approach to newborn and childhood metabolic crisis. *Emerg Med Clin North Am.* 2005;23:843–83, x.

12. Prietsch V, Lindner M, Zschocke J, et al. Emergency management of inherited metabolic diseases. *J Inherited Metab Dis.* 2002;25:531–546.

13. Sahajwalla CG, Helton ED, Purich ED, et al. Multiple-dose pharmacokinetics and bioequivalence of L-carnitine 330-mg tablet versus 1-g chewable tablet versus enteral solution in healthy adult male volunteers. *J Pharm Sci.* 1995;84:627–633.

14. Batshaw ML. Sodium benzoate and arginine: Alternative pathway therapy in inborn errors of urea synthesis. *Prog Clin Biol Res.* 1983;127:69–83.

15. Holme E, Lindstedt S. Nontransplant treatment of tyrosinemia. *Clin Liver Dis.* 2000;4:805–814.

16. Schwenk WF, Haymond MW. Optimal rate of enteral glucose administration in children with glycogen storage disease type I. *N Engl J Med.* 1986;314:682–685.

17. Shekhawat PS, Matern D, Strauss AW. Fetal fatty acid oxidation disorders, their effect on maternal health and neonatal outcome:

Impact of expanded newborn screening on their diagnosis and management. *Pediatr Res.* 2005;57:78R–86R.

18. Yoon SJ, Kim DM, Kim JU, et al. A case of thyroid storm due to thyrotoxicosis factitia. *Yonsei Med J.* 2003;44:351–354.

19. Isotani H, Sanda K, Kameoka K, et al. McCune–Albright syndrome associated with non-autoimmune type of hyperthyroidism with development of thyrotoxic crisis. *Horm Res.* 2000;53:256–259.

20. Ahmad N, Cohen MP. Thyroid storm with normal serum triiodothyronine level during diabetic ketoacidosis. *JAMA.* 1981;245:2516–2517.

21. Mouradian M, Abourizk N. Diabetes mellitus and thyroid disease. *Diabetes Care* 1983;6:512–520.

22. Charles RA, Goh SY. Not just gastroenteritis: Thyroid storm unmasked. *Emerg Med Australas.* 2004;16:247–249.

23. Dunger DB, Sperling MA, Acerini CL, et al. ESPE/LWPES consensus statement on diabetic ketoacidosis in children and adolescents. *Arch Dis Child.* 2004;89:188–194.

24. Lin M, Liu SJ, Lim IT. Disorders of water imbalance. *Emerg Med Clin North Am* 2005;23:749–770, ix.

25. Kappy MS, Bajaj L. Recognition and treatment of endocrine/metabolic emergencies in children, part II. *Adv Pediatr.* 2003;50:181–214.

26. Adrogue HJ, Madias NE. Hypernatremia. *N Engl J Med.* 2000;342:1493–1499.

CHAPTER 2

Newborn Screening

Andreas Schulze, MD, FRCPC
Dietrich Matern, MD, FACMG
Georg F. Hoffmann, MD

INTRODUCTION

Preventing children from shouldering the burden of inherited diseases is the aim of newborn screening. Prerequisites are: 1) disease detection in a presymptomatic/early stage of the disease; 2) treatability of the disease, 3) reliable start of treatment in the presymptomatic/early stage.

Screening of neonates for signs of disease or distress has several components, with the perinatal clinical evaluation being of first and foremost importance. The clinical approach is limited to the detection of symptoms, which in many disorders have been proven to be irreversible. For example, classic phenylketonuria (PKU) due to phenylalanine (Phe) hydroxylase deficiency is characterized by the insidious development of irreversible neurological damage unless treatment is initiated within the first few weeks of life. Newborn screening was first developed for the identification of this inborn error of amino acid metabolism, which was typically not diagnosed before 6 months of life when developmental delay or other nonspecific neurologic symptoms become apparent. Treatment based on a Phe-restricted diet was developed by Horst Bickel in the 1950s, but it was quickly realized that the initiation of this therapy only improved the patient's symptoms but was inadequate to reverse neurologic damage (1). Furthermore, it was recognized that a limited intake of the essential amino acid Phe requires the regular monitoring of the Phe concentration in blood. A simple method for Phe determination was developed by Robert Guthrie, a scientist initially working in cancer research and the father of a child with mental retardation (2). This test was a bacterial inhibition assay (BIA) performed on serum dried on filter paper. Guthrie then began to apply his BIA to the analysis of Phe in small blood samples also dried on filter paper with the aim of allowing the presymptomatic identification of PKU in patients and facilitating the timely initiation of dietary intervention (3). Once the efficacy of this assay was established, newborn screening began in several regions in the United States and rapidly spread around the world using the Guthrie test (4,5). A few additional disorders such as congenital hypothyroidism, galactosemia, and sickle cell disease were gradually added to many newborn screening programs, usually one new assay for each additional disorder.

The BIA was initially modified to detect other disease markers and eventually more sophisticated technologies were applied, such as fluorometric, colorimetric, and immunoassays to determine either disease metabolites or specific enzyme activities. Over the last decade, the introduction of tandem mass spectrometry (MS/MS) into newborn screening laboratories has dramatically expanded the number of disorders that can be detected in a single blood spot. More than 30 additional conditions can be detected by simultaneous acylcarnitine and amino acid analyses, including inborn errors of amino acid, organic acid, and fatty acid metabolism.

Disorders in Newborn Screening Programs

To aid in the selection of diseases to be included into screening programs, screening principles were developed by Wilson and Jungner on behalf of the World Health Organization in 1968 (6). Although these principles were not developed specifically for newborn screening, until today they represent, with some adaptation, the most commonly used selection criteria for newborn screening in almost all countries. When deciding which diseases to include in any newborn screening program careful consideration must be given to weighing the impact for affected individuals against the burden for nonaffected individuals. Detailed recommendations for screening policy will vary from country to country and region to region, depending on local economic, political, and medical factors and public health organization.

In 2002, the American College of Medical Genetics (ACMG) was commissioned by the Maternal and Child Health Bureau of the Health Resources and Services Administration of the United States Department of Health and Human Services to review the scientific basis of newborn screening and develop recommendations for which disorders should be included in newborn screening programs. The impetus for a comprehensive review of the status of newborn screening was the scattered implementation of MS/MS in screening laboratories in the United States, which led to marked discrepancies in the number of conditions included in the various screening programs. Several states provided newborn screening for only three diseases, whereas those that implemented amino acid and acylcarnitine profiling by MS/MS were screening for more than 30 conditions (a regularly updated list of conditions screened for in each state is available at: http://genes-rus.uthscsa.edu/). In 2006, the ACMG reported their conclusions: (7,8) and recommended screening for 29 diseases by all programs (core conditions; Table 2-1). These conditions were considered to fulfill three basic principles that were developed to update and replace the original Wilson and Jungner criteria: 1) each condition is identifiable in a period of time (24 to 48 hours after birth) at which it would not ordinarily be clinically detected; 2) a test with appropriate sensitivity and specificity is available; and, 3) benefits of early detection, timely intervention, and efficacious treatment have been demonstrated. Because screening tests do not primarily determine disease status, but measure analytes that in most cases are not specific for a particular disease, the ACMG report also includes 25 conditions (secondary targets) that did not meet all three selection criteria but are identified nevertheless because most of them are included in the differential diagnosis of screening results observed in core conditions (Table 2-1). Most of these secondary conditions are identified through metabolite profiling by MS/MS, which enables the determination of more than 50 analytes and analyte ratios in a small newborn screening blood spot punch. This also increases the

Newborn Screening

AT-A-GLANCE

Newborn screening is one of the best established and most important programs in preventive medicine. It represents a population-based measure for detection of newborns suffering from metabolic and endocrine disorders. Disclosure of affected individuals in the pre-symptomatic state of the disease is the prerequisite for early implementation of treatment. Timely intervention can relieve most or almost all of the burden of many of the diseases.

The screening covers a large number of rare but treatable inherited diseases. Agreement on a set of criteria such as those outlined by Wilson and Jungner (6) (Table 2-1) for inclusion of a condition into a screening program is not universal. While there is agreement that a careful balance between benefit and harm is important, the number of conditions included in newborn screening programs is variable.

Blood from newborns is taken in the first 1 to 4 days of life by a heel prick, spotted onto filter paper and sent to a screening laboratory. The laboratory investigates the dried blood spots for the diseases of the respective screening panel. In the majority of newborns (~99%), the presence of disease can be ruled out as result of the first investigation. In case of a positive result in the screening test, most screening programs request a repeated blood spot sample (re-call). Of those newborns who underwent a re-call investigation approximately 90% are not affected. In case of strong suspicion for a disease either by clearly abnormal first testing or by confirmation of abnormal test results in a re-call investigation the screening laboratory advises the sender of the specimen to initiate confirmatory testing. Because the conditions screened for are rare and confirmation and treatment are complex, care of the presumptively affected newborns should occur in close consultation and collaboration with a pediatric specialist.

Most of the population-based newborn screening programs are administered by public health services/laboratories. Screening programs must cover all parts of the screening process to achieve the goals of newborn screening.

SCREENING DISORDER	PREVALENCE*
Phenylketonuria (PKU)	1:~10,000
Galactosemia	1:~40,000
Biotinidase deficiency	1:~80,000
Congenital hypothyroidism (CH)	1:~4,000
Congenital adrenal hyperplasia (CAH)	1:~10,000
Maple syrup urine disease (MSUD)	< 1:200,000
Hepatorenal tyrosinemia type 1 (TYR-1)	1:100,000
Homocystinuria (HCY)	< 1:200,000
Citrullinemia (ASS)	1:~50,000
Argininosuccinate lyase deficiency (ASL)	1:180,000
Medium-chain acyl-CoA dehydrogenase deficiency (MCAD)	1:~15,000
(Very) long-chain acyl-CoA dehydrogenase deficiency (VLCAD)	< 1:200,000
Long-chain 3-OH-acyl-CoA dehydrogenase deficiency (LCHAD)	1:200,000
Carnitine-palmitoyl transferase I deficiency (CPT I)	< 1:200,000
Carnitine-palmitoyl transferase II deficiency (CPT II)	< 1:200,000
Carnitine-acylcarnitine-translocase deficiency (CAT)	< 1:200,000
Isovaleric aciduria (IVA)	1:~80,000
Glutaric aciduria type 1 (GA-1)	1:100,000
Propionic aciduria (PA)	1:200,000
Methylmalonic aciduria (MMA)	1:200,000
Cobalamin deficiency (CBL A,B,C,D,F)	1:200,000
3-Methylcrotonyl-CoA carboxylase deficiency (3-MCC)	1:~60,000
3-OH-methylglutaryl-CoA lyase deficiency (HMG)	< 1:200,000

*Prevalence as estimated from newborn screening in a Caucasian population, it may vary among screening populations of different ethnic background.

DISORDER	KEY METABOLITE*	COMMENTS/ CONFIRMATION ANALYSIS
PKU	↑ Phe ↓ Tyr ↑ Phe/Tyr ratio	**Confirmation:** Plasma Phe, Tyr; BH$_4$ loading test, pterins in urine, dihydropteridine reductase activity in DBS.
Galactosemia	↑ Total galactose	Galactokinase def. and UDP-gal-epimerase def. are also detected by total galactose screening. Galactosemia screening gives false negatives when baby not yet receive lactose-containing milk. **Confirmation:** Enzyme in erythrocytes.
	↓ Galactose-1-phosphate uridyltransferase (GALT)	Galactokinase def. and UDP-gal-epimerase def. are not detected by GALT screening. GALT screening is independent from feeding.
Biotinidase deficiency	↓ Biotinidase activity	**Confirmation:** Enzyme in serum.
CH	↑ TSH	Hypothalamo-hypophyseal forms of hypothyroidism are not detected by TSH screening. Citrate and EDTA blood causes false positives. **Confirmation:** Plasma thyroid hormones.
CAH	↑ 17-OH-Progesterone (17-OHP)	Screening does not reliably detect 11- and 17-hydroxylase/17,20-lyase, and 3β-OH steroid dehydrogenase deficiency. For preterm newborns cut-offs adjusted for gestational age and/or birth weight are necessary. **Confirmation:** Plasma steroids, genetic analysis.
MSUD	↑ Leucine + Isoleucine ↑ Valine ↑ (Leu+Ileu)/Phe -ratio	Screening during the first 24 hours might miss cases. **Confirmation:** Plasma amino acids and urinary organic acids.
TYR-1	↑ Tyr ↑ Succinylacetone	EDTA blood and high temperature cause false positive succinylacetone inhibition assay results. **Confirmation:** Plasma amino acids, α-fetoprotein, succinylacetone in urine, enzyme in fibroblasts.
HCY	↑ Methionine	**Confirmation:** Total homocysteine in plasma, organic acids in urine, genetic analysis, enzyme in fibroblasts.
ASS	↑ Citrulline ↓ Arginine	**Confirmation:** Plasma amino acids, orotic acid in urine.
ASL	↑ Arginino-succinate ↑ Citrulline ↓ Arginine	**Confirmation:** Plasma and urine amino acids, orotic acid in urine, enzyme in erythrocytes/fibroblasts.
MCAD	↑ C8 carnitine ↑ C8/C2 ratio ↑ C8/C10 ratio ↑ C8/C12 ratio	CD may cause non-informative acylcarnitine profile; C$_8$ may be also elevated in glutaric type II as well as C$_4$, C$_5$, C5DC, C$_{14}$ and C$_{14:1}$ acylcarnitines. **Confirmation:** Acylcarnitines in DBS/blood, urinary organic acids, enzyme in lymphocytes/fibroblasts, mutation.
VLCAD	↑ C14:1 carnitine ↑ C14 carnitine	CD or glucose infusion may cause a non-informative acylcarnitine profile. Blood for acylcarnitine profiling has to be taken prior to (not after) regular meal. **Confirmation:** Acylcarnitines in DBS/blood, urinary organic acids, enzyme in lymphocytes/ fibroblasts, mutation.
LCHAD/TFP	↑ C16OH carnitine ↑ C18OH carnitine	CD may cause a non-informative acylcarnitine profile. Fat infusion causes false positives. C16OH may be the only abnormal finding in LCHAD/TFP deficiency even with normal C2. **Confirmation:** Acylcarnitines in DBS/blood, enzyme in lymphocytes/fibroblasts, genetic analysis.
CPT I	↑ C0 (free) carnitine ↓ C16 carnitine ↓ C18 carnitine ↑ C0/(C16+C18) ratio	Carnitine supplementation (prematures) causes false positives. **Confirmation:** Acylcarnitines in DBS/blood, free carnitine in blood, enzyme in lymphocytes/fibroblasts, genetic analysis.

DISORDER	KEY METABOLITE*	COMMENTS/ CONFIRMATION ANALYSIS
CPT II and CAT	↑ C14 carnitine ↑ C16 carnitine ↑ C18 carnitine ↑ C18:1 carnitine	CD may cause a non-informative acylcarnitine profile. Special premature formula gives false positives. **Confirmation:** Acylcarnitines in DBS/blood, enzyme in lymphocytes/fibroblasts, genetic analysis.
IVA	↑ C5 carnitine	CD may cause a non-informative acylcarnitine profile. Treatment with pivalic acid containing antibiotics may cause false positive results. C5 carnitine is also elevated in SBCAD deficiency. **Confirmation:** Urinary organic acids, and acylglycines.
GA-1	↑ C5DC	CD may cause a non-informative acylcarnitine profile. **Confirmation:** Organic acids in urine (glutaric and 3-hydroxyglutaric acid by a sensitive stable isotope dilution method), enzyme in lymphocytes/fibroblasts, genetic analysis.
PA	↑ C3 carnitine ↑ C3/C0 ratio	CD may cause a non-informative acylcarnitine profile. **Confirmation:** Urinary organic acids, plasma amino acids, ammonia, enzyme in fibroblasts, mutation.
MMA	↑ C3 carnitine ↑ C3/C0 ratio	CD may cause a non-informative acylcarnitine profile. **Confirmation:** Urinary organic acids, plasma amino acids and total homocysteine, ammonia, enzyme in fibroblasts, genetic analysis.
CBL A,B,C,D,F	↑ C3 carnitine ↑ C3/C0 ratio	CD may cause a non-informative acylcarnitine profile. **Confirmation:** Urinary organic acids, plasma amino acids and total homocysteine, ammonia, enzyme in fibroblasts, genetic analysis.
3-MCC	↑ C5OH carnitine	CD may cause a non-informative acylcarnitine profile. C5OH carnitine can also be elevated in 3-methylglutaconic aciduria type I, multiple carboxylase deficiency including biotinidase and holocarboxylase deficiency, biotin deficiency, β-ketothiolase deficiency, 2-methyl 3-hydroxy butyryl-CoA dehydrogenase deficiency and **3-hydroxy-3-methylglutaryl (HMG)-CoA lyase deficiency.** **Confirmation:** Urinary organic acids, blood ammonia, enzyme in fibroblasts, genetic analysis, acylcarnitines in the mother
SCAD	↑ C4 carnitine	CD may cause a non-informative acylcarnitine profile. ↑ C4 carnitine can be also elevated in isobutyryl-CoA dehydrogenase deficiency and ethylmalonic encephalopathy. **Confirmation:** Urinary organic acids, urine acylglycines and acylcarnitines, enzyme in fibroblasts, genetic analysis.

CD = carnitine deficiency; ConfA = confirmation analysis; DBS = dried blood specimen; TSH = thyroid-stimulating hormone.

NOTE: Information and suggestions for follow up of abnormal newborn screening results is also available at: http://www.acmg.net/resources/policies/ACT/condition-analyte-links.htm.

responsibility of newborn screening laboratories to provide testing with the highest sensitivity and specificity to allow identification of affected patients while minimizing the false-positive rate.

Performance of a Newborn Screening Program

An ideal screening test would detect all newborns in a population affected with the disease with 100% sensitivity and the unaffected newborns would have normal results (100% specificity). In practice, every screening test fails

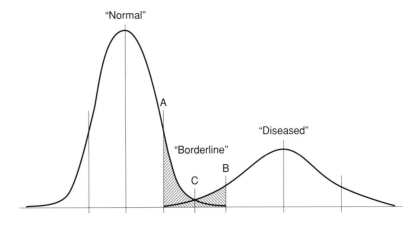

FIGURE 2-1. Bimodal distribution of a variable (e.g., the marker metabolite for a screening disease) in a population.

under certain circumstances and to a different extent. Disease-specific metabolites were used as marker(s) in most of the screening conditions (e.g., Phe in screening for PKU). These metabolites reveal usually a bimodal distribution, where the "diseased part" is separated from the "normal part" (Figure 2-1). Depending on the (patho)physiologic distribution of the metabolite(s) and the characteristic of the screening test the two parts can overlap. Diagnostic sensitivity and specificity then depends on how the decision limit ("cut-off" point) for the marker is set. In the example given in Figure 2-1, the cut-off set at point A yields 100% sensitivity but many false positives; the cut-off set at point B yields 100% specificity but many false negatives, and at point C yields some false positives and false negatives. Note that sensitivity and specificity vary reciprocally to the setting of the cut-off.

Setting the cut-off at the 99.5th percentile of healthy newborns often results in 100% sensitivity while keeping the specificity in an acceptable range. A higher cut-off is feasible when missing of disease variants (mildly affected subjects not needing treatment) is acceptable or when there is a gap between "normal" and "disease."

Applying a screening test to a population will produce four categories of results (true positives, false positives, false negatives, and true negatives; Table 2-2). If the number of cases for each category is known, the false-positive rate and positive predictive value (PPV) can be calculated. The false-positive rate should be low and the PPV, which is a measure of the proportion of persons with positive test results who are truly affected, should be high. These measures provide insight into the performance of a screening program and physicians receiving newborn screening results should be able to obtain this information from their respective screening programs. Physicians must be aware though that screening programs have different definitions of what constitutes a positive result. Some programs count any abnormal result as positive, whereas others consider only a confirmed abnormal result on a repeated blood spot test as positive (9).

To illustrate how indices help in the assessment of a screening test, consider the situation of screening for tyrosinemia type I (TYR-I). The primary marker used to identify patients with TYR-I is tyrosine (Tyr); however, Tyr levels in newborns with TYR-I can

TABLE 2-1 Newborn Screening Conditions Recommended by the ACMG, and Their Key Analytes (47).

Analyte	Core Condition	Secondary Targets
Phe	PKU	BS HPA REG
Leu/Ile, Val	MSUD	
Met	HCY	MET
Cit, Arg, ASA	ASA CIT	ARG CIT-II
Tyr	TYR-I	TYR-II TYR-III
C0	CUD	
C3	CBL A, CBL B MUT PA	CBL C, CBL D
C4		IBDH SCAD
C5	IVA	SBCAD
C5-OH	BKT HMG MCC MCD	MGA-I MHBD
C8	MCAD	GA-II MCKAT M/SCHAD
C3-DC		MAL
C10:2		DR
C5-DC	GA-I	
C14:1, C16, C18:1	VLCAD	CACT CPT-I CPT-II
C16-OH	LCHAD TFP	
Biotinidase[3,4]	BIOT	
17-OHP[4]	CAH	
TSH and/or fT4	CH	
Total Galactose and/or GALT	GALT	GALE GALK

PKU, phenylketonuria; BS, defects of biopterin cofactor biosynthesis; HPA, benign hyperphenylalaninemia; REG, defects of biopterin cofactor regeneration; MSUD, maple syrup disease; HCY, homocystinuria (doe to cystathionine beta synthase deficiency); MET, hypermethioninemia; ASA, argininosuccinic acidemia; CIT, citrullinemia; ARG, argininemia; CIT-II, citrullinemia type II (citrin deficiency); TYR-I, tyrosinemia type I; TYR-II, tyrosinemia type II; TYR-III, tyrosinemia type III; CUD, carnitine uptake defect; CBL A, methylmalonic acidemia (CBL A); CBL B, methylmalonic acidemia (CBL B); MUT, methylmalonic acidemia (mutase deficiency); PA, propionic acidemia; Cbl C, methylmalonic acidemia (CBL C); Cbl D, methylmalonic acidemia (Cbl D); IBDH, isobutyryl-CoA dehydrogenase deficiency; SCAD, short-chain acyl-CoA dehydrogenase deficiency; IVA, isovaleric acidemia; SBCAD, short branched-chain acyl-CoA dehydrogenase deficiency; BKT, β-ketothiolase deficiency; HMG, 3-hydroxy 3-methyl glutaric aciduria (HMG-CoA lyase deficiency); MCC, 3-methylcrotonyl-CoA carboxylase deficiency; MCD, multiple carboxylase deficiency; MGA-I, methylglutaconic aciduria type I; MHBD, 2-methyl 3-hydroxybutyryl-CoA dehydrogenase deficiency; MCAD, medium-chain acyl-CoA dehydrogenase deficiency; GA-II, glutaric aciduria type II (multiple acyl-CoA dehydrogenase deficiency); MCKAT, medium-chain ketoacyl-CoA thiolase deficiency; M/SCHAD, medium/short-chain 3-hydroxy acyl-CoA dehydrogenase deficiency; MAL, malonic aciduria; DR, dienoyl-CoA reductase deficiency; GA-I, glutaric acidemia type I; VLCAD, very long-chain acyl-CoA dehydrogenase deficiency; CACT, carnitine: acylcarnitine translocase deficiency; CPT-I, carnitine palmitoyltransferase I deficiency; CPT-II, carnitine palmitoyltransferase II deficiency; LCHAD, long-chain 3-hydroxy acyl-CoA dehydrogenase deficiency; TFP, trifunctional protein deficiency; BIOT, biotinidase deficiency; CAH, congenital adrenal hyperplasia (21-hydroxylase deficiency); CH, congenital hypothyroidism; GALT, classical galactosemia; GALE, galactose epimerase deficiency; GALK, galactokinase deficiency.

TABLE 2-2 The Performance of a Screening Test

	No. of Newborns w/ Positive Screening Result	No. of Newborns w/ Negative Screening Result	Total
No. of Newborns w/ Disease	True Positives (TP)	False Negatives (FN)	TP + FN
No. of Newborns w/o Disease	False Positives (FP)	True Negatives (TN)	FP + TN
Total	TP + FP	FN + TN	All Newborns Screened

$$\text{Sensitivity} = \frac{\text{Affected newborns with positive test (TP)}}{\text{All affected newborns in tested population (TP = FN)}}$$

= proportion of affected patients that have a positive test result

$$\text{Specificity} = \frac{\text{Healthy newborns with negative test (TN)}}{\text{All healthy newborns in tested population (FP + TN)}}$$

= proportion of unaffected newborns having a negative test result

$$\text{False-Positive Rate} = \frac{\text{Healthy newborns with positive test (FP)}}{\text{All newborns with positive test (TP + FP)}}$$

$$\text{PPV*} = \frac{\text{Affected newborns with positive test (TP)}}{\text{All positive tests (TP + FP)}}$$

= proportion of newborns with positive test results who are truly affected

*Positive predictive value.

with high false-positive rates and poor PPV in which biochemical or molecular genetic approaches are used (14–17). For example, screening for cystic fibrosis (CF) is performed by determining immunoreactive trypsinogen. If trypsinogen is abnormally elevated, DNA is extracted from the existing blood spot to determine whether CF mutations are present. A screening report is not issued until both tests have been completed (15,16).

Performing a screening test also requires the interpretation of the results, in particular when the test involves determination of more than a single analyte, as in amino acid and acylcarnitine profiling by tandem mass spectrometry. The result interpretation should include consideration of any available information provided on the newborn screening card to determine whether a clinically significant abnormality is present that would require follow up. Result interpretation requires knowledge of and experience with not only detectable diseases but also with typical clinical situations encountered in neonates. For example, C5 acylcarnitine is a marker for isovaleric aciduria (IVA), a classic organic aciduria that can result in a devastating outcome unless metabolic decompensation is prevented. IVA is therefore

be in the normal range. Furthermore, Tyr elevation is most often associated with benign transient hypertyrosinemia of the newborn. Assuming two patients with TYR-I were born among a screened population of 200,000 newborns and Tyr was 160 and 240 μmol/L in the patients' respective screening samples, a cut-off for Tyr chosen at the 99.5th percentile corresponding to a Tyr concentration of 180 μmol/L would yield an insufficient sensitivity of only 50%, a false positive rate of 0.5%, and a PPV of 0.1% (Table 2-3). Lowering the cut-off to the 97th percentile (150 μmol/L) raises the sensitivity to 100% but has its drawback in an increased false positive rate (3%), and further reduction of the PPV (0.03%) (Table 2-3). To overcome this untenable situation, some screening programs have stopped screening for TYR-I and others have implemented testing for succinylacetone, a specific marker for TYR-I (9,10). The latter can be performed as a primary screening test, which requires additional instrumentation and personnel, or in a second-tier approach in which any sample yielding an elevated Tyr value will be analyzed for succinylacetone (10–13). Using the two-tier approach, only samples containing both elevated analytes would be reported as abnormal.

A second-tier approach has also been introduced for several other conditions associated

TABLE 2-3 Effect on Screening Performance of Variable Cut-off Levels of Tyrosine in Detecting Two Cases of Tyr-I in a Population of 200,000 Newborns

Tyr Cut-off Set at 99.5% (180 μmol/L)	No. of Newborns w/ Positive Screening Result	No. of Newborns w/ Negative Screening Result	Total
No. of Newborns w/ Disease	1 (Tyr 240 μM)	1 (Tyr 160 μM)	2
No. of Newborns w/o Disease	999	198,999	199,998
Total	1,000	199,000	200,000

Sensitivity = 50%; Specificity = 99.5%; False-Positive Rate = 0.5%; PPV = 0.1%.

Tyr Cut-off Set at 95% (150 μmol/L)	No. of Newborns w/ Positive Screening Result	No. of Newborns w/ Negative Screening Result	Total
No. of Newborns w/ Disease	2 (Tyr 160 and 240 μM respectively)	0	2
No. of Newborns w/o Disease	5,998	194,000	199,998
Total	6,000	194,000	200,000

Sensitivity = 100%; Specificity = 97%; False-Positive Rate = 3%; PPV = 0.03%.

included in most screening panels; however, C5 acylcarnitine is also elevated in 2-methylbutyrylglycinuria and in a milder variant of IVA, both of which are of uncertain clinical significance (18,19). To further complicate the differential diagnosis of C5 acylcarnitine elevations, this analyte is also present at abnormal levels in patients treated with pivalic acid–containing antibiotics (20). Simple notification of the referring birth place about any C5 acylcarnitine elevation will therefore increase the number of false-positive results, in particular when it is encountered in premature neonates who are often treated with antibiotics.

A screening program's performance is also determined through ongoing assessment of the outcome or consequences of abnormal results. The impact of false-positive results was recently documented through an objective and quantitative assessment by Waisbren et al (21). Although it was found that expanded screening provides better long-term outcome for those patients subjected to early initiation of treatment because of early identification of their condition, infants with false-positive screening results were more often hospitalized than healthy children with normal screening results. Families who received false-positive newborn screening results were at higher risk of developing dysfunctional parent–child relationships (21). Furthermore, with the ability to identify newborns with conditions of either uncertain clinical significance (i.e., SCAD deficiency) or for which there is no effective long-term treatment (i.e., carnitine–acylcarnitine translocase deficiency), the impact of these conditions on the newborns, their families, and the healthcare system must be continuously evaluated to obtain evidence that can be used to determine whether to continue screening for specific conditions.

The Newborn Screening Process

Newborn screening programs are typically state mandated and administered. Responsibility for a successful program, however, lies with all parties involved to ensure the fundamental objectives of newborn screening are met. Therefore, newborn screening not only includes laboratory testing, but the complete process from parent education and sample collection to confirmation and initiation of treatment of identified patients. Aside from the actual laboratory analysis, interpretation, and reporting, which must be undertaken within a reasonable time frame, the healthcare provider is responsible for ensuring that screening is performed and that blood spots are properly collected at the appropriate time and sent to the screening laboratory expeditiously. Once

results become available, the healthcare provider must inform the families of the results and initiate follow up as indicated. To aid the primary care providers who receive abnormal screening results, the ACMG developed brief clinical descriptions and recommendations for clinical and laboratory follow up for each condition detectable by newborn screening (available online at: http://www.acmg.net/resources/policies/ACT/condition-analyte-links.htm).

Preanalytical Phase The preanalytical phase of the screening process consists of counseling and sampling. Healthcare providers (gynecologists, midwifes, and pediatricians) bear responsibility for this phase.

Counseling Newborn screening is mandated in most regions to ensure that all babies benefit from this preventive health measure. Written informed parental consent is required by some screening programs but voluntary opt-out is more common.

Sampling The appropriate time for blood sampling is between 24 and 72 hours post partum. The outer or inner side of the baby's heel is pricked, and blood dripped on a filter paper card ("Guthrie card") so that the marked circles on the card are completely soaked by blood (Figure 2-2). Care must be taken to ensure that blood is free-flowing and not obtained by tissue compression, which will dilute the sample and create artefactual results. The filter paper is kept at ambient temperature for 2 to 3 hours until the blood is completely dried.

In some circumstances (early discharge, blood transfusion, parenteral nutrition, treatment with corticosteroids or dopamine), an initial screening must be followed by a second screening, performed from 1 week to 3 months later depending on the circumstance. Not repeating the newborn screening in the above circumstances has resulted in a number a documented screening failures (22).

Analytical Phase The analytical phase of the screening process consists of data entry, analysis, assessment, recalling, and reporting. The screening laboratory bears the responsibility.

Data entry: Data on the newborn and the mother is provided as written information on the Guthrie card and is usually recorded by automated scanning systems. Information such as date of birth, time of blood sampling, birth weight, gestational age, feeding, medication, and so forth, is necessary for interpretation of results.

Analysis: Small dots are punched out of the dried blood spot specimen (DBS) into microtiter or filtration plates for extraction of blood. The different methods require specific extractions. Each extract is then used for the individual assay. In addition to the specimens,

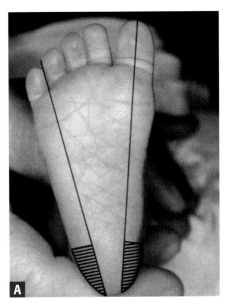

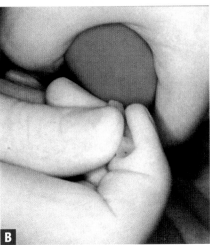

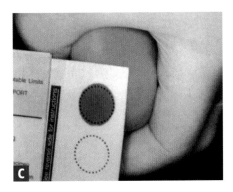

FIGURE 2-2. Technique of blood sampling in newborn screening. The heel-prick is made on the inner or outer side of the heel (hatched area) and should not exceed a depth of 2.4 mm (1.9 mm in premature infants). Blood is applied to the filter paper by completely filling the circles on both, front and back side. (Photographs with permission from Whatman GmbH).

quality controls, calibrators, and external or internal standards are analyzed depending on the assay. In the majority of assays, data transfer and processing for analysis is performed by computer systems. A schematic

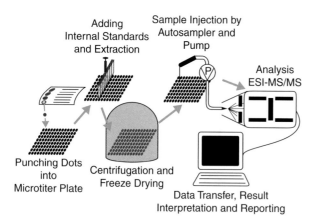

FIGURE 2-3. Schematic work flow in newborn screening laboratories exemplified for MS/MS screening.

application flow is shown for MS/MS analysis (Figure 2-3).

Assessment: Data assessment involves flagging all samples that exceed or fall below the established cut-off levels and interpretation of the results in consideration of the information provided on the screening card.

Recalling: In case of a presumptive positive screening result, the primary healthcare provider is informed of the findings and advised regarding the appropriate follow up investigations.

Reporting: Apart from the direct contact in urgent cases, screening results are sent to the provider of the sample who then informs the parents of the newborn screening results.

Postanalytical Phase In the postanalytical phase, the responsibility is shared by all parties involved in newborn screening.

Confirmation: A presumptive positive screening result should be confirmed by investigations that, with few exceptions, require specific tests in addition to repeating the screening assay. The screening laboratory has to be informed about the results of confirmatory studies.

Treatment initiation: In some conditions and under some circumstances, treatment should be initiated even before confirmation of a positive screening result becomes available. Laboratory diagnosis and treatment initiation as endpoints are integral parts of the newborn screening process and therefore both should be registered.

Laboratory Screening Methodology

The Bacterial Inhibition Assay (BIA) The BIA or original "Guthrie" Test was the impetus for newborn metabolic screening. In 1958–1959 Dr. Robert Guthrie developed a BIA to monitor blood Phe levels (23). The dried blood

spots are placed on agar plates containing a strain of *Bacillus subtilis* that requires Phe for growth. The agar also contains β-2-thienylalanine, a Phe analog, that inhibits bacterial growth. When excessive Phe is present in the blood spot, the analog's action is overcome and bacterial growth occurs, which is easily detectable. Calibrator spots allow for a rough estimate of Phe concentrations in the patient sample. Based on the success with PKU, BIAs were adopted for other inherited disorders of metabolism and were used for screening of galactosemia ('Paigen test,' see Figure 2-4), maple syrup urine disease (MSUD), and homocystinuria.

These assays were simple, inexpensive, and suited to screening large numbers of individual specimens; however, they represent semiquantitative methods with limited sensitivity, (for example, antibiotic treatment can cause false negative results) and the results must be manually entered into the laboratory information system. Therefore, different, more automatic analytical techniques for newborn screening have slowly been substituted for BIAs.

Fluorometric and Photometric Tests In the 1990s, progress toward more automated screening assays was achieved by the development and implementation of fluorometric and photometric microassays for PKU and galactosemia screening (Figure 2-5). These assays can be applied to the measurement of analyte concentrations and enzyme activities.

For example, galactosemia screening can be accomplished by determination of total galactose and galactose-1-phosphate uridyltransferase (GALT) activity. Application of enzymatic fluorometric and photometric assays is feasible for determination of metabolites and enzyme activities.

Total galactose represents the sum of free galactose and galactose fixed in galactose-1-phosphate and is measured utilizing the enzymes alkaline phosphatase and galactose dehydrogenase, both included in the commercially available assay kit (Figure 2-5). Additional estimation of galactose-1-phosphate concentration is helpful for differentiation between galactosemia and galactokinase deficiency and for therapy monitoring, is feasible by running the assay twice: once without and once with alkaline phosphatase in the assay. The difference in galactose concentration between the two assays allows an estimate of the concentration of galactose-1-phosphate. The assay for determination of GALT activity is a modification of the Beutler–Baluda test (24).

For screening of biotinidase deficiency a semiquantitative colorimetric assessment of biotinidase activity in DBSs is in use (25). Samples with biotinidase activity show a characteristic purple color upon addition of developing reagents after incubation with biotinyl *p*-aminobenzoate, whereas those with little or no activity remain straw colored. Assessment is feasible by visual interpretation but more accurate by photometric measurement.

Immunoassays Fluoroimmunometric assays are used in newborn screening to detect congenital adrenal hyperplasia (CAH) and congenital hypothyroidism. The assays use

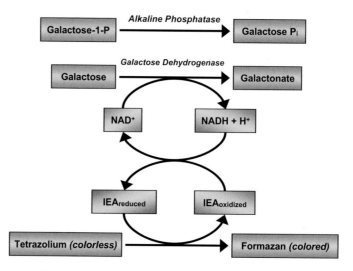

FIGURE 2-4. Reaction scheme of the enzymatic determination of total galactose. Coupling of galactose dehydrogenase with an intermediate electron acceptor (IEA) system for the colorimetric measurement.

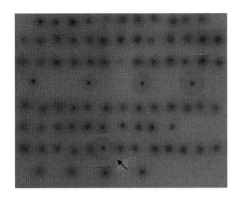

FIGURE 2-5. The Bacterial Inhibition Assay (BIA) Agar plate of a microbiological inhibition assay. The figure represents an example for adoption of the aboriginal "Guthrie test" for galactose measurement ('Paigen Test'). Control discs to which known increasing quantities of galactose were added are seen in the middle of the plate. In the lower part a positive screening sample can be found (arrow).

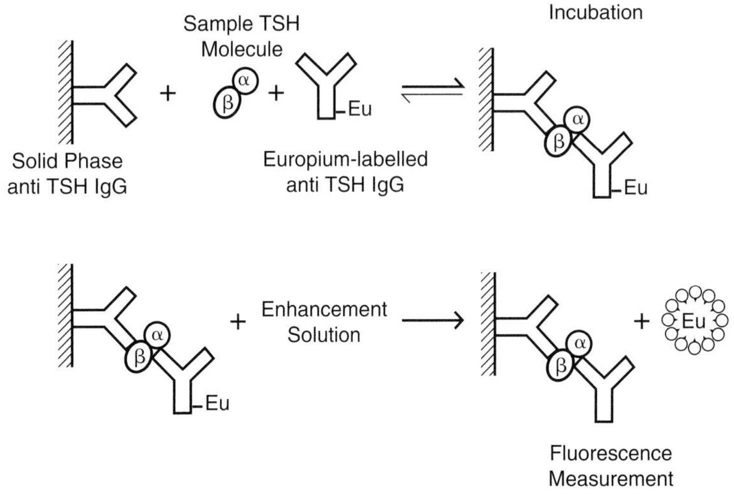

Sample TSH Molecule

Incubation

Solid Phase anti TSH IgG

Europium-labelled anti TSH IgG

Enhancement Solution

Fluorescence Measurement

FIGURE 2-6. Principle of a fluoroimmunometric assay for measurement of TSH.

mono- or polyclonal antibodies directed against distinct antigens on the analyte of interest (e.g., thyroid-stimulating hormone [TSH], 17-OH progesterone [17-OHP]). Either the antibody or the analyte is labeled with a fluorochrome, for example, europium. The antigen–antibody complexes are fixed to a solid phase in a microtiter plate before an enhancing reagent dissociates the fluochrome. The fluorescence of the resulting chelate solution is proportional to the analyte's concentration in the blood spot (Figure 2-6). The third generation assays are fully automated and their sensitivity and specificity is above 99%. The disadvantages of immunoassays derive from cross-reacting substances in blood, which is of special importance in CAH screening in which placental and fetal steroids can cross-react with the antibody directed against 17-OHP.

Newborn Screening and MS/MS Mass spectrometers are instruments measuring the weight of ions derived from a neutral compound following ionization. The mass spectrometer separates the ions based on their mass-to-charge (m/z) ratio after which they are recorded by a detector that generates a plot of m/z values over intensities, that is, a mass spectrum. The abundance of each ion in the original sample correlates to the height of each ion peak in the mass spectrum, allowing for qualitative interpretation of the ion profile. More accurate quantitative determination of the concentration of a specific ion is possible by the addition of defined concentrations of isotopically labeled internal standards early during sample preparation (Figure 2-3). In the 1980s, MS/MS was introduced into clinical laboratories because of this technology's ability to analyze acylcarnitines efficiently in complex biological samples.

Tandem mass spectrometers consist of two mass spectrometers coupled in series and separated by a "collision cell" (Figure 2-7). The first MS (MS_1) analyzes the ions in a sample (precursor ions), which are then fragmented in the collision cell by using an inert gas. The product ions resulting from fragmentation are further analyzed by the second MS (MS_2). Either MS_1 or MS_2 can be set to scan a mass range or to select one or more individual ions (26,27).

When it was recognized that acylcarnitine and amino acid analyses can be performed simultaneously on the same sample, the idea to use this technology for neonatal screening was born. Since the early 1990s, it has been proven that this technology can be applied to newborn screening because it is amenable to high-throughput, population-wide testing for a large number of disorders of fatty acid, organic acid, and amino acid metabolism (28–32). For some of these conditions effective treatment is currently not available,

which has raised many questions and concerns; however, even when treatment is not available, it can be argued that early identification is still of benefit (33).

New and future developments in MS/MS applications focus on CAH (34), TYR-I (succinylacetone) (11), and galactosemia (galactose-1-phosphate) (35). With screening for CAH, a first MS/MS application for endocrine diseases became feasible.

Molecular Genetic Analyses Mutational analysis is not feasible as a primary test in newborn screening but might be useful in a two-tier approach, in which positive tests of a primary analyte will be followed by a second, different method (e.g. mutation analysis) using the same DBS. This may increase both diagnostic sensitivity and specificity of screening. At present, such a two-tier approach is applied to CF screening where immunoreactive trypsinogen is measured in the primary test.

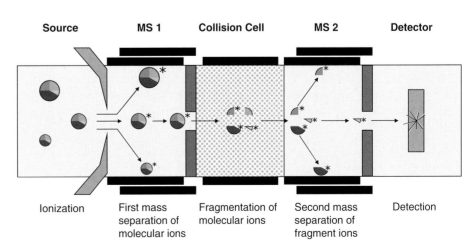

Source	MS 1	Collision Cell	MS 2	Detector
Ionization	First mass separation of molecular ions	Fragmentation of molecular ions	Second mass separation of fragment ions	Detection

FIGURE 2-7. Principle of MS/MS.

Screened Metabolic and Endocrine Conditions

Phenylketonuria PKU was the first disease for which a screening test was developed. Since the implementation of newborn screening for PKU in many countries, early detection and initiation of a Phe-restricted diet has improved the prognosis of these children significantly.

PKU, an inborn error of amino acid metabolism (see Chapter 13), is caused by deficiency of the enzyme Phe hydroxylase, which catalyzes conversion from Phe to Tyr. In PKU, the Phe level is elevated in blood, whereas the Tyr level is low. Screening for Phe allows recognition of the disease. Additional assessment of the Phe/Tyr ratio lowers the rate of false positives. In addition to PKU other forms of impaired Phe hydroxylase function, such as non-PKU hyperphenylalaninemia (HPA) and deficiency of enzymes involved in the metabolism of the cofactor tetrahydrobiopterin, can be detected by Phe (and Tyr) measurement. Detection of HPA in females, even if it does not require dietary treatment, is of importance because in adulthood their offspring may suffer from maternal PKU.

Screening method: BIA, Fluorometric and photometric microassay and MS/MS.

Key metabolite: Phe and Phe/Tyr ratio.

Differential diagnosis: HPA, cofactor deficiencies, transient benign hyperphenylalaninemia of the newborn, total parenteral nutrition, severe liver disease.

What to do if test is positive: Contact family immediately about result and report findings to newborn screening program. Consult with metabolic specialist.

Confirmatory studies: Phe and Tyr in plasma (or again in DBS); tetrahydrobiopterin loading test if available; pterins in urine, dihydropteridine reductase activity in DBS.

Prevalence (36–39): 1:10,000 (Germany); 1:20,000 (U.S.).

Galactosemia Classic galactosemia (see Chapter 9) is caused by virtually complete absence of GALT activity. Two different approaches exist to screen for galactosemia. 1) Measurement of total galactose, which is the sum of free galactose and galactose from galactose-1-phosphate. The sensitivity of the test increases when the baby receives small amounts of breast milk or lactose-containing formula, which is crucial in case of early discharge, especially if screening is done prior to the first feeding. 2) Measurement of GALT activity in DBS by a fluorometric screening test (Beutler test) has high sensitivity and is independent of diet; however, GALT testing is associated with a higher false positive rate (up to 1%) when the sample has

been exposed to higher temperatures (for example during transport in the summer) due to enzyme denaturation. Patients who have had blood transfusions may have false negative Beutler test results for as long as 2 to 3 months because of the contribution of normal GALT in the donor cells. The combined approach with measurement of total galactose and GALT has proven to be most effective. Symptoms may occur before the results of newborn screening are available.

While pending confirmation of diagnosis, patients in whom there is a high index of suspicion and urine positive for reducing substances should be on galactose-free diet and monitored for hypoglycemia, liver failure, *Escherichia coli* sepsis, and coagulopathy. Early recognition and treatment of galactosemia prevents severe liver failure and death, which otherwise might occur in the first month of life, as well as formation of cataracts. Despite strict treatment, the long-term outcome is still complicated in many patients by the development of neuropsychological and cerebellar symptoms, such as verbal dyspraxia, mental retardation, ataxia, and tremor. Females frequently develop ovarian failure.

In addition to classic galactosemia with GALT activities less than 1%, milder forms of galactosemia are identified by newborn screening as well. The most common variants are the Duarte variant and compound heterozygotes with one Duarte allele and one classic galactosemia allele. Uridine diphosphate-galactose-4'-epimerase (GALE) deficiency can also cause high total galactose at birth. The majority of patients with GALE deficiency have been asymptomatic (peripheral form), except for a few children who have had dramatic neurologic involvement. A severe generalized form of GALE deficiency exists but appears to be very rare, with only five patients from two families described to date (40).

Galactokinase deficiency, another rare condition, is characterized by extraordinarily high screening levels of free galactose, and treatment with a galactose-free diet prevents development of cataracts, the only consistent pathology in this disease.

Screening method: Fluorometric and photometric microassays.

Key metabolite: Total galactose and/or GALT activity.

Differential diagnosis: GALE deficiency, galactokinase deficiency, and severe liver disease (in case of total galactose measurement); Phosphoglucomutase, glucose-6-phosphate dehydrogenase, and 6-phosphoglycerate dehydrogenase deficiency (in case of GALT measurement).

What to do if test is positive: Contact family immediately about result and report findings to newborn screening program. Consult with metabolic specialist. If total galactose

is above 30 mg/dl stop lactose-containing milk feeding immediately until the confirmatory studies are completed.

Confirmatory studies: GALT, GALE, and galactokinase activities in erythrocytes (lysates), galactose-1-phosphate in erythrocytes (or in DBS).

Pitfalls/Attention: DBSs contaminated with breast milk or formula will cause false positive results due to high total galactose.

Prevalence (36–39): 1:40,000 (Germany); 1:70,000 (U.S.).

Biotinidase Deficiency The vitamin biotin is a coenzyme of several carboxylases. Biotinidase deficiency (see Chapter 7) leads to disturbed recycling of biotin, thus causing multiple carboxylase deficiency. Biotinidase deficiency is a model screening disease. Severe symptoms occurring weeks to months after birth are completely preventable by simple and inexpensive treatment with biotin. The disease can be detected by a simple enzyme assay amenable to newborn screening.

Differential diagnosis: None.

What to do if test is positive: Contact family immediately about result and report findings to newborn screening program. Consult with metabolic specialist. If biotinidase activity is markedly reduced, biotin supplementation (5–10 mg biotin per day PO) should be started before confirmatory studies are completed.

Confirmatory studies: Biotinidase activity in serum.

Pitfalls/Attention: Acylcarnitine analysis is not a reliable newborn screening method for biotinidase deficiency because of maternal biotin supply to the her offspring preventing the accumulation of abnormal metabolites.

Prevalence (36–39): 1:60,000 (Germany and U.S.).

Congenital Hypothyroidism Congenital hypothyroidism (CH) is the first nonmetabolic disease included in the newborn screening and in most regions it is the most prevalent disease among those for which screening is performed. CH is caused by inadequate production of thyroid hormone due to agenesis or an ectopic thyroid gland, dyshormonogenesis, endemic cretinism, and defects of the pituitary or hypothalamus (see Chapter 26). Except for hypopituitarism all cases of CH are characterized by low thyroxine (T_4) and an elevated TSH level. Most North American screening programs measure T_4 followed by TSH when T_4 values are at the lowest 5% to 10%. In Europe and Japan primary TSH screening is routine. Clinical signs of hypothyroidism, except for prolonged jaundice, may not appear for several months after birth. CH represents an ideal screening disease because of its relatively easy treatment, which prevents the development of severe cognitive delays.

Screening method: Immunoassay.

Key metabolite: T$_4$, TSH.

Differential diagnosis: Iodine deficiency.

What to do if test is positive: Contact family immediately about result and report findings to newborn screening program. Consult with pediatric endocrinologist about initiating treatment.

Confirmatory studies: Free T$_4$, TSH, radioisotope scanning (needs to be performed within 2 days of initiation of therapy), and thyroid ultrasound. Thyroid-binding globulin (TBG) in plasma may be measured if congenital TBG deficiency or TBG deficiency secondary to congenital nephrotic syndrome is suspected. Elevated reverse triiodothyronine (rT$_3$) low T$_4$ and normal TSH are characteristic of sick euthyroid syndrome.

Pitfalls/Attention: Hypothalamohypophyseal forms of hypothyroidism are not detected by TSH screening.

In practice, overtreatment and overestimation of CH may occur if hormone supplementation is started without prior initiation of adequate confirmatory studies analysis. Blood collected in citrate or EDTA tubes and then spotted onto a Guthrie card gives false-negative results. Specimens collected in the first 24 to 48 hours of life may lead to false-positive TSH elevations when using any screening approach.

Prevalence (36–39): 1:4,000 (almost uniform worldwide).

Congenital Adrenal Hyperplasia Congenital adrenal hyperplasia (CAH), the second endocrinopathy included in newborn screening programs, is caused by a defect in cortisol synthesis and in 90% of cases is due to a deficiency of the enzyme 21α-hydroxylase (21-OHD). Measurement of 17-OHP allows the diagnosis. CAH due to 17α-hydroxylase/17,20lyase and StAR deficiencies are not detected by 17-OHP screening as 17-OHP levels are low in these disorders. CAH due to 11β-hydroxylase deficiency result in elevated 17-OHP levels but the associated elevated 11-deoxycorticosterone (DOC) levels allow differentiation from 21-OHD (for details see Chapter 27). Screening assays for 17-OHP with antibodies may reveal problems in the specificity of the test because of the occurrence of cross-reactivity of steroid compounds related to 17-OHP. Premature newborns have significantly higher 17-OHP levels. Therefore in this group, reference values adjusted either for gestational age or for birth weight have to be applied.

Screening method: Immunoassay.

Key metabolite: 17-OHP.

Differential diagnosis: None.

What to do if test is positive: Contact family immediately about result and report findings

to newborn screening program. Consult with pediatric endocrinologist. If patient is symptomatic with hypoglycemia, vomiting and/or electrolyte imbalance, admit immediately, consider 25 mg IM hydrocortisone en route to hospital, and refer to pediatric endocrinologist. If patient has ambiguous genitalia, and is asymptomatic with normal electrolytes and glucose, refer immediately to pediatric endocrinologist.

Confirmatory studies: 17-OHP and other adrenal steroids in plasma and molecular genetic analysis.

Pitfalls/Attention: 17-OHP screening does not detect 17α-hydroxylase/17,20-lyase and StAR deficiencies because these disorders typically are associated with low 17-OHP levels. Additional measurement of DOC levels by NBS would lead to diagnosis of 11-11β-hydroxylase and 17α-hydroxylase/17,20-lyase deficiencies as they are associated with elevated DOC levels. For preterm newborns cut-offs adjusted for gestational age and/or birth weight are necessary. Of note, preterm infants may have falsely low levels if they are on cortisol therapy or if their mother received multiple courses of bethamethasone before delivery.

Prevalence (36–39): 1:10,000 (Germany); 1:15,000 (U.S.).

Maple Syrup Urine Disease MSUD is a disorder of branched chain amino acid (leucine, isoleucine, valine) metabolism caused by deficiency of the enzyme branched-chain ketoacid dehydrogenase. Classic MSUD presents clinically as a progressive encephalopathy within the first week of life (see Chapter 7). Immediate action must be taken if branched-chain amino acids are found distinctly elevated. Immediate hospitalization in a metabolic center is urgent. The affected children benefit greatly from life-long, dietary treatment, even if completely normal psychomotor development will not always be achieved. Screening for MSUD by leucine determination, as in former BIAs, lacks specificity. A relatively high number of newborns with benign transient hyperleucinemia tested false positive (PPV<<1%). Additional assessment of valine by MS/MS allows for more specific and sensitive screening for MSUD.

Screening method: MS/MS.

Key metabolites: Leucine + isoleucine, valine, (leucine + isoleucine)/Phe ratio.

Differential diagnosis: Intermittent and intermediary forms of MSUD, E$_3$ subunit (combined for dehydrogenase complexes) deficiency, thiamine deficiency.

What to do if test is positive: Immediately contact the family to ascertain the baby's clinical status. If any concern (ie, poor feeding, vomiting, lethargy, tachypnea), immediately initiate transport to hospital, preferably a metabolic center.

Confirmatory studies: Branched-chain amino acids and alloisoleucine in plasma, organic acids in urine.

Pitfalls/Attention: Parenteral nutrition causes false-positive results. Hyperhydroxyprolinemia causes false positive results for MSUD because standard MS/MS analysis cannot distinguish hydroxy proline from the isomers leucine and isoleucine.

Prevalence (36–39): 1:200,000 (Germany); 1:160,000 (U.S.).

Tyrosinemia Type I TYR-I is caused by deficiency of the enzyme fumarylacetoacetase, which catalyzes the last step in Tyr degradation (see Chapter 15). Untreated TYR-I can lead to liver and renal failure, rickets, porphyric and neurologic crises, and hepatocarcinoma. Some infants with severe neonatal presentation of TYR-I die within the first months of life. Since treatment with the synthetic drug NTBC became available, the disease has a favorable prognosis when treatment is initiated early. In TYR-I, blood concentrations of Tyr and succinylacetone are elevated. The latter compound is specific for TYR-I. Screening solely for Tyr lacks specificity because some other and more common conditions also cause elevation of Tyr. Increasing the cut-off point for Tyr does not circumvent this problem because newborns with TYR-I may even have normal Tyr at birth. The issue of specificity and sensitivity in Tyr screening is exemplified in Table 2-3. Only when succinylacetone is part of the newborn screen, either as a primary or second tier approach, does TYR-I screening become feasible and (10–13).

Key metabolites: Tyr and succinylacetone.

Differential diagnosis: None, if succinylacetone is part of the screen; Liver impairment, tyrosinemia types 2 and 3, and benign transient hypertyrosinemia of the newborn, in case of exclusive screening for Tyr.

What to do if test is positive: Contact family immediately about result and report findings to newborn screening program. Consult with metabolic specialist to initiate confirmatory diagnostic testing, although tyrosinemia type I typically remains asymptomatic in the newborn period.

Confirmatory studies: Plasma amino acids, serum α-fetoprotein, succinylacetone in urine.

Pitfalls/Attention: EDTA blood or exposure of the DBS to heat will give false positive results for some second tier assays (13).

Prevalence (36–39): <1:100,000; 1:20,000 (Saguenay-Lac St. Jean region of Quebec, Canada).

Homocystinuria Homocystinuria (HCY) caused by cystathionine β-synthase deficiency is an inborn error of the transsulfuration pathway (see Chapter 17). From observation in patients with HCY in whom the disease was detected early and who were treated, some evidence indicates that presymptomatic initiation of treatment can prevent cognitive impairment, lens dislocation, and thromboembolic events (41); this is of special importance in pyridoxine-responsive forms. The disorder is biochemically characterized by accumulation of homocysteine, methionine, and a variety of other metabolites of homocysteine in the body and, ultimately, excretion in the urine. Screening is done by measuring methionine. In the past, HCY was part of screening because methionine measurement was feasible by using a BIA. The fact that at present HCY is still in the panel of many screening programs is mainly historical. In the majority, figures on the frequency of HCY are derived from the number of patients in whom methionine is detected. The estimated frequencies range from 1:50,000 in Ireland to 1: 1,000,000 in Japan; the overall frequency has been reported to be between 1:200,000 and 1:335,000 (42). Several lines of evidence indicate that these frequencies are very likely to be highly underestimated. Particularly the pyridoxine-responsive form of HCY, representing the most readily treatable form, is being missed by newborn screening. This is corroborated by some studies on allele frequencies that reveal estimates for homozygote frequency of approximately 1:20,000 (43), a significantly higher prevalence than the aforementioned figure of detection by newborn screening for hypermethioninemia. In addition to insufficient sensitivity for HCY screening, methionine measurement has low specificity because several conditions other than HCY can cause increased methionine at birth. This lack of specificity for homocystinuria alone is reflected by PPVs that may be below 1% when screening relies on methionine alone.

Screening method: MS/MS.

Key metabolite: Methionine.

Differential diagnosis: Other hypermethioninemias: S-adenosylhomocysteine hydrolase deficiency, glycine N-methyltransferase deficiency, methionine adenosyltransferase deficiency, impaired liver function.

What to do if test is positive: Contact family immediately about result and report findings to newborn screening program. Consult with metabolic specialist to initiate confirmatory diagnostic testing, although homocystinuria typically remains asymptomatic in the newborn period.

Confirmatory studies: Total homocysteine in plasma, amino acids in plasma, organic (methylmalonic) acids in urine, mutation analysis, enzyme study in fibroblasts.

Prevalence (36–39): <1:250,000 (Germany), 1:270,000 (U.S.).

Citrullinemia Citrullinemia is a urea cycle defect caused by deficiency of the enzyme argininosuccinate synthase (see Chapter 11). Citrullinemia may present neonatally with hyperammonemia and coma or it may have a milder course manifesting clinically after the postnatal period. Before screening for citrullinemia became available, the clinical outcome was generally poor. Most of the patients suffered serious brain damage with global developmental delay. Treatment implemented after the first manifestation of the disease could not prevent significant neurologic sequelae. Promising evidence that timely implementation of treatment has an obvious impact on the natural course of the disease arises from the first patients detected by newborn screening (36). The disease is reliably detected in newborn screening by citrulline measurement by MS/MS. Surprisingly the number of affected newborns disclosed in newborn screening markedly exceeded expectations. That fact turned out to be due to presumably milder variants of the disease. The impact of detection and treatment in children with such milder variants has still to be elucidated.

Screening method: MS/MS.

Key metabolites: Citrulline (high), arginine (low).

Differential diagnosis: Milder, variant form of citrullinemia, citrullinemia type 2 (citrin deficiency), argininosuccinate lyase deficiency, pyruvate carboxylase deficiency.

What to do if test is positive: Immediately contact the family to ascertain the baby's clinical status. If any concern (i.e., poor feeding, vomiting, lethargy, tachypnea, seizures), immediately initiate emergency treatment with IV glucose and transport to a hospital, preferably a metabolic center.

Confirmatory studies: Amino acids in plasma and urine, blood ammonia, orotic acid in urine.

Prevalence*: 1:50,000 (Germany).

Argininosuccinate Lyase Deficiency Argininosuccinate lyase deficiency is another urea cycle defect (see Chapter 11). Affected newborns benefit from early recognition and treatment initiation; however, the long-term outcome remains to be elucidated. The condition is reliably detected in newborn screening by argininosuccinate and citrulline measurement by MS/MS.

Screening method: MS/MS.

Key metabolites: Argininosuccinate (high), citrulline (high), arginine (low).

Differential diagnosis: None.

What to do if test is positive: Immediately contact the family to ascertain the baby's clinical status. If any concern (i.e., poor feeding,

vomiting, lethargy, tachypnea, seizures), immediately initiate transport to a hospital, preferably a metabolic center.

Confirmatory studies: Amino acids in plasma and urine, blood ammonia, orotic acid in urine, enzyme studies in erythrocytes/fibroblasts.

Prevalence (36–39): 1:180,000 (Germany, U.S., Australia).

Medium-chain Acyl-CoA Dehydrogenase Deficiency In Caucasians MCAD is the most frequent inborn error of mitochondrial β-oxidation of fatty acids (see Chapter 5). Enzyme deficiency causes hypoglycemia, Reye-like episodes, and sudden unexpected death. In the prescreening era, approximately 5% of "sudden infant death syndrome" cases were thought to be caused by MCAD. The high prevalence of the disease, the simple treatment, and the reliable MS/MS-based acylcarnitine analysis make MCAD a model screening disease. Parental awareness that the child is affected and ensuring that the child avoids fasting are effective in the prevention of any sequela of the disease. In the past, a timely diagnosis was impossible to achieve because of the lack of initial symptoms, and thereafter because of often noninformative metabolic routine analysis during compensated state. Since MS/MS became available, diagnosis, even in the compensated state, is achievable. At least in Caucasian populations implementation of MS/MS in newborn screening programs is justified because of the beneficial effect on this condition alone.

Screening method: MS/MS.

Key metabolite: C8 (octanoyl carnitine), ratios C8/C2, C8/C10, C8/C12.

Differential diagnosis: Multiple acyl-CoA dehydrogenase deficiency.

What to do if test is positive: Immediately contact the family to ascertain the baby's clinical status. If any concern (ie, poor feeding, vomiting, lethargy) immediately initiate emergency treatment with IV glucose and transport to a hospital, preferably a metabolic center. Asymptomatic infants do not require emergency follow-up but should be evaluated and counseled by a metabolic specialist within days.

Confirmatory studies: Acylcarnitine profile in DBS/blood, free and total carnitine in blood, organic (dicarboxylic) acids and acylglycines in urine, enzyme studies in lymphocytes/fibroblasts, molecular genetic analysis.

Pitfalls/Attention: Carnitine deficiency might cause a noninformative acylcarnitine profile.

Prevalence (36–39): 1:15,000 (Germany, U.S.), 1:20,000 (Australia).

Very Long-chain Acyl-CoA Dehydrogenase Deficiency Very long-chain acyl-CoA dehydrogenase deficiency is an inborn error of mitochondrial β-oxidation of fatty acids causing hypoglycemia, sudden death, cardiomyopathy, liver disease, and later on recurrent rhabdomyolysis (see Chapter 5). Diagnosis is feasible by MS/MS -based acylcarnitine analysis; however, key metabolites are often only slightly increased and may become normal after a carbohydrate rich meal.

Screening method: MS/MS.

Key metabolites: C14:1 (myristoleyl-), C14 (myristoyl carnitine).

Differential diagnosis: Multiple acyl-CoA dehydrogenase deficiency.

What to do if test is positive: Immediately contact the family to ascertain the baby's clinical status. If any concern (ie, poor feeding, vomiting, lethargy) immediately initiate emergency treatment with IV glucose and transport to a hospital, preferably a metabolic center. Asymptomatic infants with mildly abnormal screening results do not require emergency follow-up but should be evaluated and counseled by a metabolic specialist within days.

Confirmatory studies: Acylcarnitine profile in DBS/blood collected prior to a regular meal, free and total carnitine in blood, serum creatine kinase, organic acids in urine (elevated dicarboxylic acids), enzyme studies in lymphocytes/fibroblasts-based acylcarnitine analysis, molecular genetic analysis.

Pitfalls/Attention: Carnitine deficiency as well as glucose infusion may cause a false-negative acylcarnitine profile, particularly in the milder variant of the disease.

Prevalence (36–39): 1:250,000 (Germany), 1:160,000 (U.S.), 1:120,000 (Australia).

Other Disorders of Mitochondrial Fatty Acid β-Oxidation and the Carnitine Cycle This group comprises conditions such as short chain acyl-CoA dehydrogenase (SCAD), medium/short chain and long chain hydroxyl-CoA dehydrogenases (M/SCHAD, LCHAD), multiple acyl-CoA dehydrogenase or glutaric acidemia type II (MADD or GAII) and carnitine cycle defects (see Chapter 5), for which a final assessment on screening properties is not yet available. Most of these have been included among the primary newborn screening targets recommended by the ACMG, others as secondary targets. Inclusion into screening panels, however, is not universal. Long-chain 3-OH-acyl-CoA dehydrogenase (LCHAD) deficiency and complete mitochondrial trifunctional protein (TFP) deficiency are β-oxidation defects that can be screened with high sensitivity and specificity. Carnitine-palmitoyl transferase 1 (CPT1) deficiency, carnitine-palmitoyl transferase II (CPT2) deficiency, and carnitine-acylcarnitine-translocase deficiency (CACT) represent inborn errors in the carnitine cycle. CPT1 is the only condition in which free carnitine is elevated, whereas it is reduced in carnitine uptake defect (CUD). CPT2 and CACT are indistinguishable by acylcarnitine analysis and outcome for CPT2 deficiency appears promising after early initiation of treatment afforded by newborn screening. A benefit of early detection of CPT1, CACT, and multiple acyl-CoA dehydrogenase (glutaric acidemia type II) deficiencies may be limited to early counseling of the affected family while successful treatment of the infant is not yet available. SCAD deficiency is of special concern as some regard it as a serious and treatable condition while others consider it merely a biochemical variant.

Screening method: MS/MS.

Key metabolites: (See Newborn Screening At-A-Glance)

What to do if test is positive: Contact family immediately about result and report findings to newborn screening program. Consult with metabolic specialist.

Confirmatory studies: Acylcarnitine profile in DBS/blood, free and total carnitine in blood (CPT1, CUD), serum creatine kinase, organic (dicarboxylic or hydroxy-dicarboxylic acids) acids in urine, urine acylcarnitines and acylglycines, enzyme studies in lymphocytes/fibroblasts, molecular genetic analysis.

Pitfalls/Attention: Carnitine deficiency might cause a noninformative acylcarnitine profile (LCHAD, CPT2, CACT); false-positive results can be caused by: fat infusion (LCHAD), carnitine supplementation in prematures infants (CPT1), premature infants with special formula and screened after first week of life (36–39) (CPT2, CACT). Maternal carnitine uptake transporter defects can be uncovered by newborn screening of offspring (44).

Combined Prevalence (36–39): app. 1:20,000.

Isovaleric Aciduria IVA is a disorder of leucine degradation that is caused by deficiency of the enzyme isovaleryl-CoA dehydrogenase (see Chapter 7). The disease is characterized clinically by severe metabolic encephalopathy presenting mostly in the neonatal period with acute, overwhelming illness, vomiting, characteristic odor of "sweaty feet," seizures, coma, intraventricular/cerebellar hemorrhage, and hyperammonemia. Fifty percent of patients die during the first episode of decompensation. Experience with affected newborns since implementation of IVA screening indicates a favorable outcome with early diagnosis and treatment. Patients with a mild, possibly benign phenotype are also being identified by newborn screening, leading to the identification of affected but asymptomatic family members (18).

Screening method: MS/MS.

Key metabolite: C5 (isovaleryl carnitine).

Differential diagnosis: 2-methylbutyryl-CoA dehydrogenase (2-MBG or SBCAD), ethylmalonic encephalopathy (increase of C4 and C5).

What to do if test is positive: Immediately contact the family to ascertain the baby's clinical status. If any concern (ie, poor feeding, vomiting, lethargy, tachypnea, odor of sweaty feet) immediately transport to a hospital, preferably a metabolic center. Asymptomatic infants with mildly abnormal screening results do not require emergency follow-up but should be evaluated and counseled by a metabolic specialist within days.

Confirmatory studies: Organic acids in urine, free and total carnitine in blood, enzyme studies in lymphocytes/fibroblasts, mutation analysis. Urine acylglycine and acylcarnitine analysis may also be informative.

Pitfalls/Attention: Carnitine deficiency might cause a noninformative acylcarnitine profile; treatment with pivalic acid containing antibiotics cause false-positive results.

Prevalence (36–39): 1:60,000 (Germany), <1:300,000 (Australia).

Glutaric Aciduria Type I Glutaric aciduria type I (GA-I) is a disorder of lysine and tryptophan metabolism caused by deficiency of the enzyme glutaryl-CoA dehydrogenase (GCDH). An encephalitis-like decompensation followed by severe dystonic–dyskinetic movement disorder represents the most common presentation of neonates with GA-I. After a presymptomatic period with only minor symptoms but frequently with progressive macrocephaly, the encephalopathic crisis occurs around the first birthday of the patient, often triggered by febrile illness/immunizations. Screening and treatment may prevent this course. Newborn screening by MS/MS-based acylcarnitine analysis requires high analytical sensitivity because the key metabolite, glutaryl carnitine, in GA-I occurs physiologically in low concentrations and is often only slightly increased in patients. In a subgroup of children with GA-I that is characterized by very low excretion of the pathognomonic organic acids glutaric and 3-hydroxyglutaric acid, MS/MS newborn screening may also be negative.

Screening method: MS/MS.

Key metabolite: C5DC (glutaryl carnitine). Some laboratories are also using ratios to other acylcarnitines.

Differential diagnosis: GA2/MADD

What to do if test is positive: Contact family immediately about result and report findings to newborn screening program. Consult with metabolic specialist.

Confirmatory studies: Organic acids in urine (glutaric and 3-hydroxyglutaric acid). If strongly consistent with GA-I treatment should be initiated immediately and molecular genetic analysis of the GCDH gene pursued. If the characteristic urine organic acid profile is not observed, exact quantification of 3-hydroxyglutaric acid should be performed by a sensitive stable isotope dilution method (if available). A normal excretion of 3-hydroxyglutaric acid will exclude the diagnosis of GA-I (false positive) otherwise. Treatment and molecular genetic confirmation should be initiated. The presence of only one known disease-causing mutation on one allele or no mutations at all should lead to the determination of GCDH activity in isolated peripheral leukocytes or cultured fibroblasts. Low enzyme activity will confirm the diagnosis of GCDH deficiency whereas normal activity will exclude the diagnosis (false positive).

Pitfalls/Attention: Carnitine deficiency might cause a noninformative acylcarnitine profile.

Prevalence (36–39): 1:80,000 (Germany), <1:300,000 (Australia).

Propionic Aciduria Among the organic acidurias, propionic aciduria (PA) has the most severe clinical phenotype. PA is caused by deficiency of propionyl-CoA carboxylase, an enzyme in the metabolism of several amino acids and in the degradation of odd-chain fatty acids. Already in the first postnatal days, many affected newborns are suffering from severe hyperammonemia requiring extracorporeal detoxification. Outcome is strongly connected with brain injury, which depends on duration, extent, and frequency of metabolic decompensation/hyperammonemia. Despite aggressive treatment recurrent metabolic decompensation is not always avoidable. The potential benefit of newborn screening for PA depends on whether the positive result comes prior to the first decompensation and clinical diagnosis—sometimes not an achievable objective. Increased propionylcarnitine is a sensitive parameter for PA screening; however, it is not specific. Some newborns not suffering from an inborn error of metabolism have high propionylcarnitine levels of, so far, unknown origin.

Screening method: MS/MS.

Key metabolite: C3 (propionylcarnitine), C3/C2 and C3/C0 ratio.

Differential diagnosis: Methylmalonic aciduria (MMA), cobalamin (CBL): A, B, C, D, F deficiencies ; vitamin B_{12} deficiency.

What to do if test is positive: Immediately contact the family to ascertain the baby's clinical status. If any concern (i.e., poor feeding, vomiting, lethargy, tachypnea) immediately transport to a hospital, preferably a metabolic center. Asymptomatic patients with mildly abnormal screening results do not require emergency follow-up but should

be evaluated and counseled by a metabolic specialist within days.

Confirmatory studies: Organic acids in urine, free and total carnitine in blood, plasma amino acids and total homocysteine, blood ammonia, enzyme studies in fibroblasts, molecular genetic analysis.

Pitfalls/Attention: Carnitine deficiency might cause a noninformative acylcarnitine profile; carnitine supplementation, sometimes applied in preterm babies, may cause a C3/C0 ratio that is not informative.

Prevalence (36–39): 1:250,000 (Germany), 1:80,000 (U.S.A), < 1:300,000 (Australia).

Methylmalonic Aciduria and Cobalamin Deficiencies MMA and CBL (A,B,C,D) deficiencies represent organic acidurias affecting the enzyme methylmalonyl-CoA mutase. Whereas MMA is caused by the primary deficiency of methylmalonyl-CoA mutase (see Chapter 7), different enzyme deficiencies in the CBL metabolism lead to disturbed synthesis of hydroxycobalamin (see Chapter 17), a cofactor of the mutase (CBL deficiency). Clinical manifestation of these diseases occur somewhat later than in PA. Newborn screening is of benefit for affected individuals.

Screening method: MS/MS.

Key metabolite: C3 (propionylcarnitine), C3/C2 and C3/C0 ratio.

Differential diagnosis: PA, transcobalamin II deficiency, Vitamin B12 deficiency.

What to do if test is positive: Immediately contact the family to ascertain the baby's clinical status. If any concern (i.e., poor feeding, vomiting, lethargy, tachypnea) immediately transport to a hospital, preferably a metabolic center. Asymptomatic infants with mildly abnormal screening results do not require emergency follow-up but should be evaluated and counseled by a metabolic specialist within days.

Confirmatory studies: Organic acids in urine, free and total carnitine in blood, amino acids and total homocysteine in plasma, blood ammonia, enzyme studies in fibroblasts, molecular genetic analysis.

Pitfalls/Attention: Carnitine deficiency might cause a noninformative acylcarnitine profile; carnitine supplementation, sometimes applied in preterm babies, may cause a C3/C0 ratio, that is not informative.

Prevalence (36–39): 1:80,000 (Germany), <1:300,000 (Australia).

3-Methylcrotonyl-CoA Carboxylase Deficiency A deficiency of 3-methylcrotonyl-CoA carboxylase (3-MCC) is caused by a defect in leucine degradation (see Chapter 7). Since introduction of screening for 3-MCC a great number of affected newborns have been found. Several concerns have to be addressed in screening for that condition. It

appears that 3-MCC is a common, mostly benign condition. Whether treatment with a low-protein diet, carnitine, and glycine supplementation has the potential to change the clinical course in severely affected patients remains to be elucidated. No evidence has so far emerged of a benefit from presymptomatic treatment. Increases of C5OH carnitine are not specific for 3-MCC deficiency because it can represent either elevations of 3-hydroxyisovalerylcarnitine or 2-methyl-3-hydroxybutyrylcarnitine. Maternal 3-MCC, was initially a surprising finding of MS/MS screening programs. Distinct increases in the baby's blood were caused by the mother who turned out to have this condition. Major concerns were raised as to how to handle the mother because her carnitine deficiency did not always have apparent clinical consequences. In addition to confirmed cases, a substantial number of positive C5OH results persist during recalls, but cannot be assigned to an underlying disease.

Screening method: MS/MS.

Key metabolite: C5OH (3-hydroxyisovalerylcarnitine).

Differential diagnosis: Multiple carboxylase deficiency (including biotinidase and holocarboxylase deficiencies), HMG-CoA lyase deficiency, β-ketothiolase, 2-methyl 3-hydroxy butyric acidemia, 3-methylglutaconic aciduria type I, and maternal 3-MCC deficiency.

What to do if test is positive: Immediately contact the family to ascertain the baby's clinical status. If any concern (i.e., poor feeding, vomiting, lethargy, tachypnea) immediately transport to a hospital, preferably a metabolic center. Asymptomatic infants with mildly abnormal screening results do not require emergency follow-up but should be evaluated and counseled by a metabolic specialist within days.

Confirmatory studies: Organic acids in urine, free and total carnitine in blood, blood ammonia, enzyme studies in fibroblasts, mutation analysis; Urine organic acids and blood acylcarnitines in the mother.

Pitfalls/Attention: Carnitine deficiency might cause a noninformative acylcarnitine profile.

Prevalence (36–39): 1:40,000 (Germany, U.S.), 1:120,000 (Australia).

HMG-CoA Lyase Deficiency HMG-CoA lyase catalyzes the last step in leucine degradation and plays an important role in ketogenesis (see Chapter 8). Patients usually present with sudden hypoketotic hypoglycemia after unremarkable development. Hypoglycemia combined with lack of ketones causes severe brain impairment. Preventing or quickly reversing catabolic states is relatively easy and efficient. Thus, HMG-CoA lyase deficiency represents a favorable screening disease; however, increases of the key metabolite C5OH may be small or even absent. Affected patients might therefore be missed by screening.

Screening method: MS/MS.

Key metabolites: C5OH (3-hydroxyisovalerylcarnitine), MeGlu (methylglutarylcarnitine).

Differential diagnosis: 3-MCC, multiple carboxylase deficiency (including biotinidase and holocarboxylase deficiencies), beta-ketothiolase, 2-methyl 3-hydroxy butyric acidemia, 3-methylglutaric acidemia type I, and maternal 3-MCC deficiency.

What to do if test is positive: Immediately contact the family to ascertain the baby's clinical status. If any concern (ie, poor feeding, vomiting, lethargy, tachypnea) immediately transport to a hospital, preferably a metabolic center. Asymptomatic infants with mildly abnormal screening results do not require emergency follow-up but should be evaluated and counseled by a metabolic specialist within days.

Confirmatory studies: Organic acids in urine, enzyme studies in fibroblasts, molecular genetic analysis.

Pitfalls/Attention: Carnitine deficiency might cause a noninformative acylcarnitine profile. Affected, well-fed newborns may be missed.

Prevalence (36–39): < 1:200,000.

Other Screened Conditions Apart from screening for inborn errors of metabolism and endocrinopathies, various programs also screen for other conditions. Among those, the most common are cystic fibrosis, sickle cell anemia and other hemoglobinopathies. In addition, hearing loss is increasingly added to individual newborn screening panels, although it is not performed by DBS testing but by electrophysiologic studies at the patient's bedside.

Cystic Fibrosis CF is a serious disorder that by disturbed functioning of a chloride channel affects excretory glands of different organs, such as lung, liver, and pancreas. Severe, recurrent pulmonary infections (*Pseudomonas*), worsening of lung function, and failure to thrive are the primary manifestations of the disease. Development and application of more aggressive therapies has allowed many CF-affected individuals to live into adulthood.

In developed industrial countries, the diagnosis based on clinical symptoms is made at a median age of 6 to 9 months (45), with screened individuals being diagnosed considerably earlier.

Newborn screening for CF is primarily based on measurement of immunoreactive trypsinogen (IRT). Because IRT screening alone has neither sufficient specificity nor sensitivity (~95%), IRT testing is often combined with analysis of a panel of CF mutations (deltaF508 is the most common mutation in

Caucasians) as a secondary test from the same DBS. The need for the secondary test arises only if IRT is above the 95th percentile. Application of this two-tier approach has increased the specificity to approximately 99%. Because of the frequency of the disorder, the remaining 1% represents a large number false positives and therefore a large number of unnecessarily burdened parents (19). For this reason, it is recommended that CF screening be performed only in the setting of a well-structured screening program in which an efficient healthcare environment with imbedded prospective outcome studies comparing screened with unscreened cohorts (46) is in place.

Hemoglobinopathies More than 5% of the world's population are carriers for one of the main hemoglobinopathies. The prevalence of disease-causing mutations of hemoglobinopathies reveals major differences in distribution, with the most affected populations in Africa, the Mediterranean region, the Middle East, India, Southeast Asia, and the black population of North America. The screening for hemoglobinopathies is widely debated. It is performed in many parts of the U.S.; however, it is not included in many screening programs of other countries, such as in Europe and Australia. The debate concerns the cost–benefit ratio and effectiveness of early treatment.

In some regions with a very high prevalence for serious hemoglobinopathies, prevention by premarital screening and counseling have been implemented as alternatives to newborn screening.

OUTLOOK

The screening criteria of Wilson and Jungner still represent the universal basis for the decision as to whether diseases with the potential to be investigated should be incorporated into a panel for population screening. Amino acid and acylcarnitine profiles of MS/MS allow detection of several additional diseases that fulfill the criteria only partially, with restriction, or not at all. It is imperative to assess each condition found by MS/MS screening for its impact as a screening disease. Such an assessment of the screening value has to be open to change because the reasoning depends on facts, which may be changing. Increasing knowledge about the natural course of diseases and their variants, new treatment options, and analytical developments improving sensitivity and/or specificity of screening tests are some of the reasons for the need to reassess expansion of screening for additional disorders. Single-case observations or reports of a positive clinical course in diseases that are classified as nontreatable conditions should not justify the decision of adding a disease to the screening panel. In contrast, timely and aggressive treatment has changed the outcome in some dis-

eases that were classified as nontreatable conditions before, thus now justifying their inclusion in a screening program (i.e., GA-1).

The implementation of the screening criteria of Wilson and Jungner is different among screening programs and countries and still a subject of debate. For example, whereas in the United Kingdom and the Netherlands only MCAD is being considered to be a potential candidate of expanded MS/MS screening; in the United States, the recent report of a task force of the ACMG recommends population screening for 29 conditions (core conditions). In addition, 25 disorders (secondary targets) that do not or only partly meet screening criteria also have to be reported (see Table 2-1) (47). An "intermediate" approach is taken in Germany, with 14 conditions agreed on and declared as screening targets (48).

Even though the current expansion of newborn screening programs is often criticized for occurring too rapidly while ignoring that many of the disorders are not fully characterized, it is unlikely that the expansion will abate. Screening for additional conditions and groups of conditions is already being either piloted, developed, or proposed, including Duchenne muscular dystrophy, Wilson disease, lysosomal storage disorders, severe combined immune deficiency, fragile X syndrome, peroxisomal disorders, and others (49–57). Most of these conditions are approached biochemically because of the sheer number of the often private mutations identified in each screened condition. However, molecular genetics analysis is expected to play a more prominent role in newborn screening sometime in the future (58).

REFERENCES

1. Bickel H, Gerrard J, Hickmans EM. Influence of phenylalanine intake on phenylketonuria. *Lancet.* 1953;II:812–823.
2. Guthrie R. The introduction of newborn screening for phenylketonuria: A personal history. *Eur J Pediatr.* 1996;155:S4–5.
3. Guthrie R. Blood screening for phenylketonuria. *JAMA.* 1961;178:863.
4. Guthrie R. Phenylketonuria screening programs. *N Engl J Med.* 1963;269:52–53.
5. Bickel H. Recent advances in the early detection and treatment of inborn errors with brain damage. *Neuropadiatrie.* 1969;1:1–11.
6. Wilson JMG, Jungner G. Principles and Practice of Screening for Disease. Public Health Papers No.34. Geneva: World Health Organization, 1968.
7. Watson MS, Lloyd-Puryear MA, Mann MY, et al. 2006. Main report. *Genet Med.* 8:12S–252S.
8. Watson MS, Lloyd-Puryear MA, Mann MY, et al. 2006. Executive Summary. *Genet Med* 8:1S–11S.
9. Frazier DM, Millington DS, McCandless SE, et al. The tandem mass spectrometry newborn screening experience in North Carolina: 1997–2005. *J Inherited Metab Dis.* 2006;29:76–85.

10. Magera MJ, Gunawardena ND, Hahn SH, et al. Quantitative determination of succinylacetone in dried blood spots for newborn screening of tyrosinemia type I. *Mol Genet Metab.* 2006;88:16–21.

11. Sander J, Janzen N, Peter M, et al. Newborn screening for hepatorenal tyrosinemia: Tandem mass spectrometric quantification of succinylacetone. *Clin Chem.* 2006;52:482–487.

12. Allard P, Grenier A, Korson MS, et al. Newborn screening for hepatorenal tyrosinemia by tandem mass spectrometry: Analysis of succinylacetone extracted from dried blood spots. *Clin Biochem.* 2004;37:1010–1015.

13. Schulze A, Frommhold D, Hoffmann GF, et al. Spectrophotometric microassay for delta-aminolevulinate dehydratase in dried-blood spots as confirmation for hereditary tyrosinemia type I. *Clin Chem.* 2001;47:1424–1429.

14. Lacey JM, Minutti CZ, Magera MJ, et al. Improved specificity of newborn screening for congenital adrenal hyperplasia by second-tier steroid profiling using tandem mass spectrometry. *Clin Chem.* 2004;50:621–625.

15. Sontag MK, Hammond KB, Zielenski J, et al. Two-tiered immunoreactive trypsinogen-based newborn screening for cystic fibrosis in Colorado: Screening efficacy and diagnostic outcomes. *J Pediatr.* 2005;147:S83–88.

16. Rock MJ, Hoffman G, Laessig RH, et al. Newborn screening for cystic fibrosis in Wisconsin: Nine-year experience with routine trypsinogen/DNA testing. *J Pediatr.* 2005;147:S73–77.

17. Kosel S, Burggraf S, Fingerhut R, et al. Rapid second-tier molecular genetic analysis for congenital adrenal hyperplasia attributable to steroid 21-hydroxylase deficiency. *Clin Chem.* 2005;51:298–304.

18. Ensenauer R, Vockley J, Willard JM, et al. A common mutation is associated with a mild, potentially asymptomatic phenotype in patients with isovaleric acidemia diagnosed by newborn screening. *Am J Hum Genet.* 2004;75:1136–1142.

19. Matern D, He M, Berry SA, et al. Prospective diagnosis of 2-methylbutyryl-CoA dehydrognase deficiency in the Hmong population by newborn screening using tandem mass spectrometry. *Pediatrics.* 2003;112:74–78.

20. Abdenur JE, Chamoles NA, Guinle AE, et al. Diagnosis of isovaleric acidaemia by tandem mass spectrometry: False positive result due to pivaloylcarnitine in a newborn screening programme. *J Inherited Metab Dis.* 1998;21:624–630.

21. Waisbren SE, Albers S, Amato S, et al. Effect of expanded newborn screening for biochemical genetic disorders on child outcomes and parental stress. *JAMA.* 2003;290:2564–2572.

22. Crombez E, Koch R, Cederbaum S. Pitfalls in newborn screening. *J Pediatr.* 2005;147:119–120.

23. Guthrie R, Susi A. A simple phenylalanine method for detecting phenylketonuria in large populations of newborn infants. *Pediatrics.* 1963;32:338–343.

24. Beutler E, Baluda MC. A simple spot screening test for galactosemia. *J Lab Clin Med* 1966;68:137–141.

25. Heard GS, Secor M Jr, Wolf B. A screening method for biotinidase deficiency in newborns. *Clin Chem.* 1984;30:125–127.

26. Chace DH. Mass spectrometry in the clinical laboratory. *Chem Rev.* 2001;101:445–477.

27. Matern D, Magera MJ. Mass spectrometry methods for metabolic and health assessment. *J Nutr.* 2001;131:1615S–20.

28. Chace DH, Millington DS, Terada N, et al. Rapid diagnosis of phenylketonuria by quantitative analysis for phenylalanine and tyrosine in neonatal blood spots by tandem mass spectrometry. *Clin Chem.* 1993;39:66–71.

29. Chace DH, Hillman SL, Millington DS, et al. Rapid diagnosis of maple syrup urine disease in blood spots from newborns by tandem mass spectrometry. *Clin Chem.* 1995;41:62–68.

30. Chace DH, Hillman SL, Millington DS, et al. Rapid diagnosis of homocystinuria and other hypermethioninemias from newborns' blood spots by tandem mass spectrometry. *Clin Chem.* 1996;42:349–355.

31. Chace DH, Hillman SL, Van Hove JL, et al. Rapid diagnosis of MCAD deficiency: Quantitatively analysis of octanoylcarnitine and other acylcarnitines in newborn blood spots by tandem mass spectrometry. *Clin Chem.* 1997;43(11):2106–2113.

32. Chace DH, DiPerna JC, Kalas TA, et al. Rapid diagnosis of methylmalonic and propionic acidemias: Quantitative tandem mass spectrometric analysis of propionylcarnitine in filter-paper blood specimens obtained from newborns. *Clin Chem.* 2001;47:2040–2044.

33. Walter JH. Arguments for early screening: A clinician's perspective. *Eur J Pediatr* 2003;162S2–4.

34. Minutti CZ, Lacey JM, Magera MJ, et al. Steroid profiling by tandem mass spectrometry improves the positive predictive value of newborn screening for congenital adrenal hyperplasia. *J Clin Endocrinol Metab.* 2004;89:3687–3693.

35. Jensen UG, Brandt NJ, Christensen E, et al. Neonatal screening for galactosemia by quantitative analysis of hexose monophosphates using tandem mass spectrometry: A retrospective study. *Clin Chem.* 2001;47:1364–1372.

36. Schulze A, Lindner M, Kohlmuller D, et al. Expanded newborn screening for inborn errors of metabolism by electrospray ionization-tandem mass spectrometry: Results, outcome, and implications. *Pediatrics.* 2003;111:1399–406.

37. U.S.A. NNSGRC. National Newborn Screening Report—2000. Electronic citation 2002; available from URL: http://genes-r-us.uthscsa.edu.

38. Zytkovicz TH, Fitzgerald EF, Marsden D, et al. Tandem mass spectrometric analysis for amino, organic, and fatty acid disorders in newborn dried blood spots: A two-year summary from the New England Newborn Screening Program. *Clin Chem.* 2001;47:1945–1955.

39. Wilcken B, Wiley V, Hammond J, et al. Screening newborns for inborn errors of metabolism by tandem mass spectrometry. *N Engl J Med.* 2003;348:2304–2312.

40. Wohlers TM, Fridovich-Keil JL. Studies of the V94M-substituted human UDP–galactose-4-epimerase enzyme associated with generalized epimerase-deficiency galactosaemia. *J Inherited Metab Dis.* 2000;23:713–729.

41. Mudd SH, Skovby F, Levy HL, et al. The natural history of homocystinuria due to cystathionine beta-synthase deficiency. *Am J Hum Genet.* 1985;37:1–31.

42. Mudd SH, Levy HL, Skovby F. Disorders of transsulfuration. In: Scriver CR, Beaudet AL, Sly WS, Valle D, eds. *The Metabolic Bases of Inherited Disease,* 6th ed. New York: McGraw-Hill; 1989:693.

43. Gaustadnes M, Ingerslev J, Rutiger N. Prevalence of congenital homocystinuria in Denmark. *N Engl J Med.* 1999;340:1513.

44. Schimmenti LA, Crombez EA, Schwahn BC, et al. Expanded newborn screening identifies maternal primary carnitine deficiency. *Mol Genet Metab.* 2007; 90: 441–445.

45. Cystic Fibrosis Foundation. Patient Registry 2004 Annual Report. Electronic citation, 2005; available at www.cff.org/publications.

46. Bonham JR, Downing M, Dalton A. Screening for cystic fibrosis: the practice and the debate. *Eur J Pediatr.* 2003;162:S42–45.

47. MCHB. Newborn screening: Toward a uniform screening panel and system. Executive summary. Electronic citation, 2005; available at www.mchb.hrsa.gov/screening/.

48. Hess R. Beschluss über eine Änderung der Richtlinien des Bundesausschusses der Ärzte und Krankenkassen über die Früherkennung von Krankheiten bei Kindern bis zur Vollendung des 6. Lebensjahres (Kinder-Richtlinien) zur Einführung des erweiterten Neugeborenen-Screenings. *Dtsch Aerztebl.* 2005;102: B970–975.

49. Zellweger H, Antonik A. Newborn screening for Duchenne muscular dystrophy. *Pediatrics.* 1975;55:30–34.

50. Drousiotou A, Ioannou P, Georgiou T, et al. Neonatal screening for Duchenne muscular dystrophy: A novel semiquantitative application of the bioluminescence test for creatine kinase in a pilot national program in Cyprus. *Genet Test.* 1998;2:55–60.

51. Kroll CA, Ferber MJ, Dawson BD, et al. Retrospective determination of ceruloplasmin in newborn screening blood spots of patients with Wilson disease. *Mol Genet Metab.* 2006; 89:134–38.

52. Meikle PJ, Grasby DJ, Dean CJ, et al. Newborn screening for lysosomal storage disorders. *Mol Genet Metab* 2006.

53. Li Y, Scott CR, Chamoles NA, et al. Direct multiplex assay of lysosomal enzymes in dried blood spots for newborn screening. *Clin Chem.* 2004;50:1785–1796.

54. Chan K, Puck JM. Development of population-based newborn screening for severe combined immunodeficiency. *J Allergy Clin Immunol.* 2005;115:391–398.

55. McGhee SA, Stiehm ER, Cowan M, et al. Two-tiered universal newborn screening strategy for severe combined immunodeficiency. *Mol Genet Metab.* 2005;86:427–430.

56. Rife M, Mallolas J, Badenas C, et al. Pilot study for the neonatal screening of fragile X syndrome. *Prenat Diagn.* 2002;22:459–462.

57. Hubbard WC, Moser AB, Tortorelli S, et al. Combined liquid chromatography–tandem mass spectrometry as an analytical method for high-throughput screening for X-linked adrenoleukodystrophy and other peroxisomal disorders: Preliminary findings. *Mol Genet Metab.* 2006;89:185–87.

58. Green NS, Pass KA. Neonatal screening by DNA microarray: Spots and chips. *Nat Rev Genet.* 2005;6:147–151.

CHAPTER 3

Molecular Testing for Endocrine and Metabolic Disorders

Johannes Zschocke, Prof. Dr. med., PhD

INTRODUCTION

Molecular genetic testing has secured an important place in the diagnostic evaluation of patients with inborn errors of metabolism and endocrine disorders. However, the benefits and limitations of this new technology have rarely been systematically assessed, and few evidence-based algorithms have been developed that would guide the use of DNA studies for individual indications. There are also myths regarding the value of molecular analyses that may lead to a waste of resources or, worse, to erroneous clinical decisions. This chapter will provide general principles that should be considered before molecular tests are requested or when interpreting results, and highlights some pitfalls in their use. Table 3-1 summarizes some questions that should be considered prior to submission of a sample for DNA analysis.

Molecular testing is only one of many approaches to identifying genetic diseases and genetic risk factors. To reach a correct diagnosis, phenotypic tests (such as biochemical or radiologic analyses or clinical examination) or even an evaluation of family history are frequently superior to "genotype analyses" with regard to sensitivity, cost, and reliability. DNA testing can be a unique tool

for clinical purposes in patients and their relatives, but only if the right questions are asked and if the molecular diagnostic reports provide correct and comprehensive information needed to guide the clinician, especially if the ordering clinician has little experience in medical genetics. Unfortunately, research studies as well as quality assessment schemes have shown that reports do not always contain all the relevant information (1).

Indications

Molecular investigations are performed most frequently for primary diagnosis or confirmation of diagnosis in a patient. The identification of a known pathogenic mutation may be the only diagnostic approach in diseases for which biochemical studies are unavailable, unreliable, or require invasive procedures (e.g., when the relevant protein is expressed in the liver or brain only). Mutation analysis can be a method of choice at very early stages of the diagnostic process when the suspected disorder is caused by one or a few common mutation(s), especially in the absence of alternative diagnostic methods. Most metabolic and endocrine disorders present a special challenge for use of these methods for primary diag

nosis because they are caused by a wide variety of different mutations (allelic heterogeneity) that differ in their impacts on protein function. In many genetic conditions, however, there are clear correlations between genotypes and phenotypes, so the results of mutation analyses may provide information on the expected disease course or the prognosis in an individual patient or family, justifying the inclusion of genetic testing as clinically relevant beyond its utility for genetic counselling alone.

DNA analysis is the most simple and reliable method for prenatal diagnosis and carrier testing in families in which the disease-causing mutations are known. It may be superior even if other methods such as enzyme studies in chorionic villi or amniotic cells, or metabolic investigations in amniotic fluid, are available. Predictive testing of asymptomatic individuals in a family in which a relative has been diagnosed with a genetic condition (usually inherited as a dominant trait) is rarely indicated in metabolic or endocrine disorders. An exception would be optimizing the monitoring of an emerging condition to prevent complications of the disorder. Carrier testing of asymptomatic underage siblings is *not* indicated until the reproductive years (2,3). Finally, there are

---

TABLE 3-1 Questions to Ask Before a Molecular Test is Requested

How sensitive is the genetic test?

Few genetic disorders are caused by single mutations that are reliably recognized with specific tests, and the sensitivity of even the most elaborate molecular methods rarely reaches 100%. Most metabolic and endocrine disorders are caused by a large number of different mutations, and the sensitivity will partly depend on the method used, for example, screening for common mutations versus. full sequence analysis.

How specific is the genetic test?

Molecular testing may provide correct information on the DNA sequence or other genetic characteristics (assuming that the laboratory

is reliable) but it may be difficult to ascertain whether the changes are causally linked with the disorder investigated. Identification of a novel missense mutation in a patient from an uncommon population background should not automatically be taken as diagnostic because the new variant may be a polymorphism in the respective gene pool.

What does a genetic test result tell me?

Most molecular tests are performed to prove or rule out a particular genetic diagnosis; however, the test may also provide information on the course or severity of a disease, or the likelihood (risk) of developing a disease (predictive test).

Could the test result change the clinical management?

A diagnostic intervention should potentially either change the management (treatment, coping strategies) of a patient or be important for other family members. This is also true for genetic tests that should be regarded as "research" if these criteria are not met.

How expensive is the test?

Molecular tests may be very expensive and the cost and benefit of the analysis should be compared with other diagnostic approaches.

some "optional" reasons to perform mutation analyses. Patients with genetic conditions often have life-long clinical problems and sometimes find it easier to relate to their illness when they know "their" individual mutations. Mutation data may help to illustrate mendelian inheritance patterns and may convince the family that nobody is "at fault" for the occurrence of a particular disease in their family.

Sample for DNA Testing

- 5–10 mL EDTA (ethylenediaminetetraacetic acid) whole blood, do not separate cells, ship by ordinary mail (within 24 hrs) or on dry ice (check with laboratory).

- If no blood sample available: filter paper card, biopsies, fibroblasts, and so forth may be used.

Methods

A large number of molecular methods are available for the examination of genetic information in which either DNA or RNA is used (4,5). Most methods are based on the polymerase chain reaction (PCR), which allows the specific amplification of small DNA sequences (usually 100–500 nucleotides, rarely up to >10,000 nucleotides). The method of choice depends on a variety of factors, some of which are depicted in Figure 3-1. Four general approaches of particular relevance to analysis of metabolic and endocrine disorders may be used.

Mutation Screening Mutation screening methods involve testing for a few specific mutations that are known to be frequent in a gene. This approach is relatively inexpensive and is the basis of most commercial mutation analysis kits. A large number of methods have been implemented in different diagnostic laboratories. The sensitivity of a mutation screening method depends on the availability of reliable mutation frequency data in the patient's ethnic background population. Examples of this kind of strategy include allele-specific oligonucleotide analysis, differential restriction enzyme digestion, and genotype microarrays, such as those used for screening of newborn bloodspots for cystic fibrosis. These methods exploit single base pair–based differences in the sequence of small fragments of DNA either by differential hybridization or response to enzyme digestion.

Mutation Scanning Mutation scanning methods examine DNA segments amplified by PCR for evidence of sequence alterations. They can detect both known and novel mutations in a gene; abnormalities identified must be further characterized or confirmed by

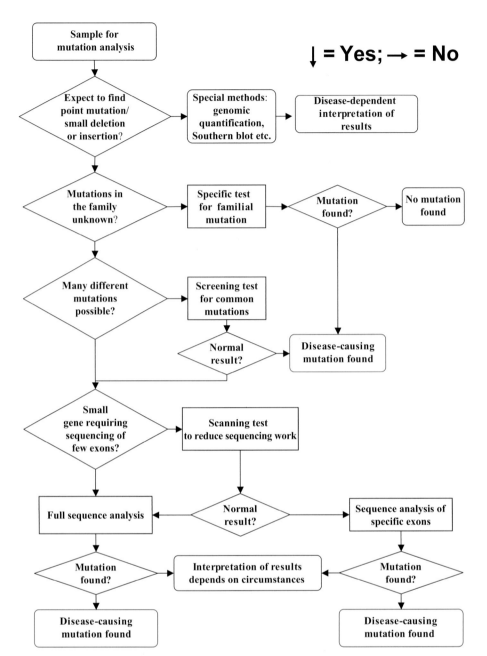

FIGURE 3-1. Flowchart of mutation analysis.

direct sequencing. Mutation scanning methods are generally less expensive than direct sequencing and may be used for investigating large genes at higher speed and lower cost. The main concern with older methods such as single-strand conformation polymorphism analysis was limited sensitivity. In contrast, modern methods such as denaturing high-performance liquid chromatography (dHPLC) or denaturing gradient gel electrophoresis have a very high sensitivity that equals direct sequencing. With fluorescent-based high-throughput capillary sequencers now widely available, many laboratories now use direct DNA sequencing as their primary diagnostic method.

Direct Sequencing Direct sequencing is the gold standard in mutation detection. For diagnostic purposes this usually involves PCR amplification of the DNA segment of interest and "cycle sequencing" amplification of the PCR products for the production of sequence-specific fragments that can be visualized by gel electrophoresis. Direct sequencing for diagnostic purposes can be automated and allows the base-specific analysis of large DNA segments in a relatively short time. Nevertheless, the clinician should be aware that incorrect sequencing results can occur due to both extrinsic and intrinsic errors in these procedures (i.e., technical errors, inexperienced laboratory staff, or heterozygosity of the patient). Even the most conscientious laboratories will occasionally miss a mutation despite full sequence analysis of a gene. To minimize this risk, sequencing should include analysis of all DNA fragments in both forward and reverse directions.

Genomic Quantification Genomic quantification may be necessary to identify large deletions or duplications that are greater than the usual exon sizes and include one or both primer recognition sites used for PCR amplification of a specific DNA segment (6). Such mutations are occasionally found in monogenic metabolic or endocrine disorders but are not usually detected by standard PCR-based methods, including direct sequencing. Recently, a novel method, multiplex ligation-dependent probe amplification (7), has been developed that is already widely used for this purpose. In this method, paired probes that hybridize to adjacent sites on the fragment to be quantitated are added to the patient sample. The probes are designed to include M13 forward and reverse tails, respectively, allowing ligation of the probes, but ligation occurs only if both probes hybridize to target sequences in the DNA to be assessed. PCR is then performed using M13 primers. The quantity of the PCR product is directly dependent on the number of copies of DNA to which the probes have hybridized.

Results

Information on DNA sequence variants identified through molecular analyses should be both comprehensive and concise. The description should follow standard nomenclature as published in print (8) and on the web (http://www.genomic.unimelb.edu.au/mdi/mutnomen/). Mutations should be described with both systematic and protein names. Systematic names describe DNA changes on the nucleotide level (bases A, C, G, or T) by using either complementary DNA or genomic reference sequences (abbreviated with the letters c. or g. to avoid confusion with amino acid numbers). They contain the nucleotide number (A in the start codon is counted as the first nucleotide in a complementary DNA) followed by the base change, for example, c.1222C.T. Systematic names have the important advantage of being unique for any given DNA change; however, the "trivial" names designating mutations at the protein level that refer to an amino acid number may be clinically more useful. Protein names are indicated by the letter p. and provide the amino acid involved in mutation (one-letter or three-letter code) followed by the residue number and finally the new amino acid produced by the mutation (e.g. p.R408W). A protein name as opposed to a systematic

name may be recognized by starting with a letter rather than a number. Protein names reflect the functional consequences of a DNA change (e.g., p.V245V in the PAH gene designates a silent mutation/polymorphism that has no functional relevance) and may be easier to remember. The starting methionine codon should be typically counted as the first residue; however, historically this has not always been the case. For example, some mutations affecting mitochondrial enzymes were first enumerated based on the amino acid number of the mature protein after cleavage (the common medium-chain acyl-coenzyme A dehydrogenase deficiency mutation K329E was initially called K304E). Indeed, many older established mutation names do not follow current guidelines in various ways, so a mixture of different names for the same mutation may cause confusion.

Extensive recommendations are available for different mutation types. Substitutions are denoted by a "." character. Deletions are denoted by the term "del" after the number of the deleted nucleotide or amino acid; a range of deleted residues is indicated by an underscore "_" by a ">" character separating the first and last affected residue. Similarly, insertions are denoted by the term "ins" after the numbers of the nucleotides flanking the insertion site (which are separated by an underscore). For deletions or duplications in single nucleotide (or amino acid) stretches or tandem repeats, the most 3' nucleotide is arbitrarily assigned to have been changed. On the protein level, frameshift deletions or insertions may be given with the abbreviation "fs," for example, fsdel or fsins. Two sequence variations in *cis* (on one chromosome) are given in a square bracket and separated by a semicolon ";". In contrast, sequence changes in *trans* (on different alleles, e.g., in recessive diseases) are separated by a plus "+" sign. The term [?] should be used when the mutation for one allele has not been identified in a recessive disorder. Intronic mutations are numbered according to their position at the beginning or end of the intron (IVS = intervening sequence). The first intronic nucleotide is described as +1, the last nucleotide as −1, either with reference to the intron number (e.g., IVS10-11G.A) or the first/last exonic nucleotide.

The terms "mutation" and "polymorphism" may be misleading as their use is not standardized. Some use the term polymorphism for a "nondisease-causing DNA change" whereas others use it to designate a "DNA change found at an allele frequency of 1% or higher in the population." A mutation may mean either "DNA change" or "disease-causing DNA change." We suggest describing rare, confirmed, disease-causing sequence variants as mutations and common

silent variants as polymorphisms and that neutral terms such as "DNA variant" should be used for other DNA changes identified.

Mutation analyses are usually regarded as "definitive" tests and thus may heavily influence diagnostic decisions. Apart from the intrinsic problems regarding the sensitivity of a test, it must be kept in mind that molecular analyses can be technically difficult, require considerable experience, and are prone to errors in principle. Quality control schemes for sequence-based DNA tests consistently show a considerable error rate in the participating laboratories; in one published study, genotyping errors occurred at a frequency of 3% to 7% (9). Mutation analyses are frequently performed in primary research laboratories as an extension of previous scientific projects, and in most countries, few laboratories have implemented strict quality control measures or have achieved accreditation. In the United States, laboratories offering molecular analyses for clinical diagnostic testing must be accredited based on federal guidelines delineated in the Clinical Laboratory Improvement Amendments (CLIA). CLIA certification cannot guarantee that errors never occur in clinical laboratory testing but it does assure the clinician that testing in a laboratory has met specified standards of accuracy and accountability. Because of CLIA regulation, any mutation ascertained in a research laboratory in the United States must be confirmed in a CLIA-approved clinical laboratory to use these data for critical clinical decisions.

If the result of a molecular test seems to be incompatible with the clinical picture, checking the results in another laboratory may be justified. Quality assessment schemes are available for molecular tests on national and international levels from a variety of sources and it is advisable to ask a laboratory if it participates in such schemes (10). Additional quality features of a diagnostic laboratory include a complete report, a limited portfolio of diagnostic tests (as comprehensive interpretation of the results requires profound knowledge of the disorder investigated), and transparent charge structures for billing.

Interpretation

The interpretation of the results is the most crucial section of a molecular report—with advances in instrumentation it is now easier to sequence a gene than to interpret the results correctly. The relevance of molecular findings may be difficult to determine for the nongeneticist and adequate interpretation requires profound knowledge of the clinical indications for testing and the spectrum and impact of mutations in a gene. There are several key questions for the clinician to keep in mind when the results of molecular testing are to be translated into patient care decisions.

How unlikely is the diagnosis when no mutation is found? There is virtually no endocrine disorder or inborn error of metabolism in which all mutations are detected, even with the most sophisticated methods. Negative results do not definitively rule out a diagnosis, particularly when the sensitivity of the method used is limited. For correct interpretation, all negative mutation reports should contain information on the sensitivity of the method used in the analysis, for example, the likelihood that a disease is caused by a mutation not recognized by the test. The results of DNA tests should be interpreted in the context of the clinical features and other relevant findings. If the sensitivity of a given analysis is high, however, the failure to identify even one mutation in an autosomal recessive disorder should prompt the clinician to reevaluate a diagnosis.

How likely is the diagnosis when a mutation is found? Related questions include: how reliable are genotype–phenotype correlations? Is the clinical picture fully explained by the genetic findings? Is the disorder fully penetrant? Are there additional, nongenetic factors of pathogenesis? Novel DNA variants can be erroneously regarded as disease causing when they are in fact silent. This is particularly true for missense mutations that cause a change in a single amino acid. It is generally unwise to speculate too much on the pathogenic impact of such a variant even if the protein structure is known and may be assessed with computer programs. It is frequently necessary to describe a novel DNA alteration as an "unknown variant" of unknown clinical relevance. In confirmed recessive disorders such variants may nevertheless be used as markers for testing of other family members or for prenatal diagnosis. Guidelines for proving disease causation of mutations have been published (11). A mutation may appropriately be judged to be deleterious if functional assays of the specific mutation can be undertaken that demonstrate altered protein function.

Cis or trans? When two mutations are found in a recessive disorder, inheritance in *trans* (on different chromosomes) should be confirmed by examining the carrier status of both parents. Two mutations may occasionally be in *cis* on the same chromosome, with another or no mutation on the second chromosome. This constellation, when unrecognized, may have disastrous consequences in prenatal diagnosis; however, caution should be exercised when initiating parental testing because of the possibility of nonpaternity.

CONCLUSION

Mutation analysis is a powerful method in clinical practice but may be expensive and is prone to methodological or interpretatory errors. Before ordering such analyses, care must be taken to define the indication and to chose the best laboratory for the test. The results of mutation studies should be explained to the patient and/or family through genetic counseling.

REFERENCES

1. Andersson HC, Krousel-Wood MA, Jackson KE, et al. Medical genetic test reporting for cystic fibrosis (deltaF508) and factor V Leiden in North American laboratories. *Genet Med.* 2002;4(5):324–327.
2. Hogben S, Boddington P. Policy recommendations for carrier testing and predictive testing in childhood: a distinction that makes a real difference. *J Genet Couns.* 2005;14(4):271–281.
3. Nelson RM, Botkjin JR, Kodish ED, et al. Ethical issues with genetic testing in pediatrics. *Pediatrics.* 2001;107(6):1451–5.
4. Nollau P, Wagener C. Methods for detection of point mutations: performance and quality assessment. IFCC Scientific Division, Committee on Molecular Biology Techniques. *Clin Chem.* 1997;43(7):1114–28.
5. Taylor GR, Day IN. *Guide to Mutation Detection.* Hoboken, NJ: John Wiley & Sons, Inc; 2005.
6. Armour JA, Barton DE, Cockburn DJ, et al. The detection of large deletions or duplications in genomic DNA. *Hum Mutat.* 2002;20(5):325–337.
7. Schouten JP, McElgunn CJ, Waaijer R, et al. Relative quantification of 40 nucleic acid sequences by multiplex ligation-dependent probe amplification. *Nucleic Acids Res.* 2002 Jun 15;30(12):e57.
8. den Dunnen JT, Antonarakis SE. Nomenclature for the description of human sequence variations. *Hum Genet.* 2001;109(1):121–124.
9. Mueller CR, Kristoffersson U, Stoppa-Lyonnet D. External quality assessment for mutation detection in the BRCA1 and BRCA2 genes: EMQN's experience of 3 years. *Ann Oncol.* 2004;15 Suppl 1:I14–I17.
10. Dequeker E, Ramsden S, Grody WW, et al. Quality control in molecular genetic testing. *Nat Rev Genet.* 2001;2(9):717–723.
11. Cotton RG, Scriver CR. Proof of "disease causing" mutation. *Hum Mutat.* 1998;12(1):1–3.

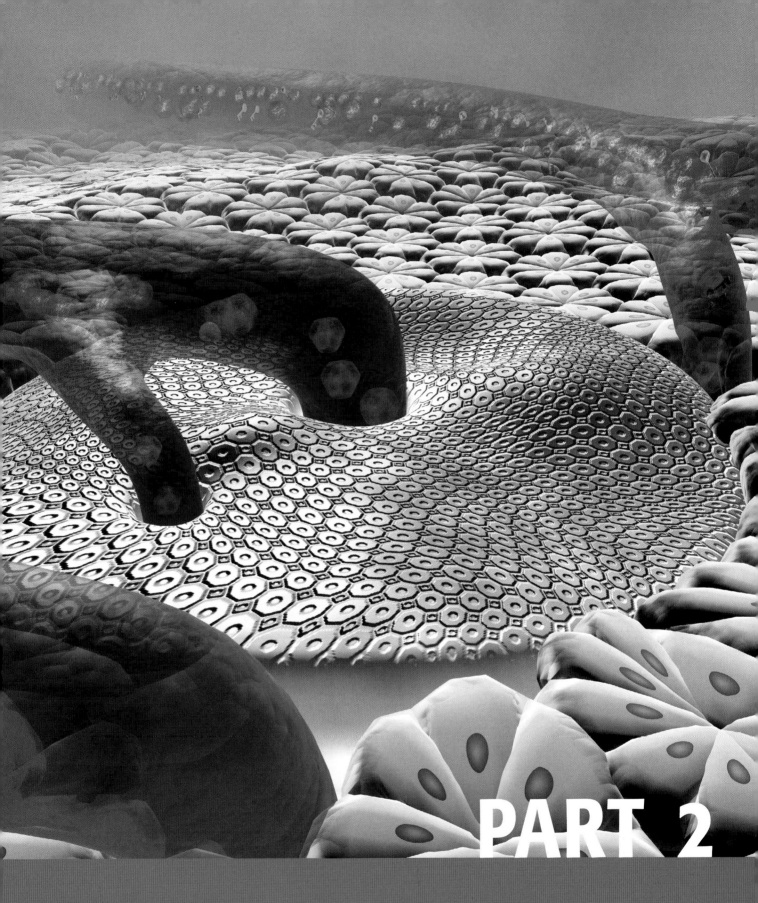

PART 2

Disorders of Fuel Metabolism

IN THIS PART

Previous page: Healthy insulin response.

CHAPTER

4

Hyperinsulinism

Andrea Kelly, MD
Charles A. Stanley, MD

Glucose homeostasis is critical for meeting the metabolic demands of the brain, and an inadequate supply of glucose can cause seizures and permanent brain damage. Because of the larger size of the infant brain relative to the rest of the body, an infant's glucose requirement of 6–8 mg/kg/minute exceeds that of an adult (2 mg/kg/minute). Since the infant brain is undergoing rapid growth and development, it is extremely vulnerable to hypoglycemia, which is defined in infants as in older children and adults as a blood glucose (BG) concentration of less than 50 mg/dL, whereas concentrations of less than 60 mg/dL are considered abnormal.

A failure of fasting adaptation generally is responsible for hypoglycemia in children. The elements of fasting include 1) glycogenolysis, 2) gluconeogenesis, 3) lipolysis, and 4) fatty acid oxidation and ketogenesis. These pathways are strictly regulated by hormones. Insulin suppresses the fasting adaptation systems, whereas counterregulatory hormones (e.g., glucagon, growth hormone, cortisol, and epinephrine) stimulate these pathways. Hyperinsulinism is the most common cause of recurrent hypoglycemia in infancy.

Etiology/Pathophysiology *Congenital hyperinsulinism* refers to inherited disorders in the pathways of insulin secretion that cause hypoglycemia. This group of disorders was referred to previously as *nesidioblastosis*. This term is considered a misnomer because nesidioblastosis is not specific for hyperinsulinism and is a common histological finding in pancreatic tissue from normal infants. With the identification of specific genetic defects responsible for congenital hyperinsulinism, a more complete description of the clinical manifestations of these disorders has become possible. In addition, the roles of these various pathways in normal insulin secretion are becoming better understood. As shown in Figure 4-1, glucose is the primary stimulant for insulin secretion. After glucose enters the β-cell via the GLUT-2 transporter, it is phosphorylated by glucokinase, the rate-limiting "glucosen-

sor" of the β-cell. Subsequent metabolism of glucose generates adenosine triphosphate (ATP), leading to an increase in the ATP:adenosine diphosphate (ADP) ratio of the β-cell. This increase closes the ATP-sensitive potassium (K_{ATP}) channel, which is composed of the sulfonylurea receptor regulatory subunit (SUR1) and the inwardly rectifying potassium pore (KIR6.2). Depolarization of the β-cell membrane ensues. Voltage-dependent calcium channels (VDCCs) open, and calcium enters the β-cell, leading to insulin release (3). A K_{ATP} channel–independent pathway for amplification of glucose-stimulated insulin secretion also exists that may depend on glutamine (4).

Amino acids stimulate insulin secretion through glutamate dehydrogenase (GDH) (see Figure 4-1), a mitochondrial enzyme responsible for the oxidative deamination of glutamate to α-ketoglutarate (5–9). GDH is allosterically activated by leucine and inhibited by guanosine triphosphate (GTP) and ATP. As with glucose, further metabolism of α-ketoglutarate generates ATP and triggers the K_{ATP} channel–dependent pathway of insulin secretion. The mechanisms by which fatty acids stimulate insulin secretion are not well understood.

In congenital hyperinsulinism, defects in any of the preceding pathways lead to dysregulated insulin secretion (10–24). Inappropriate

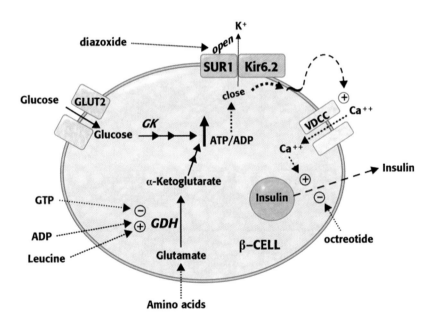

FIGURE 4-1. K_{ATP} channel–dependent pathways of insulin secretion. *Glucose* enters the β-cell through the GLUT-2 transporter and is phosphorylated by GK. Further metabolism of glucose generates ATP, leading to an increase in the β-cell ATP: ADP ratio. This increase closes the ATP-sensitive potassium (K_{ATP}) channel, and β-cell membrane depolarization ensues. VDCCs open, allowing calcium entry into the β-cell and, ultimately, insulin release. *Amino acids* stimulate insulin secretion through GDH, which deaminates glutamate to α-ketoglutarate. GDH is allosterically activated by leucine and ADP and is inhibited by GTP. As with glucose, further metabolism of α-ketoglutarate generates ATP and triggers the K_{ATP} channel–dependent pathway of insulin secretion. Diazoxide inhibits insulin secretion by maintaining the K_{ATP} channel open via SUR1. Octreotide inhibits insulin secretion downstream of the VDCC. GLUT-2 = glucose transporter 2; GK = glucokinase; K_{ATP} channel is composed of SUR1 = sulfonylurea receptor 1 and Kir6.2 = inwardly rectifying potassium pore; VDCC = voltage-dependent calcium channel; GDH = glutamate dehydrogenase.

Hyperinsulinism

AT-A-GLANCE

Hyperinsulinism (HI) refers to the group of congenital and acquired disorders of hypoglycemia that arise from dysregulated insulin secretion. Hyperinsulinism is the most common cause of persistent neonatal hypoglycemia. In the congenital forms, specific genetic defects in the pathways of insulin secretion are responsible for excess insulin secretion. Treatment of both congenital and acquired forms is intended to normalize blood glucose and hence prevent short- and long-term neurocognitive sequelae of recurrent hypoglycemia. Treatment modalities include: 1) medications that suppress endogenous insulin secretion such as diazoxide and octreotide; and, 2) pancreatectomy.

CONGENITAL HI	GENE	LOCUS	INHERITANCE	OMIM
K_{ATP} **HI**		11p15.1		256450
Diffuse	ABCC8		Recessive and dominant	
Focal	KCNJ11		Paternal K_{ATP} mutation with loss of heterozygosity of maternal allele	
GDH HI (HI/HA)	GLUD-1	10q23.3	Dominant/sporadic	606762
GK HI	GCK	7p15-13	Dominant/sporadic	602485
SCHAD deficiency	HADH	4q22-q26	Recessive	601609
CDG type 1B*	MPI	15q22-qter	Recessive	602579
Beckwith–Wiedemann	Epigenetic	11p15.5	Sporadic Epigenetic: • Loss of methylation of maternal differentially methylated region 2 (DMR2) • Gain of methylation of maternal DMR1 or H19	130650
	CDKN1C		Paternal uniparental disomy Dominant: CDKN1C, maternal DMR1	

ACQUIRED HI	GENE	LOCUS	INHERITANCE	OMIM
Transient				
Infant of diabetic mother	N/A	N/A	N/A	N/A
Peripartum stress HI	N/A	N/A	N/A	N/A
Insulinoma	MEN1	11q13		131100
Sporadic			N/A	
MEN-1			Dominant—90% of MEN-1; Sporadic—10% of MEN-1	

FORM	FINDINGS	CLINICAL PRESENTATION
K_{ATP} **HI**		
(diffuse and focal)	Fasting and protein-induced hypoglycemia	Typically present shortly after birth; often are LGA
GDH HI	Fasting and protein-induced hypoglycemia; leucine sensitivity; hyperammonemia	Presents later in infancy; not usually LGA; asymptomatic hyperammonemia
GK HI	Fasting hypoglycemia; lowering of β-cell "glucosensor"	
SCHAD	Fasting hypoglycemia; ↑ Plasma 3-hydroxylbutyryl carnitine ↑ Urine 3-hydroxyglutaric acid	
CDG type 1b	Hypoglycosylation, as determined by isoelectric focusing of serum transferrin	Protein-losing enteropathy; coagulation disorders; hepatic fibrosis
Transient neonatal HI		
Peripartum stress HI	Fasting hypoglycemia	Present shortly after birth; typically SGA, birth asphyxiated, or other "stressed" neonates
Infant of diabetic mother		Present shortly after birth; LGA
Insulinoma	Fasting hypoglycemia + leucine sensitivity	Rare in childhood; 2nd most common pancreatic tumor in MEN-1
Beckwith–Wiedemann	Fasting hypoglycemia	Hypoglycemia shortly after birth; typical features include macrosomia, macroglossia, abdominal wall defect; additional features include hemihypertrphy, embryonal tumors, adrenocortical cytomegaly, ear anomalies, visceromegaly, renal abnormalities

LGA = large for gestational age; AGA = appropriate for gestational age; CDG = carbohydrate-deficient glycoprotein syndrome.
* = single cases of hyperinsulinism associated with CDG-1d and CDG-1a have been described.

insulin secretion leads to recurrent hypoglycemia. The triggers for hypoglycemia depend on the underlying genetic defect and will be described in further detail below.

CONGENITAL HYPERINSULINISM DUE TO K$_{ATP}$ (SUR1 AND KIR6.2) CHANNEL MUTATIONS

Etiology/Pathophysiology Mutations of the ABCC8 gene encoding SUR1 and of the KCNJ11 gene encoding Kir6.2, the subunits of the β-cell K$_{ATP}$ channel, are responsible for the most common form of congenital hyperinsulinsm (HI). More than 100 mutations of the ABCC8 and 20 mutations of the KCNJ11 have been described. The SUR1 subunit is sensitive to changes in the energy state of the β-cell and regulates the opening and closing of the potassium channel pore. Diffuse disease, in which all β-cells in the pancreas have defective channels, is inherited in recessive and, less commonly, dominant fashion. The extent of K$_{ATP}$ channel dysfunction depends on the nature of the genetic defect. For instance, the common, recessive Ashkenazi SUR1 mutations delF1388 and 3992-9G→A cause complete loss of potassium channel function. Dominantly expressed K$_{ATP}$ mutations have been identified in only a few families and tend to produce milder disease due partial loss of K$_{ATP}$ channel function (15,25,26).

Because the open state of the K$_{ATP}$ channel maintains the β-cell membrane potential in a hyperpolarized state until it senses an increase in β-cell phosphate energy charge, loss of K$_{ATP}$ function leads to β-cell membrane depolarization (Figure 4-2). In this energy state, the β-cell no longer strictly regulates insulin secretion; insulin secretion cannot be down regulated appropriately at low blood glucose concentrations and also cannot be activated appropriately at increased blood glucose concentrations. In addition, exposure to fuels such as amino acids, which normally only stimulate insulin secretion in the presence of glucose (27), may be sufficient to trigger β-cell membrane depolarization and insulin secretion (28,29).

Focal K$_{ATP}$ HI suffers from the same β-cell membrane depolarization issues and hence dysregulated insulin secretion, but only a subset of pancreatic β-cells is affected. This form of congenital HI arises from inheritance of a paternal K$_{ATP}$ channel mutation (ABCC8 or KCNJ11) and a specific loss of maternal alleles of the imprinted chromosome region 11p15. The loss of the normal maternal allele occurs in a subset of pancreatic β-cells and is the result of "second hit" (30–32). This combination of an inherited K$_{ATP}$ germline mutation and the postzygotic loss of heterozygosity for the maternal allele leads to expression of the abnormal paternal allele in a clone of β-cells. Loss of normal tumor-suppressor genes on the maternal allele allows for focal expansion of these abnormal β-cells and hence the development of a focal pancreatic lesion. Because these lesions arise during fetal development, they do not disrupt the normal architecture of the pancreas and are not encapsulated, features typical of insulinomas.

In northern Europe, the incidence of severe congenital HI is approximately 1 in 40,000 (33,34), but in Saudi Arabia, where consanguinity is common, the incidence is approximately 1 in 3000 births (35).

Clinical Presentation Infants with diffuse or focal K$_{ATP}$ HI tend to be born large for gestational age and to present shortly after birth with symptomatic hypoglycemia. A typical-appearing patient is shown in Figure 4-3. The majority present within the first month of life, although in some children the diagnosis is delayed until later in infancy. Hypoglycemia may manifest as a seizure, lethargy, or cyanosis or may be asymptomatic. The hypoglycemia frequently is so severe that glucose infusion rates (GIR) up to 30 mg/kg/minute (four to five times normal) are required to prevent hypoglycemia. The volumes necessary to maintain the GIR may be so great as to cause fluid overload. Focal K$_{ATP}$ HI and recessive K$_{ATP}$ HI generally are resistant to diazoxide, a medication that activates SUR1 to maintain the K$_{ATP}$ channel in the open state. This diazoxide resistance likely reflects the underlying genetic defects that lead to complete or near-complete loss of channel function. Clinically, focal K$_{ATP}$ HI is indistinguishable from diffuse K$_{ATP}$ HI. On the other hand, children with dominant K$_{ATP}$ HI, a form identified only recently, may respond to diazoxide. This diazoxide responsiveness likely reflects partial preservation of K$_{ATP}$ channel function (25,36).

In addition to fasting hypoglycemia, some children with K$_{ATP}$ HI have postprandial hypoglycemia. Studies of this form of congenital HI reveal the presence of protein-induced hypoglycemia (Figure 4-4) (28,29). This protein sensitivity occurs in the absence of leucine sensitivity (Figure 4-5), suggesting that a

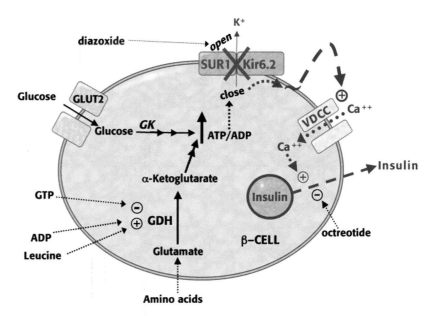

FIGURE 4-2. K$_{ATP}$ channel HI. In this form of congenital HI, recessive and dominant mutations of SUR1 and Kir6.2 lead to loss of K$_{ATP}$ channel function. The β-cell membrane is no longer hyperpolarized by the outwardly rectifying potassium current, allowing calcium influx through the VDCC. Excess insulin secretion results.

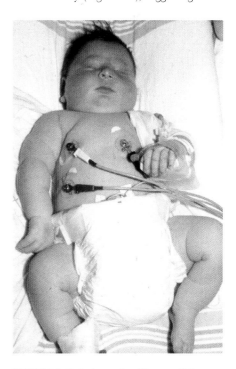

FIGURE 4-3. Typical neonate with congenital hyperinsulinism. This infant was born large for gestational age. Within the first hour of life, the infant was found with a blood glucose concentration of 19 mg/dL.

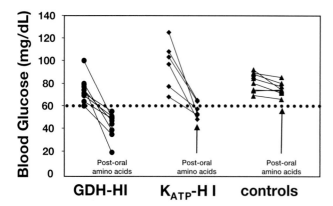

FIGURE 4-4. Protein sensitivity in congenital HI. Following an oral protein load of an amino acid hydrosylate (1.5 g/kg), patients with recessive K_{ATP} HI and GDH HI become hypoglycemic, unlike normal controls, in whom blood glucose changes little.

GDH- and K_{ATP} channel–independent pathway for amino acid–stimulated insulin secretion exists. Studies of glucose- and amino acid–stimulated insulin secretion in isolated islets from normal and SUR1 knockout mice are consistent with the ability of glutamine to amplify insulin secretion downstream of K_{ATP} channel closure (4,37). In these studies, amino acids or glutamine alone stimulated insulin secretion in SUR1 knockout islets but not in normal islets. In the SUR1 knockout islets, this insulin secretion in response to an amino acid mixture was reduced by more than 50% in the absence of glutamine. On the other hand, inhibition of glutamine production in normal islets led to significant reduction in glucose-stimulated insulin secretion that was reversed with the addition of glutamine or a nonmetabolizable glutamine analogue. Glutamine-stimulated insulin secretion likely requires β-cell depolarization and subsequent intracellular calcium elevation, conditions found in K_{ATP} HI islets. This exaggerated glutamine-stimulated insulin secretion provides a mechanism for protein-induced hypoglycemia in K_{ATP} HI.

Diagnosis Clues to the diagnosis of congenital HI include large for gestational age (LGA) birth weight and increased glucose use in a neonate with recurrent hypoglycemia. When glucose requirements exceed 10 mg/kg/min, the differential diagnosis is limited essentially to HI and hypopituitarism. The diagnosis of HI is confirmed by identifying inappropriate insulin secretion at the time of hypoglycemia. Confirmation may require a formal fasting study, which evaluates whether the normal mechanisms for fasting adaptation are intact. Measurements of plasma insulin are not always reliable in making the diagnosis of HI; insulin concentrations may be lower than the assay limit of detection yet sufficiently elevated to cause hypoglycemia. Other markers of insulin action are more sensitive in confirming the diagnosis of HI. At blood glucose concentrations of less than 50 mg/dL, free fatty acids and ketones (β-hydroxybutyrate and acetoacetate) are inappropriately suppressed, and blood glucose concentration increases by more than 30 mg/ dL in response to an injection of glucagon (1 mg). Insulin-like growth factor–binding protein 1 (IGFBP-1), a marker of insulin action at the liver, is also inappropriately suppressed in infants with HI in contrast to normal children, in whom IGFBP-1 rises tenfold in response to fasting (38). Regulation of IGFBP-1 by insulin is considered an adaptation to fasting: Suppression of IGFBP-1 increases insulin-like growth factor 1 (IGF-1) bioavailabilty,

allowing IGF-1 to have insulin-like effects, whereas an increase in IGFBP-1 with fasting limits free IGF-1, thereby minimizing the insulin-like effects of IGF-1. Frequently, cortisol and growth hormone are not elevated enough at the time of hypoglycemia to rule out deficiencies of these counterregulatory hormones (39,40). To exclude hypopituitarism as an etiology for neonatal hypoglycemia, provocative studies (e.g., growth hormone or low adrenocorticotropin hormone [ACTH] stimulation test) of these axes may be required.

Once the diagnosis of HI is made, treatment is initiated. Treatment responses provide clues to the underlying genetic defect. Diazoxide resistance suggests the presence of K_{ATP} HI, either focal or diffuse. To differentiate between focal and diffuse forms preoperatively, acute insulin-response studies (AIRs) to various secretagogues have been developed (see Figure 4-5). These also have attempted to distinguish K_{ATP} HI from other forms of HI. As a result of the presence of β-cells with unstable cell membrane potential, children with K_{ATP} HI have inappropriate insulin secretion in response to an intravenous bolus of calcium (41). Children with *diffuse* K_{ATP} HI, however, do not secrete insulin in response to tolbutamide (41) and have subnormal insulin responses to intravenous glucose (42). In contrast, children with *focal* lesions respond normally to intravenous tolbutamide and glucose (42,43), evidence that only a subpopulation of their β-cells is abnormal. Some K_{ATP} HI mutations maintain partial channel function, and thus AIRs cannot distinguish between focal and diffuse disease reliably (44,45). In addition, tolbutamide is no longer available from the manufacturer. As a result, AIRs are no longer performed routinely in the diagnostic workup of surgical HI. For children requiring surgical treatment of HI, localization of a focal lesion prior to surgery may circumvent the need for a near-total pancreatectomy. Routine imaging studies (i.e., ultrasound, computed tomographic [CT] scanning, and magnetic resonance imaging [MRI]) have not been useful in localizing these lesions because focal lesions arise during fetal development and do not disrupt normal pancreatic architecture. On the other hand, arterial stimulation venous sampling (ASVS) has been useful (45). During ASVS, calcium is injected into the three main pancreatic arteries—the gastroduodenal (GDA), which primarily serves the pancreatic head; the superior mesenteric artery (SMA), which primarily supplies the pancreatic body; and the splenic artery, which supplies the pancreatic tail. Insulin is measured at the hepatic vein. A step-up in insulin secretion following stimulation of one of the arteries suggests

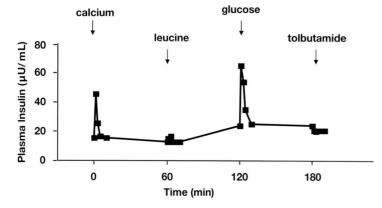

FIGURE 4-5. Acute insulin response tests in recessive K_{ATP} HI. Children with recessive K_{ATP} HI have exaggerated insulin secretion at 1 and 3 minutes in response to an intravenous bolus of calcium (0.1 mEq/kg), no insulin secretion in response to intravenous leucine (15 mg/kg) or tolbutamide (25 mg/kg), and a blunted response to intravenous glucose (0.5 g/kg). In contrast, normal individuals do not secrete insulin in response to calcium or leucine but have significant insulin secretion in response to tolbutamide and, of course, glucose.

that if a focal lesion is present, it is likely to be found in the distribution of that particular pancreatic artery. During the procedure, BG is maintained in the 60–70 mg/dL range. A potential complication of this procedure is decreased perfusion of the lower extremity due to femoral artery spasm or the dislodging of a clot following removal of the femoral artery catheter. Following the procedure, perfusion of the right lower extremity is assessed.

Transhepatic portal venous sampling (THPVS) is an alternative method of localizing a pancreatic lesion (46,47). With this procedure, BG is maintained at approximately 50 mg/dL. Venous drainage of the pancreas is accessed through the liver. Blood is collected along the length of venous drainage of the pancreas. A step-up in insulin secretion suggests the presence of a focal lesion in the area drained by that vein.

Limitations of these procedures include abnormal anatomy, normal variations in blood supply to the pancreas, and size of the patient. In addition, they are neither 100% sensitive nor specific. For these reasons, biopsies obtained intraoperatively and examined by pathologists with an expertise in HI are vital. Multiple biopsies are obtained. If all the biopsies have β-cells with enlarged nuclei, diffuse HI is most likely. If normal tissue is found, a focal lesion is suspected, and the surgeon continues to biopsy until the focal lesion is found, as shown in Figure 4-6, and completely resected (48). Complications associated with these repeated biopsies are uncommon and are similar to those occurring with routine pancreatectomy. Preliminary reports suggest that [^{18}F]dopa positron-emission tomographic (PET) scans may be able to visualize lesions in focal HI (49).

Mutational analysis of the SUR1 and Kir6.2 genes can confirm the presence of K_{ATP}

TABLE 4-1	Laboratory Findings: K_{ATP} HI	
	Decreased	**Increased**
Blood glucose < 50 mg/dL	Free fatty acids (<1.5 mmol/L)	BG response to glucagon (>30 mg/dL)
	β-Hydroxybutyrate (<1.5 mmol/L)	GH (>10 ng/mL)
	IGFBP-1 (<120 ng/mL)	Cortisol (>18 μg/dL)
		Insulin (>2 μU/mL)

channel mutations. If the likely mutation(s) is known based on an affected family member or ethnic background, mutational analysis can be directed toward these mutations preoperatively. The finding of two mutations is consistent with diffuse disease. The finding of a maternal mutation would suggest that the child has diffuse disease (either recessive or dominant) because focal lesions are associated with paternal mutations. In the setting of a paternal mutation, the affected child may have diffuse or focal disease. Mutational analysis of these HI-causing gene defects is available through research laboratories and more recently through a commercial laboratory (Table 4-1).

Treatment The goal of treatment is to maintain BG above 70 mg/dL in a safe manner that permits normal childhood development and is manageable for caretakers. Affected patients should be able to fast without becoming hypoglycemic and should demonstrate normal fasting adaptation, that is, appropriately increased free fatty acids and ketones with fasting and no glycemic response to glucagon if BG is less than 50 mg/dL. Infants should be able to fast for 18–24 hours before becoming hypoglycemic; children 2–3 years of age should tolerate 24–36 hours of fasting, whereas older children should be able to fast at least 36 hours. Because medical treatment is unlikely to completely normalize fasting adaptation, fasting tolerances that are safe are sought. An infant/child should be able to fast 10–12 hours (i.e., sleep overnight) without becoming hypoglycemic.

Medical treatment is first directed at suppressing insulin secretion. Diazoxide suppresses insulin secretion by maintaining the K_{ATP} channel in the open position. Doses of 5–15 mg/kg/day orally generally are needed. Side effects of medication are primarily cosmetic—hypertrichosis and coarsening of the face. Fluid retention can occur, particularly in preterm infants and in infants receiving large fluid volumes. Fluid retention may be significant enough to require institution of a diuretic. Rarely, leukopenia and thrombocytopenia have been reported. If a child continues to have hypoglycemia following 5 days of maximum doses of diazoxide, he or she is considered diazoxide-unresponsive, and octreotide is initiatated.

Octreotide is a somatostatin analogue and is thought to suppress insulin secretion downstream of the voltage-dependent calcium channel. Octreotide is delivered by subcutaneous injection either at 6- to 8-hour intervals or continuously through a pump at doses of 5–20 μg/kg/day. Doses larger than 20 μg/kg/day generally are no more efficacious. An effect is seen frequently with the first octreotide dose, even if the child ultimately will be declared octreotide-unresponsive. This failure arises because tachyphylaxis often occurs within 3–4 days of octreotide initiation or dose increase despite an initial hyperglycemic effect. Potential side effects include biliary sludging and altered gut motility. Growth suppression generally is not seen with prolonged octreotide use.

Glucagon antagonizes insulin action by mobilizing hepatic glycogen stores. It is delivered continuously at a dose of 1 mg/day, although some centers titrate the dose to between 5 and 10 μg/kg/hour. Glucagon is used as a temporizing measure prior to pancreatectomy. Experience with long-term outpatient use is limited; on rare occasions (i.e., when hypoglycemia persists following complete pancreatectomy, maximum octreotide doses, and continuous dextrose), continuous glucagon delivered by insulin pump has prevented hypoglycemia successfully. Side effects include vomiting and inhibition of pancreatic enzyme and gastric acid secretion.

If medical therapy fails, pancreatectomy is indicated. Focal lesions account for 30% to 70% of K_{ATP} HI cases and may be cured with focal resection. Unfortunately, focal lesions are not readily identified grossly and frequently are found in the pancreatic head, a difficult region to resect without causing damage to the bile ducts and duodenum. Multiple biopsies of the pancreas are obtained by the surgeon and examined by the pathologist intraoperatively. The identification of normal pancreas suggests the presence of a focal lesion, and the surgeon continues to biopsy until the focal lesion is isolated. The surgeon may be guided by preoperative localizing procedures such as ASVS or THPVS. An experienced surgeon and pathologist are vital to identification and complete resection of a focal lesion.

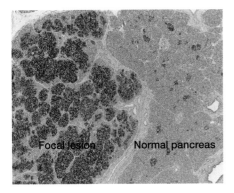

FIGURE 4-6. Pancreatic Lesion in Focal K_{ATP} channel-HI. This surgical specimen from an infant with congenital hyperinsulinism due to focal K_{ATP} channel-HI is stained for insulin. On the right is normal pancreatic tissue with islets dispersed throughout exocrine tissue. On the left is an area of adenomatosis, the site of the focal HI-causing lesion.

In the setting of diffuse HI, a 95% to 99% pancreatectomy is performed. With less than 95% pancreatectomy, sufficient β-cell mass remains to cause continued hypoglycemia. With 95% to 98% pancreatectomy, a third of patients will have persistent hypoglycemia, a third will have improved glycemic control, and a third will have diabetes. Although pancreatectomy may not cure diffuse HI, sufficient reduction in β-cell mass may occur to allow more effective medical treatment.

Immediate complications of pancreatectomy include pancreatitis, duodenal hematoma, pseudocyst formation, and injury to the bile ducts. Postoperatively, hyperglycemia is common, related to the stress of surgery, and frequently requires insulin. Only when the child is taking full feeds can a determination be made as to whether long-term insulin therapy is required. Moreover, despite the presence of hyperglycemia postoperatively, some children will have persistent hypoglycemia that is only evident when the child is on full feeds or fasts. Additional complications of pancreatectomy include obstruction of the gastrointestinal tract due adhesions and pancreatic insufficiency; the latter usually is subclinical but should be sought in the child with chronic diarrhea or poor growth. Late-onset diabetes can occur years after pancreatectomy, frequently during puberty. In the setting of pancreatectomy, diabetes has been attributed to deceased β-cell mass. However, the findings of 1) decreased insulin secretion in response to an acute glucose challenge (see Figure 4-5) and 2) hyperglycemia in three teenagers who were treated medically for recessive SUR1 HI suggest that dysregulated insulin secretion has a role in the development of late-onset diabetes (50).

Some centers do not use pancreatectomy routinely to treat HI that has failed pharmacological therapy. Instead, continuous dextrose delivered through intragastric tube is used to prevent hypoglycemia. At our center, we prefer more definitive therapy through surgery and use continuous intragastric dextrose as a last resort (i.e., significant hypoglycemia despite pancreatectomy and octreotide) because such interventions may limit normal social interaction, suppress appetite, create feeding aversions, and place the child at risk for significant hypoglycemia should the tube become disconnected.

CONGENITAL HYPERINSULINISM DUE TO GDH GAIN-OF-FUNCTION MUTATIONS

Etiology/Pathophysiology Gain-of-function mutations of the GLUD-1 gene that encodes the mitochondrial enzyme glutamate

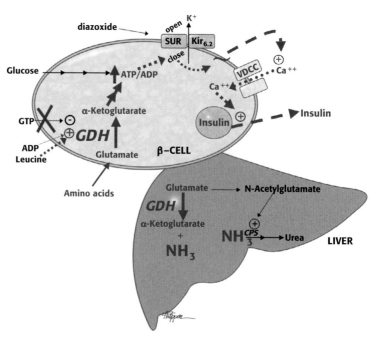

FIGURE 4-7. GDH-HI. This form of congenital HI arises as a result of dominant mutations in the mitochondrial enzyme, GDH, that cause loss of normal allosteric inhibition of GDH by GTP. These gain of function mutations lead to excess oxidation of glutamate to a-ketoglutarate, an increase in the ATP to ADP ratio, closure of the KATP-channel, and ultimately excess insulin secretion. Patients with GDH-HI have protein-induced hypoglycemia as a result of unbridled leucine activation of GDH. Hyperammonemia is thought to arise from upregulated oxidative deamination of glutamate to a-ketoglutarate in the hepatocyte. In addition, clearance of excess ammonia via ureagenesis is limited by increased conversion of glutamate to a-ketoglutarate; the glutamate pool that is necessary for the synthesis of N-acetylglutamate, a co-factor in the urea cycle, is depleted.

dehydrogenase (GDH) cause a form of hyperinsulinism associated with hyperammonemia (HI/HA, also known as GDH HI) (17,20,51–54). Inheritance of GDH HI is autosomal dominant, although up to 80% of cases represent de novo mutations. GDH is responsible for the oxidative deamination of glutamate to α-ketoglutarate (see Figure 4-1). It is allosterically activated by leucine and ADP and inhibited by GTP. It effects insulin secretion by generating α-ketoglutarate, which enters the Krebs cycle to generate ATP. The increase in ATP closes the K_{ATP} channel, β-cell membrane depolarization ensues, and insulin is secreted.

GDH HI–causing mutations impair normal inhibition of GDH by GTP and allow unchecked allosteric activation of GDH by leucine (Figures 4-7 and 4-8) (55). Enhanced leucine-stimulated insulin secretion results and manifests clinically as protein-induced hypoglycemia (56) (Figure 4-9), a hallmark of GDH HI.

Hyperammonemia, the other hallmark of and a consistent finding in GDH HI, is thought to arise from up regulated hepatic GDH activity (see Figure 4-7) (57). Up regulated GDH activity depletes the hepatocyte of glutamate, which is needed to produce N-acetylglutamate (NAG), a necessary cofactor

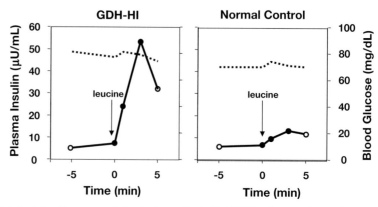

FIGURE 4-8. Acute insulin responses to leucine in a patient with GDH HI and a normal control. Exaggerated insulin secretion occurs at 1 and 3 minutes in GDH HI in response to a bolus of leucine (15 mg/kg), whereas normal controls do not respond. Blood glucose remains stable during this procedure, unlike in previous tests that required the development of hypoglycemia to identify leucine sensitivity. Insulin is shown in circles and blood glucose concentrations along the dotted line.

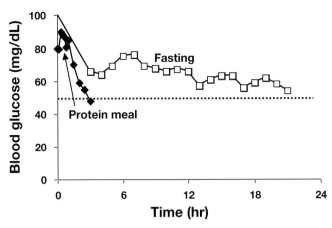

FIGURE 4-9. BG during fasting and following an oral protein challenge. In this teenager with GDH HI, fasting tolerance is shortened to 16–17 hours, as shown by blood glucose concentrations in squares. More strikingly, however, she rapidly becomes hypoglycemic following consumption of protein (1.5 g/kg). Blood glucose concentrations for the protein meal are shown in diamonds.

for the first step of ureagenesis. In addition, enhanced GDH activity leads to excess production of ammonium, disposal of which is hindered by the limited availability of NAG.

Clinical Presentation Affected newborns are of normal birth weight, and their hypoglycemia often does not manifest until later in infancy. This delayed presentation likely arises because 1) GDH HI is often associated with subtle defects in fasting, and not until later in infancy when overnight feeds are skipped is the ability to fast challenged, and because 2) protein-rich foods such as yogurt, cow's milk, and meat are not introduced into the diet until later in infancy, allowing the characteristic protein-induced hypoglycemia to be avoided until this time (see Figure 4-9). Differences in these environmental exposures likely contribute to the clinical severity. For instance, some GDH HI individuals, although having hypoglycemic symptoms, have not been diagnosed until an affected family has been identified.

GDH HI individuals appear to be asymptomatic from their hyperammonemia despite plasma concentrations two to five times normal. Protein intake, fasting, and blood glucose concentration do not affect plasma ammonia (21,22,52). Unlike with urea cycle defects, plasma amino acids and urinary amino acids are normal. In addition, hyperammonemia is not improved with benzoate, an alternate-pathway treatment used to lower plasma ammonium in urea cycle defects and liver failure (21,53,54). N-Carbamylglutamate, a NAG analogue, has been used to lower plasma ammonium by 50% (22,53), but the clinical benefit remains to be determined.

Diagnosis As with other forms of HI, the diagnosis depends on the finding of inappropriate insulin action at the time of hypogly-

cemia (i.e., suppressed free fatty acids, ketones, and IGFBP-1 and an inappropriate glycemic response to glucagon). As mentioned previously, the fasting tolerance of GDH HI may be 6–12 hours or longer. Postprandial hypoglycemia, particularly following high-protein food intake, suggests GDH HI.

Further confirming the diagnosis of GDH HI is hyperammonemia, usually in the range of 80–150 μmol/L (normal < 35 μmol/L). Spurious hyperammonemia may occur if the sample is not obtained appropriately using a free-flowing specimen that is transported on ice and assayed immediately. To exclude laboratory error, multiple plasma ammonium concentrations should be obtained appropriately.

The acute insulin response to a leucine test is particularly useful in securing the diagnosis of GDH HI (see Figure 4-8). In response to an intravenous bolus of leucine (15 mg/kg), exaggerated insulin secretion occurs. In contrast, normal controls and children with other forms of HI show little to no response to leucine (see Figures 4-5 and 4-8). In addition, following a protein meal (1–1.5 g/kg Resource protein), children with GDH HI become hypoglycemic (see Figure 4-9).

Mutational analysis for GLUD1, the gene encoding GDH, confirms the diagnosis. Mutations have been found in exons 6, 7, 10, 11, and 12 (Table 4-2).

Treatment The goal of treatment is to prevent both postprandial and fasting hypoglycemia. Patients with GDH HI respond to well to diazoxide (5–15 mg/kg/day). To monitor the efficacy of the diazoxide dose, fasting and oral protein tests are performed (Figure 4-10). If a child is not able to fast for more than 12 hours, or if significant protein-induced hypoglycemia occurs, the diazoxide dose is

- Female carriers of ornithine carbamoyltransferase deficiency, an X-linked disorder, may have asymptomatic hyperammonemia. Increased orotic acid in urine will identify such patients.

- Unlike with urea cycle defects, plasma ammonia does not increase with a protein load.

- Most mutations arise sporadically

- The hyperammonemia of GDH-HI appears to be asymptomatic. Recently, generalized seizures and behavior issues have been noted in children with GDH-HI in the absence of hypoglycemic brain damage (2). The role of chronic hyperammonemia in these seizures is not known.

increased. Patients are also instructed to avoid pure protein meals and to eat carbohydrates before protein to reduce the risk of protein-induced hypoglycemia.

CONGENITAL HYPERINSULINSM DUE TO GK GAIN-OF-FUNCTION MUTATIONS

Etiology/Pathophysiology Glucokinase (GK) catalyzes the phosphorylation of glucose, the first step in glycolysis. GK is expressed exclusively in liver and pancreatic islet β-cells, where it regulates the rate of glucose metabolism. Because of its important regulatory role in glucose metabolism, GK is considered the β-cell "glucosensor."

Because GK HI is rare, limited information is available regarding this form of HI. GK HI arises as a result of dominant gain-of-function

- Heterozygous loss of function mutations of GK increase the BG threshold for insulin secretion and lead to maturity onset diabetes of the young (MODY-2), a dominantly inherited form of diabetes (1). Homozygous loss of function mutations of GK lead to permanent neonatal diabetes

TABLE 4-2	Laboratory Findings: GDH HI		
	Decreased		**Increased**
Blood glucose < 50 mg/dL	Free fatty acids (<1.5 mmol/L)		BG response to glucagon (>30 mg/dL)
	β-Hydroxybutyrate (<1.5 mmol/L)		GH (>10 ng/mL)
	Acetoacetate		Cortisol (>18 μg/dL)
	IGFBP-1 (<120 ng/mL)		Plasma ammonia
	BG response to oral protein load		Leucine-AIR
			Glucose-AIR

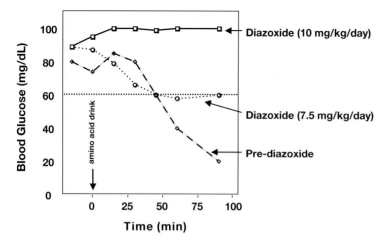

FIGURE 4-10. Diazoxide responsiveness of protein sensitivity in GDH HI. Prior to initiation of diazoxide, this patient has significant protein-induced hypoglycemia (small open circles) using an protein drink (1.5 g/kg). Treatment with diazoxide (10 mg/kg/day) prevented protein-induced hypoglycemia (squares). A year later she has outgrown her diazoxide dose (7.5 mg/kg/day), and her protein sensitivity is no longer treated adequately (large open squares).

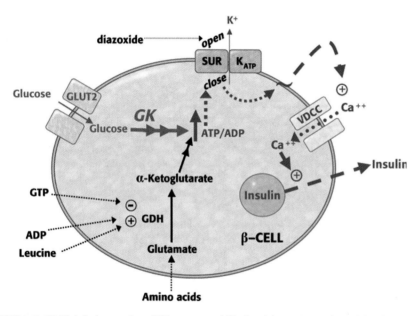

FIGURE 4-11. GK HI. Activating mutations of GK cause more avid binding of glucose to GK. Enhanced phosphorylation of glucose results, stimulating ATP production, closure of the K_{ATP} channel, β-cell membrane depolarization, opening of VDCCs, entry of calcium into the β-cell, and insulin secretion at lower blood glucose concentrations than normal.

mutations of the GCK gene encoding GK (14,58–60) (Figure 4-11). The mutations increase enzyme affinity for glucose, thereby lowering the threshold for insulin secretion.

Clinical Presentation A few reports of GK HI are available in the literature (14,58–60). In the first family, children presented late in infancy with mild hyperinsulinism and insulin secretion that was not suppressed until a BG of approximately 40 mg/dL (14). In this family and a similar family (14,58), the HI was responsive to diazoxide. More recently, a case with a de novo mutation of GK was reported (59). The GK HI was severe, unresponsive to diazoxide, and persistent despite subtotal pancreatectomy. The threshold for glucose-stimulated insulin secretion was reduced to approximately 15 mg/dL.

Diagnosis The diagnosis of GK HI depends on confirmation of HI and identification of a gain-of-function mutation in GK. Other clues suggestive of GK HI are evidence of a lowered glucose threshold.

Treatment Treatment with diazoxide has been effective in most reported cases. Some children with severe defects may not respond to diazoxide and may require pancreatectomy.

CONGENITAL HYPERINSULINSM DUE TO SCHAD DEFICIENCY

Etiology/Pathophysiology SCHAD HI is rare, with just two reports in the literature at the time of this writing (61,62). It is inherited in

an autosomal recessive fashion and arises from a defect in enzymatic activity of short-chain 3-hydroxyacyl-CoA dehydrogenase (SCHAD). SCHAD is a mitochondrial enzyme that catalyzes the conversion of 3-hydroxyacyl-CoA to 3-ketoacyl-CoA, the third step in the fatty acid β-oxidation cycle. How the defect in fatty acid oxidation causes HI is not known.

Clinical Presentation Two reports are available in the literature. Both cases were infants who presented in the neonatal period or early infancy with episodes of hypoketotic hypoglycemia. These patients did not experience the typical clinical findings associated with most fatty acid oxidation defects (i.e., episodes of Reye-like illness, hepatic dysfunction, cardiomyopathy, and/or skeletal muscle weakness).

Diagnosis The diagnosis of SCHAD deficiency is based on confirming the presence of HI, that is, hypoglycemia in the setting of excessive insulin action. To specifically diagnose SCHAD HI, elevated 3-hydroxybutyryl(C_4)-carnitine should be identified by tandem mass spectrometry on a plasma acylcarnitine profile. In addition, gas chromatography–mass spectrometry of urine reveals elevated 3-hydroxyglutaric acid.

Treatment The cases in the literature were diazoxide-responsive, suggesting that diazoxide is appropriate as a first-line agent for treating SCHAD HI.

CONGENITAL HYPERINSULINSM DUE TO CARBOHYDRATE-DEFICIENT GLYCOPROTEIN SYNDROME TYPE 1B

Etiology/Pathophysiology Carbohydrate-deficient glycoprotein syndromes (CDGs) are a heterogeneous group of disorders characterized by psychomotor and mental retardation, blood coagulation abnormalities, and hypoglycosylation of glycoproteins. CDG type 1b is unique in that a few affected children have had hypoglycemia due to hyperinsulinism (63,64). Other features of CDG-1b include protein-losing enteropathy and congenital hepatic fibrosis, but psychomotor retardation and mental retardation are absent. Mutations in phosphomannose isomerase are responsible for CDG-1b (65), but how such a defect causes hyperinsulinism is not known.

Clinical Presentation In the few cases that have been described, infants present in early infancy with protein-losing enteropathy and hypoglycemia.

Diagnosis Missing or truncated sugar chains cause hypoglycosylation of extracellular proteins that can be identified by isoelectric focusing of serum transferrin.

Treatment Mannose has been successfully to reverse the hypoglycosylation of serum glycoproteins, as well as the vomiting, diarrhea, congenital hepatic fibrosis, and hyperinsulinism of CDG-1b (64).

INFANT OF THE DIABETIC MOTHER

Etiology/Pathophysiology Because the fetus is exposed to maternal blood glucose concentrations, the infant of a mother with poorly controlled diabetes is exposed to hyperglycemia in utero. In response to this hyperglycemia, the fetus appropriately up regulates insulin secretion. Enhanced insulin secretion by the fetus manifests as macrosomia: Glycogen, protein, and fat stores are increased. At birth, the excessive glucose supply is abruptly interrupted. If insulin secretion is not down regulated sufficiently, hypoglycemia results. Glucagon deficiency may contribute to the development of hypoglycemia in the infant of a diabetic mother.

Clinical Presentation Infants typically present at birth with hypoglycemia. Maternal history of diabetes and low for gestational age (LGA) birth weight are clues to the etiology of the hypoglycemia. Hypoglycemia related to maternal diabetes generally resolves within 2 days. If hypoglycemia is prolonged, other etiologies for the hypoglycemia should be considered.

Diagnosis The diagnosis is based on maternal history. For the mother with little or no prenatal care, the diagnosis of diabetes should be entertained. In the infant, studies performed at the time of hypoglycemia (BG < 50 mg/dL) will be consistent with hyperinsulinism: suppressed free fatty acids, ketones, and IGFBP-1 and normal bicarbonate, a glycemic response to glucagon, plus or minus elevated plasma insulin.

Treatment Because the hyperinsulinemia is short-lived, the infant of the diabetic mother usually can be treated expectantly with intravenous dextrose (5–10 mg/kg/minute). Less commonly, the hyperinsulinemia is more prolonged, in which case other etiologies should be sought. If studies remain consistent with hyperinsulinemia, diazoxide can be initiated. If the preprandial BG is normal on diazoxide, a safety fast is undertaken to ensure efficacy of the diazoxide dose. The infant then can be allowed to outgrow the diazoxide dose, and BG regulation is reassessed in 3–4 months to confirm that the hyperinsulinemia was indeed transient in nature.

PERIPARTUM STRESS HYPERINSULINISM

Etiology/Pathophysiology Infants born small for gestational age (SGA), preterm, or following intrauterine/peripartum stress, such as birth asphyxia, are at risk of hypoglycemia. Excess insulin secretion, which can last for weeks to months, is the culprit (66,67). The mechanisms for dysregulated insulin secretion are not understood. Not all infants with transient neonatal HI have the typical risks for peripartum stress hyperinsulinism; some are of normal birth weight and have had no known stressors (68).

Clinical Presentation Affected infants tend to present shortly after birth with hypoglycemia. In some, prolonged intravenous dextrose or continuous feeds obligated by underlying illness can mask the hyperinsulinism for weeks. Only when intermittent bolus feeds are introduced is the hypoglycemia detected.

Diagnosis As with other forms of HI, peripartum stress HI is diagnosed by demonstrating suppressed free fatty acids, ketones, and IGFBP-1 and a glycemic response to glucagon at the time of hypoglycemia. The specific diagnosis of peripartum stress HI is suspected based on the birth history. Only when the disorder resolves weeks to months later is one assured of the transient nature of the HI.

Treatment Peripartum stress HI usually responds to diazoxide. On rare occasions, octreotide is required. Diazoxide-induced fluid retention can be a limiting factor in the use of this medication in severely ill neonates. For this reason, diuretics should be initiated empirically with diazoxide in infants who are SGA or who have lung disease. Occasionally, diazoxide causes sufficient fluid overload to compromise lung function. These patients may respond to octreotide. If octreotide is not effective, continuous feeds are introduced to maintain BG. The infant's BG regulation can be reassessed in 3–4 months to confirm that the hyperinsulinism has resolved. Uncommonly, the HI can last as long as a year (68).

INSULINOMA

Etiology/Pathophysiology Insulinomas are the most common functioning neuroendocrine tumor of the pancreas in adults, with an incidence of approximately 4 per 1 million per year (69). In the pediatric population, insulinomas are exceedingly rare. Insulinomas may arise sporadically or, less commonly, as part of multiple endocrine neoplasia type 1 (MEN-1), a disorder that causes neuroendocrine tumors of the pituitary, parathyroid, and pancreas.

Insulinomas are the second most common pancreatic tumor in MEN-1. The majority of cases of MEN-1 result from familial and sporadic dominant mutations in the coding region of the MEN1 gene located on 11q13 (70). MENIN, the protein product of the MEN1 gene, is thought to be a tumor-suppressor protein. Mutations of MEN1 alone are not sufficient to cause tumor formation. As with K_{ATP} HI, somatic loss of heterozygosity of 11q13 occurs in the lesion, unmasking the germline defect in MEN1. Mutations of MEN1 and, more commonly, loss of heterozygosity for 11q13, also have been identified in sporadically occurring insulinomas.

The mechanisms for excess insulin secretion by insulinomas are not well delineated. Gene expression studies have found increased expression of a variety of genes, including islet amyloid peptide, proprotein convertase subtilisin, α-subunit of stimulating G protein, and a large cluster of genes in the insulin secretory pathway (71–73).

Clinical Presentation Children with insulinomas present with acquired hypoglycemic symptoms beyond the first year of life. Symptoms include seizures, abnormal behavior, lethargy, and increased food consumption and weight gain in the absence of exogenous insulin or insulin secretagogues.

Diagnosis The diagnosis of insulinoma depends on identification of excess endogenous insulin secretion at the time of hypoglycemia and frequently requires a prolonged fast, up to 72 hours in older children and adults (74). As with other forms of HI, free fatty acids and ketones are suppressed, and a glycemic response to glucagon occurs at the time of hypoglycemia. Care should be taken to exclude surreptitious insulin administration by measuring C-peptide, proinsulin, and insulin antibodies, as well as insulin, at a time of hypoglycemia. Increased C-peptide (>0.2 nmol/L) and proinsulin (>5 pmol/L) at hypoglycemia confirm endogenous insulin secretion (75–77) but do not rule out administration of oral hypoglycemic agents such as sulfonylureas. When indicated clinically, plasma can be assayed for the presence of sulfonylureas; unfortunately, the second-generation sulfonylureas are more difficult to measure (76).

Once the diagnosis of HI is secured, localization procedures are performed. Endoscopic ultrasound is sensitive in experienced hands but is limited when the lesion occurs in the tail of the pancreas or is small (<8 mm); intraoperative ultrasound in combination with palpation also has been useful but, again, is limited by the experience of the staff (78). Spiral CT scanning appears to be sensitive in the detection of pancreatic neuroendocrine masses; success with MRI also has been reported. When typical imaging modalities fail to identify small lesions, ASVS and THPVS have been used successfully to localize insulinomas (78).

Treatment Surgical removal of the insulinoma is definitive treatment. Rarely, medical therapy with diazoxide is required for children in whom surgery is a high-risk procedure.

BECKWITH–WIEDEMANN

Etiology/Pathophysiology Beckwith–Wiedemann syndrome is caused by mosaic paternal isodisomy of chromosome 11p15.5. This syndrome also may arise from mutations in the p57 gene (79) or in the NSD1 gene (80) and from microdeletions in the H19 differentially methylated region (81) or in the LIT1 gene (82). Mutations in these genes disrupt normal imprinting of genes on 11p15.5. This phenomenon is similar to that found in focal HI, in which loss of heterozygosity for the maternal 11p15 causes unbalanced expression of imprinted genes that control cell growth (32,46). Hyperinsulinism has been attributed to overexpression of IGF-2 causing organ overgrowth, including β-cell hyperplasia (83). More recently, overexpression of IGF-2 has been proposed as the specific mechanism for hypoglycemia in Beckwith–Wiedeman syndrome. Overproduction of pro-IGF-2, IGF-2, or "big" IGF-2 is well described in adults with non–islet cell tumors (84–90). Increased circulation of this growth factor is thought to stimulate the insulin receptor and thus have insulin-like effects. Hence the hypoglycemia of Beckwith–Wiedemann syndrome may, at least in some cases, be a mimicker of hyperinsulinism.

Clinical Presentation Typical features of Beckwith–Wiedemann syndrome include neonatal macrosomia, macroglossia, hemihypertrophy, and abdominal wall defects (Figure 4-12) Hypoglycemia within the first few days of life is not uncommon (91,92). More persistent hypoglycemia is less common and has been attributed to hyperinsulinism (93) that is variably diazoxide-responsive and may require pancretatectomy.

Diagnosis The diagnosis of Beckwith–Wiedemann syndrome depends on the presence of clinical manifestations and paternal isodisomy of 11p15.5 or other relevant mutations. The diagnosis of HI is similar to that for other HI disorders: at the time of hypoglycemia, suppressed free fatty

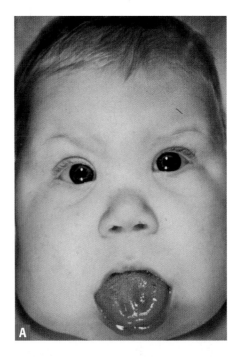
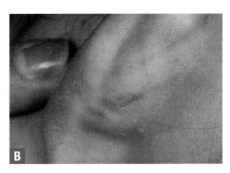
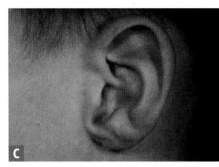
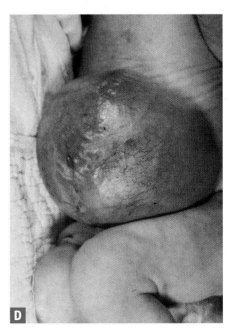

FIGURE 4-12. Features of Beckwith–Wiedemann syndrome: (A) macroglossia and microcephaly in a newborn; **(B,C)** indented ear lesions and linear groove on earlobe in a child; **(D)** omphalocele in a newborn. (Photos courtesy of Dr. Robert Gorlin, University of Minnesota Medical School.)

acids, ketones, and IGFBP-1 and a glycemic response to glucagon. Since IGF-2-related hypoglycemia will mimic HI, additional studies specifically for IGF-2, "big" IGF-2, and pro-IGF-2 should be sought in the case of Beckwith–Wiedemann syndrome. Overexpression of IGF-2 may suppress the growth hormone axis, leading to suppression of IGF-1 and IGFBP-3. Therefore, determination of these growth factors also should be done to aid in the diagnosis.

Treatment Treatment depends on the underlying etiology of the hypoglycemia. Diazoxide administration should be attempted for HI. If diazoxide fails and excess IGF-2 has not been considered previously, or if IGF-2 is known to be elevated, a trial with growth hormone may increase growth factor–binding proteins sufficiently to limit IGF-2 bioavailability and prevent hypoglycemia.

REFERENCES

1. Vionnet N, Stoffel M, Takeda J, et al. Nonsense mutation in the glucokinase gene causes early-onset non-insulin-dependent diabetes mellitus. *Nature* 1992;356:721–722.
2. Raizen DM, Brooks-Kayal A, Steinkrauss L, et al. Central nervous system hyperexcitability associated with glutamate dehydrogenase gain of function mutations. *J Pediatr* 2005;146(3):388–394.
3. Sperling MA, Menon RK. Hyperinsulinemic hypoglycemia of infancy. *Endocrin Metab Clin North Am.* 1999;28:695–708.
4. Li CH, Matter A, Buettger C, et al. A signaling role of glutamine in insulin secretion. ADA Annual Meeting, New Orleans, 2003.
5. Bryla J, Michalik M, Nelson J, et al. Regulation of the glutamate dehydrogenase activity in rat islets of langerhans and its consequence on insulin release. *Metabolism.* 1994;43:1187–1195.

6. Colman RF. Glutamate dehydrogenase (bovine liver). In: Kuby SA, ed. *A Study of Enzymes.* Boca Raton, FL: CRC Press; 1991:173–192.

7. Fahien LA, MacDonald MJ, Kmiotek EH, et al. Regulation of insulin release by factors that also modify glutamate dehydrogenase. *J Biol Chem.* 1988;263:13610–13614.

8. Fajans SS, Floyd FC, Knopf RF, et al. A difference in the mechanism by which leucine and other amino acids induce insulin release. *J Clin Endocrinol Metab.* 1967;27:1600–1606.

9. Fajans SS, Quibrera R, Peck S, et al. Stimulation of insulin release in the dog by a nonmetabolizable amino acid: Comparison with leucine and arginine. *J Clin Endocrinol Metab.* 1971;33:35–41.

10. Dunne MJ, Kane C, Shepherd RM, et al. Familial persistent hyperinsulinemic hypoglycemia of infancy and mutations in the sulfonylurea receptor. *N Engl J Med.* 1997;336:703–706.

11. Glaser B, Chiu KC, Anker R, et al. Familial hyperinsulinism maps to chromosome 11p14-15.1, 30 cM centromeric to the insulin gene. *Nat Genet.* 1994;7:185–188.

12. Glaser B, Chiu KC, Liu L, et al. Recombinant mapping of the familial hyperinsulinism gene to a 0.8 cM region on chromosome 11p15.1 and demonstration of a founder effect in Ashkenazi Jews (published erratum appears in *Hum Mol Genet.* 1995;4:2187–2188]. *Hum Mol Genet.* 1995;4:879–886.

13. Glaser B, Ryan F, Donath M, et al. Hyperinsulinism caused by paternal-specific inheritance of a recessive mutation in the sulfonylurea-receptor gene. *Diabetes.* 1999;48:1652–1657.

14. Glaser B, Kesavan P, Heyman M, et al. Familial hyperinsulinism caused by an activating glucokinase mutation. *N Engl J Med.* 1998;338:226–230.

15. Huopio H, Reimann F, Ashfield R, et al. Dominantly inherited hyperinsulinism caused by a mutation in the sulfonylurea receptor type 1. *J Clin Invest.* 2000;106:897–906.

16. Kane C, Shepherd RM, Squires PE, et al. Loss of functional K_{ATP} channels in pancreatic β-cells causes persistent hyperinsulinemic hypoglycemia of infancy. *Nat Med.* 1996;2.1344–1347.

17. MacMullen C, Fang J, Hsu BY, et al. Hyperinsulinism/hyperammonemia syndrome in children with regulatory mutations in the inhibitory guanosine triphosphate-binding domain of glutamate dehydrogenase. *J Clin Endocrinol Metab.* 2001;86:1782–1787.

18. Nestorowicz A, Inagaki N, Gonoi T, et al. A nonsense mutation in the inward rectifier potassium channel gene, Kir6.2, is associated with familial hyperinsulinism. *Diabetes.* 1997;46:1743–1748.

19. Nestorowicz A, Wilson BA, Schoor KP, et al. Mutations in the sulonylurea receptor gene are associated with familial hyperinsulinism in Ashkenazi Jews. *Hum Mol Genet.* 1996;5:1813–1822.

20. Stanley CA. The hyperinsulinism–hyperammonemia syndrome: Gain-of-function mutations of glutamate dehydrogenase. In: O'Rahilly S, Dunger DB, eds. *Genetic Insights in Paediatric Endocrinology and Metabolism.* Bristol, England: BioScientifica; 2000:23–30.

21. Weinzimer SA, Stanley CA, Berry GT, et al. A syndrome of congenital hyperinsulinism and hyperammonemia. *J Pediatr.* 1997;130:661–664.

22. Zammarchi E, Filippi L, Novembre E, et al. Biochemical evaluation of a patient with a familial form of leucine-sensitive hypoglycemia and concomitant hyperammonemia. *Metabolism.* 1996;45:957–960.

23. Thomas PM, Cote GJ, Wohllk N, et al. Mutations in the sulfonylurea receptor gene in familial persistent hyperinsulinemic hypoglycemia of infancy. *Science.* 1995;268: 426–429.

24. Thomas P, Ye YY, Lightner E. Mutations of the pancreatic islet inward rectifier Kir6.2 also leads to familial persistent hyperinsulinemic hypoglycemia of infancy. *Hum Mol Genet.* 1996;5:1809–1812.

25. Magge S, Shyng S, MacMullen C, et al. Familial leucine-sensitive hypoglycemia of infancy due to a dominant mutation of the β-cell sulfonylurea receptor. *J Clin Endocrinol Metab.* 2004;89:4450–4456.

26. Thornton PS, MacMullen C, Ganguly A, et al. Clinical and molecular characterization of a dominant form of congenital hyperinsulinism caused by a mutation in the high-affinity sulfonylurea receptor. *Diabetes.* 2003;52:2403–2410.

27. Matschinsky FM, Sweet IR. Annotated questions and answers about glucose metabolism and insulin secretion of β-cells. *Diabetes Rev.* 1996;4:130–144.

28. Kelly A, Steinkrauss L, Wanner L, et al. Amino acid–stimulated insulin secretion: lessons learned from congenital hyperinsulinism. Pediatric Academic Society's Annual Meeting, San Francisco, CA, May 1–4, 2004.

29. Fourtner S, Kelly A, Stanley C. Protein sensitivity not synonymous with leucine sensitivity (abstract). The Endocrine Society's 85th Annual Meeting, Philadelphia, PA, June 19–22, 2003.

30. Verkarre V, Fournet JC, de Lonlay P, et al. Paternal mutation of the sulfonylurea receptor (SUR1) gene and maternal loss of 11p15 imprinted genes lead to persistent hyperinsulinism in focal adenomatous hyperplasia. *J Clin Invest.* 1998;102.1286–1291.

31. Fournet JC, Verkarre V, deLonlay P, et al. Paternal SUR1 mutations and loss of imprinted genes lead to hyperinsulinism in focal adenomatous hyperplasia. Presented at ATP-Sensitive Potassium Channels and Disease symposium, St. Charles, IL, September 3–5,1998.

32. de Lonlay P, Fournet JC, Rahier J, et al. Somatic deletion of the imprinted 11p15 region in sporadic persistent hyperinsulinemic hypoglycemia of infancy is specific of focal adenomatous hyperplasia and endorses partial pancreatectomy. *J Clin Invest.* 1997;100:802–807.

33. Otonkoski T, Ammala C, Huopio H, et al. A point mutation inactivating the sulfonylurea receptor causes the severe form of persistent hyperinsulinemic hypoglycemia of infancy in Finland. *Diabetes.* 1999;48: 408–415.

34. Bruining GJ. Recent advances in hyperinsulinism and the pathogenesis of diabetes mellitus. *Curr Opin Pediatr.* 1990;2:758–765.

35. Mathew PM, Young JM, Abu-Osba YK, et al. Persistent neonatal hyperinsulinism. *Clin Pediatr.* 1988;27:148–151.

36. Henwood M, Kelly A, MacMullen C, et al. Genotype–phenotype correlations in children with congenital hyperinsulinism due to recessive mutations of the adenosine triphosphate–sensitive potassium channel genes. *J Clin Endocrinol Metab.* (in press).

37. Li C, Najafi H, Daikhin Y, et al. Regulation of leucine-stimulated insulin secretion and glutamine metabolism in isolated rat islets. *J Biol Chem.* 2003;278:2853–2858.

38. Katz LE, DeLeon DD, Zhao H, et al. Free and total insulin-like growth factor (IGF)-I levels decline during fasting: relationships with insulin and IGF-binding protein-1. *J Clin Endocrinol Metab* 2002;87(6):2978–2983.

39. Hussain K, Hindmarsh P, Aynsley-Green A. Spontaneous hypoglycemia in childhood is accompanied by paradoxically low serum growth hormone and appropriate cortisol counterregulatory hormonal responses. *J Clin Endocrinol Metab.* 2003;88: 3715–3723.

40. Hussain K, Hindmarsh P, Aynsley-Green A. Neonates with symptomatic hyperinsulinemic hypoglycemia generate inappropriately low serum cortisol counterregulatory hormonal responses. *J Clin Endocrinol Metab.* 003;88: 4342–4347.

41. Ferry RJ Jr, Kelly A, Grimberg A, et al. Calcium-stimulated insulin secretion in diffuse and focal forms of congenital hyperinsulinism. *J Pediatr* 2000;137:239–246.

42. Grimberg A, Ferry RJ, Kelly A, et al. Dysregulation of insulin secretion in children with congenital hyperinsulinism due to sulfonylurea receptor mutations. *Diabetes* 2001;50:322–328.

43. Ferry RJ Jr, Kelly A, Grimberg A, et al. Calcium-stimulated insulin secretion in diffuse and focal forms of congenital hyperinsulinism. *J Pediatr.* 2000;137:239–246.

44. Giurgea I, Laborde BK, Touati G, et al. β-Cell quiescence in focal congenital hyperinsulinism: A rational explanation for impaired acute insulin responses to calcium and tolbutamide. *J Clin Endocrinol Metab.* (in press).

45. Stanley CA, Thornton PS, Ganguly A, et al. Preoperative evaluation of infants with focal or diffuse congenital hyperinsulinism by intravenous acute insulin response tests and selective pancreatic arterial calcium stimulation. *J Clin Endocrinol Metab* 2004;89(1):288–296.

46. Giurgea I, Laborde K, Touati G, et al. Acute insulin responses to calcium and tolbutamide do not differentiate focal from diffuse congenital hyperinsulinism. *J Clin Endocrinol Metab* 2004;89(2):925–929.

47. Chigot V, DeLonlay P, Nassogne M, et al. Pancreatic arterial calcium stimulation in the diagnosis and localisation of persistent hyperinsulinemic hypoglycaemia of infancy. *Pediatr Radiol.* 2001;31:650–655.

48. Suchi M, Thornton P, Adzick N, et al. Congenital hyperinsulinism: intraoperative biopsy interpretation can direct the extent of pancreatectomy. *Am J Surg Pathol.* 2004;28:1326–1335.

49. Ribeiro MJ, De Lonlay P, Delzescaux T, et al. Characterization of hyperinsulinism in infancy assessed with PET and ^{18}F-fluoro-L-dopa. *J Nucl Med.* 2005;46:560–566.

50. Kelly A, Steinkrauss L, Bhatia P, et al. K_{ATP}–congenital hyperinsulinism and impaired glucose tolerance (abstract). Presented at the Endocrine Society's 85th Annual Meeting, Philadelphia, PA, June 19–22, 2003.

51. Stanley CA, Fang J, Kutyna K, et al. Molecular basis and characterization of the hyperinsulinism/hyperammonemia syndrome: Predominance of mutations in exons 11 and 12 of the glutamate dehydrogenase gene. HI/HA Contributing Investigators. *Diabetes.* 2000;49:667–673.

52. Miki Y, Tomohiko T, Obura T, et al. Novel misense mutations in the glutamate dehydrogenase gene in the congenital hyperinsulinism–hyperammonemia syndrome. *J. Pediatr.* 2000;136:69–72.

53. Huijmans JGM, Duran M, DeKlerk JBC, et al. Functional hyperactivity of hepatic glutamate dehydrogenase as a cause of the hyperinsulinism/hyperammonemia syndrome: Effect of treatment. *Pediatrics.* 2000;106:596–600.

54. Yorifuji T, Muroi J, Uematsu A, et al. Hyperinsulinism–hyperammonemia syndrome caused by mutant glutamate dehydrogenase accompanied by novel enzyme kinetics. *Hum Genet.* 1999; 104:476–479.

55. Kelly A, Ng D, Ferry RJ Jr, et al. Acute insulin responses to leucine in children with the hyperinsulinism/hyperammonemia syndrome. *J Clin Endocrinol Metab.* 2001;86:3724–3728.

56. Hsu BY, Kelly A, Thornton PS, et al. Protein-sensitive and fasting hypoglycemia in children with the hyperinsulinism/hyperammonemia syndrome. *J Pediatr.* 2001;138:383–389.

57. Kelly A, Stanley CA. Disorders of glutamate metabolism. *Ment Retard Dev Disabil Res Rev.* 2001;7:287–295.

58. Christesen H, Jacobsen B, Odili S, et al. The second activating glucokinase mutation (A456V): Implications for glucose homeostasis and diabetes therapy. *Diabetes.* 2002;51:1240–1246.

59. Cuesta-Munoz A, Huopio H, Otonkosk IT, et al. Severe persistent hyperinsulinemic hypoglycemia due to a de novo glucokinase mutation. *Diabetes.* 2004;53:2164–2168.

60. Gloyn AL, Noordam K, Willemsen MA, et al. Insights into the biochemical and genetic basis of glucokinase activation from naturally occurring hypoglycemia mutations. *Diabetes* 2003;52:2433–2440.

61. Molven A, Matre G, Duran M, et al. Familial hyperinsulinemic hypoglycemia caused by a defect in the SCHAD enzyme of mitochondrial fatty acid oxidation. *Diabetes.* 2004;53:221–227.

62. Clayton PT, Eaton S, Aynsley-Green A, et al. Hyperinsulinism in short-chain L-3-hydroxyacyl-CoA dehydrogenase

63. de Lonlay P, Cuer M, Vuillaumier-Barrot SB, et al. Hyperinsulinemic hypoglycemia as a presenting sign in phosphomannose isomerase deficiency: A new manifestation of carbohydrate-deficient glycoprotein syndrome treatable with mannose. *J Pediatr.* 1999;135:379–383.

64. de Lonlay P, Seta N, Barrot S, et al. A broad spectrum of clinical presentations in congenital disorders of glycosylation I: A series of 26 cases. *J Med Genet.* 2001;38:14–19.

65. Niehues R, Hasilik M, Alton G, et al. Carbohydrate-deficient glycoprotein syndrome type Ib: Phosphomannose isomerase deficiency and mannose therapy. *J Clin Invest.* 1998;101:1414–1420.

66. Collins JE, Leonard JV. Hyperinsulinsim in asphyxiated and small-for-dates infants with hypoglycaemia. *Lancet* 1984;2:311–313.

67. Collins JE, Leonard JV, Teale D, et al. Hyperinsulinaemic hypoglycaemia in small for dates babies. *Arch Dis Child.* 1990;65: 1118–1120.

68. Hoe FM, Thornton P, Steinmuller LA, et al. Perinatal stress hyperinsulinism differs from genetic hyperinsulinism due to mutations in K_{ATP} channel or glutamate dehydrogenase. Presented at the Annual Meeting of the Pediatric Academic Society, Seattle, WA, 2003.

69. Service F, McMahon M, O'Brien J, et al. Functioning insulinoma: Incidence, recurrence, and long-term survival. A 60-year study. *Mayo Clin Proc.* 1991;66:711–719.

70. Thakker R. Multiple endocrine neoplasia: Syndromes of the twentieth century. *J Clin Endocrinol Metab.* 1998;83:2617–2620.

71. Kayton M, Costouros N, Lorang D, et al. Peak stimulated insulin secretion is associated with specific changes in gene expression profiles in sporadic insulinomas. *Surgery.* 2003;134:982–987.

72. Ramanadham S, Song H, Hsu F, et al. Pancreatic islets and insulinoma cells express a novel isoform of group VIA phospholipase A2 ($iPLA_2\beta$) that participates in glucose-stimulated insulin secretion and is not produced by alternate splicing of the $iPLA_2\beta$ transcript. *Biochemistry.* 2003;42:13929–13940.

73. Wang X, Xu S, Wu X, et al. Gene expression profiling in human insulinoma tissue: Genes involved in the insulin secretion pathway and cloning of novel full-length cDNAs. *Endocr Relat Cancer* 2004;11:295–303.

74. Service F, Natt N. The prolonged fast. *J Clin Endocrinol Metab.* 2000;85:3973–3974.

75. Service F, O'Brien P, McMahon M, et al. C-peptide during the prolonged fast in insulinoma. *J Clin Endocrinol Metab.* 1993;76:655–659.

76. Service FJ. Hypoglycemic disorders (see comments). *N Engl J Med.* 1995;332:1144–1152.

77. Kao P, Taylor R, Service F. Proinsulin by immunochemiluminometric assay for the

diagnosis of insulinoma. *J Clin Endocrinol Metab.* 1994;78:1048–1051.

78. Pereira P, Wiskirchen J. Morphological and functional investigations of neuroendocrine tumors of the pancreas. *Eur Radiol* 2003;13:2133–2146.

79. Hatada I, Ohashi H, Fukushima Y, et al. An imprinted gene p57KIP2 is mutated in Beckwith–Wiedemann syndrome. *Nat Genet.* 1996;14:171–173.

80. Baujat G, Rio M, Rossignol S, et al. Paradoxical NSD1 mutations in Beckwith–Wiedemann syndrome and 11p15 anomalies in Sotos syndrome. *Am J Hum Genet.* 2004;74:715–720.

81. Sparago A, Cerrato F, Vernucci M, et al. Microdeletions in the human H19 DMR result in loss of IGF2 imprinting and Beckwith–Wiedemann syndrome. *Nat Genet.* 2004;36:958–960.

82. Niemitz EL, DeBaun MR, Fallon J, et al. Microdeletion of LIT1 in familial Beckwith–Wiedemann syndrome. *Am J Hum Genet* 2004;75:844–849.

83. Munns CF, Batch JA. Hyperinsulinism and Beckwith–Wiedemann syndrome. *Arch Dis Child.* 2001;84:F67–69.

84. Baxter RC. The role of insulin-like growth factors and their binding proteins in tumor hypoglycemia. *Horm Res.* 1996;16.195–201.

85. Kuenen BC, van Doorn J, Slee PH. Non-islet-cell tumour induced hypoglycaemia: A case report and review of literature. *Neth J Med.* 1996;48:175–179.

86. Virally ML, Guillausseau PJ. Hypoglycemia in adults. *Diabetes Metab.* 1999;25:477–490.

87. Morbois-Trabut L, Maillot F, De Widerspach-Thor A, et al. "Big IGF-II"–induced hypoglycemia secondary to gastric adenocarcinoma. *Diabetes Metab.* 2004;30:276–279.

88. Kageyama K, Moriyama T, Hizuka N, et al. Hypoglycemia associated with big insulin-like growth factor II produced during development of malignant fibrous histiocytoma. *Endocr J.* 2003;50:753–758.

89. Baig MM, Hintz MFR, Baker BB, et al. Hypoglycemia attributable to insulin-like growth factor-II prohormone–producing metastatic leiomyosarcoma. *Endocr Pract.* 1999;5:37–42.

90. Sato R, Tsujino M, Nishida K, et al. High molecular weight form insulin-like growth factor II–producing mesenteric sarcoma causing hypoglycemia. *Intern Med.* 2004;43:967–971.

91. Elliott M, Bayly R, Cole T, et al. Clinical features and natural history of Beckwith–Wiedemann syndrome: Presentation of 74 new cases. *Clin Genet.* 1994;46:168–174.

92. Martinez Y, Martinez R. Clinical features in the Wiedemann–Beckwith syndrome. *Clin Genet.* 1996;50:272–274.

93. DeBaun MR, King AA, White N. Hypoglycemia in Beckwith–Wiedemann syndrome. *Semin Perinatol.* 2000;24:164–171.

CHAPTER

5

Mitochondrial Fatty Acid Oxidation Defects

Arnold W. Strauss, MD
Brage S. Andresen, PhD
Michael J. Bennett, PhD, FRCPath, FACB

INTRODUCTION

Mitochondria can utilize either carbohydrate or fat as a source of energy. Pyruvate, derived from glucose, is transported through the mitochondrial inner membrane, decarboxylated to acetyl-coenzyme A (CoA), and thus enters the citric acid cycle producing reducing equivalents in the form of 1,5-dihydro flavin adenine dinucleotide ($FADH_2$) and nicotinamide adenine dinucleotide (NADH). These reducing equivalents are transported down the electron transport chain of inner mitochondrial membrane complexes, ultimately generating adenosine triphosphate (ATP) and consuming oxygen. Similarly, activated fatty acids (acyl-CoAs) entering the fatty acid β-oxidation (FAO) spiral generate reducing equivalents in the form of NADH and $FADH_2$, which also pass down the oxidative phosphorylation respiratory chain complexes to generate ATP.

Mitochondrial FAO represents a normal physiologic response to increased energy demands during periods of reduced caloric intake associated with fasting, reduced intake due to gastrointestinal disease, febrile illness, and increased muscular exertion. The normal endocrine response to increased energy demand results in mobilization of lipid stores and generation of free fatty acids at the plasma membrane. Long-chain fatty acids (longer than C12) and carnitine are transported by specific plasma membrane transporters such as fatty acid transporter (FAT) and fatty acid–binding protein (FABP) and the carnitine transporter (OCNT2), respectively. Short- and medium-chain fatty acids (shorter than C12) are transported directly into the cytosol (Figures 5-1 to 5-3).

At the outer mitochondrial membrane, the free fatty acids are first activated by esterification to the CoA derivative through a family of acyl-CoA synthases. Short- and medium-chain activated fatty acids can enter the mitochondrial matrix without the use of a transport system. The inner mitochondrial membrane is impermeable to activated long fatty acids and to traverse the mitochondrial membrane they must be processed through the carnitine cycle.

In the carnitine cycle (Figure 5-1), the long-chain acyl-CoA is first converted to its respective acylcarnitine species by carnitine palmitoyltransferase 1 (CPT1) at the outer mitochondrial membrane. This enzyme is the rate-limiting step for the process of FAO and is highly regulated. Carnitine:acylcarnitine translocase (CACT) is a bidirectional transporter, which carries the acylcarnitine into the mitochondrial inner membrane internal domain and transports carnitine out of the mitochondria for recycling in the pathway. At the inner aspect of the inner mitochondrial membrane carnitine palmitoyltransferase 2 (CPT2) reverses the CPT1 reaction and reforms acyl-CoA for β-oxidation. Carnitine, an essential cofactor for intramitochondrial transport of long-chain fatty acids, also requires a specific plasma membrane transport system ("transporter"-OCTN2).

The FAO pathway is the preferred metabolic energy pathway for normal cardiac muscle function. In the FAO pathway, predominantly long-chain fatty acids, with 16 and 18 carbons are sequentially broken down into 2-carbon acetyl-CoA units, which in skeletal and cardiac muscle are broken down completely by the process of oxidative

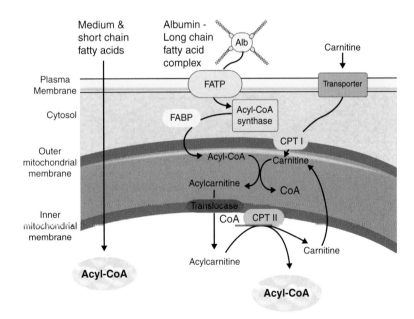

FIGURE 5-1. Uptake and Transport of Plasma Fatty Acids to the Mitochondrial Matrix. Long-chain free fatty acids are carried from the periphery bound to albumin. The initial step in their transport into cells is mediated by a family of fatty acid transport proteins (FATPs) that are expressed in a tissue-specific manner. Esterification of these fatty acids to CoA to form acyl-CoA is performed at the plasma membrane or mitochondrial outer membrane by a family of acyl-CoA synthases. After transport to mitochondria, perhaps bound to fatty acid binding proteins (FABPs), transport of long- chain fatty acids across the inner mitochondrial membrane requires (i) CPT1 to generate acylcarnitines, (ii) the carnitine:acylcarnitine translocase ("Translocase") to move the acylcarnitine across the inner membrane, and (iii) CPT2, on the matrix side of the inner membrane to recreate the long-chain acyl-CoA ester that becomes the substrate for the FAO spiral. Carnitine is transported across the plasma membrane ("Transporter"-OCTN2). Medium- and short-chain fatty acids are believed to travel by passive diffusion from plasma into the mitochondrial matrix (arrow at left of figure).

Fatty Acid Oxidation Disorders

AT-A-GLANCE

Fatty acid oxidation disorders refer to more than 20 inherited disorders of energy metabolism that represent impaired metabolic response to increased energy demands when carbohydrate metabolism is insufficient. Patients with these disorders are not able to mount an appropriate physiological response to fasting, increased muscular activity, and stress due to defects in the transporters, translocases, and enzymes that comprise the entire process of importing fatty acids into cells and, ultimately, mitochondria and their subsequent break down into acetyl-CoA. Transport of fatty acids from the plasma into highly oxidative tissues such as heart, skeletal muscle, and kidney requires fatty acid binding proteins. Upon entering the mitochondrial matrix, fatty acid metabolism efficiently produces reducing equivalents in the form of NADH and FADH that generate energy during electron transport down the respiratory chain (mitochondrial oxidative phosphorylation). FAO Disorders are broken down into three major components which include transport of fatty acids into the mitochondria (the carnitine shuttle), long-chain fatty acid oxidation at the inner mitochondrial membrane and medium/short chain fatty acid oxidation in the mitochondrial matrix. FAO disorders may become apparent during prolonged fasting, febrile illness and any stressful condition that increase energy demands and leads to metabolic decompensation. Common clinical features of these defects include fasting hypoketotic hypoglycemia and liver failure (a Reye syndrome-like picture), hepatic encephalopathy, and muscular hypotonia. Exercise induced rhabdomyolysis and cardiomyopathy are common clinical features of the disorders of carnitine shuttle and long-chain fatty oxidation defects. In some of the long-fatty oxidation disorders late clinical manifestations may include neuropathy, retinopathy and arrhythmias. The biochemical hallmarks of fatty oxidation disorders include hypoglycemia with inappropriately low ketone body formation, coagulopathy and hyperammonemia and, in the example of exercise-induced rhabdomyolysis, massive elevation of serum creatine kinase. Treatment is primarily directed at preventing the catabolic episodes by providing sufficient calories in the form of carbohydrates. Medium-chain triglycerides have been used successfully to bypass the genetic block in long-chain defects and provide a substrate for ketogenesis. Heterozygosity for disorders of the trifunctional protein in pregnancies with homozygously deficient patients may result in severe obstetric liver disease including maternal preeclapsia, acute fatty liver of pregnancy and HELLP syndrome (hemolysis, elevated liver enzymes, low platelet count). With the advent of tandem mass spectrometry for newborn screening, the combined incidence of fatty acid oxidation disorders is about one per five thousand births. Most of these disorders are treatable with a good long term outcome.

DISORDERS OF FATTY ACID UPTAKE & MITOCHONDRIAL TRANSPORT	GENE	LOCUS	OMIM
Carnitine Transporter	OCTN2, SLC22A5	5q31.1	212140
CPT1A	CPT1A	11q13.1	600528
CACT	SLC25A20	3p21.31	212138
CPT2	CPT2	1p32	600650

DISORDERS OF MITOCHONDRIAL β-OXIDATION SPIRAL	GENE	LOCUS	OMIM
SCAD	ACADS	12q22-qter	201470
MCAD	ACADM	1p31	201450
VLCAD	ACADVL	17p13	201475
SCHAD	SCHAD	4q22-26	601609
LCHAD	HADH-A	2p23	609016
TFP	HADH-A, HADH-B	2p23	609015
GAII or MADD	ETF-B, ETF-A, ETF-DH	19q13.3, 15q23-25 4q32-qter	231690, 231675

DISORDERS OF FATTY ACID UPTAKE & MITOCHONDRIAL TRANSPORT	FINDINGS	PRESENTATION
Carnitine Transporter	Fasting hypoketotic hypoglycemia, ↓*plasma carnitine*, ↑CK	*Dilated cardiomyopathy*, skeletal myopathy
CPT1A	Fasting ketotic hypoglycemia, ↑NH_3, coagulopathy, ↑plasma carnitine, ↓plasma acetyl-carnitines	Lethargy, coma, Reye syndrome/liver failure
CACT	Fasting hypoketotic hypoglycemia, ↑NH_3, coagulopathy, ↑transaminases, ↑CK, ↑plasma C16-C18-carnitines, ↓plasma carnitine	Reye syndrome/liver failure, arrhythmia, cardiomyopathy, *ventricular tachycardia*
CPT2	*Myoglobinuria, massive ↑CK*, ↓plasma carnitine, modest ↑plasma C16-C18-carnitines	*Exercise-induced skeletal myopathy*, cardiomyopathy, liver failure, cystic dysplasia of kidneys and brains

DISORDERS OF MITOCHONDRIAL β-OXIDATION SPIRAL	FINDINGS	PRESENTATION
SCAD	Acidosis, hypoglycemia ↑*urine EMA*, ↑*plasma C4-carnitine*	Lethargy, vomiting, hypotonia, seizures, developmental delay
MCAD	Fasting hypoketotic hypoglycemia, ↑urine hexanoyl-glycine, ↑*plasma C8-, C10-carnitine*	Sudden death, (hypoglycemic) seizures, lethargy, Reye syndrome, hepatomegaly
VLCAD	Fasting hypoketotic hypoglycemia, ↑CK, ↑NH_3, ↑plasma C14-, C14:1-carnitine	Cardiomyopathy, skeletal myopathy, hypotonia, Reye syndrome, *pericardial effusion*
SCHAD	Fasting hypoglycemia, ↑*insulin*, ↑urine 3-OH-glutaric acid ↑*plasma 3-OH-butyryl-carnitine*	Lethargy, seizures
LCHAD	Fasting hypoketotic hypoglycemia, ↓ cardiac ejection fraction, ↑NH_3, ↑urine C_6–C_{14} OH-dicarboxylic acids ↑plasma 3-OH-C16-carnitine	Lethargy, Reye syndrome, hepatomegaly, cardiomyopathy, *maternal liver disease*
TFP	↑CK, ↑NH_3, ↓ cardiac ejection fraction Fasting hypoketotic hypoglycemia, ↑urine C_6–C_{14} OH-dicarboxylic acids ↑plasma 3-OH-C16-carnitine	Cardiomyopathy, skeletal myopathy, Reye syndrome
GAII or **MADD**	Fasting hypoketotic hypoglycemia, ↑lactic, glutaric, ethylmalonic, dicarboxylic acids, ↑C4-C8 carnitines, ↑plasma sarcosine	Dysmorphic features, lethargy, seizures, progressive myopathy, cardiomyopathy, sweaty feet, encephalopathy

Italics indicate distinctive features of the particular disorder.

*Presenting features are usually precipitated by fasting, an intercurrent infectious illness, or prolonged exercise.

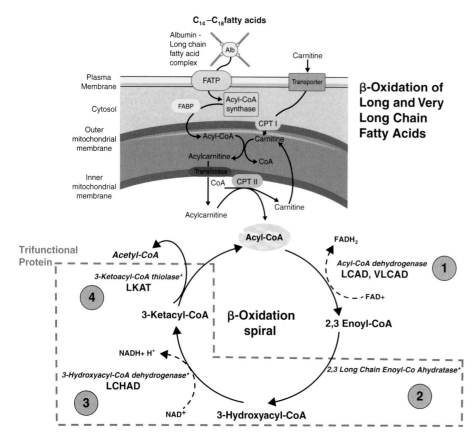

FIGURE 5-2. Long- and Very-Long-Chain Fatty Acids and Mitochondrial Fatty Acid Oxidation Spiral. This spiral consists of four enzymatic steps catalyzed by various families of enzymes that have differing specificities for fatty acids of various chain lengths. The first step is catalyzed by either LCAD or VLCAD by using FAD as a cofactor and generating 2,3-enoyl-acyl-CoA. The second step is catalyzed by long-chain 2,3-enoyl-CoA hydratase, which is part of the α-subunit of TFP. The third reaction in this spiral is catalyzed by LCHAD by using NAD as a cofactor and generating a 3-ketoacyl-CoA. LCHAD is encoded by the TFP α-subunit gene. The final step in this pathway is the thiolytic cleavage by LKAT substrate, producing a saturated acyl-CoA that is two carbons shorter and that reenters the spiral. The LKAT is encoded by the TFP β-subunit gene. Elements in the orange dotted box represent the three enzymatic activities of the TFP.

phosphorylation. In liver, the acetyl-CoA is the precursor substrate for ketone body synthesis. Ketone bodies thus generated are transported within the circulation to provide an alternative fuel for tissues with limited β-oxidation capacity such as brain. Although the pathway was first described 100 years ago, many aspects have only recently been described as genetic defects of the pathway have been identified and have emerged as significant causes of pediatric and adult morbidity and mortality.

The β-oxidation pathway consists of four sequential enzymatic steps (Figures 5-2 and 5-3). The first step, an FAD-linked acyl-CoA dehydrogenase (ACD) reaction, inserts a double bond between the α- and β-carbons of saturated, straight-chain fatty acyl-CoA substrates to form an unsaturated acyl-CoA (2,3 enoyl-CoA). Four homologous enzymes, short- (SCAD), medium- (MCAD), long- (LCAD), and very-long-chain (VLCAD) ACDs perform this reaction. The FAD-linked dehydrogenases generate electrons and the reducing equivalents from the reaction are

transferred to the respiratory chain through electron transfer flavoprotein (ETF) and its dehydrogenase (ETFQO). The second step involves hydration of the double bond by a hydratase enzyme; creating 3-hydroxyacyl-CoA species. Two hydratases (HYD) are known to perform the step: a short-chain 3-enoyl-CoA hydratase (crotonase) and a long-chain 3-enoyl-CoA hydratase. The third enzymatic step is reduction of the 3-hydroxy group to a 3-keto group by two stereospecific 3-hydroxyacyl-CoA dehydrogenases (HAD), a medium/short-chain 3-hydroxyacyl-CoA dehydrogenase (M/SCHAD) and a long-chain 3-hydroxyacyl-CoA dehydrogenase (LCHAD). M/SCHAD catalyzes 3-hydroxyl-acyl-CoA substrates, whose length is 4 to 14 carbons and contains substantial homology to LCHAD as they both catalyze the same step of FAO and share overlapping substrate specificities. Reducing equivalent here is transferred to the respiratory chain through NADH and complex 1 of the respiratory chain (Figure 5-1). Finally, there is thiolytic cleavage across the α-β position by two thio-

lases, a short-chain 3-ketoacyl-CoA thiolase (SKAT) and a long-chain 3-ketoacyl-CoA thiolase (LKAT) to form acetyl-CoA and a 2-carbon chain-shortened acyl-CoA species, which then reenters the cycle. In summary, complete oxidation of a long-chain fatty acid is accomplished by the actions of multiple enzymes at each of the four steps; each enzyme has different chain-length specificity. They include very-long-chain, medium-chain, and short-chain ACDs (VLCAD, MCAD, SCAD), long-chain and short-chain HYD, long-chain and medium/short-chain HAD (LCHAD, M/SCHAD) and long-chain and short-chain thiolase (LKAT, SKAT). The enzymatic activities of long-chain 2,3-enoyl-CoA hydratase, LCHAD, and LKAT are carried by a single protein called trifunctional protein (TFP).

Genetic defects of most of these enzymes have been characterized within the last two decades. Clinical presentation results from the individual's inability to generate energy from fatty acids and includes hepatic failure, rhabdomyolysis, cardiomyopathy and heart failure, and renal tubular acidosis reflecting on the tissues that are most dependent on the pathway. Biochemical hallmarks include hypoketosis, due to failure of hepatic ketogenesis, and hypoglycemia, due to both excessive utilization from tissues that cannot utilize fatty acids and from failure of hepatic gluconeogenesis related to liver failure. To date, all disorders of FAO are inherited autosomal recessively. The FAO pathway is fully expressed in chorionic villus and amniotic fluid cells and all of the disorders are theoretically amenable to prenatal diagnosis.

CARNITINE TRANSPORTER DEFICIENCY/ PRIMARY CARNITINE DEFICIENCY

Etiology and Pathophysiology Primary carnitine deficiency is an autosomal recessive disorder of fatty acid oxidation caused by mutations in the SLC22A5 gene encoding the high-affinity carnitine transporter, OCTN2. Plasma membrane sodium-dependent carnitine (organic cation) transporter, OCTN2, is present in cardiac and skeletal muscle and in the renal tubules. Genetic defects of this transporter result in failure of these tissues to concentrate intracellular levels of carnitine, thus reducing available cofactor for the carnitine cycle. There is also substantial renal loss of circulating carnitine leading to exacerbation of the deficiency (1). Deficiency of the muscle and kidney carnitine transporter represents the only known form of primary carnitine deficiency. Failure to transport carnitine into muscle results in lack of carnitine to supply substrate

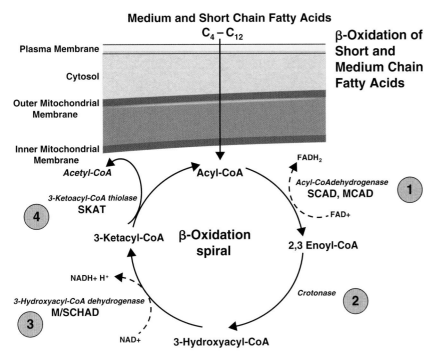

FIGURE 5-3. Short- and Medium-Chain Fatty Acids and Mitochondrial Fatty Acid Oxidation Spiral. Short- and medium-chain fatty acids do not require carnitine to enter the inner mitochondrial membrane for β-oxidation. Depending on the length of the fatty acid chain, the first step is catalyzed by SCAD or MCAD by using FAD as a cofactor and generating 2,3-enoyl-acyl-CoA. The second step in β-oxidation of short- and medium-chain fatty acids is catalyzed by 2,3-enoyl-CoA hydratase (crotonase). The third reaction is catalyzed by M/SCHAD by using NAD as a cofactor and generating a 3-ketoacyl-CoA. The final and fourth step is the thiolytic cleavage by 3-SKAT, producing a saturated acyl-CoA that is two carbons shorter and that reenters the spiral.

for the carnitine cycle, and there is impaired FAO in skeletal and cardiac muscle. In some cases, the very low plasma levels also result in reduced availability of carnitine for hepatic uptake, even though the liver carnitine transporter is present. This usually occurs at a later stage of the disease process and can result in impaired ketogenesis.

Clinical Features Most patients in whom this disorder is subsequently diagnosed present with a progressive cardiomyopathy associated with skeletal myopathy. Presentation is usually within the first year of life; and, if the patient is left untreated, the course progresses rapidly to death from heart manifestations within 2 to 4 years of age. At autopsy, the ventricular walls are extremely thickened similar to that described in endocardial fibroelastosis. Later presentations with progressive cardiac manifestations have also been described in children as old as 7 years of age.

In infants subjected to fasting stress, episodes of rapid metabolic decompensation associated with hypoketotic hypoglycemia have occasionally been described. This type of presentation may lead to sudden death, which has been attributed to hypoglycemic coma (2). There is a separate carnitine transporter in the liver that presumably functions normally in OCTN2 deficiency states, but the very low circulating carnitine levels result in

reduced availability of the substrate for hepatic uptake, resulting in secondary deficiency and insufficient hepatic carnitine to support FAO for ketogenesis.

Investigation and Diagnosis The remarkable laboratory finding in patients with the carnitine transporter defect is the marked reduction in plasma carnitine levels despite continuing renal excretion, i.e. reduced fractional clearance of carnitine. Characteristically, total carnitine will be less than 10% of the normal level, and in some patients, the level is undetectable using the most sophisticated technique of tandem mass spectrometry (MS/MS). During acute episodes of hypoketotic hypoglycemia, the urine organic acid analysis may contain modest increases of medium-chain dicarboxylic acids, but this is not a consistent finding. Serum creatine kinase (CK) levels may be modestly elevated, reflecting the skeletal muscle involvement in the disease process. Confirmation of the diagnosis can be made biochemically by monitoring the uptake of carnitine by skin fibroblasts in culture (1) or by mutational analysis of the causative SLC22A5 gene on chromosome 5q31.1-q32 (3,4). Most mutations in the SLC22A5 gene are private and confined within individual families, which means that in each new case, the entire coding region has to be sequenced. Simple molecular diagnostic strategies are not available.

Treatment and Outcomes The natural history of untreated carnitine transporter deficiency is inevitably death, either due to progressive cardiac failure, as a result of the myopathy, or an acute death due to sudden onset metabolic decompensation. Once the diagnosis is made, this is a very rewarding metabolic disorder to manage. Therapy consists of high-dose L-carnitine, which has been demonstrated in long-term follow-up to result in complete reversal of the cardiomyopathy. A recommended dose for carnitine therapy is 100 mg/kg/day divided into four doses. A good response would be to get a total plasma carnitine level of approximately 25 μmol/L (5). Patients on long-term therapy report normal skeletal muscle tone, no episodes of metabolic decompensation, and essentially normal intellect (6). Minimal residual damage may occur as a result of acute decompensation. The disorder can be detected by expanded newborn screening in which MS/MS is performed (7). Patients identified in the newborn period and treated from diagnosis would be predicted to have even better outcomes.

CARNITINE PALMITOYLTRANSFERASE 1A (CPT1A) DEFICIENCY

Etiology and Pathophysiology CPT, also known as hepatic carnitine palmitoyltransferase (CPT) 1 deficiency, is the rate-limiting enzyme for the transport of long-chain fatty acids into the mitochondria (Figure 5-2). CPT1A is specific for liver and kidney, and CPT1A deficiency presents primarily with features related to the failure of hepatic ketogenesis during periods of reduced caloric availability. Patients do not have skeletal myopathy or cardiac disease. In CPT1A deficiency, fatty acids do not enter the liver mitochondria and, therefore, cannot make ketone bodies from this source. Fatty acids that are released during the normal physiologic lipolytic phase are converted in the liver to triglycerides and result in hepatic steatosis.

Clinical Features There are three genetically distinct forms of the rate-limiting CPT1 enzyme. CPT1A is expressed in liver and kidney, CPT1B is found mainly in heart and skeletal muscle, and CPT1C is mostly expressed in brain. To date, only CPT1A deficiency has been described in humans. The clinical features of the disease are mainly those of impaired hepatic long-chain FAO and ketogenesis. Patients usually present in infancy with fasting-induced liver failure associated with hepatic encephalopathy; the laboratory findings are of hypoketonemia and hypoglycemia. Onset of symptoms is associated with poor feeding and lethargy leading to coma if the hypoglycemia is not recognized. The hepatic encephalopathy is associated with hyperammonemia, elevated liver enzymes (aspartate aminotransferase, alanine aminotransferase), and coagulopathy. The phenotype is similar to that described in MCAD deficiency and Reye syndrome (see later). Because the deficient enzyme is not expressed in muscle, the clinical features differ from those of other long-chain FAO defects in that there is no or little cardiac or skeletal muscle abnormality. Some patients with a renal tubular acidosis have been reported. Most patients present within the first year of life but less typical cases presenting as late as 7 years of age are known (8). An atypical presentation associated with a myopathy was described in a single adult individual with high residual enzyme activity. It is not yet known if the myopathy is a direct result of the enzyme defect or due to some other cause.

A single case of the severe obstetric complication of acute fatty liver of pregnancy was described in a heterozygous mother carrying a fetus who was homozygous affected with CPT1A deficiency (9).

Investigation and Diagnosis During periods of well being, patients with CPT1A deficiency appear on physical examination to be normal. Most routine laboratory tests including those for hepatic function may also be normal. The only known biochemical abnormality may be an elevated total level of serum carnitine, with almost all of the carnitine being in the free or unconjugated fraction. During periods of metabolic decompensation, the phenotype can resemble that seen in Reye syndrome with rapidly deteriorating liver function, hyperammonemia, coagulopathy, and profound hypoglycemia with hypoketonemia and hypoketonuria. Urine organic acid analysis may reveal massively increased excretion of medium-chain (C6–C12) dicarboxylic acids. This pattern of organic aciduria is nonspecific and does not distinguish from some other long-chain FAO defects.

Measuring the enzyme activity in cultured skin fibroblasts, white blood cells, and in liver confirms CPT1A deficiency. The gene for CPT1A has been cloned and it is on chromosome 11q13.1-q13.5. Most of the published CPT1A mutations identified to date are private within individual families (8,10–12), making molecular diagnosis difficult in most cases. Two interesting mutations, which are frequent in certain populations, have been identified. The first is a c.2129G>A mutation, which results in a G710E amino acid substitution in the protein, and has been identified in individuals of North American

Hutterite background (12). The second is a c.1436C>T mutation resulting in P479L, which was identified initially in an adult of Inuit background presenting with myopathy; it is common in the Alaskan and Canadian Inuit populations. Molecular strategies are feasible for these two mutations, which will be limited to individuals of these specific backgrounds.

Treatment and Outcomes The mainstay for the management of patients with all disorders of FAO remains the prevention of situations in which the pathway is mobilized as a potential energy source. In newborns and infants who do not have large glycogen reserves, it is recommended that the patient has frequent feedings and essentially a constant supply of carbohydrate as fuel even when clinically stable. Fasting duration should be limited to a maximum of 8 hours for the first 6 months, 10 hours to age 1 year, and then 10 to 12 hours maximum thereafter. At night times when there may be a longer delay between meals, a slow release source of complex carbohydrate such as uncooked cornstarch (1 g/kg body weight) may be beneficial. CPT1A deficiency is one of the least reported disorders of FAO, and there are few long-term outcome reports. Initial indications are that if catabolic events can be prevented during infancy, the outcome will be good with no long-term hepatic damage occurring (13). Because patients tend to have normal or elevated total serum carnitine levels, there is no indication for therapeutic carnitine use in this disorder. The P479L Inuit mutation is unique in that it is a genetic change, which has an effect on the postprandial malonyl-CoA inhibition of the CPT1 enzyme. In the postprandial state, when carbohydrate calories are preferentially being utilized, the intracellular level of malonyl-CoA is high. Malonyl-CoA allosterically inhibits CPT1 activity and thus reduces the flux through the FAO pathway at a time when the pathway is not required. When fasting, the malonyl-CoA levels fall and CPT1 activity is reactivated. Although when measured in vitro, the P479L mutation has only 20% residual CPT1 activity, it would appear that this activity is not switched off in response to feeding. Thus, FAO can take place even when there is adequate carbohydrate fuel. This may have important adaptive implications in a population that traditionally have eaten a high-fat diet. There is not yet sufficient cross-sectional or longitudinal information in the Inuit population to determine whether this mutation is harmful or beneficial. The initial case report was of an adult presenting with symptoms of myopathy, which may have been unrelated to the mutation.

CARNITINE: ACYLCARNITINE TRANSLOCASE DEFICIENCY

Etiology and Pathophysiology The carnitine: acylcarnitine transporter (CACT) is a bidirectional transporter protein that serves to deliver the long-chain acylcarnitines, which are generated by the activity of CPT1 into the mitochondrial matrix (Figure 5-2). Free carnitine is shuttled in the reverse direction to recycle as a substrate for CPT1. In CACT deficiency, acylcarnitines cannot be delivered to the mitochondrial matrix for oxidation, resulting in the features of a long-chain FAO defect. CACT deficiency is one of the more severe FAO defects and many patients have chronic liver disease with persistent hyperammonemia.

Clinical Features Unlike CPT1, the CACT is ubiquitously expressed in all tissues that utilize FAO as an energy source. Consequently, multiple tissues are involved in the disease process, and CACT deficiency is among the most severe disorders of the pathway. The disorder was initially described in 1992 in a patient with chronic, progressive, and eventually fatal liver failure (5). The liver failure was associated with persistent hyperammonemia that did not fully respond to the available ammonia-lowering therapies including sodium benzoate, and in one report, to exchange transfusion. Other features of CACT deficiency include hypertrophic cardiomyopathy, cardiac arrhythmias, septal heart defects, and skeletal myopathy. Laboratory findings in addition to the hyperammonemia include elevated transaminases (elevated aspartate aminotransferase and alanine aminotransferase), a coagulopathy, lactic acidosis, and increased serum CK. Acute presentation of CACT with hypoketotic hypoglycemia has been reported in a number of cases, and there is a high frequency of previous neonatal deaths in families in which a diagnosis of CACT is made.

Milder cases of CACT deficiency have been described with less severe features. These patients tend to have a modest hepatomegaly and less severe myopathy (14). There are no long-term reports of the natural history of this condition at present.

Investigation and Diagnosis A striking feature of CACT deficiency is the chronic, persistent hyperammonemia. In most long-chain FAO defects, hyperammonemia is only associated with acute exacerbation of the disease. Total carnitine levels tend to be low and the acylated fraction is disproportionately elevated. The acylcarnitine profile is abnormal in CACT deficiency with increased levels of C16 and C18 species and decreased acetyl (C2) carnitine. This pattern is not diagnostic as it is also found in patients with other long-chain FAO defects including CPT2 deficiency. Urine organic acid analysis may be normal when the patient is normoglycemic and may demonstrate a pattern of nonketotic dicarboxylic aciduria during catabolic episodes. This pattern is nonspecific but provides an important clue to the likely diagnosis.

The gene for CACT deficiency has been cloned. It is situated on chromosome 3p21. Multiple private mutations have been identified. There are no common mutations in patients with CACT deficiency; therefore, molecular analysis of patients with biochemical evidence of the defect requires full genomic sequencing (15).

Because of the nonspecific metabolite pattern seen in CACT deficiency and the lack of a common CACT mutation, it is important to exclude other FAO defects including CPT2 deficiency by using a fibroblast enzyme assay.

Treatment and Outcomes Despite a high rate of neonatal and infant mortality associated with this disorder when it was first recognized, there are a number of recent reports that suggest improved outcomes are possible. Medium-chain triglycerides (MCTs) have been used in an attempt to bypass the metabolic block associated with impaired transport of long-chain fatty acids into the mitochondrion. Medium-chain fatty acids derived from MCTs do not require the carnitine cycle to enter the inner mitochondrial compartment and produce a ketogenic effect in patients with CACT deficiency. Longer term evaluations of the beneficial effects of MCTs on this multisystemic disease are still required. As with all FAO disorders, prevention of fasting episodes by provision of adequate carbohydrate calories is an important aspect of patient management. The role for carnitine therapy has not been established but this therapy is prescribed for many patients based on low serum levels.

CARNITINE PALMITOYLTRANSFERASE 2 DEFICIENCY

Etiology and Pathophysiology CPT2 is bound to the inner aspect of the inner mitochondrial membrane (Figure 5-2). It takes the long-chain acylcarnitines that are transported into the mitochondrial matrix and reconverts them to their respective acyl-CoA species for targeting to β-oxidation. CPT2 deficiency results in failure to reform activated fatty acids and inhibition of long-chain FAO. Severe defects caused by null mutations result in multisystemic disease in the newborn with all of the hepatic, cardiac, and skeletal symptoms

as well as several congenital abnormalities including dysplastic changes in the brain and kidneys. This presentation is almost always fatal in the neonatal period. A milder form of CPT2 deficiency results in exercise-induced muscle disease. The mutations in the milder form of CPT2 deficiency are high residual activity mutations and demonstrate sufficient enzyme activity to maintain ketogenesis and cardiac function.

Clinical Features Three quite distinct clinical phenotypes have been described for CPT2 deficiency. The first and most common type of presentation is an adult presentation with exercise-induced myopathy, which may develop into frank rhabdomyolysis. This presentation is associated with myoglobinuria and portends a high risk of associated acute renal failure. The typical patient is in the late teens to early 20s and is someone who suddenly undertakes a high-energy exercise regimen and becomes ill during this exercise. In our own diagnostic practice, we have established a diagnosis of the myopathic form of CPT2 deficiency in a number of individuals who have enlisted in the military and developed symptoms while at "boot camp," this being their first exposure to intense muscular activity. Other systems including heart and liver do not appear to be effected in this form of the disease.

A much more severe neonatal form of CPT2 deficiency also exists. This is a fatal presentation in the newborn period with multisystem involvement. Patients have congenital hypertrophic cardiomyopathy, liver failure, probable skeletal muscle myopathy, dysmorphia, and congenital cystic dysplasia in the brain and kidneys. At autopsy, most of these tissues are pale due to massive lipid storage. Significant metabolic findings include hypoketotic hypoglycemia and hyperammonemia. An intermediate form of the disease presents in patients in early infancy with more classic signs of fasting intolerance due to failure to oxidize long-chain fatty acids. This form of the disease does not involve the severe dysmorphia or the severe developmental changes to brain and kidney but can present with a precipitous catabolic event leading to a Reye-like illness and, if unrecognized, to death attributable to hypoglycemia. This form is also associated with a chronic, progressive cardiomyopathy and skeletal myopathy if untreated (16).

Investigation and Diagnosis The myopathic form of CPT2 deficiency is characterized, during acute symptoms, by massive elevation of serum CK levels and frequently by myoglobinuria. It is important to monitor parameters of renal function during this phase of the disease because there is a high risk of acute renal

failure. This presentation does not involve liver or cardiac muscle. When the patient is well, the CK levels may return to normal. Plasma or serum acylcarnitine levels may show a modest elevation of long-chain species of chain lengths C16–C18 in this milder form of the disease, and the total serum carnitine level may be normal, making this a difficult diagnosis to establish. The acute neonatal form of the disease is characterized by abnormal hepatic, cardiac, skeletal, and renal function with gross laboratory findings. The serum acylcarnitine profile is more markedly abnormal, and urine organic acid analysis demonstrates nonketotic medium-chain dicarboxylic aciduria. At autopsy, there is massive lipid storage in viscera in addition to dysmorphia and cystic changes. The intermediate form of the disease produces identical laboratory findings during acute metabolic decompensation but is not always fatal. In between acute crises, many of the abnormal laboratory findings normalize. The serum acylcarnitine profile remains abnormal even when the patient is clinically well.

Enzymatic confirmation of the defect can be made usually in cultured skin fibroblasts or in white blood cells. CPT2 needs to be differentiated from other long-chain FAO defects for which the clinical presentation and laboratory findings frequently overlap.

The gene for CPT2 has been cloned. It resides on chromosome 1p32 and bears many similarities to CPT1 except that it is not regulated by diet. A strong genotype–phenotype correlation has been identified for CPT2 deficiency. The adult form of the disease is almost exclusively related to a single mutation, a c.338C>T change that results in S113L. This mutation has high residual activity when measured in vitro under optimal conditions. It is thought that this high activity spares hepatic and cardiac involvement. The mutation is also thermolabile. At high temperatures, the enzyme is further inactivated. It is believed that the increase in muscle temperature during vigorous exercise causes greater enzyme inhibition in this tissue, leading to rhabdomyolysis.

Mutations that result in the fatal neonatal presentation are generally null mutations, which result in zero enzyme activity (17,18). The dysmorphia that is associated with this presentation probably indicates an important role of fatty acid metabolism in normal development. There is a relatively common Ashkenazi Jewish mutation, c.1238-1239 del AG, which results in a frame shift change Q413fs and a highly unstable product with a very severe form of the disease. Patients with compound heterozygotes of a mild and a severe mutation tend to have the intermediate CPT2 deficiency and lack the developmental abnormalities.

Treatment and Outcomes The later onset form of CPT2 deficiency can be readily managed by restricting physical activity to levels that are not likely to precipitate an attack of rhabdomyolysis. In individuals with a relatively active lifestyle, high carbohydrate intake prior to exercise may have an effect of preventing lipolysis and the need for switching on long-chain FAO. Outcomes are generally good in patients with this disorder if the potentially life threatening events of rhabdomyolysis are prevented. The severe neonatal disease remains universally fatal. Clearly, there are a number of in utero effects that occur and result in the very severe phenotype. The intermediate form of the disease may present with acute metabolic decompensation in the neonatal period; however, if recognized in time and managed with intravenous glucose, these infants can survive the neonatal period. They are at risk for developing cardiomyopathy and skeletal myopathy and the acute effects of hepatic failure associated with fasting (Table 5-1). Long-term therapy should be directed to prevent fasting induced lipolysis with frequent feeding during infancy and provision of slow-release carbohydrate in the form of uncooked cornstarch at night if there are additional risk factors such as a febrile illness. Plasma carnitine levels are characteristically low in CPT2 deficiency, and L-carnitine is frequently prescribed. There are no convincing outcomes studies to demonstrate the benefit of carnitine therapy in any FAO disorder other than the carnitine transporter defect (19). Valproic acid (VPA), a drug that is frequently used to treat infantile convulsions, is contraindicated in CPT2 deficiency and probably other FAO defects because it triggers rhabdomyolysis.

VERY-LONG-CHAIN ACYL-CoA DEHYDROGENASE DEFICIENCY

Etiology and Pathophysiology The ACDs catalyze the initial step of the β-oxidation of the acyl-CoAs to enoyl-CoAs inside the mitochondria (Figures 5-2 and 5-3). There are three main straight-chain ACDs (VLCAD, MCAD, and SCAD), which have different but overlapping chain-length specificities. Some of the other ACDs also have partial activity with the straight-chain acyl-CoAs, but do not play an important role in straight-chain FAO.

Deficiency in dehydrogenation of long-chain acyl-CoAs, for instance palmitoyl-CoA (C16), was originally thought to be caused by a defect in LCAD, but genetic and molecular analyses have so far failed to identify any individuals with LCAD deficiency. Since the identification of the VLCAD enzyme in 1992, all patients with defective palmitoyl-CoA dehydrogenation have been proven to suffer from VLCAD deficiency instead.

VLCAD is a homodimeric enzyme that is associated with the inner mitochondrial membrane and catalyzes the dehydrogenation of C22–C12 straight-chain fatty acids, when these have been activated to their acyl-CoAs. VLCAD deficiency results in a lack of production of energy from β-oxidation of long-chain fatty acids. Because the long-chain fatty acids constitute a major proportion of the fatty acids, VLCAD deficiency is generally a more severe condition than MCAD or SCAD deficiency, and multiple tissues are affected. In particular, heart and muscle tissue depend heavily on energy from long-chain FAO, and VLCAD deficiency, therefore, affects these tissues severely. The lack of acetyl-CoA production from long-chain FAO also compromises hepatic ketogenesis, which results in fasting intolerance. The accumulat-

ing long-chain acyl-CoAs and long-chain acylcarnitines may have toxic effects and cause cardiac arrhythmias. There is a strong correlation between the severity of the enzyme defect and the clinical presentation in VLCAD deficiency.

Clinical Features The clinical features of VLCAD deficiency resemble those of CPT2 deficiency. As with CPT2 deficiency, VLCAD deficiency can also be divided into three general phenotypes: two childhood forms and one adult form (20,21). The severe childhood form is characterized by early onset of symptoms, usually in the neonatal period, and a high mortality rate or recurrent disease episodes, with low tolerance of fasting. Cardiomyopathy is frequently observed in this group of patients.

The milder childhood form is characterized by delayed onset of symptoms and a low mortality rate; often only a single episode or a few mild episodes of metabolic decompensation occur. This is frequently triggered by a metabolic stress caused by febrile illness and/or fasting. Cardiomyopathy is rare in this group, and the main clinical feature at presentation is hypoketotic hypoglycemia, resulting from failure to generate energy from long-chain FAO. Hepatomegaly and hypotonia are frequently observed in both childhood forms. As these patients get older, metabolic decompensation becomes less of a problem, but they also start to undertake more sustained exercise. Because muscle depends heavily on FAO as an energy source this leads to muscle symptoms becoming a frequent clinical symptom. In some patients, who presented with the mild childhood phenotype of the disease, the symptoms change from episodes of hypoketotic hypoglycemia to the muscular form of the disease, which is characteristic of the adult disease phenotype.

TABLE 5-1 Emergency Treatment		
Hypoketotic Hypoglycemia	**Cardiopulmonary Failure and Shock**	**Skeletal Muscle Weakness and Rhabdomyolysis**
• Intravenous glucose at 5–10 mg/kg/min through a highly reliable (usually centrally placed) line with frequent monitoring of glucose and adjustment of infusion to maintain serum glucose above 75 mg/dl.	• Intravenous glucose infusion at 5–10 mg/kg/min through a highly reliable, central line with frequent monitoring of glucose and adjustment of infusion to maintain serum glucose above 75 mg/dl.	• Intravenous glucose at 5–10 mg/kg/min through a reliable line.
• Treatment of elevated ammonia if present and not responsive to glucose infusion.	• Intubation and ventilation with consideration of paralysis to reduce muscle work.	• Full hydration if myocardial function is normal to reduce urinary stasis and induce myoglobin excretion.
• Treatment of associated infection or illness as appropriate.	• Inotropic agents as needed.	• Diuresis with possible alkalinization of the urine.
• Reduction of fever to less than 38C.	• Continuous monitoring of cardiac rhythm, systemic arterial oxygenation, and perfusion.	• Consideration of intubation, ventilation, and paralysis in life-threatening cases to reduce muscle work.
• The use of intravenous carnitine is controversial except in primary carnitine/OCTN2 deficiency.	• Extracorporal membrane oxygenation may be life saving.	
	• Frequent monitoring of cardiac function, cardiac tamponade, cardiac output.	
	• Treatment of liver failure if needed.	
	• Treatment of associated infection or illness as appropriate.	

The adult form of the disease is characterized by onset of disease after childhood. The typical presentation is that of isolated skeletal muscle involvement with recurrent episodes of muscle pain, rhabdomyolysis, and myoglobinuria. The episodes are usually triggered by exercise or fasting; however, emotional stress, cold, and menstruation may also trigger clinical manifestations. In some cases, rhabdomyolysis and myoglobinuria may result in acute renal failure (22).

Investigation and Diagnosis The clinical presentation and the findings from standard laboratory tests in patients with VLCAD deficiency show extensive overlap with other long-chain FAO defects such as CPT2 and LCHAD deficiency. A correct diagnosis may therefore be difficult. This is further complicated by the fact that many of the abnormal laboratory parameters may be normal or close to normal between episodes of metabolic decompensation.

Initial testing should include serum CK levels, glucose, ammonia, lactate, and urine organic acid analysis. If urine is collected while the child is symptomatic urine organic acid analysis will reveal dicarboxylic aciduria and, often, the presence of elevated uric acid. In contrast to MCAD deficiency, acylglycine conjugates are not present in VLCAD deficiency, as glycine conjugation is less effective with the accumulating long-chain acyl-CoA substrates. MS/MS-based screening of blood will show elevated levels of several long-chain acylcarnitines (C16:0, C14:0, and C14:1), with tetradecenoylcarnitine (C14:1) being the most prominent species. Moreover, there may be a tendency toward a higher level of accumulating longer chain length species in the severe childhood form than in the milder childhood and adult forms of the disease (23). It may be difficult to discriminate between a diagnosis of CPT2 deficiency and VLCAD deficiency based on the acylcarnitine profiles. During periods of low or no metabolic stress, the acylcarnitine profiles in patients with the milder forms of this disease may be normal (24,25).

In patients with the adult form of disease, the only presenting symptoms may be very high serum CK levels, which, during acute attacks, may exceed 10,000 U/L. Serum and urine myoglobin may be highly elevated and, if not carefully monitored, this may result in renal failure.

Autopsy usually reveals hepatomegaly with extensive macrovesicular and microvesicular steatosis in children who have died. Steatosis may also be present in skeletal and heart muscle.

In all clinical forms, the enzyme defect can be indicated by measuring the membrane-bound palmitoyl-CoA dehydrogenase activity in disrupted cultured skin fibroblasts or lymphocytes (21). Alternatively, the acylcarnitine profile from intact skin fibroblasts or lymphocytes can be measured by MS/MS analysis (26). Measurements of total β-oxidation as tritium release from intact skin fibroblasts or lymphocytes that have been cultured in the presence of tritiated oleate may also indicate the defect (27). A definitive diagnosis can be obtained by demonstration of mutations in the VLCAD gene. The gene for VLCAD is located on chromosome 17p11.13-p11.2 (28) and consists of 20 exons (29) that encode 655 amino acids (including a 40-amino acid leader peptide).

The mutation spectrum in VLCAD deficiency is very diverse, with more than 150 different mutations distributed to all 20 exons of the gene (20,30). There are no prevalent mutations, although some mutations are present in more than one family. The most frequently identified mutation is c.848T>C that results in a change from valine to alanine at position 243 of the mature protein (V243A). Mutation c.848T>C has been observed in approximately 10% of patients with the milder childhood or adult forms of the disease, and it is also the most frequently observed mutation in newborns identified by MS/MS-based screening (31).

As indicated previously, there is a clear correlation between the VLCAD genotype and clinical presentation (20,30). In the severe childhood disease phenotype, the vast majority of identified mutations are null mutations, such as frameshift, splicing, and stop mutations, that result in zero residual enzyme activity. In patients with two null mutations, the complete absence of VLCAD activity will affect many tissues, including the heart and liver, resulting in cardiomyopathy, hepatomegaly, and recurrent episodes of metabolic decompensation.

In the milder childhood and adult disease phenotypes, the vast majority of alleles harbor mutations, such as missense mutations or single amino acid deletion mutations that may result in some residual enzyme activity. Some of these mutant VLCAD proteins have been tested and, for instance, the V243A missense mutant and the delK238 one-amino acid deletion mutation both exhibit significant levels of (>20% of wild type) residual enzyme activity when recombinant mutant proteins are overexpressed in COS-7 cells (20). Patients with this type of mutation, in at least one of their alleles, may have sufficient residual VLCAD activity, when receiving adequate nourishment, to avoid liver and cardiac symptoms. Moreover, they may not undertake sufficient sustained exercise, in childhood, to precipitate severe muscle symptoms. During infections or fasting, however, the residual enzyme activity may no longer be sufficient to sustain the increasing demand on hepatic FAO, leading to hypoketotic hypoglycemia. It is also possible that, during febrile illness or due to increased temperature in exercising skeletal muscle, the partially functional mutant proteins lose all or most of their residual enzyme activity. Consistent with this, the c.848T>C mutation and several of the other mutations that have been identified in patients with the adult, mainly muscular, form of the disease show a very pronounced temperature dependence, in which all residual enzyme activity is lost at high temperature (40°C).

Treatment and Outcomes In the first days of life neonates often do not receive adequate caloric intake. This is in particular true in infants who are breastfeed. In neonates with VLCAD deficiency, the metabolic decompensation may lead to episodes of severe hypoglycemia; and, if the hypoglycemia is not recognized and corrected by intravenous glucose administration, it often leads to coma and death. Also later in life, acute episodes of metabolic decompensation may occur as a result of a fasting stress in conjunction with febrile illness. These episodes may also be corrected by intravenous glucose administration (Table 5-1).

The long-term dietary treatment for the childhood forms of VLCAD deficiency consists of avoidance of fasting by frequent feeding and reduction of the amount of long-chain fat in the diet while supplying essential fatty acids in the form of canola, walnut oil, or safflower oil. The diet should contain enough calories in the form of carbohydrates to avoid fasting-induced lipolysis and hypoglycemia and is often supplemented with extra calories in the form of MCTs (Table 5-2). Overnight continuous tube feeding or provision of a slow-release glucose source in the form of uncooked cornstarch before bedtime may be necessary in periods in which there is febrile illness or vomiting, when the child suffers from a high level of metabolic stress. The long-term dietary treatment not only prevents development of cardiomyopathy, rhabdomyolysis, muscle weakness, and hepatic symptoms, but may even reverse these symptoms if they have already occurred (32–34). Recently, trials in which MCT treatment was substituted with triheptanoin oil have been initiated in many children with VLCAD deficiency, and the results seem promising when this treatment is combined with the usual treatment regimen (35). The rationale for using triheptanoin oil is that, when metabolized, it will provide propionyl-CoA and acetyl-CoA for the tricarboxylic acid cycle. These

TABLE 5-2   Preventive Treatment of Long Chain FAO Defects

0–2 Years of Age

- Frequent feedings at intervals of every 3–4 hours.
- Assiduous avoidance of fasting for more than 6–10 hours, depending upon nutritional status and age.
- Administration of nocturnal corn starch may be needed either by nasogastric or gastrostomy tube.
- Parental monitoring of blood sugar before feedings can be considered to assess feeding intervals.
- Supplementation with essential fatty acids should be considered if a low fat formula is used.
- A formula containing medium chain triglycerides (MCT) or breast feeding with MCT supplementation.
- Consideration of supplementation with DHA.
- The use of carnitine supplementation is controversial except in primary carnitine/OCTN2 deficiency, when carnitine is essential.

Older Children and Adults

- Assiduous avoidance of fasting for more than 12 hours.
- Addition of MCT-containing oil to diet.
- Diet of 15% fat or less, but essential fatty acid supplementation.

intermediates may become limited in patients with FAO defects due to leakage from the cell. Oxidation of triheptanoin oil replenishes this loss and, thus, restores the compromised energy production from the tricarboxylic acid cycle. Just as in CPT2 deficiency, plasma carnitine levels may be low in VLCAD deficiency, and L-carnitine is frequently prescribed. As mentioned previously, there are no convincing outcomes studies to demonstrate the benefit of carnitine therapy in any FAO disorder other than the carnitine transporter defect.

VPA is a drug that is frequently used to treat infantile convulsions. VPA (dipropyl-acetic acid) is a branched, medium-chain fatty acid that can form acyl-CoA intermediates, which are subjected to limited mitochondrial β-oxidation. VPA can be conjugated to carnitine, exported out of the mitochondria, and thereby lead to mild-to-moderate carnitine deficiency. Because VPA may inhibit FAO and induce carnitine deficiency it is contraindicated in VLCAD deficiency and the other FAO defects.

The adult, muscular, form of VLCAD deficiency can be readily managed by restricting physical activity to levels that are not likely to precipitate an attack of rhabdomyolysis. In individuals with a relatively active lifestyle, high carbohydrate intake prior to exercise may have an effect of preventing lipolysis and the need for switching on long-chain FAO. Outcomes are generally good in this disorder if the potentially life threatening events of rhabdomyolysis are prevented.

Prenatal Diagnosis Prenatal diagnosis of VLCAD deficiency is frequently requested by families who have previously had an affected child who has shown the clinical symptoms of the disease. It is possible to perform prenatal diagnosis by traditional enzyme assays (21) or by analysis with the in vitro probe assay (26), but mutation analysis of DNA extracted from a chorionic villus biopsy is preferable (36). In particular, in families in which the causative mutations are already known from a previous analysis of an index case, mutation analysis is the method of choice. With the speed and accuracy of the current mutation detection methods, the causative mutations in a family that requests prenatal diagnosis can be identified in only 2 to 3 working days prior to the chorionic villus sampling, making mutation analysis feasible also in situations in which the causative mutations have not been identified beforehand.

MEDIUM-CHAIN ACYL-CoA DEHYDROGENASE DEFICIENCY

Etiology and Pathophysiology MCAD is a homotetrameric enzyme located in the mitochondrial matrix (Figure 5-3). It catalyzes the initial step in the β-oxidation of C12–C6 straight-chain acyl-CoAs, which are either directly imported from the cytosol or derived from chain-shortened long-chain-acyl-CoAs. MCAD deficiency results in a lack of production of energy from β-oxidation of medium-chain fatty acids, and hepatic ketogenesis and gluconeogenesis are compromised because the enzyme defect also results in lack of acetyl-CoA production. During periods of fasting or metabolic stress caused by illness, patients with MCAD deficiency depend heavily on energy generation from glucose oxidation, and this may rapidly lead to hypoglycemia and hypoketosis. During a metabolic crisis, the accumulating medium-chain fatty acids (like octanoate) and medium-chain acyl-CoAs may have toxic effects, which disturb ammonia metabolism and cause hyperammonemia.

The accumulating medium-chain fatty acids is also partly oxidized to dicarboxylic acids (adipic [C6], suberic [C8], sebacic [C10], and dodecanedioic [C12]) by α-oxidation; and, during acute episodes, this can be observed as dicarboxylic aciduria.

In 1976, when the first patient with MCAD deficiency was described as suffering from nonketotic dicarboxylic aciduria (37), it was believed that this was a rare condition. Since then, it has become clear that MCAD deficiency is the most common defect of FAO and one of the most common inborn errors of metabolism in populations of northern European descent. The frequency of the enzyme defect has been estimated to be 1:8,400 in Germany and 1:15,000 in the United States (38,39), based on results from MS/MS screening of newborns. Recently, it has become clear that MCAD deficiency is also present at a significant frequency (approximately 1/30,000) in Japan (40) and possibly also other Asian countries. In light of these high prevalences, it is puzzling that MCAD deficiency was considered to be a rare condition for many years. There are, however, some factors that may explain this. The majority of patients with MCAD deficiency are completely asymptomatic between episodes, and the metabolites that are looked for in traditional biochemical analysis of urine are absent between episodes. Because of this, MCAD deficiency was underdiagnosed for a long period of time. In addition, it appears that there is a reduced penetrance, and thus many affected individuals never experience clinical symptoms. It can be estimated that perhaps only approximately half of the individuals with MCAD deficiency are recognized with clinically manifest disease (41,42).

Clinical Features When MCAD deficiency manifests as disease, it has a very wide spectrum of clinical presentations. Although this is not typical, the disease may present in the first few days after birth, with symptoms ranging from benign hypoglycemia to coma and death (43–45). It could be speculated that inadequate caloric intake due to difficulties with breastfeeding plays a role in precipitating disease in neonates.

Usually the clinical presentation takes place after the neonatal period, but within the first 2 years of life (46,47). A "metabolic stress" such as prolonged fasting often in connection with viral infections (e.g., gastrointestinal and upper respiratory tract) is usually required to precipitate disease manifestation. Due to the toxicity of accumulating metabolites or simply because of the gastrointestinal infection itself, vomiting is frequently observed at disease presentation.

Many patients also present with seizures. On admission, the child may be lethargic, and, without intervention, this may rapidly progress to coma and death. The main clinical feature is hypoketotic hypoglycemia, resulting from the failure to generate energy from fatty acids. It is important to note, however, that some patients may present with lethargy and hypotonia and still have glucose levels in the normal range. This suggests that reduced consciousness and even coma are not exclusively due to low blood glucose, but may also be caused by accumulating toxic intermediates, such as octanoate and cis-4-decenoate. Hepatomegaly is frequently observed because MCAD deficiency is, for the most part, a disease of hepatic FAO. Both the clinical presentation and many of the routine laboratory findings in MCAD deficiency may resemble Reye syndrome (acute noninflammatory encephalopathy with hyperammonemia, liver dysfunction, and fatty infiltration of the liver) (48).

A typical scenario is that of the child who has suffered from an intercurrent illness with vomiting for a day or two and who is then found in a comatose state or dead after an overnight sleep. Approximately one fifth of the patients die during their first presentation (46,47). In children who have died, postmortem examination usually will reveal hepatomegaly and cerebral edema. Autopsy will show hepatomegaly with extensive macrovesicular and microvesicular steatosis. Steatosis may also be present in kidney and other tissues.

Although the majority of children survive their initial episode, it has become clear that a significant proportion of the children who have survived an acute episode, and perhaps also children who have experienced clinically unrecognized episodes, suffer from long-term sequelae (47). Approximately 40% of patients with MCAD deficiency who survive after diagnosis have been judged to be abnormal on routine developmental testing (47). A large proportion of survivors suffer from global developmental delay, but abnormalities may also be more specific and often include attention deficit, speech delay, and behavioral problems. It is likely that these symptoms are caused by minor injuries to the brain that occurred during an episode of metabolic decompensation. The number of acute episodes that occur and the severity of these episodes (indicated by the presence of seizures, encephalopathy, and coma) are probably important in determining if there will be long-term psychodevelopmental sequelae.

There are a few examples of patients with MCAD deficiency who experience the first clinical manifestation of the disease in adulthood (49–51). The initial symptoms may be vomiting and headache, which may progress to lethargy and encephalopathy. Rhabdomyolysis, muscle weakness, or cardiac symptoms (ventricular fibrillation with cardiac arrest) may also be observed, and the episodes may be life threatening. It is probable that a rather severe metabolic stress is required to precipitate disease in affected adults because this appears to be rare.

Mothers of an affected fetus may have an increased risk for pregnancy-related complications, such as hemolysis, elevated liver enzymes, and low platelets (HELLP) or acute fatty liver of pregnancy (AFLP). It is not known at present if patients with MCAD deficiency are also at risk for developing HELLP and AFLP when pregnant or whether accumulating toxic intermediates in affected mothers may harm the fetus. We have, however, observed several spontaneous abortions and a single stillborn in an affected mother (unpublished results), so when patients get pregnant their metabolic status should be followed especially carefully.

Investigation and Diagnosis Before the availability of mutation analysis and MS/MS-based acylcarnitine analysis of blood, MCAD deficiency was difficult to diagnose because the diagnosis relied on detection of diagnostic metabolites in the urine, and most of these metabolites are only present during acute illness.

In the child who is suspected of having MCAD deficiency, the initial testing should include serum CK levels, glucose, ammonia, lactate, and urine organic acid analysis. If urine is collected while the child is symptomatic, urine organic acid analysis by gas chromatography/MS will reveal C6–C10 dicarboxylic aciduria and the presence of acylglycine conjugates (hexanoyl-, suberyl-, and phenylpropionylglycine) (Cregersen et al. 1983). In contrast to the dicarboxylic acids, acylglycine conjugates are usually present even when patients are asymptomatic, although phenylpropionylglycine may be absent in children younger than 4 months of age due to lack of phenylpropionic acid–producing bacteria in the gut. In urine collected during an asymptomatic period, specific analysis for hexanoyl-, suberyl-, and phenylpropionylglycine by stable isotope dilution is a good diagnostic method (52).

Measurement of the specific MCAD enzyme activity in disrupted cultured skin fibroblasts, lymphocytes, or tissue biopsies from muscle by using octanoyl-CoA or phenylpropionyl-CoA as substrates and ETF as an electron acceptor can confirm the diagnosis of MCAD deficiency. Just as in VLCAD deficiency, MCAD deficiency can also be indicated by analysis of intact skin fibroblasts or lymphocytes by MS/MS acylcarnitine profiling (26) or by measuring total β-oxidation as tritium release after the cells have been cultured in the presence of tritiated myristate (27).

MS/MS-based acylcarnitine analysis of blood or plasma (53) is currently the preferred biochemical diagnostic method. Demonstration of an increased octanoylcarnitine (C8) concentration together with an increased C8/ and C10/carnitine ratio is highly indicative of a diagnosis of MCAD deficiency. Because MS/MS-based acylcarnitine analysis is very fast and accurate, it is also used in newborn screening for MCAD deficiency. MS/MS is readily available in many countries and regions of the world. It is important that the diagnosis based on MS/MS acylcarnitine analysis in blood is confirmed by another method because false-positive results may occur, particularly in premature babies, individuals with secondary carnitine deficiency, or individuals treated with VPA.

A definitive diagnosis for MCAD deficiency can be obtained by demonstration of known disease-causing mutations in the MCAD gene. The gene for MCAD is located on chromosome 1p31 (54) and consists of 12 exons (55) that encode 421 amino acids (including a 25-amino acid leader peptide).

The most frequently identified mutation is c.985A>G, which is located in exon 11 and results in a change from lysine to glutamic acid at position 304 (K304E) of the mature protein. The c.985A>G mutation is present in homozygous form in 80% of patients with clinically manifest disease and a further 18% are heterozygous for this mutation and one of a large variety of other mutations (56). Because of its high frequency in affected patients, the c.985A>G carrier frequency has been determined in the normal population from many countries to estimate the prevalence of MCAD deficiency. In countries such as the United States and the United Kingdom, where people of northwestern European descent make up a significant proportion of the population, the c.985A>G carrier frequency ranges from 1:40 to 1:100, whereas the mutation is virtually absent in Japan (57). Despite the absence of the c.985A>G mutation in people from Asia, MCAD deficiency caused by other mutations has been reported in children from Asia (45).

More than 100 different mutations are now known in the MCAD gene and are distributed to all exons and comprise all types (missense, nonsense, splicing, and small insertions/deletions). Gross alterations, such as deletions and insertions involving more than 10 to 20 nucleotides, are rare, with only a single example reported so far (58).

In newborns with MCAD deficiency identified by MS/MS-based screening, the common c.985A>G mutation is less prevalent than in the clinically diagnosed patients, with only 50 to 60% of newborns being homozygous for this mutation (38,39) and other mutations being more frequent. A c.199T>C mutation that causes a shift from tyrosine to histidine at position 42 (Y42H) of the mature protein is rather frequent in newborns who are identified with a less pronounced, but still diagnostic, acylcarnitine profile on MS/MS-based screening (38,59). Although this shows that there is indeed a correlation between the genotype and the biochemical phenotype in the form of the observed acylcarnitine profile, it has so far not been possible to demonstrate an obvious correlation between genotype and phenotype in patients with MCAD deficiency. Patients who are homozygous for two null mutations may remain without symptoms, whereas patients who harbor two mutations with residual enzyme activity may present with severe clinical manifestations such as sudden death (60). Moreover, numerous family studies have identified asymptomatic siblings with a genotype identical to the manifesting index patient. This clearly illustrates that nongenetic factors, such as a fasting stress often in conjunction with fever and vomiting, are the main determinants in precipitating disease episodes, and that the gene defect, regardless of it relative severity, only manifests as disease under certain circumstances. Although individuals with some genotypes, for instance compound heterozygosity for the c.985A>G mutation and the "milder" c.199T>C mutation, may have a milder biochemical phenotype, such patients must still be considered at risk for disease manifestation and should not be treated differently from other patients. The family of a newborn identified with a "mild" acylcarnitine profile by prospective screening and found to be compound heterozygous for the two mild mutations c.199T>C and c.799G>A, nicely illustrates the point that even individuals with the biochemically mildest phenotypes may still be at risk. In this family, clinical follow up revealed that an older sibling, who had the same genotype as the index patient, had suffered from a vomiting illness at 1 year of age, had become lethargic and ill quickly, and this episode had resulted in hospital admission (61).

Environmental factors, such as a higher body temperature resulting from fever, may also play a role in precipitating disease episodes, as some of the MCAD mutations, including the common c.985A>G and the c.199T>C mutations encode proteins that are temperature sensitive (61). These mutant proteins are compromised in their folding and stability and will therefore result in lower residual enzyme activity in patient cells when the body temperature increases.

Treatment and Outcomes MCAD deficiency is considered a treatable disease with a very good prognosis if recognized before clinical presentation. The mainstay of management of MCAD deficiency is to avoid prolonged fasting by instituting frequent feedings with a carbohydrate-rich diet. In young children (younger than 1 year of age), who are, of course, less tolerant to fasting, provision of supplementary nocturnal uncooked cornstarch (1–1.5 g/kg) as a source of complex carbohydrates may be needed to avoid metabolic decompensation during an overnight fast. During acute episodes of metabolic decompensation, it is crucial that hypoglycemia is corrected by intravenous glucose administration (10% at 5–8 mg/kg/min) and that this is not delayed because disease progression from lethargy to coma and death may be very rapid.

Apart from the aforementioned loss of psychodevelopmental skills in children who have experienced clinical manifestation of the disease (47), the other main long-term effect is hypotonia, which may be a result from progressive muscular damage in untreated patients.

As in other of the FAO defects, plasma carnitine levels may be low in MCAD deficiency, and L-carnitine is frequently prescribed. There are, however, no convincing studies to demonstrate the benefit of carnitine therapy. VPA therapy is contraindicated in MCAD deficiency because it may inhibit FAO and induce carnitine deficiency. Obviously, MCT supplementation, which is often recommended for the long-chain FAO defects, is contraindicated in MCAD deficiency.

Prenatal Diagnosis Although MCAD deficiency is considered relatively easy to treat, there are many examples of families that have previously had an affected child and request prenatal diagnosis (26,62,63). In 1987, the first example of prenatal diagnosis for MCAD deficiency by analysis of β-oxidation in cultured amniocytes was reported (62). Prenatal diagnosis by analysis of cultured amniocytes with the in vitro probe assay (26) is also possible; however, mutation analysis of DNA extracted from a chorionic villus biopsy is the method of choice (63). In particular, the fact that the majority of families are homozygous for the prevalent c.985A>G mutation opens the possibility for very fast and specific diagnosis by use of a mutation-specific assay. In families with other causative mutations, which have not been identified by prior prenatal diagnosis, mutation analysis is still an option because identification of unknown mutations in a family can currently be performed within a very few days prior to the chorionic villus biopsy sampling.

SHORT-CHAIN ACYL-CoA DEHYDROGENASE DEFICIENCY

Etiology and Pathophysiology SCAD is a homotetrameric enzyme located in the mitochondrial matrix (Figure 5-3). It catalyzes the initial step in the β-oxidation of C6–C4 straight-chain acyl-CoAs.

In contrast to VLCAD and MCAD deficiencies, the enzymatic block in SCAD deficiency does not in itself cause an energy deficiency because this enzyme defect only blocks the two final rounds of β-oxidation, so energy generation from all the previous oxidative steps in the degradation of long-chain fatty acids has occurred. The pathogenic consequences of SCAD deficiency are, therefore, not caused by a lack of energy production from β-oxidation, but instead are most likely caused by the toxic effects of the accumulating substrates. In particular, the toxic effects of accumulating butyric (C4) acid on neuronal and muscular tissue may explain the observed neuromuscular symptoms. The accumulating butyryl-CoA can be carboxylated to ethylmalonyl-CoA and then hydrolyzed to ethylmalonic acid (EMA), which is typically observed in the urine from patients with SCAD deficiency. It is likely that the toxic effects of accumulating EMA, for instance, inhibition of CK in the cerebral cortex, also contribute to the pathophysiology of SCAD deficiency.

Clinical Features SCAD deficiency is probably the most controversial defect of FAO. On the one hand, there have been reports on affected patients with severe disease with the biochemical markers characteristic for the disease, but who only harbor one or both of two polymorphic sequence variations in the SCAD gene. This indicates that these two polymorphic variations may be involved in disease development and that the disease, therefore, might be very frequent. On the other hand, only between 20 and 30 patients with enzymatically proven SCAD deficiency have been reported in the literature since 1987, when this defect was first described (64). This apparent enigma is hard to explain, and it suggests that SCAD deficiency is underdiagnosed due to difficulties in clinical recognition and laboratory diagnosis and/or is only one of several factors resulting in disease.

The disease can be divided into two forms on the basis of the causative mutations. In classic SCAD deficiency, the defect is caused by two inactivating mutations that result in very low or nearly undetectable residual enzyme activity. This condition seems to be very rare, and less than a dozen patients with this form of the disease have been reported. In the other form, the variant form, of the disease either of the two polymorphic variations c.511C>T or c.625G>A is present in homozygous or compound heterozygous form alone or together with heterozygosity for an inactivating mutation. Although the consequences at the molecular level of the inactivating mutations and the polymorphic variations are different and the encoded proteins have different residual enzyme activity potential, the resulting clinical phenotype of both classic and variant SCAD deficiency may be identical.

Clinically, SCAD deficiency is a very heterogeneous disease. The initial clinical presentation is usually in infancy, often in the first days of life. The first two patients with SCAD deficiency were described as having neonatal metabolic acidosis with EMA excretion (64). These patients presented after a period of poor feeding with lethargy. Although one of the neonates recovered and showed normal growth and development for 2 years thereafter, the other neonate continued vomiting, suffered hypertonia, and eventually died after a 5-day hospitalization. The extreme clinical variability of SCAD deficiency can also be illustrated by the description of a 12-year-old patient with SCAD deficiency who had suffered from recurrent episodes of vomiting since infancy without any other symptoms (65). Patients with SCAD deficiency have also been reported to present with distal upper limb weakness and hypotonia secondary to an axonal neuropathy (66).

Generally, patients with SCAD deficiency tend to present in childhood with mainly neurologic and muscular symptoms, such as hypotonia, hypertonia, myopathy, and seizures and often with developmental delay. These symptoms are probably caused by the toxic effects of accumulating butyric acid, which, due to the reduced capability of neuronal and muscular tissue to regenerate, results in more permanent and progressive damage in these tissues. SCAD deficiency is not likely to be the direct cause of an energy deficiency because the enzyme defect only blocks the last step of β-oxidation and allows energy generation from all the previous oxidative steps in the degradation of long-chain fatty acids to occur. Despite this, symptoms such as hypoglycemia and encephalopathy are also observed in patients with SCAD deficiency, most probably because the enzyme defect indirectly inhibits other energy-generating processes.

As mentioned previously, SCAD deficiency may be fatal. The results of postmortem examination of patients with SCAD deficiency may resemble those of MCAD deficiency with cerebral edema, hepato-megaly with microvesicular fat, intracanalicular cholestasis, and focal hepatocellular necrosis (64).

Similar to the other FAO defects, SCAD deficiency seems to pose an increased risk for pregnancy-related complications. It has been reported that the mother of an affected fetus, who had two severe mutations in the SCAD gene, developed HELLP during pregnancy (67), and AFLP has also been reported in the mother of a fetus homozygous for the two susceptibility polymorphisms (68).

Investigation and Diagnosis SCAD deficiency is characterized by the presence of increased urinary EMA excretion with or without accompanying methylsuccinic acid. Both EMA and succinic acid can be formed from accumulated butyryl-CoA. Butyryl-CoA can be carboxylated by propionyl-CoA carboxylase to form ethylmalonyl-CoA, which is either hydrolyzed to EMA or converted to methylsuccinyl-CoA by methylmalonyl-CoA mutase, yielding in both cases methylsuccinic acid on hydrolysis. When these metabolites, and often also butyrylglycine, are observed in urine organic acid analysis or acylglycine analysis, SCAD deficiency is indicated. Demonstration of elevated C4-carnitine by MS/MS-based acylcarnitine analysis of blood/plasma is also indicative of a diagnosis of SCAD deficiency, or alternatively, of isobutyryl-CoA dehydrogenase deficiency because butyrylcarnitine and isobutyrylcarnitine cannot be distinguished. Biochemical differentiation between these two defects may be assisted by urine organic acid analysis. In isobutyryl-CoA dehydrogenase deficiency, small amounts of isobutyrylglycine can indicate this defect, whereas demonstration of EMA, methylsuccinic acid, and butyrylglycine points toward SCAD deficiency (69,70). Ethylmalonic encephalopathy is another important differential diagnosis (see Chapter 7).

Although measurement of specific SCAD enzyme activity using butyryl-CoA as substrate in disrupted cultured cells is possible and has been used for diagnosis (64), there are examples in which the possible residual enzyme activity is highly variable and influenced by yet unidentified cellular conditions (71). In addition, the overlapping substrate specificity of MCAD and possibly other ACDs further complicates enzymatic diagnosis in fibroblasts. Demonstration of reduced enzyme activity in muscle biopsy samples, in the presence of an inactivating MCAD antibody, seems to be the best approach for enzymatic diagnosis (66); however, overall, the use of enzyme activity measurements for diagnosis is questionable. This is particularly true for the variant form of SCAD deficiency caused by a genotype with the susceptibility variations.

There are indications that analysis of intact skin fibroblasts by MS/MS acylcarnitine profiling (72) can be used for biochemical diagnosis, but a more certain diagnosis requires demonstration of inactivating mutations by full sequencing of the entire coding region of the SCAD gene.

The gene for SCAD is located on chromosome 12q22-qter and consists of 11 exons that encode 412 amino acids (including a 24-amino acid leader peptide) (73,74).

The two polymorphic susceptibility variants, c.625G>A and c.511C>T, are frequent in countries where people of northwestern European descent make up a significant proportion of the population (71,75,76). The c.625G>A variant is by far the most prevalent of the two and has so far been demonstrated to be polymorphic in various ethnic populations (75). The c.625G>A and c.511C>T variations are present in homozygous or combined heterozygous form in as much as 14% of the general population, but the variants are grossly overrepresented in patients with EMA aciduria, in whom 69% are homozygous or combined heterozygous (70,76). Based on these demographics, these two polymorphic variants are believed to confer susceptibility to disease precipitation, when present together with yet unidentified genetic and environmental factors (71). It is important to stress that the majority of the individuals who carry these susceptibility variants in both alleles will most likely remain without clinically manifest disease throughout life. Only a minority, namely those who harbor the yet unknown genetic factors and/or suffer from certain forms of environmental stress, will suffer from clinical manifestation of the enzyme defect. The finding that the residual enzyme activity from the mutant proteins, R147W (encoded by the c.511C>T variant) and G185S (encoded by the c.625G>A variant), is both critically dependent on temperature and other cellular conditions (76,77) suggests that the environmental factors, such as high body temperature from fever and/or inherited variation in cellular protein handling, determine the residual enzyme activity and, thereby, the risk for disease manifestation. Until these factors have been identified and characterized, both the management and prognosis for individuals found to harbor only the susceptibility variants is highly problematic and must mainly take into account whether they have had any clinical signs of disease.

Fewer than a dozen mutations causing classic SCAD deficiency have been reported in the literature. Surprisingly, nearly all these mutations are missense mutations that affect the folding, thermostability, and degradation of the mutant SCAD proteins (77). Because of this very skewed mutation spectrum and the observed behavior of the mutant proteins, it is likely that accumulation of aggregated, nonfunctional mutant SCAD proteins inside the mitochondria plays a role in the pathogenesis of SCAD deficiency.

It is important to remember that the nature of the mutations/susceptibility variations identified in patients with SCAD deficiency are not by themselves predictive of the disease phenotype, but they are crucial predisposing factors. A better understanding of this enigmatic disease must await identification of the additional external genetic and environmental factors that trigger disease in predisposed patients.

Treatment and Outcomes Treatment strategies and their outcome in SCAD deficiency are poorly characterized because the pathogenesis of the disease is still not well understood and the number of reported patients is low. It is, however, clear that the mainstay of management of SCAD deficiency is similar to that of the other FAO defects, namely avoiding prolonged fasting. The role of other therapeutic measures such as dietary fat restriction and carnitine supplementation is unclear. During acute episodes of metabolic decompensation intervention by intravenous glucose administration is recommended.

Prenatal Diagnosis If prenatal diagnosis for SCAD deficiency is requested, the diagnosis should be performed by mutation analysis because the present biochemical methods are slow and not sufficiently safe. Prenatal diagnosis should only be performed in families with pathogenic mutations that are known to cause classic SCAD deficiency. In light of the many unsolved questions about the possible role of the two polymorphic susceptibility variations in disease development, it is not at present advisable to perform prenatal diagnosis in families in which only c.625G>A and c.511C>T susceptibility variations have been identified.

SHORT-CHAIN 3-HYDROXYACYL-CoA DEHYDROGENASE

Etiology and Pathophysiology This enzyme catalyzes the third step of the FAO cycle, the NAD-dependent conversion of 3-hydroxyacyl-CoA substrates of 4–14 carbons in length to the 3-ketoacyl-CoA species (Figure 5-3). Thus, the enzyme has broad specificity, using both short- and medium-chain substrates. The enzyme is highly homologous across many animal species and contains substantial homology to LCHAD, consistent with the fact that both catalyze the same step of FAO and share overlapping substrate specificities. The SCHAD complementary DNA and gene (78,79) have been cloned and characterized in detail, and the crystal structure of the en-

zyme has been defined at high resolution (80). As assessed by tissue immunoblot, enzyme activity measurements, and immunocytochemistry, SCHAD is abundantly expressed in many mammalian tissues, including pancreatic islet cells, with the highest levels in the liver, skeletal muscle, and heart.

Clinical Features Because the number of patients with proven SCHAD deficiency, as documented by the presence of two SCHAD gene mutations in this recessively inherited disorder, is very small, the extent of the clinical phenotype remains uncertain. Several patients with deficiency of SCHAD enzyme activity (81,82) do not have mutations in the SCHAD gene. Although these patients may have mutations in another as yet unknown gene with SCHAD activity, these reports have resulted in confusion about the spectrum of clinical manifestations of SCHAD deficiency. Patients from the three families (83–85) with proven SCHAD mutations do exhibit recurrent and episodic hypoketotic hypoglycemia typical of many FAO defects. Thus, proven SCHAD deficiency is among the rarest of the FAO disorders. These episodes may be precipitated by stressors such as fasting and are often accompanied by seizures; however, in several patients, hypoglycemia was not precipitated by any observable stress. The unique component of clinical SCHAD deficiency is that relative hyperinsulinism is often, although not universally, present during spells of hypoglycemia, the phenotype described as persistent hyperinsulinemic hypoglycemia of infancy. To date, among cases with proven mutations, skeletal and cardiomyopathies have not been present, differentiating this disorder from the longer chain defects in trifunctional protein (see later). The SCHAD-deficient patients all presented within the first year of life, often with hypoglycemia in the neonatal period. These data suggest that among newborns with persistent hyperinsulinemic hypoglycemia of infancy, genetic screening for SCHAD deficiency should be performed. To date, SCHAD deficiency has not been detected in any patients on routine MS/MS newborn screening.

Investigation and Diagnosis At the current very limited state of knowledge, the hallmarks of SCHAD deficiency are hyperinsulinemic hypoglycemia with accumulation of 3-hydroxybutyrylcarnitine in the plasma. In general, other than the lethargy and seizures associated with episodes of hypoglycemia, the history and physical examination are normal. Family history may prove important, as consanguinity has been reported in two of the three families (83–85). The families have been of Pakistani, Asian Indian, and Norwegian origin. The keys to diagnosis include analysis of

plasma acylcarnitines on MS/MS, as elevations of hydroxybutyrylcarnitine are consistently present. Urine organic acids may show elevations of 3-hydroxybutyrate, 3,4-dihydroxybutyrate, and 3-hydroxyglutarate. Several of the documented cases are clinically normal between spells, with normal muscle tone, exercise tolerance, and cardiac function. Other laboratory testing is unrevealing, although details of liver function and plasma muscle enzymes have not been reported.

In fibroblasts from patients, expression of SCHAD protein antigen, as assessed by Western blot analysis reveals low or absent amounts. Enzyme assays in which the reverse reaction and acetoacetyl-CoA are used as substrates reveal decreased activity, but significant residual activity has usually been present, probably due to other enzymes in peroxisomes or other organelles. Because enzyme assays are not diagnostic of mutations in the known SCHAD gene, molecular genetic analysis is imperative. In the reported patients, the mutations have been homozygous for the splice consensus site mutation, IVS6-2A>G before exon 7 (84); homozygous for the missense mutation, c.733C>T changing proline-258 to leucine in exon 7 (83); and homozygous for a 6-bp deletion altering the exon 5 acceptor splice site (85). Both splice site mutations lead to exon skipping and missplicing. It is unusual among FAO disorders that all patients exhibit homozygosity, and there are two consanguineous marriages in the affected families. This suggests that carrier rates for SCHAD mutations are probably low, consistent with the rarity of this disorder.

Treatment and Outcomes As with other FAO disorders, the patients have been treated with frequent feedings and overnight infusions of cornstarch as a source of carbohydrate. In three instances, recurrent and frequent episodes of hypoglycemia with seizures persisted despite frequent feedings. One patient seemed to respond to glucagon (85); however, four patients were most successfully treated with diazoxide and chlorothiazide and became asymptomatic on this treatment regimen. In one family, two young infants died of hypoglycemia many years ago, before the diagnosis was appreciated, a 27-year-old survives with developmental delay attributed to his recurrent and resistant hypoglycemia as an infant, and a 20-year-old is normal and receiving treatment (85). Development in the recently reported and treated patients is apparently normal. Thus, in marked contrast to other FAO disorders, patients with SCHAD deficiency appear to require therapy, diazoxide, and chlorothiazide that are optimal for persistent hyperinsulinemic hypoglycemia of infancy.

ISOLATED LONG-CHAIN 3-HYDROXYACYL-CoA DEHYDROGENASE DEFICIENCY

Etiology and Pathophysiology The biochemical features of LCHAD deficiency were described in 1989 (86), before the actual isolation, purification, and characterization of the enzyme providing LCHAD activity. LCHAD catalyzes the third step in the FAO spiral, converting long-chain 3-hydroxyacyl-CoA esters into long-chain 3-keto-CoA species by using NAD as a cofactor (Figure 5-2). The first patient had accumulation of long-chain 3-hydroxy fatty acids and reduced enzymatic activity of LCHAD, as assayed in the reverse direction by using 3-keto-palmitoyl-CoA (86). In 1992, Hashimoto and colleagues (87) and Turnbull and colleagues (88) discovered that LCHAD was part of a heterooctameric protein complex with four α-subunits encoding the LCHAD activity and four β-subunits exhibiting long-chain 2,3-enoyl-CoA hydratase and LKAT activities. This protein complex, named TFP, contains enzymatic activities of the last three steps of the FAO spiral for longer chain substrates of 12–19 carbons (Figure 5-2). TFP is likely associated with the inner membrane of mitochondria, in close apposition to VLCAD and the carnitine-acylcarnitine shuttle enzymes that transport long-chain fatty acids into mitochondria across this membrane. This physical proximity probably enhances the efficiency of long-chain FAO, a process called channeling, and avoids the toxicity of free long-chain fatty acids. Both subunit genes of TFP are located head to head on chromosome 2p, and their transcription is coordinately regulated by a short intergenic region.

Clinical Features Patients with isolated LCHAD deficiency, a recessively inherited disorder, usually present in the first year of life with hypoketotic hypoglycemia and liver dysfunction, the Reye syndrome–like phenotype common among most FAO defects (89–91). This may progress to seizures, coma, and death if not promptly and vigorously treated. Unfortunately, tachycardic arrhythmias, apneic episodes, cardiopulmonary arrest, and unexplained sudden death are also common initial manifestations, occurring in up to 40% of symptomatic patients. The majority of patients have hepatomegaly and hypotonia. During an acute metabolic decompensation, hepatic dysfunction, vomiting, weakness, and respiratory insufficiency are common. A second type of patient, in whom the metabolic crisis is concomitant with severe cardiomyopathy and multiorgan failure, presents in the first month of life. More rarely, a chronic presentation with feeding difficulties and failure to thrive is noted. Other unusual manifestations are jaundice secondary to cholestasis and hypocalcemia. It is important to emphasize that relatively asymptomatic neonatal hypoglycemia may be an early manifestation. During childhood, patients with LCHAD deficiency develop ophthalmologic abnormalities including loss of visual acuity and chorioretinal atrophy (92). These eye abnormalities are unique among FAO disorders. Some patients with LCHAD may develop peripheral sensorimotor polyneuropathy.

As with all other FAO disorders, symptomatic presentations are usually precipitated by stress, most commonly reduced caloric intake for 12 or more hours, often secondary to a mild infectious illness such as gastroenteritis or a respiratory tract infection. The stress of the fetal-to-neonatal transition, as the fetus converts from using glucose as the major source of energy to using fat, but in the face of decreased feeding for 12–48 hours, often results in a neonatal presentation. This may be aggravated by breast feeding, which may result in prolonged inadequate caloric intake from colostrum. Exercise and emotional stress are also precipitants of symptoms in some cases.

It is crucial to recognize that maternal liver diseases of pregnancy (93), particularly acute fatty liver of pregnancy (AFLP) and HELLP syndromes, are associated with fetal LCHAD deficiency (91,94,95). These maternal disorders usually begin in the third trimester with hypertension and proteinuria, typical of pre-eclampsia, and then progress to jaundice (AFLP only), liver dysfunction or failure, renal dysfunction and failure, and a bleeding diathesis that may prove fatal to the mother. AFLP occurs in approximately 1:10,000 pregnancies, but HELLP syndrome is much more common (0.5–1.0% of pregnancies) (93). The appropriate treatment is immediate delivery of the fetus, and this often results in rapid improvement in the mother; however, this means that offspring of these pregnancies are often quite premature and portends a high (20–50% in various studies) mortality rate. Among women who have AFLP, 10 to 25% will be carriers for the common LCHAD mutation and carry a fetus with LCHAD deficiency. LCHAD deficiency is much rarer in patients with HELLP, occurring in less than 1% of these families. This presentation is much more common in LCHAD or general TFP deficiency than in any other disorder of FAO. It is imperative to recognize that fetuses of mothers with AFLP should always be tested for LCHAD and other FAO disorders, as they are at high risk for these genetic diseases. Deaths in unrecognized offspring of AFLP or HELLP pregnancies have, unfortunately, been common.

More recently, pediatric LCHAD deficiency has become a common presentation on abnormal MS/MS newborn screening testing (96,97). Most of these infants are asymptomatic. It is imperative to initiate prospective treatment immediately to prevent morbidity and mortality. It is also critical, however, to note that MS/MS analysis may be normal or nondiagnostic in newborn screening, such that LCHAD deficiency have been missed in rare infants by using this approach, and they may present later in metabolic crisis or die suddenly (96).

Based on diagnosis of symptomatic infants, expanded newborn screening, and the incidence of the common mutation, it is estimated that isolated LCHAD deficiency in the United States and northern Europe probably occurs in approximately 1:100,000 to 200,000 births.

Investigation and Diagnosis The most common laboratory abnormalities leading to a suspected diagnosis of LCHAD deficiency are hypoglycemia and hypoketosis in the face of a history of prolonged, reduced caloric intake (89). During acute episodes, mildly elevated plasma liver enzymes, metabolic acidosis with lactic acidemia, mildly elevated ammonia, elevated CK, and elevated uric acid are very common, occurring in 50 to 90% of patients during an acute metabolic crisis. In infants with a cardiomyopathic onset, the electrocardiogram may show supraventricular tachycardia, ventricular tachycardia, ST-T wave changes, and left ventricular hypertrophy. The echocardiogram may exhibit either hypertrophic cardiomyopathy or, more commonly, severe dilated myocardiopathy with marked left ventricular systolic dysfunction. A rare presentation is acute pulmonary edema consistent with adult respiratory distress syndrome on a chest roentgenogram. The essential diagnostic finding is elevation of long-chain acylcarnitines on plasma MS/MS, including elevated C16 (palmitoyl)-carnitine, elevated 3-hydroxypalmitoylcarnitine, elevated C18 and 3-hydroxy-C18-carnitines, and elevated C18:1-hydroxycarnitine. Free carnitine is often reduced. It is imperative and crucial to understand that acylcarnitine analysis is most diagnostic when performed in an acutely ill patient. MS/MS, unfortunately, is often completely normal when the patients recover from acute episodes.

Enzyme assays performed in cultured cells, such as skin fibroblasts or transformed lymphoblasts, using palmitoyl-CoA as the substrate and measuring the reverse activity are highly specific and usually diagnostic (98). In isolated LCHAD deficiency, activities of LKAT are usually preserved in the range of 30 to 80% of normal. The same is true for long-chain enoyl-CoA hydratase activity. Accumulation of the long-chain acylcarnitines noted above, as assayed by MS/MS in cultured cells incubated with palmitate, is also a useful confirmatory test. Immunoblot analysis of α-subunit expression is available on a research basis and usually shows reduced levels to less than 30% of normal.

In 1994, two groups showed that isolated LCHAD deficiency was secondary to a common mutation in the α-subunit of the TFP, G1528C that altered glutamic acid at position 474 of the mature subunit protein to glutamine (10,95). This mutation is common among northern Europeans and Americans of northern European ancestry, with approximately 1:150 to 1:250 individuals being carriers. Approximately 65% of patients with isolated LCHAD deficiency are homozygous for this mutation, and the remainder are compound heterozygous for G1528 and a wide variety of other missense, splice site, deletion, and insertion mutations, many of which are not as yet expressed at the messenger RNA or protein levels. LCHAD's glutamic acid-474 is homologous to the glutamic acid-170 in SCHAD, which is known to occur within the enzymatic active site, thus explaining why this missense changes alters only LCHAD activity in the TFP complex (99). Patients with suspected LCHAD deficiency should always be tested for this mutation at the molecular level.

Treatment and Outcomes Unfortunately, young patients with LCHAD deficiency who present symptomatically often die during the acute episode or suffer from sudden, unexplained death. In a large study, the initial mortality rate was between 35 and 40% (89). Survivors are usually treated acutely with intravenous infusions of 5 to 10 mg/kg/min of glucose to reverse the metabolic crisis. Although intravenous carnitine has been advocated by some, it is probably contraindicated in this long-chain defect. Other supportive measures, such as inotropic agents for cardiac dysfunction, intubation and ventilation for respiratory insufficiency, and even extracorporeal membrane oxygenation for cardiogenic shock or acute respiratory distress syndrome, are essential. Even critically ill babies do have reversible cardiopulmonary failure (Table 5-1).

After recovery from an acute crisis, surviving patients should be treated with frequent feedings during infancy, often with overnight infusions of cornstarch or other carbohydrates by nasogastric tube or gastrostomy, and avoidance of fasting. Avoiding fasting is the single most critical aspect of early treatment. Reduction in long-chain fats in the diet may prove useful but is diffi-

cult to accomplish. More important, supplementation with MCT formulae bypasses the block caused by LCHAD and is efficacious in reducing the biochemical abnormalities and frequency of recurrent metabolic crises in some infants and toddlers (Table 5-2). Treatment with oral supplements of L-carnitine is controversial and not recommended by us. Recently, Harding and coworkers (90) have specifically advocated a diet of 10% long-chain fat, some provided as a vegetable oil as a source of essential and polyunsaturated fatty acids, 10 to 20% medium-chain fat, and the remainder as protein and carbohydrate. Supplementation with multivitamins, especially fat-soluble vitamins, seems reasonable.

Most surviving patients do well, but recurrent metabolic crises induced by reduced caloric intake are common in the first years of life. Psychomotor retardation and microcephaly, believed secondary to hypoglycemia and acute crises, occur in approximately 5% of symptomatic patients (89). Later, retinopathy (up to 70%) and peripheral neuropathy (~5–10%) may be noted and can become quite debilitating due to reduced visual acuity and weakness in older patients (92). Currently, studies in which docosahexaenoic acid is used in an attempt to prevent the retinopathy and neuropathy are underway (100).

As survivors become older, episodes of skeletal myopathy with weakness, massive elevations of serum CKs (often over 100,000), hypotonia, and severe pain commence. These may be precipitated by exercise, lack of adherence to the diet, or reduced caloric intake. Very rarely, renal dysfunction secondary to severe myoglobinuria has occurred. Treatment with high-dose intravenous glucose is usually efficacious in reversing these episodes. Because the oldest survivors with known LCHAD deficiency are still younger than 30 years of age, the long-term outcomes remains unknown; however, several such young adults are leading relatively normal lives and have excellent cognitive function.

MS/MS newborn screening has detected isolated LCHAD deficiency in a few infants (97). In addition, prenatal fetal diagnosis of LCHAD deficiency in families with a previously diagnosed LCHAD-deficient sibling has occurred. To date, preventive treatment with frequent feedings, avoidance of fasting, supplementation with MCTs, and careful monitoring during infectious illnesses has documented that complete prevention of metabolic crises can be accomplished. Long term follow up will be essential to determine the degree of efficacy of this preventive treatment.

COMPLETE TRIFUNCTIONAL PROTEIN DEFICIENCY

Etiology and Pathophysiology As noted in the LCHAD section, TFP is a heterooctameric complex of four α- and four β-subunits (Figure 5-2). The subunits are encoded by two genes on chromosome 2 that are transcriptionally coordinately regulated. General or complete TFP deficiency is defined and occurs when markedly decreased activity of all three enzymatic components, LCHAD, long-chain 2,3-enoyl-CoA hydratase, and LKAT, exists.

Clinical Features We have chosen to separate descriptions of isolated LCHAD deficiency from general or complete TFP deficiency because the clinical manifestations and outcomes do differ to some extent and because TFP deficiency is much more rare, or, at least, much less commonly recognized. The most common manifestation of TFP deficiency is later-onset, episodic, recurrent skeletal myopathy with muscular pain and weakness, often induced by exercise or exposure to cold and peripheral neuropathy (98,101). The onset may be quite early, within the first 5 years of life, but is usually only diagnosed later, often after the second decade. These patients do not have hypoglycemia or cardiomyopathy. A second presentation, the one originally recognized, is neonatal onset of lethal cardiac failure or sudden death due to arrhythmias (91,98). Although some of these infants also have hypoglycemia, the cardiac manifestations predominate. Severe respiratory compromise has been observed. A few patients have presented with metabolic crises virtually identical to isolated LCHAD deficiency, within the first 6 months of life. It is noteworthy that these three types of presentations are quite similar to those of VLCAD described previously.

It is important to note that fetuses with complete TFP deficiency can cause maternal liver diseases of pregnancy, including AFLP or the HELLP syndrome (91,93,94,98). Although it appears, from limited data, that the incidence among TFP families is lower than those with LCHAD deficiency, this remains an issue and suggests that acylcarnitine MS/MS analysis should be performed in the offspring of all women with AFLP.

Investigation and Diagnosis The diagnosis should be suspected among infants with severe cardiomyopathy or unexplained tachyarrhythmias, especially with severe metabolic acidosis and hypoketotic hypoglycemia. The same abnormalities as in the infantile presentations of LCHAD and VLCAD deficiencies are present, namely metabolic and lactic acidosis, hyperuricemia, hypoglycemia, inappropriate hypoketosis, and marked elevations of CK. Tachyarrhythmias and dilated cardiomyopathy with cardiogenic shock are common. The key diagnostic test is analysis of plasma acylcarnitines, which show elevated C16 and C18 species, often with some 3-hydroxyacylcarnitine species. The profiles of general or complete TFP deficiency and isolated LCHAD deficiency overlap and may be indistinguishable. It is imperative to recognize that acylcarnitine analysis may be normal when patients are asymptomatic. For that reason, it is essential to obtain samples during the acute illness. Because of this overlap, enzymatic and molecular diagnoses are needed to distinguish isolated LCHAD deficiency from general TFP deficiency. Enzyme assays of cultured skin fibroblasts or lymphoblasts do reveal marked reductions, usually to less than 10% of normal, of LKAT and, when performed, of long-chain 2,3-enoyl-CoA hydratase (98). These assays, unfortunately, are only available on a research basis in the United States. Immunoblot studies usually confirm that there is less than 20% expression of both α-subunit (LCHAD) and β-subunit (long-chain thiolase) antigen.

Molecular analysis is only available on a research basis. Mutations in either subunit result in general or complete TFP deficiency (101). There is no common mutation; however, infantile-onset patients always exhibit at least one null mutation, usually a splicing consensus site abnormality, premature termination codon mutations, or frameshift deletion (98). Older patients with the rhabdomyolysis phenotype almost always are compound heterozygous with two missense mutations.

Treatment and Outcomes Treatment is the same as for isolated LCHAD deficiency and for VLCAD deficiency, namely, avoidance of fasting, reduced long-chain fat intake, supplementation with MCTs, supplementation with fat-soluble vitamins, and avoidance of other potential stressors such as prolonged exercise (Tables 5-1 and 5-2). The rare patients with the severe infantile onset and β-subunit have all died from myocardial failure or respiratory failure, even when the diagnosis was known prenatally in families with a previously diagnosed sibling who died. Patients with metabolic crisis do well, unless the hypoglycemia and seizures are prolonged and cause developmental delay. Older onset patients with rhabdomyolysis can usually reduce episodes significantly with dietary management and do well. As with all other FAO disorders, very few individuals older than the age of 30 exist, so the long-term outlook is uncertain.

GLUTARIC ACIDEMIA TYPE 2

Etiology and Pathophysiology The transfer of electrons from the 2,3 positions of a number of important energy-providing substrates requires the concerted activities of both ETF, a mitochondrial matrix protein, and ETF-QO, which is inner mitochondrial membrane bound and associated with coenzyme Q of the respiratory chain. Enzymes that require ETF and ETF-QO include VLCAD, LCAD, MCAD, SCAD of the FAO pathway; glutaryl-CoA dehydrogenase of the lysine- and tryptophan-metabolizing pathway at least three dehydrogenases involved with branched-chain amino acid metabolism; and two enzymes involved with N-methyl dehydrogenation of sarcosine and dimethylglycine (101). Impairment of either ETF or ETF-QO results in failure of all of these important pathways and potentially of other pathways that are not yet as well characterized (45).

With GA2 deficiency, impairment of FAO occurs at all chain lengths such that metabolic markers consistent with VLCAD, MCAD, and SCAD deficiencies may all be elevated despite normal levels and kinetics of these enzymes. Defective FAO results in hypoketotic hypoglycemia associated with the cardiomyopathy, skeletal myopathy, and hepatic encephalopathy that are seen in the FAO defects.

Impairment of glutaryl-CoA dehydrogenase in the lysine- and tryptophan-degradative pathway results in accumulation of glutaric acid, from which the name GA2 is derived. The glutarate accumulation in GA2 differs from that in primary glutaryl-CoA dehydrogenase deficiency (GA1) in that 2-hydroxyglutarate accompanies it. In GA1, the glutarate accumulation is associated with 3-hydroxyglutarate. The 2-hydroxyglutarate accumulation seen in GA2 may be a product of a separate ETF-dependent D-2-hydroxyglutarate dehydrogenase enzyme.

Accumulation of isovaleryl-CoA resulting from impaired isovaleryl-CoA dehydrogenase in the leucine-degradative pathway results in metabolic acidosis and the characteristic sweaty feet odor of isovaleric academia in patients with GA2, making this an important clinical differential to establish, as treatment for isovaleric acidemia is different to that of GA2.

Clinical Features Three distinct presentations have been described for GA2 (102). The earliest descriptions of the disease were of a fatal, neonatal presentation with multiorgan failure, hepatic encephalopathy, cardiomyopathy, muscular weakness, renal tubular acidosis, hypoglycemia, metabolic acidosis, and the characteristic odor of sweaty feet. At autopsy, dysgenesis of the brain and kidney is frequently identified, along with more cardinal signs of the failure of FAO, including massive lipid deposition in liver and other organs. This form of GA2 is known as type I. Type II describes an equally severe neonatal onset but without the profound dysmorphology. Short-term survival of these patients has been reported if a sufficiently early diagnosis can be made but these patients frequently succumb in early life to fatal metabolic decompensation (103). Type III GA2 describes a milder late-onset form of GA2, which may present with stress-induced hepatic encephalopathy, similar to that seen in some of the primary disorders of FAO. Stresses that induce a catabolic event include fasting, febrile illness, cold, and muscular exertion. Adult presentation with muscle disease including rhabdomyolysis, without hepatic involvement, has been reported for type III. All forms of GA2 are inherited in an autosomal recessive manner.

Investigation and Diagnosis GA2 typically presents with a characteristic organic aciduria with increased excretion of numerous metabolites, reflecting multiple pathway involvement. Abnormalities of FAO are reflected by C4–C18 dicarboxylic aciduria with detectable butyryl-, hexanoyl-, and suberylglycines to represent markers of the different chain lengths of fatty acids. Other metabolites include glutaric acid, for which the disorder is named, isovaleryl-, isobutyryl, and 2-methyl-butyrylglycine and, in a poorly defined variant of GA2, EMA (this variant is also known as ethylmalonic-adipic aciduria). Many of the compounds that are excreted as their acylglycine conjugates may also be found as the respective acylcarnitine derivatives in plasma. Carnitine deficiency may be present in GA2, and this may reduce the sensitivity but not the specificity of acylcarnitine measurement.

Elevated sarcosine is present in serum in the most severe cases but may be absent in type III. In some patients with type III GA2, the biochemical abnormalities may only be seen during the intermittent periods of metabolic decompensation, making it very critical to collect samples when the patient is in a catabolic phase. Both ETF and ETF-QO activities can be measured in a variety of tissues including skin fibroblasts and amniocytes. There is a clear correlation between the residual activity and clinical phenotype. In type I GA2, there is no measurable enzyme activity. In type II there is a small amount of residual activity, which appears to be sufficient to prevent developmental abnormalities but not the metabolic consequences. Type III characteristically has high residual activity; in some cases, the baseline activity has been estimated at over 50% of normal but these proteins were found to be thermolabile, resulting in more significantly reduced activity at high temperatures such as those encountered during exercise or a febrile illness.

The genes for both the α- and β- subunits of ETF and ETF-QO have been cloned. ETFA is localized to chromosome 15q23-25, ETFB to 19q13.3, and ETFQO to 4q32-ter. Mutations in all three genes that result in GA2 have been identified and a genotype: phenotype correlation has been proposed for all three proteins (104). Most families have private mutations in the genes that are involved in GA2, making a molecular diagnostic approach to diagnosis difficult. Enzymatic analysis of ETF and ETF-QO activities is presently recommended as a prerequisite to targeted molecular analysis of the abnormal enzyme.

Treatment and Outcomes Type I GA2 inevitably results in neonatal death within the first few days of life. Presently there are no treatment options. Treatment of acute symptoms in both type II and III forms is similar to treatment of acute presentations of FAO defects, described earlier in this chapter, and also of isovaleric acidemia and glutaric acidemia, which are described in Chapter 7. Long-term success has not been reported for type II, and most patients die in early infancy. The combination of multiple pathway involvement and susceptibility to acute metabolic crises make GA2 a very difficult disorder to manage. Because ETF and ETF-QO are flavoproteins, long-term treatment with high-dose riboflavin (100–300 mg/day) has been attempted and, in some of the type III cases, has been successful. High-dose carnitine is frequently given to patients but there is no evidence of improved outcome. All forms of GA2 can be diagnosed prenatally by using a combination of ultrasonography for the dysmorphic changes, metabolic flux, enzymatic and molecular assays on amniocytes, and organic acid measurement in amniotic fluid. Molecular prenatal diagnosis is the most practical in terms of gestational time course but requires prior knowledge of the mutations in an index case (105).

REFERENCES

1. Treem WR, Stanley CA, Finegold DN, et al. Primary carnitine deficiency due to a failure of carnitine transport in kidney, muscle, and fibroblasts. *N Engl J Med.* 1988; 319:1331–1336.
2. Rinaldo P, Stanley CA, Hsu BY, et al. Sudden neonatal death in carnitine transporter deficiency. *J Pediatr.* 1997;134:304–305.
3. Nezu J, Tamai I, Oku A, et al. Primary systemic carnitine deficiency is caused by mutations in a gene encoding sodium-dependent carnitine transporter. *Nat Genet.* 1999;21:91–94.
4. Wang Y, Korman SH, Ye J, et al. Phenotype and genotype variation in primary carnitine deficiency. *Genet Med.* 2001;3:387–92.
5. Stanley CA, Hale DE, Berry GT, et al. A deficiency of carnitine-acylcarnitine translocase in the inner mitochondrial membrane. *N Engl J Med.* 1992;327:19–23.
6. Cederbaum SD, Koo-McCoy S, Tein I, et al. Carnitine membrane transporter deficiency: a long-term follow up and OCTN2 mutation in the first documented case of primary carnitine deficiency. *Mol Genet Metab.* 2002;77:195–201.
7. Wilcken B, Wiley V, Sim KG, et al. Carnitine transporter defect diagnosed by newborn screening with tandem mass spectrometry. *J Pediatr.* 2001;138:581–584.
8. Brown NF, Mullur RS, Subramanian I, et al. Molecular characterization of L-CPT 1 deficiency in six patients: insights into function of the native enzyme. *J Lip Res.* 2001;42:1134.
9. Innes AM, Seargeant LE, Balachandra K, et al. Hepatic carnitine palmitoyltransferase 1 deficiency presenting as maternal illness in pregnancy. *Pediatr Res.* 2000;47:43–45.
10. IJlst L, Ruiter JP, Hoovers JM, et al. Common missense mutation G1528C in LCHAD deficiency. Characterization and expression of the mutant protein, mutation analysis on genomic DNA and chromosomal localization of the mitochondrial trifunctional protein alpha subunit gene. *J Clin Invest.* 1996;98:1028–1033.
11. Gobin S, Bonnefont J-P, Prip-Buus C, et al. Organization of the human liver carnitine palmitoyltransferase 1 gene (CPT1A) and identification of novel mutations in hypoketotic hypoglycemia. *Hum Genet.* 2002;111:179–189
12. Bennett MJ, Boriack RL, Narayan S, et al. Novel mutations in *CPT1A* define molecular heterogeneity of hepatic carnitine palmitoyltransferase 1 deficiency. *Mol Genet Metab.* 2004;82:59–63.
13. Prasad C, Johnson JP, Bonnefont JP, et al. Hepatic carnitine palmitoyltransferase 1 (CPT1A) deficiency in North American Hutterites (Canadian and American): evidence for a founder effect and results of a pilot study on a DNA-based newborn screening program. *Mol Genet Metab.* 2001;73:55–63.
14. Lopriore E, Gemke RJ, Verhoeven NM, et al. Carnitine-acylcarnitine translocase deficiency: phenotype, residual enzyme activity and outcome. *Eur J Pediatr.* 2001;160:101–104.
15. Iacobazzi V, Pasquali M, Singh R, et al. Response to therapy in carnitine/acylcarnitine translocase (CACT) deficiency due to a novel missense mutation. *Am J Med Genet.* 2004;126:150–55.
16. Sigauke E, Rakheja D, Kitson K, et al. Carnitine palmitoyltransferase II deficiency: a clinical, biochemical, and molecular review. *Lab Invest.* 2003;83:1543–1554.
17. Thuillier L, Rostane H, Droin V, et al. Correlation between genotype, metabolic data, and clinical presentation in carnitine palmitoyltransferase 2 (CPT2) deficiency. *Hum Mutat.* 2003;21:493–501.
18. Olpin SE, Afifi A, Clark S, et al. Mutation and biochemical analysis in carnitine palmitoyltransferase type II (CPT II) deficiency. *J Inherit Metab Dis.* 2003;26:543–557.
19. Walter JH. L-Carnitine in inborn errors of metabolism. What is the evidence? *J Inherit Metab Dis.* 2003;26:181–188.
20. Andresen BS, Olpin S, Poorthuis BJ, et al. Clear correlation of genotype with disease phenotype in very-long-chain acyl-CoA dehydrogenase deficiency. *Am J Hum Genet.* 1999;64(2):479–494.
21. Vianey-Saban C, Divry P, Brivet M, et al. Mitochondrial very-long-chain acyl-coenzyme A dehydrogenase deficiency: clinical characteristics and diagnostic considerations in 30 patients. *Clin Chim Acta.* 1998;269:43–62.
22. Cairns AP, O'Donoghue PM, Patterson VH, et al. Very-long-chain acyl-coenzyme A dehydrogenase deficiency—a new cause of myoglobinuric acute renal failure. *Nephrol Dial Transplant.* 2000;15(8):1232–1234.
23. Roe DS, Vianey-Saban C, Sharma S, et al. Oxidation of unsaturated fatty acids by human fibroblasts with very-long-chain acyl-CoA dehydrogenase deficiency: aspects of substrate specificity and correlation with clinical phenotype. *Clin Chim Acta.* 2001;312(1-2):55–67.
24. Browning MF, Larson C, Strauss A, et al. Normal acylcarnitine levels during confirmation of abnormal newborn screening in long-chain FAO defects. *J Inherit Metab Dis.* 2005;28(4):545–550.
25. Boneh A, Andresen BS, Gregersen N, et al. VLCAD deficiency: Pitfalls in newborn screening and confirmation of diagnosis by mutation analysis. *Mol Genet Metab.* 2006;88(2):166–170.
26. Nada MA, Vianey-Saban C, Roe CR, et al. Prenatal diagnosis of mitochondrial fatty acid oxidation defects. *Prenat Diagn.* 1996;16:117–124.
27. Olpin SE, Manning NJ, Pollitt RJ, et al. Improved detection of long-chain fatty acid oxidation defects in intact cells using [9,10-3H]oleic acid. *J Inherit Metab Dis.* 1997;20:415–419.
28. Andresen BS, Bross P, Vianey-Saban C, et al. Cloning and characterization of human very-long-chain acyl-CoA dehydrogenase cDNA, chromosomal assignment of the gene and identification in four patients of 9 different mutations within this gene. *Hum Mol Genet.* 1996;5:461–472 (erratum, p 1390).
29. Strauss AW, Powell CK, Hale DE, et al. Molecular basis of human mitochondrial very-long-chain acyl-CoA dehydrogenase deficiency causing cardiomyopathy and sudden death in childhood. *Proc Natl Acad Sci USA.* 1995;92(23):10496–10500.
30. Mathur A, Sims HF, Gopalakrishnan D, et al. Molecular heterogeneity in very-long-chain acyl-CoA dehydrogenase deficiency causing pediatric cardiomyopathy and sudden death. *Circulation.* 999;99(10): 1337–1343.
31. Spiekerkoetter U, Sun B, Zytkovicz T, et al. MS/MS-based newborn and family screening detects asymptomatic patients with very-long-chain acyl-CoA

dehydrogenase deficiency. *J Pediatr.* 2003; 143(3):335–342.

32. Cox GF, Souri M, Aoyama T, et al. Reversal of severe hypertrophic cardiomyopathy and excellent neuropsychologic outcome in very-long-chain acyl-coenzyme A dehydrogenase deficiency. *J Pediatr.* 1998;133(2):247–253.

33. Spiekerkotter U, Schwahn B, Korall H, et al. Very-long-chain acyl-coenzyme A dehydrogenase (VLCAD) deficiency: monitoring of treatment by carnitine/acylcarnitine analysis in blood spots. *Acta Paediatr.* 2000;89(4):492–495.

34. Touma EH, Rashed MS, Vianey-Saban C, et al. A severe genotype with favourable outcome in very long chain acyl-CoA dehydrogenase deficiency. *Arch Dis Child.* 2001;84(1):58–60.

35. Roe CR, Sweetman L, Roe DS, et al. Treatment of cardiomyopathy and rhabdomyolysis in long-chain fat oxidation disorders using an anaplerotic odd-chain triglyceride. *J Clin Invest.* 2002;110(2):259–269.

36. Andresen BS, Olpin S, Kvittingen EA, et al. DNA-based prenatal diagnosis for very-long-chain acyl-CoA dehydrogenase deficiency. *J Inherit Metab Dis.* 1999;22(3):281–285.

37. Gregersen N, Lauritzen R, Rasmussen K. Suberylglycine excretion in urine from a patient with dicarboxylic aciduria. *Clin Chim Acta.* 1976;70:417–425.

38. Andresen BS, Dobrowolski SF, O'Reilly L, et al. Medium-chain acyl-CoA dehydrogenase (MCAD) mutations identified by MS/MS-based prospective screening of newborns differ from those observed in patients with clinical symptoms: identification and characterization of a new, prevalent mutation that results in mild MCAD deficiency. *Am J Hum Genet.* 2001;68(6):1408–1418.

39. Maier EM, Liebl B, Roschinger W, et al. Population spectrum of ACADM genotypes correlated to biochemical phenotypes in newborn screening for medium-chain acyl-CoA dehydrogenase deficiency. *Hum Mutat.* 2005;25(5):443–452.

40. Tajima G, Sakura N, Yofune H, et al. Enzymatic diagnosis of medium-chain acyl-CoA dehydrogenase deficiency by detecting 2-octenoyl-CoA production using high-performance liquid chromatography: a practical confirmatory test for tandem mass spectrometry newborn screening in Japan. *J Chromatogr B Analyt Technol Biomed Life Sci.* 2005;823(2):122–130.

41. Wilcken B, Wiley V, Hammond J, et al. Screening newborns for inborn errors of metabolism by tandem mass spectrometry. *N Engl J Med.* 2003;348:2304–2312.

42. Derks TG, Duran M, Waterham HR, et al. The difference between observed and expected prevalence of MCAD deficiency in the Netherlands: a genetic epidemiological study. *Eur J Hum Genet.* 2005;13:947–952.

43. Andresen BS, Bross P, Jensen TG, et al. A rare disease-associated mutation in the gene for Medium Chain Acyl-CoA dehydrogenase (MCAD) changes a conserved arginine residue previously shown to be functionally essential in Short-Chain Acyl-CoA dehydrogenase (SCAD). *Am J Hum Genet.* 1993;53:730–739.

44. Korman SH, Gutman A, Brooks R, et al. Homozygosity for a severe novel medium-chain acyl-CoA dehydrogenase (MCAD) mutation IVS3-1G>C that leads to introduction of a premature termination codon by complete missplicing of the MCAD mRNA and is associated with phenotypic diversity ranging from sudden neonatal death to asymptomatic status. *Mol Genet Metab.* 2004;82(2):121–129.

45. Ensenauer R, Winters JL, Parton PA, et al. Genotypic differences of MCAD deficiency in the Asian population: novel genotype and clinical symptoms preceding newborn screening notification. *Genet Med.* 2005;7(5):339–343.

46. Touma EH, Charpentier C. Medium-chain acyl-CoA dehydrogenase deficiency. *Arch Dis Child.* 1992;67(1):142–145.

47. Iafolla AK, Thompson RJ, Roe CR. Medium-chain acyl-coenzyme A dehydrogenase deficiency: clinical course in 120 affected children. *J Pediatr.* 1994;124:409–415.

48. Waddell L, Wiley V, Carpenter K, et al. Medium-chain acyl-CoA dehydrogenase deficiency: genotype – biochemical phenotype correlations. *Mol Genet Metab.* 2006;87(1):32–39.

49. Feillet F, Steinmann G, Vianey-Saban C, et al. Adult presentation of MCAD deficiency revealed by coma and severe arrythmias [sic]. *Intensive Care Med.* 2003;29(9):1594–1597.

50. Ruitenbeek W, Poels PJ, Turnbull DM, et al. Rhabdomyolysis and acute encephalopathy in late onset medium chain acyl-CoA dehydrogenase deficiency. *J Neurol Neurosurg Psychiatry.* 1995;58(2):209–214.

51. Wilhem GW. Sudden death in a young woman from medium chain acyl-coenzyme A dehydrogenase (MCAD) deficiency. *J Emerg Med.* 2006;30(3):291–294.

52. Rinaldo P, O'Shea JJ, Coates PM, et al. Medium-chain acyl-CoA dehydrogenase deficiency: diagnosis by stable-isotope dilution measurement of urinary n-hexanoylglycine and 3-phenylpropionylglycine. *N Engl J Med.* 1988;319:1308–1313.

53. Van Hove JL, Zhang W, Kahler SG, et al. Medium-chain acyl-CoA dehydrogenase (MCAD) deficiency: diagnosis by acylcarnitine analysis in blood. *Am J Hum Genet.* 1993;52(5):958–966.

54. Matsubara Y, Kraus JP, Yang-Feng TL, et al. Molecular cloning of cDNAs encoding rat and human medium-chain acyl-CoA dehydrogenase and assignment of the gene to human chromosome 1. *Proc Nat Acad Sci USA.* 1986;83:6543–6547.

55. Zhang Z, Kelly DP, Kim J-J, et al. Structural organization and regulatory regions of the human medium-chain acyl-CoA dehydrogenase gene. *Biochemistry.* 1992;31:81–89.

56. Tanaka K, Yokota I, Coates PM, et al. Mutations in the Medium-Chain Acyl-CoA Dehydrogenase (MCAD) gene. *Hum Mutat.* 1992;1:271–279.

57. Tanaka K, Gregersen N, Ribes A, et al. A survey of the newborn populations in Belgium, Germany, Poland, Czech Republic, Hungary, Bulgaria, Spain, Turkey, and Japan for the G985 variant allele with haplotype analysis at the medium chain Acyl-CoA dehydro-

genase gene locus: clinical and evolutionary consideration. *Pediatr Res.* 1997;41:201–209.

58. Morris AA, Taylor RW, Lightowlers RN, et al. Medium chain acyl-CoA dehydrogenase deficiency caused by a deletion of exons 11 and 12. *Hum Mol Genet.* 1995;4(4):747–749.

59. Zschocke J, Schulze A, Lindner M, et al. Molecular and functional characterisation of mild MCAD deficiency. *Hum Genet.* 2001;108(5):404–408.

60. Andresen BS, Bross P, Udvari S, et al. The molecular basis of medium-chain acyl-CoA dehydrogenase (MCAD) deficiency in compound heterozygous patients: Is there correlation between genotype and phenotype? *Hum Mol Genet.* 1997;6:695–707.

61. O'Reilly L, Bross P, Corydon TJ, et al. The Y42H mutation in medium-chain acyl-CoA dehydrogenase (MCAD), which is prevalent in babies identified by MS/MS based newborn screening, is temperature sensitive. *Eur J Biochemistry.* 2004;271(20):4053–4063.

62. Bennett MJ, Allison F, Lowther GW, et al. Prenatal diagnosis of medium-chain acyl-coenzyme A dehydrogenase deficiency. *Prenat Diagn.* 1987;7:135–141.

63. Gregersen N, Winter V, Jensen PK, et al. Prenatal diagnosis of medium-chain acyl-CoA dehydrogenase (MCAD) deficiency in a family with a previous fatal case of sudden unexpected death in childhood. *Prenat Diagn.* 1995;15(1):82–86.

64. Amendt BA, Greene C, Sweetman L, et al. Short-chain acyl-coenzyme A dehydrogenase deficiency: clinical and biochemical studies in two patients. *J Clin Invest.* 1987;79: 1303–1309.

65. Seidel J, Streck S, Bellstedt K, et al. Recurrent vomiting and ethylmalonic aciduria associated with rare mutations in the short-chain acyl-CoA dehydrogenase (SCAD) gene. *J Inher Metab Dis.* 2003;26:37–42.

66. Kurian MA, Hartley L, Zolkipli Z, et al. Short-chain acyl-CoA dehydrogenase deficiency associated with early onset severe axonal neuropathy. *Neuropediatrics.* 2004;35:312–316.

67. Bok LA, Vreken P, Wijburg FA, et al. Short-chain Acyl-CoA dehydrogenase deficiency: studies in a large family adding to the complexity of the disorder. *Pediatrics.* 2003;112(5):1152–1155.

68. Matern D, Hart P, Murtha AP, et al. Acute fatty liver of pregnancy associated with short-chain acyl-coenzyme A dehydrogenase deficiency. *J Pediatr.* 2001;138(4):585–588.

69. Koeberl DD, Young SP, Gregersen N, et al. Rare disorders of metabolism with elevated butyryl- and isobutyryl-carnitine detected by tandem mass spectrometry newborn screening. *Pediatr Res.* 2003;54:219–223.

70. Pedersen CB, Bischoff C, Christensen E, et al. Variations in IBD (ACAD8) in children with elevated C4-carnitine detected by tandem mass spectrometry newborn screening. *Pediatr Res.* 2006;60(3):315–320.

71. Corydon MJ, Vockley J, Rinaldo P, et al. Role of common gene variations in the molecular pathogenesis of short-chain acyl-CoA dehydrogenase deficiency. *Pediatr Res.* 2001;49:18–23.

72. Young SP, Matern D, Gregersen N, et al. A comparison of in vitro acylcarnitine profiling

methods for the diagnosis of classical and variant short chain acyl-CoA dehydrogenase deficiency. *Clin Chim Acta.* 2003;337:103–113.

73. Naito E, Ozasa H, Ikeda Y, et al. Molecular cloning and nucleotide sequence of complementary DNAs encoding human short chain acyl-coenzyme A dehydrogenase and the study of the molecular basis of human short chain acyl-coenzyme A dehydrogenase deficiency. *J Clin Invest.* 1989;83:1605–1613.

74. Corydon MJ, Andresen BS, Bross P, et al. Structural organization of the human short-chain acyl-CoA dehydrogenase gene. *Mamm Genome.* 1997;8:922–926.

75. Nagan N, Kruckeberg KE, Tauscher AL, et al. The frequency of short-chain acyl-CoA dehydrogenase gene variants in the US population and correlation with the C(4)-acylcarnitine concentration in newborn blood spots. *Mol Genet Metab.* 2003;78:239–246.

76. Gregersen N, Winter V, Corydon MJ, et al. Identification of four new mutations in the short-chain acyl-CoA dehydrogenase (SCAD) gene in two patients: one of the variant alleles, 511C>T, is present at an unexpectedly high frequency in the normal population, as was the case for 625G>A, together conferring succptibility to cthylmalonic aciduria. *Hum Mol Genet.* 1998;7:619–627.

77. Pedersen CB, Bross P, Winter VS, et al. Misfolding, degradation, and aggregation of variant proteins. The molecular pathogenesis of short chain acyl-CoA dehydrogenase (SCAD) deficiency. *J Biol Chem.* 2003;278:47449–47458.

78. Vredendaal PJ, van den Berg IE, Malingre HE, et al. Cloning and characterization of the coding sequence. *Biochem Biophys Res Comm.* 1996;223:718–723.

79. O'Brien LK, Sims HF, Bennett MJ, et al. A mouse model for medium and short chain L-3-hydroxy-acyl-CoA dehydrogenase deficiency. *J Inherit Metab Dis.* 2000;23:127. (Abstract).

80. Barycki JJ. Biochemical characterization and crystal structure determination of human heart SCHAD provide insights into catalytic mechanism. *Biochemistry.* 1999;38:5786–5798.

81. Tein I, De Vivo DC, Hale DE, et al. SCHAD deficiency in muscle: a new cause for recurrent myoglobinuria and encephalopathy. *Ann Neurol.* 1991;30:415–419.

82. Bennett MJ, Weinberger MJ, Kobori JA, et al. Mitochondrial SCHAD deficiency. *Pediatr Res.* 1999;39:185–188.

83. Clayton PT, Eaton S, Aynsley-Green A, et al. Hyperinsulinism in short-chain L-3-hydroxy-acyl-CoA dehydrogenase deficiency reveals the importance of β-oxidation in insulin secretion. *J Clin Invest.* 2001;108:457–465.

84. Hussain K, Clayton PT, Krywawych S, et al. Hyperinsulinism of infancy associated with a novel splice site mutation in the SCHAD gene. *J Pediatr.* 2005;146:706–708.

85. Molven A, Matre GE, Duran M, et al. Familial hyperinsulinemic hypoglycemia caused by a defect in the SCHAD enzyme of mitochondrial fatty acid oxidation. *Diabetes.* 2004;53:221–227.

86. Wanders RJA Duran M, Ijlst L, et al. Sudden infant death and LCHAD. *Lancet.* 1989;2:52–53.

87. Uchida Y, Izai K, Orii T, et al. Novel fatty acid β-oxidation enzymes in rat liver. *J Biol Chem.* 1992;267:1034–1041.

88. Jackson S, Kler RS, Bartlett K, et al. Combined enzyme defect of mitochondrial fatty acid oxidation. *J Clin Invest.* 1992;90:1219–1225.

89. Den Boer MEJ, Wanders RJA, Morris AAM, et al. LCHAD deficiency: clinical Presentation and follow-up of 50 patients. *Pediatrics.* 2002;109:99–104.

90. Gillingham MB, Connor WE, Matern D, et al. Optimal dietary therapy of LCHAD deficiency. *Mol Genet Metab.* 2003;79:114–123.

91. Ibdah JA, Bennett MJ, Rinaldo P, et al. A fetal fatty acid oxidation disorder as a cause of liver disease in pregnant women. *N Engl J Med.* 1999;340:1723–1731.

92. Tyni T, Kivela T, Lappi M, et al. Ophthalmologic findings in LCHAD deficiency caused by the G1528C mutation. *Ophthalmology.* 1998;105:820–824.

93. Riely CA. Hepatic disease in the pregnant patient. *Am J Gastroenterol.* 1999;94:1728–1732.

94. Wilcken B, Leung KC, Hammond J, et al. Pregnancy and fetal LCHAD deficiency. *Lancet.* 1993;341:407–408.

95. Sims HF, Brackett JC, Powell CK, et al. The molecular basis of pediatric long chain 3-hydroxyacyl-CoA dehydrogenase deficiency associated with maternal acute fatty liver of pregnancy. *Proc Natl Acad Sci USA.* 1995;92:841–845.

96. Fearing M, Larson C, Strauss AW, et al. Normal acyl-carnitine levels during confirmation of abnormal newborn screening in long-chain fatty acid oxidation defects. *J Inherit Metab Dis.* 2005;28:1–6.

97. Sander J, Sander S, Steuerwald U, et al. Neonatal screening for defects of the mitochondrial trifunctional protein. *Mol Genet Metab.* 2005;85:108–114.

98. Spiekerkoetter U, Sun B, Khuchua Z, et al. Molecular and phenotypic heterogeneity in mitochondrial trifunctional protein deficiency due to β-subunit mutations. *Hum Mutat.* 2003;21:598–607.

99. Barycki JJ, O'Brien LK, Strauss AW, et al. Glutamate 170 of human L-3- hydroxyacyl CoA dehydrogenase is required for proper orientation of the catalytic histidine and structural integrity of the enzyme. *J Biol Chem.* 2001;276:36718–36726.

100. Harding CO, Gillingham MB, van Calcar SC, et al. Docosahexaenoic acid and retinal function in children with long-chain 3-hydroxyacyl-CoA dehydrogenase deficiency. *J Inherit Metab Dis.* 1999;22:276–280.

101. Spiekerkoetter U, Khuchua Z, Yue Z, et al. General mitochondrial trifunctional protein deficiency as a result of either α or β-subunit mutations exhibits similar phenotypes because mutations in either subunit alter TFP complex expression and subunit turnover. *Pediatr Res.* 2004;55:190–196.

102. Frerman FE, Goodman SI. Defects of electron transfer flavoprotein and electron transfer protein ubiquinone oxidoreductase: glutaric academia type II, in Scriver CR, Beaudet AL, Sly WS, Valle D (eds.): *The Metabolic and Molecular Bases of Inherited Disease*, 8th ed. New York: McGraw-Hill, 2001; pp 2357–2365.

103. Bennett MJ, Curnock DA, Engel P, et al. Glutaric aciduria type II: biochemical investigation and treatment of a child diagnosed prenatally. *J Inherit Metab Dis.* 1984;7:57–61.

104. Olsen RKJ, Andresen BS, Christensen E, et al. Clear relationship between ETF/ETFDH genotype and phenotype in patients with multiple acyl-CoA dehydrogenation deficiency. *Hum Mutat.* 2003;22:12–23.

105. Olsen RKJ, Andresen BS, Christensen E, et al. DNA-based prenatal diagnosis for severe and variant forms of multiple acyl-CoA dehydrogenation deficiency. *Prenat Diagn.* 2005;25:60–64.

CHAPTER 6

Glycogen Storage Diseases

David A. Weinstein, MD, MMSc
Karl S. Roth, MD
Joseph I. Wolfsdorf, MB, BCh

INTRODUCTION

Etiology and Pathophysiology The glycogen storage diseases (GSD) comprise several inherited diseases caused by abnormalities of the enzymes that regulate glycogen synthesis and degradation (1,2). Glycogen is stored principally in the liver and muscle. Muscle lacks glucose-6-phosphatase (G6Pase) and, therefore, is unable to release glucose for systemic use. Hypoglycemia is the primary manifestation of the hepatic glycogenoses, whereas weakness and muscle cramps are the predominant features of the muscle glycogenoses. This chapter will focus principally on clinical aspects of the hepatic glycogenoses.

After a meal, glucose is stored as glycogen, a complex, insoluble, highly branched polymer that allows efficient storage and release of glucose. The liver is freely permeable to glucose, which is rapidly phosphorylated by glucokinase to form glucose-6-phosphate. Glucose-6-phosphate is subsequently converted to glucose-1-phosphate, the starting point for glycogen synthesis. Glycogen synthase creates chains of glucose molecules by catalyzing the formation of α-1,4-linkages. A branching enzyme forms α-1,6-linkages approximately every 10 glucose units along the chain. In between meals, glycogen is degraded by the sequential action of two enzymes: hepatic glycogen phosphorylase and debranching enzyme. Debranching enzyme has two enzymatic activities: transferase and amylo-1,6-glucosidase activity. Glycogen phosphorylase is the rate-limiting enzyme in glycogenolysis, which hydrolyzes the α-1,4-linkages from the outer branches of glycogen until only four glucosyl units remain distal to the α-1,6 branch point. Then the debranching enzyme through its transferase activity transfers three of the glucosyl residues to the outer end of an adjacent chain and through its amylo-1,6-glucosidase activity of the same enzyme hydrolyses the branch point glucose residue (see Figure 6-1).

G6Pase catalyzes the terminal reaction of glycogenolysis and gluconeogenesis, the hydrolysis of glucose-6-phosphate to glucose and inorganic phosphate in hepatocytes and renal epithelial cells, allowing glucose to be released into the systemic circulation.

HEPATIC GLYCOGEN SYNTHASE DEFICIENCY (TYPE 0 GSD)

Etiology and Pathophysiology Type 0 glycogen storage disease (GSD 0) is caused by a deficiency of the hepatic isoform of glycogen synthase, which leads to a marked decrease in liver glycogen content (Figure 6-2). After consumption of carbohydrate, the inability to store glucose as glycogen in the liver results in postprandial hyperglycemia and hyperlactatemia (3). Fasting causes severe ketotic hypoglycemia.

GSD 0 is due to mutations in the GYS2 gene located on chromosome 12p12.2 and is inherited in an autosomal recessive manner (4). To date, 15 different mutations have been reported; no dominant mutation has been identified (Figure 6-3) (5).

GSD 0 has been identified throughout Europe, and North and South America. Although no high-risk population has been identified, a common mutation, R246X, has been found in people of Italian ancestry.

Clinical Presentation GSD 0 was initially described as a devastating disorder characterized by fasting hypoglycemia, seizures, and severe developmental delay (6,7). Recently, however, it has been appreciated that most children with GSD 0 have milder symptoms (8). Recurrent ketotic hypoglycemia associated with intercurrent illness often is the only manifestation, and some asymptomatic siblings have been reported (9). The physical examination is usually normal and, unlike the other hepatic glycogenoses, the liver is not enlarged.

Fasting ketotic hypoglycemia develops on cessation of nighttime feeding. Early in infancy, children are usually asymptomatic, but weaning from overnight feeding often proves to be difficult. During childhood, fasting hypoglycemia frequently is unrecognized and even significant hypoglycemia may be asymptomatic. Abundant ketonemia develops with fasting, which serves as an alternative energy source for the brain and may explain why developmental delay has been described in only 22% of children with GSD 0 (5). Whereas overnight hypoglycemia is common in infants and children, fasting is usually better tolerated with increasing age. Most children older than 7 years of age tolerate a typical overnight fast, and fasting tolerance up to 18 hours has been reported in teenagers.

Most children with GSD 0 are identified incidentally during a gastrointestinal illness or period of poor nutrition when hypoglycemia is discovered in a lethargic child. The manifestations are frequently subtle, however, and children may first come to medical attention for evaluation of short stature, failure to thrive, and hyperlipidemia. The postprandial hyperglycemia and fasting ketonuria seen in this disorder may be confused with early diabetes, and GSD 0 should be considered in any child with asymptomatic transient hyperglycemia or glucosuria (8). The postprandial hyperlactatemia may cause mild metabolic acidosis with an increased anion gap, which may account for modest growth delay.

Diagnosis A typical fasting study, performed without postprandial biochemical monitoring, demonstrates hypoglycemia with no obvious hormonal or biochemical abnormalities, leading to misdiagnosis as "ketotic hypoglycemia" or "accelerated starvation." Frequent measurements of blood glucose, lactate, and ketones (every 30 minutes for 2 hours) following consumption of a glucose (1.75 g/kg; 75 g maximum) or galactose load demonstrate the unique biochemical pattern of postprandial hyperglycemia and hyperlactatemia. Because these abnormalities are accentuated by increased concentrations of counter-regulatory hormones, it is recommended that postprandial biochemical monitoring be performed in the morning after an overnight fast.

Glycogen Storage Disease

AT-A-GLANCE

The hepatic glycogen storage diseases (GSDs) or glycogenoses comprise several inherited diseases caused by abnormalities of the enzymes that regulate the synthesis or degradation of glycogen. Hypoglycemia is the cardinal manifestation of the hepatic glycogenoses. The clinical severity of these disorders depends on numerous factors including the degree of impairment of glycogenolysis, whether gluconeogenesis is impaired, and the availability of alternative fuels (lactate, ketones) during periods of hypoglycemia. Patients with severely limited endogenous glucose production (e.g., GSD I) present with seizures, failure to thrive, or developmental delay. In contrast, patients with milder GSDs (0 or IX) often are asymptomatic until illness impairs normal dietary carbohydrate intake. All of the hepatic glycogen storage diseases are treated with individualized dietary regimens that ensure maintenance of normoglycemia, especially overnight, and minimize or prevent glucose counterregulation. Meticulous adherence to dietary therapy ameliorates the biochemical abnormalities, decreases the size of the liver, and results in normal or nearly normal physical growth and development.

There are five major types of hepatic GSDs that affect glucose homeostasis.

TYPE	ENZYMATIC DEFECT	GENE	GENE	AFFECTED TISSUES LOCATION	OMIM
Type 0	Hepatic glycogen synthase	GYS2	12p12.2	Liver	240600
Type Ia	Glucose-6-phosphatase	G6PC	17q21	Liver, kidney, intestine	232200
Type Ib/c	Glucose-6-phosphate transporter (T1)	G6PT1	11q23	Liver, kidney, intestine, neutrophils	232220
Type IIIa	Debranching enzyme	AGL	1p21	Liver, skeletal muscle, heart	232400
Type IIIb	Debranching enzyme	AGL	1p21	Liver	232400
Type VI	Glycogen phosphorylase	PYGL	14q21–22	Liver	232700
Type IX	Phosphorylase kinase	PHKA2 PHKB PHKG2	Xp22.1–22.2 16q12–13 16p12.1–11.2	Liver, blood cells, muscle	172490 172471

TYPE	LABORATORY FINDINGS	RESPONSE TO ORAL GLUCOSE	CLINICAL MANIFESTATIONS
Type 0	Fasting ketotic hypoglycemia with postprandial hyperglycemia and hyperlactatemia	↑ glucose; ↑ lactate	Normal liver size; fasting ketotic hyperglycemia;
Type Ia	Hypoglycemia; markedly elevated triglycerides; elevated uric acid and fasting lactate; low ketones	↑ glucose; ↓ lactate	Severe hepatomegaly; round "doll" face; muscle weakness; failure to thrive; short stature; progressive renal failure; pancreatitis; liver adenomas, polycystic ovarian syndrome and osteopenia may be present during adolescence
Type Ib/c	Hypoglycemia; elevated triglyceride; elevated uric acid and fasting lactate; neutropenia	↑ glucose; ↓ lactate	Same as Ia with additional consequences of neutrophilic abnormalities (multiple and recurrent infections, brain abscess, and inflammatory bowel disease: GSD enterocolitis)
Type IIIa	Ketotic hypoglycemia; elevated triglycerides; normal uric acid and fasting lactate; markedly elevated transaminases; increased creatine kinase	↑ glucose; ↑ lactate	Severe hepatomegaly; round "doll" face; muscle weakness. Liver size decreases gradually and liver enzymes normalize during childhood. Variable proximal myopathy, which may be mild in childhood but can be severe in adulthood. Liver adenomas, cirrhosis, and symptomatic cardiomyopathy are rare complications developing during adulthood
Type IIIb	Ketotic hypoglycemia; elevated triglycerides and transaminases; normal uric acid and fasting lactate	↑ glucose; ↑ lactate	Severe hepatomegaly; round "doll" face, muscle weakness. Liver size decreases gradually and liver enzymes normalize during childhood
Type VI Type IX	Hypoglycemia; normal to elevated triglycerides; normal uric acid and fasting lactate	↑ glucose; ↑ lactate	Hepatomegaly and short stature may be the only clinical manifestations

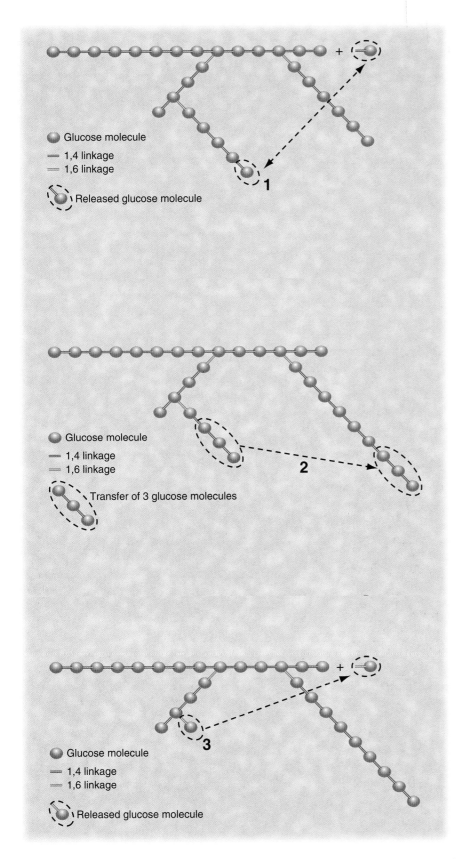

FIGURE 6-1. Schematic representation of glycogen degradation. **A.** Phosphorylase catalyzes the cleavage of glucosyl units from 1-4 glucosyl-linked chains of glycogen until only 4 glucosyl units remain before an 1,6 branch point. **B.** The branching enzyme transfers 3 glucose molecules from the short branch to the end of another branch through its transferase activity. **C.** The branching enzyme hydrolyzes the remaining glucosyl unit at the 1,6 branch point through its 1,6 glucosidase activity.

Despite the decrease in hepatic glycogen content, the glycemic response to glucagon (0.03 mg/kg; 1 mg maximum) is variable and may even be normal because some glycogen can be synthesized even with complete absence of glycogen synthase activity (8,10). In the past, confirmation of the diagnosis depended on demonstration of decreased hepatic glycogen content or abnormal enzyme activity on a liver biopsy. Mutation analysis using DNA extracted from blood or saliva is now the gold standard for making the diagnosis of GSD 0 (4,5). A few cases with no identifiable mutation in the GYS2 gene have been diagnosed by liver biopsy and enzyme assay. It is likely that the protean nature of GSD 0 and prior dependence on a liver biopsy for diagnosis account for the hitherto infrequent recognition of this condition.

Treatment The goal of treatment is to prevent hypoglycemia and minimize the associated lactic acidosis. Treatment is with a diet high in protein to provide substrate for gluconeogenesis and with low glycemic index complex carbohydrates to minimize postprandial hyperglycemia and hyperlactacidemia (11). Uncooked cornstarch (1–1.5 g/kg) administered at bedtime prevents morning hypoglycemia and ketosis. Daytime hypoglycemia tends to be mild and snacks every 2 to 4 hours prevent hypoglycemia. During illness, uncooked cornstarch is given every 6 hours, but intravenous glucose (10% dextrose administered at 1.25 times the maintenance rate of fluid administration) may be required with vomiting or gastrointestinal illness and inability to tolerate enteral intake. Before intense physical activity or participation in sports, smaller doses of cornstarch may improve stamina.

Complications and Prognosis The prognosis for patients with GSD 0 is excellent and most school-age children and adults are not limited by the condition. Short stature and osteopenia due to the chronic metabolic acidosis are common in untreated children, but improve with prevention of hypoglycemia, lactic acidosis, and ketosis. Long-term complications characteristic of other forms of GSD, such as hepatic adenomas, cirrhosis, kidney dysfunction and muscular abnormalities, have not been reported in adults with GSD 0. Nevertheless, screening for complications is recommended because very little is known about the natural history of this disease.

GLUCOSE-6-PHOSPHATASE DEFICIENCY (TYPE I GSD; VON GIERKE DISEASE)

Etiology/Pathophysiology Conversion of glucose-6-phosphate to glucose is the final step

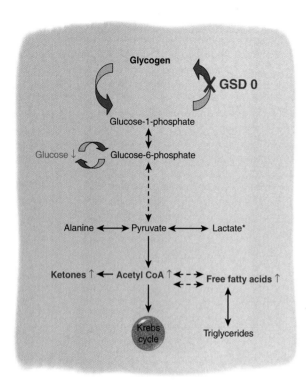

FIGURE 6-2. GSD Type 0. *Lactate is only elevated postprandially in response to oral glucose.

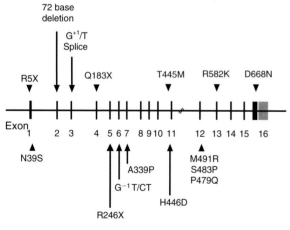

FIGURE 6-3. The mutations in GSD type 0.

in both glycogenolysis and gluconeogenesis (Figure 6-4). In normal metabolism, endogenous glucose synthesis increases during fasting or in response to counter-regulatory hormone stimulation. In type I GSD, decreased activity of the enzyme G6Pase leads to an increased concentration of glucose-6-phosphate in hepatocytes and shunting into alternative pathways with the following consequences:

1. lactic acidosis (as a result of increased glycolysis);

2. hyperuricemia (as a consequence of shunting into the pentose phosphate shunt leading to increased synthesis of uric acid; de-

creased renal excretion also occurs because lactate and uric acid share the same transporter in the kidney);

3. hypertriglyceridemia (as a result of increased synthesis of acetyl coenzyme A, the precursor of malonyl coenzyme A, which inhibits activity of carnitine palmitoyl transferase 1, leading to decreased β-oxidation of fatty acids and increased lipogenesis).

G6Pase is a complex multicomponent enzyme system located in the endoplasmic reticulum membrane and consists of a catalytic unit that faces into the endoplasmic reticulum lumen, a calcium-binding protein, and two transport proteins that facilitate transport of glucose-6-phosphate (T1), phosphate (T2), and glucose (T3) (12). The function of T1 and T2 are executed by one single protein exchanging glucose-6-phosphate and phosphate. Abnormalities of any of these components can cause abnormal enzyme function and the clinical phenotype of GSD I. There are three major subtypes of GSD I. More than 85% of patients have mutations that impair the catalytic function of the enzyme (GSD type Ia). Defects in the T1 glucose-6-phosphate transporter account for most other cases (GSD type Ib). Abnormality of the phosphate transporter (GSD type Ic) is rare.

Glycogen Storage Disease Type Ia

GSD Ia is caused by mutations in the G6PC gene located on chromosome 17q21 and is inherited in an autosomal recessive manner. The overall incidence is estimated to be 1 in 100,000 births. GSD Ia occurs in all ethnic groups, and common mutations occur in the Ashkenazi Jewish, Chinese, Japanese, and Mexican populations (13) (Table 6-1).

Clinical Presentation Patients with GSD I have impaired production of glucose from both glycogenolysis and gluconeogenesis and develop hypoglycemia within 3 to 4 hours after a meal. Lactic acid, uric acid, and triglycerides are characteristically elevated, whereas, there is inappropriate hypoketonemia in re-

sponse to hypoglycemia (14). Symptomatic hypoglycemia and hepatomegaly usually develop soon after birth. Clinical symptoms often abate once frequent feedings are commenced, and affected children may not become symptomatic again until feedings are spaced or interrupted. GSD I is occasionally diagnosed when hepatomegaly and a protuberant abdomen are discovered during a routine physical examination. When the interval between feedings increases, or when illness disrupts normal feeding, symptomatic hypoglycemia develops. The hypoglycemia is often not recognized and the disorder is discovered when the child presents with tachypnea (from lactic acidosis), seizures, lethargy, developmental delay, or failure to thrive.

Most of the clinical features of GSD I are related to the two principal metabolic abnormalities: hypoglycemia and lactic acidosis. Hypoglycemia is severe because both glycogenolysis and gluconeogenesis are impaired. Ketogenesis is impaired despite high free fatty acid concentrations. Severe hypoglycemia is especially likely to occur when serum insulin concentrations are high, such as when intravenous glucose administration or continuous intragastric feeding is abruptly discontinued. In contrast, raw cornstarch (a complex carbohydrate with a low glycemic index) administration is associated with relatively low serum insulin concentrations. When exogenous glucose delivery is interrupted in a patient treated with cornstarch, the low-insulin state allows glycogenolysis to occur resulting in increased blood lactate concentrations, thereby providing the brain with an energy substrate (15). Despite severe hypoglycemia, patients may be relatively asymptomatic.

Adaptation to hypoglycemia can occur in untreated patients, who may seek medical attention due to symptoms caused by chronic lactic acidosis. Metabolic acidosis causes tachypnea, exercise intolerance, and muscle cramping; vomiting may occur from abnormal gastric motility. Table 6-2 shows a summary of the biochemical abnormalities in untreated patients.

Diagnosis The simplest means of determining the probable defect in a child suspected of having a glycogenosis is to obtain serial blood measurements of glucose, lactate, and ketones during a fasting study. A brief fasting study (3–4 hours) in GSD I will result in hypoglycemia and development of lactic acidosis. Because glucose concentrations can fall rapidly, this test should only be performed with secure intravenous access and under close observation. During the study, glucose concentrations should be monitored every 20 to 30 minutes after 2 hours. After the plasma glucose has fallen to 50 mg/dL and a

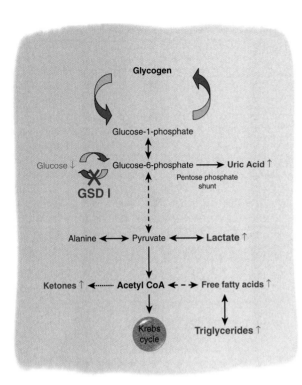

FIGURE 6-4. GSD Type 1.

sample for blood lactate determination has been obtained, glucagon (0.03 mg/kg) should be administered intravenously. In GSD I, glucagon fails to elicit a glycemic response and exacerbates lactic acidemia. When the test has been completed, intravenous glucose should be administered to restore and maintain normal blood glucose concentrations.

Mutation analysis on DNA extracted from leukocytes has become the recommended test for diagnosing GSD Ia (16,17). A total of 82 different mutations have been reported, of which 53 are missense, 10 nonsense, 16 insertion/deletion, and 3 splicing. The availability of complete gene sequencing not only allows noninvasive diagnosis of GSD I, but it has expanded the opportunities available for preimplantation screening and prenatal diagnosis. Assay of G6Pase activity on a liver biopsy should be reserved for those patients in whom GSD Ia is suspected but in whom mutation analysis is nondiagnostic.

Treatment Treatment consists of providing a continuous dietary source of glucose to prevent blood glucose from falling below the threshold for glucose counter-regulation (70–80 mg/dL) (18). In infants, the necessary amount of glucose can be delivered by frequent (every 1.5–2.5 hours) feedings during the day and continuous feeding at night through a nasogastric or gastrostomy tube and using a formula that does not contain fructose, sucrose, or galactose (e.g., Prosobee® or Lacto-free®) (19). Continuous feedings are associated with high serum insulin concentrations, and blood glucose concentrations will fall rapidly on discontinuation of the feedings if additional food or formula is not provided. Uncooked cornstarch can be gradually introduced at 6 to 12 months of age as an alternative method of glucose delivery, although some children may not tolerate it until they are older because of age-related development of amylase activity (19). The advantage of using cornstarch is that it allows feedings to be more widely spaced, minimizes glucose fluctuations and, because blood glucose levels decline more slowly, blood lactate concentrations increase and serve as an alternative fuel for the brain in the setting of hypoglycemia. An additional benefit of cornstarch is the restoration of a more normal lifestyle for older children and adults. Cornstarch typically is mixed in 3 to 4 ounces of formula, soymilk, or water, and it should be mixed just prior to administration. The cornstarch should never be heated, and it cannot be used in continuous feeding because it solidifies and obstructs the feeding tube.

Hourly glucose requirements can be estimated by calculating the basal glucose production rate by using the following formula: $y = 0.0014x^3 - 0.214x^2 + 10.411x - 9.084$ where $y =$ mg/min of glucose and $x =$ weight in kg (20). Doses of cornstarch and the interval between feedings should be individualized based on results of periodic metabolic evaluations. The goal is to maintain normal blood glucose concentrations and near-normal lactate concentrations (< mmol/L). Ideally, blood lactate should be < 1.5 mmol/l, urinary lactate < 0.06 mmol/mol creatinine, and triglycerides, uric acid, as well as liver function tests all normal. In toddlers, cornstarch is typically administered every 3 hours during the day and every 4 hours overnight. Most school-age children are maintained on six doses of cornstarch per day, whereas adults are often able to maintain adequate control on five doses of cornstarch per day (21). Most adults with GSD Ia are unable to fast for more than 5.5 to 6 hours without deterioration of metabolic control and continue to require overnight cornstarch administration (22).

Attention to both the timing and content of the diet is crucial (23). Galactose, fructose, sucrose, and lactose should be restricted because these sugars cannot be converted to glucose, and their consumption exacerbates

TABLE 6-1	Common Mutations in GSD Ia		
Mutation	**Base Change**	**Location of Mutation**	**Population**
R83C	C326T	Exon 2	Ashkenazi Jewish Eastern European
R83H	G327A	Exon 2	Chinese
130X	459insTA	Exon 3	Mexican Central American
212X	G727T	Exon 5	Japanese
Q347X	C1118T	Exon 5	Western European

TABLE 6-2	Laboratory Abnormalities in Untreated Patients with Type I GSD

- Metabolic acidosis with increased anion gap
- Hepatic transaminase (AST/ALT) levels increased
- Hyperlipidemia (particularly hypertriglyceridemia)
- Hyperuricemia
- Hyperlactatemia (lactic acidosis)
- Hypercalcemia
- Inflammatory markers (sedimentation rate and C-reactive protein) elevated
- Anemia
- Thrombocytosis
- Prolonged bleeding time

TABLE 6-3 Recommended Laboratory Screening in Patients with Type I GSD

- Electrolytes
- Renal: blood urea nitrogen/creatinine
- Liver: AST, ALT, bilirubin, alkaline phosphatase, lactate dehydrogenase
- Lipid panel
- CBC with differential
- Inflammatory: sedimentation rate +/− C-reactive protein
- Uric acid
- Lactate
- Calcium, magnesium, phosphorus
- 25-OH-Vitamin D
- Iron studies: iron, total iron binding capacity, ferritin
- Urine calcium
- Urine lactate
- Urine citrate
- Urine microalbumin
- Urine uric acid
- Serum α-fetoprotein (in presence of liver adenomatas)

the metabolic derangements through shunting into alternative pathways. Portable blood glucose and lactate meters are useful to monitor short-term control (24), and laboratory studies every 3 to 6 months are used to assess long-term biochemical control and to screen for complications (Table 6-3) (25).

During an acute illness, close monitoring of glucose and lactate concentrations is required. Despite normoglycemia, the stress response to illness can cause glycogenolysis and lead to lactic acidosis. If enteral glucose cannot be tolerated or if severe lactic acidosis causes vomiting, intravenous glucose should be commenced as soon as possible with 10% dextrose run at 1.25 to 1.5 times the usual maintenance rate of fluid administration. After the acidosis has resolved and enteral intake is again tolerated, intravenous glucose should be slowly weaned over at least 2 to 3 hours because the high insulin state will cause reactive hypoglycemia.

Complications and Prognosis Prior to the 1970s, many children with GSD I died in infancy or early childhood. Recurrent severe hypoglycemia can cause brain damage, but the prognosis has improved dramatically with early diagnosis and long-term maintenance of optimal metabolic control (21).

Both acute and long-term complications are common in GSD Ia. Lactic acid is generated as a consequence of glucose counter-regulation from hypoglycemia or stress. During illness, lactic acidosis alters gastric motility and causes vomiting. Anesthesia and the stress of surgery cause increased secretion of counter-regulatory hormones, and severe lac-

tic acidosis can develop despite maintenance of normal blood glucose concentrations. Intraoperative cardiac arrhythmias and sudden death have occurred in patients with GSD I because of inadequate glucose administration and profound lactic acidosis. Before starting a surgical procedure, the patient should receive intravenous glucose at 1.25 to 1.5 times the estimated glucose production rate to induce insulin secretion and reduce the impact of the stress response. The combination of a high glucose infusion rate and insulin resistance associated with counter-regulatory hormone secretion can cause hyperglycemia during surgery and during severe illnesses. The glucose infusion should not be decreased below the estimated hepatic glucose production rate. Any reduction in the glucose infusion rate must be done with extreme caution and with frequent monitoring of acid-base status. If acidosis develops, bicarbonate should be infused slowly to normalize the blood pH. A continuous low-dose insulin infusion may be required if severe hyperglycemia and acidosis occur.

Hepatic adenomas are detected in approximately 50% of patients by the time they complete puberty (26). The mean age at diagnosis is approximately 15 years, but adenomas occasionally develop during childhood (27). There is no gender predisposition and no difference has been found in the rate of adenoma formation in patients treated with cornstarch compared with those treated with continuous overnight intragastric drip feeding. Most adenomas remain stable over time, but they may be associated with hemorrhage or degenerate into hepatocellular carcinoma

(28). High alkaline phosphatase concentrations and elevation in the erythrocyte sedimentation rate may be seen in patients with adenomas. Ultrasonography is the preferred screening method. Magnetic resonance imaging provides greater definition when malignancy is a concern because of changes in the sonographic appearance of a lesion. Imaging is recommended at least annually after 5 years of age, and every 6 to 12 months if adenomas appear to be enlarging. Serum α-fetoprotein is normal in patients with adenomas but may be increased in some cases of hepatocellular carcinoma.

Nephromegaly was described by von Gierke in the first pathologic description of hepatorenal glycogenosis, and kidney enlargement due to glycogen storage is readily demonstrated by ultrasonography. The relative energy deficiency in renal tubular cells due to deficiency of G6Pase increases renal blood flow and glomerular filtration rate as a compensatory mechanism. Renal Fanconi syndrome with glucosuria, phosphaturia, hypokalemia, and a generalized aminoaciduria is associated with suboptimal control, but proximal tubular dysfunction is reversible when the patient's disorder is well controlled (29). Distal renal tubular dysfunction is almost universal in adolescents and adults and is associated with acidification defects, hypercalciuria, and hypocitraturia (30,31). The combination of low urinary citrate and high urinary calcium concentrations predisposes patients to nephrocalcinosis and nephrolithiasis (31). Preliminary evidence suggests that citrate supplementation may prevent these complications. With the exception of glomerular hyperfiltration, patients who are able to maintain good metabolic control usually show no significant impairment of renal function (32). Increased urinary albumin excretion may be observed in adolescents, and adults may manifest more severe renal pathology with proteinuria, hypertension, and decreased creatinine clearance due to focal segmental glomerulosclerosis and interstitial fibrosis (33). Patients with persistently elevated concentrations of blood lactate, serum lipids, and uric acid are at higher risk for development of nephropathy. Improvement of metabolic control and use of an angiotensin-converting enzyme inhibitor have been associated with decreased proteinuria and may slow the progression of renal disease. Although angiotensin-converting enzyme inhibitor therapy has been used prophylactically, treatment is usually started once persistent microalbuminuria is confirmed.

Anemia is common in patients with GSD Ia and is associated with suboptimal metabolic control (21). While anemia is usually mild, an unusual, unremitting iron-resistant anemia occurs in a subset of patients (34). The anemia can be profound, with hemoglobin concentrations as low as 4 g/dL, and it is characterized by microcytosis (mean corpuscular volume 50–70 fL), widening of the red cell distribution width, and iron studies consistent with iron deficiency. Neither erythropoietin nor treatment with oral and intravenous iron significantly improves the anemia. This form of iron-resistant anemia has been associated with large hepatic adenomas (>7 cm in diameter), which inappropriately express hepcidin, a peptide that inhibits intestinal absorption of iron and macrophage recycling of iron. Resection of hepatic adenomas has been associated with rapid correction of the anemia (34).

With patients surviving into adulthood, osteoporosis is likely to be a common cause of morbidity. Osteoporosis develops without abnormalities in calcium, phosphate, parathyroid hormone, or vitamin D metabolism (35). Poor metabolic control has been associated with decreased bone mineral content. The cause is likely multifactorial, including systemic acidosis, elevated cortisol concentrations, delayed pubertal development, inadequate dietary calcium, and lack of physical activity (36).

Other complications, seen rarely in type Ia GSD, include pancreatitis, polycystic ovaries, and a bleeding diathesis (37,38). Pancreatitis is related to hyperlipidemia, and treatment with gemfibrozil (600 mg administered twice daily) or niacin is recommended when hypertriglyceridemia persists (triglycerides >500–700 mg/dL) despite dietary modifications to improve metabolic control. Pancreatitis has been associated with use of growth hormone and glucocorticoids due to stimulation of glycogenolysis and worsening hypertriglyceridemia. Polycystic ovaries are common in poorly controlled GSD, but the condition does not appear to be inherent to the disease. Fertility appears to be unaffected, and more than 50 children have been born to mothers with GSD Ia. Platelet dysfunction associated with hyperlipidemia and acidosis is also a consequence of poorly controlled GSD. Bleeding is usually not a problem in patients in good metabolic control.

Glycogen Storage Disease Type Ib/c

GSD Ib/c is caused by defects of G6PT1, the gene that encodes the synthesis of transporter T1, which is responsible for the transport of G6P into and phosphate out of the lumen of the endoplasmic reticulum. The G6PT1 gene is located on chromosome 11q23 and is inherited in an autosomal recessive manner. The incidence is estimated to be 1 in 1,000,000 births. No high-risk ethnic group or population has been identified.

Clinical Presentation Patients with GSD Ib have symptoms similar to those of patients with GSD Ia but with the addition of neutropenia and inflammatory bowel disease (IBD) (39). Neutropenia is a consequence of disturbed myeloid maturation and is also associated with functional defects of circulating neutrophils and monocytes. The neutropenia can be either cyclic or constant, and approximately two-thirds of patients have their initial episode of neutropenia before 12 months of age. Whereas the severity of neutrophil dysfunction is variable, recurrent bacterial infections (predominantly from *Staphylococcus aureus*, *Streptococcus pneumoniae*, and *Escherichia coli*) and oral ulcers are common. An IBD resembling Crohn disease develops in the majority of patients by the teenage years and is usually the major cause of morbidity in patients with GSD Ib/c. Neutropenia and impaired neutrophil function are thought to be involved in the pathogenesis of IBD but it continues to occur frequently in patients with GSD Ib/c despite granulocyte-stimulating colony factor therapy.

Diagnosis The diagnosis of GSD Ib/c is typically made clinically when a patient with biochemical features of GSD I develops neutropenia and/or IBD. Rare cases of GSD Ia with neutropenia have been reported; therefore, mutation analysis is recommended to confirm the diagnosis. To date, approximately 65 mutations in the G6PT gene have been described. Most mutations are in exon 8, but full gene sequencing has recently become commercially available. As a result, diagnosis by liver biopsy is no longer recommended. If a liver biopsy is performed, differentiation between the types requires an analysis of G6Pase activity in both intact and fully disrupted microsomes as enzyme activity normalizes in type Ib/c when freezing disrupts the integrity of the endoplasmic reticulum.

Treatment Cornstarch therapy is individualized as described previously for type Ia. Patients with GSD Ib/c may have higher baseline glucose requirements than GSD Ia due to chronic inflammation. Hourly glucose requirements may be 25% above the calculated basal glucose production rate. Neutropenia usually responds to granulocyte-colony stimulating factor (dosed at 2-5 μg/kg/day), and the associated IBD responds to conventional therapy (40). Glucocorticoids cause adverse metabolic effects and, if possible, should not be used to treat the IBD of patients with GSD Ib/c.

Complications and Prognosis Long-term complications of GSD Ib/c appear to be less frequent than in GSD Ia. IBD is the major cause of morbidity. Life-threatening infections secondary to neutropenia are uncommon but aggressive treatment of all infections is recommended. Recently, a mother with GSD Ib/c gave birth to a healthy baby after an uneventful pregnancy.

DEBRANCHING ENZYME DEFICIENCY (TYPE III GSD; CORI DISEASE; FORBES DISEASE)

Etiology/Pathophysiology Type III GSD is caused by deficiency of glycogen debrancher enzyme (Figure 6-5). Debranching enzyme has two distinct catalytic activities. After glycogen phosphorylase has acted on the outer branches of glycogen, four glucosyl residues remain distal to the branch point. The transferase activity of debranching enzyme transfers three of the glucosyl residues to the outer end of an adjacent chain. The amylo-1,6-glucosidase activity of the same enzyme also hydrolyses the branch point glucose residue (Figure 6-1). Without normal

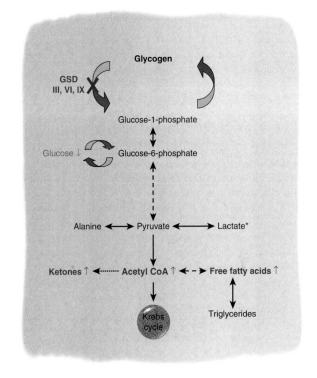

FIGURE 6-5. GSD Types III, VI, IX. *Lactate is only elevated postprandially in response to oral glucose.

debranching enzyme activity, breakdown of glycogen is arrested and an abnormal form of glycogen (limit dextrin) accumulates in affected tissues.

The gene for the debranching enzyme is located on chromosome 1p21, and GSD III is inherited in an autosomal recessive manner (2,41). The gene encodes four major nuclear RNA isoforms formed from differential splicing. Isoform 1, the predominant form in the liver, includes exon 1 but exon 2 is spliced out. Transcription starts from exon 2 in isoforms 2, 3, and 4, and these isoforms are expressed in skeletal muscle and heart. Because the isoforms are differentially expressed, the clinical phenotype depends on the location of the mutation (42). Type IIIa, which affects both liver and muscle, accounts for 85% of patients with GSD III in the United States; type IIIb affects only the liver. There are rare patients with loss of either the glucosidase activity (type IIIc) or transferase activity (type IIId) GSD.

The incidence of GSD III is estimated to be 1 in 100,000 live births. It is unusually frequent in Jews of North African descent living in Israel where the carrier frequency is 1:35.

Clinical Presentation Clinical and genetic variability is common in GSD III. In infancy and early childhood, hepatomegaly and fasting hypoglycemia may be indistinguishable from GSD I. Unlike GSD I, however, blood levels of lactate and uric acid are normal. After infancy, the hypoglycemia is usually milder than is typically seen in GSD I because the gluconeogenic pathway is intact and glucose can be derived from the outer segments of glycogen. In GSD IIIa, a variable proximal myopathy can occur, which is usually mild in childhood but can be severe in adulthood. Biochemical abnormalities include marked elevations in liver transaminase and creatine kinase concentrations (43,44). Hyperlipidemia also typically occurs. The kidneys are not enlarged, and renal function remains normal.

Diagnosis A fasting study demonstrates ketotic hypoglycemia without the hyperlactatemia characteristic of GSD I. Glucagon fails to elicit a glycemic response after a fast but does elicit a glycemic response when given 2 hours after a carbohydrate-rich meal. Until recently, definitive diagnosis depended on demonstrating abnormal glycogen (limit dextrin) and abnormal enzyme activity on a biopsy of the liver and muscle. Mutation analysis is now commercially available for the diagnosis of both type IIIa and IIIb GSD. Measurement of enzyme activity in skin fibroblasts or lymphocytes can be used to screen for GSD III but these studies may not be definitive and cannot be used for subtyping.

Treatment Provision of continuous glucose is required to maintain blood glucose above 70 mg/dL. Uncooked cornstarch (1.75 g/kg) at 6-hour intervals (both during the day and night) usually maintains normoglycemia, increases growth velocity, and decreases transaminase concentrations (45,46). The minimum amount of cornstarch necessary to prevent hypoglycemia should be used because excessive quantities may aggravate the myopathy. In some patients, more frequent administration of smaller doses of cornstarch may be beneficial in decreasing biochemical evidence of liver and muscle inflammation.

Cornstarch prevents hypoglycemia but patients with type IIIa continue to have marked elevations of their muscle enzymes. A high-protein diet has been reported to improve myopathy and growth failure (47). A diet containing at least 3 g/kg of protein is recommended, and the ideal diet should consist of approximately 55 to 60% carbohydrate, 15 to 20% protein, and 20 to 25% fat. For patients with cardiomyopathy or severe muscle disease, high-protein nocturnal enteral therapy may be beneficial. Patients need not restrict their consumption of fructose or galactose. Low–glycemic index complex carbohydrates are recommended to avoid marked postprandial hyperinsulinemia. Although amino acids can be converted to glucose via gluconeogenesis, hypoglycemia is common when protein supplementation is used without cornstarch in infants and young children.

Whereas severe hypoglycemia is less common than in type I GSD, hypoglycemia and severe ketosis can develop with illness or when enteral intake is decreased. Intravenous dextrose infused at 1.25 to 1.5 times the basal rate of glucose production is used to normalize glucose concentrations and prevent ketosis during illness.

Complications and Prognosis Hepatic adenomas occur in approximately 25% of adults with GSD III and cases of hepatocellular carcinoma have recently been reported (27). Hepatic fibrosis can occur, and some adult patients develop cirrhosis, portal hypertension, and, rarely, liver failure. Myopathy typically becomes more prominent in the third to fourth decades of life, manifesting as slowly progressive muscle weakness. Exercise causes elevations in serum creatine kinase and aldolase concentrations. Restriction of exercise may decrease progression of muscle damage. Patients with muscle involvement can develop cardiac complications. Concentric left ventricular hypertrophy, detectable by echocardiography, usually develops after puberty; however, ventricular function is usually normal (48). Severe cardiac dysfunction and arrhythmias can occur, and rare cases of severe cardiomyopathy in infants and children have been reported.

GLYCOGEN PHOSPHORYLASE DEFICIENCY (TYPE VI GSD; HERS DISEASE)

GLYCOGEN PHOSPHORYLASE KINASE DEFICIENCY (TYPE IX GSD)

Etiology/Pathophysiology Types VI and IX GSD will be considered together because both disorders result from impaired hepatic phosphorylase activity. Together, they account for approximately 25 to 30% of all cases of GSD. Although glycogen phosphorylase is the rate-limiting step in glycogenolysis, these disorders are typically mild and may be confused with "ketotic hypoglycemia." Their estimated prevalence is approximately 1 in 100,000 but this may be an underestimate.

Phosphorylase kinase of liver and muscle is a complex enzyme consisting of four subunits: α, β, δ, and γ (2). The α-subunit is encoded by the PHKA2 gene located at Xp22.2-p22.1, and mutations are associated with an X-linked disease. The β-subunit is expressed in muscle, liver, brain, and kidney and is encoded by the PHKB gene on chromosome 16q12-q13. Mutations lead to an autosomal recessive variant of GSD IX. The γ-subunit, encoded by the PHKG gene on chromosome 16p11-p12, contains the catalytic site of the phosphorylase kinase enzyme.

The hepatic glycogen phosphorylase liver gene (PYGL) gene is located at chromosome 14q21-22. Glycogen phosphorylase deficiency is inherited in an autosomal recessive manner. The disease has been estimated to affect 1 in 1,000 of the Mennonite population.

Clinical Presentation Children usually come to attention when hepatomegaly is detected on a routine physical examination or when hypoglycemia occurs as a consequence of prolonged fasting during an intercurrent illness (49). Fasting "ketotic hypoglycemia" is the cardinal manifestation and hypoglycemia is generally milder than in GSD I and III. Because gluconeogenesis, lipolysis, fatty acid oxidation, and ketogenesis are intact, blood glucose may transiently decrease to hypoglycemic levels during an overnight fast (e.g., at 2 AM), but returns to normal by morning. In older children and adults, the tendency to develop hypoglycemia often totally abates and patients can tolerate a fast of 18 to 24 hours duration. Without treatment, patients may continue to experience pronounced ketosis, and morning lethargy and nausea are common.

Hepatomegaly and short stature may be the only clinical manifestations (50). Mild hyperlipidemia and increased serum transaminase concentrations are characteristic features. Blood lactate and serum uric acid concentrations are typically normal. Muscle involvement can occur and patients may present with hypotonia, myoglobinuria, muscle weakness, and gross motor delay.

Mutations in the γ-subunit of the PHK gene lead to a more severe clinical phenotype. Frequent severe hypoglycemia similar to that seen in GSD I and GSD III may occur during infancy. Affected individuals may have severe growth retardation, muscle hypotonia, and markedly elevated hepatic transaminase concentrations. Mutations in this subunit are associated with an increased risk of cirrhosis in childhood.

Diagnosis It is possible to diagnose glycogen phosphorylase kinase deficiency by assaying the activity of the enzyme in leukocytes and erythrocytes; however, the blood assay lacks sensitivity because there are liver, muscle, heart, and brain isoforms of this enzyme. Mutation analysis for both GSD type VI and type IX has recently become commercially available.

Treatment In early childhood or in the unusual older patient with overnight hypoglycemia, uncooked cornstarch (1.5 g/kg) given at bedtime prevents nocturnal hypoglycemia (51). Even when more prolonged fasting can be tolerated without development of hypoglycemia, most children and adults report improved energy and well-being with bedtime administration of cornstarch, which prevents ketosis. A diet with a high content of protein and complex carbohydrates is recommended. No dietary restrictions are necessary. Intravenous glucose administration may be required during illness or periods of fasting; mild intercurrent illnesses are usually well tolerated.

Complications and Prognosis The prognosis for most patients with GSD VI and IX is excellent except for those with mutations in the PHKG2 gene (52). Muscle symptoms occur occasionally, and these disorders are rarely associated with a proximal renal tubular acidosis (53) and neurologic abnormalities (54). Hepatic fibrosis and cirrhosis occur commonly in patients with mutations in the γ-subunit (55). A severe cardiac-specific phosphorylase kinase variant that can lead to cardiac failure has been reported (56). Hyperlipidemia is common in untreated children and adults may be at increased risk for cardiovascular disease.

Muscle Glycogenoses

Under this general heading we will briefly consider Types IV, V, and VII GSDs for the sake of completeness, although each form is quite rare.

TYPE IV: ANDERSEN DISEASE

Etiology/Pathophysiology Andersen's disease represents less than 0.5% of all reported glycogenosis patients and has a varying phenotype. The disease results in an autosomal recessive mutation of the GBE1 gene on chromosome 3p12, which codes for the 1,4-α-glucan branching enzyme, which is the protein responsible for creating branch points in the linear glycogen strand and hence increasing water solubility. A straight-chain glycogen molecule can be cleaved; hence, severe hypoglycemia is not a part of the clinical presentation. The pathophysiology of the GBE1 mutation remains unexplained, and elucidation is complicated by the ubiquitous expression of the normal gene in many tissues. Bruno et al. have categorized clinical presentations of the neuromuscular types into four subgroups and shown a correlation between the severity of the genetic mutation and the phenotypic expression (57).

Clinical Presentation As originally described the typical presentation included failure to thrive, hepatomegaly, and progressive hepatic cirrhosis with death in early childhood. In the intervening 50 years it has become clear that the phenotype is widely variable, ranging from mild nonprogressive hepatic involvement to very severe neuromuscular involvement and an age range from fetus to adult (58). As mentioned earlier, Bruno, et al. have categorized the neuromuscular forms into four subgroups: 1) perinatal, manifesting as fetal akinesia deformation sequence and characterized by arthrogryposis multiplex congenita, hydrops and death in the perinatal period; 2) congenital, which appears as hypotonia, muscle atrophy, neuronal abnormalities affecting the respiratory centers, variable cardiomyopathy and early infant demise; 3) childhood form in which there is either a dominant myopathy or cardiomyopathy; and 4) adult, usually showing up as a generalized myopathy.

Clinical and Biochemical Findings Routine biochemical data are highly variable; liver function studies may be mildly to moderately abnormal to normal, and creatine kinase may be significantly abnormal or normal. Electromyography may show diffuse fibrillations. Urine organic acids and serum amino acids are invariably normal. Histochemical examination of muscle tissue obtained by biopsy will reveal polyglucosan bodies that will show resistance to diastase digestion. Using the polymerase chain reaction technique, gene mutations can be detected and the diagnosis of GBE1 can be confirmed.

Treatment Treatment is only symptomatic, except in those patients in whom hepatic transplant is a viable option. The disorder is so rare that little longitudinal experience with long-term follow up of the latter group is available.

TYPE V: McARDLE DISEASE

Etiology/Pathophysiology The molecular etiology of McArdle disease is an autosomal recessive mutation of the PGYM gene on chromosome 11, coding for muscle phosphorylase. This enzyme is responsible for initiation of glycogenolysis by cleaving α-1,4-glucosyl units from the outer periphery of the glycogen molecule and liberating glucose-1-phosphate monomers. Although three isoforms of the phosphorylase are known—brain/heart, liver, and muscle—but only the latter is abnormal in patients with McArdle disease. Hence, overt clinical symptoms are confined to the muscle, and neither cardiomyopathy nor encephalopathy has been reported in these patients. The inability to cleave the α-1,4-glucosyl units renders the remainder of the glycogen molecule relatively inaccessible to glycogenolysis, thus depriving the muscle of its primary fuel source. The chief energy reservoir for isometric contraction is glucose-1-phosphate released from glycogen and utilized by anaerobic glycolysis; interruption in this pathway in McArdle disease causes the symptoms of myalgia, cramping, and myoglobinuria resulting from rhabdomyolysis with isometric exercise. There has been documentation of limited mitochondrial rate of oxidative phosphorylation in muscle tissue from patients with McArdle disease, putatively from substrate delivery limitations (59). It has been suggested that decreased generation of adenosine triphosphate may affect ion transport across the sarcolemma, a process of critical importance to its function; this remains unproven, however.

Clinical Presentation Because virtually all affected individuals describe a "lifelong" exercise intolerance, it would appear logical that onset of symptoms occurs in early childhood. It is this limited exercise capacity that, especially when accompanied by cramping, will often lead the patient to seek medical advice. Characteristically, the most likely sort of exercise to cause problems is isometric, such as weight lifting; however, moderate and sustained exertion may also bring on symptoms. Patients often experience a so-called "second wind" with brief cessation of exercise, which results from increased delivery of glucose to the muscle because of enhanced blood flow. Although in itself, this presentation is more of an inconvenience than a danger, if the signs are ignored by the patient the next steps will be rhabdomyolysis and myoglobinuria with the potential for acute renal failure. A very rare variant presentation has been reported in the neonate with progressive weakness, respiratory distress, and early death.

Clinical and Biochemical Findings The most consistently abnormal laboratory test is serum creatine kinase, which, although variably increased, will be found to be elevated in virtually all affected individuals. Electromyography does not show the abnormalities that one might intuitively expect to see. The clinical *sine qua non* of McArdle disease is the demonstration of no increase or a decrease in venous lactate in the forearm after exercise. This test must be performed with scrupulous care to avoid spurious results (60). Muscle biopsy and measurement of phosphorylase activity in the sample can be avoided by DNA analysis in leukocytes (61).

Treatment Currently, no definitive treatment modality exists for McArdle disease. Low-dose creatine supplementation has been attempted in a very limited number of patients and was subjectively effective in relief of symptoms during controlled exercise testing. Oral sucrose ingestion prior to exercise improved exercise tolerance in a small study, but without lasting effect. The essential key to therapy is avoidance of rhabdomyolysis from overly stressful exercise because of the danger of myoglobinuria and consequent renal shutdown.

Type VII: Tauri Disease: Phosphofructokinase Deficiency (PFKD)

Etiology/Pathophysiology The molecular basis for Type VII GSD is an autosomal recessive mutation in the PFKM gene on chromosome 12q13.3, which codes for the M-subunit of the tetrameric enzyme protein phosphofructokinase (62). This protein in muscle is a homotetramer composed of four M-subunits; of significance is the erythrocyte isoform, which consists of tetramers of varied proportions of muscle and liver subunits. PFKM catalyzes an irreversible reaction of fructose-6-phosphate to fructose-1,6-bisphosphate, a key regulatory step in the glycolytic pathway. Given that metabolic functions of both muscle and erythrocyte are heavily reliant on glycolysis, it is clear that deficiency in a key regulatory enzyme would adversely affect both.

Clinical Presentation As in McArdle disease, patients with phosphofructokinase deficiency experience significant exercise intolerance; what sets the latter group apart, however, is characteristic absence of a "second wind" phenomenon and a tendency toward hemolysis with sustained exercise. The latter may lead to mild jaundice. Because there is a complete loss of PFK activity in muscle, the capacity for anaerobic glycolysis is correspondingly absent, which explains the absence of the "second wind" phenomenon. The erythrocyte is absolutely dependent on glycolysis for its energy requirement; hence, a partial loss of PFK activity diminishes the metabolic capacity of the red cell and renders it susceptible to damage. As in other glycogenoses, phosphofructokinase deficiency has been subclassified into various subclasses based upon age of onset, severity, and other variables (63).

Clinical and Biochemical Findings Serum creatine kinase is usually markedly elevated, as are the muscle isoforms of lactate dehydrogenase and aspartate transaminase. A mild reticulocytosis may be present as a consequence of persistent, low-grade hemolysis, together with a consequent mild hyperbilirubinemia. There is often a prominent hyperuricemia, derived from increased degradation of purine bases due to deficient generation of adenosine triphosphate secondary to impaired glycolysis. Muscle biopsy findings on histological examination are nonspecific; PFK assay shows almost complete absence of activity.

Treatment As in McArdle disease, no definitive therapy is available for phosphofructokinase deficiency. Avoidance of strenuous exercise is the key to health maintenance.

REFERENCES

1. Wolfsdorf JI, Weinstein DA. Glycogen storage diseases. *Rev Endocr Metab Disord.* 2003;4(1):95–102.
2. Elpeleg ON. The molecular background of glycogen metabolism disorders. *J Pediatr Endocrinol Metab.* 1999;12:363–379.
3. Aynsley-Green A, Williamson DH, Gitzelmann R. Hepatic glycogen synthetase deficiency. Definition of syndrome from metabolic and enzyme studies on a 9-year-old girl. *Arch Dis Child.* 1977;52(7):573–579.
4. Orho M, Bosshard N, Buist N, et al. Mutations in the liver glycogen synthase gene in children with hypoglycemia due to glycogen storage disease type 0. *J Clin Invest.* 1998;102:507–515.
5. Weinstein DA, Correia CE, Saunders AC, et al. Hepatic glycogen synthase deficiency: an infrequently recognized cause of ketotic hypoglycemia. *Mol Genet Metab.* 2006;87(4):284–288.
6. Spencer-Peet J, Norman ME, Lake BD, et al. Hepatic glycogen storage disease. Clinical and laboratory findings in 23 cases. *Q J Med.* 1971;40(157):95–114.
7. Gitzelmann R, Spycher M, Feil G, et al. Liver glycogen synthase deficiency: a rarely diagnosed entity. *Eur J Pediatr.* 1996;155:561–567.
8. Bachrach BE, Weinstein DA, Orho-Melander M, et al. Glycogen synthase deficiency (glycogen storage disease type 0) presenting with hyperglycemia and glucosuria: Report of three new mutations. *J Pediatr.* 2002;140(6):781–783.
9. Aynsley-Green A, Williamson DH, Gitzelmann R. Asymptomatic hepatic glycogen-synthetase deficiency. *Lancet.* 1978;1(8056):147–148.
10. Laberge AM, Mitchell GA, van de Werve G, et al. Long-term follow-up of a new case of liver glycogen synthase deficiency. *Am J Med Genet A.* 2003;120(1):19–22.
11. Aynsley-Green A, Williamson DH, Gitzelmann R. The dietary treatment of hepatic glycogen synthetase deficiency. *Helv Paediat Acta.* 1977;32:71–75.
12. Burchell A. The molecular basis of the type 1 glycogen storage diseases. *Bioessays.* 1992;14(6):395–400.
13. Ekstein J, Rubin BY, Anderson SL, et al. Mutation frequencies for glycogen storage disease Ia in the Ashkenazi Jewish population. *Am J Med Genet.* 2004;129A(2):162–164.
14. Binkiewicz A, Senior B. Decreased ketogenesis in Von Gierke's disease (type 1 glycogenosis). *J Pediatr.* 1973;83(6):973–978.
15. Fernandes J, Berger R, Smit GP. Lactate as a cerebral metabolic fuel for glucose-6-phosphatase deficient children. *Pediatr Res.* 1984;18(4): 335–339.
16. Rake JP, ten Berge AM, Visser G, et al. Glycogen storage disease type Ia: recent experience with mutation analysis, a summary of mutations reported in the literature and a newly developed diagnostic flowchart. *Eur J Pediatr.* 2000;159(5):322–330.
17. Matern D, Seydewitz HH, Bali D, et al. Glycogen storage disease type I: diagnosis and phenotype/genotype correlation. *Eur J Pediatr.* 2002;161 Suppl 1:S10–9.
18. Wolfsdorf JI, Plotkin RA, Laffel LMB, et al. Continuous glucose for treatment of patients with type 1 glycogen-storage disease: comparison of the effects of dextrose and uncooked cornstarch on biochemical variables. *Am J Clin Nutr.* 1990;52:1043–1050.
19. Wolfsdorf JI, Keller RJ, Landy H, et al. Glucose therapy for glycogenosis type 1 in infants: comparison of intermittent uncooked cornstarch and continuous overnight glucose feedings. *J Pediatr.* 1990;117(3):384–391.
20. Bier DM, Leake RD, Haymond MW, et al. Measurement of "true" glucose production rates in infancy and childhood with 6,6-dideuteroglucose. *Diabetes.* 1977;26(11): 1016–1023.
21. Weinstein DA, Wolfsdorf JI. Effect of continuous glucose therapy with uncooked cornstarch on the long-term clinical course of type 1a glycogen storage disease. *Eur J Pediatr.* 2002;161(Suppl 1):S35–9.
22. Wolfsdorf J, Crigler J, Jr. Biochemical evidence for the requirement of continuous glucose therapy in young adults with type 1 glycogen storage disease. *J Inherit Metab Dis.* 1994; 17:234–241.
23. Wolfsdorf JI, Ehrlich S, Landy HS, et al. Optimal daytime feeding regimen to prevent postprandial hypoglycemia in type 1 glycogen storage disease. *Am J Clin Nutr.* 1992;56:587–592.
24. Saunders AC, Feldman HA, Correia CE, et al. Clinical evaluation of a portable lactate meter

in type I glycogen storage disease. *J Inherit Metab Dis.* 2005;28(5):695–701.

25. Rake JP, Visser G, Labrune P, et al. Guidelines for management of glycogen storage disease type I - European Study on Glycogen Storage Disease Type I (ESGSD I). *Eur J Pediatr.* 2002;161(Suppl 1):S112–9.

26. Bianchi L. Glycogen storage disease I and hepatocellular tumours. *Eur J Pediatr.* 1993;152(Suppl 1):S63–70.

27. Labrune P, Trioche P, Duvaltier I, et al. Hepatocellular adenomas in glycogen storage disease type I and III: a series of 43 patients and review of the literature. *J Pediatr Gastroenterol Nutr.* 1997;24(3):276–279.

28. Franco LM, Krishnamurthy V, Bali D, et al. Hepatocellular carcinoma in glycogen storage disease type Ia: a case series. *J Inherit Metab Dis.* 2005;28(2):153–162.

29. Chen YT, Scheinman JI, Park HK, et al. Amelioration of proximal renal tubular dysfunction in type I glycogen storage disease with dietary therapy. *N Engl J Med.* 1990;323(9):590–593.

30. Restaino I, Kaplan BS, Stanley C, et al. Nephrolithiasis, hypocitraturia, and a distal renal tubular acidification defect in type 1 glycogen storage disease. *J Pediatr.* 1993;122(3):392–396.

31. Weinstein DA, Somers MJ, Wolfsdorf JI. Decreased urinary citrate excretion in type 1a glycogen storage disease. *J Pediatr* 2001;138(3):378–382.

32. Wolfsdorf JI, Laffel LMB, Crigler JF, Jr. Metabolic control and renal dysfunction in type I glycogen storage disease. *J Inherit Metab Dis.* 1997;20(4):559–568.

33. Chen YT, Coleman RA, Scheinman JI, et al. Renal disease in type I glycogen storage disease. *N Engl J Med.* 1988;318(1):7–11.

34. Weinstein DA, Roy CN, Fleming MD, et al. Inappropriate expression of hepcidin is associated with iron refractory anemia: implications for the anemia of chronic disease. *Blood.* 2002;100(10):3776–3781.

35. Lee PJ, Patel JS, Fewtrell M, et al. Bone mineralisation in type 1 glycogen storage disease. *Eur J Pediatr.* 1995;154(6):483–487.

36. Wolfsdorf JI. Bones benefit from better biochemical control in type 1 glycogen storage disease. *J Pediatr.* 2002;141(3):308–310.

37. Lee P, Leonard J. The hepatic glycogen storage diseases—problems beyond childhood. *J Inherit Metab Dis.* 1995;18:462–472.

38. Lee PJ, Patel A, Hindmarsh PC, et al. The prevalence of polycystic ovaries in the hepatic glycogen storage diseases: its association with hyperinsulinism. *Clin Endocrinol* 1995;42(6):601–606.

39. Visser G, Rake JP, Fernandes J, et al. Neutropenia, neutrophil dysfunction, and inflammatory bowel disease in glycogen storage disease type Ib: results of the European Study on Glycogen Storage Disease Type I. *J Pediatr.* 2000;137(2):187–191.

40. Visser G, Rake JP, Labrune P, et al. Granulocyte colony-stimulating factor in glycogen storage disease type 1b. Results of the European Study on Glycogen Storage Disease Type 1. *Eur J Pediatr.* 2002;161 (Suppl 1):S83–7.

41. Bao Y, Dawson TL, Jr., et al. Human glycogen debranching enzyme gene (AGL): complete structural organization and characterization of the 5' flanking region. *Genomics.* 1996;38(2):155–165.

42. Coleman RA, Winter HS, Wolf B, et al. Glycogen storage disease type III (glycogen debranching enzyme deficiency): correlation of biochemical defects with myopathy and cardiomyopathy. *Ann Intern Med.* 1992;116(11):896–900.

43. Coleman RA, Winter HS, Wolf B, et al. Glycogen debranching enzyme deficiency: long-term study of serum enzyme activities and clinical features. *J Inherit Metab Dis.* 1992;15(6):869–881.

44. Bhuiyan J, Al Odaib AN, Ozand PT. A simple, rapid test for the differential diagnosis of glycogen storage disease type 3. *Clin Chim Acta.* 2003;335(1-2):21–26.

45. Gremse DA, Bucuvalas JC, Balistreri WF. Efficacy of cornstarch therapy in type III glycogen-storage disease. *Am J Clin Nutr* 1990;52(4):671–674.

46. Borowitz SM, Greene HL. Cornstarch therapy in a patient with type III glycogen storage disease. *J Pediatr Gastroenterol Nutr.* 1987;6(4):631–634.

47. Slonim AE, Coleman RA, Moses S. Myopathy and growth failure in debrancher enzyme deficiency. Improvement with high protein nocturnal enteral therapy. *J Pediatr.* 1984;105:906–911.

48. Lee PJ, Deanfield JE, Burch M, et al. Comparison of the functional significance of left ventricular hypertrophy in hypertrophic cardiomyopathy and glycogenosis type III. *Am J Cardiol.* 1997;79(6):834–838.

49. Willems PJ, Gerver WJ, Berger R, et al. The natural history of liver glycogenosis due to phosphorylase kinase deficiency: a longitudinal study of 41 patients. *Eur J Pediatr.* 1990;149(4):268–271.

50. Schippers HM, Smit GP, Rake JP, et al. Characteristic growth pattern in male X-linked phosphorylase-b kinase deficiency (GSD IX). *J Inherit Metab Dis.* 2003;26(1):43–47.

51. Nakai A, Shigematsu Y, Takano T, et al. Uncooked cornstarch treatment for hepatic phosphorylase kinase deficiency. *Eur J Pediatr.* 1994;153:581–583.

52. Burwinkel B, Rootwelt T, Kvittingen EA, et al. Severe phenotype of phosphorylase kinase-deficient liver glycogenosis with mutations in the PHKG2 gene. *Pediatr Res.* 2003;54(6): 834–839.

53. Nagai T, Matsuo N, Tsuchiya Y, et al. Proximal renal tubular acidosis associated with glycogen storage disease, type 9. *Acta Paediatr Scand.* 1988;77(3):460–463.

54. Burwinkel B, Amat L, Gray RGF, et al. Variability of biochemical and clinical phenotype in X-linked liver glycogenosis with mutations in the phosphorylase kinase PHKA2 gene. *Hum Genet.* 1998;102:423–429.

55. Kagalwalla AF, Kagalwalla YA, al Ajaji S, et al. Phosphorylase b kinase deficiency glycogenosis with cirrhosis of the liver. *J Pediatr.* 1995;127(4):602–605.

56. Servidei S, Metlay LA, Chodosh J, et al. Fatal infantile cardiopathy caused by phosphorylase b kinase deficiency. *J Pediatr.* 1988;113(1 Pt 1):82–85.

57. Bruno C, van Diggelen OP, Cassandrini D, et al. Clinical and genetic heterogeneity of branching enzyme deficiency (glycogenosis type IV). *Neurology.* 2004;63:1053–1058.

58. Moses SW, Parvari R The variable presentations of glycogen storage disease Type IV: a review of clinical, enzymatic and molecular studies. *Curr Mol Med.* 2002;2:177–188.

59. De Stephano N, Argov Z, Matthews PM, et al. Impairment of muscle mitochondrial oxidative metabolism in McArdle's disease. *Muscle Nerve.* 1996;19:764–769.

60. Zaman Z, De Raedt S. Ischemic exercise testing in suspected McArdle disease. *Clin Chem.* 1995;46:1198–1199.

61. El-Schahawi M, Tsujino S, Shanske S, et al. Diagnosis of McArdle's disease by molecular genetic analysis of blood. *Neurology.* 1996; 47:579–580.

62. Nakajima H, Kono N, Yamasaki T, et al Genetic defect in muscle phosphofructokinase deficiency: abnormal splicing of the muscle phosphofructokinase gene due to a point mutation at the 5-prime-slice site. *J Biol Chem* 265.9392–9395, 1990.

63. Nakajima H, Raben N, Hamaguchi T, et al Phosphofructokinase deficiency; past, present and future *Curr Molec Med* 2:197–212, 2002.

CHAPTER 7

Organic Acidurias

Georg F. Hoffmann, MD
Andreas Schulze, MD, FRCPC

Organic acids occur as physiological intermediates in a variety of intracellular metabolic pathways, such as catabolism of amino acids, mitochondrial β-oxidation of fatty acids, tricarboxylic acid cycle, and cholesterol and fatty acid biosynthesis (Figure 7-1). Organic acidurias (OAs; also known as *organic acidemias*, *organic acid disorders*, or *organoacidopathies*) are a group of disorders characterized by increased excretion of non-amino organic acids in urine. Most are caused by deficiencies of enzymes in the mitochondrial metabolism of coenzyme A (CoA)–activated carboxylic acids, often derived from amino acid breakdown. These disorders result in an accumulation of precursors, which are themselves toxic or are degraded to produce toxic metabolites in the affected pathway. Analysis of organic acids by gas chromatography–mass spectrometry (GC-MS) has disclosed accumulation of organic acids due to metabolic defects of many pathways beyond amino acid degradation, especially cholesterol, fatty acid oxidation, and carbohydrate or energy metabolism (see Figure 7-1) (1). The spectrum of diseases detectable by organic acid analysis still continues to enlarge. This chapter summarizes the knowledge on classic OAs caused by defects of amino acid degradation and on the clinically overlapping subgroup termed *cerebral OAs* (2).

In defects of amino acid degradation, distal to the removal of the amino group as the initial step of amino acid degradation, characteristic organic acids, but not up to the precursor amino acid, accumulate upstream of the enzymatic block. The definitive breakdown of most amino acids occurs intramitochondrially through (β-oxidative) degradation of CoA-activated carbonic acids, the so-called acyl-CoA compounds. In contrast to aminoacidopathies such as phenylketonuria, OAs therefore frequently disturb the mitochondrial energy metabolism and predispose to acute metabolic decompensations and (lactic) acidosis. The accumulating acyl-CoA compounds are esterified with free carnitine, resulting in a diagnostically and pathophysiologically important increase of acylcarnitines. These can be reliably detected by tandem mass spectrometry (MS/MS) even in dried blood spots—the basis for the now quickly developing neonatal population screening for these disorders (3).

The clinical manifestations of these disorders are the effects of these toxic molecules on brain, liver, kidney, pancreas, retina, and other organs. In addition to different effects specific to individual organic acids, energy deficiency may evolve rapidly during metabolic decompensation and contribute to the clinical syndrome (including lactic acidosis). The catabolism of amino acids provides energy for cellular processes, and the accumulation of acyl-CoA and the concomitant decrease in free CoA disturb the mitochondrial machinery.

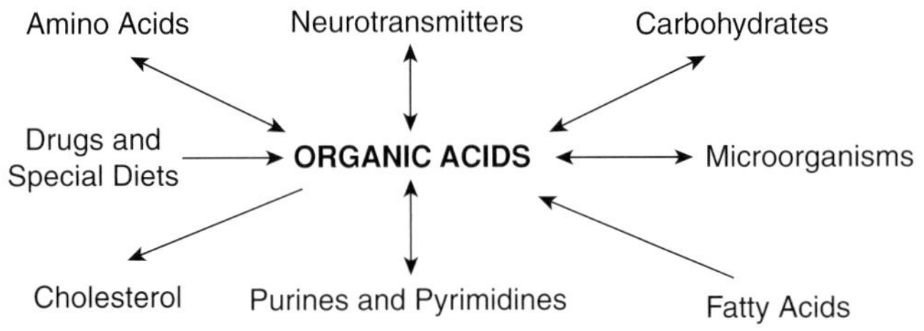

- OAs are caused by autosomal recessively inherited deficiencies of single enzymes. The cumulative frequency of the most important subgroups detectable by MS/MS neonatal screening amounts to 1 in 6000 newborns, that is, the most common acutely life-threatening inborn error of metabolism (3).

CLINICAL SPECTRUM AND DIAGNOSTIC WORKUP

Clinical Spectrum

The range of clinical and biochemical manifestations of OAs is extensive (Tables 7-1 and 7-2), depending on the pathway involved, residual enzyme activity, and individual genetic and environmental factors.

The classic OAs resulting from defects in pathways of amino acid degradation manifest in a healthy, full-term newborn usually in the first days of life with progressive irritability or drowsiness (4). However, life-threatening disease may occur as soon as a few hours after birth, or the first metabolic decompensation may occur late in infancy or even beyond. Most typically, a young infant may vomit or refuse to feed and then quickly deteriorate. The initial erroneous diagnoses usually are perinatal infection or intracranial hemorrhage. Children with milder forms may be admitted repeatedly with unusual metabolic acidosis, hypoglycemia, or neutropenia in the course of common infections, especially gastroenteritis, before it is realized that there

- Organic acid analysis should be performed on an emergency basis in every patient presenting with symptoms of unexplained metabolic crisis, intoxication, or encephalopathy.

- Metabolic derangement, such as metabolic acidosis, hypoglycemia, and leukopenia, does occur with neonatal infection, but it should be remembered that septicemia following an uneventful pregnancy and delivery from a healthy mother may be as rare as an inborn error of metabolism. The latter therefore should be sought from the beginning with equal priority. A presumptive diagnosis of a classical neonatal OA within 24–48 hours of the onset of symptoms may be indispensable for successful treatment and a satisfactory outcome.

FIGURE 7-1. Organic acids in small-molecule intermediary metabolism. (Modified from Ref. 1.)

Organic Acidurias

AT-A-GLANCE

Analysis of ninhydrin-negative, nonamino organic acids by gas chromatography–mass spectrometry (GC-MS) has allowed the identification of increasing numbers of recessively inherited disorders of small-molecule intermediary metabolism, and quantitative organic acid analysis has become the most powerful tool in the diagnostic workup of a patient suspected of suffering from an inherited metabolic disease. The disorders discovered have been referred to as

organic acidurias, organic acidemias, organic acid disorders, or organoacidopathies. The classical organic acidurias represent the pursuit of abnormalities of amino acid degradation beyond deamination, such as isovaleric, propionic, and methylmalonic acidurias. Their diagnostic hallmark is an accumulation of characteristic organic acids (and their corresponding acylcarnitines) upstream of the genetic block from dietary intake of the precursor amino

acids and/or catabolism leading to the breakdown of endogenous proteins. The clinical features result from toxicity of the accumulating metabolites. Brain, liver, and kidneys are the most frequently affected organs. Treatment usually involves 1) protein restriction, 2) supplementation of amino acids with unimpaired metabolism as well as trace elements, and 3) specific measures for detoxification if indicated.

DISEASE	ENZYME DEFECT	INCIDENCE*	GENE LOCUS	OMIM
MSUD	Branched-chain keto acid dehydrogenase (lipoamide) Type Ia E_1 component α-chain, Type Ib component β-chain, Type II dihydrolipoamide branched-chain transacylase (E_2 component)	1:215,000	19q13.1-q13.2 6p21-22 1p31, 7q31-q32, 6q14	248600 248611 248610, 608348, 238331
IVA	Isovaleryl-CoA dehydrogenase	1:80,000	15q14-q15	243500
3MCC	3-Methylcrotonyl-CoA-carboxylase α-subunit, β-subunit	1:50,000	3q25-q27, 5q12-q13	210200
MGA type 1	3-Methylglutaconyl-CoA hydratase	<1:200,000	9q22.31	250950
MGA type II (Barth syndrome)	Tafazzin	<1:200,000	Xq28	302060, 300069, 300183
MGA type III (Costeff optic atrophy)		<1:200,000	19q13.2-q13.3	258501
MGA type IV		<1:200,000		250951
MHBD	2-Methyl-3-hydroxybutyryl-CoA dehydrogenase	<1:200,000	Xp11.2	300438
PA	Propionyl-CoA carboxylase, α-chain Propionyl-CoA carboxylase, β-chain	1:200,000	13q32 3q21-q22	232000 232050
MMA (Mut⁰/Mut⁻ defects)	Methylmalonyl-CoA mutase	1:100,000	6p12.3	251000
BTD	Biotinidase	1:80,000	3p25	253260
HLCSD	Holocarboxylase synthetase	<1:200,000	21q22.1	253270
GA type I	Glutaryl-CoA dehydrogenase	1:100,000	19p13.2	231670
D2HA	D-2-hydroxyglutaric acid dehydrogenase	<1:200,000	2p25.3	600721
L2HGA	FAD-dependent L-2-hydroxyglutarate dehydrogenase	<1:200,000	14q22.1	236792
ASPA (Canavan disease)	Aspartoacylase; aminoacylase II	1:200,000	17pter-p13	271900
EE	Mitochondrial matrix protein	<1:200,000	19q13.2	602473

*Incidences as estimated in Caucasian population, varying between populations of different ethnic backgrounds. MSUD = Maple syrup urine disease; IVA = isovaleric aciduria; 3MCC = 3-methylcrotonylglycinuria; MGA type I = 3-methylglutaconic aciduria type I; MGA type II = 3-methylglutaconic aciduria type II; MGA type III = 3-methylglutaconic aciduria type III; MGA type IV = 3-methylglutaconic aciduria type IV; MHBD = 2-methyl-3-hydroxybutyryl-CoA dehydrogenase deficiency; PA = propionic aciduria; MMA = methylmalonic aciduria; BTD = biotinidase deficiency; HLCSD = holocarboxylase synthetase defiency; GA type I = glutaric aciduria type I; D2HA = D-2-hydroxyglutaric aciduria; L2HGA = L-2-hydroxyglutaric aciduria; ASPA = N-acetylaspartic aciduria; EE = ethylmalonic encephalopathy.

DISEASES	BIOCHEMICAL FINDINGS	CLINICAL PRESENTATION NEONATAL	LATER	TREATMENT
MSUD	↑ Leucine (P) ↑ Valine (P) ↑ Isoleucine (P) ↑ Alloisoleucine (diagnostic)(P) ↑ Branched-chain oxo- and hydroxyacids (U)	Poor feeding, vomiting, lethargy, somnolence, opisthotonus, seizures, cerebral edema, coma, sweat, malty, caramel-like odor	Recurrent ketoacidotic decompensations, lethargy, stupor → coma, death, ataxia, fluctuating neurological disease, progressive psychomotor retardation	Leucine-, valine-, and isoleucine-reduced diet, consider trial of thiamine
IVA	↑ Isovalerylglycine (U) ↑ 3-Hydroxyisovaleric acid (U) ↑ Isovalerylcarnitine (P, S, U, DBS) ↓ Free carnitine (P, S)	Poor feeding, vomiting, lethargy, somnolence, cerebral edema, coma, "sweaty feet" odor	Recurrent ketoacidotic decompensations, lethargy, stupor → coma, failure to thrive, chronic vomiting, anorexia, progressive psychomotor retardation.	Low-protein or leucine-reduced diet L-Carnitine (50–) 100 mg/kg/day ±L-Glycine 150–250 mg/kg/day
3MCC	↑ 3-Methylcrotonylglycine (U) ↑ 3-Hydroxyisovaleric acid (U) ↑ 3-OH-Isovalerylcarnitine (P, S, U, DBS) ↓ Free carnitine (P, S)	Poor feeding, vomiting, lethargy, ketoacidotic decompensations, lethargy, stupor → coma	Progressive psychomotor retardation, but many asymptomatic affected individuals	Low-protein or leucine-reduced diet L-Carnitine (50–) 100 mg/kg/day
MGA type I	↑ 3-Methylglutaconic acid (U) ↑ 3-Methylglutaric acid (U) ↑ 3-Hydroxyisovaleric acid (U) ↑ 3-Methylglutaconylcarnitine (P, S, U, DBS)	Variable; fasting hypoglycemia; delayed speech and progressive psychomotor retardation, but also asymptomatic affected individuals		Symptomatic; value of dietary treatment and/or carnitine substitution uncertain
MGA type II	↑ 3-Methylglutaconic acid (U) ↑ 3-Methylglutaric acid (U) ↑ 2-Ethylhydracrylic acid (U)	Dilated cardiomyopathy, neutropenia, skeletal myopathy, growth retardation		Symptomatic
MGA type III	↑ 3-Methylglutaconic acid (U) ↑ 3-Methylglutaric acid (U)	Early-onset optic atrophy, later onset of extrapyramidal symptoms, ataxia, and cognitive impairment		Symptomatic
MGA type IV	↑ 3-Methylglutaconic acid (U) ↑ 3-Methylglutaric acid (U)	Clinically heterogeneous; lactic acidosis, dysmorphic features; mostly (progressive) encephalopathy with profound psychomotor retardation, spasticity, and hypotonia		Symptomatic
MHBD	↑ 2-Methyl-3-hydroxybutyric acid (U) ↑ Ethylhydracrylic acid (U) ↑ Tiglylglycine(U) normal 2-methylacetoacetate (↑) $C_{5:1}$ Carnitine (P, S, U, DBS)	Progressive psychomotor retardation, epileptic encephalopathy, truncal hypotonia with limb spasticity, gross motor dyskinesia and athetosis, blindness, mild acidosis in catabolic states, cardiomyopathy		Symptomatic
PA	↑ Propionic acid (U) ↑ 3-Hydroxypropionic acid (U) ↑ Propionylglycine (U) ↑ Methylcitric acid (U) ↑ Glycine (P, S, U, DBS) ↑ C_3 Carnitine (P, S, U, DBS) ↓ Free carnitine (P, S) ↑ Lactic acid, (P, U) ↑ NH_3 (blood)	Poor feeding, vomiting, lethargy, ketoacidotic decompensations, lethargy, stupor, cerebral edema → coma, death	Progressive psychomotor retardation, seizures, pyramidal and extrapyramidal movement disorder, osteoporosis, pancreatitis, cardiomyopathy	Isoleucine-, valine-, methionine-, and threonine-reduced diet L-Carnitine (100–) 200 mg/kg/day Consider metronidazole or neomycin
MMA	↑ Methylmalonic acid (U) ↑ Propionic acid (P) ↑ 3-Hydroxypropionic acid (U) ↑ Propionylglycine (U) ↑ Methylcitric acid (U) ↑ Glycine (P, S, U, DBS) ↑ C_3 Carnitine (P, S, U, DBS) ↓ Free carnitine (P, S) ↑ Lactic acid, (P, U) ↑ NH_3 (blood)	Poor feeding, vomiting, lethargy, ketoacidotic decompensations, lethargy, stupor, cerebral edema → coma, death	Progressive psychomotor retardation, seizures, pyramidal and extrapyramidal movement disorder, osteoporosis, pancreatitis, cardiomyopathy	Isoleucine-, valine-, methionine-, and threonine-reduced diet L-Carnitine (50–) 100 mg/kg/day Consider metronidazole or neomycin

DISEASES	BIOCHEMICAL FINDINGS	CLINICAL PRESENTATION NEONATAL	LATER	TREATMENT
BTD	↑ Lactic acid (P, U, CSF) ↑ Propionic acid (P) ↑ 3-Hydroxypropionic acid (U) ↑ Propionylglycine (U) ↑ Methylcitric acid (U) ↑ 3-Methylcrotonylglycine (U) ↑ 3-Hydroxyisovaleric acid (U) ↑ 3-OH-Isovalerylcarnitine (P, S, U, DBS) ↓ Free carnitine (P, S) ↓ Biotinidase (diagnostic)	Progressive psychomotor retardation, ataxia, (myoclonic) seizures, skin rash and/or alopecia		Biotin 5–10 mg/day
HLCSD	↑ Lactic acid (P, U) ↑ NH₃ (blood) ↑ Propionic acid (P) ↑ 3-Hydroxypropionic acid (U) ↑ Propionylglycine (U) ↑ Methylcitric acid (U) ↑ 3-Methylcrotonylglycine (U) ↑ 3-Hydroxyisovaleric acid (U) ↑ 3-OH-Isovalerylcarnitine (P, S, U, DBS) ↓ Free carnitine (P, S) Normal biotinidase	Poor feeding, vomiting, lethargy, ketoacidotic decompensations, lethargy, stupor, cerebral edema → coma, death	Progressive psychomotor retardation, seizures, ataxia, skin rash and/or alopecia	Biotin 10–20 (–40) mg/day
GA type I	↑ Glutaric acid (U) ↑ 3-Hydroxyglutaric acid (U) ↑ Glutaconic acid (U) ↓ Free carnitine (P, S) ↑ Glutarylcarnitine (P, S, U, DBS)	Macrocephaly, frontotemporal atrophy, acute encephalopathic crisis (usually age 4–18 months) with destruction of the striatum, subsequently severe dystonic–dyskinetic disorder, leucencephalopathy in adulthood		Strict adherence to emergency protocol in early childhood Lysine- and tryptophan-reduced diet L-Carnitine (50–) 100 mg/kg/day
D2HA	↑ D-2-Hydroxyglutaric acid (U) ↑ Krebs cycle intermediates (U) ↑ GABA, protein (CSF)	Variable phenotypes from neonatal-onset epileptic encephalopathy, lack of psychomotor development, facial dysmorphia, cardiomyopathy, and early death to normal outcome		Symptomatic
L2HGA	↑ L-2-Hydroxyglutaric acid (U) ↑ Lysine, (CSF, P, U)	Progressive psychomotor retardation, ataxia, epilepsy, macrocephaly, leukodystrophy (particularly subcortical U-fibers) combined with cerebellar atrophy and signal changes in basal ganglia and the dentate nuclei		Symptomatic
ASPA	↑ N-Acetylaspartic acid (P, S, U)	Progressive psychomotor retardation, epileptic encephalopathy, macrocephaly, leukodystrophy (particularly subcortical U-fibers), optic atrophy, death		Symptomatic
EE	↑ Ethylmalonic acid, methylsuccinic acid, C₄–C₆ acylglycines (U) ↑ C₅,C₆ Acylcarnitines (P, S, U, DBS)	Progressive psychomotor retardation, multiple brain lesions on MRI, acrocyanosis, petechiae, chronic diarrhea		Symptomatic

U = urine; P = plasma; S = serum; CSF = cerebrospinal fluid; DBS = dried blood spots; MSUD = Maple syrup urine disease; IVA = isovaleric aciduria; 3MCC = 3-methylcrotonylglycinuria; MGA type I = 3-methylglutaconic aciduria type I; MGA type II = 3-methylglutaconic aciduria type II; MGA type III = 3-methylglutaconic aciduria type III; MGA type IV = 3-methylglutaconic aciduria type IV; MHBD = 2-methyl-3-hydroxybutyryl-CoA dehydrogenase deficiency; PA = proprionic aciduria; MMA = methylmalonic aciduria; BTD = biotinidase deficiency; HLCSD = holocarboxylase synthetase defiency; GA type I = glutaric aciduria type I; D2HA = D-2-hydroxyglutaric aciduria; L2HGA = L-2-hydroxyglutaric aciduria; ASPA = N-acetylaspartic aciduria; EE = ethylmalonic encephalopathy.

TABLE 7-1	Clinical Presentation of Organic Acidurias

Intoxication

Kussmaul tachypnea/acidotic breathing

Peculiar smell

Refusal of/adverse reaction to feeding

Protracted episodic vomiting

Erroneous diagnosis of pyloric stenosis (with acidosis)

Reye syndrome presentation

Hepatomegaly/ liver failure

Rhabdomyolysis

Sudden infant death syndrome (SIDS) or near-miss SIDS

Acute encephalopathy

Coma

Seizures (myoclonic, intractable)

Acute profound dyskinesia

Pseudotumor cerebri

Cerebral/intraventricular hemorrhage in full-term babies

Stroke-like episodes

Chronic encephalo(myelo)pathy

Progressive psychomotor deterioration

Macrocephaly

Ataxia (progressive)

Hypotonia

Dystonia, athetosis

Myoclonus

Seizures (myoclonic, intractable)

Peripheral neuropathy

Pyramidal signs–"cerebral palsy"

Pronounced deficiency of speech

Congenital cerebral malformations

TABLE 7-2	Clinical Chemical Indices of Organic Acidurias

Metabolic acidosis

Increased anion gap

Hyperglycemia

Ketosis and ketonuria (especially suggestive in newborns)

Lactic acidosis

Hyperammonemia

Hyperuricemia

Hypertriglyceridemia

Increase of transaminases

Granulocytopenia, thrombocytopenia, anemia

Hypoketotic hypoglycemia (fatty acid oxidation defects)

Increased creatine kinase (fatty acid oxidation defects)

Myoglobinuria (fatty acid oxidation defects)

is an underlying metabolic disease. In such patients, routine clinical chemistry may be normal in between crises.

A substantial number of patients with OAs may present differently with acute encephalopathy or chronic and fluctuating progressive neurological disease (2). These cerebral OAs characteristically present with (progressive) neurological symptoms, such as ataxia, myoclonus, extrapyramidal symptoms, metabolic stroke, and macrocephaly. The signs of classical OAs such as acidosis, hypoglycemia, myopathy, and pancreatitis are only exceptionally present. This subgroup of OAs includes glutaric aciduria type I, 4-hydroxybutyric aciduria, N-acetylaspartic aciduria (Canavan disease), malonic aciduria, and L-2- and D-2-hydroxyglutaric

acidurias. In cerebral OAs, routine clinical chemistry often is unrevealing, and elevations of diagnostic metabolites by organic acid analysis may be small and missed, particularly by semiquantitative organic acid screens. This is especially true in glutaric aciduria type I or in vitamin-responsive disorders. Important diagnostic clues, such as progressive disturbances of myelination, cerebellar atrophy, frontotemporal atrophy, hypodensities, and/or infarcts of the basal ganglia (5), can be derived from magnetic resonance imaging (MRI) or computed tomographic (CT) scans of the brain (5) (see Figure 7-14). Symmetrical, not permanent, and varying imaging changes apparently independent of defined regions of vascular supply are especially suggestive of OAs or disorders of oxidative phosphorylation. Chronic subdural effusions, hematomas, and retinal hemorrhages in infants and toddlers are characteristic findings in glutaric aciduria type I, although they are more commonly due to child abuse.

Laboratory Investigations

During exacerbations, patients with the classical OAs display metabolic acidosis (low pH and low bicarbonate), massive ketosis, and

- Testing for ketonuria is especially useful. In neonates with OAs, there is often profound ketonuria, whereas ketonuria is observed rarely even in very sick newborns suffering from nonmetabolic diseases. It is rare even in infants with neonatal diabetes.

increased anion gap (see Table 7-2). Hematological evaluation may reveal leukopenia, thrombocytopenia, and sometimes pancytopenia. Glucose concentrations may be low or sometimes even high. Hyperammonemia occurs frequently in the initial neonatal crisis. If it leads to hyperventilation, the pH may be normal or even increased. In these instances, the increased anion gap still may point toward an OA versus a urea cycle disorder. Hyperammonemia is rare in episodes after early infancy, except for propionic or methylmalonic aciduria. Lactic acid often is increased (see Table 7-2).

Organic acid analysis is best performed on early-morning urine specimens (1). The interpretation of organic acid analysis depends on key diagnostic metabolites as well as on characteristic patterns of abnormalities. Repeated analyses may be necessary, preferably during exacerbation of metabolic decompensation. Characteristic metabolites, however, also may become masked in severe metabolic decompensation and ketosis. This is particularly true for 3-oxothiolase (β-ketothiolase) deficiency, in which the diagnostic metabolites may be absent during episodes of ketosis because they are obscured by massive amounts of especially ketone bodies and lactate.

A complementary and rapid diagnostic technique for classic OAs is the analysis of acylcarnitine profiles by MS/MS. In case of sufficient availability of free carnitine, the accumulating CoA esters are in equilibrium with their corresponding acylcarnitines, which are easy to analyze, even in dried blood spots, by MS/MS. This technique has been adapted to perform neonatal screening, leading to early diagnosis and appropriate therapy (3).

Some patients with OAs may exhibit only slight elevations of diagnostic metabolites that may not be detectable by currently used organic acid analysis. This is particularly true of disorders such as defects of cobalamin metabolism, in which the elevations of methylmalonate and homocysteine are small, and of 4-hydroxybutyric aciduria, glutaric aciduria type I, and N-acetylaspartic aciduria (Canavan disease). In the latter three disorders, ordinary organic acid analysis consistently underestimates true concentrations. Specific organic acids can be quantified by stable-isotope-dilution internal standard assays (1) (Table 7-3). This is also the method of choice for prenatal diagnosis of many disorders in which direct analysis of the pathognomonic organic acid in amniotic fluid provides more rapid and precise diagnosis than analyses of organic acids or acylcarnitines in amniotic fluid or enzymatic analysis of cultured amniocytes (6,7).

TABLE 7-3 Stable Isotope Dilution Internal Standard Assays Useful in the Diagnostic Workup of Specific Organic Acidurias

Compound	Suspected Disease
N-Acetylaspartic acid	Canavan disease
Glutaric acid and 3-hydroxyglutaric acid	Glutaryl-CoA dehydrogenase deficiency
4-Hydroxybutyric acid	Succinate semialdehyde dehydrogenase deficiency
3-Hydroxyisovaleric acid	Multiple carboxylase deficiencies, isovaleric acidemia, 3-methylcrotonyl-CoA carboxylase deficiency
Methylmalonic acid	Disorders of B_{12} metabolism, including dietary deficiency, methylmalonyl CoA mutase deficiency, transcobalamin II deficiency
Succinylacetone	Hepatorenal tyrosinemia

PRINCIPLES OF TREATMENT

OAs are chronic conditions that involve various organ systems and often with a progressive pathology. A diverse multidisciplinary approach to care and treatment, including adequate consideration of individual circumstances and psychosocial support, is required. Continuous support and guidance of patients and their families are essential for optimal outcome. Beyond the specific genotype, high variability in the outcome and in the efficacy of therapeutic strategies is due to factors affecting uniformity of care, including socioeconomic variables, adequacy of information, and counseling of patients, parents, and primary physicians, as well as differences in treatment protocols and proximity to emergency facilities and centers with metabolic experience.

Patients should carry an emergency card or bracelet containing essential information and phone numbers, as well as a letter with instructions on emergency measures. Vaccinations should be carried out as recommended and should include vaccinations against varicella, hepatitis A and B, *Pneumococcus*, and influenza. Special precautions must be taken before, during, and after operations/anesthesia (4).

In classical OAs, therapy is based mainly on restriction of intake of the respective precursor amino acids, supplementation of carnitine, avoidance of catabolism, and an intensification of therapy during intercurrent illnesses.

The major principle of dietary treatment is to reduce the production of toxic organic acids by restriction of natural protein. Such a diet must meet the general, age-dependent, and individual requirements for the daily intake of energy and essential nutrients, especially amino acids and micronutrients, to ensure normal growth and development (Table 7-4).

Monitoring of plasma amino acids, prealbumin, and transferin is required to avoid protein deficiency due to overrestriction of protein. Protein deficiency induces catabolism and in its extreme life-threatening form manifests as acrodermatitis acidemia (Figure 7-2), an acro-

TABLE 7-4	Protein Requirements (g/kg/day)	
Age	Revised Safe Values (156)	German Society for Nutrition (1985)
0–3 mos.	2.7–1.6	2.7–2.1
4–12 mos.	1.4–1.1	2.1–2.0
1–3 yrs.	1.0	1.7
4–6 yrs.	0.9	1.6
7–9 yrs.	0.9	1.4
10–12 yrs.	0.9	1.1
13–15 yrs.	0.9	1.0
Adults	0.8	0.9

Note: Revised safe values from Ref. 156 are based on an intake of a high-value protein and are used, for example, for children with urea cycle disorders. Protein requirements generally are higher in the treatment of OAs where the intake of single amino acids is restricted; in these children, it is appropriate to provide more natural protein, as in the recommendations of the German Society for Nutrition (1985) (157).

dermatitis enteropathica–like skin rash (8). Supplementation of the restricted natural protein with special formulas that contain amino acids devoid of the amino acid whose breakdown is blocked (AminoAcidMixtures) and semisynthetic supplements of minerals and trace elements minimizes the risk for malnutri-

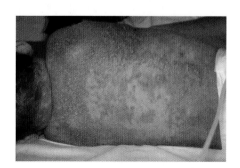

FIGURE 7-2. Acrodermatitis acidemia secondary to malnutrition in glutaric aciduria type I. Note polycyclic erythema and desquamation.

tion. Carnitine at doses of 50–200 mg carnitine per kilogram of body weight per day, or even higher, if required to maintain normal free carnitine levels, is essential for the elimination of accumulating toxic acyl-CoA compounds and for the restoration of intramitochondrial free CoA in classical OAs (9).

In vitamin-responsive disorders, enzyme activity may be restored by specific vitamins or cofactors, for example, in biotin-dependent biotinidase deficiency and holocarboxylase synthetase deficiency, vitamin B_{12}–dependent methylmalonic acidurias, and vitamin B_2–dependent multiple acyl-CoA dehydrogenase deficiency.

Emergency Treatment of Intercurrent Illness at Home

OAs often present with acute life-threatening decompensation requiring prompt decisions and measures. Since there is only a limited repertoire of pathophysiological sequences in response to metabolic illness, a limited number of therapeutic measures have to be taken immediately (10–12).

It is imperative to prevent or quickly interrupt a catabolic state at an early stage of impending decompensation. Since this usually happens at home, it is essential to educate the family about how to react adequately. Parents should be trained to calculate and manage outpatient emergency treatment. Home treatment should include adequate control of fever and vomiting, moderate protein restriction, and ample calories, glucose, and fluid to prevent catabolism and dehydration (Table 7-5). Intake of natural protein can be eliminated completely for the first 24 hours of illness, especially if the patient is treated with an AminoAcidMixture. AminoAcidMixtures help to "buffer" the metabolic capacity during intercurrent illnesses. After 24 hours, half the protein they are usually allowed must be reintroduced, the next day three-quarters, and then the full amount. One week after the intercurrent illness has resolved,

The basic principles for acute emergency therapy for OAs are:

- to suppress muscle and liver protein catabolism and ensure a glucose supply above the basal metabolic demand;

- to treat the precipitating illness;

- to reduce increased organic acid production by reduction or omission of natural protein;

- to enhance detoxifying mechanisms and urinary excretion of organic acids;

- to prevent carnitine depletion;

- to aggressively treat dehydration and acidosis.

TABLE 7-5   Home and Outpatient Emergency Treatment

A. Glucose polymer/maltodextrin solution*

Age	Percent	kcal/100 mL	Daily Amount
0–1 yrs.	10	40	150–200 mL/kg
1–2 yrs.	15	60	95 mL/kg
2–10 yrs.	20	80	1200–2000 mL/day
>10 yrs.	25	100	2000 mL/day

B. Protein intake

Natural protein	Stop (if AminoAcidMixtures are administered) or reduce to 50% of maintenance therapy (if no AminoAcidMixtures are administered). Reintroduce and increase within 1–2 days.
AminoAcidMixtures	If tolerated, AminoAcidMixtures should be administered according to maintenance therapy, e.g., 0.8–1.0 g/kg of body weight per day.

C. Pharmacotherapy

L-Carnitine	Double carnitine intake: 200 mg/kg of body weight per day orally (if tolerated)
Antipyretics†	If temperature > 35°C (101 F), e.g. ibuprofen (10–15 mg/kg of body weight per dose, 3–4 doses daily)

*Maltodextran/dextrose solutions should be administered every 2 hours day and night. If neonates and infants already receive a specific dietary treatment, protein-free food can be continued but should be fortified by maltodextran. Patients should be reassessed every 2 hours.

†Acetaminophen administration may be dangerous in acute metabolic decompensation (risk for glutathione depletion).

Note: All calculations for A, B, and C should be based on the expected and not on the actual weight!

the nutritional state should be assessed with plasma amino acid analysis because there may be a transient increase in protein requirement in order to return to positive nitrogen balance. Immediate hospital admission and intravenous treatment are indicated when vomiting persists, fluid and dextrose intake remains poor, the clinical condition deteriorates, or the disease course is prolonged. When presenting in an emergency clinic, these patients must be assessed immediately and further treatment begun without interruption. If the local metabolic center is far away, the emergency management in peripheral hospitals should be supervised by the local metabolic center, which will guide and provide the emergency protocols.

Emergency Treatment in the Hospital

Provision of ample quantities and control of fluid and electrolytes are indispensable and must be continued before any laboratory results are available. Glucose should be started via a peripheral intravenous line at 150 mL/kg/day of a 10% solution (~10 mg glucose per kilogram per minute, providing an energy supply of ~60 kcal/kg/day) in a neonate or infant. Overhydration is rarely a problem in metabolic crises because they are mostly accompanied by some degree of dehydration. Electrolytes, glucose, and acid–base balance should be checked every 6 hours, and serum sodium should be maintained at 138 mmol/L or greater.

In decompensated OAs, reversal of catabolism and of the breakdown of endogenous

protein is the major goal. During the crisis, natural protein intake is fully restricted initially but no longer than 24–48 hours. A high supply of energy is usually required (e.g., in neonates, >100 kcal/kg of body weight per day) (Table 7-6). In a sick baby, this can be accomplished only by hyperosmolaric infusions of glucose together with fat through a central venous line, which usually requires central venous catheterization. Insulin drip should be started early, especially in the presence of significant ketosis or in maple syrup urine disease (MSUD), to enhance anabolism and prevent hyperglycemia (13). One approach is to use a fixed combination of insulin to glucose (a useful combination is 1 U of insulin per 8 g of glucose). Another approach is to start with 0.1 U/kg/hour and to increase insulin dose stepwise if blood glucose concentration is higher than 150 mg/dL or if glucosuria develops. Intravenous lipids can be administered at 1–2 g/kg/day and often be increased up to 3 g/kg/day as long as serum levels of triglycerides are monitored.

Carnitine is essential for the elimination of toxic metabolites and must be administered intravenously at 100–200 mg/kg/day. Antibiotics should be started if there is any hint for an infectious cause.

After infancy, hyperammonemia develops rarely in OAs, except in propionic aciduria. The role of nitrogen-disposing drugs to treat hyperammonemia in OAs is controversial:

1. Sodium benzoate 250 mg/kg as a bolus initially over 1 hour, then 250 mg/kg/24 hours

- Treatment without adequate monitoring is dangerous because disease-specific complications, therapy-specific side effects (e.g., malnutrition), and developmental delay may be overlooked.

2. Sodium phenylacetate or phenylbutyrate 250 mg/kg as a bolus initially over 1 hour, then 250 mg/kg/24 hours

3. Arginine hydrochloride 420 mg/kg as a bolus initially over 1 hour, then 420 mg/kg/24 hours

If the response to these medicines is poor, if ammonia concentration exceeds 400 µmol/L, or if the patient is deteriorating, hemofiltration or hemodialysis needs to be considered urgently (14).

If persisting lactic acidosis is present, especially together with a history of insufficient food intake, a trial with thiamine (50–500 mg/day) should be performed (15).

After 24–48 hours, half the normal amount of natural protein must be reintroduced, the next day three-quarters, and then the full amount. This regimen of protein reintroduction is essential to minimize endogenous amino acid catabolism. The accumulation of toxic metabolites in some OAs, especially in methylmalonic and propionic acidurias, can be reduced by intestinal antibiotics (e.g., metronidazole or colistine). During treatment and after the intercurrent illness has resolved, the nutritional state should be assessed by plasma amino acids analysis as well as by measurement of prealbumin and transferrin levels because there may be a transient increase in protein requirement, especially isoleucine.

Monitoring of Treatment

Clinical monitoring should be frequent through a multidisciplinary team addressing dietary control, growth, and psychomotor development. Local services have to be involved. Growth parameters such as weight, height, and head circumference should be recorded at each visit. Psychomotor development must be assessed regularly with appropriate tests.

The development of specific recommendations for biochemical monitoring of a metabolic disorder should be based on an understanding of the pathophysiology of the

- Weight loss or insufficient weight gain in affected children is mostly caused by inadequate protein intake due to either too strict restriction of natural protein or insufficient intake of AminoAcidMixture and may herald impending metabolic decompensation!

TABLE 7-6　Inpatient Emergency Treatment

A. Energy requirement

Calories	Increase to minimum of 120% of age-dependent daily requirements			
	0–6 mos.	**7–12 mos.**	**1–3 yrs.**	**4–6 yrs.**
120% DRI (2002)* (kcal/kg of body weight per day)	108–113	108–109	106–109	94–98

B. Intravenous infusions

Glucose	(15–) 20 g/kg of body weight per day intravenously
Lipids	Start with 1–2 g/kg of body weight per day intravenously, if possible increase stepwise to 2–3 g/kg of body weight per day
Electrolytes	Electrolytes should be kept in the upper normal range
Insulin	If hyperglycemia > 150 mg/dL, start with 0.05 IE insulin/kg/h and adjust the infusion rate according to serum glucose (Note increased intracellular uptake of potassium.)
L-Carnitine	(100–) 200 mg/kg of body weight per day intravenously

C. Protein intake

Natural protein	Stop for a maximum of 24 (–48) hours, then reintroduce and increase stepwise until the amount of maintenance treatment within 3–4 days. If the child is on a low-protein diet without an amino acid mixture, increase protein within 1–2 days.
AminoAcidMixtures	If possible, AminoAcidMixtures should be administered according to maintenance therapy, e.g., 0.8–1.0 g/kg of body weight per day

D. Pharmacotherapy†

Antipyretics†	If temperature > 38.5°C (101 F), e.g. ibuprofen 10–15 mg/kg of body weight per dose
Antibiotics	Purposeful and timely administration
Antiemetics	If vomiting, ondansetron 0.1 mg/kg of body weight per dose intravenously (max. 3 doses daily)
Diuretics	If diuresis is less than 3–4 mL/kg/day, furosemide 0.5–1.0 mg/kg per dose intravenously (3–4 doses per day) (Note rebound and electrolyte loss.)
Bicarbonate	If acidosis; alkalination of urine also facilitates urinary excretion of organic acids

E. Monitoring

Blood	Glucose, blood gases, electrolytes, calcium, phosphate, complete blood cell count, creatinine, urea nitrogen, C-reactive protein, amino acids, carnitine state, blood culture, amylase/lipase (if pancreatitis)
Urine	Ketone bodies, pH

*DRI 2002, Institute of Medicine of the National Academy. Dietary reference intakes (DRI) for energy, carbohydrate, fiber, fat, fatty acids, cholesterol, protein, and amino acids. Food and Nutrition Board. Washington, DC: National Academies Press; 2002.

†Acetaminophen administration may be dangerous in acute metabolic decompensation (risk for glutathione depletion).

Note: All calculations for A–D should be based on the expected and not on the actual weight!

individual disease. The monitoring of serum phenylalanine levels in patients with phenylketonuria is perhaps the best example of this; outcome is directly related to the blood level of the phenylalanine. The same is true for the respective amino acids in MSUD. Unfortunately, the relationship between the levels of metabolites and outcome in patients with the other OAs is not quite so clear. Consequently, regular analyses of urinary organic acids or urinary amino acids or plasma and/or urinary acylcarnitines are rarely indicated.

The main aim of biochemical monitoring is to ensure that the patient's overall nutrition is not compromised. Biochemical evaluation includes blood count; serum electrolyte, calcium, phosphate, magnesium, and ferritin levels; liver and kidney function tests; alkaline phosphatase; and total protein, albumin, prealbumin, transferrin, cholesterol, triglycerides, zinc, copper, retinol (plasma), carnitine, ammonia, lactate, and plasma amino acids. The sample for the determination of plasma amino acids must be obtained in the postabsorptive state, either in the morning before breakfast or 6 hours after the last meal. Besides the essential amino acids (particularly isoleucine), other amino acids that should be monitored carefully are those that are reduced in consideration of the metabolic block. Monitoring of the essential amino acids ensures 1) that the patients has an adequate intake of natural protein, particularly if dietary treatment consists of protein restriction without the use of an AminoAcidMixture, 2) that the patient takes adequate amounts of the AminoAcidMixture, and 3) that compliance is ensured.

MAPLE SYRUP URINE DISEASE

Etiology/Pathophysiology In MSUD, branched-chain amino acids (i.e., leucine, isoleucine, and valine), their corresponding α-keto acids and hydroxyacid derivatives, as well as L-alloisoleucine are increased in physiological fluids. These amino acids and their metabolites accumulate due to inherited deficiency of the thiamine-dependent branched-chain α-keto acid dehydrogenase complex consisting of subunits $E_{1\alpha,\beta}$, E_2, and E_3 (Figure 7-3). L-Alloisoleucine results from racemization of the C_3 of L-isoleucine during transamination. Its elevation is pathognomic and diagnostic for MSUD (16).

MSUD was first reported in 1954 by Menkes, Hurst, and Craig, who noticed an unusual odor reminiscent of maple syrup in the urine of four infants who died from a rapidly progressive neurological disease (17). In general neonatal screening programs, a prevalence of 1 in 200,000 live births or fewer is encountered (18), but in the Mennonites in Pennsylvania, the prevalence is as high as 1 in 200 births (19). MSUD is caused by mutations in one of the four genes that code for proteins of the branched-chain α-keto acid dehydrogenase complex, which is analogous to the pyruvate dehydrogenase and the 2-ketoglutarate dehydrogenase multienzyme complexes. In fact, the third and last component of all three complexes is the same protein, and defects in the E_3 subunit impair the oxidative decarboxylation of pyruvate and 2-ketoglutarate, in addition to the branched-chain keto acids. The pathophysiology of E_3 deficiency, synonym *lipoamide dehydrogenase deficiency* or *2-keto acid dehydrogenase deficiency*, will be discussed further in Chapter 15.

In contrast to the classical organic acidurias, there is no accumulation of CoA metabolites (no characteristic acylcarnitines) in MSUD, and acidosis or hyperammonemia are not major features of the disease. There may be hypoglycemia. As in other aminoacidopathies, the clinical manifestations of MSUD are caused by the specific action of toxic metabolites (particularly 2-oxoisocaproic acid, the keto acid of leucine). 2-Oxoisocaproic acid has been shown to be severely neurotoxic by reducing cell respiration and inducing glial and neuronal apoptosis (20).

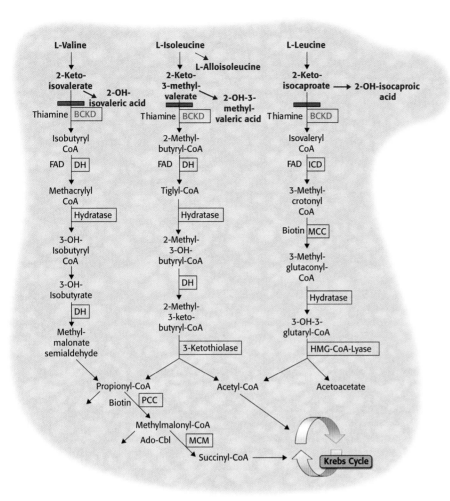

FIGURE 7-3. Metabolism of branched-chain amino acids: defect in MSUD. The metabolic block is indicated by a red line, the defective enzyme in red font; increased precursors are in blue font. Cofactors are shown beside the respective enzyme in italic. BCKDH = branched chain α-keto acid dehydrogenase, deficient in MSUD, resulting in increased concentrations of branched-chain amino-, oxo- and hydroxylacids, as well as of the diagnostically pathognomonic amino acid L-alloisoleucine; ICD = isovaleryl-CoA dehydrogenase, deficient in isovaleric acidemia; MCC = 3-methylcrotonyl-CoA carboxylase, deficient in methylcrotonylglycinuria; hydratase = 3-methylglutaconyl-CoA hydratase, deficient in 3-methylglutaconic aciduria type I; DH = dehydrogenase; PCC = propionyl-CoA carboxylase, deficient in propionic aciduria; MCM = methylmalonyl CoA mutase, deficient in methylmalonic aciduria; Ado-Cbl = adenosylcobalamin.

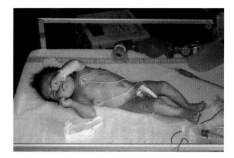

FIGURE 7-4. Opisthotonic hypertonic comatose infant with MSUD.

3–5 days and sometimes as late as 2 weeks if they are breast-feeding. If untreated, babies with the classical form of MSUD quickly deteriorate neurologically, developing lethargy, hypotonia alternating with muscular rigidity, and seizures.

A characteristic neurological presentation is of a markedly hypertonic, comatose or semi-comatose infant in an opisthotonic position (Figure 7-4). What makes MSUD challenging is that the neuroradiological, neuropathological, and electroencephalographic (EEG) findings in untreated MSUD patients are more characteristic than the name-giving odor, which even may be absent in a comatose patient who receives parental fluids but no protein. Neuroimaging shows a characteristic pattern of diffuse generalized cerebral edema, as well as localized edema affecting the cerebellar deep white matter, dorsal brain stem, cerebral peduncles, posterior limb of the internal capsule, and posterior aspect of the centrum semiovale, resulting in pseudotumor cerebri. Later on, hypomyelination develops. Convulsions appear regularly, and the electroencephalogram reveals abnormalities with comb-like rhythms (5–9 Hz) of spindle-like sharp waves over the central regions and multiple shifting spikes and sharp waves with suppression bursts. If undiagnosed and untreated, patients succumb within a few days.

Prominent neuropathological signs of untreated MSUD are cerebral atrophy and myelin deficiency, in addition to spongy degeneration and moderate astrocytic hyperplasia of the white matter. Hypodensities may be present in the globus pallidus and the thalamus. In the cerebellum, generalized necrosis of granular cells and extensive neuronal loss in pontine nuclei and substantia nigra are apparent.

Intermittent MSUD is the second most common form of MSUD, and affected patients may present repeatedly with fluctuating neurological disease such as lethargy, ataxia, and seizures that may progress quickly to coma and death during episodes of catabolic stress such as intercurrent infections or surgery/anesthesia.

Clinical Presentation Five different clinical presentations of the disease have been delineated, and they differ with respect to age of onset, clinical severity, biochemical manifestations, residual enzyme activity, and responsiveness of branched-chain α-keto acid dehydrogenase to its cofactor thiamine.

- The classical form of MSUD presents in the neonatal period, mostly on days 3–5 of life, with poor feeding, irritability, lethargy, and progressive neurological deterioration, including alternating hypertonia and hypotonia with dystonic extension of the arms.

- The intermediate form of MSUD develops slowly with progressive failure to thrive, developmental delay, and/or seizures.

- The intermittent form, which may present with ataxia, seizures, stupor, or coma, is likely to be precipitated by increased protein intake or intercurrent illnesses.

- The clinical symptomatology of the thiamine-responsive form of MSUD, in which the metabolic disturbance is ameliorated by pharmacological doses of thiamine, is similar to that seen in the intermediate form.

- Lipoamide dehydrogenase deficiency (synonyms: E_3 *deficiency*, *lipoamide dehydrogenase deficiency*, and *2-ketoacid dehydrogenase deficiency*) manifests after the neonatal period with lactic acidosis, failure to thrive, hypotonia, developmental delay, movement disorder, and progressive neurological deterioration.

Most patients with MSUD suffer from the classical form. They are normal at birth but develop feeding problems and vomiting after

Patients with intermediate MSUD variants present with failure to thrive and progressive mental retardation. In a few patients, mostly with intermittent or intermediate forms of MSUD, the metabolic defect has been corrected by pharmacological doses of thiamine (thiamine-responsive variant). However, at least two patients with classical neonatal presentation also have been shown to be thiamine-responsive. Effective doses vary greatly. As little as 10 mg and as much as 300 mg per day may be required.

These different clinical classifications overlap with one another and reflect various effects of private mutations on dysfunction of this multienzyme complex. Elevated concentrations of pathological metabolites are always demonstrable, and fulminant life-threatening clinical deterioration may occur in all variants, so the classification is only marginally useful for what is in fact a continuous spectrum of disease variants.

Diagnosis Presumptive diagnosis can be made at the bedside when the odor of maple syrup is present. Immediate confirmation by positive 2,4-dinitrophenylhydrazine (DNPH) testing is sufficient justification to initiate treatment in families at high risk. Diagnosis is confirmed by detection of the highly increased branched-chain amino acids levels via quantitative amino acid analysis and/or by increased urinary excretion of α-keto and hydroxy acids and branched-chain amino acids using GC-MS and quantitative amino acid analysis. The detection of L-alloisoleucine is pathognomonic for MSUD and helps in differentiating MSUD from conditions where branched-chain amino acids are physiologically elevated, such as during starvation and episodes of cyclic vomiting. The biochemical profile in classical MSUD patients is unmistakable.

If amino acid analysis is not readily available, addition of DNPH to urine may be carried out as a screening test, producing a yellow precipitate. Enzyme activity of the branched chain α-keto acid dehydrogenase complex can be determined in different tissues (e.g., leukocytes, lymphoblasts, cultured fibroblasts, and amniocytes) and confirms the diagnosis. Except for the common Mennonite mutation, the molecular base of MSUD is complex, and molecular testing is available in only a few research laboratories (21).

Very few patients are thiamine-responsive, and there are no good protocols to test for thiamine responsiveness. Evaluation for thiamine responsiveness with pharmacological amounts of thiamine (10 mg/kg/day) for at least 3 weeks should be performed only if the patient is in stable metabolic condition (22). However, data indicate that absorption of oral thiamine may be unreliable, and parenteral

TABLE 7-7   Laboratory Findings: MSUD
Increased
Amino acids: leucine, isoleucine, valine, alloisoleucine.
Organic acids: 2-ketoisocaproic acid, 2-keto-3-methylvaleric acid, 2-ketoisovaleric acid, 2-hydroxyisocaproic acid, 2-hydroxyisovaleric acid, 2-hydroxy-3-methylvaleric acid

administration may be necessary to judge the effect of larger doses (23) (Table 7-7).

Treatment and Outcome In MSUD, fast reduction of toxic molecules is the cornerstone of treatment (19,24). The most critical challenge is timely and correct intervention during acute metabolic decompensation in the neonatal period, as well as in later episodes. Emergency management aims to stop catabolism and initiate forced anabolism in order to lay down accumulated leucine and other branch-chain amino acids into protein. High amounts of energy are required to achieve anabolism (e.g., in neonates, more than 100 kcal/kg/day). This usually can be accomplished only by hyperosmolaric infusions of glucose (>10 mg/kg/minute), together with fat, through a central venous line and insulin drip (see "Emergency Treatment" above). Insulin should be started early. In parallel, branched-chain amino acid–free formula must be administered by orogastric perfusion to lay down branched-chain amino acids into body protein. Intravenous mixtures of amino acids lacking leucine, isoleucine, and valine can be very effective in a patient with intractable vomiting, but they are expensive and not generally available. Enteral mixtures mixed in minimal volume and dripped over 24 hours in doses of 2 g/kg of amino acids often can be tolerated even by a vomiting patient. Since plasma concentrations of isoleucine often are much lower than those of leucine, frequent quantitative analysis of plasma amino acids will determine the time to add isoleucine in the enteral mixture when the concentrations of isoleucine is lowered adequately. In many patients, valine also must be added before the leucine concentration is lowered sufficiently. Some centers would add isoleucine and valine from the beginning of emergency treatment, accepting supraphysiological levels (19).

Extracorporeal detoxification may be required if leucine levels exceed 20 mg/dL (1500 μmol/L). As in hyperammonemia, continuous arteriovenous or venovenous hemodialysis, hemofiltration, and hemodiafiltration have been shown to be effective (14).

Supplementation of carnitine is not indicated in MSUD. A liver transplant may normalize some metabolic aspects of the disease (25), and liver transplantation was suggested

recently as a reasonable treatment option for patients with classical MSUD (26).

Long-term treatment of MSUD is based on dietary restriction of branched-chain amino acids and supplementation of thiamine, if proven beneficial. Management in MSUD requires very close regulation of the diet by frequent and timely amino acid analyses (19). During rapid growth velocity (0–10 months), small infants usually require and tolerate 50–90, 30–60, and 20–50 mg/kg/day of L-leucine, L-valine, and L-isoleucine, respectively. These amounts will decrease gradually. After 1 year of age, requirements for L-leucine, L-valine, and L-isoleucine usually range around 20–40, 10–40, and 5–20 mg/kg/day, respectively. Thereafter, the tolerance of leucine decreases further with age down to 5–15 mg/kg/day in adults, whereas the requirements for L-valine and L-isoleucine usually change only little. Liver transplantation may be a reasonable long-term option for some patients (26). The decision of medical treatment versus transplantation is very complex and must be reached for each patient individually.

It is important to emphasize that strict biochemical monitoring and a branched-chain amino acid–restricted diet are recommended not only during periods of growth and development but also during one's lifetime (27) (see "Monitoring of Treatment" above). The specific amino acids to be monitored regularly are L-leucine, L-valine, and L-isoleucine.

Children with the classical form of MSUD have only a satisfactory prognosis if they are diagnosed and treated early (before age 5 days) (28). Neonatal screening had been performed in only few screening programs with modified bacterial inhibition assays (18). However, the increasing use of MS/MS neonatal screening should allow a faster, more timely, and more reliable diagnosis for affected children (3). In addition to counseling concerning treatment and prognosis, families of affected individuals should receive genetic counseling concerning recurrence risks for subsequent children. Prenatal testing is available for most of the severe forms of the disorders by enzymatic analysis of amniotic cells. Except for the Mennonites, affected families have private mutations that can be determined only rarely in research laboratories if a specific protein of the branched-chain α-keto acid dehydrogenase complex was shown to be missing by Western blot.

Optimal therapeutic target range of branched-chain amino acids in MSUD:

- Leu: 100–200 μmol/L

- Ile: 50–150 μmol/L

- Val: 150–250 μmol/L

ISOVALERIC ACIDURIA

Etiology/Pathophysiology Isovaleric aciduria (IVA) is caused by deficiency of isovaleryl-CoA dehydrogenase, an enzyme located proximally in the catabolic pathway of the essential branched-chain amino acid leucine (Figure 7-5). First descriptions of the clinical and biochemical phenotype were made by Tanaka and colleagues, and it was the first recognition of an organic aciduria (29). Tanaka and colleagues hypothesized the existence of a dehydrogenase specific for isovaleryl-CoA because of the distinct elevation of isovaleryl metabolites in the absence of elevations of other short-chain acids (29). In 1980, Rhead and Tanaka were able to prove this assumption (30). Human isovaleryl-CoA dehydrogenase was isolated from liver tissue in 1987 (31) and the corresponding gene, coding for a tetrameric 172-kDa enzyme with four identical subunits. Since then, several different mutations causing IVA have been described (32,33).

Isovaleryl-CoA dehydrogenase is a flavin enzyme containing approximately 1 mol FAD per subunit to transport electrons via coenzyme Q (CoQ) to the respiratory chain. Deficient enzyme activity can be demonstrated in fibroblasts by two different enzyme assays, and there is no correlation between the degree of enzymatic deficiency and clinical severity (30).

Due to the metabolic block, isovaleryl-CoA accumulates, and the pathognomonic metabolite isovalerylglycine is formed by conjugation of isovaleryl-CoA with the amino group of glycine through the activity of the mitochondrial enzyme glycine-N-acylase (EC 2.3.1.13). This reaction is an important detoxification pathway augmented in therapeutic intervention. Isovaleric acid, the product of hydrolysis, is quantitatively less important.

The specific pathophysiology of IVA is unclear. The accumulating CoA derivative sequesters CoA, thereby disturbing the mitochondrial energy metabolism. In bone marrow cell cultures, isovaleric acid was found to be an inhibitor of granulopoietic progenitor cell proliferation, which might be an explanation for the neutropenia seen frequently during metabolic decompensation (34).

Clinical Presentation Half the patients with IVA present in the neonatal period with severe metabolic crisis that may lead without appropriate treatment to coma and death, whereas the other half present with chronic intermittent disease consisting of episodes of metabolic acidosis and psychomotor retardation. A phenotype–genotype correlation has not been established for IVA, and both the preceding phenotypes can occur within the same family with the same mutation (35), suggesting a modifying role of environmental and epigenetic factors on the effect of the mutation on the IVA gene. In accordance with a recent publication, a mild, potentially asymptomatic phenotype exists due to a common mutation (932C-T, A282V). This mutation was detected by genetic analysis in 19 patients identified by newborn screening in 47% of mutant alleles and was also found in older, healthy siblings; thus this mutation may be associated with a mild, even asymptomatic clinical course (33).

During metabolic crisis, patients present with the typical features of an organic aciduria: acidosis, ketosis, vomiting, progressive alteration of consciousness, and finally, overwhelming illness, deep coma, and death without appropriate therapy. Children usually are healthy at birth after an uneventful pregnancy. Clinical abnormalities often develop within the first days of life. Patients refuse feeding, start to vomit, and become progressively dehydrated and lethargic. Hypothermia, tremor, twitching, and seizures can occur. A foul odor reminiscent of "sweaty feet" caused by isovaleric acid has been described and is rather pathognomonic. Abnormalities of the hematopoietic system such as thrombocytopenia, neutropenia, or pancytopenia develop during metabolic decompensation (35). Hypocalcemia and hyperglycemia also may occur. Hyperammonemia is usually mild compared with other OAs (see Table 7-2).

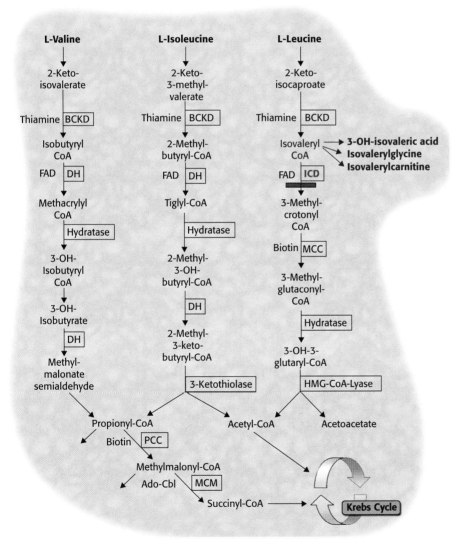

FIGURE 7-5. Metabolism of branched-chain amino acids: defect in isovaleric aciduria. The metabolic block is indicated by a red line, the defective enzyme in red font; increased precursors are in blue font. Cofactors are shown beside the respective enzyme in italic. ICD = isovaleryl-CoA dehydrogenase, deficient in isovaleric acidemia, resulting in increased concentrations of 3-OH-isovaleric acid, isovalerylglycine, and isovalerylcarnitine; BCKDH = branched chain α-keto acid dehydrogenase, deficient in MSUD; MCC = 3-methylcrotonyl-CoA carboxylase, deficient in methylcrotonylglycinuria; hydratase = 3-methylglutaconyl-CoA hydratase, deficient in 3-methylglutaconic aciduria type I; DH = dehydrogenase; PCC = propionyl-CoA carboxylase, deficient in propionic aciduria; MCM = methylmalonyl CoA mutase, deficient in methylmalonic aciduria; Ado-Cbl = adenosylcobalamin.

Acute metabolic decompensation can quickly lead to death triggered by cerebral edema, intracerebral hemorrhage, or infection. Neuropathological examination shows cerebellar edema with herniation and spongiform changes in the white matter.

In the chronic intermittent form, children slide into recurrent metabolic crises because of high intake of protein or minor infections inducing a catabolic state (35,36). Metabolic crises are characterized by vomiting, lethargy, coma, acidosis, ketosis, and the odor of "sweaty feet." Hematological abnormalities develop as described earlier, and hyperglycemia may develop most likely due to stress-induced counteregulatory hormonal effects. Pancreatitis may be a complication of acute and chronic IVA. With age, children become less sensitive to minor infections. Some patients dislike food with high protein content.

Older patients may have normal psychomotor development or mild to severe mental retardation depending on the frequency and severity of metabolic decompensations and, especially, the age of diagnosis and institution of specific metabolic therapy (35). The oldest known patient is now more than 30 years old with mild mental retardation and two episodes of dizziness, blurred vision, and walking difficulties as a teenager. She has had a pregnancy and delivery without major problems (37). Recently, a case of acute metabolic decompensation of IVA in an adult patient was described, and the authors pointed out that internists and adult neurologists also need to be aware of OAs (38).

Diagnosis The clinical symptoms of IVA are similar to those of the other OAs; even the suggestive odor of "sweaty feet" is shared by some other disorders (see Tables 7-1 and 7-2). The combination of ketoacidosis, dehydration, and hyperglycemia has led to the erroneous diagnosis of diabetic ketoacidosis (39), and the persistent vomiting in infancy has led to the erroneous diagnosis of hypertrophic pyloric stenosis and, as a result, to unnessecary surgery.

The best way to accomplish the diagnosis is quantitative analysis of urinary nonvolatile organic acids by GC-MS (1,40). Another complementary and rapid diagnostic technique is the analysis of acylcarnitine profiles by MS/MS. This technique has been adapted successfully to perform neonatal screening, leading to early diagnosis and appropriate therapy (3).

During metabolic decompensation, the urinary organic acid profile reveals high excretion of isovalerylglycine (2000–9000 mmol/mol of creatinine), which remains highly elevated in stable metabolic conditions (1000–3000 mmol/mol of creatinine). Since isovalerylglycine is

odorless, the characteristic odor is not present in the stable metabolic state. 3-Hydroxyisovaleric acid is found to be elevated only during metabolic decompensation. 4-Hydroxyvaleric acid, mesaconic acid, methylsuccinic acid, 3-hydroxyisoheptanoic acid, isovalerylglutamic acid, isovalerylglucuronide, isovalerylalanine, and isovalerylsarcosine are minor metabolites detectable in smaller amounts (20–300 mmol/mol of creatinine) (35). The acylcarnitine profile in IVA is characterized by high levels of isovalerylcarnitine in blood and urine depending on whether carnitine stores are repleted (after oral administration of 100 mg/kg L-carnitine, excretion of isovalerylcarnitine reaches 3200 mmol/mol of creatinine) (41). The diagnosis of IVA can be confirmed by enzymatic assay in cultured fibroblasts or mutation analysis, both of which are not available commercially. A practicable method for the determination of isovaleryl-CoA dehydrogenase activity as a confirmatory test using high-performance liquid chromatography (HPLC) has been described recently (42).

Several methods have been used successfully for prenatal diagnosis: stable-isotope-dilution analysis of amniotic fluid (elevated isovalerylglycine at 12 weeks of gestation in quantities of 3.5–6 μM) (6), macromolecular labeling from $(1\text{-}^{14}C)$-isovaleric acid in cultured amniocytes, or MS/MS analysis of acylcarnitines in amniotic fluid (highly elevated levels of isovalerylcarnitine, i.e., 3.12–12 μM, compared with control values from 0.59–0.99 μM) (7). Molecular diagnosis is available only in a research setting (Table 7-8).

Treatment and Outcome The main principles of therapeutic intervention are avoidance or reversal of catabolism, restriction of leucine intake, and detoxification of toxic metabolites by conjugation to glycine and/or carnitine (43). Total natural protein intake is restricted according to the patient's leucine tolerance and is adjusted to age-specific requirements. To provide a complementary source of the other amino acids, a

- Aspirin is contraindicated in patients with IVA because salicylic acid is a competing substrate for glycine-*N*-acylase, interfering with isovalerylglycine synthesis.

leucine-free formula is available. Beyond childhood, a protein-restricted diet allowing a moderate restriction of leucine intake usually is sufficient.

The other important principle of therapy is to increase the excretion of isovaleric acid as nontoxic glycine and carnitine conjugates (35). Normal tissue concentrations of glycine are already lower than the K_m concentrations for optimal enzyme functioning and tend to decrease further during metabolic decompensation. It is therefore important to ensure sufficient glycine levels to allow optimal detoxification. Therapeutic guidelines recommend a dosage of 150 mg/kg/day of glycine while the patient is stable. The dosage can be augmented up to 600 mg/kg/day during metabolic crisis. L-Carnitine is given in doses from 50–100 mg/kg/day monitored in plasma, ensuring high normal free carnitine (36,41,43).

During acute decompensation, IVA is treated like other OAs (see "Emergency Treatment" above). Measures include temporarily stopping the intake of protein and providing high energy via oral, nasogastric, or intravenous routes, 20% to 100% above the recommended daily requirements using carbohydrate (such as dextrose 20% orally or glucose intravenously) and fat (intralipid 20%). Augmented doses of glycine and high-dose L-carnitine are recommended as well as the use of soluble insulin to avoid hyperglycemia and to support intracellular glucose uptake.

Treatment has to be supervised by an experienced metabolic center and must continue for life. Special care must be taken to ensure efficient emergency procedures at all times (including travel and holidays) and to always monitor carnitine status and dietary management closely, including careful avoidance of

TABLE 7-8 Laboratory Findings: Isovaleric Aciduria	
Decreased	**Increased**
pH	Ratio of esterified to free carnitine
Free and total carnitine	Keton bodies, thrombocytopenia, neutropenia, or pancytopenia (metabolic decompensation)
	Amino acids: glycine, alanine (metabolic decompensation)
	Organic acids: isovalerylglycine (constant), 3-hydroxyisovaleric acid (metabolic decompensation), 4-hydroxyvaleric acid, mesaconic acid, methylsuccinic acid, 3-hydroxyisoheptanoic acid, isovalerylglutamic acid, isovalerylglucuronide, isovalerylalanine, isovalerylsarcosine (minor metabolites)
	Acylcarnitines: isovalerylcarnitine

overtreatment and malnutrition (see "Monitoring of Treatment" above).

Most children will survive the first life-threatening episode if correct treatment is set in place early. They have a chance to have normal psychomotor development. If efficient treatment can be accomplished before any severe metabolic decompensation, it will improve the patient's prognosis significantly up to a completely normal long-term psychomotor development and life expectancy. Therefore, early diagnosis is crucial, preferentially by extended neonatal screening (3).

3-METHYLCROTONYLGLYCINURIA

Etiology/Pathophysiology 3-Methylcrotonyl-glycinuria (MCG) is an inborn error of leucine catabolism due to deficiency of 3-α-methylcrotonyl-CoA carboxylase (Figure 7-6). Surprisingly, MCG appears to be the most frequent OA detected in MS/MS screening programs in North America, Europe, and Australia, with an overall frequency of approximately 1 in 50,000 births.

The MCG enzyme requires biotin as a cofactor, and the isolated enzymatic defect must be differentiated from other forms of methylcrotonylglycinuria caused by primary deficiencies in the biotin pathway (i.e., biotinidase and holocarboxylase synthetase deficiencies; see below). In addition to MCG, there are three other biotin-dependent carboxylases in humans: propionyl-CoA carboxylase (PCC), pyruvate carboxylase (PC), and acetyl-CoA carboxylase (ACC). The MCG enzyme, purified from bovine liver and rat liver, contains two nonidentical subunits, the biotin-binding α-subunit (73.5 kDa) and the β-subunit (61 kDa), which most likely form 6(αβ) heterodimers (44). Biotin is covalently bound to the amino group of lysine in the α-subunit. The MCG enzyme is located in the inner membrane of mitochondria, is magnesium-dependent, and can be activated by K⁺ and NH₄⁺ (44). Two complementation groups have been described corresponding to mutations in the α- and β-subunits. One mutation with a clinically asymptomatic phenotype that was identified in the Amish population in Lancaster County, Pennsylvania (USA), could be traced back to their Swiss ancestors (45,46).

The activity of 3-methylcrotonyl-CoA carboxylase measured in patient fibroblasts is severely reduced to 0% to 12% of normal without response to biotin (35). Due to the enzymatic block, 3-methylcrotonyl-CoA accumulates and is further hydrated to 3-hydroxy-isovaleryl-CoA by crotonase and deacylated to 3-hydroxyisovaleric acid. The other important pathway is the conjugation with glycine by glycine-N-acylase to form 3-methylcrotonylglycine. Secondary severe carnitine depletion, which is known to develop in the majority of patients, is caused by urinary excretion of carnitine metabolites. The most characteristic acylcarnitine is 3-hydroxyisovalerylcarnitine formed via 3-methylcrotonyl-CoA to methylcrotonylcarnitine and finally to 3-hydroxyiso-valerylcarnitine (47).

Clinical Presentation All patients with MCG show at least a short period of normal development (35). The clinical phenotype varies from asymptomatic patients, particularly women identified only by detection of abnormal metabolites in the neonatal screening samples of their healthy infants, to fulminant courses with lethality within the first year of life. No correlation between the level of residual enzyme activity and clinical presentation has been observed.

Crises, often triggered by minor infections, occur most frequently between the ages of 6 months and 3 years but also have been described in neonates and older children. Patients show vomiting, feeding difficulties, lethargy, and apnea, together with neurological symptoms such as muscular hypotonia, hyperreflexia, spasms, and seizures (focal or generalized). A few patients also were found to have neutropenia, loss of scalp hair, and fatty changes of the liver reminiscent of Reye syndrome. Death may occur from cerebral edema or cardiorespiratory arrest.

Diagnosis MCG should be considered in patients with recurrent ketoacidosis, Reye syndrome, and/or hypoglycemia, but also in patients presenting with unspecific, unexplained encephalopathies. As in other OAs, the clinical picture is common to many

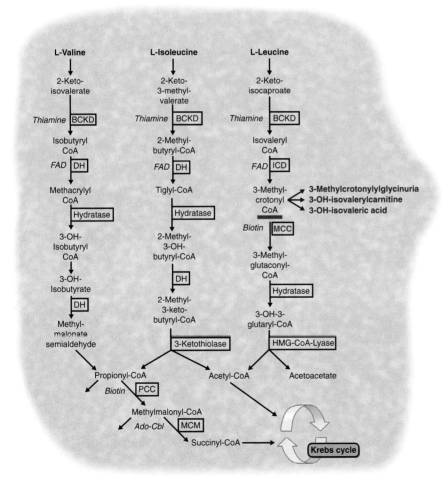

FIGURE 7-6. Metabolism of branched-chain amino acids: defect in 3-methylcrotonylglycinuria The metabolic block is indicated by a red line, the defective enzyme in red font; increased precursors are in blue font. Cofactors are shown beside the respective enzyme in italic. MCC = 3-α-methylcrotonyl-CoA carboxylase, deficient in 3-methylcrotonylglycinuria, resulting in increased concentrations of 3-hydroxyisovaleric acid, 3-methylcrotonylglycine, and 3-hydroxyisovalerylcarnitine; BCKDH = branched chain α-keto acid dehydrogenase, deficient in MSUD; ICD = isovaleryl-CoA dehydrogenase, deficient in isovaleric academia; hydratase = 3-methylglutaconyl-CoA hydratase, deficient in 3-methylglutaconic aciduria type I; DH = dehydrogenase; PCC = propionyl-CoA carboxylase, deficient in propionic aciduria; MCM = methylmalonyl CoA mutase, deficient in methylmalonic aciduria; Ado-Cbl = adenosylcobalamin.

diseases, so differentiation by laboratory workup is fundamental. The best way to accomplish the diagnosis is to study the pattern of urinary nonvolatile organic acids by quantitative GC-MS (1,35). A rapid complementary diagnostic technique is the analysis of acylcarnitine profiles by MS/MS. The key metabolites leading to diagnosis are 3-hydroxyisovaleric acid (500–7000 mmol/mol of creatinine, compared with 1–20 mmol/mol of creatinine in healthy individuals and 50–200 mmol/mol of creatinine in patients with severe ketosis of other cause) and 3-methylcrotonylglycine (50–4000 mmol/mol of creatinine) (35) in urine and 3-hydroxyisovalerylcarnitine in plasma or dried blood. Usually, the excretion via 3-hydroxyisovaleric acid is more prominent than that via 3-methylcrotonylglycine. Elevations of 3-hydroxybutyric, acetoacetic, and dicarboxylic acids can be seen in ketotic patients, but if 3-hydroxypropionic, methylcitric, and/or lactic acids are also elevated, the possibility of multiple-carboxylase deficiency should be considered.

Examination of the carnitine status reveals low free and total carnitine, an elevated ratio of esterified to free carnitine, and a high elevation of 3-hydroxyisovalerylcarnitine in plasma or dried blood spots. 3-Hydroxyisovalerylcarnitine already can be detected in newborn screening (3).

Demonstrating significantly reduced enzyme activity in fibroblasts or leukocytes without response to biotin makes the definitive diagnosis. It is important to exclude multiple-carboxylase deficiency by demonstrating normal enzyme activities of propionyl-CoA carboxylase, pyruvate carboxylase, and biotinidase.

Prenatal diagnosis is possible by stable isotope dilution analysis of amniotic fluid, which shows elevated 3-hydroxyisovaleric acid, or by enzyme activity assay in cultivated amniocytes or chorionic villi material (6). With description of the gene locus, molecular prenatal diagnosis is also possible in families with known mutations (Table 7-9).

Treatment and Outcome The main concern in patients with MCG is to prevent metabolic decompensation. The catabolic pathway of leucine degradation is challenged by increased protein intake or increased endogenous protein breakdown (35). Significant restriction of protein intake is not necessary in all patients. Moderate protein restriction of 1.5–2 mg/kg/day is often sufficient. To provide a source of the other amino acids, a leucine-free Amino-AcidMixture is available (4,35). Dietary therapy must be monitored closely, including careful avoidance of overrestriction

and malnutrition (see "Monitoring of Treatment" above).

During acute decompensation, MCG is treated like other organic acidemias (see "Emergency Treatment" above). Measures include increased provision of energy via oral, nasogastric, or intravenous routes at 20% to 100% above the recommended daily requirements using carbohydrate (such as dextrose 20% orally or glucose intravenously) and fat (intralipid 20%). Augmented doses of glycine and high-dose L-carnitine are recommended, as well as the use of soluble insulin to avoid hyperglycemia and to support intracellular glucose uptake (4,35).

Isolated 3-methylcrotonyl-CoA carboxylase deficiency has been reported repeatedly to be unresponsive to biotin until recently, when two patients were reported to be biotin-responsive (48). The first patient showed progressive psychomotor retardation and seizures, and biotin treatment resulted in a rapid and dramatic improvement in the clinical situation and correction of the biochemical phenotype. The second patient was detected by newborn screening and remained clinically asymptomatic, and the biochemical phenotype also was completely corrected by pharmaceutical doses of biotin. In both children, heterozygosity for the mutation MCCA-R385S was found, and thus this mutated allele may have a dominant-negative effect besides allowing biotin responsiveness in vivo.

MCG can be diagnosed easily in extended newborn screening programs using MS/MS, allowing for early treatment before a first severe metabolic decompensation. However, the effect of presymptomatic detection on the patient's prognosis is still uncertain (3,35). A significant number of patients are known to never develop symptoms, even without treatment.

3-METHYLGLUTACONIC ACIDURIAS

Increased urinary excretion of 3-methylglutaconic acid, usually accompanied by increased excretion of 3-methylglutaric acid, is a relatively commonly observed marker for a heterogeneous group of inborn errors of metabolism termed 3-*methylglutaconic acidurias* (see Table 7-10) (49). Only a small proportion of patients suffers from 3-methylglutaconic aciduria type I, the primary deficiency of 3-methylglutaconyl-CoA hydratase (Figure 7-7). 3-Methylglutaconic aciduria variants include 3-methylglutaconic aciduria type II, or Barth syndrome, caused by a deficiency of the mitochondrial membrane protein tafazzin (50,51), and 3-methylglutaconic aciduria type III, or Costeff optic atrophy syndrome, caused by a defect in the OPA3 gene (52). 3-Methylglutaconic aciduria is denoted type IV when the molecular defect is unknown and the other types have been excluded; this represents the largest and almost certainly the most genetically heterogeneous group of patients with the biochemical phenotype (49,53). Increased levels of 3-methylglutaconic acid also have been found in the urine of patients with primary mitochondrial disorders, for example, Pearson syndrome and ATP synthase deficiency (49), and in the plasma of patients with Smith–Lemli–Opitz syndrome (54). In the latter patients it has been speculated that 3-methylglutaconic acid arose from isoprenoid precursors via a mevalonate shunt in the cholesterol and isoprenoid pathway. However, there is as yet no substantiated explanation for the presence of elevated excretions of 3-methylglutaconic and 3-methylglutaric acids in any group of patients with normal activity of 3-methylglutaconyl-CoA hydratase.

TABLE 7-9   Laboratory Findings: 3-Methylcrotonylglycinuria

Decreased	Increased
pH	Ratio of esterified to free carnitine, ketoacidosis
Free and total carnitine	Organic acids: 3-hydroxyisovaleric acid, 3-methylcrotonylglycine
	Acylcarnitines: 3-hydroxyisovalerylcarnitine

TABLE 7-10   3-Methylglutaconic Acidurias

Combined Excretion of 3-Methylglutaconic and 3-Methylglutaric (mmol/mol of Creatinine)*	
Type I: 3-Methylglutaconyl-CoA hydratase deficiency	500–1500
Type II: Deficiency of tafazzin (Barth syndrome)	45–100
Type III: Deficiency of a mitochondrial membrane protein (Costeff syndrome)	10–100
Type IV: Unclassified (largest group, clinically heterogeneous)	40–1500
Type V: Secondary (e.g., mitochondriopathies, Smith–Lemli–Opitz syndrome)	20–200

*Normal < 10 (1).

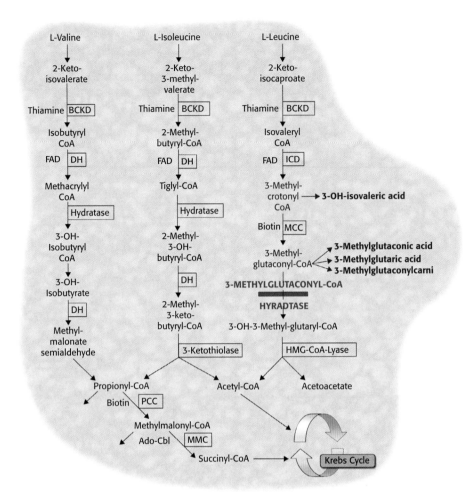

FIGURE 7-7. Metabolism of branched-chain amino acids: defect in 3-methylglutaconic aciduria type I. The metabolic block is indicated by a red line, the defective enzyme in red font; increased precursors are in blue font. Cofactors are shown besides the respective enzyme in italic. HYDRATASE = 3-methylglutaconyl-CoA hydratase, deficient in 3-methylglutaconic aciduria type I, resulting in increased concentrations of 3-methylglutaconic acid, 3-methylglutaric acid, 3-hydroxyisovaleric acid, and 3-methylglutaconylcarnitine; BCKDH = branched-chain α-keto acid dehydrogenase, deficient in MSUD; ICD = isovaleryl-CoA dehydrogenase, deficient in isovaleric academia; MCC = 3-methylcrotonyl-CoA carboxylase, deficient in methylcrotonylglycinuria; DH = dehydrogenase; PCC = propionyl-CoA carboxylase, deficient in propionic aciduria; MCM = methylmalonyl CoA mutase, deficient in methylmalonic aciduria; Ado-Cbl = adenosylcobalamin.

3-METHYLGLUTACONIC ACIDURIA TYPE I

Etiology/Pathophysiology 3-Methylglutaconic aciduria type I is caused by deficiency of 3-methylglutaconyl-CoA hydratase (see Figure 7-7) required for the conversion of 3-methylglutaconyl-CoA to 3-hydroxy-3-methylglutaryl-CoA in leucine catabolism. The hydratase is identical to a RNA-binding protein (designated AUH) possessing enoyl-CoA hydratase activity (56). The defect leads to an accumulation of 3-methylglutaconyl-CoA and its precursor, 3-methylcrotonyl-CoA. The action of a specific or nonspecific oxidoreductase on the first compound yields 3-methylglutaryl-CoA, and hydration of the latter leads to 3-hydroxyisovaleryl-CoA. Hydration of the three CoA esters results in accumulation of the diagnostic organic acids.

3-Methylglutaconic aciduria type I is a very rare disease with uncertain clinical significance. Only 11 patients from 10 families have been reported, with another 4 patients known (Dr. Zschocke, Heidelberg, personal communication).

Clinical Presentation Most patients present with variable neurological symptoms, from retardation of speech development and some delay in motor development to progressive psychomotor retardation. The causal relationship of these symptoms to the metabolic defect is uncertain. Metabolic decompensation is rare but can occur. Fasting for 18 hours in one patient but not in another was followed by hypoglycemia (55). 3-Methylglutaconic aciduria type I may present as nondisease, and more information on the clinical relevance is needed.

Diagnosis The diagnosis of 3-methylglutaconic aciduria type I due to hydratase deficiency results from a differential workup of a patient that reveals highly increased urinary concentrations of metabolites of leucine degradation (see Figure 7-7). A constellation of large amounts of 3-methylglutaconic, 3-methylglutaric, and 3-hydroxyisovaleric acids in urine with normal excretion of 3-hydroxy-3-methylglutaric acid pinpoints hydratase deficiency. Increased 3-hydroxyisovalerylcarnitine is a hint for either type of 3-methylglutaconic aciduria, and its measurement is a screening parameter in some newborn screening programs (56). The definitive diagnosis is made by demonstrating significantly reduced enzyme activity in fibroblasts or by mutation analysis. Prenatal diagnosis in general is not justified (Table 7-11).

Treatment and Outcome The need for treatment has not been established, especially for dietary treatment. Children should be monitored clinically during intercurrent illnesses. The outcome appears favorable because a significant number of patients have never developed symptoms, even without treatment.

3-METHYLGLUTACONIC ACIDURIA TYPE II (BARTH SYNDROME)

Etiology/Pathophysiology In 1983, Barth and colleagues described an extended pedigree with an unusual pediatric neuromuscular disease characterized by dilated cardiomyopathy, skeletal myopathy, retarded growth, and neutropenia (50). Since then, more than 20 patients have been reported. Pedigrees are those of an X-linked disorder of the male.

Barth syndrome is caused by a deficiency of tafazzin (a protein of the inner mitochondrial membrane) that affects mitochondrial

TABLE 7-11	Laboratory Findings: 3-Methylglutaconic Aciduria Type I
Decreased	**Increased**
Free and total carnitine	Ratio of esterified to free carnitine
	Organic acids: 3-hydroxyisovaleric acid, 3-methylglutaconic acid, 3-methylglutaric acid
	Acylcarnitines: 3-hydroxyisovalerylcarnitine, 3-methylglutarylcarnitine (inconstant)

phospholipid metabolism. Especially the phospholipid cardiolipin, in humans present almost exclusively in mitochondrial inner membranes, appears defective and deficient, disturbing the function of respiratory-chain complexes (50,51). The origin of elevated levels of 3-methylglutaconic and 3-methyl-glutaric acids in Barth syndrome, however, is unknown. The amount of the 3-methylgluta-conic aciduria appears to be independent of the severity of the clinical course.

Identification of the causative gene allowed the retrospective classification of different families labeled in the past as *X-linked endocardial fibrosis*, *severe X-linked cardiomyopathy*, or *Barth syndrome*. All these entities were shown to share the same molecular pathology (57).

Clinical Presentation The determining clinical presentation in Barth syndrome is cardiomyopathy. Patients may present at birth or during the first weeks of life, usually with congestive heart failure. With long-standing cardiac disease, endocardial fibroelastosis may develop. Additional clinical manifestations are skeletal myopathy, growth retardation, and neutropenia. Neutropenia is severe and variable but not cyclical. Bone marrow shows normal cell lines apart from the myeloid series, which usually appears to be arrested at the myelocyte stage (50). Susceptibility to severe infections is evident. Occasionally, a patient will present with neutropenia only. Muscle weakness is the main abnormal neurological sign. Delayed gross motor milestones, myopathic facies, a waddling gait, and a positive Gower sign are common. Occasionally, patients may show moderate lactic acidosis. In one patient, the plasma concentration of carnitine was low, and episodic hypoglycemia responded to carnitine supplementation.

Postnatal growth retardation may be severe, but beyond 2 years of age, deceleration of growth is ceased, and patients grow along curves paralleling 3–5 standard deviations (SDs) below normal, but with normal head circumferences.

Diagnosis Barth syndrome should be suspected in any male presenting with dilated cardiomyopathy. If neutropenia, idiopathic myopathy, and growth retardation are also present in the diagnosis of Barth syndrome is almost certain.

3-Methylglutaconic aciduria should be looked for specifically by stable-isotope-dilution methods in urine as well as in blood but is not a constant feature. Another organic acid, 2-ethylhydracrylic acid (a derivative from L-isoleucine), is also elevated in Barth syndrome. Apparently, Barth syndrome interferes with the degradation of two different branched-

chain amino acids. Muscle disease and lactic acidemia may initiate a workup for mitochondrial disorders. Muscle biopsy will reveal moderate accumulation of neutral fat, and biochemical evaluation shows involvement of two or more complexes of the respiratory chain, similar to findings caused by mitochondrial DNA mutations (e.g., MELAS). The definitive diagnosis of Barth syndrome requires determination of the cardiolipin content of thrombocytes or a positive result of mutation analysis. Mutation analysis can be used for prenatal diagnosis (Table 7-12).

Treatment and Outcome Children affected by Barth syndrome need to be managed carefully mainly by an expert cardiologist with the consistent involvement of an immunologist and neurologist. Management of cardiomyopathy includes diuretics and digitalization. Dysrhythmias are an ominous sign and may require implantation of an internal cardiac defibrillator. With time, cardiac disease may improve or deteriorate. Two children are known who received heart transplants because of progressive cardiac disease. One died suddenly 1 year after transplant; the other is surviving without evidence of recurring cardiac disease. The immunodeficiency in patients with Barth syndrome must be managed accordingly. All episodes of fever or localized infections need to be treated promptly and aggressively.

Dietary treatment with protein restriction has been employed without conclusive benefit, and children should receive a normal, varied diet. Similarly, carnitine supplementation generally does not appear to be of benefit.

About 25% of patients with Barth syndrome succumb during infancy and early childhood, mostly from either congestive cardiomyopathy or overwhelming bacterial infections. Sudden death due to ventricular dysrhythmia has been observed, even in periods of apparent well-being and absence of cardiac decompensation.

3-METHYLGLUTACONIC ACIDURIA TYPE III (COSTEFF SYNDROME)

Etiology/Pathophysiology Costeff optic atrophy syndrome is caused by mutations in the OPA3 gene resulting in a defect of a putative mitochondrial protein (52). Its specific function is unknown. The symptomatology and its evolution suggest common pathophysiological mechanisms with classical mitochondri-

opathies. The origin of elevated levels of 3-methylglutaconic and 3-methylglutaric acids is unknown, although defined mitochondrial disorders are known to also cause this biochemical constellation (e.g. Pearson syndrome and ATP synthase deficiency) (49).

Clinical Presentation The determining clinical presentation in Costeff syndrome is early-onset optic atrophy. It is associated with prolonged visual evoked potential latencies, whereas electroretinography is normal. In later childhood or adolescence, patients develop extrapyramidal signs, less commonly ataxia, and moderate cognitive impairment. In about half of patients, spasticity develops and progresses over years, whereas the other deficits remain stationary (58).

Diagnosis Costeff syndrome should be suspected in patients presenting with early-onset optic atrophy if additional neurological symptoms develop. So far the disorder has only been reported in a genetically homogeneous group of Iraqi Jews. The clinical presentation is overlapping with Behr syndrome. A difference is the presence of extrapyramidal signs in most patients, which do not occur in Behr syndrome, in which ataxia is obligatory. 3-Methylglutaconic aciduria is an indicator of the diagnosis, which now may be confirmed by molecular analysis (52).

Treatment and Outcome Treatment of Costeff syndrome is symptomatic and concentrates on the prevention of disabilities due to progressive spasticity. The disease appears non progressive, although no long-term outcome data beyond the forth decade are available (Table 7-13).

3-METHYLGLUTACONIC ACIDURIA TYPE IV (UNCLASSIFIED)

Etiology/Pathophysiology 3-Methylglutaconic aciduria type IV is surely heterogeneous. Since unexplained 3-methylglutaconic aciduria, that

TABLE 7-12   Laboratory Findings: 3-Methylglutaconic Aciduria Type II

Decreased	Increased
Leukocytes	Organic acids: 3-methylglutaconic acid, 3-methylglutaric acid, 2-ethylhydracrylic acid
Free and total carnitine (inconstant)	Acylcarnitines: none

TABLE 7-13   Laboratory Findings: 3-Methylglutaconic Aciduria Type III

Increased
Organic acids: 3-methylglutaconic acid, 3-methylglutaric acid
Acylcarnitines: none

is, type IV, also was found incidentally in asymptomatic adults, it appears doubtful that this biochemical feature by itself is of pathophysiological relevance (49). Rather, it appears to be a semispecific marker of different inborn errors of metabolism.

Clinical Presentation In 3-methylglutaconic aciduria type IV, neurological symptoms are predominant. Most identified and reported patients suffer from severe disease. The picture in many cases is one of profound retardation, neurological deterioration, spasticity with or without muscular hypertonia, and/or hypotonia (49,53). Other, less frequently observed manifestations included failure to thrive, optic atrophy with or without chorioretinal degeneration, deafness, seizures, extrapyramidal signs, and/or hepatic involvement. Individual patients have displayed self-mutilating behavior or dysmorphic features. Neuroradiological studies revealed global brain atrophy, lesions of the basal ganglia, and/or cerebellar atrophy.

In some cases, lactic acidosis was present, whereas hyperammonemia and hypoglycemia have been reported rarely. Unexplained 3-methylglutaconic aciduria, that is, type IV, can be found in completely asymptomatic individuals.

Diagnosis Diagnosis of 3-methylglutaconic aciduria type IV is by exclusion. Patients are identified because of elevated concentrations of 3-methylglutaconic and 3-methylglutaric acids in the urine without elevated 3-hydroxy-3-methylglutaric acid. Highly elevated citric acid cycle metabolites have been reported, as well as elevated urinary lactate and pyruvate and sometimes dicarboxylic aciduria. Enzyme assay of 3-methylglutaconyl-CoA hydratase is normal, as are overall in vitro evaluations of the leucine catabolic pathway (59). A workup for mitochondrial disorders is justified in the presence of significant unexplained symptoms by in vivo biochemical evaluation, mitochondrial DNA molecular analysis, and ex vivo histological and enzymatic investigations of muscular tissue. This may reveal a defined mitochondriopathy such as Pearson syndrome or mitochondrial ATP synthase deficiency. In addition, sterols should be investigated because patients with Smith–Lemli–Opitz syndrome were shown to also exhibit 3-methylglutaconic aciduria (54) (Table 7-14).

Treatment and Outcome In most patients, treatment is symptomatic and concentrates on the consequences of severe neurological manifestations. Since two as yet unresolved causes of 3-methylglutaconic aciduria, that is, types II and III, involve mitochondrial proteins, and since defined mitochondriopathies could cause 3-methylglutaconic aciduria,

TABLE 7-14   Laboratory Findings: 3-Methylglutaconic Aciduria Type IV
Increased
Lactic acid (inconstant)
Organic acids: 3-methylglutaconic acid, 3-methylglutaric acid, citric acid cycle metabolites (inconstant)
Acylcarnitines: none

and finally and most important, since the clinical manifestations are is often suggestive of a mitochondriopathy, care of patients with an identified 3-methylglutaconic aciduria should entail 1) a full assessment of muscle function with a special focus on the heart and possibly muscle ultrasound and electromyography (EMG), 2) a full neurological examination including EEG and MRI, and 3) a detailed assessment of the function of other organ systems, especially the visual system.

As in defined mitochondrial disorders, specific treatment options, that is, cofactors and vitamins, are limited and of doubtful effectiveness. If they are tried on an experimental basis, and if the condition does not improve convincingly within half a year, they should be stopped, with clinical follow-up. In one subset of patients, ubiquinone appeared to halt clinical progression (53). These patients presented with progressive predominant extrapyramidal disease and basal ganglia involvement on MRI. Dietary therapies, whether a low-protein, leucine-restricted, or ketogenic diet, are not indicated and are potentially harmful.

The identification of 3-methylglutaconic aciduria has no prognostic relevance for the individual unless a defined genetic defect can be identified. The degree of the organic aciduria does not offer any information for prognosis or patient management. However, in view of the rather precarious outcome of most patients with 3-methylglutaconic aciduria type IV, this diagnosis can be taken as an example that in some circumstances, such in patients with incidentally found unexplained 3-methylglutaconic aciduria type IV, a diagnosis may add more to confusion than to alleviating suffering.

2-METHYL-3-HYDROXYBUTYRYL-COA DEHYDROGENASE DEFICIENCY

Etiology/Pathophysiology 2-Methyl-3-hydroxybutyryl-CoA dehydrogenase deficiency is a rare cerebral OA. The defective mitochondrial enzyme is involved in the catabolism of isoleucine and the branched-chain fatty acids (Figure 7-8). The enzyme precedes 2-methylacetoacetyl-CoA thiolase, which is synonymous with β-ketothiolase and 3-oxothiolase (see Chapter 8). The latter enzyme is also involved in ketone body production, specifically ketolysis, and was recognized in the 1970s to cause recurrent ketoacidotic decompensation with dehydration and acute encephalopathy. The pattern of urinary excretion of pathological metabolites in these two disorders is identical except for the absence of 2-methylacetoacetate in 2-methyl-3-hydroxybutyryl-CoA dehydrogenase deficiency (see Figure 7-8). Retrospectively, patients with 2-methyl-3-hydroxybutyryl-CoA dehydrogenase deficiency were misdiagnosed as suffering from β-ketothiolase deficiency until Zschocke and colleagues in 2000 recognized the separate and distinct clinical and biochemical presentation and proved the defect. Since then, a dozen further patients have been described revealing a progressive neurometabolic disease with a distinct but broad spectrum of symptoms of variable onset (61–65).

Inheritance is X-chromosomal semidominant (females may be symptomatic). Mutations are found in the HADH2 gene, which had been known previously to code for an amyloid-β-binding protein (67).

The clinical consequences of 2-methyl-3-hydroxybutyryl-CoA dehydrogenase deficiency are different from those of other disorders of isoleucine breakdown, including β-ketothiolase deficiency, and appear to be related to enzyme functions outside the isoleucine catabolic pathway. The enzyme is identical to an amyloid-β-peptide-binding protein involved in Alzheimer disease (68). In addition, there appears to be significant impairment of cerebral energy metabolism (61).

Clinical Presentation 2-Methyl-3-hydroxybutyryl-CoA dehydrogenase deficiency mostly results in a progressive neurodegenerative disease (60–65). Regression usually becomes obvious in late infancy or early childhood, although two patients succumbed in infancy with severe lactic acidosis and cardiomyopathy, and another developed apparently normally up to the age of 5 years before developing a progressive movement disorder, epilepsy, and general deterioration (62). The latter patient was still alive in his midtwenties with a family history of two great uncles who had died with a diagnosis of "multiple sclerosis" at the ages of 30 and 60 years.

Affected boys usually develop truncal hypotonia with increased muscle tone and spasticity of the arms and legs, gross motor dyskinesia

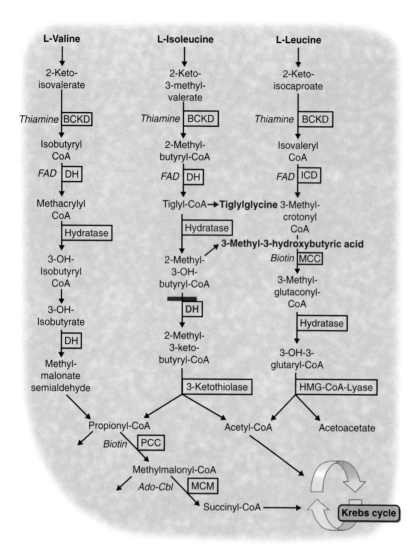

FIGURE 7-8. Metabolism of branched-chain amino acids: defect in 2-methyl-3-hydroxybutyryl-CoA dehydrogenase deficiency. The metabolic block is indicated by a red line, the defective enzyme in red font; increased precursors are in blue font. Cofactors are shown besides the respective enzyme in italic. DH = 2-methyl-3-hydroxybutyryl-CoA dehydrogenase, deficient in 2-methyl-3-hydroxybutyryl-CoA dehydrogenase, resulting in increased concentrations of 2-methyl-3-hydroxybutyric acid, tiglylglycine, and ethylhydracrylic acid; BCKDH = branched-chain α-keto acid dehydrogenase, deficient in MSUD; ICD = isovaleryl-CoA dehydrogenase, deficient in isovaleric academia; MCC = 3-methylcrotonyl-CoA carboxylase, deficient in methylcrotonylglycinuria; hydratase = 3-methylglutaconyl-CoA hydratase, deficient in 3-methylglutaconic aciduria type I; PCC = propionyl-CoA carboxylase, deficient in propionic aciduria; MCM = methylmalonyl CoA mutase, deficient in methylmalonic aciduria; Ado-Cbl = adenosylcobalamin.

and athetosis, loss of head control, a horizontal nystagmus, and retinal blindness. Ophthalmological examination at the stage of amaurosis will reveal optic atrophy and possibly retinitis pigmentosa. Motor and mental skills are lost completely, as are sensory modalities. Epilepsy is a frequent feature and may become extremely difficult to treat; children may die in status epilepticus. When hypertrophic cardiomyopathy was diagnosed, deterioration was rapid, with death due to progressive heart failure.

Neuroimaging documents progressive generalized atrophy with involvement of the basal ganglia, especially putamina, periventricular white matter abnormalities and occipital infarctions in individual patients (63,65).

Heterozygous female patients may be asymptomatic or may have variable non progressive psychomotor retardation with impaired hearing depending on X-inactivation patterns (61).

Diagnosis Clinically, 2-methyl-3-hydroxybutyryl-CoA dehydrogenase deficiency should be considered in children presenting with early-onset progressive encephalopathy, especially if there is evidence of X-linked inheritance. However, progression is not always clear, and the picture may resemble neonatal hypoxic–ischemic brain injury.

The clinical and neuroradiological presentation and evolution of 2-methyl-3-hydroxybutyryl-CoA dehydrogenase deficiency could be misdiagnosed as Leigh-like syndrome. Variably increased concentrations of lactate in blood and cerebrospinal fluid (CSF), of lactate:pyruvate ratios, and of creatine kinase also direct the diagnosis toward a primary mitochondrial disorder. Finally, reduced activity of the mitochondrial chain complex I was demonstrated in one patient (61).

The main biochemical features of 2-methyl-3-hydroxybutyryl-CoA dehydrogenase deficiency are increased urinary excretion of the isoleucine metabolites 2-methyl-3-hydroxybutyric acid and tiglyglycine (see Figure 7-8). Elevations of 2-ethylhydracrylic acid and 3-hydroxyisobutyric acid also may be found and sometimes elevations of C5:1 acylcarnitine. It is important to note that the abnormalities in urinary organic acids may only be moderate, and possibly overlooked depending on the quality of organic acid analysis.

β-Ketothiolase deficiency, the next enzyme in isoleucine degradation (see Figure 7-8), has been a well-established clinical and biochemical entity and presents with a very similar excretion pattern of urinary organic acids. However, the clinical picture of episodic severe ketoacidosis and hyperketotic hypoglycemia is completely different (see Chapter 8). The definitive diagnosis of 2-methyl-3-hydroxybutyryl-CoA dehydrogenase deficiency is achieved by demonstrating the enzymatic and/or molecular defect. If determined in an index patient, both methods can be employed for prenatal diagnosis (Table 7-15).

Treatment and Outcome Care of patients with 2-methyl-3-hydroxybutyryl-CoA dehydrogenase deficiency repeatedly should entail 1) a full assessment of muscle function with special focus on the heart and possibly muscle ultrasound and EMG, 2) a full neurological examination including EEG and MRI, and 3) a detailed assessment of the function of other organ systems, especially the visual and hearing systems. No effective treatment is known. An isoleucine-restricted diet has been implemented with questionable success (60,61,64).

TABLE 7-15	Laboratory Findings: 2-Methyl-3-hydroxybutyryl-CoA Dehydrogenase Deficiency	
Decreased	**Increased**
Free and total carnitine (inconstant)	Lactic acid (inconstant)
	Organic acids: 2-methyl-3-hydroxybutyric acid, tiglyglycine
	Acylcarnitines: tiglylcarnitine (C5:1) (inconstant)

The prognosis of 2-methyl-3-hydroxybutyryl-CoA dehydrogenase deficiency is often poor, with death in early childhood. However, in some patients without cardiomyopathy, the neurological disease may not progress for prolonged periods. This appears to be the rule in symptomatic hemizygotes, pointing to a relationship between the degree of enzyme impairment and clinical severity.

PROPIONIC ACIDURIA

Etiology/Pathophysiology The first description of a patient with propionic aciduria was in 1961, with ketosis and hyperglycinemia as the initial hallmarks (66). The disorder then was lumped together with methylmalonic aciduria as *ketotic hyperglycinemia* to distinguish it from hyperglycinemia without ketosis. Advancements in the determination of organic acids allowed the differentiation of these disorders in the 1970s (69).

Propionic aciduria is caused by autosomal recessively inherited deficiency of propionyl-CoA carboxylase (PCC), the first step in the propionate metabolism, in which propionyl-CoA is converted to methylmalonyl-CoA and then channeled into the citric acid cycle (Figure 7-9). PCC is a biotin-dependent duodecameric enzyme consisting of six α-chains (to which the biotin is covalently bound) and six β-chains (70). Over 100 disease-causing mutations have been identified in the PCCA gene (13q32) encoding for the PCC α-chain as well as in the PCCB gene (3q21-22), encoding for the PCC β-chain (71,72). Correlations between residual enzyme activity, complementation groups, or mutations and clinical features of the disorder are modest. Null mutations are more likely to lead to a classical severe clinical disease, whereas missense mutations are more likely to result in later onset of symptoms and milder clinical course (73).

Propionyl-CoA is formed from the catabolism of several branched-chain amino acids, isoleucine, threonine, methionine, and valine, of odd-numbered fatty acids, and of the three-carbon side chain of cholesterol (see Figure 7-9). Deficient PCC gives rise to accumulation of propionyl-CoA and from that of other abnormal metabolites such as methylcitrate, 3-hydroxypropionate, tiglic acid, propionylcarnitine, and propionylglycine. All these can be detected and quantified by GC-MS and/or MS/MS.

Elevated propionyl-CoA and its pathological derivatives interfere with a variety of metabolic pathways. Inhibition of the glycine cleavage enzyme leads to hyperglycinemia. Inhibition of N-acetylglutamate synthase, an enzyme of the urea cycle, causes hyperammonemia. Impairment of the activities of the pyruvate dehydrogenase complex, the ubihydroquinone:cytochrome C reductase of the respiratory chain, and several Krebs cycle enzymes results in reduced ATP synthesis, ketosis, and lactic acidosis (74,75).

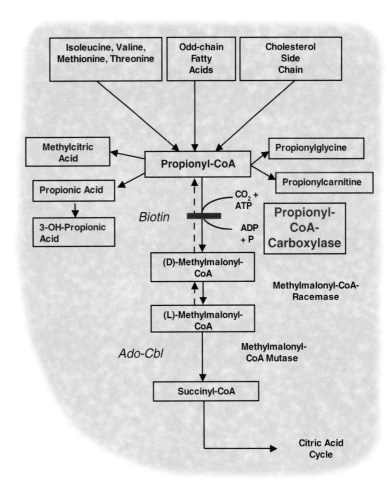

FIGURE 7-9. Metabolism of branched-chain amino acids: defect in propionic aciduria, resulting in increased concentrations of propionic, 3-hydroxypropionic and methylcitric acid, and propionylcarnitine. The metabolic block is indicated by a red line, the defective enzyme in red font; increased precursors are in blue font. Cofactors are shown beside the respective enzyme in italic. Ado-Cbl = adenosylcobalamin. (Adapted with permission from Ref. 90.)

Clinical Presentation Propionic aciduria frequently presents very early in life with life-threatening illness with severe hyperammonemia, metabolic acidosis, ketosis, lactic acidemia, hyperglycinemia/-uria, and hyperalaninemia (70,76). Patients usually are healthy at birth but quickly develop overwhelming disease, which may be misinterpreted as sepsis or ventricular hemorrhage. Both conditions in fact can be secondary complications of metabolic imbalance, and because of the extreme and rapid onset and progression, some patients may die undiagnosed. Patients may develop leukopenia, thrombocytopenia, and anemia. Massive ketosis leads to acidosis, dehydration, lethargy, and coma. Without vigorous specific therapy, death is inevitable.

Metabolic decompensations in infancy or early childhood are similar to those in the neonatal period. The first symptom is often vomiting. This has led to an erroneous diagnosis of pyloric stenosis or duodenal obstruction, resulting in a number of pyloromyotomies or other explorations. The infant also may exhibit generalized or myoclonic seizures and hepatomegaly. Liver histology has shown fatty infiltration and degeneration. Hepatomegaly can resolve following carnitine supplementation. Not all patients present with acidosis or ketosis, but the majority present with hyperammonemia. Thrombocytopenia, with or without petechiae, neutropenia, or pancytopenia can develop in the severely ill infant. Such children are unusually susceptible to infections, which may mimic an immunodeficiency disease.

Young patients often present with hypotonia, which may resolve. Many patients are anorexic, even when stable, requiring tube feeding, and may have hypochromic, normocytic anemia, especially if they suffer frequent decompensations. Chronic monoliasis can be troublesome. Over the years, growth becomes impaired, in part due to the negative effect of metabolic acidosis on growth hormone action.

- The most important key to the diagnosis of propionic aciduria is a high index of suspicion. Although the picture of an overwhelming illness in a neonate suggests sepsis, a metabolic workup should be on the list of additional investigations to be initiated at once.

A number of patients exhibit osteoporosis, and pathological fractures may occur. The increased risks of acute and recurrent pancreatitis, as well as of muscle lipidosis and cardiomyopathy, are worrisome as these complications can be rapidly fatal (77).

Neurological symptoms are frequent, including the development of chorea and dystonia. Basal ganglia hypodensities in neuroimaging indicate selective vulnerability of basal ganglia, in particular of the globus pallidus, to disordered propionate metabolism. Basal ganglia lucencies following episodes of metabolic decompensation may be transient, but metabolic stroke and basal ganglia infarction have occurred (see Figure 7-14A). Seizures tend to be generalized or of absence type, and less frequently focal. Furthermore, many patients show developmental delay and mental retardation due to cerebral atrophy. Males in particular have exhibited optic atrophy (78), and single patients have developed psychiatric disease (76).

A small subgroup of patients exhibits almost an exclusively encephalopathy and progressive neurological disease resembling of a lysosomal storage disorder (79). A milder form of propionic aciduria, reported in Japan, manifests in childhood with mild mental retardation or extrapyramidal symptoms and only occasionally with metabolic acidosis (80). Finally, a few individuals have been asymptomatic until teenage years and were diagnosed in the course of a family investigation (81).

Diagnosis Patients with propionic aciduria have highly elevated levels of glycine in plasma and urine. This is shared with other OAs, for example, methylmalonic acidurias, IVA, and 3-oxothiolase deficiency. Episodes of ketoacidosis usually exclude nonketotic hyperglycinemia. The best way to accomplish the diagnosis is by quantitative analysis of urinary nonvolatile organic acids by GC-MS (1,40). A complementary and rapid diagnostic technique is the analysis of acylcarnitine profiles by MS/MS. This technique has been adapted successfully to perform neonatal screening, leading to early diagnosis and therapy (3).

During metabolic decompensation, the urinary organic acid profile reveals high excretion of propionate metabolites such as β-hydroxypropionate, methylcitrate, tiglic acid, and propionylglycine (see Figure 7-9). Massive ketonuria can partly cover up the specific metabolites in organic acid analysis. Propionylcarnitine is readily detectable in plasma, urine, or dried blood spots. The absence of methylmalonic acid excludes methylmalonic acidurias, and the absence of β-hydroxyisovalerate and β-methylcrotonylglycine rules out multiple-carboxylase deficiency.

Propionyl-CoA carboxylase can be assayed in peripheral blood leukocytes or in cultured fibroblasts. Normal activities of 3-methylcrotonyl-CoA and pyruvate carboxylase exclude multiple-carboxylase deficiency. Molecular diagnosis has become possible and facilitates prenatal diagnosis in informative families (71,72). (For a continuously updated list of mutations, go to uchsc.edu/cbs/pcc/pccmain.htm). Prenatal diagnosis is also possible by enzyme assay, by determination of incorporation of [^{14}C]propionate in amniocytes (82), or more rapidly by quantitative stable-isotope-dilution assay of methylcitrate in amniotic fluid (6) (Table 7-16).

Treatment and Outcome Timely and effective emergency treatment is the most important determinant of outcome (76,83,84). During acute decompensation, propionic aciduria is treated like other OAs by 1) treating the precipitating illness (including the use of antibiotics), 2) reversing muscle and liver protein catabolism, 3) enhancing renal clearance of accumulating toxic compounds, and 4) ensuring a high energy intake as a calculated glucose infusion rate (see "Emergency Treatment" above). Massive ketoacidosis requires especially vigorous therapy. Large amounts of fluid, electrolytes, and bicarbonate and high doses of intravenous carnitine must be infused together with glucose. The intake of natural protein is stopped for 24–48 hours and then is reintroduced gradually. Hyperammonemia is often present and especially severe. It must be treated by providing arginine along with alternative methods of waste nitrogen excretion, that is, benzoate and phenylacetate or phenylbutyrate. If hyperammonemia is not reversed rapidly, acute hemodialysis may become necessary according to guidelines used in urea cycle disorders, especially in newborns and infants.

Long-term treatment is based on lifelong dietary restriction of isoleucine, valine, methionine, and threonine, as well as supplementation with L-carnitine (see "Principles of Treatment" and "Monitoring of Treatment" above). Patients should be taught to test for ketones in their urine. In infancy, the urine should be tested daily at home, later at intervals, but always at any sign of intercurrent illness. In individual patients, significant proprionate production occurs in the gut, which can be reduced by intermittent treatment (10 days/month) with metronidazole (10–20 mg/kg/day), colistin, or neomycin. Some patients exhibit recurrent or almost chronic hyperammonemia, especially during infancy. As hyperammonemia may be related to the rather poor intellectual outcome in many, should be checked for regularly, and if present, should be treated 1) by trying to optimize dietary therapy and 2) by providing arginine along with alternative methods of waste nitrogen excretion, that is, benzoate and phenylacetate or phenylbutyrate.

Close to 20 children with propionic aciduria who had frequent and severe metabolic compromises have undergone orthotopic liver transplantation. A larger cohort was reported by Leonard and colleagues in 2001 (85). In this series, three of eight children died following liver transplantation. Auxiliary as well as living-related liver transplantations have been performed successfully, but liver transplantation in propionic aciduria seems to be much more complicated than in patients with urea cycle disorders.

Despite early diagnosis and treatment, the neonatal-onset form of propionic aciduria is still complicated by early death in infancy or childhood. Patients with the late-onset form reach adulthood but often are handicapped by severe extrapyramidal movement disorders and mental retardation (76,83). However, progress has been achieved in survival and prevention of neurological sequelae in affected children with early diagnosis and meticulous treatment and follow up care. On an individual basis, patients can have normal intellectual outcome in adulthood.

TABLE 7-16　Laboratory Findings: Propionic Aciduria	
Decreased	**Increased**
pH	Ratio of esterified to free carnitine
Free and total carnitine	Ketone bodies, lactic acid, ammonia (metabolic decompensation)
Thrombocytopenia, neutropenia, or pancytopenia (metabolic decompensation)	Amino acids: glycine, alanine (metabolic decompensation)
	Organic acids: 3-hydroxypropionic acid, methylcitric acid, tiglic acid, propionylglycine, tiglylglycine
	Acylcarnitines: propionylcarnitine

METHYLMALONIC ACIDURIA

Etiology/Pathophysiology Methylmalonic acidurias comprise a group of diverse inherited disorders that appear with a cumulative prevalence of 1 in 100,000 in Caucasians, sharing methylmalonic acid accumulation in body fluids as the common biochemical feature (70). The disorder was first described in 1967 by Oberholzer and colleagues and by Stokke and colleagues (86,87). This section deals with methylmalonic aciduria caused by mutations in the gene encoding the apoenzyme methylmalonyl-CoA mutase (MCM). MCM alternatively can be impaired by defects in the biosynthesis of adenosylcobalamin or by deficient cobalamin transport (see Chapter 17). Methylmalonic aciduria also develops in acquired deficiency of vitamin B$_{12}$, such as pernicious anemia.

D-Methylmalonyl-CoA is formed in propionate metabolism by carboxylation of propionyl-CoA (Figure 7-10). L-Methylmalonyl-CoA is formed from D-methylmalonyl-CoA by the action of D-methylmalonyl-CoA racemase (EC 5.4.99.2). After the human gene and protein product encoding the latter enzyme have been identified, two siblings with comparatively mild methylmalonic aciduria and little if any clinical symptomatology were diagnosed with a defect in this enzyme. Isomerization of L-methylmalonyl-CoA to succinyl-CoA is catalyzed by the mitochondrial enzyme MCM, a dimer of identical subunits depending on 5-deoxyadenosylcobalamin as its cofactor (see Figure 7-10) (70).

Different genetic defects in cobalamin metabolism are known to result from a variety of mechanisms from absorption and intestinal uptake of vitamin B$_{12}$ to conversion to 5-deoxyadenosylcobalamin in the mitochondrion (see Chapter 17). In addition, defects of the apoenzyme MCM are also heterogeneous. Many disease-producing mutations of the MCM gene that differ in their pathophysiological consequences have been identified. Mut^0 patients have no enzyme activity, whereas Mut$^-$ patients have a spectrum of residual activity. Residual activity of deficient MCM corresponds to mutations in the MCM gene and translates into severe clinical presentation, reflecting a genotype–phenotype

- Methylmalonic acid is a more reliable index of body stores of cobalamin than vitamin B$_{12}$ levels in blood (88).

- In infancy, severe progressive disease may develop in breast-fed infants of mothers suffering from (undiagnosed) pernicious anemia or mothers adhering to a strict vegan diet.

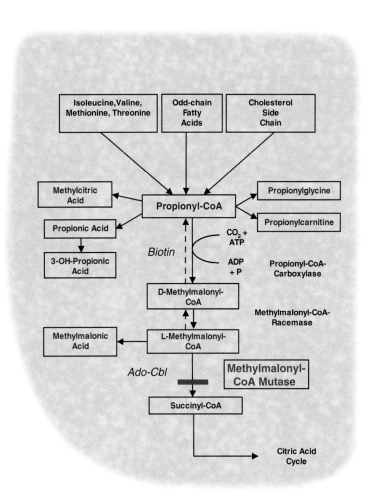

FIGURE 7-10. Metabolism of branched-chain amino acids: defect in methylmalonic aciduria, resulting in increased concentrations of methylmalonic acid in addition to propionic, 3-hydroxypropionic, and methylcitric acids and propionylcarnitine, the metabolic markers of propionic aciduria. The metabolic block is indicated by a red line, the defective enzyme in red font; increased precursors are in blue font. Cofactors are shown beside the respective enzyme in italic. Ado-Cbl = adenosylcobalamin. (Adapted with permission from Ref. 90.)

correlation in methylmalonic acidurias. The residual enzyme activity in the Mut$^-$ constellation may be stimulated further by high concentrations of hydroxycobalamin in vitro and in vivo. Despite this heterogeneity, it should be remembered that all genetic defects are rare individually and are transmitted as autosomal recessive disorders.

An impairment of energy metabolism plays a key role in the pathophysiology of methylmalonic aciduria, resulting in neurodegeneration of the basal ganglia and renal failure. It has been the subject of intense debate as to whether methylmalonic acid is the major toxin. Recently it was demonstrated that inhibition of respiratory chain and tricarboxylic acid cycle may be induced by different synergistically acting metabolites that also accumulate, particularly 2-methylcitric acid, malonic acid, and propionyl-CoA (74).

Clinical Presentation Classical methylmalonic aciduria due to deficiency of MCM presents with severe metabolic crises in the first months of life, progressive failure to thrive, feeding problems, recurrent vomiting, dehydration, hepatomegaly, lethargy, seizures, and developmental delay (70,76). Overwhelming disease in neonates is rather rare but indistinguishable from the presentation of patients with propionic aciduria with vomiting, dehydration, lethargy, and coma leading to death if not promptly recognized and treated specifically and aggressively. Presentation of MCM includes severe metabolic acidosis, ketosis, and lactic acidemia and, sometimes hypoglycemia and/or hyperammonemia. The disease course can be mistaken for sepsis or ventricular hemorrhage, both secondary complications of metabolic imbalance, and may remain undiagnosed if a metabolic workup is not included in the initial evaluation.

After the neonatal period, infants with methylmalonic aciduria develop variable clinical manifestations. In the chronic intermittent form, children slide into recurrent metabolic crises because of high intake of protein or minor infections that induce a catabolic state. Almost all these infants will present with failure to thrive, poor growth, feeding problems, developmental delay, and intermittent episodes of lethargy with clinical and laboratory findings of severe lactic and ketoacidosis. Also, infants of mothers suffering from pernicious anemia or practicing a very strict vegetarian (vegan) diet present such a picture when they are exclusively breast-fed. In these children, the clinical course is progressive, and although the biochemical derangement is rapidly reversible after initiating vitamin B_{12} therapy, neurological sequelae often are permanent. During metabolic decompensation, patients with deficiency of MCM may exhibit generalized or myoclonic seizures and hepatomegaly. Intermittent emesis may be so prominent as to suggest a primary gastrointestinal disorder. Anorexia is mostly severe and requires tube feeding. Young patients often are very hypotonic, which may resolve without sequelae. A number of skin lesions often are caused by moniliasis.

Methylmalonic aciduria carries with it a number of long-term complications (89) such as poor appetite, intermittent emesis, poor growth, and osteopenia. Chronic neurological symptoms, especially an extrapyramidal movement disorder caused by progressive destruction of the basal ganglia, are similar to those observed in other organic acid disorders, such as propionic aciduria or glutaric aciduria type I. Symmetrical necrosis of the globus pallidus in many patients results from acute stroke-like events. In other patients, often those with poor metabolic control, neurological symptoms progress slowly over several years. Pancreatitis and psychiatric disease also may occur.

Unique is the development of chronic renal failure in the second decade in 20% to 60% of patients (89), which probably is caused by chronic accumulation of methylmalonic acid (155). The risk of developing renal failure seems to correlate with the urinary level of methylmalonic acid over time and depends on the disease type. Patients with the Mut^0 form of MCM deficiency are at a higher risk to develop renal failure than patients with Mut- who are responsive to vitamin B_{12} and patients with cobalamin deficiencies. Since the pathophysiological basis of renal impairment by methylmalonic acid is still obscure, no treatment is available, and hemo- or peritoneal dialysis may become necessary.

Diagnosis The best way to accomplish the diagnosis is by quantitative analysis of urinary nonvolatile organic acid patterns by GC-MS (1,40), which will reveal elevated concentrations of methylmalonic acid and related metabolites such as propionylglycine, 3-hydroxy-

propionic acid, and methylcitrate. Quantitative analysis of plasma amino acids shows elevated concentrations of glycine, alanine, and methionine, and determinations of acylcarnitines reveal elevations of propionylcarnitine. Concomitant megaloblastic anemia and an increase in homocysteine hint at a primary disturbance of cobalamin metabolism as the cause of methylmalonic aciduria.

The level of methylmalonic acid in urine on presentation is also important in terms of overall interpretation. Excretion rates of 200 mmol/mol of creatinine or even higher may be found in asymptomatic babies and can resolve slowly in early childhood (91). The metabolic basis of this phenomenon is still not understood. On the other hand, urinary levels of methylmalonic acid may rise over 10,000 mmol/mol of creatinine during metabolic decompensation in patients with MCM deficiency.

Judgement of the response to hydroxycobalamin may be difficult. The determination of MCM in fibroblast extracts, mutation analysis of MCM (92), or investigation of labeled propionate incorporation following transfection by a vector containing cloned mutase cDNA in intact patients' fibroblasts may be required to differentiate primary defects of MCM from cblA and cblB defects.

Detection of methylmalonic acidurias is also feasible by MS/MS analysis in dried blood spots, which can be used for neonatal population screening. The acylcarnitine profile reveals increased propionylcarnitine but not methylmalonylcarnitine in newborns and is not to different from that in propionic aciduria (3).

Prenatal diagnosis is available by enzyme assay, molecular diagnosis in informative families, determination of incorporation of [^{14}C]propionate in amniocytes (82), and rap-

idly by quantitative stable-isotope-dilution assay of methylcitrate in amniotic fluid (6) (Table 7-17).

Treatment and Outcome Three decades after its recognition, major progress has been achieved in survival and prevention of neurological sequelae in children affected with methylmalonic acidurias. Prerequisite are that the diagnosis is made early and that treatment and follow-up care are performed meticulously (76). Cobalamin-dependent defects respond totally or partially to substitution with vitamin B_{12} in the form of hydroxycobalamin, not methylcobalamin (see Chapter 17).

Most patients with MCM deficiency do not respond to pharmacological doses of cobalamin and must be treated by restriction of isoleucine, valine, methionine, and threonine, together with supplementation of L-carnitine. Total natural protein intake has to be restricted according to the patient's tolerance and is adjusted to age-specific requirements (see Table 7-4). The reduction of protein intake must be monitored clinically and biochemically to prevent disturbed protein synthesis with catabolism leading acutely to metabolic decompensation and chronically to failure to thrive (see "Principles of Treatment" and "Monitoring of Treatment" above). Supplementation of the the protein-reduced diet with an AminoAcidMixture that is free of isoleucine, valine, methionine, and threonine ensures adequate protein intake, particularly during periods of growth. Often patients cannot maintain adequate nutritional intake without the use of nasogastric or gastrostomy tube feedings. The latter should be placed almost prophylactically in early infancy.

In individual patients, significant propionate production occurs in the gut, which can be reduced by intermittent treatment (10 days/month) with metronidazole (10–20 mg/kg/day), colistin, or neomycin.

Patients with methylmalonic aciduria show very low levels of free carnitine in plasma and a high percentage of esterified carnitines. As a consequence, carnitine stores become exhausted, resulting in severe

TABLE 7-17 Laboratory Findings: Methylmalonic Aciduria	
Decreased	**Increased**
pH	Ratio of esterified to free carnitine
Free and total carnitine	Ketone bodies, lactic acid, ammonia (metabolic decompensation)
Thrombocytopenia, neutropenia, or pancytopenia (metabolic decompensation)	Amino acids: glycine, alanine (metabolic decompensation)
	Organic acids: methylmalonic acid, 3-hydroxypropionic acid, methylcitric acid, tiglic acid, propionylglycine, tiglylglycine
	Acylcarnitines: propionylcarnitine (C_3), methylmalonylcarnitine (C_4 DC, inconstant)

- In the diagnostic workup of methylmalonic aciduria, it is imperative to determine homocysteine in plasma and to investigate the clinical and biochemical response to high doses of hydroxycobalamin (1–5 mg/day).

secondary metabolic consequences. L-Carnitine is given in doses of 100 mg/kg/day or more and is monitored in plasma, ensuring high-normal free carnitine levels.

Timely and effective emergency treatment is the prerequisite for a optimal outcome (see "Emergency Treatment" above) (76). During acute decompensation, methylmalonic aciduria is treated like other organic acidurias by 1) treating the precipitating illness (including the use of antibiotics), 2) controlling muscle and liver protein catabolism, 3) enhancing renal clearance of accumulating organic acids, and 4) ensuring a high energy intake by means of a calculated glucose infusion rate. Massive ketoacidosis requires especially vigorous therapy. Large amounts of fluid, electrolytes, and bicarbonate and high doses of intravenous carnitine must be infused together with glucose and possibly insulin. Forced diuresis with large amounts of fluids and furosemide is successful in removing methylmalonate from the body. The intake of natural protein is stopped for 24–48 hours and then reintroduced gradually. Hyperammonemia, if present, must be treated by providing arginine along with alternative methods of waste nitrogen excretion, that is, benzoate and phenylacetate or phenylbutyrate.

Renal insufficiency can be treated efficiently by hemo- or peritoneal dialysis, but the quality of life is compromised. In patients with renal failure requiring hemodialysis, isolated kidney transplantation becomes an issue. Only two transplant patients have been described in the literature with a follow-up of 3–4 years. Both show decreased methylmalonic acid in plasma and urine and stable renal function, with one patient still on a low-protein diet (93). The questions as to what extend the transplanted kidney can compensate the enzyme deficiency and whether the disease will recur in the transplant remain. Liver transplantation could provide enzyme activity to ameliorate the metabolic defect, and combined liver–kidney transplantation in three patients has been described. One survived, had no complications, and 16 months after surgery had a near-normal lifestyle (94), one died after transplantation, and the third patient suffered from intracranial hemorrhage (76). Isolated liver transplantation has been done in nine patients with conflicting results as successful transplantations as well as catastrophic postoperative courses have been described. Patients may develop progressive neurological disease and renal damage despite liver transplantation (95).

Despite continuous progress over the years, the overall prognosis of classical methylmalonic aciduria remains poor, whereas vitamin B_{12}–reponsive methylmalonic acidurias have a reasonable outcome (76,89).

MULTIPLE-CARBOXYLASE DEFICIENCY

The water-soluble vitamin biotin is cofactor of four important carboxylases that take part in gluconeogenesis, fatty acid synthesis, and the catabolism of several amino acids and odd-chain fatty acids (Figure 7-11). The covalent binding of biotin with apocarboxylases forming the active holocarboxylases is catalyzed by biotin holocarboxylase synthetase (HCS). In the biotin cycle, biotin is recycled after proteolytic degradation of holocarboxylases (Figure 7-12).

Biotin in small amounts is widely present in natural foods. Within the body, biotin bound to holocarboxylases represents the major source of biotin. In both dietary and endogenous sources, biotin is protein-bound as biocytin or short biotinyl peptides. Liberation of biotin from its protein conjugates is catalyzed by biotinidase (see Figure 7-12).

Deficiencies of biotinidase and HCS are the two different entities that cause multiple-carboxylase deficiency. The clinical presentation and biochemical abnormalities in multiple-carboxylase deficiency reflect deficiencies of all four carboxylases: pyruvate carboxylase, propionyl-CoA carboxylase, 3-methylcrotonyl-CoA carboxylase, and acetyl-CoA carboxylase (see Figure 7-11). The first three are mitochondrial enzymes; only the latter is a cytosolic enzyme. Pyruvate carboxylase is an essential enzyme of gluconeogenesis, propionyl-CoA carboxylase is required for the complete catabolism of several branched-chain amino acids and all odd-chain fatty acids, 3-methylcrotonyl-CoA carboxylase is required for the catabolism of the amino acid leucine, and acetyl-CoA carboxylase is required for the catalysis of the first step in fatty acid synthesis. Multiple-carboxylase deficiency can cause severe life-threatening metabolic derangements with lactic acidosis, ketosis, hyperammonemia, and a typical biochemical pattern of urinary organic acids. However, the biochemical and clinical presentation in multiple-carboxylase deficiency is very variable. In the majority of cases the age of clinical onset in biotinidase deficiency is later than in HCS deficiency, but there is an overlap in the ranges of age of onset. Most patients with HCS deficiency present acutely in the first days of life. In biotinidase deficiency, most patients become symptomatic after 3 months of age. Metabolic acidosis with Kussmaul breathing, hypotonia, seizures, impaired consciousness, and cutaneous symptoms, such as skin rash and alopecia, are characteristic manifestations. If patients are not treated immediately, irreversible hearing loss and visual impairment will follow, and subsequently, a number of infants with this disorder will die undiagnosed.

The outcome of treatment in multiple-carboxylase deficiency is favorable because both diseases, biotinidase deficiency and HCS deficiency, usually respond dramatically to oral treatment with pharmacological doses of

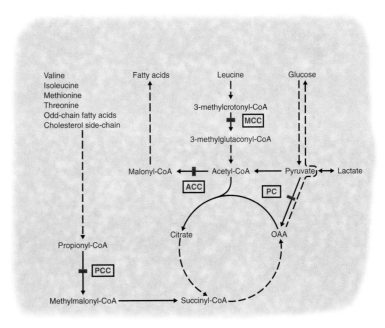

FIGURE 7-11. Location of biotin-dependent carboxylases in intermediary metabolism. The carboxylation of 3-methylcrotonyl-CoA, propionyl-CoA, acetyl-CoA, and pyruvate are all biotin-dependent. Deficient activation of the apoenzymes (holocarboxylase synthetase deficiency) and deficient release of biotin from biocytin of protein-bound biotin (biotinidase deficiency) result in a complex metabolic disturbance impairing the function of all carboxylases, as indicated by red bars. Full lines indicate one enzymatic reaction; dotted lines indicate that several enzymes are involved. ACC = acetyl-CoA carboxylase; MCC = 3-methylcrotonyl-CoA carboxylase; PC = pyruvate carboxylase; PCC = propionyl-CoA carboxylase; OAA = oxaloacetate.

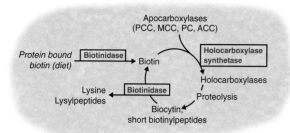

FIGURE 7-12. The biotin cycle. Biotin is cleaved from biocytin (biotinyl-lysine) or small peptides by biotinidase. Activation of the apoenzymes resulting in functioning carboxylases (3-methylcrotonyl-CoA, propionyl-CoA, acetyl-CoA, and pyruvate carboxylases) is carried out by holocarboxylase synthetase. ACC = acetyl-CoA carboxylase; MCC = 3-methylcrotonyl-CoA carboxylase; PC = pyruvate carboxylase; PCC = propionyl-CoA carboxylase. (Adapted with permission from Ref. 40.)

biotin. Prerequisite for prevention of sequelae is early diagnosis. Measurement of biotinidase activity in dried blood specimens at birth detects biotinidase deficiency reliably, and population screening for biotinidase deficiency has been integrated into many of the newborn screening programs. Introduction of expanded newborn screening with MS/MS allows for detection even of HCS deficiency, but it seems to be a very rare condition.

BIOTINIDASE DEFICIENCY

Etiology/Pathophysiology Mammalian biotinidase is detectable in most tissues, having the highest activity in liver, kidney, serum, and adrenal gland and the lowest activity in brain and CSF. Human biotinidase is a glycoprotein composed of a single polypeptide having a molecular mass of between 67 and 76 kDa. Biotinidase regenerates biotin from endogenous sources and liberates protein-bound biotin, which derives from natural foodstuff and the holocarboxylases. The first step in regeneration of biotin from endogenous sources involves proteolytic degradation of the holocarboxylases, yielding biotin covalently bound to lysine (biocytin) or short biotinylated peptides. Following degradation of carboxylases, biotinidase cleaves the amide bond of the biocytin or biotinylated peptides, releasing lysine or lysyl-peptides and free biotin. Free biotin then can be recycled and used for the reformation of holocarboxylases by the action of HCS through the so-called biotin cycle (see Figure 7-12).

The primary biochemical defect in most patients with late-onset multiple-carboxylase deficiency was shown in 1983 to be a profound deficiency of serum biotinidase (less than 10% of mean normal serum biotinidase activity) (96). Individuals with untreated late onset biotinidase deficiency eventually present with characteristic clinical manifestations and accumulation of abnormal metabolites. These patients also experience renal loss of biotin (97).

The metabolic abnormalities caused by deficiency of the respective carboxylases are as follows: lactic acidosis due to pyruvate carboxylase deficiency; hyperammonemia and accumulation of methylcitrate, 3-hydroxypropionic acid, propionylglycine, tiglylglycine, propionylcarnitine, and propionic acid due to propionyl-CoA carboxylase deficiency; and accumulation of 3-hydroxyisovaleric acid, 3-methylcrotonylglycine, and 3-hydroxyisovalerylcarnitine due to methylcrotonyl-CoA carboxylase deficiency.

Hyperammonemia is caused by secondary inhibition of N-acetylglutamate synthetase and is considered to be responsible for lethargy, somnolence, and coma. N-Acetylglutamate is the activator of carbamyl phosphate synthetase in the urea cycle (see Chapter 11).

The mode of inheritance of biotinidase deficiency is autosomal recessive. The gene that encodes for the serum enzyme has been localized to chromosome 3p25 (98). Multiple mutations have been described in symptomatic children with profound biotinidase deficiency (99). The most common mutation is a 7-base deletion/3-base insertion and is present in at least one allele in half of symptomatic children. A missense mutation, Arg-538Cys, is the second most common mutation. Two mutations have been found mainly in children identified by newborn screening: a Q456H missense mutation and a combination A171T and D444H mutation. A comparison of mutations among children identified by newborn screening versus those diagnosed symptomatically was performed by Norrgard and colleagues (100). The four mutations comprised 59% of the abnormal alleles in the two populations. Two of those occurred in the symptomatic population at a significantly greater frequency. The other two were found only in the newborn screening group. It is uncertain whether children with mutations found only in the newborn screening population may ever develop clinical symptoms. Partial biotinidase deficiency has been found to be the result of a missense mutation, D444H, in combination with a severe mutation on the second allele (101).

Clinical Presentation Symptoms of profound biotinidase deficiency can develop anytime from 1 week to 10 years of age. The mean age at presentation is between 3 and 6 months (102).

Provision of biotin by the mother in utero delays symptoms and biochemical abnormalities in newborns with biotinidase deficiency. The full clinical picture has been reported as early as 7 weeks, but discrete neurological symptoms already may be present in neonates (97). The most frequent, often episodic symptoms are lethargy, hypotonia, seizures, and ataxia, often in combination with respiratory symptoms such as stridor, episodes of hyperventilation, and apnea. If undiagnosed and untreated, the disease can be potentially fatal (see Figure 7-14B). In older children, progressive neurological disease is often the leading presentation, for example, ataxia, (myoclonic) epileptic encephalopathy, and developmental delay. Neurosensory hearing loss and eye problems, such as optic atrophy, develop in most untreated patients. Skin rash and alopecia are hallmarks of the disease, but they may develop late or not at all in half the patients (102). The pathognomonic skin lesions typically are patchy and erythematous and are localized periorificially. They may progress to cover large parts of the body as eczematoid dermatitis or as erythematous rash and may be mistaken for eczema or zinc deficiency. Some of the skin lesions are due to moniliasis. Hair loss usually is discrete but may become complete, including eyelashes and eyebrows.

Diagnosis Biotinidase deficiency presents with varying degrees of metabolic acidosis with increased anion gap, ketosis, elevated lactate, and hyperammonemia. Urinary organic acid analysis is useful for differentiating isolated carboxylase deficiencies from the multiple-carboxylase deficiencies that occur in biotinidase deficiency and holocarboxylase synthase deficiency.

Metabolic abnormalities are more likely to occur in the full-blown stage of the disease or during acute illness. However, the absence of OA or metabolic ketoacidosis does not exclude the diagnosis of biotinidase deficiency in a symptomatic child. The accumulation of abnormal organic acid metabolites such as propionate and lactate in blood and 3-hydroxypropionic acid, methylcitrate, 3-hydroxyisovaleric acid, 3-methylcrotonylglycine, and 3-hydroxybutyrate in urine, in addition to 3-hydroxyisovaleric acid and 3-methylcrotonylglycine, reflects the systemic deficiency of all affected carboxylases (see Figure 7-11). However, only 3-hydroxyisovaleric acid may be found elevated, especially in the early stages of

- The clinical vignette of biotinidase deficiency is often variable and non-specific, for example, muscular hypotonia, global developmental delay, and epilepsy. In countries where screening for biotinidase is not part of neonatal population screening, determination of biotinidase should be included in the initial diagnostic workup.

- 5–10 mg oral biotin per day promptly reverses or prevents all clinical and biochemical abnormalities in children diagnosed early with biotinidase deficiency.

TABLE 7-18 Laboratory Findings: Biotinidase Deficiency	
Decreased	**Increased**
Biotinidase	Ratio of esterified to free carnitine
Plasma or urine biotin	Lactic acid, ketone bodies
pH	Amino acids: glycine, alanine, threonine
Free and total carnitine	Organic acids: 3-hydroxyisovaleric acid, 3-methylcrotonylglycine, 3-hydroxypropionic acid, methylcitric acid, tiglic acid, propionylglycine, tiglylglycine
	Acylcarnitines: 3-hydroxyisovalerylcarnitine, propionylcarnitine (inconstant)
	Biocytin in urine

the disease, or only increased 3-hydroxyisovalerylcarnitine may be detected in dried blood specimen by MS/MS analysis. Of note, 3-hydroxyisovaleric acid is the most commonly elevated urinary metabolite not only in biotinidase deficiency but also in holocarboxylase synthetase deficiency, isolated 3-methylcrotonyl-CoA carboxylase deficiency, and acquired biotin deficiency.

Biotin is decreased in plasma and urine, and biocytin is increased in urine.

It is important to mention that all these biochemical abnormalities are absent at birth, when the patient is not yet biotin-depleted. Furthermore, some children with primarily neurological disease may have metabolic abnormalities such as elevations of lactate and/or organic acids restricted to CSF (103).

Diagnosis is made by direct measurement of serum biotinidase activity. Enzymatic activity between 0% and 10% is classified as profound biotinidase deficiency and activity between 10% and 30% as partial biotinidase deficiency. Profound biotinidase deficiency can be further divided into complete deficiency with undetectable biotinidase activity and residual activity up to 10% affinity (104,105). Besides the preceding groups, a few patients with decreased affinity of biotinidase for biocytin (K_m variants) exist. They may show erroneously high residual activity on in vitro testing. Prenatal diagnosis is feasible by measurement of biotinidase activity in cultured amniotic fluid cells and in amniotic fluid but may not be necessary because of the treatment option and favorable clinical outcome. Mutation analysis can be accomplished by direct sequencing. Specific determination of several common mutations in blood spots from newborn screening can be performed by real-time polymerase chain reacyion (PCR) of DNA (104).

In many countries, newborn screening has been established for biotinidase deficiency by measurement of biotinidase activity in dried blood specimens (Table 7-18).

Treatment and Outcome Biotinidase deficiency is treated effectively by daily oral administration of pharmacological doses of biotin. Restriction of protein is not necessary (106).

Biotin treatment has to be maintained lifelong and has no side effects. In profound biotinidase deficiency, 5–10 mg/day is sufficient and under careful biochemical monitoring the biotin dose may be reduced to 2.5 mg/day.

Most patients with biotinidase deficiency known today were detected by newborn screening. Although the diagnosis must be confirmed by measuring serum biotinidase activity, biotin supplementation has to be initiated right away to avoid symptomatic biotin deficiency, which may develop very rapidly. Patients with partial biotinidase deficiency (10% to 30% residual activity) reveal a tendency to subnormal plasma concentrations of biotin, which further decrease with age. Hypotonia, skin rash, and hair loss developed in a 6-month-old infant with partial biotinidase deficiency (30%) during an episode of gastroenteritis. The symptoms were reversed by biotin therapy (107). As a consequence, patients with partial biotinidase deficiency should be regularly monitored for biochemical abnormalities. In case of border line abnormalities small doses of biotin, e.g., 2.5 mg/week are recommended (106). However, many physicians elect to treat partial biotinidase deficiency with 5–10 mg/day at diagnosis and not await for manifestations of biochemical abnormalities. Patients with K_m variants have an increased risk to become biotin-deficient and may reveal profound or partial biotinidase deficiency. Therefore, patients with K_m variants also should be treated with biotin.

Following early detection and immediate treatment, the outcome of biotinidase deficiency is excellent.

HOLOCARBOXYLASE SYNTHETASE DEFICIENCY

Etiology/Pathophysiology The coenzyme biotin is attached to the various apocarboxylases by the enzyme holocarboxylase synthetase (HCS) (see Figure 7-12). The carboxyl group of biotin is linked by an amide bond to an epsilon-amino group of a specific lysine residue of the apoenzymes. Deficiency of HCS leads to failure of synthesis all carboxylases, causing biochemical and clinical abnormalities attributable to the dysfunction of each respective carboxylase (see Figure 7-11).

The best evidence that in humans a single HCS activates all the apocarboxylases comes from the observation of deficient acetyl-CoA carboxylase activity in addition to deficient activities of the three mitochondrial carboxylases in fibroblasts from children with HCS deficiency (108). The human enzyme is predicted to be a monomer composed of 726 amino acids with a molecular weight of 80 kDa. The cDNA of human HCS has been cloned and sequenced. The HCS gene was shown to map to chromosome 21q22.1 (109). HCS deficiency has autosomal recessive traits. Several mutations but not a predominant one have been identified. HCS deficiency is a rare condition for which 30–40 patients are known so far. Detectable residual activity has been observed in all affected individuals, suggesting that complete enzyme deficiency may be lethal in utero. The fact that there is residual enzyme activity explains why all patients with this condition responded to biotin treatment.

Clinical Presentation Although HCS deficiency initially was termed *early-onset multiple-carboxylase deficiency*, accumulative experience showed that the age at onset of symptoms varies from a few hours after birth to 6 years of age. Nevertheless, about half of patients presented acutely in the first days of life with severe metabolic decompensation, lethargy, hypotonia, vomiting, seizures, and hypothermia (106).

Patients with early-onset presentation exhibit severe metabolic acidosis with lactic acidemia, ketosis, hyperammonemia, and a typical organic aciduria. The metabolic derangement may progress quickly from lethargy, to unconsciousness, to coma and early death. Breathing problems present as tachypnea and hyperventilation (Kussmaul breathing). Skin rashes, feeding problems, vomiting, muscular hypotonia and hypertonia, seizures, and an odor of urine reminiscent of male cat urine are other commonly observed symptoms. Ataxia, tremor, and hyporeflexia or hyperreflexia are neurological manifestations of the disease. In the late-onset forms, the enzymatic defect is less severe and may present at an older age with psychomotor retardation and alopecia or with life-threatening metabolic attacks during a stressful event.

Diagnosis The full biochemical spectrum of HCS deficiency consists of lactic acidosis, ketosis, hyperammonemia, and a complex but characteristic pattern of increased organic acids, acylglycines, and acylcarnitines (see Figure 7-11). Accumulation of acyl-CoA compounds upstream of the metabolic block of each impaired carboxylase leads to the pathognomonic pattern. Organic acid analysis in urine by GC-MS reveals increased excretion of the same metabolites as in biotinidase deficiency, such as lactate; pyruvate due to pyruvate carboxylase deficiency; methylcitrate, 3-hydroxypropionic acid, propionylglycine, tiglylglycine, propionic acid, propionylcarnitine due to propionyl-CoA carboxylase deficiency; and 3-hydroxyisovaleric acid, 3-methylcrotonylglycine, and 3-hydroxyisovalerylcarnitine due to 3-methylcrotonyl-CoA carboxylase deficiency. In one patient with HCS deficiency, 3-hydroxyisovalerylcarnitine (C_5OH carnitine) was found increased in blood but not propionylcarnitine (C_3 carnitine) probably due to either a secondary deficiency of free carnitine or to different tissue concentrations of the corresponding acyl-CoA compounds (110,111). Plasma biotin is normal in HCS deficiency, as is serum biotinidase activity.

Both disorders, HCS and biotinidase deficiency, are characterized by deficient activities of carboxylases in peripheral blood leukocytes prior to biotin administration; the activities of these enzymes increase to near-normal or normal values after biotin treatment (112). Indirect confirmation of HCS deficiency and differentiation from biotinidase deficiency are feasible by measurement of activities of the mitochondrial carboxylases in skin fibroblasts under assay conditions differing in biotin concentrations. The activities of the enzymes in fibroblasts from patients with HCS deficiency vary from 0% to 30% of normal when incubated in low-biotin (10^{-10} M) medium (113) and increase or even normalize in high-biotin medium (10^{-6} to 10^{-5} M). In contrast, in biotinidase deficiency, the activity of mitochondrial carboxylases in fibroblasts is already normalized under low-biotin conditions. Definite diagnosis of HCS deficiency is achieved by direct measurement of HCS activity, but this test is not available routinely.

Prenatal diagnosis is feasible either by demonstrating decreased carboxylase activities in cultured amniocytes that increase by incubation with biotin or by demonstration of elevated 3-hydroxyisovaleric acid and/or methylcitrate in amniotic fluid by stable-isotope-dilution GC-MS. The diagnosis can be secured by performing both diagnostic procedures on the same sample of amniotic fluid. Molecular diagnosis can be offered in informative families. Affected newborns with HCS can be detected by MS/MS through newborn screening, but so far, no affected newborn has been reported (Table 7-19).

Treatment and Outcome HCS deficiency can be treated effectively with pharmacological doses of biotin (106). Children treated before irreversible neurological damage occurred generally showed resolution of the clinical symptoms and biochemical abnormalities. In some severe cases, additional restriction of protein intake seems necessary. The required dose of biotin depends on the severity of the enzyme defect and has to be assessed individually. In most patients, 10–20 mg biotin per day is sufficient, but some need higher doses (i.e., 40–100 mg/day) (114). Despite the apparently complete recovery, biochemical and clinical abnormalities persist in some patients despite very high biotin doses due to the high K_m for biotin in the defective HCS. Such children continue to excrete particularly increased concentrations of 3-hydroxyisovaleric acid in urine and eventually may develop psychomotor retardation or even the full-blown clinical spectrum (see above).

In case of acute decompensation, treatment according to the emergency protocol in OAs (see "Emergency Treatment" above) has to start without delay. Although the symptoms of holocarboxylase synthetase deficiency can appear soon after birth, it is not clear whether prenatal treatment with biotin is beneficial. Treatment of at-risk children with biotin immediately after birth until their enzyme status has been determined should be sufficient.

In the majority of affected individuals, the prognosis is good if treatment is initiated immediately and the clinical course is followed carefully by close monitoring of biochemical abnormalities.

GLUTARIC ACIDURIA TYPE I

Etiology/Pathophysiology Glutaric aciduria type I (GA-I) (synonym *glutaryl-CoA dehydrogenase deficiency*), first described by Goodman and colleagues in 1975 (115), occurs with an estimated frequency of 1 in 100,000 newborns (116) but considerably higher (up to 1 in 300) in genetically homogeneous communities, for example, the Old Order Amish of Lancaster County, Pennsylvania (117), or the Saulteaux/Ojibway Indians in Canada (118). GA-I is caused by deficiency of glutaryl-CoA dehydrogenase, a key mitochondrial enzyme in the catabolic pathway of the amino acids L-tryptophan, L-lysine, and L-hydroxylysine, catalyzing the reaction of glutaryl-CoA to crotonyl-CoA (Figure 7-13).

TABLE 7-19	Laboratory Findings: Holocarboxylase Synthetase Deficiency
Decreased	**Increased**
pH	Ratio of esterified to free carnitine
Free and total carnitine	Lactic acid, ketone bodies
Normal biotinidase	Amino acids: glycine, alanine, threonine
	Organic acids: 3-hydroxyisovaleric acid, 3-methylcrotonylglycine, 3-hydroxypropionic acid, methylcitric acid, tiglic acid, propionylglycine, tiglylglycine
	Acylcarnitines: propionylcarnitine, 3-hydroxyisovalerylcarnitine, 3-methylcrotonylcarnitine (inconstant)

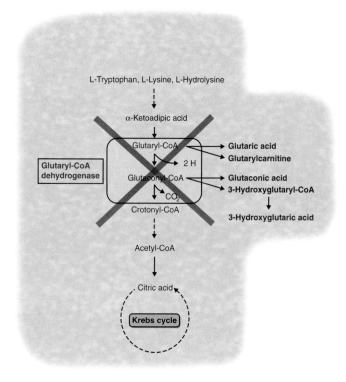

FIGURE 7-13. Metabolism of lysine, hydroxylysine, and tryptophan: defect in glutaric aciduria type I. The metabolic block is indicated by a red cross, the defective enzyme glutaryl-CoA dehydrogenase in red font, and accumulating metabolites are in blue.

The glutaryl-CoA dehydrogenase gene encodes a protein of 438 amino acids that includes a 44-amino-acid N-terminal targeting sequence that is cleaved after import into the mitochondrial matrix (119). More than 100 disease-causing mutations have been described so far, with R402W being the most frequent mutation in Caucasians, accounting for 10% to 20% of alleles. However, genotype–phenotype correlation is poor in GA-I. Therefore, disease outcome does not depend on residual enzyme activity or genotype (120) but on prevention and effective management of acute encephalopathic crises. The mature 43.3-kDa glutaryl-CoA dehydrogenase protein forms a homotetramer, each subunit containing a single molecule of flavin–adenine dinucleotide. GA-I is characterized biochemically by accumulation of the dicarbonic acids glutaric, 3-hydroxyglutaric, and glutaconic acids as well as of glutarylcarnitine.

If GA-I is not diagnosed and treated early, encephalopathic crises lead to acute striatal degeneration of the brain in the majority of patients. These crises often are precipitated by febrile illnesses or routine vaccinations during a vulnerable period of brain development in infancy or early childhood. The mechanism underlying these acute encephalopathic crises has been partially elucidated using in vitro and in vivo models (120). 3-Hydroxyglutaric and glutaric acids share structural similarities with the main excitatory amino acid glutamate. 3-Hydroxyglutaric acid induces excitotoxic cell damage specifically via activation of N-methyl-D-aspartate (NMDA) receptors. Furthermore, glutaric and 3-hydroxyglutaric acids indirectly modulate glutamatergic and GABAergic neurotransmission, resulting in an imbalance of excitatory and inhibitory neurotransmission.

Clinical Presentation Initially, affected babies show relatively mild physical signs, such as muscular hypotonia with prominent head lag, high palate, feeding difficulties, and irritability (117,122). Neuroimaging in this period typically reveals frontotemporal atrophy, widening of the Sylvian fissure due to reduced opercularization, subependymal pseudocysts, and delayed myelination, thus reflecting delayed cerebral maturation (Figure 7-14C). The importance of including GA-I in the differential diagnoses, when dealing with suspected nonaccidental trauma, cannot be overemphasized. MRI studies may reveal acute subdural hemorrhages or subdural fluid collections that in some cases may be accompanied by retinal hemorrhages. Bridging veins can be seen stretching tenuously across the space of the middle cranial fossa with the risk of distortion and rupture following minor head trauma. Of course, there is always a possibility of coexisting GA-I and nonaccidental trauma.

Posture and tone of a neonate may persist until 4–8 months of age, but as the infant gets older, the impairment of neurodevelopment may become more obvious. During febrile illnesses or after immunizations, hypotonia often is aggravated, and unusual movements and postures of hands appear. All these symptoms are reversible and of little prognostic significance. During the encephalopathic crisis, the area of injury that causes permanent disability is in the basal ganglia (especially caudate and putamen) and typically occurs between 4 and 18 months of age. The vulnerable period ends in the fourth year of life.

Encephalopathic crises usually are provoked by common infections and fever but also may develop after fasting, routine immunizations, or minor trauma. Infants typically present with acute loss of neurological functions such as head control, suck and swallow reflexes, and the ability to sit, pull to standing, or grasp toys. Examination shows an alert infant with profound hypotonia of the neck and trunk, stiff arms and legs, and twisting (athe-

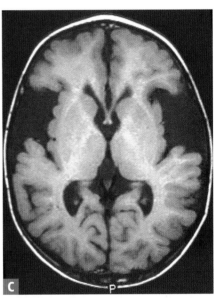

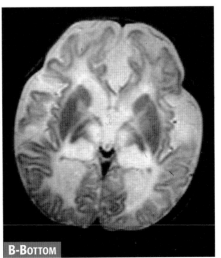

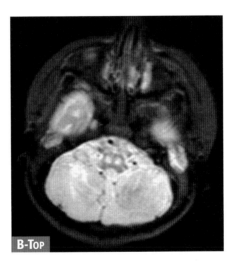

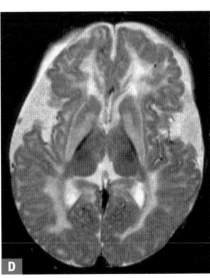

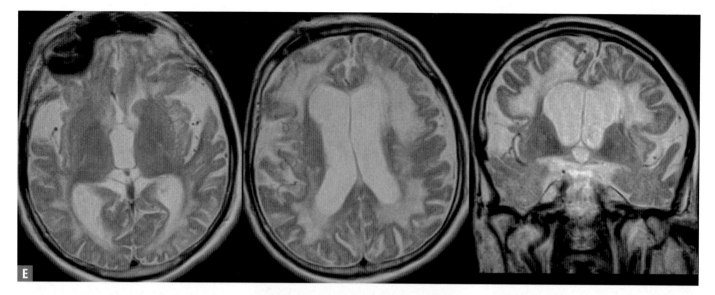

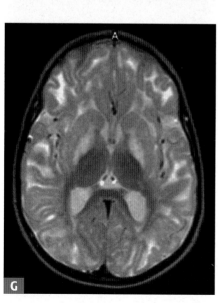

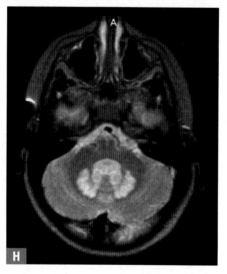

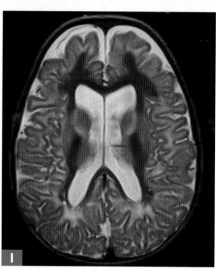

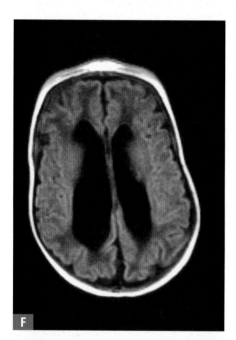

FIGURE 7-14. A to **I.** Neuroimaging findings in patients with cerebral organic acid disorders. **A.** Transveral NMR image of a 7-year-old girl who had been diagnosed with propionic aciduria in infancy and had been treated successfully since then. While in good metabolic control, she suddenly became comatose. Massive infarction of the basal ganglia had occurred, and the child died a few days later. Spin-echo technique. (Courtesy of Drs. R. Haas and W.L. Nyhan, Department of Pediatrics, University of California, San Diego, CA.) **B.** Two T2-weighted images of a 7-month-old boy with biotinidase deficiency. The image on the bottom shows absence of normal myeline signal, cerebral atrophy, and symmetrical hyperintense lesions of both thalami. The image on the top displays absence of normal myeline signal in the cerebellum as well as hyperintense signal in both pyramidal tracts. (Courtesy of Dr. T. Bast, Department of Pediatric Neurology, University of Heidelberg, Heidelberg, Germany.) **C.** Axial T1-weighted spin-echo NMR image of a 3½-year-old boy with glutaryl-CoA dehydrogenase deficiency. He was diagnosed neonatally, never suffered an encephalopathic crisis, and developed no major neurological deficits. In addition to marked extension of the Sylvian fissures (frontotemporal atrophy), the central white matter, especially around the occipital horns, appears attenuated. **D.** Axial T2-weighted spin-echo image of a 14-month-old girl with glutaryl-CoA dehydrogenase deficiency 2 months after an acute encephalopathic crisis. In addition to marked extension of the Sylvian fissures (frontotemporal atrophy), marked shrinkage and hyperintensity of the putamen and the caudate nucleus are obvious, as well as diffuse attenuation of both the central and the peripheral white matter. (Reproduced with permission from Ref. 140.) **E.** T2-weighted axial and coronal MRI images of a 66-year-old man with glutaryl-CoA dehydrogenase deficiency demonstrating confluent white matter changes, wide temporopolar and insular CSF spaces, and cortical atrophy but normal signal of basal ganglia. The previously healthy man presented from the age of 50 with slowly progressive neurological disease, including seizures, dementia, and speech problems. Aggressive behavior as well as acoustic and visual hallucinations led to the suggestion of psychiatric disease. (Reproduced with permission from Ref. 124.) **F.** Axial T1-weighted spin-echo image of a 2-month-old girl boy with D-2-hydroxyglutaric aciduria. The lateral ventricles are highly dilated, occipital more than frontal, and cerebral maturation is delayed. (Reproduced with permission from Ref. 140.) **G.** Axial T2-weighted spin-echo image of an 8½-year-old boy with L-2-hydroxyglutaric aciduria. Subcortical white matter is severely deficient, with much less involvement of the internal capsule and the periventricular white matter. Note the signal changes in the putamen. (Reproduced with permission from Ref. 140.) **H.** Axial T2-weighted spin-echo image of an 8½-year-old boy with L-2-hydroxyglutaric aciduria. Note hyperintense lesions in both dentate nuclei. **I.** Axial fast spin-echo image of an 6½-year-old girl suffering from aspartoacylase deficiency. Note the marked discrepancy between the severely affected subcortical white matter and the relatively spared central white matter, at least frontally. (Reproduced with permission from Ref. 140.)

toid) movements of hands and feet, especially when agitated. The infant also may have a generalized seizure and an acute loss of motor skills associated with dystonia. Thereafter, the patients enter a chronic phase. Further progression of neurological disease is halted if the disease is diagnosed and treated, but only rarely does substantial restitution of function occur. Around 20% of patients with GA-I follow a chronic disease course and develop the same neurological symptoms as the acutely injured children over the first 2 years of life without a readily identified crisis (122). Only single undiagnosed and never treated patients may escape the development of severe neurological disease or develop only minor motor problems (117,122).

Following the basal ganglia injury, the clinical picture is dominated by dystonic–dyskinetic posturing associated with athetoid movements with great variability within and in between patients. There is usually truncal hypotonia but also opisthotonus, spasticity, rigidity, clenched fists, and tongue thrusting. Profuse sweating is common, and some patients have repeated episodes of unexplained fever, irritability, ill-temper, anorexia, and insomnia. Fasting hypoglycemia can occur in older children and adults.

Recently, adult-onset GA-I was described in five adolescents or adults presenting with leukoencephalopathic changes of different degrees (123,124), raising the possibility of a distinct clinical manifestation in adolescence/adulthood (see Figure 7-14E).

Neuroradiological findings can be especially suggestive (117,122,125). Most characteristic is the symmetrical widening of the Sylvian fissure with poor opercularization. These findings are present in approximately 95% of all patients and usually are referred to as *frontotemporal atrophy, widened Sylvian fissures,* or less common "bat wings appearance" (see Figure 7-14C). These findings are already obvious on MRI performed in patients diagnosed by expanded neonatal screening, preceding clinical symptoms, which is suggestive of hypoplasia rather than atrophy. Ventriculomegaly and basal ganglia lesions develop after the encephalopathic crisis and are indicative of permanent damage (see Figure 7-14D). White matter changes are variable but present frequently and may become recognized as important long-term complications (see Figure 7-14E). The increased signal intensity seen on T2- and FLAIR-weighted images is localized mainly within the periventricular white matter but also in the subcortical U-fibers.

Diagnosis GA-I should be suspected in patients with macrocephaly or an extrapyramidal movement disorder beginning in child-

TABLE 7-20   Clinical Features of GA-I
1. Unspecific clinical features in pre-encephalopathic children (infancy)
• (Progressing) macrocephaly, frontal bossing
• Delayed gross motor development (poor head control, trunk hypotonicity, irritability)
• Feeding difficulties
2. Moderately suggestive clinical features
• Encephalitis-like encephalopathic crisis
• Dystonic–dyskinetic disorder associated with athetoid movements
• Sibling who died of or following an unexplained encephalopathic crisis
• Acute (metabolic) encephalopathy
• Suggestive neuroradiological findings (subdural effusions/ hemorrhages, delayed myelination, subependymal pseudocysts)
3. Highly suggestive clinical features
• Acute dystonic–dyskinetic disorder
• Acute bilateral striatal degeneration
• Specific neuroradiological findings (reduced opercularization, "frontotemporal atrophy," isolated bilateral striatal degeneration)
• Sibling who died suffering acute bilateral striatal degeneration
• Sibling with confirmed GDD

Modified from Ref. 127.

hood. The diagnostic process can be guided by further clinical features (see Table 7-20). Diagnosis is ascertained by the detection of glutaric and 3-hydroxyglutaric acids in organic acid analysis from urine, blood, or CSF and/or by the detection of elevated glutarylcarnitine. Confirmation by enzymatic analysis or demonstration of two pathogenic mutations is advisable.

Unfortunately, the diagnosis of GA-I is not always straightforward. Since a subgroup patients reveals only slight elevations of glutaric acid in urine despite severe disease progression, repeated quantitative urinary organic acid analysis or even specific determination of 3-hydroxyglutaric acid by stable-isotope-dilution techniques must be performed (126). Examination of the carnitine status mostly reveals low, often very low total and free carnitine and an elevated ratio of esterified to free carnitine. Glutarylcarnitine is elevated diagnostically in all patients with high excretion of glutaric acid and sufficient carnitine but elevated only marginally in patients with intermittently normal urinary organic acids or isolated elevation of urinary 3-hydroxyglutaric acid. Sensitivity can be improved by the evaluation of specific ratios and fortunately appears especially high in the neonatal screening setting due to the metabolic stress of the newborns (116).

The definitive diagnosis is made by demonstrating significantly reduced enzyme activity in skin fibroblasts, leukocytes, amniocytes, or chorion biopsy or two pathogenic mutations. Prenatal diagnosis is possible by determining glutaric acid with stable-isotope-dilution techniques or enzymatic and/or molecular testing (Table 7-21).

Treatment and Outcome Therapy's main aim is at preventing encephalopathic crises and neurological deterioration (11,120,127). Strict adherence to the emergency protocol is especially important in GA-I (see "Emergency Treatment" above). The most frequent mistake and thus the greatest risk for acute basal ganglia injury is a delayed or improper emergency treatment. Parents should be instructed to call their doctor if the child develops fever of 38.5°C, signs of infection, or irritability.

During the vulnerable period of brain development, that is, 0–5 years, encephalopathic crises can develop in hours to minutes without gradual or even significant metabolic derangement, leaving the child with permanent sequelae (121).

During the vulnerable period, reduction of protein (total protein 1.5–2.0 g/kg of body weight per day) or, better and more specifically, a lysine-restricted diet based on a reduced intake of L-lysine (60–100 mg/kg/day) is recommended (128). Patients receiving a

TABLE 7-21 Laboratory Findings: Glutaric Aciduria Type I	
Decreased	**Increased**
Free and total carnitine	Ratio of esterified to free carnitine
	Organic acids: glutaric acid, 3-hydroxyglutaric acid, glutaconic acid (inconstant)
	Acylcarnitines: gutarylcarnitine (C_5 DC)

lysine-restricted diet should be supplemented with a special formula such as a lysine-free AminoAcidMixture fortified with minerals and micronutrients. Additionally, L-carnitine (50–100 mg/kg/day) is prescribed to support acyl-CoA transport across the mitochondrial membrane and to prevent carnitine deficiency. Riboflavin (100 mg/day), the cofactor of glutaryl-CoA dehydrogenase, is used widely, although it is unclear how beneficial it is. Riboflavin sensitivity has been observed only anecdotally in one patient. Dietary therapy should be monitored clinically and by measurement of indices of malnutrition, including plasma concentrations of essential amino acids, micronutrients, and especially lysine and tryptophan (see "Monitoring of Treatment" above). Tryptophan is not well quantifiable by classical amino acid analysis and must be specifically requested and analyzed for and monitored carefully. Carnitine treatment should be tailored to maintain normal free carnitine concentrations in plasma. Monitoring of organic acids or glutarylcarnitine in body fluids has not an established role. Strict monitoring of weight gain, growth rate, and other anthropometrics, as well as continuous assessment of psychomotor development, should be pursued. Avoidance of malnutrition and overrestriction of protein is critical in neurologically damaged children (8).

In all patients with GA-I and neurological disease, a neurologist should be involved continuously in the care. Different neuropharmacological drugs have been used to ameliorate the severe neurological symptoms with little or no positive effect, except for baclofen and the benzodiazepines (5). Trihexyphenidyl can be efficacious and can be used safely in adolescence in high dosage for segmental and generalized dystonia. Botulinum toxin and intrathecal baclofen are valid additions for focal dystonia or very severe dystonia, especially if accompanied by spasticity, respectively.

Nonspecific multiprofessional support is of utmost importance. It must be kept in mind that despite the severe motor handicap, intellectual functions are often well preserved. Pharmacological therapy must be accompanied by daily physical therapy to prevent contractures and to alleviate pain. A simple but important prerequisite is correct positioning of the head. It should be kept in the midline position, which allows the patient the maximum of mobility and minimizes dystonia.

Special care is needed to avoid aspiration with feedings. Increased muscular tension and sweating, common findings in GA-I, increase the requirement for calories and water. Many patients need tube or gastrostomy feeding. Percutaneous gastrostomy often leads to a dramatic improvement in nutritional status,

a marked relief of psychological tension and care load in the families, and even a reduction of dyskinesia and dystonia.

Diagnosis of GA-I before the brain has been injured permanently is of utmost importance (120,127). The currently outlined current best medical practice can prevent brain degeneration in 80% to 90% of infants if they are diagnosed early and treated immediately.(5,117,118,120). Without treatment, 75% to 80% of affected children will develop severe neurological disabilities, and an additional 10%, a milder syndrome. Basal ganglia injury, once present, usually is irreversible and decreases treatment efficacy. About a fifth (21%) of patients who were diagnosed after the onset of neurological disease die due to the already developed sequelae (5,117,118). Pneumonia and respiratory failure are the usual causes of death in severely disabled patients, and patients may succumb to hyperpyrexic crises.

No information is available about pregnancies in women with GA-I. The effect of maternal metabolite levels on fetal CNS and somatic development is unknown.

D-2-Hydroxyglutaric Aciduria

Etiology/Pathophysiology D-2-Hydroxyglutaric aciduria is a rare autosomal recessively inherited cerebral OA. The metabolic origin of D-2-hydroxyglutaric acid has not been completely unraveled in mammals, but the defect was identified recently in a specific dehydrogenase converting D-2-hydroxyglutaric acid to 2-oxoglutaric acid (129,130). The enzyme is homologous to the FAD-dependent D-lactate dehydrogenase, and pathogenic mutations have been identified. The neurodegeneration in D-2-hydroxyglutaric aciduria could be linked to an excitotoxic effect. D-2-Hydroxyglutaric acid directly activates NMDA receptors, increases cellular calcium levels significantly, and inhibits ATP synthesis, but without affecting the electron-transferring complexes I–IV (120). The latter effect could trigger pathophysiological sequences identical to mitochondriopathies.

Clinical Presentation Patients with D-2-hydroxyglutaric aciduria exhibit variable phenotypes. They have been subdivided into two subgroups based on clinical and neuroradiological findings (131–133). One group includes the severely affected children who present with early-infantile-onset encephalopathy demonstrating a combination of catastrophic epilepsy, hypotonia, cerebral visual failure, and severe psychomotor retardation. Facial dysmorphism and cardiomyopathy also may be present. Both microcephaly and macro-

cephaly may occur. Moderately affected children follow a much milder clinical course with variable symptoms, including mental retardation, hypotonia, and macrocephaly. Rarely, individuals remain almost asymptomatic, that is, presenting only with well-treatable oligoepilepsy or even with no neurological symptoms (9,131).

In 2000, Muntau and colleagues reported three patients with neonatal encephalopathy, severely impaired motor and mental development, and early death (134). All showed elevated excretions of both D-2-hydroxyglutaric acid and L-2-hydroxyglutaric acid, as well as an increase in 2-oxoglutaric acid and intermittent elevations of other citric acid cycle intermediates. It is as yet unclear if these patients represent a biochemically and/or genetically distinct disorder.

Neuroimaging findings in the severely affected patient group are complex yet rather homogeneous, revealing ventriculomegaly, predominantly of the occipital horns, enlarged frontal subarachnoid spaces, subdural effusions, subependymal cysts, and signs of disturbed and delayed cerebral maturation affecting gyral development, opercularization, and myelination (see Figure 7-14F). Recently, agenesis of the corpus callosum (132), bilateral involvement of the striatum (133), and cerebral artery infarctions were added to the spectrum.

Diagnosis Clinical findings in D-2-hydroxyglutaric aciduria include facial dysmorphism, cardiomyopathy, and severe epileptic encephalopathy with varied MRI abnormalities. The clinical variability is enormous, and an overall association, if at all applicable, may be that of a mitochondrial disorder.

The biochemical hallmark of this disease is the accumulation of D-2-hydroxyglutaric acid in all body fluids, which can be detected by GC-MS. Demonstration of elevated levels of 2-hydroxyglutaric acid must be followed up by determination of blood glucose, lactate, ammonia, electrolytes, and blood gases, a complete blood count, a blood acylcarnitine profile, and especially a differential quantitation of the two isomers L- and D-2-hydroxyglutaric acid. In D-2-hydroxyglutaric aciduria, 2-oxoglutaric acid usually is elevated in urine, accompanied by variable elevations of other tricarbonic acid cycle intermediates as well as lactate. γ-Aminobutyric acid (GABA) and total protein concentrations may be elevated in CSF.

D-2-Hydroxyglutaric acid also can be elevated in multiple acyl-CoA dehydrogenase deficiency (glutaric aciduria type II), which can be distinguished by the classical urine organic acid profile of the latter disorder (see Chapter 5). Mutation analysis of the D-lactate dehydrogenase gene nowadays will provide the definitive diagnosis (130).

TABLE 7-22 Laboratory Findings: d-2-Hydroxyglutaric Aciduria
Increased
Lactic acid (inconstant)
Organic acids: D-2-hydroxyglutaric acid, 2-oxoglutaric acid and variable elevations of other tricarbonic acid cycle intermediates (inconstant)
Acylcarnitines: none

TABLE 7-23 Laboratory Findings: L-2-Hydroxyglutaric Aciduria
Increased
Amino acids: lysine (inconstant)
Organic acids: L-2-hydroxyglutaric acid
Acylcarnitines: none

Prenatal diagnosis can be performed either through genetic testing or by metabolite determination in amniotic fluid by stable-isotope-dilution GC-MS assay (Table 7-22).

Treatment and Outcome No specific therapy exists to date. Long-term care of patients should entail 1) yearly assessments of muscle function with special focus on the heart and possibly muscle ultrasound and EMG and 2) a full neurological examination, including EEG and MRI, as indicated. Since GABA usually is elevated in CSF, vigabatrin should be avoided in the treatment of seizures.

The prognosis of D-2-hydroxyglutaric aciduria is extremely variable. Severely affected children may die in infancy, whereas moderately affected patients have a better prognosis up to an unimpaired life. There is as yet no prediction of the clinical course based on biochemical, enzymatic, or molecular findings.

L-2-Hydroxyglutaric Aciduria

Etiology/Pathophysiology L-2-Hydroxyglutaric aciduria is a rare autosomal recessively inherited cerebral OA with about 50 cases reported (135–139). The metabolic origin of L-2-hydroxyglutaric acid is unknown, as is its pathogenesis (140). Recently, the defect was identified in a putative FAD-dependent L-2-hydroxyglutarate dehydrogenase converting L-2-hydroxyglutaric acid to 2-oxoglutaric acid (141,142). The enzyme is homologous to the FAD-dependent oxidoreductase, and pathogenic mutations have been identified in the corresponding gene named *Duranin*.

Clinical Presentation Like Canavan disease, L-2-hydroxyglutaric aciduria is characterized by progressive loss of myelinated arcuate fibers and a spongiform encephalopathy (135,136,139). However, time course and clinical features are different. Patients often are macrocephalic. In the first 2 years of life, mental and psychomotor development may be normal or slightly delayed. Febrile seizures, nonspecific developmental delay, and muscular hypotonia are the presenting symptoms. Progressive ataxia, variable extrapyramidal and pyramidal signs, epilepsy, and progressive mental retardation eventually develop. By adolescence, patients usually are bedridden and severely mentally retarded (IQ 40–50). Interestingly, two patients have

been reported who developed cerebral tumors, which may be a sign of an increased risk for cerebral malignancies (135).

Clinical presentation and course of L-2-hydroxyglutaric aciduria is rather uniform. No metabolic imbalance has ever been reported. However, two patients presented at birth with depressed vital signs, severe epileptic encephalopathy, and an abnormal CT showing cerebellar involvement. One of the children died after withdrawal of support at 1 month of age (137,138).

The neuroimaging findings in L-2-hydroxyglutaric aciduria are unique and mostly uniform, comprising a progressive loss of arcuate fibers combined with progressive cerebellar atrophy and signal changes in basal ganglia and the dentate nuclei (see Figure 7-14G, H). Moroni and colleagues (2000) noticed a correlation between the extent of brain lesions on MRI and clinical severity (139).

Diagnosis L-2-hydroxyglutaric aciduria results in a rather homogeneous clinical picture and abnormalities on neuroimaging. In a child presenting with a slowly progressive encephalopathy with mental retardation and ataxia from childhood, together with subcortical leukoencephalopathy, L-2-hydroxyglutaric aciduria should be high on the list of differential diagnoses. Similarly, subcortical leukoencephalopathy together with cerebellar atrophy in an adult with progressive intellectual deterioration and ataxia should prompt an investigation of urinary organic acids.

L-2-Hydroxyglutaric acid is found to be highly elevated in all body fluids and can be demonstrated by GC-MS combined with stereospecific chromatographic differentiation of the L-2- from the stereoisomeric D-2-hydroxyglutaric acid. Increased levels of L-2-hydroxyglutaric acid also can be detected in plasma and CSF, with higher levels in CSF (103). Lysine is also increased in both plasma and again even more in CSF, whereas tricarbonic acid cycle intermediates, as well as lactate, usually are normal, as is GABA, in CSF.

There is no other disease known that result in increased levels of L-2-hydroxyglutaric acid except for three patients with neonatal encephalopathy, severely impaired motor and mental development, early death, and combined D-2- and L-2-hydroxyglutaric acidurias who fall beside this categorization (134).

Prenatal diagnosis is possible by determining L-2-hydroxyglutaric acid in amniotic fluid samples (139) and now also by molecular testing (Table 7-23).

Treatment and Outcome No specific therapy exists to date. Epilepsy generally can be controlled by standard antiepileptic medications. Patients with L-2-hydroxyglutaric aciduria can be expected to reach adult life. The oldest known patients are close to 40 years of age, bedridden, and severely retarded.

N-ACETYLASPARTIC ACIDURIA (CANAVAN DISEASE)

Etiology/Pathophysiology Canavan disease is a devastating infantile neurodegenerative disorder named after Dr. Myrtelle May Moore Canavan, who described spongy degeneration of white matter of the brain of a child in 1931. N-Acetylaspartic aciduria caused by deficient aspartoacylase (N-acetylasparaginase) was recognized in 1986 in a child with a similar disease (144). In 1988, Dr. Matalon proved aspartoacylase deficiency in a child with a biopsy-proven Canavan disease, joining the pathological entity Canavan disease with the metabolic disorder N-acetylaspartic aciduria (146).

Canavan disease is found in all ethnic populations but has a much higher frequency in Ashkenazi Jews (1 in 5000 to 1 in 14,000). The frequent missense mutation E285A in the aspartoacylase gene, localized on chromosome 17p13-pter, accounts for more than 80% of alleles in Ashkenazi Jews and for 60% of alleles in patients of non-Jewish origin. A nonsense mutation, tyrosine to termination, on codon 231 (Y231X) is also frequent in Ashkenazi patients (13.4%). As a consequence of identification of the common mutations in Ashkenazi Jews, screening is being offered to Ashkenazi couples similar to screening programs for Tay–Sachs disease, and Canavan disease has become almost extinct. In the rare non-Jewish patients, mutations are more diverse, and correspondingly, more atypical clinical courses are observed (147).

In healthy individuals, high concentrations of N-acetylaspartic acid (8 mmol/g of tissue) are found exclusively in brain tissue, but its biological function still remains unclear. Its concentration in human brain is second only to glutamate. The concentration increases with brain maturation and reaches adult level at 3 years of age.

Aspartoacylase catalyzes the deacetylation of N-acetylaspartic acid to produce acetate, a substrate for the synthesis of myelin lipids, including cholesterol. In the brain, aspartoacylase is localized in oligodendrocytes (148), and its expression depends on activity of the myelination process. It has been proposed that N-acetyl-L-aspartate may function as a molecular water pump in myelinated neurons, actively transporting water from various metabolic processes in neuronal metabolism against its gradient (149). Thus deficiency of aspartoacylase may cause both accumulation of water within the oligodendrocytes, causing the spongiform white matter changes, and deficiency of acetyl groups needed for cholesterol biosynthesis, causing demyelination, both characteristic for Canavan disease.

Clinical Presentation Canavan disease mostly manifests at age 2–4 months with delayed development (146). Hypotonia with prominent head lag, epilepsy, loss of previously acquired skills, and progressive macrocephaly are found regularly. Seizures and atrophy of the optic nerve develop during the second year of life. As the disease progresses, affected children develop pyramidal signs and finally decerebration. Irritability, sleep disorders, gastroesophageal reflux, and feeding difficulties often complicate the disease course.

Neuroimaging reveals characteristic symmetrical leukodystrophic changes with loss of arcuate fibers (similar to L-hydroxyglutaric aciduria); histology demonstrates spongiform degeneration in particular of the cortex and subcortical white matter (see Figure 7-14I) with less involvement in the cerebellum and brain stem. In infancy, the changes may be subtle and misinterpreted as delayed myelination or periventricular leukomalacia. In these patients, follow-up neuroimaging studies will reveal the leukodystrophic changes.

Variant Canavan disease such as congenital, infantile, and juvenile forms have been described and have been proven in part to be caused by the same metabolic defect (147).

Diagnosis Identification of the accumulation N-acetylaspartic acid and the deficiency of aspartoacylase has obviated the need for brain biopsy for the diagnosis of Canavan disease (146). Increased urinary excretion of N-acetylaspartic acid can be detected by GC-MS. Borderline elevations are not diagnostic and usually are not confirmed. Confirmation of

TABLE 7-24	Laboratory Findings: Canavan Disease
Increased	
Organic acids: N-acetylaspartic acid	
Acylcarnitines: none	

diagnosis is by enzymatic analysis in skin fibroblasts and/or molecular diagnosis.

Prenatal diagnosis is possible by stable-isotope-dilution analysis of amniotic fluid obtained in the second trimester, which shows elevated N-acetylaspartic acid. However, borderline results have to be repeated by a follow-up amniocentesis (6). Enzyme activity in cultivated amniocytes or chorionic villous material is much lower than in fibroblasts and unsuitable for reliable prenatal diagnosis (146). With description of the gene locus, molecular prenatal diagnosis is now the method of choice in families with known mutations (Table 7-24).

Treatment and Outcome Management is symptomatic (antiepileptics) and palliative. Special care is needed to avoid aspiration with feedings. Many patients need tube or gastrostomy feeding.

Dietary therapies, for example, a ketogenic diet to replenish acetate, have not been shown to be beneficial and are potentially harmful.

A clinical protocol for gene therapy was published 2002 in New Zealand involving the transfer of a liposome-encapsulated construct containing human aspartoacylase cDNA intraventricularly (150). The clinical changes were not pronounced and were relatively transient, most likely due to inadequacies of the vector or the delivery system.

The prognosis of infantile Canavan disease is rapidly fatal, whereas milder disease courses have been described in some patients. These patients have survived beyond their early teens.

ETHYLMALONIC ENCEPHALOPATHY

Etiology/Pathophysiology Ethylmalonic encephalopathy is a devastating infantile autosomal recessive neurometabolic disorder that affects the brain, gastrointestinal tract, and peripheral vessels. The underlying metabolic defect was identified recently in a protein that is targeted to mitochondria and internalized into the matrix after energy-dependent cleavage of a short leader peptide (151). The corresponding gene was named ETHE1. The protein is required for metabolic homeostasis and energy metabolism. In 1990, Hoffmann and colleagues (152) first described this inborn error of metabolism as *ethylmalonic*

• Ethylmalonic encephalopathy is characterized by ethylmalonic and methylsuccinic aciduria, lactic acidemia resulting in severe psychomotor retardation, acrocyanosis, petechiae, and chronic diarrhea.

aciduria. Since the initial report, no more than 30 cases of ethylmalonic encephalopathy have been described worldwide, indicating that the disorder is very rare (153,154).

The etiology of increased excretion of ethylmalonic and methylsuccinic acids in ethylmalonic encephalopathy is uncertain. Ethylmalonic acid may be derived from carboxylation of elevated butyryl-CoA by propionyl-CoA carboxylase or from the R-pathway of isoleucine catabolism.

Clinical Presentation The metabolic disorder was described originally in a Mediterranean (152) and an Italian family (153). Patients present with neonatal hypotonia followed by progressive neurological deterioration, especially pyramidal dysfunction, mental retardation, orthostatic acrocyanosis with distal swelling, chronic diarrhea, and recurrent petechiae (Figure 7-15). Mild to moderate hematuria is often present. MRI may reveal areas of hyperintensity in the cerebellar white matter and lesions in the basal ganglia. The latter may appear suddenly, accompanied by acute clinical deterioration, that is, metabolic stroke (154).

Diagnosis The main biochemical features of ethylmalonic encephalopathy are increased urinary ethylmalonic and methylsuccinic acids associated with abnormal excretion of C_4 and C_5 (n-butyryl-, isobutyryl-, isovaleryl-, and 2-methylbutyryl-) acylglycines and acylcarnitines, as well as intermittent lactic acidosis. Initial laboratory studies in the investigations of ethylmalonic aciduria should include blood glucose, lactate, ammonia, electrolytes, and blood gases, a complete blood count, a blood acylcarnitine profile, and quantitative

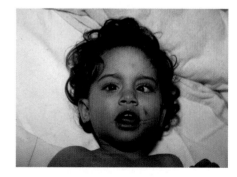

FIGURE 7-15. The index patient with ethylmalonic aciduria at the age of 22 months. The girl displayed severe hypotonia and developmental delay. Note petechial lesions together with the hemorrhagic spot.

• Hypotonia, head lag, and progressive macrocephaly in infancy are the classical clinical triad of Canavan disease.

TABLE 7-25	Laboratory Findings: Ethylmalonic Encephalopathy

Increased

Lactic acid (inconstant)

Organic acids: ethylmalonic acid, methylsuccinic acid, isobutyrylglycine, 2-methylbutyrylglycine

Acylcarnitines: butyryl/isobutyrylcarnitine (C_4) (inconstant), isovaleryl/methylbutyrylcarnitine (C_5)↑ (inconstant)

- If the biochemical diagnosis of glutaric aciduria type II is not confirmed by in vitro enzyme assays and/or molecular studies, the diagnosis of ethylmalonic encephalopathy should be high on the list.

urine organic acid analysis by GC-MS. Since respiratory chain deficiencies are an important differential diagnosis, analysis of the enzyme activities in different tissues (i.e., skin fibroblasts or muscle) may be initiated. Secondary COX-deficiency in muscle has been described in patients with ethylmalonic encephalopathy. Mutation analysis of the ETHE1 gene in available tissues nowadays will provide the definitive diagnosis (151), including prenatal diagnosis.

Ethylmalonic encephalopathy should be included in the differential diagnosis of persistent ethylmalonic aciduria caused, in addition to ethylmalonic encephalopathy, by short-chain acyl-CoA dehydrogenase deficiency, including the common variants, defects of the mitochondrial electron-transfer flavoprotein pathway or glutaric aciduria type II (sometimes also described as *ethylmalonic adipic aciduria*), some forms of respiratory chain deficiencies, and Jamaican vomiting sickness. The frequency of ethylmalonic encephalopathy may have been underestimated because the biochemical phenotype may be attributed incorrectly to one of the other metabolic disorders. Until 2004, no definitive diagnosis of ethylmalonic encephalopathy was possible (Table 7-25).

Treatment and Outcome No effective treatment of ethylmalonic encephalopathy is known. Riboflavin, carnitine, ascorbic acid, vitamin E, and/or glycine supplementations all have been tried without benefit (154), although individual patients were reported to show a slight improvement in motor function, cognitive behavior, and chronic mucoid diarrhea after treatment with riboflavin and/or coenzyme Q10. Ozand and colleagues reported one patient who remained stable on prolonged doses of methyl prednisolone (154).

Dietary therapies, for example, a diet low in branched-chain or sulfur-containing (methionine) amino acids, have not yet been shown to be beneficial and are potentially harmful.

The prognosis is poor, and ethylmalonic encephalopathy usually is lethal in early childhood.

REFERENCES

1. Hoffmann GF, Feyh P. Organic acid analysis. In: Blau N, Duran M, Blaskovics ME, Gibson KM, eds. *Physician's Guide to the Laboratory Diagnosis of Inherited Metabolic Disease*, 2nd ed. Heidelberg: Springer; 2002:27.4
2. Hoffmann GF, Gibson KM, Trefz FK, et al. Neurological manifestations of organic acid disorders. *Eur J Pedistr.* 1994;153:94.
3. Schulze A, Lindner M, Kohlmueller D, et al. Expanded newborn screening for inborn errors of metabolism by electrospray ionization-tandem mass spectrometry: Results, outcome, and implications. *Pediatrics.* 2003;111:1399.
4. Hoffmann GF, Nyhan WL, Zschocke J, et al., eds. *Core Handbook in Pediatrics: Inherited Metabolic Diseases.* Philadelphia: Lippincott Williams & Wilkins, 2002.
5. Hoffmann GF, Gibson KM. Disorders of organic acid metabolism. In: Moser HW, ed. *Handbook of Clinical Neurology*, Vol. 22. New York: Elsevier; 1996:639.
6. Jakobs C, ten Brink H, Stellard F. Prenatal diagnosis of inherited metabolic disorders by quantitation of characteristic metabolites in amniotic fluid: Facts and future. *Prenatal Diagn.* 1990;10:265.
7. Shigematsu Y, Hata I, Nakai A, et al. Prenatal diagnosis of organic acidemias based on amniotic fluid levels of acylcarnitines. *Pediatr Res.* 1996;39:680.
8. Niiyama S, Koelker S, Degen I, et al. Acrodermatitis acidemia secondary to malnutrition in glutaric aciduria type I. *Eur J Dermatol.* 2001;11:244.
9. Chalmers RA, Roe CR, Stacey TE, et al. Urinary excretion of L-carnitine and acylcarnitines by patients with disorders of organic acid metabolism: Evidence for secondary insufficiency of L-carnitine. *Pediatr Res.* 1984;18:1325.
10. Dixon MA, Leonard JV. Intercurrent illness in inborn errors of intermediary metabolism. *Arch Dis Child.* 1992;67:1387.
11. Fernandes J, Saudubray JM, Van den Berghe G, eds. *Inborn Metabolic Diseases*, 3rd ed. New York: Springer; 2000.
12. Prietsch V, Lindner M, Zschocke J, et al. Emergency management of inherited metabolic disease. *J Inherited Metab Dis.* 2002;25:531.
13. Wendel U, Langenbeck U, Lombeck I, et al. Maple syrup urine disease: Therapeutic use of insulin in catabolic states. *Eur J Pediatr.* 1982;139:172.
14. Schaefer F, Straube E, Oh J, et al. Dialysis in neonates with inborn errors of metabolism. *Nephrol Dial Transplant.* 1999;14:910.
15. Mayatepek E, Schulze A. Metabolic decompensation and lactic acidosis in propionic acidaemia complicated by thiamine deficiency. *J Inherited Metab Dis.* 1000;22:189.
16. Mamer OA, Reimer ML. On the mechanisms of the formation of L-alloisoleucine and the 2-hydroxy-3-methylvaleric acid stereoisomers from L-isoleucine in maple syrup urine disease patients and in normal humans. *J Biol Chem.* 1992;267:22141.
17. Menkes JH, Hurst PL, Craig JM. New syndrome: Progressive familial infantile cerebral dysfunction associated with an unusual urinary substance. *Pediatrics.* 1954;14:462.
18. Hoffmann GF, Machill G: 25 Jahre Neugeborenenscreening auf angeborene Stoffwechselstörungen in Deutschland. *Monatsschr Kinderheilkd.* 1994;142:857.
19. Morton DH, Strauss KA, Robinson DL, et al. Diagnosis and treatment of maple syrup disease: A study of 36 patients. *Pediatrics.* 2002;109:999.
20. Jouvet P, Rustin P, Taylor DL, et al. Branched chain amino acids induce apoptosis in neural cells without mitochondrial membrane depolarization or cytochrome C release: Implications for neurological impairment associated with maple syrup urine disease. *Mol Bio Cell.* 2000;11:1919.
21. Danner DJ, Litwer S, Herring WJ, et al. Molecular genetic basis for inherited human disorders of branched-chain α-ketoacid dehydrogenase complex. *Ann NY Acad Sci.* 1989;573:369.
22. Duran M, Wadman SK. Thiamine-responsive inborn errors of metabolism. *J Inherited Metab Dis.* 1985;8:70.
23. Haas R. Thiamine and the brain. *Ann Rev Nutr.* 1988;8:483.
24. Nyhan WL, Rice-Kelts M, Klein J, et al. Treatment of the acute crisis in maple syrup urine disease. *Arch Pediatr Adolesc Med.* 1999;152:593.
25. Wendel U, Saudubray JM, Bodner A, et al. Liver transplantation in maple syrup urine disease. *Eur J Pediatr Suppl.* 1999;2:S60.
26. Strauss KA, Mazariegos GV, Sindhi R, et al. Elective liver transplantation for the treatment of classical marple syrup urine disease. *Am J Transplant.* 2006;6:557.
27. Hoffmann B, Helbling C, Schadewaldt P, et al. Impact of longitudinal plasma leucine levels on the intellectual outcome in patients with classic MSUD. *Pediatr Res.* 2006;59:17.
28. Hilliges C, Awiszus D, Wendel U. Intellectual performance of children with maple syrup urine disease. *Eur J Pediatr.* 1993;152:144.
29. Tanaka K, Budd MA, Efron ML, et al. Isovaleric acidemia: A new genetic defect of leucine metabolism. *Proc Natl Acad Sci USA.* 1966;56:236.
30. Rhead WJ, Tanaka K. Demonstration of a specific mitochondrial isovaleryl-CoA dehydrogenase deficiency in fibroblasts from patients with isovaleric acidemia. *Proc Natl Acad Sci USA.* 1980;77:580.
31. Finocchiaro G, Ito M, Tanaka K. Purification and properties of short chain acyl CoA, medium chain acyl CoA and isovaleryl CoA dehydrogenases from human liver. *J Biol Chem.* 1987;262:7982.
32. Vockley J, Parimoo B, Tanaka K. Molecular characterization of four different classes of mutations in isovaleryl-CoA dehydrogenase

gene responsible for isovaleric acidemia. *Am J Hum Genet.* 1991;49:147.

33. Ensenauer R, Vockley J, Willard JM, et al. A common mutation is associated with a mild, potentially asymptomatic phenotype in patients with isovaleric acidemia diagnosed by newborn screening. *Am J Hum Genet.* 2004;75:1136.

34. Hutchinson RJ, Bunnell K, Thoene JG. Suppression of granulopoietic progenitor cell proliferation by metabolites of the branched-chain amino acids. *J Pediatr.* 1985;106:62.

35. Sweetman L, Williams J. Branched chain organic acidurias. In: Scriver CR, Beaudet AL, Sly WS, Valle D, eds. *The Metabolic and Molecular Bases of Inherited Disease,* 8th ed. New York: McGraw-Hill; 2001:2125.

36. Mayatepek E, Kurcynski TW, Hoppel CL. Long-term L-carnitine treatment in isovaleric acidemia. *Pediatr Neurol.* 1991;7:137.

37. Shih VE, Aubry RH, DeGrande G, et al. Maternal isovaleric acidemia. *J Pediatr.* 1984;105:77.

38. Feinstein JA, O'Brien K. Acute metabolic decompensation in an adult patient with isovaleric acidemia. *South Med J.* 2003;96:500.

39. Attia N, Sakati N, Al Ashwal A, et al. Isovaleric acidemia appearing as diabetic ketoacidosis. *J Inherited Metab Dis.* 1996;19:85.

40. Zschocke J, Hoffmann GF. Vademecum metabolicum. In: *Manual of Metabolic Paediatrics,* 2nd ed. Stuttgart: Schattauer, 2004.

41. Roe CR, Millington DS, Maltby DA, et al. L-Carnitine therapy in isovaleric acidemia. *J Clin Invest.* 1984;74:2290.

42. Tajima G, Sakura N, Yofune H, et al. Establishment of a practical enzymatic assay method for determination of isovaleryl-CoA dehydrogenase activity using high-performance liquid chromatography. *Clin Chim Acta.* 2005;353:193.

43. de Sousa C, Chalmers RA, Stacey TE, et al. The response to L-carnitine and glycine therapy in isovaleric acidemia. *Eur J Pediatr.* 1986;144:451.

44. Lau EP, Cochran BC, Fall RR. Isolation of 3-methylcrotonyl-CoA carboxylase from bovine kidney. *Arch Biochem Biophys.* 1980;205:352.

45. Baumgartner MR, Almashanu S, Suormala T, et al. The molecular basis of human 3-methylcrotonyl-CoA carboxylase deficiency. *J Clin Invest.* 2001;107:495.

46. Gallardo ME, Desviat LR, Rodriguez JM, et al. The molecular basis of 3-methylcrotonylglycinuria, a disorder of leucine catabolism. *Am J Hum Genet.* 2001; 68:334.

47. Röschinger W, Millington DS, Gage DA, et al. 3-Hydroxyisovalerylcarnitine in patients with deficiency of 3-methylcrotonyl CoA carboxylase. *Clin Chim Acta.* 1995;240:35.

48. Baumgartner MR, Dantas MF, Suormala T, et al. Isolated 3-Methylcrotonyl-CoA carboxylase deficiency: Evidence for an allele-specific dominant negative effect and responsiveness to biotin therapy. *Am J Hum Genet.* 2004;75:790.

49. Gibson KM, Elpeleg ON, Jakobs C, et al. Multiple syndromes of 3-methylglutaconic aciduria. *Pediatr Neurol.* 1993;9:120.

50. Barth PG, Scholte HR, Berden JA, et al. An X-linked mitochondrial disease affecting cardiac muscle, skeletal muscle and neutrophil leucocytes. *J Neurol Sci.* 1983;62:327.

51. Barth P, Wanders R, Vreken P, et al. X-linked cardioskeletal myopathy and neutropenia (Barth syndrome). *J Inherited Metab Dis.* 1999;22:555.

52. Anikster Y, Kleta R, Shaag A, et al. Type III 3-methylglutaconic aciduria (optic atrophy plus syndrome, or Costeff optic atrophy syndrome): Identification of the OPA3 gene and its founder mutation in Iraqi Jews. *Am J Hum Genet.* 2001;69:1218.

53. Aqeel AA, Rashed M, Ozand PT, et al. 3-Methylglutaconic aciduria: Ten new cases with a possible new phenotype. *Brain Dev.* 1994;16:23.

54. Kelley RI, Kratz L. 3-Methylglutaconic acidemia in Smith–Lemli–Opitz syndrome. *Pediatr Res.* 1995;37:671.

55. Narisawa K, Gibson KM, Sweetman L, et al. Deficiency of 3-methylglutaconyl-coenzyme A hydratase in two siblings with 3-methylglutaconic aciduria. *J Clin Invest.* 1986;77:1148.

56. Ly TB, Peters V, Gibson, KM., et al. Mutations in the AUH gene cause 3-methylglutaconic aciduria type I. *Hum Mutat.* 2003;21:401.

57. D'Adamo P, Fassone L, Gedeon A, et al. The X-linked gene G4.5 is responsible for different infantile dilated cardiomyopathies. *Am J Hum Genet.* 1997;61:862.

58. Elpeleg ON, Costeff H, Joseph A, et al. 3-Methylglutaconic aciduria type in the Iraqi Jewish "Optic atrophy plus" (Costeff) syndrome. *Dev Med Child Neurol.* 1994;36:167.

59. Gibson KM, Sherwood WG, Hoffmann GF, et al. Phenotypic heterogeneity in the syndromes of 3-methylglutaconic aciduria. *J Pediatr.* 1991;118:885.

60. Zschocke J, Ruiter JP, Brand J, et al. Progressive infantile neurodegeneration caused by 2-methyl-3-hydroxybutyryl-CoA dehydrogenase deficiency: A novel inborn error of branched-chain fatty acid and isoleucine metabolism. *Pediatr Res.* 2000;48:852.

61. Ensenauer R, Niederhoff H, Ruiter JP, et al. Clinical variability in 3-hydroxy-2-methylbutyryl-CoA dehydrogenase deficiency. *Ann Neurol.* 2002;51:656.

62. Olpin SE, Pollitt RJ, McMenamin J, et al. 2-Methyl-3-hydroxybutyryl-CoA dehydrogenase deficiency in a 23-year-old man. *J Inherited Metab Dis.* 2002;25:477.

63. Poll-The BT, Wanders RJ, Ruiter JP, et al. Spastic diplegia and periventricular white matter abnormalities in 2-methyl-3-hydroxybutyryl-CoA dehydrogenase deficiency, a defect of isoleucine metabolism: Differential diagnosis with hypoxic–ischemic brain diseases. *Mol Genet Metab.* 2004;81:295.

64. Sutton VR, O'Brien WE, Clark GD, et al. 3-Hydroxy-2-methylbutyryl-CoA dehydrogenase deficiency. *J Inherited Metab Dis.* 2003;26:69.

65. Sass JO, Forstner R, Sperl W. 2-Methyl-3-hydroxybutyryl-CoA dehydrogenase deficiency: Impaired catabolism of isoleucine presenting as neurodegenerative disease. *Brain Dev.* 2004;26:12.

66. Childs B, Nyhan WL, Borden MA, et al. Idiopathic hyperglycinemia and hyperglycinuria, a new disorder of amino acid metabolism. *Pediatrics.* 1961;27:522.

67. Ofman R, Ruiter JP, Feenstra M, et al. 2-Methyl-3-hydroxybutyryl-CoA dehydrogenase deficiency is caused by mutations in the HADH2 gene. *Am J Hum Genet.* 2003;72:1300.

68. Lustbader JW, Cirilli M, Lin C, et al. ABAD directly links Abeta to mitochondrial toxicity in Alzheimer's disease. *Science.* 2004;304:448.

69. Ando T, Rasmussen K, Nyhan WL, et al. Propionic acidemia in patients with ketotic hyperglycinemia. *J Pediatr.* 1971;78:827.

70. Fenton WA, Gravel RA, Rosenblatt DS. Disorders of propionate and methylmalonate metabolism. In: Scriver CR, Beaudet AL, Sly WS, Valle D, eds. *The Metabolic and Molecular Bases of Inherited Disease,* 8th ed. New York: McGraw-Hill; 2001:2165

71. Perez B, Desviat LR, Rodriguez-Pombo P, et al. Propionic acidemia: Identification of twenty-four novel mutations in Europe and North America. *Mol Genet Metab.* 2003;78:59.

72. Yang X, Sakamoto O, Matsubara Y, et al. Mutation spectrum of the PCCA and PCCB genes in Japanese patients with propionic acidemia. *Mol Genet Metab.* 2004;81:335.

73. Perez-Cerda C, Merinero B, Rodriguez-Pombo P, et al. Potential relationship between genotype and clinical outcome in propionic acidaemia patients. *Eur J Hum Genet.* 2000;8:187.

74. Kölker S, Okun JG: Methylmalonic acid: An endogenous toxin? *Cell Mol Life Sci.* 2005;62:621.

75. Schwab MA, Sauer SW, Okun JG, et al. Secondary mitochondrial dysfunction in propionic aciduria: a pathogenic role for endogenous mitochondrial toxins. *Biochem J.* 2006;398:107.

76. Ogier de Baulny H, Benoist JF, Rigal O, et al. Metrhylmalonic and propionic acidemias: Management and outcome. *J Inherited Metab Dis.* 2005;28:415.

77. Massoud AF, Leonard JV. Cardiomyopathy in propionic acidemia. *Eur J Pediatr.* 1993;152:441.

78. Ianchulev T, Kolin T, Moseley K, et al. Optic nerve atrophy in propionic acidemia. *Ophthalmology.* 2003;110:1850.

79. Nyhan WL, Bay C, Beyer EW, et al. Neurologic nonmetabolic presentation of propionic acidemia. *Arch Neurol.* 1999;56:1143.

80. Yorifuji T, Kawai M, Muroi J, et al. Unexpectedly high prevalence of the mild form of propionic acidemia in Japan: Presence of a common mutation and possible clinical implications. *Hum Genet.* 2002;111:161.

81. Wolf B, Paulsen EP, Hsia YE. Asymptomatic propionyl CoA carboxylase deficiency in a 13-year-old girl. *J Pediatr.* 1979;95:563.

82. Willard HF, Ambani LM, Hart AC, et al. Rapid prenatal and postnatal detection of inborn errors of propionate, methylmalonate, and cobalamin metabolism. *Hum Genet.* 1976;34:277.

83. Surtees RA, Matthews EE, Leonard JV. Neurologic outcome of propionic acidemia. *Pediatr Neurol.* 1992;8:333.

84. Wolf B, Hsia YE, Sweetman L, et al. Propionic acidemia: A clinical update. *J Pediatr.* 1981;99:835.

85. Leonard JV, Walter JH, McKiernan PJ. The management of organic acidaemias: The role of transplantation. *J Inherited Metab Dis.* 2001;24:309.

86. Oberholzer VG, Levin B, Burgess EA, et al. Methylmalonic aciduria: An inborn error of metabolism leading to chronic metabolic acidosis. *Arch Dis Child.* 1967;42:492.

87. Stokke O, Eldjarn L, Norum KR, et al. Methylmalonic acidemia: A new inborn error of metabolism which may cause fatal acidosis in the neonatal period. *Scand J Clin Lab Invest.* 1967;20:313.

88. Lindenbaum J, Savage DG, Stabler SP, et al. Diagnosis of cobalamin deficiency: II. Relative sensitivies of serum cobalamin, methylmalonic acid and total homocysteine concentrations. *Am J Hematol.* 1990;34:99.

89. Baumgartner ER, Viardot C, and 47 collegues from 39 hospitals from 7 European countries. Long-term follow-up of 77 patients with isolated methylmalonic aciduria. *J Inherited Metab Dis.* 1995;18:138.

90. Hörster F, Hoffmann GF. Pathophysiology, diagnosis, and treatment of methylmalonic aciduria: Recent advances and new challenges. *Pediatr Nephrol.* 2004;19:1071.

91. Sniderman LC, Lamber M, Giguere R, et al. Outcome of individuals with low-moderate methylmalonic aciduria detected through a neonatal screening program. *J Pediatr.* 1999;134:675.

92. Ledley FD, Rosenblatt DS. Mutations in mut methylmalonic acidemia: Clinical and enzymatic correlations. *Hum Mutat.* 1997;9:1.

93. Lubrano R, Scoppi P, Barsotti P, et al. Kidney transplantation in a girl with methylmalonic acidemia and end stage renal failure. *Pediatr Nephrol.* 2001;16:848.

94. Van't Hoff WG, Dixon M, Taylor J, et al. Combined liver–kidney transplantation in methylmalonic acidemia. *J Pediatr.* 1998;1043.

95. Nyhan WL, Gargus JJ, Boyle K, et al. Progressive neurologic disability in methylmalonic acidemia despite transplantation of the liver. *Eur J Pediatr.* 2002;161:377.

96. Wolf B, Grier RE, Allen RJ, et al. Biotinidase deficiency: The enzymatic defect in late-onset multiple carboxylase deficiency. *Clin Chim Acta.* 1983;13:273.

97. Baumgartner ER, Suormala T, Wick H, et al. Biotinidase deficiency associated with renal loss of biocytin and biotin. *Ann NY Acad Sci.* 1985;447:272.

98. Cole H, Reynolds TR, Lockyer JM, et al. Human serum biotinidase: cDNA cloning, sequence, and characterization. *J Biol Chem.* 1994;269:6566.

99. Pomponio RJ, Hymes J, Reynolds TR, et al. Mutations in the human biotinidase gene that cause profound biotinidase deficiency in symptomatic children: Molecular, biochemical, and clinical analysis. *Pediatr Res.* 1997;42:840.

100. Norrgard KJ, Pomponio RJ, Hymes J, et al. Mutations causing profound biotinidase deficiency in children ascertained by newborn screening in the United States occur at different frequencies than in symptomatic children. *Pediatr Res.* 1999;46:20.

101. Swango KL, Demirkol M, Huner G, et al. Partial biotinidase deficiency is usually due to the D444H mutation in the biotinidase gene. *Hum Genet.* 1998;102:571.

102. Wolf B, Heard GS, Weissbecker KA, et al. Biotinidase deficiency: Initial clinical features and rapid diagnosis. *Ann Neurol.* 1985;18:614.

103. Hoffmann GF, Jakobs C, Holmes B, et al. Organic acids in cerebrospinal fluid and plasma of patients with L-2-hydroxyglutaric aciduria. *J Inherited Metab Dis.* 1995;18:189.

104. Dobrowolski SF, Angeletti J, Banas RA, et al. Real time PCR assays to detect common mutations in the biotinidase gene and application of mutational analysis to newborn screening for biotinidase deficiency. *Mol Genet Metab.* 2003;78:100.

105. Suormala TM, Baumgartner ER, Wick H, et al. Comparison of patients with complete and partial biotinidase deficiency: Biochemical studies. *J Inherited Metab Dis.* 1990;13:76.

106. Baumgartner ER, Suormala T. Biotin-responsive multiple carboxylase deficiency. In: Fernandes J, Saudubray JM, van den Berghe G, eds. *Inborn Metabolic Diseases. Diagnosis and Treatment*, 3rd ed. New York: Springer; 2000:276.

107. McVoy JR, Levy HL, Lawler M, et al. Partial biotinidase deficiency: Clinical and biochemical features. *J Pediatr.* 1990;116:78.

108. Packman S, Caswell N, Gonzalez-Rios MC, et al. Acetyl CoA carboxylase in cultured fibroblasts: Differential biotin dependence in the two types of biotin-responsive multiple carboxylase deficiency. *Am J Hum Genet.* 1984;36:80.

109. Zhang XX, Leon-Del-Rio A, Gravel RA, et al. Assignment of holocarboxylase synthetase gene (HLCS) to human chromosome band 21q22.1 and to mouse chromosome band 16C4 by in situ hybridization. *Cytogenet Cell Genet.* 1997;76:179.

110. Vianey-Saban C, Guffon N, Delolne F, et al. Diagnosis of inborn errors of metabolism by acylcarnitine profiling in blood using tandem mass spectrometry. *J Inherited Metab Dis.* 1997;20:411.

111. Shigematsu Y, Bykov IL, Liu YY, et al. Acylcarnitine profile in tissues and body fluids of biotin-deficient rats with and without L-carnitine supplementation. *J Inherited Metab Dis.* 1994;17:678.

112. Suormala T, Wick H, Bonjour JP, et al. Rapid differential diagnosis of carboxylase deficiencies and evaluation for biotin responsiveness in a single blood sample. *Clin Chim Acta.* 1985;145:151.

113. Burri BJ, Sweetman L, Nyhan WL. Heterogeneity of holocarboxylase synthetase in patients with biotin-responsive multiple carboxylase deficiency. *Am J Hum Genet.* 1985;37:326.

114. Baumgartner ER, Suormala T. Multiple carboxylase deficiency: Inherited and acquired disorders of biotin metabolism. *Int J Vitam Nutr Res.* 1997;67:377.

115. Goodman SI, Markey SP, Moe PG, et al. Glutaric aciduria: A "new" disorder of amino acid metabolism. *Biochem Med.* 1975;12:12.

116. Lindner M, Kölker S, Schulze A, et al. Neonatal screening for glutaryl-CoA dehydrogenase deficiency. *J Inherited Metab Dis.* 2004;27:851.

117. Strauss KA, Puffenberger EG, Robinson DL, et al. Type I glutaric aciduria: 1. Natural history of 77 patients. *Am J Med Genet (Semin Med Genet).* 2003;121C:38.

118. Greenberg CR, Prasad AN, Dilling LA, et al. Outcome of the first 3-years of a DNA-based neonatal screening program for glutaric acidemia type 1 in Manitoba and northwestern Ontario, Canada. *Mol Genet Metab.* 2002;75:70.

119. Goodman SI, Stein DE, Schlesinger S, et al. Glutaryl-CoA dehydrogenase mutations in glutaric acidemia (type I): Review and report of thirty novel mutations. *Hum Mutat.* 1998;12:141.

120. Kölker S, Koeller, DM, Okun J, et al. Pathomechanism of neurodegeneration in glutaryl-CoA dehydrogenase deficiency. *Ann Neurol.* 2004;55:7.

121. Kölker S, Greenberg CR., Lindner M, et al. Emergency treatment in glutaryl-CoA dehydrogenase deficiency. *J Inherited Metab Dis.* 2004;27:893.

122. Hoffmann GF, Athanassopoulos S, Burlina A, et al. Clinical course, early diagnosis, treatment and prevention of disease in glutaryl-CoA dehydrogenase deficiency. *Neuropediatrics.* 1996;27:115.

123. Bähr O, Mader I, Zschocke J, et al. Adult onset glutaric aciduria type I presenting with leukoencephalopathy. *Neurology.* 2002;59:1802.

124. Külkens S, Harting I, Sauer S, et al. Late-onset neurologic disease in glutaryl-CoA dehydrogenase deficiency. *Neurology.* 2005;64:2142.

125. Twomey EL, Naughten ER, Donogue VB, et al. Neuroimaging findings in glutaric aciduria type 1. *Pediatr Radiol.* 2003;33:823.

126. Baric I, Wagner L, Feyh P, et al. Sensitivity and specificity of free and total glutaric and 3-hydroxyglutaric acids measurements by stable isotope dilution assays for the diagnosis of glutaric aciduria type I. *J Inherited Metab Dis.* 1999;22:867.

127. Baric I, Zschocke J, Christensen E, et al. Diagnosis and management of glutaric aciduria type I. *J Inherited Metab Dis.* 1998;21:326.

128. Müller E, Kölker S. Reduction of lysine intake while avoiding malnutrition: Major goals and major problems in dietary treatment of glutaryl-CoA dehydrogenase deficiency. *J Inherited Metab Dis.* 2004;903.

129. Achouri Y, Noel G, Vertommen D, et al. Identification of a dehydrogenase acting on D-2-hydroxyglutarate. *Biochem J.* 2004;381:35.

130. Struys EA, Salomons GS, Achouri Y, et al. Mutations in the D-2-hydroxyglutarate dehydrogenase gene cause D-2-hydroxyglutaric aciduria. *Am J Hum Genet.* 2005;76:358.

131. Van der Knaap MS, Jakobs C, Hoffmann, GF, et al. D-2-Hydroxyglutaric aciduria: Biochemical marker or clinical disease entity? *Ann Neurol.* 1999;45:111.

132. Wang X, Jakobs C, Bawle EV, et al. D-2-Hydroxyglutaric aciduria with absence of

corpus callosum and neonatal intracranial haemorrhage. *J Inherited Metab Dis.* 2003;26:92.

133. Wajner M, Vargas CR, Funayama C, et al. D-2-Hydroxyglutaric aciduria in a patient with a severe clinical phenotype and unusual MRI findings. *J Inherited Metab Dis.* 2002;25:28.

134. Muntau AC, Roschinger W, Merkenschlager A, et al. Combined D-2- and L-2-hydroxyglutaric aciduria with neonatal onset encephalopathy: A third biochemical variant of 2-hydroxyglutaric aciduria? *Neuropediatrics.* 2000;137.

135. Barbot C, Fineza I, Diogo L, et al. L-2-Hydroxyglutaric aciduria: Clinical, biochemical and magnetic resonance imaging in six Portuguese pediatric patients. *Brain Dev.* 1997;19:268.

136. Barth PG, Hoffmann GF, Jaeken J, et al. L-2-Hydroxyglutaric acidemia: Clinical and biochemical findings in 12 patients and preliminary report on L-2-hydroxyacid dehydrogenase. *J Inherited Metab Dis.* 1993;16:753.

137. Barth PG, Wanders RJ, Scholte HR, et al. L-2-hydroxyglutaric aciduria and lactic acidosis. *J Inherited Metab Dis.* 1998;21:251.

138. Chen E, Nyhan WL, Jakobs C, et al. L-2-Hydroxyglutaric aciduria: Neuropathological correlations and first report of severe neurodegenerative disease and neonatal death. *J Inherited Metab Dis.* 1996;19:335.

139. Moroni I, D'Incerti L, Farina L, et al. Clinical, biochemical and neuroradiological findings in L-2-hydroxyglutaric aciduria. *Neurol Sci.* 2000;21:103.

140. Kölker S, Mayatepek E, Hoffmann GF. White matter disease in cerebral organic acid disorders: Clinical implications and suggested pathomechanisms. *Neuropediatrics.* 2002;33:225.

141. Rzem R, Veiga-da-Cunha M, Noel G, et al. A gene encoding a putative FAD-dependent L-2-hydroxyglutarate dehydrogenase is mutated in L-2-hydroxyglutaric aciduria. *Proc Natl Acad Sci USA.* 2004;101:16849.

142. Topcu M, Jobard F, Halliez S, et al. L-2-Hydroxyglutaric aciduria: identification of a mutant gene C14orf160, localized on chromosome 14q22.1. *Hum Mol Genet.* 2004;13:2803.

143. Canavan MM. Schilder's encephalitis perioxalis diffusa. *Arch Neurol Psychiatry.* 1931;25:299.

144. Kvittingen EA, Guldal G, Borsting S, et al. N-Acetlaspartic aciduria in a child with a progressive cerebral atrophy. *Clin Chim Acta.* 1986;158:217.

145. Matalon R, Michals K, Sebesta D, et al. Aspartoacylase deficiency and N-acetylaspartic aciduria in patients with Canavan disease. *Am J Med Genet.* 1988;29:463.

146. Matalon R, Michals-Matalon K. Recent advances in Canavan disease. *Adv Pediatr.* 1999;6:493.

147. Toft PB, Geib-Holtorff R, Rolland MO, et al. Magnetic resonance imaging in juvenile Canavan disease. *Eur J Pediatr.* 1993;152:750.

148. Madhavaro CN, Moffett JR, Moore RA, et al. Immunhistochemical localization of aspartoacylase in the rat central nervous system. J Comp Neurol, 2004;472:318.

149. Baslow MH. Evidence supporting a role for N-acetyl-L-aspartate as a molecular water pump in myelinated neurons in the central nervous system: An analytical review. *Neurochem Int.* 2002;40:295.

150. Janson C, McPhee S, Bilaniuk L, et al. Clinical protocol gene therapy of Canavan disease:AAV-2 vector for neurosurgical delivery of aspartoacylase gene (ASPA) to the human brain. *Hum Gene Ther.* 2002;13:1391.

151. Tiranti V, D'Adamo P, Briem E, et al. Ethylmalonic encephalopathy is caused by mutations in ETHE1, a gene encoding a mitochondrial matrix protein. *Am J Hum Genet.* 2004;74:239.

152. Hoffmann GF, Hunnemann DH, Jakobs C, et al. Progressive fatal pancytopenia, psychomotor retardation and muscle carnitine deficiency in a child with ethylmalonic aciduria and ethylmalonic acidaemia. J Inherited Metab Dis. 1990;13:337.

153. Burlina A, Zacchello F, Dionisi-Vici C, et al. New clinical phenotype of branched-chain acyl-CoA oxidation defect (letter). *Lancet.* 1991;338:1522.

154. Ozand PT, Rashed M, Millington DS, et al. Ethylmalonic aciduria: An organic acidemia with CNS involvement and vasculopathy. *Brain Dev.* 1994;16:12.

155. Hörster F, Hoffmann GF. Pathophysiology, diagnosis, and treatment of methylmalonic aciduria: Recent advances and new challenges. *Pediatr Nephrol.* 2004;19:1071.

156. Dewey KG, Beaton G, Fjeld C, et al. Protein requirements of infants and children. *Eur J Clin Nutr.* 1996;50:119.

157. Deutsche Gesellschaft für Ernährung (DGE): Empfehlungen für die Nährstoffzufuhr. In: *Umschau Verlag,* 4. Frankfurt: Auflage; 1985.

CHAPTER 8

Ketone Synthesis and Utilization Defects

Claude Sansaricq, MD, PhD
Sherly Pardo-Reoyo, MD

ETIOLOGY/PATHOPHYSIOLOGY

During fasting, acetoacetate and 3-hydroxybutyrate such as ketone bodies (KB) are produced in the liver mitochondria, primarily from the oxidation of fatty acids but also from certain amino acids, among others leucine and isoleucine (Figure 8-1). KB are important sources of energy (adenosine triphosphate) for extrahepatic tissues, primarily the brain and the heart and skeletal muscles, where they are completely oxidized, or they may serve as lipogenic precursors in the liver.

Ketonemia and/or ketonuria can be due to increased production of KB, or decreased consumption and alteration of the regulatory processes. Defects in gluconeogenesis, diabetic ketoacidosis, disturbances of branched-chain amino acid metabolism, organic acidemias, congenital lactic acidosis due to multiple carboxylase deficiency, and pyruvate carboxylase deficiency are important metabolic causes of excess KB formation. The hypoglycemia seen in the ketogenic defects may result from impaired gluconeogenesis or from excessive glucose consumption due to lack of KB formation as an alternative source of energy.

The term "ketogenesis" refers to the production of KB. Defects in ketogenesis can occur due to a deficiency in one of the following hepatic mitochondrial enzymes (Figure 8-2):

1. Mitochondrial 3-hydroxy-3-methylglutaryl (HMG)-coenzyme A (CoA) synthase that catalyzes the condensation of acetoacetyl-CoA and acetyl-CoA to form HMG-CoA; or

2. HMG-CoA lyase that cleaves HMG-CoA to form acetyl-CoA and acetoacetate. HMG-CoA can also be formed from the amino acid leucine. HMG-CoA lyase deficiency also causes accumulation of leucine intermediates because complete leucine catabolism requires intact lyase activity (Figure 8-1).

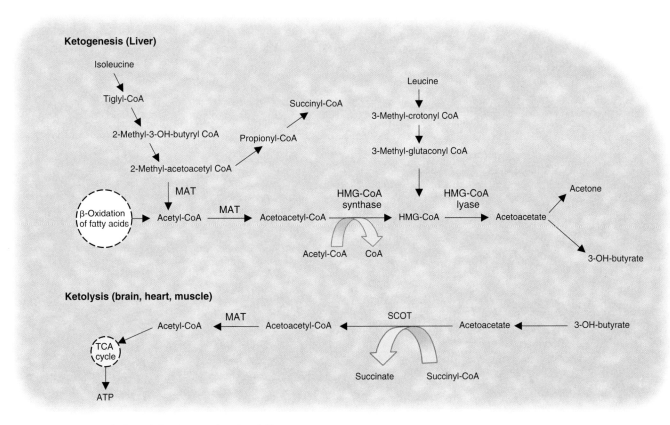

FIGURE 8-1. Normal ketone body metabolism (Ketogenesis and Ketolysis).

Ketone Synthesis and Utilization Defects

AT-A-GLANCE

Ketone synthesis and utilization defects refer to a group of metabolic disorders caused by enzymatic deficiencies in the synthesis (ketogenesis) or breakdown (ketolysis) of ketone bodies. Under normal circumstances, the ketone bodies (3-hydroxybutyrate and acetoacetate) are primarily produced in states of starvation (prolonged fasting) in all of us. Therefore the absence of ketones during such conditions can suggest a problem in ketogenesis. On the other hand ketolytic defects are primarily manifested by persistent elevation on ketone bodies even during non-fasting conditions with massive secretion during states of prolonged fasting or metabolic stress.

KETONE SYNTHESIS DEFECTS	GENE	LOCUS	OMIM
3-OH-3-methylglutaryl-CoA synthase	HMGCS2	1p13-p12	*600234
3-OH-3-methylglutaryl-CoA lyase (HMG-CoA lyase)	HMGCL	1pter-p33	+246450

KETONE UTILIZATION DEFECTS	GENE	LOCUS	OMIM
Succinyl-CoA: acetoacetate transferase (SCOT)	OXCT1	5p13	#245050
Acetoacetyl-CoA thiolase/ β-ketothiolase (MAT, T2)	ACAT1	11q22.3-q23.1	#203750

ENZYME DEFECT		FINDINGS	CLINICAL PRESENTATION BIRTH TO EARLY CHILDHOOD
HMG-CoA synthase	↓ ketones ↓ glucose Nl lactate Nl NH4	UOA: Nl ACP: Nl	Episodes of hypoglycemia and hypoketonemia/ketonuria; symptoms are non-specific and are related to the metabolic abnormalities, they include emesis, lethargy/coma.
HMG-CoA lyase	↓ glucose ↓ ketones ↑ lactate ↑ NH4	UOA: ↑ 3-OH-3methylglutaric ↑ 3-OH-isovaleric ↑ 3-methyl-glutaconic ↑ 3-methyl-glutaric (small amounts of 3-methyl-crotonylglycine) ACP: ↑ 3-methyl-glutarylcarnitine	Episodes of metabolic acidosis and hypoglycemia with absence of ketones accompanied by a typical UOA profile; symptoms are non-specific and are related to the metabolic abnormalities, they include emesis, lethargy/coma.
SCOT	Nl glucose ↑ ketones Nl lactate Nl NH4	UOA: Nl ACP: Nl	Episodes of metabolic acidosis (ketoacidosis) with normal blood glucose and ketonuria; symptoms are non-specific and are related to the metabolic abnormalities, they include emesis, lethargy/coma.
MAT	Nl glucose ↑ ketones Nl lactate Nl NH4	UOA: ↑ Tiglylglycine ↑ 2-methyl-3-OH-butyric ↑ 2-methyl-acetoacetate ACP: ↑ Tiglylcarnitine ↑ 2-methyl-3-OH-butyrylcarnitine	

Nl = normal values, NH4 = plasma ammonia, UOA = urine organic acid profile, ACP = acylcarnitine profile. In regards to the values of ketones we refer to levels present in urinalysis or urine dipsticks, although they could be measured in plasma as well.

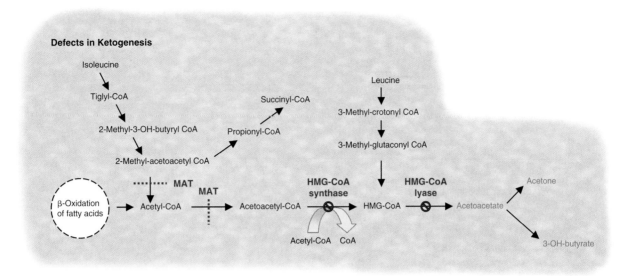

FIGURE 8-2. Abnormal ketone body metabolism (Ketogenesis).
Defects in ketogenesis are primarily caused by blocks in the metabolic pathways catalyzed by HMG-CoA synthase or HMG-CoA lyase. They are represented in this diagram as double thick red lines. MAT is involved in both ketogenesis and ketolysis but its deficiency is primarily associated with ketolysis. The enzymatic pathways blocked by MAT deficiency during ketogenesis are represented as a line of red dots.

The metabolism of KB is referred to as "ketolysis." Ketolytic defects are, for the most part, due to decreased utilization of KB in the peripheral tissues caused primarily by defects in the following mitochondrial enzymes (Figure 8-3):

1. Succinyl-CoA: acetoacetate transferase (SCOT) that transfers CoA from succinyl-CoA to acetoacetate to form acetoacetyl-CoA; and

2. Acetoacetyl-CoA thiolase/β-ketothiolase or mitochondrial acetoacetic thiolase (MAT, T2) degrades methylacetoacetyl-CoA produced in the degradation pathway of isoleucine. In the liver it also converts the reversible reaction of acetoacetyl-CoA to acetyl–CoA, which enters oxidation via the Krebs cycle. An additional mitochondrial oxothiolase located in the liver also contributes to ketogenesis by participating in the conversion of acetoacetyl-CoA in acetyl-CoA, cleaving methylacetoacetyl-CoA to a lesser degree. It is believed that

the role of the extrahepatic MAT isozyme in the pathogenesis of the ketolytic disorder is crucial.

CLINICAL PRESENTATION

The metabolic conditions resulting from failures of the enzymatic system mentioned previously often manifest themselves in the first few days of life. As in many metabolic disorders, however, some patients may present later in childhood or even as adults during states of metabolic stress such as infections, fever, dehydration, and surgeries among others. The clinical course during "stable periods," that is, the intervals between attacks, is indolent in most cases. The patients usually have normal growth and development and the frequency of episodes tends to decrease with age. A few patients have died during severe decompensation, primarily in early infancy. Several of those who have managed to survive a severe decompensation episode have had

magnetic resonance imaging (MRI) changes and developed some degree of developmental deficits or behavioral problems.

Defects of ketogenesis, show an overlapping presentation with fatty acid oxidation disorders (chapter 5) especially "hypoketotic hypoglycemia" with or without hyperammonemia, clinically symptoms of encephalopathy with vomiting and lethargy, sometimes associated with hepatomegaly.

MITOCHONDRIAL 3-HYDROXY-3-METHYLGLUTARYL-CoA SYNTHASE DEFICIENCY

Affected patients present with hypoglycemic encephalopathy rapidly progressing to coma after relatively short periods of fasting (12–18 hours) or during bouts of gastroenteritis after infancy. They have hypoglycemia, negative urine for ketones, high serum fatty acids, normal serum lactate and normal plasma ammonia levels.

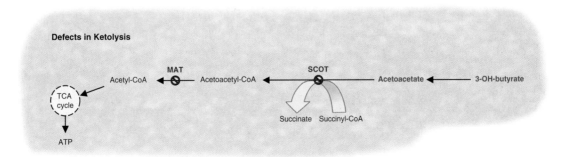

FIGURE 8-3. Abnormal ketone body metabolism (Ketolysis).
Defects in ketolysis are caused by deficiencies in the extrahepatic enzymes SCOT or MAT. The blocks in their enzymatic pathways are represented in this diagram as thick red lines.

TABLE 8-1   Summary of Laboratory Findings

	Defects in Ketogenesis		Defects in Ketolysis	
Laboratory tests	**HMG-CoA synthase**	**HMG-CoA lyase**	**SCOT**	**MAT**
Glucose	Low	Low	Normal	Low-normal
Lactate	Normal	Normal – elevated	Normal	Normal
Ammonia	Normal	Normal – elevated	Normal	Normal
Urinalysis (ketones)	Absent	Absent	Elevated	Elevated
Plasma amino acids	Normal	Normal	Normal	Normal
Urine organic acids	Nonspecific dicarboxylic aciduria.	Large amounts of : 3-OH –3 methylglutarate 3-OH isovalerate 3-methylglutaconate 3-methylglutarate Small amounts of : 3-methylcrotonylglycine	Normal	↑ Tiglylglycine ↑ 2-methyl-3-OH butyrate ↑ 2-methylacetoacetate (volatile compound usually not detected)
Acylcarnitine profile	Normal	↑ 3-methylglutarylcarnitine		↑ Tiglylcarnitine ↑ 2-methyl-3-OH-butyrylcarnitine

3-HYDROXY-3-METHYLGLUTARYL-CoA LYASE DEFICIENCY

Patients usually present with emesis, hypotonia, and lethargy. Hepatomegaly is often present. Severe metabolic acidosis, profound hypoglycemia, and elevated lactate and ammonia have been present as well. Some cases have been misdiagnosed as Reye syndrome. Pancreatitis is a recognized complication of this entity.

By contrast, defects in ketolysis present primarily with metabolic acidosis (severe ketoacidosis), ketonuria, and related symptoms such as tachypnea, vomiting, lethargy, or coma.

SUCCINYL-CoA: ACETOACETYL TRANSFERASE DEFICIENCY

Approximately 15 cases have been reported in the literature (1–16). These patients are characterized by recurrent episodes of severe ketoacidosis (elevated anion gap) and ketonuria. The presenting symptoms are tachypnea and lethargy or coma. Blood glucose, lactate, and ammonia levels are normal. Most patients still have a persistent ketonuria during stable conditions.

METHYLACETOACETYL-CoA THIOLASE DEFICIENCY

Thirty cases have been reported (17–21). All presented in ketoacidosis precipitated by intercurrent illnesses at a median age of 15 months (between 5 and 48 months old). At presentation the symptoms included episodes of emesis and tachypnea, followed by dehydration and a declining level of consciousness secondary to ketoacidosis with ketonuria and normal blood glucose, lactate, and ammonia levels.

DIAGNOSIS

Hypoketosis (ketogenesis defects) as well as hyperketosis (ketolysis defects) can only be reliably assessed in a fasting state (Table 8-1, Figure 8-4). Assessment of metabolic changes in res-ponse to controlled fasting may be helpful in cases in which extensive investigations have failed to lead to the diagnosis (Figure 8-4) (24). In some patients with fatty acid oxidation disorders, fasting can lead to the production of toxic metabolites and severe, sometimes fatal complications. It is essential to complete metabolic testing, including acylcarnitine analysis (dried blood spots) and other metabolic investigations, prior to a fasting test. In general, fasting tests for metabolic disorders should only be performed in specialized metabolic units, and only after all functional and molecular investigations have either failed to provide a diagnosis or have pointed to the need for such a study. It should also be noted that ketogenesis in the very young infant is poorly developed; hence, lack of ketones with fasting may be physiologic, whereas severe ketonuria is likely to be abnormal.

KETOGENESIS DEFECTS

Mitochondrial 3-Hydroxy-3-Methylglutaryl-CoA Synthase Deficiency (Hypoketotic Hypoglycemia). This diagnosis should be suspected when there is impaired KB formation (low KB despite high free fatty acids in serum) during prolonged fasting. The acylcarnitine profile is normal and urine organic acids reveals varying degrees of nonspecific dicarboxylic aciduria. Because the enzyme is expressed only in the liver, further studies on this tissue must be performed to confirm the diagnosis unless molecular investigations of the patient confirm two pathological mutations.

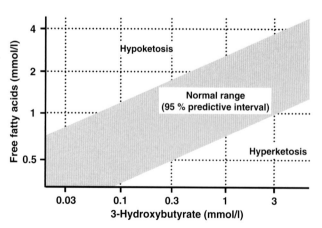

FIGURE 8-4. Graph showing the correlation between the concentrations of free fatty acids (plasma) and 3-hydroxybutyrate (deproteinized blood) in children after a 24-hour fast. Adapted from *Arch Dis Child. 1996;*75:115–119, with permission from the BMJ Publishing Group.

3-Hydroxy-3-Methylglutaryl-CoA Lyase Deficiency. The urine organic acid pattern of these patients shows massive excretion of 3-hydroxy-3-methylglutaric, 3-hydroxyisovaleric, 3-methylglutaconic, and 3-methylglutaric acids. Beta-methylcrotonylglycine may also be present. An acylcarnitine profile indicates the presence of 3-methylglutarylcarnitine in blood. The diagnosis can also be made on newborn screening by tandem mass spectrometry (MS/MS) but the elevation of the key metabolite may be very small or even absent. Enzyme studies (leukocytes, cultured fibroblasts, or liver) and/or molecular analysis must be performed to confirm the diagnosis.

Yalcinkaya et al. (22) reviewed multiple cranial studies performed using MRI and magnetic resonance spectra (MRS) in confirmed patients with HMG-CoA lyase deficiency. In this report, cranial MRI showed multiple periventricular, coalescent white matter lesions and also changes in the arcuate fibers. The authors also described involvement of the caudate and dentate nuclei. The MRS revealed decreased N-acetylaspartate and elevations of both choline and myoinositol peaks. It also revealed a peak consistent with lactate and/or 3-hydroxy-3-methylglutarate (at 1.33 ppm) and a characteristic peak at 2.42 ppm (area consistent with glutamine–glutamate) that is not present under normal conditions and has not been reported in any other disorders (22).

Succinyl-CoA: Acetoacetyl Transferase Deficiency SCOT deficiency is characterized by persistent ketonemia/uria even while the patient is clinically stable or in the fed state. Most patients develop severe episodes of ketoacidosis primarily during infections or prolonged fasting. During a prolonged fasting challenge the patient exhibits a normal glucose level in the presence of progressive ketoacidosis. Clear distinction of normal starvation ketosis, which reaches a homeostatic state from a progressive ketoacidosis, is essential to accurate diagnosis. Enzyme studies must be performed to confirm the diagnosis in skin fibroblasts.

Methylacetoacetyl-CoA Thiolase Deficiency. Patients present with intermittent episodes of ketoacidosis, but they usually excrete 2-methyl-3-hydroxybutyric acid, 2-methyl-acetoacetic acid and tiglylglycine that can be identified in urine organic acid analysis. During fasting challenges some patients have shown mild hypoglycemia but normal lactate and ammonia levels. Following isoleucine loads, all pathological metabolites increase further. 2-Methylacetoacetate is a volatile compound and hence could be missed on the organic acid analysis. Enzymatic studies from leukocytes or skin fibroblast are required for confirmation.

Ketolysis Defects

Suspect a defect in ketolysis (defects in ace-toacetyl-CoA thiolase or SCOT) in any patient who has ketosis/ketonuria with normal glucose, lactate, and ammonia levels.

Patients have been classified into two groups based on their mutation analysis and level of residual enzyme activity.

Group I: have no residual enzyme activity.

Urine organic acid analysis shows large quantities of tiglylglycine, 2-methyl-3-hydroxybutyrate, and 2-methyl-acetoacetate; both during metabolic crises and while stable.

Acylcarnitine profile indicates elevated tiglylcarnitine and 2-methyl-3-hydroxybutyrylcarnitine.

Group II: have some residual enzyme activity.

Urine organic acid analysis (during metabolic crises) demonstrates large excretion of 2-methyl-3-hydroxybutyrate with minor elevation in tiglylglycine.

Urine organic acid analysis (during stable conditions) reveals absent or mildly positive tiglylglycine, normal 2-methyl-3-hydroxybutyrate.

Acylcarnitine profile (during metabolic crises) shows elevated tiglylcarnitine and 2-methyl-3-hydroxybutyrylcarnitine.

Acylcarnitine profile (during stable conditions) demonstrates normal tiglylcarnitine and 2-methyl-3-hydroxybutyrylcarnitine.

An important differential diagnosis is 2-methyl-3-hydroxybutyryl-CoA dehydrogenase deficiency, a rare cerebral organic acid disorder due to defects in the enzyme preceding MAT in the isoleucine pathway (see chapter 7). The pattern of urinary excretion of pathologic metabolites in these two disorders is identical except for the absence of 2-methyl-acetoacetate in 2-methyl-3-hydroxybutyryl-CoA dehydrogenase deficiency. Retrospectively, patients with 2-methyl-3-hydroxybutyryl-CoA dehydrogenase deficiency were misdiagnosed as suffering from β-ketothiolase deficiency until in 2000 Zschocke and colleagues recognized the separate distinct clinical and biochemical presentation and proved the defect (25).

TREATMENT

Acute management is supportive. Key to rational management is administration of intravenous or oral glucose at least according to the glucose production rate to minimize ketone production and/or (depending on the defect) hypoglycemia. In essence, this maneuver

Summary of Lab Findings

The clinical manifestations of all the previously noted enzymatic deficiencies vary among patients and there are only weak correlations between genotype, and phenotype.

During stable periods, there may be normal laboratory findings. If the diagnosis is suspected, the tests should be repeated during metabolic decompensation or a prolonged fasting challenge.

For confirmation of these deficiencies, enzymatic and/or molecular studies are needed.

Prenatal diagnosis is possible for all these disorders. It is primarily performed via enzymatic studies in which amniocytes or chorionic villi are used. Mutation analysis may also be performed if pathogenic mutations have been previously identified in an affected individual in the family.

simply reverses any fasting component that was either causative or contributory to the acute episode. Bicarbonate administration to correct the acidosis is controversial because glucose administration should quickly reverse the pathophysioloy. Alkali should be reserved for use in patients in whom a life-threatening degree of acidosis exists. During intravenous hydration with high-concentration glucose supplementation close monitoring of electrolytes is essential. Some cases have required dialysis for correction of the severe acidosis.

Chronic management consists in dietary modifications including, moderate protein restriction (~ 1.5 g/kg/d) especially in HGM-CoA lyase deficiency, and with less well documented benefit in SCOT and aceto-acetyl-CoA thiolase deficiencies. In HMG-CoA synthase deficiency the leucine content of a normal diet could provide a source of ketogenesis independent of the defect. Evidence is lacking in support of the view that a low-fat diet will minimize ketogenesis, so that maintaining a moderate lipid intake is appropriate. Providing adequate calories from supplemental carbohydrate during intercurrent illness is critical. Most important is prevention of prolonged fasting.

As with any metabolic condition it is primarily important that the families understand the diagnosis as well as the treatment to

Rationale

Carnitine is not used routinely in these cases based on the assumption that carnitine could enhance ketogenesis through fat utilization. It should be used only in cases of proven carnitine deficiency.

minimize the impact of any decompensation that might otherwise be detrimental to the health of these patients.

Inheritance

All of the previously mentioned enzyme deficiencies are inherited in an autosomal recessive manner. Therefore, the parents of an affected child have a 25% chance at each pregnancy of having another affected child.

These metabolic disorders have been described in various ethnic groups: Saudi Arabia, the Mediterranean populations, the Northern Europeans, African-Americans, Japanese, Pakistanis, and Hispanics among others. Nonetheless, it is believed that many of these cases are missed and therefore there are not enough data to estimate an actual prevalence among the different populations.

Molecular and Prenatal Diagnosis

Succinyl-CoA: 3-Ketoacid Transferase Deficiency The SCOT gene was cloned by Fukao et al. (3) after being mapped by Kassovska-Bratinova et al. (7) to chromosome 5p13. It is a large gene that spans more than 100 kb and contains 17 exons. Fukao and colleagues have performed multiple experiments to identify pathologic mutations as well as their effects on protein structure and function. Several missense mutations in SCOT-deficient patients have been identified, and they are summarized in the Table 8-2.

Some patients reported on with an enzyme activity of less than 15% of normal had more severe episodes of decompensation and died in early infancy. One of these patients described by Berry et al. (5) had several severe episodes of ketoacidosis beginning at birth (~ 25 hospitalizations by 7 years of age). His SCOT activity was approximately 9%. He is also one of the few patients described in the literature in whom MRI abnormalities were seen. His head MRI at 19 months of age showed delayed myelination, a nonspecific finding, possibly associated with his severe

acidosis and hypoglycemic episode during the neonatal period. He had mild developmental delay and attention-deficit hyperactivity disorder (5).

Based on the structural models created by Fukao and colleagues, G324 is localized in the active site of the enzyme, whereas V221 and G219 are localized in the dimerizing surface. On the other hand G324 and G219 did not generate enzyme activity in vitro; however, V221 showed a residual enzyme activity of approximately 10% of control. In addition the patient homozygous for the V221 mutation (GS05) is known to have the milder clinical course reported to date with detectable residual enzyme activity. Therefore, it is speculated that mutation analysis could aid in predicting the severity of enzyme deficiency and thus the clinical course (3,19,20).

Three Japanese patients found to be homozygous for the T435N mutation do not show permanent ketosis. Experiments performed by Fukao et al. (6) revealed that the mutant protein derived from the T435N mutation retained significant residual activity that varied with temperature. They hypothesized that the mutant (T435N) SCOT residual enzyme activity prevented permanent ketosis in this patients, but could lose some of its activity during high temperature states seen with febrile illness, causing the patients to show severe ketonemia/uria and metabolic decompensation (6).

Mitochondrial Acetoacetyl-CoA Thiolase T2 Deficiency MAT is caused by mutations in the acetyl-CoA acetyltransferase-1 gene mapped to locus 11q22.3-q23.1 (Table 8-3). There is a poor correlation among genotype and phenotype as seen in siblings who share the same mutations. Nonetheless there are "milder mutations," which are believed to have residual activity and less accumulation of isoleucine metabolites during stable clinical conditions. Two categories of MAT-deficient patients have been described based on mutation and expression analysis. Group I comprises those patients with null mutations in either allele. Group II contains those patients with muta-

tions associated with residual MAT activity in at least one of the alleles. Fukao et al. reported that both groups have severe episodes of ketoacidosis (19). Those patients who belong to group II lack the usual markers in the urine organic acid analysis and acylcarnitine profile during stable conditions, and therefore the diagnosis in these patients could be missed.

Psychosocial Support

As with any metabolic disorder associated with severe, recurrent decompensation that may range from mild acidosis and/or hypoglycemia to coma or death, comprehensive counseling and connection to a metabolic center as well as psychosocial support for the patients and the caretakers is encouraged.

Unfortunately there are no specific support organizations available at the present time. However, the Pacific Northwest Regional Genetics Group has a free handbook for parents online at http://mchneighborhood.ichp.edu/pacnorgg/Publications.htm

TABLE 8-2   (SCOT Mutations Identified)

Ethnicity	Mutation
Spanish (GS01)	S287X
Japanese (GS02, GS08, GS09)	V133E, C456F, T435N
British (GS05)	V221M
Dutch (GS04)	G219E, G324E
American (GS06)	G324E
African-American (GS07)	G324E
Hispanic (GS15)	R217X

TABLE 8-3   MAT Mutations Identified

Ethnicity	Mutation
Japanese	
Group I : (GK01)	A333P/c.149delC
Group II : (GK19, GK19B, GK30, GK31)	N93S/ I312T; c.2T>C/ c.149delC; c.149delC/ I312T
Other ethnicities	
Group I : (GK46, GK49 GK50)	G152A/ c.52-53insC ; H397D ; IVS8+1g>t
Group II : (GK45, GK47)	A132G; G152A/ D339-V340insD
Other group II mutations	N93S, Q145E, T297M, A301P, I312T, A380T

REFERENCES

1. Niezen-Koning KE, Wanders RJA, et al. Succinyl-CoA:acetoacetate transferase deficiency: identification of a new patient with a neonatal onset and review of the literature. *Eur J Pediatr.* 1997;156: 870–873.
2. Snyderman, SE, Sansaricq C, Middleton B. Succinyl-CoA: 3-ketoacid CoA transferase deficiency. *Pediatrics.* 1998;101:709–711.
3. Fukao T, Mitchell, GA, et al. Succinyl-CoA: 3-ketoacid CoA transferase (SCOT): cloning of the human SCOT gene, tertiary structural modeling of the human SCOT monomer, and characterization of three pathogenic mutations. *Genomics.* 2000;68:144–151.
4. Fukao T, Song XQ, et al. Prenatal diagnosis of succinyl-coenzyme A: 3-ketoacid coenzyme A transferase deficiency. *Prenat Diagn.* 1996;16:471–474.
5. Berry GT, Fukao GA, et al. Neonatal hypoglycemia in severe succinyl-CoA: 3-oxoacid CoA-transferase deficiency. *J Inherit Metab Dis.* 2001;24:587–595.
6. Fukao T, Shintaku H, et al. Patients homozygous for the T435N mutation on succinyl-CoA: 3-ketoacid CoA transferase (SCOT)

do not show permanent ketosis. *Pediatr Res.* 2004;56(6):858–863.

7. Kassovska-Bratinova S, Fukao T, et al. Succinyl CoA: 3-oxoacid CoA transferase (SCOT): human cDNA cloning, human chromosomal mapping to 5p13, and mutation detection in a SCOT-deficient patient. *Am J Hum Genet.* 1996;59:519–528.

8. Song XQ, Fukao T, et al. Succinyl-CoA: 3-ketoacid CoA transferase (SCOT) deficiency: two pathogenic mutations, V133E and C456F, in Japanese siblings. *Hum Mutat.* 1998;12:83–88.

9. Tildon JT, Cornblath M. Succinyl-CoA: 3-ketoacid CoA-transferase deficiency. A cause for ketoacidosis in infancy. *J Clin Invest.* 1972;51:493–498.

10. Spence MW, Murphy MG, et al. Succinyl-CoA: 3-ketoacid CoA-transferase deficiency: a new phenotype. *Pediatr Res.* 1973;7:394.

11. Saudubray JM, Specola N, et al. Hyperketotic states due to inherited defects of ketolysis. *Enzyme.* 1987;38:80–90.

12. Middleton B, Day R, et al. Infantile ketoacidosis associated with decreased activity of succinyl-CoA: 3-ketoacid CoA-transferase. *J Inherit Metab Dis.* 1987;10:273–275.

13. Perez-Cerda C, Merinero B, et al. A new case of succinyl-CoA: acetoacetate transferase deficiency. *J Inherit Metab Dis.* 1987;15: 371–373.

14. Sakazaki H, Hirayama K, et al. A new Japanese case of succinyl-CoA: 3-ketoacid CoA-transferase deficiency. *J Inherit Metab Dis.* 1995;18:323–335.

15. Pretorius CJ, Loy Song GG, et al. Two siblings with episodic ketoacidosis and decreased activity of succinyl-coenzyme A: 3-ketoacid CoA-transferase in cultured fibroblasts. *J Inherit Metab Dis.* 1996;19:296–300.

16. Longo N, Fukao T, et al. Succinyl-CoA: 3-ketoacid transferase (SCOT) deficiency in a new patient homozygous for an R217X mutation. *J Inherit Metab Dis.* 2004;27:691–692.

17. Mitchell GA, Fukao T. (2001) Inborn errors of ketone body catabolism. In: Scriver CR, Beaudet AL, Sly WS, Valle D, Childs B, Kinzler KW, et al. eds. *The Metabolic and Molecular Bases of Inherited Disease.* 8th ed. New York: McGraw-Hill; 2001:2327–2356.

18. Fernandes J, Saudubray JM, Van Den Berghe G., et al. *Inborn Metabolic Diseases: Diagnosis and Treatment.* 4th ed. Heidelberg Springer; 2006:191–196.

19. Fukao T, Zhang GX, et al. The mitochondrial acetoacetyl-CoA thiolase (T2) deficiency in Japanese patients: urinary organic acid and blood acylcarnitine profiles under stable conditions have subtle abnormalities in T2-deficient patients with some residual T2 activity. *J Inherit Metab Dis.* 1993;26:423–431.

20. Fukao T, Scriver CR, Kondo N. The clinical phenotype and outcome of mitochondrial acetoacetyl-CoA thiolase deficiency (beta-ketothiolase or T2 deficiency) in 26 enzymatically proved and mutation-defined patients. *Mol Genet Metab.* 2001;72:109–114.

21. Zhang GX, Fukao T, et al. Mitochondrial acetoacetyl-CoA thiolase (T2) deficiency: T2-deficient patients with "mild" mutation(s) were previously misinterpreted as normal by the coupled assay with tiglyl-CoA. *Pediatr Res.* 2004;56(1):60–64.

22. Yalcinkaya C, Dincer A, et al. MRI and MRS in HMG-CoA lyase deficiency. *Pediatr Neurol.* 1999;20:375–380.

23. Vassault, A, Bonnefont JP, et al. *Techniques in Diagnostic Human Biochemical Genetics. A Laboratory Manual.* Hommes FA ed. New York: Wiley-Liss; 1991:285–308.

24. Hoffman GF, Nyhan WL, et al. *Core Handbook in Pediatrics: Inherited Metabolic Diseases.* Philadelphia: Lippincott Williams & Wilkins; 2002.

25. Zschocke J, Ruiter JP, et al. Progressive infantile neurodegeneration caused by 2-methyl-3-hydroxybutyryl-CoA dehydrogenase deficiency: a novel inborn error of branched-chain fatty acid and isoleucine metabolism. *Pediatr Res.* 2000;48:852–855.

26. Morris AAM, Thekekara A, et al. Evaluation of fasts for investigating hypoglycaemia or suspected metabolic disease. *Arch Dis Child.* 1996;75:115–119.

Karl S. Roth, MD
Claude Sansaricq MD, PhD

CHAPTER 9

The Galactosemias

INTRODUCTION

Galactose is a naturally occurring hexose, an epimer of glucose at C-4, and generally derived in the diet from intestinal hydrolysis of lactose. Although galactose can contribute to formation of glycogen through epimerization to glucose (see later), its chief role in metabolism is in formation of complex glycolipids and glycoproteins. These complex molecules are found largely in cell membranes and are vital components of cell-surface receptors, as well as myelin of the central nervous system of which galactosylceramide is a major constituent. Thus, although galactose is not considered to be an essential dietary molecule, there is plainly an absolute biosynthetic requirement for galactose. As with many similar biologic requirements, there is a pathway that normally supplies galactose for biosynthesis, even in the absence of dietary intake.

The term "galactosemia" describes a group of three disorders with elevated blood galactose concentration in common. Each results from a defect in the pathway that converts galactose into glucose. The range and severity of the phenotypes found in these disorders depend on the degree of the defect (partial or complete) and its location in the pathway, which precursors become elevated and what product(s) may become deficient as a result of the defect. It is also important to point out at the outset that much about the pathogenesis of the clinical manifestations in each of the galactosemias remains poorly understood. Thus, it is not possible to attribute sequelae directly to excess or deficiency of specific metabolites caused by the particular enzyme deficiency.

The normal metabolism of galactose to glucose occurs in a series of three reactions known as the Leloir pathway (1,2) (Figure 9-1). At the initial step, the enzyme galactokinase (GALK) adds a phosphate to the galactose to generate galactose-1-phosphate (Gal-1-P) in the process expending adenosine triphosphate (ATP). In a second, irreversible step catalyzed by the enzyme galactose-1-phosphate uridyltransferase

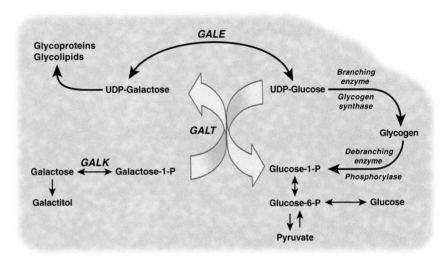

FIGURE 9-1. Leloir pathway of galactose metabolism. To convert galactose to glucose, it is first phosphorylated by GALK to produce Gal-1-P. Galactose is then exchanged with glucose group in UDPGlu to create UDPGal and release Glu-1-P. An epimerase enzyme changes the stereochemistry of in UDPGal, creating UDPGlu. This cycle allows all Gal-1-P to be converted to Glu-1-P. Once released, glucGlu-1-P is converted to glucose-6-phosphate and can enter glycolysis to generate energy. Defects of the kinase, the transferase, or the epimerase can result in deficiencies in galactose metabolism known as galactosemias.

(GALT), uridyl diphosphoglucose (UDPG) exchanges its glucose molecule for a galactose from Gal-1-P, thus producing glucose-1-phosphate (Gluc-1-P) and UDPGal. Finally, in a reaction mediated by UDP-galactose-4-epimerase (GALE) in the presence of nicotinamide adenine dinucleotide, the galactose moiety is converted to glucose, allowing the cycle to continue. When any of these three enzymes of the cycle is defective, a form of galactosemia is produced:

1. Galactosemia due to galactokinase (GALK) deficiency;

2. Galactosemia due to Gal-1-P uridyl transferase deficiency (classic galactosemia or GALT); and

3. Galactosemia due to galactose-epimerase (GALE) deficiency.

It should also be noted that there are additional, accessory pathways for galactose metabolism in humans. Through a revers-

ible reaction utilizing a uridine triphosphate (UTP)–dependent pyrophosphorylase, Gal-1-P can be converted to UDPGal; by epimerization, UDP-glucose (UDP Glc) can also be formed and both compounds used in biosynthesis of complex molecules such as glycoproteins and glycolipids (3). Recent assessment of the enzymatic activity of this pathway in mouse liver suggests that this pathway is too limited to compensate for GALT deficiency (4). Another accessory pathway that is thought to have great importance in the pathogenesis of cataracts in diabetes mellitus and galactosemia is the aldose reductase pathway (5,6). The enzyme, aldose reductase, acts on the terminal aldehydic group of glucose and hexose to produce the corresponding sugar alcohols, sorbitol and galactitol, respectively. It is thought that accumulation of impermeable sugar alcohols within cells is at least partially responsible for cataract formation and

Galactosemias

AT-A-GLANCE

Galactosemias are conditions under which tissue, serum and urine galactose concentrations are increased resulting from impaired galactose metabolism. There are three enzymatic defects in galactose metabolism such as galactokinase deficiency(GALK), galactose 1-phosphate uridyl transferase deficiency (GALT) and uridyl diphosphate 4-epimerase deficiency (GALE), each one representing a recessively-transmitted trait impairing the Leloir pathway for conversion of galactose to UDP-glucose. GALK deficiency is limited in clinical manifestations to cataracts; GALT deficiency is also known as classical galactosemia and when untreated results in cataracts, liver failure and cirrhosis, mental retardation and death; GALE deficiency appears across a spectrum of severity, from completely benign to systemic findings similar to those of classical galactosemia. Treatment is the withdrawal of milk and its replacement by a lactose-free formula. In the neonatal period patient with classical galactosemia are susceptible to gram-negative sepsis and have to be treated with a broad spectrum antibiotics until blood cultures are negative.

TYPES OF GALACTOSEMIA	INCIDENCE	LOCUS	OMIM
Galactokinase Deficiency (GALK)	1:50,000 — 1:1,000,000	17q24	230200
Galactose 1-phosphate uridyl transferase (GALT)	1:23,000 — 1:44,000	9p13	230400
Uridyl diphosphate 4-epimerase (GALE)	1:6,200 — 1:64,800	1p36-p35	230350

FORM	FINDINGS	CLINICAL PRESENTATION	
		BIRTH	CHILDHOOD & ADOLESCENCE
GALK	↑ Galactose ↑ Galactitol ↑ Galactonate	May present with pseudo tumor cerebri, or cataracts	Cataracts
GALT (Classical)	↑ Blood/Urine Galactose ↑ RBC Galactose-1-P ↑ Blood/Urine Galactitol ↑ RBC Galactonate ↑ Urinary Galactonate ↑ FSH, ↑ LH (females) ↑ LFTs, coagulopathy Hypoglycemia Direct Hyperbilirubinemia Generalized aminoaciduria No RBC GALT activity	Cataracts, jaundice; vomiting, diarrhea, failure to thrive, hepatomegaly, E Coli sepsis, liver failure, and renal Fanconi syndrome	Psychomotor delay; dyspraxia, verbal apraxia, learning difficulties, failure to thrive; cataracts; primary ovarian failure, and decreased bone mineral density.
GALE	Decreased or absent RBC GALE activity Variable GALE activity in transformed lymphoblasts ↑ RBC galactose-1-P ↑ RBC galactitol ↑ UDP-Gal ↓ UDP-Glucose	May show no symptoms, or present with cataracts, hepatomegaly, jaundice, failure to thrive, hypotonia.	Developmental delay

Lactose

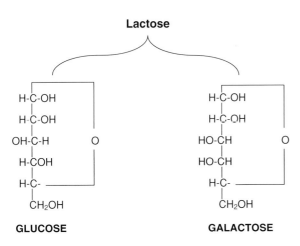

FIGURE 9-2. Lactose is a disaccharide made of glucose and galactose. It is the major source of galactose in the diet.

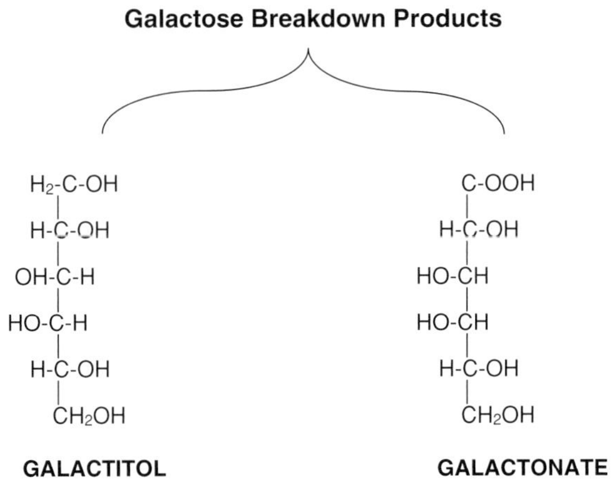

Galactose Breakdown Products

FIGURE 9-3. Galactitol is the alcohol derived from the excess galactose and galactonate in the oxidized form. Both derivatives facilitate the elimination of galactose from blood and body fluids.

pseudotumor cerebri seen in these diseases. A third accessory pathway involves the conversion of galactose to galactonate and then to xylulose by a decarboxylation reaction (7). That this is a means for galactose disposition in patients with defects in the Leloir pathway has been amply demonstrated by use of nuclear magnetic resonance detection of galactonic acid in the urine (8). All of these alternative pathways, however, even in the aggregate cannot provide sufficient metabolic disposition of accumulated galactose to offset a defect in the Leloir pathway.

Etiology/Pathophysiology The major dietary source of galactose comes from ingestion of mammalian milk. Lactose, the carbohydrate of milk, is a disaccharide comprising glucose and galactose (Figure 9-2); mammary gland synthesis of lactose requires a reversal of the epimerase step to produce galactose from glucose. After ingestion of milk hydrolysis of the constituent lactose monosaccharides takes place in the gut. The absorbed galactose (see Chapter 42) is carried to the liver and normally undergoes metabolic conversion to UDPGal for synthesis of complex molecules, glucose or glycogen; however, this conversion is interrupted in each of the galactosemias and may contribute to the long term complications of galactocemia. Galactitol, the sugar alcohol of galactose that is impermeable to biologic membranes, is synthesized (Figure 9-3), as galactose increases in the lens, a reaction mediated by aldose reductase; its accumulation is believed to account for cataract formation through osmotic swelling and consequent disruption of the crystalline structure of the lens (9–11). Gal-1-P is postulated to be responsible for the other clinical manifestations, especially liver and kidney failure; the

pathophysiologic mechanisms responsible remain enigmatic.

GALK enzyme catalyzes the phosphorylation of galactose-1-phosphate, the first step in galactose metabolism (Figure 9-4). When galactokinase is deficient, the patient will accumulate galactose that will be converted to galactitol and galactonate with effects mainly on the eyes. Conversion of galactose to galactitol is mediated by aldose reductase; there is strong evidence for down-regulation of the aldose reductase gene in the renal cortex and medulla in the presence of increased polyol concentration (12). This effect may reasonably explain the absence of renal pathology in GALK deficiency (12). There is also evidence that osmolarity plays a role in gene expression in lens epithelium in experimental animals, resulting in an increase in aldose reductase promoter activity under hypertonic conditions (13). The first GALK deficiency case was reported in 1967

by Gitzelmann in a patient with juvenile cataracts (14).

Classic galactosemia is transmitted as an autosomal recessive condition with a frequency of 1 to 23,000 to 44,000 births (15). The GALT gene has been located, and the GALT enzyme is a housekeeping enzyme in the liver and red cells as well as other tissues. In classic GALT deficiency, there is a complete to nearly complete absence of GALT activity in erythrocytes; this characteristic of the disease is a property used for newborn screening and early detection (Chapter 2).

When the GALT enzyme is missing or is altered there is accumulation of galactose, Gal-1-P, galactitol, and galactonate (Figure 9-5). As a result of the metabolic block one might assume that there is also a lack of production of UDPGal that is the precursor for glycoprotein and glycolipid formation in various tissues such as the brain. The free

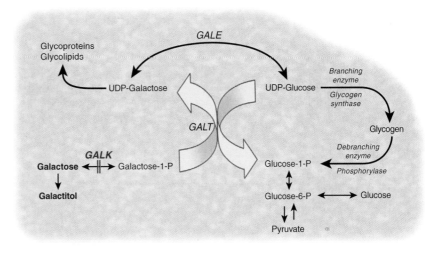

FIGURE 9-4. When the enzyme GALK is deficient then galactose accumulates and is converted to galactitol and galactonate.

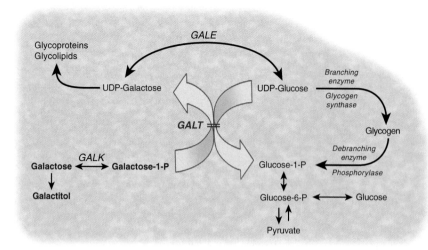

FIGURE 9-5. When the galactose-1P-Uridyl transferase enzyme is deficient, in addition to accumulation of galactose, galactitol, and galactonate, there is Gal-1-P accumulation and decreased production of UDPGal. The last two elements are likely responsible for the toxicity of the disease.

reversibility of the epimerase step at one and the same time permits treatment of the disease with a galactose-free formula and prevents galactose deficiency for important synthetic processes. Hence, endogenous production of UDPGal from glucose supplants the need for dietary galactose.

The liver is a major target organ in GALT deficiency, the early histopathology reflecting simply fatty changes, every hepatocyte being affected by these fatty droplets (16). There is also bile duct proliferation in the periportal areas, but no fibrotic changes are in evidence in the early stage. With time, in untreated patients there are diffuse fibrotic changes that mimic those seen in alcoholic cirrhosis. Precisely what produces these changes in the liver remains unknown; a recent study in GALT-deficient yeast suggests that in these cells, exposure to Gal-1-P creates a stress response consisting of down-regulation of many genes involved in RNA metabolism and practically all ribosomal protein genes. Conversely, genes involved in inositol synthesis and turnover were upregulated under these conditions (17). Nonetheless, the biochemical basis for the histopathologic changes in the galactosemic liver remain unexplained (18), and there has been a recent call from the World Congress of Pediatric Gastroenterology for more intensive investigation into this phenomenon (19).

Changes are also apparent in the central nervous system; fibrous gliosis of the white matter, with a paucity of Purkinje cells involving the cerebellum and loss of some of the granular layer has been reported (20). In an interesting series of papers, Tsakiris and coworkers (21–24) have examined the relationship between Gal-1-P, Na^+, K^+-ATPase, and Mg^{2+}-ATPase in rat brain and patient erythro-

cyte membranes. Studies in suckling rat whole-brain homogenates showed up to 500% activation of the Mg^{2+}-ATPase in the presence of concentrations of galactose, galactitol, and Gal-1-P commonly found in the blood and brain of patients with galactosemia (21). Addition of the antioxidants L-cysteine and glutathione provided a protective effect in additional studies (22). Further studies in patients with galactosemia indicated that antioxidant status was depressed by Gal-1-P and that red cell membrane ATPases as well as acetylcholinesterase were inhibited; the enzyme activities were inversely correlated with Gal-1-P levels, leading the authors to speculate that at least part of the pathophysiology of galactosemia is related to membrane damage due to insufficient antioxidant protection (23,24).

The kidneys may also be affected; there are data from experimental animals fed a galactose-rich diet, which suggest glomerular changes, including ballooning of the epithelium with increase in their absolute volume. Functionally, the animals evidenced proteinuria after ingesting the diet for 2 months (25). A study in patients with galactosemia (26) demonstrated normal galactose excretion but a 50-fold increase in urinary galactitol which, given its relative impermeability, might account for the changes seen in the experimental animals. Other functional changes, such as aminoaciduria are completely reversible.

In stages, the eye will show changes in the lens, starting with oil drop effects leading to dissociation of the orderly crystalline structure of the lens and subsequent cataract formation. Recent work in experimental animals suggests that increased reactive oxygen species, resulting from an inhibition of glutathione production results in an unfolding of the

lens proteins, increased apoptosis of the lenticular epithelial cells, and cataract formation (27). Cataracts may be present in the newborn and in the early stages are generally reversible with treatment.

The ovary is regularly impacted in classic galactosemia. Females may have streak ovaries; in some the effect appears to be prenatal whereas in others minimal function remains with drastically reduced numbers of oocytes. The net result, in any case, is ovarian failure (28). Deficient migration of embryonic germ cells to the developing gonad has been shown in galactosemic rats (29). The process of migration is postulated to depend on the unique embryonic presence of a glycoconjugate with a terminal N-acetylgalactosamine residue (30). Although these results are impossible to reproduce in humans, there is evidence that alterations in the biologic activity of follicle-stimulating hormone (FSH) occur, dependent on fluctuations in GALT expression in the anterior pituitary. Hypoglycosylated isoforms of circulating FSH has been shown in four women with galactosemia (31); it is known that hypoglycosylated FSH has a higher receptor binding affinity but is ineffective in stimulating cyclic adenosine monophosphate in response to the increased binding (32). Because the FSH molecule has glycosylated side chains intrinsic to its activity, it is postulated that GALT gene expression, in some fashion, exerts a regulatory effect on FSH. When GALT is absent or deficient, it would be reasonable to expect deficiency in FSH activity; this correlates with the data reported by Rubio-Gozalbo, et al. (33) showing isolated FSH levels elevated in females with galactosemia in proportion to the level of galactosemic dietary control.

In the neonatal period the white cell may show a deficiency in the bactericidal protein, bactericidal/permeability-increasing protein. This protein has a very high affinity for the lipopolysaccharide capsule of Gram-negative bacteria to which it binds and enhances permeability, causing lysis (34). These data help to explain the earlier observations by Kobayashi et al. (35) that galactose impairs neutrophil function, rendering the naturally susceptible newborn with classical galactosemia still more liable to develop severe sepsis due to Gram-negative organisms, mainly Escherichia coli.

GALE catalyzes the interconversion of UDP-galactose and UDP-glucose; it is encoded by GALE gene that is mapped on 1p36-p35 chromosomal region (Figure 9-6). GALE has been reported as a benign "peripheral defect," with the enzyme deficiency confined to circulating blood cells (RBC), or a clinically severe, rare, "generalized defect" in which the defect is present in many tissues and

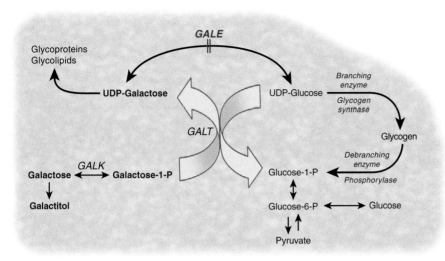

FIGURE 9-6. When the GALE deficiency is total, there is mainly accumulation of UDPGal and some Gal-1-P and galactose as in the classic galactosemia.

causes significant morbidity and permanent impairment. Molecular studies in various mutated cell lines from reported patients suggest that the mutations all result in unstable proteins (36,37). Erythrocytes in both types of affected patients have decreased to nearly absent of GALE and because red cells lack DNA, deficient UDPGal metabolism is equally severe. There is detectable GALE activity in transformed lymphoblasts and fibroblasts in both benign and systemic forms; it is postulated that because there is a spectrum of detectable activity, only those mutations that result in extremely unstable protein will present as the systemic variant (37).

Clinical Presentation

Galactokinase Deficiency In the newborn, galactosemia due to GALK deficiency causes cataract formation as the only consistent abnormality (38). Rarely, a picture of pseudotumor cerebri with distention of the cranial sutures secondary to cerebral edema has been observed. Galactitol, derived from the excess galactose, has been postulated to be responsible for this clinical manifestation, which appears to be only transitory. Older, untreated patients with GALK deficiency continue to manifest cataracts as the sole major manifestation of this disease.

Classic Galactosemia In classic galactosemia, Gal-1-P accumulation and abnormal glycosylation of glycoproteins and glycolipids are presumed to be causative for most clinical manifestations. This is based on the observation that although GALK-deficient patients, who are unable to synthesize Gal-1-P, are healthy with the exception of cataracts, classic galactosemic patients accumulate Gal-1-P and are severely affected. Consequently, the sooner the baby starts milk feeding the earlier

the symptoms appear; they have been seen as early as the second day of life. Clinical findings include feeding intolerance (as vomiting, diarrhea, bloating), anorexia, failure to thrive, possible hypoglycemia, bleeding manifestations, prolonged jaundice, hemolytic anemia, hyperchloremic acidosis, albuminuria and aminoaciduria (renal Fanconi syndrome), cataracts, liver failure, and sepsis due to Gram-negative organisms, mainly E.coli. The patient becomes hypoalbuminemic, develops ascites and anasarca, and may die if the diagnosis is not recognized. The early clinical changes in the lens have been described as "oil drop changes" leading to cataract formation.

Early predictions following the initial treatment of galactosemia with a galactose-free diet were very positive in favor of an excellent long-term prognosis. Careful long-term follow up of patients with this disorder, however, has shown that despite consequent galactose restriction in the diet, patients with classical galactosemia may still be at risk for impaired motor development, progressive neurological disease and abnormalities that lead to a poor neuropsychological outcome (39,40,41,42). Causes for these observations remain elusive, while theories abound (43–45). Defective galactosylation of sphingolipids due to low UDPGal may be responsible for the neurological sequelae. Diagnosis after 2 months of age is associated with poor long term outcomes (45). Above-average intelligence, as measured by intelligence quotient testing, is possible for any given affected individual; however, most patients exhibit an intelligence quotient in the range of 70 to 90, placing them in the mildly impaired to low-normal category. It is unclear whether the intellectual deficits are cumulative with time because published follow-up studies of specific individuals over

lifetimes are not available. Visual spatial disturbances are extremely common among these patients and may lead to poor school performance even with normal intelligence. In addition, a relatively frequent complication of classic galactosemia is developmental verbal dyspraxia, a sensory motor disturbance leading to great difficulty in word pronunciation (41,42). In some children, this may be severe enough to render them mute. Because of these significant cognitive difficulties, it is extremely important to maintain a close watch on development in an affected infant, and especially to evaluate language development on a frequent basis.

Affected females are at risk of ovarian failure (46); if ovarian failure develops early they may not develop secondary sex characteristics and may have a decrease in growth velocity secondary, as estrogens along with growth hormone are responsible for the growth spurt during puberty. Parents of affected females must be advised early of the risk of primary ovarian failure. Abnormal glycosylation of hormones and toxic damage to the ovaries has also been reported (29,31). The question remains whether the premature depletion of the ovarian follicular reserve is due to an in utero effect depleting the initial pool of follicles or due to an accelerated rate of degradation as a result of galactose toxicity. In contrast to females, testicular function appears not to be affected.

A final aspect of the clinical presentation of GALT deficiency is growth, which was noted by Waggoner, et al. (42) to be adversely affected in many patients in childhood and early adolescence. In a recent study, Panis, et al. (47) examined the growth patterns in 40 individuals with classic galactosemia, including prenatal growth and adjusted for gestational age. Prenatal growth was within reference ranges for all 40 patients, including weight, length, and head circumference. Postnatally, there was a decreased height and weight velocity in girls, and both genders failed to achieve their target, midparental heights; females showed greater deficits than boys. The authors speculated that decreased growth factors or inadequate hormone replacement might explain the gender differences. In an ancillary study, Panis and coworkers (48) described a decrease in a number of markers, signifying diminished bone metabolism in these galactosemic patients. No dietary deficiencies or serum deficits in calcium, phosphate, and bone-related hormones, including parathyroid hormone and calcitriol could be demonstrated. These findings can be correlated with an earlier study showing, unexpectedly, that bone mineral density was diminished in males as well as females (49). This suggests that a basis for poor growth and bone metabolism exists outside of that created by ovarian failure, although it remains unclear what these factors are.

Galactose-Epimerase Deficiency Patients affected with a clinically benign variant of GALE deficiency are usually asymptomatic. Whereas the metabolic defect, an unstable enzyme protein, is demonstrable in the red cells, it does not functionally affect the liver or fibroblasts because the unstable protein can be rapidly replenished. Moreover, patients in this category may be shown to have normal or near-normal GALE activity in their lymphoblasts, which represents nonperipheral enzyme activity (37). By contrast, the severe form is due to the systemic loss of the epimerase enzyme activity in red cells, transformed lymphoblasts, fibroblasts, liver, and other tissues. Of note, there is no correlation between the degree of impairment of GALE activity in RBCs compared to lymphoblasts; as a result RBC GALE activity level cannot be used to distinguish the clinically benign form from the severe form of GALE deficiency and further raises the possibility of tissue-specific factors that influence either expression or function of GALE. Patients affected with the severe form may present in the neonatal period with symptoms suggestive of classic galactosemia, such as vomiting, jaundice, hypotonia, weight loss, hepatomegaly, galactosuria, generalized aminoaciduria, and delayed motor and intellectual development. Only a few cases of the systemic variant have thus far been reported, although Opena and colleagues have demonstrated that there is a spectrum of GALE activity in many patients who are clinically unaffected when unstressed (37).

Variant Forms of Classic Galactosemia More than 300 mutations in the GALT gene have been recorded from population groups throughout the world; these include missense and nonsense mutations, as well as base substitutions distributed in exons and introns. As with many genes that are subject to numerous mutations (notably cystic fibrosis), most clinically recognizable phenotypes are due to a few specific mutations, whereas the remainder of the mutations are far less significant in causation of disease. The impact of the nonsense mutations is predictably most severe, although this can be somewhat attenuated by the nature of the mutation on the paired gene. In this regard, it should be noted that the number of known mutations would predict a high frequency of mixed heterozygotes in most Western countries where racial intermarriage is more a rule than an exception.

The most frequent among the less severe GALT gene mutations have been recognized by the stability of the uridyltransferase protein in various buffer systems or its electrophoretic mobility, or to stability with temperature changes. These include the Duarte, the Los Angeles, the Black, the Indiana, the Chicago, the Muenster, and the Rennes variants. The Duarte variant contains a base substitution of A → G at c.940 (resulting in aspartate substituted for asparagine), a mutation shared with the Los Angeles variant (50–51). Both have electrophoretic mobility on the gel that is more rapid than normal but opposite changes from normal in enzymatic activity. The Duarte has approximately half of the normal enzyme activity whereas that of the Los Angeles variant is higher than normal. It is now understood that the A → G mutation alone does not change enzymatic activity of the protein product. There is, however, an additional abnormality that consists of a 4-bp deletion in the 5′ promoter region of the GALT gene in the Duarte allele, which impairs transcription (52). By contrast, in the Los Angeles variant there is a codon alteration for leucine, which, it is postulated, results in more efficient translation of messenger RNA and thus, enhanced enzymatic activity through increased protein synthesis (51).

The Duarte variant (N314D) is quite common around the world, averaging in various studies a frequency of approximately 6% in white individuals and a slightly lower average incidence in non-Caucasians. The relatively high frequency of the Q188R and K285N mutations, which account for 70 percent of mutations causing classic galactosemia in Caucasians, would predict a relatively high incidence of compound heterozygosity. Double heterozygote patients with the Duarte and the classic types (compound heterozygotes, D/G) have approximately 25% of normal GALT enzyme activity while homozygous patients (D/D) and heterozygotes (D/N) for Duarte have approximately 50% and 75% activity. Evidence accumulates that there is no deleterious effect of continuing normal feeding in patients with the Duarte variant, even in neonates. To ensure the infant can metabolize galactose appropriately, regular measurements of Gal-1-P are recommended. Gal-1P usually sinks below 2mg/dl after a few months. Further monitoring would not be necessary. Some centers still maintain these infants on low-galactose intake at least over the period of rapid brain growth. A baby homozygous for the Duarte or the Los Angeles variant would not be expected to need treatment as these conditions are asymptomatic. Homozygosity for Q188R mutation is associated with near complete absence of GALT activity and a severe clinical and biochemical phenotype.

The Black variant (S135L), the most frequently reported mutation (50%) in the African American population is characterized by residual enzyme activity in the liver and intestines in the range of 10% of normal. Although this is generally insufficient to prevent clinical symptoms, it is often enough to ameliorate the onset and make it more insidious than that in a Caucasian infant. For this reason alone, a false-negative screening result in such a patient may cause a disastrous outcome. The other 130 mutations that cause decrease in the GALT activity, may alllow for up to 30% remaining enzymatic activity (53).

Diagnosis Affected newborns with classical galactosemia or with the severe epimerase deficiency may have elevated liver enzyme tests, direct hyperbillirubinemia, abnormal coagulation studies, generalized aminociduria, glycosuria and hypoglycemia. Although galactose is a reducing sugar excreted in urine, determination of the disorder by measurement of reducing substances in urine should only be used as a simple first screening test for classic galactosemia and not confirm or reject the diagnosis. Special points to remember:

- Intravenous fluids typically given to neonates in crisis can dilute the presence of galactose in urine.
- After discontinuing milk feeding galactose will be cleared from body fluids within a few hours even in a baby with classical galactosemia.
- GALT activity must be measured before any blood transfusion is performed.
- Other reducing substances (i.e., glucose) may give a false positive result.
- Galactosuria may be found in patients with liver disease.

Urinary excretion of galactitol is elevated in all forms of galactosemia; urinary galactitol remains elevated in patients with GALT deficiency, even after galactose restriction, or after blood transfusion. GALT activity is measured in RBC hemolysates and decreased GALT enzymatic activity is diagnostic of classical galactosemia; elevated galactose-1-P levels in the presence of normal GALT activity suggests epimerase deficiency and appropriate enzymatic testing should be initiated. Measurement of epimerase in red cells and transformed lymphoblasts as well as UDPGalactose and UDPglucose in red cells, would differentiate between the peripheral versus generalized form of GALE deficiency. Genetic testing for GALT deficiency is clinically available.

Prenatal Diagnosis Prenatal detection has been performed by enzyme analysis on amniocytes, by assay of galactitol in amniotic

- Q188R and K285N account for 70 percent of mutations in Caucasians. S135L is most common in African-Americans (62%). Heterozygotes are normal.

fluid or DNA analysis. Although available, the ethical considerations raised generally mimic similar concerns as in phenylketonuric pregnancy regarding termination of what is essentially a normal pregnancy and conceptus; this has tended to discourage open discussion with families. In reality the issues are more difficult to confront in GALT deficiency because of our lack of understanding about the variable outcomes and/or means of prevention.

Usually within a week after birth the test results will be made available. Any infant showing symptoms as described earlier should be placed on a lactose-free formula as a precaution until results are provided. Mothers wishing to breastfeed should be encouraged to continue pumping their breasts until a definitive diagnosis is made. Differential diagnosis in a newborn with persistent galactosemia should include patent ductus venosus with hypoplasia of the intrahepatic portal vein, hepatic hemangioendothelioma with portovenous shunting and citrin deficiency; the latter three conditions are associated with elevated plasma total bile acids and α-fetoprotein. Heterozygosity for GALE and GALT deficiency, delayed closure of the ductus venosus may account for some of the cases of transient galactosemia (galactosemia resolves within a month). In a series of 100 patients, the etiology of transient galactosemia in 55 newborns was unknown (55).

Treatment A galactose-free formula must be prescribed to infants with GALK deficiency. If classic galactosemia (GALT deficiency) is suspected a lactose-/galactose-free feeding regimen should be initiated without delay, even before the diagnosis has been confirmed enzymatically or by DNA analysis. Breast feeding and formulas containing lactose must be stopped immediately. If present, hypoglycemia is treated by intravenous administration of glucose (6 to 9 mg/kg/min). Fresh frozen plasma may be necessary if there are signs of hemorrhage secondary to hepatic failure.

If the patient is not vomiting, a lactose-free formula should be started. In practice a soy-based formula such as "Isomil or Prosobee", or proprietary lactose-free formulas "Elecare," or "Nutramigen" is appropriate, although the cost of Nutramigen is significantly greater than Isomil without therapeutic advantage. Treatment of hyperbilirubinemia may necessitate the use of phototherapy as indirect bilirubin is usually elevated. When table food is introduced restriction in fruits and vegetables is not recommended.

Erythrocyte Gal-1-P accumulation assay is used to monitor compliance with the diet as the red cells in galactosemia are deprived of the GALT enzyme and therefore they tend to retain high levels of this compound if the patient is noncompliant. However, endogenous galactose-1-P production may contribute to galactose-1-P concentration explaining why some patients in spite of a strict diet continue having high levels. Gitzelmann (54) has proposed a theory of self-intoxication based on the fact that red cells from well-treated, affected infants contain Gal-1-P concentrations substantially higher than those of normal infants. It was proposed that there is a futile cycle of galactose phosphorylation—dephosphorylation with inorganic phosphate sequestered, as well. If, as is generally accepted but unproven, Gal-1-P is the responsible metabolic toxin, this could actually explain why central nervous system manifestations of the disease and other long term sequelae may develop even in early treated patients. All treated patients should have their diet supplemented with calcium and have calcium and vitamin D levels monitored annualy. IgF-1, IgFBP3 levels and free T_4 and TSH should be evaluated in children with growth failure or, whose predicted height is below their target height. Neuropsychological evaluation at frequent intervals for early detection of motor, speech and cognitive deficiencies is recommended. Annual eye evaluations should be obtained, and speech therapy should be started as soon as possible if there is speech delay.

Females should be monitored annually for signs of ovarian failure by measuring gonadotropins levels starting at 10 years of age. Estrogen therapy at small doses gradually increased in growing children may start at 12 years of age (see Chapter 36).

Uridine, once attempted as a means of treatment for classic GALT deficiency, has been essentially discarded. No significant effect of additional treatment with uridine could be demonstrated on long-term parameters of development in patients.

In severe forms of UDPGal-4-epimerase deficiency a narrow balance in dietary galactose needs for biosynthesis (galactosylated compounds) and excess causing accumulation of Gal-1-P should be aimed for. Monitoring Gal-1-P and UDPGalactose levels in red cells may be of use in this regard.

Psychosocial Support

As with any disorder associated with chronic metabolic disease, consultation with a psychologist may help the family cope with the emotional and practical problems intrinsic to treatment. Parents should be referred for genetic counseling as well.

REFERENCES

1. Leloir LF. Enzymatic transformation of uridine diphosphate glucose into a galactose derivative. *Arch Biochem.* 1951;33:186–190.
2. Leloir LF, Cardini CE. Carbohydrate metabolism. *Annu Rev Biochem.* 1953;22:179–210.
3. Shin YS, Niedermeier HP, Endres W, et al. Agarose gel isofocusing of UDP galactose pyrophosphorylase and galactose-1-phosphate uridyltransferase. Developmental aspect of UDP-galactose pyrophosphorylase. *Clin Chim Acta.* 1987;166:27–35.
4. Leslie N, Yager C, Reynolds R, et al. UDP-galactose pyrophosphorylase in mice with galactose-1-phosphate uridyltransferase deficiency. *Mol Genet Metab.* 2005;85:21–27.
5. Yabe-Nishimura C. Aldose reductase in glucose toxicity: a potential target for the prevention of diabetic complications. *Pharmacol Rev.* 1998;50:21–34.
6. Ai Y, Zheng Z, O'Brien-Jenkins A, et al. A mouse model of galactose-induced cataracts. *Hum Mol Genet.* 2000;9:1821–1827.
7. Cuatrecasus P, Segal S. Galactose conversion to D-xylulose: an alternative route of galactose metabolism. *Science.* 1966;153:549–551.
8. Wehrli S, Berry GT, Palmieri M, et al. Urinary galactonate in patients with galactosemia: quantitation by NMR spectroscopy. *Pediatr Res.* 1997;42:855–861.
9. Murata M, Ohta N, Sakurai S, et al. The role of aldose reductase in sugar cataract formation: aldose reductase plays a key role in lens epithelial cell death (apoptosis). *Chem Biol Interact.* 2001;130:617–625.
10. Kador PF, Sun G, Rait VK, et al. Intrinsic inhibition of aldose reductase. *J Ocul Pharmacol Ther.* 2001;17:373–381.
11. Kador PF, Betts D, Wyman M, et al. Effects of topical administration of an aldose reductase inhibitor on cataract formation in dogs fed a diet high in galactose. *Am J Vet Res.* 2006;67:1783–1787.
12. McGowan MH, Iwata T, Carper DA: Characterization of the mouse aldose reductase gene and promoter in a lens epithelial cell line. 1998. Available at: http://www.emory.edu/molvis/v4/p2. Accessed
13. Edmands SD, Hughs KS, Lee SY, et al: Time-dependent aspects of osmolyte changes in rat kidney, urine, blood and lens with sorbinil and galactose feeding. *Kidney Int.* 1995;48:344–353.
14. Gitzelmann R. Hereditary galactokinase deficiency, a newly recognized cause of juvenile cataracts. *Pediatr Res.* 1967;1:14–23.
15. Schweitzer-Kranz S. Early diagnosis of inherited metabolic disorders towards improving outcome: the controversial issue of galactosemia. *Eur J Pediatr.* 2003;162:S50–S53.
16. Medline A, Medline NM. Galactosemia: early structural changes in the liver. *Can Med Assoc J.* 1972;107:877–878.
17. Slepak T, Tang M, Addo F, et al. Intracellular galactose-1-phosphate accumulation leads to environmental stress response in yeast model. *Mol Genet Metab.* 2005;86:360–371.

18. Tanner MS. Mechanisms of liver injury relevant to pediatric hepatology. *Crit Rev Clin Lab Sci.* 2002;39:1–61.

19. Perlmutter D, Azevedo RA, Kelly D, et al. Metabolic liver disease: working group report of the first world congress of pediatric gastroenterology, hepatology, and nutrition. *J Pediatr Gastro Nutr.* 2002;35:S180–S186.

20. Crome L. A case of galactosemia with the pathological and neuropathological findings. *Arch Dis Child.* 1962; 37:415–421.

21. Tsakiris S, Marinou K, Schulpis KH. The in vitro effects of galactose and its derivatives on rat brain Mg^{2+}-ATPase activity. *Pharmacol Toxicol.* 2002;91:254–257.

22. Tsakiris S, Schulpis KH, Marinou K, et al. Protective effect of L-cysteine and glutathione on the modulated suckling rat brain Na^+, K^+-ATPase and Mg^{2+}-ATPase activities induced by the in vitro galactosemia. *Pharmacol Res.* 2004;49:475–479.

23. Schulpis KH, Michelakakis H, Tsakiris T, et al. The effect of diet on total anti-oxidant status, erythrocyte membrane Na^+, K^+-ATPase and Mg^{2+}-ATPase activities in patients with classical galactosemia. Clin Nutr 24:151–157, 2005.

24. Tsakiris S, Michelakakis H, Schulpis KH. Erythrocyte membrane acetylcholinesterase, Na^+, K^+-ATPase and Mg^{2+}-ATPase activities in patients with classical galactosemia. *Acta Paediatr.* 2005; 94:1223–1226.

25. Daniels BS, Hostetter TH. Functional and structural alterations of the glomerular permeability barrier in experimental galactosemia. *Kidney Int.* 1991;39:1104–1111.

26. Schadewaldt P, Killius S, Kamalanathan L, et al. Renal excretion of galactose and galactitol in patients with classical galactosemia, obligate heterozygous parents and healthy subjects. *J Inherit Metab Dis.* 2003;26:459–479.

27. Mulhern ML, Madson CJ, Danford A, et al. The unfolded protein response in lens epithelial cells from galactosemic rat lenses. *Invest Ophthalmol Vis Sci.* 2006;47:3951–3959.

28. Kaufman FR, XU YK, Ng WG, et al. Gonadal function and ovarian galactose metabolism in classic galactosemia. *Acta Endocrinol.* (Copen) 1989;120:129–133.

29. Bandyopadhyay S, Chakrabarti J, Banerjee S, et al. Prenatal exposure to high galactose adversely affects initial gonadal pool of germ cells in rats. *Hum Reprod.* 2003;18:276–282.

30. Alonso E, Saez FJ, Madrid JF, et al. GalNAc moieties in O-linked oligosaccharides of the primordial germ cells of Xenopus embryos. *Histochem Cell Biol.* 2002;117:345–349.

31. Prestoz LLC, Couto AS, Shin YS, et al. Altered follicle stimulating hormone isoforms in female galactosaemia patients. *Eur J Pediatr.* 1997;156:116–120.

32. Combarnous Y. Molecular basis of the specificity of binding of glycoprotein hormones to their receptors. *Endocr Rev.* 1992;13:670–691.

33. Rubio-Gozalbo ME, Panis B, Zimmermann LJ, et al. The endocrine system in treated patients with classical galactosemia. *Mol Genet Metab.* 2006;89:316–322.

34. Levy O, Martin S, Eichenwald E, et al. Impaired innate immunity in the newborn: Newborn neutrophils are deficient in bactericidal/permeability-increasing protein. *Pediatrics.* 1999;104:1327–1333.

35. Kobayashi RH, Kettelhut BV, Kobayashi AL. Galactose inhibition of neonatal neutrophil function. *Pediatr Infect Dis.* 1983;2:442–445.

36. Timson DJ. Functional analysis of disease-causing mutations in human UDP-galactose 4-epimerase. *FEBS J.* 2005;272:6170–6177.

37. Openo KK, Schulz JM, Vargas CA, et al. Epimerase-deficiency galactosemia is not a binary condition. *Am J Hum Genet.* 2006;78:89–102.

38. Bosch AM, Bakker HD, Van Gennip AH, et al. Clinical features of galactokinase deficiency: a review of the literature. *J Inherit Metab Dis.* 2002;25:629–634.

39. Kaufman FR, McBride-Chang C, Manis FR, et al. Cognitive functioning, neurologic status and brain imaging in classic galactosemia. *Eur J Pediatr.* 1995;154(supplement 2):S2–S5.

40. Nelson D. Verbal dyspraxia in children with galactosemia. *Eur J Pediatr.* 1995;154(supplement 2):S6–S7.

41. Schweitzer S, Shin Y, Jacobs C, et al. Long-term outcome in 134 patients with galactosemia. *Eur J Pediatr.* 1993;152:36–43.

42. Waggoner DD, Buist NRM, Donnell GN. Long-term prognosis in galactosemia: results of a survey of 350 cases. *J Inherit Metab Dis.* 1990;13:802–818.

43. Berry GT, Moate PJ, Reynolds RA, et al. The rate of de novo galactose synthesis in patients with galactose-1-phosphate uridyltransferase deficiency. *Mol Genet Metab.* 2004;81:22–30.

44. Lai K, Langley SD, Khwaja FW, et al. GALT deficiency causes UDP hexose deficit in human galactosemia cells. *Glycobiology.* 2003; 13:285–294.

45. Lebea PJ, Pretorious PJ. The molecular relationship between deficient UDP-galactose uridyltransferase (GALT) and ceramide galactosyltransferase (CGT) enzyme function: a possible cause for poor long-term prognosis in classic galactosemia. *Med Hypotheses.* 2005;65:1051–1057.

46. Forges T, Monnier-Barbarino P, Leheup B, et al. Pathophysiology of impaired ovarian function in galactosaemia. *Hum Reprod Update.* 2006;12:573–584.

47. Panis B, Gerver WJ, Rubio-Gozalbo ME. Growth in treated classical galactosemia patients. *Eur J Pediatr.* 2007;166:443–446.

48. Panis B, Forget PPh, van Kroonenburgh MJPG, et al. Bone metabolism in galactosemia. *Bone.* 2004;35:982–987.

49. Rubio-Gozalbo ME, Hamming S, van Kroonenburgh MJPG, et al. Bone mineral density in patients with classic galactosemia. *Arch Dis Child.* 2002; 87:57–60.

50. Elsas LJ, Dembure PP, Langley S, et al. A common mutation associated with the Duarte galactosemia allele. *Am J Hum Genet.* 1994;54:1030–1036.

51. Elsas LJ, Lai K, Saunders CJ, et al. Functional analysis of the human galactose-1-phosphate uridyltransferase promoter in Duarte and LA variant galactosemia. *Mol Genet Metab.* 2001;72:297–305.

52. Kozak L, Francova H, Pijackova A, et al. Presence of a deletion in the 5-prime upstream region of the GALT gene in Duarte(D2) alleles. *J Med Genet.* 1999;36:576–578.

53. Elsas LJ, Lai K. The molecular biology of galactosemia. *Genet Med.* 1998;1:40–48.

54. Gitzelmann R. Galactose-1-phosphate in the pathophysiology of galactosemia. *Eur J Pediatr.* 1995;154:S45–S49.

55. Nishimura Y, Tajima G, Bahagia A, et al. Differential diagnosis of neonatal mild hypergalactosaemia detected by mass screening: Clinical significance of portal vein imaging. J. Inherit Metab Dis. 2004;27:11.

CHAPTER 10

Disorders of Fructose Metabolism

Claude Sansaricq, MD, PhD
Manisha Balwani, MD, MS

INTRODUCTION

Fructose is a quantitatively important source of carbohydrates, especially in the Western diet. It is a component of table sugar (sucrose, Glc-Fru disaccharide) and is contained in large amounts in honey, fruits and various vegetables. Fructose, sucrose and sorbitol (metabolised mainly via fructose) are frequent food additives. A special concern are sucrose-containing infant formula. Fructose also constitutes the main carbohydrate in seminal fluid. Our average daily dietary intake is around 100g. In the last century fructose and sorbitol were used as carbohydrates in parental nutrition, e.g. equimolar solutions of glucose and fructose prepared by hydrolysis of sucrose as "invert sugar". As IV solutions containing fructose or sorbitol have significant disadvantages for every individual and can be deadly for patients with fructose intolerance they should not be used any longer.

Oral fructose is absorbed in the small intestine and mainly metabolized in the liver. Significant fructose metabolism also takes place in the kidney and the small intestine, explaining the organ manifestations of genetic diseases of fructose metabolism.

Normal fructose metabolism comprises three enzymes (Figure 10-1). The irreversible phosphorylation of fructose by fructokinase yields fructose-1-phosphate which is cleaved by aldolase B into phosphorylated C3-metabolites that enter glycolysis or gluconeogenesis.

HEREDITARY FRUCTOSE INTOLERANCE

Etiology/Pathophysiology Hereditary fructose intolerance (HFI) is an autosomal recessive inborn error of fructose metabolism that results from a deficiency of class 1 aldolase B, which is predominantly found in the liver (also called 'hepatic' or 'liver' aldolase, fructose 1-aldolase B). This isoenzyme is also expressed in the kidney and intestinal mucosa, which are subsidiary sites for metabolism of exogenous fructose (1). Patients with HFI are sensitive to any source of fructose, including dietary or parenteral sucrose, sorbitol, and fructose. Early diagnosis and treatment can prevent acute and long-term metabolic derangement and hepatic and renal toxicity.

Aldolase B catalyzes two separate reactions:

1. Reversible splitting of fructose 1-phosphate (F-1-P) to D-glyceraldehyde (GAH) and dihydroxyacetone phosphate (DHAP), which then enters the glycolytic pathway;

2. Reversible splitting of fructose-1,6-biphosphate into D-glyceraldehyde-3-phosphate (GAH3-P) and DHAP.

There are another two isoenzymes of aldolase (A and C) that are also responsible for the cleavage of fructose-1,6-biphosphate into DHAP and GAH-3P. All three isoenzymes, A, B, and C share 68–78% homology with each other but are located on different chromosomes (A is located at 16q22-q24, B is located at 9q22.3 and C at 17 cen-q12 loci). Aldolase A is mainly expressed in muscle cells and red cell and aldolase C in brain; however, it seems that there may be sufficient residual activity of these two isoenzymes in the liver cells that allows glycolysis and gluconeogenesis to take place in patients with HFI as long as their diet does not contain fructose.

Fructose biphosphate is an intermediary of both glycolysis and gluconeogenesis. Because the reaction catalyzed by aldolase B is reversible depending on cellular conditions, fructose biphosphate can be split to the triose phosphate compounds (glycolysis) or during fasting, more fructose biphosphate can be produced through the condensation of triose phosphates with increased endogenous glucose production through gluconeogenesis. Reduced activity of aldolase B results in

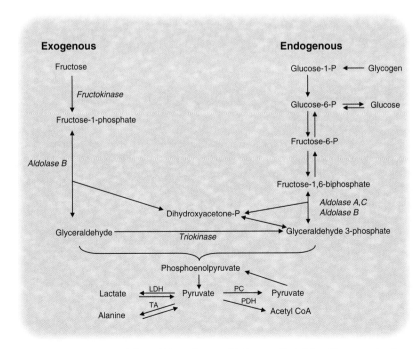

FIGURE 10-1. Normal fructose metabolism. Aldolase B is responsible for reversible splitting of fructose 1-phosphate (F-1-P) to D-glyceraldehyde and dihydroxyacetone phosphate as well as reversible splitting of fructose-1,6-biphosphate into D-glyceraldehyde-3-phosphate and dihydroxyacetone phosphate.

Disorders of Fructose Metabolism

AT-A-GLANCE

Hereditary fructose intolerance (HFI) and fructose 1,6-biphosphatase (FBP1) deficiency are two distinct disorders of fructose metabolism. HFI results from deficiency of aldolase B, which is found in liver, kidney, and intestine. Ingestion of fructose results in gastrointestinal symptoms and secondary hypoglycemia, which may be life threatening. Diagnosis is established by detailed history and mutation analysis. Management of this condition is by avoidance of fructose/sucrose/sorbitol in the diet. Prompt identification of this condition is essential to avoid complications. The long-term effects of untreated HFI result in growth failure and liver failure and can lead to death.

FBP1 deficiency is also considered an inborn error of fructose metabolism although it is not a part of the fructose pathway. It results in hypoglycemia and acidosis often already in the neonatal period and can be potentially life threatening. Management includes avoidance of fasting and fructose in the diet, and treatment of acidosis if present should be initiated.

DISORDER	INHERITANCE	ENZYME	LOCUS	OMIM
HFI	autosomal recessive	Aldolase B	9q 22.3	+229600
FBP1	autosomal recessive	Fructose 1,6-biphosphatase	9q 22.2-22.3	*229700

DISORDER	FINDINGS	CLINICAL PRESENTATION INFANCY	CLINICAL PRESENTATION CHILDHOOD/ADOLESCENCE
HFI	Hypoglycemia Fructosuria Proteinuria Aminoaciduria Hypophosphatemia Metabolic acidosis Reduced clotting factors Anemia thrombocytopenia Hyperuricemia	Vomiting Failure to thrive Anemia Jaundice Hepatomegaly Seizures Liver Failure Hemorrhagic diathesis	Epigastric pain Nausea Bloating Vomiting Diarrhea Growth retardation Chronic liver disease Aversion to sweets Absence of dental caries
FBP1	Metabolic acidosis Hypoglycemia Lactic acidosis Ketonuria ↑ 2-Oxoglutaric acid (U)	Hyperventilation Tachycardia Apneic spells Irritability Lethargy Coma Vomiting Hepatomegaly Jaundice Seizures Hypotonia	Anorexia Vomiting

hypoglycemia and acidosis due to impaired gluconeogenesis as well as glycogenolysis through inhibition of glycogen phosphorylase by the accumulated F-1-P. The accumulation of F-1-P also causes sequestering of inorganic phosphate, leading to a decrease in adenosine triphosphate (ATP) and inorganic phosphate. This increases the activity of the liver adenosine monophosphate deaminase enzyme and catabolism of the hepatic adenine nucleotide pool, resulting in increased uric acid levels. The free fructose concentration in the blood is elevated due to inhibition of fructokinase (the enzyme that phosphorylates fructose) by the accumulated F-1-P. The cause of the hepatic and renal tubular dysfunction is not well understood.

Clinical Presentation There is a broad spectrum of clinical manifestations in patients with HFI (1,2). The manifestations vary with age, level of enzyme activity, amount, and duration of fructose ingestion. Some patients are very sensitive to fructose and will be symptomatic with even small doses whereas others are able to tolerate moderate amounts.

Exclusively breast fed infants remain symptom free. Symptoms appear with the introduction of sucrose supplementation to formula or fruits or fruit juices. Infants may present with abdominal discomfort, nausea, anorexia, vomiting, failure to thrive, hypoglycemia, apneic spells, and seizures. Acutely ill children may have jaundice and hepatomegaly.

If undiagnosed and the fructose is continued in the diet, these patients present with failure to thrive, proximal renal tubular acidosis (RTA), bleeding tendency, and hepatomegaly, which may progress to liver failure with hypoalbuminemia and ascites. Rarely, they can develop severe metabolic acidosis due to renal tubular dysfunction and lactic acidosis. In younger children the severity of the clinical presentation is proportional to the fructose intake in the diet.

In older children and adults, this disorder can present with vomiting, epigastric pain, nausea, and bloating and an aversion to fructose-containing foods. These episodes may or may not be associated with hypoglycemia. The physical signs include growth failure and hepatomegaly. Adult patients may sometimes be diagnosed only after fructose infusions result in severe hypoglycemia. Often patients will develop an adaptive response by avoiding certain sweet foods that contain fructose. As a consequence a large number of adults with HFI will be free of dental caries.

Genetics

HFI is inherited as an autosomal recessive trait. The frequency of HFI is estimated as 1:20,000 in Germany and 1:30,000 in England. It is caused by a deficiency of aldolase B. The aldolase B gene has been localized to chromosome 9 and cloned (3).

Diagnostic Tests

Laboratory evaluation typically shows hypoglycemia, liver impairment with abnormal coagulation studies, elevated tyrosine and methionine, increased billirubin and abnormal liver function tests. Generalized aminoaciduria, proximal tubular acidosis and hypophosphatemia may be present due to development of renal Fanconi syndrome. Hyperuricemia, anemia and thrombocytopenia are also common. Intravenous fructose challenge has been historically used as a primary diagnostic test but intravenous fructose is not available in most countries and the test is potentially life-threatening. Oral fructose challenge has not been evaluated, is unpleasant for the patient, and may also have serious complications. Fructose challenge has therefore become contraindicated as the primary diagnostic approach when this diagnosis is suspected; mutation analysis should be used.

Urine-reducing Substances Fructosuria is present after ingestion of fructose in diet and can be detected by checking the urine for reducing substances. Specific determination of fructose is possible in metabolic laboratories, by thin-layer chromatography, for example.

Enzyme Activity Analysis The aldolase B activity, as determined in liver or small intestine cells by using both F-1,6 biphosphate and F-1-P as substrates is usually increased in patients with HFI. Normal levels are approximately 1 IU/g wet weight liver tissue. In patients with HFI the ratio is usually more than 3 IU/g.

DNA Diagnosis This is available clinically by sequencing of the aldolase B gene. Three of the most common mutations (A149D, A174D and N334K), account for approximately 75% of alleles (4–7). Negative results do not rule out the diagnosis because there might be unidentified mutations.

Treatment Patients with HFI can be treated very satisfactorily with the elimination of fructose/sucrose/sorbitol and fructose-containing foods in the diet (Table 10-1). Care should be taken to avoid infant formulas or medications that contain fructose. Tolerance to fructose may increase with age. There is a normalization of laboratory parameters after a fructose-restricted diet is instituted. Infusions containing fructose or sorbitol can be life threatening. Intravenous glucose should be used for management of hypoglycemia.

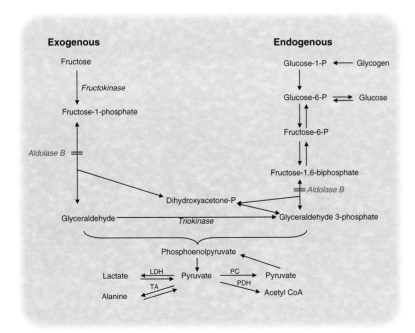

FIGURE 10-2. Hereditary fructose intolerance. Deficiency of Aldolase B results in accumulation of fructose 1- phosphate and impaired gluconeogenesis and glycolysis.

TABLE 10-1 Diet for patients with HFI and FDP*

Permitted	Not Permitted/Special Considerations
Poultry, beef, lamb, veal, pork, game meats	Lunch meats, ham, bacon, hot dogs, sausages that used sugar in the curing/smoking process
Fish, shellfish	Smoked fish that used sugar in the curing/smoking process
Cheese	Specialty cheeses that have additional ingredients such as cheese soaked in wine or beer, and flavored cheeses (honey, maple syrup, etc)
Eggs	No special considerations
Milk	Milk products with sugar (i.e., chocolate, milk)
Potatoes, pasta, rice	Sweet potato, yam, pastas containing prohibited ingredients (i.e., stuffed ravioli, tomato pasta)
Only certain vegetables (asparagus, beans, cabbage, cauliflower, peppers, lettuce, spinach)	All other vegetables (some examples include carrot, tomato, corn and any canned/frozen vegetable that contains sugar)
Only bread or crackers that are made without fructose, sugar or sorbital	Nearly all breads and crackers
	Fruits (including dehydrated and extracted)
Cereal that do not contain fructose, sugar or sorbital	Sweetened cereals or any cereal that contains, fructose, sugar or sorbitol
Butter, margarine, cooking oils	No special considerations
Plain yoghurt, sugarless ice cream, sugarless pudding	Most desserts as they contain sugar or fruit.
Salt, pepper, cinnamon, poppy seeds, salad dressings made without sugar	Mayonnaise, ketchup, jellies, jams, mustards or salad dressings made with sugar

*Free of fructose, sucrose and sorbitol.

Notes: most chewing gums are made with sorbitol; many "Children's" medicines contain fructose.

FRUCTOSE 1,6-BIPHOSPHATASE-1 DEFICIENCY

Etiology/Pathophysiology Fructose 1,6-biphosphatase-1 (FBP1) catalyzes the conversion of fructose 1-6-biphosphate to fructose-6-phosphate (Figure 10-3), an essential enzymatic step in gluconeogenesis. This step is responsible for production of endogenous glucose from gluconeogenic precursors including fructose. FBP1 deficiency is not a true defect of the fructose metabolism pathway, rather it is a defect of gluconeogenesis. In patients with FBP1 deficiency maintenance of euglycemia is dependent on intake of exogenous glucose or galactose and breakdown of hepatic glycogen. At times of stress or fasting, when glycogen stores are depleted, affected individuals are unable to utilize gluconeogenic substrates (e.g., amino acids, lactate, ketones, and glycerol), developing hypoglycemia, ketosis, lactic acidosis and elevated glycerol levels with concomitant glyceroluria (8,9). Patients with deficiency of FBP1, when challenged with D-fructose, tend to accumulate F-1-P. The consequence is a decrease of the intracellular concentration of ATP and inorganic phosphate and impaired glycogenolysis through inhibition of glycogen phosphorylase. The mechanism of this inhibition remains somewhat enigmatic, because F-1-P has been found to inhibit liver phosphorylase only at nonphysiologic concentrations. Decreased glycogenolysis and impaired gluconeogenesis lead to hypoglycemia, lactic acidosis and glyceroluria during loading tests with fructose as in HFI, although at much higher doses. During metabolic derangement the decrease in ATP and inorganic phosphate increases the activity of the liver adenosine monophophate deaminase enzyme, leading to increased catabolism of the hepatic adenine nucleotide pool and an increase in the uric acid level.

Clinical Presentation Most patients with FBP1 present in the first week of life with a severe, life-threatening metabolic acidosis and hypoglycemia (10). Affected newborns who undergo fasting or decreased intake in the first few days of life rapidly exhaust their glycogen stores and develop symptoms such as hyperventilation, irritability, lethargy and eventually coma, seizures, and respiratory

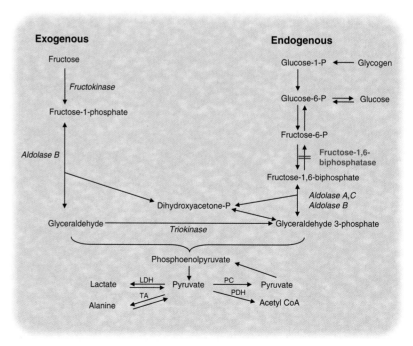

FIGURE 10-3. Fructose-1,6-bisphosphatase deficiency. Fructose-1,6-bisphosphatase catalyzes the splitting of fructose-1,6-bisphosphate into fructose 6-phosphate and inorganic phosphate. FBP deficiency results in impaired gluconeogenesis.

or cardiac arrest. Physical examination may show tachycardia, tachypnea, muscle weakness and hepatomegaly. Organic acid analysis reveals increased 2-oxoglutarate, deriving from metabolism of excessive pyruvate to large quantities of 2-oxoglutarate.

In some patients symptoms do not develop for months or even years later and are usually triggered by stress (i.e., infections) and episodes of fasting. Children may present with anorexia, vomiting, hypoglycemia, and metabolic acidosis. In infants, even a fast of a few hours may provoke hypoglycemia, whereas in older children and adults fasting for up to 14 to 20 hours may be tolerated. Urine is usually positive for ketones. Between the episodes patients are metabolically stable with mild, intermittent, or chronic metabolic acidosis. Patients develop severe hypoglycemia with metabolic acidosis on ingestion of fructose. Fatal hepatic or renal injury following ingestion of fructose has been reported. Patients with FBP1, unlike those with HFI, do not have an aversion to sweets. They are usually developmentally normal unless there has been prolonged untreated hypoglycemia. In contrast to HFI, renal tubular function and coagulation is normal. Liver function is usually normal.

Laboratory Evaluation Laboratory findings in patients with FBP1 deficiency include hypoglycemia (blood glucose concentration of less than 40 mg/dL), anion gap metabolic acidosis, elevated glycerol in blood and urine, elevated alanine, and elevated lactate and pyruvate. The lactate:pyruvate ratio is increased (up to 30) due to insufficient oxidation of nicotinamide adenine dinucleotide oxidase. Free fatty acids and uric acid are also elevated. Ketones are elevated but in some patients ketone elevation can be modest or absent (11). In patients with FBP1 deficiency, a fructose or glycerol challenge test or a prolonged fast (>12–14 h) induces hypoglycemia and an increase in lactate levels (>2 standard deviations above mean). It should be noted that in any patient in whom this diagnosis is suspected, both of these tests are absolutely contraindicated because the test is potentially life-threatening.

Fructose-induced hypoglycemia cannot be reversed by glucagon administration; however, in the fed state patients have a normal hyperglycemic response to glucagon. Feeding a diet excessively high in protein or fat can also provoke hypoglycemia and metabolic acidosis. The mechanism for each substrate's effect is different: in the case of protein, the additional intake of amino acids encourages gluconeogenesis,

which provokes the appearance of the defect, whereas excessive fat intake enhances malonyl-CoA production, which inhibits carnitine palmitoyl-CoA transferase. This impairs entry of fatty acids into the mitochondria, impairs ketone synthesis and promotes hypoglycemia.

Confirmation of the diagnosis can be established with measurement of the FBP1 activity in the liver. Liver biopsy usually reveals fatty infiltration of the liver and elevated lipid content in patients with hepatomegaly. Other tissues, in which one can measure the FBP activity are kidney cortex and jejunum. FBP1 activity is variably present in leukocytes; however, normal activity in the peripheral leukocyte does not rule out hepatic FBP1 deficiency (12–14).

Genetic Testing The disease is transmitted as an autosomal recessive trait, the true incidence of which is not yet known. The FBP1 gene has been cloned and localized to chromosome 9q22.2-22.3. The gene contains 7 exons and 6 introns and a promoter region. A variety of mutations have been described (15–17). The majority of these are nucleotide substitutions; no relationship of genotype to phenotypic expression of the disease has yet been elucidated. There may be unidentified mutations in the promoter regions or mutations in the physiologic regulators of this enzyme that account for this disorder.

Treatment Patients with FBP1 deficiency should avoid fructose/sucrose/sorbitol and fructose-containing products in the diet, especially in childhood (see Table 10-3). Prolonged fasting should be avoided as it can induce hypoglycemia. Hypoglycemia should be managed with intravenous dextrose, the amounts sufficient to maintain a normal blood glucose concentration until the patient is once again able to eat a usual diet. Liver size will usually diminish following an acute episode. Acidosis can be corrected by intravenous bicarbonate solution. Patients should be carefully monitored during periods of stress for hypoglycemia.

Psychosocial Support/ Genetic Counseling

Patients should be provided genetic counseling as with any genetic or metabolic disorder. The autosomal recessive nature of inheritance should be explained including recurrence risks for future pregnancies (i.e., 25%). Enzyme analysis cannot be used for prenatal diagnosis because the enzyme is not deficient in amniocytes, but molecular testing remains an option.

REFERENCES

1. Cox TM. Aldolase B and fructose intolerance. *FASEB.* 1994;8:62–71.
2. Wong D. Hereditary fructose intolerance. *Mol Genet Metab.* 2005;85:165–167.
3. Rottman WH, Tolan DR, Penhoet EE. Complete amino acid sequence for human aldolase B derived from cDNA and genomic clones. *Proc Natl Acad Sci.* 1984;81:2738–2742.
4. Cross NC, de Franchis R, Sebastio G, et al: Molecular analysis of aldolase B genes in hereditary fructose intolerance. *Lancet.* 1990;335:306–309.
5. Brooks CC, Tolan DR. Association of the widespread A149P hereditary fructose intolerance mutation with newly identified sequence polymorphism in the aldolase B gene. *Am J Hum Genet.* 1993;52:835–840.
6. Rellos P, Segusch J, Cox TM. Expression, purification and characterization of natural mutants of aldolase B. *J Biol Chem.* 2000;2675:1145–1151.
7. DR Tolan. Molecular basis of heretidary fructose intolerance: Mutations and polymorphisms in the human aldolase B gene. *Hum Mutat.* 1995;6:210–218.
8. Baker L, Winegrad AI. Fasting hypoglycaemia and metabolic acidosis associated with deficiency of hepatic fructose-1,6-diphosphatase activity. *Lancet.* 1970;II:13–16.
9. Green HL, Stifel FB, Herman RH. "Ketotic hypoglycemia" due to hepatic fructose-1,6-diphosphatase deficiency. *Am J Dis Child.* 1972;124:415–429.
10. Pagliara AS, Karl IE, Keating JP, et al. Hepatic fructose-1,6-diphosphatase deficiency. A cause of lactic acidosis and hypoglycemia in infancy. *J Clin Invest.* 1972; 51:2115–2123.
11. Morris AAM, Deshpande S, Ward-Platt MP, et al. Impaired ketogenesis in fructose-1,6-biphosphatase deficiency: a pitfall in the investigation of hypoglycemia. *J Inherit Metab Dis.* 1995; 18:28–32.
12. Melancon SB, Nadler HL. Detection of fructose-1,6-diphosphatase deficiency with the use of white blood cells. *N Engl J Med.* 1972;286:731–732.
13. Burdhel P, Bohme H-J, Didt L. Biochemical and clinical observations in four patients with fructose-1,6-diphosphatase deficiency. *Eur J Pediatr.* 1990;149:574–576.
14. Besley GTN, Walter JH, Lewis MA, et al. Fructose-1,6-bisphophatase deficiency: severe phenotype with normal leukocyte enzyme activity. *J Inherit Metab Dis.* 1994;17:333–335.
15. El-Maghrabi MR, Lange AJ, Jiang W, et al. Human fructose-1,6-bisphosphatase gene (FBP1): exon-intron organization, location to chromosome 9q22.2-q22.3, and mutation screening in subjects with fructose-1,6-bisphosphatase deficiency. *Genomics* 1995;27:520–525.
16. Kikawa Y, Inuzuka M, Jin BY, et al. Identification of genetic mutations in Japanese patients with fructose-1,6-biphosphatase deficiency. *Am J Hum Genet.* 1997;61:852–861.
17. Herzog B, Wendel U, Eschrich K. Novel mutations in patients with fructose-1,6- bisphosphatase deficiency. *J Inherit Metab Dis.* 1999;22:132–138.

CHAPTER
11

Urea Cycle Disorders

Marshall L. Summar, MD

INTRODUCTION

The urea cycle was first described in 1932 by Krebs and Henseleit (1) (Figure 11-1). This biochemical pathway, with a great capacity for production of urea from free ammonia, provides an effective defense against the latter's extreme neurotoxicity. The proteins and corresponding DNA sequences have been gradually described since that time (2–8). The cycle is composed of five catalytic enzymes, a regulatory compound-producing enzyme, and at least two transport proteins. Like most metabolic pathways, the urea cycle interdigitates with several other pathways such as the citric acid cycle and the nitric oxide synthase (NOS) pathway (Figure 11-1). The cycle is the principal mechanism for the clearance of waste nitrogen produced by protein turnover, the metabolism of other compounds such as adenosine monophosphate, and dietary intake.

The urea cycle disorders (UCD) result from inherited molecular defects that compromise this clearance. They represent one of the most challenging disease groups from both treatment and diagnostic standpoints. The aggregate incidence of these disorders is estimated to be at least 1 in 25,000 births but partial defects may make this number much higher. Severe deficiency or total absence of activity of any of the first four enzymes—carbamyl phosphate synthetase I (CPSI), ornithine transcarbamylase (OTC), argininosuccinic acid synthetase (ASS), argininosuccinic acid lyase (ASL)—or the enzyme N-acetyl glutamate synthase (NAGS) which facilitates production of the regulatory compound N-acetyl glutamate results in the accumulation of ammonia and other precursor metabolites during the first few days of life. In milder (or partial) urea cycle enzyme deficiencies, ammonia accumulation may be triggered by illness or stress at almost any time of life, resulting in repeated elevations of plasma ammonia concentration. The hyperammonemia may be less severe and the symptoms more subtle. Defects in the fifth enzyme in the pathway, arginase (ARGI), also result in a more subtle disease with predominant progressive neurologic symptoms. Defects in the transporter proteins for ornithine (hyperornithinemia-hyperammonemia-homocitrullinuria [HHH] syndrome) and aspartate (Citrullinemia II) also have presentations different from the classic disorders.

Biochemical and Molecular Aspects of the Urea Cycle

The urea cycle is a model system for studying biochemical disease, because it is the sole processing mechanism for waste nitrogen, has a limited number of components, and is amenable to *in vitro* and *in vivo* testing of functional changes. As shown in Figure 11-1, the urea cycle is composed of five primary enzymes, one regulatory cofactor producing reaction, and at least two transport molecules across the mitochondrial membrane. Inborn errors of metabolism are associated with each step in the pathway and have been well described over the years. The cycle has the interesting property of having a subset of the enzymes participate in another metabolic pathway that produces all of the body's nitric oxide (NO). The urea cycle as a nitrogen clearance system is limited primarily to the human liver and intestine with carbamyl phosphate synthetase and ornithine transcarbamylase limited exclusively to those tissues. The enzymes downstream that process citrulline into arginine are ubiquitous in their distribution although their role in nitrogen clearance is mainly limited to the liver. As the rate-limiting enzyme in the urea cycle, a decreased function of CPSI would have the greatest impact on cycle function under conditions where environmental stress causes increased demand. We have identified a number of polymorphisms in CPSI that appear to have functional significance, and affect NO production under environmental stress (9–12). Other changes should also affect both the processing of ammonia and the ability to generate NO. A brief review of the five enzymes and cofactor producer of the urea cycle follows.

CARBAMYL PHOSPHATE SYNTHETASE I

CPSI is the rate-limiting enzyme catalyzing the first committed step of the urea cycle (Figure 11-2), the primary system for removing waste nitrogen produced by protein metabolism. Expression of CPSI is limited to high levels in the liver and smaller amounts in the intestinal mucosa. It is compartmentalized within the mitochondria although it is genomically (2q35) encoded. Of note, a cytosolic CPS II exists in the hepatocyte as a part of the pyrimidine biosynthetic pathway and which is independent of NAG regulation.

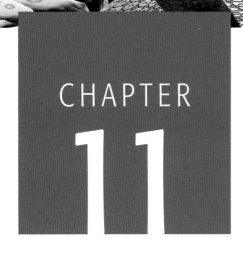

FIGURE 11-1. Urea Cycle. For abbreviations see "At A Glance".

Urea Cycle Defects

AT-A-GLANCE

The urea cycle disorders (UCDs) result from defects in the metabolism of waste nitrogen produced by the breakdown of protein and other nitrogen-containing molecules. The waste nitrogen is converted into ammonia and transported to the liver where it is processed via the urea cycle. The urea cycle is composed of five catalytic enzymes, a cofactor producer, and at least two transport proteins. Lysinuric protein intolerance, a transport defect of the dibasic amino acids resulting in a secondary impairment of the urea cycle, is discussed in Chapter 42. The incidence of these disorders is estimated to be at least 1 in 25,000 births but partial defects may make this number higher. Deficiency of any of the first four enzymes (CPSI, OTC, ASS, ASL) in the urea cycle or the cofactor producer NAGS results in the accumulation of ammonia and other precursor metabolites during the first few days of life. Severity of the disease is influenced by the position of the defective enzyme in the pathway and the severity of the enzyme defect. All UCDs have autosomal recessive inheritance except for OTC, which is an x-linked disorder in which female carriers may be symptomatic depending on the skewed inactivation of the X chromosome. The initial symptoms of a newborn with UCD are non-specific: failure to feed, loss of thermoregulation with a low core temperature, and somnolence. They can rapidly develop cerebral edema and the related signs of lethargy, anorexia, hyperventilation or hypoventilation, hypothermia, seizures, neurologic posturing, coma, and death. Defects in the fifth enzyme in the pathway, arginase (ARGI), result in progressive neurologic symptoms. Defects in the transporter proteins for ornithine (Hyperornithinemia-hyperammonemia-homocitrullinuria syndrome) and aspartate (Citrullinemia II) also have presentations different from the classic disorders. The mainstays of treatment are: 1) reducing plasma ammonia concentration; 2) pharmacologic management to allow alternative pathway excretion of excess nitrogen; 3) reducing the amount of nitrogen in the diet; 4) avoiding or reversing catabolism through the introduction of calories supplied by carbohydrates and fat; and, 5) reducing the risk of neurologic damage.

TYPES OF UCD	OCCURRENCE	GENE	LOCUS	OMIM
Carbamyl phosphate synthetase I (CPSI)	1/50,000	CPSI	2q35	#237300
Ornithine transcarbamylase (OTC)	1/30,000	OTC	Xp21.1	#311250
Argininosuccinate synthetase or citrullinemia type I (ASS or CTLNI)	1/50,000	ASS	9q34.1	#215700
Argininosuccinate lyase (ASL)	1/50,000	ASL	7cen-q11.2	#207900
Arginase (ARGI)	1/100,000	ARGI	6q23	#207800
N-Acetyl glutamate synthase (NAGS)	1/100,000	NAGS	17q21.31	#237310
Hyperornithinemia-hyperammonemia-homocitrullinuria (HHH)	1/100,000	SLC25A15	13q14	#238970
Citrullinemia Type II (CTLNII)	1/100,000	SLC25A13	7q21.3	#603471, #605814

DISORDER	FINDINGS	CLINICAL PRESENTATION
CPSI	Hyperammonemia, cerebral edema. Low citrulline and arginine levels.	Encephalopathy, cerebral edema–associated respiratory changes (hyper- and hypoventilation) and hepatomegaly. Seizures, vomiting, anorexia, and dilated pupils. Patients with ASL may have dry and brittle hair showing trichorrhexis nodosa microscopically; Approximately 15% of females carriers of OTC deficiency may develop hyperammonemia at some point in their lives, due to random X-inactivation in liver cells. Acrodermatitis enteropathica has been described and is probably due to low arginine levels.
OTC	Hyperammonemia, cerebral edema. Low citrulline and arginine levels. Elevated orotic acid levels in urine.	
ASS	Hyperammonemia, cerebral edema. Very high citrulline and low arginine levels.	
ASL	Hyperammonemia, cerebral edema. High citrulline, argininosuccinic acid. Chronic elevation of hepatic enzymes.	
NAGS	Hyperammonemia, cerebral edema. Low citrulline and arginine levels.	
ARGI	Elevated arginine, variable, often mild hyperammonemia.	Progressive spasticity. Loss of motor milestones. Seizures. Can present with hyperammonemic encephalopathy.
HHH	Hyperornithinemia, hyperammonemia, and homocitrullinuria.	Loss of milestones, spasticity, seizures, delay in growth and development.
CTLNII	Elevated citrulline, mild-to-severe hyperammonemia, and acidosis.	Adult-onset form presents with psychiatric and neurologic dysfunction. Can present with hyperammonemic encephalopathy. Patients often avoid carbohydrates in diet.

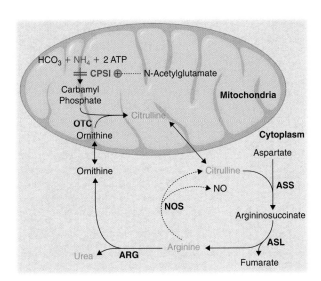

FIGURE 11-2. Carbamyl phosphate synthetase I deficiency. Carbamyl phosphate, citrulline, arginine, and urea are decreased and NH₃ is increased.

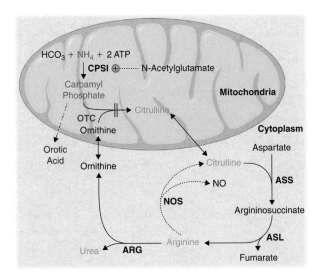

FIGURE 11-3. Ornithine transcarbamylase deficiency. Citrulline, arginine, and urea are decreased and carbamyl phosphate, orotic acid, and NH₃ are increased.

The gene locus for CPS is coincidentally also on the 2nd chromosome (2p21). CPS II is the source of the urinary orotic acid which is a diagnostic feature of OTC deficiency. Mature CPSI is a 160-kDa protein monomer that catalyzes the conversion of ammonia and bicarbonate to carbamyl phosphate (CP) with the expenditure of two adenosine triphosphates. This reaction incorporates the first of two ammonia groups in synthesis of urea. Posttranslational modification is currently unknown beyond cleavage of the first 38 residues after entry into the mitochondria (13–19).

ORNITHINE TRANSCARBAMYLASE

OTC catalyzes the condensation of CP and ornithine to citrulline. This homotrimer is encoded on the X-chromosome and is the most common of the classically presenting UCDs (20–22). Its location on the X-chromosome results in a significant number of clinically affected carrier females. Unlike CPSI, human OTC can be successfully expressed in bacteria from recombinant plasmid. The crystalline structure for the gene has been determined (Figure 11-3).

ARGININOSUCCINIC ACID SYNTHETASE

ASS catalyzes the condensation of aspartate and citrulline to form argininosuccinate. The transfer of an ammonia group from glutamate to aspartate and subsequent formation of argininosuccinate accounts for the second ammonia group of urea. In addition to its critical role in the urea cycle, ASS is involved in the cycling of arginine and citrulline in the production of NO. Its distribution and regulation are tied into two systems, and this enzyme is found in most cells. The enzyme is found in the cytoplasm and it requires the transport of citrulline out of the mitochondria to perform its function for the urea cycle. For NO synthesis it is located in calveolar complexes with ASL and nitric oxide synthase (23). This enzyme also depends on the production of aspartate from either the tricarboxylic acid cycle or protein catabolism. There are 10 nonfunctional, widely dispersed pseudogenes for this enzyme, which suggests some method for repeated duplication within the genome (24). Defects in this gene can present with hyperammonemia as severe as OTC and CPSI defects (Figure 11-4).

ARGININOSUCCINIC ACID LYASE

ASL catalyzes the cleavage of argininosuccinate into arginine and fumarate (Figure 11-5). Like ASS it serves two masters and has a similar ubiquitous distribution and expression pattern. Of note the enzyme resembles the δ-crystalline gene in the eye and is a homotetramer (25). This enzyme also demonstrates alternative splicing in a fraction of its product, which could be influenced by regional polymorphisms (26–28).

ARGINASE I

The enzyme arginase I (ARGI) is distributed throughout the body with high concentrations in the liver, kidney and gut as described by Cedarbaum et al (29–33). There is an ARG II isozyme that has a more limited distribution and does not appear to play a significant role in ureagenesis (30). There are a number of studies ongoing looking at the role of ARGI and its polymorphisms in asthma and NO metabolism (34–36). The crystalline structure of this enzyme is known and will be helpful in elucidating the role of functional polymorphisms (Figure 11-6).

N-ACETYL GLUTAMATE SYNTHETASE

This enzyme and gene were recently characterized by Tuchman and colleagues (37–40). The distribution of this enzyme is being studied at this time but appears to match that of CPSI. This enzyme catalyzes the formation of N-acetylglutamate from glutamate and acetyl-coenzyme A (CoA). This molecule is the essential allosteric cofactor for CPSI function. The production of NAG and CPSI's

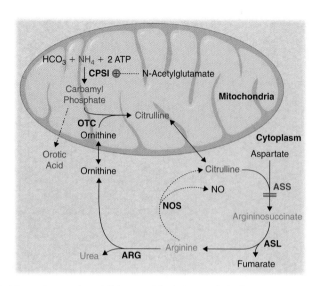

FIGURE 11-4. Argininosuccinate synthase deficiency. Arginine is decreased; citrulline, carbamyl phosphate, orotic acid, and NH_3 are increased.

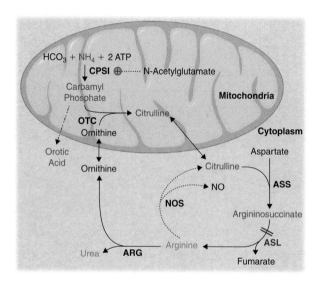

FIGURE 11-5. Argininosuccinate lyase deficiency. Arginine is decreased and citrulline, carbamyl phosphate, orotic acid, argininosuccinate, and NH_3 are increased.

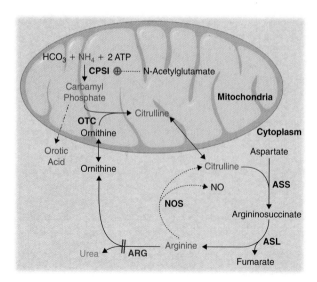

FIGURE 11-6. Arginase deficiency. Arginine, citrulline, NH_3, and orotic acid may be mildly increased.

reliance on it may represent a key vulnerability to environmental factors in urea cycle function (Figure 11-7).

ORNITHINE TRANSPORTER MITOCHONDRIAL 1

The liver-expressed enzyme ornithine transporter mitochondrial 1 (ORNT1) is responsible for the transport of ornithine across the mitochondrial membrane in the liver. Its absence or defective function is associated with a hyperammonemia disorder known as HHH syndrome.

CITRIN

Citrin (SLC25A13) or Solute Carrier Family 25 has been reported as the mutated causative gene for citrullinemia II almost exclusively in Asian patients. The citrin transporter is a calcium-binding mitochondrial transporter that is thought to exchange aspartate and glutamate across the mitochondrial membrane. Defects in this gene would affect the ability of ASS to produce argininosuccinate. Beyond the effects on the urea cycle, defects in this transporter also appear to cause generalized hepatic disease (41–46,55).

CLINICAL PRESENTATION

CPSI, OTC, ASS, ASL, or NAGS

Key to clinical diagnosis is the fact that, within given age groups, the constellation of symptoms is directly related to the neurotoxicity of ammonia. Thus, the presenting symptoms of urea cycle defects are primarily neurologic. The acute disease presentation is brought about by cerebral edema and progressive neurocognitive dysfunction. Elevations in ammonia are thought to have a direct effect on cerebral edema whereas elevations in brain glutamine levels (a buffer for excess nitrogen) are thought to effect neurotransmission and perhaps the edema as well (47–51). Depending on the age of the patient, the outward manifestations of cerebral edema can vary from ataxia, confusion, increased agitation or somnolence to neurologic posturing as pressure is brought to bear on the brain stem. After fusion of the sutures in the skull, the closed space of the skull magnifies the effect of the swelling, and unchecked, progressive swelling will typically result in complete venous stasis or herniation of the brainstem. The cerebral dysfunction that results from the elevations in glutamine, ammonia, and effects on other aspects of neuronal function often results in seizures. This increase in cerebral metabolism during a phase of decreased

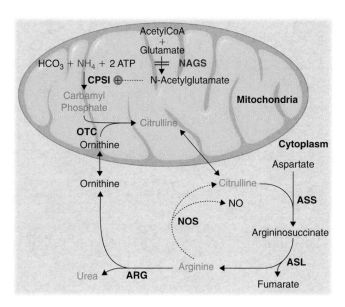

FIGURE 11-7. N-Acetyl glutamate synthase deficiency. Citrulline, arginine, carbamyl phosphate, and urea are decreased and NH_3 is increased.

venous flow complicates the clinical course for these patients. Without aggressive treatment the prognosis for a patient with hyperammonemia and cerebral edema is poor. The exceptions to this clinical presentation are the disorders in the transporters (HHH syndrome and Citrin deficiency) and ARGI deficiency, which will be described separately.

Neonatal Onset This presentation typically is the result of a severe defect in urea cycle capacity. When the protein of the first feedings is added to the already existing stress and catabolism of the neonatal period it creates an additional ammonia burden, and there is clinical evidence that these patients will become hyperammonemic under even ideal conditions (52). The difficulty with recognizing these patients is the similarity of their symptoms to other more common problems such as neonatal sepsis or birth hypoxia. Infants with a UCD usually appear normal at birth but deteriorate as the ammonia accumulates. This typically occurs within the first 48 to 72 hours of life as the infant's intake increases, but may be delayed by 1 to 2 weeks. As these patients develop cerebral edema they may manifest some irritability, diminished oral intake and vomiting but then progress to somnolence and lethargy. As their somnolence increases their oral intake will continue to diminish and the rate of intrinsic protein catabolism will accelerate. Most patients will develop some degree of dehydration from their decreased intake, since normal infants take in fluid with nutrition. Although the decrease in oral intake will reduce the amount of exogenous protein for ammonia production, the catabolism induced by poor intake and

the stress of the neonatal period results in enough tissue protein breakdown to overwhelm this. As the cerebral edema and vascular stasis progress the patient will develop hyperventilation to adapt to the perceived blood flow changes resulting in an elevation in the blood pH from respiratory alkalosis As the pressure increases on the brain stem and central nervous system (CNS) function fails, the patient's respiratory rate will decrease and eventually respiratory drive will disappear. Some patients will develop seizures, although these can be difficult to detect in the context of decreasing CNS function. Unchecked the patients will become comatose and eventually die from CNS failure accompanied by brain stem herniation (5). In OTC deficiency, male infants are especially at risk of acute metabolic decompensation with hyperammonemia and subsequent encephalopathy, coma and death. The symptoms in female carriers vary both in time of onset and severity due to non-random X-inactivation in the liver cells (53). Female carriers presenting during the first year of life with severe hyperammonemia have skewed X-inactivation, expressing more of the mutated allele in the liver cells (54). Infants with CPSI, OTC and citrullinemia type I, all UCD associated with low arginine, can present with acrodermatitis eneteropathica, even in the presence of normal zinc levels (55).

Delayed Onset Patients not presenting in the neonatal period usually have some partial function of their urea cycle. The onset of their symptoms is a summation of their residual enzyme activity, diet, and environmental stressors. These patients can manifest an acute severe hyperammonemic episode similar to the neonatal patients if they undergo a significant catabolic stress such as during an infection or after trauma. These episodes can occur anywhere from just outside the newborn period to quite late in life (6–7th decade). It should be noted that delayed onset of OTC may also be seen in affected males late in life, despite the

absence of a compensating normal X chromosome. Many of these patients will experience numerous mild hyperammonemic episodes, which can result in cumulative neurologic damage. The diagnosis of these cases is often delayed because the symptoms and signs can be quite subtle. As a probable result of physical discomfiture due to mild hyperammonemia from dietary exposure, many of these patients will subconsciously avoid protein in their diet, which can be an important historical clue. These patients can also have episodes triggered by drugs that decrease urea cycle function such as valproic acid and chemotherapeutic agents, or pregnancy (56–63). A characteristic example of delayed presentation is seen in females carriers with OTC deficiency. Some female carriers with OTC can be asymptomatic with orotic aciduria (spontaneous or after protein intake) but others can have delayed presentation due to various degrees of enzymatic activity and symptomatology (skewed X chromosome inactivation); symptoms may range from protein aversion to chronic vomiting, growth retardation, hypotonia, psychomotor retardation, hyperammonemic coma, or psychiatric disorders. Mutations that allow for residual OTC enzyme activity may cause hyperammonemic coma in males, during adolescence or adulthood.

Clinical Presentation of Other Urea Cycle Defects

HHH Syndrome The HHH syndrome is an autosomal recessive inherited disorder caused by a defect in the ornithine transporter protein (ORNT1) due to mutations in SLC25A15 gene (64). ORNT1 carries ornithine across the inner mitochondrial membrane from cytosol to matrix. Impaired transport of ornithine not only disrupts the urea cycle at the level of OTC reaction, but would also prevent ornithine degradation in the reaction catalyzed by a second mitochondrial matrix enzyme, ornithine aminotransferase resulting in the accumulation of both ammonia and ornithine. The clinical symptoms are related to hyperammonemia and resemble those of the other UCDs. Plasma ornithine concentrations are extremely high, ranging from 380 to 630 umol on a self-restricted protein diet. The defect in ornithine translocase results in diminished ornithine transport into the mitochondria, ornithine accumulation in the cytoplasm and reduced intramitochondrial ornithine. The results are impaired ureagenesis and orotic aciduria, the latter resulting from accumulated CP leaking from the mitochondrion and converted by CPS II to orotate. Homocitrulline, thought to originate from transcarbamylation of lysine, in the absence of intramitochondrial ornithine, is excreted in urine. Most patients have intermittent hyperammonemia accompanied by vomiting, lethargy, and coma (in extreme cases). Growth is abnormal and intellectual development is affected. Spasticity is common, as are seizures (64,65). Retinal depigmentation and chorioretinal thinning has been reported in one patient (66). Adult patients are found with partial activity of the enzyme. They typically self-select low-protein diets. Diagnosis is complicated because plasma ornithine levels can normalize on a protein-restricted diet. The presence of hyperammonemia and homocitrullinuria are helpful for diagnostic purposes.

Citrin Deficiency Citrullinemia II is an autosomal disorder caused by citrin deficiency. Citrin is an aspartate glutamate carrier located on the inner mitochondrial membrane and catalyzes an important step in both the urea cycle and the aspartate/malate NADH shuttle. Deficiency of citrin results in decreased aspartate transport and limitation of the ASS enzymatic activity, which combines aspartate and citrulline to make ASS in the urea cycle. In addition citrin deficiency causes an increased NADH/NAD+ ratio through its impact on the aspartate/malate shuttle, which may affect several cell functions, such as aerobic glycolysis, glyconeogenesis, UDP-galactose epimerase activity, fatty acid synthesis and utilization (67). Citrullinemia type II has a neonatal form and an adult form, both caused by recessive mutations of the SLC25A13 gene. The neonatal form presents with neonatal intrahepatic cholestasis, which is characterized by metabolic derangements in gluconeogenesis, aerobic glycolysis, urea synthesis, UPD-galactose epimerase activity and possibly in fatty acid synthesis and utilization. Patients may have hypergalactosemia, hypermethioninemia, tyrosinemia without elevated urinary succinylacetone, elevated serum bile acids, low levels of vitamin K-dependent coagulation factors, hypercitrullinemia, hemolytic anemia, hypoglycemia, and develop cataracts. Liver histology shows markedly fatty changes and fibrosis. The disease spontaneously remits by 12 months of age (41–45,47,68–70). Only one patient had progressive liver disease requiring liver transplantation at the age of 10 months (46). The adult form is more likely to present with insidious neurologic findings in adulthood (44,45). The majority of patients reported have been Japanese or Asian who share a common mutation. These patients can also have the dietary peculiarity of avoiding carbohydrates rather than protein. This probably is due to the overlap of this disorder with glucose metabolism and the physical discomfiture endured upon carbohydrate intake. Treatment for hyperammonemia is the same as in the other UCDs.

Arginase Deficiency Initial presentation of ARGI deficiency is not typically characterized by rapid-onset hyperammonemia. These patients often present with the development of progressive spasticity with greater severity in the lower limbs (71,72). They also develop seizures and gradually lose intellectual attainments. Growth is usually slow and without therapy they usually do not reach normal adult height. Other symptoms that may present early in life include episodes of irritability, anorexia, and vomiting. Severe episodes of hyperammonemia are seen infrequently with this disorder but can be fatal. Diagnosis is made by elevated levels of arginine in the blood and by analysis of enzymatic activity in red blood cells. Treatment is identical to that for other UCDs, with limitation of protein, use of essential amino acid supplements, and diversion of ammonia from the urea cycle with sodium benzoate or sodium phenylbutyrate.

Diagnosis The most important step in diagnosing UCDs is clinical suspicion of hyperammonemia (see Figure 11-8). A blood ammonia level is the first laboratory test in evaluating a patient with a suspected urea cycle defect. However, because as emphasized repeatedly in this chapter, there are no characteristic routine laboratory abnormalities besides elevated ammonia, therefore the importance of clinical suspicion is paramount to diagnosis. Particular care should be taken in drawing a blood ammonia because there is significant variability depending on proper technique and handling. The blood sample for ammonia determination should be placed on ice and ideally run within 15 minutes of collection in order to avoid false elevation of ammonia levels. The false increase in ammonia levels due to delay of sample processing is attributed to the generation and release of ammonia from red blood cells and the deamination of amino acids, especially glutamine. The clinician should remember that treatment should not be delayed in efforts to reach a final diagnosis, and that later stages of treatment should be tailored to the specific disorder. In addition to plasma ammonia laboratory data useful in the diagnosis of UCDs include, pH, CO_2, the anion gap, blood lactate, acylcarnitines, plasma and urine amino acids, and urine organic acid analyses including the specific determination of orotic acid (73,74). Patients with true urea cycle defects will typically have normal glucose and electrolyte levels. The pH and CO_2 can vary with the degree of cerebral edema and hyper- or hypoventilation. In neonates it should be remembered that the basal ammonia level is elevated over that of adults, which typically is less than 35 μmol/L. An elevated plasma ammonia level of 150 μmol/L (>260 μg/dL) or higher in neonates and more than 100 μmol/L (175 μg/dL) in older children and adults, associated with a normal anion gap and a normal blood glucose level, is a strong indication for the presence of a urea cycle defect. Quantitative amino acid analysis can be used to evaluate these patients and arrive at a tentative diagnosis. Elevations or depressions of the intermediate amino-containing molecules arginine, citrulline, and argininosuccinate (Figure 11-8) will give clues to the point of defect in the cycle. The amino acid profile in sick newborns can be quite different from those in children and adults; this should be taken into account (74). The levels of the nitrogen-buffering amino acid glutamine will also be quite high and can serve as confirmation of the hyperammonemia. Other amino acids that are frequently elevated in USDs are alanine and asparagine as they serve as storage forms of waste nitrogen. Plasma arginine may be decreased in all UCDs except for ARGI where arginine levels are 10 to 20 times higher than normal. Plasma citrulline levels are low in NAGS, CPSI and OTC deficiencies as citrulline is the product of the CPS and OTC activities. A 100-fold elevation in plasma citrulline suggests ASS deficiency or citrullinemia type I. A 10-fold elevation of citrulline in association with large amounts of ASA suggests ASL deficiency.

In HHH syndrome plasma ornithine and urine homocitrulline are elevated, whereas in lysinuric protein intolerance (LPI) urinary lysine, arginine and ornithine levels are elevated and blood levels may be normal or low. If a defect in NAGS, CPSI, or OTC is suspected, the presence of the organic acid orotate in the urine can help distinguish the diagnosis (Figure 11-8). Orotic acid is produced when there is an overabundance of CP, which spills into the pyrimidine biosynthetic system and the cytosolic CPS II converts it to orotate. Urinary orotic acid is elevated in OTC, ASS, ASL, and arginase deficiencies (the elevation may be minimal in ASL deficiency) as well as in LPI and HHH syndrome. Orotic acid is normal in NAGS, CPSI, transient hyperammonemia and variable in heterozygous (female) OTC deficiency. The determination of urine organic acids and acylcarnitines will also herald the presence of an organic aciduria. Other genetic defects of ammonia detoxification are LPI (see Chapter 42), the hyperinsulinism-hyperammonemia syndrome (see Chapter 4), hypoprolinemia (paradoxical fasting hyperammonemia), and pyruvate carboxylase deficiency (see Chapter 19). All of them are very rare and important hints are obtained through the investigations outlined above.

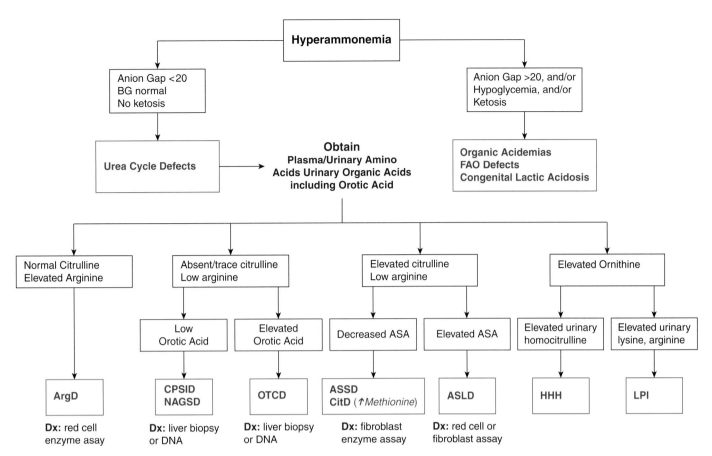

FIGURE 11-8. Hyperammonemia diagnostic algorithm. CPSID: Carbamyl phosphate synthetase I deficiency; NAGSD: N-Acetylglutamate synthase deficiency; OTCD: Ornithine transcarbamylase deficiency; ASSD: Argininosuccinic acid synthase deficiency; CitD: Citrin deficiency (citrullinemia type II); ASLD: Argininosuccinic acid lyase deficiency; ArgD: Arginase deficiency; HHH: Homocitrullinuria, hyperornithinemia, hyperammonemia.

Enzymatic and genetic diagnosis is available for all of these disorders. For CPSI, OTC, and NAGS, enzymatic diagnosis is made on a liver biopsy specimen freshly frozen in liquid nitrogen (75). Enzymatic testing for ASS and ASL can be done on fibroblast samples, and ARGI as well as ASL can be tested on red blood cells (73). However enzymatic testing for ASL or ASS is usually not required as the plasma and urine aminoacid analysis is definitive. Clinically approved DNA sequence analysis is only available for OTC at the time of this printing, but its availability for the other disorders is anticipated soon, as it is available outside the United States. Genetic testing for OTC deficiency will identify 80% of the asymptomatic carriers. For the remaining 20% of the carriers whose mutations can not be detected carrier risk estimation must rely on biochemical data such as elevated glutamine levels and increased orotic acid excretion after allopurinol challenge. Oxypurinol, an allopurinol metabolite enhances the excretion of orotate by inhibiting orotidine decarboxylase. The allopurinol test is performed as following: After collection of the first morning urine, a single oral dose of allopurinol is given (children un-

der 6 years, 100 mg; children 6–10 years, 200 mg, and adult women 300 mg). Urine is then collected during four 6-h periods during 24 hrs and stored frozen. During the test, soft drinks and alcoholic beverages are not allowed because of the presence of benzoate or caffeine. Menstruating females should have the test 7–12 days after the beginning of their menses. An increased orotate value of 12 mmol/mol creatinine has 0.8 sensitivity and 0.92 specificity in detecting carrier status for OTC deficiency (76).

Prenatal testing for USD includes measurement of substrate accumulation in the amniotic fluid, like ASA in ASL, enzyme analysis in chorionic villi, amniocytes, or fetal red blood cells and DNA testing.

Current extended newborn screening panels using tandem mass spectrometry detect abnormal concentrations of analytes associated with ASS deficiency and ASL deficiency, but the sensitivity and specificity of such screening for these disorders is unknown.

Newborn screening by tandem mass spectometry does not detect NAGS, CPSI or OTC deficiency and cannot be expected to reliably detect all cases of arginase deficiency. A frequently updated web resource for testing infor-

mation can be found at the National Institutes of Heath (NIH)–sponsored site: http://www.geneclinics.org.

TREATMENT OF UREA CYCLE DISORDERS

This section provides an overview of UCD management (74,77–80,82). The treatment of these patients requires a highly coordinated team of specialists trained in caring for patients with inborn errors of metabolism. An NIH-sponsored website with links to experts in urea cycle management and treatment protocols is available at: http://www.rarediseasesnetwork. org/ucdc.

Emergency management of patients in a UCD-based hyperammonemic coma is dependent on three interdependent principles: 1) physical removal of the ammonia by dialysis or some form of hemofiltration; 2) reversal of the catabolic state through caloric supplementation and in extreme cases, hormonal suppression (glucose/insulin drip); and 3) pharmacologic scavenging of excess nitrogen. These are not consecutive but should be pursued independently in parallel as quickly as possible (74,80–81).

Central venous access should be established at once and dialysis begun immediately at the highest available flow rate if plasma ammonia is higher than 500 μmol/L or if ammonia does not fall with high-calorie infusion plus pharmaceutical measures. Dialysis is very effective for the removal of ammonia and the clearance is dependent on the flow through the dialysis circuit (74,81). In severe cases of hyperammonemia, provision for hemofiltration should be made to follow the dialysis until the patient is stabilized and the catabolic state is reversed. Some patients will reaccumulate ammonia after their initial round of dialysis and may require additional periods of dialysis. Most patients will have a slight rise in ammonia after dialysis because removal by scavengers and the liver will not be as effective. This slight rise usually does not necessitate repeated dialysis. Dialysis seems to become less effective when plasma ammonia levels are less than 200 μmol/L and can be discontinued.

The importance of the management of the catabolic state cannot be overstressed (49,84–88). Because the catabolism of protein stores is often the triggering event for hyperammonemia, the patient will not stabilize and ammonia will continue to rise until it is reversed or death supervenes. Fluids, dextrose, and Intralipid® should be given to blunt the catabolic process. The patient should be assessed for dehydration and the fluid deficit should be replaced. Because these patients suffer from cerebral edema, care should be taken with overhydration. The nitrogen-scavenging drugs are usually administered in a large volume of fluid, which should be taken into consideration. A regimen of 80 to 120 kcal/kg/d is a reasonable goal. The administration of insulin and glucose at 6–8 mg/kg/min, helps in catabolism reversal. The presence of glycosuria is an indication for continuation of the insulin drip at a rate that keeps glucose levels between 120 and 170 mg/dl. At the same time, protein must be temporarily (no more than 24 to 48 hours) removed from intake (PO or TPN) to avoid adding exogenous protein catabolism and nitrogen release. Supplementation of arginine serves to replace arginine not produced by the urea cycle (in addition to the partial cycle function it can stimulate) and prevents its deficiency from causing additional protein catabolism. Refeeding the patient as soon as practicable is useful because more calories can be administered this way. The use of essential amino acid formulations in feeding can reduce the amount of protein necessary to meet basic needs. Table 11-1 is extracted from Singh et al. (78) and lists the proposed protein and caloric needs for patients with UCDs.

Emergency pharmacologic management with ammonia scavengers and arginine is initiated as soon as possible by using the drug combination phenylacetate and benzoate (Ammonul; Ucyclyd Pharma), ideally while the dialysis is being arranged and the diagnostic work up is under way. These two agents are used in combination to trap nitrogen in excretable forms and are administered in 25 to 35 ml/kg of 10% dextrose in water as an initial loading dose over a period of 90 to 120 minutes. Sodium benzoate combines with glycine to make hippurate, which is excreted by the kidneys (or removed in the dialysate), and sodium phenylacetate combines with glutamine to make phenacetylglutamine, which is excreted in the urine (82,83). The body replaces these amino acids by using excess nitrogen. It is suspected that the removal of glutamine by phenylacetate has the additional benefit of removing a compound suspected of having a major role in the neurotoxicity of these disorders (49, 84–88). If dialysis is used extensively, reloading the drugs is worth considering because they are dialyzable. Arginine must also be administered continuously in the acute phase of treatment of UCDs. In addition to replenishing circulating amino acid levels, arginine can utilize those parts of the cycle not affected by genetic blocks and incorporate some nitrogen. Because arginine is the precursor for NO production, it is worth considering modification of the arginine dose downward if the patient develops vasodilation and hypotension. Table 11-2 lists doses for the acute management of these patients according to the diagnosis at the time of treatment (information extracted from Food and Drug Administration package insert). Because of the potential for toxicity of these drugs, consultation with an experienced metabolic physician is recommended before starting treatment. A resource for finding these physicians and other treatment suggestions is the NIH-sponsored Urea Cycle Disorders Consortium found at http://www.rarediseasesnetwork.org/ucdc.

After the initial loading phase and dialysis, maintenance infusions of the same dose of the ammonia scavengers listed in Table 11-2 should be given over a period of 24 hours. If the exact enzyme defect is known the amount of arginine administered can be adjusted downward in patients with NAGS, CPSI, or OTC deficiency. Citrulline should be started in patients who tolerate nasogastric feedings if NAGS, CPSI, or OTC deficiency is diagnosed.

OTHER TREATMENT ISSUES

In all instances intensive care treatment must be meticulous. Ventilator or circulatory support may be required as well as anticonvulsive medication. Antibiotic therapy and a septic work up are recommended because sepsis is an important consideration in the differential diagnosis in the primary presentation and may be present leading

TABLE 11-1	Recommended Daily Nutrient Intakes (Ranges) for Infants, Children, and Adults With UCDs			
Age	Protein (g/kg)	Nutrient Patient Intake (kcal/kg)	Kcal Energy (kcal/kg)	Fluid (mL/kg)
Infants				
0 to < 3 mo	2.20–1.25	150–101	150–125	60–130
3 to < 6 mo	2.00–1.15	100–80	140–120	160–130
9 to < 12 mo	1.60–0.90	80–75	120–110	130–120
Girls and Boys	(g/d)	(kcal/d)	(kcal/d)	(mL/d)
1 to < 4 yr	8–12	800–1040	945–1890	945–1890
4 to < 7 yr	12–15	1196–1435	1365–2415	1365–2445
7 to < 11 yr	14–17	1199–1693	1730–3465	1730–3465
Women				
11 to < 15 yr	20–23		1575–3150	1575–3150
15 to < 19 yr	20–23		1260–3150	1260–3150
≥ 19 yr	22–25		1785–2625	1875–2625
Men				
11 to < 15 yr	20–23		2100–3885	2100–3885
15 to < 19 yr	21–24		2200–4095	2200–4095
≥ 19 yr	23–32		2625–3465	2625–3465

TABLE 11-2 Ammonul Dosage and Administration Summary Table

Patient Population	Ammonul	Components of Infusion Solution			Dosage Provided		
		Arg HCl Injection, 10%	Dextrose Injection, 10%	Sodium Phenylacetate	Sodium Benzoate	Arg HCl
Neonates to Young Children							
NAGS, CPS, and OTC Deficiency							
Loading Dose (90 min)	2.5 mL/kg	2.0 mL/kg	$\geq$ 25 mL/kg	250 mg/kg	250 mg/kg	200 mg/kg
Maintenance Dose	2.5 mL/kg/24 h	2.0 mL/kg/24 h	$\geq$ 25 mL/kg	250 mg/kg/24 h	250 mg/kg/24 h	200 mg/kg/24 h
Unknown, ASD, and ASL Deficiency							
Loading Dose (90 min)	2.5 mL/kg	6.0 mL/kg	$\geq$ 25 mL/kg	250 mg/kg	250 mg/kg	600 mg/kg
Maintenance Dose	2.5 mL/kg/24 h	6.0 mL/kg/24 h	$\geq$ 25 mL/kg	250 mg/kg/24 h	250 mg/kg/24 h	600 mg/kg/24 h
Older Children and Adults:							
NAGS, CPS, and OTC Deficiency							
Loading Dose (90 min)	55 mL/m^2	2.0 mL/kg	$\geq$ 25 mL/kg	5.5 g/m^2	5.5 g/m^2	200 mg/kg
Maintenance Dose	55 mL/m^2/24 h	2.0 mL/kg/24 h	$\geq$ 25 mL/kg	5.5 g/m^2/24 h	5.5 g/m^2/24 h	200 mg/kg/24 h
Unknown, ASD and ASL Deficiency							
Loading Dose (90 min)	55 mL/m^2	6.0 mL/kg	$\geq$ 25 mL/kg	5.5 g/m^2	5.5 g/m^2	600 mg/kg
Maintenance Dose	55 mL/m^2/24 h	6.0 mL/kg/24 h	$\geq$ 25 mL/kg	5.5 g/m^2/24 h	5.5 g/m^2/24 h	600 mg/kg/24 h

to further catabolism. Electrolytes and acid base balance are to be checked every 6 hours. The use of osmotic agents such as mannitol is not thought to be effective in treating the cerebral edema from hyperammonemia but this is mainly anecdotal. In canines, opening the blood–brain barrier with mannitol resulted in cerebral edema by promoting the entry of ammonia into the brain fluid compartment (50,89). Intravenous steroids (because of their catabolic properties) and valproic (due to its mitochondrial toxicity) acid must be avoided. Measures to reduce cerebral metabolism to protect the brain, such as head cooling, have been proposed but their efficacy is untested. Other measures include physiologic support (pressors, buffering agents to maintain pH and buffer arginine HCl, etc.) and maintenance of renal output, particularly if ammonia scavengers are being used. Finally, it is imperative to reassess continuation of care after the initial phase of treatment.

Rapid response to the hyperammonemia is indispensable for a good outcome (2,48). Symptomatology centers around cerebral edema and pressure on the brainstem. The resulting decrease in cerebral blood flow plus prolonged seizures, when they occur, are poor prognostic factors. In adults, because the sutures of the skull are fused, sensitivity to hyperammonemia appears considerably greater than in children. Thus treatment should be aggressive and intensified at a lower ammonia concentration than in children.

Neurologic Evaluation

Cerebral studies should be conducted to determine the efficacy of treatment and whether continuation is warranted. Electroencephalography should be performed because so many of these patients develop status epilepticus. If available, magnetic resonance imaging–determined cerebral blood flow can be used to establish whether venous stasis has occurred from cerebral edema. Evaluation of brain stem function and higher cortical function is useful to assess outcome. Finally, the decision about continuation of treatment is dependent on baseline neurologic status, duration of the patient's coma and potential for recovery, and whether the patient is a candidate for transplantation. If the basic urea cycle defect is severe enough then liver transplantation should be considered. Criteria for transplantation are of course linked back to neurologic status, duration of coma, and availability of a suitable organ. Diagnostic samples of DNA, liver, and skin should be obtained because they can be essential in family counseling and future treatment issues.

MAINTENANCE THERAPY

Long-term maintenance therapy of UCD consists of protein restriction provided by a mix of intact dietary protein and medical foods made up primarily of essential amino acids and appropriate titration of nitrogen-scavenging medications, energy intake, and vitamin and mineral supplements. Maintenance of protein intake should address the specific enzyme defect (patients with OTC or CPS may require the most protein restriction, and be tailored to the clinical picture of the patient (i.e., growth rate; weight gain; head circumference; plasma ammonia and amino-acids; hematocrit; total protein and albumin; serum prealbumin and transferrin) (78,90). The physician and nutritionist should be aware that even the most carefully created nutritional treatment plan will often be confounded by the individual patient's noncompliance which can be due to a host of external factors such as lifestyle, eating behaviors, socio-economic issues, etc. A protein and caloric intake by age nutritional plan is outlined in general terms in Table 11-1, as the intake will need to be adjusted depending on the defect. In addition to very low protein foods, non-protein energy sources such as protein-free diet powder (e.g. Product 80,056; Mead Johnson) and protein-free diet powder with iron (e.g. ProPhree) play an important role in ensuring caloric intake. G-tube placement may be required in an infant who eats poorly.

Chronic therapy with ammonia scavenger drugs includes the administration of the oral prodrug of phenylacetate, phenylbutyrate (Buphenyl). The usual total daily dose of Buphenyl tablets and powder for patients with UCDs is 450 to 600 mg/kg/day in patients weighing less than 20 kg or 9.9 to 13 g/m^2/day in larger patients. The tablets and powder are to be taken in equally divided amounts with each meal or feeding (i.e., three to six times per day).

Phenylbutyrate should be used with caution during pregnancy. Citrulline supplementation is recommended for patients diagnosed with NAGS, CPSI or OTC deficiency; citrulline daily intake is recommended at 0.17 g/kg/day or 3.8 g/m^2/day; some argue that patients may require higher citrulline dosage or supplementation with arginine in order to maintain acceptable glutamine levels (91). The drawback of using arginine instead of citrulline in patients with OTC or CPS is that the waste nitrogen atom from aspartate (the second nitrogen atom normally incorporated into urea) used in the ASS reaction is not used. Arginine supplementation is needed for patients diagnosed with ASL or ASS deficiency; arginine (free base) daily intake is recommended at 0.4 to 0.7 g/kg/day or 8.8 to 15.4 g/m^2/day; larger doses of up to 0.7 g/kg/day may be given to neonates but it is unclear whether such large doses are necessary in older patients (92). In ASL deficiency arginine supplementation not only maintains adequate arginine levels but also increases production of ASS, thus enhancing urinary excretion of waste nitrogen in the form of ASS. In patients with NAGS, the use of carbamyl glutamate has been demonstrated to be very effective (93).

LONG-TERM MANAGEMENT

Every effort should be made to avoid triggering events. It is imperative to prevent or quickly interrupt a catabolic state at an early stage of impending decompensation during subsequent illnesses or surgeries, as well as during any event resulting in significant bleeding or tissue damage. In addition, growth spurt, menses, pregnancy, childbirth, and the use of valproic, chemotherapy or glucocorticoids may induce catabolic state and precipitate a hyperammonemic episode. It is essential to educate the family to recognize the earliest signs and symptoms of hyperammonemia such as anorexia, vomiting, confusion, altered behavior, headache, ataxia, lethargy and visual disturbances and how to react adequately. During times of stress and increased catabolism due to acquired illness, such as febrile viral syndrome, some of the measures taken by the family in addition to calling their pediatrician and the metabolic specialist, may include a decrease in protein intake by 50% to 100% , an increase of non-protein calories by 25% to 50%, an increase in the dosage of the scavenging medications by 50%, an increase in fluid intake from 1 × to 1.5 × normal maintenance levels and aggressive treatment of the underlying illness. The threshold for seeking emergency room attention should be low. If symptoms do not disappear within 24 to 48 hours, the patient should be evaluated at the ER; if there is any progression of these symptoms, help should be sought immediately. (78,80,94,95,99–101, 115). During elective surgeries the patient should be admitted to the hospital on the day before the surgery. At this time a plasma ammonia and quantitative aminoacids should be requested to ensure that the patient is in good metabolic control before surgery. During surgery intravenous fluids containg 10% glucose solution at 1.5 times maintenance should be used. If the surgery is prolonged intralipids and aminoacids(at 0.7g/kg/day) should be administered along with glucose and maintenance dose of intravenous sodium benzoate and sodium phenylacetate (Ammonul) as well as arginine chloride. All patients should carry an emergency card or bracelet containing essential information and phone numbers as well as instructions on emergency measures. Every patient should be attached to a hospital with a dedicated team of metabolic specialists that can be reached at any time. For holidays it is prudent to enquire about metabolic services in the respective region.

Clinical and laboratory monitoring at regular intervals is important to ensure adequate protein intake and optimal metabolic control. Clinical parameters to be monitored include weight gain, growth rate, head circumference, liver size, appearance of the hair, skin and nails, and neuropsychological evaluation starting at one year of age. In severe ALS deficiency the enlargement of the liver may persist in spite of adequate treatment and may eventually become cirrhotic. Laboratory evaluation usually includes plasma ammonia, quantitative aminoacids, liver enzymes and total protein, albumin, prealbumin and transferrin. Hematocrit should be assessed yearly. The biochemical targets for optimal control includes a plasma ammonia level of less tan 40 µmol/L and a plasma glutamine level of less than 1000 µmol/L, normal levels of the essential aminoacids, especially the branched chain aminoacids such as leucine,valine and isoleucine and normal transferrin and prealbumin levels; decreased levels of the two latter proteins signal incipient protein deficiency. Of note, some patients appear to maintain good metabolic control with higher than 1000 µmol/L glutamine levels. The ideal level of plasma arginine is said to be between 50–200 µmol/L (90) but some physicians advocate 90–200 µmol/L levels. Patients should also avoid dehydration, an especially common occurrence among adults in connection with alcohol intake, hiking, and airline flights. Not all adult patients who recover from a hyperammonemic episode require chronic nitrogen scavengers, but they ought to be considered because many of these patients can become more brittle as time goes on. In particular, intravenous steroids for asthma or valproic acid are contraindicated.

Should psychiatric problems occur over the long term, caregivers should be alert to the possibility of hyperammonemia, either acute requiring attention or chronic and the damage done thereby. In addition, many patients with citrullinemia II have presented with mental disturbance (44,45).

Clinical observation of patients with ASL demonstrate that they have a high incidence of chronic, progressive cirrhosis with eventual fibrosis of the liver. This finding is not commonly seen in the other UCDs (although there are allegorical reports of such events in ARG1 deficient patients) and studies are underway to better determine the exact pathophysiology. It is important to provide genetic counseling to assess risk to other family members. Liver transplantation is considered in patients with severe disease as in OTC or CPS deficiencies, and very poor prognosis, progressive liver disease leading to cirrhosis and liver failure as may be seen in neonatal ASL deficiency, recurrent episodes of decompensation and life threatening complications that are not well controlled by medical means (97).

NEW DIRECTIONS IN UREA CYCLE RESEARCH

Polymorphisms and mutations in CPSI, the rate-limiting portion of the urea cycle, are an excellent model with which to apply the concept of environmental–genetic interaction (103). As shown in Figure 11-1, the urea cycle interacts with the production of NO and is the major source for arginine, which is NO's direct precursor. The effect of these changes on intermediates and subsequent NO formation modifies a number of pathophysiologic systems (97,8,9,11,12). This idea of genetic and environmental interaction is not new; however, CPSI provides an excellent example of this concept. Commonly distributed functional polymorphisms in CPSI may not result in hyperammonemia, but instead affect the production of downstream metabolic intermediates during key periods of need. Under duress, shortages of these precursor molecules uncouple NO synthase from the generation of NO. In addition to resulting in a paucity of NO, the enzyme can continue to donate electrons and generate more free radicals resulting in further damage. These findings may play a role in the pathophysiology of surgically related pulmonary hypertension, bone marrow transplant toxicity, blood pressure regulation, and asthma (97,9,11,12,34,98).

SUMMARY

The urea cycle provides an excellent model for the understanding of inborn errors of metabolism. Defects throughout the cycle affect a variety of molecular mechanisms including catalytic enzymes, cofactor producers, and transport proteins. The timely diagnosis and treatment of these diseases directly affects the outcome of the patient, and awareness by the clinician is paramount. In addition to their clinical impact as inborn errors, mild defects in the urea cycle may also affect the production of NO under physiologically stressful conditions. The availability of urea cycle intermediates, developed for the treatment of the rare diseases, in the treatment of these more common conditions may have consequences well beyond the limited number of urea cycle–deficient patients.

REFERENCES

1. Krebs HA, Henseleit K. Untersuchungen uber die harnstoffbildung im tierkorper. Hoppe-Seyler's Z Physiol Chem. 1932;210:325–332.
2. Brusilow SW. Disorders of the urea cycle. Hosp Pract. (Office Edition) 1985;20:65–72.
3. Caldovic L, Morizono H, Gracia PM, et al. Cloning and expression of the human N-acetylglutamate synthase gene. Biochem Biophys Res Commun. 2002;299(4):581–586.
4. Cederbaum SD, Yu H, Grody WW, et al. Arginases I and II: do their functions overlap? Mol Genet Metab. 2004;81 (Suppl 1):S38–S44.
5. Jackson MJ, Beaudet AL, O'Brien WE. Mammalian urea cycle enzymes. [Review]. Annu Rev Genet. 1986;20:431–464.
6. Saheki T, Kobayashi K, Iijima M, et al. Adult-onset type II citrullinemia and idiopathic neonatal hepatitis caused by citrin deficiency: involvement of the aspartate glutamate carrier for urea synthesis and maintenance of the urea cycle. Mol Genet Metab. 2004;81 (Suppl 1):S20–S26.
7. Shambaugh GE. Urea biosynthesis I. The urea cycle and relationships to the citric acid cycle. [Review]. Am J Clin Nutr. 1977;30:2083–2087.
8. Summar ML, Hall LD, Eeds AM, et al. Characterization of genomic structure and polymorphisms in the human carbamyl phosphate synthetase I gene. Gene. 2003;311:51–57.
9. Pearson DL, Dawling S, Walsh WF, et al. Neonatal pulmonary hypertension—urea-cycle intermediates, nitric oxide production, and carbamoyl-phosphate synthetase function. N Engl J Med. 2001;344(24):1832–1838.
10. Summar M. Molecular genetic research into carbamyl phosphate synthetase. I: Molecular defects, prenatal diagnosis, and cDNA sequence. J Inherit Metab Dis. 1998;21:30–39.
11. Summar ML, Hall L, Christman B, et al. Environmentally determined genetic expression: clinical correlates with molecular variants of carbamyl phosphate synthetase I. Mol Genet Metab. 2004;81Suppl:12–19.
12. Summar ML, Gainer JV, Pretorius M, et al. Relationship between carbamoyl-phosphate synthetase genotype and systemic vascular function. Hypertension. 2004;43(2):186–191.
13. Britton HG, Garcia-Espana A, Goya P, et al. A structure-reactivity study of the binding of acetylglutamate to carbamoyl phosphate synthetase I. Eur J Biochem. 1990;188:47–53.
14. Guy HI, Evans DR. Function of the major synthetase subdomains of carbamyl-phosphate synthetase. J Biol Chem. 1996;271:13762–13769.
15. Guy HI, Evans DR. Substructure of the amidotransferase domain of mammalian carbamyl phosphate synthetase. J Biol Chem. 1995;270:2190–2197.
16. Mareya SM, Raushel FM. Mapping the structural domains of E. coli carbamoyl phosphate synthetase using limited proteolysis. Bioorg Med Chem. 1995;3:525–532.
17. Powers-Lee SG, Corina K. Domain structure of rat liver carbamoyl phosphate synthetase I. J Biol Chem. 1986;261:15349–15352.
18. Rubio V, Cervera J. The carbamoyl-phosphate synthase family and carbamate kinase: structure-function studies. [Review]. Biochem Soc Trans. 1995;23:879–883.
19. Rubio V. Structure-function studies in carbamoyl phosphate synthetases. [Review]. Biochem Soc Trans. 1993;21:198–202.
20. Tuchman M, McCullough BA, Yudkoff M. The molecular basis of ornithine transcarbamylase deficiency. Eur J Pediatr. 2000;159(Suppl 3):S196–S198.
21. Tuchman M, Jaleel N, Morizono H, et al. Mutations and polymorphisms in the human ornithine transcarbamylase gene. Hum Mutat. 2002;19(2):93–107.
22. Yeh SJ, Hou WL, Tsai WS, et al. Ornithine transcarbamylase deficiency. J Formosan Med Assoc. 1997;96(1):43–45.
23. Solomonson LP, Flam BR, Pendleton LC, et al. The caveolar nitric oxide synthase/arginine regeneration system for NO production in endothelial cells. J Exp Biol. 2003;206 (Pt 12):2083–2087.
24. Beaudet AL, Su TS, O'Brien WE, et al. Dispersion of argininosuccinate-synthetase-like human genes to multiple autosomes and the X chromosome. Cell. 1982;30(1):287–293.
25. Takiguchi M, Matsubasa T, Amaya Y, et al. Evolutionary aspects of urea cycle enzyme genes. Bioessays. 1989;10(5):163–166.
26. Abramson RD, Barbosa P, Kalumuck K, et al. Characterization of the human argininosuccinate lyase gene and analysis of exon skipping. Genomics. 1991;10(1): 126–132.
27. Barbosa P, Cialkowski M, O'Brien WE. Analysis of naturally occurring and site-directed mutations in the argininosuccinate lyase gene. J Biol Chem. 1991;266(8):5286–5290.
28. Linnebank M, Tschiedel E, Haberle J, et al. Argininosuccinate lyase (ASL) deficiency: mutation analysis in 27 patients and a completed structure of the human ASL gene. Hum Genet. 2002;111(4-5):350–359.
29. Ash DE, Scolnick LR, Kanyo ZF, et al. Molecular basis of hyperargininemia: structure-function consequences of mutations in human liver arginase. Mol Genet Metab. 1998;64(4):243–249.
30. Cederbaum SD, Spector EB. Arginase activity in fibroblasts. Am J Hum Genet. 1978;30(1):91–92.
31. Dizikes GJ, Grody WW, Kern RM, et al. Isolation of human liver arginase cDNA and demonstration of nonhomology between the two human arginase genes. Biochem Biophys Res Commun. 1986;141(1):53–59.
32. Dizikes GJ, Spector EB, Cederbaum SD. Cloning of rat liver arginase cDNA and elucidation of regulation of arginase gene expression in H4 rat hepatoma cells. Somat Cell Mol Genet. 1986;12(4):375–384.
33. Grody WW, Dizikes GJ, Cederbaum SD. Human arginase isozymes. Isozymes Curr Top Biol Med Res. 1987;13:181–214.
34. Meurs H, Maarsingh H, Zaagsma J. Arginase and asthma: novel insights into nitric oxide homeostasis and airway hyper-responsiveness. Trends Pharmacol Sci 2003; 24(9):450–455.
35. Ricciardolo FL. cNOS-iNOS paradigm and arginase in asthma. Trends Pharmacol Sci. 2003;24(11):560–561.
36. Rudmann DG, Moore MW, Tepper JS, et al. Modulation of allergic inflammation in mice deficient in TNF receptors. Am J Physiol Lung Cell Mol Physiol. 2000;279(6): L1047–L1057.
37. Caldovic L, Tuchman M. N-acetylglutamate and its changing role through evolution. Biochem J. 2003;372(Pt 2):279–290.
38. Caldovic L, Morizono H, Yu X, et al. Identification, cloning and expression of the mouse N-acetylglutamate synthase gene. Biochem J. 2002;364(Pt 3):825–831.
39. Tuchman M, Holzknecht RA. Human hepatic N-acetylglutamate content and N-acetylglutamate synthase activity. Determination by stable isotope dilution. Biochem J. 1990;271(2):325–329.
40. Ben Shalom E, Kobayashi K, Shaag A, et al. Infantile citrullinemia caused by citrin deficiency with increased dibasic amino acids. Mol Genet Metab. 2002;77(3):202–208.
41. Naito E, Ito M, Matsuura S, et al. Type II citrullinaemia (citrin deficiency) in a neonate with hypergalactosaemia detected by mass screening. J Inherit Metab Dis. 2002;25(1):71–76.
42. Ohura T, Kobayashi K, Abukawa D et al. A novel inborn error of metabolism detected by elevated methionine and/or galactose in newborn screening: neonatal intrahepatic cholestasis caused by citrin deficiency. Eur J Pediatr. 2003;162(5):317–322.
43. Saheki T, Kobayashi K, Iijima M, et al. Adult-onset type II citrullinemia and idiopathic neonatal hepatitis caused by citrin deficiency: involvement of the aspartate glutamate carrier for urea synthesis and maintenance of the urea cycle. Mol Genet Metab. 2004;81 (Suppl 1):S20–S26.
44. Saheki T, Kobayashi K. Mitochondrial aspartate glutamate carrier (citrin) deficiency as the cause of adult-onset type II citrullinemia (CTLN2) and idiopathic neonatal hepatitis (NICCD). J Hum Genet. 2002;47(7): 333–341.
45. Tamamori A, Okano Y, Ozaki H et al. Neonatal intrahepatic cholestasis caused by citrin deficiency: severe hepatic dysfunction in an infant requiring liver transplantation. Eur J Pediatr. 2002;161(11):609–613.
46. Yamaguchi N, Kobayashi K, Yasuda T, et al. Screening of SLC25A13 mutations in early and late onset patients with citrin deficiency and in the Japanese population: Identification of two novel mutations and establishment of multiple DNA diagnosis methods for nine mutations. Hum Mutat. 2002;19(2):122–130.

47. Batshaw ML. Hyperammonemia. Curr Prob Pediatr. 1984;14:1–69.
48. Brusilow SW. Urea cycle disorders: clinical paradigm of hyperammonemic encephalopathy. Prog Liver Dis. 1995;13:293–309.
49. Butterworth RF. Effects of hyperammonaemia on brain function. [Review]. J Inherit Metab Dis. 1998;21 (Suppl 1):6–20.
50. Fujiwara M. Role of ammonia in the pathogenesis of brain edema. Acta Med Okayama. 1986;40(6):313–320.
51. Takahashi H, Koehler RC, Hirata T, et al. Restoration of cerebrovascular CO2 responsivity by glutamine synthesis inhibition in hyperammonemic rats. Circ Res. 1992;71(5):1220–1230.
52. Tuchman M, Mauer SM, Holzknecht RA, et al. Prospective versus clinical diagnosis and therapy of acute neonatal hyperammonaemia in two sisters with carbamyl phosphate synthetase deficiency. J Inherit Metab Dis. 1992;15:269–277.
53. Rowe PC, Newman SL, Brusilow SW. Natural history of symptomatic partial ornithine transcarbamylase deficiency. New Eng. J. Med. 1986; 314: 541–547.
54. Yorifuji T, Muroi J, Uematsu A, et al. X-inactivation pattern in the liver of a manifesting female with ornithine transcarbamylase (OTC) deficiency. Clin. Genet. 1998; 54: 349–353.
55. Lee JY, Chang SE, Suh CW, et al. A case of acrodermatitis enteropathica-like dermatosis caused by ornithine transcarbamylase deficiency. J. Am. Acad. Derm. 2002; 46: 965–967.
56. Mitchell RB, Wagner JE, Karp JE, et al. Syndrome of idiopathic hyperammonemia after high-dose chemotherapy: review of nine cases [see comments]. Am J Med. 1988;85:662–667.
57. Batshaw ML, Brusilow SW. Valproate-induced hyperammonemia. Ann Neurol. 1982;11:319–321.
58. Bourrier P, Varache N, Alquier P, et al. [Cerebral edema with hyperammonemia in valpromide poisoning. Manifestation in an adult, of a partial deficit in type I carbamylphosphate synthetase]. [French]. Presse Med. 1988;17:2063–2066.
59. Castro-Gago M, Rodrigo-Saez E, Novo-Rodriguez I, et al. Hyperaminoacidemia in epileptic children treated with valproic acid. Childs Nerv Syst. 1990;6:434–436.
60. Elgudin L, Hall Y, Schubert D. Ammonia induced encephalopathy from valproic acid in a bipolar patient: case report. Int J Psychiatry Med. 2003;33(1):91–96.
61. Kugoh T, Yamamoto M, Hosokawa K. Blood ammonia level during valproic acid therapy. Jpn J Psychiatry Neurol. 1986;40(4):663–668.
62. Vainstein G, Korzets Z, Pomeranz A, et al. Deepening coma in an epileptic patient: the missing link to the urea cycle. Hyperammonaemic metabolic encephalopathy. Nephrol Dial Transplant. 2002;17(7):1351–1353.
63. Cordero DR, Baker J, Dorinzi D , et al. Ornithine transcarbamylase deficiency in pregnancy. J. Inherit. Metab. Dis.2005;28:237–240.

64. Camacho JA, Obie C, Biery B, et al. Hyperornithinaemia-hyperammonaemia-homocitrullinuria syndrome is caused by mutations in a gene encoding a mitochondrial ornithine transporter. Nature Genet. 1999;22: 151–158.
65. Salvi S, Santorelli FM, Bertini E, et al. Clinical and molecular findings in hyperornithinemia-hyperammonemia-homocitrullinuria syndrome. Neurology 57 2001; 911–914.
66. Lemay JF, Lambert MA, Mitchell, GA, et al. Hyperammonemia-hyperornithinemia-homocitrullinuria syndrome: neurologic, ophthalmologic, and neuropsychologic examination of 6 patients. J. Pediat. 1992;121: 725–730.
67. Saheki T, Kobayashi K. Physiological role of citrin , a liver-type mitochondrial aspartate-glutamate carrier, and pathophysiology of citrin sdeficiency. Recent Res. Devel Life Sci.2005;3:1–15.
68. Tazawa Y, Kobayashi K, Abukawa D, et al. Clinical heterogeneity of neonatal intrahepatic cholestasis caused by citrin deficiency: case reports from 16 patients. Mol Genet Metab. 2004;83:213–219.
69. Hashisu m, Oda Y, Goto m, et al. Citrin deficiency presenting with ketotic hypoglycemia and hepatomegaly in chilhood. Eur J Pediatr.2005;164:109–110.
70. Lee NC, Chien YH, Kobayashi K, et al. Time course of acylcarnitine elevation in neonatal intrahepatic cholestasis caused by citrin deficiency. J Inherit Metab Dis. 2006;29:551–555.
71. Cederbaum SD, Shaw KN, Valente M. Hyperargininemia. J Pediatr. 1977;90(4): 569–573.
72. Iyer R, Jenkinson CP, Vockley JG, et al. The human arginases and arginase deficiency. J Inherit Metab Dis. 1998;21 (Suppl 1):86–100.
73. Steiner RD, Cederbaum SD. Laboratory evaluation of urea cycle disorders. J Pediatr. 2001; 138(1 Suppl):S21-S29.
74. Summar M. Current strategies for the management of neonatal urea cycle disorders. J Pediatr 2001; 138(1 Suppl):S30–S39.
75. Tuchman M, Tsai MY, Holzknecht RA, et al. Carbamyl phosphate synthetase and ornithine transcarbamylase activities in enzyme-deficient human liver measured by radiochromatography and correlated with outcome. Pediatr Res. 1989; 26(1):77–82.
76. Arranz JA, Riudor E, Rodes M, et al. Optimization of allopurinol challenge: Sample purification, protein intake control, and the use of oritidine response as a discriminative variable improve performance of the test for diagnosing ornithine carbamoyltransferase deficiency. Clin Chemistry 1999; 45:995–1001.
77. Summar ML. Presentation and management of urea cycle disorders outside the newborn period. Crit Care Clin. 2005;21(4 Suppl):ix.
78. Singh RH, Rhead WJ, Smith W, et al. Nutritional management of urea cycle disorders. Crit Care Clin. 2005;21(4 Suppl): S27–S35.
79. Lee B, Singh RH, Rhead WJ, et al. Considerations in the difficult-to-manage urea cycle disorder patient. Crit Care Clin. 2005; 21(4 Suppl):S19–S25.
80. Summar ML, Barr F, Dawling S, et al. Unmasked adult-onset urea cycle disorders in

the critical care setting. Crit Care Clin. 2005;21(4 Suppl):S1–S8.
81. Summar M, Pietsch J, Deshpande J, et al. Effective hemodialysis and hemofiltration driven by an extracorporeal membrane oxygenation pump in infants with hyperammonemia. J Pediatr. 1996;128(3):379–382.
82. Batshaw ML. Sodium benzoate and arginine: alternative pathway therapy in inborn errors of urea synthesis. Prog Clin Biol Res. 1983;127:69–83.
83. Batshaw ML, Brusilow SW. Evidence of lack of toxicity of sodium phenylacetate and sodium benzoate in treating urea cycle enzymopathies. J Inherit Metab Dis. 1981;4(4):231.
84. Batshaw ML, Brusilow SW. Treatment of hyperammonemic coma caused by inborn errors of urea synthesis. J Pediatr. 1980;97(6):893–900.
85. Brusilow SW, Valle DL, Batshaw M. New pathways of nitrogen excretion in inborn errors of urea synthesis. Lancet. 1979;2(8140):452–454.
86. Brusilow SW. Phenylacetylglutamine may replace urea as a vehicle for waste nitrogen excretion. Pediatr Res. 1991;29(2):147–150.
87. Connelly A, Cross JH, Gadian DG, et al. Magnetic resonance spectroscopy shows increased brain glutamine in ornithine carbamoyl transferase deficiency. Pediatr Res. 1993;33(1):77–81.
88. Willard-Mack CL, Koehler RC, Hirata T, et al. Inhibition of glutamine synthetase reduces ammonia-induced astrocyte swelling in rat. Neuroscience. 1996;71(2):589-599.
89. Fujiwara M, Watanabe A, Shiota T et al. Hyperammonemia-induced cytotoxic brain edema under osmotic opening of blood-brain barrier in dogs. Res Exp Med. (Berl) 1985;185(6):425–427.
90. Berry GT, Steiner RD. Long-term management of patients with urea cycle disorders. Jour Pediatr. 2001; 138: S56–S60.
91. Wilcken B; Problems in the managenment of urea cycle disorders. Mol Genet Metabol. 2004;81:S86–91.
92. Brusilow SW, Batshaw ML. Arginine therapy of arginosuccinate deficiency. Lancet 1979;1:124–7.
93. Morizono H, Caldovic L, Shi D, et al. Mammalian N-acetylglutamate synthase. Mol Genet Metab. 2004;81(Suppl 1):S4–11.
94. Smith W, Kishnani PS, Lee B, et al. Urea cycle disorders: clinical presentation outside the newborn period. Crit Care Clin. 2005;21(4 Suppl):S9–17.
95. Dixon MA, Leonard JV. Intercurrent illness in inborn errors of intermediary metabolism. Arch Dis Child. 1992;67:1387–1391.
96. Leonard JV, McKiernan PJ, et al. The role of liver transplantation in urea cycle disorders. Mol Genet Metabol.2003;81:s74–78.
97. Barr FE, Beverley H, VanHook K, et al. Effect of cardiopulmonary bypass on urea cycle intermediates and nitric oxide levels after congenital heart surgery. J Pediatr. 2003;142(1):26–30.
98. Williams SM, Ritchie MD, Phillips III JA, et al. Multilocus analysis of hypertension: a hierarchical approach. Hum Hered. 2004;57(1):28–38.

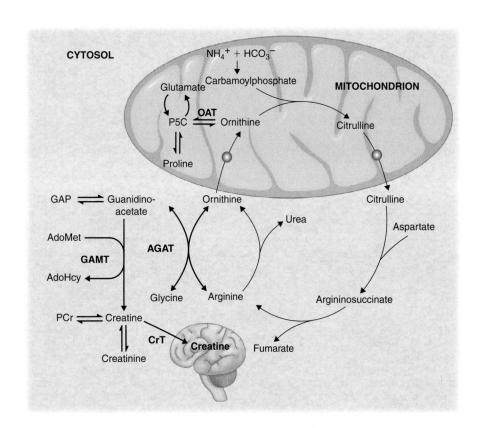

CHAPTER 12

Creatine Deficiency Syndromes

Andreas Schulze, MD, FRCPC

INTRODUCTION

Hereditary defects of creatine (Cr) synthesis or transport of Cr into the brain are described as Cr deficiency syndromes (CDSs). The group of CDSs consists of three different diseases: arginine:glycine amidinotransferase (AGAT), guanidinoacetate methyltransferase (GAMT), and Cr transporter (CrT) deficiency. The common denominator of all these diseases is the virtually complete absence of Cr and phosphocreatine (PCr) mainly in brain. All CDSs have been discovered recently. Gyrate atrophy of choroid and retina represents an additional condition that may be added on to the CDSs because Cr deficiency is part of clinical appearance in gyrate atrophy.

Etiology/Pathophysiology The Cr/PCr system plays an important role in energy buffering and transmission. In addition to the mitochondrial and cytosolic Cr kinase system for shuttle of high-energy phosphates, synthesis and transport of Cr are integral parts of cellular energy metabolism.

Cr is taken up from the food by intestinal absorption and is synthesized endogenously, mainly in the kidneys, pancreas, and liver. Endogenous cytosolic Cr synthesis consists of two enzyme reactions (Figure 12-1). In the first step, the L-arginine:glycine amidinotransferase (AGAT) catalyzes the reversible transamidination of the guanidino group from arginine to glycine yielding guanidinoacetate and ornithine. The AGAT reaction is the rate-limiting step in Cr biosynthesis. Guanidinoacetate formation by AGAT is negatively controlled by high concentrations of guanidinoacetate, Cr, and ornithine. In the second step, the S-adenosylmethionine: guanidinoacetate N-methyltransferase (GAMT) catalyzes the S-adenosyl-L-methionine–dependent methylation of guanidinoacetate to yield Cr and S-adenosyl-L-homocysteine. Cr is transported through the blood and is taken up into Cr-requiring tissues against a large concentration gradient (plasma [Cr]

$\sim$50 μM; intracellular [Cr + PCr] up to 40 mM). Uptake into the tissues is accomplished by a Na$^+$- and Cl$^-$-dependent Cr transporter (CrT). Cr and PCr are nonenzymatically converted at an almost constant rate ($\sim$1.7%/d) into creatinine, which passively diffuses out of the cells and is excreted by the kidneys into the urine. The urinary creatinine excretion therefore represents a convenient indicator of the total Cr stores in the body. A 70-kg man contains approximately 120 g Cr, of which more than 90% is found in muscle tissue (1). For maintenance of the body Cr concentration, 1 to 2 g of Cr, which is equivalent to the amount of urinary excreted creatinine, must be provided through diet and endogenous synthesis.

ARGININE:GLYCINE AMIDINOTRANSFERASE DEFICIENCY

Etiology/Pathophysiology AGAT deficiency is a recently recognized, rare, autosomal recessive inborn error of creatinine metabolism caused by a defect in the AGAT gene, which has been mapped to chromosome 15q15.3 (2).

FIGURE 12-1. The metabolic pathway of Cr/PCr. AdoHcy, S-adenosylhomocysteine; AdoMet, S-adenosylmethionine; AGAT, arginine:glycine amidinotransferase; CrT, creatine transporter; GAMT, guanidinoacetate methyltransferase; GAP, guanidino-acetophosphate; OAT, Ornithine-Δ-aminotransferase; P5C, Δ1-pyrroline-5-carboxylate; PCr, phosphocreatine. Adapted with permission from Schulze (1).

Creatine Deficiency Syndromes

AT-A-GLANCE

Hereditary defects of creatine synthesis or transport of creatine into the brain are described as creatine deficiency syndromes (CDSs). The group of CDSs consists of three different diseases: AGAT, GAMT, and CrT deficiency. The common denominator of all these diseases is the virtually complete absence of creatine and phosphocreatine, mainly in the brain. Developmental delay, severe speech disturbance, and mental retardation are common symptoms. GAMT deficiency has the most severe clinical phenotype, additionally presenting with an extrapyramidal movement disorder and drug-resistant seizures. Replenishment of creatine and (in GAMT deficiency) lowering of guanidinoacetate are the goals of treatment. Gyrate atrophy of the choroid and retina represents an additional condition that may be added to the CDSs because creatine deficiency is part of the clinical appearance. Gyrate atrophy is a metabolic disease of the eyes with slowly progressive chorioretinal degeneration and hyperornithinemia. Treatment is directed toward lowering of ornithine.

All CDSs are inherited monogenic diseases with autosomal recessive traits except for CrT deficiency, which is X-linked.

TYPES OF CDS	OCCURRENCE	GENE	LOCUS	OMIM
Arginine:glycine amidinotransferase def. (AGAT)	Very Rare	AGAT	15q15.3	602360
Guanidinoacetate methyltransferase def. (GAMT)	Rare	GAMT	19p13.3	601240
X-linked Creatine transporter def. (CrT)	Rare	SLC6A8	Xq28	300352
Gyrate atrophy due to ornithine Δ-aminotransferase def. (OAT)	Rare	OAT	10q26	258870

FORM	FINDINGS	CLINICAL PRESENTATION	TREATMENT
AGAT	↓ GAA (P,U,CSF*) ↓ Cr/PCr (brain MRS) ↓ Cr (P,24-h-U,CSF*) ↓ Crn (24-h-U,CSF*) Nl- ↓ Crn (S) ↑ organic acids (U)	Developmental delay, speech disturbance, and mental retardation.	Creatine monohydrate 400 mg/kg/d
GAMT	↑ GAA (P,U,CSF) ↓ Cr/PCr (brain MRS) ↓ Cr (P,U,CSF) ↓ Crn (24-h-U,CSF) Nl- ↓ Crn (S) ↑ organic acids (U)	Developmental delay, severe speech disturbance, severe mental retardation are obligatory. Drug-resistant epilepsy, dystonic-dyskinetic movements, autistic self aggressive behavior are facultative.	Creatine monohydrate 400 mg/kg/d; GAA lowering by arginine-restricted diet + ornithine supplementation
CrT	↑ Cr-to-Crn ratio (U) ↑ Cr (24-h-U) Nl- ↑ Cr (P) Nl- GAA (P,U,CSF) Nl- Crn (P,U)	In males, developmental delay, severe speech disturbance, severe mental retardation, and focal epilepsy. In females, learning disabilities or no symptoms	No treatment available.
OAT	↑ Orn (P,U,CSF) ↓ GAA (U) ↓ Cr (P,U) ↓ Crn (24-h-U) ↑ Arg,Lys,Cys (U) Nl- ↓ Lys (P)	Slowly progressive chorioretinal degeneration with myopia, night-blindness, tunnel vision, and blindness in 4th and 5th decade.	Vitamin B$_6$, and/or, ornithine lowering by arginine-restricted diet

Cr = creatine; Crn = creatinine; GAA = guanidinoacetate; MRS = magnetic resonance spectroscopy; PCr = phosphocreatine; Orn = ornithine; Arg = arginine; Lys = lysine; Cys = cystine; CSF* = no data available for patients so far; NI = normal.

The disease is caused by deficiency of AGAT. The highest concentration of the immunoreactive AGAT protein has been shown to be in the proximal tubules of the kidney; it is also present in hepatocytes and in α cells of the pancreas of the rat (3). In situ hybridization studies in adult rat brain revealed a ubiquitous neuronal and glial expression of AGAT (4). AGAT catalyzes the first and rate-limiting step in Cr biosynthesis, the reversible transamidination of the guanidino group from arginine to glycine to yield guanidinoacetate and ornithine (Figure 12-1). The block of AGAT reaction leads to decreased formation of guanidinoacetate and deficient endogenous Cr synthesis. Cr depletion is not compensated by intake of Cr with food and results in the lack of PCr mainly in brain (Figure 12-2). The symptoms in AGAT-deficient patients can be assumed to be caused by impairment of the Cr/PCr system.

Clinical Presentation Only a few patients with AGAT deficiency have been described thus far. Their symptoms are nonspecific and include developmental delay during the 1st year of life, followed by severe speech delay and mild-to-moderate mental retardation (Table 12-1).

The first cases, 4- and 6-year-old sisters, presented with mild mental retardation and severe language delay. The results of magnetic resonance imaging (MRI) of their brains were normal but proton-magnetic resonance spectroscopy (^{1}H-MRS) disclosed generalized depletion of Cr in the brains. Guanidinoacetate was low in blood and urine but plasma Cr was normal. Cr monohydrate oral administration led to almost complete brain Cr level restoration along with improvement of developmental scores (5). AGAT enzymatic activity tested in lymphoblasts was undetectable and genetic testing showed a homozygous mutation (W149X) of the AGAT gene (2). An affected cousin presented at 2 years of age with severe developmental delay, mild generalized hypotonia, poor social contact, short attention span, stereotypic movement of the hands, and speech delay. He had the same laboratory findings as the two index cases and showed clinical improvement on treatment (6). Another patient presented at 10 months of age with moderate central hypotonia, failure to thrive, and speech delay (Kathreen Johnston, personal communication).

Diagnosis Laboratory evaluation shows decreased Cr concentration in the blood and decreased guanidinoacetate in both blood and urine. There are no data available about the concentrations of Cr, creatinine, and guanidinoacetate in the cerebrospinal fluid (CSF) but they are suspected to be low. ^{1}H-MRS of the brain shows a virtually absent Cr/PCr signal. Urinary organic acid analysis

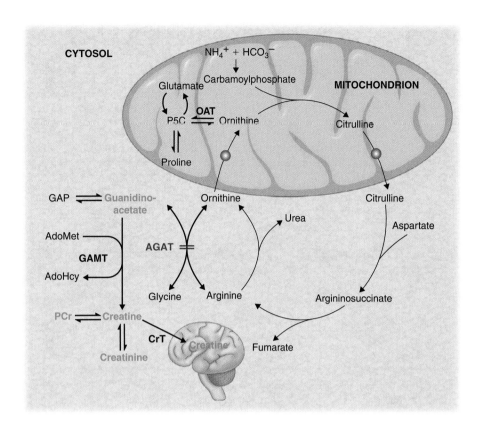

FIGURE 12-2. Snapshot AGAT (green indicates decreased).

may show elevated concentrations of organic acids and other metabolic compounds due to the fact that concentration of organic acids is expressed in millimoles per mole of creatinine and the latter is decreased because of deficient Cr synthesis. ACAT enzymatic activity can be measured in stimulated lymphocytes or fibroblasts. Genetic testing is also available. Prenatal diagnosis seems feasible by AGAT measurement in chorionic villi or

by mutation analysis if mutations are known from the index case. The diagnostic algorithm for AGAT deficiency is shown in Figure 12-3 (Table 12-2).

Treatment AGAT deficiency is treated by supplementation of Cr monohydrate (400 mg/kg/d) given with fluids or food and evenly spread over three to six times a day (7). Treatment (in two children) led to nearly

TABLE 12-1	Comparison of Symptoms in Creatine Deficiency Syndromes			
Chacteristic		GAMT-D	AGAT-D	CrT-D
Speech disturbance				
	Expressive	+++	+++	++
	Comprehensive	++	++	+
Mental retardation		+++	++	++
Therapy-refractory epilepsy		+/−	−	−
Mild epilepsy/EEG abnormalities		+	+/−	+/−
Dystonic-dyskinetic movement		+	−	−
Autistic, self-aggressive behavior		+	+/−	+/−
MRI changes *(especially of globus pallidus)*		+/−	−	−
Muscular hypotonia		+/−	+/−	+/−
Midface hypoplasia		−	−	+/−
Mild learning disability in carrier females		−	−	+/−
X-chromosomal trait		−	−	+

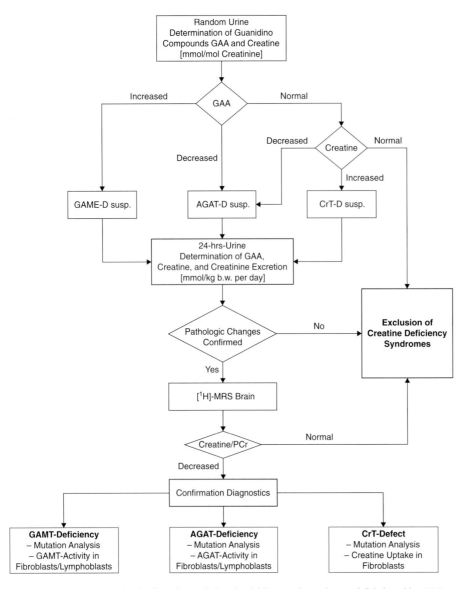

FIGURE 12-3. Diagnostic flowchart for diagnosis or exclusion of Cr deficiency syndromes in case of clinical suspicion. AGAT, arginine:glycine amidinotransferase; CrT, creatine transporter; D, deficiency; GAA, guanidinoacetate; GAMT, guanidinoacetate methyltransferase; MRS, magnetic resonance spectroscopy; PCr, phosphocreatine. Adapted with permission from Schulze (22).

complete replenishment of Cr/PCr in brain after 1.5 years of treatment and has been associated with clinical improvement, although general cognitive and language development remains delayed. Early diagnosis and initiation of treatment in the first months of life might prevent development of symptoms.

TABLE 12-2	Laboratory Findings in AGAT
Decreased	**Increased**
Guanidinoacetate (P, U, CSF*)	Organic acids (U)
Cr (P, 24-h-U, CSF*)	
Creatinine (24-h-U)	
Creatinine (P) (nl- ↓)	

CSF*: no data available for patients so far

GUANIDINOACETATE METHYLTRANSFERASE DEFICIENCY

Etiology/Pathophysiology GAMT deficiency was the first detected inborn error of Cr biosynthesis in humans (8). The GAMT gene is mapped to chromosome 19p13.3 and several mutations have been identified. The inheritance is autosomal recessive.

The disease is caused by deficiency of S-adenosyl-L-methionine:N-guanidinoacetate methyltransferase (GAMT). GAMT is most abundant in the liver, kidneys, and pancreas (9) and to a lesser extent in the brain, lymphocytes, fibroblasts, and other tissues. In situ hybridization studies in adult rat brain revealed a ubiquitous neuronal and glial expression of GAMT (4). GAMT catalyzes the S-adenosyl-L-methionine–dependent meth-

ylation of guanidinoacetate to yield Cr and S-adenosyl-L-homocysteine (Figure 12-1). The block of GAMT reaction leads to deficient endogenous Cr synthesis, accumulation of guanidinoacetate, and PCr depletion mainly in brain (Figure 12-4). Developmental delay, speech disturbance, mental retardation, muscular hypotonia, and autistic behavior of varying degrees are common to all CDSs and are probably due to the impairment of the Cr/PCr system. Severe epilepsy refractory to antiepileptic drug treatment and dyskinetic movement disorder are exclusively found in GAMT deficiency and are probably caused by accumulation of guanidinoacetate (1). Activation of γ-aminobutyric acid-A receptors, inhibition of cerebral Na$^+$/K$^+$-adenosine triphosphatase, inhibition of Cr uptake, and generation of reactive oxygen species are possible ways in which guanidinoacetate acts as neurotoxic agent (10).

The combined impact of creatine/PCr deficiency and accumulation of guanidinoacetate is responsible for the more severe clinical phenotype in GAMT deficiency.

Clinical Presentation The first patient with GAMT-D was described in 1994 (8). The clue to diagnosis was the finding of virtually absent Cr/PCr in the brain by ^{1}H-MRS. Immediately after this first description additional patients were diagnosed through in vivo ^{1}H-MRS (11,12).

Among the CDSs, GAMT deficiency is the disease with the most severe clinical phenotype (Table 12-1). The clinical presentation of GAMT-deficient patients is characterized by developmental delay at 6 to 12 months of age, developmental regression in the 2nd year of life, severe mental retardation and speech disability, muscular hypotonia, dyskinetic/dystonic involuntary movements, and seizures resistant to antiepileptic drugs. In older patients, autism with self-aggressive behavior develops. Patients who suffer milder affected of GAMT deficiency present with developmental delay, speech delay, and mild epilepsy or electroencephalographic (EEG) changes. In some patients MRI of the brain showed delayed myelination or increased signal intensity in T2-weighted images of the globus pallidus (13).

Diagnosis Guanidinoacetate is increased in urine, blood, and CSF, whereas Cr is decreased in urine, blood, and CSF. Creatinine is decreased in CSF and may be decreased or normal in blood. Creatinine excretion measured in 24-hour urinary collection is decreased.

^{1}H-MRS of the brain shows a virtually absent Cr/PCr signal (Figure 12-5). Phosphorus MRS reveals decreased PCr and appearance of a new

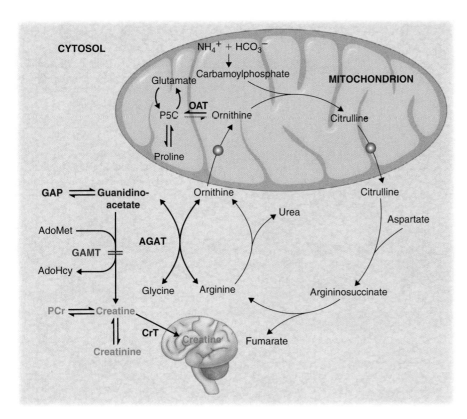

FIGURE 12-4. The defect in GAMT (Blue indicates increased precursors due to block and green indicates decreased metabolites).

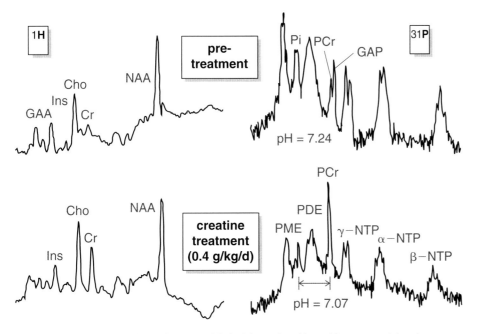

FIGURE 12-5. *In vivo* proton and phosphorus MRS of the brain in a patient with guanidinoacetate methyltransferase deficiency. GAA, guanidinoacetate; Ins, inositols; Cho, choline-containing compounds; Cr, total Cr (mainly Cr and phosphocreatine); NAA, N-acetyl-L-aspartate; Pi, inorganic phosphate; PCr, phosphocreatine; GAP, guanidinoacetophosphate; PME, phosphomonoester; PDE, phosphodiester; NTP, nucleoside 5′-triphosphate. Reproduced with permission from Schulze (1).

TABLE 12-3	Laboratory Findings in GAMT
Decreased	**Increased**
Cr (P, U, CSF)	Guanidinoacetate (P, U, CSF)
Creatinine (24-h-U, CSF)	
Creatinine (P) (NI- ↓)	Organic acids (U)
	Amino acids (U)

born screening for GAMT deficiency appears feasible by measurement of guanidinoacetate in dried blood specimens (14). Genetic testing is available. The diagnostic algorithm of GAMT deficiency is shown in Figure 12-3 (Table 12-3).

Increased guanidinoacetate in urine is pathognomonic for GAMT deficiency.

Treatment Treatment in GAMT deficiency is directed toward the replenishment of the cerebral Cr pool and reduction of guanidinoacetate (10).

Cr is supplemented as Cr monohydrate (400 mg/kg/d). Cr is given with food evenly spread in three to six portions over the day (7). Even with pharmacologic doses of Cr, replenishment of the cerebral Cr pool is not complete and takes months to years (10). The clinical response to Cr supplementation includes resolution of extrapyramidal signs and improvement of epilepsy and behavior. None of the patients assumed normal development, however, and in all patients, mental retardation and severe speech delay persisted, probably due to irreversible brain damage.

Reduction of guanidinoacetate is achieved by a semisynthetic arginine-restricted diet and supplementation of low doses of ornithine (100 mg/kg/d) and sodium benzoate (100 mg/ kg/d) (15). To restrict arginine intake, the amount of natural protein is limited to 0.4 to 0.7 g/kg/day. To meet the minimal protein requirements the patients receive a synthetic, arginine-free mixture of essential amino acids (0.7 g/kg/d in infants and children and 0.2 g/kg/d in adults). The treatment results in significant reduction of guanidinoacetate in plasma, urine, and CSF and in distinct improvement of epilepsy and behavior (15).

Further attempts to improve the clinical course or even to prevent handicaps of the disease in affected children include high-dose ornithine treatment (800 mg/kg/d) to lower guanidinoacetate levels (16) and presymptomatic disease detection and treatment initiation (14). The first results of presymptomatic treatment are very encouraging.

resonance assigned to guanidinoacetophosphate in brain and muscle (Figures 12-5 and 12-6).

Urinary organic acid analysis may reveal elevated concentrations of organic acids and other metabolic compounds because the concentration of organic acid is expressed in millimoles per mole of creatinine and the latter is decreased due to of deficient Cr.

GAMT enzymatic activity can be measured in stimulated lymphocytes or fibroblasts. New-

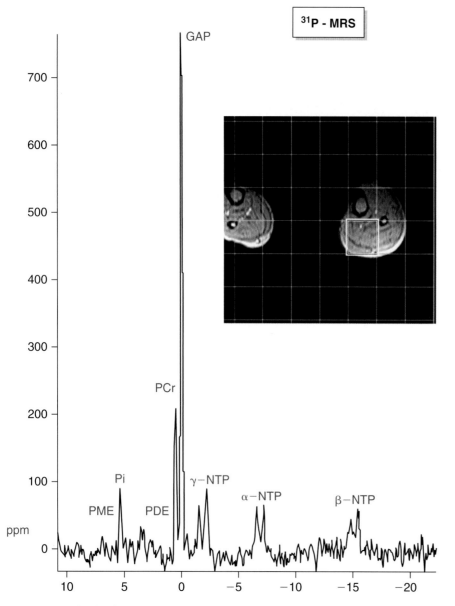

FIGURE 12-6. *In vivo* phosphorus MRS of the calve muscle in a patient with guanidinoacetate methyltransferase deficiency. PME, phosphomonoester; Pi, inorganic phosphate; PDE, phosphodiester; PCr, phosphocreatine; GAP, guanidinoacetophosphate; NTP, nucleoside 5'-triphosphate. Reproduced with permission from Schulze (1).

X-LINKED CREATINE TRANSPORTER DEFICIENCY

Etiology/Pathophysiology In 2001, the first patient having CrT deficiency was described (17) and the underlying molecular defect was identified (18).

The disease is caused by an inherited deficiency of the Na^+- and Cl^--dependent X-linked CrT. The CrT1 gene is mapped to chromosome Xq28 (19), and several mutations have been described. The CrT is a member of Solute Carrier Family 6 (neurotransmitter transporters), a sodium-dependent plasma membrane transporter family. The CrT1 gene (SLC6A8) is expressed in most tissues, with the highest levels in skeletal muscle and kidney and somewhat lower levels in colon, brain, heart, testis, and prostate (20,21). In situ hybridization studies in adult rat brain revealed the presence of the CrT1 in neurons and oligodendrocytes but not in astrocytes (4). A second CrT gene, CrT2, is expressed in testis only. The CrT is responsible for cellular Cr uptake against a huge concentration gradient of Cr. The deficiency of the CrT results in depletion of Cr and PCr mainly in brain and in increased renal Cr excretion (Figure 12-7).

- CrT deficiency is an X-linked mental retardation syndrome. In case of a family history of mental retardation in males the CrT deficiency must be considered.

Clinical Presentation Hemizygous males present with severe mental retardation and severe speech disorder. Focal seizures, failure to thrive, behavioral abnormalities, muscular hypotonia, and midface hypoplasia are additional features in some cases. Speech disorder is characterized as expressive dysphasia with impaired comprehensive speech to a lesser extent. Children learn some single words but attain no further language skills. Their behavioral abnormality is described as compulsive and in part aggressive, with some autistic features in their social contact. Facial dysmorphia presented in five adults of one family as midface hypoplasia and in one case as protrusive forehead, short nose, and low-set eye brows. The results of MRIs are normal in the majority of cases except in three patients who presented with generalized brain atrophy. Symptoms in CrT deficiency are developing during infancy and childhood with no obvious progression thereafter. A variety of other organ manifestations develop only in elderly people (e.g., chronic constipation, megacolon, gastric and duodenal ulcers, and myopathic facies). Females may be asymptomatic or may have mild cognitive delays and behavioral problems (22).

Diagnosis There is only one laboratory finding but it is highly specific and sensitive: substantially increased urinary Cr (Table 12-4). The molar ratio of Cr-to-creatinine in random urine of affected males is greater than 3.0 (normal < 1.7 in children).

^{1}H-MRS of the brain reveals a virtually absent Cr/PCr signal in brain. Cr uptake studies in fibroblasts are used for confirmation of diagnosis and to differentiate among patients, carriers, and controls. Prenatal analysis seems only feasible by mutation analysis and only if mutations are known from the index case. Genetic testing is available. The diagnostic algorithm for CrT deficiency is shown in Figure 12-3.

Treatment There is no effective treatment available for the CrT defect (7). Cr therapy fails because the transport of Cr from blood into the brain is impaired. Only in affected females, who may have different residual Cr transport capacity, supplementation with Cr (200–400 mg/kg/d) might be of benefit.

Antiepileptic treatment with valproate or carbamazepine is successful in seizure control.

TABLE 12-4	Laboratory Findings in CrT
Increased	**Normal**
Cr-to-creatinine ratio (U)	Guanidinoacetate (P, U, CSF)
Cr (24-h-U)	
Cr (P) (n−↑)	Creatinine (P, U)

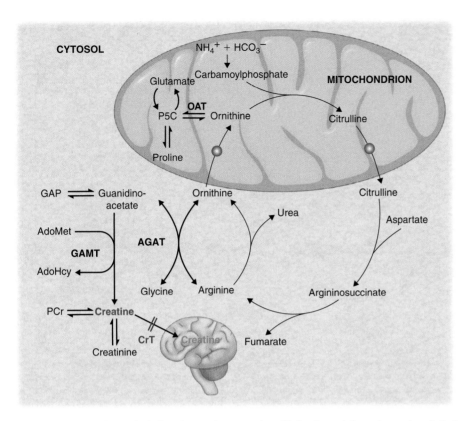

FIGURE 12-7. The defect in CrT (Blue indicates increased precursors due to block and green indicates decreased metabolites).

GYRATE ATROPHY DUE TO ORNITHINE AMINOTRANSFERASE DEFICIENCY

Etiology/Pathophysiology Hyperornithinema due to deficiency of ornithine aminotransferase (OAT) was first described in nine patients with gyrate atrophy of the choroid and retina (23).

Gyrate atrophy of choroid and retina is caused by deficiency of the L-ornithine:2-oxoacid aminotransferase (OAT) (24). The inheritance is autosomal recessive, with a higher prevalence in the Finish population. OAT is a pyridoxal phosphate–requiring enzyme that catalyzes the reversible conversion of ornithine and α-ketoglutarate to Δ1-pyrroline-5-carboxylate (P5C) and glutamate. OAT, a mitochondrial matrix enzyme, is most abundant in the liver, followed by kidney, retina, and intestine (25). The ornithine metabolism is closely linked to the urea cycle and the synthesis of Cr, polyamines, and proline (Figure 12-1); however, hyperammonemia is not found during fasting, after meals, or stress testing. The block of the OAT reaction results in a 10- to 20-fold increase of plasma ornithine (Figure 12-8). Ornithine also accumulates in other body fluids and tissues (26). Gyrate atrophy of the choroid and retina is a metabolic disease of the eyes.

Deficiency of OAT combined with the inhibitory effect of ornithine on several enzymes is most probably the cause for the pathophysiology of chorioretinal degeneration.

The analysis of the rat gene structure revealed a single expressed gene and three pseudogenes (27). The OAT gene is mapped to 10q26 (28). To date more than 60 disease-causing mutations have been reported, but there is an extensive allelic heterogeneity. Three alleles are known to produce mutant enzymes that are pyridoxine responsive.

Clinical Presentation Night blindness and myopia are usually the first symptoms in late childhood or around puberty, the time when the retinal degeneration seems to accelerate. Funduscopic appearance of chorioretinal atrophy as illustrated in Figure 12-9 is pathognomonic for gyrate atrophy.

The results of standard tests of visual function become abnormal, and there are periods of rapid progression interspersed with periods of stable function. Visual acuity (myopia) decreases gradually over decades in some patients and abruptly over a few years in others. The visual field is constricted and progresses by its concentric reduction to a "tunnel-vision." Electrophysiological examination reveals elevated dark-adaptation thresholds and very small or nondetectable electroretinographic responses. The electroretinogram may be normal at the early time when only a few focal lesions are present, and then it becomes diminished in amplitude and is usually totally extinguished well before the atrophy becomes complete.

Posterior subcapsular cataracts occurring late in the second decade of life combined with the restricted visual field result in severe impairment in the third decade of life. At this time much of the fundus is involved while the optic disc, cornea, and iris remain normal in appearance. Patients become virtually blind between the ages 40 years and 55 years when chorioretinal degeneration is complete.

In addition to the ocular findings, some patients present systemic abnormalities. Most

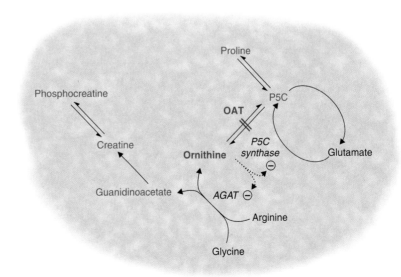

FIGURE 12-8. The defect in OAT (Blue indicates increased precursors due to block and green indicates decreased metabolites).

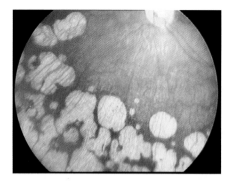

FIGURE 12-9. Funduscopy in a 9-year-old child with gyrate atrophy of the choroid and retina. It is characterized by sharply demarcated, circular areas of chorioretinal degeneration in the midperiphery of the ocular fundus with increased pigmentation around the margins of these lesions. These lesions start as punctate yellowish dots, which gradually enlarge to circular areas, coalesce, and extend toward the posterior pole of the fundus. (Courtesy of Dr. P. Mueller, Children's Hospital Leipzig, Germany)

patients have normal intelligence. MRI findings include degenerative lesions in the white matter and premature atrophic changes. EEG findings consist of abnormal slow background activity, focal lesions, or high-amplitude β rhythm (29). Tubular aggregates and selected

- The clinical course in gyrate atrophy is from slowly progressive ophthalmological changes in childhood to blindness in the fifth decade. Other organs are less affected.

atrophy of the type II fibers of skeletal muscle do not cause muscle weakness, although muscle performance of affected patients may be impaired when speed or acute strength is required. Only a small number of patients have clinical evidence of muscle weakness. Peculiar fine, sparse, straight hair is a rare finding.

Diagnosis Laboratory evaluation reveals elevated plasma ornithine values ranging from 400 to 1400 μmol/L (normal $<$ 80 μmol/L). Urinary excretion of ornithine and other dibasic amino acids (arginine, lysine, cystine) is elevated, particularly at plasma ornithine concentrations greater than 600 μmol/L. Funduscopy shows characteristic chorioretinal degeneration and ^{1}H-MRS reveals decreased PCr in muscle and decreased Cr/PCr in brain. Enzyme analysis is feasible in stimulated lymphocytes, but it is not necessary to confirm the diagnosis. Prenatal diagnosis is

TABLE 12-5	Laboratory Findings in OAT	
Decreased	**Increased**
Cr (P, U)	Ornithine (P, U, CSF)
Creatinine (24-h-U)	Arginine, lysine, cystine (U)
Guanidinoacetate (U)	
Lysine (P) (↓ or NI)	

potentially possible by OAT measurement in amniotic fluid cells or chorionic villi or by mutation analysis if mutations are known from the index case (Table 12-5).

Treatment Permanent reduction of plasma ornithine to values less than 200 μmol/L slows or stops the chorioretinal degeneration (30). The main treatment goal is to achieve as far as possible reduction of ornithine. Target ranges are between 200 and 400 μmol/L.

Few patients respond to pharmacologic doses of vitamin B$_6$ (40–200 mg/d in children and 40–500 mg/d in adults). Vitamin B$_6$-responsiveness has to be investigated prior to other treatment options (Figure 12-10). Some patients respond to ornithine reduction. It requires a natural protein–restricted

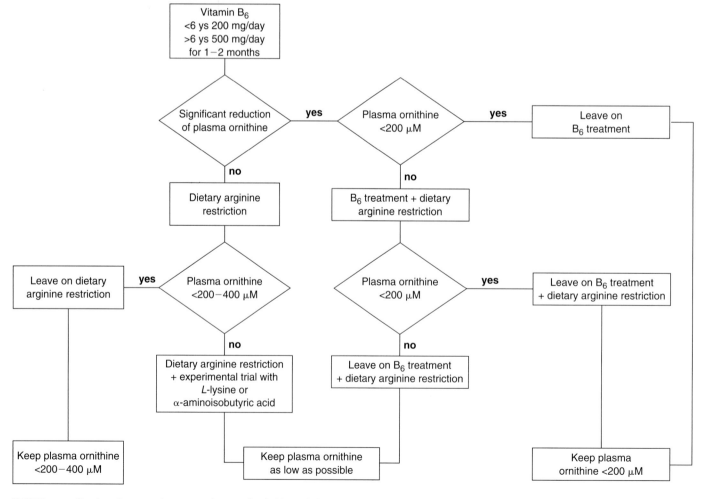

FIGURE 12-10. Flowchart of treatment in gyrate atrophy. Reproduced with permission from Hoffmann and Schulze (31).

diet (0.3–0.5 g/kg/d in children and 0.25 g/kg/d in adults). Protein requirements are met by supplementation with an arginine-free essential amino acid mixture (0.3–0.5 g/kg/d in children and 0.25–0.3 g/kg/d in adults) (31).

Other therapeutic trials include pharmacologic doses of lysine (5 g/m^2/d) or the nonmetabolizable amino acid α-aminoisobutyrate (0.1 g/kg/d) to enhance renal clearance of ornithine or supplementation with proline. The efficacy has not been proved and there are a limited number of observations. Cr administration at 1.5 to 20 g/day in adults corrects histologic muscle changes but does not halt the progress of chorioretinal degeneration (32).

Combined treatment approaches seem necessary in most patients because no form of therapy is unequivocally effective. Adequacy of treatment is monitored by measuring of plasma ornithine concentration and funduscopy.

REFERENCES

1. Schulze A. Creatine deficiency syndromes. *Mol Cell Biochem.* 2003;244(1-2):143–150.
2. Item CB, Stockler-Ipsiroglu S, Stromberger C, et al. Arginine-glycine amidinotransferase deficiency: the third inborn error of creatine metabolism in humans. *Am J Hum Genet.* 2001;69(5):1127–1133.
3. McGuire DM, Gross MD, Elde RP, et al. Localization of L-arginine-glycine amidinotransferase protein in rat tissues by immunofluorescence microscopy. *J Histochem Cytochem.* 1986;34:429–435.
4. Braissant O, Henry H, Loup M, et al. Endogenous synthesis and transport of creatine in the rat brain: an in situ hybridization study. *Mol Brain Res.* 2001;86 (1-2):193–201.
5. Bianchi MC, Tosetti M, Fornai F, et al. Reversible brain creatine deficiency in two sisters with normal blood creatine level. *Ann Neurol.* 2000;47(4):511–513.
6. Battini R, Leuzzi V, Carducci C, et al. Creatine depletion in a new case with AGAT deficiency: clinical and genetic study in a large pedigree. *Mol Genet Metab.* 2002;77(4): 326–331.
7. Stoeckler-Ipsiroglu S, Battini R, DeGrauw T, et al. Disorders of creatine metabolism. In: Blau N, Hoffmann GF, Leonard J, Clarke JTR, eds. *Physician's Guide to the Treatment and Follow-Up of Metabolic Diseases.* New York: Springer-Verlag; 2006:255–265.
8. Stöckler S, Holzbach U, Hanefeld F, et al. Creatine deficiency in the brain: a new, treatable inborn error of metabolism. *Pediatr Res.* 1994;36(3):409–413.
9. Walker JB. Creatine: biosynthesis, regulation, and function. *Adv Enzymol.* 1979;50:177–242.
10. Schulze A. Strategies in the treatment of GAMT deficiency. In: Jakobs C, Stoeckler-Ipsiroglu S, Verhoeven NM, Salomons GS, eds. *Clinical and Molecular Aspects of Defects in Creatine & Polyol Metabolism.* 1st ed. Heilbronn: SPS Verlagsgesellschaft; 2005:19–33.
11. Schulze A, Hess T, Wevers R, et al. Creatine deficiency syndrome caused by guanidinoacetate methyltransferase deficiency: diagnostic tools for a new inborn error of metabolism. *J Pediatr.* 1997;131(4):626–631.
12. Ganesan V, Johnson A, Connelly A, et al. Guanidinoacetate methyltransferase deficiency: new clinical features. *Pediatr Neurol.* 1997;17(2):155–157.
13. Schulze A, Bachert P, Schlemmer H, et al. Lack of creatine in muscle and brain in an adult with GAMT deficiency. *Ann Neurol.* 2003;53(2):248–251.
14. Schulze A, Hoffmann GF, Bachert P, et al. Successful pre-symptomatic diagnosis and treatment from birth in GAMT deficiency. *Neurology.* 2006;67:719–721.
15. Schulze A, Ebinger F, Rating D, et al. Improving treatment of guanidinoacetate methyltransferase deficiency: reduction of guanidinoacetic acid in body fluids by arginine restriction and ornithine supplementation. *Mol Genet Metab.* 2001;74(4):413–419.
16. Schulze A, Anninos A, Hoffmann GF, et al. AGAT enzyme inhibition by high-dose ornithine: a new approach in treatment of GAMT deficiency. *J Inherit Metab Dis.* 2005; 28[Suppl. 1]:227.
17. Cecil KM, Salomons GS, Ball WS, Jr, et al. Irreversible brain creatine deficiency with elevated serum and urine creatine: a creatine transporter defect? *Ann Neurol.* 2001;49(3):401–404.
18. Salomons GS, van Dooren SJ, Verhoeven NM, et al. X-Linked creatine-transporter gene (SLC6A8) defect: a new creatine-deficiency syndrome. *Am J Hum Genet.* 2001;68(6): 1497–1500.
19. Gregor P, Nash SR, Caron MG, et al. Assignment of the creatine transporter gene (SLC6A8) to human chromosome Xq28 telomeric to G6PD. *Genomics.* 1995;25:332–333.
20. Nash SR, Giros B, Kingsmore SF, et al. Cloning, pharmacological characterization, and genomic localization of the human creatine transporter. *Recept Channels.* 1994;2:165–74.
21. Sora I, Richman J, Santoro G, et al. The cloning and expression of a human creatine transporter. *Biochem Biophys Res Commun.* 1994;204:419–274.
22. Schulze A. Angeborene Störungen des Kreatinstoffwechsels (Kreatinmangelsyndrome). In: Hoffmann GF, Grau JG, eds. *Stoffwechselerkrankungen in der Neurologie.* 1 ed. Stuttgart, New York: Georg Thieme Verlag; 2004:102–108.
23. Simell O, Takki K. Raised plasma-ornithine and gyrate atrophy of the choroid and retina. *Lancet.* 1973;1(7811):1031–1033.
24. Valle D, Kaiser-Kupfer MI, Del Valle LA. Gyrate atrophy of the choroid and retina: deficiency of ornithine aminotransferase in transformed lymphocytes. *Proc Natl Acad Sci USA.* 1977;74(11):5159–5161.
25. Rao GN, Cotlier E. Ornithine delta-aminotransferase activity in retina and other tissues. *Neurochem Res.* 1984;9(4):555–562.
26. Seiler N, Daune G, Bolkenius FN, et al. Ornithine aminotransferase activity, tissue ornithine concentrations and polyamine metabolism. *Int J Biochem.* 1989;21(4):425–432.
27. Shull JD, Pennington KL, George SM, et al. The ornithine aminotransferase-encoding gene family of rat: cloning, characterization, and evolutionary relationships between a single expressed gene and three pseudogenes. *Gene.* 1991;104(2):203–209.
28. Barrett DJ, Bateman JB, Sparkes RS, et al. Chromosomal localization of human ornithine aminotransferase gene sequences to 10q26 and Xp11.2. *Invest Ophthalmol Vis Sci.* 1987;28(7):1037–1042.
29. Valtonen M, Nanto-Salonen K, Jaaskelainen S, et al. Central nervous system involvement in gyrate atrophy of the choroid and retina with hyperornithinaemia. *J Inherit Metab Dis.* 1999;22(8):855–866.
30. Kaiser-Kupfer MI, Caruso RC, Valle D. Gyrate atrophy of the choroid and retina. Long-term reduction of ornithine slows retinal degeneration. *Arch Ophthalmol.* 1991;109(11): 1539–4815.
31. Hoffmann GF, Schulze A. Disorders of ornithine, lysine, and tryptophan. In: Blau N, Hoffmann GF, Leonard J, Clarke JTR, eds. *Physician's Guide to the Treatment and Follow-Up of Metabolic Diseases.* New York: Springer-Verlag; 2006:129–138.
32. Vannas-Sulonen K, Sipila I, Vannas A, et al. Gyrate atrophy of the choroid and retina. A five-year follow-up of creatine supplementation. *Ophthalmology.* 1985;92(12):1719–1727.

CHAPTER 13

Phenylketonuria

Peter Burgard, PD Dr. Phil.
Xiaoping Luo, MD
Georg F. Hoffmann, MD

ETIOLOGY/PATHOPHYSIOLOGY

Classic phenylketonuria (PKU) is an autosomal recessive disorder of phenylalanine metabolism. It results in severe mental retardation and additional neurologic problems when treatment is not started within the first few weeks of life. When a very strict diet is begun early and well maintained, affected children can expect normal development and a normal life span. The worldwide overall incidence is 1:10,000 with a large national/ethnic variability (1:20,000 live births in South America, 1:4,500 in Ireland, 1:2,600 in Turkey, and 1:200,000 in Finland). In Europe, the estimated prevalence in the general population is 1:10,000 (1). Because of the severity of the disease if untreated and the excellent outcome when children are treated early and well, newborn screening for PKU is performed in most countries.

PKU is caused by a defect of a single enzyme, phenylalanine hydroxylase, that converts the essential amino acid phenylalanine into tyrosine (a nonessential amino acid that becomes essential in PKU) (Figure 13-1). Failure of the conversion to take place results in a buildup of phenylalanine. Through a mechanism that is not well understood, the excess phenylalanine is toxic to the central nervous system.

The range and severity of the phenotypes found in PKU depends on the degree of the defect (partial or complete). In normal metabolism the apoenzyme phenylalanine hydroxylase (PAH) and its cofactor tetrahydrobiopterin (BH₄) regulate phenylalanine degradation. The gene coding for phenylalanine hydroxylase is located on the long arm of chromosome 12. Phenylalanine hydroxylase is produced in the liver and its activity is regulated by the blood concentration of phenylalanine. When blood levels of phenylalanine are increased, the genetic transcription of phenylalanine hydroxylase is activated, resulting in a reciprocal decrease of blood phenylalanine concentration. In patients with PKU, because of the enzymatic defect/deficiency of phenylalanine hydroxylase, protein intake by natural food or protein catabolism during fasting or febrile illness leads to increased blood phenylalanine concentration in most body tissues including the brain.

In the developing organism increased phenylalanine levels interfere with the processes of myelination, synaptic sprouting, and dendritic pruning. The mechanism(s) by which these events take place have not yet been elucidated. In addition, elevated phenylalanine levels competitively inhibit the transport through the blood–brain barrier and the neuronal uptake of other neutral amino acids, leading to reduced cerebral intracellular tyrosine and 5-hydroxytryptophan concentrations. These reductions limit the production of serotonin and the catecholamines dopamine, noradrenaline, and adrenaline; melanin concentrations are also reduced. Although diminished quantities of an inhibitory neurotransmitter substance such as

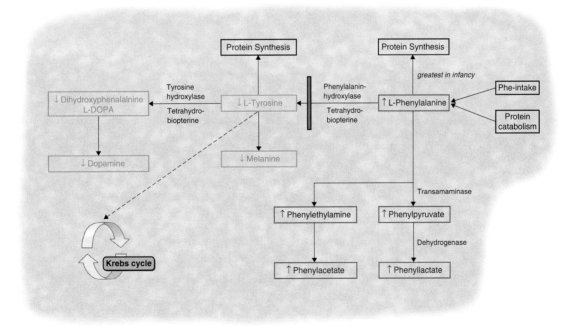

FIGURE 13-1. Defect and accumulating metabolites in phenylketonuria.

Phenylketonuria

AT-A-GLANCE

Phenylketonuria (PKU) is the most frequent inherited disorder of amino acid metabolism (prevalence 1:10.000). Approximately 500 mutations of the phenylalanine hydroxylase (PAH) gene on chromosome 12 have been identified so far, resulting in partial to complete inactivity of the hepatic enzyme PAH and consequently in increased phenylalanine (Phe) concentrations in blood (hyperphenylalaninemia [HPA]) and tissues. PKU causes structural and functional ab-

normalities of the brain, resulting in progressive neurologic impairments such as seizures, ataxia, paresis, severe mental retardation. and behavioral problems. The range and severity of the phenotypes found in PKU depend on the degree of the enzyme deficiency. The disorder can be detected by neonatal screening and treated successfully with a semisynthetic low Phe diet resulting in a nearly normal development. Experimental trials suggest efficacy of an alternative

treatment in a number of patients with type II and exceptional ones with type I with pharmacologic doses of BH_4 (~ 20 mg/kg/d); however long-term experience is not available. Non-PKU HPA or mild hyperphenylaninaemia (MHP) does not require therapy. Maternal PKU causes a fetopathy in pregnant mothers with PKU (Phe > 360 μmol/L). Strict dietary treatment must be started before conception and maintained throughout pregnancy.

TYPES OF PKU		DEFINITION	OCCURRENCE	GENE	LOCUS	OMIM
Classic PKU	Type I	Phe > 1200 μmol/L	~ 50%	PAH	12q24.1	261600
Mild PKU	Type II	360-600 μmol/L $\leq$ Phe $\leq$ 1200 μmol/L	~ 30%	PAH	12q24.1	261600
Non-PKU HPA/MHP	Type III	Phe < 360-600 μmol/L	~ 20%	PAH	12q24.1	261600
BH_4-PAH	Types II+III	Phe < 1200 μmol/L + BH_4 response	~35%	PAH	12q24.1	261600

FORM	FINDINGS		BIRTH	CLINICAL PRESENTATION CHILDHOOD TO ADULTHOOD	TREATMENT
Type I **Classic**	↑ Phe (PS, U) ↓ Tyrosine (PS)	↑ Phe-Pyruvate (U) ↑ Phe-Lactate (U) ↑ Phe-Acetate(U)	normal	Mousy odor, eczema, microcephaly, seizures, spasticity, paresis, mental retardation, behavioral abnormalities	Lifelong
Type II **Mild**	↑ Phe (PS, U) ↓ Tyrosine (PS)	↑ Phe-Pyruvate (U) ↑ Phe-Lactate (U) ↑ Phe-Acetate (U)	normal	Similar presentation as Type I if untreated. Less dietary restriction of Phe to achieve metabolic control.	At least until adulthood
Type III **Non-PKU-** **HPA/MHP**	↑ Phe (PS) ↓ Tyrosine (PS)		normal	Normal	Only for women during pregnancy if Phe $\geq$ 360 μmol/L
BH_4-PAH	Depending on Type		normal	Depending on type	Depending on type

PS = plasma and serum; U = urinary organic acids
BH_4-PAH = BH_4-responsive PAH deficiency

serotonin may have clearly defined clinical consequences resulting in hyperreflexia seen in children with severe hyperphenylalaninemia, it remains unclear what the aggregate effects of these reductions might be.

The defect in phenylalanine hydroxylase activity can be total or partial, resulting in different metabolic and clinical phenotypes. Side pathways partially degrade phenylalanine to phenyllactate and the phenylketones, phenylpyruvate, and phenylacetate but are not sufficient for phenylalanine homeostasis (for an overview, see Reference 1). The pathway for phenylalanine breakdown in phenylketonuria and the biosynthetic products of tyrosine (which is further catabolized to fumarate, an intermediate in the Krebs Cycle, and acetoacetate, a ketone body) is shown in Figure 13-1.

CLINICAL PRESENTATION

The newborn with PKU appears normal because the phenylalanine level of the fetus is regulated by the mother's intact metabolism, unless the mother herself has either untreated classic PKU or severe hyperphenylalaninemia. Without treatment and after regular normal intake of natural protein, the child will present with constitutional, intellectual and neurologic abnormalities and signs. Constitutional abnormalities (80%–100% of patients) such as hypopigmentation of the skin and hair (fair) and iris (blue) develop rapidly due to impaired metabolism of melanin. These may or may not be apparent in Black or Asian children. Elevated phenylacetate excretion gives the urine of the PKU infant a "mousy odor" and can cause eczema. If untreated by the 3rd month of life neurologic and intellectual development can be impaired with manifestations including microcephaly, hyper- and hypoexcitability, movement disorders, abnormal pattern on electroencephalography and seizures. Retrospectively, a physician will often find in a review of history that an affected infant had been especially irritable with an erratic sleep pattern.

Speech and intellectual development become severely impaired (IQ < 40) by the end of early childhood in the untreated classic PKU patient, with apraxia by age 18 to 24 months a very frequent finding. Mildly depressed IQ is common in suboptimally treated PKU. In addition children, adolescents, and adults can present with increased but also decreased muscle tone and reflexes (70%), ataxia (5%), tremor (30%), di- or tetraparesis (5%) as well as erratic behavior, aggressiveness, extreme anxiety, and withdrawal and autism-like behavior. In most cases untreated adolescents and adults with classic PKU can-

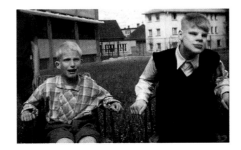

FIGURE 13-2. Untreated patients with classic PKU.

not be managed by their families and require institutional care (2) (Figure 13-2).

DIAGNOSIS

Neonatal Screening Neonatal screening measurements of phenylalanine can be performed by a bacterial inhibition assay (Guthrie test), enzymatic or fluorometric methods, or tandem mass spectrometry (MS/MS). The implementation of MS/MS in newborn screening has significantly improved the efficacy as well as the specificity by decreasing the false-positive rate. A positive screening result of hyperphenylalaninemia, that is, a blood phenylalanine level above the cut off value for screening (usually in the range of 120–150 μmol/L) has to be confirmed by a quantitative amino acid analysis, which measures phenylalanine and tyrosine in plasma, with a phenylalanine/tyrosine ratio greater than or equal 3 being diagnostic (see Chapter 2). In patients with PKU, plasma tyrosine is decreased and urinary organic acid analysis shows elevated excretion of phenylpyruvate, phenyllactate, and phenylacetate.

Differential Diagnoses Defects in the cofactor metabolism of BH_4 have to be differentiated from primary monogenic defects of phenylalanine hydroxylase by urinary pterin analysis and determination of enzyme activity of dihydropteridine reductase, which can be performed in dried blood spots. In many centers, approximately 30 minutes before a feeding a dose of 20 mg/kg BH_4 is administered orally to children with a positive screening result for phenylalanine. To perform this test the initial plasma phenylalanine concentration should be greater than 400 μmol/L (6.7 mg/dL). Combination with single-dose phenylalanine loading prior to BH_4 administration is not recommended as the results are difficult to interpret. Following BH_4 administration plasma samples are collected for phenylalanine and tyrosine at 0, 4, 8, and 24 hours as well as a urine sample 4 to 8 hours after BH_4 administration for pterin analysis (this must be protected from light). When there is a primary disorder of BH_4 metabolism, plasma phenylalanine

falls to normal (usually by 8 hours) with an increase in tyrosine (also see Chapter 11). This test may also identify BH_4-responsive phenylalanine hydroxylase. In such children the drop in phenylalanine and the increase in tyrosine are often only partial and/or delayed. In any case the diagnostic work up of a positive neonatal screening result of hyperphenylalaninemia requires the determination of pterins in urine and enzyme activity of dihydropteridine reductase, whereas BH_4 loading is only supplementary and optional. The identical work up is also required for any individual in whom hyperphenylalaninemia is identified in later life for the first time.

Dietary treatment of hyperphenylalaninemia due to phenylalanine hydroxylase deficiency is always indicated at phenylalanine levels greater than 360 to 600 μmol/L (cut off for treatment). Unfortunately national guidelines recommend different cut offs as the indication of starting dietary treatment ranging from 400 μmol/L in the United Kingdom (6), to 360 to 600 μmol/L in the United States (7), to 600 μmol/L in Germany (8) and France (9), and there is no logical explanation for these differences. Newborn screening with MS/MS technology often detects hyperphenylalaninemia very early in life when protein intake or neonatal catabolism can still be insufficient to make a clear decision for treatment. Particularly during the 1st year of life hyperphenylalaninemia near the treatment cut-off level (Mild PKU vs. Non-PKU HPA/MHP) can be ambiguous due to a high rate of protein synthesis (Figure 13-1) (1). In these cases normal feeding is continued but phenylalanine concentrations are regularly monitored, and treatment is begun once concentrations exceed the cut off for treatment. The gold standard for deciding for or against the necessity of dietary treatment is a standardized protein challenge at the age of 5 months when the child is given 100 to 180 mg phenylalanine/kg/day during 3 consecutive days. The 72-hour phenylalanine level is interpreted as the phenotypic peak level, which is used to establish the indication for treatment (cut off for treatment) as well as to determine the subtype of PKU (Table 13-1) (1). Alternatively, an approach of gradually increasing the daily phenylalanine intake can be used to define the subtype. This approach determines the individual phenylalanine tolerance, that is, the daily amount of phenylalanine intake that still allows maintaining plasma phenylalanine levels in the age appropriate recommended range (Table 13-2). Phenylalanine tolerance is an estimate and reflection of the residual activity of phenylalanine hydroxylase.

TABLE 13-1 Enzymatic and Metabolic Phenotypes, Phenylalanine Tolerance, and Therapy of Different Subtypes of Hyperphenylalaninemias

HPA Subtype	Residual PAH in Vivo Activity Estimated by Liver Biopsy (enzymatic phenotype)	Blood Phenylalanine Level (standardized protein challenge; metabolic phenotype)	Phenylalanine Tolerance at Age 5 Years	Therapy
Type I Classic PKU	< 1 %	> 1200 μmol/L	<21 mg/kg/d	Dietary treatment for life
Type II Mild PKU	1-3 %	360/600-1200 μmol/L	21-50 mg/kg/d	Dietary treatment at least until adulthood
Type III Non-PKU HPA/MHP	> 3%	< 360-600 μmol/L	>115 mg/kg/d	Treatment only in case of MPKU

HPA = hyperphenylalaninemias; MHP = mild hyperphenylalaninemias; PAH = phenylalanine hydroxylase.

TABLE 13-2 Treatment Recommendations for PKU

Age	Protein Requirement (g /kg)	Phe Tolerance (mg/d)	Biochemical Monitoring Phe & Tyr	Phe Tolerance (mg/d)	Target Blood Phe (μmol/L)				Phe-free AAM	
					Germany	UK	USA	France	Type	g/d***
0 – 3 mo	2.3-2.1	~ 130-400	weekly	~ 130-400	40-240	120-360	120-360	120-300	1	3-10
4 – 12 mo	2.1-2.0	~ 130-400	weekly	~ 130-400	40-240	120-360	120-360	120-300	1	3-10
1 – 3 y	1.7	~ 130-400	weekly to biweekly	~ 130-400	40-240	120-360	120-360	120-300	2	20-50
4 – 6 y	1.6	~ 200-400	weekly to biweekly	~ 200-400	40-240	120-360	120-360	120-300	2	20-50
7 – 9 y	1.4	~ 200-400	biweekly to monthly	~ 200-400	40-240	120-480	120-360	120-300	2	20-50
10 – 12 y	1.1	~ 350-800	1 to 3 mo	~ 350-800	40-900	120-480	120-360	<900	2	50-90
13 – 15 y	1.0	~ 350-800	1 to 3 mo	~ 350-800	40-900	120-700	120-600	<900	2	50-90
Adolescents	0.9	~ 450-1000	1 to 3 mo; yearly**	~ 450-1000	40-1200	120-700	120-900	<900-1200	3	60-150
Adults	0.9	~ 450-1000	1 to 3 mo; yearly**	~ 450-1000	40-1200	120-700	120-900	<1200-1500	3	60-150

*Protein requirement for PKU diet is assigned higher than actual recommendations of DACH, Recommended Dietary Allowance, and World Health Organization for healthy people because bioavailability of amino acids mixtures seems to be not equivalent to natural protein.

** France

*** Spread as evenly as possible through the 24 hours.

Phe-free AAM = phenylalanine-free mixture.

Liver biopsy and measurement of the hepatic enzyme activity is never indicated; however, mutation analysis can be helpful for decision making about treatment and for further genetic counseling of the family. Approximately 500 mutations of the phenylalanine hydroxylase gene have been described so far (http://pahdb.mcgill.ca), resulting in total or partial impairment of the enzyme activity predicting the metabolic phenotype (4) according to the three subtypes (Table 13-1). Most mutations are null mutations in which there is no detectable phenylalanine hydroxylase activity. As in most autosomal recessive traits, mutations are not spontaneous; however, they are associated with geographic and/or ethnic origin.

Prenatal diagnosis of PKU homozygotes and heterozygotes can be achieved through genetic testing in informative families or restriction fragment length polymorphisms related to the phenylalanine hydroxylase gene but is usually not indicated (3).

- Untreated PKU has become very rare in countries in which neonatal screening is performed; however, it does exist in individuals immigrating from countries in which screening is not performed or when screening has failed, e.g., false-negative screening.

TREATMENT AND OUTCOME

Phenylketonuria

National guidelines recommend different cut offs for the indication to start dietary treatment ranging from 400 μmol/L in the United Kingdom (6), to 360 to 600 μmol/L in the United States (7), to 600 μmol/L in Germany (8) and France (9). With regard to the appropriate time for starting treatment there is consensus that treatment should start as early as possible and not later than after 4 weeks

of life. Dietary therapy of hyperphenylalaninemias, the PKU diet, eliminates all of the very high protein foods because all protein contains phenylalanine. A synthetic formula that is entirely devoid of phenylalanine but includes all other amino acids is used as a nutritional substitute for the eliminated foods (5). The phenylalanine-deficient diet is then supplemented with natural foods containing an appropriate amount of phenylalanine to supply the child's needs for normal growth. Not every child has the same degree of enzyme deficiency; some have enough enzyme activity that the diet can be quite liberal, whereas most must adhere to a very strict diet. In classic PKU the diet should be maintained for a lifetime to keep blood phenylalanine levels in the age appropriate range (Table 13-2). This is especially important in infancy and early childhood, although it is sometimes quite difficult to maintain especially during intercurrent illness. The implementation of the diet should be monitored by an expert team consisting of a pediatric metabolic specialist and a dietician with training and experience in disorders of amino acid metabolism. Phenylalanine requirements and tolerance change with somatic growth and age, and frequent, periodic blood monitoring as well as oversight and monitoring of normal growth and development are essential to therapeutic success.

During infancy, administration of the diet is relatively simple: breast milk has a relatively low phenylalanine content, so that dietary treatment can be initiated by feeding the baby half breast milk and half a phenylalanine-free infant formula. The diet of older patients has four components: 1) complete avoidance of food containing high amounts of phenylalanine (i.e., meat, poultry, fish, milk, cheese, pulses and cereals, nuts, etc.); 2) calculated intake of low-protein/phenylalanine natural food (vegetables and fruit) and specially manufactured product foods containing very low amounts of protein (special bread, biscuits, pasta, cream, milk, etc.) summing up to the individual daily phenylalanine tolerance; 3) sufficient intake of fat and carbohydrates to fulfill the energy requirements of the patient; 4) calculated intake of a phenylalanine free amino acid mixture supplemented with vitamins, minerals, and trace elements as the main source of protein. During periods of fasting and/or intercurrent illnesses (febrile infections) catabolism can result in a rapid increase of phenylalanine concentration and must be counteracted by dietary reduction of phenylalanine intake. In addition, during growth spurts in childhood and adolescence phenylalanine requirements can increase and must be balanced by adjustment of the dietary components. It is worthwhile to point out that phenylalanine requirements per kilogram of body weight generally decrease with age.

Treatment must be monitored by regular measurement of blood phenylalanine concentrations. Published national guidelines differ again and are available from the United States, United Kingdom, Germany, and France (6–10) (Table 13-2).

Experimental trials using pharmacologic doses of BH$_4$ (5–20 mg/kg of body weight/day) suggest that for approximately 70% of PKU types II and III (phenylalanine levels without diet <1200 μmol/L) or 35 % of all patients, respectively, oral treatment with the cofactor BH$_4$ might be an alternative to dietary treatment (11,12). BH$_4$-responsive phenylalanine hydroxylase deficiency is defined by a 30% reduction of blood phenylalanine levels within 15 hours after BH$_4$ monotherapy. Little is known about the mechanism of BH$_4$ responsiveness but five functional hypotheses have been suggested (13): 1) increased BH$_4$ levels compensate a reduced binding affinity of phe-

nylalanine hydroxylase for the cofactor; 2) BH$_4$ chaperones the stability of phenylalanine hydroxylase; 3) BH$_4$-driven change in regulation of BH$_4$ biosynthesis; 4) up-regulation of phenylalanine hydroxylase enzyme expression; and 5) phenylalanine hydroxylase messenger RNA stabilization. There is no doubt that this treatment can reduce blood phenylalanine levels into the therapeutic range in some individuals; however, data on long-term efficacy and possible side effects are not available.

Particularly during infancy, childhood, and adolescence close monitoring of nutrition, growth, neurologic, and neuropsychologic development are mandatory (14). Psychologic monitoring should measure milestones of development during the first 2 years of life, speech (2 years) and intellectual development (at 5 and 10 years) as well as information processing and reaction times (in adolescence and adulthood).

When treatment is started early (not later than 4 weeks of age) and performed strictly (mean blood phenylalanine level ≤ 400 μmol/L during infancy and childhood), motor and intellectual development can be expected to be near to normal. For each 4-week delay in the initiation of treatment, IQ at the age of 4 years is reduced by 0.25 standard deviation. For each increase of mean blood phenylalanine level by 300 μmol/L, IQ during school age is reduced by 0.5 standard deviation. After the age of 10 years IQ remains stable even when dietary treatment is stopped (15–18). Compared with healthy controls neuropsychologic parameters of choice reaction time, attention, and executive functions are impaired in these individuals. Adverse effects on these parameters are correlated with concurrent phenylalanine levels. Study designs with experimental variation of phenylalanine levels revealed that these effects are reversible even after longer periods of high blood levels (19,20). Contrary to a scholastic and professional career that can be expected to be normal, even early and strictly treated patients have an increased risk for psychiatric abnormalities, predominantly with introversive symptoms of anxiety, social withdrawal, and depressive mood or attention deficits. Compared with normative data antisocial and aggressive behaviors appear to be reduced, possibly related to the introversive

symptoms. The etiology of psychiatric symptoms is unclear and has been explained by a combination of psychosocial and metabolic causes (21). A therapeutic trial of reducing blood phenylalanine levels by intensified dietary therapy is indicated in adults who develop psychiatric symptoms. Neurologic symptoms of resting tremor, intention tremor, and increased muscle reflexes can be observed in adolescent and adult patients but longitudinal data are lacking to demonstrate progressive disease. Parietal and occipital MRI abnormalities of deep white matter on T2-weighted images have been reported in patients with overt neurologic symptoms (22,23) but all of these patients have had a history of poor treatment during childhood. In addition most early and strictly treated patients show similar MRI changes unrelated to neurophysiologic functions (visual evoked potentials, sensory evoked potentials, and nerve conduction velocity) and improve after longer periods of low phenylalanine levels (24,25). At present, such MRI abnormalities are interpreted as reversible dysmyelination. It remains unclear whether abnormal imaging, neurologic, and neuropsychologic data have to be interpreted as early signs of late-onset deterioration but are seen to favor a risk-minimizing policy of lifelong treatment (18).

Maternal PKU

Maternal PKU (MPKU) is a condition that endangers the pregnancy outcome of women with PKU and blood phenylalanine levels greater than 360 μmol/L, resulting in intrauterine conditions analogous to fetal alcohol syndrome. The severity of the manifestations depend on the maternal phenylalanine level and can include cardiac defects (usually conotruncal), microcephaly dysmorphic features, intrauterine growth retardation, neuronal migration disorders, and corpus callosum agenesis. The etiology is not well understood. Phenylalanine concentrations in every fetus are increased by an inwardly directed placental gradient by 1.5. According to a study by Lenke and Levy (26), maternal phenylalanine levels greater than 1200 μmol/L severely increase the risk for congenital abnormalities as shown by Table 13-3.

TABLE 13-3 Congenital Abnormalities in MPKU		
Congenital Abnormalities	**MPKU**	**Unaffected Mothers**
Mental retardation	92%	5%
Microcephaly	73%	4.8%
Intrauterine retardation	40%	9.6%
Congenital heart defects	12%	0.8%

Based on the report by Lenke and Levy (26).

Lowering maternal phenylalanine levels during pregnancy to a level between 60 and 360 μmol/L results in a favorable outcome in virtually all cases (27–29). Preconception dietary training and reduction of phenylalanine levels into the safe range are strongly recommended. Increased phenylalanine levels of the father (paternal PKU) at time of conception (30) are not related to any adverse effect on the fetus.

Legal and Institutional Support

Dietary treatment of PKU is expensive and family subsidy depends on the national or local regulations concerning reimbursement. In most of the United States, any state subsidy of treatment cost ends at the age of majority (legal adulthood). The exception to this is that many states will reinstate support during pregnancy; often, however, bureaucratic procedures delay the support until well into the first trimester. Legal counseling may help the family to deal with social welfare institutions and health insurance companies.

Psychosocial Support

During infancy treatment of PKU is a task for the whole family. During childhood and adolescence responsibility is gradually transferred to the patient, and adult patients should be trained to care for themselves independently. Overall, as for all chronic diseases, the rate of compliance with recommendations for PKU is approximately 50% (31,32). Consultation with a pediatric psychologist trained in behavioral medicine may help the family and the patient to cope with the cognitive, emotional, and behavioral aspects of the disease and the treatment. In addition parent and patient organizations can offer social, informational, and practical support.

REFERENCES

1. Scriver CR, Kaufman S. Hyperphenylalaninemia: phenylalanine hydroxylase deficiency. In: Scriver CR, Beaudet AL, Sly WS, Valle D eds. *The Metabolic and Molecular Bases of Inherited Disease.* 8th ed. New York: McGraw-Hill; 2001:1667–1724.
2. Pietz J: Neurological aspects of adult phenylketonuria. *Curr Opin Neurol.* 1998;11:679–688.
3. Lidsky AS, Ledley FD, DiLella AG, et al. Extensive restriction site polymorphism at the human phenylalanine hydroxylase locus and application in prenatal diagnosis of phenylketonuria. *Am J Hum Genet.* 1985;37:619–634.
4. Guldberg P, Rey F, Zschocke J, et al. A European multicenter study of phenylalanine hydroxylase deficiency: classification of 105 mutations and a general system for genotype-based prediction of phenotype *Am J Hum Genet.* 1998;63:71–79.
5. Poustie VJ, Rutherford P. Dietary interventions for phenylketonuria. *Cochrane Database Systematic Reviews.* 2000;2 CD001304.
6. Medical Research Council Working Party on Phenylketonuria. Recommendations on the dietary management of phenylketonuria. *Arch Dis Child.* 1993;68:426–427.
7. National Institutes of Health Consensus Development Conference Statement. Phenylketonuria: screening and management. October 16-18, 2000. *Pediatrics.* 2001;108:972–982.
8. Burgard P, Bremer HJ, Bührdel P, et al. Rationale for the German Recommendations for Phenylalanine Level Control in Phenylketonuria 1997. *Eur J Pediatr.* 1999;158:46–54.
9. Abadie V, Berthelot J, Feillet F, et al. Consensus national sur la prise en charge des enfants dépistés avec une hyperphénylalaninémie. *Arch Pédiatr.* 2005;12:594–601.
10. Blau N, Burgard P. Disorders of phenylalanine and tetrahydrobiopterin metabolism. In: Blau N, Hoffmann GF, Leonard, J, Clarke, J eds. *Physician's Guide to the Treatment and Follow-up of Metabolic Diseases.* Heidelberg: Springer; 2005:25–34.
11. Bernegger C, Blau N. High frequency of tetrahydrobiopterin-responsiveness among hyperphenylalaninemias: a study of 1,919 patients observed from 1988 to 2002. *Mol Genet Metab.* 2002;77:304–313.
12. Muntau A, Röschinger W, Habich M, et al. Tetrahydrobiopterin as an alternative treatment for mild phenylketonuria. *N Engl J Med.* 2002;247:2122–2132.
13. Blau N, Erlandsen H. The metabolic and molecular bases of tetrahydrobiopterin-responsive phenylalanine hydroxylase deficiency. *Mol Genet Metab.* 2004;82:101–111.
14. NSPKU. Management of PKU: A consensus document for the diagnosis and management of children, adolescents and adults with PKU. National Society for Phenylketonuria, 1999. Available at: http://web.ukonline.ca.uk/nspku. Accessed August 15, 2007.
15. Smith I, Beasley MG, Ades AE. Intelligence and quality of dietary treatment in phenylketonuria. *Arch Dis Child.* 1990;65:472–478.
16. Smith I, Beasley MG, Ades AE. Effect on intelligence of relaxing the low phenylalanine diet in phenylketonuria. *Arch Dis Child.* 1991;66:311–316.
17. Burgard P. Development of intelligence in early treated phenylketonuria. *Eur J Pediatr.* 2000;159:74–79.
18. Koch R, Burton B, Hoganson G, et al. Phenyketonuria in adulthood: a collaborative study. *J Inherit Metab Dis.* 2002;25:333–346.
19. Schmidt E, Rupp A, Burgard P, et al. Sustained attention in adult phenylketonuria: the influence of the concurrent phenylalanine blood-level. *J Clin Exp Neuropsychol.* 1994;16:681–688.
20. Griffiths P. Neuropsychological approaches to treatment policy issues in phenylketonuria. *Eur J Pediatr.* 2000;2:82–86.
21. Smith I, Knowles J. Behaviour in early treated phenylketonuria (PKU). A systematic review. *Eur J Pediatr.* 2000;159:89–93.
22. Villasana D, Butler IJ, Williams JC, et al. Neurological deterioration in adult phenylketonuria. *J Inherit Metab Dis.* 1989;12:451–457.
23. Thompson AJ, Smith I, Brenton D, et al. Neurological deterioration in young adults with phenylketonuria. *Lancet.* 1990;336:602–605.
24. Cleary MA, Walter JH, Wraith JE, et al. Magnetic resonance imaging in phenylketonuria: Reversal of cerebral white matter change. *J Pediatr.* 1995;127:251–255.
25. Walter JH, White F, Wraith JE, et al. Complete reversal of moderate/severe brain MRI abnormalities in a patient with classical phenylketonuria. *J Inherit Metab Dis.* 1997;20:367–369.
26. Lenke RR, Levy HL. Maternal phenylketonuria and hyperphenylalaninemia. *N Engl J Med.* 1980;303:1202–1208.
27. American Academy of Pediatrics. Maternal phenylketonuria. *Pediatrics.* 107: 2001;427–428.
28. Koch R, Hanley W, Levy H et al. The Maternal Phenylketonuria International Study: 1984-2002. *Pediatrics.* 2003;112:1523–1530.
29. Widaman KF, Azen C. Relation of prenatal phenylalanine exposure to infant and childhood cognitive outcomes: results from the international maternal PKU collaborative study. *Pediatrics.* 2003;112:1537–1543.
30. Fisch RO, Matalon R, Weisberg S, et al. Children of fathers with phenylketonuria: An international survey. *J Pediatr.* 1991;118:739–741.
31. Osterberg L, Blaschke, T. Adherence to medication. *N Engl J Med.* 2005;353:487–497.
32. Walter JH, White FJ, Hall SK, et al. How practical are recommendations for dietary control in phenylketonuria? *Lancet.* 2002;360:55–57.

CHAPTER 14

Hyperphenylalaninemias: Disorders of Tetrahydrobiopterin Metabolism

Nenad Blau, PhD
Beat Thöny, PhD

BIOSYNTHESIS AND FUNCTION OF TETRAHYDROBIOPTERIN

Tetrahydrobiopterin (BH$_4$) is essential for diverse processes and is ubiquitously present in all tissues of higher organisms. The best investigated functions of BH$_4$ is as a natural cofactor of the following enzymes:

Aromatic amino acid hydroxylases:
   Phenylalanine-4-hydroxylase (PAH)
   Tyrosine-3-hydroxylase (TH)
   Tryptophan-5-hydroxylase (TPH)

All three forms of nitric oxide synthase (NOS) (For a review, see Refs. 9 and10).

In addition, BH$_4$ is required by the enzyme glyceryl-ether monooxygenase for hydroxylation of the α-carbon atom of the lipid carbon chain of glyceryl ether to form α-hydroxyalkyl glycerol (11).

BH$_4$ biosynthesis proceeds in the de novo pathway in a Mg^{2+}-, Zn^{2+}-, and NADPH-dependent reaction from guanosine triphosphate (GTP) via the two intermediates, 7,8-dihydroneopterin triphosphate (NH$_2$TP) and 6-pyruvoyl-5,6,7,8-tetrahydropterin (PTP) (Figure 14-1). The three enzymes GTP cyclohydrolase I (GTPCH), 6-pyruvoyl-tetrahydropterin synthase (PTPS), and sepiapterin reductase (SR) are required and sufficient to carry out the proper stereospecific reaction to 6R,L-erythro-5,6,7,8-tetrahydrobiopterin (BH$_4$). The committing and rate-limiting step is carried out by GTPCH, a homodecamer containing a single zinc ion in each subunit and consisting of a tightly associated dimer of two pentamers (12,13). The reaction from NH$_2$TP to PTP is catalyzed by PTPS in a Zn^{2+}- and Mg^{2+}-dependent reaction without consuming an external reducing agent. Crystallographic analysis revealed that PTPS is composed of a pair of trimers arranged in a head-to-head fashion to form the functional hexamer (14). The final step is the NADPH-dependent reduction of the two side-chain keto groups of PTP by homodimeric SR.

Besides the involvement in the de novo biosynthesis of BH$_4$, SR also may participate

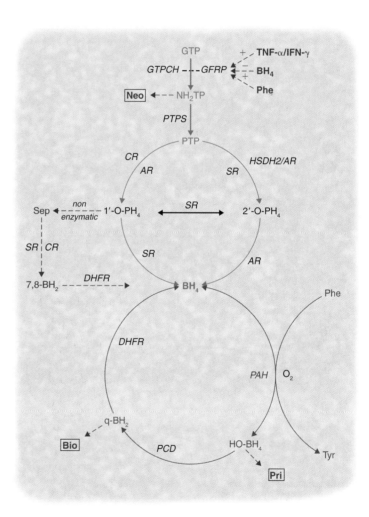

FIGURE 14-1. Phenylalanine hydroxylating system (purple), tetrahydrobiopterin (BH$_4$) biosynthesis (orange), and salvage pathway (brown). Enzymes involved in the biosynthesis of BH$_4$: GTP cyclohydrolase I (GTPCH) converts GTP to dihydroneopterin triphosphate (NH$_2$TP), 6-pyruvoly-tetrahydropterin synthase (PTPS) converts NH$_2$TP to 6-pyruvoly-tetrahydropterin (PTP), and sepiapterin reductase (SR) catalyzes the final two steps of reduction of PTP to BH$_4$. PTP can be reduced to BH$_4$ either by alternative reductases, carbonyl reductase (CR), aldose reductase, and 3β-hydroxysteroid dehydrogenase 2 (HSDH2) via 1'-keto-tetrahydropterin (1'-O-PH$_4$) and 2'-keto-tetrahydropterin (2'-O-PH$_4$) or through the salvage pathway via sepiapterin (Sep) and 7,8-dihydrobiopterin (7,8-BH$_2$). This reaction involves dihydrofolate reductase (DHFR). The phenylalanine hydroxylating system consists of the apoenzyme phenylalanine hydroxylases (PAH), cofactor BH$_4$, molecular oxygen (O$_2$), and two regenerating enzymes, pterin-4α-carbinolamine dehydratase (PCD) and dihydropteridine reductase (DHPR). 4α-Hydroxy-terahydropterin (HO-BH$_4$), product of the PAH reaction, is dehydrated to the quinonoid dihydrobiopterin (q-BH2) by PCD and subsequently reduced back to BH$_4$ by DHPR. Neopterin (Neo), biopterin (Bio), and primapterin (Pri) are metabolites (in red) found in different body fluids and used as makers for disorders in BH$_4$ metabolism. In pink, regulation of the BH$_4$ biosynthesis at the level of the GTPCH-GFRP complex through cytokines (positive), BH$_4$ (negative), and phenylalanine (Phe) (positive).

Disorders of Tetrahydrobiopterin Metabolism

AT-A-GLANCE

Tetrahydrobiopterin (BH_4) deficiencies, a group of rare inherited neurological diseases with monoamine neurotransmitter deficiency, may present phenotypically with or without hyperphenylalaninemia (HPA). It is a heterogenous group of diseases affecting either all organs, only the peripheral hepatic phenylalanine hydroxylase system, or only the central nervous system. Common but variable symptoms found in autosomal recessive variants of BH_4 deficiency are mental retardation, convulsions, disturbance of tone and posture, abnormal movements, hypersalivation, and swallowing difficulties. Onset of symptoms is in the first months of life.

Generalized BH_4 deficiency can be caused by mutations in genes encoding the enzymes involved in its biosynthesis (GTP cyclohydrolase I [GTPCH] and 6-pyruvoly-terahydropterin synthase [PTPS]) or regeneration (pterin-4α-carbinolamin dehydratese/dimerization cofactor of hepatocyte nuclear factor 1α [PCD/DCoH] and dihydropteridine reductase [DHPR]). The mutations are all inherited autosomal recessively. Biochemical, clinical, and DNA data on patients with BH_4 deficiencies are tabulated in the BIODEF and BIOMDB databases and are available on the Internet (www.bh4.org). Depending on the enzyme defect and the mode of inheritance, patients are diagnosed by different analytical and biochemical approaches. Early diagnosis and immediate treatment are essential for a good outcome.

Two forms of cerebral BH_4 deficiency may occur without HPA and are described in Chapter 45: the autosomal dominantly inherited form of GTPCH deficiency (dopa-responsive dystonia [DRD], initially described as Segawa disease) and sepiapterin reductase (SR) deficiency.

Patients presenting *with* HPA usually are detected through the neonatal screening programs for PKU, whereas those presenting *without* HPA are recognized by the development of "typical" neurological signs and symptoms and/or by analysis of neurotransmitter metabolites and pterins in CSF (see Chapter 45). In most neonatal screening programs, BH_4 deficiency with HPA comprises 1% to 2% of patients detected with HPA.

TYPES OF BH$_4$ DEFICIENCY (WITH HPA)	OCCURRENCE	GENE	LOCUS	OMIM
GTP cyclohydrolase I (GTPCH)	4%*	*GCH1*	14q22.1-22.2	233910
6-Pyruvoly-tetrahydropterin synthase (PTPS)	61%*	*PTS*	11q22.3-23.3	261640
Pterin-4α-carbinolamine dehydratase (PCD)	4%*	*PCBD*	10q22	264070
Dihydropteridine reductase (DHPR)	31%*	*QDPR*	4p15.3	261630

*Of all BH_4 deficiencies.

FORM	URINE	FINDINGS BLOOD*	CSF	BIRTH	CLINICAL PRESENTATION INFANCY - ADOLESCENCE
GTPCH	↓ Neo ↓ Bio	nl–↑ Phe ↓ Neo ↓ Bio	↓ Neo ↓ Bio ↓ 5-HIAA ↓ HVA	Increased prematurity, abnormal tonus, and feeding difficulties	Progressive dystonia, hypotonia of the trunk, hypertonia of extremities, hypersalivation, choreoatethosis, seizures, and mental retardation
PTPS	↑ Neo ↓ Bio	↑ Phe ↑ Neo ↓ Bio	↑ Neo ↓ Bio ↓ 5-HIAA ↓ HVA	Increased prematurity, abnormal tonus, and feeding difficulties; low birth weight	Progressive dystonia, hypotonia of the trunk, hypertonia of extremities, hypersalivation, choreoatethosis, seizures, and mental retardation
PCD	↑ Neo nl–↓ Bio ↑ Pri	↑ Phe (transient)	↑ Neo nl Bio nl 5-HIAA nl HVA	Transient alterations in tone (hypotonia/ hypertonia)	No symptoms
DHPR	nl Neo ↑ Bio	↑ Phe ↓ DHPR nl Neo ↑ Bio	nl Neo ↑ Bio ↓ 5-HIAA ↓ HVA ↓ 5-MTHF	Possibility of prematurity, abnormal tonus, and feeding difficulties.	Progressive dystonia, hypotonia of the trunk, hypertonia of extremities, hypersalivation, choreoaatethosis, seizures, calcification of basal ganglia, and mental retardation

*Dried blood on filter paper (Guthrie card).
Bio = total biopterin; 5-HIAA = 5-hydroxyindoleacetic acid; HVA = homovanillic acid; Neop = neopterin; Phe = phenylalanine; Pri = primapterin; 5-MTHF = 5-methyltetrahydrofolate; nl = normal.

in the pterin salvage pathway by catalyzing the conversion of sepiapterin (Sep) to 7,8-dihydrobiopterin ($7,8\text{-}BH_2$) that is then transformed to BH_4 by dihydrofolate reductase (DHFR) (15). Both reactions consume NADPH. Although SR is sufficient to complete the BH_4 biosynthesis, a family of alternative NADPH-dependent aldo-keto reductases, including carbonyl reductases (CR), aldose reductases (AR), and the 3β-hydroxysteroid dehydrogenase type 2 ($HSDH_2$) may participate in the diketo reduction of the carbonyl side chain in vivo (16–18). Moreover, based on the discovery of the autosomal recessive deficiency for SR, which presents with neurotransmitter deficiency but without overt hyperphenylalaninemia (19), different routes for the final two-step reaction of BH_4 biosynthesis involving these alternative reductases were proposed. CR converts 6-pyruvoyl tetrahydropterin (PTP) to both, the 2'-oxo-tetrahydropterin (2'-O-PH_4) and the lactoyl tetrahydropterin (1'-O-PH_4); however, the rate of production is much more favorable for the 1'-oxo-tetrahydropterin intermediate. On the other hand, the 3β-hydroxysteroid dehydrogenase type 2 efficiently converts PTP to 2'-O-PH_4. AR can convert 6-PTP to 6-lactoyl tetrahydropterin, or to 2'-oxo-tetrahydropterin to BH_4. In summary, alternative routes for BH_4 biosynthesis in the absence of SR involve either the 2'-oxo-tetrahydropterin intermediate via the concerted action of 3β-hydroxysteroid dehydrogenase type 2 and AR or the 1'-oxo-tetrahydropterin intermediate via the concerted action of AR, CR, and dihydrofolate reductase. It was proposed that due to low expression or activity of dihydrofolate reductase and 3β-hydroxysteroid dehydrogenase type 2 in human brain, the biosynthesis from 6-pyruvoyl tetrahydropterin to BH_4 in the absence of SR cannot be completed. This leads to central BH_4 deficiency with accumulation of the unstable 1'-oxo-tetrahydropterin and its degradation products, detected as "abnormal" pterin metabolites, that is, $7,8\text{-}BH_2$ in the CSF.

Regeneration of BH_4 is an essential part of the phenylalanine hydroxylating system. During the catalytic event of aromatic amino acid hydroxylases, molecular oxygen is transferred to the corresponding amino acid, and BH_4 is oxidized to BH_4–4β-carbinolamine (HO-BH_4) (see Figure 14-1) (20). Two enzymes are involved in its subsequent dehydratation and reduction to BH_4: pterin–4α-carbinolamine dehydratase (PCD) and dihydropteridine reductase (DHPR). Enzymatic recycling of BH_4 is essential for phenylalanine metabolism 1) to ensure a continuous supply of reduced cofactor and 2) to prevent accumulation of harmful metabolites produced by rearrangement of HO-BH_4. The primary structure of PCD is identical with a protein of the cell nucleus that has transcription function named *dimerization cofactor* (DCoH) of hepatocyte nuclear factor 1α (HNF-1α), recently reported to have general transcriptional function (21–23). In the following, PCD will be designated as the dual-function protein PCD/DCoH. Furthermore, a functional homologue, DCoH2, was identified that partially complements PCD/DCoH mutants in mice and humans (24,25).

TETRAHYDROBIOPTERIN DEFICIENCIES

The BH_4 deficiencies are a heterogeneous group of diseases, and different clinical and biochemical criteria define and characterize the variants (1). The primary enzyme defect, its severity, outcome of the BH_4 challenge, type of mutation, and responses to therapy are some of the criteria used to define a specific defect. The terms *severe* or *mild/peripheral* should be used according to the actual need for treatment with neurotransmitter precursors. Accordingly, the nomenclature used here applies. Older terms such as *atypical PKU* and *malignant PKU* should be avoided.

In addition to classical BH_4 deficiencies, for example, autosomal recessive GTP cyclohydrolase I deficiency, 6-pyrovuly-tetrahydropterin synthase (PTPS) deficiency, carbinolamine-4α-dehydratase (PCD) deficiency, and dihydropteridine reductase (DHPR) deficiency, there are genetic disorders related to BH_4 deficiency presenting without hyperphenylalaninemia (HPA), for example, dopa-responsive dystonia (DRD, [autosomal dominant] adGTPCH deficiency, initially described as Segawa disease), and sepiapterin reductase (SR) deficiency (see Chapter 45).

Because classical BH_4 deficiencies are a group of diseases that can be detected but not identified through neonatal mass screening for HPA, specific investigations for BH_4 deficiency is essential in every newborn detected with even slightly elevated phenylalanine levels (26,27). Screening for BH_4 deficiency should be done in all newborns with plasma phenylalanine levels higher than 120 μmol/L, as well as in older children with suggestive neurological signs and symptoms (28). The following tests are recommended:

1. Analysis of pterins in urine

2. Measurement of DHPR activity in blood from a Guthrie card

3. Loading test with BH_4

4. Analysis of pterins, folates, and neurotransmitter metabolites in cerebrospinal fluid (CSF)

5. Enzyme activity measurement

6. Mutation analysis

The first two tests are essential and enable all BH_4 defects presenting with HPA to be differentiated. With some limitations, the BH_4 loading test is an additional, useful diagnostic tool for the rapid differentiation between classic phenylketonuria (PKU) and BH_4 variants. This test alone cannot differentiate between some patients with the mild form of PKU/HPA and BH_4 variants. Analysis of neopterin, biopterin, 5-methyltetrahydrofolic acid (5-MTHF) and the neurotransmitter metabolites 5-hydroxyindoleacetic acid (5-HIAA) and homovanillic acid (HVA) is necessary in every infant identified with BH_4 deficiency and also enables differentiation between severe and mild forms of BH_4 deficiencies Table 14-1.

GTP Cyclohydrolase I Deficiency

Etiology/Pathophysiology GTP cyclohydrolase I (GTPCH) catalyzes the first step in the biosynthesis of BH_4 from GTP (see Figure 14-1) (10). The GTPCH enzyme, a homodecamer consisting of a tightly associated dimer of two pentamers, converts GTP to 7,8-dihydroneopterin triphosphate, a precursor of neopterin. GTPCH activity can be regulated at the transcriptional and post-translational levels. BH_4 and phenylalanine modulate the enzymatic activity via GTPCH feedback regulatory protein GFRP, which binds to GTPCH, thereby inducing a yet unknown conformational change. GFRP mediates the end-product feedback inhibition by BH_4. The inactive complex can be reverted to an active form by phenylalanine. The regulation on the transcriptional level by cytokines, phytohemagglutinin, and endotoxin (lipopolysaccharide) in a cell- and tissue-specific mode is probably predominant. In humans, a biochemical consequence of this immunostimulation is the excretion of both neopterin and 7,8-dihydroneopterin by activated macrophages and, consequently, accumulation in plasma and urine.

GTPCH activity is not detectable in liver biopsies of patients with GTPCH deficiency and is very low in cytokine-stimulated fibroblasts (29).

Clinical Presentation GTPCH deficiency is a rare form of HPA, with only few cases listed in the BIODEF database. The clinical course of illness is similar in all untreated patients and to other severe forms of BH_4 deficiencies. The variable but common symptoms are mental

• Autosomal recessive GTPCH deficiency without HPA was described in few patients presenting with dopa-responsive dystonia.

TABLE 14-1   Laboratory Diagnosis of BH₄ Deficiencies

Test	Protocol	Interpretation
Phenylalanine (B)	Blood spots on filter paper (Guthrie test or tandem mass spectrometry [MS/MS])	Normal < 120 μmol/L
BH₄ loading test (20 mg/kg)	Blood spots on filter paper or plasma for Phe and Tyr at times 0, 4, 8, and 24 h after administration	a) Normalization of blood Phe 4–8 h after administration in patients with GTPCH, PTPS, and PCD deficiency b) Significant reduction (almost normalization) of blood Phe 4–8 h after administration in patients with DHPR deficiency. c) Significant reduction (>30%) of blood Phe 4–8 h after administration in patients with BH₄-responsive PAH deficiency (mild PKU)
Pterins (neopterin, biopterin, and primapterin) in urine	Urine spot sample before the BH₄ loading test and 4–8 hours after BH₄ administration; protect from light; keep frozen.	Abnormal pterins pattern
DHPR activity*	Blood spots on filter paper	Normal 1.0–3.5 mU/mg Hb
Neurotransmitter metabolites in CSF (5-HIAA and HVA)	CSF (1–2 mL); discard first 0.5 mL; keep frozen at −80°C	Very low in most BH₄-deficient patients
Folates in CSF (5-MTHF)	CSF (1–2 mL); discard first 0.5 mL; keep frozen at −80°C	Very low in patients with DHPR deficiency

*Some DHPR-deficient newborns may present with normal urinary pterins in the first weeks of life.

retardation, convulsions (grand mal or myoclonic attacks), disturbance of tone and posture, drowsiness, irritability, abnormal movements, recurrent hyperthermia without infections, hypersalivation, and swallowing difficulties. Diurnal fluctuation of alertness and neurological symptoms are also reported. The most prominent clinical signs and symptoms are summarized in Table 14-2.

Diagnosis Most of the patients were detected trough the neonatal screening for PKU, but at least four patients with GTPCH deficiency passed the newborn PKU screening program because of initially normal blood phenylalanine values. Neopterin and biopterin are very low or not detectable in urine, blood, and CSF. The BH₄ loading test is positive (fast reduction of blood phenylalanine after administration of 20 mg BH₄ per kilogram of body weight). Neurotransmitter metabolites 5-HIAA and HVA in CSF are very low (HVA is more reduced than 5-HIAA). Very low production of

neopterin and biopterin and very low GTPCH activity are seen in cytokine-stimulated fibroblasts. Four patients were found to be homozygotes (R184H, M211I, M211V, and M213T) and one was a compound heterozygote (Q110X, second allele not defined) for mutations in the GCH1 gene. Two patients with homozygous mutations (P199A and R249S) presented without HPA (Table 14-3).

Treatment Blood phenylalanine concentrations should be more rigidly controlled than in classical PKU patients. In patients with GTPCH deficiency, administration of BH₄ appears to be the most efficient therapy in controlling blood phenylalanine levels. Higher doses (>10 mg/kg/day) are required for BH₄ to cross the blood–brain barrier.

L-Dopa (3–15 mg/kg/day) and 5-hydroxytryptophan (2–9 mg/kg/day) administration in combination represents a common therapeutic approach to all BH₄-deficiency variants. Carbidopa (10% or 25% of L-Dopa), an

- Prenatal diagnosis is possible by measuring pterin metabolites in amniotic fluid or through mutation analysis in informative families.

inhibitor of peripheral aromatic amino acid decarboxylase, reduces the therapeutic requirements of L-Dopa. Use of L-dopa/25% carbidopa, as a slow-release preparation (Sinemet Depot), seems to be beneficial in patients with the severe form of BH₄ deficiency. Good results have been obtained recently in similar cases with the concurrent administration of L-Deprenyl (0.2–0.3 mg/kg/day), a selective monoamine oxidase (MAO) B inhibitor or Entacapone (10–15 mg/kg/day), a catechol-O-methyltransferase (COMT) inhibitor, allowing dosage reduction of the administered precursors by slowing down their catabolism. The dosages of medications should be adjusted to the individual needs of each patient, with careful monitoring of adverse effects and reversal of neurological manifestations. Biochemically, therapy is monitored by regular investigations of neurotransmitter metabolites (5-HIAA and HVA) and pterins in CSF.

TABLE 14-2   Signs and Symptoms in Patients with Autosomal Recessive GTPCH Deficiency (n = 18)

Symptoms	Neonatal, <30 days	Infancy, <18 mos.	Childhood, <10 yrs.
Progressive psychomotor retardation despite treatment for PKU	±	+	+
Hypotonia/hypertonia/dystonia	+	+	+
Temperature instability	+	+	+
Seizures—myoclonic		+	+
Microcephaly	+	+	+
Hypersalivation	+	+	+
Mental retardation		+	+
Feeding difficulties	+	+	+

TABLE 14-3   Laboratory Findings GTPCH

Decreased	Increased
Neopterin (U, B, CSF)	Phenylalanine (B)
Biopterin (U, B, CSF)	
5-HIAA (CSF)	
HVA (CSF)	

TABLE 14-4   Signs and Symptoms in Patients with PTPS ($n = 230$) and DHPR ($n = 138$) Deficiencies

Symptoms	Neonatal, <30 days	Infancy, <18 mos.	Childhood, <10 yrs.	Adolescence, >11 yrs.
Progressive mental and physical retardation despite dietary phenylalanine restriction	±	+	+	+
Myoclonic or tonic–clonic seizures		+	+	+
Temperature instability	+	+	+	
Hypersalivation	+	+	+	+
Lethargy and irritability		+	+	
Hypotonia/hypertonia/dystonia	+	+	+	
Retardation and regression	+	+	+	+
Choreoathetosis		+	+	
Calcification of basal ganglia[†]		+	+	+
Feeding difficulties		+	+	+

[†]Primarily DHPR deficiency.

Note: Low birth weight can be associated with PTPS.

6-Pyruvoyl-tetrahydropterin Synthase Deficiency

Etiology/Pathophysiology 6-Pyruvoyl-tetrahydropterin synthase (PTPS) catalyzes a Zn^{2+}- and Mg^{2+}-dependent reaction from 7,8-dihydroneopterin triphosphate to 6-pyruvoyl-tetrahydropterin (see Figure 14-1). PTPS is considered to be constitutively expressed but is not ubiquitously present in higher animals. However, following immunostimulatory induction of GTPCH by cytokines, PTPS can become the rate-limiting step in BH_4 biosynthesis at least in humans, where PTPS activity is much lower than in rodents. Human PTPS also was shown to be subject to regulatory phosphorylation, and it appears to be essential because a phosphorylation-deficient mutant of PTPS was identified from a patient with a defect in BH_4 biosynthesis.

PTPS activity is very low or absent is red blood cells and fibroblasts from patients with PTPS deficiency.

- A central form of PTPS deficiency may present with only mild HPA or even normal blood phenylalanine levels.

Clinical Presentation PTPS deficiency is the most common form of BH_4 deficiency, with more than 316 cases listed in the BIODEF database. About 80% of all patients with PTPS deficiency are referred to as having *severe* manifestations with characteristic truncal hypotonia and increased limb tone with pronated hand posture. A decrease in activity or loss of head control may precede the onset of a progressive neurological degenerative disease, and usually these patients become hypertonic, especially in the lower extremi-

ties. There may be bradykinesia and episodic "lead pipe" or "cogwheel" rigidity. Symptoms of generalized dystonia with marked diurnal fluctuations were reported in some adult patients. Difficulty in swallowing, oculogyric crises, somnolence, irritability, hyperthermia, seizures, and impaired neurophysiological development may occur, as in other BH_4 deficiencies (Table 14-4).

Patients with the mild "peripheral" forms of PTPS deficiency may have phenotypic changes with increasing age and present with normal CSF neurotransmitters in the first months of life. However, they may become progressively neurologically abnormal between 1 and 2 years of age, with very low CSF neurotransmitter levels and, therefore, may need substitution treatment with neurotransmitter precursors.

- Prenatal diagnosis is possible by the measurement of pterin metabolites in amniotic fluid; PTPS activity in fetal erythrocytes or cultured amniocytes, or through mutation analysis in informative families.

Diagnosis Patients are detected through the neonatal screening for PKU (Phe > 120 μmol/L). In severe PTPS deficiency, neopterin is very high and biopterin very low or not detectable in urine, blood, CSF, or cytokine-stimulated fibroblasts. Neurotransmitter metabolites 5-HIAA and HVA are very low in CSF, and PTPS activity is very low in unstimulated fibroblasts (Table 14-5). A positive BH_4 loading test (fast reduction of blood phenylalanine after administration of 20 mg BH_4 per kilogram of body weight) is characteristic of PTPS deficiency. A total of 43 known mutations are distributed across all six exons and

the first three introns of the PTS gene. No hot spots for mutations are found, although two mutations, N52S and P87S, appear to be relatively frequent in the Asian population. Among the exonic mutations, there are 1 insertion (R16ins), 5 deletions (K38fs, F40fs, V57del, K120fs, and K131fs), and 33 substitutions. The three splice-site mutations are distributed in the first three introns, and two of them lead to skipping of exon 3 (IVS2-7TnA and IVS3+1GnA). For more details, see the BIOMDB database (www.bh4.org).

Treatment Treatment of patients with the severe form of PTPS deficiency includes correction of elevated blood phenylalanine levels by BH_4 and substitution with neurotransmitter precursors (for details, see the GTPCH-deficiency section and Chapter 45). Patients with the mild peripheral phenotype require only BH_4 monotherapy to correct HPA.

Pterin-4α-carbinolamine Dehydratase Deficiency

Etiology/Pathophysiology Dehydratation of 4α-OH-BH_4, the first product of the reaction of aromatic amino acid hydroxylases, is catalyzed by the enzyme pterin-4α-carbinolamine dehydratase (PCD) (see Figure 14-1). The human cytoplasmic PCD/DCoH, whose sequence is identical to the rat protein, is a homotetramer. In the absence of PCD/DCoH, dehydratation of 4α-OH-BH_4 also occurs

TABLE 14-5   Laboratory Findings PTPS

Decreased	Increased
Biopterin (U, B, CSF)	Phenylalanine (B)
5-HIAA (CSF)	Neopterin (U, B, CSF)
HVA (CSF)	

TABLE 14-6 Laboratory Findings PCD	
Subnormal	**Increased**
Biopterin (U)	Phenylalanine (B)
	Neopterin (U)
	Primapterin (U)

TABLE 14-7 Laboratory Findings DHPR	
Decreased	**Increased**
5HIAA (CSF)	Phenylalanine (B)
HVA (CSF)	Biopterin (U, B, CSF)
5MTHF (CSF)	
DHPR activity in Gurthrie cards	

- Prenatal diagnosis is possible by the measurement of pterin metabolites in amniotic fluid, DHPR activity in fetal erythrocytes or cultured amniocytes, or through mutation analysis in informative families.

nonenzymatically, but at a rate that is, at least in the liver, insufficient to maintain BH$_4$ in the reduced state. As a consequence, liver PCD/DCoH deficiency in humans causes 4α-OH-BH$_4$ to be rearranged via an intermediate to primapterin (7-substituted biopterin) that is excreted in the urine. A biopsy of duodenal mucosa from a patient with a homozygous E96K mutation had 17% of normal activity. Since subjects with mutant PCD have only a transient form of HPA and, to our knowledge, no transcription factor HNF-1α-related expression defects, it was speculated that this may be explained at least in part by a compensatory activity of the DCoH$_2$ isoenzyme.

Clinical Presentation This is a benign form of BH$_4$ deficiency. In the early neonatal period, some patients present with neurological impairments, such as transient abnormality on electroencephalogram and progressive hypotonia with delay in motor development or slight upper limb tremors after stimulation. Mostly, these patients show no significant clinical abnormalities other than transient alterations in tone and need no treatment. Only 1 of 22 patients listed in the BIODEF database needed a substitution with BH$_4$ and neurotransmitter precursors.

Diagnosis Patients with PCD deficiency present with HPA only in the early neonatal period. HPA seems to be a transient condition. Increased neopterin (only in the early neonatal period), subnormal biopterin, and increased primapterin are found in urine (Table 14-6). The BH$_4$ loading test is positive (fast reduction of blood phenylalanine after administration of 20 mg BH$_4$ per kilogram of body weight). Neurotransmitter metabolites 5-HIAA and HVA in CSF are normal. So far, nine different mutations have been detected in patients with PCD deficiency, most of them located in exon 2.

Treatment BH$_4$ monotherapy (5–10 mg/kg/day) is given during the first months of life; thereafter, no treatment is required but patients should be followed by a developmental pediatrician throughout childhood.

Dihydropteridine Reductase Deficiency

Etiology/Pathophysiology The final conversion of quinonoid dihydrobiopterin (q-BH$_2$) to BH$_4$ is carried out by the dimeric dihydrop-

teridine reductase (DHPR) (see Figure 14-1). DHPR deficiency is the second most common form of BH$_4$ deficiency.

The relatively high levels of DHPR, compared with those of aromatic amino acid hydroxylases, and its presence in tissues lacking these enzymes imply that DHPR may be involved in other metabolic processes. For example, there is evidence that DHPR, in the presence of NADH, could preserve tetrahydrofolate levels in brain, where the concentrations of dihydrofolate reductase are rather low. The exact mechanism is not known.

Clinical Presentation The clinical course of illness is similar to that seen in severe forms of GTPCH and PTPS deficiencies (see Table 14-4). In addition, extensive neuronal loss, calcification (due to cerebral folate deficiency), and abnormal vascular proliferation were noted in the central cortex, white matter, basal ganglia, and thalamus. DHPR deficiency is considered to be the most severe form of BH$_4$ deficiency. The control of blood phenylalanine levels needs to be more strict than in other forms of BH$_4$ deficiency.

- Mild forms of DHPR deficiency may present without neurological abnormalities and with reduced serotonin biosynthesis only.

Diagnosis Patients are detected through the neonatal screening for PKU (Phe > 120 µmol/L). Neopterin is normal or slightly elevated and biopterin is very high in urine, blood, and CSF (Table 14-7). The BH$_4$ loading test is positive (fast to moderate reduction of blood phenylalanine after administration of 20 mg BH$_4$ per kilogram of body weight). Neurotransmitter metabolites 5-HIAA, HVA, and 5-methyltetrahydrofolate (5-MTHF) are very low in CSF. DHPR activity is very low in blood spots (Guthrie card) and fibroblasts. Neopterin production is normal and biopterin production is elevated in cytokine-stimulated fibroblasts. So far, the 33 different reported mutant alleles are spread over all coding exons and two introns of the QDPR gene. Two mutations were found to be associated with a mild form of DHPR deficiency, that is, affecting only serotonin metabolism in the brain (G151S, F212C). For more details, see BIOMDB database (www.bh4.org).

Treatment In contrast to patients with other forms of BH$_4$ deficiency, these patient generally should not use BH$_4$ to control blood phenylalanine levels. Instead, they need a low-phenylalanine diet. Only a few DHPR-deficient patients are on BH$_4$ therapy, mostly in a combination with diet. Neurotransmitter precursor substitution therapy is identical to that for patients with GTPCH and PTPS deficiency (for more details, see the GTPCH-deficiency section). Administration of folinic acid (Leucovorin) is essential to restore normal CSF folate levels. This therapy (10–20 mg/day) may reverse and at least halt both the demyelinating processes and the calcification of the basal ganglia in patients with DHPR deficiency.

REFERENCES

1. Blau N, Thöny B, Cotton RGH, et al. Disorders of tetrahydrobiopterin and related biogenic amines. In: Scriver CR, Beaudet AL, Sly WS, et al., eds. *The Metabolic and Molecular Bases of Inherited Disease.* New York: McGraw-Hill; 2001:1725–1776.
2. Blau N, Bonafé L, Thöny B. Tetrahydrobiopterin deficiencies without hyperphenylalaninemia: Diagnosis and genetics of dopa-responsive dystonia and sepiapterin reductase deficiency. *Mol Genet Metab.* 2001; 72:172–185.
3. Thöny B, Blau N. Mutations in the GTP cyclohydrolase I and 6-pyruvoyl-tetrahydropterin synthase genes. *Hum Mutat.* 1997; 10:11–20.
4. Thöny B, Neuheiser F, Kierat L, et al. Mutations in the pterin-4α-carbinolamine dehydratase gene cause a benign form of hyperphenylalaninemia. *Hum Genet.* 1998;103:162–167.
5. Smooker PM, Howells DW, Dianzani I, et al. The spectrum of mutations in dihydropteridine reductase deficiency. In: Ayling JE, Nair MG, Baugh CM, eds. *Chemistry and Biology of Pteridines and Folates.* New York: Plenum Press; 1993:135–138.
6. Blau N, Barnes I, Dhondt JL. International database of tetrahydrobiopterin deficiencies. *J Inherited Metab Dis.* 1996;19:8–14.
7. Ichinose H, Ohye T, Takahashi E, et al. Hereditary progressive dystonia with marked diurnal fluctuation caused by mutation in the GTP cyclohydrolase I gene. *Nat Genet.* 1994;8:236–241.
8. Bonafé L, Thöny B, Penzien JM, et al. Mutations in the sepiapterin reductase gene cause a novel tetrahydrobiopterin-dependent

monoamine neurotransmitter deficiency without hyperphenylalaninemia. *Am J Hum Genet.* 2001;69:269–277.

9. Thöny B. Tetrahydrobiopterin and its function. In: Blau N, ed. *PKU and BH4: Advances in Phenylketonuria and Tetrahydrobiopterin Research.* Heilbronn: SPS Publications; 2006:503–554.

10. Thöny B, Auerbach G, Blau N. Tetrahydrobiopterin biosynthesis, regeneration, and functions. *Biochem J.* 2000;347:1–26.

11. Taguchi H, Armarego WLF. Glyceryl-ether monooxygenase (EC 1.14.16.5): A microsomal enzyme of ether lipid metabolism. *Med Res Rev.* 1998;18:43–89.

12. Nar H, Huber R, Meining W, et al. Atomic structure of GTP cyclohydrolase I. *Structure.* 1995;3:459–466.

13. Auerbach G, Herrmann A, Bracher A, et al. Zinc plays a key role in human and bacterial GTP cyclohydrolase I. *Proc Natl Acad Sci USA.* 2000;97:13567–13572.

14. Nar H, Huber R, Heizmann CW, et al. Three-dimensional structure of 6-pyruvoyl-tetrahydropterin synthase, an enzyme involved in tetrahydrobiopterin synthesis. *EMBO J.* 1994;13:1255–1262.

15. Nichol CA, Smith GK, Duch DS. Biosynthesis and metabolism of tetrahydrobiopterin and molybdopterin. *Annu Rev Biochem.* 1985;54:729–764.

16. Milstien S, Kaufman S. The biosynthesis of tetrahydrobiopterin in rat brain: Purification and characterization of 6-pyruvoyl tetrahydropterin (2′-oxo)reductase. *J Biol Chem.* 1989;264:8066–8073.

17. Park YS, Heizmann CW, Wermuth B, et al. Human carbonyl and aldose reductases: New catalytic functions in tetrahydrobiopterin biosynthesis. *Biochem Biophys Res Commun.* 1991;175:738–744.

18. Iino T, Tabata M, Takikawa S, et al. Tetrahydrobiopterin is synthesized from 6-pyruvoyl-tetrahydropterin by the human aldo–keto reductase AKR1 family members. *Arch Biochem Biophys.* 2003;416:180–187.

19. Bonafe L. Tetrahydrobiopterin deficiency without hyperphenylalaninemia: Sepiapterin reductase deficiency. In: Blau N, ed. *PKU and BH4: Advances in Phenylketonuria and Tetrahydrobiopterin Research.* Heilbronn: SPS Publications; 2005:533–611.

20. Lazarus RA, Benkovic SJ, Kaufman S. Phenylalanine hydroxylase stimulator protein is a 4α-carbinolamine dehydratase. *J Biol Chem.* 1983;258:10960–10962.

21. Mendel DB, Khavari PA, Conley PB, et al. Characterization of a cofactor that regulates dimerization of mammalian homeodomain protein. *Science.* 1991;254:1762–1767.

22. Citron BA, Davis MD, Milstien S, et al. Identity of 4α-carbinolamine dehydratase, a component of the phenylalanine hydroxylation system, and DCoH, a transregulator of homeodomain proteins. *Proc Natl Acad Sci USA.* 1992;89:11891–11894.

23. Hauer CR, Rebrin I, Thony B, et al. Phenylalanine hydroxylase–stimulating protein/pterin-4α-carbinolamine dehydratase from rat and human liver: Purification, characterization, and complete amino acid sequence. *J Biol Chem.* 1993; 268:4828–4831.

24. Bayle JH, Randazzo F, Johnen G, et al. Hyperphenylalaninemia and impaired glucose tolerance in mice lacking the bifunctional DCoH gene. *J Biol Chem.* 2002; 277:28884–28891.

25. Hevel JM, Stewart JA, Gross KL, et al. Can the DCoHα isozyme compensate in patients with 4α-hydroxy-tetrahydrobiopterin dehydratase/DCoH deficiency? *Mol Genet Metab.* 2006;88:38–46.

26. Blau N, Bonafé L, Blaskovics M. Disorders of phenylalanine and tetrahydrobiopterin. In: Blau N, Duran M, Blaskovics M, Gibson KM, eds. *Physician' Guide to the Laboratory Diagnosis of Metabolic Disease.* Heidelberg: Springer; 2002:89–106.

27. Dhondt JL. Strategy for the screening of tetrahydrobiopterin deficiency among hyperphenylalaninaemic patients: 15-years experience.*J Inherited Metab Dis.* 1991;14:117–127.

28. Blau N, Thöny B, Spada M, et al. Tetrahydrobiopterin and inherited hyperphenylalaninemias. *Turk J Pediatr.* 1996;38:19–35.

29. Bonafé L, Thöny B, Leimbacher W, et al. Diagnosis of dopa-responsive dystonia and other tetrahydrobiopterin disorders by the study of biopterin metabolism in fibroblasts. *Clin Chem.* 2001;47:477–485.

CHAPTER 15

Tyrosinemia and Other Disorders of Tyrosine Degradation

James V. Leonard, PhD, FRCP, FRCPCH
Andrew A. M. Morris, PhD, FRCPCH

INTRODUCTION

Tyrosine is derived from the diet, from metabolism of phenylalanine, and from the body's proteins during catabolic stress. Tyrosine degradation is catalyzed by a series of five enzymatic reactions with end products being acetoacetate and fumarate. The hepatocyte and renal proximal tubules are the only two cell types that express the complete pathway and contain sufficient quantities of all enzymes required for tyrosine catabolism (Figure 15-1). Normal plasma tyrosine concentrations are between 30 and 120 μmol/L. Increased concentrations of tyrosine in plasma are common and may be the result of a primary inherited metabolic disorder but they may also be secondary. The most common causes are listed in

TABLE 15-1   Causes of Hypertyrosinemia

Primary	Secondary
Tyrosinemia type 2 (tyrosine aminotransferase deficiency)	Any cause of acute liver disease, including galactosemia
Tyrosinemia type 3 (4-hydroxyphenylpyruvate dioxygenase deficiency)	Transient neonatal tyrosinemia, including prematurity
Tyrosinemia type 1 (fumarylacetoacetase deficiency, hepatorenal tyrosinosis)	Nitisinone (NTBC) therapy
	Scurvy (rare)
	Hyperthyroidism (rare)

Table 15-1. The primary disorders are all defects in the tyrosine degradation pathway. The first is tyrosine aminotransferase deficiency (tyrosinemia type 2) and the second is 4-hydroxyphenylpyruvate dioxygenase deficiency (tyrosinemia type 3). The most common disorder in the pathway, however, is a defect of the last enzyme, namely fumarylacetoacetase, which causes tyrosinemia type 1 (also known as hepatorenal tyrosinosis). The most common secondary causes of high plasma tyrosine concentrations are acute liver disease and transient neonatal tyrosinemia.

Initial Investigations

Patients with high plasma tyrosine concentrations will generally need the examination and tests listed in Table 15-2. The dietary protein intake should also be assessed. These tests should identify those causes of tyrosinemia that require urgent treatment, namely tyrosinemia type 1 and galactosemia. Further testing will be needed to confirm these diagnoses or to establish the diagnosis of tyrosinemia type 2 or 3. Figure 15-2 gives a diagnostic algorithm for a neonate with a high tyrosine concentration.

TYROSINEMIA TYPE 1

Fumarylacetoacetase deficiency (also known as hepatorenal tyrosinosis).

Clinical Features Tyrosinemia type 1 is an autosomal recessive disorder caused by reduced or absent activity of fumarylacetoacetase. As

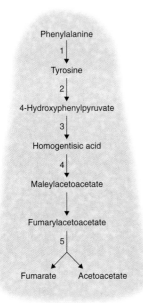

Figure 15-1. Normal tyrosine catabolism. 1 = Phenylalanine hydroxylase; 2 = Tyrosine aminotransferase; 3 = 4-Hydroxyphenylpyruvate dioxygenase; 4 = Homogentisate dioxygenase; 5 = Fumaryl acetoacetase.

TABLE 15-2   Initial Investigations for Elevated Plasma Tyrosine Concentrations

Liver function tests

Clotting studies

Plasma aminoacids (quantitative)

Erythrocyte galactose-1-phosphate uridyl transferase[a] (quantitative or Beutler screening test)

Urine organic acids (including succinylacetone and phenolic acids)

[a]neonates and infants only

Tyrosinemia and Other Disorders of Tyrosine Degradation

AT-A-GLANCE

Raised tyrosine concentrations are seen in three disorders of tyrosine metabolism (tyrosinemia types 1–3). Secondary causes of raised plasma tyrosine concentrations include acute liver failure and transient neonatal tyrosinemia. Transient tyrosinemia is common in neonates, particularly those born prematurely, probably due to immaturity of the enzyme 4-hydroxyphenylpyruvate dioxygenase. In a neonate with high tyrosine concentrations and liver failure, it is particularly important to exclude galactosemia because it requires urgent dietary treatment. Tyrosinemia type 1 can also cause liver failure. Most cases of this disorder respond to nitisinone but patients need monitoring for hepatocellular carcinoma. Adults with alkaptonuria have progressive arthritis and an increased risk of heart disease; tyrosine concentrations are normal. Hawkinsin is a tyrosine derivative found in the urine of a few families; its excretion is inherited as an autosomal dominant trait.

TYPES	ENZYME DEFECT	INCIDENCE	GENE	LOCUS	OMIM
Tyrosinaemia type 1	Fumarylacetoacetase	1:17,000 (Quebec) 1:100,000 (Sweden) Lower elsewhere	FAH	15q23-q25	2767000
Tyrosinaemia type 2	Tyrosine aminotransferase	Unknown	TAT	16q22.1-q22.3	276600
Tyrosinaemia type 3	4-Hydroxyphenylpyruvate dioxygenase	Unknown	HPD	12q24-qter	276710
Alkaptonuria	Homogentisate 1,2-diogygenase	Unknown	HGD	3q21-q23	203500
Hawkinsinuria	4-Hydroxyphenylpyruvate dioxygenase	Unknown	HPD	12q24-qter	140350

FORM	FINDINGS	CLINICAL PRESENTATION		TREATMENT
		INFANCY	LATER	
Tyrosinemia type 1	↑ tyrosine (P) ↑ methionine (P) ↑ succinylacetone (U & P) ↑ δ-aminolevulinate (U) ↑ α-fetoprotein (S)	Poor feeding, vomiting failure to thrive, bleeding due to liver failure, hepatosplenomegaly, porphyria-like crises	Growth retardation, rickets, bruising, hepatomegaly	Nitisinone (NTBC) and low-phenylalanine and -tyrosine diet OR Liver transplantation Liver transplantation
Tyrosinemia type 2	↑ tyrosine (P) = methionine (P) no succinylacetone (U & P)	Painful red eyes due to corneal erosions, painful hyperkeratotic lesions on hand or sole, cognitive or behavioral problems		Low-phenylalanine and -tyrosine diet
Tyrosinemia type 3	↑ tyrosine (P) = methionine (P) no succinylacetone (U & P)	Variable, some patients have learning difficulties or neurologic problems		Low-phenylalanine and -tyrosine diet but maybe not essential
Alkaptonuria	↑ homogentisic acid (U)	Ochronosis, arthritis, and heart disease starting in adolescence and adulthood		As yet, none of proven benefit
Hawkinsinuria	hawkinsin (U) ↑ pyroglutamate (U)	Uncertain, failure to thrive and metabolic acidosis have been reported in some infants		Possibly low-phenylalanine and -tyrosine diet in infancy, none thereafter.

U = urine; P = plasma; S = serum.

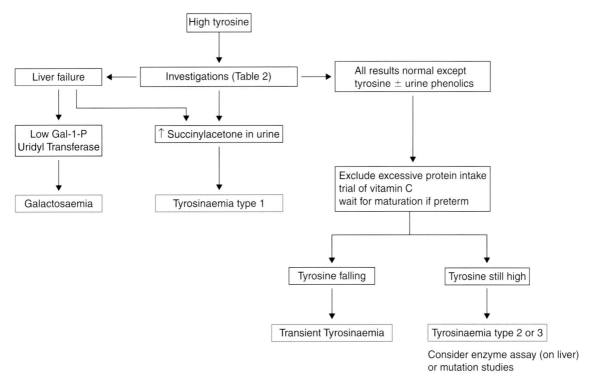

Figure 15-2. Diagnostic algorithm for neonates with high plasma tyrosine concentrations. Note that there are many other causes of neonatal liver failure besides galactosaemia and tyrosinaemia type 1.

a result, fumarylacetoacetate and maleylacetoacetate accumulate in the liver and kidney. These metabolites are highly toxic, probably acting as alkylating agents, and cause serious, progressive tissue damage. Succinylacetone is formed from these and can be detected in blood and urine (Figure 15-3).

There is wide phenotypic variation in tyrosinemia type 1 and patients may present at any age from birth to adult life. An international survey of 108 patients showed that 90% of patients present in infancy, 36% in the first 2 months (1). The initial symptoms are usually non-specific, such as irritability, poor feeding, vomiting, or failure to thrive. Examination at this stage reveals firm hepatomegaly, which may be accompanied by splenomegaly, edema, and ascites. Investigations show predominantly abnormalities of hepatic synthetic function with severe abnormalities of clotting that are not corrected by vitamin K. Typically, plasma aminotransferase levels are only mildly elevated and plasma bilirubin concentrations are normal. A renal tubular disorder is almost always present, often with striking hypophosphatemia, which is responsible for bone disease.

Additional problems soon appear. Some patients present with bleeding and are initially examined for a hematologic problem. Others have hypoglycemia, which may be related to pancreatic islet hypertrophy as well as liver disease (2). Sepsis is a frequent complication and often precipitates an 'acute hepatic crisis'.

When in crisis, the child is often irritable and febrile. Abdominal examination reveals a hard liver, spleen, and ascites. Gastrointestinal bleeding is common. In addition to severe coagulopathy, there may be markedly raised plasma aminotransferase levels and moderate jaundice. Hepatic crises may resolve spontaneously but some proceed to liver failure and hepatic encephalopathy.

Older patients may present with more chronic disease, the symptoms and signs of which are more subtle. There may only be

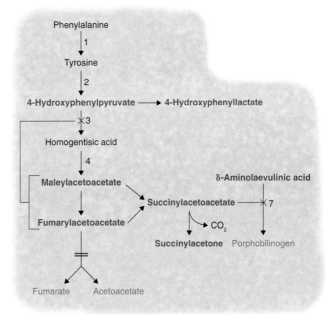

Figure 15-3. Defect and accumulating metabolites in tyrosinemia type 1. In tyrosinemia type 1, the immediate precursor, fumarylacetoacetate (FAA) is diverted into succinylacetoacetate and succinylacetone. Succinylacetone reduces the activity of the parahydroxyphenylpyruvic acid dioxygenase resulting in elevation of plasma tyrosine concentration and similarly the activity of the δ-Aminolaevulinic acid dehydratase in liver and circulating red blood cells resulting in decreased heme synthesis and increased urinary excretion of aminolevulinic acid (ALA). 1 = Phenylalanine hydroxylase; 2 = Tyrosine aminotransferase; 3 = 4-Hydroxyphenylpyruvate dioxygenase; 4 = Homogentisate dioxygenase; 7 = δ-Aminolaevulinic acid dehydratase.

mild hepatomegaly, bruising, or growth retardation. All patients have some degree of cirrhosis, which is usually (but not always) seen on imaging. Almost all patients have renal tubular dysfunction with hypophosphatemic rickets. The rickets may be subclinical but sometimes it is the main clinical problem in patients with a chronic course (3). Glomerular function is also affected (4) and a few patients progress to end-stage renal failure, requiring renal transplantation (3).

Hepatocellular carcinoma is the most serious complication of tyrosinemia type 1. The pathogenesis is thought to be the induction of mutations by maleylacetoacetate and fumarylacetoacetate through their action as alkylating agents (5). Hepatocellular carcinoma has been reported in patients as young as 15 months but it is more frequent in older patients. In the international survey, 18% of children surviving beyond 2 years developed hepatocellular carcinoma (1). This study was conducted before the introduction of treatment with nitisinone ([NTBC] 2-(2-nitro-4-trifluoromethylbenzoyl) cyclohexane-1,3-dione); a similar frequency of malignancy is still seen in patients who start nitisinone after 2 years of age but it is much lower if nitisinone is started by the age of 1 year (see later). On rare occasions, however, a patient will present with a hepatoma and few symptoms of liver disease.

Patients with tyrosinemia may also have porphyria-like crises, often following minor infections (6). After a prodromal period of lethargy and irritability, the patient develops severe pain, often in the legs. The patient may adopt an opisthotonic posture to alleviate the pain. Autonomic signs are common, including tachycardia, hypertension, ileus, and vomiting. One third of patients develop weakness, which may progress to acute respiratory failure. Patients may require ventilation for up to 3 months before they recover, and they may be left with a chronic polyneuropathy. The crises are caused by succinylacetone inhibiting the enzyme δ-aminolevulinic acid dehydratase (7). As a result, there is accumulation of δ-aminolevulinic acid, the neurotoxic chemical implicated in acute intermittent porphyria. Cardiomyopathy is a rare complication (8).

Investigations and Diagnosis As already mentioned, patients generally have a severe clotting disorder with milder abnormalities of standard liver function tests. Serum α-fetoprotein (AFP) is usually strikingly elevated. Prior to treatment, most patients have biochemical evidence of rickets and decreased renal tubular reabsorption of phosphate. The extent of the renal tubular disorder varies: generalized aminoaciduria is common but fewer patients have glycosuria or renal tubular acidosis.

Imaging of the kidney often shows nephromegaly and/or nephrocalcinosis (4). Imaging of the liver shows patchy changes with focal abnormalities. This represents cirrhosis with regenerative nodules that may later become malignant.

The plasma amino acid profile shows elevated tyrosine, phenylalanine, and methionine concentrations with low levels of branched-chain amino acids. The high tyrosine concentration is caused by secondary inhibition of 4-hydroxyphenylpyruvate dioxygenase (9). Urine organic acid analysis reveals succinylacetone, 4-hydroxyphenyllactate, and 4-hydroxyphenylpyruvate and non-specific compounds characteristic of liver disease.

The key metabolite is succinylacetone and the presence of this in urine or plasma is diagnostic. It is important to use a sensitive and specific test for succinylacetone because the concentrations may be very low in some patients, particularly those with late-onset disease (10). The diagnosis can be confirmed by measuring enzyme activity in cultured skin fibroblasts. The diagnosis should not, however, be based solely on enzyme studies because there is a genetic variant that causes no clinical problems but has a low enzyme activity in vitro (pseudodeficiency) (11). The diagnosis can also be confirmed by identifying mutations in the FAH gene. The two most common mutations are IVS12+5G>A and IVS6-1G>T. The former accounts for 94% of the alleles in the isolated Saguenay-Lac St Jean area of Quebec (12). Together the two mutations account for approximately 60% of alleles in those of European descent. Common mutations have also been identified in the Finnish, Pakistani, and Turkish populations (13). A mutation R341W is responsible for the pseudodeficiency and 2.2% of Norwegians are carriers (14).

Treatment and Outcomes For many years, the mainstay of treatment for tyrosinemia type 1 was a low tyrosine and phenylalanine diet. Although there was some improvement in many patients, dietary treatment did not prevent progression of the disease. The only alternative was liver transplantation.

Over the last decade, the management of tyrosinemia type 1 has been completely altered by the introduction of nitisinone. This compound is a potent inhibitor of 4-hydroxyphenylpyruvate dioxygenase (15). It almost completely arrests flux through the tyrosine degradation pathway, such that there is almost no formation of the toxic metabolites. Treatment with nitisinone should start as soon as the diagnosis is made. The standard dose is 1 mg/kg/day but a few patients require a higher dose. The response should be assessed by monitoring urine succinylacetone

as well as liver function (including blood clotting), renal tubular function, plasma amino acids (quantitative), and serum AFP. Succinylacetone should disappear from the urine within 1 week of starting nitisinone and subsequently its presence is an indication for increasing the dose. Some centers also measure plasma succinylacetone or erythrocyte δ-aminolevulinic acid dehydratase: these may take longer to return to normal. Monitoring of AFP is discussed later. In most patients there is a rapid improvement in liver and renal function. A few patients with liver failure do not respond. An initial plasma bilirubin concentration greater than 100 μmol/L is a poor prognostic sign. If there is no improvement in liver function (particularly clotting) after 7 to 14 days, urgent transplantation is necessary.

Plasma tyrosine concentrations increase in patients given nitisinone, as a result of the enzyme inhibition. Very high tyrosine concentrations can have adverse effects on the eye, skin, and brain (see tyrosinemia type 2). It is, therefore, necessary to treat patients with a diet low in phenylalanine and tyrosine at the same time that nitisinone is introduced. The available data do not yet indicate how strictly plasma tyrosine concentrations need to be controlled; most centers aim to keep levels between 250 and 500 μmol/L with an otherwise normal amino acid profile. The cognitive outcome is sometimes disappointing but this may be due to factors other than the tyrosine concentration (P.T. Clayton, personal communication).

The low phenylalanine and tyrosine diet used in patients receiving nitisinone is analogous to that used in phenylketonuria. A small, measured amount of natural protein is given each day, along with an amino acid mixture that is free from phenylalanine and tyrosine. Blood tyrosine concentrations are measured regularly and the natural protein intake adjusted as necessary. The restriction of phenylalanine often leads to low blood concentrations, particularly in the afternoon, when levels tend to be lowest (16). Phenylalanine supplements may be needed to avoid very low concentrations but they do, of course, raise tyrosine levels so the minimum possible dose should be used.

Few adverse effects of nitisinone have been reported apart from the rise in tyrosine concentrations. Some patients develop transient eye problems (soreness, photophobia, or erosions), presumably related to the raised tyrosine concentrations, although levels were no higher than in asymptomatic patients (17). Initial thrombocytopenia and neutropenia have been reported but long-term withdrawal of the drug has never been necessary.

Treatment with nitisinone abolishes the acute hepatic and porphyric crises (18).

Cirrhosis may also improve but it is unlikely to resolve completely. The risk of liver cancer mainly depends on the age at which nitisinone is started. The risk appears to be low in patients starting treatment by 6 months of age. Among 180 such patients in the International nitisinone Trial (currently aged 2–13 years), there has been one hepatic malignancy (E. Holme, personal communication, 2004). Unfortunately, late-diagnosed patients have a much higher risk. Hepatocellular carcinoma has occurred in 25% of the 91 patients in the International nitisinone Study who started nitisinone after the age of 2 years (E. Holme, personal communication, 2004). This is probably due to their cirrhosis and also the mutagenic effects of previous fumarylacetoacetate exposure. Thus, late-diagnosed patients need to be followed very carefully. It is not yet clear whether the risk of malignancy falls with duration of nitisinone treatment in late-diagnosed patients. If nitisinone is not taken regularly, the risk appears to increase dramatically.

All patients with tyrosinemia type 1 should undergo regular monitoring of serum AFP. In most patients, a frequency of every 3 months seems to be appropriate. The concentration usually decreases to normal following the introduction of nitisinone and an increase indicates the need for immediate assessment, including liver imaging (17). A number of late-diagnosed patients have persistent elevation of AFP and some of these patients have hepatomas. Normal AFP concentrations have been reported in the presence of a hepatoma but this appears to be rare (19). Lectin-reactive AFP may be a better predictor (20). Many centers undertake routine hepatic imaging. One regimen is to perform ultrasonography every 6 months, with magnetic resonance imaging if a nodule is seen or if the AFP value causes concern. Unfortunately, no imaging technique can distinguish reliably between all benign and malignant nodules.

The possibility of malignancy is now the main indication for transplantation in tyrosinemia type 1. If there is any suggestion of malignant change, liver transplantation is necessary. There may also be a place for elective transplantation in late-diagnosed patients, particularly those starting nitisinone (NTBC) after 2 years of age. Although AFP monitoring and imaging will identify most cases of hepatocellular carcinoma in time for transplantation, a few will already have metastases. The 5-year survival for pediatric liver transplantation is now more than 90% in some centers and elective transplantation for tyrosinemia has a better outcome than average. Complications do still occur and patients need lifelong immunosuppressive drugs, which are associated with significant morbidity. Decisions about elective transplantation will depend on the individual circumstances of each patient.

Liver transplantation prevents the neurologic and hepatic complications of tyrosinemia and it is standard practice to stop nitisinone (NTBC). The enzyme defect persists, however, in the kidney and patients continue to excrete succinylacetone (21). Although renal tubular function improves in many (21), there is a risk of progressive renal disease, even though less nephrotoxic immunosuppression is now used.

Prenatal Diagnosis Prenatal diagnosis of tyrosinemia type 1 is possible by using various techniques. Molecular studies are used if the mutations are known in the index case or if there are informative linkage markers. Otherwise, fumarylacetoacetase can be measured in cultured chorionic villus cells or amniocytes (22). If this technique is used, the pseudodeficiency mutation should previously have been excluded in the parents. Succinylacetone can be measured directly in amniotic fluid by using a sensitive assay, such as stable isotope dilution (23). Some centers use a combination of the latter two techniques if molecular studies are not possible.

TYROSINEMIA TYPE 2

Tyrosine aminotransferase deficiency (Figure 15-4 also known as Richner–Hanhart syndrome).

Clinical Features Tyrosinemia type 2 is a rare autosomal recessive disorder. More than 50 cases have been reported, nearly half of these having an Italian ancestry (24). Tyrosinemia type 2 can affect the eye, skin, and brain. Ophthalmologic symptoms occur in approximately 70%, skin lesions in 80%, and learning difficulties in 50% of patients in whom the diagnosis is established. Manifestations may differ within the same pedigree. It is uncertain how many patients remain undiagnosed—a number are probably asymptomatic.

The first symptoms are usually ophthalmologic. Patients often present with photophobia, pain, redness, and lacrimation, typically within the 1st year, although adult-onset has been reported. Severe photophobia may make it difficult to examine the child. Slit lamp examination shows bilateral dendritic corneal erosions that are readily confused with herpetic ulcers. Without treatment, corneal scarring may lead to permanent visual loss and glaucoma.

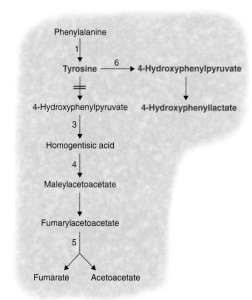

Figure 15-4. Defect and accumulating metabolites in tyrosinemia type 2. In tyrosinemia type 2 because of tyrosine aminotransferase deficiency, tyrosine accumulates which subsequently is converted by the aspartate aminotransferase enzyme to 4-hydroxyphenylpyruvate and 4-hydroxyphenyllactate. 1 = Phenylalanine hydroxylase; 3 = 4-Hydroxyphenylpyruvate dioxygenase; 4 = Homogentisate dioxygenase; 5 = Fumaryl acetoacetase; 6 = Aspartate aminotransferase.

The skin lesions are painful hyperkeratotic plaques on the palms and soles, including the digits. They are usually found at pressure points, such as the fingertips. The lesions may start as blisters and may ulcerate (Figure 15-5 A and B). Typically, skin problems appear after the 1st year. The neurologic problems are predominantly cognitive and behavioral. Some patients are mildly affected with poor fine coordination that varies with the metabolic status. Other patients have more severe impairment, with marked retardation and difficult, aggressive behavior.

Investigation and Diagnosis Tests of liver and kidney function are normal. Patients with tyrosinemia type 2 usually have a marked increase in plasma tyrosine, often above 1200 μmol/L (24). In some patients, however, concentrations may be as low as 400 μmol/L on a normal diet. The true proportion of patients who develop symptoms is, therefore, uncertain. Urine contains a wealth of tyrosine metabolites, including some formed distal to the metabolic block, such as 4-hydroxyphenylpyruvate, 4-hydroxyphenyllactate, and 4-hydroxyphenylacetate. This paradoxical finding is explained by the ability of aspartate aminotransferase to convert tyrosine to 4-hydroxyphenylpyruvate when it is present at high concentrations (Figure 15-4); several tissues, notably muscle, contain aspartate aminotransferase but lack

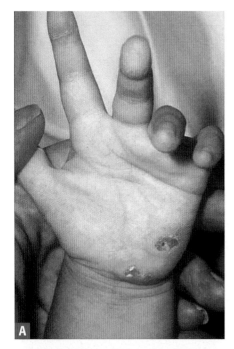

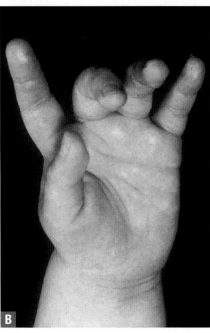

Figure 15-5. A and **B.** Hyperkeratotic lesion on palm of child **(A)** with tyrosinemia type 2 and the resolution **(B)** after treatment.

the enzymes to metabolize 4-hydroxyphenylpyruvate further, leading to its excretion. Thus, tyrosinemia types 2 and 3 cannot be distinguished by organic acid analysis. The diagnosis of tyrosinemia type 2 may be confirmed either by measuring the enzyme activity in liver or by molecular genetic studies. The R57W mutation is frequent in Italian patients (25).

The ophthalmologic problems in tyrosinemia type 2 are thought to result from tyrosine crystals precipitating in corneal epithelial cells,

disrupting lysosomes and leading to inflammation (26). In contrast, skin biopsies show no tyrosine crystals and minimal inflammation (27).

Treatment and Outcomes The mainstay of treatment is a diet low in tyrosine and phenylalanine (as described previously for patients with tyrosinemia type 1 who receive NTBC). In some patients, acceptable tyrosine concentrations have been achieved using a low-protein diet (in which the natural protein intake is adequate without the need for a tyrosine and phenylalanine-free amino acid supplement). Tyrosine aminotransferase requires pyridoxine as a cofactor and, although no pyridoxine-responsive patient has been described, a trial of oral pyridoxine (50–150 mg/d) has been recommended. With good control of plasma tyrosine concentrations, the eye and skin problems will resolve. Unfortunately, the neurologic and behavioral complications are much less likely to improve. Patients do not develop eye or skin lesions if the plasma tyrosine concentrations are maintained below 800 μmol/L but neurologic abnormalities may deteriorate at this concentration. At present it is not possible to give a precise target for tyrosine concentrations. Most centers aim to keep the plasma tyrosine concentration at least below 500 μmol/L.

It is not yet certain whether high maternal tyrosine concentrations have effects on the fetus. Two affected mothers have had children with learning difficulties and other problems (24) but a number of other mothers with tyrosinemia type 2 have had healthy children. Until more data are available, it seems prudent to keep tyrosine concentrations particularly well controlled during pregnancy.

TYROSINEMIA TYPE 3

4-Hydroxyphenylpyruvate dioxygenase deficiency (Figure 15-6).

Clinical Features This autosomal recessive disorder appears to be rare but it is possible that most patients remain undiagnosed. The phenotype has not been clearly defined. There is a suspicion, however, that the condition may be associated with mental retardation and possibly other neurologic complications (28). Several cases have been identified during the investigation of children with neurologic problems, such as developmental delay, seizures, or ataxia. More recently, patients have been identified in neonatal screening programs and most of these have also had learning difficulties. A few patients identified by neonatal screening are asympto-

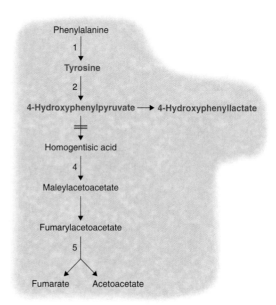

Figure 15-6. Defect and accumulating metabolites in tyrosinemia type 3. In tyrosinemia type 3 because of the p-hydroxyphenylpyruvic acid dioxygenase deficiency, tyrosine accumulates as well as 4-hydroxyphenylpyruvic acid and 4-hydroxyphenyllactate. 1 = Phenylalanine hydroxylase; 2 = Tyrosine aminotransferase; 4 = Homogentisate dioxygenase; 5 = Fumaryl acetoacetase.

matic and developing normally but this could be because of their dietary treatment. The patients do not have the eye or skin problems found in tyrosinemia type 2; this is partly because the plasma tyrosine concentrations are generally lower but there is considerable overlap so this cannot be the whole explanation (28).

Investigation and Diagnosis The biochemical findings are similar to those in tyrosinemia type 2 but the plasma tyrosine concentrations are usually less that 1200 μmol/L. Tyrosine levels may fall spontaneously over the first few months. Enzyme studies in liver tissue have been used for a number of years to establish the diagnosis. Molecular genetic studies now provide an alternative means to confirm the diagnosis (29) so it is increasingly difficult to justify a liver biopsy.

Treatment and Outcomes Most patients have received dietary treatment to lower their blood tyrosine concentrations. Target levels have varied and some patients have had a low-phenylalanine and -tyrosine diet whereas others have had a low-protein diet. Because the phenotype is poorly understood, it is not known whether treatment is necessary and whether it influences the long-term outcome. As a compromise, it has been suggested that the diet could be relaxed after the first few years of life. Ascorbic acid (vitamin C) is the natural co-factor for the enzyme and supplements have been tried but as yet there are no reports of improved tyrosine concentrations.

SECONDARY TYROSINEMIA

Secondary tyrosinemia is seldom a problem except in neonates and infancy. Any acute parenchymal liver disease may increase certain plasma amino acid concentrations, notably phenylalanine, tyrosine, and sometimes methionine. Galactosemia is the most frequent cause of this in the newborn period and cases are often detected in neonatal screening programs for phenylketonuria.

Transient Tyrosinemia in the Newborn

Transient tyrosinemia in the newborn is the most common disorder of tyrosine metabolism. Blood tyrosine concentrations in this condition usually reach a peak by 14 days, when they may exceed 1000 μmol/L. Affected babies are generally asymptomatic but lethargy has been reported. Subsequently concentrations fall to normal, generally by the age of 1 month. In premature babies, the condition is more common and tyrosine concentrations may remain elevated for longer. Transient tyrosinemia was much more common in the past, when babies were given milk with a higher protein content.

Most cases of transient tyrosinemia are thought to result from immaturity of 4-hydroxyphenylpyruvate dioxygenase. The theory has not been proven because liver biopsies cannot be justified. In typical cases of transient tyrosinemia, urine contains 4-hydroxyphenylpyruvate, 4-hydroxyphenyllactate, and 4-hydroxyphenylacetate, which would be consistent with 4-hydroxyphenylpyruvate dioxygenase deficiencies. Moreover, the fall in tyrosine concentration can usually be accelerated by ascorbic acid, which is a cofactor for 4-hydroxyphenylpyruvate dioxygenase. If a patient does not respond to ascorbic acid, the protein intake should be reduced and the assessments listed in Table 15-2 should be considered. Transient tyrosinemia is probably benign but there have been reports of subtle long-term cognitive and behavioral abnormalities (30).

Neonatal Screening for Tyrosinemia

Several newborn screening programs have evaluated patients with raised tyrosine concentrations. This has not proved a satisfactory way to detect cases of tyrosinemia type 1 because blood tyrosine concentrations are often only slightly elevated, particularly if screening is undertaken within a few days of birth. Moreover, it is relatively common to find raised tyrosine concentrations, particularly in premature babies, due to transient tyrosinemia. Thus, there are unacceptable numbers of false positives and/or false negatives, depending on the threshold concentration chosen. To increase the specificity, screening laboratories have used other tests for tyrosinemia type 1, such as AFP, succinylacetone, or δ-aminolevulinic acid dehydratase (31). In Quebec, succinylacetone is now the primary screening test rather than tyrosine (32). Screening is probably only cost-effective in regions with a high incidence of tyrosinemia type 1. The value of screening for tyrosinemia types 2 and 3 is unknown.

ALKAPTONURIA

Despite its relatively low prevalence, alkaptonuria was the first disorder to be recognized as an inborn error of metabolism more than 100 years ago (33). Deficiency of homogentisate dioxygenase leads to the accumulation of homogentisic acid and its oxidized derivative, benzoquinone acetic acid (Figure 15-7). This can then be polymerized to form a dark pigment, which is deposited in connective tissue.

Clinical Features Urine from patients with alkaptonuria darkens when exposed to air, particularly if it is alkalinized. Alkaptonuric patients usually excrete acid urine of normal color that does not darken for several hours. Cloth diapers may, however, turn black when washed, as may contaminated clothes and sheets. Some patients develop visible

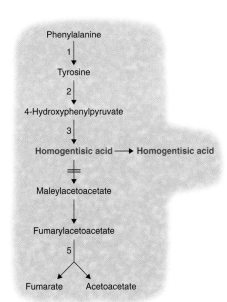

Figure 15-7. Defect and accumulating metabolites in alkaptonuria. In alkaptonuria, deficiency of homogentisate dioxygenase leads to accumulation of homogentisic acid. 1 = Phenylalanine hydroxylase; 2 = Tyrosine aminotransferase; 3 = 4-Hydroxyphenylpyruvate dioxygenase; 5 = Fumaryl acetoacetase.

pigmentation (ochronosis) of the sclerae or the cartilage of the ears after 30 years of age. Pigment may also be seen in the buccal mucosa and nails and as dusky coloration of the skin.

Patients with alkaptonuria generally have no symptoms as children or young adults but from adolescence onward they develop "ochronotic arthritis," usually starting in the hip or knee (34). It can be difficult to differentiate between common injuries (for example from sports) and the disorder. The clinical picture may resemble rheumatoid arthritis, with episodes of acute inflammation. Older patients may become bedridden due to severe limitation of movement. The early radiographic features resemble osteoarthritis; later, there may be ankylosis of the lumbosacral spine.

Patients with alkaptonuria may develop heart disease with generalized arteriosclerosis and calcification of the heart valves (34).

Investigation and Diagnosis Plasma tyrosine concentrations are normal in alkaptonuria. Organic acid analysis demonstrates the presence of homogentisic acid and establishes the diagnosis. Quantification of homogentisate is possible using high-performance liquid chromatography or specific enzymatic methods. Mutation analysis has been undertaken in a number of patients (34).

Treatment and Outcomes No treatment has been shown to prevent the long-term complications of alkaptonuria. The production of homogentisic acid can be reduced by dietary restriction of phenylalanine and tyrosine but there are major difficulties with compliance because the symptoms are so long delayed (35). Homogentisic acid production can also be reduced by use of NTBC (34); however, unless dietary phenylalanine and tyrosine are restricted, high tyrosine concentrations may lead to long-term complications (see Tyrosinemia type 1) but low dose nitisinone may be an alternative (36). Treatment with ascorbic acid has also been used to reduce the oxidation of homogentisate and pigment formation but as yet there is no evidence of benefit.

REFERENCES

1. van Spronsen FJ, Thomasse Y, Smit GP, et al. Hereditary tyrosinemia type I: a new clinical classification with difference in prognosis on dietary treatment. *Hepatology.* 1994;20:1187–1191.
2. Russo P, O'Regan S. Visceral pathology of hereditary tyrosinemia type I. *Am J Hum Genet.* 1990;47:317–324.
3. Kvittingen EA, Talseth T, Halvorsen S, et al. Renal failure in adult patients with hereditary tyrosinaemia type I. *J Inherit Metab Dis.* 1991;14:53–62.

4. Forget S, Patriquin HB, Dubois J, et al. The kidney in children with tyrosinemia: sonographic, CT and biochemical findings. *Pediatr Radiol.* 1999;29:104–108.

5. Kvittingen EA, Rootwelt H, Berger R, et al. Self-induced correction of the genetic defect in tyrosinemia type I. *J Clin Invest.* 1994;94:1657–1661.

6. Mitchell G, Larochelle J, Lambert M, et al. Neurologic crises in hereditary tyrosinemia. *N Engl J Med.* 1990;322:432–437.

7. Sassa S, Kappas A. Hereditary tyrosinemia and the heme biosynthetic pathway. Profound inhibition of delta-aminolevulinic acid dehydratase activity by succinylacetone. *J Clin Invest.* 1983;71:625–634.

8. Edwards MA, Green A, Colli A, et al. Tyrosinaemia type I and hypertrophic obstructive cardiomyopathy. *Lancet.* 1987;1:1437–1438.

9. Lindblad B, Lindstedt S, Steen G. On the enzymic defects in hereditary tyrosinemia. *Proc Natl Acad Sci USA.* 1977;74:4641–4645.

10. Haagen AAM, Duran M. Absence of increased succinylacetone in the urine of a child with hereditary tyrosinaemia type 1. *J Inherit Metab Dis.* 1987;10:323–325.

11. Kvittingen EA, Borresen AL, Stokke O, et al. Deficiency of fumarylacetoacetase without hereditary tyrosinemia. *Clin Genet.* 1985;27:550–554.

12. Grompe M, St Louis M, Demers SI, et al. A single mutation of the fumarylacetoacetate hydrolase gene in French Canadians with hereditary tyrosinemia type I. *N Engl J Med.* 1994;331:353–357.

13. St Louis M, Tanguay RM. Mutations in the fumarylacetoacetate hydrolase gene causing hereditary tyrosinemia type I: overview. *Hum Mutat.* 1997;9:291–299.

14. Rootwelt H, Brodtkorb E, Kvittingen EA. Identification of a frequent pseudodeficiency mutation in the fumarylacetoacetase gene, with implications for diagnosis of tyrosinemia type I. *Am J Hum Genet.* 1994;55:1122–1127.

15. Lindstedt S, Holme E, Lock EA, et al. Treatment of hereditary tyrosinaemia type I by inhibition of 4-hydroxyphenylpyruvate dioxygenase. *Lancet.* 1992;340:813–817.

16. Wilson CJ, Van Wyk KG, Leonard JV, et al.: Phenylalanine supplementation improves the phenylalanine profile in tyrosinaemia. *J Inherit Metab Dis.* 2000;23:677–683.

17. Holme E, Lindstedt S. Tyrosinaemia type I and NTBC (2-(2-nitro-4-trifluoromethylbenzoyl)-1,3-cyclohexanedione). *J Inherit Metab Dis.* 1998;21:507–517.

18. Gibbs TC, Payan J, Brett EM, et al. Peripheral neuropathy as the presenting feature of tyrosinaemia type I and effectively treated with an inhibitor of 4-hydroxyphenylpyruvate dioxygenase. *J Neurol Neurosurg Psychiatry.* 1993;56:1129–1132.

19. Paradis K, Weber A, Seidman EG, et al. Liver transplantation for hereditary tyrosinemia: the Quebec experience. *Am J Hum Genet.* 1990;47:338–342.

20. Baumann U Duhme V, Auth MK, McKiernan PJ, et al. Lectin-reactive alphafetoprotein in patients with tyrosinemia type I and hepatocellular carcinoma. *J Pediatr Gastroenterol Nutr.* 2006;43:77–82

21. Laine J, Salo MK, Krogerus L, et al. The nephropathy of type I tyrosinemia after liver transplantation. *Pediatr Res.* 1995;37:640–645.

22. Kvittingen EA, Guibaud PP, Divry P, et al. Prenatal diagnosis of hereditary tyrosinaemia type I by determination of fumarylacetoacetase in chorionic villus material. *Eur J Pediatr.* 1986;144:597–598.

23. Jakobs C, Kvittingen EA, Berger R, et al. Prenatal diagnosis of tyrosinaemia type I by use of stable isotope dilution mass spectrometry. *Eur J Pediatr.* 1985;144:209–210.

24. Fois A, Borgogni P, Cioni M, et al. Presentation of the data of the Italian registry for oculocutaneous tyrosinaemia. *J Inherit Metab Dis.* 1986;9:262–264.

25. Natt E, Kida K, Odievre M, et al. Point mutations in the tyrosine aminotransferase gene in tyrosinemia type II. *Proc Natl Acad Sci USA.* 1992;89:9297–9301.

26. Bienfang DC, Kuwabara T, Pueschel SM. The Richner-Hanhart syndrome: report of a case with associated tyrosinemia. *Arch Ophthalmol.* 1976;94:1133–1137.

27. Bohnert A., Anton-Lamprecht I. Richner-Hanhart's syndrome: ultrastructural abnormalities of epidermal keratinization indicating a causal relationship to high intracellular tyrosine levels. *J Invest Dermatol.* 1982;79:68–74.

28. Ellaway CJ, Holme E, Standing S, et al. Outcome of tyrosinaemia type III. *J Inherit Metab Dis.* 2001;24:824–832.

29. Ruetschi U, Cerone R, Perez-Cerda C, et al. Mutations in the 4-hydroxyphenylpyruvate dioxygenase gene (HPD) in patients with tyrosinemia type III. *Hum Genet.* 2000;106:654–662.

30. Rice DN, Houston IB, Lyon IC, et al. Transient neonatal tyrosinaemia. *J Inherit Metab Dis.* 1989;12:13–22.

31. Schulze A, Frommhold D, Hoffmann GF, et al. Spectrophotometric microassay for delta-aminolevulinate dehydratase in dried-blood spots as confirmation for hereditary tyrosinemia type I. *Clin Chem.* 2001;47:1424–1429.

32. Mitchell GA, Grompe M, Lambert M, et al. Hypertyrosinemia. In: Scriver CR, Beaudet AL, Sly WS, Valle D, eds. *The Metabolic and Molecular Basis of Inherited Disease.* 8th ed. vol 2. New York: McGraw-Hill; 2001:1777–1805.

33. Garrod AE. The incidence of alkaptonia: a study in chemical individuality. *Lancet.* 1902;2:1616.

34. Phornphutkul C, Introne WJ, Perry MB, et al. Natural history of alkaptonuria. *N Engl J Med.* 2002;347:2111–2121,

35. de Haas V, Carbasius Weber EC, de Klerk JB, et al. The success of dietary protein restriction in alkaptonuria patients is age-dependent. *J Inherit Metab Dis.* 1998;21:791–798.

36. Suwannarat P, O'Brien K, Perry MB, et al. Use of nitisinone in patients with alkaptonuria. *Metabolism.* 2005;54:719–728.

CHAPTER 16

Disorders of Transsulfuration

Brian Fowler, PhD

INTRODUCTION

Transsulfuration is a major metabolic route for the catabolism of methionine in humans and involves the formation of S-adenosylmethionine (SAM), S-adenosylhomocysteine (SAH), homocysteine (Hcy), cystathionine, and cysteine (1–3). The methionine transamination pathway is also involved in methionine metabolism but is a minor pathway that occurs only when methionine levels are abnormally high (>350 μmol/L) (2,3) and leads to the formation of 4-methylthio-2-oxobutyrate, 3-methylthiopropionate, methanethiol, and dimethylsulphide.

Inborn errors of transsulfuration result from mutant alleles leading to severe loss of function of enzymes involved in the conversion of the essential amino acid methionine to cysteine (1). Cysteine is a key component of the glutathione cycle, linking this cycle to methionine metabolism. Methionine originating from the diet or from protein catabolism undergoes a number of metabolic transformations. Besides its role in protein synthesis, methionine's major function is in the formation of SAM. SAM is the donor of a methyl group (1-C unit) in a wide range of vital biologic methylation reactions, including the methylation of DNA and RNA, and the formation of neurotransmitters, hormones, creatine, and phospholipids. SAM also provides the propylamino group for the synthesis of polyamines, which as polycations, are important in the stabilization of intracellular structures containing negatively charged species such as negatively charged DNA or in membranes. In the polyamine synthesis pathway SAM is first decarboxylated by SAM decarboxylase and then donates a propylamino group to putrescine, which is formed from ornithine, yielding spermidine and 5-methylthioribose 1-phosphate (1). This latter compound can be reconverted to methionine.

The conversion of methionine to cysteine (Figure 16-1) begins with the methionine adenosyltransferase (MAT) catalyzed activation to SAM. The donation of the methyl group of SAM, in any of the many SAM-dependent methyltransferase reactions, results in the formation of SAH. In the reaction catalyzed by the highly abundant glycine methyltransferase, SAM is converted to SAH by transferring the methyl group to glycine, which is thereby converted to sarcosine (N-methylglycine) (4). Glycine methyltransferase (GMT) fulfils the need for a high-capacity utilization of SAM and can be considered an integral enzyme in the transsulfuration sequence. SAH, through competitive inhibition of many SAM-dependent methyltransferases, plays a critical role in the regulation of biologic methylation. SAH is then hydrolyzed by SAH hydrolase to adenosine and Hcy (5). The equilibrium constant of this reaction strongly favors SAH synthesis but so long as Hcy and adenosine are efficiently removed hydrolysis predominates. In the remethylation pathway Hcy is converted to methionine through either the 5-methyltetrahydrofolate and cobalamin-dependent reaction catalyzed by methionine synthase (see Chapter 17) or the betaine methyltransferase catalyzed reaction (6). Alternatively, Hcy is condensed in transsulfuration with serine by cystathionine β-synthase (CBS) to form cystathionine. CBS is a pyridoxal phosphate-requiring enzyme that has a SAM-binding activation site, and it also binds heme but the role of heme in the function of the enzyme is unclear (7). The CBS gene has been fully characterized (8) and over 140 disease-causing mutant alleles have been identified (9). Cystathionine is then broken down to cysteine and α-oxobutyrate by γ-cystathionase, which also requires pyridoxal 5'phosphate (vitamin B_6). The γ-cystathionase gene has also been characterized and mutant alleles identified in subjects with cystathioninuria. Cysteine is an important precursor of the antioxidant glutathione. Glutathione is important in a number of cellular processes: as a reductant in the scavenging of free radicals; in the metabolism of xenobiotics; in the transport of amino acids; and in the synthesis of proteins and DNA.

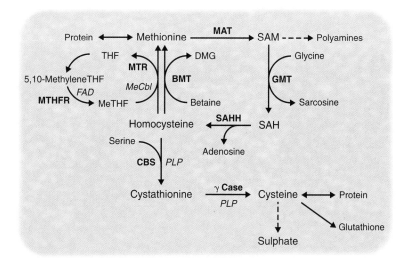

FIGURE 16-1. Outline of Methionine Metabolism. BMT = betaine methyltransferase, γ Case = gamma-cystathionase, CBS = cystathionine ß-synthase, DMG = dimethylglycine, FAD = flavin adenine dinucleotide, GMT = glycine methyltransferase, MAT = methionine adenosyltransferase, MeCbl = methylcobalamin, MeTHF = 5-methyltetrahydrofolate, MTHFR = methylenetetrahydrofolate reductase, MTR= methionine synthase, PLP= pyridoxal phosphate, SAH(H) = S-adenosylhomocysteine (hydrolase), SAM = S-adenosylmethionine, THF = tetrahydrofolate.

Transsulfuration

AT-A-GLANCE

Disorders of transsulfuration include deficiencies of enzymes involved in the conversion of the essential sulfur-containing amino acid methionine to cysteine. Biochemical features are mainly related to the pathologic alterations of concentrations of the main amino acid substrates of the pathway itself as well as important closely related metabolites such as methylated compounds. Cystathionine ß-synthase (CBS) deficiency, the classic form of homocystinuria, is the second most common inherited disorder of amino acid metabolism in some populations and causes multisystem progressive disease of varying severity. Treatment of this disorder centers on the reduction of elevated homocysteine (Hcy) by one or a combination of high-dose pyridoxine in responsive patients, betaine administration, or restriction of dietary methionine intake. Glycine N-methyltransferase (GMT) has been described in three patients with mild liver disease and S-adenosylhomocysteine hydrolase (SAHH) deficiency has been reported in three patients with neurologic and liver abnormalities. The clinical manifestation of methionine adenosyltransferase (MAT) deficiency is poorly understood; most patients appear to be symptom free although exceptional patients have shown evidence of brain demyelination or cognitive impairment. γ-Cystathionase deficiency is considered to be a benign condition.

DISORDER	OCCURRENCE	GENE	LOCUS	OMIM
MAT deficiency	>60 patients	MAT1A	10q22	250850
GMT deficiency	3 patients	GMT	6p12	606664
SAHH deficiency	3 patients	SAHH	20cen-q13.1	180960
CBS deficiency	~1:50'000 − 1:300'000	CBS	21q22.3	236200
γ-Cystathionase deficiency	~1:100,000	CTH	1p31.1	219500

DISEASE	FINDINGS		CLINICAL PRESENTATION	
			CHILDHOOD	JUVENILE/ADULT
MAT deficiency	↑ Met N/↓SAM N/↑ Hcy		Unpleasant odor due to excretion of methionine metabolites. Majority of patients without other clinical features: rarely neurologic involvement.	
GMT deficiency	↑ Met ↑ SAM N Hcy N SAH	N Sarc	Only 3 patients described with mild hepatomegaly and elevated transaminases at 1, 2, and 5 years of age.	
SAHH deficiency	↑ Met ↑ SAM ↑ SAH ?↑ Hcy	↑ Sarc	First patient presented in 1st year with severely delayed psychomotor development, muscular hypotonia, lack of tendon reflexes, elevated creatinine kinase, transaminases, and delayed myelination.	
CBS deficiency	↑ UHcy ↑/N Met ↑ Hcy	↑ CyHcy ↓ Cy	Severe presentation at 2-5 years with lens dislocation and myopia, skeletal abnormalities, mental retardation, cerebrovascular accidents, arteriovenous thrombosis.	Later presentation even in adulthood with milder abnormalities and sometimes involvement of just one organ
γ-Cystathionase deficiency	↑ Ca ↑ UCa	N/↑ UHcy N/↑ MMA	Most likely a benign disorder. Transiently seen in newborns, secondary finding in liver disease, neural tumors, and severe vitamin B₆ deficiency.	

Ca = cystathionine; Cy = cystine; CyHcy = cysteine homocysteine disulfide; Met = methionine; N = normal; Sarc = sarcosine; UHcy = urinary Hcy.

Oxidation of the sulfur atom and further breakdown of cysteine occurs through a number of enzymatic reactions ultimately yielding inorganic sulfate (10). First cysteine sulphinic acid is formed by the action of cysteine dioxygenase, and then transamination with α-oxoglutarate yields pyruvate and sulphite. The oxidation of sulphite to sulphate is catalyzed by the molybdenum-containing enzyme sulphite oxidase. Cysteine sulphinic acid can also be decarboxylated, yielding hypotaurine which is oxidized by a nicotinamide adenine dinucleotide–requiring enzyme resulting in the formation of taurine, an important amino acid with neurotransmitter function. In normal male adults approximately 70% of sulfur administered as methionine is excreted as inorganic sulfate, illustrating the major quantitative importance of this pathway in humans.

DISORDERS OF TRANSSULFURATION

Methionine-S-Adenosyltransferase Deficiency (MAT I/III)

Etiology/Pathophysiology MAT exists in three distinct forms: I, II, and III. The MAT I/III forms, encoded by the MAT1A gene, are expressed only in the liver, whereas the MAT II form, encoded by the MAT2A gene (1), is mainly expressed in fetal liver and in nonhepatic tissues such as kidney, brain, testis, and lymphocytes. Deficiency of MATI/III results in persistent hypermethioninemia without homocystinuria. SAM, the essential product of this enzyme reaction, appears to be normal or slightly reduced in plasma (11) (Figure 16-2). Inheritance in the majority of patients with persistent hypermethioninemia due to MAT1A gene mutations is autosomal recessive. A dominant form of inheritance has been described in patients with hypermethioninemia associated with the R264H mutation (12). Although only the MAT2A gene is expressed in brain it has been postulated that severe deficiency of MAT I/III may be associated with demyelination in those patients showing neurologic features (13). It has been suggested that there may be a relationship between the severity of the MAT2A gene mutation, the degree of elevation of methionine, and the occurrence of disease (14).

Clinical Presentation The great majority of patients with deficiency of MAT I/III have shown no clinical abnormalities except for unpleasant, sulfurous breath odor. When the plasma methionine concentration ex-

ceeds approximately 300 μM, transamination of methionine may lead to formation of 4-methylthio-3-oxobutyrate and dimethyl sulfide, causing the distinct pungent odor of the breath.

A few patients have shown neurologic abnormalities such as nystagmus, dysdiadochokinesis, increased tendon reflexes, mental retardation, dystonia, and dysmetria associated with demyelination of the brain seen on magnetic resonance imaging (MRI) studies. Because the total number of patients is small and long-term follow-up data are not yet available, a link between MAT I/III deficiency and manifestation of disease in at least some patients remains to be excluded.

Diagnosis First-line testing includes plasma amino acids and total plasma Hcy. Biochemical features of the MAT I/III deficiency include elevated plasma methionine, which can be detected on newborn screening, low-to-normal plasma SAM and normal-to-mildly elevated plasma total Hcy.

The finding of high plasma methionine needs to be interpreted carefully as it can occur in severe liver disease, hepatorenal tyrosinemia, CBS deficiency, or in infants fed a high-protein diet. High methionine can also be caused by rarer defects due to enzyme deficiencies downstream from MAT, such as GMT or S-adenosyl-homocysteine hydrolase (SAHH) deficiencies. Mildly elevated plasma total Hcy of 19.7 and 28.6 μmol/L (reference values 5–15 μmol/L) has been reported in two patients with MAT I/III and severely inactivating mutations of the MAT1A gene (15) might

lead to erroneous diagnosis of CBS deficiency. It is suggested that the elevated Hcy is due to decreased SAM levels (SAM stimulates CBS activity). Plasma SAM levels are normal to low in patients with MAT I/III deficiency, differentiating them from patients with CBS and GMT deficiency in whom SAM levels are elevated. Cystine levels are lowered in patients with CBS deficiency.

Confirmation of the diagnosis by enzyme assay requires liver tissue and therefore is not routinely performed. Differentiation of the primary hypermethioninemias (Figure 16-3) is aided by measurement of plasma levels of SAM and SAH. SAM levels in 13 patients ranged from below the reference values to within the reference range (48.2–120 nmol/L, reference 92.8 ± 16.2). SAH levels were also on the low side, ranging from undetectable to 36 nmol/L (reference range 15–45 nmol/L) (11).

The MAT1A gene has been localized to chromosome 10q22 and loss of function mutations have been described in several patients (14). Heterozygosity for the relatively common R264H mutant allele is associated with elevated methionine levels (12); however, the majority of described mutations are private. Prenatal diagnosis is theoretically possible by mutation analysis in chorionic villous material.

Mutations causing severe loss of enzyme activity and leading to extremely high methionine levels are associated with neurologic abnormalities, cognitive deficits, and MRI changes of white or gray matter in some but not all cases (Table 16-1).

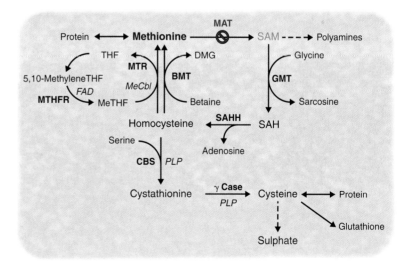

FIGURE 16-2. Methionine adenosyl transferase deficiency and its laboratory consequences (elevated levels in blue, decreased levels in green). BMT = betaine methyltransferase, γ Case = gamma-cystathionase, CBS = cystathionine ß-synthase, DMG = dimethylglycine, FAD = flavin adenine dinucleotide, GMT = glycine methyltransferase, MAT = methionine adenosyltransferase, MeCbl = methylcobalamin, MeTHF = 5-methyltetrahydrofolate, MTHFR = methylene-tetrahydrofolate reductase, MTR = methionine synthase, PLP = pyridoxal phosphate, SAH(H) = S-adenosylhomocysteine (hydrolase), SAM = S-Adenosylmethionine, THF = tetrahydrofolate.

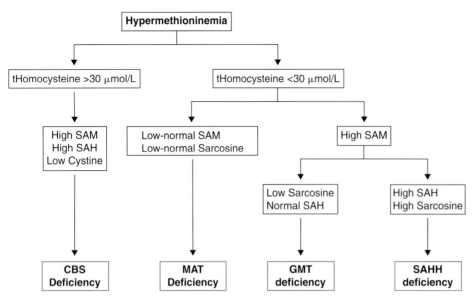

FIGURE 16-3. Diagnostic flowchart of hypermethioninemia. tHomocysteine = total homocysteine, CBS = cystathionine ß-synthase, GMT = glycine methyltransferase, MAT = methionine adenosyltransferase, SAH = S-adenosylhomocysteine, SAM = S-Adenosylmethionine.

TABLE 16-1	Laboratory Findings in MAT I/III Deficiency	
Decreased	**Increased**	
MAT I/III activity in liver	Plasma methionine	
+/− SAM	+/− plasma total Hcy	
+/−SAH		

Treatment The majority of patients have developed normally without treatment; however, administration of SAM (400 mg of the toluene sulphonate, twice daily) corrects deficiency of this compound in patients with evidence of demyelination and can reverse this process (16). Treatment with SAM may be advisable in cases with specific mutations leading to a severe enzyme deficiency and very high methionine levels.

GLYCINE N-METHYLTRANSFERASE DEFICIENCY (GMT)

Etiology/Pathophysiology This very rare disorder is caused by deficiency of GMT (17,18). GMT is found in liver and exocrine pancreas and carries out the transfer of a methyl group from SAM to glycine with the formation of sarcosine (N-methylglycine) and SAH (Figure 16-4). Because this methyltransferase plays an important quantitative role in through put of methyl groups, its deficiency causes elevated concentrations of methionine and SAM in tissues and physiologic fluids. Pathogenic effects in this disorder may be related to SAM elevation rather than hypermethioninemia per se.

Clinical Presentation Only three patients have been described (17,19), presenting at 1, 2, and 5 years of age with mild hepatomegaly, slightly elevated transaminases, persistent hypermethioninemia (10 x normal), elevated SAM (20 x normal), low sarcosine, and normal total Hcy levels.

Diagnosis First-line screening in this disorder includes quantitative plasma amino acids and total Hcy. Biochemical and laboratory features of GMT deficiency include elevated plasma methionine, elevated plasma SAM, and elevated transaminases. Normal plasma

TABLE 16-2	Laboratory Findings in GMT Deficiency	
Decreased		**Increased**
+/−SAH		Plasma methionine
+/− Sarcosine		SAM

SAH and low sarcosine levels differentiate GMT deficiency from SAHH deficiency. Normal total Hcy levels rule out CBS deficiency. The elevated methionine levels in this disorder possibly result from down regulation of the conversion of methionine to SAM by the accumulated SAM.

Although direct measurement of GMT enzymatic activity in the liver or pancreas has not been possible, a mutation of the GMT gene in one patient was associated with greatly reduced activity when expressed in E. Coli (19). Confirmation of the diagnosis by enzyme assay in liver tissue is not routinely justified.

The GMT gene has been localized to chromosome 6p12 and mutations leading to deficient enzyme activity have been described in each of the three patients (Table 16-2).

Treatment Dietary restriction of methionine together with added cysteine to guard against possible glutathione deficiency has been speculated to be beneficial.

S-ADENOSYL-HOMOCYSTEINE HYDROLASE DEFICIENCY (SAHH)

Etiology/Pathophysiology SAHH catalyzes the reversible hydrolysis of SAH to adenosine and Hcy and sustains the flux of methionine

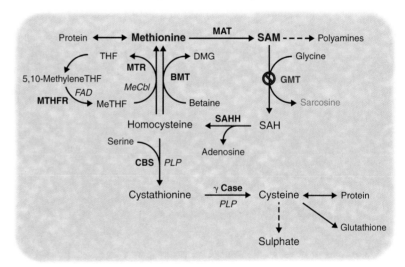

FIGURE 16-4. Glycine N-methyltransferase deficiency and its laboratory consequences (elevated levels in blue, decreased levels in green). BMT = betaine methyltransferase, γ Case = gamma-cystathionase, CBS = cystathionine ß-synthase, DMG = dimethylglycine, FAD = flavin adenine dinucleotide, GMT = glycine methyltransferase, MAT = methionine adenosyltransferase, MeCbl = methylcobalamin, MeTHF = 5-methyltetrahydrofolate, MTHFR = methylenetetrahydrofolate reductase, MTR = methionine synthase, PLP = pyridoxal phosphate, SAH(H) = S-adenosylhomocysteine (hydrolase), SAM = S-Adenosylmethionine, THF = tetrahydrofolate.

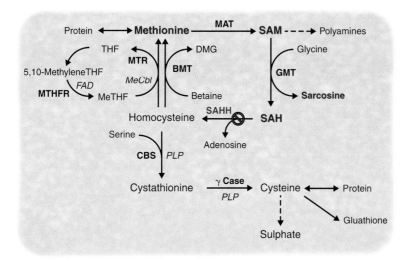

FIGURE 16-5. S-Adenosylhomocysteine hydrolase deficiency and its laboratory consequences (elevated levels in blue). BMT = betaine methyltransferase, γ Case = gamma-cystathionase, CBS = cystathionine ß-synthase, DMG = dimethylglycine, FAD = flavin adenine dinucleotide, GMT = glycine methyltransferase, MAT = methionine adenosyltransferase, MeCbl = methylcobalamin, MeTHF = 5-methyltetrahydrofolate, MTHFR = methylenetetrahydrofolate reductase, MTR = methionine synthase, PLP = pyridoxal phosphate, SAH(H) = S-adenosylhomocysteine (hydrolase), SAM = S-Adenosylmethionine, THF = tetrahydrofolate.

TABLE 16-3	Laboratory Findings in SAHH Deficiency
Decreased	**Increased**
SAHH enzyme activity	Plasma methionine
Choline	Plasma SAH
Phosphatidyl choline	Plasma SAM
	+/− plasma total Hcy

to the transsulfuration pathway (Figure 16-5). Marked deficiency of liver, erythrocyte, and cultured skin fibroblast SAHH activity has been demonstrated in a single patients see footnote (20). This defect causes massively increased plasma and cerebrospinal fluid levels of SAH, which is a well-established inhibitor of numerous SAM-dependent methyltransferases. This inhibition likely leads to disrupted levels of several substrates and/or products of methylation reactions with marked pathophysiologic consequences.

Clinical Presentation

The single male patient described had exhibited psychomotor delay since birth and regression of attained developmental milestones after 5 months of age. He had also exhibited marked muscular hypotonia and lack of tendon reflexes. Concomitant, convergent strabismus was observed at 11 months of age. Muscle histology revealed abnormal myelin figures within the muscle fibers and extracellularly. Electromyography showed myopathic potentials. Histological examination of a liver biopsy indicated the presence of mild, active chronic hepatitis with moderate portal fibrosis, and electron microscopy revealed hyperplasia of the smooth endoplasmic reticulum. Plasma transaminases and creatine kinase were elevated with low levels of albumin and fibrinogen and a prolonged prothrombin time. At 1 year of age, MRI revealed atrophy of white matter and delayed myelination. MR spectroscopy of white matter revealed a reduced ratio of choline to creatine with normal gray matter.

Diagnosis

First-line testing in the SAHH deficiency includes plasma amino acids, and plasma total Hcy. As for MAT I/III and GMT deficiencies, diagnosis is aided by measurement of plasma levels of SAM and SAH. In the one patient diagnosed with SAHH deficiency, the methionine level was markedly elevated by 10- to 15-fold of the normal range, with SAH being 150-fold and SAM 30-fold above the mean of the reference range. Total Hcy was slightly elevated as was cystathionine. Liver enzymes were elevated and partial prothrombin time was prolonged. Additional altered metabolite levels included elevations of sarcosine, guanidinoacetate, betaine, dimethylglycine, and cystathionine with low levels of choline and phosphatidyl choline.

The finding of only mildly elevated plasma total Hcy (14.5–15.9 μmol/L, reference < 10.7) differentiates this condition from CBS deficiency and the elevated SAM levels rule out MAT I/III deficiency. Elevated SAH and sarcosine levels provide strong evidence against GMT deficiency. The elevation of sarcosine in SAHH is attributed to an increased rate of SAM-dependent methylation of glycine. Assay of the enzyme in erythrocytes, cultured skin fibroblasts, and liver extracts is possible for confirmation of the diagnosis.

The SAHH gene has been localized to chromosome 20cen-q13.1 and paternally and maternally inherited mutations were found in the single described patient. Prenatal diagnosis is theoretically possible by mutation analysis in chorionic villous material (Table 16-3).

Treatment The treatment approach in the first patient consisted of a low-methione diet supplemented with egg yolk (a source of phosphatidyl choline) and creatine monohydrate (5 g/d). Short-term results showed improved muscle strength and mental function.

Miscellaneous Clinical Information SAHH deficiency suspected in three previously reported siblings is more likely to be secondary to liver disease than to a primary enzyme deficiency. One previous case described with hypermethioninemia, myopathy, delayed psychomotor development, mild liver disease, and elevated creatine kinase may also have SAHH deficiency. Two additional cases of SAHH deficiency have been described with essentially similar clinical and biochemical findings (21, 22).

CYSTATHIONINE β-SYNTHASE DEFICIENCY (CBS)

Etiology/Pathophysiology Classic homocystinuria due to CBS deficiency is an autosomal recessive disorder with significant phenotypic heterogeneity. CBS, the key enzyme of transsulfuration, converts Hcy to cystathionine and requires pyridoxal 5'-phosphate as coenzyme (Figure 16-6). In vitro studies have shown that SAM acts as a switch between the transsulfuration and remethylation pathways. As concentrations of SAM increase, CBS activity is enhanced but 5,10-methylenetetrahydrofolate reductase and betaine methyltransferase are inhibited, thereby limiting the remethylation of Hcy to methionine.

CBS deficiency leads to accumulation of Hcy, methionine, SAH, and reduced formation of cystathionine and cysteine in body fluids and tissues. The exact pathophysiologic mechanisms are not fully understood but likely ones include the following. Elevated Hcy, in this and other forms of severe hyperhomocysteinemia, is thought to cause vascular damage through endothelial damage, interference with platelet function and coagulation, and increased oxidative stress. Neurologic damage is a likely consequence of cerebrovascular accidents and in addition

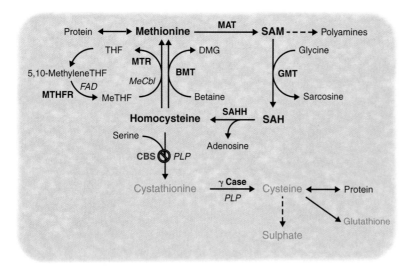

FIGURE 16-6. Cystathionine β-synthase deficiency and its laboratory consequences (elevated levels in blue, decreased levels in green). BMT = betaine methyltransferase, γ Case = gamma-cystathionase, CBS = cystathionine ß-synthase, DMG = dimethylglycine, FAD = flavin adenine dinucleotide, GMT = glycine methyltransferase, MAT = methionine adenosyltransferase, MeCbl = methylcobalamin, MeTHF = 5-methyltetrahydrofolate, MTHFR = methylenetetrahydrofolate reductase, MTR = methionine synthase, PLP = pyridoxal phosphate, SAH(H) = S-adenosylhomocysteine (hydrolase), SAM = S-Adenosylmethionine, THF = tetrahydrofolate.

may be due to disturbances of neurotransmission by Hcy itself and the related metabolites, Hcy sulphinic acid and homocysteic acid (Figure 16-6). The elevated concentrations of SAH may interfere with essential transmethylation reactions. Hcy alone is unlikely to cause skeletal changes and lens dislocation because these are not seen in homocystinuria due to remethylation defects. A possible mechanism for lens dislocation is disruption of the cysteine-rich zonular fibers as a consequence of cystine depletion (23). The disruption of the zonular fibers often causes bilateral dislocation of the lens inferiorly or nasally, increases the curvature of the lens, and leads to lenticular myopia and astigmatism. Iridodonesis (quivering of the iris on movement of the eye ball) is another sign of instability of the lens. Glaucoma may result from acute papillary obstruction due to the anterior dislocation of the lens.

Clinical Presentation CBS deficiency is a progressive, multiorgan disorder with involvement of the ocular, skeletal, central

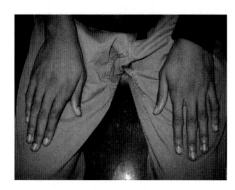

FIGURE 16-7. Arachnodactyly in an adolescent with homocystinuria.

nervous, and vascular systems (24). Patients are born normal but in the untreated, severe form they develop the full constellation of clinical abnormalities within 2 to 5 years of life. Ocular changes such as downward dislocation of the optical lens (ectopia lentis) and rapidly progressive myopia, which may precede lens dislocation, are consistent clinical findings in CBS deficiency. Ectopia lentis, although rarely seen before 2 years of age, is present in 70% of the patients by 10 years of age. Iridodonesis, glaucoma, detachment and degeneration of the retina, cataracts, and optical atrophy may also occur in some patients. Genu valgum and pes cavus are usually the first signs of skeletal changes. During peripubertal years the skeletal changes manifest as tall stature with decreased upper to lower segment ratios, elongation and thinning of the long bones, enlargement of the epiphyses and metaphyses, especially around the knees and arachnodactyly (Figure 16-7). These skeletal changes give the patients a similar appearance to that of patients with Marfan syndrome. The presence of osteoporosis, particularly of the spine, distinguishes patients with CBS from those patients with Marfan. This occurs earlier in pyridoxine-nonresponsive cases and has been described as early as 1 year of age. Generalized osteoporosis almost invariably occurs, at least after childhood, and may result in collapse of the vertebrae and scoliosis.

The most frequent abnormality of the central nervous system is mental retardation, although it is not usually seen during the first 2 years of life. Other neurologic manifestations include seizures, psychiatric disorders (episodic depression, behavioral disorders, obsessive-compulsive disorders, and personal-

TABLE 16-4   Central Nervous System Disease

- Mental Retardation:
  IQ ~ 65% (10–138)
- Neurological Abnormalities:
  Seizures (grand mal) (~20%)
  Abnormal EEG
  Extrapyramidal Disturbances
- Psychiatric Abnormalities (~50%)

ity disorders) and focal changes due to cerebrovascular accidents (Table 16-4).

Thromboembolic complications of the central nervous system may occur from the 1st year of life. Arteriovenous thromboembolic events can occur in all vessels and are often a cause of early death and less commonly ischemic heart disease (Table 16-5).

Hypopigmentation of the skin and hair as well as coarse hair are other features of homocystinuria. In treated patients with pyridoxine-responsive homocystinuria, a clear demarcation is observed between the darker, newly growing hair and the old blond hair. After initiation of pyridoxine therapy, hair consistency has been noted to change from coarse to a softer texture (25). Less severely affected patients present later in life, sometimes well into adulthood and without the full constellation of clinical signs but severe vascular complications, especially cerebrovascular thromboemboli (Table 16-5).

Diagnosis The diagnosis of CBS deficiency (26) is based on clinical findings and results of biochemical analysis. First-line testing includes fasting quantitative plasma amino acids, urinary amino acids, plasma total Hcy and, in some situations the cyanide nitroprusside screening test. Total Hcy refers to the total amount of Hcy present after the quantitative reductive cleavage of all disulfide bonds. Hcy exists in various forms in plasma (Table 16-6) and total Hcy measurement reflects the sum of nonoxidized Hcy (–SH form), disulfide forms (-S-S), and protein-bound Hcy. The cyanide nitroprusside urinary screening test (Brandt test) for homocystinuria is a qualitative test with low

TABLE 16-5   Vascular Disease

1	Arterial and venous thromboembolism
2	A major cause of morbidity and the most frequent cause of death in CBS deficiency
3	Peripheral veins (~50%)
4	Cerebrovascular (~30%)
5	Peripheral arteries (~10%)
6	Myocardial infarction (~5%)

TABLE 16-6   Structure and Forms of Hcy in Plasma

Term	Structure	Mean Normal Plasma Concentration
Hcy	$H-S-CH_2-CH_2-CH(NH_2)-COOH$	0.2 μmol/L
Protein-bound Hcy	$Albumin-Cys-S-CH_2-CH_2-CH(NH_2)-COOH$	8 μmol/L
Cysteine-Hcy mixed disulphide	$Cys-S-CH_2-CH_2-CH(NH_2)-COOH$	2 μmol/L
Hcy disulfide	$Hcy-S-CH_2-CH_2-CH(NH_2)-COOH$	not detectable
Total Hcy	All forms released by chemical reduction	10 μmol/L

sensitivity and false-negative results in up to approximately 30% of cases and cannot be used alone to exclude homocystinuria. Elevated plasma methionine, markedly elevated plasma total Hcy (usually > 200 μmol/L), elevated urinary Hcy, elevated SAM and SAH, and low cystine are highly suggestive of CBS deficiency. Biochemical and laboratory features of CBS deficiency include elevated plasma methionine (can be detected on newborn screening), markedly elevated plasma total Hcy, elevated urinary Hcy and elevated plasma SAM and SAH.

Exceptional cases may have only slightly increased total Hcy and could be confused with MAT deficiency but plasma SAM and SAH measurement distinguishes these two defects. Sensitivity of elevations of methionine to detect CBS deficiency in newborn screening samples is insufficient, particularly in pyridoxine-responsive cases (24).

- Results of urine screening for homocystinuria by the cyanide nitroprusside test can be falsely negative.

Confirmation of the diagnosis by enzyme assay can be performed using cultured skin fibroblasts or stimulated lymphocytes. Exceptional patients with typical biochemical and clinical features may show high residual enzyme activity (26).

The CBS gene has been localized to chromosome 21q22.3 (8), and so far more than 140 disease-causing mutant alleles have been described (9). Molecular genetic testing is of limited use for diagnosis because many mutations are private. The relatively common I278T and G307S amino acid changes are generally associated with pyridoxine responsiveness and nonresponsiveness, respectively. Prenatal diagnosis is possible by mutation analysis in chorionic villous material or by enzyme assay in cultured amniocytes (26) (Tabel 16-7).

Treatment Lifelong treatment can undoubtedly ameliorate the sequelae of the disease and optimal long-term outcome depends on its earliest possible introduction (27). Treatment is focused on normalizing Hcy levels, although this is difficult to achieve in most patients. Approximately half of patients show a clear response to pyridoxine (B_6) in doses from as low as 25 up to 1000 mg/day with normalization of Hcy levels in just a few cases (28). Pyridoxine responsiveness generally correlates with the presence of residual CBS activity in cultured fibroblasts. B_6 responsiveness, which must be tested in the presence of normal folate and B_{12} levels, is indicated by a fall of total Hcy and methionine levels. Pyridoxine (50 mg three times a day in the neonate and 100–200 mg three times a day in older children) can be prescribed to assess pyridoxine responsiveness and achieve metabolic control. So far no side effects have been reported, such as ataxia and sensory neuropathy, for high doses of pyridoxine up to 500 mg/day. Nevertheless careful neurologic follow up is indispensable in patients on high-dose pyridoxine.

Pyridoxine response may be prejudiced by folate status so that 5 to 10 mg/day of folic acid should also be given. In patients who are partially or nonresponsive to pyridoxine a low-methionine diet based on an amino acid mixture and natural protein can effectively reduce Hcy and methionine levels but compliance can be difficult. Administration of betaine, the substrate for betaine methyltransferase, can also lower Hcy but at the expense of raising methionine. The maximum effective dose of betaine appears to be 150 mg/kg/day. Cerebral edema has been recently reported in two patients receiving betaine (29). Although the mechanism

TABLE 16-7   Laboratory Findings in CBS Deficiency

Decreased	Increased
CBS enzyme activity	Plasma methionine
Plasma cystine	Plasma total Hcy
	Plasma SAH
	Plasma SAM
	Urinary Hcy

is unclear and hundreds of patients receive betaine without this complication, careful monitoring of methionine levels is indicated. Plasma cystine should be maintained within the normal range and supplemented accordingly up to 200 mg/kg/day.

Administration of vitamin C is reported to improve endothelial function in CBS-deficient patients. The use of antithrombotic agents such as aspirin and/or dipyridamole has no proven long-term benefit and should be considered on an individual basis (28).

Screening and Prevalence To date newborn screening based on measurement of plasma methionine has revealed an incidence ranging from 1:65,000 in Ireland to an average of 1:344,000 worldwide. There are a number of factors that point to this being a significant underestimate of the true frequency of this condition. First, screening so far has almost exclusively detected pyridoxine-nonresponsive patients in populations with an approximately equal distribution of responsive and nonresponsive clinically detected patients. Second, the sensitivity of detection of hypermethioninemia may be inadequate due to a delay in the appearance of increased methionine at the time of newborn screening at an early age and difficulties in selecting cutoff values. Third, studies of the frequency of heterozygosity for common CBS mutations within Danish and Norwegian populations suggest a much higher frequency of homozygosity for these pyridoxine-responsive mutant alleles of approximately 1:20,000 and 1:6,000, respectively (30, 31).

Pregnancy Outcome Information from more than 100 pregnancies in women with CBS deficiency suggests that there is no significant risk of malformations in the offspring in those with the pyridoxine-responsive form of the disorder. Experience in nonresponsive women is less but suggests that complications during pregnancy and abnormalities in offspring are infrequent events and are not related to the degree of biochemical abnormalities during pregnancy. Nevertheless, pregnancies in CBS-deficient women should be carefully monitored and awareness of increased risk of maternal thromboembolism, especially postpartum, is necessary (27).

Hcy as Risk Factor for Common Vascular Disease A large number of retrospective and prospective studies have established that a moderate increase of total Hcy is an independent risk factor for various forms of cardiovascular disease, including peripheral arterial occlusive, coronary artery disease, cerebrovascular disease and venous thrombosis (32). The exact cause for increased Hcy levels in patients with vascular disease and if and how moderate hyperhomocysteinemia results in vascular damage remains to be elucidated. Genetic factors as well as nutritional factors such as folate, vitamin B_{12}, and B_6 are also implicated.

γ-CYSTATHIONASE DEFICIENCY

Etiology/Pathophysiology γ-Cystathionase, the second enzyme of transsulfuration, converts cystathionine to cysteine and like CBS requires pyridoxal 5'-phosphate as coenzyme. Cystathioninuria caused by γ-cystathionase deficiency is an autosomal recessive inborn error of metabolism with an estimated in-cidence of 1:73,000. Deficient activity leads to greatly elevated levels of cystathionine and N-acetyl cystathionine in urine and plasma. In contrast to CBS deficiency plasma cystine levels are normal. The natural history of γ-cystathionase deficiency suggests that the disorder is benign.

Clinical Presentation The great majority of patients with deficiency of γ-cystathionase have no associated clinical abnormalities. Ascertainment bias explains the early observations of an association of this disorder with mental retardation. Patients with cystathionase deficiency and mental retardation either had siblings with the same biochemical disorder but no mental retardation or with mental retardation but no cystathionase deficiency.

Diagnosis First-line testing includes quantitative plasma amino acids and urinary amino acids. Biochemical findings suggestive of γ-cystathionase deficiency include elevated plasma cystathionine, elevated urinary cystathionine, and normal plasma methionine, cystine, and total Hcy. Elevated levels of cystathionine in urine are of the order of a few millimoles per day, and in plasma range from 6 to 80 µmol/L (reference < 0.3). Transient increases of urinary cystathionine may be seen in premature and some full-term infants, probably because this enzyme is absent in fetal liver and is expressed after birth. In transient cystathionuria of infancy the elevation of urinary cystathionine is mi-nor and disappears by the age of 3 months. Elevated urine and plasma levels have also been observed in patients with thyreotoxicosis, generalized liver disease, neural tumors (neuroblastoma, ganglioblastoma), hepatoblastoma, vitamin-B_6 deficiency, and in patients with elevated Hcy due to a re-methylation defect, although plasma levels in these patients are not so high as in primary cystathioninuria (1).

TABLE 16-8	Laboratory Findings in γ-Cystathionase	
Decreased	**Increased**
γ-Cystathionase	Plasma cystathionine
	Urine cystathionine

The CTH gene has been identified and mutations have been described in several patients with cystathioninuria (33) (Table 16-8).

Treatment The majority of individuals show a dramatic response of urinary cystathionine concentrations to administration of pyridoxine in high doses of 100 mg/day or more. Theoretically a low-methionine diet should also reduce accumulation of cystathionine but its use is highly questionable due to the benign nature of the disorder.

REFERENCES

1. Mudd SH, Levy HL, Kraus JP. Disorders of Transsulfuration. In: Scriver CR, Beaudet AL, Sly WS, et al. eds. *The Metabolic and Molecular Basis of Inherited Disease*. 8th ed. New York: McGraw-Hill; 2001:2007–2056.
2. Fowler B: Disorders of homocysteine metabolism. *J Inherit Metab Dis.* 1997;20:270–285.
3. Finkelstein JD. Pathways and regulation of homocysteine metabolism in mammals. *Semin Thromb Hemost.* 2000;26:219–225.
4. Yeo E, Wagner C. Tissue binding of glycine N- methyltransferase, a major folate-binding protein of liver. *Proc Natl Acad Sci USA.* 1994;91:210–214.
5. Hershfield MS, Aiyar VN, Premakumar R, et al. S-adenosylhomocysteine hydrolase from human placenta. Affinity purification and characterisation. *Biochem J.* 1985;230:43–52.
6. Garrow TA. Purification, kinetic properties, and cDNA cloning of mammalian betaine-homocysteine methyltransferase. *J Biol Chem.* 1996;271:22831–22838.
7. Kery V, Bukovska G, Kraus JP. Transsulfuration depends on heme in addition to pyridoxal 5'-phosphate - cystathionine beta-synthase is a heme protein. *J Biol Chem.* 269: 1994; 25283–25288.
8. Kraus JP, Oliveriusova J, Sokolova J, et al. The human cystathionine beta-synthase (CBS) gene: complete sequence, alternative splicing, and polymorphisms. *Genomics.* 1998;52:312–324.
9. Miles EW, Kraus JP. Cystathionine beta-synthase: structure, function, regulation, and location of homocystinuria-causing mutations. *J Biol Chem.* 2004;279:29871–29874.
10. Johnson JL, Duran M: Molybdenum cofactor deficiency and isolated sulfite oxidase deficiency. In: Scriver CR, Beaudet AL, Sly WS, et al. eds. *The Metabolic and Molecular Basis of Inherited Disease*. 8th ed. New York: McGraw-Hill; 2001:3163–3177.
11. Stabler SP, Steegborn C, Wahl MC, et al. Elevated plasma total homocysteine in severe methionine adenosyltransferase I/III deficiency. *Metabolism.* 2002;51:981–988.
12. Chamberlin ME, Ubagai T, Mudd SH, et al. Dominant inheritance of isolated hypermethioninemia is associated with a mutation in the human methionine adenosyltransferase 1A gene. *Am J Hum Genet.* 1997;60:540–546.
13. Chamberlin ME, Ubagai T, Mudd SH, et al. Demyelination of the brain is associated with methionine adenosyltransferase I/III deficiency. *J Clin Invest.* 1996;98:1021–1027.
14. Chamberlin ME, Ubagai T, Mudd SH, et al. Methionine adenosyltransferase I/III deficiency: novel mutations and clinical variations. *Am J Hum Genet.* 2000;66:347–355.
15. Kim SZ, Santamaria E, Jeong TE, et al. Methionine adenosyltransferase I/III deficiency: two Korean compound heterozygous siblings with a novel mutation. *J Inherit Metab Dis.* 2002;25:661–671.
16. Surtees R, Leonard J, Austin S. Association of demyelination with deficiency of cerebrospinal-fluid S-adenosylmethionine in inborn errors of methyl-transfer pathway. *Lancet.* 1991;338:1550–1554.
17. Mudd SH, Cerone R, Schiaffino MC, et al.: Glycine N-methyltransferase deficiency: a novel inborn error causing persistent isolated hypermethioninaemia. *J Inherit Metab Dis.* 2001;24:448–64.
18. Luka Z, Cerone R, Phillips JA 3rd, et al. Mutations in human glycine N-methyltransferase give insights into its role in methionine metabolism. *Hum Genet.* 2002;110:68–74.
19. Augoustides-Savvopoulou P, Luka Z, Karyda S, et al. Glycine N -methyltransferase deficiency: a new patient with a novel mutation. *J Inherit Metab Dis.* 2003;26:745–759.
20. Baric I, Fumic K, Glenn B, et al. S-adenosylhomocysteine hydrolase deficiency in a human: a genetic disorder of methionine metabolism. *Proc Natl Acad Sci USA.* 2004;101:4234–4239.
21. Buist NR, Glenn B, Vugrek O, et al. S-adenosylhomocysteine hydrolase deficiency in a 26-year-old man. *J Inherit Metab Dis.* 2006;29:538–545.
22. Baric I, Cuk M, Fumic K, et al. S-Adenosylhomocysteine hydrolase deficiency: a second patient, the younger brother of the index patient, and outcomes during therapy. *J Inherit Metab Dis.* 2005;28:885–902.
23. Fowler B: Homocystinuria due to cystathionine ß-synthase deficiency. In: Baxter P, ed. *Vitamin Responsive Conditions in Paediatric Neurology*. London: International Child Neurology Association, Mac Keith Press;2001:30–46.
24. Mudd SH, Skovby F, Levy HL, et al. The natural history of homocystinuria due to cystathionine ß-synthase deficiency. *Am J Hum Genet.* 1985;37:1–31.
25. Reish O, Townsend D, Berry S, et al. Tyrosinase inhibition due to interaction of homocyst(e)ine with copper: the mechanism for reversible hypopigmentation in homocystinuria due to cystathionine beta-synthase deficiency. *Am J Genet.* 1995;57:127–13.
26. Fowler B, Jakobs C. Post- and prenatal diagnostic methods for the homocystinurias. *Eur J Pediatr.* 1998;157:S88–93.
27. Yap S, Naughten E. Homocystinuria due to cystathionine b-synthase deficiency in Ireland:

25 years experience of anewborn screened and treated population with reference to clinical outcome and biochemical control. *J Inherit Metab Dis.* 1998;21:738–747.

28. Andria G, Sebastio G. Fowler B. Disorders of sulfur amino acid metabolism, in Fernandes J, Saudubray J-M, van den Berghe G, eds. *Inborn Metabolic Diseases, Diagnosis and Treatment.* 3rd ed. Heidelberg: Springer-Verlag: 2000:225–231.

29. Yaghmai R, Kashani AH, Geraghty MT, et al. Progressive cerebral edema associated with high methionine levels and betaine therapy in a patient with cystathionine beta-synthase (CBS) deficiency. *Am J Med Genet.* 2002;108:57–63.

30. Gaustadnes M, Ingerslev J, Rutiger N. Prevalence of congenital homocystinuria in Denmark. N *Engl J Med.* 1999;340:1513.

31. Refsum H, Fredriksen A, Meyer K, et al. Birth prevalence of homocystinuria. *J Pediatr.* 2004;144:830–832.

32. Homocysteine Studies Collaboration: Homocysteine and risk of ischemic heart disease andstroke: a meta-analysis. *JAMA.* 2002;288:2015–2022.

33. Wang J, Hegele RA. Genomic basis of cystathioninuria (MIM 219500) revealed by multiple mutations in cystathionine ß-lyase (CTH). *Hum Genet.* 2003;112:404–408.

CHAPTER 17

Inborn Errors of Folate and Cobalamin Transport and Metabolism

Chantal F. Morel, MD, FRCP(C), FCCMG
David S. Rosenblatt, MDCM, FCCMG, FRCPC, FCAHS

INTRODUCTION

The inborn errors of folate and cobalamin (Cbl) transport and metabolism, resulting from either defects in a transport system or from enzymatic deficiency, lead to decreased availability of vitamin coenzymes. Inherited disorders of folate metabolism include those characterized by abnormal absorption and transport and those caused by enzyme deficiencies (either primary or secondary due to Cbl coenzyme defects (Figure 17-1)). Inherited disorders of Cbl metabolism are also classified as those involving absorption and transport (Figure 17-2) and those involving intracellular utilization (Figure 17-3).

NORMAL FOLATE TRANSPORT AND METABOLISM

Folate metabolism involves absorption, transport, and intracellular reactions that result in the formation and interconversion of folate coenzymes (Figure 17-1). Reduced folates act as coenzymes, which serve as 1-C acceptor or donor units in a variety of reactions: methionine synthesis, histidine catabolism, purine ring synthesis, serine–glycine interconversion, and thymidylate synthesis (a key reaction in pyrimidine synthesis) (1–3).

- 10-Formyl-tetrahydrofolate (THF) is the folate precursor essential for purine synthesis.
- 5,10-Methylene-THF is the folate precursor essential for pyrimidine synthesis.
- Histidine catabolism results in the formation of 5,10-methenyl-THF, which can then be converted to either 5,10-methylene-THF or 10-formyl-THF.
- Serine to glycine conversion requires THF.
- 5,10-Methylene-THF reductase (MTHFR) converts 5,10-methylene-THF to 5-methyl-tetrahydrofolate (MeTHF). This reaction is irreversible in the cell.
- MeTHF, the principal form of folate in extracellular fluids, serves as the folate transport substrate in the body.

- MeTHF transfers its methyl group to methylcobalamin (MeCbl) to generate methionine from homocysteine. This reaction is mediated by the enzyme methionine synthase. The transfer of the methyl group to yield methionine leads to the regeneration of THF.
- When the activity of the methionine synthase is impaired, folates become "trapped" in the MeTHF form because the MTHFR reaction is irreversible in vivo (see Cobalamin section later).

Folate coenzymes thus play a vital role in DNA metabolism through two different pathways: 1) the formation of precursors required for DNA synthesis and 2) the synthesis of methionine, which is subsequently required for the synthesis of S-adenosylmethionine (SAM). SAM is a methyl group (1-C unit) donor used in many biologic methylation reactions, including the methylation of DNA and RNA.

Relatively few of the potentially numerous disorders of folate metabolism have been identified in patients, reflecting the likelihood that many deficiencies in this pathway may be incompatible with life (1). Folate deficiency leads to impaired purine and pyrimidine synthesis, which directly leads to an impairment of DNA synthesis (3). The rapidly dividing cells of the bone marrow are affected earlier than other cells, resulting in megaloblastic anemia. Other hematologic abnormalities occur, including macrocytosis

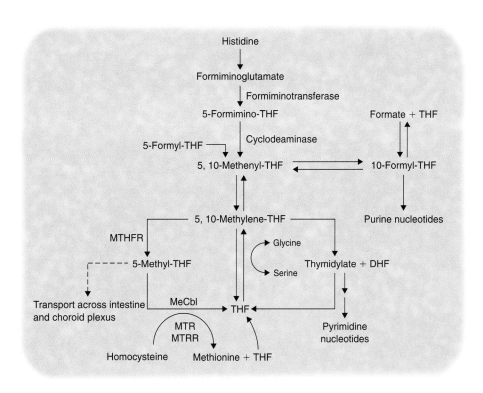

FIGURE 17-1. Summary of folate pathway. DHF= dihydrofolate, MeCbl= methylcobalamin, MTHFR= 5,10-methylenetetrahydrofolate, MTR= methionine synthase, MTRR= methionine synthase reductase, THF= tetrahydrofolate.

Inborn errors of folate and cobalamin transport and metabolism

AT-A-GLANCE

The inborn errors of folate and cobalamin (Cbl) transport and metabolism result from either defects in a transport system or from enzymatic deficiency and they lead to decreased availability of vitamin-derived coenzymes. Biochemical features depend on which part of the pathway is affected. Functional deficiencies of methionine synthase (folate pathway) lead to homocystinuria and hyperhomocysteinemia, whereas functional deficiencies of methylmalonyl-CoA mutase lead to methylmalonic aciduria and acidemia. Combined functional deficiencies lead to both biochemical abnormalities. Severe methylene-tetrahydrofolate reductase (MTHFR) deficiency is the most common inborn error of folate metabolism, and the cblC disorder is the most common defect of Cbl metabolism. When the folate pathway is involved, megaloblastic anemia is frequently part of the clinical presentation, along with various other hematologic abnormalities (severe MTHFR deficiency is the exception). Neurologic manifestations of varying degrees of severity are seen in many of these conditions. The goal of treatment is to normalize the biochemical abnormalities by administering pharmacologic doses of Cbl and/or folate. Betaine has become a useful therapeutic agent when the folate pathway is impaired.

DISORDER*	OCCURRENCE	GENE	LOCUS	OMIM
Hereditary folate malabsorption	~ 30 patients	PCFT	17q11.2	229050
Glutamate FTCD deficiency	~ 20 patients	FTCD	21q22.3	229100
Severe MTHFR deficiency	> 100 patients	MTHFR	1p36.3	236250
Hereditary intrinsic factor deficiency	~ 100 patients	GIF	11q13	261000
Imerslund-Gräsbeck syndrome	> 250 patients	CUBN, AMN	10p12.2, 14q32	261100
Transcobalamin (TC) deficiency	~ 50 patients	TC2	22q11.2	275350
cblC	~ 300 patients	MMACHC	1p34.1	277400
cblG	> 35 patients	MTR	1q43	236270
cblE	~ 20 patients	MTRR	5p15.3-p15.2	250940
cblA	~ 60 patients	MMAA	4q31.1-31.2	251100
cblB	~ 50 patients	MMAB	12q24	251110

DISEASE	FINDINGS		CLINICAL PRESENTATION	
			FIRST YEAR OF LIFE	CHILDHOOD & ADOLESCENCE
Hereditary folate malabsorption	↓ Folate N/↓ M	↑ UFGA ↑ UOA	Megaloblastic anemia +/− pancytopenia, diarrhea, stomatitis, FTT, neurologic deterioration, seizures, ataxia, partial immunodeficiency, neuropathy.	Presents in first few months of life.
Glutamate FTCD deficiency	↑ UFGA N/↓ M N/↑ F	N/↑ H ↓ FTCD	Presents from infancy to adulthood. Mild: no or mild mental retardation, no hematologic problems, may have hypotonia, speech delay, + +UFGA. Severe: megaloblastic anemia, mental retardation, growth deficiency, hypotonia, abnormal EEG, cortical atrophy.	
Severe MTHFR deficiency	HC/UHC N/↓ M N/↓ SAM	↓ MTHFR	Progressive encephalopathy, apnea, seizures, microcephaly, brain atrophy, mental retardation.	Later presentation may manifest up to adulthood as encephalopathy, ataxia, psychiatric problems, thrombosis.
Hereditary IF deficiency	↓ Cbl ↓ IF	N/↑ UHC N/↑ MMA N/↑ B	Usually presents after 1 year of age. Megaloblastic anemia, failure to thrive, vomiting, anemia, diarrhea, constipation, anorexia, irritability. May have pancytopenia.	Usually presents before 5 years of age. Nonclassic form may present in childhood or adolescence.

DISEASE	FINDINGS		CLINICAL PRESENTATION	
			FIRST YEAR OF LIFE	CHILDHOOD & ADOLESCENCE
Imerslund-Gräsbeck syndrome	↓ Cbl	N/↑ UHC N/↑ MMA	Megaloblastic anemia +/− pancytopenia, non-progressive proteinuria, neurological abnormalities such as paresthesias, spasticity, ataxia, cerebral atrophy.	Usually presents before 1 year of age. Rare late-onset cases reported.
TC deficiency	↓ TC N/↓ IG	N/↑ UHC N/↑ MMA +/− PCP	Megaloblastic anemia, lethargy, vomiting/diarrhea, weakness, severe infections, absence of neurological abnormalities (present if diagnosis delayed).	Usually presents in infancy. Rare adult cases where TC binds Cbl but cannot deliver to tissues.
cblC/cblD/cblF	↓ AdoCbl	↑ HC/UHC ↑ MMA ↓ MeCbl	Acute neurological deterioration, multisystem disease, retinopathy (*cblC*), MR, megaloblastic anemia +/− pancytopenia.	Confusion, ataxia, extrapyramidal symptoms, usually mild mental retardation.
cblG/cblE	↓ MeCbl ↑ HC/UHC N/↓ C	↓ M	Lethargy, feeding difficulties, vomiting, abnormal tonus, mental retardation, FTT, seizures, blindness, ataxia, cerebral atrophy, delayed myelination, megaloblastic anemia.	Usually presents before 1 year of age. Rare late-onset cases reported.
cblA/cblB	↓ AdoCbl ↑ MMA MA	N/↑ NH4 N/↑ G N/↑ K	Acidotic crisis within 1st year of life, FTT, lethargy, vomiting, hypotonia, encephalopathy, mental retardation, metabolic strokes, bone marrow failure.	Usually presents in infancy. Rare late-onset cases reported.

AdoCbl = adenosylcobalamin, B = hyperbilirubinemia, C = cystathionine, CVA = cerebrovascular accidents, EEG = electroencephalogram, F = folate, FTCD = formiminotransferase-cyclodeaminase, FTT = failure to thrive, G = glycine, H = histidine, Hcy = homocysteine, IF = intrinsic factor, IG = immunoglobulins, K = ketonuria, M = methionine, MA = metabolic acidosis, MeCbl = methylcobalamin, MMA = methylmalonic aciduria, N = normal, NH₄ = ammonia, SAM = S-adenosylmethionine, TC = transcobalamin, UFGA = urinary formiminoglutamic acid, UHC = urinary homocystine, UOA = urinary orotic acid.

*cblD and cblF not included due to their rarity and unidentified gene loci.

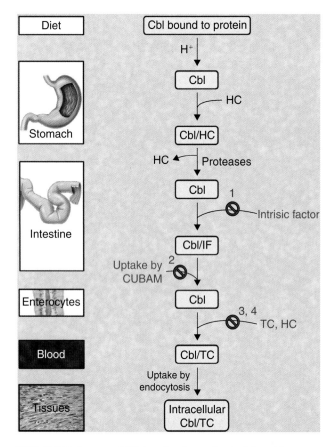

FIGURE 17-2. Summary of Cbl absorption, transport and cellular uptake. Cbl= cobalamin, Cbl/HC= Cbl–haptocorrin complex, Cbl/IF= Cbl–intrinsic factor complex, Cbl/TC= Cbl– transcobalamin complex, CUBAM= ileal receptors made up of cubulin and amnionless proteins, HC= haptocorrin, TC= transcobalamin. 1: Intrinsic factor deficiency, 2: Imerslünd–Grasbeck disease, 3: Trans–Cbl deficiency, 4: Haptocorrin deficiency. Adapted from European Journal of Pediatrics, 157;S60–S66, 1998, Genetic Defects of folate and cobalamin metabolism, B. Fowler, Figure 1 ©Springer-Verlag; with kind permission of Springer Science and Business Media.

and hypersegmented neutrophils on blood smear, leukopenia, and thrombocytopenia. Digestive problems such as failure to thrive, vomiting, diarrhea, mouth ulcers, and weight loss are frequently seen. In addition, neurologic disturbances such as hypotonia, seizures, lethargy, mental retardation, and ataxia occur, reflecting the importance of folate in the function of the central nervous system (CNS) (1–3).

Homocystinuria with or without hyperhomocysteinemia and megaloblastic anemia can be caused by various conditions, including inborn errors of folate metabolism (Table 17-1).

NORMAL COBALAMIN TRANSPORT AND METABOLISM

Cbl metabolism involves several steps including absorption, transport, and intracellular processing and utilization (Figures 17-2 and 17-3) (1,2,4).

- Dietary Cbl is mostly acquired from animal sources, including meat and milk. Therefore, individuals with strict vegan diets are at risk Cbl for deficiency, especially infants, and resulting persistent damage.

- Cbl is absorbed through a series of steps, including proteolytic release from associated proteins, binding to intrinsic factor ([IF], a gastric secretory protein), recognition of the Cbl–IF complex by CUBAM receptors on ileal mucosal cells, transport across these cells, and release into the portal circulation by binding to transcobalamin (TC).

- Intracellular processing of Cbl follows endocytosis of the Cbl–TC complex bound to its cell-surface receptor: intralysosomal degradation of TC, release of Cbl into the cytoplasm, and enzyme-mediated reduction of Cbl's central cobalt atom.

- The end result of the intracellular processing is the formation of Cbl coenzymes: methylcobalamin (MeCbl) and adenosylcobalamin (AdoCbl).

These Cbl coenzymes are needed for only two reactions in humans: those catalyzed by the mitochondrial methylmalonyl-CoA mutase (AdoCbl) and the cytosolic, folate-dependent enzyme methionine synthase (MeCbl).

Activity of methionine synthase is required for the synthesis of methionine from homocysteine. When MeCbl is lacking or the activity of methionine synthase is low due to mutations in the MTR gene, hyperhomocysteinemia and homocystinuria ensue. Decreased activity of methionine synthase in inherited vitamin B_{12} deficiencies inhibits the regeneration of THF and traps folate as MeTHF, a form of folate that is not available for purine and pyrimidine biosynthesis, resulting in symptoms of folate deficiency even in the presence of adequate folate levels (the folate trap hypothesis). Thus, in both folate and vitamin B_{12} deficiency, folate is unavailable for synthesis of purine and pyrimidine substrates required for DNA synthesis. In addition to the decreased availability of folate, elevated levels of homocysteine and/or low levels of methionine and SAM presumably contribute to the neurologic abnormalities seen in patients with defective MeCbl formation.

The second Cbl coenzyme, Adocbl, is required by L-methylmalonyl-CoA mutase (MUT), which catalyzes the conversion of L-methylmalonyl-CoA to succinyl-CoA. When AdoCbl is unavailable or MUT activity is decreased similar to gene mutations affecting the MUT enzyme itself, the resulting biochemical consequences are methylmalonic acidemia and methylmalonic aciduria, and metabolic acidosis (although the acidosis is not always present) (see Chapter 7).

In conditions simultaneously impeding the synthesis of MeCbl and AdoCbl (cblC, cblD, cblF), both methionine synthase and MUT activities are decreased due to the unavailability of their cofactors. The clinically detectable consequences include homocystinuria and methylmalonic aciduria, accompanied by hyperhomocysteinemia, low methionine and methylmalonic acidemia.

Homocystinuria/hyperhomocysteinemia, methylmalonic aciduria/acidemia, and megaloblastic anemia can be caused by various conditions, including inborn errors of Cbl metabolism. Table 17-1 summarizes the differential diagnoses to consider when confronted with low serum Cbl levels and increased homocysteine or methylmalonic acid levels. Figure 17-4 provides a flow diagram for patients presenting with neurologic abnormalities and hyperhomocysteinemia in the 1st year of life, and Figure 17-5 illustrates the sequential clinical work up of a patient thought to have an inherited form of megaloblastic anemia.

DISORDERS OF FOLATE ABSORPTION AND METABOLISM

Hereditary Folate Malabsorption

Etiology/Pathophysiology Also referred to in the literature as congenital malabsorption of folate because of its early clinical onset, this rare condition has been reported in approximately 30 patients. It is inherited in an autosomal recessive fashion. All patients have severely decreased intestinal absorption of oral folic acid or reduced .folates, such as 5-formyltetrahydrofolic acid (folinic acid) or methyltetrahydrofolic acid, as well as decreased choroid plexus transport of folate into the CNS (2,3). The gene mutated in this

- Severe pancytopenia has been reported and is also due to bone marrow impairment, which can potentially affect all hematologic cell line precursors.
- Low serum, red blood cell, and CSF folate levels are found.
- Low or normal methionine levels: a decrease is due to MeTHF deficiency, which in turn impsairs the remethylation of homocysteine to methionine. Plasma homocysteine is normal.
- Urinary excretion of forminimoglutamic and orotic acids may occur.

Folate absorption may be directly looked for by measuring serum folate levels following an oral dose of between 5 mg and 100 mg of folic acid (8,9).

A gene coding for the folate transporter defective in this condition has been identified; however, disease-causing mutations have only been described in one family, rendering this test likely research-based at present.

Because the defect in hereditary folate malabsorption is not expressed in amniocytes or chorionic villus cells, prenatal diagnosis is not an option.

Treatment Neurologic outcome is thought to be poor in general unless the condition is diagnosed early and treated aggressively. The goal of therapy is to maintain folate levels in the serum, red blood cells, and CSF above levels associated with folate deficiency: 4, 150, and 15 ng/mL, respectively (2). It is essential to monitor folate levels in CSF (3). High-dose oral folic acid (up to 60 mg/d) or lower parenteral doses in the physiologic range correct the hematologic abnormalities; however this is much less effective in raising the CSF folate level and in correcting the neurologic findings. Both MeTHF and folinic acid (5 mg intramuscularly twice

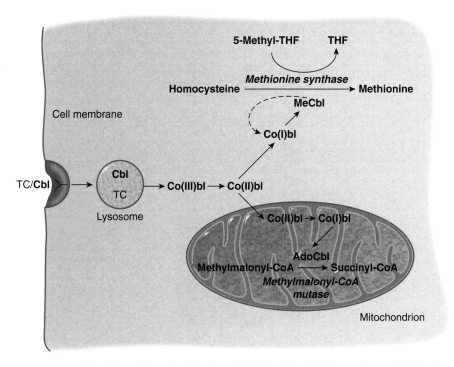

FIGURE 17-3. Intracellular Cbl metabolism. AdoCb l= adenosylcobalamin, Cbl= cobalamin, MeCbl= methylcobalamin, MTRR= methionine synthase reductase, TC/Cbl= transcobalamin–Cbl complex, TC= transcobalamin, THF= tetrahydrofolate.

condition encodes for a proton-coupled folate transporter (PCFT/HCP1) required for folate homeostasis in humans (5). It is thought that this transporter acts both at the level of the choroid plexus and the intestine, although rare reports of patients with isolated defects of folate transport into the cerebrospinal fluid (CSF) do exist and contradict this theory (6). Transport of folates across other cell membranes is not affected in this disorder. The hematologic and gastrointestinal manifestations are corrected by oral administration of relatively low amounts of folate in comparison to the higher amounts needed to raise CSF folate levels. Folate metabolism in cultured fibroblasts is not abnormal.

Clinical Presentation Patients typically present in the first months of life. Severe megaloblastic anemia is the hallmark of this condition. Diarrhea, stomatitis, and failure to thrive frequently occur, and most patients have progressive neurologic deterioration. Seizures, ataxia, and movement abnormalities can occur. Intracranial calcifications and peripheral neuropathy have been seen, as have partial defects in humoral and cellular immunity (2,3,7–9).

Diagnosis Biochemical and laboratory features of hereditary folate malabsorption include:

- Severe megaloblastic anemia due to bone marrow impairment secondary to folate deficiency.

TABLE 17-1	Causes of low serum cobalamin and elevated serum and/or methylmalonic acid and homocysteine levels		
↓ **Cobalamin**	↑ **Methylmalonic Acid**	↑ **Homocysteine**
Idiopathic	Renal insufficiency	Incorrect sample or processing
Pregnancy	Infancy	Renal insufficiency
Chronic diseases	Methylmalonyl-CoA mutase deficiency	MTHFR polymorphisms
Folate deficiency	cblA/cblB	Folate deficiency
Drugs (i.e., anticonvulsants, oral contraceptives)	cblC/cblD/cblF	Vitamin B6 deficiency
Imerslund–Gräsbeck syndrome	Other inborn errors of cobalamin metabolism	Chronic diseases (i.e., thyroid disease, leukemia)
Intrinsic factor deficiency	? Mild methylmalonic acid– related enzyme defects	Drugs (i.e. isoniazid)
Transcobalamin deficiency	? Bacterial gut contamination	Severe MTHFR deficiency
? Haptocorrin deficiency	? Volume contraction	cblC/cblD/cblF
		cblE/cblG
		Other inborn errors of cobalamin metabolism

cbl = colabamin; MTHFR = methylenetetrahydrofolate reductase.

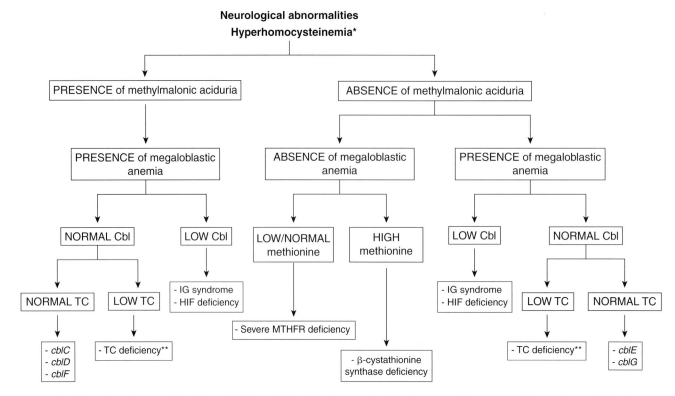

FIGURE 17-4. Flow diagram for patients presenting with neurologic abnormalities and hyperhomocysteinemia in the 1st year of life. FTCD= formiminotransferase-cyclodeaminase, HF malabsorption= hereditary folate malabsorption, HIF deficiency= hereditary intrinsic factor deficiency, IG syndrome= Imerslund–Gräsbeck syndrome, TC= transcobalamin.

*Disorders that can also present with normal total homocystine levels include: Hereditary IF deficiency, Imerslund–Gräsbeck syndrome, and TC deficiency.

**Presence of neurologic abnormalities only if diagnosis is delayed.

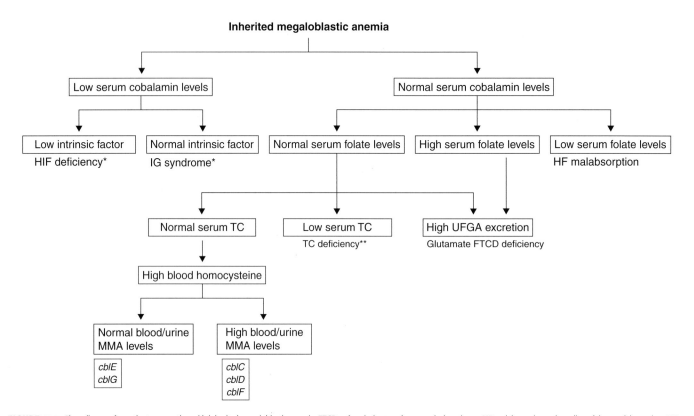

FIGURE 17-5. Flow diagram for patients presenting with inherited megaloblastic anemia. FTCD= formiminotransferase-cyclodeaminase, HF malabsorption= hereditary folate malabsorption, HIF deficiency= hereditary intrinsic factor deficiency, IG syndrome= Imerslund–Gräsbeck syndrome, MMA= methylmalonic acidemia, TC= transcobalamin, UFGA= urinary formiminoglutamic acid.

*Can also present with slight elevations in serum homocysteine, urine homocystine, and serum MMA.

**Presence of neurological abnormalities only if diagnosis is delayed.

weekly) may be more effective in raising CSF levels and either one can be given in combination with high-dose (40 mg/d) oral folic acid. Folinic acid can also be administered subcutaneously, intravenously, or orally. A recent report states that in some cases, high doses of folinic acid (up to 400 mg orally daily) may eliminate the need for parenteral therapy (7).

The clinical response to folates has varied among patients and, in some cases, seizures worsened after folate therapy initiation. Oral doses of folate may be increased to 100 mg/day if necessary. If oral therapy fails to raise CSF folate levels, parenteral therapy should be used. Intrathecal folate therapy should be considered if CSF folate levels cannot be raised by other treatments, although there is no experience with the dose of folate that may be required.

Glutamate Formiminotransferase-Cyclodeaminase Deficiency

Etiology/Pathophysiology Glutamate formiminotransferase-cyclodeaminase (FTCD) deficiency (Figure 17-6) is a rare autosomal recessive disorder of folate metabolism that has been described in fewer than 20 patients (2). It is associated with a deficiency of the enzyme by the same name. This bifunctional enzyme is involved in the catabolism of histidine. The transfer of a

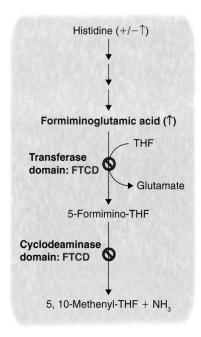

FIGURE 17-6. Glutamate formiminotransferase-cyclodeaminase deficiency and its laboratory consequences (indicated in parentheses). FTCD = glutamate formiminotransferase-cyclodeaminase, THF = tetrahydrofolate.

formimino group from formiminoglutamate to tetrahydrofolate (THF) is catalyzed by its glutamate formiminotransferase domain, and the subsequent release of ammonia and the formation of 5,10-methenyltetrahydrofolate is catalyzed by its formiminotetrahydrofolate cyclodeaminase domain. 5,10-methenyltetrahydrofolate can either be converted to 5,10-methylenetetrahydrofolate or to 10-formyltetrahydrofolate (Figure 17-1). The latter is required for purine synthesis (and is also converted to methylenetetrahydrofolate, making it available for other folate-dependent reactions). The hematologic abnormalities that can be seen in this condition may be related to impaired purine synthesis, due to the nature of the rapidly dividing cells of the bone marrow.

FTCD activity is found only in the liver and kidney, and defects in either the formiminotransferase domain or in the cyclodeaminase domain will result in formiminoglutamate excretion due to the accumulation of the enzyme's substrate. The gene that encodes this enzyme has been identified on chromosome 21q22.3 and named FTCD (10).

Clinical Presentation Two different phenotypes are associated with deficiency of the FTCD enzyme: a severe phenotype and a mild phenotype. The severe form of FTCD deficiency is characterized by mental and growth retardation, hypotonia, abnormal electroencephalograms, and dilation of cerebral ventricles with cortical atrophy. Several of the patients had a folate-responsive megaloblastic anemia with macrocytosis and hypersegmentation of neutrophils. Patients ranged in age from 3 months to 42 years (2,9).

The mild form of this condition presents with either mild or no mental retardation, isolated speech delay, absence of hematologic abnormalities, but a greater excretion of formiminoglutamate. Hypotonia may also be a presenting feature (11).

Diagnosis Biochemical and laboratory features of FTCD deficiency include:

- Elevated urinary excretion and serum levels of formiminoglutamate: this compound is proximal to the enzyme block, and therefore accumulates in FTCD deficiency.

- Elevated urinary excretion of 4-amino-5-imidazolecarboxamide, an intermediate of purine synthesis, may occur. Because purine synthesis is defective, there may be a build up of other compounds that are required for their synthesis.

- Elevated urinary excretion of hydantoin propionic acid (stable oxidation product of the formiminoglutamate precursor 4-imidazole-5-propionate) may occur: because formiminoglutamate levels are in-

creased, it gets shunted to an alternative pathway.

- Normal or high serum folate levels: a histidine-rich load will increase folate levels.

- Normal Cbl levels: the Cbl pathway and formation of Cbl cofactors are not affected in FTCD deficiency.

- Low or normal serum methionine levels: low methionine can occur as a direct consequence of decreased formation of MeTHF due to decreased synthesis of 5,10-methylenetetrahydrofolate.

- May have hyperhistidinemia and histidinuria because deficiency of FTCD impairs histidine catabolism, leading to its potential build up in body fluids.

A histidine load can help to establish the diagnosis by provoking formiminoglutamate elevation in blood and urine (9,11).

FTCD activity is expressed only in the liver and the kidneys. It is not expressed in cultured fibroblasts, and there is doubt as to whether it is expressed in red blood cells. The residual activity that has been measured in the livers of five patients has varied from 14% to 54% of control values. It has generally not been possible to confirm the diagnosis by enzyme assay from liver biopsies.

Because the gene has been identified, it has been possible to find disease-causing mutations. Three mutations have been identified to date in mildly affected patients: c403C->T (R135C), c896G->C (R299P), and c990dupG (11).

The enzyme is not expressed in cultured cells, making prenatal diagnosis by enzymatic activity impossible. Directly measuring formiminoglutamate levels in amniotic fluid may be an option, but this has not been reported (9). If the mutations have been identified in the affected sibling, molecular prenatal diagnosis can be accomplished. Alternatively, if the mutations are not known, linkage analysis could be attempted in informative families.

Treatment It is not clear whether reducing formiminoglutamate excretion is of any clinical value. Although two patients in one family responded to folate therapy by reducing excretion of formiminoglutamate, six other unrelated patients did not. One of two patients responded to methionine supplementation. Pyridoxine and folic acid have been used to correct megaloblastic anemia in one infant (9).

Severe Methylenetetrahydrofolate Reductase Deficiency

Etiology/Pathophysiology Severe MTHFR deficiency (Figure 17-7) is a rare autosomal recessive disorder causing decreased production of

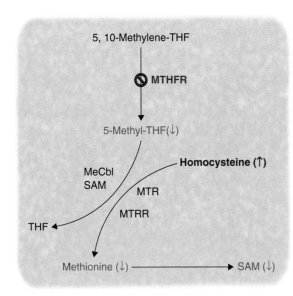

FIGURE 17-7. Severe 5,10-methylene-tetrahydrofolate reductase deficiency and its laboratory consequences (indicated in parentheses). MeCbl= methylcobalamin, MTHFR=,5,10-methylene-tetrahydrofolate reductase, MTR= methionine synthase, MTRR= methionine synthase reductase, SAM= S-adenosylmethionine, THF= tetrahydrofolate.

MeTHF. With close to 100 patients identified, it is the most common and most studied inherited disorder of folate metabolism (12). It is caused by mutations in the MTHFR gene. 5-Methyltetrahydrofolate is the methyl donor for the vitamin B_{12}-dependent remethylation of homocysteine to methionine, a reaction catalyzed by methionine synthase. Methionine is then converted to SAM, the predominant methyl donor in humans. The absence or reduction in MTHFR activity results in an increased total plasma homocysteine, low or normal methionine levels, low or normal SAM levels, and neurologic manifestations of varying degree. It is not clear whether the neuropathology in this disease results from the elevated homocysteine levels, from decreased methionine and resulting interference with methylation reactions, or from some other metabolic effect. The clinical severity is proportional to the degree of enzyme activity: the most severe phenotypes are seen with little or no residual enzyme activity (2,3,9,12).

Clinical Presentation Most reported patients have been diagnosed in infancy. The predominant early manifestations are progressive encephalopathy with apnea, seizures, and microcephaly. Coma and death have ensued in some cases. Some infants were born with hydrocephalus internus (13) and several were shown to have progressive brain atrophy; some of them also demonstrated demyelination on magnetic resonance imaging (MRI). Individual patients have presented at any time from infancy to adulthood. In the older patients, ataxic gait, motor

abnormalities, psychiatric disorders (schizophrenia), and symptoms related to cerebrovascular events have been reported. Interestingly, at least one adult with severe enzyme deficiency was completely asymptomatic. CNS autopsy findings have included: dilated cerebral vessels, microgyria, hydrocephalus, perivascular changes, demyelination, gliosis, astrocytosis, and macrophage infiltration (9,12). In some patients, thrombosis of both cerebral arteries and veins was the cause of death. There have been reports of patients with findings similar to those seen in subacute degeneration of the spinal cord due to Cbl (vitamin B_{12}) deficiency (2). Severe MTHFR deficiency is not associated with megaloblastic anemia or methylmalonic aciduria.

Diagnosis Biochemical and laboratory features of severe MTHFR deficiency include:

- Hyperhomocysteinemia and homocystinuria: because of decreased bioavailability of MeTHF, the remethylation of homocysteine to methionine reaction will be impaired, leading to an accumulation of homocysteine.

- Low or normal folate levels.

- Low or normal methionine levels: methionine synthesis is expected to be impaired when MeTHF levels are reduced.

- Low or normal SAM levels: methionine is the precursor to SAM. If methionine levels are low, less SAM will be produced.

- Absence of megaloblastic anemia. The block in the conversion of 5,10-methylene-tetrahydrofolate to MeTHF does not result in the trapping of folates as MeTHF: there is no interference with the availability of reduced folates for purine and pyrimidine synthesis.

- Absence of methylmalonic aciduria. The formation of the Cbl cofactor AdoCbl and the functioning of the enzyme MUT are not affected in MTHFR deficiency: methylmalonic acid is normally converted to succinyl-CoA, thus it does not accumulate in body fluids.

The definitive diagnosis of severe MTFHR deficiency is made by assaying MTHFR enzyme activity in liver, leukocytes, lymphocytes, or cultured fibroblasts (2,9,12). Mildly affected patients (i.e., presenting in adulthood) may have residual enzyme activity as

- Clinical presentation in infancy: acute encephalopathy

- Clinical presentation in childhood: progressive encephalopathy, late stages resembling adulthood onset disease

- Clinical presentation in adulthood: ataxia, motor abnormalities, psychiatric symptoms, subacute degeneration of spinal cord, and cerebrovascular events

high as 20% of control values, whereas severely affected individuals (i.e., presenting in infancy) usually have little or no detectable enzyme activity.

The MTHFR gene has been localized to chromosome 1p36.3. More than 50 disease-causing mutations have been reported. Because most are private, molecular diagnosis is not routinely available (12).

Prenatal diagnosis can be offered by measuring MTHFR enzyme activity in cultured amniocytes or chorionic villus cells (14). In addition, linkage analysis using common MTHFR gene polymorphisms has recently been reported for prenatal diagnosis purposes (15). Direct mutation analysis, if the disease-causing mutations are known within a family, can also be offered.

Treatment Early diagnosis is essential in the infantile form of the disease, because the best outcome has been in patients treated from birth with oral doses of betaine (20–150 mg/kg/d) following prenatal diagnosis (12). Experiments in which mouse MTHFR knockout models have been used have shown dramatic phenotype improvement when betaine was administered throughout pregnancy and lactation (16). Betaine is a substrate for betaine methyltransferase, a liver-specific enzyme (it is also found in the kidney) that converts homocysteine to methionine. Thus, betaine may be doubly beneficial by lowering homocysteine levels and raising methionine levels. Because betaine methyltransferase is not present in the brain, the CNS effects must be mediated through the effects of the circulating levels of metabolites (9). The dose of betaine should be titrated according to plasma levels of homocysteine and methionine. It has been suggested that the therapeutic threshold is reached when the serum betaine level approaches 400 μM (2,12). Other therapeutic agents have been used in MTHFR deficiency but, when administered without betaine, have not been effective. These include folic acid or reduced folates, methionine, pyridoxine, Cbl (vitamin B_{12}), carnitine, and riboflavin.

Miscellaneous Clinical Information Nine common polymorphisms have been identified in the MTHFR gene (17). One particular polymorphism, 677C>T, leads to an intermediate level of enzyme activity, and an enzyme that is thermolabile compared with control when present in the homozygous state (12,18). It has been argued that this polymorphism is a risk factor for hyperhomocysteinemia and subsequent vascular disease and coronary heart disease. Patients with this polymorphism do not have severe enzyme deficiency nor any of the clinical findings associated with severe MTHFR deficiency. The 677C>T polymorphism has also been identified as a risk factor for neural tube defects.

DISORDERS OF COBALAMIN ABSORPTION AND TRANSPORT

Absorption of dietary Cbl initially involves its binding to the glycoprotein haptocorrin (HC) (also referred to as R binder, transcobalamin I) in the saliva. In the intestine, HC is digested by proteases, allowing Cbl to bind to IF, which is produced by the parietal cells of the stomach. A specific receptor complex, CUBAM, recognizes the IF–Cbl complex, which is then taken up by enterocytes. Cbl bound to transcobalamin (TC, previously referred to as transcobalamin II), the physiologically important circulating Cbl-binding protein, enters the portal circulation. Inherited defects of several of these steps are known (Figure 17-2).

Current values that define "normal" serum Cbl levels are in the range of 200 to 1000 pg/mL (150–750 pmol/L). Cbl deficiency is usually defined as a serum Cbl level of less than 200 pg/mL (150 pmol/L) (4,18,29). However it is recognized that only 90% to 95% of Cbl-deficient patients (i.e. with hematologic and/or neurologic signs and symptoms extremely suggestive of Cbl deficiency) have values corresponding to this cut off. It is estimated that 5% to 10% of Cbl-deficient patients will have values in the 200 to 300 pg/mL range (150–220 pmol/L), and 0.1% to 1% have values greater than 300 pg/mL (220 pmol/L) (19). Many studies have suggested that measuring the characteristic metabolites of Cbl deficiency (total plasma homocysteine and serum and/or urine methylmalonic acid levels) may assist in identifying Cbl-deficient patients (4,18,19). These pretreatment values can also be used to monitor metabolic response to Cbl supplementation.

In addition, it is important to note that most studies attempting to define normal and abnormal serum Cbl levels studied adult, especially elderly, populations in whom decreased dietary Cbl intake was the main cause of the deficiency. Serum Cbl levels in children and infants with intrinsic defects in Cbl malabsorption and intracellular metabolism may differ from that of the adult populations studied.

Hereditary Intrinsic Factor Deficiency

Etiology/Pathophysiology This condition is also misleadingly called congenital pernicious anemia. It is a rare autosomal recessive cause of Cbl deficiency, due to the absence or nonfunctionality of IF (Figure 17-2). Fewer than 100 patients with this condition have been reported. A polymorphism thought to be linked to a disease-causing mutation has been identified in the GIF (gastric intrinsic factor) gene localized to 11q13 (20). Yassin et al. (21) identified a 4-bp deletion (c183_186delGAAT) in the coding region of the GIF gene as the cause of IF deficiency in an 11-year-old girl with severe anemia and Cbl deficiency. Recently, mutations in GIF were identified in patients from four families with likely Imerslund-Gräsbeck syndrome (see next section), demonstrating potential for phenotypic overlap between the two conditions (22).

Some patients produce no IF, whereas in others it may be detectable immunologically. There have been reports of IF with reduced affinity for Cbl, reduced affinity for the IF–Cbl receptor, or increased susceptibility to proteolysis (9).

In absence of IF, Cbl absorption by the ileal cells is much less efficient (only 1% of ingested Cbl) since the ileal receptor recognizes the Cbl–IF complex (1). This leads to low serum Cbl levels. In turn, there is decreased Cbl available for intracellular processing, leading to decreased levels of MeCbl and AdoCbl. When these cofactors are reduced, methionine synthase (which relies on MeCbl for its normal functioning) and MUT (which relies on AdoCbl for its normal functioning) activities are impaired. The biochemical abnormalities include hyperhomocysteinemia, homocystinuria and methylmalonic aciduria. Folate trapping as MeTHF occurs, resulting in megaloblastic anemia and other hematologic abnormalities. Neurologic symptoms are likely due to combined effects of the unavailability of physiologically usable folate as well as the Cbl deficiency.

Clinical Presentation Megaloblastic anemia is the main finding and usually presents after

the 1st year of life but before the age of 5 years. In cases of partial deficiency, clinical presentation has been delayed until adolescence or adulthood (9). The patients present with failure to thrive, often with vomiting and alternating diarrhea and constipation, jaundice, anorexia, and irritability. They are anemic and several have presented with pancytopenia. There may be hepatosplenomegaly, stomatitis or atrophic glossitis, developmental delay, arthritis, and myelopathy or peripheral neuropathy.

Diagnosis Biochemical and laboratory features of hereditary IF deficiency include:

- Megaloblastic anemia due to folate trapping with deficient DNA synthesis.
- Low serum Cbl: in the absence of IF, ileal uptake of Cbl is much less effective.
- Hyperhomocysteinemia, homocystinuria, and methylmalonic aciduria may be present due to functional deficiencies of methionine synthase and MUT, respectively.
- Hyperbilirubinemia may occur.

A deoxyuridine-suppression test on marrow cells is useful but is not easily available in most clinical laboratories. This test measures the DNA incorporation of label from thymidylate (dTMP) into a trichloroacetic acid precipitate before and after incubation of washed bone marrow cells in an excess of deoxyuridine. In the presence of folate or Cbl deficiency, this preincubation reduces incorporation to only 30% to 40% of that observed in the absence of deoxyuridine, as compared with approximately 10% when there is no folate or Cbl deficiency.

In contrast to acquired forms of pernicious anemia, there is normal gastric acidity and normal gastric cytology in hereditary IF deficiency. Pancreatic function is normal and there are no IF autoantibodies. The Schilling test demonstrates abnormal Cbl absorption but this is normalized when the labeled Cbl is mixed with a source of normal IF, such as gastric juice from an unaffected individual. Some patients may have a lack of immunologically reactive IF.

Molecular diagnosis is possible although not widely available.

Treatment An initial dose of 1 mg/day of hydroxycobalamin (OHCbl) is administered intramuscularly to replenish body stores until biochemical and hematologic values normalize (9). The maintenance OHCbl dose required to maintain normal values may be as low as 0.25 mg (250 µg) every 3 months. To prevent persistence of neurologic abnormalities, it is imperative that treatment be started in a timely manner.

Defective Transport of Cbl by Enterocytes (Imerslund–Gräsbeck Syndrome, or Megaloblastic Anemia 1)

Etiology/Pathophysiology Also called juvenile congenital megaloblastic anemia, this is an autosomal recessive condition identified in more than 250 patients caused by defective uptake of IF–Cbl by enterocytes (Figure 17-2). Most patients are found in Norway, Finland, or Saudi Arabia, and among Sephardic Jews. It displays locus heterogeneity: it is caused by mutations in one of at least two genes, CUBN (10p12.1) encoding a protein called cubulin, or AMN (14q32) encoding a protein called amnionless. Amnionless and cubulin form the functional receptor complex (CUBAM) essential for endocytosis of IF–Cbl at the level of enterocytes (23). This complex is responsible for endocytosis of various other ligands (albumin, transferrin, vitamin D–binding proteins, etc.) and has also been identified in several other tissues including the renal parenchyma. Interestingly, some patients have normal IF–Cbl uptake in homogenates of ileal biopsy specimens, suggesting that potentially a third defect (i.e., in intraenterocyte processing) may result in the same phenotype. Haplotype analysis has excluded both CUBN and AMN in five families studied, strengthening the likelihood that at least one more gene locus can lead to this condition (24). The same group has recently identified homozygous nonsense and missense mutations in the GIF gene (associated with hereditary IF deficiency) in four of the five families with likely Imerslund–Gräsbeck syndrome, with no identified mutations in CUBN and AMN. The clinical phenotype in these patients was typical for Imerslund–Gräsbeck syndrome, thus demonstrating an overlap between these two conditions (22).

Clinical Presentation Malabsorption of Cbl results in megaloblastic anemia through the same pathophysiologic process as the one discussed in IF deficiency. The anemia usually manifests once fetal hepatic Cbl stores have been depleted (9). Although the disease usually appears between the ages of 1 year and 5 years, later onsets have been reported. Pancytopenia has been associated with this condition. In addition, inadequate functioning of the CUBAM complex at the level of the kidneys results in proteinuria, due to defective protein reabsorption. Most patients present with varying degrees of proteinuria. In patients with onset of proteinuria in childhood, the renal pathology is not progressive and remains stable into adulthood. Neurologic abnormalities may be present as a consequence of Cbl deficiency. These include paresthesias, sensory deficits, spasticity, truncal ataxia, cerebral atrophy, confusion, and dementia.

Diagnosis Biochemical and laboratory features of defective transport of Cbl by enterocytes include:

- Megaloblastic anemia with occasional pancytopenia due to folate trapping and defective DNA synthesis.
- Low serum Cbl levels due to decreased ileal absorption.
- Proteinuria due to deficient protein reabsorption at the level of the renal tubules.
- Hyperhomocysteinemia, methylmalonic aciduria, and homocystinuria may occur due to functional deficiencies of MUT and methionine synthase, but the levels are not usually as high as those seen in intracellular Cbl metabolism defects.

As with hereditary IF deficiency, gastric morphology and pancreatic function are normal and there are no IF autoantibodies. In contrast to patients with IF deficiency: 1) the Schilling test is not corrected by providing a source of human IF with the labeled Cbl and 2) IF levels are normal.

Molecular confirmation of the diagnosis is possible now that two genes have been characterized. GIF mutation analysis should also be undertaken, because phenotypic overlap between Imerslund–Gräsbeck syndrome and hereditary IF deficiency has recently been demonstrated (22). Given the likelihood of a potential fourth locus, this may not be successful in all families.

Treatment An initial dose of 1mg/day of hydroxycobalamin (OHCbl) is administered intramuscularly to replenish body stores until biochemical and hematologic values normalize. As with hereditary IF deficiency, once the Cbl stores are replete, the maintenance OHCbl dose required to maintain normal values may be as low as 0.25 mg (250 μg) every 3 months. Treatment with OHCbl corrects the neurologic and hematologic findings but not the proteinuria (9).

Transcobalamin I/R Binder/ Haptocorrin Deficiency

Etiology/Pathophysiology Although this entity is mentioned in many books and cited as being an autosomal dominant condition (Figure 17-2) on OMIM, it is not clear that it is associated with a distinct phenotype. HC's exact role in not known, but it may act as a transport system to remove noxious Cbl analogs from the brain and other tissues by carrying them to the liver for excretion into the bile. The HC gene has been cloned and mapped to chromosome 11q11-q12. No mutations have been described in any patient with HC deficiency. Currently, five cases are reported in the literature, all with adult onset and neurologic rather than hematologic findings (26).

Clinical Presentation Hematologic abnormalities are not seen in this condition, because TC, the physiologically important Cbl transporter, is present in normal quantities. Neurologic findings reportedly associated with HC deficiency are subacute combined degeneration of the spinal cord, optic atrophy, ataxia, paresthesias, sensory changes, decreased deep tendon reflexes, and dementia (9).

Diagnosis Biochemical and laboratory features of HC deficiency include:

- Low serum Cbl because most circulating Cbl is bound to HC.
- Deficient or absent HC in plasma, saliva, and leukocytes.
- Normal or low levels of TC–Cbl.

Treatment Because it has not been possible to reliably assign a phenotype to the biochemical finding of low or absent HC, it is uncertain whether treatment is warranted.

Transcobalamin (TC/TCII) Deficiency

Etiology/Pathophysiology TC deficiency (Figure 17-2) is a rare autosomal recessive condition characterized by absent or abnormally functioning TC with resultant deficiency in physiologically available Cbl. It has been described in fewer than 50 patients. The gene has been identified and is localized to chromosome 22q11.2 (2). Because there is intracellular Cbl depletion, this disorder results in clinical signs of Cbl deficiency. Partial TC deficiency, transmitted in an autosomal dominant fashion and resulting in neurologic, mental, and hematologic abnormalities in 20 members of a 4-generation family (children and adults) has recently been described (27).

Clinical Presentation Clinical presentation of the autosomal recessive disorder typically occurs in the 1st or 2nd month of life with nonspecific symptoms such as pallor, failure to thrive, weakness, vomiting, and diarrhea. Mouth ulcerations may be found. Megaloblastic anemia (due to folate trapping) is usually present, but pancytopenia or isolated erythroid hypoplasia have been described. Neutropenia can lead to severe infections. The presence of immature white

- Clinical presentation: in first few months of life, lethargy, vomiting/diarrhea, weakness, megaloblastic anemia, immunodeficiencies, usually absence of neurologic abnormalities at onset.

cell precursors in an otherwise hypocellular marrow may mistakenly lead to the diagnosis of leukemia. Immunologic deficiencies such as defective humoral and cellular immunity and granulocyte dysfunction have been seen. Neurologic abnormalities are infrequent but may be associated with delayed diagnosis, treatment with folate in the absence of Cbl, or inadequate Cbl treatment. When present, neurologic abnormalities have consisted of ataxia, developmental delay, neuropathy, myelopathy, and encephalopathy (2,9).

Diagnosis Biochemical and laboratory features of transcobalamin deficiency include:

- Megaloblastic anemia: caused folate trapping with impaired DNA synthesis in bone marrow cells.

- Normal serum Cbl levels (majority bound to HC, not to TC).

- Low unsaturated Cbl–binding capacity (measures capacity of unsaturated TC to bind Cbl).

- No immunologically detectable circulating TC (using anti-TC antibodies).

- Decreased Immunoglobulin (Ig) G, IgM, IgA.

- Hyperhomocysteinemia, methylmalonic aciduria, and homocystinuria may occur due to functional decreased activity of MUT and methionine synthase, but levels are not usually as high as those seen in intracellular Cbl metabolism defects.

It is important to perform the unsaturated Cbl–binding capacity test before initiating Cbl treatment. Because TC is involved in the transport of Cbl through the enterocyte, the Schilling test may be abnormal in TC-deficient patients. Patients with abnormally functioning but present TC have normal Schilling test results. It is possible to study TC synthesis in cultured cells such as fibroblasts, allowing for diagnosis in patients who do not synthesize TC.

Mutations have been identified in fewer than 10 patients. Several types of mutations have been identified, including a single nucleotide deletion, a larger deletion, a nonsense mutation, defective RNA editing (28), and activation of a cryptic exonic splice site. Once mutations have been identified in a particular family, molecular diagnosis is a potential option.

Prenatal diagnosis is possible by three methods. The first consists of studying TC synthesis in cultured amniocytes in families in which the affected sibling's disorder is characterized by absence of TC (15,30). The second consists of molecular studies in those families in which disease-causing mutations have been identified (14). Many polymor-phisms have been described in this gene, making the option of gene tracking linkage a third possibility for families in which specific mutations have not been identified.

Treatment It is recommended to begin with a daily dose of systemic OHCbl, 1 mg/day, to replenish intracellular Cbl reserve. The dose can then be decreased to once or twice weekly when the hematologic profile has been corrected. Treatment of TC deficiency requires that serum Cbl levels be kept very high: a value in the range of 1000 to 10,000 pg/ml (750–7400 pmol/L) is necessary for successful treatment. These levels have been achieved with doses of oral or systemic (intramuscular) OHCbl or cyanocobalamin (CNCbl) of 500 to 1000 μg twice weekly. Intravenous Cbl is not recommended because of the rapid loss of the vitamin in the urine. Folic acid or folinic acid can reverse the megaloblastic anemia. Doses up to 15 mg orally four times daily have been used. Of importance, folates must never be given as the sole therapy in TC deficiency because of the danger of hematologic relapse and neurologic deterioration (9).

DISORDERS OF INTRACELLULAR UTILIZATION OF COBALAMIN

Cultured fibroblasts are usually used in the diagnosis of intracellular Cbl metabolism defects. The incorporation of [^{14}C]propionate into macromolecules is a good screen for the integrity of the MUT reaction, whereas the incorporation of [^{14}C]MeTHF serves as a good indicator for the function of methionine synthase. Complementation analysis is used to define the specific intracellular defect of Cbl metabolism. Cells from an undiagnosed patient are cocultivated with cells from patients with known defects, and replicate cultures are either treated or not treated with polyethylene glycol (a cell fusing agent). If the defects from the patient under study and from the patient with a known condition belong to different classes (in other words, affect different genes), fusion results in partial correction of the defect in incorporation, because both gene products are present in the fused cells. This partial correction is termed "complementation." If, however, the defect in the two cell lines belongs to the same class (affects the same gene), complementation does not occur. Thus, patient cells complement with cells from all complementation groups except that to which the patient belongs.

The complementation classes of intracellular Cbl metabolism are named cblA, cblB, cblC, cblD, cblE, cblF, cblG and cblH.

cblF

Etiology/Pathophysiology The cblF complementation group (Figure 17-8) is a very rare disorder of intracellular Cbl metabolism described in only two siblings and seven other unrelated patients. It is most likely inherited

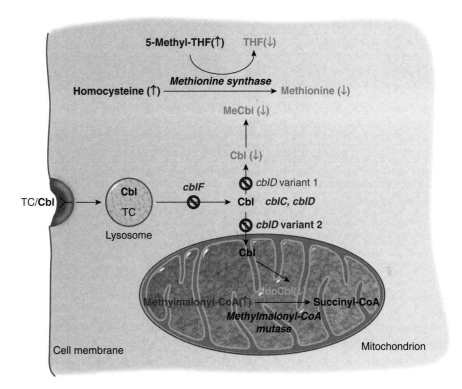

FIGURE 17-8. Summary of cblF, cblC and cblD deficiencies and their laboratory consequences (in parentheses). AdoCbl= adenosylcobalamin, Cbl= cobalamin, MeCbl= methylcobalamin, MTRR= methionine synthase reductase, TC/Cbl= transcobalamin–Cbl complex, TC= transcobalamin, THF= tetrahydrofolate.

- Clinical presentation in infancy, failure to thrive, stomatitis/glossitis, hypotonia, lethargy, hematologic abnormalities including anemia, recurrent infections, and developmental delay.

in an autosomal recessive manner. The defect in cblF appears to be due to trapping of endocytosed Cbl in the lysosomes following degradation of TC. Cbl accumulates in the lysosomes and is not available for conversion to either AdoCbl or MeCbl. The consequence is a functional deficiency of both enzymes that require the Cbl coenzymes for their normal functioning: methionine synthase and MUT. In addition, cblF patients fail to absorb oral Cbl, suggesting that the putative lysosomal defect affects ileal Cbl transcytosis as well (9).

Clinical Presentation Clinical signs and symptoms are usually evident in the 1st year of life (2,9). These are the consequences of Cbl deficiency as well as folate trapping as MeTHF. Presentation has included stomatitis, glossitis, hypotonia, hematologic abnormalities (anemia, macrocytosis and hypersegmented polymorphonuclear neutrophils, pancytopenia, neutropenia, or thrombocytopenia), failure to thrive, recurrent infections, developmental delay, lethargy, hypotonia, aspiration pneumonia, hepatomegaly, and encephalopathy. Minor facial anomalies have been described in two patients. Severe feeding difficulties requiring tube feeding, tooth abnormalities, and dextrocardia were seen in one patient. One infant died suddenly at home in the 1st year of life. A boy diagnosed at the age of 11 years had recurrent stomatitis in infancy, arthritis at the age of 4 years, and confusion and disorientation at 10 years. He also had a pigmentary skin abnormality.

Diagnosis Biochemical and laboratory features of cblF include:

- Low intracellular MeCbl and AdoCbl levels; there is decreased formation of both Cbl coenzymes because Cbl cannot be released from the lysosomes once it has been dissociated from TC.
- Accumulation of Cbl in lysosomes.
- Hyperhomocysteinemia and homocystinuria: there is low MeCbl formation, resulting in a functional deficiency in methionine synthase activity.
- Low or normal methionine levels; there is low MeCbl formation, resulting in a functional deficiency in methionine synthase activity.
- Methylmalonic aciduria and methylmalonic acidemia; there is low AdoCbl formation, resulting in a functional deficiency in MUT activity

- Normal or high cystathionine because homocysteine is elevated, some of it is shunted to make cystathionine through the enzyme β-cystathionine synthase.
- Low or normal serum Cbl levels: There may be defective ileal transcytosis, resulting in low Cbl levels; however if transcytosis is only partially affected or normal, serum Cbl levels are expected to be unaffected because Cbl–TC and Cbl–HC complexes form normally.
- Presence of megaloblastic anemia due to folate trapping. May have severe pancytopenia due to generalized bone marrow depression.

The Schilling test has been abnormal in all the patients studied.

Fibroblast studies show decreased incorporation of labeled propionate and of labeled MeTHF, reflecting decreased function of Cbl-dependent enzymes. Total cellular uptake of labeled CNCbl is elevated, but virtually the entire label is found as free CNCbl in lysosomes. Consequently, there is no conversion of CNCbl to either AdoCbl or MeCbl. The definitive diagnosis of cblF is made by genetic complementation analysis.

Molecular investigations are not an option given that the genetic defect remains unknown.

Prenatal diagnosis has been performed by measuring accumulation of intracellular CNCbl as well as incorporation of both labeled propionate and labeled MeTHF in cultured amniocytes (14,29).

Treatment Treatment with parenteral OHCbl (first daily and then biweekly) at a dose of 1 mg/day seems to be effective in correcting the metabolic and clinical findings (9). Oral betaine at 250 mg/kg/day has also been used. Experience in the treatment of this condition is quite limited.

cblC

Etiology/Pathophysiology The cblC complementation group (Figure 17-8) is the most common inborn error of vitamin B_{12} metabolism with approximately 300 patients diagnosed. It is inherited in an autosomal recessive manner and it has been suggested that a defect in the cytosolic reduction of Cbl once it leaves the lysosome is responsible for this condition (9). If the reduction of Cbl does not occur, there is impairment of synthesis of both Cbl coenzymes, MeCbl and AdoCbl. Atkinson et al. mapped the gene for this defect to chromosome 1 in 2002 (30), and Lerner-Ellis et al. identified the gene in 2005 (31). The gene was named MMACHC, for methylmalonic aciduria cblC type with homocystinuria. This disor-

- Clinical presentation in early-onset subgroup: acute neurologic deterioration, multisystem pathology, retinopathy, pancytopenia or megaloblastic anemia, and moderate-to-severe cognitive disability.
- Clinical presentation in late-onset subgroup: confusion, disorientation, gait abnormalities, extrapyramidal symptoms, megaloblastic anemia (seen less than in early-onset subgroup), and mild-to-moderate cognitive disability.

der presents with both neurologic and systemic metabolic abnormalities due to folate trapping and Cbl deficiency, and recent data show subgroups of early-onset and late-onset occurrence with potentially different clinical outcomes. Recent findings suggest that high CSF levels of homocysteine may be associated with neurotoxicity in cblC patients.

Clinical Presentation Many patients in the early-onset subgroup became acutely ill in the first year of life, and most were diagnosed prior to 1 year of age (2,9,13). The symptoms are those of severe Cbl deficiency. The presentation may resemble bacterial or viral sepsis (32). The clinical course in this subgroup is initially characterized by feeding difficulties, hypotonia, and lethargy. Progressive neurologic deterioration follows, and coma may ensue. Hypotonia, hypertonia, or a combination of both may be accompanied by the onset of abnormal movements and/or seizures. These patients usually have moderate-to-severe cognitive disability. Hematologically, there is severe pancytopenia or a nonregenerative megaloblastic anemia, the consequences of folate trapping leading to impaired DNA synthesis. Multisystem involvement develops in many patients, with renal failure, hepatic dysfunction, cardiomyopathy, interstitial pneumonia, or hemolytic uremic syndrome, secondary to widespread microangiopathy. Ophthalmologic examination frequently reveals an unusual retinopathy characterized by perimacular hypopigmentation surrounded by a hyperpigmented ring, and a more peripheral salt-and-pepper appearance. Nystagmus is also observed. Visual impairment is not infrequent. Microcephaly and hydrocephaly both occur. Many patients in the early-onset subgroup died within the 1st year of life.

The late-onset subgroup can present at any time during childhood and even in adulthood. The clinical course is characterized by milder hematologic abnormalities, confusion and disorientation, extrapyramidal symptoms, gait abnormalities, and milder cognitive disability (33). Neurologic manifestations have usually been prominent, regardless of the age of onset.

There is one recent report of two siblings who presented at the ages of 12 and 4 years with renal biopsy-confirmed chronic thrombotic microangiopathic nephropathy, absence of neurologic symptoms, mild pigmentary retinal abnormalities, and fibroblast studies compatible with a mild cblC disorder (34).

Diagnosis Biochemical and laboratory features of cblC include:

- Low intracellular MeCbl and AdoCbl levels: there is decreased formation of both Cbl coenzymes.

- Hyperhomocysteinemia and homocystinuria: there is low MeCbl formation, resulting in a functional deficiency in methionine synthase activity.

- Low or normal methionine levels: there is low MeCbl formation, resulting in a functional deficiency in methionine synthase activity.

- Methylmalonic aciduria and methylmalonic acidemia: there is low AdoCbl formation, resulting in a functional deficiency in MUT activity

- Normal serum Cbl levels and TC levels.

- Normal or high cystathionine because homocysteine is elevated, some of it is shunted to make cystathionine through the enzyme β-cystathionine synthase.

- Presence of megaloblastic anemia due to folate trapping. May have severe pancytopenia due to generalized bone marrow depression.

- Normal acid/base status or metabolic acidosis.

Fibroblast studies show decreased uptake of label from both propionate and MeTHF. Uptake of CNCbl is decreased and there is reduced synthesis of both MeCbl and AdoCbl. The definitive diagnosis of cblC is made by genetic complementation analysis.

Molecular diagnosis is an option for this condition. When both mutations have been identified in a patient, molecular analysis can be used for carrier detection in the family, for clinical diagnosis of other at-risk family members, and for prenatal diagnosis.

Molecular investigations have revealed 42 different mutations in MMACHC in 204 patients (31). One mutation, c.271dupA, accounted for 40% of all the mutant alleles. Patients who are homozygous for this mutation invariably have the early-onset phenotype, whereas patients who are homozygous for a different mutation, c.394C>T, belong to the late-onset group. In addition, seven mutations identified showed clustering by population of origin. Mutation analysis therefore allows for genotype–phenotype correlations.

Prenatal diagnosis can be performed by measuring the incorporation of labeled propionate and labeled MeTHF, by measuring the synthesis of MeCbl and AdoCbl in cultured chorionic villus cells or amniocytes and by measuring methylmalonic acid levels in amniotic fluid (14,29). Cultured chorionic villus cell studies should always be confirmed by cultured amniocyte studies (29). Mutation analysis is possible if the disease-causing mutations have been identified in the proband.

Treatment Treatment with 1mg/day parenteral OHCbl decreases methylmalonic acid and homocysteine levels; however, these are usually not completely normalized. Daily oral betaine, 250 mg/kg/day, with twice weekly intramuscular 1 mg OHCbl, results in normalization of methionine and homocysteine levels and decreases urinary methylmalonic acid. Oral hydroxycobalamin is insufficient, and both carnitine and folinic acid were ineffective. Despite normalization of biochemical parameters, permanent neurologic sequela may not be preventable. Moderate-to-severe impairment seems to be the norm in the patients with onset of disease in the 1st year of life, whereas mild-to-moderate disability is seen in patients with later onset. Of a group of 44 patients with early onset, 13 died and only one was neurologically intact (9).

cblD

Etiology/Pathophysiology The cblD complementation group (Figure 17-8) is the rarest intracellular Cbl metabolism defect with a total of five patients now described (9). All five patients are male, making both X-linked recessive and autosomal recessive inheritance possibilities. The defect has been postulated to be in the reduction of cytosolic Cbl upon its exit from the lysosomes, similar to the defect causing cblC. In fact, the biochemical features of the two original and, until recently, only known patients were identical to those of cblC patients. Authors of a recent report have described three additional patients with complementation studies indicative of cblD comprising features that differ from the original two patients and from cblC patients (24). Two of these three patients presented with functional impairment of methionine synthase but no evidence of dysfunction of MUT (named cblD variant 1), whereas the third patient demonstrated the opposite results, functional deficiency of MUT with normal function of methionine synthase (named cblD variant 2). Despite these differences, fibroblast studies

- Clinical presentation: normal-to-severe cognition delays, neurologic dysfunction, behavioral abnormalities, changes on MRI, megaloblastic anemia

for these three patients clearly assign them to the cblD group. Thus, heterogeneity exists within the cblD complementation group, and these recent results indicate further complexity in the intracellular Cbl metabolism.

Clinical Presentation Of the two original patients, who were brothers and products of a consanguineous union, the older one had mild mental retardation, behavioral abnormalities, ataxia and nystagmus, whereas the youngest was developmentally and neurologically normal. Both exhibited a mild megaloblastic anemia (2,9). The three newly described patients have many neurologic features including: mild to severe developmental delay and mental retardation, spastic ataxia, dystonic movements, nystagmus, severe hypotonia and seizures. Behavioral abnormalities have included hyperactivity, aggressivity and abnormal sleep patterns. MRI has shown cerebral and/or cerebellar atrophy, demyelination, and cerebellar vermis hypoplasia. Only one of these three patients had megaloblastic anemia (24).

Diagnosis Biochemical and laboratory features of the originally described combined cblD defect are quite similar to those seen in cblC complementation group, whereas the findings seen in the cblD variant 1 are similar to the cblE/cblG complementation groups and the cblD variant 2 resembles the cblA/cblB complementation groups.

Fibroblast complementation studies confirm the diagnosis of cblD, whether it is the combined defect, the variant 1, or the variant 2.

The gene for cblD has recently been discovered (25); however, genetic testing is not yet clinically available.

Prenatal diagnosis has not been reported in cblD; however, it is theoretically possible by studying cultured amniocytes or chorionic villus cells for incorporation of labeled propionate and MeTHF and intracellular synthesis of MeCbl and AdoCbl. If the family mutation is known, prenatal diagnosis could be done on DNA extracted from amniocytes or chorionic villus cells.

Treatment Treatment for this condition would resemble that of cblC. The authors who recently reported 3 new cases of cblD state that there was an overall improvement, but not reversal, of the neurologic abnormalities upon initiation of treatment. Biochemical and hematologic abnormalities resolved. The regimen used involved betaine (9–15 g/d or 200 mg/kg/day), folic acid (15 mg/d) and OHCbl (1 mg IM daily followed by 1 mg IM weekly) in 2 patients and OHCbl with carnitine in the other patient. In vitro, these patients' cells had a dramatic response to OHCbl administration (24).

Functional Methionine Synthase Deficiency (cblE: Methionine Synthase Reductase Deficiency, and cblG: Methionine Synthase Deficiency)

Etiology/Pathophysiology These conditions are both autosomal recessive in inheritance and rare (Figure 17-9). They will be discussed together because their clinical and biochemical presentations are virtually identical.

cblG: The *cblG* disorder is caused by mutations in the methionine synthase gene, MTR, itself (35). At least 33 patients have been diagnosed with this form of intracellular Cbl metabolism defect (9).

cblE: The cblE disorder is due to mutations in the methionine synthase reductase, MTRR, gene (36). Methionine synthase reductase is necessary to keep the methionine synthase–bound Cbl in a functional state. At least 27 patients have been diagnosed with this disorder (9).

Both these disorders cause isolated functional methionine synthase deficiency with resultant megaloblastic anemia due to folate trapping and neurologic defects, which may be caused by elevated levels of homocysteine and/or low levels of methionine and SAM.

Clinical Presentation Most individuals with cblE and cblG are symptomatic in the 1st year of life, but one cblG patient was not diagnosed until age 26 years and had been misdiagnosed with multiple sclerosis at the age of 21 years.

Another cblG patient presented with mainly psychiatric symptoms in the fourth decade (9). Megaloblastic anemia occurred in almost all these patients. The neurologic dysfunctions include lethargy, poor feeding, vomiting, failure to thrive, developmental delay, nystagmus, hypotonia or hypertonia, ataxia, seizures, and blindness. Cerebral atrophy is a frequent finding, and delayed myelination may also be seen on imaging studies of the CNS (2,9,13).

Diagnosis Biochemical and laboratory features of cblE and cblG include:

- Megaloblastic anemia due to folate trapping and defective DNA synthesis in erythropoietic bone marrow precursors.

- Low intracellular MeCbl due to decreased formation of the coenzyme, secondary to methionine synthase deficiency or methionine synthase reductase deficiency.

- Hyperhomocysteinemia and homocystinuria: there is reduced methionine synthase activity, leading to a build up of the substrate.

- Hypomethioninemia due to decreased methionine synthase activity.

- Normal or high cystathionine because homocysteine is elevated, some of it is shunted to cystathionine through the enzyme β-cystathionine synthase.

- Normal serum and urinary methylmalonic acid, intracellular AdoCbl: AdoCbl synthesis is not affected in this condition, therefore the activity of MUT is not impaired.

- Normal serum Cbl levels and folate levels.

Methionine synthase enzyme activity assays on fibroblast extracts allows differentiation between cblE and cblG defects: whereas cblG cells have decreased methionine synthase activity in the standard assay, cblE cells require specific reducing conditions to demonstrate the deficient enzyme activity.

Cultured fibroblasts from both cblE and cblG patients have decreased incorporation of labeled MeTHF and decreased intracellular synthesis of MeCbl following incubation in labeled CNCbl. In some cblG patients (cblG variants) no Cbl forms are bound to methionine synthase following incubation in labeled CNCbl.

Genetic complementation studies in which MeTHF is used as the substrate will distinguish cblE from cblG patients.

Molecular diagnosis is an option for both these conditions. When both mutations have been identified in a patient, molecular analysis can be used for carrier detection in the family, for clinical diagnosis of other at-risk family members, and for prenatal diagnosis.

cblG: Mutations in the MTR gene encoding methionine synthase have been identified in many patients with cblG, and include nonsense, missense, and splice site mutations (35). P1173L is a frequently encountered missense mutation in patients with cblG.

cblE: Mutations in the MTRR gene encoding methionine synthase reductase have been identified in patients with cblE and tend to be private (36).

Prenatal diagnosis has been accomplished in both disorders by measuring MeCbl levels in cultured amniocytes (14,29). Cultured chorionic villus cells can also be used but negative results ascertained with this type of cell line should always be confirmed by cultured amniocyte studies (29). Molecular diagnosis is possible in those families in which disease-causing mutations have been identified.

Treatment Successful correction of nearly all the metabolic abnormalities has been accomplished with 1 to 2 mg OHCbl or MeCbl in daily intramuscular injections until Cbl levels have been replenished, and then injections once or twice weekly (9). It has, however, proven difficult to reverse the neurologic findings once they have developed. Treatment with betaine (250 mg/kg/d) has been used, and one cblG patient treated with L-methionine (40 mg/kg/d) had neurologic improvement. Despite therapy, many patients with cblG and cblE do not do well. Prenatal therapy has been successful in one case.

Miscellaneous Clinical Information One known case exemplifies the benefits of prenatal therapy. In one family with a previous child diagnosed with cblE, cultured amniocyte studies

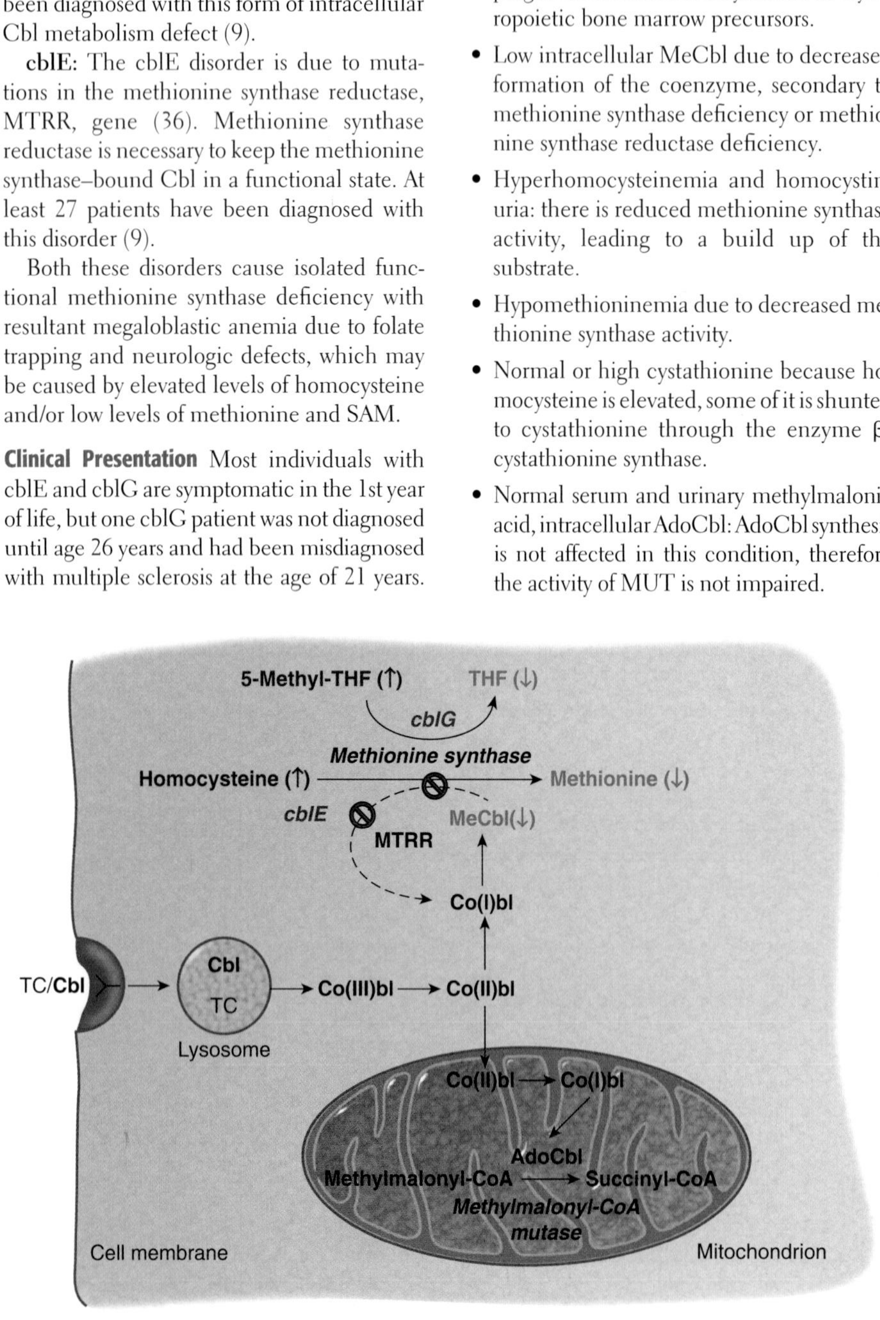

FIGURE 17-9. Summary of cblE and cblG deficiencies and their laboratory consequences (in parentheses). AdoCbl= adenosylcobalamin, Cbl= cobalamin, MeCbl= methylcobalamin, MTRR= methionine synthase reductase, TC/Cbl= transcobalamin–Cbl complex, TC= transcobalamin, THF= tetrahydrofolate.

showed an affected fetus in an at-risk pregnancy. OHCbl therapy twice weekly was initiated in the mother during the second trimester, and the baby was treated with OHCbl starting at birth. This child has developed normally to age 14 years. In contrast, his older brother, who was not treated until after his metabolic decompensation in infancy had significant developmental delay at 18 years of age (9,14).

Adenosylcobalamin Deficiency cblA cblB

These conditions are both autosomal recessive in inheritance and rare (Figure 17-10). They will be reviewed together because of the similarities seen at the clinical and biochemical levels.

cblA: The cblA disorder is caused by mutations in the MMAA gene on chromosome 4q31.1-q31.2 (37). The role of this mitochondrial protein remains unknown but there are several hypotheses: 1) it may be involved in Cbl transport into the mitochondria; 2) it may play a role in maintaining the integrity of the MUT enzyme; 3) it may be involved in intramitochondrial reduction reactions. At least 60 patients have been diagnosed with this form of intracellular Cbl metabolism defect (9).

cblB: The cblB disorder is due to mutations in the MMAB gene located on chromosome 12q24 (38). The protein encoded by this gene is an adenosyltransferase (39), which catalyzes the final intramitochondrial step in the syn-

thesis of AdoCbl. Fewer than 50 patients with cblB have been identified (9).

Methylmalonic acid is normally derived from propionic acid as part of the catabolic pathways for isoleucine, valine, threonine, methionine, cholesterol, and odd-chain fatty acids. Both these disorders cause isolated functional MUT deficiency due to decreased AdoCbl formation with resultant methylmalonic aciduria, elevated serum methylmalonic acid levels, and organic acidemia. The phenotype is similar to MUT deficiency (see Chapter 7).

Clinical Presentation Most patients present with an acidotic crisis in the 1st year of life, many in the neonatal period. Vomiting, dehydration, tachypnea, lethargy, failure to thrive, developmental retardation, hypotonia, and encephalopathy are presenting symptoms. Bone marrow abnormalities such as anemia, leukopenia, and thrombocytopenia may occur when toxic levels of methylmalonic acid are reached. Other biochemical abnormalities that can be seen are hyperammonemia, hyperglycinemia, and ketonuria. There have been reports of "metabolic strokes" and extrapyramidal signs following episodes of metabolic decompensation. Chronic renal failure may be a long-term complication of patients with methylmalonic acidemia (9).

From a prognostic perspective, cblA patients generally do better than cblB patients (see Treatment section).

There have been reports of cblA late-onset cases in which children have selectively avoided protein in their diets.

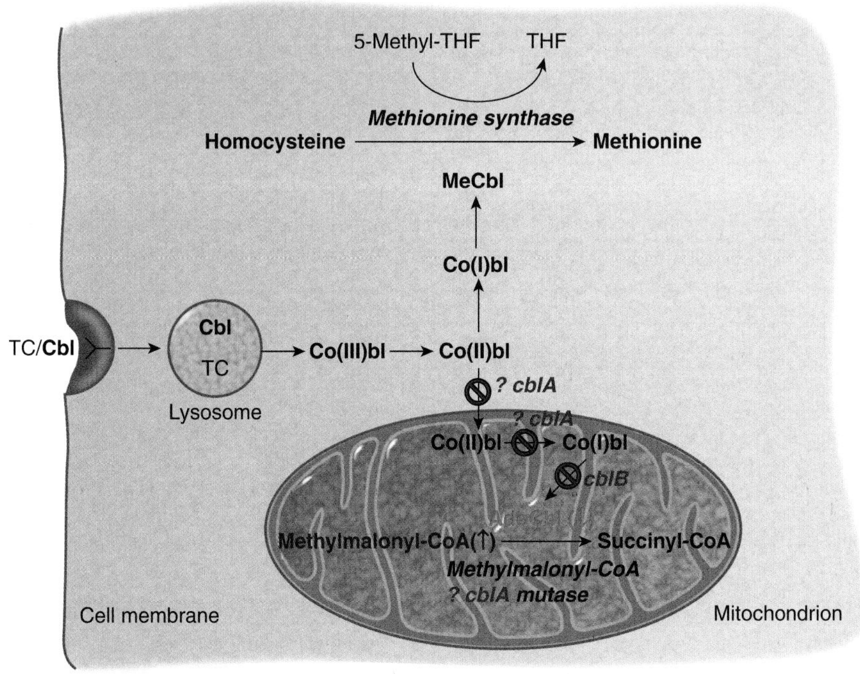

- Clinical presentation: acidotic crisis in neonatal period or 1st year of life, developmental retardation, hypotonia, failure to thrive, encephalopathy, anemia, leukopenia, thrombocytopenia, and pancytopenia. Metabolic strokes, extrapyramidal signs, and chronic renal failure are long-term complications.

Diagnosis Biochemical and laboratory features of cblA and cblB include:

- Low intracellular AdoCbl due to inability to form this Cbl coenzyme.
- Methylmalonic acidemia and methylmalonic aciduria due to functional deficiency of L-methylmalonic-CoA reductase.
- Propionic acid and its metabolites 3-hydroxypropionate and methylcitrate are also found in the urine: methylmalonic acid is normally the catabolic product of propionic acid. When methylmalonic acid cannot be broken down, propionic acid and its metabolites accumulate.
- Severe secondary carnitine deficiency develops, with especially reduced levels of free carnitine.
- The following acylcarnitine species accumulate diagnostically and can be used for neonatal screening programs: C_3-acylcarnitine and C_4-dicarboxylic acylcarnitine.
- No homocystinemia, no homocystinuria: there is no functional deficiency of the methionine synthase enzym, nor are there decreased levels of the coenzyme, MeCbl.
- Normal intracellular MeCbl levels: formation of this coenzyme is unaffected in cblA and cblB.
- Metabolic acidosis, hyperammonemia, hyperglycinemia, and ketonuria may be seen: the hyperammonemia is believed to result from inhibition of the carbamyl phosphate synthetase I by methylmalonic acid. The pathogenesis of hyperglycinemia in these disorders is not fully understood, but methylmalonic acid may inhibit the glycine cleavage enzyme system.
- Normal serum Cbl levels and folate levels.
- Absence of megaloblastic anemia because the function of methionine synthase is not impaired in these disorders, folates are not trapped under the MeTHF form, and there is no interference with the availability of reduced folates for purine and pyrimidine synthesis.

The differentiation of cblA and cblB from mutase deficiency can be made by finding normal levels of MUT in fibroblast extracts or by the failure of intact cblA or cblB fibroblasts to increase labeled propionate incorporation following transfection by a vector containing

FIGURE 17-10. Summary of cblA and cblB deficiencies and their laboratory consequences (in parentheses). AdoCbl= adenosylcobalamin, Cbl= cobalamin, MeCbl= methylcobalamin, MTRR= methionine synthase reductase, TC/Cbl= transcobalamin–Cbl complex, TC= transcobalamin, THF= tetrahydrofolate.

cloned mutase cDNA. Both tests are only available on a research basis. A useful clinical tool to attempt differentiation is to administer Cbl and follow the response by measuring the excretion of methylmalonic acid: patients in the cblA and cblB groups will usually exhibit decreased excretion (9).

Cultured fibroblasts from both cblA and cblB patients have decreased incorporation of labeled propionate but this defect is responsive to the addition of OHCbl to the culture medium. Decreased synthesis of AdoCbl following incubation with labeled CNCbl is observed.

Complementation studies will distinguish cblA, cblB and MUT patients.

Molecular diagnosis is an option for both these conditions. When two pathogenic mutations have been identified in a patient, molecular analysis can be used for carrier detection in the family, for clinical diagnosis of other at-risk family members, and for prenatal diagnosis.

cblA: Mutations in the MMAA gene have been identified in approximately 40 patients with cblA (40,41), and include premature stop codons, splice site defects, and missense mutations. R145X is a frequently encountered premature stop mutation identified in 21 of 37 patients in a recent study.

cblB: Mutations in the MMAB gene encoding for a Cbl adenosyltransferase have been identified in patients with cblB (41).

Prenatal diagnosis has also been accomplished by 1) measuring methylmalonic acid levels in amniotic fluid or less reliably, in maternal urine, 2) by measuring methylmalonic acid levels in amniotic fluid and activity of MUT in amniocytes, and 3) by studying the metabolism of propionate and methylmalonic acid in amniocytes (14,29). Results of cultured chorionic villus cells studies should be confirmed by cultured amniocyte studies (29). Molecular diagnosis is possible in those families in which disease-causing mutations have been identified.

Treatment There are two components to the treatment of patients with cblA and cblB: the first is dietary restriction of protein (see Chapter 7) and the second is Cbl therapy. OHCbl at a dose of 1 mg can be given orally daily or intramuscularly once or twice per week (9). In addition, carnitine (50–100 mg/kg/d) supplementation is essential. Close monitoring of plasma amino acids, blood pH, ammonia, serum and urinary concentrations of methylmalonic acid, and clinical parameters is necessary to ensure proper balance in the diet and the success of therapy.

Some patients have become resistant to Cbl therapy, and AdoCbl may or may not be effective. cblA patients generally improve on Cbl therapy (success rate of 90%), with 70%

doing well long term; however, cblB patients are less responsive to Cbl therapy (success rate of 40%) and their long-term outcome is poorer (2). Prenatal therapy has been attempted (see Miscellaneous Clinical Information).

Miscellaneous Clinical Information There is one report of a patient with clinical and biochemical features of cblA, but with genetic complementation studies showing complementation with cblA control cell lines, suggesting the possibility of a new complementation group, designated cblH (OMIM 606169). "This patient has recently been found to have CblD variant 1 (42).

There are several reports of prenatal therapy for Cbl-responsive forms of methylmalonic aciduria. With Cbl administration, the levels of methylmalonic acid, which were initially elevated in the maternal urine, decreased (14).

REFERENCES

1. Fowler B. Genetic defects of folate and cobalamin metabolism. *Eur J Pediatr.* 1998;157:S60–S66.
2. Rosenblatt DS, Fenton WA. Inherited disorders of folate and cobalamin transport and metabolism. In: Scriver CR, Beaudet AL, Sly WS, et al. eds. *The Metabolic & Molecular Basis of Inherited Disease.* 8th ed. New York: McGraw-Hill; 2001:3897–3933.
3. Zittoun J. Congenital errors of folate metabolism. In: Wickramasinghe SN, ed. *Bailliere's Clinical Hematology* London: W.B. Saunders; 1995:603–616.
4. Carmel R. Cobalamin deficiency. In: Carmel R, Jacobsen DW, eds. *Homocysteine in Health and Disease.* London: Cambridge University Press; 2001:289–305.
5. Qiu A, Jansen M, Sakaris A, et al. Identification of an intestinal folate transporter and the molecular basis for hereditary folate malabsorption. *Cell.* 2006; 127:917–928.
6. Wevers RA, Hansen SI, van Hellenberg et al. Folate deficiency in cerebrospinal fluid associated with a defect in folate binding protein in the central nervous system. *J Neurol Neurosurg Psychiatry.* 1994; 57(2):223–226.
7. Geller J, Kronn L, Somasundaram J, et al. Hereditary folate malabsorption: family report and review of the literature. *Medicine.* 2002;81:51–68.
8. Jebnoun S, Kacem S, Mokrani C, et al. A family study of congenital malabsorption of folate. *J Inherit Metab Dis.* 2001; 24:749–750.
9. Rosenblatt DS, Fowler B. Disorders of cobalamin and folate transport and metabolism. In: Fernandez J, Saudubray J-M, van den Berghe B, eds. *Inborn Metabolic Diseases: Diagnosis and Treatment.* 4th ed. Berlin: Springer; 2006:343–351.
10. Solans A, Estivill X, de la Luna S. Cloning and characterization of human FTCD on 21q22.3, a candidate gene for glutamate formiminotransferase deficiency. *Cytogenet Cell Genet.* 2000; 88:43–49.

11. Hilton JF, Christensen KE, Watkins D, et al. The molecular basis of glutamate formiminotransferase deficiency. *Hum Mutat.* 2003; 22:67–73.
12. Thomas MA, Rosenblatt DS. Severe Methylenetetrahydrofolate reductase deficiency. In: Ueland PM, Rozen R, eds. *MTHFR Polymorphisms and Disease.* Georgetown, TX: Landes Bioscience/Eurekah.com; 2005:41–53.
13. Ogier de Baulny H, Gérard M, Saudubray JM, et al. Remethylation defects: guidelines for clinical diagnosis and treatment. *Eur J Pediatr.* 1998;157(Suppl. 2):S77–S83.
14. Rosenblatt DS. Prenatal diagnosis of miscellaneous biochemical disorders. In: Milunsky A, ed. *Genetic Disorders of the Fetus: Diagnosis, Prevention and Treatment.* 5th ed. Baltimore: Johns Hopkins University Press; 2004:630–644.
15. Morel CF, Scott P, Christensen E, et al. Prenatal diagnosis for severe methylenetetrahydrofolate reductase deficiency by linkage analysis and enzymatic assay. *Mol Genet Metab.* 2005;85:115–120.
16. Schwahn BC, Laryea MD, Chen Z, et al. Betaine rescue of an animal model with methylenetetrahydrofolate reductase deficiency. *Biochem J.* 2004; 382:831–840.
17. Leclerc D, Sibani S, Rozen R. Molecular biology of methylenetetrahydrofolate reductase (MTHFR) and overview of mutations/polymorphisms. In: Ueland PM, Rozen R, eds. *MTHFR Polymorphisms and Disease.* Georgetown, TX: Landes Bioscience/Eurekah.com; 2005:1–20.
18. Carmel R, Green R, Rosenblatt DS, et al. Update on cobalamin, folate and homocysteine. Hematology. Am Soc Hematol Educ Program. 2003: 62–81.
19. Stabler S, Allen RH, Savage DG, et al. Clinical spectrum and diagnosis of cobalamin deficiency. *Blood.* 1990;76:871–881.
20. Gordon MM, Brada N, Remacha A, et al. A genetic polymorphism in the coding region of the gastric intrinsic factor gene (GIF) is associated with congenital intrinsic factor deficiency. *Hum Mutat.* 2004;23:85–91.
21. Yassin F, Rothenberg,SP, Rao S, et al. Identification of a 4-base deletion in the gene in inherited intrinsic factor deficiency. *Blood.* 2004;103:1515–1517.
22. Tanner SM, Li Z, Perko JD, et al. Hereditary juvenile cobalamin deficiency caused by mutations in the intrinsic factor gene. *Proc Natl Acad Sci USA.* 2005;102:4130–4133.
23. Fyfe JC, Madsen M, Hojrup P, et al. The functional cobalamin (vitamin B12)-intrinsic factor receptor is a novel complex of cubilin and amnionless. *Blood.* 2004;103:1573–1579.
24. Suormala T, Baumgartner M.R, Coelho D, et al. The cblD defect causes either isolated or combined deficiency of methyl adenosylcobalamin synthesis. *J Biol Chem.* 2004;279:42742–42749.
25. Coelho D, Suormala T, Stucki M, et al. Gene identification of the cblD defect of vitamin B12 metabolism. *N Engl J Med.* 2008;358:1454–1464.
26. Carmel R. Mild transcobalamin I (haptocorrin) deficiency and low serum cobalamin concentrations. *Clin Chem.* 2003;49:367–374.
27. Teplitsky V, Huminer D, Zoldan J, et al. Hereditary partial transcobalamin II deficiency with neurologic, mental and hematologic abnormalities in children and adults. *Isr Med Assoc J.* 2003;5:868–872.

28. Qian L, Quadros EV, Regec A, et al. Congenital transcobalamin II deficiency due to errors in RNA editing. *Blood Cells Mol Dis.* 2002;28:134-142, 143–145.

29. Morel CF, Watkins D, Scott P, et al. Prenatal diagnosis for methylmalonic acidemia and inborn errors of B12 metabolism and transport. *Mol Genet Metab* 2005;86:160–171.

30. Atkinson JL, Paterson A, Renaud D, et al. Genetic mapping of Cobalamin C deficiency: putative linkage to 1q. *Am J Hum Genet.* 2002;71(Suppl):452 (Abstract 1652).

31. Lerner-Ellis JP, Tirone JC, Pawelek PD, et al. Identification of the gene responsible for methylmalonic aciduria and homocystinuria, cblC type. *Nat Genet.* 2006;36:93–100.

32. Harding CO, Pillers D-AM, Steiner RD, et al. Potential for misdiagnosis due to lack of metabolic derangement in combined methylmalonic aciduria/hyperhomocystinemia (CblC) in the neonate. *J Perinatol.* 2003;23:384–386.

33. Bodamer OAF, Rosenblatt DS, Appel SH, et al. Adult-onset combined methylmalonic aciduria and homocystinuria (cblC). *Neurology.* 2001;56:1113.

34. Van Hove JLK, Van Damme-Lombaerts R, Grunewald S, et al. Cobalamin disorder cbl-C presenting with late-onset thrombotic microangiopathy. *Am J Med Genet.* 2002;111: 195–201.

35. Watkins D, Ru M, Hwang H-Y, et al. Hyperhomocysteinemia due to methionine synthase deficiency, cblG: structure of the MTR gene, genotype diversity, and recognition of a common mutation, P1173L. *Am J Hum Genet.* 2002;71:143–153.

36. Wilson A, Leclerc D, Rosenblatt DS, et al. Molecular basis for methionine synthase reductase deficiency in patients belonging to the cblE complementation group of disorders in folate/cobalamin metabolism. *Hum Mol Genet.* 1999;8:2009–2016.

37. Dobson CM, Wai T, Leclerc D, et al. Identification of the gene responsible for the cblA complementation group of vitamin B12-responsive methylmalonic acidemia based on analysis of prokaryotic gene arrangements. *Proc Natl Acad Sci USA.* 2002; 99:15554–15559.

38. Dobson CM, Wai T, Leclerc D, et al, Identification of the gene responsible for the cblB complementation group of vitamin B12-dependent methylmalonic aciduria. *Hum Mol Genet.* 2002;11:3361–3369.

39. Johnson CL, Pechonick E, Park SD, et al. Functional genomic, biochemical, and genetic characterization of the Salmonella pduO gene, an ATP:cob(I)alamin adenosyltransferase gene. *J Bacteriol.* 2001;183:1577–84.

40. Lerner-Ellis JP, Dobson CM, Wai T, et al. Mutations in the MMAA gene in patients with the cblA disorder of vitamin B12 metabolism. *Hum Mutat.* 2004;24:509–516.

41. Yang X, Sakamoto O, Matsubara Y, et al. Mutation analysis of the MMAA and MMAB genes in Japanese patients with vitamin B12-responsive methylmalonic acidemia: identification of a prevalent MMAA mutation. *Mol Genet Metab.* 2004;82:329–33.

42. Watkins D, Matiaszuk N, Rosenblatt DS. Complementation studies in the cblA class of inborn error of cobalamin metabolism: evidence for interallelic complementation and for a new complementation class (cblH). *J Med Genet.* 2003;37:510–513.

CHAPTER 18

Oxidative Phosphorylation Diseases and Mitochondrial DNA Depletion Syndrome

Mark A. Tarnopolsky, MD, PhD, FRCP(C)
Sandeep Raha, PhD

INTRODUCTION

This chapter will provide a general overview of mitochondrial cytopathies presenting in the pediatric age group. Although there are a variety of disorders in which mitochondrial dysfunction is a secondary phenomenon (Prader-Willi syndrome, Friedreich's ataxia, etc.), we will focus predominantly on the disorders that result from direct mutations to mitochondrial DNA (mtDNA), those that alter mtDNA content and quality (depletion and deletions, respectively), and those that alter the composition and assembly of the electron transport chain (ETC) complexes. Although the pyruvate dehydrogenase (PDH) complex disorders are often considered within the mitochondrial cytopathy framework, these will be covered separately in Chapter 13. Given the complexities of the ETC and the uniqueness of the mitochondrial genome, a background on the normal physiology and general principles of mtDNA replication and general mitochondrial biology is essential for understanding the phenotypic and biochemical consequences of mitochondrial dysfunction and to rationally plan diagnostic and therapeutic strategies. Although the focus will be on the pediatric mitochondrial cytopathies, there is a very wide clinical spectrum and a number of the disorders discussed in this chapter can also present in adulthood, particularly the mtDNA point mutations. A classic example of this is the 8993 mutation in which a lower mutational burden can result in adult onset neuropathy, ataxia, retinitis, and pigmentosa (NARP) or a higher mutational burden can result in fatal infantile maternally inherited Leigh syndrome.

NORMAL PHYSIOLOGY

The cascade of enzymes referred to as the ETC can generate up to 38 adenosine triphosphate (ATP) molecules per molecule of glucose. The production of this energy requires a system of regulatory and signaling mechanisms whose complexity has only begun to be appreciated over the last decade. Not surprisingly, a number of diseases have been identified in which the cause is a defect in the signaling pathways or structural elements within the functional framework of this complex organelle. These diseases not only result due to decreased energy supply but also from macromolecular damage incurred from an elevated level of reactive oxygen species. The clinical challenge in diagnosing and treating mitochondrial dysfunction is complicated by the broad presentation of the symptoms (phenotype). Any alteration in the ATP output of the mitochondria has the potential to impact on all cellular pathways that are dependent upon ATP. It is therefore important to gain a rudimentary understanding of the elements involved in oxidative phosphorylation and its control as well as the role of mitochondria within the cell. This chapter will attempt to briefly outline the function of the mitochondria in maintaining cellular homeostasis as well as review the clinical impact of disorders of oxidative phosphorylation. It should be kept in mind that a large number of cellular processes do involve the mitochondria given their critical role in energy homeostasis.

Mitochondrial Respiratory Chain

Mitochondria contain their own circular DNA (16,569 bp) encoding 13 mitochondrial proteins, 22 mitochondrial tRNAs and the 12S and 16S mitochondrial rRNA (Figure 18-1); however, the vast majority of mitochondrial proteins are encoded for by the nuclear genome. These extramitochondrially encoded proteins must be targeted and chaperoned into the proper compartment of the mitochondria.

The mitochondrial respiratory chain consists of five major enzymes termed complexes I through V. Each of these complexes is a multi-subunit assembly consisting of nuclear and mitochondrially encoded subunits (except for complex II, which has no subunits encoded by mtDNA). The first four complexes contain metal centers as well as ubiquinone or cytochrome c binding sites to facilitate electron transfer from nicotinamide adenine dinucleotide hydrogenase (NADH) or flavin adenine dinucleotide hydrogenase (FADH) to oxygen (complex I also contains a flavin mononucleotide moiety). Figure 18-2 demonstrates the sequence of electron flow through the respiratory chain cascade. The primary objective of this electron flow is to couple the transfer of electrons from high-energy compounds (such as NADH and FADH) to the generation of a proton motive force by translocating protons from the cytosol to the intermembrane space via complexes I, III, and IV. Briefly, electrons accepted from $NADH + H^+$ are shuttled through complex I via a flavin mononucleotide moiety and through a pair of iron sulfur centers to ubiquinone. Ubiquinone shuttles the electrons to complex III. In a similar manner, $FADH + H^+$ transfers its electrons into the system at complex II. The crucial difference between these two entry points is that complex I is able to translocate protons into the intermembrane space whereas the complex II does not. As a consequence $NADH + H^+$ is more effective, on a molar basis, for (net) ATP synthesis. Cytochrome c shuttles the electrons to cytochrome c oxidase (COX), which is the terminal enzyme complex in the electron cascade. Complex IV is then oxidized by molecular oxygen, forming water in the process. The net proton gradient can be utilized by complex V in the synthesis of ATP, a compound that is used as the energy currency of the cell. The ATP synthase complex is composed of two major segments an F_0 and F_1. The F_1 segment is situated in the mitochondrial matrix, whereas the F_0 segment sits within the inner mitochondrial membrane. These individual segments are composed of functional regions including a proton channel (subunits A and C), a molecular ratchet used to couple the conformational change associated with proton flux to the molecular rotor (subunit α). Finally, the molecular rotor is coupled to conformational changes in the α and β subunits evoking the ATP synthase

Disorders of Oxidative Phosphorylation

AT A GLANCE

The oxidative phosphorylation disorders are a result of mutations that alter either the respiratory chain enzymes directly or the assembly or transcriptional machinery involved in mitochondrial structure and function. These defects result in an impressive array of diverse clinical phenotypes; organs that rely heavily on oxidative phosphorylation are often more severely affected (skeletal muscle, brain, heart, and liver). The defects that directly alter mtDNA show maternal inheritance; however, an increasing number of "sporadic" mutations are now shown to be due to autosomal recessive nuclear mutations. The diagnosis of mitochondrial cytopathies requires a combination of enzymology, histopathology, blood, and urine metabolomics (lactate and organic acids), magnetic resonance imaging, magnetic resonance spectroscopy, and DNA mutation analysis. There are no proven therapies; however, based on case series and knowledge of the pathophysiology, patients often receive a combination of cofactors (coenzyme Q10, riboflavin, and α-lipoic acid), antioxidants (vitamins E and C), and other treatments (creatine monohydrate and dichloroacetate).

TYPES	COMMON MUTATIONS	OMIM
LHON	G11778A, T14484C, G3460A, G14459A	535000, 516006, 516000, 516006
MELAS	G1642A, A3243G, A3260G, T3271C	540000, 590050
MERRF	A8344G, T8356C, G8363A	545000, 509006
NARP/MILS	T8993C, T8993G, T9176C	516060
KSS	single large mtDNA deletion	530000
MNGIE	thymidine phosphorylase	603041
Leigh Disease	NDUFB1, NDUFS7, SDHA, SURF1, PDH$_C$	256000
mtDNA depletion	thymidine kinase (TK2), deoxy-Guanosine kinase (dGK)	188250, 601465
cardiomyopathy	SCO2, COX10, A4295G, A4300G, A8296G	604272, 602125, 590045, 590060

FORM	LABORATORY FINDINGS	CLINICAL PRESENTATION (all have some muscle weakness, fatigue, hypotonia depending on age)	TREATMENT
LHON	H: often normal E: often normal S: lactate +/−	Painless loss of vision More common in men Onset: teens and 20s	Acute - ? high-dose vitamin E Chronic (+/−) – COQ10, creatine, vitamin E, lipoic acid, riboflavin
MELAS	H: RRF, SSV, COX-ve E: often mixed ETC defect S: lactate +, ++	Any combination of hearing loss, ataxia, exercise intolerance, diabetes, stroke, dementia at any age	Acute - ? IV arginine (stroke) Chronic (+/−) – COQ10, creatine, vitamin E, lipoic acid, riboflavin.
MERRF	H: RRF (COX-ve), COX-ve E: often mixed ETC defect S: lactate +, ++	Any combination of ataxia, neuropathy, lipomas, myoclonic epilepsy Onset: child > teen.	Chronic (+/−) – COQ10, creatine, vitamin E, lipoic acid, riboflavin
KSS	H: RRF, COX-ve E: often mixed ETC defect S: lactate +, ++	Ataxia, retinitis pigmentosa, heart block, high CSF protein, ptosis, ophthalmoplegia Onset < 25 years of age.	Chronic (+/−) – COQ10, creatine, vitamin E, lipoic acid, riboflavin,
MNGIE	H: RRF, COX-ve (+/−) E: often mixed ETC defect S: lactate +	Abdominal pain, bloating, malabsorption, neuropathy, encephalopathy (during stress) Onset: teens	Chronic (+/−) – COQ10, creatine, vitamin E, lipoic acid, riboflavin, + TPN in most cases
Leigh Disease	H: complex IV: general ↓ COX, may be N otherwise E: I or II or III or IV or PDH ↓ S: lactate +, ++	Psychomotor regression, ataxia, apneas, tremor, optic atrophy, dystonia, Onset: infantile Death: 2–4 years of age	Acute: ? value of dichloroacetate Chronic (+/−) – COQ10, creatine, vitamin E, lipoic acid, riboflavin ? ketogenic diet.

FORM	LABORATORY FINDINGS	CLINICAL PRESENTATION (all have some muscle weakness, fatigue, hypotonia depending on age)	TREATMENT
mtDNA Depletion	H: EM –homogeneous material in mitochondria E: often mixed defect S: lactate +/−, +, ++	Hepatoencephalopathy: liver failure, psychomotor regression, encephalopathy, hypotonia Encephalomyopathic: as above – liver failure. Onset: 1st y, early childhood	Chronic (+/−) – COQ10, creatine, vitamin E, lipoic acid, riboflavin
Cardiomyopathy	H: low COX in SURF, SCO2, may be normal in others E: ↓↓ COX in SURF, SCO2 S: lactate ++	Severe infantile (SCO2, COX15) – hypotonia, cardiac failure, respiratory failure Older child: dyspnea with exercise, may be asymptomatic early in course.	Chronic (+/−) – COQ10, creatine, vitamin E, lipoic acid, riboflavin, + + afterload reduction.

H = muscle histology; E = enzymology; S = serum or plasma; LHON = Leber hereditary optic neuropathy; MELAS = mitochondrial myopathy, encephalopathy, lactic acidosis, and stroke-like episodes; MERRF = myoclonic epilepsy associated with ragged-red fibers; KSS = Kearns-Sayre syndrome; MNGIE = mitochondrial neurogastrointestinal encephalopathy; COX = cytochrome c oxidase, SURF = Surfeit; SCO2 = synthesis of cytochrome c oxidase; RRF = ribosome-recycling factor; SSV = strongly SDH-reactive blood vessels; PDH = pyruvate dehydrogenase; NDUFB1 = NADH dehydrogenase (ubiquinone) 1 beta subcomplex; NDUFS7 = NADH ubiquinone oxidoreductase Fe S protein 7; SDHA = succinate dehydrogenase complex, subunit A, flavoprotein; CSF = cerebral spinal fluid.

EXAMPLES OF SOME COMPONENTS OF A MITOCHONDRIAL COCKTAIL*

Medication	Mechanism of Action	Dose
Coenzyme Q10	Bypass complex I and II	2-5 mg/kg/d
Coenzyme Q10	(COQ10 deficiency)	7.5-30 mg/kg/d
Creatine	Alternative energy source, neuroprotection	100 mg/kg/d
Thiamine	Cofactor for PDH	3-9 mg/kg/d
Riboflavin	Bypass complex I (via II)	3-5 mg/kg/d
Vitamin E	Antioxidant	5-10 mg/kg/d
Vitamin C	Antioxidant	5-10 mg/kg/d
L-carnitine	Treat secondary deficiency	30-50 mg/kg/d
Succinate	Bypass complex I defects	30-70 mg/kg/d
α-Lipoic acid	Antioxidant, component of mitochondria	3-5 mg/kg/d
Dichloroacetate	Activate PDH and reduce lactate	25 mg/kg/d

*It is important to start with the lowest possible dosage of any medication and titrate the dosage to effect and as tolerated. The main side effect with all of the above medications is gastrointestinal upset, which can often be treated by dividing the dosage into a two or three time per day dosing regimen.

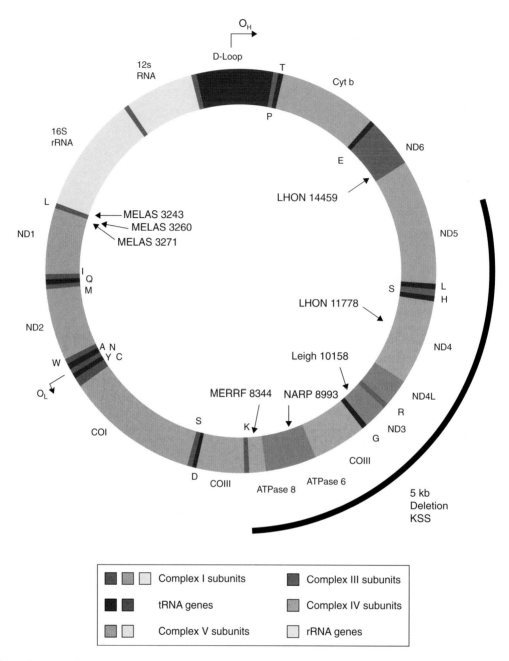

FIGURE 18-1. Morbidity map for mtDNA. The positions of the mitochondrially encoded proteins, tRNAs and rRNAs are indicated on the map. Only a few of the known mtDNA mutation have been denoted. The complete list of mitochondrial DNA mutations known to date is available from *Neuromuscul Disord.* 2004;14:107–116. The table summarizes some of the clinical symptoms associated with each of the mutations listed on the morbidity map.

activity. The flow of electrons through the F_0 segment induces a counterclockwise rotation of the "head" of the F_1 ATPase. This rotation evokes conformation changes within the α and β subunits, which contain the adenosine diphosphate/ATP binding sites. This results in catalytic activity such that the flow of three protons through this complex results in the synthesis of one molecule of ATP. Clearly the large number of subunits required for the proper coordination of enzyme activity in these multi-subunit structures suggests that mutations in any one of these components could result in a loss of function of not only the specific enzyme complex but the entire respiratory chain (RC) cascade. Therefore defects in either electron flow or proton pumping will result in an inability of the system to generate an ample proton gradient for effective ATP synthesis.

In addition to the composition of the individual subunit, these large, multi-subunit structures need to be imported into the mitochondria and properly assembled. For example, complex I is composed of approximately 43 subunits and totals to a mass of greater than 900 kDa. Although the pathway or its assembly has not been fully elucidated as of yet, factors such as GRIM 19 (1) are thought to play an important role in guiding the assembly of this multi-subunit complex. GRIM 19 was originally thought to have a proapoptotic activity in interferon- and retinoic acid–induced tumorigenesis (2) and therefore has given rise to the speculation about whether there are more such assembly factors that could form part of the link between respiratory enzyme dysfunction and programmed cell death.

More definitive links between ETC assembly/chaperones and mitochondrial disorders come from recent evidence for defects in those associated with complex IV assembly/function.

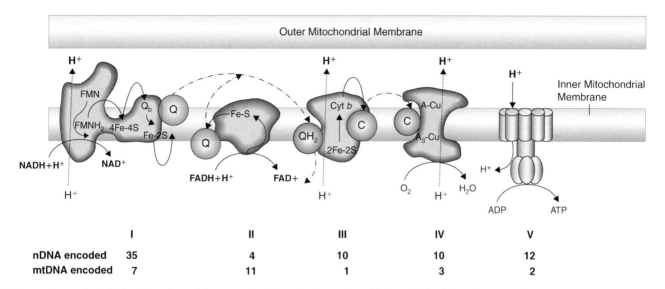

FIGURE 18-2. The cascade of mitochondrial respiratory chain enzymes. Complexes I through V are situated the inner mitochondrial membrane. Complex I accepts electrons from NADH and shuttles them to ubiquinone (Q) through flavin mononucleotides (FMN) and iron-sulfur centers (Fe-S). This electron movement results in the translocation of protons from the cytosol to the intermembrane space. The ubiquinone then delivers the electrons to complex III, where they are transferred to cytochrome c through an iron-sulfur center and cytochrome b. Complex III also translocates protons from the cytosol to the intermembrane space. Complex IV facilitates the oxidation of cytochrome c by oxygen.
Complex II reduces Q by transferring electrons from FADH₂; however it does not translocate any protons across the inner mitochondrial membrane and therefore does not contribute to the proton motive force. The channelling of protons from the intermembrane space through complex V results in the synthesis of ATP.

For example, Leigh disease can be caused by mutations in SURF1 (3), a factor required for the functional assembly of COX (4). Hypertrophic cardiomyopathy can also be associated with mutations in SCO2 (5), an assembly factor responsible for the insertion of copper into COX during its maturation (6). Additionally, defects in peptides such as the leucine-rich pentracticopeptide repeat cassette, a nuclear-encoded transcriptional factor that is thought to enhance the stability of COX subunits, can also result in disease. Specifically, a mutation in this gene has been shown to affect the stability of COXI and COXIII, two mitochondrially encoded subunits, in a French-Canadian variant of Leigh disease (7). It is therefore important to appreciate that mutations in transcriptional factors, chaperones as well as the functional enzyme units involved in oxidative phosphorylation, can contribute to the onset of disease.

mtDNA mutations can also occur from free radical generation resulting from oxygen radicals formed during routine operation of the ETC. It is estimated that under basal operation, the ETC liberates 1% to 2% of its electrons as radicals, which can result in cumulative damage to DNA. Although lipids and proteins are also damaged they are subjected to molecular turnover and are not so consequential in the long run. Such damage is considered to be a normal part of aging and is thought to be responsible for some of its characteristic phenotype (8). In fact it has been demonstrated, in a mouse model (9), that removing the ability of mtDNA polymerase to proofread during replication

(thereby preserving damaged DNA bases and allowing these to accumulate more rapidly) results in significantly accelerated onset of the aged phenotype. In cases in which preexisting mutations in mtDNA result in attenuated RC activity and increased formation of free radicals, and the ensuing damage to the mtDNA can accelerate the clinical pathology, a process known as a "vicious cycle" is established. Enzymes designed to dissipate superoxides, such as manganese superoxide dismutase (MnSOD) and Cu/Zn superoxide dismutase (Cu/ZnSOD), normally respond to changes in the level of reactive oxygen species production and may form part of an adaptation response for dealing with elevated levels of radical formation within the cell. In light of such adaptive responses, there has been much discussion focused around the question of whether these so called destructive radicals are essential signaling molecules (10) (Figure 18-3).

Mitochondrial Biogenesis and Heteroplasmy

Classically the mitochondrion has been portrayed as an isolated "ovoid" shaped organelle, primarily resulting from electron micrographic representations. The advent of fluorescence technology along with the development of microscopes that impart low photon damage have resulted in a dramatic change in the way individual mitochondria are visualized. Within the context of a live cell, mitochondria form highly reticulated structures that are continuously fusing and breaking apart. Such dynamic motions are

an important component of "good cellular health." Recent evidence suggests that mutations in the mfn2 gene (a gene important for the maintenance of mitochondrial morphology) results in a form of Charcot-Marie-Tooth syndrome (11).

Mitochondrial dynamics also play an important role in mitotic segregation of mitochondrial mutations and contribute to the concept of heteroplasmy and polyplasmy. Unlike nuclear genes that contain two alleles, there are multiple copies of mtDNA within a single cell. There are thought to be between 2 and 10 copies of mtDNA within each mitochondrion and between 100 and 1,000 mitochondria per cell (depending on the type of cell). More important, because mitochondria replicate independently of cell division, individual cells can contain different numbers of mutant and wild-type mitochondria (this ratio is referred to as the percentage of heteroplasmy). During cell division, there is generally a random distribution of mitochondria resulting in shuffling of the mitochondrial population. If some of these mitochondria contain mutant DNA while others contain wild-type DNA, then this heterogeneous population will become distributed randomly (Figure 18-4). Depending on the energetic demands of the tissue, the percentage of heteroplasmy may result in pathogenesis. The threshold for the mutation is a combination of these two variables. In general, the threshold is defined as the point of disease onset or where mitochondrial enzyme activity declines as a result of sufficient mutated mtDNA. The range of heteroplasmy for disease onset can be quite

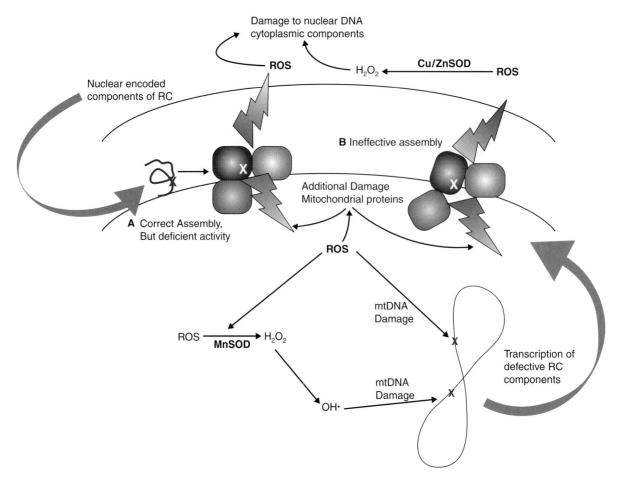

FIGURE 18-3. Mutations in respiratory chain subunits result in elevated formation of reactive oxygen species. A damaged component of the respiratory chain complex (marked with an "**X**") can result in either **(A)** correct assembly of the complex, but the activity of the enzyme will be hampered; alternatively, the mutation can result in **(B)** the incorrect assembly of the complex, also resulting in attenuation of the activity. In either case, the disruption in electron flow through the enzyme cascade will result in a net increase in the formation of reactive oxygen intermediates. These reactive molecules have the potential to damage other molecules including mitochondrial or nuclear DNA or other proteins. Damage to mtDNA can result in the production of additional damaged subunits for components of the respiratory chain complexes. This may result in further attenuation of electron flow and subsequently an increase in reactive oxygen species generation. Therefore this becomes a "vicious cycle." Antioxidant defense enzymes such as mitochondrial manganese superoxide dismutase and the cytosolic Cu/Zn superoxide dismutase are involved in dissipating the elevated levels of superoxide.

broad. In general, a relatively high mutant load is required (usually >80%); however, there are reports of quite low levels of heteroplasmy having a profound phenotypic impact (12). Chinnery and colleagues documented the case of two brothers with the mtDNA A3243G mutation, in which one of the brothers had only a 5.95% mutant load within single fibers of the gastrocnemius muscle and rate of mitochondrial ATP production was reduced to 35% of the normal mean value (12). Consequently, enzyme activity levels in vitro and/or heteroplasmy levels cannot be rigidly applied to a prediction of the phenotypic consequences.

CONSEQUENCES OF MITOCHONDRIAL DYSFUNCTION

The most obvious pathologic consequence of mitochondrial dysfunction is a decrease in aerobic energy transduction. This reduction in ATP production is understandable

when considering that the aerobic oxidation of glucose yields approximately 14-fold more ATP molecules per mol of glucose compared with that derived from anaerobic glycolysis. As a consequence, cells such as the retina, basal ganglia, cardiac muscle, and skeletal muscle are particularly sensitive to mitochondrial dysfunction and these tissues commonly display clinical and biochemical features in the presence of mitochondrial dysfunction. Due to the increased reliance on anaerobic glycolysis, there is an increase in the use of alternative energy sources such as phosphocreatine hydrolysis. Depletion of phosphocreatine has been seen in brain and skeletal muscle (13) from patients with mitochondrial disease. We have also frequently seen an increase in myoadenylate deaminase activity at the tissue level, which is likely another strategy to maintain cellular energy charge via the adenylate kinase/myoadenylate deaminase pathway. Enhanced anaerobic glycolysis leads to an increase in

lactate generation and/or an elevated lactate/pyruvate (L/P) ratio.

In response to the decreased aerobic energy transduction, a variety of signaling pathways leading to mitochondrial biogenesis can cause excessive proliferation of mitochondria in the subsarcolemmal and intramyofibrillar regions of the cell. The massive accumulation in the subsarcolemmal region leads to the classic rimlike histologic feature of ragged red fibers (RRF) (Figure 18-5). As a consequence of the mitochondrial proliferation and the increased attempt to flux energy through the phosphocreatine creatine system, there is an up-regulation of mitochondrial creatine kinase that, in the presence of oxidative stress, can dimerize and form paracrystalline inclusions thereby altering the three-dimensional structure of the mitochondria (Figure 18-6). Dysfunction of the ETC, particularly at complexes I and III, leads to an increased generation of free radicals, which induces the up-regulation of antioxidant enzymes such

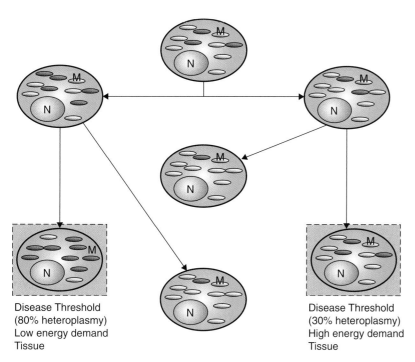

FIGURE 18-4. The level of mutant mtDNA defines the tissue-specific disease threshold. A cell originally containing 30% mutant mtDNA (red) replicates to form two daughters cells, one with 50% mutant mtDNA, and the other with only 20%. These daughter cells can then replicate to form two new cells (80% and 10% heteroplasmy). In tissues that have a low energy demand (such as fibroblasts) a much higher level of heteroplasmy is required to observe the onset of disease. In contrast, tissues that demand a great deal of aerobic energy, such as muscle, a significantly lower level of heteroplasmy will cause pathogenesis.

Disease Threshold
(80% heteroplasmy)
Low energy demand
Tissue

Disease Threshold
(30% heteroplasmy)
High energy demand
Tissue

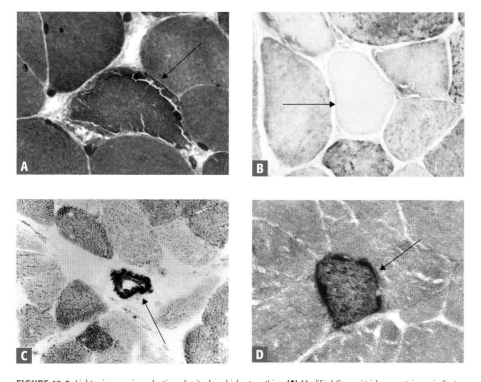

FIGURE 18-5. Light microscopic evaluation of mitochondrial cytopathies. **(A)** Modified Gomori trichrome stain → indicates a classic ragged red fiber in a patient with MELAS A3243G; **(B)** Cytochrome oxidase stain → indicates COX-negative fiber in a patient with Kearn–Sayre syndrome; **(C)** Succinate dehydrogenase stain → indicates strongly SDH-positive fiber (SSV) in a patient with MELAS A3243G; **(D)** Myoadenylate deaminase stain → indicates significant accumulation in a ragged red fiber in a patient with MELAS A3260G.

as Cu/ZnSOD, and MnSOD. Eventually the endogenous ability of the body to adapt to the excess of free radical production is overwhelmed and cellular oxidative stress occurs. Another consequence of mitochondrial dysfunction is an induction of cellular apoptosis in nerve and possibly skeletal muscle. At the extreme end of energy dysfunction, tissue necrosis can be seen such as in bilateral striatal necrosis (Figure 18-7). The therapies that have been devised to enhance mitochondrial function have been based on ameliorating the aforementioned pathologic consequences, and this will be discussed in more detail in a subsequent section.

Demographics of Mitochondrial Disease

Epidemiologic data related to mitochondrial disorders are a difficult topic to discuss because of the heterogeneity of diseases that are manifested as a result of the dysfunction of this organelle. Oxidative phosphorylation disorders can be regarded as among the most common group of inborn errors of metabolism. As of 2004, pathogenic mutations had been identified in 30 of the 37 genes encoded for by mtDNA (14). It was suggested by these authors that almost 25% of oxidative phosphorylation disorders are caused by mtDNA mutations. Based on Australian statistics, Thorburn and colleagues have estimated that birth prevalence of disorders related to oxidative phosphorylation dysfunction may be as high as 1/5,000 (14). One of the great difficulties of obtaining good epidemiologic data for mitochondrial disorders is that there are large numbers of specialized centers to which samples are referred. Therefore individual centers quite often have incomplete regions of coverage (14). North American (15) and European (12) epidemiologic studies all suggest that oxidative phosphorylation disorders are far from rare diseases. These studies report estimated the prevalence of ETC disorders to be between 1/7,000 and 1/2,000. These birth prevalence rates are comparable to those of Duchenne muscular dystrophy and amyotrophic lateral sclerosis, diseases that are much more familiar to the general public. There are, however, subpopulations, such as the Lebanese population in Australia and the Saguenay-Lac St. Jean population in Quebec in which the incidence of mitochondrial disorders is significantly higher than that within the general population. Because part of the problem related to obtaining accurate birth prevalence data has been the lack of clear cut guidelines for defining mitochondrial disease, it has been suggested that the utilization of the modified Walker,

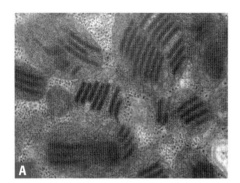
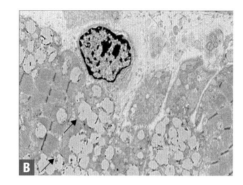
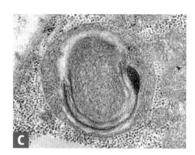

FIGURE 18-6. Electron microscopic evaluation of mitochondrial cytopathies. **(A)** Electron micrograph demonstrating multiple paracrystalline inclusions in a patient with a cytochrome B mutation (G15497A). **(B)** Electron micrograph of a child with fatal encephalomyopathic DNA depletion syndrome → indicates mitochondrial proliferation with a fine granular appearance; inset shows a higher power of a single rounded mitochondria with homogeneous-appearing material in the center.

Nijmegen, Nonaka, or Wolfson criteria be used in the future to derive more concrete epidemiologic data (15).

GENERAL DIAGNOSTIC TESTING

Blood

The hallmark of mitochondrial dysfunction is an elevation of serum lactate. In adults, an isolated serum lactate has a sensitivity of only 0.62 and a specificity of greater than 0.9 (16). Recently, a study in the pediatric age group has found a very similar sensitivity of 0.60 for those with "definite" mitochondrial cytopathies (17). As a consequence, an elevated lactate level can be helpful to rule in (high specificity) the disease but a normal lactate cannot be used to rule out (modest sensitivity) mitochondrial disease. In the pediatric age group, specificity is likely to be lower than in the adult population due to a greater number of variables that induce false-positive results (i.e, elevated lactate in the absence of disease) compared with the adult population. Common causes of a false-positive elevation in lactate include a struggling child with a difficult blood draw, blood that was not put on ice and separated rapidly and assayed, and the presence of other conditions known to increase lactate (critical illness, hypoxemia, diabetes, and immediate postprandial period). For these reasons, we recommend a careful review of the blood drawing experience and the drawing of three samples while the patient is in a fasted state without extensive struggling if a single questionable blood result was obtained. A CSF lactate level is also helpful in that some conditions result in disproportionate involvement of the central nervous system. Furthermore, the lumbar puncture is helpful to rule in or rule out alternative diagnosis such as infection, leukodystrophy, acute disseminating encephalomyopathy, and multiple sclerosis in children and adolescents with a central nervous system presentation. An elevated CSF

protein can also be seen in Kearns-Sayre syndrome (KSS), mtDNA depletion syndrome, and some cases of mitochondrial myopathy, encephalopathy, lactic acidosis, and stroke-like episodes (MELAS). In fact, the highest CSF protein level that our service has seen is 4.5 g/L in a child with mtDNA depletion syndrome.

The L/P ratio is sometimes used as an indicator of mitochondrial disease and in most cases an elevated L/P ratio can be helpful in ruling in disease but a normal L/P ratio cannot be used to rule out disease. The L/P ratio in serum is a crude indicator of intracellular redox potential and we find that the L/P ratio in fibroblasts and other cells is much more sensitive and a specific indicator of ETC dysfunction. L/P ratios are a first line of investigation for RC defects when assessing cultured fibroblasts. This determination can be problematic as a result of technical considerations such as the increased level of growth hormones found in current stocks of fetal bovine serum (18). In our experience, the serum L/P ratio is quite variable and we have had several patients with MELAS 3243 who have low normal and high L/P ratios on consecutive months with no change in clinical signs or symptoms. In general, a high L/P ratio is associated with mitochondrial cytopathies, pyruvate carboxylase, or α-ketoglutarate dehydrogenase deficiency; whereas, a normal or low L/P ratio is more consistent with PDH deficiency (see Chapter 13). Nevertheless, one must be careful not to rule out RC defects in the case of near normal L/P ratios using cultured cells for the test can yield false negative results (i.e, a normal L/P ratio can be seen in Leber hereditary optic neuropathy (LHON), MELAS, and other mitochondrial disorders).

Other blood tests that are helpful in the evaluation of mitochondrial cytopathies include the complete blood count (CBC), creatine kinase (CK) activity, and liver function tests. The CBC is helpful in cases such as

Pearson bone marrow syndrome in which sideroblastic anemia is noted. The CBC is also helpful to rule out anemia from other causes that can exacerbate or mimic a preexisting mitochondrial cytopathy (i.e, a severe vitamin B12 deficiency). Approximately, 11% of our patients with definite mitochondrial cytopathy also have a coexistent B12 and/or red blood cell folate deficiency, which can ultimately lead to neurologic symptoms and megaloblastic anemia (Tarnopolsky et al. unpublished data, 2005).

The serum CK activity is often normal in patients even with skeletal muscle involvement but frequently elevated during periods of illness and can signal rhabdomyolysis. The measurement of CK is particularly important in differentiating mitochondrial disease from congenital muscular dystrophy, Duchenne muscular dystrophy, and inflammatory myopathies, which can mimic mitochondrial cytopathies. Occasionally, patients with mitochondrial cytopathies have a low-grade (less than two times the upper limit of normal) baseline elevation of CK activity but this occurs in the minority of patients. During an acute illness, it is important to monitor CK activity for a significant increase as this can signal a risk of rhabdomyolysis, and added monitoring and precautions are required during this period to prevent possible renal tubular dysfunction. Although rhabdomyolysis during fasting or metabolic stress is less common in the mitochondrial cytopathies compared with fatty oxidation defects, strenuous activity or illness can cause rhabdomyolysis and myoglobinuria, particularly in patients with cytochrome *b* mutations, COX, and can be the sole manifestation of a mtDNA point mutation (A3260G), although it may occur rarely with other mutations. Consequently, urine myoglobin should be assessed in patients with pigmenturia or during any metabolic crisis in a patient with an elevated CK level. In addition to CK, the transaminases, aspartate aminotransferase and alanine

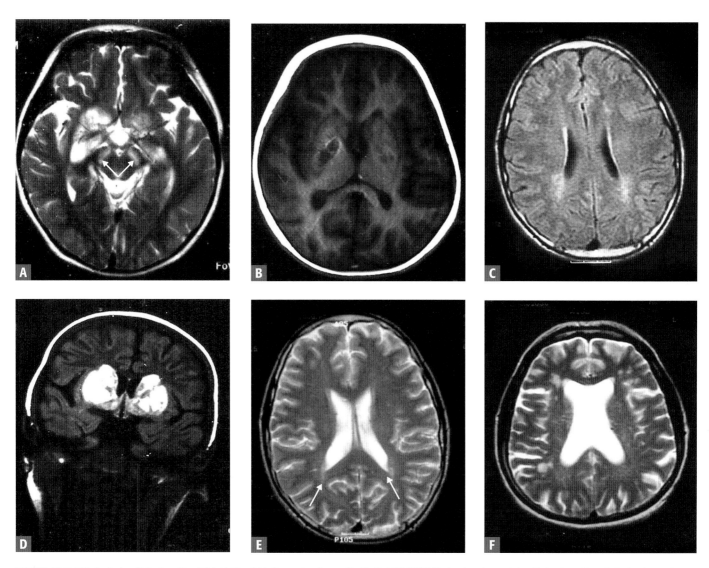

FIGURE 18-7. MRI of mitochondrial cytopathies. **(A)** Axial T2-weighted image in a 2-year-old girl with MILS (T8993C), showing abnormal signal in basal ganglia → indicates changes in substantia nigra. **(B)** Axial T1 image showing cystic change in the basal ganglia in the patient in panel A. **(C)** Axial FLAIR image showing occipital periventricular white matter changes in a patient with Kearn–Sayre syndrome. **(D)** Coronal T2 image showing symmetric involvement of the globus pallidus and putamen in a female with maternally inherited Leigh syndrome. **(E)** Axial T2-weighted image of a 16-year-old boy with MNGIE syndrome, showing symmetric subtle occipital white matter changes (→). **(F)** Axial T2-weighted image from a teenager with MELAS A3243G, showing asymmetric multiple white matter high signal regions.

aminotransferase, will increase concurrent with an elevation in CK given their presence in skeletal muscle; however, isolated elevation of the transaminases, usually with the concurrent elevation of bilirubin and γ-glutamyltranspeptidase, can indicate a primary hepatic presentation of mitochondrial disease. Predominantly hepatic involvement is seen in one subgroup of mtDNA depletion and Alper syndrome (see later).

Urine

Patients with mitochondrial cytopathies can have elevations of several organic acids in the urine, which can also fluctuate during periods of metabolic crisis. The more common organic acids that are elevated in the urine include lactate, alanine, malate, fumarate, 3-methyl glutaconic acid, and ethylmalonic acid. The organic acid profile is particularly helpful in the work up of a child with suspected mitochondrial disease because other primary organic acidurias can present with a mitochondrial phenotype. For example, glutaric aciduria type 2 and 3-methyl glutaconic aciduria type 3 can both mimic mitochondrial cytopathies. Interestingly, a recent study found that urine lactate and all Krebs cycle intermediates (except for malate and fumarate) were not useful discriminators of mitochondrial disease (19).

Although rhabdomyolysis with concurrent fasting or metabolic stress is less common in the mitochondrial cytopathies compared with fat oxidation defects, we have had several patients with clear evidence of pigmenturia during strenuous activity or concurrent illness. We and others have seen rhabdomyolysis with cytochrome *b* mutations, COX deficiency, and more recently, we have seen it in several patients with a mtDNA point mutation at A3260G. Consequently, urine myoglobin should be assessed in anyone reporting pigmenturia and during any metabolic crisis in a patient with mitochondrial cytopathy with an elevated CK level.

Muscle Biopsy

The muscle biopsy is critically important for the evaluation of a suspected mitochondrial cytopathy. We and others have published articles specifically looking at procurement of samples and proper handling, and readers are encouraged to obtain more details from these references (20,21). Details of the histologic and structural abnormalities in mitochondrial disease, as well as the needle method of muscle biopsy technique, are found in a recent review[7]. Other details regarding general aspects of the muscle biopsy procedure can be found on the World Wide Web at http://www.neuro.wustl.edu/neuromuscular/lab/mbiopsy.htm.

The acquisition of a high-quality muscle biopsy is very important. Our service has had numerous referrals in which a muscle biopsy was taken in a peripheral hospital and placed into formalin; consequently a very limited assessment can be done on such a sample. Anyone suspected of mitochondrial cytopathy requires that a muscle biopsy be taken by an experienced individual and the samples have to be prepared and stained appropriately. The choice of a needle or an open muscle biopsy has been a debate over the years; the downside of the needle muscle biopsy has traditionally been a very small sample size. We have created a hybrid Bergström muscle biopsy needle from a commercially available 5-mm needle (Stille; Stockholm, Sweden). With the addition of a custom-made metal insert into the end of the needle and application of hand suction through a 60-mL syringe, a much larger sample is possible and our success rate for obtaining all samples (~200 mg) required for mitochondrial assessment is greater than 98%.

Whichever method is chosen, one piece must be placed in liquid nitrogen or immediately on dry ice and transported to the laboratory for ETC assessment using muscle homogenates or, if isolated mitochondria are required, the sample must be placed in buffer and taken immediately to the laboratory where the isolation is completed. A second sample is mounted in optimal cutting temperature media for frozen section analysis. Another sample should be placed into chilled glutaraldehyde (2%) and rapidly processed for electron microscopy. There are some who advocate fixing a large strand of tissue to a clamp prior to fixation; however, it requires quite a large amount of tissue and the mitochondrial architectural changes as described later are very well visualized with immediate placement in 2% glutaraldehyde. This substantially cuts down on the volume of tissue that is required and eliminates the need for a large, open biopsy. We usually place another piece of muscle into an RNase/DNase-free tube for possible DNA, RNA, or protein quantification.

At the light microscopic level, there are a number of stains that are essential (modified Gomori trichrome, COX, succinate dehydrogenase (SDH), hematoxylin and eosin) and several that are helpful (NADH–tetrazolium reductase, oil red-O, myoadenylate deaminase, periodic-acid Schiff). Modified Gomori trichrome staining highlights the classic RRF where the proliferated mitochondria stain red and characteristic cracking can occur due to sheer forces during sectioning consequent to the proliferated intramyocellular lipid (Figure 18-5A). The RRF represents one of the major diagnostic criteria in most disease classifications schemes (15,22). The proportion of RRF increases with age and, in general, its prevalence is less common in pediatric disorders, with less than 1% as a minor category in pediatric disorders and greater than 2% as a major category in pediatric disorders and greater than 2% as a major diagnostic category in adult mitochondrial disease (15,22). COX stain shows three major patterns in mitochondrial disease, the first being complete absence, which can be seen in severe COX deficiency in infancy such as SCO2 deficiency and in cases of SURF-1 mutations (Leigh disease). A patchy reduction in COX staining (COX-negative fibers) is seen in normal human aging, but these are in greater abundance in a variety of mitochondrial cytopathies (MELAS, myoclonic epilepsy associated with ragged red fibers [MERRF], KSS, chronic progressive external ophthalmoplegia [CPEO]) and can be the only finding in some of the mtDNA deletion syndromes (KSS, CPEO) (Figure 18-5B). In MELAS syndrome the RRF also stain COX positive, whereas COX staining is often negative in the RRFs from patients with MERRF, KSS, and CPEO. Other oxidative stains (SDH and NADH–TR) tend to show enhanced staining in the RRFs and often the proportion that is strongly positive is higher than with the modified Gomori trichrome stain. Stains such as SDH can also highlight mitochondrial proliferation in blood vessels such as the strongly succinate dehydrogenase–positive blood vessel (Figure 18-5C).

As a general rule, the histologic abnormalities seen in pediatric mitochondrial cytopathies are less prevalent and/or intense than those seen in adult cases. General, nonspecific findings in mitochondrial cytopathy include a variation in fiber size, atrophic angular fibers with fiber type grouping in the presence of associated neuropathy, and nonspecific increases in lipid staining (oil red-O). Myoadenylate deaminase staining strongly highlights the RRFs, which probably represents a compensatory up-regulation for the anaerobic energy defect in these dysfunctional fibers (Figure 18-5D).

At the electron microscopic level, there are several hallmarks including paracrystalline inclusions that represent an up-regulation of mitochondrial CK that has dimerized and crystallized. The paracrystalline inclusion is seen in a variety of other conditions including structural and inflammatory myopathies as well as with advanced age (Figure 18-6A). Nevertheless, these latter conditions are often readily apparent by the history, physical examination, and other histologic features. Other features seen in mitochondrial cytopathy include electron densities in the mitochondria, pleomorphic and enlarged mitochondria, and the obvious mitochondrial proliferation in a subsarcolemmal and intramyofibrillar region. Homogeneous and granular staining within mitochondria has also been seen in the mtDNA depletion syndrome (Figure 18-6B).

Magnetic Resonance Imaging

Magnetic resonance imaging (MRI) is extremely important in the work up of a patient with suspected mitochondrial cytopathy. Further details regarding the MRI characteristics in mitochondrial disease can be found in a recent review (23). In addition to identifying changes suggestive of mitochondrial cytopathy, MRI is also very important in the evaluation of other neurologic disorders that can mimic mitochondrial cytopathies. T1-weighted images predominantly show anatomy and can yield nonspecific structural findings such as thinning or absence of the corpus callosum or migration defects that can be seen in a variety of conditions including an epiphenomenon in mitochondrial cytopathies. More helpful, however, are the T2-weighted and fluid attenuated inversion recovery imaging sequences, which can often highlight focal lesions in specific mitochondrial disorders. MRI is particularly helpful in the diagnosis of Leigh disease, a chronically progressive or relapsing remitting neurologic disorder in the presence of elevated lactate and high signal seen in brainstem, cerebellum, and/or basal ganglia (particularly the putamen) and in the globus pallidus and striatum. Other areas include the midbrain, thalamus, and occasionally even the white matter, with nonspecific leukodystrophy type changes. Occasionally the corpus striatum involvement can be quite striking, which has been labeled in some cases as bilateral striatal necrosis (Figure 18-7A, 18-7B, and 18-7D). In a number of the mitochondrial cytopathies there is often a nonspecific atrophy that is present and usually progresses with age.

Many of the mitochondrial cytopathies show periventricular white matter changes, particularly in the occipital region, which can have a similar appearance to the various leukodystrophies (Figures 18-7C and 18-7E). One of the diseases that often demonstrates quite substantial leukoencephalopathy changes is mitochondrial neurogastrointestinal encephalomyopathy (MNGIE) syndrome (Figure 18-7E).

In MELAS syndrome there can be nonspecific periventricular white matter changes (Figure 18-7C); however, during an acute strokelike episode high T2 and fluid attenuated inversion recovery signal regions often crossing artery watershed regions are characteristic. With techniques such as diffusion-weighted imaging, defects are usually noted in the area of the strokelike episode.

Magnetic Resonance Spectroscopy

The two main nuclei that are used in MR spectroscopy (MRS) evaluation of mitochondrial cytopathy are phosphorus (^{31}P) and hydrogen (^{1}H). In brain imaging with ^{31}P-MRS, the findings that are suggestive of mitochondrial cytopathy include a reduction in phosphocreatine and an increase in organic phosphate and occasionally a low ATP content[3]. The coupling of MRS with exercise of skeletal muscle usually shows a delayed phosphocreatine resynthesis rate that indicates impaired mitochondrial function (24).

Proton MRS (^{1}H-MRS) takes advantage of the choline, lactate, creatine, and N-acetylaspartate peaks. There can be variable reductions in choline and N-acetylaspartate with variable appearance of lactate. The increase in lactate is often seen in areas that are abnormal on MRI. In the case of MELAS syndrome, high levels of ventricular CSF lactate are associated with more severe neurologic impairment (25).

Exercise Testing

Most patients with mitochondrial cytopathy who are ambulatory note a decrease in work capacity, especially during aerobic-type activity. Most children report difficulties in keeping up with their peers, and this is particularly evident during endurance-type activity, such as long walks, cycling, jogging, and soccer, due to the impaired aerobic energy transduction. In general, reproducible exercise testing in children younger than 6 years of age is difficult and cognitive involvement as well as peripheral neuropathy and severe muscle weakness can limit the ability to perform exercise. In older children and teenagers who are pauci symptomatic, exercise testing can add information in the diagnostic work up. For full details of exercise testing in mitochondrial cytopathies the reader is referred to a recent review (26). Exercise testing can also be helpful in the evaluation of other conditions that can mimic mitochondrial cytopathies including disorders of glycogenolysis (McArdle disease), myoadenylate deaminase deficiency, and fat oxidation defects.

Forearm exercise testing coupled with measurements of venous lactate and ammonia can help to rule in and rule out adenosine monophosphate deaminase deficiency (failure of ammonia rise postexercise) and disorders of glycolysis (failure of lactate rise postexercise). The resting lactate appears to be as sensitive and specific as the forearm ischemic, semiischemic, and aerobic exercise paradigms. When a forearm exercise test is coupled with venous oxygen determination and/or near infrared spectroscopy, the pattern of attenuated to zero deoxygenation of venous blood and/or myoglobin/hemoglobin is characteristic of mitochondrial cytopathy (27). It is important for this to be completed in an experienced laboratory with well-established control values to establish standard deviation cut offs for the expected changes.

Endurance exercise protocols performed on a cycle ergometer can yield characteristic patterns of mitochondrial cytopathy. Generally, the maximal oxygen consumption (VO_{2max}) is lower in patients with mitochondrial cytopathy; however, this finding is not specific because it can also be seen in a variety of cardiopulmonary disorders. Patients with mitochondrial cytopathies usually show an elevated respiratory exchange ratio ($RER = VCO_2/VO_2$), which indicates the increased reliance on anaerobic energy transduction. In addition, there is a hyperdynamic circulation with greater than expected increases in heart rate and cardiac output for a given exercise workload. It is important again that each laboratory establish their normal criteria for a particular age group. Using a variety of reports and literature and exercise tests for a set time period can differentiate mitochondrial cytopathy patients from controls with a sensitivity ranging from 0.63 to 0.75 and a specificity of 0.7 to 0.9 (26). The following protocol is suggested: 2-hour fast prior to the test, 10 minutes of quiet rest before initiating exercise, initiate pedaling at 60 rpm at 0 W for 5 minutes, and the stepwise increase to 15 or 30 W (depending on the age and strength of the child) for 10 minutes. During this time record the heart rate, RER, VO_2, VCO_2, and pre- and postexercise lactate. In general, patients with mitochondrial cytopathy will show elevations in RER, heart rate, pre- and postexercise lactate with a decrease in VO_2 with such a protocol.

Enzymatic and Molecular Analysis

Because of the diversity of mitochondrial disorders, the biochemical diagnosis needs to be performed using a number of different approaches and evaluated using consistent guidelines. Suggestions tabled by a number of mitochondrial centers adapted the modified Walker criteria (17,28,29). If an RC defect is suspected, then enzyme activity assessment is usually the primary biochemical marker in the diagnosis. In general, the coupled activity of complexes I and III, complexes II and III as well as complex IV are readily performed in whole cell homogenates. All three of these tests involve the monitoring of cytochrome c reduction or oxidation and are relatively robust in cell homogenates from a variety of target tissue. These three assays along with the monitoring of mitochondrial citrate synthase activity, as a reference for normalization purposes, are usually the primary means of determining the functional status of the mitochondrial oxidative phosphorylation system. The measurement of isolated complex I or III in cell homogenates derived from patient skin fibroblasts becomes impractical because of the background interference from intracellular diaphorases (1,18). Alternative strategies here include the isolation of mitochondria from a small batch of cultured cells (30) or effective permeabilization of the cell so as to allow for removal of the interfering enzyme activity (31). In all cases the preparation of mitochondria from sample tissue would, in theory, allow for substantially more consistent data; however the amounts of tissue available do not usually allow for effective isolation procedures. As a result there is great need to adapt these molecular assessments to small (~50 mg) amounts of tissues.

In addition to looking at enzyme activity, whole cell homogenates or isolated mitochondria from patient samples can be subjected to Western blot analysis for a variety of mitochondrial proteins including specific respiratory enzyme chain components. The primary objective of this method is to look for relative abundance of specific mitochondrial proteins in comparison to controls. The definition of normal ranges can be difficult because there are a number of subjective steps during the overall assessment. Nevertheless this method is quite effective for examining the abundance of individual proteins and therefore can provide useful information on defects in individual RC subunits, assembly factor–related deficits, and deficits in other mitochondrial proteins.

Genetic analysis for mtDNA mutations can be performed from biopsy tissue, cultured cells, or blood. In general, it is preferable to obtain tissue from skeletal muscle for most of the mtDNA defects because they can be present in low levels in blood (white blood cells) due to mitotic segregation and selection against the mutation in rapidly turning over tissues. Several cases in which an mtDNA mutation was ruled out by mtDNA mutation analysis on DNA derived from peripheral blood mononuclear cells and we subsequently demonstrated a pathologic mutation in skeletal muscle. In the majority of cases the tests are performed using conventional mutation detection strategies such as restriction fragment length polymorphisms (RFLP) or sequencing of the entire mitochondrial genome. There are now a plethora of publications addressing the assessment of most mtDNA mutations. With the advent of single nucleotide polymorphism detection technologies it will likely not be very much longer before these systems are routinely used in mitochondrial mutation detection in a high-throughput format. These technologies need to be quantitative to allow for determination of heteroplasmy, which is an important diagnostic criterion. It is important to note the need for more sensitive detection methodologies as a heteroplasmy of less that 10% is difficult to detect using the conventional methodologies mentioned previously.

In addition to methods for the targeted monitoring of specific mutations, it is necessary to scan the patient's mtDNA for unknown mutations. The most commonly utilized approach for this is mtDNA sequencing. A number of diagnostic centers have taken the approach of sequencing the entire mitochondrial genome. With the advent of automated sequencing and even nucleic acid extraction the challenge of high-throughput mitochondrial genome sequence does not appear to be so overwhelming. One caveat that must be borne in mind is that while a positive mtDNA mutation supports the mitochondrial nature of the disease, the converse is not true; mtDNA mutations can be unstable, especially in culture. Therefore the inability to detect a mutation does not rule out a potential mtDNA mutation (32).

Exploratory Analytical Methods

Relatively new techniques, such as blue native gel electrophoresis, have made important contributions toward mitochondrial RC complex (33) diagnostics. Blue native gel electrophoresis separates the entire enzyme complex as one migratory unit and deficits in one or more of the components can be detected as a result of the change in mobility of the entire supramolecular enzyme complex. In cases in which an RC deficiency has been demonstrated, there is almost a complete absence of the protein species in question from the gel. Admittedly, the primary drawback to this technique is the amount of sample that is required. Between 20 and 70 μg of solubilized membrane protein from a mitochondrial fraction is required for conclusive results. Even then, the results from muscle tissue provide the

most lucid results with those from cultured fibroblasts not being very effective.

Additional techniques are also under investigation and development for the more robust diagnosis of mitochondrial disorders. Robinson and colleagues have begun to implement the examination of ^{14}C-whole cell oxidation in lieu of the difficulties with obtaining consistent L/P ratios with cultured cells (18).

Denaturing high-performance liquid chromatography, which relies on the chromatographic differences between perfectly matched and multiple mismatched sequences has also been recognized as a means of determining whether mtDNA contains mutations (34). In fact this technology may serve as a rapid prescreen for mtDNA prior to sequencing to ensure a cost-effective analysis of mtDNA.

Prenatal Diagnosis of Mitochondrial Disease

Prenatal diagnosis of mitochondrial cytopathies in cases in which the defect is an identified nuclear-encoded mutation (i.e, SCO2, thymidine phosphorylase, thymidine kinase 2 [TK2], etc.) is no different from any other disorder that is inherited through classic mendelian inheritance. In cases of mtDNA mutations, or when a mitochondrial disease is strongly suspected but a mutation is not found, the situation becomes far more complex and very few centers have experience in providing prenatal diagnosis (30,35,36). Prenatal diagnosis is usually performed on amniocytes or chorionic villous cells (CVS). The measurement of RC components in either of these two cell types is difficult because mitochondrial isolates are the most accurate but difficult to prepare due to the limited amount of starting material available (37). One of the problems associated with prenatal diagnosis is the contamination of fetal tissue with that from the mother. Perhaps more important in cases of mtDNA mutations it is very difficult to predict the phenotype from prenatal studies for several reasons: 1) the mutational load in the mother's tissues and in the fetal tissues sampled (i.e, amniocytes and chorionic villi) may not correspond to that of other fetal tissues and 2) the mutational load in tissues sampled prenatally may shift *in utero* or after birth because of random mitotic segregation. Despite these inherent difficulties, there is some progress in providing reasonably accurate prenatal diagnosis for the 8993 (neurogenic, ataxia, and retinitis pigmentosa) mutation (38). For the 8993 mutation, it appears that some prediction about all other tissues can be made from the percentage of heteroplasmy determined from a CVS sample, and one center has had experi-

ence with 56 pedigrees and has constructed predictive clinical outcome tables based on mutational load in the CVS samples (38). Limited preliminary evidence is also emerging that for the MELAS 3243 mutation, a similar prediction can be made for the level of the mutational burden (39); however, given that adult patients with apparently low mutational burdens can have significant symptoms (12), it will be some time before predictions can be made with confidence. At the current time, it is critically important that prenatal diagnosis for mitochondrial disorders be done only at centers with experience in the area. Several publications have discussed the risks and benefits of prenatal diagnosis as well as other reproductive options (oocyte donation, cytoplasmic transplant, etc.) (30,32,35,36).

Putting it all Together: Suggested Diagnostic Criteria

There are several proposed criteria put forth for the diagnosis of mitochondrial cytopathies (22,28,29). In general, these use combinations of major and minor criteria that consist of the clinical phenotype, muscle histology and electron microscopy, blood and CSF lactate, pathogenic mitochondrial mutations, MRI, MRS, and urine organic acid abnormalities in the presence of a family member with proven mitochondrial disease. These categories usually place the diagnosis into definite, probable, and possible categories. It should be noted that each criterion has specific and unique criteria, and acceptance of one criterion rather than another should be made by each center based on the availability of, and experience with, the various testing measurements. The two criteria schemes that are particularly relevant to the pediatric population are the modified Walker (22), and the Nijmegen (28), criteria. Recently, the application of the modified Walker criteria to a group of 400 pediatric patients referred for evaluation of mitochondrial disease revealed that 28% had definite mitochondrial disease (17).

Essentially, the Nijmegen criteria are based on a point system and the modified Walker criteria are a combination of major and minor criteria. From a clinical perspective we use a blend of these two systems.

Major Criteria:

1. classic mitochondrial clinical phenotype (see later) with variable combinations of strong family history, unexplained newborn infant death, exercise intolerance, muscle weakness, ptosis, and progressive external ophthalmoplegia;

2. greater than 2% COX-negative fibers or global reduction of COX activity in the presence of adequate controls;

3. residual activity of RC complex less than 20% in a tissue and less than 30% in a cell line;

4. nuclear mtDNA mutation of proven pathogenicity;

5. classic MRI or pathology changes consistent with Leigh disease.

Minor Criteria:

1. movement disorder, failure to thrive, neonatal hypotonia, still birth associated with a paucity of *in utero* movement, or global developmental delay;

2. histology shows RRFs to be more than 2%, any RRFs in patients younger than 16 years of age, and more than 2% subsarcolemmal accumulation of mitochondria in patients younger than 16 years of age;

3. enzymology shows antibody-based demonstration of RC defect or residual activity of RC complex 20% to 30% in one tissue, 30% to 40% in a cell line, and 30% to 40% in two or more tissues;

4. fibroblast ATP synthesis rate 2 to 3 standard deviations below mean or inability to grow in a galactose media;

5. nuclear mtDNA mutation of probable pathogenicity;

6. elevated blood lactate on three occasions, elevated CSF lactate, elevated blood alanine, elevated CSF alanine, elevated trichloroacetic acid intermediates (fumarate or malate), ethylmalonic, or 3 methyl-glutaconic acid in urine;

7. paracrystalline inclusion or abnormal mitochondrial morphology;

8. abnormal T2 signal in basal ganglia, abnormal T2 signal during acute metabolic crisis crossing vascular territories, elevated brain lactate peak, abnormal ^{31}P MRS in muscle with reduced phosphocreatine/inorganic phosphate ratio.

We follow a modified Walker type protocol in which definite mitochondrial disease = two major, or one major + two minor and probable mitochondrial disease = one major + one minor, or three minor, and possible = one major.

CATEGORIES OF PEDIATRIC MITOCHONDRIAL DISEASE

Mitochondrial DNA Disorders

The first mutations in the mtDNA were described in 1988 with the finding of pathogenic mutations associated with LHON (11778) and MELAS (3243) as well as single large scale deletions being responsible for KSS. Since 1988, over a 100 pathologic mutations in the mitochondrial genome associated with a variety of phenotypes ranging from Leigh disease, Alper disease, MELAS syndrome, MERFF, NARP, and LHON have been elucidated. In general, the mtDNA mutations are responsible for the majority of those found in adult patients and only 11% to 25% of pediatric patients. In the infant/neonate group the more common mtDNA point mutations responsible for disease include A3243G (infantile encephalopathy, MELAS syndrome) maternally inherited Leigh disease (T8993C, T8993G, T9176C), bilateral striatal necrosis (T8851C, T9176C) and more recently, new mutations have been found to be responsible for some cases of complex 1 deficiency of Leigh syndrome (40–42). The family history is particularly important in the work up of suspected mitochondrial cytopathy. In the mtDNA-associated disorders a careful history taking from the mother often reveals exercise intolerance or more substantial neurologic findings including episodic encephalopathy, strokelike episodes, migraine, retinitis pigmentosa, and episodic ataxia, and there is often a family history of similar conditions. In most cases of pediatric mitochondrial disease the inheritance appears to be sporadic, autosomal recessive or autosomal dominant, and nuclear defects are more commonly suspected/inferred or proven in pediatric RC diseases.

Nuclear DNA Disorders

The majority of pediatric patients with mitochondrial disorders have definite or presumed nuclear DNA defects. As a consequence, Mendelian patterns of inheritance are more commonly seen, with an increasing number of "sporadic" cases being attributed to autosomal recessive conditions. The vast spectrum of mutations have been identified in genes encoding for proteins involved in pyrimidine degradation, mtDNA transcription, adenine nucleotide translocase, DNA helicases, subunit assembly, and in ETC subunits. Despite the recent expansion of the known mutations identified previously, there are still several major categories of disease in which the specific gene mutation is unknown (i.e, KSS). There is a large proportion of patients with mitochondrial cytopathy who meet definite criteria for disease and are often categorized on the basis of the specific enzyme deficiency. The most common isolated enzyme deficiency is complex I deficiency, which accounts for at least 30% of all cases, with complex IV deficiency being the second most common isolated deficiency. In children, combined complex I, II, and IV deficiencies are usually the second most commonly identified RC deficit (17,43).

PEDIATRIC MITOCHONDRIAL DISORDERS

Leigh Disease

Pathophysiology/Presentation Leigh disease is one of the quintessential mitochondrial cytopathies first described by Dennis Leigh in 1951 based on the neuropathologic findings of cystic cavitation, demyelination, and vascular proliferation in neuronal loss predominantly in the thalamus, brain stem, and posterior columns of the spinal cord 29. Clinically, Leigh disease is a rapidly progressive encephalopathy occurring in infancy or childhood with a mean age of onset of approximately 2 years. It is characterized clinically by any one of a number of features including, psychomotor regression, optic atrophy, ophthalmoplegia, dystonia, tremor, corticospinal tract signs, ataxia, and respiratory abnormalities usually with apneas. Leigh disease is caused by complex I deficiency (~25%–35% of all cases), complex II deficiency (~10% of all cases), complex IV deficiency (~20% of all cases), PDH deficiency (~ 20% of cases) and mtDNA mutations (~15%–20% of all cases) (44).

Often there is a history of some neurologic involvement during periods of concurrent illness and other metabolic stressors; however, occasionally the disease can present precipitously during a minor concurrent illness. The progression of neurologic dysfunction can be extremely rapid and devastating. In one of our patients, a previously healthy female who during an upper respiratory tract infection developed a masklike face, rigidity, and within 6 hours experienced hypopnea requiring intubation from which she did not recover (T8993C mutation). A 3-year-old boy with slight ataxia and optic atrophy suddenly developed hypopnea with somnolence and was found to have a PCO_2 level of 90 mm Hg, which required ventilation until his death 6 months later (complex I deficiency, NDUFS2 mutation). In patients with Leigh disease, prompt hospitalization and assessment of respiratory status are critical during periods of concurrent illness.

Diagnosis The clinical history and MRI pattern in the presence of an elevated serum and/or CSF lactate are essentially pathognomonic for Leigh disease. Nevertheless, specific mutation analysis is extremely helpful from a genetic counseling and prenatal diagnostic perspective. The first step is a muscle biopsy to determine which of the ETC enzymes are affected; however, some of these can be detected in fibroblasts as well (44). If a specific defect is not identified in the muscle biopsy, fibroblast analysis for assessment of the PDH complex is the next step in a male infant. The finding of a DNA mutation can allow for prenatal diagnosis. Our group has been involved in two successful prenatal diagnostic scenarios with a known mutation in NDUFS2 in a case of complex I deficiency Leigh syndrome and a SURF1 mutation in a case of complex IV deficiency Leigh syndrome. In selected cases in which the biochemical defect is expressed in fibroblasts the opportunity for prenatal diagnosis on cultured amniocytes or CVS sample can be considered. The complex IV deficiency SURF1 mutation case showed the most striking abnormalities in fibroblasts, with profound reductions of complex IV activity and extremely high L/P ratios. The group currently with the most experience with this technique is the Nijmegen group in the Netherlands.

Cardiomyopathies

Pathophysiology/Presentation Cardiomyopathy is a common finding in pediatric and adult mitochondrial cytopathy, with a recent study demonstrating that 40% of pediatric mitochondrial cytopathies involve cardiomyopathy (17). Of these, the majority have hypertrophic cardiomyopathy (58%), dilated cardiomyopathy (29%), with the remainder showing signs of left ventricular noncompaction (13%). The diagnosis of cardiomyopathy in a child with mitochondrial cytopathy is very important from a counseling standpoint because the prognosis is particularly grim, with a survival rate at age 16 years of only 18%; this is in contrast to children with mitochondrial cytopathy and neuromuscular features without cardiomyopathy, for whom the survival rate at age 16 years was 95% (17).

Hypertrophic cardiomyopathy is the predominant and/or exclusive feature in children with defects in COX assembly including SCO2, COX10, and COX15. Most children with SCO2 deficiency also show significant hypotonia due to alpha motor neuron involvement, usually have very elevated lactate concentrations and have an invariably fatal outcome; the vast majority of children die before 2 years of age, many in the first few months of life (5,45,46). Cardiomyopathies can also be seen in isolated ETC complex defects with the most common in our practice being complex I deficiency. Cardiomyopathy can be seen as a coexisting phenomenon in several point mutations including the MELAS A3243G gene mutation; it can be seen as a predominant symptom in a variety of mtDNA mutations (A1555G, A4295G, A4330G, A8296G, T9997C, G15243A, A4269G, C4320T, G8363A). Although not a cardiomyopathy per se, patients with KSS often show progressive conduction block. The finding of a conduction block is essential because prophylactic pacing can be life saving.

The cardiomyopathy is often asymptomatic and is picked up as part of the work up in a child with suspected mitochondrial disease. Every child with mitochondrial cytopathy as an infant should be screened for cardiomyopathy because there may be an opportunity for therapies (i.e, after-load reduction) and it also helps from a prognostic standpoint, as noted previously. Older children can present with exercise-induced shortness of breath and cyanosis, and in younger children cyanosis during periods of stress or at night when sleeping can be a presenting symptom.

Diagnosis Infants with hypertrophic cardiomyopathy and very elevated serum lactate and documented cytochrome IV deficiency on muscle biopsy should be assessed for SCO2 deficiency (in all cases E140K is a common mutation that can be assessed using polymerase chain reaction [PCR]-RFLP analysis) (45). If this is negative, sequencing of the SCO2 gene and assessment of COX10 and COX15 can be considered. Specific point mutation analysis for some of the known mtDNA point mutations can also be undertaken using PCR-RFLP. Obviously, echocardiography is critically important; the most common thing that has been missed in patients referred from hospitals where there is less experience with metabolic cytopathies is a noncompaction cardiomyopathy.

Mitochondrial DNA Depletion

Pathophysiology/Presentation mtDNA depletion syndrome is generally categorized into two groups, namely the encephalomyopathy form and the hepatoencephalopathic form. mtDNA depletion was first characterized by reduction in mtDNA copy number in the affected tissues (47). More recently mutations have been demonstrated in the deoxyguanosine kinase (dGK) gene in patients with hepatoencephalopathic form (48), and mutations in TK2 in children with the encephalomyopathic form of mitochondrial depletion syndrome (49). These mutations interrupt the deoxyribose nucleotide metabolic pathway and inhibit incorporation of the deoxyribonucleotide triphosphates into the mtDNA, resulting in a reduction in mtDNA copy number. So far, mutations in dGK are found in only 10% to 15% of all patients with the hepatoencephalopathic form of mtDNA depletion, with approximately 20% of those with the encephalomyopathic form showing mutations in TK2 (48,50). These results clearly demonstrate that there are a number of genes responsible for mtDNA depletion in liver, muscle, and brain. The discovery of these

mutations is extremely helpful in understanding the pathogenesis of the syndrome and for accurate genetic and prenatal counseling.

The mtDNA depletion syndrome is a disorder that usually presents in the first few months of life, often with a rapidly progressive and fatal outcome. Within a given mutation, there can be significant clinical heterogeneity. For example, in mutations in TK2, variable levels of encephalopathy and hypotonia can be seen with some even showing evidence of spinal muscular atrophy (lower motor neuron disease) (50). With the dGK mutations, liver failure is present and usually progressive. These children usually have variable degrees of encephalopathy; however, some can have isolated liver failure and interestingly one patient with isolated liver failure apparently showed a good response to liver transplantation (48). From a clinical perspective, some cases of Alper hepatopathic polio dystrophy can present with severe hypotonia and progressive renal failure, which has a significant overlap with and may even show evidence of mtDNA depletion in the liver. Several cases of Alper disease have recently been described with mutations in the polymerase gamma gene (51).

Diagnosis A diagnosis of mtDNA depletion is made by measuring the copy number of mtDNA relative to a nuclear DNA "housekeeping" gene (i.e, 18S). The depletion is very often tissue specific and for the hepatoencephalopathic form, liver is the gold standard tissue, whereas in the encephalomyopathic form it is skeletal muscle that invariably shows the depletion, with brain tissue showing the depletion when available at autopsy. As mentioned, only a minority of patients will show the mutations and in general, if there is hepatic involvement the dGK mutations should be first assessed and if they are negative, recent evidence suggest that perhaps DNA polymerase gamma should also be assessed (51). In the encephalomyopathic form, the TK2 gene mutation should be assessed. From a biochemical perspective, all of the ETC complexes are usually uniformly below normal. The skeletal muscle is occasionally normal on histological examination but can show some evidence of mitochondrial proliferation with pleomorphism and accumulation of homogeneous material within the mitochondria (Figure 18-6B). In addition, children can present with a renal Fanconi syndrome, seizures, congestive heart failure, and progressive external ophthalmoplegia. Occasionally the disease can present in early childhood when psychomotor regression and/or progressive weakness can be presenting features.

Mitochondrial DNA Disorders

Pathophysiology/Presentation By definition, these disorders are maternally inherited and are due to specific point mutations in either tRNA or specific subunit regions of the mtDNA. There are mutations in essentially every region noted in almost every region of the mtDNA with over 100 specific point mutations being considered pathogenic. An updated list of all known mitochondrial and nuclear DNA mutations resulting in mitochondrial disease is available in the journal Neuromuscular Disorders (volume 14, pages 107–116, 2004).

MELAS is the most common of the mtDNA point mutations and can have an extremely wide range of phenotypic presentation from asymptomatic hearing loss to ataxia, dementia, ophthalmoplegia, encephalopathy, strokelike episodes, exercise intolerance, proximal myopathy, and type 2 diabetes. The progression of MELAS can be chronically progressive or relapsing and remitting. The age at onset of symptoms is as variable as the clinical phenotypes, with presentations starting in infancy through to teenage years.

MERRF can present as isolated myoclonic epilepsy with and without ataxia, myopathy, peripheral neuropathy, and multiple lipomas (particularly in the head and neck) and, in several cases with neuropsychiatric manifestations including severe obsessive-compulsive disorder and psychotic features. The time of onset again can range from infancy to teenage years and there is usually a progressive decline in function.

LHON usually results in painless, rapidly progressive visual loss with centrocecal scotoma. The onset is usually in teens and 20s and is more common in males than females. The basis for the sex difference in prevalence is unclear but could relate to the antioxidant properties of the female sex hormone, 17-β-estradiol.

There are a host of other mtDNA point mutations that can present in the pediatric age group including lethal infantile mitochondrial disorder (A15923G, A15924G), complex I deficiency Leigh disease (T10191C, T10158C, T12706C, G13513A, G14459A), isolated myopathy (T618C, T3250C, A3302G, G5521A, A12320G, C15990T), and exercise intolerance (predominantly cytochrome *c* mutations such as G14846A, G15059A, G15084A) (40–42,52).

Diagnosis The mtDNA mutations are suspected with a family history suggestive of maternal inheritance or with a classic phenotypic presentation (i.e, multiple strokelike episodes in the pediatric age group). The point mutations in the transfer RNA regions of the mitochondrial genome often result in

variable combinations of ETC enzyme activity reduction, whereas isolated enzyme activity reductions can point to specific protein subunit DNA regions (i.e, complex I = ND subunits, complex III = cytochrome *b*). Targeted PCR-RFLP is the most common method used to screen for the "common mutations," whereas exploratory analysis for new mutations can be done with DNA sequencing, denaturing high-performance liquid chromatography and other methods, as noted previously.

Other Mitochondrial Disorders

Pathophysiology/Presentation/Diagnosis There are three nuclear disorders that can present in the pediatric age group (MNGIE, KSS, and coenzyme Q10 deficiency), and one that presents usually in later adulthood (CPEO).

MNGIE is an autosomal recessive condition characterized by severe gastrointestinal cramps, malabsorption, and weight loss in combination with a peripheral neuropathy and an often pauci- or oligo-symptomatic leukoencephalopathy (53). The onset is often in the early-to-late teenage years with relentless progression of the gastrointestinal problems often leading to total parental nutritional requirement and progressive peripheral neuropathy with distal weakness and painful dysesthias. The leukodystrophy is often not clinically apparent except during periods of concurrent illness when a delirium/encephalopathic picture can appear. Work up in these patients demonstrates variable elevations of lactate with evidence of demyelinating peripheral neuropathy (sometimes mimicking chronic inflammatory demyelinating polyneuropathy), invariant leukodystrophic changes on MRI, and often multiple mtDNA deletions in skeletal muscle samples. The gene responsible for this disorder is thymidine phosphorylase, which is involved in the initial degradation pathway of thymidine. The recommended testing for this condition involves measurement of plasma thymidine concentrations (elevated) or white blood cell–derived measurements of thymidine phosphorylase activity (reduced) (54).

KSS is a multisystem mitochondrial disorder characterized by progressive external ophthalmoplegia, myopathy, heart block, elevated CSF protein, and onset before the age of 25. These patients often show elevation in lactate in the plasma, the skeletal muscle samples showing variable reduction in ETC enzyme activity and a single deletion of 4977 bp. The specific nuclear gene responsible for this condition has not yet been identified and the diagnosis is based on the aforementioned clinical features.

Coenzyme Q10 deficiency has been reported in several cases of childhood-onset ataxia with cerebellar atrophy (55). These children had other clinical features including combinations of seizures, developmental delay, mental retardation, and pyramidal signs. This condition is suspected when linked muscle enzyme assays (I + III and II + III) show low activity, yet the individual components do not show reductions. The importance of making the diagnosis comes from the fact that some of the children have shown a clinical response to very high doses of coenzyme Q10 (55).

There are some overlap between KSS and CPEO, with some patients showing intermediate variants with features more severe than classic CPEO but not severe enough to meet the criteria for KSS. Many of these cases are autosomal recessive; however, an autosomal dominant inheritance pattern has been seen. CPEO usually starts as an insidious ptosis and restriction of extraocular eye movements in the fourth to fifth decade that may often go unnoticed in the earliest stages. Skeletal muscle fatigue and weakness is occasionally present and some patients go on to develop a progressive peripheral neuropathy. Serum lactate is variably elevated, which can be normal, and a muscle biopsy can show variable reductions in ETC enzyme activity and often multiple mtDNA deletions.

In several cases of autosomal dominant and autosomal recessive CPEO, specific mutations have been identified in the polymerase gamma gene, adenine nucleotide translocase 1, and twinkle (C10Orf2, a DNA helicase) (56,57). The constellation of sensory ataxic neuropathy, dysarthria, and ophthalmoparesis (SANDO) can present in childhood or middle age and can be diagnosed by the presence of multiple mtDNA deletions, RRF, and the constellation of clinical symptoms from which its name is derived. The SANDO phenotype has been associated with mutations in the polymerase gamma gene and more recently an apparent germ line mosaicism has been suggested in a case showing a twinkle mutation (56). In many cases, however, no specific gene mutation has been identified in the aforementioned genes and there are clearly a number of other mutations yet to be identified.

TREATMENT OF MITOCHONDRIAL DISORDERS

Cofactors, Antioxidants and Drugs

The rationale for treatment of mitochondrial disorders is derived from the known pathologic consequences of the disease as described previously: 1) due to the increase in oxidative stress, antioxidant compounds have been recommended (vitamin E, vitamin C, coenzyme Q10, alpha lipoic acid); 2) to enhance ETC flux and/or bypass a specific defect compounds such as succinate, coenzyme Q10, vitamin K3, riboflavin, and thiamine have been proposed and evaluated as treatments; 3) to provide alternative energy sources to the cell some studies have evaluated the use of creatine monohydrate to increase intracellular phosphocreatine stores with some evidence of success in vivo and in vitro; 4) dietary manipulation with a high-fat diet to increase the flux through complex II for a complex I defect has been proposed and these may also be of some benefit in PDH mutations, particularly with difficult to control seizures where ketogenesis may be secondarily useful as an antiseizure intervention; 5) supplementation with L-carnitine has also been proposed by some because a secondary carnitine deficiency can occur, yet in the absence of a carnitine deficiency the efficacy remains somewhat questionable. A list of some of the treatments and their doses is presented in the At-A-Glance page. A more complete discussion of each of these compounds can be found in review papers (58,59).

Given the fact that dihydroorotate is essential in maintaining the purine nucleotide pool in mitochondria and its function is dependent on ETC activity and to the fact that mitochondrial cells in vitro often require an exogenous source of uridine, treatment with uridine prodrugs such as triacetyluridine and magnesium orotate has been proposed. To date, however, there has been one abstract suggesting potential benefit of triacetyluridine in a few cases of Leigh disease but randomized trials have not yet been completed for either of these compounds. There is certainly biological rationale for further research in this area.

Dichloroacetate has been proposed as a treatment for mitochondrial cytopathies because it invariably reduces serum lactate concentrations by activating the PDH complex. Several trials have been completed and a few are still continuing; however, the overall efficacy has not been dramatic and one of the side effects is the development of peripheral neuropathy (60). Our approach has been to use dichloroacetate in cases of acute metabolic crisis in which the serum lactate concentrations are acutely elevated above 10 mmol/L, and to use it only for the short term during these periods of metabolic crisis.

In summary, most of the constituents of the "mitochondrial cocktail" are based on biological rationale and many have been shown to be well tolerated with a few side effects in mitochondrial and nonmitochondrial disease states. As a single agent, studies with coenzyme Q10 and creatine monohydrate have probably have been the most

extensive (58,59), and on balance, there does appear to be some degree of efficacy and they are well tolerated. Ultimately, a "complete" mitochondrial cocktail strategy will likely be most effective because it would target many of the multiple final common pathways of cellular dysfunction induced by mitochondrial disorders. The difficulty will be to evaluate the infinite possible combinations in an extremely heterogeneous group of individuals by using a prospective, randomized, double-blind methodology. The development of animal models of mitochondrial disease will certainly be extremely useful in identifying isolated and combination therapies for mitochondrial cytopathies and this should significantly advance the development of clinical studies with these compounds.

Other Therapies

At this time, there are no genetic therapies for mitochondrial cytopathy although interesting strategies have been demonstrated in vitro by using mutation-specific peptide nucleotide acids for mtDNA mutations and deletons[9]. With the increasing recognition of nuclear DNA mutations the potential for viral vector and other DNA-based strategies as well as possible small interfering RNA strategies may be possible in the future.

Exercise has also been demonstrated to be of benefit in mitochondrial cytopathies, with endurance and resistance type exercise showing evidence of efficacy (61). At the genetic level, the sporadic mitochondrial mutation may be more amenable to therapy because exercise-induced muscle damage can activate satellite cells, which often show no or very low levels of mutational burden. This activation of the satellite cells can result in a mitochondrial "DNA shifting," which can potentially reduce the mutant percentage of heteroplasmy in the skeletal muscle (62,63). The difficulty with exercise in the pediatric population is that compliance and accessibility are difficult. In general, we recommend that children be as active as possible in school and play-based activities provided that they work "within their limit" and do not push to the point at which they become nauseated, vomit, or develop encephalopathic features. We have had several patients who have experienced vertigo, nausea, vomiting, and even exercise-induced deafness if they overexert themselves. For this reason, we advise people to "listen to your body" but have noted that with very careful and progressive activity the threshold for the onset of these symptoms is increased and most people are better able to tolerate activities of daily living without adverse affects.

GENERAL CARE ISSUES

In addition to the provision of a mitochondrial "cocktail," a number of other aspects of the diet are important. Many children do not tolerate prolonged periods of fasting and in general, ingesting more frequent meals throughout the day is preferable. In children who are particularly vulnerable to fasting, it may be necessary to add complex carbohydrates such as Polycose or cornstarch. Polycose is generally much easier to blend into food but does not have as long a duration of action as cornstarch. Cornstarch, however, is difficult to add to formula but can be mixed into pabulum. Care must be taken with cornstarch when using percutaneous endoscopic gastrostomy and G-tubes because it can clog the tube. As mentioned previously, a high-fat diet may be of benefit in complex I deficiency especially when severe seizures are a feature, given the potential benefit from the ketosis. Given that many infants and children have limited exercise capacity, energy expenditure can be quite low and care must be taken not to overfeed children and induce obesity, which can further impair mobility and lead to other chronic health care issues.

From an anesthetic perspective, probably the most important issue is to avoid prolonged periods of fasting. The provision of calories from dextrose and/or a total parenteral nutrition solution is important to prevent fasting-induced metabolic stress. It is also important to postpone any surgical procedure during a period of even minor concurrent illness. With respect to specific anesthetic agents, there does not appear to be a particular predisposition toward true malignant hyperthermia in patients with mitochondrial cytopathy; however, malignant hyperthermia-like situations can arise with a metabolic crisis induced by additional metabolic stress, which then can mimic some aspects of malignant hyperthermia. It is important to maintain euthermia throughout the anesthetic period to avoid an increase in shivering-induced thermogenesis. For brief procedures such as a needle muscle biopsy, electromyography, or lumbar puncture we have found that propofol and local anesthetic has been well tolerated without a single adverse reaction in several hundred procedures. Given that propofol only induces the form of conscious sedation we always use a local anesthestic, often with preapplication of a topical patch such as EMLA cream.

From a physical activity perspective, we encourage participation in recreational activities, play, and gym class, provided the teacher and patient are aware of the signs and symptoms of "pushing too hard." We usually advise that they do not perform any vigorous physical activity if they are experiencing a migraine headache or have a concurrent illness such as an upper respiratory tract infection. We usually have occupational and physiotherapy involved with most of our children with mitochondrial cytopathy to assess and treat possible contracture formation, which is more common in children with peripheral neuropathy and severe spasticity. Participation in formal physical activity is usually well tolerated provided that there is a very gradual introduction to the activity, and we have found that activities such as Tai Chi, karate, and ballet are particularly helpful in children with dyscoordination and/or ataxia because essentially no other therapy has any beneficial affect on these neurologic symptoms.

Peripheral neuropathy and other types of neurogenic pain can be a feature of mitochondrial cytopathy especially in MNGIE syndrome and SANDO in which the peripheral neuropathy can be quite dysesthetic. Gabapentin is generally well tolerated and one of our first-line therapies among the anticonvulsants for neuropathic pain; however, we do find that it is best to start this in the evening and gradually titrate the dose to avoid somnolence. More recently, we have had success with pregabalin in those patients who cannot tolerate gabapentin. We have also found that a combination of capsicin cream and EMLA (50/50 mix) is often effective for mild-to- moderate dysesthesias from peripheral neuropathy and has the advantage of being a nonsystemic therapy.

For severe spasticity, baclofen is a good first-line medication and in children with a seizure disorder the benzodiazepines are quite helpful in this regard. We have had a few patients who have used tizanidine with varying levels of success. We do not advocate the use of dantrolene in patients with mitochondrial disorders because it can result in significant weakness and fatigue of skeletal muscle. In children with severe spasticity that is limiting hygiene or activities of daily living, Botulinum toxin injections can be of benefit. Seizures are very common in children with mitochondrial cytopathy and in general, standard anticonvulsants for the given seizure types should be used as in any other seizure disorder with a few caveats. Valproic acid should not be used except as a last resort because it may trigger Reye syndrome–like hepatic dysfunction in children with mitochondrial cytopathy. We have also found that Topamax is particularly sedating in children with mitochondrial cytopathy but still can be used in selective cases.

A number of patients experience significant gastrointestinal problems, particularly those with MNGIE syndrome in whom abdominal pain, cramps and diarrhea predominate. These symptoms may be improved with elemental or total parenteral nutrition diets if necessary. Buscopcan is sometimes helpful in alleviating abdominal cramps and pain and if there is a lot of gas production, simethicone can be tried. In a variety of other conditions (particularly MELAS) severe constipation, in some cases leading to intestinal pseudoobstruction, can be seen. A high fluid and fiber intake is the first-line therapy followed by stool softeners or other lactulose and glycerin suppositories if there is no bowl movement in 3 days. Finally, prokinetic agents can be tried as a last resort. We do not recommend the use of mineral oil–based laxatives because reflux is quite common and can lead to an oil-based pneumonitis.

Psychologic support is very important for patients with mitochondrial cytopathy and their family. We have frequently seen a high degree of anxiety and marital strife in maternally inherited disorders, with individuals blaming themselves or their spouse for the condition. A high degree of family stress is present in the families of children with severe mitochondrial cytopathy because of frequent doctor's appointments, multiple hospitalizations, and the complexities and intensity of care. Psychologic and emotional support for the caregivers is very important and often people find comfort and support through a group such as the United Mitochondrial Disease Foundation who have a great deal of educational information as well as a yearly conference for scientists and patients and their families. As children get older and gain insight into their disorder, they frequently experienced depression and despair, particularly those who are oligo- or paucisymptomatic who have older siblings or other their family members who have died of a mitochondrial cytopathy. This latter issue is extremely important to identify because early intervention with counseling and possibly antidepressant medications may be of benefit. We have also seen cases of anger and in one case persistent suicidal ideation in a teenager with MERRF syndrome and severe obsessive-compulsive disorder.

In summary the diagnosis, treatment and long-term care of patients with mitochondrial cytopathies is extremely complicated and requires a dedicated team and a variety of specialists including medical (genetics, neurology, respirology, cardiology, physical medicine and rehabilitation, gastroenterology, and psychiatry) and paramedical (nursing, social work, occupational therapy, physical therapy, genetic counseling, and nutrition) personnel to deal effectively with all of the complexities of this disorder. It is usually best to have one physician as the "quarterback" and it is very important to be cognizant of the anxiety and occasional despair experienced by patients in their late teens when they are transferred to adult clinics where often there is not the same level of comprehensive support and care for mitochondrial cytopathies.

REFERENCES

1. Huang G, Lu H, Hao A, et al. GRIM-19, a cell death regulatory protein, is essential for assembly and function of mitochondrial complex I. *Mol Cell Biol.* 2004;24: 8447–8456.
2. Fearnley IM, Carroll J, Shannon RJ, et al. GRIM-19, a cell death regulatory gene product, is a subunit of bovine mitochondrial NADH:ubiquinone oxidoreductase (complex I). *J Biol Chem.* 2001;276:38345–38348.
3. Pequignot MO, Dey R, Zeviani M, et al. Mutations in the SURF1 gene associated with Leigh syndrome and cytochrome C oxidase deficiency. *Hum Mutat.* 2001;17:374–381.
4. Zhu Z, Yao J, Johns T, et al. SURF1, encoding a factor involved in the biogenesis of cytochrome c oxidase, is mutated in Leigh syndrome. *Nat Genet.* 1998;20:337–343.
5. Tarnopolsky MA, Bourgeois JM, Fu MH, et al. Novel SCO2 mutation (G1521A) presenting as a spinal muscular atrophy type I phenotype. *Am J Med Genet A.* 2004;125:310–314.
6. Glerum DM, Shtanko A, Tzagoloff A. SCO1 and SCO2 act as high copy suppressors of a mitochondrial copper recruitment defect in Saccharomyces cerevisiae. *J Biol Chem.* 1996;271:20531–20535.
7. Xu F, Morin C, Mitchell G, et al. The role of the LRPPRC (leucine-rich pentatricopeptide repeat cassette) gene in cytochrome oxidase assembly: mutation causes lowered levels of COX (cytochrome c oxidase) I and COX III mRNA. *Biochem J.* 2004;382:331–336.
8. Raha S, Robinson BH. Mitochondria, oxygen free radicals, disease and ageing. *Trends Biochem Sci.* 2000;25:502–508.
9. Trifunovic A, Wredenberg A, Falkenberg M, et al. Premature ageing in mice expressing defective mitochondrial DNA polymerase. *Nature.* 2004;429:417–423.
10. Raha S, Robinson BH. Metabolic actions of free radicals: walking the tightrope. *Heart Metab.* 2003;19:4–10.
11. Zuchner S, Mersiyanova IV, Muglia M, et al. Mutations in the mitochondrial GTPase mitofusin 2 cause Charcot-Marie-Tooth neuropathy type 2A. *Nat Genet.* 2004;36:449–451.
12. Chinnery PF, Taylor DJ, Brown DT, et al. Very low levels of the mtDNA A3243G mutation associated with mitochondrial dysfunction in vivo. *Ann Neurol.* 2000; 47:381–384
13. Tarnopolsky MA, Parise G. Direct measurement of high-energy phosphate compounds in patients with neuromuscular disease. *Muscle Nerve.* 1999;22:1228–1233.
14. Thorburn DR, Sugiana C, Salemi R, et al. Biochemical and molecular diagnosis of mitochondrial respiratory chain disorders. *Biochim Biophys Acta.* 2004;1659:121–128.

15. Naviaux RK. Developing a systematic approach to the diagnosis and classificationn of mitochondrial disease. *Mitochondrion.* 2004;4:351–361.

16. Tarnopolsky M, Stevens L, MacDonald JR, et al. Diagnostic utility of a modified forearm ischemic exercise test and technical issues relevant to exercise testing. *Muscle Nerve.* 2003;27:359–366.

17. Scaglia F, Towbin JA, Craigen WJ, et al. Clinical spectrum, morbidity, and mortality in 113 pediatric patients with mitochondrial disease. *Pediatrics.* 2004;114:925–931.

18. Cameron JM, Levandovskiy V, MacKay N, et al. Respiratory chain analysis of skin fibroblasts in mitochondrial disease. *Mitochondrion.* 2004;4:387–394.

19. Barshop BA. Metabolomic approaches to mitochondrial disease: correlation of urine organic acids. *Mitochondrion.* 2004;4:521–527.

20. Bourgeois JM, Tarnopolsky M. Pathology of skeletal muscle in mitochondrial disorders. *Mitochondrion.* 2004;4:441–452.

21. Vogel H. Mitochondrial myopathies and the role of the pathologist in the molecular era. *J Neuropathol Exp Neurol.* 2001;60:217–227.

22. Bernier FP, Boneh A, Dennett X, et al. Diagnostic criteria for respiratory chain disorders in adults and children. *Neurology.* 2002;59:1406–1411.

23. Haas R, Dietrich R. Neuroimaging of mitochondrial disorders. *Mitochondrion.* 2004;4:471–490.

24. Arias-Mendoza F. In vivo magnetic resonance spectroscopy in the evaluation of mitochondrial disorders. *Mitochondrion.* 2004;4:491–501.

25. Kaufmann P, Shungu DC, Sano MC, et al. Cerebral lactic acidosis correlates with neurological impairment in MELAS. *Neurology.* 2004;62:1297–1302.

26. Tarnopolsky M. Exercise testing as a diagnostic entity in mitochondrial myopathies. *Mitochondrion.* 2004;4:529–542.

27. van Beekvelt MC, van Engelen BG, Wevers RA, et al. Quantitative near-infrared spectroscopy discriminates between mitochondrial myopathies and normal muscle. *Ann Neurol.* 1999;46:667–670.

28. Wolf NI, Smeitink JA. Mitochondrial disorders: a proposal for consensus diagnostic criteria in infants and children. *Neurology.* 2002;59:1402–1405.

29. Nissenkorn A, Zeharia A, Lev D, et al. Multiple presentation of mitochondrial disorders. *Arch Dis Child.* 1999;81:209–214.

30. Pitkanen S, Raha S, Robinson BH. Diagnosis of complex I deficiency in patients with lactic acidemia using skin fibroblast cultures. *Biochem Mol Med.* 1996;59:134–137.

31. Faivre L, Cormier-Daire V, Chretien D, et al. Determination of enzyme activities for prenatal diagnosis of respiratory chain deficiency. *Prenat Diagn.* 2000;20:732–737.

32. Amiel J, Gigarel N, Benacki A, et al. Prenatal diagnosis of respiratory chain deficiency by direct mutation screening. *Prenat Diagn.* 2001;21:602–604.

33. Van Coster R, Smet J, George E, et al. Blue native polyacrylamide gel electrophoresis: a powerful tool in diagnosis of oxidative phosphorylation defects. *Pediatr Res.* 2001;50:658–665.

34. Frueh FW, Noyer-Weidner M. The use of denaturing high-performance liquid chromatography (DHPLC) for the analysis of genetic variations: impact for diagnostics and pharmacogenetics. *Clin Chem Lab Med.* 2003;41:452–461.

35. Jacobs LJ, de Wert G, Geraedts JP, et al. The transmission of OXPHOS disease and methods to prevent this. *Hum Reprod Update.* 2006;12:119–136.

36. Thorburn DR, Dahl HH. Mitochondrial disorders: genetics, counseling, prenatal diagnosis and reproductive options. *Am J Med Genet.* 2001;106:102–114.

37. Robinson BH. Prenatal diagnosis of disorders of energy metabolism. *Semin Neurol.* 2001;21:269–273.

38. Dahl HH, Thorburn DR, White SL. Towards reliable prenatal diagnosis of mtDNA point mutations: studies of nt8993 mutations in oocytes, fetal tissues, children and adults. *Hum Reprod.* 2000;15 Suppl 2:246–255.

39. Chou YJ, Ou CY, Hsu TY, et al. Prenatal diagnosis of a fetus harboring an intermediate load of the A3243G mtDNA mutation in a maternal carrier diagnosed with MELAS syndrome. *Prenat Diagn.* 2004;24:367–370.

40. Kirby DM, Boneh A, Chow CW, et al. Low mutant load of mitochondrial DNA G13513A mutation can cause Leigh's disease. *Ann Neurol.* 2003;54:473–478.

41. Kirby DM, Kahler SG, Freckmann ML, et al. Leigh disease caused by the mitochondrial DNA G14459A mutation in unrelated families. *Ann Neurol.* 2000;48:102–104.

42. McFarland R, Kirby DM, Fowler KJ, et al. De novo mutations in the mitochondrial ND3 gene as a cause of infantile mitochondrial encephalopathy and complex I deficiency. *Ann Neurol.* 2004;55:58–64.

43. Leigh D. Subacute necrotizing encephalomyopathy in an infant. *J Neurol Neurosurg Psychiatry.* 1951;14:216–221.

44. Rahman S, Blok RB, Dahl HH, et al. Leigh syndrome: clinical features and biochemical and DNA abnormalities. *Ann Neurol.* 1996;39:343–351.

45. Jaksch M, Paret C, Stucka R, et al. Cytochrome c oxidase deficiency due to mutations in SCO2, encoding a mitochondrial copper-binding protein, is rescued by copper in human myoblasts. *Hum Mol Genet.* 2001;10: 3025–3035.

46. Sue CM, Karadimas C, Checcarelli N, et al. Differential features of patients with mutations in two COX assembly genes, SURF-1 and SCO2. *Ann Neurol.* 2000;47:589–595.

47. MacMillan CJ, Shoubridge EA. Mitochondrial DNA depletion: prevalence in a pediatric population referred for neurological evaluation. *Pediatr Res.* 1996;14:203–210.

48. Salviati L, Sacconi S, Mancuso M, et al. Mitochondrial DNA depletion and dGK gene mutations. *Ann Neurol.* 2002;52:311–317.

49. Mancuso M, Filosto M, Bonilla E, et al. Mitochondrial myopathy of childhood associated with mitochondrial DNA depletion and a homozygous mutation (T77M) in the TK2 gene. *Arch Neurol.* 2003; 60:1007–1009.

50. Mancuso M, Salviati L, Sacconi S, et al. Mitochondrial DNA depletion: mutations in thymidine kinase gene with myopathy and SMA. *Neurology.* 2002;59:1197–1202.

51. Ferrari G, Lamantea E, Donati A, et al. Infantile hepatocerebral syndromes associated with mutations in the mitochondrial DNA polymerase-gammaA. *Brain.* 2005;128:723–731.

52. Andreu AL, Hanna MG, Reichmann H, et al. Exercise intolerance due to mutations in the cytochrome b gene of mitochondrial DNA. *N Engl J Med.* 1999;341:1037–1044.

53. Hirano M, Silvestri G, Blake DM, et al. Mitochondrial neurogastrointestinal encephalomyopathy (MNGIE): clinical, biochemical, and genetic features of an autosomal recessive mitochondrial disorder. *Neurology.* 1994;44: 721–727.

54. Marti R, Spinazzola A, Tadesse S, et al. Definitive diagnosis of mitochondrial neurogastrointestinal encephalomyopathy by biochemical assays. *Clin Chem.* 2004;50:120–124.

55. Lamperti C, Naini A, Hirano M, et al. Cerebellar ataxia and coenzyme Q10 deficiency. *Neurology.* 2003;60:1206–1208.

56. Hudson G, Deschauer M, Busse K, et al. Sensory ataxic neuropathy due to a novel C10Orf2 mutation with probable germline mosaicism. *Neurology.* 2005;64:371–373.

57. Kaukonen J, Juselius JK, Tiranti V, et al. Role of adenine nucleotide translocator 1 in mtDNA maintenance. *Science.* 2000;289:782–785.

58. Mahoney DJ, Parise G, Tarnopolsk MA y. Nutritional and exercise-based therapies in the treatment of mitochondrial disease. *Curr Opin Clin Nutr Metab Care.* 2002;5:619–629.

59. Tarnopolsky MA, Beal MF. Potential for creatine and other therapies targeting cellular energy dysfunction in neurological disorders. *Ann Neurol.* 2001;49:561–574.

60. Barshop BA, Naviaux RK, McGowan KA, et al. Chronic treatment of mitochondrial disease patients with dichloroacetate. *Mol Genet Metab.* 2004;83:138–149.

61. Taivassalo T, De Stefano N, Argov Z, et al. Effects of aerobic training in patients with mitochondrial myopathies. *Neurology.* 1998;50:1055–1060.

62. Clark KM, Bindoff LA, Lightowllers RN, et al. Reversal of a mitochondrial DNA defect in human skeletal muscle. *Nat Genet.* 1997;16: 222–224.

63. Taivassalo T, Fu K, Johns T, et al. Gene shifting: a novel therapy for mitochondrial myopathy. *Hum Mol Genet.* 1999; 8:1047–1052.

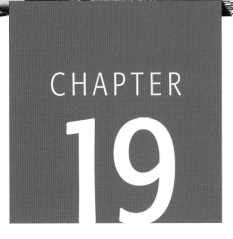

CHAPTER 19

Disorders of Pyruvate Metabolism and the Tricarboxylic Acid Cycle

Douglas S. Kerr, MD, PhD
Arthur B. Zinn, MD, PhD

INTRODUCTION

Disorders of pyruvate metabolism and the tricarboxylic acid (TCA) cycle represent a major subset of recognized disorders of energy metabolism, including especially a large number of defects of mitochondrial ETC and oxidative phosphorylation (see Chapter 18) along with defects of fatty acid β-oxidation and gluconeogenesis. Many of these defects of energy metabolism are associated clinically with lactic acidemia. Inherited disorders of pyruvate metabolism, gluconeogenesis, the TCA cycle, the electron transport chain (ETC) and oxidative phosphorylation are commonly referred to as primary genetic lactic acidemias. Other groups of genetic disorders can also lead to lactic acidemia, especially during states of severe metabolic decompensation, and are commonly referred to as the secondary genetic lactic acidemias, including defects of fatty acid β-oxidation and organic acid catabolism. In addition, lactic acidemia commonly is caused by a range of acute or chronic acquired conditions that produce impaired peripheral oxygenation. Clinical differentiation among the primary genetic lactic acidemias, secondary lactic acidemias, and acquired conditions associated with ischemia is not simple and ultimately may require detailed biochemical, enzymatic, and/or genetic testing.

PYRUVATE DEHYDROGENASE COMPLEX DEFICIENCY

Etiology/Pathophysiology In the normal fed state, in the presence of oxygen and increased insulin, glucose is converted to pyruvate via the glycolytic pathway in the cytosol, transported into mitochondria, and irreversibly decarboxylated to acetyl-coenzyme A (CoA) by the activated pyruvate dehydrogenase complex (PDC). PDC thereby serves as the gateway for pyruvate into the TCA cycle, permitting complete oxidation of pyruvate to carbon dioxide and maximum energy production via oxidative

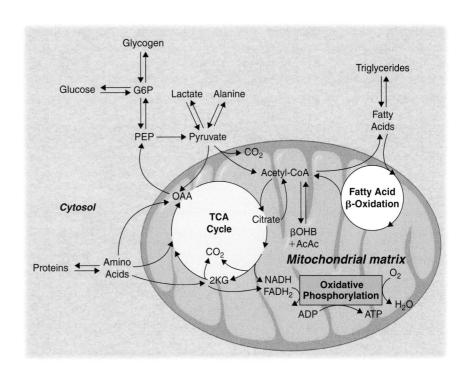

FIGURE 19-1. Overview of energy metabolism, showing relationships between carbohydrate, fatty acid, and amino acid oxidation, acetyl-CoA formation, the TCA cycle, oxidative phosphorylation, gluconeogenesis, and fatty acid synthesis. The relative locations of cytosolic and mitochondrial reactions are indicated in this simplified metabolic diagram. Not shown are specific anaplerotic and gluconeogenic amino acids that are potential sources of TCA cycle intermediates, including glutamate (converted to 2-ketoglutarate), aspartate (transaminated to oxaloacetate), and isoleucine, valine, methionine, and threonine (catabolized to succinyl-CoA via propionyl-CoA).

phosphorylation (Figures 19-1 and 19-2). Alternatively, excess acetyl-CoA generated under these conditions can be exported (via citrate) from the mitochondria to the cytosol, where it is used as a substrate for fatty acid synthesis, providing for storage of energy. In the fasting state with diminished insulin, PDC is inactivated by phosphorylation of the pyruvate dehydrogenase component (E1) by pyruvate dehydrogenase kinase, thus conserving pyruvate for gluconeogenesis and replenishment of the TCA cycle.

PDC is a mitochondrial complex consisting of five enzyme activities, three of which catalyze the conversion of pyruvate to acetyl-CoA (E1 - pyruvate dehydrogenase, a thiamine pyrophosphate (TPP)-dependent

enzyme formed from two subunits, α and β, which catalyzes decarboxylation of pyruvate to form hydroxyethyl-TPP; E2 - dihydrolipoamide transacetylase, which transfers this 2-C fragment to acetyllipoate and then to CoA to form acetyl-CoA and reduce lipoate; and E3 - dihydrolipoamide dehydrogenase, which reoxidizes reduced lipoic acid with nicotinamide adenine dinucleotide (NAD), forming a reduced form of NAD (NADH), a substrate for complex I of the ETC). The additional two specific regulatory enzymes are pyruvate dehydrogenase phosphatase and kinase, which remove or add phosphate to E1, thereby activating or inactivating the overall complex (Figure 19-3). E2 forms the core of the complex, binding multiple copies of

Disorders of Pyruvate Metabolism and the Tricarboxylic Acid Cycle

AT-A-GLANCE

Inherited disorders of pyruvate metabolism and the tricarboxylic acid (TCA) cycle are uncommon conditions that interfere with critical transformations of energy substrates (fuels) required for gluconeogenesis or adenosine triphosphate production. The pyruvate dehydrogenase complex (PDC) is the gateway for entry of carbohydrate into the TCA cycle and fatty acid synthesis. Pyruvate carboxylase (PC) and phosphoenolpyruvate carboxykinase (PEPCK) are initial steps in gluconeogenesis and replenishment of TCA

intermediates. The TCA cycle generates reduced NAD and FAD for oxidative phosphorylation. Several TCA cycle disorders have been described including 2-ketoglutarate dehydrogenase complex (KDC) deficiency, succinate dehydrogenase (SDH) deficiency, and fumarase deficiency (Figure 1). Genetic deficiencies of PDC, PC, PEPCK, or the TCA cycle primarily affect the developing nervous system and may result in lactic acidosis, hypoglycemia, and/or accumulation of specific metabolic intermediates useful for initial

diagnosis. Diagnostic confirmation depends on assay of specific enzymes or mutational analysis. Treatment opportunities are limited, but dietary modification can be helpful for pyruvate metabolism disorders. In addition to these classic genetic deficiency states, partial deficiencies associated with germ line or somatic mutations of two of the TCA cycle enzymes, fumarase and succinate dehydrogenase, predispose to specific cancer syndromes.

AFFECTED PROTEINS	OCCURRENCE	GENE	LOCUS	OMIM
Pyruvate dehydrogenase, α-subunit (E1α)	More common	PDHA1	Xp22.2-22.1	300502
Pyruvate dehydrogenase, β-subunit (E1β)	Very Rare	PDHB	3p13-q23	179060
Dihydrolipoamide transacetylase (PDC E2)	Rare	DLAT	11q23.1	608770
Dihydrolipoamide dehydrogenase (E3)	Rare	DLD	7q31-q32	246900
E3 binding protein (E3BP)	Rare	PDHX	11p13	245349
Pyruvate dehydrogenase phosphatase	Very Rare	PDP1	8q22.1	605993
Pyruvate carboxylase (PC)	Rare	PC	11q13.4-13.5	608786

Phosphoenolpyruvate carboxykinase (PEPCK)
  Mitochondrial
  Cytosolic
	
	Very Rare
	" "
		
		PCK2
		PCK1
			
			14q11.2
			20q13.31
				
				261650
				261680

2-Ketoglutarate dehydrogenase (KDC E1)	Very Rare	OGDH	7p14-p13	203740
Dihydrolipoamide transuccinylase (KDC E2)	Very Rare	DLST	14q24.3	126063

Succinate dehydrogenase (SDH)
  SDH Subunit A
  SDH Subunit B
  SDH Subunit C
  SDH Subunit D
  SDH + Aconitase
	
	Rare
	Rare
	Rare
	Rare
	Rare
		
		SDHA
		SDHB
		SDHC
		SDHD
		?
			
			5p15
			1p36.1-p35
			1q21
			11q23
			?
				
				600857
				185470
				602413
				602690
				255125

Fumarase (Fumarate hydratase, FH)	Rare	FH	1q42.1	606812

DEFECT	LAB FINDINGS	CLINICAL PRESENTATION	
		INFANCY	CHILDHOOD & ADOLESCENCE
PDC (E1α, E1β, E2, E3BP, PDP)	↑ Lactate, ↑ pyruvate, Nl lactate/pyruvate ratio, ↑ Alanine	Severe lactic acidosis (aggravated by glucose), microcephaly, brain malformations, feeding difficulty, hypotonia, seizures, developmental delay, Leigh syndrome	Mental retardation, seizures, hypotonia, ataxia, peripheral neuropathy, Leigh syndrome
E3	↑ Lactate and pyruvate, Nl lactate/pyruvate ratio, ↑ alanine ↑ leucine, ↑ isoleucine, ↑ valine, ↑ urine 2-ketoglutarate and branched keto acids	Developmental delay, microcephaly, seizures, ataxia, Leigh syndrome ± hepatomegaly with liver dysfunction ± hypoglycemia	Mental retardation, seizures, ataxia, Leigh syndrome ± liver failure
PC	↓ Glucose, ↑ ketones, ↑ lactate, ↑ pyruvate, Nl- ↑ lactate/pyruvate ratio, ↑ alanine, ↑ ammonia	Hypoglycemia with severe lactic acidosis, hyperammonemia, and ketosis, hepatomegaly, hypomyelination, difficult to manage, frequently fatal	Fasting hypoglycemia with lactic acidemia, mental retardation, seizures
PEPCK	↓ Glucose, ↑ lactate and pyruvate, nl lactate/pyruvate ratio, ↑ alanine, N ammonia	Hypoglycemia and lactic acidemia aggravated by fasting hepatomegaly	Prognosis uncertain
KDC (E1 or E2)	Nl- ↑ Blood lactate and pyruvate, Nl- ↑ L/P ratio, ↑ Urine 2-ketoglutarate	Developmental delay and hypotonia, with or without lactic acidemia	Prognosis uncertain, except for some degree of mental retardation
SDHA	Nl Urine succinate, ↑ CSF succinate (?)	Encephalomyopathy, isolated hypertrophic cardiomyopathy, cardiomyopathy and skeletal myopathy, Leigh syndrome, Kearns-Sayre syndrome, cerebellar ataxia	Late-onset optic atrophy, ataxia, and dementia
Fumarase	Nl- ↑ Blood lactate and pyruvate, ↑ urine fumarate, succinate, and 2-ketoglutarate	Hypotonia, encephalomyopathy, developmental delay, structural malformations of the brain	Mental retardation ranging from mild to severe, survival variable
SDHB, SDHD	None	Generally none	Paraganglioma, pheochromocytoma, renal cell carcinoma
Fumarase	None	None	Multiple cutaneous and uterine leiomyomatosis, renal cancer

Nl = normal; CSF = cerebral spinal fluid.

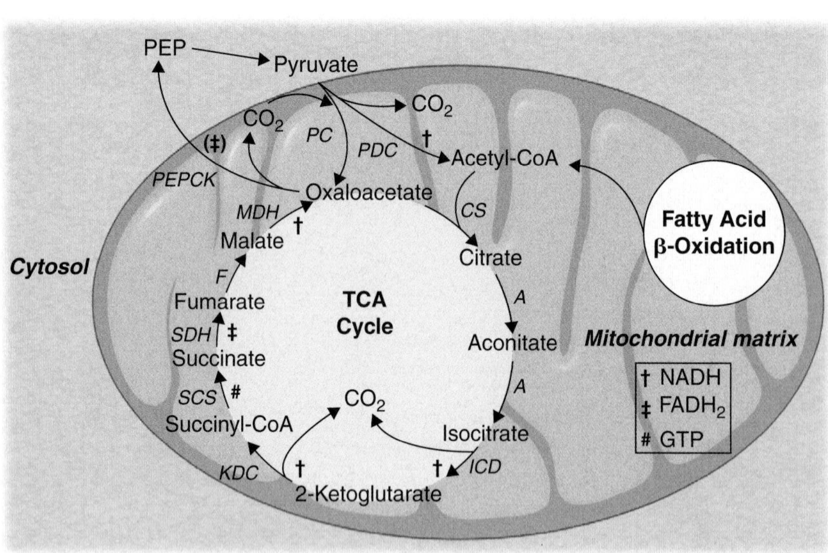

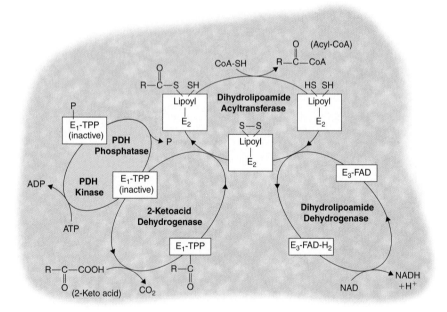

FIGURE 19-2. Detailed view of relationships of pyruvate metabolism, acetyl-CoA, and the TCA cycle. Abbreviations used for enzyme names are: PDC = pyruvate dehydrogenase complex; PC = pyruvate carboxylase; PEPCK = phosphoenolpyruvate carboxykinase (the two different locations of PEPCK, cytosolic and mitochondrial, are not shown); CS = citrate synthase; A = aconitase; ICD = isocitrate dehydrogenase; KDC = 2-ketoglutarate dehydrogenase complex; SCS = succinyl-CoA synthase; SDH = succinate dehydrogenase; F = fumarase; and MDH = malate dehydrogenase. High-energy products produced by these metabolic enzymes that are potential intermediates for oxidative phosphorylation (NADH and 1,5-dihydroflavin adenine dinucleotide[FADH]) and guanosine triphosphate (GTP), are indicated by the symbols shown in the inset. The malate shuttle, which allows for trafficking of dicarboxylic acids and reducing equivalents between the mitochondrial cytosol and matrix, is shown in Figure 19-4.

FIGURE 19-3. Component reactions within the PDC and the KDC (as well as the branched-chain 2-ketoacid dehydrogenase complex). Abbreviations used for the catalytic components are: E_1, first component of pyruvate or 2-ketoglutarate dehydrogenase; E_2, dihydrolipoamide transacetylase or trans-succinylase; and E_3, dihydrolipoamide dehydrogenase, which is common to all three enzyme complexes. The regulatory enzymes PDH (E1) kinase and phosphatase are specific for PDC. The R- in the ketoacid substrates and CoA products of these reactions are CH_3- for PDC and $COOH-CH_2-CH_2$- for KDC. Additional abbreviations are: TPP = thiamine pyrophosphate; lipoyl-$(SH)_2$ = reduced covalently bound lipoamide; CoA-SH = coenzyme A; and $FADH_2$ = reduced flavin adenine dinucleotide. Pyruvate is initially decarboxylated by dephospho-E1 with noncovalently bound TPP, then hydroxyethyl-TPP is oxidized by E2 with covalently bound lipoic acid, and the acetyl moiety transferred to CoASH, leaving reduced lipoic acid, which is oxidized by FAD bound to E3, producing FADH, that in turn reduces NAD to NADH.

E1 and E3 (the latter via an E3-binding protein). When PDC activity is deficient due to mutations of any of the subunits required for activity, pyruvate oxidation is impaired, and pyruvate and lactate accumulate in the carbohydrate-fed state, as it does in anaerobic glycolysis. In contrast to the increased L/P ratio seen in anaerobic conditions or defects of the ETC, the L/P ratio is generally normal in patients with PDC deficiency because the respiratory chain is not impaired and NADH oxidation is preserved. The overall effect of PDC deficiency is that the potential energy production from carbohydrate is severely limited, whereas the oxidation of fatty acids or β-hydroxybutyrate and acetoacetate derived from fasting endogenous lipolysis or dietary fat is not impaired. The preservation of fatty acid oxidation in patients with PDC deficiency forms the rationale for use of the ketogenic diet as therapy.

PDC deficiency can be caused by mutations of the α or β subunits of pyruvate dehydrogenase (E1), dihydrolipoamide transacetylase (E2), the E3-binding protein, pyruvate dehydrogenase phosphatase, or dihydrolipoamide dehydrogenase (E3) 1-8. The clinical consequences of defects of E1α, E1β, E2, E3-binding protein, or E1-phosphatase are not qualitatively distinct because each of these defects has the common biochemical effect of impairing function of the overall complex. The E3 protein is unique in that it is common to all three of the 2-ketoacid dehydrogenase complexes, as discussed in a separate section later.

Mutations of the E1α subunit, which is encoded on the X chromosome, account for approximately 70% of cases of PDC deficiency. In affected males the E1α subunit has a missense mutation, which allows the PDC to have some residual function. Complete disruption of this gene is lethal for embryonic male mice, and no mutations that completely abolish PDC activity have been described in surviving affected human males. Females who are heterozygous for an E1α mutation are generally less severely affected than males who are hemizygous for the same mutation because of random X chromosome inactivation in females. For the same reason, affected females appear able to survive with more severe mutations than males, as they have some residual enzymatic activity.

The clinical manifestations of mutations affecting different components of PDC are similar (except for E3 deficiency). The cells in the body that are most affected are in tissues that depend heavily on energy from glucose oxidation, including the central and peripheral nervous systems, especially the developing brain and basal ganglia. A wide range of clinical heterogeneity, in both the spectrum and severity of disease, has been observed in patients with PDC deficiency. The clinical heterogeneity does not correlate well with measurements of enzyme activity in vitro or the nature of the causative mutations.

Clinical Presentation The clinical presentation of PDC deficiency is quite variable,

TABLE 19-1   Approach to Differentiation of Primary Lactic Acidemias*

| Clinical Feature | Group of Disorders | | | |
	PDC	Gluconeogenesis	TCA Cycle[†]	ETC
Metabolic:				
Peripheral pO$_2$ #	Normal	Normal	Normal	Normal
L/P ratio	Normal	Normal	Variable	High
Effect of fasting on blood lactate	Decreased	Increased	None or decreased	None or decreased
Effect of Cho intake on blood lactate	Increased	Decreased	None or increased	None or increased
Hypoglycemia	No	Yes	No	Occasionally
Hyperalaninemia	Yes	Yes	Yes	Occasionally
Systemic:				
CNS dysfunction	Yes	Variable	Yes	Common
Abnormal brain MRI	Common	Uncommon	Occasionally	Common
Peripheral neuropathy	Occasionally	No	No	Occasionally
Skeletal myopathy	No	No	No	Common
Cardiomyopathy	No	No	Occasionally	Common
Hepatic dysfunction	No	Yes	No	Occasionally
Renal disease	Occasionally	(in G6Pase def.)	No	Occasionally
Visual dysfunction	No	No	No	Occasionally
Deafness	No	No	No	Occasionally
Diabetes mellitus	No	No	No	Occasionally

PDC = pyruvate dehydrogenase complex; TCA = tricarboxylic acid; ETC = electron transport chain; CNS = central nervous system; L/P ratio = lactate/pyruvate ratio.

*No single feature is absolute or diagnostic. Confirmation of a diagnosis depends on additional laboratory testing.

#Low pO$_2$ suggests acute or chronic nonmetabolic illness.

[†]SDH deficiency behaves like an ETC defect.

ranging from fatal congenital lactic acidosis to relatively mild ataxia or neuropathy compatible with extended survival. The clinical consequences fall into two major categories: metabolic and neurologic. The metabolic consequences may include severe lactic acidosis in the newborn period or early infancy, usually leading to death. Neurologic manifestations that appear in those who survive the neonatal period may include developmental delay, hypotonia, seizures, microcephaly, ataxia, and peripheral neuropathy. Virtually all of the neurologic manifestations of PDC deficiency are the consequences of impaired central or peripheral nervous system function, without primary myopathy, cardiomyopathy, or systemic dysfunction. Less commonly seen manifestations are congenital brain defects, particularly affecting the corpus callosum, or degenerative changes, including Leigh syndrome (which also may be associated with several other mitochondrial disorders). Facial dysmorphism has been noted in some cases of PDC deficiency with features similar to the fetal alcohol syndrome (9).

Diagnosis The most common laboratory abnormalities associated with PDC deficiency are increased blood lactate and pyruvate, with a normal L/P ratio (10–20 in venous blood) because respiratory chain activity is not impaired and NADH oxidation is preserved. Although a normal L/P ratio is neither unique to, nor invariably found in, patients with PDC deficiency, the ratio can be an important feature to distinguish lactic acidemia caused by hypoxemia or defects of the ETC, in which the L/P ratio is typically high. Alanine is also increased in patients with PDC deficiency, but this is less distinctive. In some cases, blood lactate is normal or only intermittently increased, especially after a carbohydrate meal. Measurement of lactate and pyruvate in the cerebrospinal fluid or estimation of brain lactate by magnetic resonance spectroscopy are useful additional tests if blood lactate is normal. A guide to an initial clinical approach to distinguishing among the primary lactic acidemias is provided in Table 19-1. This table incorporates a range of metabolic features, including the blood lactate/pyruvate (L/P) ratio, the effect of fasting and carbohydrate ingestion on blood lactate, the presence of hypoglycemia and/or hyperalaninemia, and various systemic manifestations to distinguish among the groups of disorders.

The diagnosis of PDC deficiency depends on measuring enzyme activity in cells or tissues (Figure 19-3). The most common approach is to assay PDC in cultured skin fibroblasts. Fibroblast PDC activity may be normal in some cases of PDC deficiency, especially in affected females, depending on lyonization of the X-linked PDC E1α gene (*PDHA1*), and less commonly in males. If the possibility of PDC deficiency is strongly suspected, assays in additional cells (such as blood lymphocytes), tissues, or a muscle biopsy are recommended. If overall PDC activity is low, its catalytic components (E1, E2, and E3) also can be assayed. Some diagnostic laboratories utilize immunoblotting or immunocytochemistry for further definition of which subunit is affected. The latter method is particularly useful for detecting a small subpopulation of cells lacking immunoreactive E1α. Because approximately 70% of cases of PDC deficiency are caused by mutations within the E1α gene, PDHA1, mutational analysis of cDNA (or preferably both cDNA and genomic DNA) for this gene may provide final diagnostic confirmation. Genetic testing is limited by the observation that more than 70 different *PDHA1* mutations have been described in less than 200 published cases that have been analyzed, none of which account for more than 10% of the cases.

Treatment Successful treatment of PDC deficiency remains limited; however, the options are better than for most mitochondrial disorders. In principle, it should be possible to bypass the lack of PDC activity by providing a ketogenic diet to generate acetyl-CoA (Figures 19-1 and 19-2). There has now been considerable experience with this approach. To replace blood glucose with sufficient amounts of β-hydroxybutyrate and acetoacetate to serve as alternate energy sources for the nervous system and sufficient amounts of fatty acids to serve as fuel for skeletal muscle and heart, it is necessary to maintain a strict ketogenic diet by providing an extremely low intake of dietary carbohydrate. A strict ketogenic diet means less than 10% of energy from carbohydrate, not more than 15% of energy from protein, and at least 75% of energy from fat. In infants and younger children, this can best be accomplished by liberal use of a commercial carbohydrate-free formula that is otherwise nutritionally complete. Comparison of outcomes of affected brothers or unrelated males with the same mutation indicated that the earlier the diet is started and the greater the restriction of dietary carbohydrate, the better are the prospects for mental development and survival (10). Strict ketogenic diets have been used effectively with younger infants, but are difficult to maintain as children get older. Children with more severe forms of PDC deficiency show very limited benefit from this therapy. Supplementation with L-carnitine (~ 25–50 mg/kg/d to normalize plasma free carnitine) may be beneficial for patients on ketogenic diets to prevent secondary carnitine deficiency. Sustaining ketosis during intravenous feeding is very difficult, but can be accomplished by using fat emulsions and providing all potassium as the acetate salt. Other reported therapies have included administration of high doses of thiamine, in the range of 100 to 3,000 mg/day. Although there are case reports suggesting that thiamine may be of benefit, no controlled trials have been performed, and the mechanism by which thiamine may be of benefit remains uncertain. Dichloroacetate (DCA), an analog of pyruvate, activates PDC by inhibiting pyruvate dehydrogenase kinase. A controlled clinical crossover trial of DCA administration to children with congenital lactic acidosis failed to show evidence of clinical benefit, including a subset of cases with PDC deficiency (11). Because DCA is not an approved drug and is potentially toxic, its use should be confined to approved clinical trials.

Prenatal Diagnosis Parents of severely affected PDC-deficient children frequently inquire about prenatal diagnosis. It is useful to note that less than 10% of known cases have had an affected sibling. Measurement of PDC activity in amniotic cells or chorionic villus samples is not a reliable method for prenatal testing. In principle, the optimal method of diagnosis would be mutational analysis of amniotic or chorionic villus cells, provided the mutation has been identified in the proband. Successful diagnosis of a fetus with PDC deficiency has not yet been reported.

PYRUVATE CARBOXYLASE DEFICIENCY

Etiology/Pathophysiology Pyruvate carboxylase (PC) catalyzes the carboxylation of pyruvate to oxaloacetate, replenishing this key intermediate of the TCA cycle (anaplerosis) and providing the first step in conversion of pyruvate to glucose (gluconeogenesis) (Figures 19-1 and 19-2). The PC reaction is an energy (adenosine triphosphate [ATP])-dependent mitochondrial reaction, which involves enzyme-bound biotin and is activated by acetyl-CoA. The enzyme is made up of identical subunits encoded by a single gene located on chromosome 11.

Deficiency of PC impairs the carboxylation of pyruvate to oxaloacetate, resulting in pyruvate being shunted to lactate and alanine. Due to lack of oxaloacetate, acetyl-CoA cannot enter the TCA cycle to produce citrate, and excess acetyl-CoA leads to increased ketone body synthesis in the liver. At the same time, lack of oxaloacetate hinders gluconeogenesis via phosphoenolpyruvate carboxykinase (PEPCK), resulting in fasting hypoglycemia and enhanced lactic acidemia, features that distinguish PC (or PEPCK) deficiency from PDC deficiency.

In defects of gluconeogenesis, carbohydrate administration usually reverses the hypoglycemia and lactic acidemia; whereas in PDC deficiency fasting decreases the degree of lactic acidemia, does not lead to hypoglycemia, and carbohydrate administration can result in increased lactate levels. Energy depletion resulting from dysfunction of the TCA cycle and hypoglycemia contributes to CNS dysfunction. Glycerol production from "glyceroneogenesis" may be disrupted, leading to impaired lipid synthesis and myelin formation, and inadequate white matter development. The urea cycle may also be disrupted because oxaloacetate deficiency leads to aspartate deficiency, which disrupts the conversion of citrulline and aspartate to argininosuccinate via the activity of argininosuccinate synthetase and leads to increased plasma ammonia and citrulline levels. Finally, PC is needed for formation of oxaloacetate, an intermediate in the malate–aspartate shuttle that, first, serves to transfer reducing equivalents from the cytosol into the mitochondria (via malate) for oxidation by the ETC, and second, serves to transfer oxaloacetate to the cytosol, by transamination to aspartate (Figure 19-4). The malate–aspartate shuttle also provides a means of exporting intramitochondrial amino groups into the cytosol for urea synthesis. Disruption of the malate cycle due to severe lack of oxaloacetate leads to a more reduced state in the cytosol, and disruption of the urea cycle. As a result, the ratio of lactate/pyruvate and ammonia may be increased in severe PC deficiency (but not in milder forms of the disease).

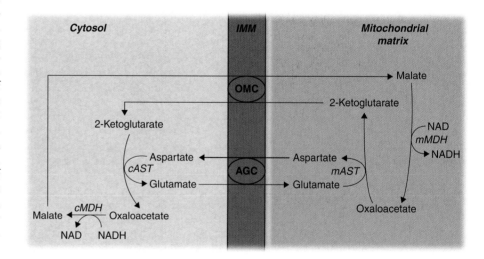

FIGURE 19-4. The aspartate malate shuttle. The outer mitochondrial membrane and intermembrane space are not indicated. This shuttle allows NADH generated in the cytosol to enter the mitochondria via malate, where NADH is regenerated and oxidized by the ETC, and provides a mechanism for transporting aspartate out of the mitochondria to the cytosol, as a substrate for argininosuccinate synthase in the formation of urea. Deficiency of citrin, which is one form of AGC, is a cause of hyperammonemia (see Chapter 11). AGC = aspartate glutamate carrier; cAST and mAST = cytosolic and mitochondrial aspartate aminotransferases; cMDH and mMDH = cytosolic and mitochondrial malate dehydrogenases; IMM = inner mitochondrial membrane; NAD = nicotinamide adenine dinucleotide; NADH = reduced nicotinamide adenine dinucleotide; and OMC = oxoglutarate (ketoglutarate) malate carrier.

Clinical Presentation   The age of onset and degree of severity of PC deficiency have been characterized as severe neonatal, usually fatal (type B); less severe infantile, compatible with survival but with impaired neurologic development (type A); and milder, later onset, usually with some developmental delay (type C) (1). The latter group includes a so-called "benign" form, but because these cases have clinically significant symptoms, they should instead be considered relatively mild forms. As more cases of PC deficiency have been identified, it appears that there is a spectrum of phenotypes overlapping these clinical categorizations (12). Overall, the clinical presentation may include neurologic manifestations of hypotonia, hypertonia, ataxia, choreoathetosis, microcephaly, and other manifestations of impaired white matter development. Hypomyelination of the brain may be detectable by magnetic resonance imaging. The liver may be enlarged with abnormal liver function tests.

In the newborn, mild-to-moderate PC deficiency is likely to present with hypoglycemia, lactic acidemia, and a normal L/P ratio. These patients may improve with feeding or intravenously administered glucose. In more severe (type B) PC deficiency, the neonate also invariably has elevated citrulline and may develop hyperammonemia, ketosis, and an increased L/P ratio, frequently associated with tremor and bizarre ocular behavior (13). These infants do not respond well to feeding or intravenous glucose. Even with anaplerotic treatment (see later), the prognosis in these severe cases is poor, with high mortality rates.

Children who survive with milder PC deficiency are frequently developmentally delayed and may develop a seizure disorder. As affected children get older, they are less likely to develop acute metabolic crises because it takes longer to deplete their glycogen reserves, but prolonged fasting and intercurrent infectious illnesses increase the risk of metabolic decompensation.

Diagnosis   Clinical suspicion of PC deficiency in the newborn period depends on recognition of the combination of acute metabolic features described previously, most commonly including hypoglycemia, lactic acidemia, and ketosis (Table 19-2). The combination of hypoglycemia, lactic acidemia, hyperammonemia, hypercitrullinemia, and ketosis is virtually pathognomonic for severe PC deficiency. When glucose is provided, correcting hypoglycemia, blood lactate may typically (but not always) decrease. In milder cases the L/P ratio is normal, but in severe neonatal cases the L/P ratio may be increased (disrupting the cytosolic/mitochondrial redox balance). Plasma amino acid analysis may show increased alanine and

Clinical Feature	PC	PEPCK	Fructose-1, 6-Bisphosphatase*	Glucose-6-Phosphatase*
Fasting aggravated:				
Hypoglycemia	+	+	+	+
Lactic acidosis	+	+	+	+
Ketosis	+ +	+	±	±
Nl lactate/pyruvate	±	+	±	+
Hyperalaninemia	+	+	+	+
Hyperammonemia	±			
Hypercitrullinemia	±			
Hypoaspartatemia	±			
Hyperaspartatemia		±?		
Hepatomegaly	+	+	+ +	+ +
Nephromegaly				+
Hyperlipidemia			+	+ +
Hyperuricemia			+	+
Hypophosphatemia			+	
Abnl fructose test			+	+
Abnl glucagon test				+
Abnl galactose test				+
Platelet dysfunction				+
Neutropenia				±**

TABLE 19-2   Differentiation of Disorders of Gluconeogenesis

Nl = normal; Abnl = abnormal; PC = pyruvate carboxylase; PEPCK = phosphoenolpyruvate carboxykinase.

*These disorders are included in Chapters 6 and 10.

**Present in glucose-6-phosphate translocase deficiency (GSD Type Ib,c).

citrulline, with decreased aspartate and glutamate. The differential diagnosis includes other defects of gluconeogenesis (e.g., PEPCK deficiency (see later), fructose bisphosphatase deficiency, and glucose-6-phosphatase deficiency (see Table 19-2 and Chapters 10 and 6), as well as defects of biotin metabolism (e.g., biotinidase or holocarboxylase synthase deficiencies; see Chapter 7). Biotinidase and holocarboxylase deficiencies are not likely to be confused with PC deficiency because they result in multiple carboxylase deficiencies with urinary excretion of organic acids derived from their respective substrates (including lactate, 3-hydroxypropionate, methylcitrate, and β-methylycrotonylglycine); furthermore, the more common biotinidase deficiency should be detected by extended newborn screening programs that include assays for biotinidase and an expanded panel of acylcarnitines (see Chapter 2). Confirmation of PC deficiency depends on assay of enzyme activity in cultured skin fibroblasts or a liver (not skeletal muscle) biopsy, and distinction from these other disorders. Mutational analysis is currently difficult due to the large size of the gene and the genetic heterogeneity that has been found in cases examined to date. The exception is in specific population isolates (e.g., certain native North

American tribes) that have a high incidence of specific mutations (14).

Treatment   The first step in treatment of metabolic crises associated with PC deficiency is control of hypoglycemia, lactic acidosis, ketosis, and hyperammonemia by providing intravenous glucose, followed, if hyperammonemia (>200 μM) persists, by the addition of intravenous sodium phenylacetate and sodium benzoate (without arginine), similar to the standard protocol for treating urea cycle defects (see Chapter 8 for details). In these severe situations with hyperammonemia and unresponsive lactic acidosis, intravenous administration of sodium or potassium citrate would be expected to help provide an anaplerotic source of cytosolic oxaloacetate (via citrate lyase) for transamination to aspartate as a substrate for argininosuccinate synthetase, opening up the urea cycle (13). The efficacy of this approach and amount of citrate needed are not established, but it appears reasonable to give 1000 to 1500 mg/kg/day as a constant infusion of sodium/potassium citrate (excess citrate can produce symptomatic lowering of ionized calcium). Hemodialysis may be indicated if lactic acidosis and/or hyperammonemia are severe (e.g., >15 mM or 400 μM, respectively), the patient is encephalopathic, or there is poor response to these medical measures (with appropriate recognition that the prognosis in such situations is very poor). If the patient's blood ammonia is not elevated, administration of aspartate and other gluconeogenic amino acids, via standard parenteral nutrition, can provide "anaplerotic" sources for replenishment of oxaloacetate. Recently, triheptanoate, a nitrogen/sodium/potassium-free anaplerotic source of oxaloacetate (via propionyl-CoA), has been reported to be beneficial in treating acute metabolic crises due to PC deficiency; the starting dose was 2 g/kg, followed by up to 35% of total dietary energy, administered enterally (15).

Long-term management requires avoiding fasting, provision of a high-carbohydrate (70%–80% of energy) diet containing sources of oxaloacetate (as dietary protein, (10%–15% of energy, if not hyperammonemic, or citrate, or triheptanoate), and home monitoring for fasting hypoglycemia and ketosis. Liver transplantation has been reported to improve systemic metabolic control (lactic acidemia and ketosis), but failed to improve pre-existing neurologic dysfunction; PC may play a critical anaplerotic role in brain metabolism (16). Although biotin is sometimes given to patients with primary PC deficiency, there is no convincing evidence of its efficacy, as distinguished from its benefit in multiple carboxylase deficiencies.

Prenatal Diagnosis Prenatal diagnosis has been successfully performed in a few cases by measurement of PC activity in cultured amniocytes (17). Mutational analysis of products of conception could enhance the reliability of prenatal diagnosis, if the mutation had been identified previously in the proband (12).

PHOSPHOENOLPYRUVATE CARBOXYKINASE DEFICIENCY

Etiology/Pathophysiology PEPCK catalyzes the decarboxylation of oxaloacetate to phosphoenolpyruvate (PEP). Like PC, PEPCK is an energy-dependent reaction, but requires guanosine triphosphate instead of ATP. Oxaloacetate can be formed from pyruvate via PC, or from gluconeogenic amino acids or other sources of propionyl-CoA, via the TCA cycle (Figure 19-2). PEP, in turn, can be converted to glucose (gluconeogenesis), glycerol (glyceroneogenesis), or pyruvate (for oxidation or "futile recycling"). There are two forms of PEPCK, a cytosolic and a mitochondrial form, which are encoded by two distinct genes (located on chromosomes 20 and 14, respectively). The relative amounts and functions of these two forms vary among different tissues and species. Hormonal regu-

lation of expression of the cytosolic form by insulin, cortisol and counter-regulatory hormones that increase cyclic AMP, has been extensively investigated (18). PEPCK deficiency is uncommon and not well characterized. The predicted consequences of PEPCK deficiency are similar to those for PC deficiency, resulting in impairment of fasting gluconeogenesis and accumulation of lactate and pyruvate, but not impairment of ureagenesis or the TCA cycle (L/P ratio is normal). Impaired glyceroneogenesis may interfere with triglyceride or phospholipid synthesis and fatty acid recycling in adipose tissue.

Clinical Presentation In the few reported cases of PEPCK deficiency that presented in infancy, clinical manifestations have included hepatomegaly associated with lactic acidemia and hypoglycemia, which were aggravated by fasting (19,20). Death occurred in early infancy or childhood. Unlike PC deficiency, hyperammonemia has not been described in severe cases of PEPCK deficiency, presumably because lack of aspartate would not be an expected consequence of this disorder. Because so few cases have been described, it is not clear what the degree of clinical heterogeneity is and whether milder cases of PEPCK deficiency exist.

Diagnosis The diagnosis of PEPCK deficiency should be considered in infants with hepatomegaly, fasting hypoglycemia, and lactic acidemia, without hyperammonemia. These metabolic features are common to other defects of gluconeogenesis (PC, fructose-1,6-bisphosphatase, glucose-6-phosphatase; see Table 19-2). PEPCK activity can be assayed in cultured skin fibroblasts, in which the activity is predominantly mitochondrial. If a liver biopsy can be obtained, mitochondrial and cytosol fractions should be isolated, and PEPCK activity assayed separately in the two fractions. Mutations causing PEPCK deficiency have not yet been characterized.

Treatment Successful treatment of PEPCK deficiency has not been reported. In principle, the approach described previously for treating patients with PC deficiency should be helpful, including avoiding fasting and providing parenteral glucose or oral carbohydrate feedings. All of these measures are aimed at enhancing glycogen storage. On the other hand, it should not be necessary to provide patients with PEPCK deficiency a source of oxaloacetate; a supplemental source of glycerol (other than glucose) conceivably might be beneficial, but has not been reported.

Prenatal Diagnosis Prenatal diagnosis of PEPCK deficiency has not been reported.

2-KETOGLUTARATE DEHYDROGENASE COMPLEX DEFICIENCY

Etiology/Pathophysiology The 2-ketoglutarate dehydrogenase complex (KDC) catalyzes oxidative decarboxylation of 2-ketoglutarate to succinyl-CoA and CO_2. 2-Ketoglutarate is an intermediate of the TCA cycle, formed from aconitic acid or by deamination/transamination of glutamate (Figure 19-2). KDC is a multienzyme complex that is analogous to PDC, with three catalytic subunits (Figure 19-3). E1 (a thiamine pyrophosphate-dependent enzyme) and E2 (contains lipoic acid) are specific to this complex, whereas E3 is common to PDC, KDC, and the branched-chain 2-ketoacid dehydrogenase complex. Unlike PDC, KDC activity is not regulated by phosphorylation or dephosphorylation. KDC deficiency disrupts overall energy metabolism via the TCA cycle because this step is required for oxidation of substrates derived from carbohydrate, fat, and protein.

Clinical Presentation The few cases of KDC deficiency that have been reported are typically associated with developmental delay, hypotonia, progressively severe encephalopathy, pyramidal symptoms, and failure to thrive (21,22). Some of these children exhibited permanent lactic acidosis with acute episodes during stress and infections. In infancy, KDC deficiency may cause acute lactic acidosis, with an elevated L/P ratio. The clue to diagnosis usually comes from urine organic acid analysis, which shows significant increases of 2-ketoglutaric and 2-hydroxyglutaric acids, that frequently (but not necessarily) are persistent. Several cases of DOOR syndrome (onycho-osteodystrophy, dystrophic thumbs, sensorineural deafness) have been reported as having KDC deficiency.

Diagnosis The diagnosis of KDC deficiency may be suspected after finding increased urinary 2-ketoglutaric acid. Moderately increased urinary excretion of 2-ketoglutaric acid is seen fairly commonly and is a nonspecific finding, so investigation of possible KDC deficiency has usually (not always) depended on persistence of this finding, without increases of downstream TCA intermediates (e.g., succinic or fumaric acids). KDC activity can be assayed in cultured skin fibroblasts, lymphocytes, or skeletal muscle. Variability of cell/tissue expression of KDC deficiency has not been described. Enzymatic analyses have suggested probable deficiencies of the E1 or E2 components. Specific mutations have not yet been reported.

Treatment No effective treatment of KDC deficiency has been described, other than supportive care.

Prenatal Diagnosis Prenatal diagnosis has not been reported for KDC deficiency.

DIHYDROLIPOAMIDE DEHYDROGENASE (E3) DEFICIENCY

Etiology/Pathophysiology The E3 component (dihydrolipoamide dehydrogenase) of PDC and KDC is the same gene product (Figure 19-3). E3 is also a necessary component of the branched-chain 2-ketoacid dehydrogenase complex, which is defective in maple syrup urine disease (see Chapter Organic Acid Disorders). Typically, deficiency of E3 has the effect of producing multiple 2-ketoacid dehydrogenase complex deficiencies. The predicted consequences of this multiple deficiency state are accumulation of all the metabolites that characterize the individual deficiencies including lactic and pyruvic acidemia; increased urinary excretion of lactic, pyruvic, 2-ketoglutaric, 2-ketoisocaproic, 2-ketomethylvaleric, 2-ketoisovaleric, and the 2-hydroxy analogs of each of these ketoacids; and increased plasma alanine, glutamate, leucine, isoleucine, and valine. In reality, however, actual observations in E3-deficient cases have not shown this full spectrum of findings, but a variable combination of these metabolic abnormalities. A phenotype has been described that is similar to KDC deficiency. The gene that encodes for E3 is on chromosome 7.

Clinical Presentation The clinical features of E3 deficiency are predominantly neurologic, and variably include microcephaly, developmental delay, ataxia, Leigh syndrome, and lactic acidosis (23–25). Some cases have had liver dysfunction with hepatomegaly, sometimes progressing to liver failure; other cases have also had hypoglycemia or hypocalcemia.

Diagnosis The diagnosis of E3 deficiency should be considered in patients who have multiple metabolic abnormalities that reflect a combined deficiency of PDC, KDC, and the branched-chain 2-ketoacid dehydrogenase complex. The key metabolic tests are blood lactate and pyruvate, plasma amino acid, and urine organic acid analysis. It is important to keep in mind that these abnormalities are not evident in a consistent manner, and one may need to consider the possibility of E3 deficiency in patients who exhibit only a subset of these abnormal findings. E3 can be assayed in blood lymphocytes, cultured skin fibroblasts, or various tissues. The diagnostic laboratory should be able to distinguish heterozygotes from homozygous-deficient cases. Normal PDC activity in cultured skin

fibroblasts has been reported in a case of E3 deficiency. Several pathogenetic mutations have been identified. A common mutation has been reported in Arab and Jewish subpopulations. Prenatal testing is possible, optimally with a combination of assaying enzyme activity and mutational analysis (23).

Treatment Treatment options for E3 deficiency are very limited because of the multiple pathways affected. Dietary carbohydrate and branched-chain amino acids can be restricted, as they would be for PDC deficiency and maple syrup urine disease, but there is no known method of avoiding substrates that do not depend on the TCA cycle, as carbohydrate, fat, and protein metabolism all lead to products that enter the TCA cycle. D,L-lipoic acid supplementation has been reported to be of benefit in a few patients, but these reports have not been substantiated. The rationale for the use of lipoic acid is weak because reduced lipoic acid is a substrate for E3, not a cofactor.

SUCCINATE DEHYDROGENASE DEFICIENCY

Etiology/Pathophysiology Succinate dehydrogenase (SDH) is unique among the TCA cycle enzymes because in addition to its role in the TCA cycle, it is also a component of complex II (succinate:ubiquinone oxidoreductase) of the mitochondrial ETC. SDH/complex II catalyzes the irreversible conversion of succinate to fumarate and reduction of flavin adenine dinucleotide (FAD) to reduced flavin adenine dinucleotide ($FADH_2$), providing electrons to the respiratory chain ubiquinone pool (Figure 19-2). Complex II is composed of four subunits. The SDH component of complex II is composed of two of these subunits: subunit A (SDHA), a flavoprotein, and subunit B (SDHB), an iron sulfur protein. The other two subunits, subunit C (SDHC) and subunit D (SDHD), are integral membrane proteins that contain a single heme group and the ubiquinone-binding site. Complex II is unique among the five complexes that make up the mitochondrial oxidative phosphorylation system in that it is composed exclusively of nuclear-encoded components, whereas the other complexes are composed of some components encoded by the mitochondrial genome and others by the nuclear genome. In addition to these four nuclear-encoded subunits, there is growing evidence that there are other proteins that play a role in complex II synthesis or stabilization.

Initially, the reported cases of SDH deficiency relied on enzyme analysis to establish a diagnosis and generally did not determine unambiguously whether affected patients had SDH deficiency, complex II deficiency, or a

combined deficiency of SDH and complex II. More recently described cases have also been characterized by mutational analysis of the genes that encode the four subunits of complex II, thereby permitting more precise diagnosis. It now appears that genetic deficiencies of *SDHA* (and very rarely, *SDHB*) produce neuromuscular problems that resemble those associated with defects of the other TCA cycle enzymes or respiratory chain complexes (26–28), whereas mutations of *SDHB*, *SDHC*, or *SDHD* produce an unusual cancer predisposition syndrome characterized by the development of pheochromocytoma or paraganglioma. The neurologic disorders associated with *SDHA* mutations will be discussed in this section, whereas the tumorigenesis disorders will be discussed later (see Cancer Predisposition Syndromes Associated with TCA Cycle Enzyme Defects).

The pathogenesis of SDH deficiency is uncertain, although it is generally accepted that it leads to impaired TCA function and impaired ATP production. These impairments do not explain the variable tissue-specific expression or the variable age of onset of the associated clinical disorders. Similarly, the role of several complex II subunits in tumorigenesis is unexplained by this traditional view of complex II function.

Clinical Presentation SDH deficiency, whether an isolated deficiency or associated with complex II deficiency, accounts for a very small proportion of patients ($< 5\%$) identified with respiratory chain complex deficiencies. Only a handful of patients with genetically defined SDH/complex II deficiency have been reported. This small group of patients has had a highly variable clinical phenotype including Leigh syndrome, Kearns-Sayre syndrome, optic atrophy and cerebellar ataxia, isolated cardiomyopathy, combined cardiomyopathy and skeletal myopathy, and late-onset optic atrophy and ataxia. In the subset of patients in whom mutational analysis was performed, all the cases except one were found to have *SDHA* mutations. The majority of these patients had Leigh syndrome associated with homozygous *SDHA* mutations. Another set of cases (two siblings) presented with an adult-onset neurodegenerative disorder characterized by optic atrophy, ataxia, and myopathy. These two patients were found to be heterozygous for a single *SDHA* mutation. To date, only one patient with a neurologic disorder (i.e., myopathy) has been found to have a mutation in *SDHB*. No cases of *SDHC* or *SDHD* deficiency have been found among neurologically affected patients.

Diagnosis As opposed to the other TCA cycle defects described in this chapter, SDH deficiency is not typically characterized by increased urinary excretion of metabolites proximal to the enzyme deficiency, in this case, succinate. In some cases, however, succinate was shown by magnetic resonance spectroscopy to be elevated in cerebrospinal fluid and the brain. Many cases of SDH deficiency, but not all, are associated with lactic acidosis. Thus, standard metabolic analysis of the commonly collected body fluids does not provide useful clues to the presence of an underlying SDH defect. The diagnosis can be made by polarographic analysis of isolated skeletal muscle mitochondria, but this approach is not widely available. Most commonly, the diagnosis of SDH deficiency is established by enzyme analysis of cultured skin fibroblasts or skeletal muscle biopsy. All tissues should be analyzed for both SDH activity and succinate: ubiquinone oxidoreductase (complex II) activity to establish and help localize the deficiency. Mutational analysis can confirm the diagnosis, but such testing is not clinically available.

Treatment Specific treatment for SDH deficiency, either isolated or as part of complex II deficiency, is not currently available.

Prenatal Diagnosis Prenatal diagnosis of SDH deficiency by measurement of metabolites in amniotic fluid or by enzyme analysis of fetal cells is not reliable. Prenatal diagnosis has been accomplished using mutational analysis of chorionic villus samples for a family in which the proband had previously been shown to have two missense mutations in the *SDHA* gene. The use of genetic testing for prenatal diagnosis of SDH deficiency should be possible for other families in which the genetic defect has been established in the proband.

SUCCINATE DEHYDROGENASE/ ACONITASE DEFICIENCY

Etiology/Pathophysiology Nearly two dozen patients from several families have been reported with a combined deficiency of SDH and aconitase. The initial biochemical and immunochemical studies of these patients demonstrated that the impaired SDH activity was accompanied by a more generalized deficiency of complex II, reduced amounts of immunoreactive SDH subunit B (the iron-sulfur cluster containing subunit of SDH), and aconitase deficiency. Aconitase is a TCA cycle enzyme that also contains an iron-sulfur cluster (Figure 19-2). Further studies showed a more generalized defect, with milder abnormalities of two other respiratory chain complexes, complex I and complex III, which also contain iron-sulfur clusters. Immunoblots showed a selective decrease in the amount of the Rieske iron-sulfur–containing protein of complex III in

the mitochondria, but increased amounts of its precursor in the cytosol. These findings suggested that these patients had a generalized defect in the synthesis, mitochondrial importation, processing, or stabilization of a family of mitochondrial proteins that contain iron-sulfur clusters. The disorder appears to be inherited as an autosomal recessive trait, with a common founder effect. The genetic basis of this disorder has not been determined.

Clinical Presentation Patients with combined SDH/aconitase deficiency typically present in childhood with exercise intolerance accompanied by episodes of marked muscle fatigue, weakness and swelling, myoglobinuria, and occasionally, cardiac palpitations (29,30). No clinical follow up has been published recently on patients with this disorder.

Diagnosis The biochemical hallmarks of combined SDH/aconitase deficiency are few. The blood lactate and pyruvate concentrations are normal at rest, but markedly increased with exercise. There have been no reports of abnormal urinary organic acid findings in these patients. A skeletal muscle biopsy specimen stains negatively for SDH, and ultrastructural studies show paracrystalline mitochondrial inclusions and amorphous, iron-rich storage material. Measuring the activity of the iron-sulfur cluster–containing enzymes of the TCA cycle (aconitase) and the respiratory chain (complex I, complex II, and complex III) in a skeletal muscle biopsy will permit the diagnosis to be made.

Treatment No specific treatment for combined SDH/aconitase deficiency is currently available.

Prenatal Diagnosis Combined SDH/aconitase deficiency has not been diagnosed prenatally.

FUMARASE DEFICIENCY

Etiology/Pathophysiology Fumarase (fumarate hydratase; FH) catalyzes the reversible interconversion between fumarate and malate. The enzyme is a homotetramer. It exists in two isoforms: a cytosolic form and a mitochondrial form, which are encoded by the same gene located on chromosome 1q42.1. Within the mitochondrion, fumarate is an intermediate of the TCA cycle, irreversibly formed from succinate by the action of SDH or reversibly formed from malate (Figure 19-2). Fumarate is formed from three sources in the cytosol: 1) fumarylacetoacetate hydratase, in the tyrosine catabolic pathway; 2) argininosuccinate lyase, in the urea cycle; and 3) adenosylsuccinase, in the purine nucleotide cycle. Fumarate itself cannot be

transported across the mitochondrial membrane, but can be indirectly transported from the cytosol to the mitochondrion via the malate shuttle (Figure 19-4). The presumed pathogenetic basis of fumarase deficiency is that it disrupts flux through the TCA cycle, which leads to impaired aerobic metabolism. It is also thought that fumarase deficiency can have secondary metabolic consequences by leading to increased fumarate concentrations in the cytosolic and/or mitochondrial compartments of the cell, which impair other enzymatic reactions (e.g., SDH or glutamate dehydrogenase) or succinylpurine metabolism.

Clinical Presentation Approximately two dozen cases of fumarase deficiency have been described since the disorder was first reported in 1986 (31,32). The clinical manifestations of the disorder primarily involve the CNS, but are quite variable in scope and severity. Patients generally present in infancy and in the mildest cases, fumarase deficiency is associated with relatively mild learning disability. Milder cases manifest with developmental delay and hypotonia. More severe cases can be associated with severe encephalopathy, seizures, and, in a few cases, structural malformations of the brain including hydrocephalus or agenesis of the corpus callosum. The most severe cases, that is, those associated with CNS malformations, can manifest prenatally with polyhydramnios. As expected, survival is also variable, ranging from death in the early childhood to survival into adulthood. Most patients do not present with a profound metabolic acidosis or hyperammonemia, but they might have lactic acidemia. The biochemical hallmark of fumarase deficiency is an abnormal urine organic acid pattern characterized by increased excretion of fumarate and, to a milder extent, succinate and 2-ketoglutarate.

Diagnosis Fumarase deficiency is initially diagnosed by urine organic acid analysis, which invariably shows increased fumarate excretion and, more variably, increased succinate and 2-ketoglutarate. The degree of fumarate excretion is relatively mild (~ 100–200 mg/g creatinine) compared with many of the other organic acidurias (e.g., methylmalonic acidemia) in which excretion of the characteristic metabolites is often 100 to1,000-fold greater than normal during an acute metabolic crisis. Once suspected, the diagnosis can be confirmed by enzyme analysis of white blood cells, cultured skin fibroblasts, or whole tissue biopsy (e.g., liver or skeletal muscle). Mutational analysis of the fumarase gene has recently become available on a clinical basis. Heterozygote detection can be accomplished by enzyme analysis or by mutational analysis (in those cases wherein the mutational defect has been determined for the proband).

Treatment No effective treatment for patients with fumarase deficiency has been demonstrated to date. The suggestion has been made that patients might respond to supplementation with citrate or aspartate, both of which are anaplerotic precursors that are converted to oxaloacetate and might serve to "reprime" the TCA cycle. To date, the efficacy of this approach has not been reported.

Prenatal Diagnosis Prenatal diagnosis of fumarase deficiency has been accomplished by enzyme analysis of cultured amniotic fluid cells or chorionic villus cells alone or in combination with mutational analysis of either cultured amniotic fluid cells or chorionic villus (33,34).

CANCER PREDISPOSITION SYNDROMES ASSOCIATED WITH TCA CYCLE ENZYME DEFECTS

The genetic enzyme deficiencies discussed so far in this chapter have all been autosomal recessive disorders that are expressed by homozygous individuals, with the exception of PDC E1 deficiency, which is an X-linked disorder. All these disorders cause principally neurologic manifestations, albeit with a highly variable range and severity of effects. As would be predicted, the heterozygous (carrier) state for these autosomal recessive disorders has not been found to cause any neurologic problems, either milder or later in onset than those found in the homozygously affected patients. Recently, a rather remarkable association between the heterozygous state for two of the TCA cycle defects, SDH deficiency and fumarase deficiency, has been found to cause predisposition for unique cancer syndromes. In the case of both enzymes, the predisposition is inherited as an autosomal dominant trait. SDH deficiency is associated with pheochromocytoma, paraganglioma, and renal cell carcinoma, whereas fumarase deficiency is associated with multiple cutaneous and uterine leiomyomatosis and renal cancer.

SDH DEFECTS

Etiology/Pathophysiology As discussed above, none of the patients identified with SDH deficiency associated with neurologic manifestations has been found to have homozygous mutations affecting SDHB (except for one case), SDHC or SDHD. However, patients carrying heterozygous germ-line mutations in these genes have been identified as having predisposition for a unique cancer syndrome associated with paragangliomas, pheochromocytomas and/or renal cell carcinoma (35–38).

Paraganglioma and pheochromocytoma are tumors of the autonomic nervous system.

The term paraganglioma is generally used to refer to tumors of the head and neck, whereas the term pheochromocytoma refers to tumors in other sites, such as the adrenal gland, abdomen, and thorax. Most paraganglioma are not endocrinologically active, whereas pheochromocytomas are almost always so.

Four genetically distinct forms of hereditary paraganglioma/pheochromocytoma have been identified: PGL-1, PGL-2, PGL-3, and PGL-4. Genetic studies have shown that PGL-1, PGL-3, and PGL-4 are associated with mutations in SDHD, SDHC, and SDHB, respectively. The genetic basis for PGL-2 has not been identified, but it is thought that it might be caused by mutations in a gene that encodes for a protein involved in SDH assembly or stabilization. SDHD mutations are the most commonly identified cause of hereditary paraganglioma, followed by mutations of SDHB and, much less commonly, mutations of SDHC. SDH mutations have also been identified in cases of sporadic paraganglioma, but the precise frequency of such mutations has not yet been determined.

SDHB, SDHC, and SDHD appear to function as tumor suppressor genes, which act through the classic two-hit model of tumorigenesis. The first "hit" is associated with a germ-line mutation, and the second mutation is a somatic mutation that affects the wild-type allele and occurs later in life. Thus, hereditary SDH-associated paraganglioma syndromes are inherited as autosomal dominant traits, as opposed to the genetic SDHA-associated neurologic disorders that are inherited as autosomal recessive traits.

In addition to this distinction between the SDHA-associated neurologic disorders and the SDH-associated paraganglioma, parent-of-origin studies have demonstrated that SDHD, but not SDHB and SDHC mutations, might be subject to parental imprinting. Paraganglioma only develop in patients who inherited their SDH mutation from their father, whereas the somatic mutation has been identified in the maternally derived wild-type allele. Thus, SDHD appears to undergo maternal imprinting. Recent studies have shown that SDHD expression is biallelic, suggesting that the imprinting is only functional in tissues that develop the characteristic tumors.

Clinical Presentation Paragangliomas are tumors that generally develop in adolescence or young adulthood. In one recent study of the role of SDHB and SDHD mutations in the pathogenesis of these tumors, the mean age of onset for SDHB mutation–positive and SDHD mutation–positive patients was approximately 39 years; the earliest age of onset was 5 years and the oldest age of onset was 65 years (38). Paraganglioma of the head and

neck were more common among patients with SDHD mutations than among patients with SDHB mutations, whereas the reverse was true for extraadrenal abdominal tumors. Patients with SDHD mutations were more likely to have multiple tumors, but less likely to have malignant tumors than were patients with SDHB mutations. SDHB mutations are more likely to be associated with other types of tumors, namely, renal carcinoma or thyroid papillary carcinoma. SDHB and SDHD mutations have also been identified in a substantial proportion of patients who have sporadic paraganglioma.

Diagnosis The diagnosis of paraganglioma, pheochromocytoma, or renal carcinoma is beyond the scope of this chapter. Once the appropriate tumors have been diagnosed, especially in patients with a family history of the same or related tumors, mutational analysis of the SDHB, SDHC, and SDHD genes can confirm the underlying cause of the disorder. Given the relative incidence of mutations of these three genes in these tumors, mutational analysis should begin with SDHD testing, followed by testing for SDHB and SDHC. Patients who present with pheochromocytoma and a family history of multiple endocrine neoplasia type 2, von Hippel–Lindau syndrome or neurofibromatosis type 1, should be evaluated for mutations in the corresponding genes before being evaluated for a possible SDH mutation. Classic metabolic testing is not useful in diagnosing these patients.

Treatment Treatment for the tumors associated with SDH mutations does not entail any effort to manipulate the presumed metabolic basis of the disorder. Genetic testing for the various causative SDH genes will play a role in the treatment of these tumors because different mutations influence the clinical expression of these tumors. Similarly, patients with apparently "sporadic" cases will also need to undergo genetic testing, as they and other members of their families have a considerable risk of being mutation carriers.

Prenatal Diagnosis Prenatal diagnosis of heterozygous SDHB, SDHC, or SDHD mutations is theoretically possible by genetic testing. This has not been accomplished to date and the relative merits of doing so are problematic.

FUMARASE DEFECTS

Etiology/Pathophysiology Classic fumarase deficiency, which produces a range of neurologic problems, is an autosomal recessive disorder. Affected patients inherit one functionally significant mutation from each parent, and the parents have no evidence of neurologic disease. In recent years, heterozygous mutations of the *FH* gene have been shown to cause a very different phenotype—a marked predisposition to develop a highly unusual constellation of tumors, the multiple cutaneous and uterine leiomyomatosis (MCUL) syndrome (39–41).

As opposed to classic fumarase deficiency, MCUL syndrome is transmitted as an autosomal dominant trait, which follows the two-hit model of cancer formation. Thus, fumarase appears to be acting as a tumor suppressor gene. The initial germ-line mutation affects one of the fumarase alleles, whereas the second mutation is a somatic mutation affecting the wild-type fumarase allele. There does not appear to be any difference between the spectrum of mutations seen in classic fumarase deficiency and the germ-line mutations seen in MCUL syndrome. Fumarase activity is very low or absent in affected tissues, consistent with the two-hit hypothesis for the pathogenesis of these syndrome. The mechanism by which the fumarase gene acts as a tumor suppressor gene is not understood.

Clinical Presentation Leiomyomata are tumors composed of smooth muscle fibers. The MCUL syndrome is characterized by multiple small tumors that develop in the skin and uterus. The disorder can develop in late adolescence, but does not usually begin until adulthood. The disorder is characterized by incomplete penetrance.

Diagnosis The diagnosis of the various tumors that have been found in association with fumarase mutations is beyond the scope of this chapter. Once the appropriate tumors have been diagnosed, especially in patients with a family history of the same or related tumors, mutational analysis of the fumarase gene can confirm the underlying cause of the disorder.

Treatment The treatment for the tumors associated with fumarase mutations does not entail any effort to manipulate the presumed metabolic basis of the disorder.

Prenatal Diagnosis Prenatal diagnosis of heterozygous fumarase mutations is theoretically possible by genetic testing for families that have a recognized mutation. This has not been accomplished to date and the relative merits of doing so are problematic.

REFERENCES

1. Robinson BH. Lactic acidemia: disorders of pyruvate carboxylase and pyruvate dehydrogenase. In: Scriver CR, Sly WS, Valle D, et al. eds. *The Metabolic and Molecular Basis of Inherited Disease*. New York: McGraw-Hill; 2001:2275–2295.

2. Kerr DS, Wexler ID, Zinn AB. The pyruvate dehydrogenase complex and tricarboxylic acid cycle. In: Fernandes J, Saudubray J-M, van Berghe GV, eds. *Inherited Metabolic Diseases. Diagnosis and Treatment*. Berlin: Springer-Verlag; 2000:109–120.

3. De Meirleir L. Defects of pyruvate metabolism and the Krebs cycle. *J Child Neurol.* 17 Suppl 3;2002;:3S26–3S33.

4. Lissens W, De Meirleir L, Seneca S, et al. Mutations in the X-linked pyruvate dehydrogenase (E1) alpha subunit gene (PDHA1) in patients with a pyruvate dehydrogenase complex deficiency. *Hum Mutat.* 2000;15:209–219.

5. Brown RM, Head RA, Boubriak II, et al. Mutations in the gene for the E1beta subunit: a novel cause of pyruvate dehydrogenase deficiency. *Hum Genet.* 2004;115:123–127.

6. Brown RM, Head RA, Brown GK. Pyruvate dehydrogenase E3 binding protein deficiency. *Hum Genet.* 2002;110:187–191.

7. Dey R, Aral B, Abitbol M, et al. Pyruvate dehydrogenase deficiency as a result of splice-site mutations in the PDX1 gene. *Mol Genet Metab.* 2002;76:344–347.

8. Maj MC, MacKay N, Levandovskiy V, et al. Pyruvate dehydrogenase phosphatase deficiency: identification of the first mutation in two brothers and restoration of activity by protein complementation. *J Clin Endocrinol Metab.* 2005;90:4101–4107.

9. Robinson BH, MacMillan H, Petrova-Benedict R, et al. Variable clinical presentation in patients with defective E1 component of pyruvate dehydrogenase complex. *J Pediatr.* 1987;111:525–533.

10. Wexler ID, Hemalatha SG, McConnell J, et al. Outcome of pyruvate dehydrogenase deficiency treated with ketogenic diets. Studies in patients with identical mutations. *Neurology.* 1997;49:1655–1661.

11. Stacpoole PW, Kerr DS, Barnes C, et al. Controlled clinical trial of dichloroacetate for treatment of congenital lactic acidosis in children. *Pediatrics.* 2006;117:1519–31.

12. Wexler ID, Kerr DS, Du Y, et al. Molecular characterization of pyruvate carboxylase deficiency in two consanguineous families. *Pediatr Res.* 1998;43:579–584.

13. Garcia-Cazorla A, Rabier D, Touati G, et al. Pyruvate carboxylase deficiency: metabolic characteristics and new neurological aspects. *Ann Neurol.* 2006;59:121–127.

14. Carbone MA, MacKay N, Ling M, et al. Amerindian pyruvate carboxylase deficiency is associated with two distinct missense mutations. *Am J Hum Genet.* 1998;62:1312–1319.

15. Mochel F, Delonlay P, Touati G, et al. Pyruvate carboxylase deficiency: clinical and biochemical response to anaplerotic diet therapy. *Mol Genet Metab.* 2005;84:305–312.

16. Nyhan WL, Khanna A, Barshop BA, et al. Pyruvate carboxylase deficiency—insights from liver transplantation. *Mol Genet Metab.* 2002;77:143–149.

17. Van Coster RN, Janssens S, Misson JP, et al. Prenatal diagnosis of pyruvate carboxylase deficiency by direct measurement of catalytic activity on chorionic villi samples. *Prenat Diagn.* 1998;18:1041–1044.

18. Hanson RW, Patel YM. Phosphoenolpyruvate carboxykinase (GTP): the gene and the enzyme. *Adv Enzymol Relat Areas Mol Biol.* 1994;69:203–281.

19. Vidnes J, Sovik O. Gluconeogenesis in infancy and childhood. III. Deficiency of the extramitochondrial form of hepatic phosphoenolpyruvate carboxykinase in a case of persistent neonatal hypoglycaemia. *Acta Paediatr Scand.* 1976;65:307–312.

20. Clayton PT, Hyland K, Brand M, et al. Mitochondrial phosphoenolpyruvate carboxykinase deficiency. *Eur J Pediatr.* 145:46–50. 1986;

21. Dunckelmann RJ, Ebinger F, Schulze A, et al. 2-ketoglutarate dehydrogenase deficiency with intermittent 2-ketoglutaric aciduria. *Neuropediatrics.* 2000;31:35–38.

22. Surendran S, Michals-Matalon K, Krywawych S, et al. DOOR syndrome: deficiency of E1 component of the 2-oxoglutarate dehydrogenase complex. *Am J Med Genet.* 2002;113:371–374.

23. Hong YS, Kerr DS, Liu TC, et al. Deficiency of dihydrolipoamide dehydrogenase due to two mutant alleles (E340K and G101del). Analysis of a family and prenatal testing. *Biochim Biophys Acta.* 1997;1362:160–168.

24. Grafakou O, Oexle K, van den HL, et al. Leigh syndrome due to compound heterozygosity of dihydrolipoamide dehydrogenase gene mutations. Description of the first E3 splice site mutation. *Eur J Pediatr.* 2003;162:714–718.

25. Odievre MH, Chretien D, Munnich A, et al. A novel mutation in the dihydrolipoamide dehydrogenase E3 subunit gene (DLD) resulting in an atypical form of alpha-ketoglutarate dehydrogenase deficiency. *Hum Mutat.* 2005;25:323–324.

26. Bourgeron T, Rustin P, Chretien D, et al. Mutation of a nuclear succinate dehydrogenase gene results in mitochondrial respiratory chain deficiency. *Nat Genet.* 1995;11:144–149.

27. Parfait B, Chretien D, Rotig A, et al. Compound heterozygous mutations in the flavoprotein gene of the respiratory chain complex II in a patient with Leigh syndrome. *Hum Genet.* 2000;106:236–243.

28. Rustin P, Rotig A. Inborn errors of complex II-unusual human mitochondrial diseases. *Biochim Biophys Acta.* 2002;1553:117–122.

29. Hall RE, Henriksson KG, Lewis SF, et al. Mitochondrial myopathy with succinate dehydrogenase and aconitase deficiency. Abnormalities of several iron-sulfur proteins. *J Clin Invest.* 1993;92:2660–2666.

30. Haller RG, Henriksson KG, Jorfeldt L, et al. Deficiency of skeletal muscle succinate dehydrogenase and aconitase. Pathophysiology of exercise in a novel human muscle oxidative defect. *J Clin Invest.* 1991;88:1197–1206.

31. Zinn AB, Kerr DS, Hoppel CL: Fumarase deficiency: a new cause of mitochondrial encephalomyopathy. *N Engl J Med.* 1986;315:469–475.

32. Kerrigan JF, Aleck KA, Tarby TJ, et al. Fumaric aciduria: clinical and imaging features. *Ann Neurol.* 2000;47:583–588.

33. Manning NJ, Olpin SE, Pollitt RJ, et al. Fumarate hydratase deficiency: increased fumaric acid in amniotic fluid of two affected pregnancies. *J Inherit Metab Dis.* 2000;23:757–759.

34. Coughlin EM, Christensen E, Kunz PL, et al. Molecular analysis and prenatal diagnosis of human fumarase deficiency. *Mol Genet Metab.* 1998;63:254–262.

35. Astuti D, Latif F, Dallol A, et al. Gene mutations in the succinate dehydrogenase subunit SDHB cause susceptibility to familial pheochromocytoma and to familial paraganglioma. *Am J Hum Genet.* 2001;69:49–54.

36. Gimenez-Roqueplo AP, Favier J, Rustin P, et al. Functional consequences of a *SDHB* gene mutation in an apparently sporadic pheochromocytoma. *J Clin Endocrinol Metab.* 2002;87:4771–4774.

37. Aguiar RC, Cox G, Pomeroy SL, et al. Analysis of the *SDHD* gene, the susceptibility gene for familial paraganglioma syndrome (PGL1), in pheochromocytomas. *J Clin Endocrinol Metab.* 2001;86:2890–2894.

38. Neumann HP, Pawlu C, Peczkowska M, et al. Distinct clinical features of paraganglioma syndromes associated with *SDHB* and *SDHD* gene mutations. *JAMA.* 2004;292.943–951.

39. Alam NA, Bevan S, Churchman M, et al. Localization of a gene (*MCUL1*) for multiple cutaneous leiomyomata and uterine fibroids to chromosome 1q42.3-q43. *Am J Hum Genet.* 2001;68:1264–1269.

40. Tomlinson IP, Alam NA, Rowan AJ, et al. Germline mutations in FH predispose to dominantly inherited uterine fibroids, skin leiomyomata and papillary renal cell cancer. *Nat Genet.* 2002;30:406–410.

41. Alam NA, Rowan AJ, Wortham NC, et al. Genetic and functional analyses of *FH* mutations in multiple cutaneous and uterine leiomyomatosis, hereditary leiomyomatosis and renal cancer, and fumarate hydratase deficiency. *Hum Mol Genet.* 2003;12:1241–1252.

CHAPTER 20

Diabetes Mellitus

Constantin Polychronakos, MD
Costa Voulgaropoulos, MD
Zubin Punthakee, MD

NORMAL PYSIOLOGY: CONTROL OF SUBSTRATE FLUX

Overview

Long term health depends on insulin mediated availability of glucose, amino acids and fatty acids to cells as substrates for energy production and cell growth. Diabetes mellitus is the clinical condition of hyperglycemia accompanied by inadequate insulin effect (due to insulin deficiency or impaired insulin action). The metabolic abnormalities in diabetes mellitus are due to a pathologic shift in energy substrate control. Carbohydrates, amino acids, and lipids are all used as forms of energy that must be stored when there is abundance and released for consumption when needed. While energy flux is a complex, multifactorial process, it is largely regulated by a balance between insulin and counterregulatory hormones (glucagon, cortisol, catecholamines and growth hormone) during fasting or in the postprandial state. Insulin's main functions in energy homeostasis are to promote uptake of glucose by muscle and adipose tissue, inhibit glucose production by the liver, and inhibit triglyceride release from adipose tissue. The counterregulatory hormones serve the opposite function during fasting or starvation. During a carbohydrate containing meal, circulating insulin levels rise while glucagon secretion is suppressed by glucagon-like peptide-1 (GLP-1) and amylin. Although most cell types require insulin for optimal glucose uptake, glucose itself can drive some of its own uptake into cells such as muscle (termed "glucose-mediated glucose uptake"), and some tissues, such as the brain, take up glucose independently of insulin or other hormones. Glucose uptake into cells is mediated by specific glucose transporters (GLUTs) (Table 20-1). While glucose is the most important energy substrate, ketones generated from fat breakdown provide a key alternative cellular energy source when intracellular glucose availability is low; fasting, insulin deficiency or

impairment of insulin action result in decrease of intracellular glucose and an increase in ketones production.

Insulin sensitivity and its opposite, insulin resistance, refer to the relative concentration of insulin required to achieve normal extracellular glucose levels. Excessive elevation of counterregulatory hormones as occurs with the stress response to severe illness is associated with insulin resistance. Exercise increases insulin-independent glucose uptake in skeletal muscle (by increasing translocation of GLUT4 to the muscle cell membrane) and in this way induces a state of increased insulin sensitivity.

The liver is the primary storage site of carbohydrate as glycogen, with muscle storing a small amount of glycogen; adipose tissue stores lipid and muscle stores protein that can be liberated for gluconeogenesis.

The liver is primarily responsible for the exchange of these energy forms from one to another. In the presence of a healthy β-cell mass, precise metabolic control of insulin secretion overrides all other hormones to maintain blood glucose within a narrow normal range. In the absence of insulin there is an uncontrollable release of substrate from storage tissues to the extracellular space. Glucose is the substrate most easily detectable and useful for clinical monitoring, but amino acids, lipids, and free fatty acids also rise. Unregulated β-oxidation of fatty acids leads to ketone formation with consequent acidosis, a life-threatening complication of insulin deficiency.

Insulin Synthesis and Secretion

Insulin is produced and secreted by the β-cells of the pancreatic islets of Langerhans. The signal peptide of preproinsulin is cleaved, resulting in proinsulin. Mature insulin is then formed when the C-peptide is removed through cleavage at amino acids 30 and 63, leaving the A chain (21 amino acids) and B chain (30 amino acids) cross-linked to each other through disulfide bonds (Figure 20-1). Equimolar quantities of insulin and C-peptide are stored in vesicles for secretion. Moreover, amylin, a peptide hormone that potentiates insulin action is also synthesized by insulin producing islet cells and is secreted in a 1:20 molar ratio with insulin.

TABLE 20-1 Glucose Transporters

Glucose Transporter	Tissue Distribution	Primary Function
GLUT1	Widespread	General basal glucose transport including across blood–brain barrier, insulin independent
GLUT2	Pancreatic β cells	Glucose concentration–dependent regulation of insulin secretion
	Hepatocytes	Control of glucose homeostasis
	Intestinal mucosa	Glucose absorption
	Renal proximal tubule	Glucose reabsorption
GLUT3	Neurons	Glucose uptake into brain
GLUT4	Adipose tissue	Insulin stimulated glucose uptake
	Skeletal muscle	
	Cardiac muscle	
GLUT5	Intestinal mucosa	Fructose absorption

Diabetes Mellitus

AT-A-GLANCE

Diabetes mellitus is the common end-point of a variety of disorders of insulin production and/or insulin action resulting in hyperglycemia. Diabetes typically presents with increased urination, increased thirst, fatigue, and weight loss, although youth with type 2 diabetes may be asymptomatic. It may present with acute metabolic decompensation with hyperosmolar dehydration and/or ketoacidosis.

Diabetes results from inadequate insulin secretion, which can be absolute or relative to increased requirements because of defects of insulin action. The American Diabetes Association classifies diabetes into type 1 (T1DM), type 2 (T2DM), gestational, and other, which encompasses a wide range of congenital and acquired disorders. The most common form of diabetes in pediatrics is T1DM. Destruction of the β-cells of the pancreas, usually autoimmune (type 1A), eventually leads to complete lack of insulin secretion. The second most common form of diabetes in children is T2DM, which accounts for 8% to 45% of newly diagnosed diabetes in North American children depending on the population studied. T2DM has been increasing worldwide in children since the 1980's concurrent with rising obesity. It results from peripheral and hepatic resistance to insulin coupled with inability of the pancreatic β-cells to compensate. Single gene mutations are responsible for 1–5% of diabetes in children and fall into two categories: neonatal diabetes and maturity onset diabetes of the young (MODY). Gestational diabetes is a temporary form of diabetes that is due to the decline in insulin sensitivity during pregnancy. It is often the harbinger of permanent T2DM or T1DM in the years following pregnancy.

TYPE	PATHOPHYSIOLOGY/INSULIN SECRETION/ INSULIN RESISTANCE	GENETICS	OMIM
Type 1	Autoimmune destruction of β-cells; genetic predisposition plus unknown environmental trigger; eventually absent IS; mild IR in poorly controlled diabetes; IR caused by hyperglycemia rather than being a cause of hyperglycemia	Polygenic, 40–50% of genetic clustering related to HLA DR/DQ	+222100
Type 2	IR plus β-cell insufficiency both required; in youth, invariably associated with obesity; absolute IS increases early (but still a "relative insufficiency" since hyperglycemia is present), with gradual, progressive decline; marked IR due to obesity, genetic or other factors	Multifactorial, strong genetic predisposition, higher prevalence in non-Causasian populations	#125853
Gestational	As with type 2; IR exacerbated by human placental lactogen; IS increases to compensate for IR, but not enough, suggesting the IR has "unmasked" a β-cell defect; marked IR due to placental hormones	As with type 2	N/A
MODY	Impaired β-cell development or glucose stimulated IS; IR not a feature	AD; 6 known types	#606391
Neonatal (Permanent)	Impaired β-cell development or glucose stimulated IS; IR not a feature	AR (including MODY genes) or dominant KCNJ11 gene	#606176
Neonatal (transient)	Transient β-cell defect; decreased IS in infancy, then normal; decreased IS again in early adulthood; IR not a feature	Double dose of paternally expressed gene(s) at 6q24	%601410
Mitochondrial	β-cell defect; decreased IS; IR not a feature	Mitochondrial genes and maternal inheritance	Many
Abnormal insulin	Bioinactive insulin; increased secretion of inactive insulin or proinsulin; IR not a feature	AR	+176730
Abnormal insulin receptor	Abnormal synthesis, trafficking, degradation, binding or phosphorylation of the insulin receptor; markedly increased IS initially; in some cases IS decreases with time; very severe IR	AR	+14760 #246200 #262190
Lipoatrophic	Paucity of adipose tissue leads to lipid accumulation in muscle and liver causing IR; increased IS initially to compensate for IR; severe IR	AR; multiple genes	Many
Cystic Fibrosis Related	Inflammation and fibrosis of exocrine pancreas progresses to affect islet fuction; IS decreases progressively; increased IR with inflammation	CF is AR (CFTR gene)	#219700 *602421
Drugs	Various; transient or permanent damage of β-cells; some drugs cause IR	N/A	N/A
Syndromes	Various; IS decreases eventually in most syndromes; most syndromes have increased IR	Various	Many
Endocrine Disorders	Mostly increase counterregulatory hormone effects; some lead to decreased IS; some endocrine disorders have increased IR	N/A	N/A

AR = autosomal recessive; AD = autosomal dominant; IR = insulin resistance; IS = insulin secretion; MODY = maturity-onset diabetes in the young; CFTR = cystic fibrosis transmembrane conductance regulator.

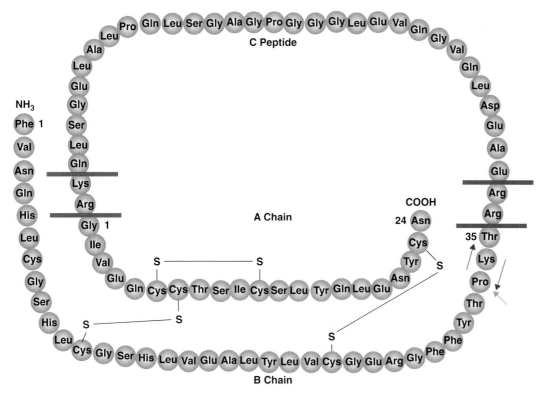

FIGURE 20-1. Structure of the human proinsulin peptide and the cleavage sites that generate the two disulfide-linked chains. Amino acid substitutions in synthetic, rapid-acting insulins are indicated: red arrows show the Lys and Pro residues whose sequence is swapped in Lispro and the green arrow indicates the Pro that is mutated in Aspart.

Glucose-stimulated insulin release is a multistep process that has clinical implications in certain forms of diabetes and hypoglycemic disorders. Glucose enters the β-cell via (GLUT) 2 (Table 20-1) and is then phosphorylated by glucokinase to glucose-6-phosphate. The formation of glucose-6-phosphate by glucokinase in the cytoplasm is the rate stimulating step in the pathway of glucose-stimulated insulin release and supports that glucokinase is the glucose sensor for the β-cell. Glucose-6-phosphate is metabolized in the mitochondria via the Krebs cycle to produce ATP, which raises the cytosolic ratio of ATP:ADP and results in binding of ATP to the ATP-dependent potassium channel. The ATP-dependent potassium channel is an octameric membrane structure consisting of four Kir6.2 subunits, which form a pore for potassium flux across the cell membrane, and four regulatory SUR (sulfonylurea receptor) subunits. In the absence of ATP binding, the channel is open and allows potassium to flow out of the cell across a concentration gradient. When ATPs bind to the Kir6.2 subunits, a conformational change closes the pore to potassium egress, depolarizes the cell membrane and triggers calcium influx via the L-type voltage-gated calcium channels. The increase in intracellular calcium causes

migration of secretory vesicles to the cell membrane and release of insulin (Figure 20-2). Pharmacologic agents make use of this cell physiology to influence insulin secretion. Sulfonylureas bind to the SUR subunit, resulting in channel closure and insulin secretion for treatment of type 2 diabetes and in some forms of neonatal diabetes (1). Diazoxide, a medication used in hyperinsulinism, acts in the opposite manner, stabilizing the channel so it remains open and insulin secretion is suppressed. Other factors can stimulate insulin secretion when glucose levels are not low. Fatty acids acutely enhance glucose-stimulated insulin secretion (2), however chronic fatty acid elevation impairs insulin secretion. Amino acids such as leucine or arginine stimulate insulin secretion by acting as substrate in the Krebs cycle to raise intracellular ATP levels. Incretins are intestinal peptide hormones that are

released during the ingestion of glucose or amino acids and stimulate a substantially greater rise in insulin levels than attributable to the effect of glucose or amino acids (the incretin effect). The incretin effect is responsible for approximately 50% of the insulin response to a meal. Glucagon-like peptide (GLP-1) and glucose-dependent insulinotropic polypeptide are the most important (3), but gastrin, secretin, and cholecystokinin also have minor roles. The GLP-1 mimetic, exenatide and inhibitors of GLP-1 degradation by the protease dipeptidyl peptidase (DPP-IV inhibitors, such as sitagliptin) have been available since 2005 for treatment of type 2 diabetes. In addition to improved glycemic control, these medications may have added benefits of weight loss and preservation of islet cell mass (4), but long term safety has not yet been established.

There are two phases to insulin secretion in response to a glucose infusion. The first phase insulin response (FPIR) is the immediate release of preformed insulin from mature granules, which peaks at approximately 5 minutes and lasts 10 minutes. The second phase starts at 10 to 20 minutes and lasts as long as the glucose infusion continues

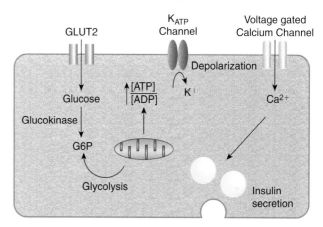

FIGURE 20-2. Insulin release by the β cell is subject to precise regulation, mostly by ambient glucose concentrations. After constitutive entry in the β cell, glucose is phosphorylated by glucokinase, the rate-limiting enzyme that is believed to be an important part of the glucose sensing mechanism. The resulting increase in the ATP/adenosine diphosphate ratio causes depolarization of the membrane by closing K^+ channels, which results in the opening of voltage-gated Ca^{++} channels and insulin release from secretory granules. The K^+ channel is the target of sulfonylureas and mutations of SUR and KIR 6.2, its two protein components, have been involved in both diabetes and hyperinsulinemia.

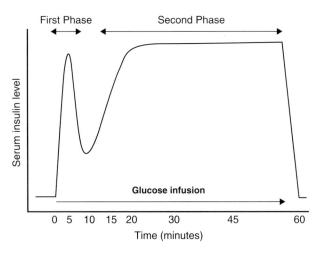

FIGURE 20-3. Illustration of a profile of the two phases of insulin release in response to glucose.

(Figure 20-3). Loss of FPIR occurs prior to development of fasting hyperglycemia and is a marker of β-cell damage. Amino acids such as arginine also stimulate FPIR. These and other tests useful for evaluation of β-cell function are described in the Chapter on Endocrine Testing.

Insulin Action

The insulin receptor is a tetrameric cell-surface receptor composed of two extracellular α-subunits and two transmembrane β-subunits linked by disulfide bridges. The α-subunits form the insulin-binding pocket and the β-subunits are tyrosine kinases, which phosphorylate one another. The activated insulin receptor phosphorylates tyrosine residues on second messenger molecules to activate two major intracellular signaling pathways. The phosphoinositide-3 kinase (PI3 kinase) pathway is mediated primarily by phosphorylation of the insulin receptor substrates 1 through 4, and is responsible for most of insulin's metabolic effects on glucose such as glycogen synthesis in the liver and glucose uptake in muscle. The mitogen-activated protein kinase pathway is mediated by phosphorylation of Shc and is responsible for most of the protein synthesis and cellular growth effects of insulin (5) (Figure 20-4).

Insulin is an anabolic hormone with effects on carbohydrate, lipid, and protein metabolism (Figure 20-5). One of insulin's main functions is to facilitate cellular uptake of glucose, particularly in muscle cells, but also in adipocytes and other cells. It does this by trafficking vesicles containing the glucose transporter GLUT4 to the cell membrane. In the liver, insulin inhibits glycogenolysis and gluconeogenesis, and stimulates glycogen synthesis by upregulating hexokinase, phosphofructokinase, and glycogen synthase. Insulin also stimulates hepatic fatty acid synthesis from glucose and is critical for suppressing hepatic ketogenesis from malonyl-coenzyme A (CoA). In the adipocytes, insulin promotes uptake and prevents release of triglycerides by upregulating lipoprotein lipase and downregulating hormone-sensitive lipase, respectively. Insulin is protein anabolic, primarily by inhibiting protein breakdown.

Another important effect of insulin is increased cell membrane Na⁺K⁺ATPase activity. The consequent shift of potassium into cells makes monitoring hypokalemia critical in the management of diabetic ketoacidosis.

Counterregulatory Hormones

In the management of diabetes, it is important to be aware of the effects of the counterregulatory hormones, which are important for the sensing and avoidance of hypoglycemia. When they are not properly balanced with insulin levels, they contribute to the development of diabetic ketoacidosis. They include glucagon, growth hormone, epinephrine, and cortisol (Table 20-2).

The pancreatic α-cell hormone glucagon stimulates hepatic glycogenolysis, gluconeogenesis from amino acids and glycerol, and ketogenesis. Glucagon acts at the adipocyte to upregulate hormone-sensitive lipase, thereby enhancing lipolysis and free fatty acid delivery to the liver. Catecholamines promote adipocyte lipolysis, hepatic glycogenolysis, and peripheral insulin resistance. Cortisol promotes protein catabolism to provide amino acid substrate for gluconeogenesis, and also impairs peripheral insulin-mediated glucose uptake. Growth hormone increases gluconeogenesis and glycogenolysis and adipocyte lipolysis.

In the infant, cortisol and growth hormone are extremely important for maintenance of fasting blood glucose levels, and their deficiency leads to hypoglycemia. Cortisol deficiency due to autoimmune adrenal insufficiency is a life-threatening condition that occurs more often in type 1 diabetes and typically presents with hypoglycemia. The glucagon response to hypoglycemia is lost for unknown reasons after several years of type 1 diabetes (T1DM). These individuals are able to counterregulate normally, only if their catecholamine response remains intact. If the catecholamine response is lost because of autonomic neuropathy, they are at high risk for life-threatening hypoglycemia.

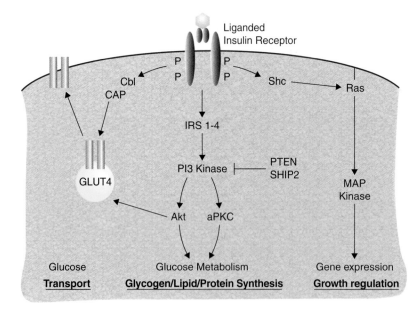

FIGURE 20-4. Mediators of insulin action at the target cell. Ligand binding of the insulin receptor causes a conformational change that allows tyrosine autophosphorylation of the receptor and phosphorylation of substrate proteins. Phosphorylation of cobalamin allows interaction with CAP to initiate trafficking of GLUT4-containing vesicles to the cell membrane for glucose uptake. Phosphorylation of the insulin receptor substrates (IRS) activates the phosphoinositide 3 kinase (PI3 kinase) pathway that, via Akt also traffics GLUT4 to the cell membrane. PI3 kinase also activates the atypical protein kinase Cs (aPKC), which mediates the metabolic effects of insulin. The PI3 kinase pathway is inhibited by PTEN and SHIP2. Finally, the mitogenic and trophic effects of insulin are initiated by sequential phosphorylation of Shc, Ras, and mitogen-activated protein kinase (MAPK), which leads to altered gene expression.

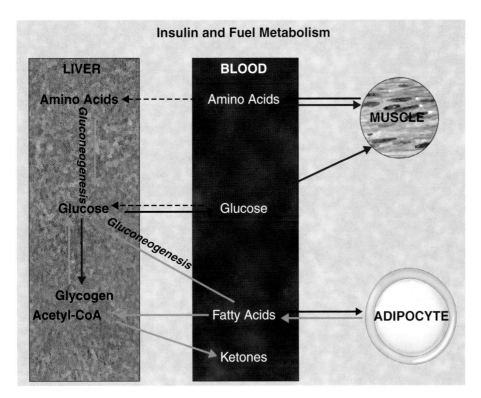

Insulin and Fuel Metabolism

FIGURE 20-5. In the postprandial state, insulin is the major stimulus to peripheral organs to take up substrate for use or storage (blue arrows). During fasting the process is reversed by a reduction in the insulin levels and secretion of counterregulatory hormones, which both result in a catabolic mode that involves release of stored substrate to the circulation (green arrows).

TABLE 20-2	Counterregulatory Hormone Actions		
Counterregulatory Hormone	Effect on Muscle	Effect on Adipose Tissue	Effect on Liver
Glucagon	–	↑ lipolysis	↑ gluconeogenesis
			↑ glycogenolysis
			↑ ketogenesis
Catecholamines	↓ glucose uptake	↑ lipolysis	↑ glycogenolysis
Cortisol	↓ glucose uptake		
	↑ proteolysis		
Growth Hormone	↓ glucose uptake	↑ lipolysis	↑ gluconeogenesis
			↑ ketogenesis

TYPE 1 DIABETES

Epidemiology of Type 1 Diabetes

T1DM is one of the most common chronic diseases in the pediatric age group in populations of European descent, occurring in childhood with an overall prevalence of 0.2% to 0.5%. Although the majority of cases are diagnosed before the age of 18, with peaks at 3 to 6 years of age and the midteens (6), the disease can present as late as the fourth or fifth decade of life. Seasonal variation in new-onset cases has been reported but the most striking epidemiologic feature relates to geographic distribution. T1DM is predominantly a disease of European/Middle Eastern populations. It is less common in Asians and Native Americans. The incidence of T1DM in Africans has likely been underestimated due to scarcity of epidemiologic data and medical care in many areas of Africa (6). In Europe a striking North to South gradient exists with the incidence in Finland as high as 40/100,000 per year, down to 5 to 10/100,000 in southern Europe with a high-incidence "hot spot" in the island of Sardinia (6). Migration studies suggest both genetic and environmental factors as the basis of these geographic differences.

Equally striking is a well-documented secular trend that has seen the incidence of T1DM double in the space of two generations in some countries (7,8). Unknown environmental factors have been postulated to account for this increase. Based on recent patterns, it has been projected that the worldwide incidence of T1DM may be 40% higher in 2010 than in 1998 (7).

Pathophysiology of Type 1 Diabetes

Immunology It is now generally accepted that most cases of T1DM are due to T cell–mediated autoimmune destruction of the pancreatic β-cells (9). From limited autopsy data (10), combined with what is known from the animal models, the non-obese diabetic (NOD) mouse and the Bio-Breeding Diabetes Prone (BB-DP) rat, it has been shown that this destruction is due to infiltration of the pancreatic islets by macrophages, dendritic cells, and lymphocytes (insulitis). Both CD4+ (helper) and CD8+ (cytotoxic) T lymphocytes are involved. Autoantibodies to islet antigens do not cause β-cell damage, but apparently develop secondary to β-cell damage, and are useful as disease markers. The rate of β-cell destruction varies widely between individuals, and not all antibody-positive individuals will develop diabetes. Risk of progression to disease increases with each positive antibody (11,12). The first easily detectable evidence of compromised β-cell function is blunting of FPIR, which is measured by an intravenous glucose tolerance test (described in detail in Chapter 49).

The fact that autoantibodies appear several years prior to the clinical onset of disease indicates that the process of destruction is gradual and long (13). Insulin secretion is initially normal in autoantibody-positive individuals, which provides a window of opportunity to predict and potentially prevent T1DM before much of the β-cell mass has been destroyed (Figure 20-6). Trial-Net, a large multicenter study sponsored by the National Institutes of Health, and its precursor, the Diabetes Prevention Trial (DPT-1), use diabetes antibody screening of first degree relatives of patients with T1DM combined with measurement of FPIR to identify high-risk individuals who might be eligible for diabetes prevention studies.

Autoantibodies can be detected against whole islet preparations (islet cell antibodies), and this has been the standard test for diabetes autoantibody screening for many years. Autoantibodies to insulin, glutamic acid decarboxylase (GAD), and IA2 (also called ICA512, an intracellular phosphatase), may be more specific and sensitive. It is not known how many more autoantigens are involved in T1DM, which one may be the primary trigger of autoimmunity, or if indeed one antigen can be singled out as such.

Stages in Development of Type 1A Diabetes

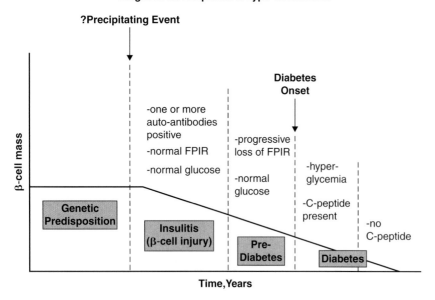

FIGURE 20-6. Schematic diagram of the stages in the development of β-cell autoimmunity and type 1 diabetes.

Genetics Familial clustering and twin studies clearly point to genetic predisposition as a major contributor to T1DM risk. Concordance in monozygotic twins is greater than 40% for clinical T1DM and approaches 70% for islet autoimmunity (12). In dizygotic twins it falls to approximately 5%, the same as that of any siblings, which is again an order of magnitude higher than the general population. Interestingly, offspring of affected fathers have a 6% to 7% risk, more than double that of affected mothers (14). Possible explanations are parental imprinting (silencing of either the maternal or the paternal allele) at one or more genetic loci or the effects of the maternal environment in utero.

T1DM is a multifactorial genetic disease because it does not fit any mendelian pattern of inheritance. Many different susceptibility genes have been identified. Carrying a susceptibility gene places an individual at risk for diabetes compared with noncarriers but does not automatically mean that person will get the disease.

By far the most important diabetes susceptibility genes are found in the HLA region located on chromosome 6p21 in the major histocompatibility complex. Almost half of the genetic risk of T1DM maps to this area. Members of this family of highly homologous proteins involved in antigen presentation are by far the most polymorphic in the human genome, meaning that there are multiple differences among individuals at each gene. This confers a heterozygosity advantage to the host by allowing the presentation of a larger variety of antigens to the immune system to provide greater protection from emerging new pathogens (15).

The major histocompatibility complex is divided into three regions (classes I, II, and III), that contain the different HLA genes.

The terminology for these genes can be confusing. Type 1 diabetes is mostly associated with the HLA class II region, which encodes three proteins called DR, DQ, and DP. Each has α and β chains, encoded by genes A or B, molecules that are expressed on the surface of cells (Figure 20-7) and present antigens to CD4+ T lymphocytes. Each gene encodes a protein and, within the same gene, different protein sequences among individuals are called alleles. Each allele is assigned a number preceded by an asterisk. Thus, DQB1*0302 refers to the allele designated as 0302 at the β chain of the DQB1 locus. Often, single-digit numbers are used instead, referring to results of serologic typing rather than molecular sequences. Thus, the DQB1*0302, sequence corresponds to serotype DQ8 and DQB1*0201 to DQ2. At the DR locus, DRB1*0401 corresponds to DR4 and DRB1*0301 to DR3. T1DM susceptibility is mapped mainly to variants in the DR and DQ genes. Originally it was noted that the great majority of T1DM patients carry the DR3 or DR4 antigens. In Caucasians, the highest diabetes risk is found in individuals who are heterozygous for DR3/DR4, followed

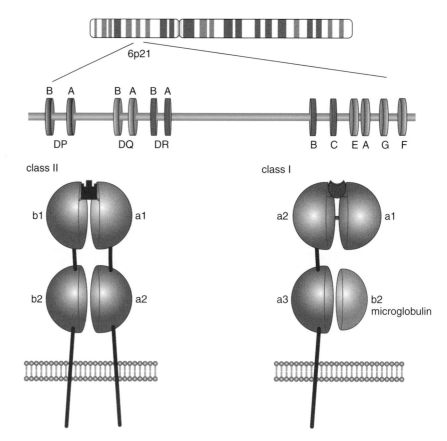

FIGURE 20-7. Position of the class I and class II HLA genes on chromosome 6 and their molecular structure. Class II proteins are dimers of homologous A and B chains, encoded by distinct but adjacent genes. The extracellular portion of each chain has two subunits of which a1 and b1 form the groove that holds the antigenic epitope being presented. Class I molecules have a single chain, two of whose three subunits (a1 and a2) form the groove, stabilized by association with a β2-microglobulin molecule. Antigen can only be recognized by T cells if presented in that groove. Although not as specific as T-cell receptors, grooves of different molecules within each class, and different alleles of each, preferentially bind and present different peptides.

by those who are homozygous for DR4 or for DR3. Although the DR gene almost certainly has independent biologic effects of it own, most of the classically known predisposing effects of DR3 and DR4 are actually due to linkage disequilibrium with DQ, which has now been shown to be the most strongly associated with T1DM susceptibility. Linkage disequilibrium means that these alleles are inherited together, such that DR3 goes almost always together with DQ2 and DR4 with DQ8. The amino acid at position 57 of the β chain of DQ appears to be of critical importance. Alleles encoding an amino acid other than aspartate in that position confer a high risk of T1DM. The most important are DQB1*0302 and DQB1*0201, which correspond to DR4 and DR3, respectively. Aspartate-encoding alleles are generally either neutral or protective. The strongly protective DQB1*0602 (associated with the antigen DR2) is found in 15% to 20% of Europeans but in less than 1% of T1DM-affected individuals. The mechanism by which HLA modulates T1DM risk is the subject of an intense research effort. It is hypothesized that predisposing alleles are poor presenters of T1DM-related autoantigens, which results in inefficient development of self-tolerance. For a concise recent review see reference (16).

The HLA class II locus (IDDM1) is the most significant genetic locus conferring risk or protection for T1DM because it accounts for approximately 40% to 50% of familial clustering. Important as it is, it cannot account for all of the genetic predisposition to T1DM. Most individuals with predisposing HLA genotypes (20%–25% of the European population) are unaffected and the risk to HLA-identical siblings is a fraction of the risk to monozygotic twins, suggesting that additional genes are important. Conversely, the 25% of siblings who share no HLA haplotype with the proband still have a sixfold higher risk of T1DM than the general population (17). This non-HLA component of genetic susceptibility to T1DM is due to cumulative effects of a yet unknown number of other genes. Attempts to discover such loci with genome-wide linkage analysis have ruled out the presence of another locus with a magnitude of effect approaching that of the HLA region, but there are undoubtedly many loci with smaller effects.

Of the 20 or so other loci reported in the literature to be linked to T1DM, only one has been confirmed beyond doubt. Designated IDDM2, it involves the insulin gene and accounts for approximately 5% to 10% of familial clustering. Long alleles at an upstream repeat polymorphism on the insulin gene (called "variable number of tandem repeats") are associated with a two- to threefold reduced

T1DM risk and probably act by enhancing insulin expression in the thymus (18). As with other tissue-specific self-antigens, insulin needs to be expressed in the thymus to induce self-tolerance (19). In parallel to the linkage studies, the candidate-gene approach has also been pursued, again with only two results confirmed beyond doubt. An amino acid substitution in LYP, a phosphatase important in controlling lymphocyte function, has an almost equal effect (20), whereas a much smaller but statistically significant effect has been attributed to noncoding polymorphisms modulating expression levels of cytotoxic T lymphocyte–associated-4 (CTLA4), a gene that encodes important molecules involved in T cell regulation (21,22).

Environmental factors Incomplete concordance in identical twins and a trend over the last couple of generations of increased incidence of T1DM in the absence of changes in ethnic composition are strong arguments in favor of environmental risk factors for T1DM. In experimental animals, no amount of environmental manipulation can induce diabetes in the absence of a susceptible genetic background but, in its presence, risk can be modulated several-fold by manipulations of microbial exposure, diet, and other factors.

Many infectious agents have been proposed to cause diabetes but only congenital rubella is solidly confirmed: 20% of patients will develop T1DM later in childhood, and many will also develop thyroiditis (23). Other infections like cytomegalovirus and Coxsackie virus have an undetermined role in the development of autoimmune T1DM. One postulated but unproven mechanism for this is "molecular mimicry," whereby viral antigens trigger an immune response that cross-reacts with similarly structured β-cell antigens. If an infection is involved in the etiology of T1DM, there is probably a long time interval between the infection and subsequent development of diabetes. Early exposure to a wide variety of pathogens is protective in animal models and such a mechanism has been proposed as an explanation for the lower T1DM incidence in southern compared with northern Europe, where there is less exposure to environmental pathogens (hygiene hypothesis).

Nutritional factors have been incriminated as well, although data are conflicting. In the rodent models, elimination of cow's milk or introduction of fish oil (24) significantly decreases the incidence of diabetes. It has been postulated that exposure to cow's milk antigens in early infancy may directly increase the risk of T1DM, or, alternatively, that it is the absence of breast milk, with its associated antibodies, which is harmful. The Trial to Reduce Insulin-Dependent Diabetes in the

Genetically at Risk (TRIGR) study, a prospective randomized trial of eliminating cow's milk in the first 6 months of life, will define the relevance of this nutritional factor in human T1DM. TrialNet is studying the effect of omega-3-fatty acid supplementation during the last trimester of the mother's pregnancy and/or the first 3 years of life for children at high risk of developing T1DM. The hypothesis is that omega-3-fatty acids have a protective effect on development of autoimmunity by suppressing inflammation.

Next to nothing is known with any degree of certainty about other types of environmental influences on risk for T1DM. Discordance in monozygotic twins, most of whom share the same macroenvironment, indicates that much of the nongenetic component of T1DM etiology is stochastic, that is, the random probability of contracting an infectious disease or the random recombination of the immunoglobulin and T-cell receptor genes in individual lymphocytes.

Diagnosis of Type 1 Diabetes

Clinical presentation The clinical manifestations of diabetes reflect the metabolic abnormalities that arise from insulin deficiency. The earliest clinical stage of diabetes is isolated compensated hyperglycemia with minimal or no symptoms. Insulin is produced at adequate amounts to meet basal needs, but cannot completely rise to meet the increased needs of meals or illness. Blood sugars are mostly in the normal range, but may rise for brief periods into the 200–300 range. Patients at this stage are usually discovered by elevated glucose in screening urine or blood testing done as part of a general physical examination or medical visit for a minor illness.

With further loss of insulin production, a patient will develop persistent hyperglycemia (150 to 400 mg/dl range) which results from excessive hepatic glucose release and unregulated gluconeogenesis. Adipose tissue and muscle are steadily broken down to provide substrate for gluconeogenesis and virtually all patients experience weight loss despite usual or increased food intake. Patients may experience headaches, abdominal pains and fatigue from hyperglycemia. Circulating glucose levels over 180 mg/dl result in osmotic glucose diuresis with symptoms of nighttime urination (nocturia) and urinary incontinence (bedwetting), increased thirst (polydipsia) and increased urination (polyuria). Genital yeast infection may develop due to glucosuria. Eventually a patient is unable to compensate for net loss of body water and chronic dehydration develops, compounding weight loss from tissue wasting and leading to variable degrees of lactic acidosis. Due to the slow and non-specific onset patients typically seek medical attention after 2 to 6 weeks of symptoms. There is initially sufficient pancreatic insulin to limit ketogenesis, however, if insulin treatment is not started, the stress of dehydration or coexisting illness will soon lead to a rise in counterregulatory hormones, unrestrained ketogenesis, and rapid progression to diabetic ketoacidosis (DKA). Diabetic ketoacidosis (DKA) is the most severe and life-threatening stage of type 1 diabetes presentation. DKA occurs in conditions of low insulin levels and elevated counterregulatory hormones (especially glucagon). The importance of glucagon elevation in DKA is underscored by the observation that patients with absence of both insulin and glucagon (as in pancreatic agenesis or cystic fibrosis related diabetes) will develop severe hyperglycemia, but rarely ketoacidosis. In DKA, accumulation of ketoacids and lactic acid leads to a metabolic acidosis, which stimulates an increase in respiratory drive. This causes the characteristic rapid deep breathing of DKA (Kussmaul respirations). Dehydration (typically 10%) results in tachycardia, dry mucous membranes and poor perfusion of extremities. Nausea, vomiting and abdominal cramps are characteristic sign of moderate to severe DKA. It is important to be vigilant to the possibility of co-existing infectious gastroenteritis, acute appendicitis, pneumonia, kidney stones or genitourinary infection, especially if gastrointestinal symptoms, acidosis, urinary ketones and blood count do not improve steadily with the first 6 to 12 hours of rehydration and insulin therapy. DKA results in fatigue and lethargy or irritability, but patients are arousable and oriented. Coma and disorientation are ominous signs and warrant emergency assessment for cerebral edema or other cause of neurological deterioration. Without treatment, diabetic ketoacidosis will result in death within days. With appropriate insulin treatment, T1DM causes little or no short-term symptomatology. Lost weight is rapidly regained and growth continues normally, with a catch-up in the rare cases that have gone untreated long enough to show growth deceleration. Some polyuria and polydipsia may recur during periods of excessive hyperglycemia. Wide glycemic fluctuations may cause transient visual blurring.

Differential diagnosis Transient benign hyperglycemia due to stress may occasionally reach levels of 250 to 350 mg/dL (15–20 mmol/L), a range that overlaps levels seen in new T1DM cases. A negative history for the signs of diabetes (weight loss, polydipsia, polyuria, nocturia), absence of ketosis and presence of acute illness justifies monitoring blood glucose and urine ketones closely for one to several days

to clarify if hyperglycemia is persistent. Hemoglobin A1c is typically elevated in new onset type 1 diabetes mellitus, but will be in the normal range in transient stress-induced hyperglycemia. Insulin or c-peptide levels during stress hyperglycemia will be appropriately elevated, but in new onset T1DM will be inappropriately normal or mildly low. Measurement of diabetes autoantibodies with or without assessment of β-cell integrity by measuring FPIR can rule out early T1DM. Patients who have T2DM may present with hyperglycemia and mildly elevated or normal HbA1c, but will usually have very high insulin levels. The possibility of T2DM should be considered in overweight adolescents, especially from non-Caucasian ethnic backgrounds. Still, it is sometimes unclear at initial presentation if a patient has T1DM or T2DM. In these cases, measurement of c-peptide levels, diabetes autoantibodies (especially GAD65 and IA2) and genetic testing for MODY (especially if there is a family history of dominant inheritance and negative antibodies) will clarify diagnosis and guide long term management recommendations. In a patient with significant hyperglycemia of uncertainty etiology, it is safer to assume early T1DM and begin insulin therapy than to risk serious patient morbidity of untreated T1DM. It is important to keep in mind that ketoacidosis occus in both T1DM and T2DM.

Management of Type 1 Diabetes

The healthcare team Receiving a diagnosis of diabetes is extremely stressful for patients and families and often leads to prolonged anger, grief, and dysfunction regarding diabetes. Diabetes is a demanding chronic health condition that can result in poor quality of life, early, debilitating organ damage, impaired reproductive function and shortened life span. Despite advances in diabetes care technology, many patients (especially adolescents) suffer from poorly controlled diabetes leaving them at risk for emotional problems, episodes of preventable DKA, and long-term complications developing in early to mid adult years. A small percentage (about 10–20%) of patients will readily adapt to having diabetes, maintain healthy self-care habits and have very low risk of having long term complications.

The currently accepted approach to providing successful care is through a multidisciplinary diabetes team in order to provide access to the wide range of services needed to support long term diabetes care. At the center of this healthcare team is the patient (and the family); professional members include physician, nurse educator, dietitian, and social worker, psychologist, child life specialist and pharmacist. The team exists to serve the

patient; the healthcare team should avoid playing the role of 'authoritarian expert' as this creates an obstacle to effective communication. The patient should be guided toward being a 'motivated expert of their own diabetes care' and work collaboratively with the professional members of their healthcare team.

The healthcare team helps the patient master insulin dosing, maintain healthy habits, and cope with feelings of anger, fear, sadness and frustration. The first step is to establish a non-threatening collaborative relationship. Long term diabetes management is a process of rehabilitation and requires continued assessment and anticipatory management of medication regimen, psychological and functional state, social condition. Motivation to adhere to diabetes care tasks (checking blood sugars, taking insulin or other medication, counting carbohydrates) and healthy life habits (sleep, exercise, weight control and avoiding smoking) often needs to be supported by targeted social work and psychological interventions. While diabetes education is essential, it alone does not ensure satisfactory glycemic control.

In addition to assisting patients achieve a high quality of daily living, a large part of the work of the healthcare team is secondary prevention of long-term complications. Most patients experience no hyperglycemic symptoms even when blood sugars are chronically high enough to cause complications. This makes it easy for patients to discontinue healthy diabetes care habits, and makes it a formidable challenge for the healthcare team to maintain patient motivation long term. The Diabetes Control and Complications Trial (DCCT), a randomized controlled trial of intensive management, demonstrated remarkably reduced complication risk in patients maintaining glucose values closer to normal (25,26).

Diabetes management tools The basic tools needed in caring for diabetes are insulin, insulin delivery devices, glucose measuring method and ketone measuring method.

Insulins All insulins currently sold in the United States are based on recombinant human insulin. Regular insulin is unmodified 'short acting' insulin; it begins acting about 30 minutes after injection into subcutaneous fat, peaks after 2 to 3 hours and lasts for 6 to 8 hours. NPH, an isophane suspension of insulin, has a broad absorption peak from 5 to 8 hours after injection and duration of about 10 hours, but unacceptably wide variability in day to day absorption (25 to 45%).

Synthetic insulins have been created by modifying the insulin amino acid sequence or side chain molecules involved in self aggregation. These insulins have altered dissociation kinetics which either consistently delay absorption (basal insulins) or accelerate absorption (bolus or 'rapid acting' insulins). The currently available rapid acting insulins are lispro, aspart, and glulisine; these insulins peak in 30 minutes and have a 3 hour duration of action (though aspart has a slight tail effect extending to 5 hours after injection). The basal insulins are glargine and detemir; these generally have a broad low peak from 2 to 12 hours after injection and subsequently decline with duration from 20 to 24 hours. Glargine insulin, which aggregates at neutral pH, is packaged in acidic solution and as a result, patients may experience brief pain or stinging with injection. Detemir, which acts by binding of its myristic acid moiety to albumin in the interstitial fluid, is in neutral solution and painless on injection.

All insulins will act immediately and equivalently when injected intravenously. In general, all insulins will have a longer duration of action if a very large dose of insulin is taken and conversely, a shorter duration if a much smaller than usual dose is taken. Reducing a 24 hour basal insulin dose by 50% will shorten duration of action to about 12 hours.

Insulin delivery devices These are devices used to inject insulin into the subcutaneous fat for absorption. Insulin syringes provide reliable delivery within the volume error of the syringe size. Syringes are available with 0.5 unit markings to allow for smaller pediatric doses (to estimate 0.25 unit increments, for example). While all patients and families should be taught to use insulin syringes, insulin pens (which deliver doses in 1 unit or in 0.5 unit increments) provide a portable, convenient tool for insulin dosing that appeals to many teens and adults. For younger children (<5 yrs), who because of size have very small insulin requirements, diluted insulin (U-10, U-50, etc.) should be considered. Although this necessitates additional training of family and staff to prevent medication error, diluted insulin allows for reliable administration of very small doses and lowers the risk of hypoglycemia.

Insulin pumps allow for reliable microdosing of insulin (basal rates as low as 0.025 units/hour for the Animas pump and 0.05 units/hour for the Minimed and Deltec pumps and in all pumps, bolus dosing in 0.1 unit increments) that is not possible with U-100 insulin and syringes or insulin pens. Insulin pumps provide flexibility in duration of insulin delivery, insulin dosage calculators that factor blood sugar value and carbohydrate amount, and keep a log of insulin delivered.

Insulin pumps are an excellent method of managing insulin in closely supervised infants and young children. Older children and adolescents who are motivated to use an insulin pump can achieve very good glycemic control, but most find it difficult to consistently change infusion sets every 2 to 3 days and not intermittently miss meal or snack bolus doses. A patient who does not like the idea of using an insulin pump or a patient who is deliberately undermining their insulin regimen should not be started on insulin pump therapy.

Glucose measuring methods Blood sugar measurement by glucometer is essential for assessing insulin doses and determining if symptoms are due to blood sugar extremes. It is important that a patient maintain correct date and time on their glucometer to facilitate downloading data. It is best for patients to maintain a logbook of blood sugars with commentary about activity and meals. Continuous glucose monitoring sensors are devices that consist of a subcutaneous electrode that measures nearly continuous interstitial fluid glucose values but requires at least several glucometer blood sugars values to calibrate the device to real blood sugar range. These are most helpful when coupled with insulin pump therapy to allow titration of basal and bolus dosing and to prevent hypoglycemia.

HbA1c The A1c fraction of nonenzymatically glycosylated hemoglobin (A1C) is the most frequently used indicator of long term glycemic control and a reliable correlate of integrated glucose levels (area under the curve) in the preceding 2 to 3 months. The ADA recommends the measurement of HbA1C levels every 3 months (is that for children and adults??). It should be noted that HbA1c levels do not provide information about the degree of blood glucose variability (amplitude and frequency of glycemic excursions), which can provide information regarding the risk of long term sequelae. Glycemic variability can be estimated by glucometer data but is best assessed by analysis of continuous glucose monitoring. A large discrepancy between hb and glucometer data or patient's blood glucose logs, may be considered evidence of falsification of blood glucose levels by a patient.

Ketone measuring methods During times of illness, measurement of ketones allows assessment of severity of illness and adequacy of hydration state, insulin dosing, and carbohydrate intake. Strips measure acetoacetate in urine and reflect ketogenesis in the 4 to 6 hour period preceding urine void. Capillary blood ketone measurement using a home ketone meter (Precision Xtra™ from Abbott labs) that measures β-hydroxybutyrate provides more immediate information about generation of ketones. Blood ketone measurement can show a decline in ketone level within 30 minutes of effective treatment rather than waiting hours to see the result of a urine ketone test strip. This is a very useful tool for very young children in whom illness may rapidly progress to ketoacidosis and obtaining urine samples may be difficult.

Insulin regimens While there are many different insulin regimens possible, older NPH based insulin regimens have been mostly supplanted by nearly physiologic insulin regimens made possible by short rapid acting insulins, insulin pump technology and basal insulins. Physiologic, or basal/bolus, insulin administration aims to mimic the normal mealtime insulin release (bolus insulin) that matches up to carbohydrate absorption and degree of hyperglycemia and provide a steady, lower level (basal insulin) to suppress catabolism and hepatic glucose output between meals and overnight. The appeal of a basal/bolus regimen from a patient's perspective is decreased hypoglycemia and flexibility of schedule and carbohydrate amount of meals. A basal/bolus regimen requires more diabetes care tasks (injections or insulin pump operations) during the course of the day and may not be feasible for patients with adherence problems. Moreover, in a non-adherent patient, insulin pump therapy often leads to more frequent episodes of diabetic ketoacidosis than an NPH based regimen. In patients who are unable to take a lunchtime bolus dose, a regimen using basal bolus dosing combined with morning NPH may be recommended, though glycemic control will be compromised. Likewise, premixed insulins (70/30 or 75/25) dosed twice a day may be used in patients with poor adherence who require a simpler, though less precise regimen. However, premixed formulations offer much less flexibility with respect to timing and amount of meals. With all insulin dosing plans, it is best to calculate a low dose estimate and titrate upward over days to weeks based on blood sugar response. A summary of the main insulin protocols is depicted in Figure 20-8.

Dose calculation of basal bolus regimens (including CSII) begins with an estimate of total daily insulin (TDI) followed by calculation of the distribution of basal and bolus doses. TDI is based on body mass and is influenced by age, activity levels, degree of insulin deficiency and insulin resistance. Relative basal insulin dose may be low in younger children and in patients with significant endogenous insulin production but can be quite high in patients with insulin resistance. Bolus dosing has two components: carbohydrate grams in a meal or snack and corrective dosing (or insulin sensitivity) which is the amount of insulin needed to bring down current hyperglycemia. The relative amounts of insulin needed for basal and bolus dosing

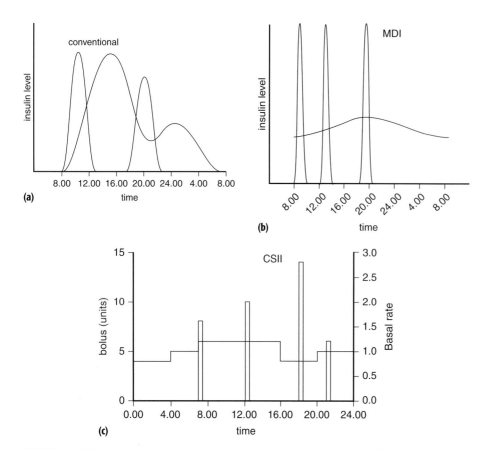

(a) conventional

(b) MDI

(c) CSII

FIGURE 20-8. Schematic representation of the three most commonly used regimes for insulin administration. Top panel: conventional two-dose regime of mixtures of short-acting (regular, lispro, or aspart, dark curve) and intermediate-acting (NPH) insulin (light curve). Insulin administration is planned so that the expected peaks coincide with planned meals. Meals must be fixed in timing and amount of carbohydrate. Middle panel: multiple doses of insulin (MDI) for which rapid-acting insulin (Lispro or Aspart, dark curve) is administered prior to each meal and, sometimes, snack. Coverage between meals is ensured by a steady state of long-acting insulin, such as Glargine (light-colored curve). Insulin dose may vary according to the amount of carbohydrate to be eaten, allowing flexible meal times and amounts. Glargine cannot, however, be adjusted to hour-by-hour changes in insulin needs between meals, such as for exercise, down phenomenon, and so forth. Bottom panel: constant subcutaneous infusion of insulin (CSII) provides the greatest flexibility as, in addition to adjusting insulin boluses (light histogram) as in MDI, it allows programming of the basal rate (dark histogram) to fit the patient's empirically determined insulin-requirement pattern.

have been determined empirically and are summarized in these dosing guidelines for starting a newly diagnosed patient:

1. Calculate total daily insulin (TDI) requirement by age:

    0–7 years: TDI = weight in kilograms * 0.5 = __ units per day

    8–11 years: TDI = weight in kilograms * 0.6 = __ units per day

    12–18 years: TDI = weight in kilograms * 0.7 = __ units per day

2. Calculate basal insulin dose = (TDI * 0.3 to 0.5) units basal insulin once daily

3. Calculate bolus carbohydrate dose by using the '500 rule' (500 ÷ TDI) or the '450 rule' (450 ÷ TDI). The 500 rule estimates grams carbohydrate covered by one unit of Novolog or Humalog insulin; the 450 rule is used with Regular insulin. For example, a patient whose TDI is 30 units and uses Regular insulin, it is estimated by using

the 450 rule that he requires 1 unit per 15 grams carbohydrate; if the patient is preparing to eat a 45 gram carbohydrate meal, then 3 units short acting insulin should be taken 5–10 minutes prior to eating the 45 grams of carbohydrate.

4. Calculate correction dose by using the '1800 rule' (1800 ÷ TDI) or '1500 rule' (1500 ÷ TDI). The 1800 rule estimates the

point drop in blood glucose in mg/dl for every unit of Novolog or Humalog insulin given to correct for hyperglycemia; the 1500 rule is used with Regular insulin. The calculated correction insulin dose is generally not given more frequently than every 3 hours (in order to avoid late hypoglycemia) and is usually added to the meal dose whenever premeal blood sugar is elevated. For example, in a patient whose TDI dose is 30 units and uses Humalog insulin, a 60 mg/dl point drop in blood glucose per unit of Humalog is estimated. If the patient's blood glucose is 270 mg/dl, then 2 units of insulin would be expected to bring blood sugar down to 150. However, if in this example 2 units of insulin lowered the blood sugar to 200, then this would indicate the correction dose is actually 1 unit per 25 mg/dl (Table 20-3).

NPH based regimens are accompanied by a fixed carbohydrate meal plan that includes breakfast, lunch, mid-afternoon snack, supper and bedtime snack. Dosing calculation for twice daily NPH based regimens is also based on kilogram body weight:

1. calculate total daily insulin requirement (TDI) as shown above

2. calculate morning insulin dose (AMI): AMI = TDI * 0.667

3. calculate morning NPH (amNPH): amNPH = AMI * 0.667

4. calculate morning rapid or short acting insulin: amReg = AMI–amNPH

5. calculate evening (pre-supper) insulin dose (PMI): PMI = TDI − AMI

6. calculate evening NPH (pmNPH; given with supper dose or at bedtime): pmNPH = PMI * 0.5

7. calculate evening rapid or short-acting insulin: pmReg = PMI * 0.5

As an alternative to the fixed carbohydrate dose for rapid- or short-acting insulin at breakfast and supper meal described above, these doses may be calculated using the 500 and 1800 rule. If a patient is experiencing overnight

TABLE 20-3   Approximate Insulin to Carbohydrate and Correction Ratios per Age Group

Age Group	Insulin to Carbohydrate Ratio (1 unit per X grams)	Correction Ratio (1 unit per X mg/dl BG)
Adolescents	1:5 to 1:15	1:25 to 1:50
Older children	1:10 to 1:30	1:50 to 1:100
Younger children	1:20 to 1:60	1:120 to 1:300
Infants*	1:100 to 1:300	1:300 to 1:1000

*Infants often require diluted insulin either as injections, or by insulin pump. A 1:10 dilution factor typically provides readily measured volumes in the infant dosing range. Care must be taken to carefully instruct the family on proper dilution technique using diluent made by the same pharmaceutical company that makes the insulin, according to their guidelines. BG = blood glucose.

hypoglycemia, one can substitute the evening NPH with basal insulin, though this substitution would require a rapid or short acting insulin dose for a bedtime snack. The advantage of the NPH regimen is that a child does not need to take insulin at school or for a mid-afternoon snack, but this comes at the cost of increased risk of hypoglycemia if intensive insulin therapy is attempted.

Mealtime insulin administration should be calculated in each instance on the basis of the carbohydrate content of the anticipated meal (meal coverage) and then adjusted to compensate for off-target premeal blood glucose (correction). Rapid-acting insulin for each meal can be prescribed as one unit of insulin per x grams of carbohydrate. This insulin to carbohydrate ratio is approximately 1 U of rapid-acting insulin for every 5 to 15 g carbohydrate for older children and 1 unit for every 15 to 30 g carbohydrate for young children. Such adjustment is straightforward with CSII and MDI but impractical and not recommended for conventional regimens, which must rely instead on a fixed carbohydrate intake for each meal.

Insulin dosages must be constantly re-evaluated because of growth, change of season and activity patterns, school holidays, and so forth. Adjustments are often needed more frequently than every three months during clinic visits. Thus, it is important to keep communication channels open to provide support between visits. Electronic mail and web-based, password-protected uploading of monitoring results are emerging as the most efficient communication means between clinic visits but they cannot replace telephone availability for more complex problems. Adjustments should take into account patterns over several days and should almost never be done on the basis of a single result.

Blood glucose monitoring Daily self-monitoring of blood glucose (SMBG) prandially and at bedtime is mandatory for young T1DM patients. Preprandial checks allow calculation of the correction dosage to be added to the meal dosage. Ideally, 3 hour postprandial glycemia should also be checked, at least occasionally, to evaluate the efficacy of the insulin: carbohydrate ratio. While most current glucometers have similar precision, there are differences in size of blood drop, ability to be downloaded, and stability of time and date settings. Families should be instructed to keep a written blood sugar and food intake log (or alternatively to keep and electronic logbook record) and to frequently check that the date and time settings on their glucometer are correct.

For treatment adjustments, SMBG logs should be viewed column-wise (e.g., all A.M.

tests, because they are all determined by the overnight infusion rate or HS injection) rather than row-wise (good days vs. bad days). Weekly column averages should be compiled and compared with target.

Patients can easily fabricate handwritten records and they often do. Patients may generate false data in their meter as well by using control solution, testing family members or friends, etc. With increasingly tamper-proof meters, memory uploads are much more reliable and patients should be asked to always bring their meters along with the logbook for possible verification. Fingertips should be tactfully inspected for lancet marks commensurate with the number of tests reported. Evidence of deception should be pointed out to the patient in a nonconfrontational, empathic manner (an important skill that takes time to master) the physician should explore the patient's circumstances that motivates fabrication (for example to avoid punishment from parents or feelings of self-disappointment).

It should be kept in mind that conventional SMBG only captures distinct time points, between which large glycemic fluctuations might occur. Constant glucose monitoring is now possible with disposable subcutaneous sensors connected to a portable device. These devices measure interstitial glucose levels and require calibration with blood glucoses (from fingerstick testing) a minimum of twice per day. Some systems give the results in retrospect at the end of 72 h, useful for pattern analysis and long-term adjustments. Recently introduced real-time monitoring improves insulin dose adjustment. Glucose sensors reliable enough to be used for automatic control of "smart" CSII pumps will enable feedback control similar to that of the cell and represent the most realistic hope for a true breakthrough in diabetes management over the coming years. In the meantime, conventional SMBG remains indispensable. Evaluated against constant glucose monitoring, testing four times a day was found to provide a good overall picture (25).

Routine testing for ketones is not necessary. Ketones should be tested when blood glucose levels are high on two or more consecutive tests or when patients are ill, regardless of blood sugar. Continued elevation of ketones despite insulin treatment of blood sugars indicates inadequate carbohydrate intake or ongoing systemic inflammation. Persistent large elevation of ketones in an apparently well, euglycemic patient can be the first sign of an impending acute severe illness, such as influenza and appendicitis; ketogenesis can begin 1 to 2 days prior to the onset of clinical symptoms. Measurement of blood ketone by ketometer can also distinguish if an

unexpected high blood sugar is due to missed insulin doses (ketones elevated) or overeating (ketones normal).

Other aspects of monitoring Physical examination for growth and weight gain, pubertal development, presence of goiter or other signs of hypothyroidism, hydration status, blood pressure, and lipohypertrophy at injection sites should be done at each visit. A decline in growth rate warrants evaluation for hypothyroidism, celiac disease, or systemic cause of growth failure. Poorly controlled diabetes can impair normal growth. Mauriac syndrome, originally described in the 1930s and seldom seen anymore, is an extreme example of this and consists of growth retardation, truncal obesity, round facies, and hepatomegaly. Annual laboratory testing for dyslipidemia with a fasting lipid profile, autoimmune hypothyroidism with thyroid stimulating hormone (TSH) and celiac disease with serum markers (e.g., tissue transglutaminase IgA) may detect these conditions at an early stage. Screening for markers of autoimmune thyroiditis (antithyroglobulin and thyroid peroxidase antibodies) should also be part of the initial screening effort.

Patients over the age of 10 years who have had diabetes for at least 3 to 5 years should have an annual retinal screening examination and random urinary microalbumin/creatinine measurement. Although foot problems are rare before adult years, an annual foot examination in adolescence is recommended, in part to promote good foot care habits. Screening for depression should be routinely performed on all children over age 10 years. Lastly, because the prevalence of eating disorders are greater in the pediatric diabetes population, providers should consider this diagnosis in patients and refer to a treatment program when a clinical history is suspicious.

Nutrition Highly regimented eating (being forced to eat when not hungry or being denied food when hungry) can often lead to enduring anger and resentment in the pediatric patient. A flexible meal and insulin regimen that accommodates a child's appetite can lessen food conflicts.

Diabetes nutrition management for patients on basal bolus dosing regimens is largely an effort to match insulin dose to carbohydrate intake. Carbohydrate counting is a method of determining the total carbohydrate content of a meal then calculating the corresponding insulin dose based on insulin to carbohydrate ratio. Carbohydrate counting is a core component of diabetes education and allows for tighter glycemic control and systematic dose adjustment. Patients who are illiterate or have math learning difficulties, however, may not be able to master carbohydrate counting and may do better with fixed meal plans.

In general, children with diabetes are instructed to avoid foods with high sugar content. Unfortunately, most foods successfully mass marketed to children are quite high in sugar. The absorption curve of rapid acting insulin is a relatively slow process (0.5–3 hours) compared to glucose absorption (10–30 minutes) This difference often leads to early post prandial hyperglycemia followed by late and potentially serious post prandial hypoglycemia, particularly in young children who are given their insulin after meals. Unless closely supervised and taught prudent eating habits, children with easy access to sugar containing foods will have frequent hyperglycemia due to inability to limit their sugar intake.

For routine meal planning, selecting foods with high fiber, low glycemic index carbohydrates and low total fat content is the best choice for T1DM and T2DM (26). The absorption curve of carbohydrate from unprocessed foods (for example, whole grains and legumes) and mixed meals is closer to the action time of insulin and leads to smoother blood sugar control. High fat foods, such as pizza, cause hyperglycemia 3 to 5 hours after a meal requiring 10-20% higher meal insulin dosing; in patients using an insulin pump, square or dual wave insulin dosing is recommended for high fat meals. If using an insulin pump, may use square or dual wave dosing. Low carbohydrate diets lead to excessive elevation in fatty acids and ketonemia and are not recommended.

A population of children with T1DM and obesity are becoming increasingly observed in clinics. In these children excess caloric intake and appropriate matching with insulin can lead to exogenous obesity and insulin resistance. The addition of metformin to standard insulin requires insulin regulation and tightening of glycemic control (27–29). Perhaps most importantly, preventative changes to diet by using caloric restriction may be necessary to prevent exogenous obesity and insulin resistance. Lastly, since diabetic adolescents are at higher risk of deficiencies in other nutrients such as calcium and magnesium, presumably due to intermittent hyperglycemic diuresis, a daily multivitamin or calcium supplement is generally recommended.

In NPH based regimens, the timing and carbohydrate content of meals should be matched with the anticipated peaks of insulin doses.

Exercise Physical activity, and particularly resistance training with weights, increases insulin sensitivity independently of its effect on adiposity and for this reason is encouraged in all patients with diabetes. Patients in the honeymoon phase and young children in the first 2 years of their diabetes are at risk for developing hypoglycemia within 30 to 60 minutes of starting exercise. These children may be provided a small snack with start of exercise. In patients who no longer have endogenous insulin production, however, blood sugar will rise sharply in the first 15 to 20 minutes of vigorous exercise due to catecholamine release, then by 45 to 60 minutes of exercise return to pre-exercise level, and then drop to hypoglycemia range by 90 minutes after initiation of exercise. In order to prevent exercise-associated hypoglycemia, an 'exercise snack' of 15 to 25 grams carbohydrate—without a corresponding insulin dose—should be taken after every hour of strenuous exercise. For prolonged physical activity, such as hiking or long bicycle trips, an exercise snack should be taken after every hour of activity. Late hypoglycemia due to muscle glycogen depletion may occur 6 to 12 hours after prolonged physical activity and can be prevented by lowering basal insulin doses by 20 to 50%.

Discontinuing insulin during exercise is not recommended. During activities that prohibit wearing a pump, patients should be taught to take a 'disconnection bolus' of insulin prior to every hour of pump disconnection. The amount of the disconnection bolus is typically equivalent to 50 to 100% of the amount of basal insulin that will be missed during the subsequent hour of disconnection. Athletic patients may benefit from using a pump that includes the disconnection bolus as an option on the dosing display.

The importance of long-term exercise, especially in sedentary individuals, should be emphasized—a goal of the healthcare team is to motivate patients to exercise 60 minutes daily. This may include chores, organized sports and home play or exercise sessions. For patients who are not involved in a rigorous organized sport, physicians may prescribe evaluation and training sessions by an exercise physiologist. Adolescents who are involved in demanding sports such as wrestling or long distance running will often experience a significant reduction in insulin need and improvement in HbA1c values for the duration of the sport season.

Overall treatment goals The fundamental treatment goal for all patients and families is smooth transition back to normal life after initial diagnosis and long term functioning with diabetes. Children with diabetes should not miss school more often than non diabetic peers. They should be provided with age-appropriate supervision at school for blood glucose monitoring before meals or if feeling ill, and insulin dosing with meals. It is essential for children to have their classmates and teachers educated in the facts of diabetes in an engaging way to establish a supportive atmosphere at school. In this way, a child with diabetes will not feel isolated or flawed and will not be subject to maltreatment in school.

Treatment goals for glucose levels and hemoglobin A1c The basic glycemic treatment goal for all patients with T1DM is to achieve blood glucose levels as close to normal without excessive hypoglycemia and without an unreasonably complex medication regimen.

The proximity to near normal blood sugars can be influenced by the type of treatment regimen used. Selection of treatment regimen depends on patient preference and medical assessment of appropriateness. A motivated patient following a carbohydrate prudent diet, exercising regularly and using a basal bolus regimen via pump or subcutaneous injections can reach HbA1c goals in the 6.5 to 7 range without significant hypoglycemia. Moreover, the addition of Symlin (pramlintide), a human amylin analog, can prevent the 2 hour prandial blood sugar peaks that frequently accompany insulin only regimens (30). A HbA1c of under 7.5% in patients on premixed insulins (such as Humalog or Novolog with NPH or Novolog 70:30 or Humalog 75:25 preparations) may be difficult to achieve without incurring excessive hypoglycemia. Patients suspected of non-adherence to diabetes care tasks, but who nonetheless achieve HbA1C values below 7.5%, may have an intercurrent disorder of malabsorption such as celiac disease. Glycemic goals set by the American Diabetes Association (ADA) vary according to age range (see Table 20-4).

Reducing A1C from 9% to 7% over a few years was found by the DCCT to reduce risk of nephropathy by half and retinopathy by three quarters and significant cardiovascular events by 42% (31,32). The benefit of

TABLE 20-4	Glycemic Goals By Age		
Years	**Preprandial BG**	**Bedtime BG**	**HbA1c**
0–6	100–180	110–200	7.5–8.5%
6–12	90–180	100–180	<8%
13–19	90–130	90–150	<7.5%

BG = blood glucose.

reducing A1C below 7% has not been validated and raises the issue of exceeding the range given the exponentially increasing effort and risk of hypoglycemia associated with further reducing A1C levels. An A1C result should only be interpreted if the method and reference range are known. Methods certified by the DCCT standard (33) can be cautiously used to estimate complications risk and compare results from different centers but, ultimately, A1C levels are most useful in monitoring patients in comparison to themselves over time.

Diabetic Ketoacidosis (DKA)

DKA is a life-threatening emergency and occurs in three clinical circumstances: new onset type 1 diabetes mellitus, complete insulin omission in an individual with established diabetes and in acute severe illness with inadequate insulin dosing. Progression of DKA is usually preventable if recognized early and treated with increased oral fluids, insulin and carbohydrate. Home management of hyperglycemia and ketosis may include using 1.5 to 2 times the usual corrective insulin dose, providing oral fluids of 10 to 20 ml/kg every 4 to 6 hours and frequent carbohydrate snacks with corresponding insulin. Mild to moderate DKA (bicarbonate 10 to 15) in a patient who is not vomiting may be managed with oral or intravenous fluid therapy and subcutaneous insulin. Antiemetics, such as ondansetron (Zofran) may be helpful to curtail emesis and allow rehydration therapy to reverse ketoacidosis. A patient who has been repeatedly vomiting and has reached severe dehydration of DKA will typically have a bicarbonate level of <10 and pH of ≤7.2. Sodium, calcium, phosphorus and potassium wasting occurs and necessitates intravenous fluid and electrolyte therapy. Standard practice is to use intravenous insulin therapy (insulin drip) which allows for finer titration of insulin, fluid and glucose delivery to control time course of recovery. DKA is the leading cause of morbidity and mortality in children and vigilant monitoring for cardiovascular collapse, electrolyte disturbances and cerebral edema are paramount at the initiation and throughout the course of therapy.

Treatment should aim to restore fluid volume and electrolyte balance and reverse the metabolic derangement over a 24 to 48 hour period by the judicious use of insulin, glucose and IV fluid therapy. Reliable intravenous access is a must and for critically ill patients, central venous line, arterial line and foley urine cather may be necessary.

DKA treatment protocols consist of 3 sequential overlapping phases: rehydration,

insulin therapy and glucose delivery via IV route. A bolus of saline (10 to 20 ml/kg over 1 hour) will stabilize circulation while the intravenous insulin infusion is being prepared. Tachycardia is a finding correlated with low intravascular volume. In a patient who has massive diuresis equal to or exceeding the volume of the initial rehydration bolus and remains very tachycardic or showing signs of poor perfusion, it is necessary to repeat this initial saline bolus. Potassium should be added as soon as it has been established that the patient has urine output, even if K is on the high side of normal, to anticipate the massive intracellular shift as insulin reverses the catabolic state. After normal saline bolus, hydration and electrolyte replacement is continued by switching to IV fluids to 0.45% NS with 20 mEq/L KAcetate and 20mEq/L KPhosphate at a rate of 3000 to 3500 ml/m2/24 hours. The risk of osmotic complications can increase with accelerated reduction of serum sodium concentration, thus it is preferable to let a patient maintain upper normal or even slightly elevated serum sodium levels in the first 24 hours. Providing excessive chloride by using KCl may lead to development of hyperchloremic metabolic acidosis, especially in young patients.

After the initial rehydration bolus, serum glucose will drop several hundred points (to approximately 400 mg/dl) due to enhanced renal perfusion and glucosuria. Regular insulin is started as an infusion of 0.05 units/kg/hour in very young children to 0.1 U/kg/hour for adolescents. Blood glucose should be monitored hourly and when levels reach 300, 5% dextrose added to the IV fluid. Dextrose and insulin delivery should be titrated upward to produce slow steady rise of bicarbonate value (about 0.5 to 1 mmol/L rise per hour) while keeping serum glucose in the 200 to 300 range until bicarbonate is normalized. If acidosis persists despite apparently appropriate insulin therapy one needs to consider other causes of acidosis (and appropriate intervention): for example, inadequate glucose delivery to stop ketogenesis (treat by increasing insulin and glucose administration); continued severe dehydration with lactic acidosis (give additional fluid bolus); unrecognized underlying infection (evaluate CBC with differential, CXR etc.); or another acute inflammatory condition (such as cholelithiasis or nephrolithiasis), hyperchloremic acidosis (remove excess chloride from IV fluids; see above), urinary or stool bicarbonate losses (obtain nephrology or gastroenterology consultation, respectively).

Acute cerebral edema, a complication of DKA that occurs more often in the pediatric

age group remains a potential neurosurgical emergency in the first 24 to 36 hours of treatment. A review of 69 cases of intracerebral complications of DKA found that children younger than 5 years of age, and especially children younger than 3 years of age with new-onset diabetes are particularly at risk (34). Although still debated, the rate of hydration, tonicity of administered fluid, rate of correction of glycemia, and degree of serum sodium decrease have not consistently linked to increased rates of cerebral edema. Nevertheless, most clinicians feel that until the etiology of cerebral edema is better understood, it is best to avoid rapid changes in hydration or osmolality. Another study suggested that treatment with bicarbonate increases the risk for cerebral edema, but this retrospective review was flawed by the fact that the children who received bicarbonate were more acidotic and dehydrated at presentation than those who did not (35). Perhaps more important is to provide immediate intervention when there are definite signs of neurologic deterioration as this has been associated with better outcomes (36). Thus, the patient should be closely monitored with mental status evaluation and vital signs. Treatment for suspected cerebral edema is with infusion of mannitol at dosages as high as 1 g/kg of body weight. The value of hyperventilation is questionable. A sample protocol for the management of DKA is given in Table 20-5. An alternative approach using subcutaneous insulins is available from the ADA (37).

In established patients, it is important to involve the diabetes healthcare team once the patient is nearly ready for discharge in order to clarify the cause of dysfunction that led to DKA and to provide targeted education, counseling and follow up support. Social and psychiatric evaluation is mandatory in recurrent DKA cases.

Special Circumstances in Type 1 Diabetes

Hypoglycemia Hypoglycemia is the most common acute complication in T1DM. The symptoms of mild hypoglycemia (glucose <60 mg/dL or 3.3 mmol/L) are due mostly to compensatory sympathetic stimulation: tremors, pallor, cold sweat, and palpitations. With progressively lower glucose levels, symptoms of neuroglycopenia predominate: fatigue, lightheadedness, confusion, loss of consciousness, and convulsions. Severe hypoglycemia is generally defined as that requiring assistance from another person due to profound confusion or loss of consciousness. Frequent bouts of hypoglycemia can result in "hypoglycemia unawareness," in

TABLE 20-5   Sample DKA Protocol

DIABETIC KETOACIDOSIS ORDERS
(pH < 7.30, bicarbonate < 15 mmol/L)

DATE: _____   TIME: _____   PATIENT WEIGHT: _____

1) INVESTIGATIONS:

Blood Glucose, Urea, Creatinine, Blood Gas

Electrolytes, CBC

Urine glucose + ketones

S
T
A
T

2)   INITIAL FLUID BOLUS -NORMAL SALINE

Dehydration   < 5%:   no bolus

Dehydration   5%:   5 mL/kg

Dehydration   10%:   10 mL/kg

SHOCK: 20 mL/kg

Bolus: _____mL

3) POST-BOLUS FLUID ORDERS – NORMAL SALINE*:

(1/2 Deficit _____ mL - Bolus _____ mL) / 12 (based on 12 hr) = _____ mL/hr

+ Insensible loss _____ mL/hr

+ Urine output _____ mL/hr

= Subtotal: _____ mL/hr

Minus insulin infusion (** see below): _____ mL/hr

HOURLY FLUID RATE: _____ mL/hr

4) MEDICATIONS: INSULIN: Regular

**Infusion 0.1 U/kg/hr = _____ mL/hr IV

Mix 10 U in 100 mL of normal saline = 0.1 U/ mL

Therefore infusion rate (mL/hr) = weight in kg/hr

5) ADDITIONAL GUIDELINES:

A)   After 2 to 3 hr of 0.9% saline, consider switching to 0.45% saline at same rate if patient is not hyperosmolar.

B)   When blood glucose < 17 mmol/L (300 mg/dL), add 5% or 10% dextrose to IV fluid. *

C)   When K^+ < 5.5 mmol/L and child is voiding, add 20mEq KAc/L and 20mEqKPhos/L to IV fluid.

D)   After 12 hr, recalculate the fluid orders to correct the remaining deficit over the next 24 hr.

* Use at least D5% regardless of starting blood sugars if <5 years old.

6) MONITORING:

A)   Vital signs q 30 to 60 min., including GCS.

B)   100% oxygen by mask, if patient is in shock.

C)   Cardiac monitor.

D)   Diabetic flow sheet - strict hourly Ins and Outs.

E)   Bedside glucose every 1 to 2 hr.

F)   Blood glucose, electrolytes, blood gases every 3 to 4 hr.

G)   If patient is unconscious, insert a Foley catheter.

H)   If patient is vomiting, insert an N/G tube and/or give anti-emetic.

Signature _____

which progressively lower blood glucose levels are needed to elicit a catecholamine counterregulatory response. Without catecholamine symptoms as a warning signal, patients with hypoglycemia unawareness are at risk for severe hypoglycemia.

Rates of severe hypoglycemia are higher in children younger than 6 years of age, likely related to the age at which a child is able to recognize and articulate symptoms of hypoglycemia. There is concern that recurrent or severe hypoglycemia might lead to cognitive impairment in very young children with T1DM, but this has not been shown conclusively. Occasional mild hypoglycemia that does not impair the patient's ability to self-treat by taking some readily absorbable glucose might be considered the "price to pay" for good glycemic control.

Patients and families should be taught to recognize and appropriately treat hypoglycemia and to anticipate and prevent it under high-risk situations (such as increased activity, decreased carbohydrate intake). Glucagon should be available in the home and at school for prompt treatment of severe hypoglycemia. Some adolescents will develop anxiety and phobic behavior regarding hypoglycemia. If not recognized and openly addressed, it can lead to chronic emotional distress as well as uncontrolled diabetes; these patients benefit from counseling by a diabetes knowledgeable psychologist, sometimes in conjunction with anti-anxiety medication as well as being encouraged to use a low hypoglycemia risk regimen, such as CSII with real-time continuous glucose sensor.

Honeymoon At the time of diagnosis, a sufficient residual β-cell mass is still present in most T1DM patients, to be capable of regulated secretion of some insulin. Acutely, hyperglycemia inhibits insulin secretion ("glucotoxicity"), but once good near normal glycemic control has been established with exogenous insulin, those cells that have not been destroyed by the autoimmune process are able once again to secrete insulin. As a result, diabetes can be managed with lower doses of exogenous insulin.

It is important to prepare the family and patient for the eventual end of the honeymoon phase. When meeting with families, discuss insulin dosing in terms of estimated total daily insulin requirement (~ 80% of kilogram body weight), then explain what portion of TDI is being recommended as injected insulin. In this way, patient and family will not become alarmed when insulin needs increase and will have a sense of what range of dosing their child may need when the honeymoon phase ends. Families that do not understand the limited time frame of honeymoon dosing recommendations will often continue giving inappropriately small insulin doses for months or years after the honeymoon phase has ended.

Unfortunately, the honeymoon phase can reinforce unhealthy adaptation to diabetes for many children. Adolescents patients who are not closely supervised will test the limits of self-diabetes care and find they can skip insulin doses and blood sugar checks without any apparent penalty to health or HbA1c. An attitude of denial and poor adherence often becomes established during this time and is then complicated by despair, anger and frustration when the honeymoon phase ends. The healthcare team should be alert to this pattern and provide anticipatory support.

Illness and surgery During acute intercurrent illness, glucose levels may rise through the counterregulatory action of stress hormones or fall because of reduced food intake. For all ill patients, it is important that adequate fluid, insulin and carbohydrate be provided to prevent progression to secondary DKA. Skipping carbohydrate and insulin is a common mistake for patients who experience loss of appetite during illness but have (initially) near normal blood sugars. Over a periods of 6 to 8 hours, the lack of insulin and ingested carbohydrate leads to an exponential rise in hepatic glucose release, ketogenesis and ultimately, DKA. The correct approach in a patient with loss of appetite is to recommend small doses of insulin along with carbohydrate (which may be taken as sips of sugar-containing soda pop or juice) every few hours to prevent ketogenesis. Adequate water must also be taken throughout the day to prevent dehydration, which can interfere with insulin absorption and raise counterregulatory hormone levels.

Patients on insulin pump therapy who are experiencing hyperglycemia during illness may try using a temporary basal rate increase of 20 to 30%, but will typically need to switch to injections during moderate or severe illness. CSII and MDI dosing schedules can easily scale insulin amount to adjust for reduced intake but patients following NPH-based regimens should be warned not to take their usual insulin dose if they feel they will not be able to eat their fixed meals. Such patients can be managed ad hoc, on an improvised MDI schedule that errs on the side of underdosing. A small amount of ketones is normal even in nondiabetic ill children but its presence indicates that insulin must be given, in however small amounts.

Training families to manage sick days should be part of initial diabetes management and reinforced at outpatient visits. Nausea and vomiting are problematic because they can rapidly lead to dehydration and ketoacidosis that requires emergency department intravenous rehydration or hospitalization. Using Ondansetron (Zofran) (at doses of 2 mg for children weighing 8 to 15 kg, 4 mg for children weighing more than 15 kg and up to 30 kg, and 8 mg for children weighing more than 30 kg) at the start of nausea or emesis can prevent dehydration and allow a child to recover from a viral gastrenteritis or other minor acute illness at home. If there are any questions, however, as to the etiology of emesis or if the child continues having emesis despite Ondansetron, then emergency medical evaluation is indicated. Other antiemetics, such as Tigan (trimethobenzamide) and Phenergan (promethazine) carry higher risks of adverse effects of Ondansetron; Phenergan is sedating and should be avoided.

For the child in whom unrelenting vomiting or food refusal is interfering with the ability to deliver sufficient insulin because of hypoglycemia, a "mini-dose" glucagon rescue has been proposed (38). A typical U100 insulin syringe is used and children 2 years and younger receive two "units" (20 g) of subcutaneous glucagon, and those older than 2 years receive one unit per year of age up to 15 units (150 g). This dose can be doubled and given again 30 minutes later if hypoglycemia does not resolve. The reason a standard dose of glucagon (500–1000 g) is not given is that the higher dose might make the vomiting worse.

Much the same considerations apply during surgery. Frequent glucose monitoring and frequent or continuous administration of short-acting insulin must be instituted, according to any of a number of protocols, until the patient returns to oral intake.

Travel Patients and families should be sensitized to the need for planning T1DM management during travel ahead of time and for assuring that all diabetes-care equipment and supplies are packed in carryon luggage. Traveling across time zones shortens or lengthens the duration of the day or night, which is a problem for patients on conventional regimes. Patients on insulin pump therapy can simply adjust the time on their pump to whatever the local time is whenever they are in a new time zone. The decreased activity of long distance travel typically leads to higher blood sugars. Adjustments to the NPH dose and/or improvised MDI schedules should be planned with the care team as soon as the itinerary is available. If insulin must be purchased in another country it should be kept in mind that all insulin in the United States is bottled as 100 unit/cc (U100); the concentration is not necessarily the same in other countries.

"Brittle" diabetes This is a condition of uncontrolled diabetes characterized by erratic wide fluctuations in blood sugar and repeated episodes of DKA and/or hypoglycemic seizure. The majority of individuals who develop brittle diabetics have psychological problems and use diabetes disruption (with frequent need for emergency medical care) for secondary gain. In addition, chronic recurrent emotional stress may lead to catecholamine elevations that result in unexpected hyperglycemia and DKA. Non-psychological causes include irregular insulin absorption due to injection into lipohypertrophied sites, variable intestinal carbohydrate absorption due to celiac disease or autonomic gastropathy, alcohol or other substance abuse, and adrenal insufficiency should all be considered.

Psychosocial problems Psychosocial problems are very common in children with diabetes and their families and almost always interfere with adherence to diabetes care recommendations. Up to half of children with diabetes may develop depression, anxiety, or conduct disorder (39). Eating disorders are a serious and common problem in adolescents with diabetes and are characterized by skipped insulin doses in an effort to control weight and purge for binge eating. This type of diabetes bulimia most often occurs in intelligent, otherwise highly functioning girls and often leads to recurrent DKA and chronic poor control.

It is recommended that parents do not relinquish complete responsibility for diabetes care regimen to children under age 16 years, but instead stay closely involved in a supportive way. Nonetheless, a minor who is intent on undermining their diabetes regimen can find numerous ways to deceive supervising adults and conceal skipped insulin doses—such as reporting fabricated blood sugars, altering glucometer readings by using glucometer control solution or diluents, or even testing on non-diabetic friends. A patient can deftly mislead a supervising adult into believing that they have given an insulin injection when in fact they have not—for example, one patient recounted that whenever her mother supervised her injections, she would pretend to draw up insulin but actually draw up only air from her insulin vial, show the apparently dosed insulin syringe to her mother, then inject herself with the syringe of air, all in a matter of seconds. Another patient revealed that after his physician had requested that his mother supervise all insulin doses, he would sit at the end of the same sofa for all his insulin doses and while his mother sat next to him, he would reach across to his opposite arm as if injecting insulin, but actually inject into a potted plant next to the sofa. In differentiating psychological causes of poor glycemic control in an adolescent, it necessary to have a reliable adult actually administer all insulin doses for one to two weeks then meet with healthcare team to review the blood sugar data for this period. In cases where a reliable adult is not available, consideration may be given to hospitalization for metabolic control and insulin dosing assessment.

All members of the healthcare team should be familiar with psychological, non-confrontational interviewing techniques (such as motivational interviewing) and involve a mental health professional when it is apparent that psychological dysfunction is causing poor glycemic control. It is imperative that social work and child protective services be involved without delay in cases of poor diabetes control due to neglect or an abusive environment.

Pregnancy Planned pregnancies in intensively managed diabetes have similar outcomes to pregnancies in nondiabetics (40). However, pregnancy in the pediatric age group is seldom planned. Poorly controlled preconception diabetes, be it type 1 or type 2, can have severe consequences both for the mother and the baby. Therefore, adolescent diabetic girls should be counseled about contraception and the risks of unplanned pregnancy.

Diabetic mothers have decreased hypoglycemia awareness in the first trimester and are therefore at increased risk of severe hypoglycemia. During the second half of pregnancy, human placental lactogen levels are high enough to cause significant insulin resistance, so that doses of insulin have to be adjusted frequently. Preexisting retinopathy or nephropathy can progress and lead to visual loss or renal insufficiency. Therefore prepregnancy or at latest upon discovery of pregnancy, an ophthalmology examination and assessment of urinary protein excretion and creatinine clearance are important. Spontaneous abortion and preeclampsia are more common in uncontrolled diabetes. Risks to the baby are twofold. The risk of malformations including neural tube, renal, and cardiac defects and caudal regression syndrome is two- to threefold in poorly controlled diabetes and is greater with higher maternal A1C at conception (41). Angiotensin converting enzyme (ACE) inhibitors are associated with fetal renal agenesis so they must be stopped preconception in hypertensive or albuminuric girls. Later in pregnancy, poorly controlled blood glucose levels can lead to either poor fetal growth due to nutritional compromise (weight gain is often inadequate in adolescent pregnancies), or macrosomia due to excessive insulin production by the fetus as it strives to control the large concentrations of glucose it receives from the hyperglycemic mother.

Diabetes management in pregnancy is very intensive. Plasma glucose targets recommended by the ADA (42) are:

- ≤ 105 mg/dL (5.8 mmol/L) fasting
- ≤155 mg/dL (8.6 mmol/dL) 1 hour after meals
- ≤130 mg/dL (7.2 mmol/L) 2 hours after meals

The Canadian Diabetes Association (43) and International Diabetes Foundation (44) recommend targets that are 5 to 15 mg/dL (0.3 to 0.8 mmol/L) lower.

Meal planning with three meals and three snacks to maintain adequate weight gain is very important. Insulin pumps are often the most effective means of safely achieving tight metabolic control in pregnancy. Aspart and glargine insulins are not used due to theoretical concerns about insulin growth factor receptor cross reactivity. Management of pregnancy in diabetes requires an experienced multidisciplinary team.

Insulin edema Rarely, severe edema can occur in patients with diabetes following initiation of insulin treatment or in patients with long-standing poorly controlled diabetes following intensification of insulin treatment. It has mostly been reported in T1DM, although it has also been seen in T2DM. It is usually self-limited and can be effectively treated with diuretics. It is perhaps related to insulin-induced sodium retention or to increased vascular permeability leading to loss of albumin from the circulation (45,46).

Pancreas and islet transplantation Pancreas transplantation currently offers the most physiologic therapy for diabetes. The procedure is reserved for those who have long-standing, very poorly controlled diabetes despite best efforts where there is a major impact on social functioning. It is a rare procedure in children and adolescents. Less than 1% of transplant recipients at the University of Minnesota from 1978 to 2000 were younger than 18 years of age (47). Although there are no prospective studies, pancreas transplantation does appear to stabilize nephropathy and neuropathy; however, retinopathy can deteriorate initially because of rapid blood glucose control. Because of the high risk of the surgery and long-term risks of immunosuppression, pancreas transplantation alone is less common than pancreas after kidney transplantation performed for uremic patients already taking immunosuppressive agents or simultaneous pancreas and kidney transplant. Seventy-nine to 88% of these pancreata remain functional after 1 year with current steroid-free immunosuppressive regimens (47). There are variations of the surgery with drainage of the exocrine pancreas to the bladder or the intestine and the venous drainage to the systemic or hepatic portal system.

Islet transplant is a simpler procedure with an infusion of islets into the hepatic portal vein; however, preparation of the graft is much more complicated. This procedure has only recently become viable, with 80% insulin independence after 1 year achieved using the Edmonton protocol (48). Unfortunately, longer term results have been less encouraging. Islet transplantation is in its early stages and is not widely available but has promise to reduce blood glucose lability and reduce hypoglycemic episodes. Risks include portal vein thrombosis or perihepatic bleeding. Hypercholesterolemia and hypertension have been observed in more than half of recipients. Raised creatinine and oral ulcers are other side effects of the immunosuppression.

The problem with both pancreas and islet allotransplantation is availability of donor organs. An obvious extension of islet infusion would be β-cell infusion. With advances in stem cell biology, ex vivo differentiation and culture of autologous or allogeneic β cells with subsequent portal infusion is the best hope for a universally applicable cure in the future.

Autoimmune Conditions Associated with Type 1 Diabetes

As an autoimmune disease, T1DM diabetes is associated with other autoimmune diseases. It can occur as part of a syndrome. Autoimmune polyglandular syndrome type 1 (APS 1) also known as autoimmune polyendocrinopathy, candidiasis and ectodermal dystrophy is an autosomal recessive disease with mucocutaneous candidiasis, hypoparathyroidism, and adrenal insufficiency as its hallmarks, and 10% will develop autoimmune diabetes mellitus. Other features include teeth and nail dystrophies, gonadal failure, hypothyroidism, pernicious anemia, atrophic gastritis, and autoimmune hepatitis. The onset is usually in infancy, often with chronic mucocutaneous candidiasis as the presenting symptom.

The most common polyglandular syndrome, APS 2 (Schmidt syndrome) has adrenal insufficiency and hypothyroidism as its main features, and 40% of patients develop diabetes. Alopecia, GI manifestations and myasthenia gravis are also seen in APS 2. The various endocrinopathies can develop over years or decades.

X-linked immunodeficiency, polyendocrinopathy (T1DM and hypothyroidism), and diarrhea is a rare syndrome that is usually fatal due to infection.

In the absence of syndromes, hypothyroidism is present in 5% of children with T1DM (49) and annual thyroid-stimulating hormone screening should be part of routine diabetic care. The prevalence of celiac disease in T1DM is 5% to 10% (50). Most are asymptomatic and screening is controversial, but for those who have gastrointestinal complaints, poor growth, or unexplained hypoglycemia or poor glucose control, screening with tissue transglutaminase and antigliadin antibodies is warranted. Adrenal insufficiency is less common in people with diabetes, but it must also be considered as a cause of poor diabetes control, especially hypoglycemia.

TYPE 2 DIABETES MELLITUS

Epidemiology of Type 2 Diabetes

T2DM is the most common type of diabetes if all age groups are considered. In North America it is the second most common type of diabetes in children and adolescents with prevalence estimates of 1 to 50/1,000 during the 1990s. Proportions observed in Native populations are at the higher end of the range (1). In Japanese school children, T2DM is now more common than type 1 (51). The diagnosis of T2DM diabetes in children is made on average between 12 and 16 years of age, and rarely before age 10; however, the youngest patient reported was diagnosed at 4 years of age (1).

Obesity is the main risk factor in the development of T2DM in children and adolescents. The obesity epidemic has been accompanied by an increased incidence of T2DM in this age group. Most children with T2DM have a body mass index (BMI) above the 85th percentile.

Non-European ethnicity is another risk factor. In North America, Blacks, Hispanics, Asians, and Native Americans are at increased risk. Some of this risk is due to the greater prevalence of obesity in these groups, but among Asians for example, smaller increments in BMI confer higher risks of diabetes than in the general population.

Family history is a significant risk factor. Between 74% and 100% of children with T2DM have an affected first or second degree relative (1). Maternal history of gestational diabetes has also been shown to be a strong predictor of obesity and T2DM in childhood. This may reflect genetic predisposition but also appears to be related at least in part to the intrauterine metabolic environment. In addition, adults who were born large- or small-for-gestational age or as twins have a higher risk of T2DM, and adolescents who were born large-for-gestational age or small-for-gestational age have a higher risk of insulin resistance (52). It is hypothesized that this is a result of early metabolic imprinting to compensate for the in utero nutritional environment.

Pathophysiology of Type 2 Diabetes

T2DM is a heterogeneous disorder with a common endpoint of hyperglycemia. There are two components. First is insulin resistance and this can be divided into peripheral resistance (muscle and fat) and hepatic resistance. Second is β-cell failure. The homeostatic response to insulin resistance is to increase insulin secretion, and diabetes results when this mechanism fails. A person with little pancreatic reserve will become diabetic at a lower degree of insulin resistance than a person with greater pancreatic reserve (Figure 20-9). The relationship between insulin sensitivity and insulin secretion is hyperbolic, such that the product of insulin sensitivity and insulin secretion is a constant (53) called the insulin disposition index. The implication is that regulatory feedback exists to maintain steady glucose disposal in the face of changing insulin sensitivity. The majority of insulin-resistant people do not become diabetic because their

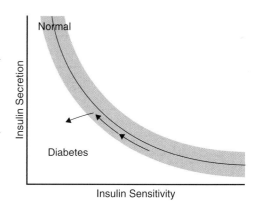

FIGURE 20-9. Schematic of insulin sensitivity vs. insulin secretion. For each individual in the steady state, insulin sensitivity × insulin secretion is a constant. Curves in the gray area will maintain normal blood sugars. The arrows show how, initially with decreased insulin sensitivity (increased insulin resistance), insulin secretion increases to maintain a constant blood sugar, and then worsening insulin resistance and progressive β-cell failure lead to diabetes.

pancreas can compensate, thus maintaining the insulin disposition index. When the pancreas is unable to compensate, the insulin disposition index decreases, and beyond a certain threshold, diabetes develops. If this occurs at a young age and diabetes onset is in childhood or adolescence, one can imagine that the degree of insulin resistance or the pancreatic defect is severe.

Insulin resistance There is a highly complex system regulating the effect that insulin has on its target tissues. Alterations at any step can contribute to insulin resistance. This is a field of active research.

Although obesity is only present in approximately 70% of adults with T2DM, it is found in virtually all youth with T2DM. Obesity contributes to insulin resistance in many ways. First, excess adiposity leads to high circulating levels of triglycerides and free fatty acids that are taken up by various cells. Accumulation of triglycerides in muscle cells (intramyocellular lipid) is directly associated with insulin resistance. In the muscle cells, fatty acids impair glucose oxidation by competing for the metabolic machinery, and their metabolites decrease insulin-mediated glucose uptake by inhibiting PI3 kinase signaling (54).

Adipose tissue secretes many hormones and cytokines (collectively called adipokines) that alter insulin sensitivity. Two beneficial adipokines, leptin and adiponectin, enhance insulin-stimulated glucose uptake. In obesity, leptin resistance is common and adiponectin levels are decreased, both of which are associated with insulin resistance and diabetes (55). Adipose tissue secretes tumor necrosis factor-α and interleukin-6, which promote inflammation and insulin resistance. Tumor necrosis factor-α also acts to increase serine phosphorylation of the insulin receptor and decrease its signaling ability (54). Visceral fat seems to confer more risk than subcutaneous fat due to different secretory patterns of the two depots (55).

Independently of fat mass, the excessive caloric intake of obese individuals is directly responsible for part of the resistance, through down-regulation of the insulin receptor secondary to hyperinsulinemia. Short-term fasting improves insulin resistance in the absence of direct effect on adiposity (56).

Puberty is a well-known cause of insulin resistance. Glucose uptake in response to insulin is 30% less in pubertal children than in prepubertal children or adults (3). This is a transient phenomenon and is most likely due to the pubertal surge of growth hormone and not sex steroids (57). Although the insulin resistance of puberty is a normal physiologic phenomenon seen in all healthy children, when it is combined with the insulin resistance of obesity and perhaps an additional genetic component, extreme insulin resistance occurs that requires a vigorous β-cell response. Patients with an insulin secretory defect are unable to compensate and will develop diabetes.

Even when an adaptive increase in insulin secretion prevents hyperglycemia, severe insulin resistance has health consequences of its own, and is often as part of a larger metabolic derangement called the insulin resistance syndrome, the metabolic syndrome, or syndrome X. As defined by the National Cholesterol Education Program for adults it includes abdominal obesity, impaired fasting glucose, dyslipidemia with low HDL-cholesterol and high triglycerides, and hypertension. The inflammatory marker C-reactive protein is also often elevated (58), reflecting its status as a metabolic-vascular-inflammatory condition with risk of premature cardiovascular disease (59). Features of the metabolic syndrome are similar in children except that blood glucose levels are generally normal until late in the progression. In girls, it is associated with premature adrenarche and polycystic ovary syndrome. This condition is discussed further in Chapter 21.

Insulin secretory defect Early changes leading to T2DM have not been studied in children, but in adults, FPIR is decreased before onset of overt diabetes (60) whereas the second phase is augmented in level and duration. As β-cell dysfunction progresses, the second phase diminishes to the point it can no longer compensate for the increased needs. Progressive β-cell failure in the face of insulin resistance leads to diabetes (61). This is generally a slow process, and years can pass

between the development of clinical hyperglycemia and diagnosis.

The underlying problem is loss of β cells due to unknown factors through apoptosis, which is progressive and irreversible (62). After a point, a vicious circle develops whereby the effects of inadequate insulin secretion lead to increased circulating glucose and free fatty acids that further impair β-cell function. These phenomena are called glucotoxicity and lipotoxicity, respectively. Chronically elevated levels of glucose alter gene expression in the β cell, resulting in both decreased insulin transcription and cellular oxidative stress. Lipotoxicity is the inhibition of glucose-stimulated insulin secretion due to accumulation of fatty acid metabolites in the β cell. Glucotoxicity and lipotoxicity are partially reversible if circulating glucose and free fatty acid levels are reduced by treating the diabetes (63).

Genetics Twin and family studies have shown strong heritability of T2DM, with monozygotic twins having 63% concordance, and first degree relatives having an absolute risk of 30% to 40% compared with 7% in the general population (64). African-American adolescents have higher insulin levels and lower insulin-stimulated glucose disposal than BMI-matched white adolescents (1), suggesting ethnic differences in the genetic factors that determine insulin response. In adults, several gene polymorphisms have been associated with T2DM. Associations that have been replicated in several populations include genes encoding PPARγ, which is important for adipocyte differentiation and fatty acid metabolism, SUR and Kir6.2, which together make up the ATP-dependent potassium channel of the β cell, glucokinase, which regulates glucose handling in the β cell, the glucagon receptor, and GLUT1, the glucose transporter responsible for noninsulin-mediated glucose uptake in many tissues (64). Some of these gene products are involved in insulin sensitivity and others in insulin secretion.

Environment There is no doubt that the rapid increase in incidence of diabetes over one generation is not due to changes in genetic makeup of the population. Increased availability of fat and carbohydrate calorie-rich foods and decreased opportunity for physical activity are contributing to obesity and insulin resistance and are applying a "stress" to genetic predispositions. The epidemic of obesity and type 2 diabetes has occurred during an era of high exposure to endocrine disruptor toxins in the environment and food supply. A recent review has suggested that the surge in metabolic obesity may be due to these chemical obesogens ad-

versely influencing adipocyte differentiation and metabolism (65).

Diagnosis of Type 2 Diabetes

Clinical presentation Symptoms are similar to those of T1DM, and include polyuria, polydipsia, fatigue, blurry vision, and possible weight loss (in the setting of baseline overweight); however, in T2DM the progression is more insidious, so the symptoms may go unnoticed for some time before presentation. Diagnosis is sometimes made incidentally when blood tests are done for other reasons, often after the patient seeks medical attention as a result of obesity or other complications. It is a common misconception that DKA is rare in T2DM—in fact, one study reported that 33% of T2DM adolescents presented with DKA (25).

Diagnostic criteria The diagnostic criteria for diabetes are the same regardless of the type. Fasting blood glucose levels ≥ 126 mg/dL (7.0 mmol/L) or casual levels ≥ 200 mg/dL (11.1 mmol/L) on two separate days or once with metabolic decompensation are diagnostic. The oral glucose tolerance test (OGTT) has more of a place in the diagnosis of T2DM than in T1DM. In addition to identifying diabetes per se, the OGTT can identify the prediabetic states of impaired fasting glucose and impaired glucose tolerance by using the criteria shown in Table 20-6. The significance of these categories in children has not been investigated.

Distinguishing T1DM from T2DM is becoming increasingly difficult given that the prevalence of obesity is increasing even in children with autoimmune β-cell destruction. Fortunately, the acute intervention for poorly controlled diabetes of both types is the same and there is no urgency to make the distinction. In general, signs of insulin resistance such as acanthosis nigricans or polycystic ovary syndrome suggest T2DM. The absence of islet cell antibodies points to T2DM, but their presence does not necessarily rule it out. In one study, antibodies to GAD, autoantibodies to insulin, and islet cell antibodies were present in 35%, 30%, and 8% of 48 children and adolescents diagnosed with T2DM, respectively (66). In large studies in the United States and Europe, approximately 4% of adult patients characterized as having T2DM are GAD antibody positive (67). Compared with other patients with T2DM, these individuals are less insulin resistant, have more favorable lipid levels, and have a lower prevalence of the metabolic syndrome. Some have called this type of diabetes "type 1½" or latent autoimmune diabetes of adults.

The assessment of insulin and/or C-peptide levels may be suggestive of T2DM if levels are

TABLE 20-6   Diagnosis of Diabetes and Dysglycemic States

Dysglycemic state	Diagnostic Criteria
Impaired Fasting Glucose (IFG)	Fasting glucose 100-125 mg/dL (5.6-6.9 mmol/L)
Impaired Glucose Tolerance (IGT)	Plasma glucose 140-199 mg/dL (7.8-11.0 mmol/L) 2 h after a 75-g oral glucose load
Diabetes	*Fasting glucose ≥ 126 mg/dL (7.0 mmol/L) Or *Random glucose ≥ 200 mg/dL (11.1 mmol/L) Or *Plasma glucose ≥ 200 mg/dL (11.1 mmol/L) 2 hr after a 75-g oral glucose load *In the absence of metabolic decompensation, confirm with the same or another test on a different day
Cystic Fibrosis–Related Diabetes without fasting hyperglycemia	As above for diabetes with fasting glucose < 126 mg/dL (7.0 mmol/L)
Cystic Fibrosis–Related Diabetes with fasting hyperglycemia	As above for diabetes with fasting glucose ≥126 mg/dL (7.0 mmol/L)
Gestational Diabetes	During a 1-hr 50-g glucose load screen: 1-hr glucose ≥ 185 mg/dL (10.3 mmol/L) Or During a 2-hr 75-g OGTT, at least two of: fasting glucose ≥ 95 mg/dL (5.3 mmol/L) 1-hr glucose ≥ 180 mg/dL (10.0 mmol/L) 2-hr glucose ≥ 155 mg/dL (8.6 mmol/L)

high. Low values are not helpful at the time of initial presentation because they may indicate absolute insulin deficiency with permanent β-cell failure, or they may be a transient consequence of glucotoxicity. Therefore, if C-peptide is to be used as a marker, it is best done after glucose control is achieved and past the period of possible honeymoon for T1DM.

Management of Type 2 Diabetes

Treatment Goals Treatment goals for T2DM include normalization of fasting blood glucose levels (as nearly as possible) with A1C <7.0% while avoiding hypoglycemia to prevent long-term microvascular complications. Additional goals are to manage the components of metabolic syndrome including obesity, dyslipidemia, and hypertension and other co-morbidities of obesity such as fatty infiltration of liver and PCOS. The United Kingdom Prospective Diabetes Study was a landmark study in T2DM adults that showed aggressive control of blood glucose reduced the incidence and progression of retinopathy and nephropathy by 21% to 33%; however, reduction in macrovascular complications was not significant (68).

Management Strategy

Patients with T2DM should be followed by the diabetes team every 3 to 4 months. Inten-

sive involvement with a dietitian to work on weight loss is an important component of the visit. Blood glucose records, diet and physical activity, and additional health problems should be discussed. Physical examination including blood pressure should be done at each visit. Retinopathy screening should be performed at diagnosis and every 1 to 2 years thereafter by an experienced professional. Foot examination including assessment of neuropathy with Semmes–Weinstein filament should be done once a year. Liver enzymes should be measured at diagnosis, A1C should be monitored at each visit, and fasting lipid profile and urine albumin/creatinine ratio assessed every year. Children with T2DM are candidates for influenza and pneumococcal vaccinations.

Monitoring

Self-monitoring of blood glucose is an essential part of T2DM treatment. Depending on the degree of hyperglycemia and treatment regimen, monitoring frequency may vary. The main difference between monitoring in T1DM and T2DM is that postprandial monitoring is often more frequently used in T2DM. In non-pharmacologically treated children, monitoring may be limited to times of symptoms or acute illness. Those on medication should check more frequently, and those on insulin or sulfonylureas should be monitoring before each

meal and at bedtime to avoid asymptomatic hypoglycemia. A1C should be evaluated every 3 to 4 months to assess long-term blood glucose control.

Lifestyle Modification

Nonpharmacological measures should always be part of the management of T2DM, whether or not medications are also prescribed. If hyperglycemia is mild and the patient is asymptomatic and otherwise metabolically stable, nonpharmacological means may be sufficient. In adults, lifestyle modifications alone are successful in only 10% of people with T2DM (1).

Diet and exercise are cornerstones of treatment to reduce obesity and improve insulin sensitivity. These are discussed further in Chapter 21. Exercise improves insulin resistance and diabetic control in adults with T2DM (69). Weight loss (or weight maintenance in premenarchal girls or boys before Tanner V) is the goal (70). Low-calorie, low-fat diets are best instituted with the help of a dietician knowledgeable in the treatment of diabetic children. Physical activity can be increased by limiting sedentary activities like television and computer use. The objective is to create healthy habits in a child that will persist throughout life. Children and, to a lesser extent, adolescents are not likely to make major changes in their diet and exercise patterns without concomitant changes in the whole family's lifestyle, and thus it is critical that the parents be actively engaged in this process.

Medication

FDA approved pharmacologic treatments for T2DM in children are limited in comparison to all the oral antidiabetic agents available for use in adults (Table 20-7); only metformin is approved for use in children with T2DM. The others are also briefly mentioned because current studies with some of these classes of drugs are underway. In adults, metformin, sulfonylureas, and thiazolidinediones are equally effective and meglitinides and α-glucosidase inhibitors slightly less so. These agents are used in combinations with each other and with insulin. Most oral agents can be divided into the general classes of insulin sensitizers, which reduce hepatic or peripheral insulin resistance, and insulin secretagogues, which stimulate insulin secretion.

Insulin sensitizers: Metformin is a biguanide. Although its mechanism of action is not entirely clear, it seems to affect primarily hepatic insulin sensitivity by inhibiting the flux of glucogenic substrates through the mitochondria in the liver. The net effect is largely

TABLE 20-7   Oral Antihyperglycemic Agents

	Biguanides	Sulfonylureas	Thiazolidenediones	Meglitinides	α-Glucosidase inhibitors	GLP-1	DPP-4
Agents	Metformin	Gliclazide	Pioglitazone	Nateglinide	Acarbose	Exenatide	Sitagliptin
		Glimepiride	Rosiglitazone	Repaglinide	Miglitol	Liraglutide	Vidagliptin
		Glipizide					
		Glyburide					
Molecular target	Unknown	SUR/Kir6.2	PPARγ	SUR/Kir6.2	α-Glucosidase	GLP-1R	DPP-4
Main effect	↓ hepatic glucose output	↑ insulin secretion	↑ insulin sensitivity in fat and muscle	↑ insulin secretion	Slows intestinal glucose absorption	↑ Glucose, ↑ insulin secretion	↑ Glucose, ↑ insulin secretion
Lowers A$_1$c (%)[a]	1.5–2	1.5–2	0.7–1	1.5–2	0.7–1	1-2	0.5-1.5
Postprandial effect	−	−	−	+	+	+	+
Side effects	Lactic acidosis[b] ↓ Vit. B$_{12}$ levels	Hypoglycemia[a] Weight gain	Edema Weight gain ↑ liver enzymes	Hypoglycemia[a]	GI	GI	
Contraindications	Renal failure Liver disease Heart failure Hypoxia/acidosis	Renal failure	Liver disease Heart failure	IBD Cirrhosis Renal failure			

[a]when used as monotherapy

[b]theoretical; GLP-1R = GLP-1 receptor; GI = gastrointenstinal; IBD = inflammatory bowel disease.

to reduce hepatic glucose production, but metformin also has a minor role in improving peripheral insulin sensitivity (71). A randomized, controlled trial in which up to 1,000 mg metformin was given twice daily in 82 children with T2DM aged 10 to 16 years showed that after 16 weeks, fasting blood glucose decreased 49 mg/dL (2.4 mmol/L) and A1C decreased 1.1% compared with the placebo group (72). Approximately 25% of children experience abdominal pain, nausea and vomiting, or diarrhea, but in the majority the symptoms resolve after 2 to 3 weeks and can be minimized by building up from low doses over 1 or 2 months. There is also a theoretical risk of lactic acidosis with this medication, so metformin is contraindicated in those with liver or renal disease (decreased metabolism or excretion may lead to toxic levels) or heart failure (risk of acidosis), and it should be stopped temporarily during radiocontrast procedures (renal compromise leading to less excretion). Metformin does not cause hypoglycemia when used as monotherapy.

Thiazolidinediones: These agents are under study for treatment of T2DM in children. Currently available drugs in this class are rosiglitazone and pioglitazone. They are ligands for PPARγ in adipose tissue and improve peripheral insulin sensitivity. The main side effects in adults are weight gain (which may be quite significant and may be related to the PRARγ role in adipocyte differentiation) and edema. The prototype, troglitazone, was associated with fulminant hepatic failure so the thiazolidinediones are contraindicated in liver disease. Rosiglitazone has been associated with increased risk of myocardial infarction in adults, but the cardiac risks to adolescents using rosiglitazone have not yet been defined.

Insulin secretagogues: Sulfonylureas, the first of the insulin secretagogues to be developed, act at the K$^+$-ATP channel of the β cell at the SUR (sulfonylurea receptor) subunit to depolarize the membrane and trigger insulin release. They are long acting and insulin secretion is independent of blood glucose levels, so the primary side effect is fasting hypoglycemia. They also may cause weight gain, in part simply because of improved metabolic control, but hyperinsulinism may also play a role. The most widely used sulfonylurea is glyburide. Other agents, such as gliclazide, glipizide and glimepiride cause less hypoglycemia and are safer in renal insufficiency (73).

Meglitinides: These agents are newer secretagogues that also act at the K$^+$-ATP channel. They have a short duration of action and they are particularly useful for control of postprandial hyperglycemia. They too cause weight gain, but, importantly, there is much less risk of hypoglycemia than with sulfonylureas. They are safe in patients with renal

and liver disease. These drugs are generally given before meals three times a day, in combination with either an insulin sensitizer or the basal insulin glargine. Currently, repaglinide, nateglinide, and mitiglinide are in clinical use. Nateglinide has been shown to be safer and more effective in MODY3 than sulfonylureas (74).

Incretin mimetics: Agonist analogs of the incretin glucagon-like peptide 1 (GLP-1 analogs) and drugs that block the degradation of incretins by the enzyme dipeptidyl peptidase 4 (DPP-4 inhibitors) are currently in clinical use in adults. They improve meal stimulated insulin secretion and are postulated to improve beta-cell regeneration or to decrease apoptosis. In clinical trials, they improve glycemic control to the same extent as other available medications. The GLP-1 analogs have the additional advantage of causing weight loss, but they are administered as subcutaneous injections and cause gastrointestinal side effects in a significant proportion of patients. These medications have not been studied in children.

Alpha-glucosidase inhibitors: These agents inhibit digestion of sugars to monosaccharides in the gut lumen and thereby delay absorption and control postprandial hyperglycemia. Acarbose and miglitol cause gastrointestinal side effects that are unacceptable to most adolescents, including flatulence and diarrhea. Because they do not enter the circulation, they have no systemic side effects and are safe in renal and liver disease. Their effect on glycemic control is only modest.

Insulin: Often, oral agents will not be sufficient in youth with T2DM, and insulin is the treatment of choice, especially if the fasting blood glucose exceeds 250 mg/dL (13.9 mmol/L) or if there are symptoms or ketones (70). Insulin is used as it is in T1DM, and can be given as combinations of short- and intermediate-acting insulin in twice-a-day or multiple daily injection regimens, keeping in mind that the rapid-acting insulin analogs aspart and lispro are very useful for controlling postprandial hyperglycemia. Starting doses of 0.5 to 1 U/kg/day as the total daily insulin dose are appropriate, but, due to insulin resistance in T2DM, much more than 1 U/kg/day may be needed. Metformin is usually started at the same time as insulin therapy. Insulin requirements may decline rapidly during the first weeks of treatment as glucotoxicity improves and endogenous insulin secretion increases. Some children can regain acceptable metabolic control and stop the insulin after 2 to 6 weeks or more (70).

Prevention of Type 2 Diabetes

In adults, several prevention studies have demonstrated that overweight individuals with impaired glucose tolerance or women with a history of gestational diabetes can reduce their 3-year risk of T2DM by up to 58% (75,76) with lifestyle modification. These interventions included 150 minutes of moderate-intensity physical activity per week and a mean weight loss of 7%.

Pharmacologic agents have also been used in adults to prevent progression to diabetes in high-risk patients with impaired glucose tolerance or severe insulin resistance. The drug metformin was able to decrease the risk of diabetes by 31% in the Diabetes Prevention Program trial (75). Troglitazone, a thiazolidinedione insulin sensitizer that is no longer on the market, reduced diabetes risk by 56% (77,78), and acarbose reduced the risk by 25% (79).

There are no medications approved for prevention of T2DM in high-risk children. Given the success of lifestyle modifications in adults, dietary and exercise programs at the community or individual level for children seem the prudent choice. Several school programs are being evaluated, particularly in Native American communities in the United States and Canada. Studies are underway evaluating the safety and efficacy of metformin in youth with prediabetes.

Preventive interventions should be targeted to those at risk. In adults, the OGTT seems to be a more sensitive test of abnormal glucose homeostasis than fasting blood glucose (80), but in children there are no formal recommendations available for screening for impaired fasting glucose or impaired glucose tolerance. Although these conditions have a high rate of progression to diabetes in adults, their natural history in children has not been studied. "Case finding" for diabetes in children has been recommended by the ADA in high-risk individuals, including overweight or at-risk-of-overweight children older than 10 years of age or younger if puberty has started, and who have two of the following: family history of T2DM in first or second degree relatives, race other than Caucasian, or signs of insulin resistance or associated conditions (acanthosis nigricans, polycystic ovary syndrome, hypertension, or dyslipidemia). It is debatable whether these individuals should be tested with the OGTT or simply with fasting glucose and insulin levels.

Hyperglycemic Hyperosmolar Syndrome

Although youth with T2DM may present with DKA, another potentially fatal acute complication is the hyperglycemic hyperosmolar nonketotic syndrome (HHONK). It often results from a delay in diagnosis and treatment of T2DM. Because patients with T2DM may have a relative, rather than an absolute insulin deficiency, there is the potential to develop hyperglycemia and dehydration while maintaining suppression of ketogenesis. In fact, the lack of ketosis usually delays presentation to a point at which dehydration and concomitant electrolyte loss is severe. (81)

HHONK in youth presents with dehydration, vomiting, headache, or other neurologic signs, in the setting of obesity with or without the typical symptoms of polydipsia and polyuria. The presentation can be strikingly similar to that of cerebral edema. The diagnostic criteria are blood glucose greater than 600 mg/dL (33 mmol/L), pH greater than 7.3, bicarbonate greater than 15 mEq/L, absent or minimal ketonemia or ketonuria, effective serum osmolality ($2 \times [Na^+](mEq/L) + [glucose](mg/dL)/18$ or $2 \times [Na^+](mmol/L) + [glucose](mmol/L)$) greater than 320 mOsm/kg, and stupor or coma (37). Treatment is like that of DKA with intravenous insulin infusion and fluids as a bolus and then an infusion to replace the water deficit over 48 hours (37), although patients with HHONK typically require more fluid replacement than patients with DKA. Despite treatment, the case fatality rate is approximately 12% (81).

ATPYICAL DIABETES MELLITUS

Not all cases of diabetes can be neatly classified as type 1 or type 2 (Table 20-8). Ketosis, although much more frequent in T1DM, can also occur in patients whose previous and/or subsequent course fits the clinical definition of T2DM. This phenomenon was first described in individuals of African descent (82) but it can occur in other ethnic groups (83,84). Most of these patients have a T2DM profile of insulin resistance and negative autoantibodies (84); however, a significantly increased frequency of diabetes-predisposing HLA alleles (82,84) suggests that autoimmunity may play a role in the acute β-cell dysfunction responsible for the ketoacidosis.

OTHER TYPES OF DIABETES

Gestational Diabetes

Gestational diabetes mellitus (GDM) is the onset of diabetes after 20 weeks gestation. Gestational diabetes can be considered in the spectrum of T2DM because the risk factors are the same. Additional risk factors include significant weight gain during pregnancy, previous GDM, and previous macrosomic infant. The main reason for GDM is inability of the pancreas to compensate for the increased insulin resistance mediated by placental hormones, particularly human placental lactogen.

Most often glucose metabolism returns to normal after delivery, but at 3 to 6 months, 16% to 20% of women still have abnormal glucose metabolism (85). Subsequent risk of T2DM is even higher. Therefore, 6 weeks to 6 months postpartum, screening for T2DM with an OGTT is indicated. Pregnancy per se may contribute to development of T2DM because risk increases with number of pregnancies, but the association may primarily be a reflection of the insulin resistance of pregnancy "unmasking" an underlying β-cell defect.

The main risks of GDM to the baby are macrosomia (which can lead to traumatic delivery), hypoglycemia, hypocalcemia, and respiratory distress. Macrosomia occurs because when the fetus is exposed to high levels of maternal glucose it secretes large amounts of insulin in response. Insulin is a potent growth factor in utero. Because organogenesis is complete by the time GDM develops, risk of malformations is generally not thought to be increased; however, as children, adolescents, and adults, these offspring have increased prevalence of obesity, insulin resistance, and diabetes. Some of this may be related to genetic susceptibility, but it also appears to be related, at least in part, to the metabolic consequences of the in utero environment.

TABLE 20-8   Classification of Diabetes Mellitus

Type 1 diabetes (β-cell destruction)

  Immune mediated

  Idiopathic

Type 2 diabetes (insulin resistance with insulin deficiency)

Other specific types

  Genetic defects of β-cell function

    1. **HNF-1α (MODY3)**
    2. **glucokinase (MODY2)**
    3. HNF-4a (MODY1)
    4. insulin promoter factor-1 (MODY4)
    5. HNF-1b (MODY5)
    6. NeuroD1 (MODY6)
    7. Mitochondrial DNA
    8. SUR/Kir6.2
    9. Others

  Genetic defects in insulin action

    1. Type A insulin resistance
    2. Leprechaunism
    3. Rabson–Mendenhall syndrome
    4. Lipoatrophic diabetes
    5. Others

  Diseases of the exocrine pancreas

    1. Pancreatitis
    2. Trauma/pancreatectomy
    3. Neoplasia
    4. **Cystic fibrosis**
    5. Hemochromatosis
    6. Fibrocalculous pancreatopathy
    7. Others

  Endocrinopathies

    1. Acromegaly
    2. Cushing syndrome
    3. Glucagonoma
    4. Pheochromocytoma
    5. Hyperthyroidism
    6. Somatostatinoma
    7. Aldosteronoma
    8. Others

  Drug or chemical induced

    1. Vacor
    2. Pentamidine
    3. Nicotinic acid
    4. **Glucocorticoids**
    5. Thyroid hormone
    6. Diazoxide
    7. β-adrenergic agonists
    8. Thiazides
    9. Dilantin
    10. α-interferon
    11. **L-asparaginase**
    12. Others

  Infections

    1. Congenital Rubella
    2. Cytomegalovirus
    3. Others

  Uncommon forms of immune-mediated diabetes

    1. Stiff-man syndrome
    2. Antiinsulin receptor antibodies
    3. Others

  Other genetic syndromes sometimes associated with diabetes

    1. **Down syndrome**
    2. **Klinefelter syndrome**
    3. **Turner syndrome**
    4. Wolfram syndrome (DIDMOAD)
    5. Friedreich ataxia
    6. Huntington chorea
    7. Laurence–Moon syndrome
    8. Bardet–Biedl syndrome
    9. Myotonic dystrophy
    10. Porphyria
    11. **Prader–Willi syndrome**
    12. Others

Gestational Diabetes

More common causes in pediatrics are in bold green type. Modified with permission of the American Diabetes Association from Diabetes Care. 2004;27(Suppl. 1):S5–S10.

All pregnant women should be evaluated for GDM at 24 to 28 weeks of gestation. Women with risk factors should be screened in the first trimester and rescreened if negative at 24 to 28 weeks. Two strategies may be used. One is to start with a 50-g oral glucose screen. If the 1 hour blood glucose is greater than or equal to 185 mg/dL (10.2 mmol/L), GDM is diagnosed. If the 1-hour value is 140 to 185 mg/dL (7.8–10.2 mmol/L) then one must continue to a 75-g OGTT with measurements at 0, 60, and 120 minutes. If any two values exceed the cut offs of 95 mg/dL (5.3 mmol/L), 190 mg/dL (10.6 mmol/L), and 160 mg/dL (8.9 mmol/L) at the respective time points, then GDM is diagnosed.

Depending on the degree of hyperglycemia, management may begin with diet and exercise but if targets are not achieved in 2 weeks, insulin must be started. Glucose monitoring should be done in the fasting state and 1 or 2 hours after each meal. Glucose targets are the same as for pregnancies in women with T1DM. The ADA recommends the following plasma glucose targets:

- ≤ 105 mg/dL (5.8 mmol/L) fasting
- ≤155 mg/dL (8.6 mmol/dL) 1 hour after meals
- ≤130 mg/dL (7.2 mmol/L) 2 hours after meals.

The Canadian Diabetes Association (86) recommends targets that are 10 to 15 mg/dL (0.5–0.8 mmol/L) lower.

TABLE 20-9   Types of MODY

	OMIM number	Gene mutated	Chromosome
MODY1	125850	Hepatocyte nuclear factor-4-α (HNF4A)	20q12-q13.1
MODY2	125851	Glucokinase (GCK)	7p15-p13
MODY3	600496	Hepatic transcription factor-1 (TCF1, or HNF1A)	12q24.2
MODY4	606392	Insulin-promoter factor 1 (IPF1)	13q12.1
MODY5	604284	Hepatic transcription factor 2 (TCF2 or HNF1α)	17cen-q21.3
MODY6	606394	*NEUROD1*	2q32

Insulin can be given as NPH and regular or lispro insulin. If insulin needs are high, the number of injections becomes burdensome, or glucose control is difficult to safely achieve, an insulin pump should be considered. There is not enough safety evidence to recommend oral agents in pregnancy, particularly in adolescents. GDM must be managed by professionals experienced in treating diabetes during pregnancy with the support of an experienced obstetric team.

Monogenic Diabetes

In a small proportion of cases, diabetes has a simple inheritance pattern, suggesting causation by a single gene. Clinical manifestations depend on the gene involved.

Maturity-onset Diabetes in the Young (MODY)

The term maturity-onset diabetes in the young (MODY refers to an autosomal dominant condition that involves hyperglycemia of young onset, often in the pediatric age group, that resembles T2DM in that it is relatively mild and does not usually require insulin treatment. Here, however, the similarities end. MODY patients are usually not obese and not insulin resistant, the diabetes being due to pure β-cell failure. Linkage analysis has demonstrated locus heterogeneity and has allowed the positional cloning of no fewer than six genes, all involved in some way in β-cell development or function (MODY1–MODY6, Table 20-9). Regardless of which gene is responsible, the disease is due to loss-of-function mutations in the heterozygous state, leading to haploinsufficiency (phenotype due to reduction of the protein product level to 50% of normal).

The diagnosis is usually suspected because of a clear family history of dominant inheritance. One of the parents is affected, at the very least, but did not necessarily had genetic testing for MODY at the time the proband comes to medical attention. Insulin-taking patients with this type of family history should be tested for antibodies and, if negative, for HNF-1α mutations, because MODY3 is by far the most frequent type of MODY likely to require insulin at an early age. Children with what appears to be T2DM, whether lean or overweight, should also be tested for MODY if the family history is suggestive. Although insulin needs will severity of glycemic disorder and not genotype, this is an important diagnosis to make for the purpose of family counseling.

Management is individualized and includes the same lifestyle considerations aimed at maximizing insulin sensitivity as for T2DM. Insulin sensitizers and sulfonylureas can be used, with insulin as the ultimate solution if these fail.

Neonatal Diabetes

Persistent hyperglycemia requiring insulin and starting at birth is rare, estimated at 1:400,000 live births (87). Neonatal diabetes mellitus (NDM) is due to β-cell dysfunction in the absence of insulin resistance. In approximately half the cases it is transient (TNDM) and insulin requirements drop to zero by a few weeks or months of age. The compromised β-cell mass and/or function remanifests itself in a large proportion of patients later in life as mild diabetes that can be managed usually without insulin.

Virtually all TNDM cases have been traced to a parentally imprinted locus on chromosome 6q24. Two genes there, HYMA1 and ZAC, are normally expressed only from the paternal copy. A double dose of one or both of these genes appears to cause TNDM.

Simple molecular diagnosis is available for the two most common causes of the double dose: 1) paternal uniparental disomy, in which both copies of chromosome 6 derive from the father, is nonheritable and seen in sporadic cases; 2) paternal duplication of a small segment that includes 6q24, which is seen in familial cases in which transmission is strictly paternal. In rare cases, the disease may be due to disruption of the DNA methylation that silences the maternal copy (88,89). Molecular diagnosis allows prediction that the case is transient and can distinguish sporadic from familial ones, for future family counseling.

Permanent neonatal diabetes has a more diverse etiology. Approximately half of the European cases are due to a mutation of the KCNJ11 gene, encoding a β-cell potassium channel crucial in the regulation of insulin release. Gain-of-function mutations inhibit insulin secretion (presumably by stabilizing the potassium flux across the cell membrane and preventing depolarization), whereas homozygous loss of function of KCNJ11 is a known cause of hyperinsulinism. Molecular diagnosis is straightforward because the gene only has two exons and mutations cluster in "hot spots," as is customary with gain of function (there is an infinite number of ways to destroy a protein, but only certain amino acid substitutions will enhance it). Diagnosis is important, as these patients respond to sulfonylureas and can be taken off insulin (90,91). Permanent neonatal diabetes has been found due to homozygosity for the MODY genes glucokinase (92) and IPF-1 (insulin-promoter factor-1). In the latter case there was complete absence of the pancreas and exocrine deficiency as well, demonstrating that this transcription factor is necessary for pancreas development (93). In almost half of cases of permanent neonatal diabetes, the cause of remains unknown.

Interestingly, common polymorphisms in three MODY/NDM genes (KCNJ11, IPF-1, and glucokinase) have been associated with ordinary T2DM (94,95), an illustration of how rare diseases can sometimes provide insights important in understanding common ones.

Mitochondrial Diabetes

Because of their high rate of metabolism, β-cells are particularly vulnerable to disorders disrupting the function of the mitochondria. As nerve and muscle have the same vulnerability, diabetes due to a mitochondrial disorder is often part of a syndrome with neurologic or muscular manifestations. Some mitochondrial proteins are encoded by regular nuclear genes but a number of crucial ones are encoded by the 15-kb mitochondrial genome (mDNA) that occurs in hundreds of copies in every cell and is transcribed and translated inside the mitochondria with the use of transfer RNAs that are also encoded in mDNA.

Insulin-deficient diabetes is a well-known feature of the syndrome characterized by myoclonus, epilepsy, lactic acidosis and strokelike episodes, due to mutations in the mitochondrial leucine transfer RNA (96). It can also occur with the Kearns–Sayre syndrome (cardiomyopathy, ophthalmoplegia, retinal degeneration), due to large mDNA deletions (97). Depending on the percentage of copies of mDNA that carry the mutation in the affected tissues (heteroplasmy), severity of manifestations can vary. Deafness may be the only other manifestation other than diabetes. Inheritance is maternal and molecular confirmation is straightforward once the diagnosis is suspected on the basis of the accompanying features. Mitochondrial DNA sequencing, starting with the leucine transfer RNA, should be done in patients with diabetes and deafness with no other explanation (a situation that accounts for as many as 2% of individuals diagnosed as T2DM).

Mutations in Wolframin, a mitochondrial gene encoded in the nucleus (4p16.1) in the homozygous state cause Wolfram syndrome (diabetes insipidus, diabetes mellitus, optic atrophy, and deafness) (98).

Abnormal Insulins and Insulin Receptors

Several rare monogenic forms of diabetes are caused by abnormalities of insulin itself. These include mutations that prevent cleavage of C-peptide, leading to hyperproinsulinemia, and structural mutations of insulin that make it less bioactive (e.g., insulin Chicago and insulin Wakayama). These patients respond to exogenous insulin.

Mutations of the insulin receptor gene can lead to impairment of biosynthesis, translocation to the membrane, insulin binding or tyrosine phosphorylation, or increased degradation. The nature of the mutation and the degree to which it impairs insulin signaling often determines the severity of the insulin resistance, the syndromic category and the life expectancy (99). The clinical syndromes all include severe insulin resistance with acanthosis and in girls, and varying degrees of hyperandrogenism and virilization. They often present with postprandial hyperglycemia and fasting hypoglycemia due to excessive production of insulin by the pancreas. Children with type A insulin resistance are otherwise phenotypically normal. Diabetes and hypoglycemia present from the 1st year to the 2nd decade of life. Treatment is with high-dose insulin (1000–30000 U/d) and/or metformin. Severe diabetic complications can develop but these patients live well into adulthood (100).

Severe insulin receptor defects lead to marked abnormalities in utero. Insulin levels are significantly elevated. Leprechaunism, the most severe of these syndromes, is characterized by marked intrauterine growth retardation, a wizened appearance with thick skin and a lack of subcutaneous fat, elfin-like facies with prominent eyes, thick lips, upturned nostrils and low-set posteriorly rotated ears, protuberant abdomen, enlarged ovaries in females, and enlarged heart and kidneys (due to insulin cross-reacting with insulin-like grow factor-I receptors), failure to grow, and usually death by 1 year of age (99). Their main metabolic problem is fasting hypoglycemia. Rabson–Mendenhall syndrome is similar in presentation but the dysmorphic features are different and include premature dysplastic teeth. There is an association with pineal hyperplasia (99). The insulin binding is not as severely affected as in Leprechaunism so children with Rabson–Mendenhall survive, on average, 10 years (99). They develop severe and intractable ketoacidosis, which may be due to a decline in insulin secretory capacity (101). The diabetes is difficult to control even with high doses of insulin and metformin or thiazolidinediones (100). Leptin is another potential therapy that has shown preliminary success (102).

Lipoatrophic Diabetes

Lipoatrophies are a heterogeneous group of disorders that have in common the partial or complete absence of adipose tissue. Absence of subcutaneous fat gives these patients a muscular appearance. Seemingly paradoxically, this leads to severe insulin resistance, as is seen in obesity. It is possible that the cause is absence of "beneficial" substances secreted by adipocytes such as leptin and adiponectin. In congenital generalized lipoatrophy due to SEIPIN or AGPAT-2 gene mutations, it is the marked deficiency of visceral and subcutaneous fat that gives the patients a muscular appearance. Its prevalence is estimated at less than 1:1,000,000 (103). Familial partial lipodystrophy due to LMNA gene mutation and late-onset familial partial lipodystrophy due to PPARγ mutation usually present in later childhood or adolescence with loss of subcutaneous fat over the limbs, buttocks, and trunk but an increase in fat around the face and neck and visceral fat. The prevalence of partial lipodystrophies is estimated at less than 1:15,000,000 (103). Acquired lipodystrophies like those associated with autoimmune juvenile dermatomyositis and aggressively treated HIV appear similar to the partial lipodystrophies (104). All lipodystrophies share common features including hyperin-

sulinemia, hyperglycemia, hypertriglyceridemia, acanthosis, female hyperandrogenism, hepatomegaly with steatosis, cardiomyopathy, hyperphagia, and heat intolerance. Depending on the degree of fat loss, diabetes may present from preteen years to adult life. These patients are prone to all the micro- and macrovascular complications of diabetes.

Treatments remain limited. Extremely high doses of insulin may be needed (1,000 U/d) and the volumes required may be difficult to tolerate, especially for young children. Metformin may provide some benefit by reducing the high amount of hepatic glucose production. Thiazolidinediones have been shown to increase subcutaneous fat mass and decrease A1C and triglycerides in adults with lipoatrophy. Treatment with subcutaneous leptin has been shown in a few patients to decrease A1C, triglycerides, and liver size. (104)

Cystic Fibrosis–Related Diabetes

Cystic fibrosis (CF) is a multisystem disease caused by deficiency of the cystic fibrosis transmembrane conductance regulator (CFTR) chloride channel, which leads to inspissated secretions of the lungs, pancreas, intestine, and male reproductive tract. As treatments for the lung disease have improved, patients are surviving long enough to develop cystic fibrosis–related diabetes (CFRD). Although CF first affects exocrine pancreatic function, as obstruction, inflammation and fibrosis progress, the islets are also damaged. Both insulin and glucagon responses are affected (105). The absence of glucagon's counterregulatory effect may put these patients at higher risk of hypoglycemia when treated for their diabetes, although for the most part, they are able to compensate for glucagon deficiency with a robust catecholamine response. DKA is much less common and slower to develop than in T1DM. If ketoacidosis develops in a CF patient, T1DM should always be considered.

Up to 50% of CF patients will develop CFRD. The median age of onset is approximately 20 years, but it can occur at any age, including infancy (106). Risk factors include pancreatic insufficiency, recurrent pulmonary infection, corticosteroid treatment, and supplemental feeding (107). According to a North American consensus conference in 1998 (108), diagnostic criteria are the same as for T1DM and T2DM with the additional distinction between diabetes with and without fasting hyperglycemia. They recommend screening all CF patients annually with a random blood glucose. If the random glucose is 126 mg/dL (7.0 mmol/L) or higher, then assess fasting glucose and apply 126 mg/dL (7.0 mmol/L) as a diagnostic cutoff. They recommend an OGTT for those with polyuria or polydipsia, poor weight gain, linear growth, or pubertal progression or unexplained chronically worsening pulmonary function. European recommendations are for annual OGTT in all those older than age 10 (107).

Compared with CF patients with no diabetes, CFRD patients have more weight loss, more rapid decline in lung function, and increased mortality. Interestingly, some of these differences appear years before development of the diabetes and have been postulated to be due to subclinical insulin deficiency with resultant protein catabolism. Microvascular diabetic complications have also been described in 5% to 21% of CFRD patients (108). It is not clear if the incidence of microvascular complications is different from that in T1DM and T2DM. Treatment of CFRD with insulin significantly improves body weight, slows the decline in lung function, and may reduce the incidence of lung infections. There are no data regarding the effect of treatment on microvascular complications.

Insulin is the treatment of choice. There has been some success in the early stages with sulfonylureas, which may be more acceptable and convenient for the patients (109). Use of oral diabetes agents in CFRD is controversial. Treatment practices vary between treating all diagnosed CFRD or treating only once fasting hyperglycemia develops. Because the consequences of insulin deficiency on lung function and nutritional status occur before any overt hyperglycemia, lower thresholds for treatment may provide more benefit. Twice daily mixed short- and intermediate-acting insulin are seldom effective because of the need for frequent feeding in CF and the erratic eating pattern of many of these patients. Meal time rapid-acting insulin using insulin to carbohydrate ratios is considered the standard of care. Neither calories nor fat should be restricted, but sugar-containing drinks should be avoided between mealtimes. There is no evidence to support particular treatment targets, but generally, near-normal glucose levels should be achieved if possible to do so safely, as in other forms of diabetes. A1C measurement is of limited value because it is spuriously low in CF due to increased red blood cell turnover time. Self-monitoring of blood glucose is recommended three to four times a day, and 2-hour postprandial measurements are useful for determining adequacy of meal time insulin doses.

Drugs and Conditions Predisposing to Diabetes

Several drugs and toxins can exacerbate a predisposition to diabetes. L-asparaginase, interferon-α, pentamidine, didanosine, Vacor (a rat poison), and several immunosuppressive agents damage the β-cell and may cause temporary or permanent diabetes. Diazoxide, Dilantin, and somatostatin analogs reversibly impair insulin secretion. Glucocorticoids, β-adrenergic agonists, protease inhibitors, and possibly niacin and thiazides cause insulin resistance.

Syndromic diabetes is either due to insulin secretory defects as in Wolfram or primary insulin resistance with subsequent β-cell failure as in Turner, Klinefelter, Lawrence–Moon, Bardet–Biedl, Prader–Willi, and myotonic dystrophy. Treatments include insulin, and for those with obesity-related insulin resistance, weight loss.

Conditions that damage the islets, such as pancreatitis or hemolytic uremic syndrome, not uncommonly cause diabetes. Diabetes in hemolytic uremic syndrome may be permanent, transient, or may resolve for a time only to reappear a few years later. Iron overload due to transfusions in thalassemia major also causes islet damage and diabetes.

Endocrinopathies listed in Table 20-8 are primarily diseases of adults and are rare in children. Somatostatinomas directly inhibit insulin secretion (but may also cause hypoglycemia by inhibiting glucagon secretion, or by cosecretion of insulin). The other endocrinopathies cause significant increases of metabolic counterregulatory hormones (or their effects in the case of thyroid hormone facilitating adrenergic activity) and insulin resistance. Treatment starts by correcting the underlying disease. Diabetes may persist in a large minority and insulin or insulin-sensitizing agents may be needed.

DIABETES COMPLICATIONS AND COMORBIDITIES

Overview

The chronic complications of diabetes are due to longstanding hyperglycemia so they are the same regardless of the type of diabetes. The duration and severity of hyperglycemia alter the risk, so persons with mild forms of diabetes such as MODY2, and short-duration forms such as GDM generally do not develop complications. Most of the available data on complications come from studies of type 1 and type 2 diabetes.

Complications can be divided into microvascular and macrovascular. Microvascular complications include retinopathy, ne-phropathy, and neuropathy. Macrovascular complications including cardiovascular, cerebrovascular, and peripheral vascular disease are more common in T2DM because of the other cardiovascular risk factors of the metabolic syndrome, but are the leading cause of death in patients with both forms of diabetes.

At one time, it was believed that children were protected from diabetes complications and that the prepubertal period did not contribute to future risk. We now know this is not true. Prepubertal duration of diabetes and degree of hyperglycemia contribute to postpubertal microalbuminuria (110), and both prepubertal and pubertal duration of diabetes play a role in the development of retinopathy (111).

In the DCCT, adolescents with less than 5 years duration of T1DM developed significant retinopathy at a rate of 3.2 per 100 person-years with a cumulative incidence of approximately 16% after 5 years, and microalbuminuria at a rate of 5.8 per 100 person-years or approximately 28% after 5 years. Clinical neuropathy developed in 3.2% over an average of 7.8 years (32). In Pima Indians with T2DM, incidence of retinopathy in those whose diabetes began before age 20 was less than half that of those whose onset was after age 20, but development of nephropathy was not different (112). There are no data about clinical cardiovascular outcomes in children with diabetes. Given that the metabolic profile of these children with T2DM is similar to that of adults with T2DM, the adult literature is cautiously extrapolated to pediatrics.

Macrovascular Complications

Atherosclerotic cardiovascular disease is rare in childhood, but its precursors are present in the young. Autopsy studies have demonstrated that the extent of early atherosclerosis of the aorta and coronary arteries is directly associated with levels of lipids, blood pressure, and obesity in childhood and adolescence (113–115).

Although clinical macrovascular disease has not been described in children with diabetes, diabetes (especially type 2) is a risk factor for future cardiovascular, cerebrovascular, and peripheral vascular disease. Neither the DCCT nor the UKPDS were able to show significant improvement in cardiovascular risk with aggressive blood glucose control; however, studies in adults have shown that patients with diabetes benefit greatly from control of hypertension (116) and dyslipidemia (117,118). Therefore screening is part of routine care and treatment and with dietary and activity measures should be instituted early. Pharmacologic treatment of children has no basis in evidence but may be considered in very high risk individuals. Antismoking education should be provided as part of the routine diabetes visit.

Hypertension

Hypertension is a common complication of both type 1 and type 2 diabetes. For macrovascular disease, the UKPDS showed that hypertension is a stronger risk factor than hyperglycemia, and treating hypertension is more beneficial than treating hyperglycemia (116,119). Blood pressure must be measured using an appropriate size cuff. In adults, blood pressure targets are lower than in the general population but there is no evidence to support different targets in diabetic children from the usual 95th percentile cut off for abnormality. Weight loss and decreased salt intake should be attempted first. If drug therapy is necessary, ACE inhibitors are the first line because of their blood pressure–independent renal and cardiovascular protective effects in diabetes. If ACE inhibitors cannot be tolerated or are insufficient alone, diuretics, nondihydropyridine calcium channel blockers, or β-blockers may be substituted or added. There is a small risk of worsening blood glucose control or hypoglycemia unawareness with β-blockers. Women taking ACE inhibitors who are contemplating pregnancy or become pregnant need to discontinue the drug due to teratogenicity.

Dyslipidemia

T2DM is associated with an atherogenic lipid profile with high triglycerides, low HDL cholesterol, and small, dense LDL. Among young adults aged 15 to 34 years, diabetes was a risk factor for early atherosclerotic disease (120). Although adults with both forms of diabetes are considered at high risk of cardiovascular disease and, target lipid levels reflect this, there is no evidence that target lipids for children with diabetes should be different from those for other children. Nonetheless, the ADA made recommendations that children with diabetes have the same target lipids as adults with diabetes, that is LDL less than 100 mg/dL (2.6 mmol/L), HDL more than 40 mg/dL (1.02 mmol/L), and triglycerides less than 150 mg/dL (1.7 mmol/L). Treatment is nonpharmacologic if the LDL is 100 to 129 mg/dL (2.6–3.34 mmol/L). They suggest to "consider" medication if LDL is 130 to 159 mg/dL (3.35–4.09 mmol/L) and there are other cardiovascular risk factors such as obesity, hypertension, smoking, or family history of premature cardiovascular disease. They recommend starting medication if LDL higher than 160 mg/dL (4.1 mmol/L). Exercise, diet, weight loss, and improved glycemic control are the initial treatment measures. Although the American Heart Association Step-One Diet (< 30% of total calories from fat, <10% of total calories from saturated fat, <10% of total calories from polyunsaturated fat, and <100 mg of cholesterol/1,000 kcal) can be attempted, current recommendations are to go straight to the Step-Two diet (< 10% of calories from saturated fat and <67 mg cholesterol/1,000 kcal). Pharmacologic therapy includes bile acid–binding resins for children older than 10 years of age or 5-hydroxy-3-methylglutaryl–CoA reductase inhibitors for postmenarchal girls or for boys who are at or beyond Tanner II (121). Elevated liver enzymes and muscle pain or rhabdomyolysis are infrequent side effects. Adolescent girls should be aware that these drugs are not approved in pregnancy.

Microvascular Complications

Retinopathy Diabetic retinopathy is common in both type 1 and type 2 diabetes and is the most frequent cause of new cases of blindness in individuals age 20 years and older. Nonproliferative retinopathy progresses from microaneurysms and small dot hemorrhages to larger hemorrhages and hard exudates to retinal infarcts (cotton-wool spots). Macular edema from small-vessel leakage in the macula can lead to central vision loss. Macular edema can be treated by focal retinal laser photocoagulation to prevent further vision loss. Proliferative retinopathy develops as a result of retinal ischemia and involves growth of new retinal vessels. New vessels that extend into the vitreous cavity can hemorrhage and cause vision loss. Fibrosis can lead to retraction and retinal detachment. Proliferative disease is amenable to panretinal scatter laser photocoagulation. (122) Because these are treatable, it is important to have regular follow up with an experienced professional.

Clearly, prevention is better than treatment. The DCCT and UKPDS demonstrated that intensive glucose control can reduce the incidence and progression of retinopathy by 76% and 21% to 54%, respectively (31,68). Tight blood pressure control can also reduce progression by 34%, at least in T2DM (116).

Nephropathy

Diabetic nephropathy occurs in 20% to 40% of adults with diabetes and is the leading cause of end-stage renal disease. Even with modern diabetes management, a 2003 Swedish study showed that approximately 40% of patients in whom with diabetes was diagnosed at 15 to 34 years of age developed renal involvement within 10 years of diabetes onset (123). Among the earliest clinical signs of nephropathy is microalbuminuria, defined as urine albumin of 30 to 300 mg/day. The spot urine for albumin:creatinine ratio is a reliable alternative to timed collections. An albumin:creatinine ratio of 30 to 300 μg/mg is in the microalbuminuric range. The natural history is progression to overt proteinuria, hypertension, glomerulosclerosis, and renal insufficiency ending in end-stage renal disease.

Children and youth with T1DM should be screened yearly starting 5 years after diagnosis or 5 years after onset of puberty, whichever comes later. Annual screening should start at the time of diagnosis in T2DM because true duration is usually unknown. Once microalbuminuria is detected, it should be confirmed with a first morning void albumin:creatinine ratio or a split-time 24-hour urine collection because there is a high prevalence of orthostatic and exercise-induced proteinuria in adolescents. Improvement in glycemic control can often reverse microalbuminuria in adolescents. Before starting any treatment, persistence should be documented every 3 to 4 months over 1 year.

The DCCT and UKPDS demonstrated that intensive glucose control can reduce the progression of nephropathy by 54% and 48%, respectively (31,68). Tight blood pressure control can also reduce progression by 39%, at least in T2DM (116). After instituting modest salt restriction, in the pediatric age group, ACE inhibitors are the drugs of choice. ACE inhibitors have been shown to be renal protective independent of their blood pressure–lowering effect (124). They are contraindicated in pregnancy. Protein restriction, which has been used in adults with advanced nephropathy, is not advisable in children although excessive protein intake should be avoided. Primary renal disease must always be considered and is particularly common in some Native American populations with high incidences of T2DM (125).

Neuropathy

There are many forms of neuropathy in diabetes, the most common being symmetric peripheral neuropathy that causes decreased sensation, sweating, and muscle tone and contributes to pain and foot ulcers and deformities. Autonomic neuropathy can affect the gastrointestinal, cardiovascular, genitourinary, and sudomotor systems and cause gastroparesis and diarrhea, arrhythmia, erectile and female sexual dysfunction, and dry skin. Other types include cranial mononeuropathies, radicular neuropathy, amyotrophy, and insulin neuritis.

Neurological disorders, including peripheral neuropathy and cerebellar ataxia occur in 10% of individuals with celiac disease and have an autoimmune etiology (126). Clinical neuropathy in diabetic children and adolescents is rare (127), but its occurrence warrants investigation for coexisting celiac disease. Screening foot examinations should begin after 5 years in the postpubertal child with T1DM and at diagnosis in T2DM. Tight glycemic control can decrease the incidence of diabetic neuropathy by 60% (31). Established diabetic neuropathy is disabling and its treatment symptomatic.

Skin Changes

Diabetes is associated with several skin diseases. The classic one is necrobiosis lipoidica diabeticorum. Others include diabetic dermopathy, granuloma annulare, diabetic bullae, yellow skin, and diabetic ulcers. It is uncommon to see these in children. Diabetic thick skin is seen in poorly controlled diabetic children and usually presents as limited joint mobility. This is diagnosed by having the patient place the hands together in a "prayer" position. Normally, the fingers should fit tightly together. Limited joint mobility is documented when thickened skin tethers the fingers downward into a curved position, so that there is a space when the fingers are put together. The most common lesion, lipohypertrophy of injections sites, can be prevented and minimized by rotating sites and avoiding overuse of any particular site. Lipoatrophy of injection sites used to be common but is seldom seen now that animal insulins are no longer used.

Skin infections are not uncommon. Fungal infections including vaginitis, balanitis, and paronychia can be treated topically and with improved glucose control. Bacterial infections, particularly staphylococcal, but also pseudomonal occur. Poor leukocyte chemotaxis and wound healing predispose to infections (128).

CONCLUSION

Diabetes is a major, multifaceted health problem whose impact on personal and public health justifies major effort by all involved, from political decision makers to public health authorities to healthcare professionals to affected individuals and their families. Effective long term pediatric diabetes care requires specialized staffing, clinical equipment and training, and can be difficult to manage in a general primary care setting. In the pediatric age groups, the importance of the team approach makes care by a secondary or tertiary care facility the optimal choice.

For the less common forms of diabetes, the variety and complexity of causes can be intimidating; however, the clinician must keep in mind that the individual patient's metabolic status is what will ultimately determine the best management strategy, regardless of etiology.

REFERENCES

1. American Diabetes Association. Type 2 diabetes in children and adolescents. *Pediatrics*. 2000;105(3 Pt 1):671–680.
2. Amery CM, Nattrass M. Fatty acids and insulin secretion. *Diabetes Obes Metab*. 2000;2(4):213–221.
3. Vilsboll T, Holst JJ. Incretins, insulin secretion and type 2 diabetes mellitus. *Diabetologia*.2004;47(3):357–366.
4. Combettes M, Kargar C. Newly approved and promising antidiabetic agents. *Therapie*. 2007;62(4):293–310.
5. Zick Y. Insulin resistance: a phosphorylation-based uncoupling of insulin signaling. *Trends Cell Biol*. 2001;11(11):437–441.
6. Viik-Kajander M, Moltchanova E, Libman I, et al. Incidence of childhood type 1 diabetes worldwide. Diabetes Mondiale (DiaMond) Project Group. *Diabetes Care*. 2000;23(10):1516–1526.
7. Onkamo, P. Vaananen S, Karvonen M, et al. Worldwide increase in incidence of type I diabetes—the analysis of the data on published incidence trends. *Diabetologia*. 1999;42(12):1395–1403.
8. Gale EA. The rise of childhood type 1 diabetes in the 20th century. *Diabetes*. 2002;51(12):3353–3361.
9. Eisenbarth GS. Type 1 diabetes: molecular, cellular and clinical immunology. *Adv Exp Med Biol*. 2004;552:306–310.
10. Foulis AK, and e. al. The histopathology of the pancreas in type 1 (insulin-dependent) diabetes mellitus: a 25-year review of deaths in patients under 20 years of age in the United Kingdom. *Diabetologia*. 1986;29(5):267–274.
11. LaGasse JM, Brantley MS, Leech NJ, et al. Successful prospective prediction of type 1 diabetes in schoolchildren through multiple defined autoantibodies: an 8-year follow-up of the Washington State Diabetes Prediction Study. *Diabetes Care*. 2002;25(3):505–511.
12. Verge, CF, Gianani R, Kawasaki E, et al. Prediction of type I diabetes in first-degree relatives using a combination of insulin, GAD, and ICA512bdc/IA-2 autoantibodies. *Diabetes*. 1996;45(7):926–933.
13. Atkinson MA, Eisenbarth GS. Type 1 diabetes: new perspectives on disease pathogenesis and treatment. *Lancet*. 2001;358(9277):221–229.
14. Warram, JH, Krolewski AS, Gottlieb MS, et al. Differences in risk of insulin-dependent diabetes in offspring of diabetic mothers and diabetic fathers. *N Engl J Med*. 1984;311(3):149–152.
15. Hughes AL, Nei M. Pattern of nucleotide substitution at major histocompatibility complex class I loci reveals overdominant selection. *Nature*. 1988;335(6186):167–170.
16. Melanitou E, Fain P, Eisenbarth GS. Genetics of type 1A (immune mediated) diabetes. *J Autoimmun*. 2003;21:93–98.
17. Risch N. Assessing the role of HLA-linked and unlinked determinants of disease. *Am J Hum Genet*. 1987;40(1):1–14.
18. Vafiadis P, Bennett SP, Todd JA, et al., Insulin expression in human thymus is modulated by INS VNTR alleles at the IDDM2 locus. *Nat Genet*. 1997;15(3):289–292.
19. Derbinski J, Schulte A, Kyewski B, et al. Promiscuous gene expression in medullary thymic epithelial cells mirrors the peripheral self. *Nat Immunol*. 2001;2(11):1032–1039.
20. Bottini N, Musumeci L, Alonso A, et al. A functional variant of lymphoid tyrosine phosphatase is associated with type I diabetes. *Nat Genet*. 2004;36(4):337–338.
21. Ueda H, Howson JM, Esposito L, et al. Association of the T-cell regulatory gene CTLA4 with susceptibility to autoimmune disease. *Nature*. 2003;423(6939):506–511.
22. Anjos SM, Tessier MC, Polychronakos C. Association of the cytotoxic T lymphocyte-associated antigen 4 gene with type 1 diabetes: evidence for independent effects of two polymorphisms on the same haplotype block. *J Clin Endocrinol Metab*. 2004;89(12):6257–6265.
23. Robles DT, Eisenbarth GS. Type 1A diabetes induced by infection and immunization. *J Autoimmun*. 2001;16(3):355–362.
24. Scott FW, Cloutier HE, Kleemann R, et al. Potential mechanisms by which certain foods promote or inhibit the development of spontaneous diabetes in BB rats: dose, timing, early effect on islet area, and switch in infiltrate from Th1 to Th2 cells. *Diabetes*. 1997;46(4):589–598.
25. Zavalkoff SR, Polychronakos C. Evaluation of conventional blood glucose monitoring as an indicator of integrated glucose values using a continuous subcutaneous sensor. *Diabetes Care*. 2002;25(9):1603–1606.
26. Rendell M. Dietary Treatment of Diabetes Mellitus. *N Engl J Med*. 2000. 342:1440–1441.
27. Hamiton J, Cummings E, Zdravkovic V, et al. Metformin as an adjunct therapy in adolescents with type 1 diabetes and insulin resistance: a randomized controlled trial. *Diabetes Care*. 2003; 26:138–143.
28. Särnblad S, Kroon M, Aman J. Metformin as additional therapy in adolescents with poorly controlled type 1 diabetes: randomised placebo-controlled trial with aspects on insulin sensitivity. *Eur J Endocrinol*. 2003;149:323–329.
29. Khan AS, McLoughney CR, Ahmed AB. The effect of metformin on blood glucose control in overweight patients with Type 1 diabetes. *Diabet Med*. 2006;23:1079–1084.
30. Heptulla RA, Rodriguez LM, Bomgaars L, et al. The role of amylin and glucagon in the dampening of glycemic excursions in children with type 1 diabetes. *Diabetes*. 2005;54:1100–1107.
31. The Diabetes Control and Complications Trial Research Group. The effect of intensive treatment of diabetes on the development and progression of long-term complications in insulin-dependent diabetes mellitus. *N Engl J Med*. 1993;329(14):977–986.
32. Diabetes Control and Complications Trial Research Group Effect of intensive diabetes treatment on the development

and progression of long-term complications in adolescents with insulin-dependent diabetes mellitus: Diabetes Control and Complications Trial. *J Pediatr.* 1994;125(2):177–188.

33. Little RR. Glycated hemoglobin standardization: National Glycohemoglobin Standardization Program (NGSP) perspective. *Clin Chem Lab Med.* 2003;41(9):1191–1198.

34. Rosenbloom AL. Intracerebral crises during treatment of diabetic ketoacidosis. *Diabetes Care.* 1990;13(1):22–33.

35. Glaser N, Barnett P, McCaslin I, et al. Risk factors for cerebral edema in children with diabetic ketoacidosis. The Pediatric Emergency Medicine Collab-orative Research Committee of the American Academy of Pediatrics. *N Engl J Med.* 2001;344(4):264–269.

36. Muir AB, Quisling RG, Yang MC, et al. Cerebral edema in childhood diabetic ketoacidosis: natural history, radiographic findings, and early identification. *Diabetes Care.* 2004;27(7):1541–1546.

37. Kitabchi AE, Umpierrz GE, Murphy MB, et al. Hyperglycemic crises in diabetes. *Diabetes Care.* 2004;27 Suppl 1:S94–102.

38. Haymond MW, Schreiner B. Mini-dose glucagon rescue for hypoglycemia in children with type 1 diabetes. *Diabetes Care.* 2001;24(4):643–645.

39. Kovacs M, Goldston D, Obronsky DS, et al. Psychiatric disorders in youths with IDDM: rates and risk factors. *Diabetes Care.* 1997;20(1):36–44.

40. Howorka K, Pumpria J, Gabriel M, et al. Normalization of pregnancy outcome in pregestational diabetes through functional insulin treatment and modular out-patient education adapted for pregnancy. *Diabet Med.* 2001;18(12):965–972.

41. Suhonen L, Hiilesmaa V. Teramo K. Glycaemic control during early pregnancy and fetal malformations in women with type I diabetes mellitus. *Diabetologia.* 2000;43(1):79–82.

42. American Diabetes Association. Gestational diabetes mellitus. *Diabetes Care.* 2003;26 Suppl 1:S103–105.

43. Canadian Diabetes Association Clinical Practice Guidelines Expert Committee. Pre-existing Diabetes and Pregnancy. *Can J Diabetes.* 2003;27(S2):S94–S98.

44. European Diabetes Policy Group. Guidelines for Diabetes Care. International Diabetes Federation Brussesls; Walter Wirtz Druck & Verlag, 1998.

45. Hirshberg B, Muszkat M, Marom T, et al. Natural course of insulin edema. *J Endocrinol Invest.* 2000;23(3):187–188.

46. Konrad D, Daneman D, Kirby M, et al. Cardiac failure after initiation of insulin treatment in diabetic patients with beta-thalassemia major. *J Pediatr.* 2003;143(4):541–542.

47. Sutherland DE, Gruessner RW, Dunn DL, et al. Lessons learned from more than 1,000 pancreas transplants at a single institution. *Ann Surg.* 2001;233(4):463–501.

48. Ryan EA, Lakey JR, Play BW, Successful islet transplantation: continued insulin reserve provides long-term glycemic control. *Diabetes.* 2002;51(7) 2148–2157.

49. Kordonouri O, Klinghammer A, Lang EB, et al. Thyroid autoimmunity in children and adolescents with type 1 diabetes: a multicenter survey. *Diabetes Care.* 2002;25(8):1346–1350.

50. Barera G, Bonfanti R, Viscardi M, et al. Occurrence of celiac disease after onset of type 1 diabetes: a 6-year prospective longitudinal study. *Pediatrics.* 2002;109(5):833–838.

51. Kitagawa T, Owada M, Urakami T, et al. Increased incidence of non-insulin dependent diabetes mellitus among Japanese schoolchildren correlates with an increased intake of animal protein and fat. *Clin Pediatr.* 1998;37(2):111–115.

52. Murtaugh MA, Jacobs DR Jr, Moran A, et al. Relation of birth weight to fasting insulin, insulin resistance, and body size in adolescence. *Diabetes Care.* 2003;26(1):187–92.

53. Kahn SE, Prigeon RL, mcCulloch DK, et al. Quantification of the relationship between insulin sensitivity and beta-cell function in human subjects. Evidence for a hyperbolic function. *Diabetes.* 1993;42(11):1663–1672.

54. Ruan H, Lodish HF. Insulin resistance in adipose tissue: direct and indirect effects of tumor necrosis factor-alpha. *Cytokine Growth Factor Rev.* 2003;14(5):447–455.

55. Guerre-Millo M. Adipose tissue and adipokines: for better or worse. *Diabetes Metab.* 2004;30(1):13–19.

56. Belfiore F, Iannello S, Rabuazzo AM, et al. Metabolic effects of short-term fasting in obese hyperglycaemic humans and mice. *Int J Obes.* 1987;11(6):631–640.

57. Moran A, Jacobs DR Jr, Steinberger J, et al. Association between the insulin resistance of puberty and the insulin-like growth factor-I/growth hormone axis. *J Clin Endocrinol Metab.* 2002;87(10):4817–4820.

58. Lambert M, Delvin EE, Paradis G, et al. C-Reactive protein and features of the metabolic syndrome in a population-based sample of children and adolescents. *Clin Chem.* 2004;50(10):1762–1768.

59. Ten, S. and N. Maclaren, Insulin resistance syndrome in children. *J Clin Endocrinol Metab.* 2004;89(6):2526–2539.

60. Hanley AJ, D'Agostino R Jr, Wagenknecht LE, et al. Increased proinsulin levels and decreased acute insulin response independently predict the incidence of type 2 diabetes in the insulin resistance atherosclerosis study. *Diabetes.* 2002;51(4):1263–1270.

61. Kahn SE. The relative contributions of insulin resistance and beta-cell dysfunction to the pathophysiology of Type 2 diabetes. *Diabetologia.* 2003;46(1):3–19.

62. Steppel JH, Horton ES. Beta-cell failure in the pathogenesis of type 2 diabetes mellitus. *Curr Diabet Rep.* 2004;4(3):169–175.

63. Poitout V, Robertson RP. Minireview: Secondary beta-cell failure in type 2 diabetes—a convergence of glucotoxicity and lipotoxicity. *Endocrinology.* 2002;143(2):339–342.

64. Florez JC, Hirschhorn J, Altshuler D. The inherited basis of diabetes mellitus: implications for the genetic analysis of complex traits. *Annu Rev Genom Hum Genet.* 2003;4:257–291.

65. Grün F, Blumberg B. Environmental Obesogens: Organotins and Endocrine Disruption via Nuclear Receptor Signaling. *Endocrinology.* 2006;147:S50–S55.

66. Halhout EH, Thomas W, El-Shahawy M, et al. Diabetic autoimmune markers in children and adolescents with type 2 diabetes. *Pediatrics.* 2001;107(6):E102.

67. Zinman B, Kahn SE, Haffner SM, et al. Phenotypic characteristics of GAD antibody-positive recently diagnosed patients with type 2 diabetes in North America and Europe. *Diabetes.* 2004;53(12):3193–3200.

68. United Kingdom Prospective Diabetes Study (UKPDS) Group. Intensive blood-glucose control with sulphonylureas or insulin compared with conventional treatment and risk of complications in patients with type 2 diabetes (UKPDS 33). *Lancet.* 1998;352(9131):837–853.

69. Bloomgarden ZT. American Diabetes Association Annual Meeting, 1998. Insulin resistance, exercise, and obesity. *Diabetes Care.* 1999;22(3):517–522.

70. Gahagan S, Silverstein J. Prevention and treatment of type 2 diabetes mellitus in children, with special emphasis on American Indian and Alaska Native children. American Academy of Pediatrics Committee on Native American Child Health. *Pediatrics.* 2003;112(4) e328.

71. Kirpichnikov D, McFarlane SI, Sowers JR. Metformin: an update. *Ann Intern Med.* 2002;137(1):25–33.

72. Jones KL, Arslanian S, Peterokova VA, et al. Effect of metformin in pediatric patients with type 2 diabetes: a randomized controlled trial. *Diabetes Care.* 2002;25(1):89–94.

73. Gottschalk M, Danne T, Vlajnic A, et al. Glimepiride versus metformin as monotherapy in pediatric patients with type 2 diabetes: a randomized, single-blind comparative study. *Diabetes Care.* 2007;30:790–794.

74. Tuomi T, Honkanen EH, Isomaa B, et al. Improved prandial glucose control with lower risk of hypoglycemia with nateglinide than with glibenclamide in patients with maturity-onset diabetes of the young type 3. *Diabetes Care.* 2006 Feb;29:189–194.

75. Tuomilehto J, Lindstrom J, Eriksson JG, et al. Prevention of type 2 diabetes mellitus by changes in lifestyle among subjects with impaired glucose tolerance. *N Engl J Med.* 2001;344(18):1343–1350.

76. Knowler WC, Barreett-Connor E, Fowler SE, et al. Reduction in the incidence of type 2 diabetes with lifestyle intervention or metformin. *N Engl J Med.* 2002;346(6):393–403.

77. Buchanan TA, Xiang AH, Peters RK, et al. Preservation of pancreatic beta-cell function and prevention of type 2 diabetes by pharmacological treatment of insulin resistance in high-risk hispanic women. *Diabetes.* 2002;51(9):2796–2803.

78. Gerstein HC, Yusuf S, Bosch J, et al. Effect of rosiglitazone on the frequency of diabetes in patients with impaired glucose tolerance or impaired fasting glucose: a randomised

controlled trial. *Lancet* 2006;368(9541): 1096–1105.

79. Chiasson JL, Josse RG, Gomis R, et al. Acarbose for prevention of type 2 diabetes mellitus: the STOP-NIDDM randomised trial. *Lancet*. 2002; 359(9323):2072–2077.

80. Harris MI, Eastman RC, Cowie CC, et al. Comparison of diabetes diagnostic categories in the U.S. population according to the 1997 American Diabetes Association and 1980–1985 World Health Organization diagnostic criteria. *Diabetes Care*. 1997;20(12):1859–1862.

81. Morales AE, Rosenbloom AL. Death caused by hyperglycemic hyperosmolar state at the onset of type 2 diabetes. *J Pediatr*. 2004;144(2):270–273.

82. Banerji MA, Chaiken RL, Huey H, et al. GAD antibody negative NIDDM in adult black subjects with diabetic ketoacidosis and increased frequency of human leukocyte antigen DR3 and DR4. *Flatbush diabetes*. *Diabetes*. 1994;43:741–745.

83. Tan KC, Mackay IR, Zimmet PZ, et al. Metabolic and immunologic features of Chinese patients with atypical diabetes mellitus. *Diabetes Care*. 2000;23:335–338.

84. Maldonado M, Hampe CS, Gaur LK, et al. Ketosis-prone diabetes: dissection of a heterogeneous syndrome using an immunogenetic and b-cell functional classification, prospective analysis and clinical outcomes. *J Clin Endocrinol Metab*. 2003;88:5090–5098.

85. Pallardo, F., et al., Early postpartum metabolic assessment in women with prior gestational diabetes. *Diabetes Care*. 1999;22(7):1053–1058.

86. Canadian Diabetes Association Clinical Practice Guidelines Expert Committee. Gestational diabetes mellitus. *Can J Diabetes*. 2003;27(S2):S99–S105.

87. von Muhlendahl KE, Herkenhoff H. Long-term course of neonatal diabetes. *N Engl J Med*. 1995;333(11):704–708.

88. Temple, I.K. and J.P. Shield., Transient neonatal diabetes, a disorder of imprinting. *J Med Genet*. 2002;39(12):872–875.

89. Gardner RJ, MacKay DJ, Mungall AJ, et al. An imprinted locus associated with transient neonatal diabetes mellitus. *Hum Mol Genet*. 2000;9(4):589–596.

90. Vaxillaire M, Populaire C, Busiah K, et al. Kir6.2 mutations are a common cause of permanent neonatal diabetes in a large cohort of French patients. *Diabetes*. 2004;53(10):2719–2722.

91. Sagen JV, Raeder H, Hathout E, et al. Permanent neonatal diabetes due to mutations in KCNJ11 encoding Kir6.2: patient characteristics and initial response to sulfonylurea therapy. *Diabetes*. 2004;53(10):2713–2718.

92. Njolstad PR, Sovik O, Cuesta-Munoz A, et al. Neonatal diabetes mellitus due to complete glucokinase deficiency. *N Engl J Med*. 2001;344(21):1588–1592.

93. Stoffers DA, Zinken NT, Stanojevic V, et al. Pancreatic agenesis attributable to a single nucleotide deletion in the human IPF1 gene coding sequence. *Nat Genet*. 1997;15(1):106–110.

94. Gloyn AL, Weedon MN, Owen KR, et al. Large-scale association studies of variants in genes encoding the pancreatic beta-cell KATP channel subunits Kir6.2 (KCNJ11) and SUR1 (ABCC8) confirm that the KCNJ11 E23K variant is associated with type 2 diabetes. *Diabetes*. 2003;52(2):568–572.

95. Hani EH, Stoffers DA, Chevre JC, et al. Defective mutations in the insulin promoter factor-1 (IPF-1) gene in late-onset type 2 diabetes mellitus. *J Clin Invest*. 1999; 104(9):R41–48.

96. Goto Y, Nonaka I, Horai S. A mutation in the tRNA(Leu)(UUR) gene associated with the MELAS subgroup of mitochondrial encephalomyopathies. *Nature*. 1990;348(6302):651–653.

97. Morais CT, DiMauro S, Zeviani M, et al. Mitochondrial DNA deletions in progressive external ophthalmoplegia and Kearns-Sayre syndrome. *N Engl J Med*. 1989;320(20):1293–1299.

98. Inoue H. A gene encoding a transmembrane protein is mutated in patients with diabetes mellitus and optic atrophy (Wolfram syndrome). *Nat Genet*. 1998;20(2):143–148.

99. Longo N, Wang Y, Smith SA, et al. Genotype-phenotype correlation in inherited severe insulin resistance. *Hum Mol Genet*. 2002;11(12):1465–1475.

100. Musso C, Cochran E, Moran SA, et al. Clinical course of genetic diseases of the insulin receptor (type A and Rabson-Mendenhall syndromes): a 30-year prospective. *Medicine*. 2004;83(4): 209–222.

101. Longo N, Wang Y, Pasquali M. Progressive decline in insulin levels in Rabson-Mendenhall syndrome. *J Clin Endocrinol Metab*. 1999;84(8):2623–2629.

102. Coehran E, Young JR, Sebring N, et al. Efficacy of recombinant methionyl human leptin therapy for the extreme insulin resistance of the Rabson-Mendenhall syndrome. *J Clin Endocrinol Metab*. 2004;89(4):1548–1554.

103. Mantzoros C, Flier JS. Lipodystrophic syndromes. In: Rose BD, ed. UpToDate. Wellesley, MA: *UpToDate*; 2005:xxx-xxx.

104. Oral EA. Lipoatrophic diabetes and other related syndromes. *Rev Endocr Metab Disord*. 2003;4(1):61–77.

105. Moran A, Diem P, Klein DJ, et al. Pancreatic endocrine function in cystic fibrosis. *J Pediatr*. 1991;118(5):715–723.

106. Lombardi F, Raia V, Spagnudo MI, et al. Diabetes in an infant with cystic fibrosis. *Pediatr Diabetes*. 2004;5(4):199–201.

107. Mackie AD, Thornton SJ, Edenborough FP. Cystic fibrosis-related diabetes. *Diabet Med*. 2003;20(6):425–436.

108. Moran A, Hardin D, Rodman D, et al. Diagnosis, screening and management of cystic fibrosis related diabetes mellitus: a consensus conference report. *Diabetes Res Clin Pract*. 1999;45(1):61–73.

109. Rosenecker J, Eichler I, Barmeir H, et al. Diabetes mellitus and cystic fibrosis: comparison of clinical parameters in patients treated with insulin versus oral glucose-lowering agents. *Pediatr Pulmonol*. 2001;32(5):351–335.

110. Schultz CJ, Konopelska-Bahu T, Dalton RN, et al. Microalbuminuria prevalence varies with age, sex, and puberty in children with type 1 diabetes followed from diagnosis in a longitudinal study. Oxford Regional Prospective Study Group. *Diabetes Care*. 1999;22(3):495–502.

111. Holl RW, Iang GE, Grabert M, et al. Diabetic retinopathy in pediatric patients with type-1 diabetes: effect of diabetes duration, prepubertal and pubertal onset of diabetes, and metabolic control. *J Pediatr*. 1998;132(5):790–794.

112. Krakoff J, Lindsay RS, Looker HC, et al. Incidence of retinopathy and nephropathy in youth-onset compared with adult-onset type 2 diabetes. *Diabetes Care*. 2003;26(1):76–81.

113. Berenson GS, Srinivasan SR, Bao W, et al. Association between multiple cardiovascular risk factors and atherosclerosis in children and young adults. The Bogalusa Heart Study. *N Engl J Med*. 1998;338(23):1650–1656.

114. McGill HC Jr, McMahan CA, Herderick EE, et al. Obesity accelerates the progression of coronary atherosclerosis in young men. *Circulation*. 2002;105(23): 2712–2718.

115. McGill HC Jr, McMahan CA, Zieske AW, et al. Association of Coronary Heart Disease Risk Factors with microscopic qualities of coronary atherosclerosis in youth. *Circulation*. 2000;102(4):374–379.

116. United Kingdom Prospective Diabetes Study Group. Tight blood pressure control and risk of macrovascular and microvascular complications in type 2 diabetes: UKPDS 38. *Br Med J*. 1998;317(7160):703–713.

117. Miettinen TA, Pyorala K, Olsson AG, et al. Cholesterol lowering with simvastatin improves prognosis of diabetic patients with coronary heart disease. A subgroup analysis of the Scandinavian Simvastatin Survival Study (4S). *Diabetes Care*. 1997;20(4):614–620.

118. The Long-Term Intervention with Pravastatin in Ischaemic Disease (LIPID) Study Group. Prevention of cardiovascular events and death with pravastatin in patients with coronary heart disease and a broad range of initial cholesterol levels. *N Engl J Med*. 1998;339(19):1349–1357.

119. Adler AI, Stratton IM, Neil HA, et al. Association of systolic blood pressure with macrovascular and microvascular complications of type 2 diabetes (UKPDS 36): prospective observational study. *Br Med J*. 2000;321(7258): 412–419.

120. McGill HC Jr, McMahan CA, Zieske AW, et al. Effects of nonlipid risk factors on atherosclerosis in youth with a favorable lipoprotein profile. *Circulation*. 2001;103(11):1546–1550.

121. American Diabetes Association. Management of dyslipidemia in children and adolescents with diabetes. *Diabetes Care*. 2003;26(7):2194–2197.

122. Frank RN. Diabetic retinopathy. *N Engl J Med.* 2004;350(1) 48–58.

123. Svensson M, Sundkvist G, Amgvist HJ, et al. Signs of nephropathy may occur early in young adults with diabetes despite modern diabetes management: results from the nationwide population-based Diabetes Incidence Study in Sweden (DISS). *Diabetes Care.* 2003;26(10): 2903–2909.

124. Lewis, EJ, Hunsicker LG, Brain RP, et al. The effect of angiotensin-converting-enzyme inhibition on diabetic nephropathy. The Collaborative Study Group. *N Engl J Med.* 1993;329(20): 1456–1462.

125. Bulloch B, Postl BD, Ogborn MR, Excess prevalence of non diabetic renal disease in native American children in Manitoba. *Pediatr Nephrol.* 1996;10(6):702–704.

126. Alaedıni A, Green PH, Sander HW, et al. Ganglioside reactive antibodies in the neuropathy associated with celiac disease. *J Neuroimmunol.* 2002 Jun;127:145–148.

127. Donaghue KC, Fung AT, Fairchild JM, et al. Prospective assessment of autonomic and peripheral nerve function in adolescents with diabetes. *Diabet Med.* 1996; 13(1):65–71.

128. Paron NG, Lambert PW. Cutaneous manifestations of diabetes mellitus. *Prim Care.* 2000;27(2):371–383.

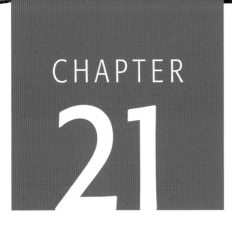

CHAPTER 21

Overweight and Obesity

Stephen B. Sondike, MD

NORMAL REGULATION OF ENERGY, METABOLISM, AND APPETITE

Energy requirements are highest in infants and decrease slowly to adult levels throughout childhood. Typical energy requirements for children and adolescents are listed in Table 21-1.

The Components of Energy Expenditure

Basal Metabolic Rate, Resting Energy Expenditure The major use of food energy in the body is for the basal metabolic rate (BMR), which is the energy required to maintain the basic autonomic functions, such as heartbeat, respiration, and basic metabolic and cellular functions. Because BMR is difficult to measure in free-living conditions, most clinicians use resting energy expenditure (REE), which is BMR plus energy required for arousal. REE usually is 3% higher and is approximately 2.94 kJ/minute in the average child (4). The BMR can be approximated by the Harris–Benedict equation or measured directly by indirect calorimetry, which calculates REE by measuring oxygen consumption and carbon dioxide production. The REE is responsive to changes in body weight, and following weight loss, a person may have an REE up to

15% lower than a person of the same body composition with a stable weight (5).

Thermic Effect of Eating The thermic effect of eating (TEE) describes the increase in metabolic rate following the ingestion of food that is necessary to digest, metabolize, and store micro- and macronutrients. Typically, the metabolic rate is increased by 10% after an average meal, although the increase can be as high as 30% during episodes of starvation, such as in anorexia nervosa, and is lower in obese children than in normal-weight controls (6). There is no evidence that differences in TEE lead to weight gain in the long term (7).

Physical Activity Physical activity energy expenditure is the energy required to move skeletal muscle and is the most variable of the components of energy expenditure. Other components of energy expenditure include that required for growth and to maintain a thermoneutral environment, but these are relatively insignificant outside the neonatal period. Non exercise activity thermogenesis (NEAT) is the energy expended for everything that is not sleeping, eating, or sportslike exercise. Recent studies regarding NEAT reveal that the amount of this kind of activity may be detemined genetrically, and those with obesity may be more "efficient" with

everyday movements, whereas thin people may fidget more (8).

Maintenance of Fat Mass by Regulation of Energy Expenditure Metabolic regulation of adipocyte homeostasis is a complex interaction that involves the brain, nervous system, gut, and adipocyte. New pathways are still being elucidated. Fasting leads to adiposity maintenance by mechanisms that include but are not limited to an increase in orexigenic hormones and a decrease in anorexic hormones, a decrease in the thermic effect of eating, a decrease in BMR, a suppression of thermogenesis, and psychological disturbance that leads to cravings for food. These effects have been shown to persist for up to 12 weeks after refeeding. Overfeeding has the reverse effect. These processes are active in both short- and long-term fasting and overfeeding.

Neuroendocrine Regulation of Appetite

The appetite center in the brain generally is regarded as being in the paraventricular nucleus (PVN). The PVN contains two powerful neurotransmitters, neuropeptide Y (NPY) and agouti-related protein (AgRP), that are synthesized in the adjacent arcuate nucleus (ACN) and transferred to the PVN by fibers. NPY and AgRP are both potent appetite stimulators, known in both animal and human models to stimulate uncontrolled eating when ingested (9,10) (Figure 21-1). Galanin is a hypothalamic hormone that is believed to stimulate appetite by increasing cravings for fat (11). Orexigenic hormone A and B (A–B) are other peptide hormones secreted by the lateral hypothalamus that increase appetite (12).

α-Melanocyte-stimulating hormone (α-MSH) is the primary central appetite-suppressing neurotransmitter and is the primary antagonist for AgRP (13). α-MSH, like other melanocortins, is cleaved from proopiomelanocortin (POMC) by prohormone

Age	Total kcal	Basal	Activity	Growth	Thermic Waste
1	100	50	15	20	15
3	95	50	17	18	15
6	80	40	20	10	10
9	70	38	20	5	8
12	60	35	10	10	5
15	48	38	7	7	8
18	40	25	5	2	5

TABLE 21-1 Approximate Energy Requirements by Age (kcal/kg)

Adapted from Behrman et al. *Nelson's Textbook of Pediatrics,* 16th ed. W. B. Saunders, 2000:142.

Overweight and Obesity
AT-A-GLANCE

Obesity is a multifactorial disorder of energy balance characterized by increased adiposity. The Centers for Disease Control and Prevention no longer recommend the use of the term *obese* in children and adolescents (ages 2–20 years). The preferred definitions are *at risk* for overweight for children with body mass index (BMI, kg/m^2) between the 85th to 95th percentile for age and o*verweight* for those with a BMI above the 95th percentile for age. The age- and gender-specific BMI growth charts can be found on the CDC Web site at www.cdc.gov. For adults, a BMI > 25 kg/m^2 is considered overweight, and a BMI >30 kg/m^2 is considered obese. The American

Obesity Association (AOA) still uses the terms *overweight* and *obese* for children as well as adults. For this review, I will use the CDC definitions of *at risk* and *overweight* to refer to individuals and *overweight* and *obese* to refer to populations.

Regardless of the cause of obesity, it is always the result of positive energy balance. Whether it is due to a genetic abnormality, hormonal imbalance, or medication or the cause is unknown, the end result of the abnormality is an increase in energy intake or a decrease in energy use or both.

Pediatric and adolescent obesity is increasing at epidemic proportions in American society and worldwide, as are complications due to childhood obesity. Although many factors are implicated, increased portion sizes, unhealthy food choices, and increases in sedentary activity are most likely causative. Hormonal and genetic causes (endogenous obesity) do occur, but exogenous obesity is much more common. Treatment involves decreasing sweetened beverages, making healthy food choices, and decreasing sedentary lifestyle, with family involvement being essential.

ENDOGENOUS OBESITY

Cause	Pathophysiology
Genetic predisposition	High concordance in twins; BMI in adopted children correlates with BMI of birth parents; however, genetic predisposition not sufficient itself to cause obesity
Monogenic obesity	Monogenic causes of overweight and obesity are rare; most monogenic causes involve central impairment of satiety, and the majority are caused by mutations of the POMC, PC1, MC4R, SIM1, leptin, and leptin receptor genes. 3% to 4% of people with morbid obesity have a defect in the melanocortin-4 receptor (the most common monogenic form of obesity) leading to uncontrolled appetite; a defect in PPAR-γ may increase adipocyte differentiation—this is the only known defect that acts on the end organ rather than centrally to cause obesity
Alternations in the fetal environment	Intrauterine growth retardation: risk of central adiposity; infants of poorly-controlled diabetic mothers: risk of obesity
Endocrinopathies associated with obesity	Hypothalamic hyperphagia due to brain injury from tumor, surgery, or trauma; cortisol excess from excessive central (or rarely ectopic) ACTH production or adrenal cancer is associated with poor growth; typical adult body habitus may be absent in children, who may have more diffuse obesity; hyperinsulinism due to a genetic defect in insulin secretion or, rarely, insulinoma; affected infants in particular have increased overall body size, including length and weight
Syndromes with associated obesity	Subjects with Prader–Willi syndrome have hyperphagia, most likely due to ghrelin excess; obesity is common in Down syndrome and fragile X; other syndromes and associated physical findings are presented in Table 24-3
Medications	Glucocorticoids cause obesity and growth failure; some antipsychotics cause obesity by increasing appetite; thiazolidinediones can cause obesity in adults; effect in children is unknown
Too many calories consumed	↑ Portion size ↑ Availability of sweetened beverages ↑ Availability of processed and "fast" foods that are high in fat and total calories
Too little exercise	↑ TV and computer time ↓ School and extracurricular physical activity ↓ Neighborhood play physical activity

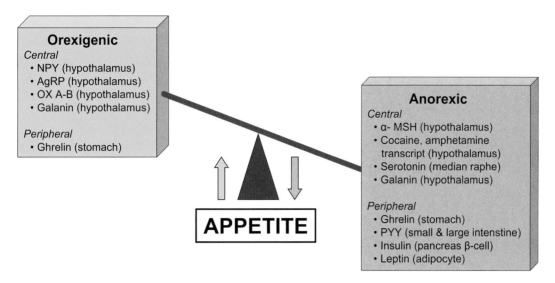

FIGURE 21-1. Major neurotransmitters and hormones involved in appetite regulation. Orexigenic factors are released in response to a fast to increase energy intake; anorexic factors are released in response to overfeeding and decrease energy intake. The site where each factor is produced is indicated in parentheses. NPY = neuropeptide Y, AgRP = Agouti-related peptide, OX A–B = orexigenic hormone A and B, α-MSH = α-melanocyte stimulating hormone, CCK = cholecystikinin, PYY = peptide YY.

convertase enzyme (PC1). α-MSH is co-transported with cocaine and amphetamine transcript (CORT), also a product of POMC and another appetite suppressor (14). Mutations in the POMC and PC1 genes, which decrease these inhibitory hormones, lead to early-onset massive obesity. These and other monogenic mutations will be discussed below. Serotonin (5-HT) has been associated with appetite suppression, particularly of carbohydrate intake (15). 5-HT is released into the bloodstream during meals. Dopamine has been associated with the pleasure of eating, and subjects with a dopamine receptor defect may be prone to obesity (16).

Gut Hormone Regulation of Appetite

Possibly the most important orexigenic hormone released by the gut is ghrelin. Ghrelin is a peptide hormone released by oxyntic mucosal cells in the antrum of the stomach. Ghrelin levels rise rapidly in the fasting state and reach a peak before a meal, especially when a meal is expected (17). Ghrelin has been shown to be reduced in subjects who have had roux-en-Y gastric bypass surgery and is felt to contribute to weight loss in these subjects independent of the mechanical effects of bariatric surgery (18). Ghrelin levels are increased in those with Prader–Willi syndrome, perhaps explaining their hyperphagia (19). Ghrelin may function by blocking the action of the anorexic hormone leptin.

Insulin acts via the bloodstream on central regulators to reduce food intake (20). Insulin levels are increased after a meal. However, unlike leptin deficiency, insulin deficiency does not result in obesity. In fact, in untreated type 1 diabetes, where there is a near-absolute deficiency in insulin, weight loss is the rule despite a large caloric intake (diabetic hyperphagia). This is so because one of the functions of insulin is lipogenesis—fat deposition is impossible without it. Cholecystikinin (CCK) is a peptide that is secreted from the I cells of the pancreas in response to a recent meal. Functions of CCK include stimulation of pancreatic enzyme secretion and inhibition of gastric emptying and secretion bile acids (21). CCK is also the most prominent mediator of short-term satiety. CCK feeds back by both vagal nerve and hormonal methods to the central nervous system (CNS) to decrease appetite in response to food intake.

Peptide YY (PYY) is expressed by L mucinic cells in the small and large intestine. Another modulator of short-term energy balance, PYY is released in response to a large meal to decrease appetite (22).

Adipocyte-Derived Hormones and Cytokines

Adipocyte Factors Associated with Insulin Resistance Until recently, it was believed that the adipocyte was an inert organ, involved only with the storage of energy. With the discovery of *leptin*, a hormone released exclusively by the adipocyte to regulate appetite, we now know that adipose tissue functions as a very active endocrine organ. This seminal discovery about the genetic nature of obesity occurred when a single-base defect was discovered in the obese *ob/ob* mouse on chromosome 6 (analogous to chromosome 7 in humans) that codes for an abnormal version of leptin (23). Circulating leptin acts on neurotransmitters in the PVN of the hypothalamus to

suppress appetite by reducing NPY and AgRP and increasing α-MSH (24). Leptin levels are directly related to the fat mass of the individual and thus may serve as a signal to the brain of overall nutritional status.

The discovery of leptin caused great excitement because it was speculated that obese individuals might be leptin-deficient, suggesting potential pharmacological intervention. However, it became apparent that most obese humans, rather than being leptin-deficient, are in fact leptin overproducers—implying a feedback loop that functions as expected (25). Leptin resistance, rather than leptin deficiency, may play a role in the development of obesity. Although occasional mutations causing leptin deficiency are found in humans, these conditions are rare. Most obese humans do not have a deficiency in leptin. Leptin levels are significantly related to fasting insulin levels and insulin resistance in heavy children and to fasting insulin levels in thin children (26). Since the discovery of leptin, several other adipocyte hormones have been discovered (Table 21-2).

High levels of the adipocyte hormone *resistin* are associated with the development of insulin resistance (27,28). Proinflammatory

TABLE 21-2 Hormones and Cytokines Produced by the Adipocyte

Associated with Insulin Sensitivity	Associated with Insulin Resistance
Adiponectin	Leptin
Acylation-stimulating hormone	Resistin
	Interkeukin 6
	Tumor necrosis factor-α

cytokines, such as *interleukin 6* (IL-6) and *tumor necrosis factor* α (TNF-α), are produced in the adipocyte and increase subacute systemic inflammation and cause endothelial damage (29,30). There appears to be a link between inflammation and the metabolic syndrome. C-reactive protein (CRP), a systemic inflammatory marker that is produced in the liver in response to IL-6, is currently in widespread use in identifying cardiovascular risk in adults, but its use has not been established in children. CRP is modulated by physical activity, with active obese individuals having lower levels than weight-matched sedentary individuals. In children and adolescents, CRP levels clearly are linked to adiposity. A recent paper has linked CRP and features of the metabolic syndrome in children and adolescents, although it is not clear if this is a direct association or is related to the fact that both CRP and the metabolic syndrome are each closely linked to obesity (31).

Adipocyte Factors that Increase Insulin Sensitivity *Adiponectin* is an adipocyte hormone that may have a beneficial effect on cardiovascular risk and features of the metabolic syndrome (32). Low adiponectin levels are associated with increased insulin resistance. Adiponectin deficiency also has been associated with increased vascular inflammation and the development of nonalcoholic fatty liver disease (NAFLD) and nonalcoholic steatorrheic hepatitis (NASH).

Acylation-stimulating hormone (ASP) acts in a paracrine manner on the adipocyte to increase postprandial lipid clearance. ASP also increases insulin sensitivity and acts centrally to increase satiety (33).

Peripheral Hormones

Peripheral hormones involved in energy balance by directly affecting rates of lipogenesis and lipolysis include catecholamines, insulin, cortisol, and growth hormone (GH). Catecholamines such as epinephrine and norepinephrine exert lipolytic effects both by themselves and as messangers for hormones such as thyroid hormone (34). Insulin, discussed previously as an anorexic agent, works directly as a potent inhibitor of lipolysis, promoting fat accumulation (35). The actions of cortisol are more complex, being reported as promoting lipolysis, inhibiting lipolysis, or having no effect (36–38). It has been suggested that in vivo, cortisol suppresses lipolysis in visceral adipose tissue but encourages lypolysis in peripheral tissue, a theory that is supported by observation of the cushingoid phenotype of central obesity and peripheral wasting. Cortisol is released during stress and fasting and may increase fatty acid oxidation in this state but not in the fed, non emergent state. The observation that individuals with cortisol excess are overweight, whereas those with chronic cortisol deficiency are wasted (Addison disease), suggests that the long-term effect of cortisol stimulation is lipogenic. GH is also released during times of stress, and its action is lipolytic (39). Some studies suggest that GH and cortisol are additive in times of fasting and stress, promoting the availability of fat stores for energy (40).

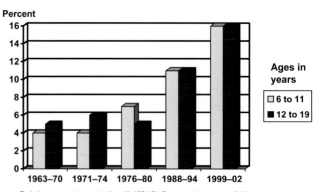

Prevalence of Overweight Among Children and Adolescents Ages 6–19 years

Excludes pregnant women starting with 1971–74. Pregnancy status not available for 1963–70. Data for 1963–65 are for children 6–11 years of age; data for 1966–70 are for adolescents 12–17 years of age, not 12–19 years.
SOURCE: CDC/NCHS, NHES, NHANES

FIGURE 21-2. Prevalence of overweight among children and adolescents ages 6–19 years.

EPIDEMIOLOGY OF OBESITY

The recent increase in weight in the American population, particularly in children, is nothing less than staggering (Figure 21-2). According to the most recent National Health and Nutrition Examination Surveys (NHANES 1999–2000), 65.7% of adults are overweight or obese. Among children aged 6–19 years, 31.5% are overweight or at risk for overweight (41). When compared with the NHANES II survey (1976–1980), the prevalence of overweight has doubled in children aged 6–11 years and tripled in children aged 12–17 years (42). The rates of increase are highest in children above the 95th percentile for weight, so not only is the population in general becoming heavier, but the fattest children are becoming even heavier (41,42). These increases represent the public health crisis for the 21st century; the costs related to obesity and obesity-related disease are approaching and likely will soon surpass those of tobacco (43). Because of these alarming trends, it has been suggested that our current generation of children may be the first in the modern age to have a life expectancy lower than that of their parents.

Urban communities and minorities are more likely to suffer from overweight. Among non-Hispanic blacks, 35.4% of children aged 6–19 years are overweight; among Mexican Americans, the rate is 39.9% (41). The obesity epidemic is not unique to the United States or even only Western cultures; in fact, the World Health Organization has declared that overweight soon will overtake underweight as a worldwide problem (44). Among European populations, data from the MONICA (monitoring cardiovascular) disease study suggest that at least 15% of men and 22% of women are obese (45). Data from the Far East, Middle East, and Africa also show a trend toward increasing obesity (46–50). In Western cultures, usually those in lower socioeconomic status suffer from obesity, but in some third-world nations the reverse is the case (51). Currently, more than 1 billion people are overweight, and more than 300 million people are estimated to be obese worldwide (52).

Since the 1970s, there has been an alarming increase in the rate of weight-related disease in children. The prevalence of hypertension has shown a concordant increase (53). Type 2 diabetes has shown an even more alarming trend, increasing by at least tenfold since 1974 and comprising over 40% of new pediatric diabetes diagnoses in some centers (54). Especially concerning is the lowered quality of life and self-esteem of overweight children (55). Since overweight in children has been shown to track well into adulthood, (56), primary prevention in children and adolescence is of paramount importance.

Although occasionally a specific genetic, hormonal, or metabolic anomaly may be identified during evaluation of the overweight child, these causes are exceedingly rare. A large majority of overweight in children is exogenous, and workup in search of a cause is almost always fruitless. Treatment failures and recidivism are common in weight management treatment centers. Many centers report 50% or greater dropout rate, and up to 85% of those who do lose weight in a treatment program fail to maintain their weight long term (57–59).

PATHOGENESIS OF ENDOGENOUS OBESITY

The causes of overweight and obesity are multifactorial. Adoption and twin studies reveal between 50% and 90% genetic concordance. Other risk factors include choosing high-fat and high-sugar foods, large portion size, and increased television viewing and video game playing. Protective factors include breast-feeding, slower eating, and increased physical activity.

Genetic Factors

Twin and Adoption Studies Two Scandinavian twin studies reveal high concordance for body mass index (BMI). The Finnish Twin Registry studied 7000 pairs of twins and found that 55% to 74% percent of the total variance in BMI was explained by genetic factors (60). The Swedish Twin Study of 362 sets of twins also showed high BMI heritability that was slightly greater for males (0.74) than for females (0.69) (61). In a recent study of children in New York City, 66 pairs of twins, including 41 monozygotic and 25 dizygotic pairs, from 3–17 years of age were analyzed for BMI and body fat (62). Analyses indicated significant genetic influence on percentage body fat, with genes estimated to account for 75% to 80% of the phenotypic variation. The Danish Adoption Register reported height and weight data on 540 nonfamilial adoptees. They found a lower BMI correlation between the adoptee and the adopted parents (0.03–0.10) compared with the child and the biological parent (0.16–0.17) (63).

Monogenic Causes of Nonsyndromic Obesity Although the heritability of overweight and obesity has been firmly established, monogenic causes are rare. Most of these involve central impairment of satiety, and the majority are caused by mutations of the POMC, PC1, MC4R, leptin, and leptin-receptor genes.

POMC neurons in the hypothalamus are important regulators of energy homeostasis, with POMC-derived peptide α-MSH and brain melanocortin receptors playing a key role in this process. Defects in the melanocortin-4 receptor (MC4R) has been shown to result in decreased satiety and uncontrolled eating beginning in the first year of life. MC4R is a G protein–coupled receptor expressed mainly in the hypothalamus and is the most common genetic defect, comprising up to 3% to 4% of cases of nonsyndromic morbid obesity (64). The mode of transmission usually is autosomal dominant with incomplete penetrance; patients homozygous for the defect develop extremely severe forms of obesity. Affected patients, in addition to increased fat mass, have increased lean mass and a marked increase in bone density. Reproductive function and fertility are normal. Defects in the prohormone convertase 1 (PC1) gene have been reported to cause extreme childhood obesity, abnormal glucose tolerance and postprandial hypoglycemia, hypogonadotropic

hypogonadism, hypocortisolism, elevated plasma proinsulin and POMC concentrations, but very low insulin levels (65). PC1 is involved in proinsulin and POMC cleavage; deficiency in PC1 activity results in high plasma concentrations of proinsulin, whose partial insulin-like action and its long biological half-life account for the impaired glucose tolerance and postprandial hypoglycemia. Patients with homozygous or compound heterozygous mutations of the POMC gene develop early-onset obesity and hyperphagia due to loss of α-MSH signaling at the MC4R, acute adrenal insufficiency with hypoglycemia at birth due to adrenocorticotropic hormone (ACTH) deficiency, and ginger hair as a result of the lack of α-MSH action at MC1Rs in the skin and hair follicles (66,67). Defects in the MC3R are associated with obesity in rat models, but studies on MC3R mutations in humans are inconclusive (68,69). A balanced translocation in the SIM1 gene, a locus on chromosome 6 whose function is associated with development of the PVN, has been associated with hyperphagia and early-onset obesity (70). This phenotype may be due to hypocellularity of the PVN because it has been found in mice heterozygous with a null SIM1 gene defect (PVN neurons express the MC4R and appear to be physiological targets of α-MSH, which inhibits food intake).

Isolated cases of obese patients with leptin receptor defects and leptin protein defects have been reported. Affected patients, homozygous for the leptin receptor defect, present with morbid obesity in the first months of life, normal birth weights, hyperphagia, highly emotional and social disability, but no mental retardation. Fasting glucose levels and oral glucose tolerance tests are normal. Leptin levels are elevated (600–670 ng/mL). GH deficiency, hypothalamic hypothyroidism, and hypogonadotropic hypogonadism are associated endocrinopathies, suggesting that leptin and the leptin receptor are a critical link between energy stores and hypothalamic–pituitary function (71).

Patients with the leptin gene defect are markedly obese and hyperphagic and have low levels of serum leptin in relation to their elevated BMI, hypogonadotropic hypogonadism, high rates of childhood infections due to abnormalities of T-cell number and function, and elevated insulin levels and can become hyperglycemic as they get older (72). A defect in the peroxisome proliferator–activated receptor (PPAR)γ-2 may cause increased adipocyte differentiation from preadipocytes, more commitment to the adipocyte line from pluripotent stem cells, and adipocyte growth. This is the only known genetic defect that may act directly on the end organ rather than on central

mechanisms to cause obesity (73). In general, monogenetic obesity is associated with early-onset extreme obesity.

Genetic Syndromes Where Obesity Is a Central Characteristic The genetic syndromes for which obesity is a defining characteristic are nearly always associated with mental retardation. Prader–Willi syndrome (PWS) is by far the most common. PWS often presents in the neonatal period with hypotonia, hypogenitalism, and failure to thrive during the first months of life. Muscle weakness may persist throughout life. Persistent obsessive-type behaviors are common, and hyperphagia is the rule (74). A recent study revealed that PWS subjects have higher levels of the orexigenic hormone ghrelin (75). Approximately 75% of patients have a deletion of the 15q11-q13 paternal chromosome, 20% have maternal uniparental disomy (two maternal copies and no paternal copies of the 15 chromosome), and 5% have a mutation of the imprinting center or a chromosomal translocation involving proximal 15q. All the preceding molecular defects can be detected with methylation studies. If the methylation studies are abnormal, fluorescence in situ hybridation (FISH) studies to document deletion, or uniparental disomy (UPD) studies to confirm maternal UPD can follow. An abnormal methylation test in the presence of normal FISH and UPD studies indicates a mutation in the imprinting center. Treatment of PWS requires limiting access to food, often by employing drastic measures such as locking the refrigerator and cabinets. GH has been shown to be effective in ameliorating some of the symptoms of PWS. GH therapy is associated with improved linear growth, lower BMI, and increased physical strength and agility (76). However, recent concerns have arisen over sudden deaths associated with GH therapy, likely related to impaired ventilation secondary to body composition changes in children already at risk for apnea. Polysonography before initiation of GH treatment is recommended (77).

A summary of the other most common syndromes is given in Table 21-3. Mental retardation syndromes that are often but not always associated with obesity include fragile X syndrome and Down syndrome. A recent review of anthropomorphics of children with fragile X syndrome revealed that more than a third have a BMI greater than 2 standard deviations (SDs) above the mean (78). Studies show that between 40% and 70% of adults with Down syndrome are obese. Obesity in Down syndrome is not related to the degree of developmental delay but is positively correlated with living at home rather than in an assisted-living facility (79).

TABLE 21-3 Genetic Syndromes Associated with Obesity

Syndrome	Rate	Heredity	GENE	Locus	OMIM
Prader-Willi	1/10,000-15,000	Non-Mendelian (imprinting)	SNRPN, Necdin	15q12, 15q11-q13	#176270
Bardet-Biedl	1/13,000- Middle East; 1/160,000- Europe	Autosomal recessive	Genetically heterogeneous	20p12, 16q21, 15q22.3-q23, 14q32.1, 12q21.2, 11q13, 9q31-q34.1, 7p14, 4q27, 4q27, 3p12-q13, 2q31	#209900
Albright Hereditary OsteoDystrophy	3-7/1,000,000 (Japan); 2:1 female/male	Sex influenced autosomal dominant	GNAS1	20q13	#103580
Borjeson-Forssman-Lehmann	5 families reported	X-Linked	PHF6	Xq26.3	#301900
Cohen	~ 100 reported cases	Autosomal recessive	COH1	8q22-q23	#216550
Alstrom	~50 families	Autosomal recessive	ALMS1	2p13	#203800
Carpenter	~ 140 cases	Autosomal recessive	RAB23	6p11	#201000

Syndrome	Typical Features Other than Obesity	Level of Retardation
Prader-Willi	Neonatal hypotonica / failure to thrive; characteristic behaviorial disorder (tantrums, obsessive-compulsive, discomfort with change in routine); narrow bifrontal diameter, almond shaped palpebral fissures, down-turned mouth, small, narrow hands and feet, hypogonadism	Usually mild
Bardet-Biedl	Hypogonadism, postaxial polydachtyly; rod cone dystrophy; renal disease	Mild
Albright I lereditary Osteo-Dystrophy	Short, stocky build; round face; short neck, brachydactyly, hormonal disorders, ectopic calcifications; pseudohypoparathyriodism	Moderate to none
Borjeson-Forssman-Lehmann	Hypogonadism, large thick, ears, short stature, prominent supraorbital ridges, deep set eyes, ptosis, and narrow palpebral fissures	Severe
Cohen	Infantile hypotonia, narrow hands and feet with long tapering fingers, downslanting palpebral fissures, high nasal bridge, short philtrum, high narrow palate, prominent central incisors, open mouth, progressive retinochoroidal dystrophy, defective vision in bright light, optic atrophy	Mild to moderate
Alstrom	Obesity, insulin resistance, retinitis pigmentosa, with nystagmus and early loss of central vision, neurosensory deafness, ancanthosis nigracans, type II diabetes, dilated cardiomyopatthy	May have delayed early milestones
Carpenter	Craniosynostosis, polysyndactyly, congenital heart disease, mental retardation, hypogenitalism, cryptorchidism, obesity, umbilical hernia and bony abnormalities	Mild to moderate

Alterations in the Fetal Environment

Intrauterine growth retardation (IUGR), defined as birth weight and/or length of less than the 10th percentile, is usually caused by maternal or fetal factors or placental insufficiency. Biological changes that occur in utero in IUGR children lead to later insulin resistance, cardiovascular disease, and metabolic syndrome (80). Although the exact mechanisms are unknown, it is believed that an intrauterine insult leads to permanent alterations in the set points of the hypothalamic–pituitary–adrenal axis. These adaptations, though beneficial to the malnourished fetus, become maladaptive in the energy-abundant environment of postnatal life. Adrenal glucocorticoid secretion and disorders of insulin and insulin-like growth factor 1 (IGF-1) secretion have been implicated. Although IUGR children, on average, do not have higher BMIs than children of normal birth weight, they do have visceral adiposity, and those who do become overweight have more obesity-related metabolic disease than weight-matched children with normal birth weight. Likely this is due to metabolic alterations related to catch-up growth, sometimes referred to as the *thrifty phenotype* (81).

Infants of diabetic mothers (IDMs) may be particularly prone to develop obesity in childhood, although the results of population studies are conflicting (82). Recent studies reflect only a small role for intrauterine environment in the development of obesity in IDMs because there is little effect when corrected for BMI of the mother (83).

Endocrinopathies That Present with Obesity

As described previously, much of the control system related to energy balance is located in the hypothalamus; therefore, injury to this section of the brain often leads to disordered feeding behaviors and the development of obesity (hypothalamic hyperphagia). Injury can be caused by tumor, surgery, radiation, infiltrative, inflammatory diseases of the hypothalamus, or trauma; craniopharyngioma and its subsequent removal are a common cause. Craniopharyngiomas are benign tumors found in the hypothalamus and pituitary. They are common in children, constituting between 6% and 9% of pediatric brain tumors. The peak incidence is at ages 5–10 years, but they can occur throughout childhood and in adults. Obesity is present postoperatively in up to 52% of patients, with at least half of these patients having severe difficulty controlling their desire to eat (84,85). Despite the high incidence of GH deficiency, most patients with hypothalamic obesity continue to grow at a normal growth rate, most likely due to the effects of insulin on the IGF-1 receptor. What complicates the picture is that some of the patients with hypothalamic obesity are on hydrocortisone replacement and

TABLE 21-4 Medications Commonly Used in Children that Are Associated with Weight Gain

Class	Examples	Common Uses	Other
Corticosteroids	Prednisone, methylprednisolone	Asthma, rheumatoid disease, cancers	Up to 13-kg gain after 1 year chronic use
Atypical antipsychotics	Olanzipine, risperidone	Schizophrenia, oppositional-defiant disorder, mood disturbance	16-kg weight gain per year or greater; some report as much as 85-kg weight gain; worse with olanzipine than risperidone
Thiazolidinediones	Rosiglitazone, pioglitazone	Type 2 diabetes	2- to 3-kg weight gain over 6 months
Injectible progesterones	Depot medroxyprogesterone (Depo-Provera)	Contraception, cessation of menses	Up to 10 lb/year; overweight at baseline greater risk for weight gain
Anticonvulsants	Valproate, carbamazipine, gabapentin	Seizure control, mood stabilization	Up to 15–20 lb/year weight gain; consider topirimate in those at risk

sometimes a patient's weight may be attributed to the hydrocortisone dose instead of to hypothalamic obesity; however, patients who have weight gain secondary to hydrocortisone dose also will have decreased growth velocity. Octreotide has been shown in some clinical trials to be effective in reducing obesity in hypothalamic hyperphagia (86).

Cortisol excess, whether from an exogenous source or excessive central or peripheral ACTH production or from an adrenal tumor, causes obesity. These conditions are described in detail in Chapter 28. Signs and symptoms in adults include truncal obesity. Increased fat in the dorsal neck and above the supraclavicular fossa, along with kyphosis due to osteopenia, cause the well-described "buffalo hump." Progressive rounding of the facies (moon facies) and a florid, ruddy appearance of the face may be noted. In children, the obesity may be more diffuse with less peripheral wasting and no obvious buffalo hump. Hirsutism, virilization, and irregular menses in women are common findings and may be seen in postmenarchal girls. Short stature and growth failure, as in most endocrine causes of obesity, usually are seen (87). Impaired glucose tolerance occurs in 80% of patients (88). Pseudo-Cushing syndrome is a transient increase in cortisol that is caused by stress or depression (89). Obesity develops because cortisol is lipogenic and because it stimulates appetite.

Hyperinsulinemia occurs secondary to obesity, but in cases of primary insulin excess it may lead to obesity. Insulin is a significant growth factor in utero and in young children. Elevated insulin levels due to genetic defects in insulin secretion or, rarely, tumor, result in hypoglycemia, excessive growth and obesity. Newborn infants of poorly controlled diabetic mothers may present with hypoglycemia and may have seizures. Infants with Beckwith–Wiedeman syndrome present with macroglossia, exophthalmos, hyperinsulinism, and hypoglycemia. These conditions of primary insulin excess are all to be differentiated from hyperinsulinism that is secondary to insulin resistance, which will be discussed below (90) (for more details see Chapter 4).

GH deficiency or hypothyroidism rarely cause significant overweight in children but should be considered in children who have poor linear growth (91).

Medications Associated with the Development of Obesity

Several medications have been shown to increase weight in children and adolescents (Table 21-4). Chronic oral glucocorticoids (e.g., for asthma treatment) can lead to profound weight gain, as described earlier. Antipsychotics such as olanzipine and risperidone cause significant weight gain (92,93). Although the mechanism for this weight gain is unclear, olanzipine has been shown to increase serum ghrelin concentrations (94). Injectible progesterone can cause weight gain, particularly in those with a higher baseline weight (95). Thiozolidenediones cause considerable weight gain in some adults with type 2 diabetes; there are not enough data available to know if the risk of obesity with these PRAR-γ agonists is similar in youth (96). Anticonvulsants, particularly valproic acid, are a common cause of weight gain in children (97).

PATHOGENESIS OF EXOGENOUS OBESITY

The "Toxic Environment"

Exogenous obesity is the term used when no specific underlying cause is found. By far the vast majority of cases of obesity are exogenous. The etiology of exogenous obesity is polymorphic, caused by a variety of interactions among the external environment, heredity and genetics, and hormonal response. However, with the increase in obesity in recent years being far too great to be attributable to a change in genetic or biological responses, it is clear that the environment is playing the largest role. It has been said that modern society is obesogenic: If one has the predisposition, development of obesity is nearly unavoidable. This is also known as the "toxic environment."

Increased Caloric Intake During the early days of human existence, humans could do well just to find enough energy for basic survival. Hunter-gatherers would forage for berries and hunt for food. They would have to survive barren winters and long famines. Hence humans became efficient at storing energy. In the modern world, food is abundant, even often for the most impoverished. Overnutrition is now overtaking undernutrition as a worldwide problem (98). We are eating more and more energy with each meal (99). An American cooking recipe book in its first edition in the 1950s had recipes that served six people; the same recipes in the same proportions now are recommended to serve four people. Fast-food restaurants provide "extra value" by providing larger portions at only a slightly increased price. Extremely large sweetened beverages are the rule, with some stores selling 64-ounce (1.9-L) fountain beverage cups meant to be finished in one serving. Eating in front of the television, where cues to terminate eating are lost, has become more common. Because of these and other causes, the average American takes in about 15% more energy in 2004 than he or she did in 1970 (100).

Decreased Physical Activity Despite increased caloric intake, physical activity is less than in the past. Television and computer time has been implicated in reducing physical activity in children and youth. Since the introduction of television in the 1950s, when television viewing was a family event, the amount of time spent watching television has increased steadily. Today, an American child watches an average of 4 hours of television per day. Television viewing has been positively correlated with the development of obesity (101). Children view approximately 20,000 television commercials per year, many for high-fat or high-sugar foods. Thus, besides being less physically active, children are more likely to ingest high-fat and high-sugar foods while viewing television.

With the improvements in computer performance and increasing quality of video games, as well as the social possibilities of the Internet, children are spending more time in front of the computer. Computer games may be preferable entertainment to playing sports for many children, particularly those who are deconditioned.

Opportunities for physical activity are also less. With movement away from both cities and rural areas to suburban areas, the amount of walking has decreased. Often these neighborhoods have no sidewalks or walking paths, and stores are located on busy streets, far away from residences and with abundant parking (102). Sports have become more competitive, so often children who do not have the desire, financial means, or parental commitment to become involved at a very young age may find their opportunities to participate in organized sports limited as they get older. For many children, the schools may be their primary source of physical activity. With only one state in the United States (Illinois) requiring daily physical education, and with increased emphasis on academics and standardized testing, physical education, recess, and free play time all continue to decrease (103).

COMORBIDITIES DUE TO CHILDHOOD OBESITY

It is a common but incorrect assumption that treating overweight in childhood is an exercise in primary prevention, and the goal is to prevent adult disease. To the contrary, childhood obesity has many morbidities that are manifested in the child (Table 21-5).

Insulin Resistance and the Metabolic Syndrome

Insulin resistance is found in the majority of subjects with obesity. Common physical manifestations include *acanthosis nigricans*, a velvety hyperpigmentation found in skin folds and on the back of the neck. Interaction between excessive amounts of circulating in-

TABLE 21-5   Childhood and Adult-Onset Morbidities Associated with Childhood Obesity

Childhood-Onset Morbidities	Adult-Onset Morbidities
Insulin resistance, prediabetes, type 2 diabetes	Type 2 diabetes
Dyslipidemia (↑ triglycerides, ↓ HDL)	Atherosclerotic cardiovascular disease
Hypertension (especially systolic)	Diabetic microvascular disease
Asthma	Pickwickian syndrome: left-sided heart failure, pulmonary hypertension
Obstructive sleep apnea	
Fatty liver and steatorrheic hepatitis	Cirrhosis
Gastroesophageal reflux	Osteoarthritis
Cholecystitis	Cancer
Orthopedic: SCFE, Blount disease, flatfoot	Lower wages, lower academic achievement
Pseudotumor cerebri	
Low self-esteem	

sulin with IGF receptors on keratinocytes and dermal fibroblasts leads to the characteristic hyperpigmented, thickened plaques (104). Often this pigmentation is mistaken for dirt by patients and parents.

Originally described by Reaven in 1988, the *metabolic syndrome* (syndrome X, dysmetabolic syndrome, insulin resistance syndrome) increasingly is becoming recognized as the primary risk factor for the development of cardiovascular disease (CVD) in adults (105). The metabolic syndrome (MS) is composed of a number of factors that are independently correlated with CVD but cluster together and increase risk to a greater degree than the factors do individually. The main features of the MS are dyslipidemia, insulin resistance, obesity, and hypertension. Development of one component of the MS increases the risk for development of the others. For example, obesity, hypertension, and dyslipidemia are seen in more than 30% of subjects with impaired glucose tolerance but in fewer than 10% of subjects with normal glucose tolerance (106). Microalbuminuria is a late finding in the MS but is highly correlated with mortality (107).

Data are emerging demonstrating that the relations that comprise the MS in adults are also present in children, even if the full-blown syndrome is not present. Obese youth are more likely than normal-weight youth to have increased systolic blood pressure, increased triglycerides, and decreased high-density lipoprotein (HDL) cholesterol (although these parameters still may be within the normal range) (108). The magnitude of the impact of these changes on adult cardiovascular risk is unknown. The Bogalusa Heart Study showed that *atherosclerotic plaques* may begin developing as early as age 5 (109). Among the major risk factor for the development of early CVD, increased low-density lipoprotein (LDL) cholesterol and reduced HDL cholesterol are associated with increased fatty streak

formation in children who have had autopsies for death from other causes. Obesity increases rates of *dyslipidemia* between two- and eightfold. Suggested diagnostic criteria for MS for both adults and children are shown in Table 21-6.

Obesity and Type 2 Diabetes

Type 2 diabetes is an emerging epidemic in pediatric populations. Until recently, it was commonly referred to as "adult-onset" diabetes (to contrast with type 1 "juvenile-onset" diabetes). With type 2 diabetes comprising up to 40% of new childhood diabetes diagnoses in some centers, the term is clearly a misnomer and now seldom used (110). Unlike type 1 diabetes, which is caused by complete failure of the pancreas to produce insulin, type 2 diabetes is characterized by increased insulin levels and insulin resistance in combination with a partial defect in insulin secretion. Type 2 diabetes has shown a tenfold increase in recent years, surpassing even the increase in rates of overweight (54). Childhood type 2 diabetes is even more common in non-Caucasian ethnic groups, affecting Native Americans (particularly Pima Indians), Hispanics (particularly Mexican Americans), and African Americans at much higher rates (111). Long term, it is associated with blindness, renal failure, amputation, atherosclerotic CVD, and death.

Unlike type 1 diabetes, the development of type 2 diabetes is often insidious, and it may be discovered during routine screening. Those with type 2 diabetes may present with polydipsia, polyuria, or unexplained weight loss, but more often, glucosuria or vaginal candidiasis discovered on screening exams. Diagnosis is confirmed by random or fasting blood glucose and insulin measurement or a 2-hour oral glucose tolerance test (OGTT). Diagnosis and treatment of type 2 diabetes are discussed in Chapter 20.

TABLE 21-6   Diagnostic Criteria for the Metabolic Syndrome in Children and Adults (Must Have Three or More)

	Adult Criteria	**Childhood Criteria**
Dyslipidemia	Fasting triglycerides > 150 mg/dL	Fasting triglycerides >110 mg/dL
	HDL < 40 mg/dL in men or < 50 mg/dL in women	HDL < 40 mg/dL
Insulin resistance	Fasting plasma glucose > 110 mg/dL	Fasting plasma glucose > 110 md/dL
Abdominal obesity	Waist circumference > 102 cm in men or 88 cm in women	Waist circumference > 90th percentile
Hypertension	SBP > 130 mm Hg or DSP > 85 mm HG	SBP or DBP > 90th percentile for height

From Cook S, Weitzman M, Auinger P, et al. Prevalence of a metabolic syndrome phenotype in adolescents: Findings from the Third National Health and Nutrition Examination Survey 1994–1998. *Arch Pediatr Adolesc Med.* 2003;147:821–827.

Before the development of frank diabetes, many overweight children have hyperinsulinism and normal random glucose levels. An OGTT at this point may show glucose intolerance. This state is commonly called *prediabetes*. Lifestyle modification is indicated. Although there is no definitive evidence that the insulin sensitizer metformin can prevent the onset of disease at this point, clinical trials are now underway, and many clinicians are offering this treatment.

Association of Fat Distribution and Cardiovascular Risk

Recent studies have confirmed that there is a relationship between body fat distribution and CVD risk that is independent of the relationship between obesity and CVD risk (112–114). Fat distribution usually is described as being in one of two patterns. An *android* pattern describes a higher ratio of fat in the upper body segment, particularly the abdomen. A *gynoid* pattern refers to a higher distribution of fat in the lower body, particularly the hips and thighs. These patterns are commonly referred to as an "apple" (android) or "pear" (gynoid) shape. The android shape has been shown to increase CVD risk in adults. Daniels and colleagues confirmed this effect in children and adolescents, showing an association between visceral fat and increased triglycerides and decreased HDL cholesterol, as well as increased blood pressure and increased left ventricular mass (115). These effects are independent of total body fat percentage. The mechanisms of increased CVD risk with increased visceral fat are not well understood but likely are related to insulin resistance, cortisol, and adipocyte hormones.

Gastrointestinal Complications

Nonalcoholic Fatty Liver Disease (NAFLD) and Nonalcoholic Steatorrheic Hepatitis (NASH)

NAFLD and NASH are emerging diseases in the obese population and are becoming more prevalent in children. A recent study showed that 77% of obese children in a Chinese sample had some degree of hepatic steatosis (116). It is uncertain whether the benign NAFLD is a precursor to NASH or whether they are separate entities. NASH progresses to cirrhosis and liver failure in up to 10% of cases (117). The diagnosis is suspected in obese children who have elevated liver functions and no history of hepatic disease or alcohol abuse and is confirmed by liver biopsy. First, however, type 2 diabetes should be ruled out because untreated diabetes is a treatable cause of fatty liver and liver function abnormalities. No specific treatment other than lifestyle modification has been shown to be effective for NAFLD or NASH. Liver enzymes improve with subsequent weight loss.

Cholelithiasis (Gallstones)
Cholelithiasis is fourfold more common in the obese than in nonobese populations (118). Gallstones are more common in females than in males and more common during or after pregnancy. Usually they are cholesterol gallstones in the obese. The diagnosis of gallstones should be entertained in an overweight child with unexplained abdominal pain and can be confirmed by ultrasound. Treatment can be medical, with dissolution of stones, or surgical, by laparoscopic cholecystectomy.

Gastroesophageal Reflux Disease (GERD)
GERD is a common condition resulting in increased acid in the distal esophagus. GERD leads to a variety of symptoms, including chest pain and hoarseness. Long-term complications include Barrett esophagus and esophageal adenocarcinoma. GERD has been associated with high-fat diet as well as overweight, but overweight appears to be more important. A recent NHANES report showed increased hospitalizations for GERD related to increased BMI but no association with a high-fat diet (119). A Scandinavian study showed a definite and dose-related increase in GERD with increasing BMI and also associations with female gender and hormone-replacement therapy, which may implicate estrogen as a causative agent (120).

Neurological Complications

Pseudotumor Cerebri (Benign Intracranial Hypertension)
Pseudotumor cerebri is a condition defined by severe headache and increased intracranial pressure with normal or small ventricles. The later in childhood it occurs, the higher is the association with obesity. With younger children, the association is as low as 10%, but up to 90% of older teenagers with pseudotumor cerebri are obese (121). The mechanism for pseudotumor cerebri in the obese is obscure but is likely due to either decreased cerebrospinal fluid (CSF) absorption by the arachnoid villi or increased intracranial venous pressure. Another theory suggests that central obesity raises intra-abdominal pressure, which increases pleural pressure and cardiac filling pressure, which impede venous return from the brain, leading to increased intracranial venous pressure (122).

The diagnosis is suspected by the observation of papilledema on funduscopic examination and confirmed by lumbar puncture, which is both a diagnostic and therapeutic procedure.

Orthopedic Complications

Blount's Disease (Idiopathic Tibia Vera)
Blount's disease is bowing inward of the lower extremity associated with the increased forces from excess weight causing injury to the growth plate, growth suppression, and angulation. Diagnosis is made radiographically. Infantile Blount's disease, a congenital condition not associated with weight bearing, may respond to bracing, but the correction in obese older children is usually surgical (123).

Slipped Capital Femoral Ephysis (SCFE)
SCFE is caused by mechanical damage to the growth plate. The epiphysis of the proximal femur slips through the growth plate in a posterior direction (124). Typically, SCFE is related to periods of rapid growth, such as during puberty or during GH therapy. It presents with hip pain on external rotation of the hip. Treatment is surgical, with in situ fixation by a single screw. About 40% of cases are

bilateral. The cause is unknown, although SCFE is associated with several endocrine disorders, including GH deficiency and hypothyroidism. Endocrinopathy causes an imbalance in the growth plate of the hip leading to greater susceptibility for slippage. For example, GH stimulates epiphyseal hypertrophy, whereas gonadotropins stimulate fusion. While uncomplicated SCFE is bilateral in 25% of cases, SCFE due to endocrinopathy usually is bilateral. Sequelae include avascular necrosis and may result in permanent deformity if not discovered and treated early.

Flatfoot Flatfoot is a collapse of the normal arch of the foot. Flatfoot is common in overweight adolescents (125). Preexisting flatfoot often is exacerbated by obesity, where increased weight bearing puts extra stress on the already taxed posterior tibial tendon and ligaments that support the arch. Flatfoot usually presents with atraumatic chronic foot pain, and correction usually is surgical.

Osteoarthritis (OA) OA, particularly of the knee, is associated with obesity (126). More common in women than men, OA usually presents in the fourth decade of life or later. Recent investigations suggest that the relationship between OA and obesity is mechanical rather than metabolic in nature. It is unknown whether the effects of OA are present in childhood or adolescence.

Pulmonary Complications

Asthma Both asthma and obesity are on the rise in current populations, although the association is unproven. In our obesity referral population, a recent chart review revealed a 32% prevalence of asthma (127). It is unknown whether treatment of obesity will improve asthma.

Obstructive Sleep Apnea (OSA) OSA is a breathing disorder characterized by repeated collapse of the upper airway during sleep, with cessation of airflow at night and daytime sleepiness due to nonrestful sleep caused by the persistent nighttime awakenings. OSA is a major independent risk factor for CVD and stroke. Up to 50% of morbidly obese children may have some degree of OSA (128). OSA should be suspected in overweight individuals who snore loudly and fall asleep during the day. Diagnosis is made through sleep studies, and treatment is by continuous positive airway pressure (CPAP) during sleeping hours. In its most severe form, chronic daytime hypoxemia and hypercapnia may develop *Pickwickian syndrome*, a sleep apnea disorder in moderately to severely obese people, named after a character in the Charles Dickens novel The Pickwick Papers. Once blood gas abnormalities occur, pulmonary hypertension and right-sided heart failure may follow (129).

Reproductive Complications

Obese males suffer from reproductive abnormalities, including decreased sperm motility, decreased libido, and impotence. These conditions may be linked through a mild hypogonadotrophic hypogonadism (130) likely due to negative feedback on the pituitary from the increased estrogens produced in adipocytes.

Polycystic ovarian syndrome (PCOS, Stein–Leventhal syndrome) is a multifactorial condition that in some cases is characterized by overstimulation of the ovaries secondary to increased luteinizing hormone (LH) production, leading to cystic changes. The condition is associated with androgenic and hyperinsulinemic changes, including obesity, acne, hirsutism, and acanthosis nigricans. Over the long term, PCOS has been associated with infertility, CVD, type 2 diabetes, and endometrial cancer. Not all women with PCOS are obese, and it is most likely that obesity contributes to the etiology of PCOS rather than that PCOS causes obesity (131).

Psychological Complications

Overweight status in childhood and adolescence is associated with *low self-esteem* and the development of *eating disorders*. Overweight children suffer from stigmatization, teasing, and stereotyping. Media images portray larger people as sloppy, unclean, and morally undesirable. Obese children often are singled out in physical education classes. In one study, first graders were shown pictures of children with a variety of handicaps, as well as one who was obese, and the children ranked the obese child as the least desirable friend (132).

It is uncertain whether *major depression* is a cause or effect in the development of obesity. Some reports show that lean adolescents who suffer from depression discordantly develop obesity as adults (133). Also, those who suffer from sexual abuse are more likely to become obese (134). A recent study shows that children suffering from overweight have as low a quality of life as those undergoing chemotherapy for leukemia (55).

Neoplastic Associations

Several cancers have been shown to be related to long-term obesity. Postmenopausal breast cancer is increased in obese women, although obesity seems to be somewhat protective in premenopausal breast cancers. However, mortality is high for all obese woman with breast cancer likely because breast masses are more difficult to detect in obese compared with lean women (135,136). Obesity consistently has been associated with uterine (endometrial) cancer (137). Obese women have two to four times greater risk of developing the disease than do women of a healthy weight regardless of menopausal status. Obesity has been shown to be associated with *colon cancer*, with a stronger link for men than for women (138). *Renal cell carcinoma* and obesity consistently have been linked in women but not in men (139). *Adenoma of the esophagus*, *gastric cancer*, and *cancer of the gallbladder* also have been linked to obesity in some studies (140–142). Although much attention has been focused on the connection between *prostate cancer* and obesity, a link has not been firmly established (143). Whether obesity in childhood contributes to adult cancer risk is unknown.

MEDICAL EVALUATION OF AN OVERWEIGHT CHILD

Measurement of Adiposity

Body Mass Index BMI is a commonly used measurement in practice settings. It is calculated by taking the weight in kilograms and dividing by the square of the height in meters (kg/m^2). BMI relates well to morbidity and mortality in adults (64). In children, BMI is limited by its inability to differentiate adiposity from lean body mass. Thus, for example, a muscular, athletic adolescent may have the same BMI as on overweight youth with poor muscle mass. BMI also does not differentiate between metabolically active visceral fat and less active subcutaneous fat (144). Another limitation is its steep rise on growth charts in childhood, so a child who develops more quickly or more slowly may have a BMI that does not reflect his or her actual habitus. In general, however, BMI correlates reasonably well with adiposity, and because of its ease of use and the fact that there exist standard, easily available percentiles and cutoff values, BMI is a useful tool in practice.

Anthropometrics Skinfold thickness measurements can be obtained from different sites in the body, most commonly triceps, subscapular, and suprailiac, and compared with age-, sex-, and race-matched controls to estimate adiposity. Although used reliably in research settings, this technique is limited by intraobserver variability and requires specialized training (145).

Waist:hip ratios and waist circumference are common, easily obtained measures of body shape and visceral adiposity. High visceral fat, as demonstrated by a high weight:height (W:H) ratio (>0.9) implies increased CVD risk in adults (146). Studies in the pediatric population, however, show that the W:H ratio correlates poorly with visceral fatness. Waist circumference (WC), in contrast, correlates well with visceral fat as measured by dual-energy x-ray absorptiometry (DEXA)

and other methods. The conicity index, which is a ratio that incorporates waist circumference with height and weight, performs better than W:H ratio in children but still not as well as WC alone (147–149). It is likely that changing skeletal structure and body habitus associated with normal childhood growth makes ratios less useful in children than in adults. Distributions and percentiles of WC for different ethnic groups have been published recently (150).

Other methods of measuring adiposity, largely used in research settings, are described in Table 21-7 (151–157).

Clinical Assessment

Every child who presents for a primary-care visit should have height and weight measured and BMI calculated. The BMI should be plotted on the standard Centers for Disease Control and Prevention (CDC) growth charts. Those above the 85th percentile

TABLE 21-7	Measurement of Adiposity	
Method	**How Its Done**	**Pros/Cons**
Body mass index (BMI)	Weight in kilograms divided by the square of the height in meters (kg/m^2)	Easy to use, pediatric standards with percentiles exist; correlates reasonably well with adiposity; "weight" does not differentiate fat from lean mass (such as muscle in an athlete leading to high BMI)
Skinfold thickness	Usually obtained from triceps, subscapular, and suprailiac skinfolds; calculated from age-, sex-, and race-adjusted formulas	Used reliably in research settings; technique is limited by intraobserver variability and requires specialized training
Waist:hip ratio (W:H), waist circumference (WC)	Measurement of the narrowest point of the waist and the widest point of the hip while standing	Easily obtained; W:H ratio correlates poorly with visceral fatness in children; compared to W:H ratio or the conicity index (which uses WC, height, and weight), WC has superior correlation with visceral fat as measured by DEXA; pediatric percentiles for WC are published (16)
Bioelectric impedance analysis (BIA)	Electrodes are placed on the bare feet of a lying-down subject, supplying an alternating current that is conducted by body water and dissolved electrolytes; impedance values rise sharply within the first 10 minutes after assuming the supine position and then continue to rise more gradually for up to 4 hours, so length of recumbent time should be standardized	The procedure is quick and painless; limitations include variations due to state of hydration and inaccuracy at extremes of body weight, overestimating fatness in the underweight, and underestimating fatness in the obese
DEXA	Estimates fat and fat-free mass by measuring differential attenuation of x-rays passing through tissue	DEXA is accurate and reproducible; radiation exposure is trivial and procedure takes < 5 minutes; strong correlation between trunk fat by DEXA and intra-abdominal fat measured by CT/MRI; it is expensive and does not differentiate between intra-abdominal and subcutaneous fat
CT and MRI	CT and MRI can be used to calculate body fat and fat-free mass and to specifically measure visceral fat	Expensive and require specialized personnel to evaluate; CT requires a much higher dose of radiation than DEXA, whereas MRI is not associated with radiation exposure
Total-body electrical conductivity (TOBEC)	Total-body electrical conductivity (TOBEC) measures fat-free mass by passing the body through a coil, generating a magnetic field; disruption of the field by electrolytes is measured and used to estimate adiposity; FFM contains water and electrolytes, but fat; does not and therefore does not contribute to TOBEC measurement; a calibration equation is used to calculate LBM	Technique is quick and noninvasive; Extremely expensive; mostly used with neonates in research settings, although TOBEC has been validated in older children
Air-displacement plethysmography (BodPod)	Air-displacement plethysmography uses air-pressure differences inside a small chamber to estimate body fat	Very accurate for adults; not approved for children under age 7, and its cost limits clinical utility
Underwater weighing	Hydrostatic weighing (HW) is the "gold standard" for body fat measurements in research settings (23); HW involves measuring lung residual volume and requires the subject to completely submerge and empty the lungs under wate	Extremely expensive and requires a specialized area with room for a pool; technique may be difficult for younger children

TABLE 21-8 Suggested Workup of the Overweight Child

Clinical Parameter	Workup
BMI > 85th percentile for age	• Careful history and physical exam looking for associated signs and symptoms • Diet and activity logs • Blood pressure • Fasting lipid profile • Fasting glucose, insulin • Hemoglobin A1c • AST, ALT
If fasting glucose > 100 mg/dL, insulin > 15 mU/mL or hemoglobin A1c > 6.0%, add	• Oral glucose tolerance test
If growth rate is decreased, add	• Free T$_4$, TSH • 24-hour urine for free cortisol and creatinine • IGF-1, IGFBP-3 • Bone age • MRI of the pituitary if GH deficiency or more than one endocrine abnormality is present
If female with irregular menses, acanthosis nigricans and/or signs of hyperandrogenism, add	• FSH, LH, DHEA-S, free testosterone, androstenedione, pelvic US to evaluate for polystic ovarian disease
If early onset of obesity with or without syndromic features, retinitis pigmentosa, pubertal delay, add	• Genetic testing for the appropriate monogenic or syndromic causes of obesity

for age and sex should be further evaluated (see Table 21-8). A careful history and physical examination would distinguish children with exogenous obesity from children with endocrine or genetic causes of obesity, which represent only 5% of the obese population (Figure 21-3). Patients with endocrine causes usually have decreased growth velocity despite increased weight gain. Children with hypothyroidism, hypercortisolism, or GH deficiency present with decreased growth rate, delayed bone age, and increased weight gain. Of note, children with hypercortisolism may present with generalized obesity instead of developing the characteristic central fat distribution. Laboratory evaluation of patients suspected of having an endocrinopathy should include free triiodothyroxine (T$_4$), thyroid-stimulating hormone (TSH), 24-hour urine for free cortisol and creatinine, IGF-1, insulin-like growth factor-binding protein-3 (IGFBP-3), and a bone age. If more than one

endocrine abnormality or GH deficiency is present, magnetic resonance imaging (MRI) of the pituitary with gadolinium contrast material is suggested. A history of CNS injury, tumor, severe nocturnal headaches, and emesis suggests hypothalamic obesity.

In the presence of facial dysmorphism, cognitive delays, hypotonia, hypogonadism, retinitis pigmentosa, and other associated finding characteristic of specific syndromes, appropriate testing, including genetic testing, should be initiated (see Table 21-3). Genetic testing also may be considered in patients with early-onset extreme obesity.

Evaluation for obesity comorbidities should be performed in all obese children regardless of etiology. In an oversweight child without dysmorphisms, normal intelligence, and normal growth velocity, a workup is unlikely to be fruitful. Instead, search for comorbidities. A fasting lipid profile, including LDL, HDL, and total cholesterol and triglycerides, should be checked as well as liver function tests. Fasting insulin and glucose levels are helpful for evaluating insulin resistance. If either is abnormal, a 2-hour OGTT is indicated. Hemoglobin A1C measurement should be obtained to evaluate for asymptomatic type 2 diabetes and particularly if there is history of polydipsia and polyuria. In overweight female patients with irregular menses, hyperandrogenism, and/or acanthosis nigricans, laboratory evaluation should include measurement of LH/FSH, DHEAS, free testosterone, and D4A and a pelvic ultrasound to evaluate for PCOS. Suspicion of sleep apnea warrants a sleep study.

For a large majority of patients, no specific cause will be found for obesity. In this case, a careful evaluation of lifestyle habits should be undertaken. A 3-day self-reported dietary history is useful, usually done on two weekdays and one weekend day. A food-frequency questionnaire and activity logs are also helpful. These logs should be reviewed, if possible, by a registered dietitian in order to recommend changes that fit in culturally and within the confines of the family environment.

TREATMENT OF OBESITY

It is important to remember that in prepubertal children, because they are growing taller, it may not be necessary to actually lose weight to improve health status. Most experts recommend that before the age of 7, weight maintenance or a slowed rate of weight gain is appropriate for management. Above 7 years of age, slow weight loss of approximately 1 kg/month usually is recommended (158). In my clinical practice, I subscribe to the practice of "health at every size," which adheres to the philosophy that overall physical and psychological health, rather a number on a scale, is

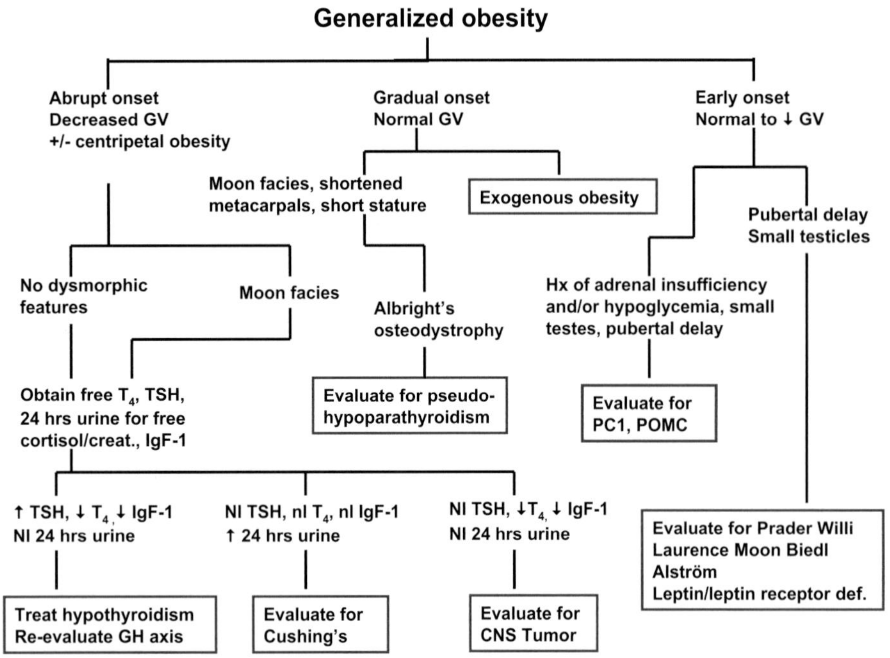

FIGURE 21-3. Diagnostic algorithm for child or adolescent presenting with obesity.

TABLE 21-9 Treatment of the Overweight Child

At risk or mild and moderate overweight (BMI > 85th percentile without serious comorbidities)

Dietary:

- Remove sweetened beverages
- Do not skip meals
- Eliminate eating while viewing television
- Increase fiber in diet
- Five-a-day fruit and vegetable practices
- Slow down eating (put down fork between bites)

Physical activity:

- 30 minutes of aerobic activity three times per week
- Encourage walking in everyday activities
- Do not remove from gym class
- Limit screen time to 1–2 hours/day
- Family-oriented activities

Severe obesity (Z-scores > 2), above approach has failed

Dietary (specialized programs):

- Ketogenic diet
  Protein-sparing modified fasts
  "Atkins diet"
- Low glycemic index diet

Physical activity:

- Involve kinesthesiologist for severely deconditioned children
- Non-weight-bearing exercise (e.g., swimming)

Extremely severe obesity (BMI > 40 with morbidity or > 50)

Surgical approaches:

- Roux-en-Y
- Laproscopic gastric banding
- Implantible gastric stimulator

the best measure of treatment outcome (159). Therefore, even in overweight teenagers, I often will use weight maintenance as a goal, and often, just by slowing or stopping weight gain in these children, normalization of laboratory values and improvement in self-esteem occur. Often small lifestyle changes that can be followed by the whole family are enough to impart a return to health. The changes should be both dietary and related to physical activity (Table 21-9).

Dietary Changes

For mildly and moderately overweight children, "diets" usually are not necessary. Diets have the disadvantage of making children feel deprived, putting an unwanted focus on food, lowering metabolic rate, and stigmatizing the child. The first step is often to remove sweetened beverages and fruit drinks from the diet and replace them with water and sugar-free beverages. Skipping meals is common in overweight children and coun-terproductive; it often leads to unhealthful choices later in the day. This practice should be discouraged. High-fiber foods have been shown to improve lipids and decrease appetite and should be encouraged (160). Switching to whole-grain pasta and breads and incorporating "five-a-day" practices for fruit and vegetable servings can increase dietary fiber. Snacking in front of the television leads to overeating and should be discouraged. Healthful eating at restaurants should be discussed.

Physical Activity

Increased physical activity can be encouraged in small increments. Although 30 minutes of aerobic exercise often is recommended, this may be an unreasonable expectation for deconditioned children. School physical education is important—do not write notes to remove children from gym class without a medical contraindication. Limit screen time (i.e., TV, computer, and video games) to 2 hours per day. Include walking in everyday life activities. Encourage the stairs rather than the elevator. Suggest getting off the school bus one stop earlier than usual and walking to the destination. Have the child agree to walk the dog. Encourage family activities that involve physical activity.

Treatment of Extreme Obesity

Some children may suffer from significant complications secondary to being overweight or may be so overweight that more interventional methods may be required. The following programs have been used to increase the rate of weight loss. These are all related to dietary management, medication, or surgery, but increased physical activity is recommended in all of them.

Ketogenic Diets Very low carbohydrate diets (VLCDs) have been reported in the literature for the treatment of both obesity and diabetes. These approaches are so low in carbohydrate that the body metabolizes fatty acids as its primary energy source. The fatty acids are metabolized incompletely, and they are reduced to the ketone bodies acetoacetate and β-hydroxybutyrate, which are circulated in the bloodstream and excreted through the urine, breath, and skin. Because of the ketosis involved, these diets are known as *ketogenic diets*. The two types of VLCDs reported most commonly are those with extreme restriction of total energy intake and those that restrict energy intake from specific nutrients.

The most common ketogenic diets reported in the literature are the protein-sparing modified fasts (PSMFs). These are very low energy ketogenic diets, usually restricted to 600–800 kcal/day composed almost entirely of protein. These plans usually are instituted in an impatient setting for 8–12 weeks. Potential advantages of a PSMF include increased nitrogen sparing and improvement in maintenance of lean body mass when compared with nonketogenic very low energy diets. Suskind and colleagues report weight loss in an uncontrolled trial using a PSMF in children (161). Willi and colleagues reported increased weight loss in obese adolescents on a PSMF and showed that the weight lost was predominately fat and not lean body mass (162). The other type of ketogenic diet commonly used in treatment centers is a non-energy-restricted VLCD. This is the type of diet represented by the lay publications *Dr Atkins' Diet Revolution* and *Protein Power*, among others. Despite the extreme popularity of these diets, there have been very few reports until recently, with very promising results in adults (163–165). In the only trial of a non-energy-restricted ketogenic diet in children and adolescents, increased weight loss and improved non-HDL cholesterol was shown in 12 weeks (166). Although a VLCD appears to be very effective in short-term trials, long-term efficacy has not yet been established, and further studies are needed before recommending a VLCD as first-line treatment of obesity.

Glycemic Index Approach The glycemic index describes the rise of blood glucose occurring after consuming a given quantity of a carbohydrate-containing food (167). The glycemic index of a carbohydrate is determined primarily by dietary factors affecting food digestibility, gastrointestinal motility, or insulin secretion (including carbohydrate type, food structure, fiber, and associate protein and fat). It is an experimentally derived value where test subjects are given 50 g of a test food, and the rise in blood glucose is measured at 15-minute intervals for 2 hours. The area under the glucose response curve then is calculated and compared with that of the same subject under test conditions with 50 g of a standard food, usually glucose or white bread. Increased weight loss, greater satiety, and improved HDL cholesterol have been reported in subjects on a low-glycemic-index diet (168–170). Since the glycemic index does not represent the quantity of carbohydrate intake but only the quality of those carbohydrates, these diets are not expected to result in ketosis. Recent trials by Speith, Ebberling, and others show improved weight loss in low glycemic approaches in children compared with low-fat approaches in randomized, controlled trials (171,172). Although widely used in Europe and Australia, the glycemic index approach is still controversial, with many critics commenting that glycemic index measures only pure foods, and the metabolic effect of a mixed diet, where many different types of foods are eaten at the same time, is unknown.

Pharmacotherapy Currently, two medications are approved for weight loss in adolescents: sibutramine (Meridia) and orlistat (Xenical) (Table 21-10). Sibutramine is a central inhibitor of uptake of norepinephrine, serotonin, and dopamine and works by decreasing appetite. It has been shown to be effective over 1 year in adults in double-blind, controlled trials. Side effects include increased pulse rate and blood pressure, insomnia, anxiety, and sleep disturbance (173). Sibutramine cannot be used in conjunction with serotonin reuptake inhibitors or monoamine oxidase (MAO) inhibitors. Sibutramine is approved for ages 16 and older.

Orlistat, a fat-absorption inhibitor, has been show to reduce body weight over 1 year in adolescents. Side effects are mostly related to fat malabsorption and include steatorrhea, diarrhea, flatulence, and fat-soluable vitamin malnutrition (174). These side effects increase with greater fat intake. Although in some adolescents the negative conditioning associated with fat intake is a benefit, many discontinue the medication due to discomfort rather than decreased fat intake.

Off-label use of medications that have been associated with weight loss include metformin, an insulin sensitizer; topiramate, an anticonvulsant; and fluoxitine, a serotonin reuptake inhibitor (175–177). Herbal medications such as ephedra and ma huang (often used in conjunction with caffeine) have been shown to improve weight loss but are too dangerous to be recommended and in fact have been removed from the market. Potential adverse

TABLE 21-10	Medications Used for Weight Loss	
Medication	**Type**	**Side Effects**
Sibutramine (Merida)*	Psychostimulant with some serotonin-enhancing activity	Nervousness, irritability, headache, dry mouth, nausea, constipation
Orlistat (Xenical)*	Lipase inhibitor	Steatorrhea, bloating, anal leakage
Phenylpropanolamine (Dexatrim, Accutrim)	Psychostimulant	Nervousness, irritability, headache, dry mouth, nausea, constipation
Ephedrine/caffeine (usually sold in combination, currently off the market)	Psychostimulant	Insomnia, jitteriness, high blood pressure, agitation, arythmias, sudden death
Diethylproprion (Tenuate, Tenuate Dospan)	Psychostimulant	Nervousness, irritability, headache, dry mouth, nausea, constipation
Phenteramine (Ionamin)	Psychostimulant	Nervousness, irritability, headache, dry mouth, nausea, constipation
Phendimetrazine (Bontril, Prelu-2)	Psychostimulant	Nervousness, irritability, headache, dry mouth, nausea, constipation
Benzphetamine (Didrex)	Psychostimulant	Nervousness, irritability, headache, dry mouth, nausea, constipation
Fluoxetine (Prozac): Off-label	Selective serotonin reuptake inhibitor	Fatigue, diarrhea, sweating, insomnia, thirst, nausea, constipation
Topirimate (Topamax): Off-label	Antiepileptic	Fatigue, dizziness, ataxia, dysarthria, parasthesia, nausea, somnolence, nervousness
Combinations of various herbs and minerals including guarana, ginseng, green tea leaf, cromium, and others (TrimSpa, Metabolife, Stacker 2, and others)	Mostly psychostimulants	Not evaluated; likely psychomotor excitation

*Indicates approved for use in adolescents.
Modified from Sondike et al. *Contemp Pediatr.* 2000;17.

TABLE 21-11   Criteria for Bariatric Surgery in Adolescents

All the following should be present when considering bariatric surgery in an adolescent:

- Youth has failed at least 6 months of organized attempts at weight management, as determined by primary care provider.
- Has attained or nearly attained sexual maturity.
- Severely obese (BMI > 40) with serious obesity-related comorbidites or BMI >50 with less severe comorbidities.
- Demonstrated commitment to comprehensive medical and psychologic evaluation both before and after surgery.
- Females agree to avoid pregnancy for at least 1 year postoperatively.
- Capable of and willing to adhere to nutritional guidelines postoperatively.
- Able to provide informed assent to surgical treatment.
- Demonstrated decisional capacity.
- Supportive family environment.

From Inge et al. *Pediatrics.* 2004;114:217–223.

reactions include hypertension, arrhythmia, stroke, and sudden death (178). Chromium has long been believed to contain weight-loss properties, but scientific studies have shown it to be ineffective (179). In general, weight-loss supplements or medications for children are not recommended because of risk of side effects and lack of evidence for long-term benefit.

Bariatric Surgery Bariatric surgery can be considered as a last resort for adolescents so overweight that they are suffering from life-threatening health complications (Table 21-11). The roux-en-Y gastric bypass procedure has shown excellent long-term weight loss but high morbidity and mortality (180). The expert panel convened by the American Pediatric Surgical Association recommended that surgery be considered only in those most at risk, who have achieved skeletal maturity, have had at least 6 months of compliance in a weight management program, and agree not to become pregnant for 1 year (181). The procedure used in adolescents is the roux-en-Y gastroplasty, which has shown most effectiveness but is also the most highly morbid of weight-loss surgical procedures. Nutritional deficiencies are common, particularly low levels of iron, vitamin B_{12}, vitamin D, and calcium. Thiamine deficiency is common in patients with frequent vomiting, and a case of beriberi was reported recently in a young adult after undergoing roux-en-Y gastroplasty (182).

Adjustable laparoscopic gastric banding (LGB) has the advantage of being reversible but has shown less long-term success than roux-en-Y and has not been approved by the Food and Drug Administration (FDA) for use in adolescents. Possible device-related complications include port malposition or malfunction, tubing leaks, band slippage leading to gastric prolapse, foreign-body infection, and band erosion into the stomach or esophagus. Moreover, because these mechanical devices have a finite lifetime, adolescent patients may need to undergo replacement of the device someday (183).

Gastric pacing (implantable gastric stimulator [IGS]) is a new modality in which a device creating electrical stimulation is placed in the smooth muscle of the stomach, decreasing appetite (184). IGS placement is a significantly less morbid procedure than other forms of bariatric surgery. Early results using IGS are promising, and further study is needed (184,185).

REFERENCES

1. Centers for Disease Control and Prevention Web site, www.cdc.gov; accessed August 2005.
2. American Obesity Association Web site, www.obesity.org/subs/childhood/prevalence.html; accessed August 2005.
3. Dietz WH. Health consequences of obesity in youth: Childhood predictors of adult disease. *Pediatrics.* 1998;101:518–525.
4. Goran MI, Treuth MS. Energy expenditure, physical activity, and obesity in children. *Pediatr Clin North Am.* 2001;48:931–953.
5. Doucet E, St.-Pierre S, Almeras N, et al. Evidence for the existence of adaptive thermogenesis during weight loss. *Br J Nutr.* 2001;85:715–723.
6. Maffeis C, Schutz Y, Pinelli L. Postprandial thermogenesis in obese children before and after weight reduction. *Eur J Clin Nutr.* 1992;46:577–583.
7. Tataranni PA, Larson DE, Snitker S, et al. Thermic effect of food in humans: Methods and results from use of a respiratory chamber. *Am J Clin Nutr.* 1995;61:1013–1019.
8. Levine JA, Lanningham-Foster LM, McCrady SK, et al. Interindividual variation in posture allocation: Possible role in human obesity. *Science.* 2005;307:584–586.
9. Chronwall BM, Zukowska Z. Neuropeptide Y, ubiquitous and elusive. *Peptides.* 2004;25:359–363.
10. Charbonneau C, Bai F, Richards BS, et al. Central and peripheral interactions between the agouti-related protein and leptin. *Biochem Biophys Res Commun.* 2004;319:518–524.
11. Gundlach AL, Burazin TC. Galanin–galanin receptor systems in the hypothalamic paraventricular and supraoptic nuclei: Some recent findings and future challenges. *Ann NY Acad Sci.* 199821;863:241–251.
12. Rodgers RJ, Ishii Y, Halford JC, et al. Orexins and appetite regulation. *Neuropeptides.* 2002;36:303–325.
13. Fehm HL, Smolnik R, Kern W, et al. The melanocortin melanocyte-stimulating hormone/adrenocorticotropin (4–10) decreases body fat in humans. *J Clin Endocrinol Metab.* 2001;86:1144–1148.
14. Hunter RG, Philpot K, Vicentic A, et al. CART in feeding and obesity. *Trends Endocrinol Metab.* 2004;15:454–459.
15. Simansky KJ. Serotonergic control of the organization of feeding and satiety. *Behav Brain Res.* 1996;73:37–42.
16. Small DM, Jones-Gotman M, Dagher A. Feeding-induced dopamine release in dorsal striatum correlates with meal pleasantness ratings in healthy human volunteers. *Neuroimage.* 2003;19:1709–1715.
17. Kojima M, Hosoda H, Kangawa K. Clinical endocrinology and metabolism: Ghrelin, a novel growth-hormone-releasing and appetite-stimulating peptide from stomach. *Best Pract Res Clin Endocrinol Metab.* 2004;18:517–130.
18. Morinigo R, Casamitjana R, Moize V, et al. Short-term effects of gastric bypass surgery on circulating ghrelin levels. *Obes Res.* 2004;12:1108–1116.
19. DelParigi A, Tschop M, Heiman ML, et al. High circulating ghrelin: A potential cause for hyperphagia and obesity in Prader–Willi syndrome. *J Clin Endocrinol Metab.* 2002;87:5461–5464.
20. Baskin DG, Figlewicz Lattemann D, Seeley RJ, et al. Insulin and leptin: Dual adiposity signals to the brain for the regulation of food intake and body weight. *Brain Res.* 1999;848:114–123.
21. Hayes MR, Moore RL, Shah SM, et al. 5-HT3 receptors participate in CCK-induced suppression of food intake by delaying gastric emptying. *Am J Physiol Regul Integr Comp Physiol.* 2004;287:R817–823.
22. Batterham RL, Cohen MA, Ellis SM, et al. Inhibition of food intake in obese subjects by peptide YY3–36. *N Engl J Med.* 2003;349:941–948.
23. Green ED, Maffei M, Braden VV, et al. The human obese (OB) gene: RNA expression pattern and mapping on the physical, cytogenetic, and genetic maps of chromosome 7. *Genome Res.* 1995;5:5–12.
24. Baskin DG, Blevins JE, Schwartz MW. How the brain regulates food intake and body weight: the role of leptin. *J Pediatr Endocrinol Metab.* 2001;14:1417–1429.
25. Hassink SG, Sheslow DV, de Lancey E, et al. Serum leptin in children with obesity: Relationship to gender and development. *Pediatrics.* 1996;98:201–203.
26. Steinberger J, Steffen L, Jacobs DR Jr. Relation of leptin to insulin resistance

syndrome in children. *Obes Res.* 2003;11:1124–1130.

27. Heilbronn LK, Rood J, Janderova L, et al. Relationship between serum resistin concentrations and insulin resistance in nonobese, obese, and obese diabetic subjects. *J Clin Endocrinol Metab.* 2004;89:1844–1848.

28. Vozarova de Courten B, Degawa-Yamauchi M, et al. High serum resistin is associated with an increase in adiposity but not a worsening of insulin resistance in Pima Indians. *Diabetes.* 2004;53:1279–1284.

29. Hotamisligil GS, Spiegelman BM. Tumor necrosis factor α: A key component of the obesity–diabetes link. *Diabetes.* 1994;43:1271–1278.

30. Kim HJ, Higashimori T, Park SY, et al. Differential effects of interleukin 6 and 10 on skeletal muscle and liver insulin action in vivo. *Diabetes.* 2004;53:1060–1067.

31. Lambert M, Delvin EE, Paradis G, et al. C-reactive protein and features of the metabolic syndrome in a population-based sample of children and adolescents. *Clin Chem.* 2004;50:1762–1768.

32. Lopez-Bermejo A, Botas P, Funahashi T, et al. Adiponectin, hepatocellular dysfunction and insulin sensitivity. *Clin Endocrinol (Oxf).* 2004;60:256–263.

33. Walsh MJ, Sniderman AD, Cianflone K, et al. The effect of ASP on the adipocyte of the morbidly obese. *J Surg Res.* 1989;46:470–473.

34. Arner P, Wennlund A, Ostman J. Thyroid hormone regulation of the catecholamine effects in human adipose tissue. *Acta Endocrinol (Copenh).* 1981;96:65–69.

35. Moustaid N, Jones BH, Taylor JW. Insulin increases lipogenic enzyme activity in human adipocytes in primary culture. *J Nutr.* 1996;126:865–870.

36. Djurhuus CB, Gravholt CH, Nielsen S, et al. Effects of cortisol on lipolysis and regional interstitial glycerol levels in humans. *Am J Physiol Endocrinol Metab.* 2002;283:E172–177.

37. Rask E, Walker BR, Soderberg S, et al. Tissue-specific changes in peripheral cortisol metabolism in obese women: Increased adipose 11β-hydroxysteroid dehydrogenase type 1 activity. *J Clin Endocrinol Metab.* 2002;87:3330–3336.

38. Hauner H, Entenmann G, Wabitsch M, et al. Promoting effect of glucocorticoids on the differentiation of human adipocyte precursor cells cultured in a chemically defined medium. *J Clin Invest.* 1989;84:1663–1670.

39. Ottosson M, Lonnroth P, Bjorntorp P, et al. Effects of cortisol and growth hormone on lipolysis in human adipose tissue. *J Clin Endocrinol Metab.* 2000;85:799–803.

40. Djurhuus CB, Gravholt CH, Nielsen S, et al. Additive effects of cortisol and growth hormone on regional and systemic lipolysis in humans. *Am J Physiol Endocrinol Metab.* 2004;286:E488–494.

41. Hedley AA, Ogden CL, Johnson CL, et al. Prevalence of overweight and obesity among US children, adolescents, and adults, 1999–2002. *JAMA.* 2004;291:2847–2850.

42. Troiano RP, Flegal KM. Overweight children and adolescents: Description, epidemiology, and demographics. *Pediatrics.* 1998;101:497–504.

43. Finkelstein EA, Fiebelkorn IC, Wang G. National medical spending attributable to overweight and obesity: How much, and who's paying? *Health Aff (Millwood).* 2003;W3:219–226.

44. Chopra M, Galbraith S, Darnton-Hill I. A global response to a global problem: The epidemic of overnutrition. *Bull WHO.* 2002;80:952–958.

45. Dobson AJ, Evans A, Ferrario M. Changes in estimated coronary risk in the 1980s: Data from 38 populations in the WHO MONICA Project. World Health Organization. Monitoring Trends and Determinants in Cardiovascular Diseases. *Ann Med.* 1998;30:199–205.

46. Hsieh PL, FitzGerald M. Childhood obesity in Taiwan: Review of the Taiwanese literature. *Nurs Health Sci.* 2005;7:134–142.

47. Gu D, Reynolds K, Wu X, et al. Prevalence of the metabolic syndrome and overweight among adults in China. *Lancet.* 2005;365:1398–1405.

48. Azizi F, Azadbakht L, Mirmiran P. Trends in overweight, obesity and central fat accumulation among Tehranian adults between 1998–1999 and 2001–2002: Tehran lipid and glucose study. *Ann Nutr Metab.* 2005;49:3–8.

49. Manios Y, Kolotourou M, Moschonis G, et al. Macronutrient intake, physical activity, serum lipids and increased body weight in primary schoolchildren in Istanbul. *Pediatr Int.* 2005;47:159–166.

50. Mukuddem-Petersen J, Kruger HS. Association between stunting and overweight among 10–15-year-old children in the North West Province of South Africa: The THUSA BANA Study. *Int J Obes Relat Metab Disord.* 2004;28:842–851.

51. Monteiro CA, Conde WL, Lu B, et al. Obesity and inequities in health in the developing world. *Int J Obes Relat Metab Disord.* 2004;28:1181–1186.

52. World Health Organization. Overweight and Obesity, www.who.int/dietphysicalactivity/publications/facts/obesity; accessed August 15, 2005.

53. Sorof JM, Lai D, Turner J, et al. Overweight, ethnicity, and the prevalence of hypertension in school-aged children. *Pediatrics.* 2004;113:475–482.

54. Pinhas-Hamiel O, Dolan LM, Daniels SR, et al. Increased incidence of non-insulin-dependent diabetes mellitus among adolescents. *J Pediatr.* 1996;128:608–615.

55. Schwimmer JB, Burwinkle TM, Varni JW. Health-related quality of life of severely obese children and adolescents. *JAMA.* 2003;289:1813–1819.

56. Guo SS, Wu W, Chumlea WC, et al. Predicting overweight and obesity in adulthood from body mass index values in childhood and adolescence. *Am J Clin Nutr.* 2002;76:653–658.

57. Zeller M, Kirk S, Claytor R, et al. Predictors of attrition from a pediatric weight management program. *J Pediatr.* 2004;144:466–470.

58. Skender ML, Goodrick GK, Del Junco DJ, et al. Comparison of 2-year weight loss trends in behavioral treatments of obesity: diet, exercise, and combination interventions. *J Am Diet Assoc.* 1996;96:342–346.

59. Kramer FM, Jeffery RW, Forster JL, et al. Long-term follow-up of behavioral treatment for obesity: Patterns of weight regain among men and women. *Int J Obes.* 1989;13:123–136.

60. Kaprio J, Pulkkinen L, Rose RJ. Genetic and environmental factors in health-related behaviors: Studies on Finnish twins and twin families. *Twin Res.* 2002;5:366–371.

61. Stunkard AJ, Harris JR, Pederson N, et al. An adoption study of human obesity. *N Engl J Med.* 1990;322:1483–1487.

62. Faith MS, Pietrobelli A, Nunez C, et al. Evidence for independent genetic influences on fat mass and body mass index in a pediatric twin sample. *Pediatrics.* 1999;104:61–67.

63. Herskind AM, McGue M, Sorensen TI, et al. Sex and age specific assessment of genetic and environmental influences on body mass index in twins. *Int J Obes Relat Metab Disord.* 1996;20:106–113.

64. Vaisse C, Clement K. Melanocortin-4 receptor mutations are a frequent and heterogeneous cause of morbid obesity. *J Clin Invest.* 2000;106:253–262.

65. Jackson RS, Creemers JW, Ohagi S, et al. Obesity and impaired prohormone processing associated with mutations in the human prohormone convertase 1 gene. *Nat Genet.* 1997;16:303–306.

66. Wabitsch M. The acquisition of obesity: Insights from cellular and genetic research. *Proc Nutr Soc.* 2000;59:325–330.

67. Krude H, Biebermann H, Luck W, et al. Severe early-onset obesity, adrenal insufficiency and red hair pigmentation caused by POMC mutations in humans. *Nat Genet.* 1998;19:155–157.

68. Butler AA, Kesterson RA, Khong K, et al. A unique metabolic syndrome causes obesity in the melanocortin-3 receptor–deficient mouse. *Endocrinology.* 2000;141:3518–3521.

69. Lee YS, Poh LK, Loke KY. A novel melanocortin 3 receptor gene (MC3R) mutation associated with severe obesity. *J Clin Endocrinol Metab.* 2002;87:1423–1426.

70. Holder JL Jr, Butte NF, Zinn AR. Profound obesity associated with a balanced translocation that disrupts the SIM1 gene. *Hum Mol Genet.* 2000;9:101–108.

71. Montague CT, Farooqi IS, Whitehead JP, et al. Congenital leptin deficiency is associated with severe early-onset obesity in humans. *Nature.* 1997;387:903–908.

72. Clement K, Vaisse C, Lahlou N, et al. A mutation in the human leptin receptor gene causes obesity and pituitary dysfunction. *Nature.* 1998;392:398–401.

73. Ristow M, Muller-Wieland D, Pfeiffer A, et al. Obesity associated with a mutation in a genetic regulator of adipocyte differentiation. *N Engl J Med.* 1998;339:953–959.

74. Gunay-Aygun M, Cassidy SB, Nicholls RD. Prader-Willi and other syndromes associated with obesity and mental retardation. *Behav Genet.* 1997;27:307–324.

75. Tauber M, Conte Auriol F, Moulin P, et al. Hyperghrelinemia is a common feature of

Prader–Willi syndrome and pituitary stalk interruption: A pathophysiological hypothesis. *Horm Res.* 2004;62:49–54.

76. Myers SE, Carrel AL, Whitman BY, et al. Sustained benefit after 2 years of growth hormone on body composition, fat utilization, physical strength and agility, and growth in Prader–Willi syndrome. *J Pediatr.* 2000;137:42–49.

77. Eiholzer U. Deaths in children with the Prader–Willi syndrome. *Horm Res.* 2005;63:33–39.

78. de Vries BB, Fryns JP, Butler MG, et al. Clinical and molecular studies in fragile X patients with a Prader–Willi-like phenotype. *J Med Genet.* 1993;30:761–766.

79. Rubin SS, Rimmer JH, Chicoine B, et al. Overweight prevalence in persons with Down syndrome. *Ment Retard.* 1998;36:175–181.

80. Arends NJ, Boonstra VH, Duivenvoorden HJ, et al. Reduced insulin sensitivity and the presence of cardiovascular risk factors in short prepubertal children born small for gestational age (SGA). *Clin Endocrinol (Oxf).* 2005;62:44–50.

81. Bavdekar A, Yajnik CS, Fall CH, et al. Insulin resistance syndrome in 8-year-old Indian children: Small at birth, big at 8 years, or both? *Diabetes.* 1999;48:2422–2429.

82. Plagemann A, Harder T, Kohlhoff R, et al. Overweight and obesity in infants of mothers with long-term insulin-dependent diabetes or gestational diabetes. *Int J Obes Relat Metab Disord.* 1997;21:451–456.

83. Gillman MW, Rifas-Shiman S, Berkey CS, et al. Maternal gestational diabetes, birth weight, and adolescent obesity. *Pediatrics.* 2003;111:e221–6.

84. Muller HL, Emser A, Faldum A, et al. Longitudinal study on growth and body mass index before and after diagnosis of childhood craniopharyngioma. *J Clin Endocrinol Metab.* 2004;89:3298–3305.

85. Skorzewska A, Lal S, Waserman J, et al. Abnormal food-seeking behavior after surgery for craniopharyngioma. *Neuropsychobiology.* 1989;21:17–20.

86. Lustig RH, Hinds PS, Ringwald-Smith K, et.al. Octreotide therapy of pediatric hypothalamic obesity: A double-blind, placebo-controlled trial. *J Clin Endocrinol Metab.* 2003;88:2586–2592.

87. Kirk LF Jr, Hash RB, Katner HP, et al. Cushing's disease: Clinical manifestations and diagnostic evaluation. *Am Fam Phys.* 2000;62:1119–1127, 1133–1134.

88. Friedman TC. Carbohydrate and lipid metabolism in endogenous hypercortisolism: Shared features with metabolic syndrome X and NIDDM. *Endocr J.* 1996;43:645–655.

89. Papanicolaou DA, Yanovski JA, Cutler GB Jr, et al. A single midnight serum cortisol measurement distinguishes Cushing's syndrome from pseudo-Cushing states. *J Clin Endocrinol Metab.* 1998;83:1163–1167.

90. Munns CF, Batch JA. Hyperinsulinism and Beckwith–Wiedemann syndrome. *Arch Dis Child Fetal Neonatal Ed.* 2001;84:F67–69.

91. Styne DM. Childhood and adolescent obesity: Prevalence and significance. *Pediatr Clin North Am.* 2001;48:823–854, vii.

92. Graham KA, Perkins DO, Edwards LJ, et al. Effect of olanzapine on body composition and energy expenditure in adults with first-episode psychosis. *Am J Psychiatry.* 2005;162:118–123.

93. Farwell WR, Stump TE, Wang J, et al. Weight gain and new onset diabetes associated with olanzapine and risperidone. *J Gen Intern Med.* 2004;19:1200–1205.

94. Murashita M, Kusumi I, Inoue T, et al. Olanzapine increases plasma ghrelin level in patients with schizophrenia. *Psychoneuroendocrinology.* 2005;30:106–110.

95. Bonny AE, Britto MT, Huang B, et al. Weight gain, adiposity, and eating behaviors among adolescent females on depot medroxyprogesterone acetate (DMPA). *J Pediatr Adolesc Gynecol.* 2004;17:109–115.

96. Derosa G, Cicero AF, Gaddi A, et al. Metabolic effects of pioglitazone and rosiglitazone in patients with diabetes and metabolic syndrome treated with glimepiride: A twelve-month, multicenter, double-blind, randomized, controlled, parallel-group trial. *Clin Ther.* 2004;26:744–754.

97. Easter D, O'Bryan-Tear CG, Verity C. Weight gain with valproate or carbamazepine: A reappraisal. *Seizure.* 1997;6:121–125.

98. de Onis M, Blossner M. Prevalence and trends of overweight among preschool children in developing countries. *Am J Clin Nutr.* 2000;72:1032–1039.

99. Rolls BJ. The supersizing of America: Portion size and the obesity epidemic. *Nutr Today.* 2003;38:42–53.

100. Center for Disease Control and Prevention. Trends in intake of macronutrients—United States, 1971–2000. *MMWR* 2004;53(4);80–82.

101. Halford JC, Gillespie J, Brown V, et al. Effect of television advertisements for foods on food consumption in children. *Appetite.* 2004;42:221–225.

102. Vandegrift D, Yoked T. Obesity rates, income, and suburban sprawl: An analysis of US states. *Health Place.* 2004;10:221–229.

103. Centers for Disease Control and Prevention (CDC). Participation in high school physical education—United States, 1991–2003. *MMWR.* 2004;53:844–847.

104. Cruz PD Jr, Hud JA Jr. Excess insulin binding to insulin-like growth factor receptors: Proposed mechanism for acanthosis nigricans. *J Invest Dermatol.* 1992;98:82–85S.

105. Reaven GM. The role of insulin resistance in human disease. *Diabetes.* 1988;37:1495.

106. Isomaa B, Almgren P, Tuomi T, et al. Cardiovascular morbidity and mortality associated with the metabolic syndrome. *Diabetes Care.* 2001;24:683–689.

107. Palaniappan L, Carnethon M, Fortmann SP. Association between microalbuminuria and the metabolic syndrome: NHANES III. *Am J Hypertens.* 2003;16:952–958.

108. de Ferranti SD, Gauvreau K, Ludwig DS, et al. Prevalence of the metabolic syndrome in American adolescents: Findings from the Third National Health and Nutrition Examination Survey. *Circulation.* 2004;110:2494–2497.

109. Berenson GS, Srinivasan SR, Nicklas TA. Atherosclerosis: A nutritional disease of childhood. *Am J Cardiol.* 1998;82:22–29T.

110. Weiss R, Dziura J, Burgert TS, et al. Obesity and the metabolic syndrome in children and adolescents. *Obstet Gynecol Surv.* 2004;59:822–824.

111. Dagogo-Jack S. Ethnic disparities in type 2 diabetes: Pathophysiology and implications for prevention and management. *J Natl Med Assoc.* 2003;95:1115–1116.

112. Snijder MB, Zimmet PZ, Visser M. Independent and opposite associations of waist and hip circumferences with diabetes, hypertension and dyslipidemia: The AusDiab Study. *Int J Obes Relat Metab Disord.* 2004;28:402–409.

113. von Eyben FE, Mouritsen E, Holm J, et al. Intra-abdominal obesity and metabolic risk factors: A study of young adults. *Int J Obes Relat Metab Disord.* 2003;27:941–949.

114. Onat A, Avci GS, Barlan MM, et al. Measures of abdominal obesity assessed for visceral adiposity and relation to coronary risk. *Int J Obes Relat Metab Disord.* 2004;28:1018–1025.

115. Daniels SR, Morrison JA, Sprecher DL, et al. Association of body fat distribution and cardiovascular risk factors in children and adolescents. *Circulation.* 1999;99:541–545.

116. Chan DF, Li AM, Chu WC, et al. Hepatic steatosis in obese Chinese children. *Int J Obes Relat Metab Disord.* 2004;28:1257–1263.

117. McCullough AJ. The clinical features, diagnosis and natural history of nonalcoholic fatty liver disease. *Clin Liver Dis.* 2004;8:521–533, viii.

118. Schweizer P, Lenz MP, Kirschner HJ. Pathogenesis and symptomatology of cholelithiasis in childhood: A prospective study. *Dig Surg.* 2000;17:459–467.

119. Ruhl CE, Everhart JE. Overweight, but not high dietary fat intake, increases risk of gastroesophageal reflux disease hospitalization. The NHANES I Epidemiologic Follow-up Study. *Ann Epidemiol.* 1999;9:424–435.

120. Nilsson Johnsen R, Ye W, Hveem K, et al. Obesity and estrogen as risk factors for gastroesophageal reflux symptoms. *JAMA.* 2003;290:66–72.

121. Balcer LJ, Liu GT, Forman S, et al. Idiopathic intracranial hypertension: Relation of age and obesity in children. *Neurology.* 1999;52:870–872.

122. Sugerman HJ, DeMaria EJ, Felton WL 3d, et al. Increased intra-abdominal pressure and cardiac filling pressures in obesity-associated pseudotumor cerebri. *Neurology.* 49:507–511.

123. Thompson GH, Carter JR. Late-onset tibia vara (Blount's disease). *Curr Concepts Clin Orthop.* 1990;255:24–35.

124. Poussa M, Schlenzka D, Yrjonen T. Body mass index and slipped capital femoral epiphysis. *J Pediatr Orthop B.* 2003;12:369–371.

125. Luhmann SJ, Rich MM, Schoenecker PL. Painful idiopathic rigid flatfoot in children and adolescents. *Foot Ankle Int.* 2000;21:59–66.

126. Powell A, Teichtahl AJ, Wluka AE, et al. Obesity: a preventable risk factor for large

joint osteoarthritis which may act through biomechanical factors. *Br J Sports Med.* 2005;39:4–5.

127. Children's Hospital of Wisconsin Nutrition, Exercise and Weight Management Program. Unpublished data, compiled 2003–2004. NEW Kids Program, unpublished data.

128. Ray RM, Senders CW. Airway management in the obese child. *Pediatr Clin North Am.* 2001;48:1055–1063.

129. Weitzenblum E, Chaouat A, Kessler R, et al. Daytime hypoventilation in obstructive sleep apnoea syndrome. *Sleep Med Rev.* 1999;3:79–93.

130. Strain GW, Zumoff B, Kream J, et. al. Mild hypogonadotropic hypogonadism in obese men. *Metabolism.* 1982;31:871–875.

131. Chang RJ. A practical approach to the diagnosis of polycystic ovary syndrome. *Am J Obstet Gynecol.* 2004;191:713–717.

132. Lerner RM, Gellart E. Body build indentification, preference, and aversion in children. *Dev Psychol.* 1969;5:456.

133. McElroy SL, Kotwal R, Malhotra S, et al. Are mood disorders and obesity related? A review for the mental health professional. *J Clin Psychiatry.* 2004;65:634–651.

134. Gustafson TB, Sarwer DB. Childhood sexual abuse and obesity. *Obes Rev.* 2004;5:129–135.

135. van den Brandt PA, Spiegelman D, Yuan SS, et al. Pooled analysis of prospective cohort studies on height, weight, and breast cancer risk. Am J Epidemiol. 2000;152:514–527.

136. Petrelli JM, Calle EE, Rodriguez C, et al. Body mass index, height, and postmenopausal breast cancer mortality in a prospective cohort of U.S. women. Cancer Cause Control. 2002;13:325–332.

137. Goodman MT, Hankin JH, Wilkens LR, et al. Diet, body size, physical activity, and the risk of endometrial cancer. Cancer Res. 1997;57:5077–5085.

138. Ford ES. Body mass index and colon cancer in a national sample of adult U.S. men and women. Am J Epidemiol. 1999;150:390–398.

139. Chow WH, McLaughlin JK, Mandel JS, et al. Obesity and risk of renal cell cancer. Cancer Epidemiol Biomark Prevent. 1996;5:17–21.

140. Brown LM, Swanson CA, Gridley G, et al. Adenocarcinoma of the esophagus: Role of obesity and diet. J Natl Cancer Inst. 1995;87:104–109.

141. Lagergren J, Bergström R, Nyrén O. Association between body mass and adenocarcinoma of the esophagus and gastric cardia. Ann Intern Med. 1999;130:883–890.

142. Moerman CJ, Bueno-de-Mesquita HB. The epidemiology of gallbladder cancer: Lifestyle-related risk factors and limited surgical possibilities for prevention. Hepatogastroenterology. 1999;46:1533–1539.

143. Rodriguez C, Patel AV, Calle EE, et al. Body mass index, height, and prostate cancer mortality in two large cohorts of adult men in the United States. Cancer Epidemiol Biomark Prevent. 2001;10:345–353.

144. Daniels SR, Khoury PR, Morrison JA. The utility of body mass index as a measure of body fatness in children and adolescents: Differences by race and gender. *Pediatrics.* 1997;99:804–807.

145. Reilly JJ, Wilson J, Durnin JV. Determination of body composition from skinfold thickness: A validation study. *Arch Dis Child.* 1995;73:305–310.

146. Megnien JL, Denarie N, Cocaul M, et al. Predictive value of waist-to-hip ratio on cardiovascular risk events. *Int J Obes Relat Metab Disord.* 1999;23:90–97.

147. Taylor RW, Jones IE, Williams SM, et al. Evaluation of waist circumference, waist-to-hip ratio, and the conicity index as screng tools for high trunk fat mass, as measured by duel x-ray absorptiometry, in children aged 3–19 years. *Am J Clin Nutr.* 2000;72:490–495.

148. Slyper AH. Childhood obesity, adipose tissue distribution, and the pediatric practitioner. *Pediatrics.* 1998;102:e4.

149. Neovius M, Linne Y, Rossner S. BMI, waist-circumference and waist-hip-ratio as diagnostic tests for fatness in adolescents. *Int J Obes Relat Metab Disord.* 2005;29:163–169.

150. Fernandez JR, Redden DT, Pietrobelli A, et al. Waist circumference percentiles in nationally representative samples of African–American, European–American, and Mexican–American children and adolescents. *J Pediatr.* 2004;145:439–444.

151. Sun G, French CR, Martin GR, et al. Comparison of multifrequency bioelectrical impedance analysis with dual-energy x-ray absorptiometry for assessment of percentage body fat in a large, healthy population. *Am J Clin Nutr.* 2005;81:74–78.

152. Prior BM, Cureton KJ, Modlesky CM, et al. In vivo validation of whole body composition estimates from dual-energy x-ray absorptiometry. *J Appl Physiol.* 1997;83:623–630.

153. Ohsuzu F, Kosuda S, Takayama E, et al. Imaging techniques for measuring adipose-tissue distribution in the abdomen: A comparison between computed tomography and 1.5-tesla magnetic resonance spin-echo imaging. *Radiat Med.* 1998;16:99–107.

154. Van Loan M. Assessment of fat-free mass in teenagers: Use of TOBEC methodology. *Am J Clin Nutr.* 1990;52:586–590.

155. Cochran WJ, Klish WJ, Wong WW, et al. Total body electrical conductivity used to determine body composition in infants. *Pediatr Res.* 1986;20:561–564.

156. Wells JC, Fuller NJ. Precision of measurement and body size in whole-body air-displacement plethysmography. *Int J Obes Relat Metab Disord.* 2001;25:1161–1167.

157. Oppliger RA, Looney MA, Tipton CM. Reliability of hydrostatic weighing and skinfold measurements of body composition using a generalizability study. *Hum Biol.* 1987;59:77–96.

158. Schwimmer JB. Managing overweight in older children and adolescents. *Pediatr Ann.* 2004;33:39–44.

159. Bacon L, Stern JS, Van Loan MD, et al. Size acceptance and intuitive eating improve health for obese, female chronic dieters. *J Am Diet Assoc.* 2005;105:929–936.

160. Liu S, Willett WC, Manson JE, et al. Relation between changes in intakes of dietary fiber and grain products and changes in weight and development of obesity among middle-aged women. *Am J Clin Nutr.* 2003;78:920–927.

161. Suskind RM, Blecker U, Udall JN. Recent advances in the treatment of childhood obesity. *Pediatr Diabetes.* 2000;1:23–33.

162. Willi SM, Oexmann MJ, Wright NM, et al. The effects of a high-protein, low-fat, ketogenic diet on adolescents with morbid obesity: Body composition, blood chemistries, and sleep abnormalities. *Pediatrics.* 1998;101:61–67.

163. Westman EC, Yancy WS, Edman JS, et al. Effect of 6-month adherence to a very low carbohydrate diet program. *Am J Med.* 2002;113:30–36.

164. Sharman MJ, Volek JS. Weight loss leads to reductions in inflammatory biomarkers after a very-low-carbohydrate diet and a low-fat diet in overweight men. *Clin Sci (Lond).* 2004;107:365–369.

165. Volek J, Sharman M, Gomez A, et al. Comparison of energy-restricted very-low-carbohydrate and low-fat diets on weight loss and body composition in overweight men and women. *Nutr Metab (Lond).* 2004;1:13.

166. Sondike SB, Copperman N, Jacobson MS. Effects of a low-carbohydrate diet on weight loss and cardiovascular risk factor in overweight adolescents. *J Pediatr.* 2003;142:253–258.

167. Jenkins DJ, Kendall CW, Augustin LS, et al. Glycemic index: Overview of implications in health and disease. *Am J Clin Nutr.* 2002;76:266–273S.

168. Ludwig DS, Majzoub JA, Al-Zahrani A, et al. High glycemic index foods, overeating, and obesity. *Pediatrics.* 1999;103:E26.

169. Gilbertson HR, Thorburn AW, Brand-Miller JC, et al. Effect of low-glycemic-index dietary advice on dietary quality and food choice in children with type 1 diabetes. *Am J Clin Nutr.* 2003;77:83–90.

170. Luscombe ND, Noakes M, Clifton PM. Diets high and low in glycemic index versus high monounsaturated fat diets: Effects on glucose and lipid metabolism in NIDDM. *Eur J Clin Nutr.* 1999;53:473–478.

171. Spieth LE, Harnish JD, Lenders CM, et al. A low-glycemic index diet in the treatment of pediatric obesity. *Arch Pediatr Adolesc Med.* 2000;154:947–951.

172. Ebbeling CB, Leidig MM, Sinclair KB, et al. Effects of an ad libitum low-glycemic load diet on cardiovascular disease risk factors in obese young adults. *Am J Clin Nutr.* 2005;81:976–982.

173. Poston WS, Foreyt JP. Sibutramine and the management of obesity. *Exp Opin Pharmacother.* 2004;5:633–642.

174. O'Meara S, Riemsma R, Shirran L, et al. A systematic review of the clinical effectiveness of Orlistat used for the management of obesity. *Obes Rev.* 2004;5:51–68.

175. Mogul HR, Peterson SJ, Weinstein BI, et al. Metformin and carbohydrate-modified diet: a novel obesity treatment protocol: Preliminary findings from a case series of nondiabetic women with midlife weight gain and hyperinsulinemia. *Heart Dis.* 2001;3:285–292.

176. Wilding J, Van Gaal L, Rissanen A, et al. A randomized, double-blind,

placebo-controlled study of the long-term efficacy and safety of topiramate in the treatment of obese subjects. *Int J Obes Relat Metab Disord.* 2004; 28:1399–1410.

177. Goldstein DJ, Rampey AH Jr, Roback PJ, et al. Efficacy and safety of long-term fluoxetine treatment of obesity: Maximizing success. *Obes Res.* 1995; 3:481–490S.

178. Shekelle PG, Hardy ML, Morton SC, et al. Efficacy and safety of ephedra and ephedrine for weight loss and athletic performance: a meta-analysis. *JAMA.* 2003;289:1537–1545.

179. Pittler MH, Stevinson C, Ernst E. Chromium picolinate for reducing body weight: Meta-analysis of randomized trials. *Int J Obes Relat Metab Disord.* 2003;27:522–529.

180. Inge TH, Zeller M, Garcia VF, et al. Surgical approach to adolescent obesity. *Adolesc Med Clin.* 2004;15:429–453.

181. Inge TH, Krebs NF, Garcia VF, et al. Bariatric surgery for severely overweight adolescents: Concerns and recommendations. *Pediatrics.* 2004;114:217–223.

182. Towbin A, Inge TH, Garcia VF, et al. Beriberi after gastric bypass surgery in adolescence. *J Pediatr.* 2004;145:263–267.

183. Horgan S, Holterman MJ, Jacobsen GR, et al. Laparoscopic adjustable gastric banding for the treatment of adolescent morbid obesity in the United States: A safe alternative to gastric bypass. *J Pediatr Surg.* 2005;40:86–90.

184. Cigaina V. Long-term follow-up of gastric stimulation for obesity: The Mestre 8-year experience. *Obes Surg.* 2004;14:S14–22.

185. Luca M, Segato G, Busetto L, et al. Progress in implantable gastric stimulate on: Summary of results of the European multicenter study. *Obes Surg.* 2004;14:S33–39.

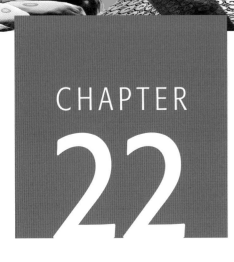

CHAPTER 22

Lipids and Lipoprotein Abnormalities

Juergen R. Schäfer, PD, Muhidien Soufi, MD
Julia Steinberger, MD, MS and Ertan Mayatepek, MD

INTRODUCTION

More than two decades ago Brown and Goldstein discovered the mechanisms of cholesterol uptake by the low-density lipoprotein (LDL) receptor pathway (1–3). In 1985 they received the Nobel Prize in Medicine for unravelling this puzzle (4). The investigators identified the progressive accumulation of cholesterol due to a defect of the LDL receptor (LDLR), and its role within the pathologic process causing atherosclerosis (5,6), which leads to the clinical manifestations of myocardial infarctions and strokes (7–9). Cholesterol is a vital compound required for cell proliferation and integrity and steroid hormone and bile acid synthesis, whereas triglycerides and fatty acids are necessary for energy supply and storage. Brown and Goldstein addressed the problems we face with cholesterol by saying "Cholesterol is a Janus-faced molecule. The very property that makes it useful in cell membranes, namely its absolute insolubility in water, also makes it lethal."

The water-insoluble lipids are carried in highly specialized lipoproteins that regulate the transport to various tissues (10–12). Lipoprotein particles contain esterified and unesterified cholesterol, triglycerides, phospholipids, and proteins. Lipoprotein-associated proteins are so-called apolipoproteins that are structural components of these particles (i.e., apoB-100, apoA-I), cofactors for enzymes (i.e., apoC-II, apoA-I, apoA-IV), or specific ligands for receptors (i.e., apoB-100, apoE) (13–15). In this complex system LDLs, the major carrier of blood cholesterol has been implicated in the storage of cholesterol in atherosclerotic plaques. Models for the mechanism of cholesterol accumulation in atherosclerotic plaques emphasize increased LDL uptake into the vessel wall or increased retention of LDL that has already entered the vessel wall (16–18).This chapter will review the pathways of lipids and lipoproteins, especially cholesterol entry and removal, the metabolism, and the physical changes of cholesterol as well as genetic defects of the lipoprotein metabolism. The formation of atherosclerosis in the vessel wall (18–20) and the treatment of hyperlipidemia will be also discussed.

Apolipoproteins

In recent years the central role of apolipoproteins in lipid metabolism became evident. Apolipoproteins have three key functions: 1) structural for the integrity of the particle, 2) cofactor for enzymes, and 3) ligands to very specific receptors. Several mutations and defects of apolipoproteins with major implications for lipid metabolism have been discovered (21,22), demonstrating the overwhelming role of these components for intact lipid and lipoprotein metabolism in humans (Table 22-1A and 22-1B).

Exogenous Pathway of Lipid Metabolism

The lipid transport systems can be seen as three distinct but interacting entities, which are: the exogenous, the endogenous, and the reverse lipoprotein pathways. The exogenous lipid metabolism refers to the intestinal absorption of dietary fat and cholesterol. Chylomicrons carry the exogenously delivered triglycerides from the gut and are very rich in fatty acids (Tables 22-2 and 22-3). Chylomicrons have the apolipoproteins B-48, C-II, E, and A-IV and at a lower content A-I, A-II, A-V, C-I, and C-III. Cholesterol uptake as well as the uptake of plant sterols is regulated by the Niemann Pick C 1–like protein, an integral membrane protein expressed mainly in small intestine, stomach, and muscle (23,24). Intracellularly the sterols are esterified by the action of Acyl-coenzyme A:cholesterol acyltransferase-2, whereas unesterified sterols (mainly phytosterols) will be secreted back into the intestine by two proteins called ABC G5 and G8 transporters (25,26). Sitosterolemia is considered to be a rare disease associated with elevated plant sterols in plasma (27) due to a defect of the ABC G5 or G8 genes (28). These genes are expressed primarily in the intestine and play a major role in limiting intestinal sterol absorption. This is because the encoded proteins can eject cholesterol from the intestinal cell and prevent it from getting into the blood stream. In the enterocyte the free fatty acids form triglycerides with glycerol, whereas free cholesterol is esterified by the action of acyl:cholesterol acyltransferase to cholesterol esters (Table 22-4).

Triglycerides and cholesterol are assembled intracellularly as chylomicrons with the most prominent apolipoprotein B-48. Apo B-48 does not bind to the LDLR. Thus, there is no premature clearance of chylomicrons by the LDLR before the particle is delipidated sufficiently by the action of lipases. Lipoprotein lipase is activated by apo C-II, which is an important cofactor (29,30). In this fashion, chylomicrons are delipidated and become smaller (thus, denser) by releasing free fatty acids from the core, resulting in formation of chylomicron remnants. These particles can be eliminated via apo E by the hepatic chylomicron remnant receptors for which apo E is a high-affinity ligand (31–33). Fatty acids are used as an energy source, for synthesis of important biomolecules, or are converted to triglyceride and can be stored in adipose tissue (29,34).

Endogenous Pathway of Lipid Transport and Metabolism

Very low density lipoprotein (VLDL) carries endogenously produced, liver-derived triglycerides and to a lesser degree cholesterol. VLDL contains mainly apo B-100, E, and to a lesser degree C and A. VLDL is converted by the action of lipoprotein lipases to intermediate density lipoprotein (IDL), which carries cholesterol esters and triglycerides. IDL again is converted by delipidation of specific lipases to LDL particles which carry most of the circulating cholesterol and cholesterol esters. The structural protein component of LDL is apoB-100, which binds specifically to the so-called LDL or apoB/E receptor.

Lipids and Lipoprotein Abnormalities
AT A GLANCE

Lipid and lipoprotein abnormalities are a major factor in the formation of the atherosclerotic plaque. There is increasing evidence that these abnormalities are present as early as in childhood and track into adulthood. Early prevention and intervention may slow the progression of atherosclerosis and decrease the morbidity and mortality from cardiovascular disease.

DISORDER	GENE	PRIMARY ORGAN/TISSUE	CHROMOSOME	OMIM
Lipoprotein lipase deficiency	Lipoprotein lipase (LPL)	Adipose, Muscle	8p22	238600
Apolipoprotein C-II deficiency	Apolipoprotein C-II (apoC-II)	Liver	19q13	207750
Familial dysbetalipoproteinemia (FD)	Alipoprotein E (apo E)	Liver	19q13	107741
Hepatic lipase deficiency	Hepatic lipase (HL)	Liver	15q22	151670
Familial hypercholesterolemia (FH) (homozygous)	Low-density lipoprotein receptor (LDLR)	Liver	19p13	143890
Familial hypercholesterolemia (FH) (heterozygous)	Low-density lipoprotein receptor (LDLR)	Liver	19p13	143890
Defective apolipoprotein B-100 (FDB)	Apolipoprotein B-100 (apo B-100)	Liver	2p24	107730
Apolipoprotein A-I deficiency (familial)	Apolipoprotein A-I (apo A-I)	Liver, intestine	11q23	107680
Apolipoprotein A-I deficiency (structural mutations)	Apolipoprotein A-I (apo A-I)	Liver, intestine	11q23	107680
Tangier disease	ATP-binding cassette protein AI (ABCAI)	All tissues	9q31	205400
LCAT deficiency (complete)	Lecithin:cholesterol acyltransferase (LCAT)	Liver	16q22	245900
LCAT deficiency (partial)	Lecithin:cholesterol acyltransferase (LCAT)	Liver	16q22	245900
Abetalipoproteinemia	Microsomal transfer protein (MTP)	Liver, intestine	4q22-q24	200100
Hypobetalipoproteinemia (homozygous)	Apolipoprotein B-100 (apo B-100)	Liver	2p24	107730
Hypobetalipoproteinemia (heterozygous)	Apolipoprotein B-100 (apo B-100)	Liver	2p24	107730
Autosomal recessive hypercholesterolemia (AHR)	Low-density lipoprotein receptor adaptor protein	Liver	1p35	605747

DISORDER	ROUTINE LABORATORY	MAJOR CLINICAL SYMPTOMS
Lipoprotein lipase deficiency	Triglycerides and cholesterol increased, HDL cholesterol decreased	Abdominal pain, lipemia retinalis, eruptive xanthomas
Apolipoprotein C-II deficiency	Triglycerides and cholesterol increased, HDL cholesterol decreased	Abdominal pain, lipemia retinalis, eruptive xanthomas
Familial dysbetalipoproteinemia (FD)	Adults: Triglycerides and cholesterol increased, HDL cholesterol normal	Adults: palmar xanthomas, tuberoeruptive xanthomas, claudication, coronary artery disease
Hepatic lipase deficiency	Adults: Triglycerides, cholesterol, and HDL cholesterol increased	Adults: Carotid/femoral bruits, coronary artery disease
Familial hypercholesterolemia (FH) (homozygous)	Total and LDL cholesterol increased, triglycerides normal, HDL cholesterol decreased	Cutaneous and tendon xanthomas, arcus corneae, carotid/femoral bruits, coronary artery disease

DISORDER	ROUTINE LABORATORY	MAJOR CLINICAL SYMPTOMS
Familial hypercholesterolemia (FH) (heterozygous)	See homozygous FH, broad range (levels lower than in homozygous FH)	Adults: Tendon xanthomas, arcus corneae, carotid/femoral bruits, coronary artery disease
Defective apolipoprotein B-100 (FDB)	Triglycerides normal, total and LDL cholesterol increased, HDL cholesterol decreased or normal	Adults: Tendon xanthomas, arcus corneae, carotid/femoral bruits, coronary artery disease
Apolipoprotein A-I deficiency (familial)	Triglycerides increased or normal, cholesterol normal, HDL cholesterol decreased	Adults: Carotid/femoral bruits, coronary artery disease
Apolipoprotein A-I deficiency (structural mutations)	Triglycerides decreased or normal, cholesterol normal, HDL cholesterol decreased	No symptoms (except in single cases: systemic amyloidosis)
Tangier disease	Triglycerides increased, cholesterol normal, HDL cholesterol decreased	Enlarged orange tonsils later in life, hepatosplenomegaly, peripheral neuropathy
LCAT deficiency (complete)	Triglycerides and cholesterol increased, HDL cholesterol decreased, urea and creatinine increased, in some cases (adults) urine protein increased	Adolescents and adults: Arcus corneae, corneal deposits
LCAT deficiency (partial)	Triglycerides decreased or normal, cholesterol normal, HDL cholesterol decreased	Adolescents and adults: Arcus corneae, corneal deposits
Abetalipoproteinemia	Triglycerides, cholesterol, and HDL cholesterol decreased, acanthocytosis	Malabsorption, Adolescents/Adults: Ataxia, retinal degeneration
Hypobetalipoproteinemia (homozygous)	Triglycerides, cholesterol, and HDL cholesterol decreased, acanthocytosis	Malabsorption, Adolescents/Adults: Ataxia, retinal degeneration
Hypobetalipoproteinemia (heterozygous)	Triglycerides and HDL cholesterol normal, cholesterol decreased	No clinical symptoms
Autosomal recessive hypercholesterolemia (AHR)	Cholesterol and LDL cholesterol increased, triglycerides normal	Tendon xanthoma, coronary artery disease

The catabolism of apo B–containing lipoproteins, such as VLDL, IDL, and LDL, occurs by receptor-mediated endocytosis. The receptor that is responsible for this uptake is the well-defined LDLR (3,35). This receptor is a transmembrane protein consisting of 860 amino acids that are encoded by an mRNA of 5.3 kb. The LDLR gene locus is found on chromosome 19 and spans 45 kb, with 18 exons and 17 introns (36). Many of the exons from the LDLR have similarity with exons from other genes, indicating that this gene was assembled by exon shuffling (Figure 22-1).

The LDLR has a typical domain structure that is related to the exon organization of the gene (36–38). The apo B/E ligand–binding domain is encoded by exons 2 to 6 and contains clusters of negatively charged amino acids that bind the lipoprotein particles via basic amino acids in the ligands apo B-100 and apo E (39,40). Exons 7 to 14 encode a 400–amino acid domain that has 33% identity with the human epidermal growth factor precursor (37). This domain is called the epidermal growth factor precursor homology domain and it plays an important role in the process of acid-dependent dissociation of the lipoprotein after the endocytosis (41,42). This domain is also involved in positioning the ligand-binding domain at the cell surface so that the receptor can bind the lipoprotein. The transmembranic domain that anchors the protein in the cellular membrane is encoded by exons 16 and 17. The cytoplasmic tail of the receptor is encoded by exons 17 and 18 (43). As mentioned previously the catabolism of apo B/E–containing lipoproteins is mediated by endocytosis. In this process the lipoprotein particles are endocytosed in coated pits at the cellular surface (44). Once the receptor–ligand complex enters the acidic internal environment of endosomes, the lipoprotein dissociates from the LDLR and is then catabolized in secondary lysosomes. The receptor itself is recycled and moves to the cell surface where it can be used for another round of endocytosis (Figure 22-2) (41,42,45). The amount of receptor synthesis in cells is strongly regulated by the availability of cholesterol. (46,47) When intracellular cholesterol rises, the expression of LDLRs is down regulated. Excess cholesterol also down regulates the expression of ß-hydroxy ß-methylglutaryl CoA reductase, the major rate-limiting enzyme in cholesterol biosynthesis. Both of these regulatory mechanisms contribute to the maintenance of intracellular cholesterol concentrations (48,49).

Reverse Cholesterol Transport

Beyond low LDL cholesterol levels, recent epidemiologic study revealed the important role of decreased high-density lipoprotein (HDL) cholesterol as a risk factor for atherosclerosis. The reverse cholesterol pathway is considered to be vasoprotective and is driven by HDL. HDL is a protein-rich particle and carries cholesterol esters from peripheral tissue back to the liver. HDL contains apo A-I and A-II and at a lower content apo C-I, C-II, C-III, D, A-V, and E.

In the last decade we learned much about the molecular basis of those mechanisms mediating the protective effect of HDL. HDL is the central effector of reverse cholesterol transport (50–52). It is able to transfer cholesterol from peripheral tissues as well as from atheromas of the artery wall back to the liver. The precursors of HDL are produced by the intestine and liver as lipid lipoproteins, named lipid-free apoA-I or lipid-poor pre-β1-HDL-particles. These particles have the ability to take up cholesterol and other lipids from peripheral tissues. This interaction is mediated by a specific receptor, the adenosine triphosphate–binding cassette transporter-A1 (ABC-A1), which interacts with apo A-I (53,54). After transferring those lipids to the HDL precursors, the so-formed

Apo	Chromosome	MW. (KDa)	Concentration (mg/dL)	Fraction	Site of production	Function
A-I	11q23-q24	28.5	120-140	HDL, Chylomicron	Liver, gut	Activation of LCAT, binding to SR-BI and HDL-receptor
A-II	1q21-q23	17	35-50	HDL	Liver	Activation of HL
A-IV	11q23	46	< 5	HDL, Chylomicron	Gut	Activation of LCAT, binding to LDLR
A-V	11q23	38	< 2	VLDL, HDL	Liver	Activation of hepatic triglyceride lipase
B-100	2p24-p23	550	70-90	Chylomicron, VLDL, IDL, LDL	Liver	Structural protein of VLDL, IDL, and LDL, ligand for the LDLR
B-48	2p24-p23	265	< 5	Chylomicron, VLDL	Gut	Structural protein of CM, binding to LRP
C-I	19q13.2	6.5	5-8	HDL, Chylomicron, VLDL	Liver	Activation of LCAT
C-II	19q13.2	8.8	3-7	HDL, Chylomicron, VLDL	Liver	Activation of LPL
C-III	11q23.1-q23.2	8.9	10-12	HDL, Chylomicron, VLDL	Liver	Inhibitor of LPL
D	3q26.2	29	8-10	HDL	Liver	Activation of LCAT
E	19q13.2	34	3-5	VLDL, IDL, HDL, Chylomicron,	Liver	Ligand of the LDL/VLDL-receptor and LRP
H	17q23-qter	50	5-30	VLDL, HDL, Chylomicron	Liver	Participation in different physiologic pathways (lipoprotein metabolism, coagulation, and production of antiphospholipid autoantibodies)
Apo (a)	6	350900	Variable	Lp(a)	Liver	Function unknown

TABLE 22-1A   The Specifications and Functions of Different Apolipoproteins

TABLE 22-1B	Description of Apolipoproteins
Apo A-I	Apo A-I is the structural and most important protein component of HDL particles in plasma (25-27). Apo A-I is crucial for cholesterol efflux from peripheral tissue back to the liver as "reverse cholesterol transport." The molecule is synthesized in the liver as well as in the small intestine. Apo A-I is a cofactor for lecithin cholesterol acyltransferase (LCAT), which is responsible for the formation of most plasma cholesteryl esters. Few mutations of apo A-I are known that cause hypoalphalipidemia, and one mutation (Apo A-1 Iowa) has been identified to cause systemic nonneuropathic amyloidosis (28).
Apo A-II	Apo A-II is also an important protein component of HDL particles. Apo A-II may stabilize the HDL structure by its association with lipids, thereby affecting HDL metabolism (29).
Apo A-IV	Apo A-IV is synthesized primarily in the intestine and is associated with chylomicrons, VLDL, and HDL. Apo A¬IV is an activator of LCAT and may have a role in chylomicron and VLDL metabolism (30–32).
Apo A-V	The apo A-V gene is located on chromosome 11q23. Apo A-V is an important determinant of plasma triglyceride levels, and might be a risk factor for coronary artery disease. Apo A-V is found in very low concentrations on chylomicrons, as well as in VLDL and HDL (33–35).
Apo B (Apo B-100, Apo B-48)	There are two different isoforms of apo B in the plasma, the shorter form apo B-48 and the full form of apo B-100. The apo B gene is localized on chromosome 2p24-p23 (36,37). Apo B is the structural apolipoprotein of chylomicrons (apo B-48), VLDL (apo B-100), IDL (apo B-100), LDL (apo B-100), and Lp(a) (apo B-100 in combination with apo(a)). Apo B-100 functions as a recognition signal for the cellular binding and internalization of LDL particles by the LDLR (38,39). Apo B-48 is synthesized exclusively by the gut, whereas apo B-100 is synthesized by the liver. Interestingly both the intestinal apo B-48 and hepatic apo B-100 are coded by a single gene and by a single mRNA transcript. Both proteins share a common amino terminal sequence. ApoB-100 has 4,563 amino acids. Apo B-48 is homologous to apo B-100 over its entire length for approximately 2,130 amino acid residues with the amino terminal portion of B-100 but contains no sequence from the carboxyl end of B-100. ApoB-48 seems to represent the amino terminal 47% of apo B-100. Apo B-48 may be the product of an intestinal mRNA with an in-frame UAA stop codon resulting from a C-to-U change in the codon CAA encoding Gln (2153) (40) in apo B-100 mRNA. Apo B-48 is created by RNA editing by the apo B mRNA–editing enzyme (catalytic polypeptide 1), which is located on chromosome 12p13.1 (41). Apo B–containing lipoproteins are assembled in the liver (apo B-100: VLDL, IDL, LDL, Lp(a)), and intestine (apoB-48: chylomicron). Microsomal triglyceride transfer protein (MTP) transfers lipids to apo B (42). It is worthwhile to note that apo B as well as MTP genes were found in the heart, suggesting that the heart might be able to secrete apo B–containing lipoproteins (43-45). This mechanism could represent a thus far poorly understood pathway of "reverse fatty acid transport" enabling cardiac myocytes to unload surplus fatty acids not required for their energy supply. Defects of the apo B-100 gene cause familial defective apo B-100 (FDB) (46,47). FDB causes hypercholesterolemia and an increased risk for CAD. Cholesterol levels are elevated in FDB due to the impaired clearance of LDL particles (48,49).
Apo C-I	Apo C-I is synthesized mostly in the liver and comprises up to 10% of the VLDL protein content (2% of HDL) (50-52); however, apo C-I can be produced in macrophages as well. Apo C-I seems to modulate the interaction of apo E with VLDL and IDL particles by inhibiting their binding to the VLDL receptor and LDLR-related protein (59,60).
Apo C-II	Apo C-II is found on triglyceride-rich particles (chylomicrons, VLDL) and HDL. Apo C-II is an activator of several triacylglycerol lipases such as the enzyme lipoprotein lipase (61). Lipoprotein lipase is able to hydrolyze triglycerides and provide free fatty acids for the energy supply of peripheral cells. Mutations of the apo C-II gene are rather rare but defects of apo C-II can cause severe hyperchylomicronemia with extremely elevated triglycerides, eruptive xanthomas, and a high risk of acute pancreatitis (22,62).
Apo C-III	Apo C-III is synthesized in liver and (to a lesser degree) in the intestine. Apo C-III is found on VLDL and comprises up to 50% of the VLDL protein composition (and ~ 2% of the HDL). Apo C-III inhibits several lipases such as the lipoprotein and HL. Thus, apo C-III decreases the uptake of lymphatic chylomicrons by hepatic cells and inhibits the catabolism of triglyceride-rich particles (63,64).
Apo D	Apo D is found within the HDL fraction and is associated in the macromolecular complex with the enzyme LCAT but has otherwise no similarity with other apolipoproteins. In contrast apo D is highly homologous to the plasma retinol-binding protein and other proteins of the α-2-microglobulin superfamily of carrier proteins, also known as lipocalins.
Apo E	Apo E is produced in most organs with significant amounts in liver, brain, spleen, lung, adrenal, ovary, kidney, and muscle. Apo E is crucial for the metabolism of triglyceride-rich particles such as chylomicron remnants and VLDL remnants and constitutes up to 20% of the protein content of VLDL (and ~2% that of the HDL). The triglyceride-rich particles are modified by the interaction with lipases and are finally removed from the circulation by receptor-mediated endocytosis in the liver by binding to the LDLR or in adipose tissue or muscle by binding to the VLDL receptor. Apo E is a main apoprotein of chylomicrons and VLDL. There are three different apo E alleles: apo E-2, which has two cysteine residues, one at position 112 and another at position 158; the most common (in Caucasians 60%–80%) apo E-3 allele has only one cysteine at position 112 and an arginine at position 158; and apo E-4 allele, which has two arginine but no cysteine residues at positions 112 and 158. Apo E-2 has reduced binding affinity compared with apo E-3 (53-54). In contrast apo E-4 has a higher affinity for the LDLR or apo B/E receptor. Apo E binds to specific receptors such as the LDLR (apo B/E) or VLDL receptor on liver cells and peripheral tissues. Apo E is essential for the normal catabolism of triglyceride-rich lipoproteins and defects in apo E cause hypertriglyceridemia such as familial dysbetalipoproteinemia or type III hyperlipoproteinemia (HLP III). Hyperlipoproteinemia type III is typically found in patients homozygous for the apo E 2 alleles. Clinically these patients can have xanthomas or yellowish lipid deposits in the palmar crease. Most persons with the apo E 2/2 genotype are normolipidemic and have even lower LDL levels by which they seem to be protected against CAD. Obviously, certain comorbidities may be necessary for patients with apo E 2/2 to develop hypertriglyceridemia (55,56). The comorbidities include factors such as diabetes mellitus, renal diseases, hypothyroidism, certain drugs, as well as mutations of other apolipoproteins such as the apo A-V S19W mutation (57). Individuals with the common apo E 4 variant are at higher risk for both CAD and the early onset of Alzheimer disease (52,58).

(Continued)

TABLE 22-1B Description of Apolipoproteins *(Continued)*

Apo H (Apo H, beta-2-glycoprotein I)	Apo H may participate in a variety of different physiologic pathways such as lipoprotein metabolism, coagulation, and the production of antiphospholipid autoantibodies. Apo H may also be a cofactor for anionic phospholipid binding by the antiphospholipid autoantibodies in patients with lupus and primary antiphospholipid syndrome. In contrast apo H seems not to be necessary for the reactivity of antiphospholipid autoantibodies associated with infections. Apo H binds to various kinds of negatively charged substances such as heparin, phospholipids, and dextran sulfate. Apo H may prevent activation of the intrinsic blood coagulation cascade by binding to phospholipids on the surface of damaged cells.
Lip(a)	Lip(a) is an atherosclerogenic particle that is composed of LDL in combination with an apo (a) LDL and apo (a) bound by a disulfide bridge. Apo (a) has five domains that are called "kringles" (40,65). Part of the apo (a) (kringle 4) is highly homologous to plasminogen. This similarity to plasminogen enables Lp(a) to interfere with the fibrinolytic system as it competes with plasminogen to bind to the plasminogen receptors. In this way Lp(a) leads to an impaired plasminogen activation and thus to a decrease in plasmin generation at the site of a thrombus, resulting in a decrease in thrombolytic activity. Lp(a) is a fascinating structure combining both the atherogenic properties of LDL and the prothrombotic properties of apo (a) by inhibiting plasminogen activation (66,67). In certain situations of vessel injuries a particle like Lp(a) could be useful, because it delivers cholesterol (by its LDL part) for cell membrane repair and it prevents extended bleeding by inhibiting fibrinolysis (by its apo (a) part). Nevertheless, Lp(a) seems to be a proatherosclerogenic structure (67,68). The therapeutic options to lower this particle are very limited. There might be some minor decrease under treatment with nicotinic acid, whereas most other lipid-lowering drugs failed to lower Lp(a) sufficiently. In special cases LDL apheresis appears to be the only reliable treatment currently available to lower Lp(a) (69,70).

HDL-3-particles are modulated under the influence of different enzymes, such as lecithin: cholesterol acyltransferase (LCAT), cholesteryl ester transfer protein (CETP), and phospholipid transfer protein (PLTP) (Table 22-5).

Enzymatic modulation results in maturation of the particles, forming larger HDL-2-particles. These particles are then removed from the circulation by different pathways. The contained lipids can be transferred selectively to hepatocytes and cells of steroid hormone–producing tissues under mediation of a specific surface receptor called scavenger receptor B1 (SR-B1) (55). The mechanism by which SR-B1 achieves the dissociation of lipids and proteins and the incorporation of cholesteryl esters to the plasma membrane is not completely understood. Unlike other receptors SR-B1 does not act as a holoparticle receptor. It has been suggested that SR-B1 forms a hydrophobic channel through which cholesterol may diffuse to the plasma membrane (51,55). In addition, it seems that some cofactors such as hepatic lipase (HL) are required to be present. It is interesting to note that the lack of SR-B1 in SR-B1 knock out animals leads to a modest increase of HDL; however, these animals develop severe atherosclerotic lesions. In contrast, animal models with an SR-B1 overexpression show extremely low levels of HDL but seem to be protected against HDL (56,57). An alternative pathway involved in the clearance of HDL is an indirect one, through the action of CETP, HL, and endothelial lipase (EL) (58,59). This indirect pathway acts through the transfer of cholesteryl esters from HDL-2 to apo B–containing lipoproteins such as VLDL, IDL, and LDL via the action of CETP (60,61). The lipoproteins are then removed from the circulation through the LDLR pathway. In return, CETP mediates the transfer of triglycerides

TABLE 22-2 The Properties, Electrophoresis Mobility and Apolipoprotein Composition of Lipoprotein Particles

Lipoprotein	Density (g/mL)	Electrophoresis	Seize (nm)	Apoprotein
Chylomicron	< 0.95	No mobility	75-1200	A-I, A-IV, B-48
VLDL	0.95-1.006	pre-β	30-80	B-100, C-I-III, E AV
IDL	1.006-1.019	slow pre-β	25-35	B-100, C-III, E
LDL	1.019-1.063	β	18-25	B-100
HDL2	1.063-1.125	α	9-12	A-I, A-II, A-IV, AV,C-I-III, E
HDL3	1.125-1.210	α	5-9	
Lp(a)	1.040-1.090	slow pre-β	25-30	B-100, apo (a)

TABLE 22-3 Lipid Composition of Different Lipoprotein Particles

Lipoprotein	Cholesterol (%)	Phospholipid (%)	Protein (%)	Triglyceride (%)	Cholesterol ester (%)
Chylomicron	2	7	2	86	3
VLDL	7	18	8	55	12
IDL	9	19	19	23	29
LDL	8	22	22	6	42
HDL2	5	33	40	5	17
HDL3	4	35	55	3	13

TABLE 22-4 The Function of Intracellular Enzymes and Transporter Proteins

Protein	Function
Acyl-CoA-cholesterol-acyltransferase	Intracellular esterification of cholesterol from free cholesterol and oleate (cholesterololeat)
HMG-CoA reductase	Key enzyme of the de novo synthesis of cholesterol (transforms HMG-CoA to mevalonate)
ABC A1	Secretion of cholesterol from cells to newly synthesized pre ß–HDL
Niemann Pick diseaselike protein 1 (NPC1L1)	Transporter for diet-derived cholesterol into the enterocytes of the gut
ABC G 4/G 8	Secretion of cholesterol and plant sterols from enterocytes into the lumen of the gut

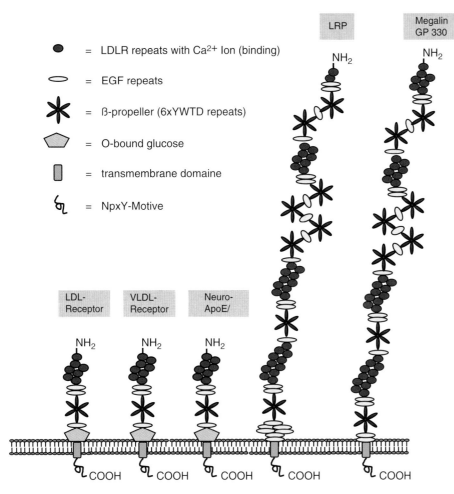

FIGURE 22-1. Structure of the LDLR superfamily.

includes total cholesterol, triglycerides, and HDL cholesterol. Either plasma or serum samples can be used; however, serum cholesterol is somewhat lower (approximately 3%) compared with plasma. After food intake triglycerides have a substantial increase, whereas there is only a small effect on cholesterol concentrations. The major lipid effect occurs 3 to 4 hours after a meal. Once the total cholesterol, triglycerides, and HDL cholesterol values are known, LDL cholesterol can be estimated by the Friedewald formula: LDL cholesterol = Total cholesterol – HDL cholesterol – triglyceride/5. In patients with triglycerides above 400 mg/dL the cholesterol subfractions should not be calculated and instead determined by sequential ultracentrifugation (63). Direct measurement of HDL and LDL cholesterol is available for routine laboratory diagnostics (10,64).

FAMILIAL HYPERCHOLESTEROLEMIA

Primary Causes of Hyperlipidemia

Etiology/Pathophysiology Familial hypercholesterolemia (FH) is a prevalent autosomal codominant inherited disorder of lipid metabolism resulting in the development of premature atherosclerosis. LDLR deficiency is the primary defect of FH. The frequency of heterozygous FH in the general population is approximately 1:300 to 500 persons (65, 66) whereas the number of homozygous FH carriers is 1:1,000,000 persons.

The mechanisms underlying FH are mutations in the gene encoding the LDLR, which cause an abnormal function of the LDLR.

from the apo B–containing lipoproteins to the HDL. Triglycerides in HDL are hydrolyzed by HL. The concerted action of CETP and HL leads to a conversion of the larger HDL-2 to smaller HDL-2 and to the release of lipid-free apo A-I and/or lipid-poor pre-β1-HDL. These particles can again interact with peripheral tissues, and so the circle of reverse cholesterol transport is closed.

Classification of Dyslipidemias

The clinical classification of dyslipidemia was introduced many years ago by Fredrickson (62) and is still very useful. Despite the fact that a variety of different genetic defects can produce identical phenotypes and despite the fact that several disturbances such as low HDL or high Lp(a) are not included in Fredrickson's classification, it is a useful and practical system enabling the appropriate drug or diet treatment (Table 22-6).

Routine Evaluation of Dyslipidemias

Baseline lipid analysis should be performed after a fasting period of 12 to 14 hours before

blood is drawn so that the influence of postprandial hyperlipidemia, chiefly on triglycerides, is minimized. The routine lipid profile

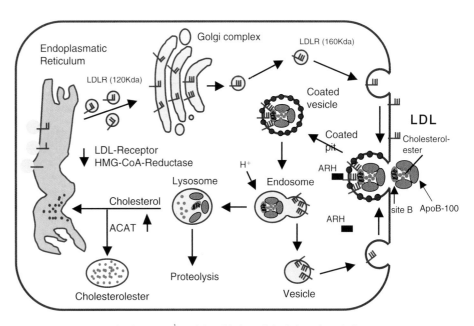

FIGURE 22-2. LDL uptake by the LDLR and regulation of the intracellular cholesterol metabolism.

TABLE 22-5   The Function of Plasmatic and Cell-Associated Enzymes of the Lipoprotein Metabolism

Enzyme	Function
Lipoprotein lipase (endothelial-associated LPL)	Hydrolysis of triglycerides from VLDL and chylomicrons
Hepatic triglyceride lipase (liver-associated HTGL)	Hydrolysis of triglycerides and phospholipids of IDL and HDL
Endothelial lipase	Hydrolysis of phospholipids and triglycerides of HDL
LCAT	Esterification of cholesterol from free cholesterol and lecithin (generates > 80% of all cholesterol esters)
CETP	Transfer of cholesterol ester from HDL to VLDL and LDL in exchange of triglycerides from VLDL
PLTP	Transfer of phospholipids between HDL and VLDL / IDL

LCAT = lecithin:cholesterol acyltransferase; CETP = choleseryl ester transfer protein; PLTP = phospholipid transfer protein.

TABLE 22-6   The Classification of Lipid Disorders by Fredrickson

Phenotype	Chylomicron	VLDL	IDL	LDL	Chol	TG	Plasma
I	↑↑↑			↓	↑	↑↑↑	creamy overlay
II a		↑↑		↑↑	↑↑		clear
II b		↑		↑↑	↑↑	↑	clear
III		↑	↑↑	↓	↑↑	↑↑	clear
IV		↑↑↑		↓		↑↑	clear or opalescent
V	↑↑↑	↑↑↑		↓	↑	↑↑↑	opalescent

Mutations in the LDLR gene affect synthesis, binding, internalization, and recycling of the LDLR protein, thereby leading to elevated plasma LDL cholesterol levels. Mutations in the LDLR gene that produce abnormal receptors can be divided into five different classes (Figure 22-3). Class 1 mutations (null alleles) affect the receptor synthesis. In these individuals no receptor is detectable. Class 2 mutations (transport-defective alleles) are the most common LDLR gene mutations. In these individuals the intracellular transport between endoplasmic reticulum and Golgi apparatus is either completely blocked (Class 2 A) or delayed (Class 2 B), resulting in a relative LDLR deficiency at the cellular surface (5,6,67). Class 3 mutations (binding-defective alleles) produce receptors that are unable to bind LDL normally via the ligands apoB/E. Class 4 mutations (internalization-defective alleles) produce receptors that are able to bind LDL particles normally but fail to internalize the bound LDL. Class 5 mutations (recycling-defective alleles) produce receptors that bind and internalize LDL normally but fail to discharge the LDL in endosomes thereby failing to recycle to the cellular surface.

FH heterozygotes carry one mutant and one normal allele; thus, their cells are able to bind and catabolize LDL at half of the normal rate. Cells of FH homozygotes are nearly or completely unable to take up LDL.

Clinical Presentation Typical clinical signs of FH are deposition of LDL-derived cholesterol in corneal arcus, tendinous xanthomas, and in arteries (atheromas). In heterozygous carriers coronary atherosclerosis develops by the third decade. In homozygous FH carriers planar xanthomas may already be evident at birth in the web between the first two digits. In homozygotes xanthomas and the development of coronary artery disease (CAD) starts in the first 4 years of life, mostly causing death from myocardial infarction or stroke before they reach the age of 15 years (Figure 22-4). Further clinical findings in homozygous familial hypercholesterolemia includes carotid/femoral bruits and aortic flow murmur.

In individuals with homozygous FH, the severity of the clinical phenotypes, especially of coronary atherosclerosis, vary even among individuals who are homozygous for the same mutation. This is also due to the concentration of plasma LDL. The clinical manifestations of heterozygous FH are also modified by environmental factors, especially by diet (e.g., low-fat Mediterranean diet).

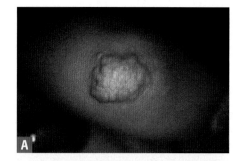

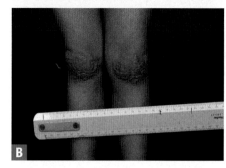

FIGURE 22-4. **A** and **B** Illustrate severe xanthomata of the elbow (**A**) and knees (**B**) of a 4-year-old boy with a homozygous defect of the LDLR (homozygote FH). His total cholesterol was at 1200 mg/dL. This young boy and his brother (identical twins) were discovered at the age of 3 years at the childrens hospital in Marburg and were started on weekly LDL apheresis at the age of 4 years.

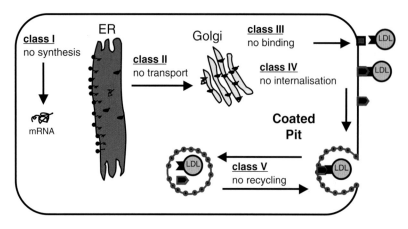

FIGURE 22-3. Classification of the various LDLR mutations. The mutations are divided into five different classes relative to their phenotypic effects on the protein and affect: I) receptor synthesis, II) transport, III) ligand binding, IV) clustering, and V) recycling of the LDLR.

Diagnosis FH is characterized by an elevated plasma LDL cholesterol concentration, as LDL is the major cholesterol-transporting lipoprotein in human plasma. Heterozygous carriers have nearly twofold elevations in plasma cholesterol ranging from 350 to 550 mg/dL. Homozygous FH carriers have severe hypercholesterolemia with cholesterol values ranging from 600 up to more than 1,000 mg/dL (68), with some positive correlation with age. Triglycerides are within normal ranges in both groups of carriers.

Due to the large number of LDLR gene mutations (>400) DNA analysis is only performed in selected populations in which the incidence of a particular mutant allele is high.

Treatment One of the main aims in the treatment of FH individuals is to lower the plasma LDL level to the maximum degree possible. In heterozygous individuals this can be achieved most effectively by administration of lipid-lowering drugs such as statins. These drugs raise the LDLR mRNA expression of the single intact gene, thereby leading to increased LDL uptake (69). In prepubertal children as well as in postpubertal individuals with heterozygous FH a low-saturated-fat (<7%–10% of energy intake) and low-cholesterol diet (<200 mg/d) should be initially started and carefully monitored. Sitosterol/sitostanol margarines may supplement the low-saturated-fat, low-cholesterol diet. Drug therapy (cholestyramine or colestipol in prepubertal patients: initial dose 1 g/d, maximum dose 20 g/d; and statins in postpubertal patients: initial dose 5–20 g/d, maximum dose 40–80 m/d) should be initiated if the LDL cholesterol remains elevated.

Most homozygote FH individuals with two defective alleles are resistant to treatment attempts that are effective in heterozygotes, especially with regard to lipid-lowering drugs, which stimulate LDLRs. Initially the same diet as that for heterozygous FH and a statin with or without ezetimibe should be introduced. Nevertheless, in these individuals LDL can be significantly decreased only by LDL apheresis (weekly or bimonthly) or if necessary even by surgery (liver transplantation) (70). In general, treatment and subsequent reduction of LDL levels in FH is the major route toward reaching a slower progression, stabilization, or even regression in the development of CAD.

FAMILIAL DEFECTIVE APO B

Etiology/Pathophysiology Ligands of the LDLR, namely apo B-100 and apo E can have abnormal binding capacities that are caused by mutations in their genes. Such mutations create

a clinical picture consistent with that seen in FH, but with a different genotypic etiology. As apo B-100 is a protein constituent of LDL and VLDL, binding of apo B-100 to the LDLR is necessary for the removal of these particles from plasma.

The gene locus for apo B is located on chromosome 2. It is 43 kb in length and consists of 29 exons. Exons 26 and 29 are the largest containing 7,572 and 1,906 bases respectively (35,71). One of the most frequent mutations, transmitted as an autosomal codominant has been reported for codon 3500 of apo B-100. It is caused by a single nucleotide exchange (CGG to CAG) in exon 26 of the apo B-100 gene. The mutation leads to a glutamine to arginine exchange and has been termed familial defective apo B-100 (FDB). The frequency of this mutation in the European population is similar to that observed in heterozygous FH and occurs in 1:500 persons (43,44,72). Besides this mutation, two other mutations in this gene region have been identified (73,74), whose overall frequency in the European population is less than the observed frequency for FDB. Most recently a new apoB mutation was identified, the apo B-100 His 3543 Tyr, with a frequency of 0.47% compared with 0.12% for the known Arg 3500 Gln mutation (four times more frequent than "classic" FDB and therefore the most common apo B mutation). (75).

All of these defective apo B100 proteins show decreased binding to the LDLR and a delayed catabolism as demonstrated by *in vivo* kinetic studies. The binding capacities of these variants range from 5% to 27%. The molecular mechanism that leads to this reduced binding has been resolved by Boren et al. (36). In this model apo B wraps around the LDL particle as a belt and specifically interacts via the carboxyl tail of apo B with amino acid arginine 3500, thereby allowing apo B100 to bind via site B (residues 3359–3369), which is the binding site to the LDLR (36). It is thus not an amino acid exchange that directly affects the binding site to the LDLR, instead it affects a modulator element that unmasks site B and by this interacts with the LDLR binding (76).

Presentation and Diagnosis Individuals carrying mutations in apo B-100 show phenotypes as in a mild form of FH. The hyperlipidemia is usually less severe than that observed with LDLR defects because LDL precursors can be endocytosed via the ligand in apo E. In these individuals the LDL plasma levels may be moderately elevated or markedly increased between 250 and 350 mg/dL in the heterozygote form. Approximately 5% of affected patients present with tendon xanthomas. The number of patients with premature

CAD is less than 1%. In the few patients reported so far with a homozygote defect of apo B (77), the cholesterol levels are less severely elevated compared with those in FH and also the clinical course is less severe (78).

Treatment Treatment of FDB carriers with a special diet and lipid-lowering drugs is similar to that used for heterozygous FH patients (cholestyramine or colestipol in prepubertal patients: initial dose 1 g/d, maximum dose 20 g/d; and statins in postpubertal patients: initial dose 5–20 g /d, maximum dose 40–80g/d). The mechanism of the lipid-lowering drugs is via an increased extraction of IDL via the ligand apo E by upregulated LDLRs, thus decreasing the conversion of IDL into LDL particles.

AUTOSOMAL RECESSIVE HYPERCHOLESTEROLEMIA

Etiology/Pathophysiology Autosomal recessive hypercholesterolemia (ARH) was recently described by Garcia et al. in a Lebanese family (79). The primary defect was identified in the year 2001, representing a defective gene encoding for the ARH 1 protein, which is located on chromosome 1. The ARH 1 gene is 45 Kb and has 16 exons encoding for a 20-kDa protein. Studies on lymphocytes of ARH patients demonstrated that ARH 1 is an adaptor protein that is necessary for the LDLR to internalize the LDL–LDLR complex. ARH1 interacts specifically by a phosphotyrosine-binding domain with the NPxY motif of the LDLR and thus enables the internalization of the receptor–ligand complex into the coated pits (80). Interestingly ARH 1 is required only for the function of LDL uptake into lymphocytes and hepatocytes, but not for fibroblasts. It is speculated that fibroblasts have their own compensating adapter protein that is able to replace ARH 1 (81,82,83).

Presentation and Diagnosis So far, ARH deficiency has been identified in only a few cases, all of them originating from the Mediterranean region and each seeming to be rather infrequent. Despite a normal binding and uptake of LDL in cultured fibroblasts affected patients present with typical signs of FH, such as very large tendon xanthomata, increased risk for premature CAD and elevated LDL cholesterol. Plasma LDL levels tend to be lower (350–600 mg/dL) and the onset of symptomatic CAD somewhat later in these probands than in FH homozygotes. There is no cosegregation, either with the LDLR or with the apo B genes.

Treatment Treatment of affected patients should, besides dietary attempts, be initiated with lipid lowering drugs as outlined for heterozygous FH subjects (cholestyramine or colestipol in prepubertal patients: initial dose 1 g/d, maximum dose 20 g/d; and statins in postpubertal patients: initial dose 5–20 g/d, maximum dose 40–80 g/d).

Genetic Defects Leading to Hypertriglyceridemia

Triglyceride levels are modulated by lipoprotein ligands such as apo E and enzymes such as lipoprotein lipase, HL, and CETP. There are numerous inherited as well as acquired disorders of triglyceride metabolism (84). The serum triglyceride concentrations are considered to be normal at less than 150 mg/dL (1.7 mmol/L), borderline high at 150 to 199 mg/dL (1.7–2.2 mmol/L), high at 200 to 499 mg/dL (2.2–5.6 mmol/L), and very high at greater than 500 mg/dL (>5.6 mmol/L). Serum triglyceride values higher than 1,000 mg/dL (11 mmol/L) are rare and occur in fewer than 1:5,000 individuals. In these patients serum is opalescent or even milky due to high levels of chylomicrons (85).

MIXED HYPERTRIGLYCERIDEMIA

Etiology/Pathophysiology Mixed hypertriglyceridemia (type V hyperlipoproteinemia) is characterized by triglyceride levels above the 99th percentile in association with a creamy plasma supernatant and increases in chylomicrons and VLDL. Most patients have a secondary form in which some other dyslipidemia (e.g., familial hypertriglyceridemia due to partial LPL deficiency) is exacerbated by other factors. There is also a primary form of type V hyperlipoproteinemia in which there is no deficiency in LPL or its ligand apo C-II. The underlying defect in this disorder is uncertain but apo E, which is a ligand for the hepatic chylomicron and VLDL remnant receptor, may play a role (13).

Clinical Presentation The clinical manifestations include hepatosplenomegaly and occasional eruptive xanthomas. Patients with marked hypertriglyceridemia (>1000 mg/dL [11.3 mmol/L]) may develop the hyperchylomicronemia syndrome. The clinical manifestations of the more severe form include abdominal pain and/or pancreatitis, dyspnea, eruptive xanthoma, and lipemia retinalis (Figure 22-5) (86).

Diagnosis Mixed hypertriglyceridemia can be diagnosed by confirming the presence of chylomicrons and excess VLDL on agarose gel electrophoresis or ultracentrifugal analysis (87). A rough but simple approach to severe hypertriglyceridemia is the "refrigerator test." In this test the plasma is stored in the refrigerator overnight and examined the next

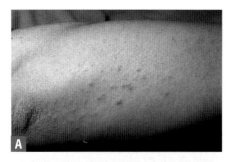

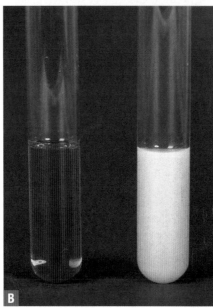

FIGURE 22-5. A Illustrates eruptive xanthomas in a 24-year-old woman with severe HLP V due to a defect of lipoprotein lipase. The patient was admitted to our hospital with acute pancreatitis during pregnancy due to triglyceride levels of up to 11,500 mg/dL. We treated this life-threatening disease by eliminating the triglycerides, applying the extracorporal lipid elimination with LDL apheresis once (within 30 min after treatment started the triglycerides dropped to 6,000 mg/dL and the patient was almost pain free). **B** Illustrates the serum of this patient with HLP V in comparison to normal plasma.

day. Chylomicrons in excess form a creamy supernatant. The presence of a turbid infranatant is caused by the VLDL-rich particles, a typical finding in patients with type V hyperlipidemia. Type V hyperlipidemia is different from type I hyperlipidemia, as in type I only chylomicrons are elevated but the infranatant is clear. Because the delipidation process is almost identical for chylomicrons and VLDL, a true type I pattern is extremely rare, and usually patients will present with a type V hyperlipidemia due to a defect of either LPL activity or apo C-II (the ligand for lipoprotein lipase on chylomicrons and VLDL) (88).

Treatment Patients with mixed hypertriglyceridemia are treated with fibric acid derivatives and nicotinic acid as described later in the Chapter (Therapy of Hyperlipidemias).

FAMILIAL DYSBETALIPOPROTEINEMIA

Etiology/Pathophysiology Apo E is a constituent of several plasma lipoproteins including chylomicrons, VLDL, IDL, and a subclass of HDL (HDL-E). The major physiologic role of apo E is its interaction with lipoprotein receptors such as LDLR and LDLR-related protein. In this process apo E mediates the catabolism of chylomicron remnants and VLDL remnants that underwent lipolytic processing by lipoprotein lipases. The gene for apo E is 3.7 Kb in length and is located on chromosome 19. The mature apo E protein consists of 299 amino acids and is a polymorphic protein (13). This results from the existence of three alleles E2, E3, and E4 at a single gene locus. The normal apo E form apo E3 differs from the mutated apo E2 allele in a cysteine for arginine substitution at position 158. The apo E2 mutation is found in most patients with recessive type III hyperlipoproteinemia (89).

The molecular basis for type III hyperlipoproteinemia lies in defective binding of apo E to the LDLR and subsequent accumulation of β-VLDL and chylomicron remnants, which are taken up afterward by macrophages in peripheral tissues and are converted to foam cells, the progenitors of cholesterol—laden cells in the atherosclerotic plaque. Mapping studies of apo E have localized the LDLR binding site of apo E between amino acids 136 and 150, a region that is rich in basic amino acids and similar to the corresponding binding region in apo B. Naturally occurring mutations at different residues in this region of apo E also cause type III hyperlipoproteinemia in a dominant inherited way. It is interesting that residue 158, which causes type III hyperlipoproteinemia in apo E2 patients is not directly involved in receptor binding. Instead this mutation structurally alters the conformation of region 136 to 150 and prevents binding to the LDLR (90).

Diagnosis This disease is characterized by elevated cholesterol and triglyceride levels (91). The VLDL cholesterol/triglyceride ratio is greater than 0.3 (the normal ratio is 0.2). Apo E isoform analysis is performed by isoelectric focusing or apo E genotyping can be performed by restriction fragment length polymorphism of the apo E gene (92,93).

Clinical Presentation Peripheral clinical signs of this disease are tuberoeruptive xanthomas at the elbows and xanthomas of the palmar creases (xanthomata palmare striatum). In one third of affected patients premature atherosclerosis occurs, but this atherosclerosis is unlike that in FH, which is predominantly located in peripheral vessels.

Treatment Most patients with type III hyperlipoproteinemia are treated with dietary intervention; however, in some cases drug therapy is necessary and requires the use of statins or nicotinic acid or fibric acid derivatives.

FAMILIAL HYPERTRIGLYCERIDEMIA

Etiology/Pathophysiology Familial hypertriglyceridemia (type IV hyperlipoproteinemia) is an autosomal dominant disorder associated with moderate elevations in the serum triglyceride concentration (200–500 mg/dL [2.3–5.6 mmol/L]). The diagnosis can only be made once the lipid levels of direct relatives are known. Patients with familial hypertriglyceridemia are frequently heterozygous for inactivating mutations of the lipoprotein lipase gene (94). As in most patients with hypertriglyceridemia, in familial hypertriglyceridemia the serum HDL cholesterol levels are low. The most common LPL mutations raise serum triglycerides by 20% to 80%. The effect on CAD progression of the Asp 9 Asn mutation (aspartic acid to asparagine at position 9) within the LPL gene has been studied by the REGRESS study (95).

Diagnosis Heterozygosity for the Asp 9 Asn mutation causes a defect of the LPL activity with a mild elevation of serum triglycerides and low HDL cholesterol. Carriers of Asp 9 Asn mutation more often had a history of CAD, lower HDL cholesterol, and a slightly higher triglyceride and LDL cholesterol levels. CAD progressed in carriers more rapidly than in noncarriers, but lipid-lowering therapy with pravastatin was able to delay the CAD progress in carriers (96).

Treatment The treatment is similar to that of other forms of hypertriglyceridemia with the potential of adding pravastatin.

GENETIC CAUSES LEADING TO HYPOLIPIDEMIA

Familial Hypobetalipoproteinemia and Abetalipoproteinemia

Etiology/Pathophysiology Abetalipoproteinemia (or Bassen–Kornzweig syndrome) is a rare, autosomal recessive disease. The primary defect is a mutation of the microsomal triglyceride transfer protein gene. The assembling and secretion of apo B–containing lipoproteins is severely disturbed in liver and intestinal cells and results in fat absorption and impaired transport (97,98).

Clinical Presentation Due to severely reduced levels of apo B lipoproteins, which are essential in the transport of fat-soluble vitamins and thus critical for the normal functioning of the nervous system and retina, patients with abetalipoproteinemia suffer from peripheral neuropathy, ataxia and progressive retinal degeneration. Some of these clinical signs and symptoms may not be present in childhood.

Diagnosis Due to the lack of apo B–containing lipoproteins the concentration of VLDL (pre-β lipoprotein) is extremely low and LDL cholesterol (β lipoprotein) is virtually absent.

Treatment Early supplementation with vitamin E and other fat-soluble vitamins may improve the clinical course of this rare disease.

FAMILIAL HYPOALPHALIPOPROTEINEMIA AND HDL CHOLESTEROL DEFICIENCY

Etiology/Pathophysiology Low HDL levels are defined as HDL cholesterol below 40 mg/dL (< 1.03 mmol/L) in males or below 50 mg/dL (< 1.29 mmol/L) in females. Very low HDL cholesterol is defined as HDL below 20 mg/dL (< 0.52 mmol/L) and occurs in 1:200 adult men or 1:400 adult women. Complete HDL deficiency, however, is very rare and occurs in 1:20,000 persons. Complete HDL deficiency is mostly due to a defect of one of these three genes: ABC A1, Apo A-I, or LCAT. This entity was first described as Tangiers disease by Fredrickson in a family from Tangier Island. The primary defect for Tangier disease is a defect of ABC A1, which is a transporter protein of the ABC group (53,99). These transporter proteins are involved in the transport of various substances across the cell membranes, including ions, peptides, vitamins, and hormones. The ABC A1 transporter is crucial for the initial phase of reverse cholesterol transport from extrahepatic cells including vascular wall macrophages. So far more than 50 mutations of ABC A1 have been identified. ABC A1 gene variants cause moderately low HDL cholesterol in the heterozygous state as familial hypoalphalipoproteinemia.

The defect of apo A-I is another rare cause for hypoalphalipoproteinemia (100). Apo A-I is an important ligand for HDL to cellular receptors such as the SR-BI and ABC A1.

LCAT is associated with HDL. LCAT esterifies cholesterol in plasma, a process for which apo A-I is an important cofactor.

Clinical Presentation Homozygous ABC A1 mutations cause HDL cholesterol deficiency in Tangier disease with cholesterol ester deposition in reticuloendothelial organs.

Diagnosis Patients with Tangier disease have large orange tonsils (due to the cholesterol ester deposition), hepatosplenomegaly, no measurable HDL cholesterol, extremely low apoA-I, low LDL cholesterol, and elevated triglycerides.

Apo A-I deficiency due to defects of the apo A-I gene has been associated with premature CAD.

Complete LCAT deficiency results in free cholesterol and phosphatidylcholine deposition in membranes, leading to corneal opacification, anemia, and renal failure. The corneal opacification caused this rare disease to be named "fish eye disease" (101).

Treatment Little is known about the efficacy of triglyceride lowering therapy in these patients.

SECONDARY CAUSES FOR DYSLIPIDEMIA

Etiology/Pathophysiology There are numerous factors by which patients might develop secondary dyslipidemia. Elevated total and LDL cholesterol and low HDL cholesterol may be secondary to a diet rich in saturated fatty acids, hypothyroidism, chronic liver disease, chronic renal failure, cholestasis, Cushing syndrome, anorexia nervosa, acute intermittent porphyria, or the use of certain drugs such as oral contraceptives.

Hypertriglyceridemia can be caused by a diet rich in carbohydrates, alcohol consumption, obesity and metabolic syndrome, pregnancy, diabetes mellitus, hypothyroidism, pancreatitis, nephrotic syndrome, bulimia, Cushing syndrome, hypopituitarism, glycogen storage disease, lipodystrophy syndrome, acute intermittent porphyria, systemic lupus erythematosus, or the use of certain drugs such as beta-blockers, diuretics, estrogens (contraceptive or replacement) or glucocorticoids.

Human immunodeficiency virus–infected children treated with highly active antiretroviral therapy that includes protease inhibitors may develop lipoprotein abnormalities, most commonly increased total and LDL cholesterol levels.

Lipid abnormalities, particularly high triglycerides and low HDL cholesterol, are strongly associated with insulin resistance (79). This may result from an increased production of VLDL (102). Insulin administration in healthy adults results in a rapid decline in plasma free fatty acid levels and VLDL triglyceride production (81). Insulin-resistant individuals with type 2 diabetes mellitus are resistant to this inhibitory effect and have increased rates of VLDL production (80). Studies in rats have shown that hyperinsulinemia stimulates the synthesis of fatty acids by increasing the transcription of genes for lipogenic enzymes in the liver (82). In addition, the contribution of free fatty acids from visceral adipose tissue could increase their flux to the liver, providing substrate for VLDL production. The low HDL cholesterol levels found in patients with insulin resistance may be due to an accelerated catabolic rate of HDL cholesterol, as demonstrated in individuals with type 2 diabetes (83). Lipid abnormalities are frequently found also in overweight and obese children. Data from the Bogalusa Heart Study have shown that overweight children have significantly higher levels of total cholesterol, LDL cholesterol, triglycerides, and lower HDL cholesterol when compared with normal weight children (103).

Diagnosis The medical history, family history, and physical examination are of critical importance in these patients. Assessment of body habitus, fasting blood glucose, thyroid function, and renal function constitute a reasonable first-line battery of tests to evaluate the common causes of secondary dyslipidemia and target specific therapies.

Treatment The treatment of secondary dyslipidemia is based on LDL cholesterol and triglyceride levels as further detailed below.

THERAPY OF HYPERLIPIDEMIAS

Existing pediatric guidelines are based on a consensus report originally published in 1992 from the National Cholesterol Education Program (NCEP) Expert Panel on Blood Cholesterol Levels in Children and Adolescents (104).

Dietary Therapy

Dietary recommendations and/or alterations are basic and fundamental for the treatment of all patients with hyperlipidemia. To lower elevated cholesterol levels in children and adolescents, the panel recommended that all healthy children older than 2 years of age adopt a fat- and cholesterol-restricted diet that contains the appropriate number of calories to support growth and development and to maintain a "desirable" body weight. Consumption of a wide variety of foods was recommended to achieve nutrient needs and with a goal to achieve an average daily intake of no more than 10% of total calories from saturated fat, no more than 30% from total fat, and intake of no more than 300 mg of dietary cholesterol per day. For those children whose LDL cholesterol level remains above 130 mg/dL while compliant with the fat- and cholesterol-restricted diet recommended for the general population, a more restrictive diet is recommended. The increased restriction further limits saturated fat intake to less than 7% of total caloric intake and cholesterol intake to less than 200 mg/day. In some severe forms of familial hypercholesterolemia and in some cases of secondary hyperlipidemias, the preventive effect of diet might not be sufficient and additional drug treatment will be necessary to support the dietary intervention.

Drug Therapy

If life style changes and dietary intervention are not able to achieve the cholesterol target values, drug therapy might be indicated. This section will summarize the pharmaceutical options to treat elevated lipids. These include resins (such as bile acid–binding substrates), specific cholesterol uptake inhibitors (ezetimibe), fibrates, nicotinic acid and 3-hydroxy-3-methylglutaryl (HMG)–CoA reductase inhibitors.

Bile acid sequestrants (resins)

Cholestyramine and colestipol are able to bind bile acids in the intestine. The drugs are not absorbed and function in the intestine only. Usually there is no interference with fat absorption and no malabsorption of dietary fat with this treatment. The binding of bile acids by the bile acid sequestrants requires an increase in bile production to keep the normal enterohepatic function. Usually only small amounts of cholesterol are oxidized to bile acids by the key-enzyme 7-α-hydroxylase. The loss of bile acids increases the transfer of cholesterol to bile acids within the liver. Subsequently the intrahepatic cholesterol biosynthesis as well as the hepatic LDLR expression increases. The increase of the LDLR leads to an increase in LDL cholesterol uptake within the liver and lowers plasma cholesterol levels. The increase of the intrahepatic cholesterol biosynthesis is an undesired side effect of this therapy and can be eliminated by the combination with HMG-CoA reductase inhibitors (statins). Bile acid sequestrants are the drugs with which we have the longest experience and they produce the lowest systemic effects. Nevertheless, given the high prevalence of gastrointestinal complaints, poor palatability, low compliance, and limited effectiveness, it is unlikely that the bile acid–binding resins will be sufficient to achieve target LDL cholesterol levels in children who meet the criteria for lipid-lowering drug therapy. The starting dose of cholestyramine and colestipol is 1 mg/day and the maximum dose is 20 g/day (see Table 22-7 for more information).

Ezetimibe

Ezetimibe is a selective cholesterol absorption inhibitor and has been available since the year 2002. Ezetimibe acts primarily within the intestine and inhibits the intestinal uptake of cholesterol from both sources: nutritional and enterohepatic. Recently a specific cholesterol receptor was identified, the so-called Niemann-Pick C-1 like protein (NPC1L1) (24). This protein is concentrated in the intestine and seems to be the primary target of ezetimibe. Ezetimibe is almost completely glycosylated and is eliminated by the gut. There is no interaction with the cytochrome P450 system and the half-life time of ezetimibe and its functional metabolites is 22 hours. A single dose of 10 mg/day is sufficient. The cholesterol-lowering effect is at approximately 10% to 15% of initial levels when used as a monotherapeutic drug. As with the sequestrant resins, ezetimibe treatment increases intrahepatic cholesterol biosynthesis, which is why ezetimibe should be used in combination with HMG-CoA reductase inhibitors (105). In this way, the lowest dose of any available statin in combination with ezetimibe achieves the same LDL reduction as the maximal available statin dose used as single-drug therapy. Furthermore ezetimibe not only lowers serum cholesterol but also plant sterols and can be used for the treatment of patients with phytosterolemia (106). Ezetimibe is very well tolerated with only few side effects, such as mild increase of liver enzymes or creatinine kinase. Ezetimibe is approved for the use in children with FH who are older than 10 years of age. The ezetimibe dose is 10 mg/day (see Table 22-7 for more information).

Fibric acid derivates (Fibrates)

Clofibrate and its derivates bezafibrate, fenofibrate, and gemfibrozil are lipid-lowering drugs with the most effective triglyceride-lowering and HDL cholesterol–increasing properties (107). Because in a recent World Health Organization trial clofibrate was associated with a high mortality rate and an increase in some rare types of cancers, fibrates are seldom used in the United States. There are only very few studies demonstrating beneficial effects of fibrates in patients with low HDL cholesterol or diabetes mellitus. Fibrates interact with specific transcriptional factors, the so-called peroxisomal proliferators activated receptor α (PPAR α), which is instrumental in regulation of a broad array of key genes. The interaction with PPAR-α increases the lipoprotein lipase activity and the production of several factors such as apo A-I, apo A-II, ABC 1, and SR-B1 (108,109). Furthermore there is a (minor) inhibition of the HMG-CoA reductase. All together there is

TABLE 22-7   Lipid Lowering Drugs in Children

Drug Class	DRUG EFFECT			SUGGESTED DRUG DOSE		
	LDL	HDL	Triglycerides	Initial	Maximum	Side effects
Bile acid–binding resins	↓	0	↑			
Cholestyramine				1 g/d	20 g/d	Gastrointestinal
Colestipol				1 g/d	20 g/d	May increase triglycerides
Colesevelam				1.5 g/d	3.75 g/d	May interfere with absorption of fat-soluble vitamins/ some medications
Nicotinic acid	↓	↑	↓			
Niacin				500 mg/d	2-6 g/d	Flushing
						Hepatic failure
						Glucose intolerance
						Myopathy
						Hyperuricemia
						Gastrointestinal
Fibric acid derivatives*	0	↑	↓↓			
Gemfibrozil				600 mg/d	1,200 mg/d	Gastrointestinal
Fenofibrate				54-160 mg/d	160 mg/d	Cholelithiasis
						Potentiate warfarin
						Anemia
HMG-CoA reductase inhibitors+	↓↓	↑	↓			
Simvastatin				5-20 mg/d	4-80 mg/d	Elevated liver enzymes
Pravastatin						Muscle soreness
Lovastatin						Rhabdomyolysis
Fluvastatin						
Atorvastatin						
Cholesterol absorption inhibitors#	↓	0	0			
Ezetimibe				10 mg/d		Elevated liver enzymes

*-In combination with statins or renal insufficiency can lead to myopathy.
+-Contraindicated for liver disease and pregnancy.
#-Contraindicated for fibrates and liver disease.

a minor cholesterol-lowering effect but a more pronounced triglyceride lowering together with a mild increase of HDL. Fibrates are usually well tolerated and side effects, such as nausea, abdominal pain, elevated liver enzymes, increase of creatinine kinase, myositis, or cholelithiasis, are rare. Most troublesome is the interaction of some fibrates with other drugs and the cytochrome P450 3A4 system. The competitive inhibition of the cytochrome P450 system especially by gemfibrozil has a major impact on the catabolism of other lipid-lowering drugs such as statins. The interaction of gemfibrozil with cerivastatin, an HMG-CoA reductase inhibitor, resulted in severe forms of myositis and ended disastrously for several patients. Therefore cerivastatin was withdrawn from the market. Fenofibrate is preferred once the coadministration of statins with fibrates is required. Due to the potential and serious side effects on CYP 3A4, independent statins such as pravastatin or fluvastatin are preferred and

close patient monitoring is necessary. Since the introduction of statins with their overwhelming beneficial effects demonstrated in almost all statin trials, fibrates have been used rather rarely. In a randomized, crossover trial of bezafibrate in children with FH (110) the medication was well tolerated with no impact on growth or development. This class of drugs should be used preferentially for children with severe elevations in triglyceride levels who are at risk for pancreatitis. Gemfibrozil starting dose is 600 mg/day and the maximum dose is 1200 mg/day. Fenofibrate starting dose is 54 to 160 mg/day and the maximum dose is 160 mg/day (see Table 22-7 for more information).

Nicotinic acid and nicotinic acid derivates

Nicotinic acid has been used as a lipid-lowering agent mostly in the United States before statins became available. Nicotinic acid

lowers triglycerides more efficiently than cholesterol. Despite the fact that nicotinic acid was used as a lipid-lowering drug for more than 40 years it was only most recently that a G-protein–related receptor for nicotinic acid was identified. The nicotinic acid receptor had been known before as a "protein upregulated in macrophages by interferon-γ" receptor as well as an HM74 protein in macrophages. Nicotinic acid prevents the liberation of free fatty acids from the adipose tissue as well as their uptake in the liver. Thus, the production of triglycerides and VLDL (and subsequently LDL) is decreased by the action of nicotinic acids (111). Furthermore nicotinic acids are able to increase HDL cholesterol by up to 30%. The HDL increase is found at lower nicotinic acid doses (1 g/d), whereas most of the LDL-lowering effect is seen at higher doses of nicotinic acids (3 g/d) only (112). With high doses of nicotinic acids there are reports of Lp(a)-lowering effects as well. The most disturbing side effects of nicotinic acids are prostaglandin mediated and include episodes of flush, itching, and nausea. Recently a new formula was developed (Niaspan) that permits a slow release of nicotinic acid with significantly lower rates of side effects. Liver and muscle enzymes should be monitored, especially when nicotinic acid is given in combination with other lipid-lowering drugs such as statins. Given the poor tolerance and the potential for very serious adverse effects, this class of drugs is not routinely recommended for use in the pediatric age groups. Niacin starting dose is 500 mg/day and the maximum dose is 2 to 6 g/day (see Table 22-7 for more information).

HMG CoA reductase inhibitor (statin, CSE-inhibitor)

HMG-CoA reductase inhibitors are the most efficient and best-characterized cholesterol-lowering drugs currently available. Numerous studies (4S, CARE, LIPID, HPS, WOSCOP, AFCAPS/TexCAPS, PROVE-IT, TNT) with HMG-CoA reductase inhibitors (such as pravastatin, simvastatin, lovastatin, and atorvastatin) have demonstrated beneficial effects on mortality and morbidity rates in primary and secondary CAD prevention (111,112,113,114). The inhibition of the key enzyme of endogenous cholesterol synthesis, the HMG-CoA reductase, is highly efficient in lowering LDL cholesterol. The first HMG-CoA reductase inhibitor was Compactin, which was discovered in 1976. After treatment with an HMG-CoA reductase inhibitor we find an inhibition of intrahepatic cholesterol synthesis and subsequently an increase of hepatic LDLR. This results in an increase in LDL uptake in the liver, which ends up with a LDL cholesterol–lowering effect (115,116). The potential side effects of HMG-CoA reductase inhibitors are elevated liver and muscle enzymes and gastrointestinal problems. Myositis and myopathy are the most serious side effects of statins, which need to be observed and require immediate interruption of statin treatment. Troublesome is the combination of HMG-CoA reductase inhibitors with drugs such as fibrates, which interfere with the catabolism by the cytochrome P450 system. HMG-CoA reductase inhibitors are considered to be safe and therefore in England low-dose statins can be bought as over the counter drugs without prescriptions. The combination with fibrates, cyclosporine A, calcium channel blockers, and other drugs might be troublesome and requires careful monitoring. For these combinations, statins such as pravastatin or fluvastatin seem to have a lower potential for side effects because these statins are not catabolized by the P450 system. There has been increasing experience with the statins in the context of clinical trials in children. A number of trials have shown the efficacy as well as short- and intermediate-term safety of these drugs in children (117–123). Adverse effects do not appear to be increased over those noted in clinical studies in adults; however, long–term safety and compliance remain concerns, as well as demonstration of an impact on clinical disease. Guidelines for initiation, titration, and monitoring of statin therapy in children are given by manufacturers of HGM-CoA reductase inhibitors, with starting doses of 5 to 20 mg/day and maximum doses of 40 to 80 mg/day (see Table 22-7 for more information).

Special considerations in children

In children of high-risk families for CAD cholesterol levels should be determined in early childhood for prompt intervention. In children with hypercholesterolemia, diet treatment should have highest priority, whereas lipid-lowering drugs should only be used if no other options are available. LDL cholesterol levels higher than 190 mg/dL should also be treated in children without a strong family history of CAD, whereas in children with CAD in the core family, LDL cholesterol should be lower than 160 mg/dL. Because the widest experience is presently available with use of bile acid–binding agents these drugs are currently recommended as first-line lipid-lowering drugs in children. Because these drugs have several intestinal side effects, especially in children, statins such as pravastatin or cholesterol absorption inhibitors such as ezetimibe might be more practical.

LDL cholesterol–lowering drug therapy is only recommended for those children 10 years of age and older in whom LDL cholesterol remains extremely elevated after an adequate 6 to 12 month trial of diet therapy. Drug therapy should be considered for children with LDL cholesterol levels at or above 190 mg/dL, or whose levels are at or above 160 mg/dL together with either the presence of two or more other cardiovascular disease risk factors or a positive family history of premature cardiovascular disease (104). Pravastatin has been approved in children with FH who are older than 8 years of age and ezetimibe in children who are older than 10 years. In contrast fibrates are not recommended for children (65–70,124).

LDL apheresis

LDL apheresis is a procedure by which specifically LDL cholesterol, apoB, and Lp(a) are separated from the blood. Several systems of LDL apheresis are available, such as immunoadsorption columns, dextran sulfate cellulose columns, and the heparin precipitation system (77). The U.S. Food and Drug Administration in 1996 approved the use of these systems in patients who despite diet and maximum tolerated drug therapy have an LDL cholesterol level greater than 300 mg/dL (>7.8 mmol/L) if coronary heart disease is absent or an LDL cholesterol level greater than 200 mg/dL (>5.2 mmol/L) once coronary heart disease is present. These LDL cholesterol levels are clearly above those levels that newer cholesterol interventional trials would recommend and need a careful reevaluation. Because LDL apheresis is a rather complex procedure it is usually performed only in specialized centers. The expected lipid-lowering effects of a single treatment must be more than 50% of the starting level of LDL cholesterol and Lp(a). There should be no significant reduction in HDL cholesterol. Some systems, especially the heparin precipitation system (59), are able to lower factors such as fibrinogen as well. Side effects are rare and include most commonly hypotension. Hypotension can be severe in patients taking an angiotensin-converting enzyme inhibitor, especially in treatment with high flux membrane plasma filters and the dextran sulphate system. LDL apheresis is able to stabilize coronary atherosclerosis and might reduce the risk for restenosis after percutaneous transluminal carotid angioplasty and the risk for graft vessel disease after heart transplantation (78). LDL apheresis should only be performed in patients after all medical options to lower LDL cholesterol, such as a high-dose atorvastatin (80 mg/d) in combination with the cholesterol absorption inhibitor ezetimibe (10 mg/d), have been exhausted.

SUMMARY

The treatment of hyperlipidemia has changed dramatically within the past 10 years. The discovery of HMG-CoA reductase inhibitors has revolutionized lipid-lowering therapy. Since the publication of the 4S study in 1994 there is convincing evidence that HMG-CoA reductase inhibitors can prevent atherosclerosis and myocardial infarction in humans (71,72). Subsequently numerous lipid-lowering interventional studies, mostly using pravastatin or simvastatin, demonstrated the need to lower LDL cholesterol to prevent coronary events (112,113,73). The recommended LDL cholesterol levels dropped dramatically in recent years. The generally accepted cholesterol level in the 1960s was approximately 300 mg/dL, in the 1980s it was 250 mg/dL, and at the end of the 1990s it was below 190 mg/dL. At present the recommended LDL level in patients with CAD (or CAD equivalent such as diabetes mellitus) is well below 100 mg/dL and in patients with the highest risk LDL cholesterol should be lower than 70 mg/dL. There is no question that for LDL cholesterol "the lower the better" is the appropriate approach (74). At the same time drug treatment has improved dramatically by using potent HMG-CoA reductase inhibitors and the introduction of specific cholesterol absorption inhibitors such as ezetimibe (75). With these agents, it is possible to lower LDL cholesterol by more than 60%. In patients with hypertriglyceridemia, fibrates, nicotinic acid, omega 3 fatty acids, and medium chain fatty acids can be used in addition to appropriate diet recommendations. Secondary CAD prevention is rather simple, and usually most of the patients need to be treated with a lipid-lowering drug, preferably HMG-CoA reductase inhibitors (126).

Primary prevention is by far the more complex issue. For this, in recent years risk calculators such as the PROCAM Risk Score calculator (www.chd-taskforce.com) were developed and can be used easily (76). This implies a shift from the simple analysis of a laboratory level such as cholesterol to the total risk score of an individual, which goes far beyond the sole measurement of lipid levels. There is no question that a better understanding of the genetic and metabolic mechanisms leading to hyperlipidemia will improve our therapeutic options within the next several years. Furthermore new lipid-lowering drugs and gene therapy will enable us to fight one of the most important cardiovascular risk factors more efficiently. Despite all the fascinating discoveries especially in the field of CAD prevention and clinical lipid metabolism, we should not forget that our current knowledge of a "healthy lifestyle" (stop smoking, eat healthfully, engage in physical activities, and keep blood pressure, body weight, and LDL cholesterol low) is good enough that we could easily reduce CAD morbidity and mortality by more than 50%. Changes in lifestyle are difficult to implement and remain a major barrier to effective prevention of lipid-related cardiovascular disease.

REFERENCES

1. Goldstein JL, Brown MS. The low-density lipoprotein pathway and its relation to atherosclerosis. *Annu Rev Biochem.* 1977;46:897–930.
2. Brown MS, Goldstein JL. Familial hypercholesterolemia: a genetic defect in the low-density lipoprotein receptor. *N Engl J Med.* 1976;294:1386–1390.
3. Brown MS, Herz J, Goldstein JL. LDL-receptor structure. Calcium cages, acid baths and recycling receptors. *Nature.* 1997;388:629–630.
4. Brown MS, Goldstein JL. 1985 Nobel laureates in medicine. *J Invest Med.* 1996; 44:14–23.
5. Hobbs HH, Russell DW, Brown MS, et al. The LDL receptor locus in familial hypercholesterolemia: mutational analysis of a membrane protein. *Annu Rev Genet.* 1990;24:133–170.
6. Hobbs HH, Brown MS, Goldstein JL. Molecular genetics of the LDL receptor gene in familial hypercholesterolemia. *Hum Mutat.* 1992;1:445–466.
7. Berger K, Schulte H, Stogbauer F, et al. Incidence and risk factors for stroke in an occupational cohort: the PROCAM Study. Prospective Cardiovascular Muenster Study. *Stroke.* 1998;29:1562–1566.
8. Gordon T, Kannel WB, Castelli WP, et al. Lipoproteins, cardiovascular disease, and death. The Framingham study. *Arch Intern Med.* 1981;141:1128–1131.
9. Kannel WB, Castelli WP, Gordon T. Cholesterol in the prediction of atherosclerotic disease. New perspectives based on the Framingham study. *Ann Intern Med.* 1979;90:85–91.
10. Friedewald WT, Levy RI, Fredrickson DS. Estimation of the concentration of low density lipoprotein cholesterol without use of the preparative ultracentrifuge. *Clin Chem.* 1972;18:499–502.
11. Alaupovic P. Apolipoproteins and lipoproteins. *Atherosclerosis.* 1971;13:141–146.
12. Alaupovic P, Lee DM, McConathy WJ. Studies on the composition and structure of plasma lipoproteins. Distribution of lipoprotein families in major density classes of normal human plasma lipoproteins. *Biochim Biophys Acta.* 1972;260:689–707.
13. Mahley RW, Rall SC, Jr. Apolipoprotein E: far more than a lipid transport protein. *Annu Rev Genomics Hum Genet.* 2000;1: 507–537.
14. Innerarity TL, Mahley RW, Weisgraber KH, et al. Familial defective apolipoprotein B-100: a mutation of apolipoprotein B that causes hypercholesterolemia. *J Lipid Res.* 1990;31:1337–1349.
15. Schaefer EJ, Zech LA, Jenkins LL, et al. Human apolipoprotein A-I and A-II metabolism. *J Lipid Res.* 1982;23:850–862.
16. Goldstein JL, Brown MS. Molecular medicine. The cholesterol quartet. *Science.* 2001;292:1310–1312.
17. Steinberg D. Underlying mechanisms in atherosclerosis. *J Pathol.* 1981;133:75–87.
18. Steinberg D. Lipoproteins and the pathogenesis of atherosclerosis. *Circulation.* 1987;76:508–514.
19. Schaefer JR, Klumpp S, Maisch B, et al. Why does atherosclerosis occur where it occurs? *Atherosclerosis.* 2005;180:417–418.
20. Hufnagel B, Dworak M, Soufi M, et al. Unsaturated fatty acids isolated from human lipoproteins activate protein phosphatase type 2Cbeta and induce apoptosis in endothelial cells. *Atherosclerosis.* 2005;180:245–254.
21. Mar R, Pajukanta P, Allayee H, et al. Association of the APOLIPOPROTEIN A1/C3/A4/A5 gene cluster with triglyceride levels and LDL particle size in familial combined hyperlipidemia. *Circ Res.* 2004;94:993–999.
22. Farese RV, Jr., Linton MF, Young SG. Apolipoprotein B gene mutations affecting cholesterol levels. *J Intern Med.* 1992;231:643–652.
23. Altmann SW, Davis HR Jr, Zhu LJ, et al. Niemann-Pick C1 Like 1 protein is critical for intestinal cholesterol absorption. *Science.* 2004;303:1201–1204.
24. Davis HR Jr, Zhu LJ, Hoos LM, et al. Niemann-Pick C1 Like 1 (NPC1L1) is the intestinal phytosterol and cholesterol transporter and a key modulator of whole-body cholesterol homeostasis. *J Biol Chem.* 2004;279:33586–33592.
25. Graf GA, Yu L, Li WP, et al. ABCG5 and ABCG8 are obligate heterodimers for protein trafficking and biliary cholesterol excretion. *J Biol Chem.* 2003;278: 48275–48282.
26. Lee MH, Lu K, Hazard S, et al. Identification of a gene, ABCG5, important in the regulation of dietary cholesterol absorption. *Nat Genet.* 2001;27:79–83.
27. Bhattacharyya AK, Connor WE. Beta-sitosterolemia and xanthomatosis. A newly described lipid storage disease in two sisters. *J Clin Invest.* 1974;53:1033–1043.
28. Lu K, Lee MH, Hazard S, et al.Two genes that map to the STSL locus cause sitosterolemia: genomic structure and spectrum of mutations involving sterolin-1 and sterolin-2, encoded by ABCG5 and ABCG8, respectively. *Am J Hum Genet.* 2001;69:278–290.
29. Tacken PJ, Hofker MH, Havekes LM, et al. Living up to a name: the role of the VLDL receptor in lipid metabolism. *Curr Opin Lipidol.* 2001;12:275–279.
30. Beisiegel U, Heeren J. Lipoprotein lipase (EC 3.1.1.34) targeting of lipoproteins to receptors. *Proc Nutr Soc.* 1997;56:731–737.
31. Krapp A, Ahle S, Kersting S, et al. Hepatic lipase mediates the uptake of chylomicrons and beta-VLDL into cells via the LDL receptor-related protein (LRP). *J Lipid Res.* 1996;37:926–936.
32. Herz J, Kowal RC, Goldstein JL, et al. Proteolytic processing of the 600 kd low density lipoprotein receptor-related protein (LRP) occurs in a trans-Golgi compartment. *EMBO J.* 1990;9:1769–1776.
33. Krieger M, Herz J. Structures and functions of multiligand lipoprotein receptors: macrophage scavenger receptors and LDL receptor-related protein (LRP). *Annu Rev Biochem.* 1994;63:601–637.
34. Goudriaan JR, Espirito Santo SM, Voshol PJ, et al. The VLDL receptor plays a major role in chylomicron metabolism by enhancing LPL-mediated triglyceride hydrolysis. *J Lipid Res.* 2004;45:1475–1481.
35. Sappington TW, Raikhel AS. Ligand-binding domains in vitellogenin receptors and other LDL-receptor family members share a common ancestral ordering of cysteine-rich repeats. *J Mol Evol.* 1998;46:476–487.
36. Sudhof TC, Goldstein JL, Brown MS, et al. The LDL receptor gene: a mosaic of exons shared with different proteins. *Science.* 1985;228:815–822.
37. Russell DW, Lehrman MA, Sudhof TC, et al. The LDL receptor in familial hypercholesterolemia: use of human mutations to

dissect a membrane protein. *Cold Spring Harb Symp Quant Biol.* 1986;51 Pt 2:811–819.

38. Wessel GM. A protein of the sea urchin cortical granules is targeted to the fertilization envelope and contains an LDL-receptor-like motif. *Dev Biol.* 1995;167:388–397.

39. Schneider WJ, Beisiegel U, Goldstein JL, et al. Purification of the low density lipoprotein receptor, an acidic glycoprotein of 164,000 molecular weight. *J Biol Chem.* 1982;257:2664–2673.

40. Schneider WJ, Goldstein JL, Brown MS. Purification of the LDL receptor. *Methods Enzymol.* 1985;109:405–417.

41. Davis CG, Goldstein JL, Sudhof TC, et al. Acid-dependent ligand dissociation and recycling of LDL receptor mediated by growth factor homology region. *Nature.* 1987;326:760–765.

42. Innerarity TL. Structural biology. LDL receptor's beta-propeller displaces LDL. *Science.* 2002;298:2337–2339.

43. Russell DW, Schneider WJ, Yamamoto T, et al. Domain map of the LDL receptor: sequence homology with the epidermal growth factor precursor. *Cell.* 1984;37:577–585.

44. Anderson RG, Brown MS, Goldstein JL. Role of the coated endocytic vesicle in the uptake of receptor-bound low density lipoprotein in human fibroblasts. *Cell.* 1977;10:351–364.

45. Brown MS, Herz J, Goldstein JL. LDL-receptor structure. Calcium cages, acid baths and recycling receptors. Nature. 1997;388:629–630.

46. Brown MS, Dana SE, Goldstein JL. Regulation of 3-hydroxy-3-methylglutaryl coenzyme A reductase activity in human fibroblasts by lipoproteins. *Proc Natl Acad Sci USA.* 1973;70:2162–2166.

47. Brown MS, Goldstein JL. A receptor-mediated pathway for cholesterol homeostasis. *Science.* 1986;232:34–47.

48. Brown MS, Goldstein JL. A proteolytic pathway that controls the cholesterol content of membranes, cells, and blood. *Proc Natl Acad Sci USA.* 1999;96:11041–11048.

49. Horton JD, Goldstein JL, Brown MS. SREBPs: activators of the complete program of cholesterol and fatty acid synthesis in the liver. *J Clin Invest.* 2002;109:1125–1131.

50. von Eckardstein A, Nofer JR, Assmann G. High density lipoproteins and arteriosclerosis. Role of cholesterol efflux and reverse cholesterol transport. *Arterioscler Thromb Vasc Biol.* 2001;21:13–27.

51. Rigotti A, Miettinen HE, Krieger M. The role of the high-density lipoprotein receptor SR-BI in the lipid metabolism of endocrine and other tissues. *Endocr Rev.* 2003;24: 357–387.

52. Fredenrich A, Bayer P. Reverse cholesterol transport, high density lipoproteins and HDL cholesterol: recent data. *Diabetes Metab.* 2003;29:201–205.

53. Rust S, Rosier M, Funke H, et al. Tangier disease is caused by mutations in the gene encoding ATP-binding cassette transporter 1. *Nat Genet.* 1999;22:352–355.

54. Schmitz G, Langmann T, Heimerl S. Role of ABCG1 and other ABCG family members in lipid metabolism. *J Lipid Res.* 2001;42:1513–1520.

55. Cao G, Garcia CK, Wyne KL, et al. Structure and localization of the human gene encoding SR-BI/CLA-1. Evidence for transcriptional control by steroidogenic factor 1. *J Biol Chem.* 1997;272:33068–33076.

56. Rigotti A, Trigatti BL, Penman M, et al. A targeted mutation in the murine gene encoding the high density lipoprotein (HDL) receptor scavenger receptor class B type I reveals its key role in HDL metabolism. *Proc Natl Acad Sci USA.* 1997;94:12610–12615.

57. Trigatti B, Rayburn H, Vinals M, et al. Influence of the high density lipoprotein receptor SR-BI on reproductive and cardiovascular pathophysiology. *Proc Natl Acad Sci USA.* 1999;96:9322–9327.

58. Armstrong VW, Schleef J, Thiery J, et al. Effect of HELP-LDL-apheresis on serum concentrations of human lipoprotein(a): kinetic analysis of the post-treatment return to baseline levels. *Eur J Clin Invest.* 1989;19:235–240.

59. Dugi KA, Brandauer K, Schmidt N, et al. Low hepatic lipase activity is a novel risk factor for coronary artery disease. *Circulation.* 2001;104:3057–3062.

60. Czarnecka H, Yokoyama S. Lecithin:cholesterol acyltransferase reaction on cellular lipid released by free apolipoprotein-mediated efflux. *Biochemistry.* 1995;34: 4385–4392.

61. Ji Y, Jian B, Wang N, et al. Scavenger receptor BI promotes high density lipoprotein-mediated cellular cholesterol efflux. *J Biol Chem.* 1997;272:20982–20985.

62. Fredrickson DS. Phenotyping. On reaching base camp (1950–1975). *Circulation.* 1993;87:III1–III15.

63. Gofman JW, DeLalla O, Glazier F, et al. The serum lipoprotein transport system in health, metabolic disorders, atherosclerosis and coronary heart disease. Plasma (Milano) 1954;2:413–428.

64. Norum RA, Lakier JB, Goldstein S, et al. Familial deficiency of apolipoprotein A-I and C-III and precocious coronary-artery disease. *N Engl J Med.* 1982; 306:1513–1519.

65. Rodenburg J, Vissers MN, Trip MD, et al. The spectrum of statin therapy in hyperlipidemic children. *Semin Vasc Med.* 2004;4:313–320.

66. Wiegman A, Hutten BA, de Groot E, et al. Efficacy and safety of statin therapy in children with familial hypercholesterolemia: a randomized controlled trial. *JAMA.* 2004;292:331–337.

67. Stein EA. Statins in children. Why and when. *Nutr Metab Cardiovasc Dis.* 11 Suppl 2001;5:24–29.

68. Ose L. Diagnostic, clinical, and therapeutic aspects of familial hypercholesterolemia in children. *Semin Vasc Med.* 2004;4:51–57.

69. Black DM. Statins in children: what do we know and what do we need to do? *Curr Atheroscler Rep.* 2001;3:29–34.

70. Hoeg JM, Brewer HB Jr. 3-Hydroxy-3-methylglutaryl–coenzyme A reductase inhibitors in the treatment of hypercholesterolemia. *JAMA.* 1987;258:3532–3536.

71. Rosenson RS. Mechanisms of benefit of lipid lowering in patients with coronary heart disease. In: Rose BD, ed. *UpToDate.* Waltham, MA: UpToDate; 2005.

72. Rosenson RS. Clinical trials of cholesterol lowering in patients with coronary heart disease. In: Rose BD, ed. *UpToDate.* Waltham, MA: UpToDate; 2005.

73. Gould AL, Rossouw JE, Santanello NC, et al. Cholesterol reduction yields clinical benefit: impact of statin trials. *Circulation.* 1998;97:946–952.

74. Third Report of the National Cholesterol Education Program (NCEP) Expert Panel on Detection, Evaluation, and Treatment of High Blood Cholesterol in Adults (Adult Treatment Panel III) final report. *Circulation.* 2002;106:3143–3421.

75. Rosenson RS. Lipid lowering with drugs other than statins and fibrates In: Rose BD, ed. *UpToDate.* Waltham, MA: UpToDate; 2005.

76. Assmann G, Cullen P, Schulte H. Simple scoring scheme for calculating the risk of acute coronary events based on the 10-year follow-up of the prospective cardiovascular Munster (PROCAM) study. *Circulation.* 2002;105:310–315.

77. Gordon BR, Saal SD. Immunoadsorption and dextran sulfate cellulose LDL-apheresis for severe hypercholesterolemia: the Rogosin Institute experience 1982–1992. *Transfus Sci.* 1993;14:261–268.

78. Koga N, Watanabe K, Kurashige Y, et al. Long-term effects of LDL apheresis on carotid arterial atherosclerosis in familial hypercholesterolaemic patients. *J Intern Med.* 1999;246:35–43.

79. Lewis GF, Carpentier A, Adeli K, et al. Disordered fat storage and mobilization in the pathogenesis of insulin resistance and type 2 diabetes. *Endocr Rev.* 2002;23:201–229.

80. Malmstrom R, Packard C, Caslake M, et al. Defective regulation of triglyceride metabolism by insulin in the liver in NIDDM. *Diabetologia.* 1997;40:454–462.

81. Lewis GF, Uffelman KD, Szeto LW, et al. Interaction between free fatty acids and insulin in the acute control of very low density lipoprotein production in humans. *J Clin Invest.* 1995;95:158–166.

82. Assimacopoulos-Jeannet F, Brichard S, Rencurel F, et al. In vivo effects of hyperinsulinemia on lipogenic enzymes and glucose transporter experssion in rat liver and adipose tissues. *Metabolism.* 1995;44:228–233.

83. Golay A, Shi M-Z, Chiou Y-AM, et al. High density lipoprotein (HDL) metabolism in noninsulin-dependent diabetes mellitus: measurement of HDL turnover using tritiated HDL. *J Clin Endocrinol Metab.* 1987;65(3):512–518.

84. Grundy SM. Hypertriglyceridemia, atherogenic dyslipidemia, and the metabolic syndrome. *Am J Cardiol.* 1998;81:18B–25B.

85. Santamarina Fojo S, Brewer HBJ. The familial hyperchylomicronemia syndrome. New insights into underlying genetic defects [clinical conference]. *JAMA.* 1991;265: 904–908.

86. Chait A, Brunzell JD. Chylomicronemia syndrome. *Adv Intern Med.* 1992;37: 249–273.

87. Gofman JW, Lindgreen FT, Elliot H. Ultracentrifugal studies of lipoproteins of human serum. *J Biol Chem.* 1949;179:973–978.

88. Nevin DN, Brunzell JD, Deeb SS. The LPL gene in individuals with familial

88. combined hyperlipidemia and decreased LPL activity. *Arterioscler Thromb*. 1994; 14:869–873.

89. Mahley RW, Huang Y, Rall SC Jr. Pathogenesis of type III hyperlipoproteinemia (dysbetalipoproteinemia). Questions, quandaries, and paradoxes. *J Lipid Res*. 1999;40: 1933–1949.

90. Innerarity TL, Hui DY, Bersot TP, et al. Type III hyperlipoproteinemia: a focus on lipoprotein receptor- apolipoprotein E2 interactions. *Adv Exp Med Biol*. 1986;201:273–288.

91. Weisgraber KH, Innerarity TL, Rall SCJ, et al. Atherogenic lipoproteins resulting from genetic defects of apolipoproteins B and E. *Ann NY Acad Sci*. 1990;598:37–48.

92. Hackler R, Schaefer JR, Motzny S, et al. Rapid determination of apolipoprotein E phenotypes from whole plasma by automated isoelectric focusing using PhastSystem and immunofixation. *J Lipid Res*. 1994;35:153–158.

93. Hixson JE, Vernier DT. Restriction isotyping of human apolipoprotein E by gene amplification and cleavage with HhaI. *J Lipid Res*. 1990;31:545–548.

94. Razzaghi H, Aston CE, Hamman RF, et al. Genetic screening of the lipoprotein lipase gene for mutations associated with high triglyceride/low HDL-cholesterol levels. *Hum Genet*. 2000;107:257–267.

95. Kastelein JJ, Groenemeyer BE, Hallman DM, et al. The Asn9 variant of lipoprotein lipase is associated with the -93G promoter mutation and an increased risk of coronary artery disease. The Regress Study Group. *Clin Genet*. 1998;53(1):27–33.

96. Jukema JW, van Boven AJ, Groenemeijer B, et al. The Asp9 Asn mutation in the lipoprotein lipase gene is associated with increased progression of coronary atherosclerosis. REGRESS Study Group, Interuniversity Cardiology Institute, Utrecht, The Netherlands. Regression Growth Evaluation Statin Study. *Circulation*. 1996;94:1913–1918.

97. Wetterau JR, Aggerbeck LP, Bouma ME, et al. Absence of microsomal triglyceride transfer protein in individuals with abetalipoproteinemia. *Science*. 258:999–1001, 1992.

98. Rader DJ, Brewer HB Jr. Abetalipoproteinemia. New insights into lipoprotein assembly and vitamin E metabolism from a rare genetic disease. *JAMA*. 270:865–869, 1993.

99. Schmitz G, Langmann T, Heimerl S. Role of ABCG1 and other ABCG family members in lipid metabolism. *J Lipid Res*. 2001;42: 1513–1520.

100. Nakata K, Kobayashi K, Yanagi H, et al. Autosomal dominant hypoalphalipoproteinemia due to a completely defective apolipoprotein A-I gene. *Biochem Biophys Res Commun*. 1993;196:950–955.

101. Kuivenhoven JA, Pritchard H, Hill J, et al. The molecular pathology of lecithin:cholesterol acyltransferase (LCAT) deficiency syndromes. *J Lipid Res*. 1997;38:191–205.

102. Lewis GF, Steiner G. Hypertriglyceridemia and its metabolic consequences as a risk factor for atherosclerotic cardiovascular disease in non-insulin-dependent diabetes mellitus. *Diabetes Metab Rev*. 1996;12:37–56.

103. Freedman DS, Dietz WH, Srinivasan SR, et al. The relation of overweight to cardiovascular risk factors among children and adolescents: The Bogalusa Heart Study. *Pediatrics*. 1999;103:1175–1182.

104. American Academy of Pediatrics. National Cholesterol Education Program: Report of the Expert Panel on Blood Cholesterol Levels in Children and Adolescents. *Pediatrics*. 1992;89:525–584.

105. Dujovne CA, Ettinger MP, McNeer JF, et al. Efficacy and safety of a potent new selective cholesterol absorption inhibitor, ezetimibe, in patients with primary hypercholesterolemia. *Am J Cardiol*. 2002;90:1092–1097.

106. Salen G, von Bergmann K, Lutjohann D, et al. Ezetimibe effectively reduces plasma plant sterols in patients with sitosterolemia. *Circulation*. 2004;109:966–971.

107. Watts GF, Dimmitt SB. Fibrates, dyslipoproteinaemia and cardiovascular disease. *Curr Opin Lipidol*. 1999;10:561–574.

108. Schoonjans K, Staels B, Auwerx J. Role of the peroxisome proliferator-activated receptor (PPAR) in mediating the effects of fibrates and fatty acids on gene expression. *J Lipid Res*. 1996;37:907–25.

109. Roglans N, Vazquez-Carrera M, Alegret M, et al. Fibrates modify the expression of key factors involved in bile-acid synthesis and biliary-lipid secretion in gallstone patients. *Eur J Clin Pharmacol*. 2004;59:855–861.

110. Wheeler KA, West RJ, Lloyd JK, et al. Double blind trial of bezafibrate in familial hypercholesterolaemia. *Arch Dis Child*. 1985;60:34–37.

111. Gould AL, Rossouw JE, Santanello NC, et al. Cholesterol reduction yields clinical benefit: impact of statin trials. *Circulation*. 1998;97:946–952.

112. Barringer TA. WOSCOPS. West of Scotland Coronary Prevention Group. *Lancet*. 1997;349:432–433.

113. Scandinavian Simvastatin Survival Study Group. Randomised trial of cholesterol lowering in 4444 patients with coronary heart disease: The Scandinavian Simvastatin Survival Study (4S). *Lancet*. 1994;344:1383–1389.

114. Schaefer JR, Schweer H, Ikewaki K, et al. Metabolic basis of high density lipoproteins and apolipoprotein A-I increase by HMG-CoA reductase inhibition in healthy subjects and a patient with coronary artery disease. *Atherosclerosis*. 1999;144:177–184.

115. Shepherd J, Cobbe SM, Ford I, et al. Prevention of coronary heart disease with Pravastatin in men with hypercholesterolemia. *N Engl J Med*. 1995;333:1301–1307.

116. Furberg CD, Byington RP, Crouse JR, et al. Pravastatin, lipids, and major coronary events. *Am J Cardiol*. 1994;73:1133–1134.

117. Ducobu J, Brasseur D, Chaudron JM, et al. Simvastatin use in children. *Lancet*. 1992;339:1488.

118. de Jongh S, Ose L, Szamosi T, et al. Efficacy and safety of statin therapy in children with familial hypercholesterolemia: a randomized, double-blind, placebo-controlled trial with simvastatin. *Circulation*. 2002;106:2231–2237.

119. Knipscheer HC, Boelen CC, Kastelein JJ, et al. Short-term efficacy and safety of pravastatin in 72 children with familial hypercholesterolemia. *Pediatr Res*.1996;39:867–871.

120. Firth JC, Marais AD, Byrnes P, et al. Fluvastatin in heterozygous familial hypercholesterolemia. *Cardiol Young*. 2000; 10[Suppl 2]:35. (abstract).

121. Lambert M, Lupien PJ, Gagne C, et al. Treatment of familial hypercholesterolemia in children and adolescents: effect of lovastatin. Canadian Lovastatin in Children Study Group. *Pediatrics*. 1996;97:619–628.

122. Stein EA, Illingworth DR, Kwiterovich PO Jr, et al. Efficacy and safety of lovastatin in adolescent males with heterozygous familial hypercholesterolemia: a randomized controlled trial. *JAMA*. 1999;281:137–144.

123. McCrindle BW, Ose L, Marais AD. Efficacy and safety of atorvastatin in children and adolescents with familial hypercholesterolemia or severe hyperlipidemia: a multicenter, randomized, placebo-controlled trial. *J Pediatr*. 2003;143:74–80.

124. Holmes KW, Kwiterovich PO Jr. Treatment of dyslipidemia in children and adolescents. *Curr Cardiol Rep*. 2005;7:445–456.

CHAPTER 23

Defects of Cholesterol Biosynthesis

Dorothea Haas, MD
Richard I. Kelley, MD, PhD
Georg F. Hoffmann, MD

INTRODUCTION

Cholesterol plays an essential role in many cellular and developmental processes. In addition to being a structural lipid in membranes and myelin, cholesterol is the precursor for bile acids, steroid hormones, neurosteroids, and oxysterol synthesis. Subcellular organelles such as caveolae and lipid rafts are enriched in cholesterol. Finally, cholesterol is necessary for the modification and the function of several hedgehog signaling proteins that control embryonic development. Most defects of cholesterol synthesis are caused by enzyme deficiencies in the post-squalene portion of the pathway (Figure 23-1). Only mevalonic aciduria (MVA) and Hyperimmunoglobulinemia D syndrome (HIDS), both due to mevalonate kinase deficiency, are found in the proximal part of the pathway (Figure 23-2).

The 27-carbon cholesterol molecule is synthesized from lanosterol, the first sterol in the cholesterol synthesis pathway, via a series of approximately 30 enzymatic reactions. Defects of cholesterol biosynthesis result in congenital malformation syndromes. Many of the malformations in Smith-Lemli-Opitz syndrome (SLOS), lathosterolosis, and desmosterolosis are consistent with impaired function of sonic hedgehog (SHH), which plays a major role in the patterning of forebrain and limb development. Mutations in the SHH gene result in holoprosencephaly, a malformation sequence also found in some patients with SLOS. Because cholesterol was thought to be essential for the autoprocessing of SHH, a splitting of the protein in an inactive part and a signaling part, the apparent dysfunction of SHH in SLOS was assumed to be caused by the interference of 7-dehydrocholesterol (7-DHC) in this process. It was later found that 7-DHC has the same effect on SHH autoprocessing as cholesterol, and it also did not impair the signaling function of sterol-modified SHH. It is now thought that decreased intracellular cholesterol levels impair the SHH signaling cascade in SLOS and lathosterolosis downstream of the SHH

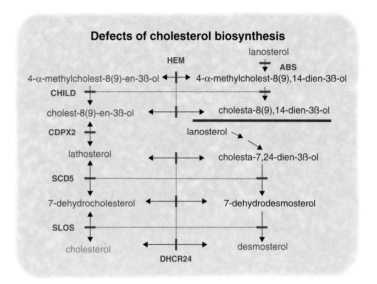

FIGURE 23-1. Defects of the distal cholesterol biosynthesis pathway. Red bars represent enzyme blocks, the corresponding disorders are given in red next to the bars. ABS = Antley-Bixler syndrome; HEM = Greenberg dysplasia; CHILD = CHILD syndrome; CDPX2 = Conradi-Hünermann syndrome; SCD5 = Lathosterolosis; SLOS = Smith-Lemli-Opitz syndrome; DHCR24 = Desmosterolosis; Accumulating metabolites are printed in blue. Metabolites that may be deficient are printed in green.

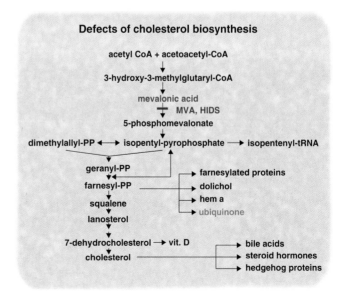

FIGURE 23-2. Defects of the proximal cholesterol biosynthesis pathway. Red bars represent enzyme blocks, the corresponding disorders are given in red next to the bars. MVA = Mevalonic aciduria; HIDS = Hyper-IgD syndrome. Accumulating metabolites are printed in blue. Metabolites that may be deficient are printed in green.

Defects of Cholesterol Biosynthesis

AT-A-GLANCE

Defects of cholesterol biosynthesis comprise a heterogeneous group of disorders. Congenital skeletal malformations, facial dysmorphic features, psychomotor retardation, and failure to thrive are common to most of the defects. Mevalonic aciduria (MVA) and hyperimmunoglobulin D syndrome (HIDS) present with recurrent febrile crises. CHILD syndrome and Conradi–Hünermann syndrome have ichthyosiform skin involvement in addition to skeletal abnormalities. In Smith-Lemli-Opitz syndrome, desmosterolosis, and lathosterolosis the malformations involve many different organ systems. Antley–Bixler syndrome and Greenberg dysplasia are lethal in early life in most patients.

DISORDERS	OCCURRENCE	GENE	LOCUS	OMIM
Smith-Lemli-Opitz syndrome (SLOS)	1:10.000–1:60.000	DHCR7	11q13	270400
Mevalonic aciduria (MVA)	Rare	MVK	12q24	251170
Hyper-IgD syndrome (HIDS)	Rare	MVK	12q24	260920
Conradi-Hünermann syndrome (CDPX2)	Rare	EBP	Xp11.23-p11.22	302960
CHILD syndrome	Very Rare	NSDHL	Xq28	308050
Greenberg dysplasia (HEM)	Very Rare	LBR	1q42.1	215140
Pelger–Huët anomaly (PHA)	Rare	LBR	1q42.1	169400
Antley–Bixler syndrome (ABS)	Rare	POR	7q11.2	207410
Lathosterolosis (SC5D)	Very Rare	SC5D	11q23.3	607330
Desmosterolosis (DHCR24)	Very Rare	DHCR24	1p33-p31.1	602398

DISORDER	LABORATORY FINDINGS	CLINICAL PRESENTATION BIRTH	CHILDHOOD & ADOLESCENCE
SLOS	↑ 7-DHC ↑ 8-DHC nl-↓ Cholesterol	Facial abnormalities: microcephaly, blepharoptosis, anteverted nares, retromicrognathia, low-set posteriorly rotated ears, high palate, palatal clefts; skeletal abnormalities: syndactyly toes 2/3, postaxial polydactyly, foot deformities; genital and organ malformations (CNS, cardiac, renal and ureteral, gastrointestinal, pulmonary)	Feeding difficulties, failure to thrive, psychomotor retardation, behavioral abnormalities, autism
MVA	↑ Mevalonic acid ↑ LTE₄ NL-↑ IgD	Facial abnormalities: microcephaly, dolichocephaly, wide irregular, fontanels low-set and posteriorly rotated ears, down slanted palpebral fissures, blue sclerae	Mild-to-severe psychomotor retardation, autism; recurrent crises (fever, vomiting and diarrhea, hepatosplenomegaly), failure to thrive, hypotonia, myopathy, ataxia due to cerebellar atrophy, cataracts, retinal dystrophy
HIDS	↑ IgD ↑ Mevalonic acid	No morphologic abnormalities	Recurrent episodes of fever, abdominal distress, lymphadenopathy, skin rashes; normal psychomotor development
CDPX2	↑ 8(9)Cholestenol ↑ 8-DHC	Asymmetric rhizomelic shortening of the limbs, ichthyotic skin lesions following Blaschko lines, punctate calcification of cartilaginous structures, cataracts	Growth retardation, mild-to-moderate mental retardation, resolution of cutaneous inflammation
CHILD	↑ 4-Methylsterols ↑ 4-Carboxysterols	Unilateral ichthyosiform erythroderma, hemidystrophia, unilateral limb defects, punctate calcifications of cartilaginous structures, malformations of brain, heart, or kidney	Regional improvement of cutaneous inflammation
HEM	↑ 8,14-Cholestadienol ↑ 8,14,24-Cholestatrienol	Fetal hydrops, extramedullary hematopoiesis, short-limbed dwarfism, abnormal chondroosseous mineralization, rarely malformation of internal organs	Intrauterine death
PHA		Abnormally shaped granulocytic nuclei; homozygotes ("pince-nez"); mild skeletal abnormalities	Homozygotes: rarely mental retardation or epilepsy
ABS	↑ Lanosterol ↑ Dihydrolanosterol	Limb anomalies: radiohumeral synostosis, bowing of femora, neonatal femoral fractures; facial dysmorphism: multiple craniosynostosis, midface hypoplasia, urogenital malformation (under virilized males)	Early death due to respiratory failure in 50% of the patients; surviving patients: normal intelligence
SC5D	↑ Lathosterol	Facial abnormalities: Microcephaly, micrognathia, anteverted nares, high palate; postaxial hexadactyly, syndactyly; genital malformations	Progressive cholestatic liver disease, psychomotor retardation, muscular hypotonia, conductive deafness
DHCR24	↑ Desmosterol	Facial abnormalities; microcephaly; limb anomalies; ambiguous genitalia; malformations of brain and internal organs	Early death in patients with severe malformations; surviving profound developmental delay in surviving patients

CNS = Central nervous system; 7-DHC = 7-dehydrocholesterol; 8-DHC = 8-dehydrocholesterol; IgD = immunoglobulin D; LTE₄ = leukotriene E₄; NL = normal.

receptor Patched at the level of Smoothened, a G-protein-linked protein.

SMITH-LEMLI-OPITZ SYNDROME

Etiology/Pathophysiology SLOS is an autosomal recessively inherited disorder. The underlying defect is a deficiency of microsomal 7-dehydrocholesterol reductase (DHCR7), the enzyme that converts 7-DHC to cholesterol in the last step of cholesterol biosynthesis. This results in an accumulation of 7-DHC and its isomer 8-dehydrocholesterol (8-DHC) in plasma and all tissues and, in most patients, a marked deficiency of cholesterol (1). The human DHCR7 gene is located on chromosome 11q13 (2,3,4). Of the more than 100 different DHCR7 mutations that have been identified, the majority are missense mutations, and more than 30% of the known mutations are in exon 9 (5). The most frequent mutation, representing approximately 30% of known alleles is the splice site mutation, IVS8-1G>C, which results in an inactive, truncated protein.

There is a correlation of the DHCR7 genotype with the severity of the SLOS phenotype (6). Many of the severely affected patients are homozygous or compound heterozygous for null mutations, the most common being IVS8-1G>C and W151X. Severity is also influenced by the maternal apo E genotype. Certain apo E genotypes associated with increased cholesterol transport are speculated to cause higher cholesterol levels in the embryo, resulting in a less severe phenotype than predicted by the genotype (7).

Clinical Presentation SLOS shows wide clinical variation, ranging from intrauterine or neonatal death to patients with minimal facial dysmorphism and near-normal mental development (1). Severely affected fetuses with SLOS typically have nuchal edema, growth retardation, polydactyly, cleft palate, and structural abnormalities of brain, heart, or kidneys. Typically affected newborns show characteristic facial features, including microcephaly, narrow bifrontal diameter, ptosis, anteverted nares, retrognathia, and low-set, posteriorly rotated ears. Ocular defects include mainly congenital and occasionally postnatal cataracts, strabismus, and nystagmus. Congenital sensorineural hearing deficits may affect as many as 10% of the patients. During the first months SLOS patients often have striking glabellar and other midline capillary hemangiomas, which usually fade with age. The mouth is large and broad, and the palate is highly arched. Midline clefts ranging from a bifid uvula to lip and palatal clefts are common. Because of the muscular hypotonia, the mouth is sometimes described as "tent-shaped" (Figure 23-3). Older children have broad alveolar ridges with irregularly erupted teeth.

More than 95% of SLOS patients have unilateral or bilateral syndactyly of toes 2 and 3, typically Y-shaped (1). Various foot deformities ranging from clubfoot to valgus deformities can also occur. The thumb is often short and proximally placed (Figure 23-3). Less frequent are clinodactyly or brachydactyly. Many of the more severely affected patients have postaxial polydactyly, and in some children there is rhizomelic shortening of the limbs.

Genital abnormalities usually occur even in relatively mildly affected boys and range from cryptorchidism to severe hypospadias and, in more severely affected patients, apparent complete sex reversal. In females, hypoplastic labia minora and majora can occur, but usually the external genitalia are normal (8).

Many patients are growth retarded at birth. Feeding is difficult from birth in most patients and sometimes becomes almost impossible in later infancy. These feeding problems include weak or poorly coordinated sucking, swallowing difficulties, lack of interest in feeds, volume intolerance, gastroesophageal reflux, poor intestinal motility, and an increased incidence of protein allergies. Often the patients are intolerant of oral stimulation and refuse solid food in later months. More than 50% require nasogastric tube feeding or gastrostomy feeding for several years.

With rare exceptions global psychomotor retardation is characteristic of SLOS. In most patients, gross motor development is more severely delayed than fine motor development, and expressive language is more impaired than receptive language.

Behavioral problems are another common feature. In the 1st year of life, children with SLOS are usually quiet and sleep a lot. Later in infancy inconsolable screaming, especially at night, is a major characteristic of SLOS. Many patients develop behavioral characteristics of autism such as rocking, hand flapping, abnormal obsessions, insistence on routine, and some fulfill standard diagnostic criteria for autism. In older children, aggressive and self-injurious behavior such as hand biting and head banging is typical. Insomnia and sleep cycle disturbances are also common features and often correlate with cholesterol deficiency.

Severe photosensitivity occurs in many patients and requires effective sun protection. More than 50% of the patients have marked tactile hypersensitivity of the hands and feet and do not tolerate walking barefoot on grass or sand.

- Approximately 10% of children with biochemically confirmed SLOS have mental development in the mildly retarded range (IQ 50–70).

- Patients with just borderline mental retardation or even normal intelligence have been described in single reports.

More severely affected patients, formerly classified as SLOS type II, are distinguished from "classic" SLOS by the number and severity of organ malformations. Structural abnormalities of the central nervous system usually consist of midline defects and holoprosencephaly sequence, but enlarged ventricles and frontal lobe hypoplasia also occur. Endocardial cushion defects are the most frequent cardiac abnormalities and often are life limiting. Even in mildly affected patients, atrial septal defects are often found. Malformations of the urinary tract include renal hypoplasia or aplasia, renal cortical cysts, hydronephrosis, and ureteral duplication. In most patients, intestinal motility is impaired, either due to identified structural abnormalities such as intestinal aganglionosis or pyloric stenosis or less well-defined functional dysmotility. Pulmonary hypoplasia with abnormal pulmonary lobation can occur in severe cases and limit life expectancy.

Diagnosis

Laboratory findings

- The levels of 7-DHC and 8-DHC are elevated in plasma, as typically measured by gas chromatography/mass spectrometry (GC/MS).

- A low maternal estriol level (<0.5 multiples of the median) can be an early sign of a fetus with SLOS and should lead to further investigations, especially when associated with sonographic evidence of SLOS-type malformation

- Prenatal diagnosis is possible by either determination of the 7-DHC/cholesterol ratio in amniotic fluid or chorionic villi or by molecular testing, if the mutations in the index patient are known

- Even patients with a classic SLOS phenotype may have only slightly elevated or borderline levels of 7-DHC and 8-DHC. Sterol analysis of lymphoblasts or fibroblasts grown in delipidated culture medium and molecular analysis should be performed in those patients

- Treatment of non-SLOS patients with psychoactive medications, such as Risperdal or buspirone, is a common cause of mildly increased levels of 7-DHC and 8-DHC in plasma

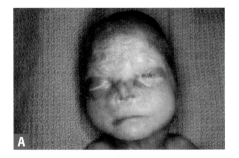

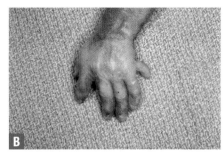

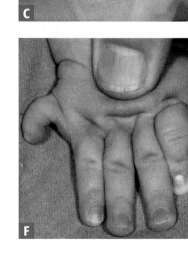

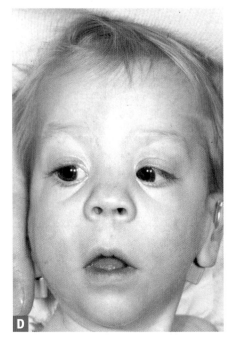

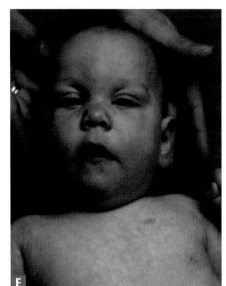

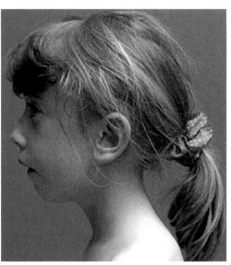

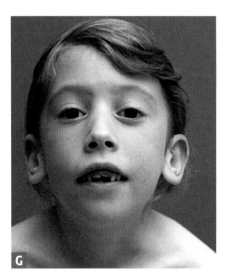

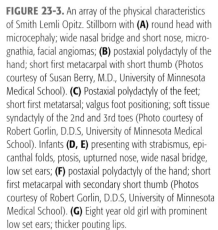

FIGURE 23-3. An array of the physical characteristics of Smith Lemli Opitz. Stillborn with **(A)** round head with microcephaly; wide nasal bridge and short nose, micrognathia, facial angiomas; **(B)** postaxial polydactyly of the hand; short first metacarpal with short thumb (Photos courtesy of Susan Berry, M.D., University of Minnesota Medical School). **(C)** Postaxial polydactyly of the feet; short first metatarsal; valgus foot positioning; soft tissue syndactyly of the 2nd and 3rd toes (Photo courtesy of Robert Gorlin, D.D.S., University of Minnesota Medical School). Infants **(D, E)** presenting with strabismus, epicanthal folds, ptosis, upturned nose, wide nasal bridge, low set ears; **(F)** postaxial polydactyly of the hand; short first metacarpal with secondary short thumb (Photos courtesy of Robert Gorlin, D.D.S., University of Minnesota Medical School). **(G)** Eight year old girl with prominent low set ears; thicker pouting lips.

- The plasma cholesterol level is decreased in most patients; however, because approximately 10% of SLOS patients have normal cholesterol levels, routine measurement of cholesterol alone is not a suitable screening method.
- Mutations in the DHCR7 gene.

Additional investigations

- Echocardiography (cardiac defects?)
- Abdominal sonography (renal or urinary tract malformations?)

- Ophthalmological examination (cataracts?)
- Hearing assessment

Treatment Dietary cholesterol supplementation results in improved growth and behavior in most patients (9,10). Photosensitivity and polyneuropathy improve significantly. Cholesterol can be given as purified cholesterol powder in suspension (Table 23-1), or as egg yolk (cooked or, preferably, in pasteurized, liquid form). Treatment with supple-

ments of bile acids has not been effective (10) except in severely affected patients with cholestasis or when there is clinically evidence of bile acid deficiency. Unfortunately, an effect of cholesterol supplementation on intrinsic cognitive abilities has not been found (11); most likely because cholesterol cannot be transported across the blood–brain barrier and because the developmental disabilities are largely determined by irreversible prenatal cerebral maldevelopment. Plasma sterol levels often improve slowly over many months

TABLE 23-1   Well-Day Treatment Recommendation SLOS

7-DHC+8-DHC Cholesterol	Age/indication	Medication	Dosage (mg/kg/d)#
< 0.5	0-10 y	Cholesterol	100
	Adults		500-1000*
	All ages	Simvastatin	0.5-1
≥ 0.5	0-2 y	Cholesterol	150-200
	>2 y		100-150
	Cholestasis	Ursodeoxycholate	15-25

*mg/d

#Dosage for purified cholesterol powder. Cholesterol is more efficiently absorbed when given as egg yolk.

or years after initiation of cholesterol supplementation; however, effects on behavior often are evident already after only several days of cholesterol treatment (1), possibly because of changes in levels of adrenal steroids, many of which, unlike cholesterol, can cross the blood–brain barrier. Treatment of mildly affected SLOS patients with simvastatin, an inhibitor of 3-hydroxy-3-methyl-glutaryl–coenzyme A (HMG-CoA) reductase, causes a rapid fall of 7- and 8-DHC and a rise of cholesterol (12), probably via augmentation of residual DHCR7 activity, allowing more complete conversion of the abnormal sterols to cholesterol. Mental, motor, and social development as well as weight, length, and head circumference reportedly improved in two patients who were not pretreated with cholesterol (12), but others, even those whose cholesterol levels normalized on simvastatin, have shown no change in cognitive function. The clinical benefit of additional simvastatin also varies in patients who are pretreated with cholesterol. In some patients, irritability, auto-aggression, social behavior, and autistic features improve. In others, the addition of simvastatin shows no measurable clinical improvement. Simvastatin should not be used in severely affected patients (ratio of [7-DHC+8-DHC]/cholesterol > 0.5) expected to have no or minimal residual DHCR7 activity, because the residual DHCR7 activity is too low, and simvastatin could further lower cholesterol levels with severe side effects (hepatotoxicity and reversible increase of creatine kinase) (13). Studies in a larger group of SLOS patients are needed to evaluate the potential benefits and risks of simvastatin treatment (Table 23-1).

Emergency treatment For acute illnesses, when enteral cholesterol supplementation cannot be continued, or under conditions of severe stress likely to deplete low-density lipoprotein (LDL) cholesterol, such as surgical procedures, fresh frozen plasma can be given as an emergency parenteral source of LDL cholesterol (1). Acute respiratory distress syndrome appears to be a relatively common if unpredictable complication in severe SLOS, typically associated with lower respiratory infections and anesthesia, and may be treated with fresh frozen plasma and/or surfactant.

Supportive treatment A large proportion of SLOS patients require nasogastric tube

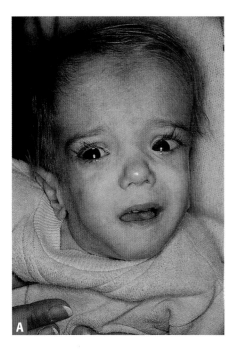

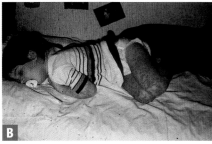

FIGURE 23-4. (A) Infant with MVA presenting with microcephaly, dolichocephaly, low set and posteriorly rotated ears, epicanthal folds, depressed nasal bridge and blue sclerae. **(B)** Child with MVA and morbilliform rash which develop in some patients during crisis.

feeding or gastrostomy to provide adequate caloric intake. It is important not to overfeed the children simply to achieve better growth. Most SLOS patients have a genetically determined short stature and, because of their muscle hypoplasia, their normal well-nourished weight during infancy typically is 1 to 2 standard deviations less than their length. Trying to achieve arbitrary and inappropriately high weight goals based on age or length alone only increases adipose tissue and thereby limits the availability of cholesterol to the organs (8). The reduced muscle mass and limited motor activity of SLOS infants may also reduce their caloric requirements, which can be as much as 20 to 30 kcal/kg/day less than predicted for age and size. Furthermore, for the more severely affected SLOS infants, weight gain often follows a slow linear curve from birth, unlike the more usual asymptotic curve of infancy. As a result, the weight z-score deviates even further from length between birth and 2 to 3 years.

Follow-up investigations

Laboratory investigations

- Serum sterols, transaminases, albumin, Fe, ferritin, folate, vitamin B_{12}
- For biochemically severely affected children: coagulation studies, assessment of adrenal function
- Patients on simvastatin: creatine kinase, transaminases, and sterols 4 and 12 weeks after start of the treatment, then every three months

General investigations These assessments should consist of body growth, general health (6 monthly), detailed psychomotor and neurobehavioral examinations and testing every 2 years until the age of 6 starting from the age of 24 months, such as with the Bayley Scales of Infant Development.

An autism assessment should be made in patients with a developmental quotient (DQ) greater than 18 months.

Outcome Life expectancy in SLOS is primarily determined by the severity of already prenatally acquired internal malformations and the quality of general supportive care. Severely affected patients may die in the newborn period from cardiac, renal, or gastrointestinal malformations. Acute respiratory distress syndrome or adrenal insufficiency during minor infections is frequently found as a cause of death during early infancy. The vast majority of mildly and moderately affected children survive with various degrees of developmental delay and failure to thrive. In later infancy and adolescence behavioral problems may become prominent for parents and caretakers.

MEVALONIC ACIDURIA AND HYPERIMMUNOGLOBULINEMIA D SYNDROME

Etiology/Pathophysiology MVA and HIDS are autosomal recessively inherited disorders due to a deficiency of mevalonate kinase. The location of the gene encoding mevalonate kinase, MVK, is chromosome 12q24 (14). In classic MVA, seven mutations could be identified in 10 of 20 known patients, most of which cluster in the C-terminal region of the protein (15). Most patients with HIDS are compound heterozygotes for missense mutations in the gene for mevalonate kinase. One mutation, V337I, is present in more than 80% of HIDS patients (16), almost always in combination with a null or other very low activity mutation in the other allele. The V337I mutation results in a slight reduction of the stability and in the catalytic activity of the enzyme. The activity of mevalonate kinase is reduced to 5% to 15% in HIDS patients, whereas it is below 5% in patients with MVA (17).

Clinical Presentation MVA shows considerable clinical heterogeneity. Severely affected patients present from birth with congenital malformations such as microcephaly, dolichocephaly, and wide irregular fontanels, low set and posteriorly rotated ears, down slanted palpebral fissures, blue sclerae, and central cataracts. Stillbirths with skeletal malformations have been observed in affected families, possibly a result of the same genetic defect. The cardinal manifestations include mild-to-severe psychomotor retardation, recurrent crises (fever, vomiting, and diarrhea), failure to thrive, hypotonia, and myopathy. Short stature, ataxia due to a progressive cerebellar atrophy, and ocular involvement with cataracts and retinal dystrophy become predominant findings after preschool age and can be the major manifestations in milder cases (17,18). Severely affected patients may suffer from cholestatic liver disease.

Most MVA patients suffer from frequent crises characterized by fever, vomiting, and diarrhea. These episodes appear to be noninfectious and are accompanied by arthralgia, subcutaneous edema, and a morbilliform rash in some patients. Two patients developed uveitis, which worsened during crises. In childhood, episodes occur as often as 25 times per year, lasting on average 4 to 5 days, but 3- or 4-weekly spells are most common, and some patients have very few spells. Over years the severity and the frequency of these attacks decline.

In HIDS, recurrent febrile attacks that usually start before the end of the 1st year of life dominate the clinical course (19). The fever lasts 4 to 6 days and can be unprovoked or initiated by vaccination, minor trauma, surgery, or even emotional stress. The crises usually are associated with abdominal pain, vomiting, diarrhea, and cervical lymphadenopathy. Other common symptoms include hepatosplenomegaly, headache, backache, arthralgia, and rashes. After the attack the patients are largely free of symptoms, although skin and joint symptoms disappear more slowly than fever and gastrointestinal complaints (20). Most patients display neither malformations nor neurologic abnormalities.

Diagnosis

Laboratory findings

- Elevated mevalonic acid in urine and plasma (MVA and HIDS).
- Elevated immunoglobulin Ig D (HIDS).
- Elevated leukotriene E_4 (MVA).
- Mutations in the MVK gene (MVA and HIDS).
- Reduced enzymatic activity in fibroblasts (MVA and HIDS)

Additional investigations (MVA)

- Cranial magnetic resonance imaging (cerebellar atrophy)
- Ophthalmologic examination: slit lamp examination, funduscopy, electroretinography (cataracts? retinal dystrophy?)

Outcome The prognosis for patients with MVA is restricted (17,18). Approximately half of the patients die within the 1st years of life. Beyond school age, the clinical picture is often stable; however, patients may succumb to a progressive myopathy. Retinal dystrophy may become another important long-term manifestation of the disease. HIDS is considered to be a relatively benign condition. Life expectancy may be reduced in some patients due to severe infections or the development of renal amyloidosis (21).

Treatment There is no established therapeutic regime for patients with MVA. Long-term administration of coenzyme Q_{10} together with vitamins C and E to treat an intrinsic deficiency in the synthesis of coenzyme Q_{10}

- In some HIDS patients the excretion of mevalonic acid may only be slightly elevated between febrile crises. The sensitivity of organic acid analysis is inadequate to recognize these concentrations. Therefore isotope-dilution GC/MS is the method of choice.

- Prenatal diagnosis is possible by isotope-dilution GC/MS (in classic MVA), by determination of mevalonate kinase activity in cultured amniocytes and chorionic villus, and by mutational analysis

and to treat a possible increased sensitivity to reactive oxygen species seems to stabilize the clinical course and improve somatic and psychomotor development (8). Dietary supplementation of cholesterol may reduce the frequency and severity of febrile attacks in some mildly affected patients but has further compromised more severely affected patients (17), possibly by excessive downregulation of HMG-CoA reductase activity. An experimental trial with lovastatin in two patients with classic MVA resulted in clinical decompensation manifesting as elevated body temperature, acute myopathic changes, highly elevated creatine kinase, and worsened ataxia, diarrhea, and vomiting (17).

Despite these severe adverse effects of HMG-CoA reductase inhibitors in classic MVA, a recently completed study has shown a highly beneficial effect of simvastatin in HIDS (22). Similarly a beneficial effect of anakinra was described (23) (Table 23-2).

Emergency treatment Intervention with corticosteroids (prednisone 2 mg/kg/d) is beneficial during clinical crises in patients with MVA and HIDS, with resolution of the crises within 24 hours. The severity of attacks can also be reduced with the leukotriene receptor inhibitors, montelukast and zafirlukast.

Follow-up Investigations (MVA) These assessments should consist of CK, cholesterol, coenzyme Q_{10}, vitamin E, hepatic function, and renal function.

TABLE 23-2	Well-Day Treatment Recommendation		
MVA		**HIDS**	
Medication	**Dosage (mg/kg/d)**	**Medication**	**Dosage (mg/kg/d)**
Coenzyme Q_{10}	5–10	Coenzyme Q_{10}	5–10
Tocopherol	25	Simvastatin	0.5–1.0
Ascorbic acid	50–60	Anakinra	1–2 (sc)
Cholesterol*	50–100		
Alpha-lipoic acid	15		

*Positive effects in mildly affected patients, but clinical deterioration in more severely affected patients.

General investigations These assessments should consist of body growth, general health (6 monthly), detailed psychomotor and neurobehavioral examinations and testing every 2 years until the age of 6 starting from the age of 24 months, such as with the Bayley Scales of Infant Development. Cranial magnetic resonance imaging should be performed every 2 years until the age of 6 years. Ophthalmological monitoring yearly.

CONRADI–HÜNERMANN SYNDROME

Etiology/Pathophysiology Conradi–Hünermann syndrome (CDPX2) is an X-linked dominant disorder with skeletal, skin, and ocular manifestations that is usually a lethal prenatal disorder in hemizygous males. Biochemically, CDPX2 patients have elevated concentrations of 8(9)-cholestanol and 8-DHC in plasma and tissues due to a defect of 3β-hydroxysteroid-Δ8, Δ7-isomerase (24). Mutations in the emopamil binding protein (EBP) gene encoding for the 3β-hydroxysteroid-Δ8,Δ7-isomerase have been demonstrated in CDPX2 patients (25). At least 41 different mutations spread throughout the EBP gene have been reported to date. Most are predicted to be null mutations. In females there are no clear genotype–phenotype correlations, probably because clinical severity is mainly determined by the individual's random X-inactivation pattern.

Clinical Presentation Affected females show bilateral asymmetric shortening of the long bones, scoliosis, punctate calcification of cartilaginous structures, cataracts, and ichthyotic skin lesions that typically follow the lines of Blaschko. The lesions usually resolve during infancy although variable ichthyosis, alopecia, and residual pigmentary abnormalities may remain. A few patients also have polydactyly and dysmorphic facial features and renal or cardiac malformations. Intelligence is normal except in severely affected individuals.

At least four hemizygous male CDPX2 patients with apparently hypomorphic EBP mutations are known. The phenotype includes chondrodysplasia punctata and ichthyosiform erythroderma, but severe mental retardation, microcephaly, and Dandy–Walker variant have been present in all or most. Two 46,XY males resembling classic female CDPX2 have been shown to be mosaic for a normal EBP allele and an apparent postzygotic EBP mutation.

CHILD SYNDROME

Etiology/Pathophysiology Congenital hemidysplasia, ichthyosiform erythroderma, and limb defects (CHILD) syndrome is a second X-linked dominant disorder in cholesterol biosynthesis with presumed male lethality and clinical similarity to CDPX2. A few affected males probably due to somatic mosaicism have been described. Most cases of CHILD syndrome are caused by mutations in the NSDHL (NAD[P]H steroid dehydrogenase-like) gene. NSDHL encodes a subunit of the sterol-4-demethylase complex, the enzymatic step just prior to 3β-hydroxysteroid-Δ8,Δ7-isomerase (26). In these patients elevated levels of 4-methylsterols and 4-carboxysterols have been detected.

In two females with clinical features of CHILD syndrome a sterol pattern suggestive of CDPX2 has been found. Subsequently those patients were found to have mutations in the EBP gene (27). These observations indicate that there is clinical overlap between the two X-linked disorders.

Clinical Presentation CHILD syndrome is characterized by striking unilateral psoriasiform skin lesions with a sharp demarcation at the midline of the trunk, typically with sparing of the face (Figure 23-5) (28). The

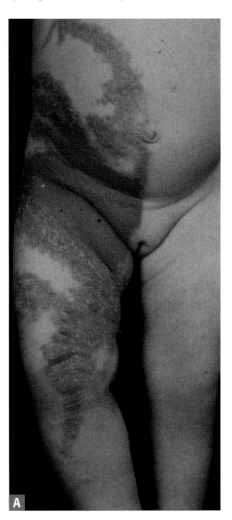

skin lesions are usually present at birth and persist throughout life, although there may be some amelioration during childhood, and new lesions sometimes arise in areas of skin trauma. Additional features like alopecia or nail involvement typically occur on the affected side. Unilateral punctate calcifications similar to those in CDPX2 are present in the epiphyses and other cartilaginous structures. In some patients, unilateral internal malformations including central nervous system, kidneys, and heart have been reported. The right side is involved twice as often as the left side. Cataracts are not found in CHILD syndrome.

GREENBERG DYSPLASIA AND PELGER-HUËT ANOMALY

Etiology/Pathophysiology Greenberg dysplasia (also called Hydrops-ectopic calcification-"moth-eaten" skeletal dysplasia, HEM), is an autosomal recessively inherited lethal in utero disorder. It is allelic with Pelger-Huët anomaly (PHA), a benign autosomal dominant hematologic trait. Both are caused by mutations in the lamin B receptor (LBR) gene, a gene that encodes the LBR along with having separate functions in sterol biosynthesis and the structure of the nuclear envelope. The LBR, a member of the sterol reductase family, is evolutionarily conserved and targets heterochromatin and lamins to the nuclear membrane. The detection of increased levels of 8,14-cholestanol in tissues

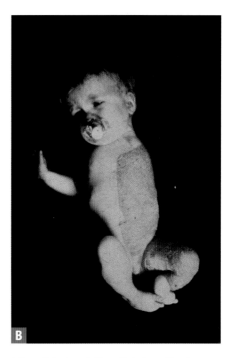

FIGURE 23-5. CHILD syndrome (**A** and **B**) is characterized by striking unilateral psoriasiform skin lesions with a sharp demarcation at the midline of the trunk, typically with sparing of the face (Photos courtesy of Robert Gorlin, D.D.S, University of Minnesota Medical School).

and fibroblasts of fetuses with HEM, suggested a deficiency of sterol-Δ^{14} reductase encoded by the LBR gene (29). Subsequently, mutations in both alleles of the LBR gene were found in several HEM cases and heterozygous mutations in this gene were later shown to cause PHA (30). Although homozygous PHA patients have short stature and other skeletal abnormalities, they are phenotypically different from those with HEM, suggesting that these two distinct disorders may be two extremes of one clinical spectrum (31).

Clinical Presentation All nine cases of HEM reported to date have had nonimmune hydrops fetalis, short limbs, and severe chondroosseous calcifications with a moth-eaten appearance. Postaxial polydactyly has been reported in some patients and additional organ malformations were found in one patient. All cases have been lethal prenatally (31). PHA is a disorder characterized by abnormally shaped blood granulocytes and now associated with heterozygosity from mutations in LBR. Homozygous PHA patients do not display a well-defined syndrome. In some individuals mental retardation, epilepsy, short stature, and hand abnormalities have been described, but generalized skeletal dysplasia and severe congenital malformations have not been found.

ANTLEY–BIXLER SYNDROME

Etiology/Pathophysiology Antley Bixler syndrome (ABS) has both genetic and teratogenic etiologies. Mutations of the fibroblast growth factor receptor-2 gene have been reported in sporadic cases of ABS or ABS-like syndromes. In some cases, an ABS-like phenotype was caused by an early in utero exposure to fluconazole, an inhibitor of lanosterol-14α demethylase. This led to the evaluation of sterol metabolism in fibroblasts of ABS patients, and in one patient with ambiguous genitalia increased levels of lanosterol (the first sterol in the cholesterol synthesis pathway) and dihydrolanosterol were found (32). These metabolites suggested a functional deficiency of lanosterol-14α demethylase, a cytochrome P450 enzyme, encoded by CYP51. Mutation analysis of CYP51, however, disclosed no obvious pathogenic mutation. Instead, mutations in the POR gene encoding P450 oxidoreductase, the obligate electron donor for all cytochrome P450 enzymes, have been identified in patients with ABS (33).

Clinical presentation ABS is a rare multiple anomaly syndrome with limb anomalies, craniofacial dysmorphisms, organ malformations, ambiguous genitalia (a few cases), and

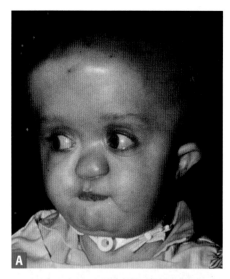

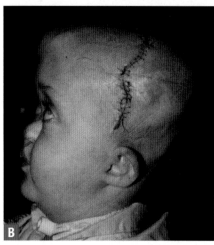

FIGURE 23-6. A and **B.** Infant with ABS presenting with craniosynostosis and brachycephaly, frontal bossing, ocular proptosis, low nasal bridge, pear-shaped nose, long philtrum, severe midface hypoplasia, and low-set malformed ears. (Photos courtesy of Robert Gorlin, DDS, University of Minnesota Medical School).

a high mortality rate. The craniofacial abnormalities include multiple craniosynostoses, severe midface hypoplasia, proptosis, and choanal atresia (Figure 23-6). Malformations of the limbs include radiohumeral synostosis, bowed femora, arachnodactyly, multiple joint contractures, and fractures of the long bones. Intelligence in most patients appears to be normal.

LATHOSTEROLOSIS

Etiology/Pathophysiology Lathosterol 5-desaturase (SC5D) catalyzes the conversion of lathosterol to yield 7-DHC in the cholesterol synthetic pathway. In the subsequent enzymatic step, 7-DHC is reduced by DHCR7 to yield cholesterol. The two patients with lathosterolosis described to date had abnormal sterol profiles with accumula-

tion of lathosterol in plasma and/or cultured fibroblasts. In both patients, missense mutations were found in both alleles of the SC5D gene (34,35). Detection of residual conversion of labeled mevalonate to cholesterol in cultured cells from both patients confirmed that these mutations act as hypomorphs, at least in vitro (35). A mouse model (SC5D$^{-/-}$) for lathosterolosis by targeted disruption of the murine SC5D gene in embryonic stem cells was developed mainly to examine whether some of the phenotypic features of SLOS are caused by a lack of cholesterol or by an accumulation of 7-DHC (35). There were phenotypic similarities between the lathosterolosis patients and the SC5D$^{-/-}$ mouse with the exception that the prolonged survival of the patients compared with the knock-out mouse was probably related to the presence of hypomorphic alleles with residual enzyme activity. Hypomorphic alleles are those in which function is reduced but not completely lost.

Clinical presentation Both patients exhibited an SLOS-like phenotype (34,35). They had craniofacial abnormalities with microcephaly and micrognathia, and limb abnormalities with postaxial polydactyly and syndactyly. The second patient had genital abnormalities and the first patient developed progressive cholestatic liver disease, conductive deafness, and severe psychomotor retardation.

DERMOSTEROLOSIS

Etiology/Pathophysiology In the four known patients with desmosterolosis (DHCR24) in three families, an accumulation of desmosterol was found in plasma, tissue, and cultured cells. Mutations in both alleles of the DHCR24 gene were demonstrated in all patients (36). The DHCR24 gene catalyzes the reduction of the -24 double bond of sterol intermediates during cholesterol biosynthesis and acts as an antiapoptotic factor in neurons. It has a role in protecting cells against amyloid beta peptide toxicity and oxidative stress and might be involved in the molecular events of adrenocortical tumorigenesis by facilitating steroid synthesis and cell growth as shown by overexpression in adrenal cancer cells.

Clinical Presentation Desmosterolosis patients have had remarkably different clinical phenotypes. The first patient was a dysmorphic female who died shortly after birth at 34 weeks of gestation. She had macrocephaly, cleft palate, total anomalous pulmonary venous return, clitoromegaly, short limbs, and generalized osteosclerosis (37). The second patient had a milder but still very abnormal phenotype consisting of severe microcephaly, a submucous cleft of the palate, mild contractures of the hands, bilateral clubfeet, and intrauterine and postnatal growth retardation. In addition he had a patent ductus arteriosus and complete agenesis of the corpus callosum (38). At the age of 40 months, his psychomotor development was severely retarded but slowly progressing. Two additional patients, both fetal demises in the second trimester, had severe microcephaly and other brain malformations as dominant characteristics.

REFERENCES

1. Kelley RI, Hennekam RCM. The Smith-Lemli-Opitz syndrome. *J Med Genet.* 2000;37:321–355.
2. Fitzky BU, Witsch–Baumgartner M, Erdel M, et al. Mutations in the D7-sterol reductase gene in patients with the Smith-Lemli-Opitz syndrome. *Proc Natl Acad Sci USA* 1998;95:8181–8186.
3. Wassif CA, Maslen C, Kachilele-Linjewile S, et al. Mutations in the human sterol D7-reductase gene at 11q12 – 13 cause Smith-Lemli-Opitz syndrome. *Am J Hum Genet.* 1998;63:55–62.
4. Waterham HR, Wijburg FA, Hennekam RCM, et al. The Smith-Lemli-Opitz syndrome is caused by mutations in the 7-Dehydrocholesterol reductase gene. *Am J Hum Genet.* 1998;63:329–338.
5. Jira PE, Waterham HR, Wanders RJA, et al. Smith-Lemli-Opitz syndrome and the DHCR7 gene. *Ann Hum Genet.* 2003;67:269–280.
6. Witsch-Baumgartner M, Fitzky BU, Ogorelkova M, et al. Mutational spectrum in the Delta7-sterol reductase gene and genotype-phenotype correlation in 84 patients with Smith-Lemli-Opitz syndrome. *Am J Hum Genet.* 2000;66:402–412.
7. Witsch-Baumgartner M, Gruber M, Kraft HG, et al. Maternal apo E genotype is a modifier of the Smith-Lemli-Opitz syndrome. *J Med Genet.* 2004;41:577–584.
8. Haas D, Kelley RI, Hoffmann GF. Inherited disorders of cholesterol biosynthesis. *Neuropediatrics.* 2001;32: 113–122.
9. Elias ER, Irons MB, Hurley AD, et al. Clinical effects of cholesterol supplementation in six patients with the Smith-Lemli-Opitz syndrome (SLOS). *Am J Med Genet.* 1997;68:305–310.
10. Irons M, Elias ER, Abuelo D, et al. Treatment of Smith-Lemli-Opitz syndrome: results of a multicenter trial. *Am J Med Genet.* 1997;68:311–314.
11. Sikora DM, Ruggiero M, Petit-Kekel K, et al. Cholesterol supplementation does not improve developmental progress in Smith-Lemli-Opitz syndrome. *J Pediatr.* 2004;144:783–791.
12. Jira PE, Wevers RA, de Jong J, et al. Simvastatin. A new therapeutic approach for Smith-Lemli-Opitz syndrome. *J Lipid Res.* 2000;41:1339–1346.
13. Starck L, Lovgren-Sandblom A, Bjorkhem I. Simvastatin treatment in the SLO syndrome: a safe approach? *Am J Med Genet.* 2002;113:183–189.
14. Gibson KM, Hoffmann GF, Tanaka RD, et al. Mevalonate kinase map position 12q24. *Chromosome Res.* 1997;5:150.
15. Houten SM, Koster J, Romeijn GJ, et al. Organisation of the mevalonate kinase (MVK) gene and identification of novel mutations causing mevalonic aciduria and hyperimmunoglobulinaemia D and periodic fever syndrome. *Eur J Hum Genet.* 2001;9:253–259.
16. Cuisset L, Drenth JPH, Simon A, et al. Molecular analysis of MVK mutations and enzymatic activity in hyper-IgD and periodic fever syndrome. *Eur J Hum Genet.* 2001;9:260–266.
17. Hoffmann GF, Charpentier C, Mayatepek E, et al. Clinical and biochemical phenotype in 11 patients with mevalonic aciduria. *Pediatrics.* 1993;91:915–921.
18. Prietsch V, Mayatepek E, Krastel H, et al. Mevalonate kinase deficiency –enlarging the clinical and biochemical spectrum. *Pediatrics.* 2003;111:258–261.
19. Frenkel J, Houten SM, Waterham HR, et al. Clinical and molecular variability in childhood periodic fever with hyperimmunoglobulinaemia D. *Rheumatology.* 2001;40:579–584.
20. Drenth JPH, van den Meer JWM. Hereditary periodic fever. *N Engl J Med.* 2001;345:1748–1757.
21. D'Osualdo A, Picco P, Caroli F, et al. MVK mutations and associated clinical features in Italian patients affected with autoinflammatory disorders and recurrent fever. *Eur J Hum Genet.* 2005;13:314–320.
22. Simon A, Drewe E, van der Meer JVM, et al. Simvastatin treatment for inflammatory attacks of the hyper-IgD and periodic fever syndrome. *Clin Pharmacol Ther.* 2004;75:476–483.
23. Bodar EJ, van der Hilst JC, Drenth JP, et al. Effect of etancrcept and anakinra on inflammatory attacks in the hyper-IgD syndrome: introducing a vaccination provocation model. *Neth J Med.* 2005;63:260–264.
24. Kelley RI, Wilcox WG, Smith M, et al. Abnormal sterol metabolism in patients with Conradi-Hünermann-Happle syndrome and sporadic lethal chondrodysplasia punctata. *Am J Med Genet.* 1999;83:213–219.
25. Braverman N, Lin P, Moebius FF, et al. Mutations in the gene encoding 3beta-hydroxysteroid-delta8,delta7-isomerase cause X-linked dominant Conradi-Hunerman syndrome. *Nat Genet.* 1999;22:291–294.
26. König A, Happle R, Bornholdt D, et al. Mutations in the NSDHL gene, encoding a 3beta-hydroxysteroid dehydrogenase, cause CHILD syndrome. *Am J Med Genet.* 2000;90:339–346.
27. Grange DK, Kratz LE, Braverman NE, et al. CHILD syndrome caused by deficiency of 3beta-hydroxysteroid-delta8, delta7-isomerase. *Am J Med Genet.* 2000;90:328–335.
28. Happle R, Koch H, Lenz W. The CHILD syndrome: Congenital hemidysplasia with ichthyosiform erythroderma and limb defects. *Eur J Ped Surg.* 1980;134:27–33.
29. Waterham HR, Koster J, Mooyer P, et al. Autosomal recessive HEM/Greenberg skeletal dysplasia is caused by 3beta-hydroxysterol delta14-reductase deficiency due to mutations in the Lamin B receptor gene. *Am J Hum Genet.* 2003;72:1013–1017.
30. Hoffmann K, Dreger CK, Olins AL, et al. Mutations in the gene encoding the lamin B receptor produce an altered nuclear morphology in granulocytes (Pelger-Huet anomaly). *Nat Genet.* 2002;31:410–414.
31. Oosterwijk JC, Mansour S, van Noort G, et al. Congenital abnormalities reported in Pelger-Huët homozygosity as compared to Greenberg/HEM dysplasia: highly variable expression of allelic phenotypes. *J Med Genet.* 2003;40:937–941.
32. Kelley RI, Kratz LE, Glaser RL, et al. Abnormal sterol metabolism in a patient with Antley-Bixler syndrome and ambiguous genitalia. *Am J Med Genet.* 2002;110:95–102.
33. Flück CE, Tajima T, Pandey, AV, et al. Mutant P450 oxidoreductase causes disordered steroidogenesis with and without Antley-Bixler syndrome. *Nat Genet.* 2004;36:228–230.
34. Brunetti-Pierri N, Corso G, Rossi M, et al. Lathosterolosis, a novel multiple-malformation/mental retardation syndrome due to deficiency of 3beta-hydroxysteroid-delta5-desaturase. *Am J Hum Genet.* 2002;71:952–958.
35. Krakowiak PA, Wassif CA, Kratz L, et al. Lathosterolosis: an inborn error of human and murine cholesterol synthesis due to lathosterol 5-desaturase deficiency. *Hum Mol Genet.* 2003;12:1631–1641.
36. Waterham HR, Koster J, Romeijn GJ, et al. Mutations in the 3beta-hydroxysterol delta24-reductase gene cause desmosterolosis, an autosomal recessive disorder of cholesterol biosynthesis. *Am J Hum Genet.* 2001;69:685–694.
37. FitzPatrick DR, Keeling JW, Evans MJ, et al. Clinical phenotype of desmosterolosis. *Am J Med Genet.* 1998;75:145–152.
38. Andersson HC, Kratz L, Kelley R. Desmosterolosis presenting with multiple congenital anomalies and profound developmental delay. *Am J Med Genet.* 2002;113:315–319.

Inborn Errors of Peroxisome Biogenesis and Function

Ronald J.A. Wanders, PhD

PEROXISOME BIOGENESIS

The essential features of peroxisome biogenesis have been elucidated in recent years. These features are: 1) peroxisomes are not autonomously multiplying organelles but are derived from the endoplasmic reticulum; 2) all peroxisomal proteins, including peroxisomal matrix and membrane proteins, are encoded by the nuclear genome and synthesized on free polyribosomes; 3) the newly synthesized proteins are posttranslationally imported from the cytosol into preexisting peroxisomes; and, 4) import of new peroxisomal proteins into peroxisomes leads to an expansion of the size of peroxisomes, which makes them grow until a critical size is reached. Subsequently, the peroxisomes divide into two daughter peroxisomes that can then undergo the same cycle of events. Figure 24-1 presents a simplified scheme of peroxisome biogenesis. Correct targeting of proteins to peroxisomes is achieved via so-called peroxisome targeting signals (PTSs). Peroxisomal matrix proteins are targeted to peroxisomes via one of two different targeting signals which are short, conserved stretches of amino acids at the C-terminal (PTS1) or N-terminal (PTS2) end of peroxisomal matrix proteins. PTS sequences are recognized in the cytosol by receptor proteins. The loaded receptors are then recognized specifically by the peroxisomal protein import machinery, after which the matrix proteins are translocated across the peroxisomal membrane, whereas the receptors are released back into the cytosol for another round of import.

In principle, peroxisomal membrane proteins follow a similar pathway, although the targeting signal is different as well as the receptor recognizing this signal. Correct targeting of peroxisomal proteins to peroxisomes has turned out to require a complex network of proteins, which are all essential for peroxisome biogenesis. These proteins are called *peroxins* and the corresponding genes PEX genes. So far, 32 different PEX genes have been identified in different organisms. In humans, 16 PEX genes are known now, and mutations in 12 PEX genes have been described in

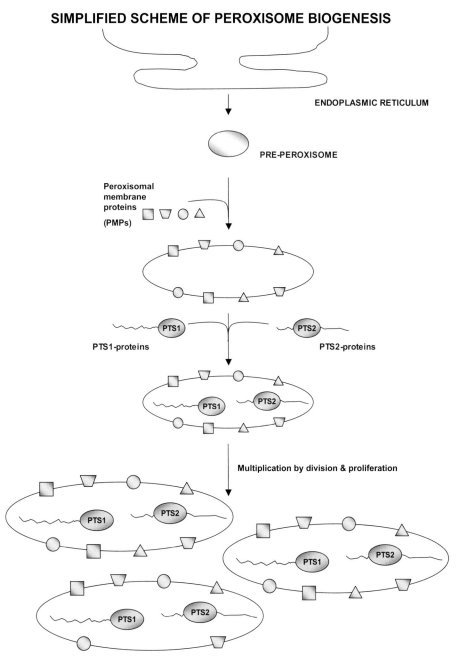

SIMPLIFIED SCHEME OF PEROXISOME BIOGENESIS

FIGURE 24-1. Schematic depicting the mechanism of peroxisome biogenesis: peroxisomes can originate from pre-existing peroxisomes by division of one peroxisome into two daughter peroxisomes, but can also be derived from the endoplasmic reticulum in the form of a pre-peroxisome, which is converted into a mature peroxisome by import of peroxisomal membrane proteins (PMPs), followed by uptake of peroxisomal matrix proteins, containing either a PTS1 or PTS2 signal.

Inborn Errors of Peroxisome Biogenesis and Function

AT-A-GLANCE

The inborn errors of peroxisome function and/or biogenesis, in short named *peroxisomal disorders,* comprise a group of 15 different diseases characterized by autosomal recessive inheritance with the exception of X-linked adrenoleukodystrophy. Although different classifications have been proposed through the years, there is now consensus to subdivide the group of peroxisomal disorders into two subgroups, including: 1) the peroxisome biogenesis disorders (PBDs); and, 2) the single-peroxisomal-enzyme/transporter deficiencies.

The PBD group is characterized by a defect in peroxisome biogenesis, either partial or generalized, and includes Zellweger syndrome (ZS), neonatal adrenoleukodystrophy (NALD), infantile Refsum disease (IRD), and rhizomelic chondrodysplasia punctata type 1 (RCDP-1). Because there is overlap in clinical signs and symptoms, the first three disorders are often referred to as *Zellweger spectrum disorders* (ZSDs), with ZS being the most severe form and NALD and IRD the less severe forms. In ZS, NALD, and IRD, peroxisome biogenesis is fully defective, caused by mutations in a number of different so-called PEX genes. RCDP-1, although belonging to the PBD group, is characterized by a partial defect in peroxisome biogenesis resulting in a distinct clinical picture and a distinct set of peroxisomal abnormalities in plasma and tissues.

The group of single-peroxisomal-enzyme/transporter deficiencies includes at least 10 disorders in which the defect involves a single peroxisomal protein, but the peroxisome structure is intact, with X-linked adrenoleukodystrophy as most frequent. For all peroxisomal disorders, post- and prenatal laboratory methods are available, whereas therapeutic options are limited. The different peroxisomal disorders with information about their occurrence, enzyme defect, mutated gene, and OMIM classification are listed below.

DISORDER	OCCURRENCE[+]	GENE	LOCUS	OMIM
Zellweger syndrome (ZS)	>500	*PEX1, PEX2,*	7q21-q22, 8q21.1	214100
Neonatal adrenoleukodystrophy (NALD)	>200	*PEX3, PEX5*	6q23-q24, 12p13.3	214100
Infantile Refsum disease (IRD)	>200	*PEX6, PEX10*	6p21.1, 1p36.32	202370
		PEX12, PEX13	17q21.1, 2p14-p16	
		PEX14, PEX16	1p36.22, 11p11.11	
		PEX19, PEX26	1q22, 22q11.21	
Rhizomelic chondrodysplasia punctata Type 1 (RCDP Type 1)	>200	PEX7	6q22-q24	215100
X-linked adrenoleukodystrophy (X-ALD)	>2000	*ABCD1*	Xq28	300100
Acyl-CoA oxidase deficiency (ACOXI-deficiency)	>20	*ACOX1*	17q25.1	264470
D-bifunctional protein deficiency (DBP-deficiency)	>200	*HSD17B4*	5q2	261515
2-Methylacyl-CoA racemase deficiency (AMACR-deficiency)	>5	*AMACR*	5q13.2-p.12	604489
Rhizomelic chondrodysplasia punctata Type 2 or DHAPAT deficiency (RCDP Type 2)	>10	*GNPAT*	1q42.1-42.3	222765
Rhizomelic chondrodysplasia punctata Type 3 or alkylDHAP synthase deficiency (RCDP Type 3)	>5	*AGPS*	2q33	600121
Refsum disease or phytanoyl-CoA hydroxylase deficiency (ARD/CRD)	>200	*PHYH / PAHX*	10p15-p14	266500
Hyperoxaluria Type 1 or alanine glyoxylate aminotransferase deficiency (PH1)	>200	*AGXT*	2q37.3	259900
Glutaric acidemia Type 3 (GA3)	1	?	?	231690
Acatalasaemia	>5	*CAT*	11p13	115500
Mulibrey nanism (MUL)	>20	*TRIM*	17q22-23	253250

*In addition to the disorders of peroxisome biogenesis described above (ZS, NALD, IRD, RCDP type1), some cases with hyperpipecolic acidaemia (HPA) have been described in literature of which at least the four original cases described by Gatfield et al., Burton et al., and Thomas et al. (see Wanders, 2004, for references) turned out to be affected by a true disorder of peroxisome biogenesis. In addition, a number of cases have been described with hyperpipecolic acidaemia, but no defect in peroxisome biogenesis. The defect in these patients has remained obscure. All peroxisomal disorders are rare, therefore, given are estimates of worldwide diagnoses.

+ = Number of reported cases.

PEROXISOMAL DISORDER	BIOCHEMICAL ABNORMALITIES					CLINICAL SIGNS AND SYMPTOMS
Biogenesis Defects	VLCFA	PRIS	PHYT	D/THCA	PL	
ZS, NALD, IRD	↑	↑[b]	↑[b]	↑	↓	ZS, NALD, and IRD represent a spectrum of disease severity with ZS being the most and IRD the least severe disorder. Common to ZS, NALD, and IRD are liver disease, variable neuro-developmental delay, retinopathy, and perceptive deafness. ZS patients are usually hypotonic from birth and die before one year of age, whereas NALD patients show neonatal onset hypotonia and seizures and have progressive white matter disease, usually dying in late infancy. IRD patients may survive beyond infancy, and some may even reach adulthood
RCDP type 1	N	N	↑[b]	N	↓	Patients have a disproportionally short stature primarily affecting the proximal parts of the extremities. Other symptoms include typical facial abnormalities, congenital contractures, ocular abberations, severe growth deficiency, and mental retardation
Single Enzyme Deficiencies	VLCFA	PRIS	PHYT	D/THCA	PL	
X-ALD	↑	N	N	N	N	Two major forms, including childhood cerebral adrenoleukodystrophy (CCALD) and adrenomyeloneuropathy (AMN); in the severe form (CCALD) normal development until 6 years of age is followed by rapid deterioration and death within two years
ACOX1D	↑	N	N	N	N	Hypotonia, early onset seizures, hearing loss, retinopathy, neurological abnormalities
DBP-deficiency	↑	↑[b]	↑[b]	↑	N	Craniofacial abnormalities; neurological disturbances; Zellweger-like phenotype, including neuronal migration defect
AMACR deficiency	N	↑[b]	↑[b]	↑	N	Slow, progressive loss of vision; neurological deterioration; in some patients marked hepatopathy
RCDP2 (DHAPAT deficiency)	N	N	N	N	↓	Severe growth retardation, mental retardation, rhizomelia, early death
RCDP3 (ADHAPS deficiency)	N	N	N	N	↓	Severe growth retardation, mental retardation, rhizomelia, early death
Refsum disease (ARD/CRD)	N	N	↑	N	N	Loss of vision, cerebellar ataxia, anosmia, ichtyosis, cardiac problems
Hyperoxaluria type 1 (AGT deficiency)	N	N	N	N	N	Progressive loss of kidney function
Acatalasaemia	N	N	N	N	N	Increased tendency to develop oral gangrene

[a]ZS, Zellweger syndrome; NALD, neonatal adrenoleukodystrophy; IRD, infantile Refsum disease; RCDP, rhizomelic chondrodysplasia punctata; X-ALD, X-linked adrenoleukodystrophy; VLCFA, very-long-chain FAs; PRIS, pristanic acid; PHYT, phytanic acid; D/THCA, di- and trihydroxycholestanoic acid; PL, plasmalogens; N, normal; ↑, elevated; ↓, decreased.

[b]Levels may vary from normal to elevated because phytanic acid and pristanic acid are derived from exogenous (dietary) sources only.

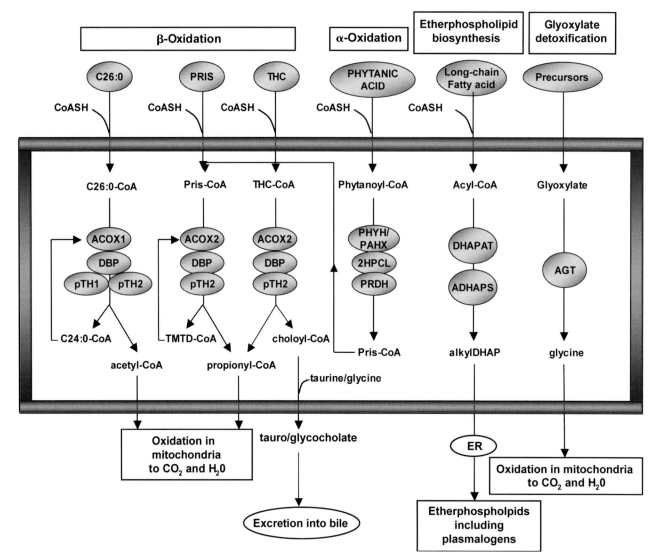

FIGURE 24-2. Schematic scheme depicting the four most important functions of peroxisomes in humans: (1) fatty acid beta-oxidation; (2) fatty acid alpha-oxidation; (3) etherphospholipids (plasmalogen) biosynthesis, and (4) glyoxylate detoxification plus the enzymes involved in the different metabolic pathways. Abbreviations used are: PRIS = pristanic acid; THC = trihydroxycholestanoic; FA = fatty acid; ACOX1 = straight-chain acyl-CoA oxidase; ACOX2 = branched-chain acyl-CoA oxidase; DBP = D-bifunctional protein; pTH1 = peroxisomal thiolase 1; pTH2 = peroxisomal thiolase 2 (SCPx); TMTD-CoA = 4,8,12-trimethyltridecanoyl-CoA; PHYH/PAHX = phytanoyl-CoA hydroxylase; 2-HPCL = 2-hydroxyphytanoyl-CoA lyase; PRDH = pristanal dehydrogenase; DHAPAT = dihydroxyacetonephosphate acyltransferase; ADHAPS = alkyl-DHAP synthase; AGT = alanine-glyoxylate aminotransferase; ER = endoplasmic reticulum

peroxisome biogenesis disorder (PBD) patients, as discussed below. Most PEX genes have orthologues in other species with only a few exceptions. This agrees with the notion that the mechanism of peroxisome biogenesis is highly conserved among eukaryotic species.

PEROXISOME FUNCTION

Peroxisomes catalyze a number of essential metabolic functions. The most important, at least in humans, are: 1) fatty acid β-oxidation; 2) etherphospholipid biosynthesis; 3) fatty acid α-oxidation; and, 4) glyoxylate detoxification (Figure 24-2). β-Oxidation of fatty acids in peroxisomes occurs via a similar mechanism as in mitochondria and involves a set of four consecutive reactions, which are the follow-

ing: 1) dehydrogenation through the two acyl-CoA oxidases, one specific for the coenzyme A esters of straight-chain fatty acids such as C26:0 (ACOX1), and the other one specific for the coenzyme A esters of 2-methyl branched-chain fatty acids such as pristanic acid and di- and trihydroxycholestanoic acid (DHCA and TCHA) (ACOX2); 2) hydration (of the double bond); 3) dehydrogenation again (note that both reactions 2 and 3 are handled by a single bifunctional enzyme called D-*bifunctional protein* [DBP], alternatively named *multifunctional enzyme II* [MFE-II] or *multifunctional protein 2* [MFP-2]); and, 4) thiolytic cleavage. Human peroxisomes contain two thiolases, pTH1 and pTH2. Both thiolases are involved in C26:0 oxidation, whereas pTH2, also named *SCPx*, is indispensable in the oxidation of the

2-methyl branched-chain fatty acids (see Figure 24-2). Of note, the enzymes just described are sufficient for the β-oxidation of straight-chain fatty acids and 2-methyl branched-chain fatty acids with the methyl group in the (2S) configuration. However the β-oxidation of (2R)-methyl branched-chain fatty acids requires the participation of 2-methylacyl-CoA racemase (AMACR), the enzyme that can convert (2R)-methylacyl-CoAs into the corresponding (2S)-methylacyl-CoAs and vice versa (Figure 24-3). Peroxisomes also are able to oxidize mono- and polyunsaturated fatty acids, which requires the active presence of a number of auxiliary enzymes to remove the double bonds.

Although the mechanisms are similar, the physiological roles of the mitochondrial and peroxisomal β-oxidation systems are

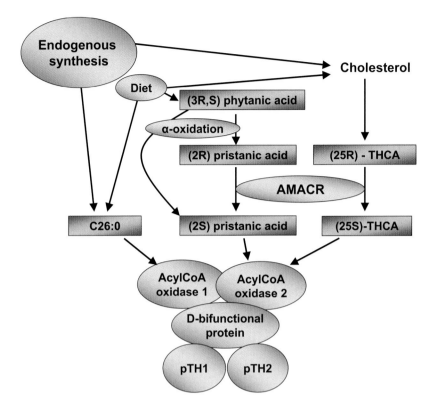

FIGURE 24-3. Schematic depicting the central role of the enzyme 2-methylacyl-CoA racemase (AMACR) and the organization of the peroxisomal beta-oxidation system and its main substrates including C26:0, pristanic acid, and trihydroxycholestanoic acid, as derived from dietary sources or via endogenous synthesis.

completely different. Indeed, whereas mitochondria oxidize the bulk of the long-chain fatty acids as derived from lipolysis and dietary sources, peroxisomes play a crucial role in the degradation of a variety of different fatty acids, including: 1) very-long-chain fatty acids (notably C26:0); 2) pristanic acid; and, 3) di- and trihydroxycholestanoic acid. The latter compounds are the direct precursors of the primary bile acids cholic acid and chenodeoxycholic acid, respectively, and are synthesized from cholesterol in the liver. In addition, the peroxisomal fatty oxidation system is only able to chain-shorten fatty acids and is not able to degrade fatty acids to completion, as can the mitochondrial oxidation system. The distinct physiological roles of the mitochondrial and peroxisomal β-oxidation systems become also clear from the marked differences in clinical signs and symptoms in patients with a defect in either mitochondrial or peroxisomal β-oxidation.

The *second* major function of peroxisomes involves etherphospholipid synthesis, which is fully dependent on peroxisomes because the first part of the etherphospholipid synthesis pathway, as mediated by the enzymes acyl-CoA reductase, dihydroxyacetonephosphate acyl-transferase (DHAPAT), and alkyldihydroxyacetonephosphate synthase (ADHAPS), is strictly localized in peroxisomes (see Figure 24-2). In humans, etherphospholipid

synthesis is crucial not only for the formation of platelet-activating factor (PAF) but also for the formation of plasmalogens, a group of ether-linked phospholipids present in heart and skeletal muscle, kidney, brain, and red blood cells. Liver has a very low content of plasmalogen. The two single-enzyme deficiencies that have been identified so far involve the first two enzymes in the etherphospholipid pathway. The first enzyme is DHAPAT, which catalyzes the esterification of dihydroxyacetone phosphate (DHAP) with a long-chain acyl-CoA ester. The second enzyme is ADHAPS, which is responsible for the formation of the characteristic ether bond at the sn-1 position of etherphospholipids by the replacement of the sn-1 fatty acid in acyl-DHAP with a long-chain alcohol to produce alkyl-DHAP. Enzymatic defects of the two enzymes result in decreased plasmalogen levels and the phenotype of rhizomelic chondrodysplasia punctata (RCDP). So far, the true physiological role of etherphospholipids in general and plasmalogens in particular has remained unresolved. The unique importance of etherphospholipids is stressed by the fact that a single defect in etherphospholipid synthesis is associated with severe clinical signs and symptoms, as observed in RCDP types 2 and 3, as discussed below.

Fatty acid α-oxidation is an alternative mechanism allowing the breakdown of fatty

acids. Most fatty acids can be degraded by β-oxidation, except for some fatty acids with a methyl group at the 3-position, such as phytanic acid, which can be degraded only via α-oxidation. The key enzyme in fatty acid α-oxidation is phytanoyl-CoA hydroxylase. The product of the hydroxylase reaction is 2-hydroxyphytanoyl-CoA, which is split into formyl-CoA and pristanal through the action of the enzyme 2-hydroxyphytanoyl-CoA lyase (see Figure 24-2). The subsequent step in the pathway, that is, the conversion of pristanal to pristanic acid remains ill-defined. α-Oxidation is strictly peroxisomal, which explains the accumulation of phytanic acid in Zellweger spectrum disorders (see Figure 24-2). Finally, peroxisomes are also indispensable for glyoxylate detoxification, which is due to the fact that the enzyme alanine glyoxylate aminotransferase is localized in peroxisomes, at least in humans (see Figure 24-2). In case of a deficiency of this enzyme, as in hyperoxaluria type 1, glyoxylate accumulates in peroxisomes and gets converted into either glycolate or oxalate, followed by precipitation of oxalate in multiple tissues as the insoluble calcium oxalate salt. In addition to the functions of peroxisomes listed earlier, peroxisomes are involved in a number of additional metabolic functions not covered here. Recent data have shown that peroxisomes are not involved in the formation of isoprenoids and cholesterol despite earlier thoughts to the contrary.

Peroxisomes play an essential role in many cellular processes with obvious consequences for embryonic and fetal development, as exemplified by the clinical signs and symptoms associated with specific disorders belonging to one of the two groups of peroxisomal disorders, including 1) the peroxisome biogenesis disorders (PBDs) and 2) the single-peroxisomal-enzyme/transporter deficiencies. The PBD group actually is composed of two subgroups; within the *first* subgroup are disorders in which peroxisome formation is fully deficient, with the subsequent loss of most, if not all, peroxisomal functions. This subgroup is referred to as the *Zellweger spectrum disorders* (ZSDs), which include Zellweger syndrome (ZS), neonatal adrenoleukodystrophy (NALD), infantile Refsum disease (IRD), and other variants not easily assignable to either disease category. The *second* subgroup includes only a single entity, called *rhizomelic chondrodysplasia punctata type 1* (RCDP1), which is characterized by a partial defect in peroxisome biogenesis at the level of the PTS2 import pathway, whereas the PTS1 import pathway functions normally. What follows is a description of the etiology/pathophysiology, presentation, diagnosis, and treatment of the peroxisomal disorders identified so far, except for: 1) glutaric aciduria type 3, which has been described in a single patient only; **2**) Mulibrey nanism, which remains to be established as a true peroxisomal disorder; and, **3**) acatalasemia. The At-A-Glance page summarizes the clinical and biochemical abnormalities in the different peroxisomal disorders, which will be discussed in more detail below.

PEROXISOME BIOGENESIS DISORDERS

PBD Subgroup 1: Zellweger Syndrome (ZS), Neonatal Adrenoleukodystrophy (NALD), and Infantile Refsum Disease (IRD)

Etiology/Pathophysiology In ZS and the other ZSDs, the fundamental problem is the inability to synthesize peroxisomes, which is caused by mutations in one of the many genes whose correct expression is required for proper peroxisome formation. As a consequence, most, if not all, peroxisomal functions are lost in ZSD patients, leading to: **1**) the accumulation of a range of metabolites, including very-long-chain fatty acids (VLCFAs), phytanic acid, pristanic acid, and pipecolic acid; and, **2**) a deficiency of other compounds, including etherphospholipids. The exact pathophysiological mechanism underlying the different ZSDs is unclear, although the pathophysiological role of the peroxisomal β-oxidation system seems clear from the fact that patients with an isolated defect in the peroxisomal β-oxidation system at the level of

D-bifunctional protein also may present with a Zellweger-like syndrome.

Literature data indicate that there is a distinct correlation between the extent of peroxisomal dysfunction and the phenotype of ZSD patients. Furthermore, there appears to be a correlation between certain genotypes and the severity of the clinical signs and symptoms, as exemplified by the G843D mutation, which, at least in its homozygous form, is associated with a less severe phenotype, such as infantile Refsum disease.

Clinical Presentation ZS is dominated by: **1**) the typical craniofacial dysmorphia, including a high forehead, large anterior fontanel, hypoplastic supraorbital ridges, epicanthal folds, and deformed earlobes; and, **2**) profound neurological abnormalities (see Figure 24-4). ZS children show severe psychomotor retardation, profound hypotonia, neonatal seizures, glaucoma, retinal degeneration, and impaired hearing (1). There is usually calcific stippling of the epiphyses and small renal cysts. Brain abnormalities in ZS include not only cortical dysplasia and neuronal heterotopias but also regressive changes. There is dysmyelination rather than demyelination (1). Patients with NALD have hypotonia, seizures, possibly polymicrogyria, and progressive white matter disease, and they usually die in late infancy. Patients with IRD may have external features reminiscent of ZS but do not show disordered neuronal migration and no progressive white matter disease. Their cognitive and motor development varies between severe global handicaps and moderate learning disabilities

with deafness and visual impairment due to retinopathy. Their survival is variable. Most patients with IRD reach childhood, and some even reach adulthood. Clinical distinction between the different PBD phenotypes is not very well defined. Common to all three are liver disease, variable neurodevelopmental delay, retinopathy, and perceptive deafness with onset in the first months of life. In addition to ZS, NALD, and IRD, overlapping phenotypes as well as additional phenotypes have been described in the literature that do not belong to either disease category.

Diagnosis/Laboratory Findings As a consequence of the inability to synthesize peroxisomes, most, if not all, peroxisomal functions are lost, which results in multiple biochemical abnormalities in plasma and tissues of ZSD patients (see Figure 24-2 and the At-A-Glance page). These include:

- Nonspecific laboratory findings such as (conjugated) hyperbilirubinemia, elevated liver transaminases, hypoprothrombinemia, and elevated serum iron levels

- Elevated plasma/serum very-long-chain fatty acid levels as a result of an impaired peroxisomal β-oxidation. The most important diagnostic parameters are the absolute level of C26:0 and the C26:0/C22:0 ratio. Both parameters are elevated in virtually all ZSD patients.

- Elevated plasma/serum levels of the bile acid intermediates di- and trihydroxycholestanoic acids (DHCA and THCA), which are elevated in most, if not all, ZSD patients.

- Elevated plasma/serum levels of the branched-chain fatty acids, phytanic acid, and pristanic acid. Because phytanic acid and pristanic acid are derived from exogenous (dietary) sources only, levels in plasma may vary wildly from normal to markedly abnormal.

- Elevated plasma/serum and urinary levels of L-pipecolic acid. Note that L-pipecolic acid levels may vary wildly from normal to markedly abnormal.

- Abnormal profile of urinary organic acids, including (nonketotic) dicarboxylic aciduria with an elevated sebacic acid/adipic acid ratio, epoxydicarboxylic aciduria, and elevated 2-hydroxysebacic acid. Urinary organic acids are abnormal in most, but not all, ZSD patients.

- Reduced plasmalogen levels in erythrocytes and tissues because of deficient etherphospholipid biosynthesis. Note that erythrocyte plasmalogen levels are deficient (<10% of control) only in the severe forms of ZSD, including classical ZS, whereas levels usually are mildly reduced (30% to 50% of control)

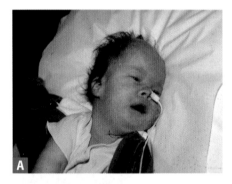

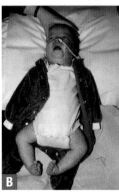

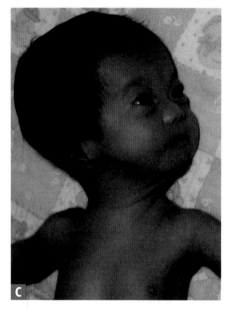

FIGURE 24-4. A to **C.** Characteristic phenotype of infants presenting with Zellweger (photos used by permission of Susan Berry, M.D. and Robert Gorlin, D.D.S., M.S., D.Sc., University of Minnesota Medical School).

to normal in NALD and IRD patients. Subsequent to the analysis in plasma and erythrocytes, as described earlier, fibroblasts studies should be done with the ultimate aim of pinpointing the molecular defect, which requires complementation analysis. The abnormalities in fibroblasts include:

- Deficient formation of etherphospholipids, including plasmalogens

- Deficient activity of the two peroxisomal enzymes, dihydroxyacetonephosphate acyltransferase (DHAPAT) and alkyl-dihydroxyacetonephosphate synthase (ADHAPS)

- Accumulation of the very-long-chain fatty acid C26:0 with an elevated C26:0/C22:0 ratio

- Deficient peroxisomal β-oxidation of C26:0 and pristanic acid

- Deficient α-oxidation of phytanic acid

- Absence of several peroxisomal proteins, as shown by immunoblot analysis

- Absence of peroxisomes as assessed by immunofluorescence microscopy analysis

The set of abnormalities listed above is found only in fibroblasts from patients with a severe type of ZSD, such as ZS. In fibroblasts of milder affected patients, the abnormalities may be much less pronounced, with only partial deficiencies for most parameters measured. In such cases, growth of fibroblasts at 40°C, rather than at 37°C, may help because at 40°C, the abnormalities found tend to be more severe (2). In exceptional cases, no abnormalities are found in fibroblasts.

If fibroblast studies have shown that the patient is truely affected by a ZSD, complementation studies need to be done to determine the complementation group to which the patient belongs. Complementation analysis involves the fusion of fibroblasts of two different ZSD patients to yield heterokaryons, which contain the DNA from the two different ZSD patients. This implies that if the mutated genes in the two patients are different, peroxisome biogenesis will be restored in the heterokaryons, whereas no restoration of peroxisome biogenesis will take place if the mutated genes in the two patients are identical. Large-scale complementation studies have been performed that have led to identification of 12 different complementation groups, which are now known to be caused by mutations in the following genes: PEX1, PEX2, PEX3, PEX5, PEX6, PEX10, PEX12, PEX13, PEX14, PEX16, PEX19, and PEX26. Molecular analysis of these PEX genes is carried out in a few centers around the world.

If clear-cut abnormalities have been detected in fibroblasts from an index patient in a particular family requesting prenatal diagnosis, prenatal diagnosis can be done using biochemical and/or molecular methods. Molecular analysis is definitely the method of choice, but it requires prior determination of mutation(s) in the relevant PEX gene.

- First-line testing should include (Figure 24-5 presents a flowchart) fasting plasma/serum VLCFA analysis, preferably by gas chromatography–mass spectrometry (GC-MS). If abnormal, one can be sure that the patient is suffering from a ZSD or some other peroxisomal disorder, including acyl-CoA oxidase deficiency or D-bifunctional protein deficiency. Additional studies in fibroblasts have to be done to resolve whether the patient is affected by a disorder of peroxisome biogenesis or a defect in peroxisomal β-oxidation. If plasma VLCFAs are normal, a peroxisomal disorder including a ZSD in general is excluded, although in exceptional cases the VLCFA profile may be deceptively normal. Additional studies in plasma (notably analysis of bile acid intermediates) and fibroblasts are warranted in such cases (see Figure 24-5).

Definitive diagnosis of a ZSD is obtained by detailed studies in fibroblasts, including complementation analysis (see Figure 24-5). Molecular analysis is possible if complementation studies have identified the complementation group. Prenatal diagnosis is possible using biochemical and/or molecular methods.

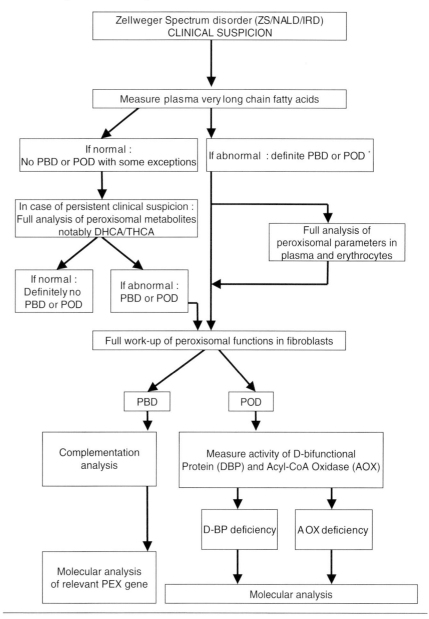

FIGURE 24-5. Flowchart for the differential diagnosis of patients with clinical signs and symptoms suggestive of a Zellweger spectrum disorder. Modified from Wanders and Waterham (2005) Clin. Genet 67, 107–133.

Treatment There is no curative therapy presently available for the ZSDs. Treatment has focused on symptomatic therapy and should include evaluation of feeding, hearing, vision, liver function, and neurological and developmental function. All patients benefit from the use of hearing aids and other assistive devices. Appropriate educational programs also are recommended. It is important that the child be provided adequate calories, which often includes feeding by means of a gastrostomy tube. The use of a specific diet low in phytanic acid is advocated by avoiding cow's milk and products derived from it to reduce exposure to phytanic acid. Since many children have some degree of malabsorption, elemental formulas may be better tolerated. Coagulation and other synthetic liver functions should be monitored, and supplementation of vitamin K and other fat-soluble vitamins is recommended. Liver dysfunction may lead to varices that respond to sclerosing therapies. Bile acid therapy involving cholic acid (100 mg/day) plus chenodeoxycholic acid (100 mg/day) may improve liver function by reducing the accumulation of the bile acid synthesis intermediates DHCA and THCA (3).

Seizures are present in many patients and sometimes are difficult to control. Standard antiepileptic drugs may be used. The use of docosahexaenoic acid (DHA) has been suggested, notably by Martinez and coworkers (4), who have administered DHA to ZSD patients in the form of docosahexaenoic acid ethyl ester at 100–500 mg/day. DHA is important for brain and retina function and is low in patients affected by a severe ZSD. The efficacy of DHA supplementation in ZSD patients is still under debate.

PDB Subgroup 2: Rhizomelic Chondrodysplasia Punctata Type 1

Etiology/Pathophysiology RCDP type 1 is caused by mutations in the PEX7 gene, which codes for the PTS2 receptor (see Figure 24-6 which depicts the normal pathway). If the PTS2 receptor is absent or dysfunctional, correct import of PTS2 proteins such as alkyl-DHAP synthase and phytanoyl-CoA hydroxylase fails, which leads to a block in: 1) the formation of etherphospholipids, including plasmalogens; and, 2) the oxidation of phytanic acid (see Figure 24-7 for clarification). Our own experience in more than 100 RCDP type 1 patients has shown that plasmalogen levels in erythrocytes, when analysed, in tissues are always markedly deficient, whereas phytanic acid levels may vary from normal to elevated depending on the age of the patient and the

amount of phytanic acid taken in via the diet. Although the exact pathophysiological mechanism is not known at present, it is clear that the clinical signs and symptoms of RCDP are related directly to the inability to synthesize etherphospholipids. This is concluded from the fact that a single deficiency at the level of DHAPAT or alkyl-DHAP synthase, as in RCDP types 2 and 3, is associated with the same clinical signs and symptoms.

Clinical Presentation In its classical form, RCDP is clinically characterized by a disproportionally short stature primarily affecting the proximal parts of the extremities, facial features as a broad nasal bridge, highly arched palate, dysplastic ears, micrognathia, congenital contractures, and severe mental retardation with spasticity (5) (see Figure 24-8). Roentgenological studies have shown symmetrical shortening of femur and humerus with irregular and broad metaphyses, calcific stippling mainly of the epiphyses, absent femur head nucleus, coronal clefts of vertebrae, increased intervertebral disk spaces, cupping of dorsal ribs, and a barrel-formed thorax. Review of unpublished cases from our center and patients described in literature shows that calcific stippling of the epiphyses and periarticular areas is present in all patients younger than 18 months of age and disappears in older patients. The femoral heads remain severely deformed, and all patients also lack a clear nucleus of the femur head. No coronal cleft was noted in the majority of patients older than 3 years of age. In most cases, the spinal column showed irregular and/or small disks with increased distances between the vertebrae. In patients older than 10 years of age, x-rays of the chest show signs of chronic infections and a barrel-shaped thorax with severe torsion scoliosis.

Diagnosis/Laboratory Findings As a consequence of mutations in the PEX7 gene, which codes for the PTS2 receptor, peroxisome biogenesis is impaired in RCDP type 1 at the level of the PTS2 import pathway. This results in a functional deficiency of all PTS2 proteins, including alkyl-DHAP synthase, phytanoyl-CoA hydroxylase, and peroxisomal thiolase (pTH1) (see Figure 24-7), and the subsequent inability to synthesize etherphospholipids, including plasmalogens, and α-oxidize phytanic acid. The deficiency of peroxisomal thiolase 1 (pTH1) has no consequences because the function of pTH1 is taken over by the other peroxisomal thiolase, pTH2 (SCPx) (see Figure 24-2). This results in the following laboratory abnormalities:

- Deficiency of erythrocyte plasmalogens. Note that erythrocyte plasmalogens are

deficient in all RCDP type 1 patients, including those with a mild form of disease, typified by lack of rhizomelia and survival into the second or third decade.

- Deficiency of platelet-activating factor (PAF). Note that PAF may be normal in mild RCDP type 1 patients.

- Accumulation of phytanic acid but not pristanic acid in plasma. Note that since phytanic acid is derived from exogenous dietary sources only, phytanic acid levels may vary from normal to markedly abnormal. Since β-oxidation of pristanic acid is normal in RCDP type 1, plasma pristanic acid levels are normal in RCDP type 1 patients.

If fibroblasts studies are performed subsequent to analyses in plasma and erythrocytes, the following abnormalities are found:

- Deficient formation of etherphospholipids, including plasmalogens
- Deficiency of ADHAPS
- Partial deficiency of DHAPAT
- Deficient α-oxidation of phytanic acid
- Mislocalization of peroxisomal thiolase in its abnormal 44-kDa precursor form to the cytosol
- Mutations in the PEX7 gene

First-line testing should include analysis of plasmalogen levels in erythrocytes of candidate patients (Figure 24-9 presents a flowchart). If normal, one of the peroxisomal forms of RCDP, including type 1, type 2, or type 3, is excluded. If abnormal, one can be sure of either RCDP type 1, type 2, or type 3. Differentiation between the three types requires detailed studies in fibroblasts, followed by molecular testing of either PEX7, GNPAT, or AGPS (see Figure 24-9).

Plasma phytanic acid analysis should not be used as a first-line test because it is normal in RCDP types 2 and 3 and also may be normal in type 1 patients depending on their age and dietary intake of phytanic acid and its precursors. If both erythrocyte plasmalogens and plasma phytanic acid are abnormal, the patient is almost definitely suffering from RCDP type 1, which may prompt direct molecular analysis of PEX7. Prenatal diagnosis is possible for RCDP type 1 using biochemical and/or molecular methods, with preference for the latter.

Treatment At this moment, there are no realistic options for treatment in RCDP type 1 patients except for a diet restricted in phytanic acid in milder affected patients. Phytanic acid is especially high in ruminant (i.e., cow, sheep, and goat) products and some fish (e.g., cod).

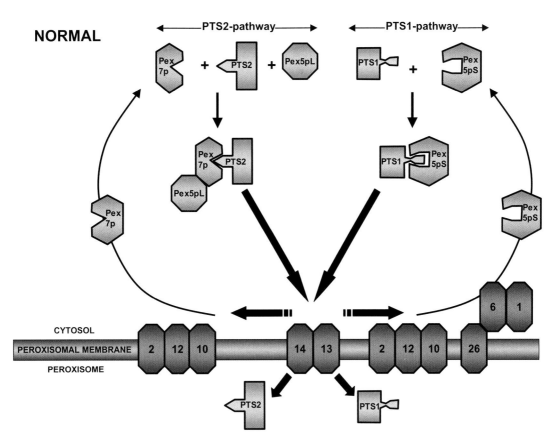

FIGURE 24-6. Peroxisome biogenesis in humans and its essential features in which the presumed roles of the different peroxins is shown within the frame work of the original peroxisome biogenesis model. Modified from Wanders and Waterham (2005) Clin. Genet 67, 107–133.

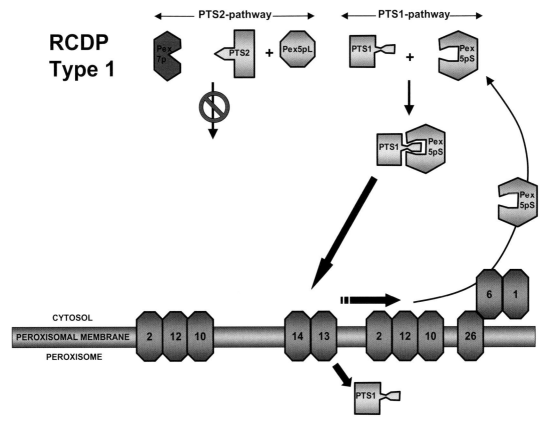

FIGURE 24-7. RCDP type 1 is depicted, in which the *PEX7* gene is mutated, causing the functional loss of the PTS2 receptor; as a result PST2-containing proteins can not be imported into peroxisomes; peroxisomal matrix proteins, containing the PTS1 signal, are imported as PTS1 receptor remain normal. Modified from Wanders and Waterham (2005) Clin. Genet 67, 107–133.

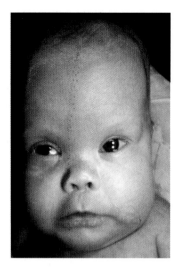

FIGURE 24-8. Infant presenting with Chondrodysplasia, rhizomelic type I.

DISORDERS OF PEROXISOME FUNCTION

X-Linked Adrenoleukodystrophy (X-ALD)

Etiology/Pathophysiology The key biochemical abnormality in X-ALD is the accumulation of saturated VLCFAs in plasma, fibroblasts, and other cell types. Excess hexacosanoic acid (C26:0) is the most striking and characteristic feature of X-ALD. The accumulation of VLCFAs is due to the deficient capacity to degrade these fatty acids, a function normally carried out by peroxisomes. The protein involved in X-ALD is called *ALDP* and is encoded by the *ABCD1* gene and belongs to the family of ABC proteins. Importantly, ALDP is a so-called half-ABC transporter, which implies that ALDP is probably active only after homodimerization (with ALDP) or heterodimerization (with one of the three other peroxisomal half-ABC transporters). ALDP has been claimed to carry VLCFAs across the peroxisomal membrane, although definitive proof is still lacking.

The mechanism behind the toxicity of VLCFAs has remained obscure so far. Pathological changes in X-ALD are restricted to the brain and spinal cord white matter, the adrenal cells, and the Leydig cells in the testis. The adrenal dysfunction may be a direct consequence of the accumulation of VLCFAs. The cells in the zona fasciculata are distended with abnormal lipids, which may interfere directly with the production of active steroids. In addition, C26:0 excess increases the viscosity of membranes, and this, in turn, may interfere with adrenal cell function.

Whether VLCFAs affect the nervous system in the same way is unclear. The nervous system of patients with childhood cerebral ALD (CCALD) shows acute and relatively symmetrical demyelinative lesions that involve the parieto-occipital regions most severely. In addition to the myelin breakdown, there is perivascular infiltration of lymphocytes, resembling that seen in multiple sclerosis. Most other tissues are intact. A third or more of patients with adrenoleukodystrophy are free of nervous system involvement or develop a milder disability in childhood. Thus nervous system involvement may depend on some factors beyond the VLCFA excess, such as autoimmune or cytokine-mediated reactions somehow triggered by the abnormal accumulation of VLCFAs. The interplay among these metabolic rearrangements, immunological factors, and demyelination remains unclear (6).

Clinical Presentation X-ALD is the most common single peroxisomal disorder, with a minimum incidence of 1 in 21,000 males in the United States and 1 in 15,000 males in France. The phenotype varies widely. At present, seven relatively distinct phenotypes are distinguished, of which three present in childhood (Table 24-1). The two most frequent phenotypes are childhood cerebral

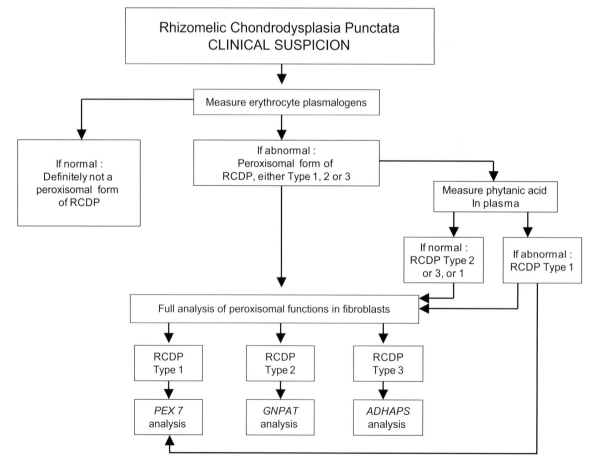

FIGURE 24-9. Flowchart for the differential diagnosis of patients with clinical signs and symptoms suggestive of rhizomelic chondrodysplasia punctata.

TABLE 24-1	Frequency of Phenotypes in X-ALD
Phenotype	**Frequency (%)**
Childhood cerebral	31–39
Adolescent cerebral	0–4.8
Adult cerebral	1–2.8
Adrenomyeloneuropathy	26.4–46
Addison only	6–14
Asymptomatic	3.6–8.6

Adapted from Ref. 15.

ALD (CCALD) and adrenomyeloneuropathy (AMN). In CCALD, symptoms are first noted most commonly at between 4 and 8 years of age. The most common initial manifestations are hyperactivity, which is often mistaken for an attention deficit disorder, and worsening school performance in a child who previously had been a good student. Auditory discrimination is often impaired, although tone perception is preserved. Spatial orientation is often impaired. Other initial symptoms include visual disturbances, ataxia, poor handwriting, seizures, and strabismus. Seizures occur in nearly all patients and in fact may represent the first manifestation of the disease. CCALD tends to progress rapidly with increasing spasticity and paralysis, visual and hearing loss, and loss of the ability to speak or swallow. The mean interval between the first neurological symptom and apparently vegetative state is 1.9 ± 2 years (range 0.5–10.5 years). The cerebral phenotype is observed not only in childhood but may also present later in adolescence (adolescent cerebral ALD) or adulthood (adult cerebral ALD). AMN is the second most frequent phenotype of X-ALD (6). The onset of neurological symptoms in this phenotype usually occurs in the third and fourth decades. Neurological deficits are due primarily to myelopathy and to a lesser extent neuropathy. Patients gradually develop a progressive spastic paraparesis due to low-tracked degeneration in the spinal cord, often in combination with a disturbed vibration sense in the legs and sphincter dysfunction. The mean age of onset of AMN is 28 ± 9 years. At least 40% of AMN patients do develop some cerebral involvement associated with a more rapid downhill progression.

X-ALD can present with Addison disease and/or crisis and should be investigated in boys as well as in adults with Addison disease. It is important to emphasize that approximately 40% of women heterozygous for X-ALD develop AMN-like symptoms in middle age or later. Cerebral involvement and adrenocortical insufficiency are rare, however.

First-line testing should include:

- VLCFA analysis in plasma, which is fully reliable for detection of hemizygotes.

Molecular testing of ABCD1 is possible. >200 different mutations have been identified so far. Prenatal diagnosis is possible using biochemical or preferably molecular methods.

Diagnosis/Laboratory Findings Biochemical abnormalities can be summarized as follows:

- Accumulation of VLCFAs, notably C26:0, in plasma
- Deficient peroxisomal β-oxidation of C26:0 in lymphocytes and fibroblasts
- Mutations in ABCD1

It should be noted that plasma VLCFA analysis is a very reliable method for diagnosis with very few, if any, false-negative results. Plasma VLCFA analysis is less robust in the case of carrier detection, as concluded from studies in obligate heterozygotes showing normal values in 20% of patients. Now that molecular analysis of ABCD1 has become available, molecular testing is the preferred diagnostic modality.

Treatment It is crucially important to provide adrenal steroid hormone therapy for every ALD patient with adrenal cortical insufficiency. Almost all affected boys and 60% of men with AMN have impaired adrenal reserve (6). Most X-ALD patients have increased plasma adrenocorticotropin (ACTH) levels and impairment of cortisol responsiveness to a 0.25-mg intravenous dose of cosyntropin (Cortrosyn) after 60 minutes. Moser and colleagues (6) recommend that at least one of these tests be performed yearly. All diagnosed patients should undergo an ACTH stimulation test to detect frank adrenal failure or subclinical decreased adrenal cortical reserve. If left untreated, these patients may succumb to adrenal crises. Adrenal steroid hormone therapy does not appear to alter the course of neurological deterioration, however. Based on the success of dietary restriction of phytanic acid in Refsum disease, a diet low in C26:0 was tried in X-ALD patients without success. Subsequently, dietary therapy based on supplementation with oleic acid and erucic acid (GTO/GTE) was tried, again without success. Current evidence suggests that bone-marrow transplantation is still the only effective treatment of X-ALD, provided that graft-versus-host reactions do not occur, immunosuppressive drugs are tolerated, and transplantation is performed early in the course of the disease.

Acyl-CoA Oxidase Deficiency

Etiology/Pathophysiology Peroxisomes contain two different acyl-CoA oxidases called ACOX1 and ACOX2. ACOX1 is involved in the β-oxidation of saturated fatty acids, whereas ACOX2, also called *branched-chain acyl-CoA oxidase*, is involved in the oxidation of 2-methyl branched-chain fatty acid such as pristanic acid and di- and trihydroxycholestanoic acid. So far, only patients with a deficiency at the level of ACOX1 have been described in the literature. Since ACOX1 is only involved in the oxidation of saturated fatty acids, the only abnormality in ACOX1-deficient patients is the accumulation of VLCFAs, notably C26:0.

The pathological mechanism behind the clinical signs and symptoms of acyl-CoA oxidase deficiency has remained obscure. Interestingly, although VLCFAs accumulate both in X-ALD and acyl-CoA oxidase deficiency, the clinical signs and symptoms associated with the two diseases are quite different. Whether or not this has to do with the more marked accumulation of VLCFAs in acyl-CoA oxidase–deficient patients remains to be established.

Clinical Presentation So far, only very few patients have been described in the literature (7). In general, the clinical presentation of acyl-CoA oxidase deficiency mimics that of NALD in many respects. Most patients show neonatal-onset hypotonia, failure to thrive, sensory deafness, hepatomegaly, delayed motor development, absent reflexes, retinopathy with extinguished electroretinograms, and frequent convulsions. Although dysmorphic features usually are absent, some patients with acyl-CoA oxidase deficiency have been described with dysmorphic features. Some patients do show some development, as exemplified by head control at 5 months, crawling at 12 months, and walking without assistance at 32 months in one patient described in literature.

Diagnosis/Laboratory Findings The deficient activity of acyl-CoA oxidase gives rise to a number of biochemical abnormalities, including:

- Accumulation of VLCFAs in plasma.
- Deficient oxidation of C26:0 but not of pristanic acid in fibroblasts. This follows logically from the fact that the CoA-esters of C26:0 and pristanic acid are handled by different acyl-CoA oxidases (see Figure 24-2).
- Mutations in ACOX1, the gene coding for acyl-CoA oxidase 1.

Treatment At this time, no realistic options for therapy have been described for acyl-CoA oxidase deficiency.

D-Bifunctional Protein Deficiency

Etiology/Pathophysiology D-Bifunctional protein (DBP), alternatively called *multifunctional protein 2* (MFP-2), *multifunctional enzyme II* (MFE-II), or D-*specific peroxisomal bifunctional enzyme* (D-PBE), catalyzes the second and third steps of peroxisomal β-oxidation and plays a key role in the oxidation of all fatty acids oxidized in peroxisomes. A deficiency of DBP leads to a block in the peroxisomal β-oxidation of all fatty acids and fatty acid derivatives, including: **1)** VLCFAs; **2)** pristanic acid; **3)** di- and trihydroxycholestanoic acid; **4)** long-chain dicarboxylic acid; and, **5)** certain thromboxanes and prostaglandins. The pathological mechanisms behind the devastating consequences of a defect in DBP have remained unresolved. Especially interesting is that the clinical signs and symptoms of patients deficient in DBP strongly resemble those observed in the ZSDs, including central nervous system (CNS) abnormalities, such as disordered neuronal migration leading to characteristic cytoarchitectonic abnormalities involving the cerebral hemispheres, cerebellum, and inferior olivary complex (8). The absence of these abnormalities in X-ALD patients may exclude VLCFAs as pathogenetic factors, although it must be emphasized that VLCFA levels usually are much higher in DBP-deficient patients (5- to 10-fold higher compared with controls) than in X-ALD patients (3- to 5-fold higher compared with controls). On the other hand, it is also difficult to imagine that pristanic acid and the bile acid intermediates are important in the pathophysiology of DBP deficiency because patients suffering from 2-methylacyl-CoA racemase deficiency, in which pristanic acid and the bile acid intermediates also accumulate, show no CNS involvement, as observed in DBP deficiency. Clearly, much remains to be learned about the pathogenic factors involved.

Clinical Presentation The clinical signs and symptoms of DBP deficiency are in general very severe (8). This is immediately clear if it is realized that, in retrospect, the first case of DBP deficiency was described as pseudo–Zellweger syndrome. In general, children with DBP deficiencies show severe CNS involvement with profound hypotonia, uncontrolled seizures, and failure to acquire any significant developmental milestones. Infants usually are full-term and show no evidence of intrauterine growth retardation. Dysmorphic features, including macrocephaly, high forehead, flat natal bridge, low-set ears, large open fontanelles, and micrognathia are found in most children. As described earlier, neuronal migra-

First-line testing should include:

- VLCFA analysis in plasma. If abnormal, the levels of pristanic acid and di- and trihydroxycholestanoic acid should be measured, followed by detailed studies in fibroblasts to pinpoint the enzymatic defect.

Prenatal diagnosis of DBP deficiency is possible using biochemical and preferably molecular methods.

tion is disturbed in most cases with areas of polymicrogyria and heterotopic neurons in the cerebrum and cerebellum. Only very few patients with a milder clinical course have been described in literature. In these patients, cranial facial dysmorphia is absent, and the clinical picture resembles that observed in IRD patients.

Diagnosis/Laboratory Findings The deficient activity of DBP leads to a number of biochemical abnormalities, including:

- Elevated plasma VLCFA levels.

- Elevated plasma pristanic acid level. Note that pristanic acid is derived from dietary sources only, which explains that levels may vary from normal to markedly abnormal.

- Accumulation of the bile acid intermediates di- and trihydroxycholestanoic acid.

- Deficient β-oxidation of C26:0 and pristanic acid in fibroblasts.

- Deficient activity of either the enoyl-CoA hydratase and/or 3-hydroxyacyl-CoA dehydrogenase components of DBP.

- Mutations in HSD17B4, the gene encoding DBP.

Treatment At this time, no realistic options for therapy have been described for DBP deficiency.

2-Methyl-acyl-CoA Racemase Deficiency

Etiology/Pathophysiology 2-Methyl-acyl-CoA racemase plays a crucial role in the oxidation of 2-methyl branched-chain fatty acids such as pristanic acid and di- and trihydroxycholestanoic acids. The reason is that the peroxisomal β-oxidation system only reacts with 2-methyl branched-chain fatty acids in which the methyl group has the right (2S) configuration (see Figure 24-3) (9). Since pristanic acid, as well as di- and trihydroxycholestanoic acids, also occurs in the wrong (2R) configuration, 2-methyl-acyl-CoA racemase is required to convert a (2R)-methyl group into the correct (2S)-methyl group. With respect to the patho-

genesis of 2-methyl-acyl-CoA racemase deficiency, there is currently no information in the literature.

Clinical Presentation So far, only very few patients have been described with 2-methyl-acyl-CoA racemase deficiency (10). Although only four patients have been described so far, it is already clear that the clinical signs and symptoms of 2-methyl-acyl-CoA racemase deficiency may differ markedly. Indeed, the first two patients were characterized by an adult-onset sensorimotor neuropathy, whereas a recently identified patient presented very early in life with fulminant liver failure. At this time, it is too early to tell what the dominant phenotype of 2-methyl-acyl-CoA racemase deficiency will be.

Diagnosis/Laboratory Findings The following abnormalities are found in 2-methyl-acyl-CoA racemase deficiency:

- Accumulation of both pristanic acid and the bile acid intermediates di- and trihydroxycholestanoic acids

- Partial block in the peroxisomal β-oxidation of pristanic acid

- Mutations in AMACR, the gene coding for 2-methyl-acyl-CoA racemase

Treatment Given the fact that patients with 2-methyl-acyl-CoA racemase deficiency accumulate both pristanic acid and phytanic acid, and knowing that these two fatty acids are derived from dietary sources only, a diet reduced in phytanic acid seems advisable in 2-methyl-acyl-CoA racemase–deficient patients, following the same guidelines as used for the dietary treatment of adult Refsum disease patients. Cholic acid should be substituted.

Refsum Disease, Adult Form

Etiology/Pathophysiology The exact pathogenetic mechanism explaining the toxicity of phytanic acid to neuronal, cardiac, and bone tissue has remained obscure. Retinal degeneration seems to be due to the excess deposition of phytanic acid in ocular tissue. Pathological examinations have revealed an almost complete loss of photoreceptors, thinning of the inner nuclear layer, and reduction of the number of ganglion cells of the retina. It could be that these phenomena are due to the deleterious effect of phytanic acid itself because phytanic acid is readily incorporated into phospholipids. In this respect, it should be noted that photoreceptor cells are rich in docosahexaenoic acid (DHA), and recent studies have shown that rat retina photoreceptor cells depend on DHA for there survival and differentiation because in the absence of DHA, photoreceptor cell apoptosis is markedly increased. Although DHA is normal in Refsum patients, it could well be that phytanic acid, through its incorporation in phospholipids, disturbs photoreceptor membranes. Whether this membrane distortion hypothesis is also responsible for the polyneuropathy observed in Refsum patients, which is of the mixed motor and sensory type and mainly affects the distal part of the lower limbs with muscular atrophy, weakness, and sensory disturbances, remains to be established. Finally, it is very likely that the biochemical abnormalities in Refsum disease are not restricted to the accumulation of phytanic acid only, which is due to the deficiency of phytanoyl-CoA hydroxylase (see Figure 24-2). Instead, it is more likely that the α-oxidation pathway plays a much broader role in the degradation of fatty acids, not restricted to the oxidation of phytanic acid only.

Clinical Presentation Patients in whom adult Refsum disease (ARD) is destined to develop are perfectly normal as infants, show no obvious defects in growth and development, and usually present in late childhood with progressive loss of night vision, a decline in visual capacity, and anosmia (11,12). After 10–15 years or more, patients may develop additional abnormalities, including deafness, ataxia, polyneuropathy, icthyosis, and cardiac disturbances. Short metacarpals and/or metatarsals are found in around 30% of patients. The full constellation of cardinal features as defined by Refsum in the 1940s, which includes retinitis pigmentosa (RP), cerebellar ataxia, and chronic polyneuropathy, is seen rarely in single ARD patients. Indeed, whereas RP is an early clinical sign present in all ARD patients, ataxia and polyneuropathy develop later and are observed in only around 70% and 50% of patients, respectively. Virtually every individual ultimately diagnosed as having ARD experiences visual symptoms first. The delay between first ophthalmological evaluation and the diagnosis of ARD is enormous, ranging from 1–28 years with a mean of 11 years. Night blindness and loss of visual capacity, especially when combined with anosmia, should lead to prompt analysis of plasma phytanic acid in order to start therapy. Furthermore, electroretinography (ERG) should be done, which shows either a reduction or a complete loss of rod and cone responses. Over the years, a concentric visual field constriction develops, and finally, only tubular vision remains.

The polyneuropathy is of a mixed motor and sensory type that is asymmetrical, chronic, and progressive in untreated ARD patients. Initially, symptoms often wax and wane. Later, the distal lower limbs are affected with muscular atrophy and weakness. Over the course of years, muscular weakness can become widespread and disability involving not only the limbs but also the trunk. Almost without exception, individuals with Refsum disease have peripheral sensory disturbances, most often impairment of deep sensation, particularly perception of vibration and position/motion in the distal legs.

Diagnosis/Laboratory Findings The following abnormalities are found in ARD:

- Elevated phytanic acid levels in plasma and tissues
- Deficient α-oxidation of phytanic acid in cultured skin fibroblasts and deficient activity of the enzyme phytanoyl-CoA hydroxylase
- Mutations in the PAHX/PHYH gene

Rhizomelic Chondrodysplasia Punctata Types 2 and 3

Etiology/Pathophysiology RCDP types 2 and 3 are caused by mutations in the two genes GNPAT and AGPS, which code for the first (DHAPAT) and second (ADHAPS) enzymes involved in etherphospholipid biosynthesis. A deficiency of either DHAPAT or ADHAPS leads to a block in etherphospholipid biosynthesis, which results in deficient formation of all etherphospholipids, including plasmalogens and platelet-activating factor (PAF). As a result of a deficiency of either DHAPAT or ADHAPS, plasmalogen levels are deficient in erythrocytes and tissues of RCDP type 2 and type 3 patients.

Although the exact physiological role of etherphospholipids, including plasmalogens, remains to be established, it is clear that the clinical signs and symptoms of RCDP, as dominated by shortening of the extremities, facial abnormalities, mental retardation, and spasticity, are caused by the inability to synthesize etherphospholipids.

Clinical Presentation In the literature, only very few cases of RCDP types 2 and 3 have been described. The clinical signs and symptoms of all patients described resemble those observed in RCDP type 1 in all respects. Accordingly, all RCDP type 2 and type 3 patients show disproportionally short stature, primarily affecting the proximal parts of the extremities; facial features such as a broad nasal bridge, highly arched palate, dysplastic ears, and micrognathia; congenital contractures; and severe mental retardation with spasticity. RCDP type 2 and type 3 patients also show the roentgenological abnormalities described for RCDP type 1, with a symmetrical shortening of the femur and humerus with irregular and broad metaphyses, calcific stippling mainly of the epiphyses, absent femur head nucleus, coronal clefts of vertebrae, increased intravertebral disk spaces, cupping of the dorsal ribs, and a barrel-formed thorax.

Diagnosis/Laboratory Findings A deficiency of either DHAPAT or ADHAPS causes distinct biochemical abnormalities, including:

- Deficiency of erythrocyte (and tissue) plasmalogens
- Impaired de novo synthesis of etherphospholipids, including plasmalogens, in fibroblasts and a deficiency of either DHAPAT or ADHAPS
- Mutations in either GNPAT or AGPS, the genes coding for DHAPAT and ADHAPS, respectively

Treatment In the literature, no therapeutic options for either RCDP type 1, type 2, or type 3 have been described. Especially in milder affected patients a therapeutic trial of a diet restricted in phytanic acid appears reasonable.

Hyperoxaluria Type 1

Etiology/Pathophysiology Primary hyperoxaluria type 1 (PH-1) is caused by a deficiency of the enzyme alanine glyoxylate aminotransferase (AGT), which is localized in peroxisomes and converts the toxic metabolite glyoxylate into glycine (13) (see Figure 24-10 for the normal pathway). In contrast, primary hyperoxaluria type 2 (PH-2) is caused by deficiency of the enzyme glyoxylate reductase, which is located in the cytosol, and therefore, PH-2 is not a peroxisomal disorder. If glyoxylate is not detoxified immediately by AGT as in PH-1, glyoxylate will accumulate in peroxisomes and will be either reduced to glycolate or oxidized to oxalate (Figure 24-11). Glycolate is water soluble and can be excreted via the urine. This is not true, however, for oxalate, which precipitates as calcium oxalate. Deposition of calcium oxalate within the kidney parenchymatous tissue (nephrocalcinosis) or the renal pelvis/urinary tract (urolithiasis) continues until, eventually, renal function is impaired, causing subsequent sequelae, such as uremia and systemic oxalosis. The failure to clear oxalate from the body leads to its further deposition in almost all areas of the body, affecting multiple tissues in addition to the kidneys and urinary tract, including: 1) the myocardium with heart block, myocarditis, and cardioembolic stroke; 2) the nerves (peripheral neuropathy); 3) bone (bone pain, multiple fractures,

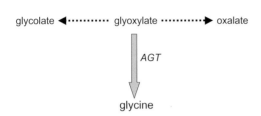

FIGURE 24-10. Simplified scheme depicting the metabolism of glyoxylate in normal human beings. Under normal conditions glyoxylate is rapidly degraded by the peroxisomal enzyme alanine-glyoxylate aminotransferase (AGT) with little formation of glycolate and oxalate.

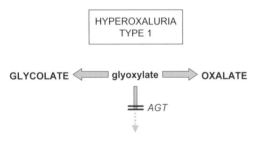

FIGURE 24-11. In hyperoxaluria type 1 patients, peroxisomal AGT is deficient and the glyoxylate, which accumulates in peroxisomes, is converted into oxalate and glycolate.

and osteosclerosis); **4)** the eyes (retinopathy and optic atrophy); **5)** bone marrow; and, **6)** other organs.

Clinical Presentation *Primary hyperoxaluria* is a collective term that encompasses an indeterminate number of genetically inherited conditions, of which only PH-1 and PH-2 have been characterized. PH-1 is clinically variable both in symptoms and in timing. In most patients, first symptoms start before 5 years of age. There is an enormous spread, however, in the ages at which the disease becomes apparent, which can be as early as the first year of life or may happen much later in life, even beyond the fifth decade. In its severe neonatal presentation, PH-1 is characterized by rapidly progressive oxalosis, renal failure, and early death.

Diagnosis/Laboratory Findings The most common method of diagnosing PH-1 is by measuring urinary oxalate excretion. Markedly elevated urinary oxalate levels usually are indicative for either PH-1 or PH-2. For differential diagnosis, urinary glycolate and L-glycerate must be measured. It should be noted that a significant number of PH-1 patients (up to 25%) with proven AGT deficiency have hyperoxaluria but no hyperglycolic aciduria. At the other extreme, some PH-1 patients have extreme hyperglycolic aciduria with only mildly elevated oxalate excretion. In addition, isolated hyperglycolic aciduria and concomitant hyperoxaluria and hyperglycolic aciduria have been found in patients with normal AGT levels.

Definitive diagnosis of PH-1 and PH-2 requires enzymatic studies and subsequent molecular analysis. Enzymatic diagnosis of PH-2 is straightforward because the enzyme glyoxylate reductase can be measured reliably in lymphocytes. Enzymatic diagnosis of PH-1 is much less straightforward for two reasons. First, in contrast to glyoxylate reductase, AGT is expressed only in liver, which requires a percutaneous liver needle biopsy. Second and more important, although AGT can be measured reliably in minimal amounts of liver material, the results of AGT enzyme testing are not unequivocal. The reason is that AGT activity may be quite normal, as measured in a human liver homogenate, but may be inactive under in vivo conditions because of its mislocalization to the mitochondrion. This astonishing phenotype of an enzyme being functionally inactive because of its localization in the wrong compartment obviously complicates the results of the AGT enzyme assay. Since this peroxisome-to-mitochondrion-mistargeting phenotype is quite frequent, there is a strong case for direct molecular analysis of the AGXT gene, because the underlying cause for the mistargeting of AGT to the mitochondrion has been established now. Indeed, a Gly170Arg substitution on the background of the minor allele (frequency in the normal population 4%) leads to mistargeting of 90% of AGT to the mitochondrion. The same is true for the Phe152Ile mutation. In addition to these two mutations, more than 50 additional mutations in the AGXT gene have been identified that, in general, render the enzyme inactive without changing its subcellular localization.

Treatment Overall, the management of PH-1 greatly depends on the degree of renal function. Treatment is directed toward: **1)** decreasing oxalate production by inhibiting oxalate synthesis; and, **2)** increasing oxalate solubility at a given urinary concentration of oxalate. Most of the efforts have concentrated on ways to increase the solubility of calcium oxalate. High fluid intake and alkalinization of the urine remain the mainstays of this approach. Indeed, excessive volume is necessary to help excrete the enormous amounts of endogenously produced oxalate. Other helpful therapies may include the use of magnesium oxide (650–1300 mg/day). Furthermore, hemodialysis can remove large quantities of oxalate and its precursors. Attempts to try to reduce the production of oxalate with succinimide, allopurinol, calcium carbimide, and isocarbazide have been unsuccessful.

Importantly, pyridoxine should be tried in every patient. A third of patients with PH-1 respond to pharmacological doses of pyridoxine. Indeed, pyridoxine at the usual daily dose of 1000 mg/m^2 of body surface area can bring about a substantial reduction in the production and excretion of oxalate, except in patients with a pyridoxine-resistant form of the disease. The efficacy of pyridoxine probably is related directly to the extent to which AGT is deficient. Indeed, if there is some residual enzyme activity, high levels of pyridoxal phosphate, which is the obligatory cofactor in the AGT enzyme reaction, may allow residual enzyme activity to operate optimally. In this way, flux through AGT may be stimulated considerably, leading to a reduced production of oxalate. Recent studies have shown a clear association between homozygosity for the two mistargeting mutations Gly170Arg and Phe152Ile and pyridoxine responsiveness, the reason being that pyridoxine is able to interfere with the mistargeting of AGT to the mitochondrion, thereby increasing the residual activity of AGT in peroxisomes from 5% to 10%. In our experience, all patients homozygous for the Gly170Arg substitution who had a preserved renal function at the time of diagnosis were able to preserve renal function throughout the follow-up period when treated accordingly with pyridoxine, a high fluid intake, and potassium citrate (14).

In patients in whom AGT is fully deficient, pharmacological doses of pyridoxine show no effect. These patients usually develop renal failure, requiring renal transplantation. The overall success rate of this treatment, however, is low because the biochemical defect resides in the liver and not in the kidney. As a consequence, a renal transplantation gives only temporary relief, the new organ inevitably becoming obstructed by further deposition of calcium oxalate. Definite correction of the metabolic lesion requires liver transplantation. Mutation analysis also may be useful in the decision as to whether to perform combined liver–kidney or isolated kidney transplantation in PH-1 patients with end-stage renal disease (ESRD). We believe that even in those PH-1 patients who already have developed ESRD, AGXT mutation analysis can be very useful. It would seem advisable to perform only an isolated kidney transplantation in patients homozygous for Gly170Arg or Phe152Ile. On the other hand, the adverse outcome of pyridoxine-negative mutations would provide a strong argument for a combined liver–kidney transplantation or a timely planned liver transplantation in such patients.

ACKNOWLEDGMENTS

I gratefully acknowledge Mrs. Maddy Festen for expert preparation of the manuscript, Mr. Jos Ruiter for the artwork, and the European Union for financial support (EU "Peroxisome" Project Number LSHG-CT-2004-512018).

REFERENCES

1. Powers JM. The pathology of peroxisomal disorders with pathogenetic considerations. *J Neuropathol Exp Neurol.* 1995;54:710–719.
2. Gootjes J, Schmohl F, Mooijer PA, et al. Identification of the molecular defect in patients with peroxisomal mosaicism using a novel method involving culturing of cells at 40°C: Implications for other inborn errors of metabolism. *Hum Mutat.* 2004;24:130–139.
3. Setchell KD, Heubi JE, Bove KE, et al. Liver disease caused by failure to racemize trihydroxycholestanoic acid: Gene mutation and effect of bile acid therapy. *Gastroenterology.* 2003; 124:217–232.
4. Martinez M, Mougan I, Roig M, et al. Blood polyunsaturated fatty acids in patients with peroxisomal disorders: A multicenter study. *Lipids.* 1994;29:273–280.
5. Spranger JW, Opitz JM, Bidder U, Heterogeneity of chondrodysplasia punctata. *Humangenetik.* 1971;11:190–212.
6. Moser HW, Loes DJ, Melhem ER, et al. X-linked adrenoleukodystrophy: Overview and prognosis as a function of age and brain magnetic resonance imaging abnormality. A study involving 372 patients. *Neuropediatrics.* 2000;31:227–239.
7. Poll-The BT, Roels F, Ogier H, et al. A new peroxisomal disorder with enlarged peroxisomes and a specific deficiency of acyl-CoA oxidase (pseudo-neonatal adrenoleukodystrophy). *Am J Hum Genet.* 1988; 42:422–434.
8. Ferdinandusse S, Ylianttila MS, Gloerich J, et al. Mutational spectrum of D-bifunctional protein deficiency and structure based genotype–phenotype analysis. *Am J Hum Genet.* 2006;78:112–124.
9. Wanders RJA. Peroxisomes, lipid metabolism, and peroxisomal disorders. *Mol Genet Metab.* 2004;83:16–27.
10. Ferdinandusse S, Denis S, Clayton PT, et al. Mutations in the gene encoding peroxisomal α-methylacyl-CoA racemase cause adult-onset sensory motor neuropathy. *Nat Genet.* 2000;24:188–191.
11. Wierzbicki AS, Lloyd MD, Schofield CJ, et al. Refsum's disease: A peroxisomal disorder affecting phytanic acid α-oxidation. *J Neurochem.* 2002;80:727–735.
12. Wanders RJA, Jansen GA, Skjeldal OH, Refsum disease, peroxisomes and phytanic acid oxidation: A review. *J Neuropathol Exp Neurol.* 2001;60:1021–1031.
13. Danpure CJ, Purdue PE. Primary hyperoxaluria. In: Scriver CR, Beaudet AL, Sly WS, et al., eds. *The Metabolic and Molecular Bases of Inherited Disease.* New York: McGraw-Hill; 1995:2385–2426.
14. van Woerden CS, Groothoff JW, Wijburg FA, et al. Clinical implications of mutation analysis in primary hyperoxaluria type 1. *Kidney Int.* 2004;66:746–752.
15. Moser HW, Smith KD, Watkins PA, et al. X-linked adrenoleukodystrophy. In: Scriver CR, Beaudet AL, Sly WS, et al., eds. *The Metabolic and Molecular Bases of Inherited Disease.* New York: McGraw-Hill; 2002:3257–3301.

CHAPTER 25

Congenital Disorders of Glycosylation

Christian Körner, PhD
Christian Thiel, PhD
Georg F. Hoffmann, MD

INTRODUCTION

Etiology/Pathophysiology Congenital disorders of glycosylation (CDG) comprise an ever-growing group of 17 autosomal recessive inherited diseases that affect the de novo biosynthesis of glycoproteins (Figure 25-1, (1)). The transfer of oligosaccharide chains onto newly synthesized proteins is one of the most widespread forms of co- and posttranslational modifications that is found in animals, plants, and bacteria. Glycoproteins are mainly located in subcellular organelles and in cellular membranes, and most abundantly in extracellular fluids and matrices. The oligosaccharide moieties of glycoproteins affect their folding, their transport, and their biologic activity and

stability. The complex process of protein glycosylation requires more than 100 glycosyltransferases, glycosidases, and transport proteins. Oligosaccharide moieties are connected to glycoproteins predominantly by either N-glycosidic linkages, in which glycans are linked to amino groups of asparagine residues, or by O-glycosidic linkage, where the glycans are bound to hydroxyl groups of serine or threonine residues (2). Because the deficiencies in O-glycosylation known so far are not yet integrated into the group of CDG (1), this chapter will focus on N-glycosylation defects.

CDG present with multiorgan involvement, mostly accompanied by neurologic symptoms (Table 25-1). CDG are subdivided into two groups. CDG-I comprise deficiencies that

either affect the biosynthesis of dolichol-linked oligosaccharides or the transfer of oligosaccharides onto newly synthesized proteins by the oligosaccharyltransferase complex in the endoplasmic reticulum. CDG-II affect the subsequent trimming and elongation of N-glycans in the endoplasmic reticulum and the Golgi apparatus (3) (Figure 25-2). CDG types, in which a glycosylation defect could clearly be proven by isoelectric focusing of serum transferrin but the specific genetic defect has not yet been identified, are termed CDG-Ix or CDG-IIx.

Due to its uniform glycan structures (Figure 25-3) serum transferrin remains the standard protein in initial CDG diagnostics, which is conducted by isoelectric focusing. CDG-I is characterized by an increased amount of di- and asialotransferrin at the expense of tetrasialotransferrin due to the loss of complete N-glycan chains, whereas in most cases of CDG-II shortened N-glycans accumulate (4). Combined isoelectric focusing investigations on other glycoproteins such as α1-antitrypsin and α1-antichymotrypsin may help to identify CDG in case of unclear transferrin patterns (5) (Figure 25-1).

CLINICAL SPECTRUM AND DIAGNOSTIC WORK UP OF CDG

In view of the extremely broad clinical spectrum, it can almost be recommended to consider CDG in any unexplained clinical presentation. CDG affects all organs but neurologic symptoms often dominate. All patients with unexplained multiorgan disease and especially a combination of mental and psychomotor retardation, strabismus, cerebellar atrophy, and coagulopathy should raise clinical suspicion. In addition to neurologic symptoms (psychomotor retardation, epilepsy, ataxia, cerebellar atrophy, neuronal migration disorder, stroke-like episodes, cerebral thrombosis, hypotonia, abnormal eye movements, and polyneuropathy) the following clinical features have been described

Defect	CDG	Enzyme/Transporter

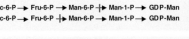

| | Ia | phosphomannomutase |
| | Ib | phosphomannose isomerase |

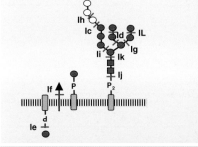

	Ic	Dol-P-Glc:α1,3-glucosyltransferase
	Id	Dol-P-Man:α1,3-mannosyltransferase
	Ie	dolichyl-phosphomannose synthase
	If	MDPU1 (Dol-P-Man/Dol-P-Glc utilization)
	Ig	Dol-P-Man:α1,6-mannosyltransferase
	Ih	Dol-P-Glc: α1,3-glucosyltransferase
	Ii	GDP-Man: α1,3-mannosyltransferase
	Ij	UDP-GlcNAc: Dol-P-GlcNAc transferase
	Ik	GDP-Man: β1,4-mannosyltransferase
	IL	Dol-P-Man: β1,2-mannosyltransferase

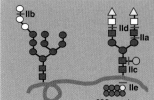

	IIa	β1,2-GlcNAc-transferase II
	IIb	α1,2-glucosidase I
	IIc	GDP-fucose transporter
	IId	β1,4-galactosyltransferase I
	IIe	COG-7 (Golgi trafficking defect)

FIGURE 25-1. Molecular defects in CDG. Molecular defects in CDG known so far affect biochemical processes in the biosynthesis of GDP-mannose in the cytosol (CDG-Ia and Ib), in the elongation of dolichol-linked glycans at the outer and the inner leaflet of the endoplasmic reticulum (CDG-Ic-IL), and in trimming and elongation of the oligosaccharide moiety of newly synthesized glycoproteins in the endoplasmic reticulum and in the Golgi apparatus (CDG-IIa-IIe). The affected reaction step for each CDG type is marked by a red bar. The symbols represent: light green rectangle = dolichol; blue square = N-acetylglucosamine; red circle = mannose; white circle = glucose; green circle = fucose; white square = galactose; yellow triangle = sialic acid. Additional abbreviations: Glc, glucose; Fru, fructose; Man, mannose; GlcNAc, N-acetylglucosamine; Dol, dolichol; GDP, guanosine diphosphate; UDP, uridine diphosphate; P, phosphate; COG, conserved oligomeric Golgi complex.

Congenital Disorders of Glycosylation
AT-A-GLANCE

Congenital disorders of glycosylation (CDG), formerly termed carbohydrate-deficient glycoprotein syndromes (7), are a rapidly expanding group of autosomal recessive multisystem disorders associated with deficiencies in the biosynthesis of glycoproteins. Common clinical presentations in CDG patients are mental retardation, seizures, hypotonia, cerebellar hypoplasia and ataxia, liver disease, coagulopathy, and dysmorphism. Less common symptoms include microcephaly, pericarditis, failure to thrive, and protein-losing enteropathy. CDG are classified into two groups. CDG type I comprise deficiencies that either affect the biosynthesis of dolichol-linked oligosaccharides or the transfer of oligosaccharides onto newly synthesized proteins by the oligosaccharyl-transferase complex in the endoplasmic reticulum. CDG type II affect the subsequent trimming and elongation of N-glycans in the endoplasmic reticulum and the Golgi apparatus. Treatment is symptomatic but must be carefully tailored in most CDG types. In two types of CDG, CDG-Ib and CDG-IIc, treatment of patients with an oral monosaccharide therapy leads to partial normalization of the defects (3).

CDG-TYPE	AFFECTED PROTEIN (REFERENCE)	OCCURRENCE	GENE	LOCUS	OMIM
CDG-Ia	Phosphomannomutase 2 [8,9]	80%	PMM2	16p13	212065 601785
CDG-Ib	Phosphomannose isomerase [19]	5%	MPI	15q22	154550 602579
CDG-Ic	Dolichol-P-glucose:$Man_9GlcNAc_2$-PP-dolichol glucosyltransferase [20,21]	5%	hALG6	1p22	604566 604655
CDG-Id	Dolichol-P-mannose: $Man_5GlcNAc_2$-PP-dolichol mannosyltransferase [23]	Very rare	hALG3	3q27	601110
CDG-Ie	Dolichol-P-mannose synthase-1 [24,25]	Very rare	DPM1	20q13	608789
CDG-If	Lec35/MPDU1 (Utilization of dolichol-P-mannose and dolichol-P-glucose [26,27])	Very rare	MPDU1	17p13	604041
CDG-Ig	Dolichol-P-mannose:$Man_7GlcNAc_2$-PP-dolichol mannosyltransferase [28–30]	Very rare	hALG12	22q13	607143
CDG-Ih	Dolichol-P-glucose:$Glc_1Man_9GlcNAc_2$-PP-dolichol-α1,3-glucosyltransferase [31]	Very rare	hALG8	11p15	608104
CDG-Ii	GDP-mannose:$Man_1GlcNAc_2$-PP-dolichol mannosyltransferase [33]	Very rare	hALG2	9q22	607906
CDG-Ij	UDP-GlcNAc:dolichol phosphate N-Acetylglucosamine-1-phosphotransferase [34]	Very rare	DPAGT1	11q23	608093
CDG-Ik	GDP-Man:$GlcNAc_2$-PP-dolichol mannosyltransferase [35–37]	Very rare	hALG1	16p13	608540
CDG-IL	Dolichol-P-mannose:α1,2 mannosyltransferase [38]	Very rare	hALG9	11q23	608776
CDG-IIa	Golgi N-acetyl-glucosaminyltransferase II [39,40]	Very rare	MGAT2	14q21	212066
CDG-IIb	Endoplasmic reticulum glucosidase I [41]	Very rare	GCS1	2p13	606056
CDG-IIc	Golgi GDP-fucose transporter [42,43]	Very rare	FUCT1	11p11	605881 266265
CDG-IId	Golgi UDP-galactose:N-acetylglucosamine β-1,4-galactosyltransferase [46]	Very rare	ß4GALT1	9p13	607091
CDG-IIe	Subunit 7 of COG complex in Golgi trafficking [48]	Very rare	COG7	16p12	608779 606978

CDG TYPE	LABORATORY FINDINGS	CLINICAL PRESENTATION BIRTH	CLINICAL PRESENTATION CHILDHOOD & ADOLESCENCE
Ia	↓ antithrombin III ↓ factor XI, ↓ protein C ↓ thyroxine-binding globulin ↑↑ liver transaminases ↑ serum transaminases ↓ cholesterol, ↓ cholinesterase ↓ tetrasialotransferrin ↑ disialotransferrin ↑/↑↑ asialotransferrin	psychomotor retardation, hypotonia, inverted nipples, cerebellar atrophy, coagulation abnormalities, abnormal subcutaneous fat distribution	psychomotor retardation, osteopenia, thorax and vertebral column abnormalities, sexual infantilism
Ib	↓ antithrombin III ↓ factor XI, ↓ protein C ↓ thyroxine-binding globulin ↑ aminotransferases ↓ tetrasialotransferrin ↑ disialotransferrin ↑/↑↑ asialotransferrin	protein-losing enteropathy hepatomegaly, congenital fibrosis of the liver, coagulation abnormalities	thromboses, hepatic fibrosis, protein-losing enteropathy, hypoglycemia
Ic	↓↓ antithrombin III ↓↓ factor XI ↑ ammonia level ↓ tetrasialotransferrin ↑ disialotransferrin ↑/↑↑ asialotransferrin ↑ dolichol-linked $Man_9GlcNAc_2$	hepatogastrointestinal symptoms, psychomotor retardation, strabismus, coagulation abnormalities	psychomotor retardation, strabismus
Id	↓ antithrombin III ↓ apolipoprotein B ↓ tetrasialotransferrin ↑ disialotransferrin ↑/↑↑ asialotransferrin ↑ dolichol-linked $Man_5GlcNAc_2$	psychomotor retardation, hypsarrhythmia, postnatal microcephaly	psychomotor retardation, hypsarrhythmia, postnatal microcephaly
Ie	↓↓ factor XI ↑ creatine kinase ↑ transaminases ↓ tetrasialotransferrin ↑ disialotransferrin ↑ asialotransferrin not increased dolichol-linked $Man_5GlcNAc_2$	psychomotor retardation, seizures, axial hypotonia, dysmorphic features, hepatosplenomegaly, coagulation abnormalities	epilepsy, hypotonia, psychomotor retardation, dysmorphic features
If	↓ antithrombin III ↓ liver transaminases not elevated tetrasialotransferrin ↑ asialotransferrin, ↑ disialotransferrin ↑ dolichol-linked $Man_5GlcNAc_2$ ↑ dolichol-linked $Man_9GlcNAc_2$	psychomotor retardation, muscular hypotonia, hypertonia, contractures, seizures, skin disease	ataxia, profound psychomotor retardation
Ig	↓ antithrombin III ↓ immunoglobulins (IgA, IgG, IgM) ↑ partial thromboplastin time ↓ tetrasialotransferrin ↑↑ disialotransferrin ↑ asialotransferrin ↑ dolichol-linked $Man_7GlcNAc_2$	psychomotor retardation, mental retardation, hypotonia, facial dysmorphism, convulsions, feeding problems	microcephaly, muscular hypotonia, prolonged partial thromboplastin time, supragluteal fat pads, facial dysmorphism
Ih	↓ antithrombin III ↓ factor XI, ↓ protein C ↓ severe hypoalbuminia tetrasialotransferrin ↑ asialotransferrin, ↑ disialotransferrin ↑ dolichol-linked $Man_9GlcNAc_2$	gastrointestinal symptoms, hepatomegaly, coagulation abnormalities, severe diarrhea	diarrhea, protein-losing functions resolve, mild hyperechogenic, hepatomegaly, without portal hypertension

CDG TYPE	LABORATORY FINDINGS	CLINICAL PRESENTATION BIRTH	CLINICAL PRESENTATION CHILDHOOD & ADOLESCENCE
Ii	↑ partial thromboplastin time ↓↓ factor XI ↓ tetrasialotransferrin ↑ disialotransferrin ↑ asialotransferrin ↑ dolichol-linked $Man_1GlcNAc_2$ ↑ dolichol-linked $Man_2GlcNAc_2$	normal at birth, ophthalmological abnormalities, seizures, hypomyelinization, hepatomegaly, coagulation abnormalities, psychomotor delay	no data available
Ij	↓ antithrombin III ↓ tetrasialotransferrin ↑ disialotransferrin ↑ asialotransferrin ↓ dolichol-linked $Glc_3Man_9GlcNAc_2$	normal at birth, infantile spasms, development delay, microcephaly, arched palate, micrognathia, exotropia severe hypotonia	minimal linguistic ability
Ik	↓↓ circulating B cells ↓↓ immunoglobulin G ↓ tetrasialotransferrin ↑↑ disialotransferrin ↑ asialotransferrin ↑ dolichol-linked $GlcNAc_2$	fetal hydrops, psychomotor retardation, seizures, coagulation abnormalities, hepatosplenomegaly, multiple dysmorphic features, large fontanel, hypertelorism, micrognathia, hypogonadism, cardiomyopathy, muscular hypotonia	no data available
IL	↓ tetrasialotransferrin ↑ disialotransferrin ↑ asialotransferrin ↑ dolichol-linked $Man_6GlcNAc_2$ ↑ dolichol-linked $Man_8GlcNAc_2$	normal at birth, development delay, severe microcephaly, central hypotonia, seizures, hepatomegaly, asthma	no data available
IIa	↑ AST, ↓↓ factor IX, ↓ factor XII ↓ antithrombin III ↓↓ tetrasialotransferrin ↑↑ disialotransferrin	severe psychomotor retardation but no, neuropathy or cerebral hypoplasia, coagulation abnormalities, facial dysmorphism, seizures	severe psychomotor retardation, facial dysmorphism, seizures
IIb	↑ AST ↑↑ tetrasaccharides in urine Inconspicious isoelectric focusing pattern	psychomotor retardation, hypotonia, hepatomegaly, craniofacial dysmorphism, epilepsy, hypoventilation, feeding problems, seizures	psychomotor retardation, hypotonia, hepatomegaly craniofacial dysmorphism, epilepsy, hypoventilation, seizures
IIc	high leukocytes counts without pus formation, normal isoelectric focusing pattern bacterial infections, lack of Sialyl-Lewis X on neutrophils affected inflammation, absence of ABO blood groups (Bombay phenotype)	dysmorphism, psychomotor retardation, severe infections, therapy	psychomotor and physical retardation
IId	↑ partial thromboplastin time ↓↓ factor XI, ↓ antithrombin III ↓ fibrinogen ↑ serum creatine kinase ↓↓ cholinesterase ↓↓ tetrasialotransferrin ↑ trisialotransferrin ↑/↑↑ disialotransferrin ↑↑ monosialotransferrin ↑/↑↑ asialotransferrin	macrocephaly, hydrocephalus, hypotonia, coagulation abnormalities, myopathy	muscular hypotonia marked with reduced muscle mass but sitting and standing alone possible
IIe	↓ tetrasialotransferrin ↑ trisialotransferrin ↑ disialotransferrin ↑ monosialotransferrin ↑ asialotransferrin	dysmorphism, skeletal dysplasia, hypotonia, hepatosplenomegaly, jaundice, epilepsy, death in infancy	no data available

TABLE 25-1   Initial Investigations After Diagnosing CDG

- **Extended neurological examination** including formal developmental/IQ testing
- **Orthopedic evaluation**
- Cerebral nuclear MRI
- **Electrophysiologic studies**
- **Kidney ultrasonography**
- **Liver ultrasonography**
- **Fasting blood sugar**
- **Kidney function test**
- **Liver function tests**
- **Endocrinological evaluation, especially thyroid hormones, including thyreoglobulin, and gonadotropins**
- Clotting studies including individual factor IX, factor XI, proteins C and S, AT III, heparin cofactor II, and complement system
- Full blood count including reticulocytes
- Genetic counseling

Investigations in **bold** should be repeated at regular intervals, yearly or at least every other year.

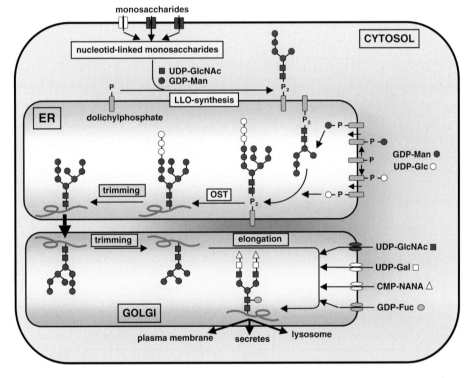

FIGURE 25-2. Assembly and processing of N-linked glycans. The biosynthesis of N-linked glycans starts with the transfer of the nucleotide-activated sugars N-acetylglucosamine and mannose onto the lipid-carrier dolichol (LLO) at the outer leaflet of the endoplasmic reticulum up to an oligosaccharide with the structure GlcNAc₂Man₅. Following the transfer into the lumen of the endoplasmic reticulum by a flippase mechanism, the nascent glycan is further elongated with mannose and glucose residues, which are transferred from dolichol-mannose and dolichol-glucose donors at the luminal side of the endoplasmic reticulum. All elongation reactions inside and outside the endoplasmic reticulum are catalyzed by a subset of different glycosyltransferases. The oligosaccharide GlcNAc₂Man₉Glc₃ is transferred by the multisubunit enzyme complex oligosaccharyltransferase (OST) onto glycosylation consensus sequences of nascent proteins. After removal of the three glucose residues and one mannose residue, which plays a central part in protein folding quality control, the newly synthesized glycoprotein is transferred to the Golgi apparatus by vesicular transport. In the Golgi apparatus a series of trimming reactions lead to the shortened oligosaccharide structure GlcNAc₂Man₃. At this point a broad variety of N-acetylglucosaminyl transferases, galactosyltransferases, sialyltransferases, and fucosyltransferases can elongate the oligosaccharide to its mature form, which shows a tremendous heterogeneity. The symbols for monosaccharide residues represent: blue square = N-acetylglucosamine; red circle = mannose; white circle = glucose; green circle = fucose; white square = galactose; yellow triangle = sialic acid. Glc, glucose; Man, mannose; GlNAc, N-acetylglucosamine; Gal, galactose; NANA, sialic acid; Fuc, fucose; GDP, guanosine diphosphate; UDP, uridine diphosphate; CMP, cytidine monophosphate; P = phosphate.

in CDG, and reading this list gives a feeling of the variability and complexity of the clinical situation but also when to initiate a diagnostic cascade:

- General symptoms (hydrops fetalis, failure to thrive, microcephaly, recurrent infections)
- Skin manifestations (inverted nipples, abnormal fat pads, progeria-like syndrome, ichthyosis)
- Ophthalmologic symptoms (strabismus, retinitis pigmentosa, optical atrophy, coloboma, cataract)
- Hormonal imbalances (retarded growth, hypogonadism, delayed or missing puberty, hyperinsulinism)
- Orthopedic problems (osteopenia, contracted joints, exostosis)
- Disturbed coagulation (thrombosis, bleeding tendency, phlebitis)
- Cardiac disease (cardiomyopathy, pericardial effusion, pericarditis in the neonatal period)
- Gastrointestinal disease (ascites, cyclic vomiting, chronic diarrhea, protein-losing enteropathy, hepatomegaly, hepatitis-like disease; liver histology shows fibrosis and lipid and glycogen vacuoles)
- Renal disease (proteinuria, congenital nephrotic syndrome, microcysts, proximal tubulopathy in the neonatal period)

The diagnostic work up for CDG should start with the analysis of the glycosylation pattern of transferrin by isoelectric focusing (Figure 25-3). It must, however, be kept in mind that isoelectric focusing of transferrin might give false-negative results prenatally as well as during the 1st weeks of life (6). It is therefore not applicable for prenatal diagnosis and, if negative, should be repeated after 2 to 3 months in a young infant in whom CDG is suspected. Later on in life, the degree of abnormalities of transferrin can vary sometimes up to a false normal pattern. On the other hand secondary disturbances of glycosylation result in an abnormal glycosylation pattern and must be differentiated (chronic alcoholism, classic galactosemia, or fructose intolerance). If the clinical picture is very suggestive of CDG, repeat isoelectric focusing of transferrin or enzymatic or molecular testing is recommended. It should be obvious that even cruder screening tests such as carbohydrate-deficient transferrin (CDT) determination, which is a method to quantify the amount of CDT in serum, are valuable if positive, but should not be considered an appropriate diagnostic method for CDG.

The isoelectric focusing needs to be performed on serum because EDTA plasma

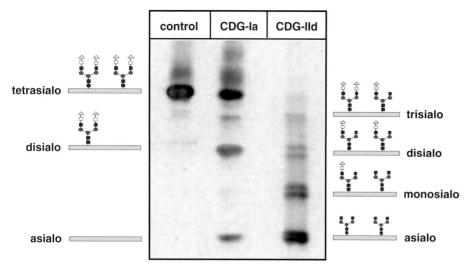

FIGURE 25-3. Transferrin isoelectric focusing (IEF). The pattern of Fe₂-isotransferrin obtained by IEF of a control serum shows the highest intensity for the tetrasialotransferrin band (lane 1). A CDG type I pattern (lane 2) is characterized by increased asialo- and disialotransferrin bands, whereas the tetrasialotransferrin band is decreased. In the CDG type II pattern (lane 3) the tri-, di-, mono-, and asialotransferrin bands are all elevated at the expense of the tetrasialotransferrin band. The symbols for monosaccharide residues represent: blue square = N-acetylglucosamine; red circle = mannose; white circle = glucose; and yellow triangle = sialic acid. Double bands in case of the CDG-IId patient are due to an isoform of human transferrin.

may cause false negative results due to iron chelation. Genetic protein variants of transferrin can also cause a shift in isoelectric focusing and can be differentiated from CDG by repeating the isoelectric focusing after neuraminidase treatment, which removes the sialic acid residues from the protein. Studying the parents will further aid in the differentiation because they are carriers of the same genetic protein variant without being affected. Investigation of other glycoproteins in addition to transferrin can either substantiate or dismiss the diagnosis in patients with clinical suspicion of CDG (5).

Isoelectric focusing of transferrin does not detect diseases of fucose metabolism (CDG-IIc). This disorder can be detected in a first attempt by blood group determination because the patients lack a detectable ABO blood group on their erythrocytes (Bombay blood group).

In summary the diagnostic workup of CDG can be an especially complex process. In contrast to most other inborn errors of metabolism, repeated investigations and additional enzymatic or molecular studies may be warranted despite primarily normal biochemistry. It is advisable to perform the studies in laboratories with expertise in CDG.

Care of Patients with CDG

Although in most CDG types no specific therapy is available, the symptomatic treatment of the patient is complex and requires pathophysiologic knowledge of the disorder. CDG are chronic conditions that involve different organ systems and often show progressive pathology, which seems to stabilize in mid childhood.

A carefully balanced interdisciplinary approach to care and treatment is needed. Psychosocial support and genetic counseling for prenatal or preimplantation diagnosis are important to help the family cope with the disease and make informed decisions. Physiotherapy, developmental, and speech therapy are indispensable for almost any patient. Orthopedic equipment is often helpful and advice and help from a social worker may be needed to obtain all necessary financial and medical support. Families may get valuable emotional support and practical advice from meeting other affected families.

Following the diagnosis of CDG a number of additional investigations should be initiated to detect other associated manifestations (see At-A-Glance and Table 25-1). These investigations should be repeated at regular intervals, that is, yearly or every other year.

The coagulation abnormalities require special awareness. In CDG there is a combination of increased tendency of bleeding and thrombosis. If patients develop recurrent strokes they should be given small doses of acetylsalicylic acid (~1 mg/kg body weight/d).

Dehydration is to be strictly avoided and intravenous fluid substitution should be initiated early, especially during intercurrent illnesses such as gastrointestinal infections and during anesthesia and surgery. During such episodes electrolytes, blood glucose, coagulation factors (especially factor IX and factor XI) as well as proteins C, S, and antithrombin (AT) III and heparin cofactor II should be monitored, if partial thromboplastin time is normal.

CDG-Ia: PHOSPHOMANNOMUTASE 2 DEFICIENCY

Etiology/Pathophysiology CDG-Ia is the most frequent form of CDG with more than 400 patients world wide, (approximately 80% of all diagnosed patients). The molecular defect of CDG-Ia is caused by mutations in the *PMM2* gene located at chromosome 16p13, which encodes for phosphomannomutase 2 (8). The cytosolic enzyme catalyzes the conversion of mannose-6-phosphate to mannose-1-phosphate (Figure 25-1). Reduced enzyme activity leads to a decrease of the downstream product GDP-mannose (9), which is required for the assembly of dolichol-linked oligosaccharides outside and inside the endoplasmic reticulum. In contrast to fibroblasts from healthy controls, which produce mainly $Glc_3Man_9GlcNAc_2$ oligosaccharides linked to the dolichol carrier (Figure 25-2), fibroblasts of CDG-Ia patients show an accumulation of shortened dolichol-linked oligosaccharides such as $Man_3GlcNAc_2$ and $Man_5GlcNAc_2$ (10). These represent bad substrates for the oligosaccharyltransferase complex, thereby leading to the loss of oligosaccharide side chains linked to glycoproteins. The complex clinical phenotype of CDG-Ia remains poorly understood. Further insight is expe+cted from a CDG-Ia mouse model.

Clinical Presentation The disorder presents at birth in most cases (11) with somatic stigmata such as inverted nipples and abnormal subcutaneous adipose tissue distribution. Development delay, poor feeding, strabismus, axial hypotonia, and cerebellar hypoplasia are common findings (Figures 25-4 and 25-5). After birth, cardiac effusion may be detectable as a result of hypertrophic obstructive cardiomyopathy. A reduction of nerve conduction velocity, especially at the lower limbs, may manifest at the age of 6 to 8 months. Disappearance of tendon reflexes has been observed by 1 year of age (12). After infancy, retinitis pigmentosa develops. Other features include hepatomegaly with fibrosis and steatosis, nephrotic syndrome due to multiple microcysts, joint contractures, and skeletal abnormalities. Defective hemostasis, due to the reduced amounts of factor XI and the anticoagulation factors protein C and AT III, leads to thromboembolic complications. Strokelike episodes occur often during pyretic infections.

Endocrine abnormalities have also been described. The lack of pubertal development and primary ovarian failure in CDG females resembles the phenotype in galactosemia (13).

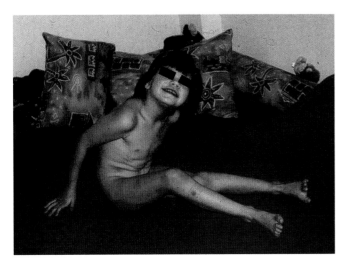

FIGURE 25-4. Eight-year-old girl with CDG-Ia (phosphomannomutase 2 deficiency). Obvious features are muscular hypotonia, impaired coordination, and disproportionately long extremities.

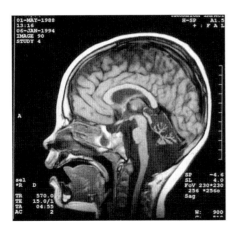

FIGURE 25-5. Sagittal NMR displaying severe cerebellar atrophy in a nearly 6-year-old CDG-Ia patient.

This may result from either reduced follicle-stimulating hormone (FSH) bioactivity and bioavailability due to abnormal glycosylation of FSH or to abnormal glycosylation of the FSH receptor affecting its ability to bind FSH. Males with CDG have been described as having normal or delayed puberty with normal virilization, small or normal testes, and testosterone values in the low-to-normal range (14,15). Cryptorchidism has been associated with males affected by CDG-Ia, with reports as high as 56% in participants in a small study (13).

Children with CDG in general are clinically euthyroid but may present with the biochemical picture of partial thyroxine-binding globulin deficiency (low total T_4, normal free T_4, normal thyroid-stimulating hormone [TSH]). The cause is still being debated; however, these patients require no treatment unless they present with elevated TSH and low free T_4.

Feeding problems such as anorexia, vomiting, and diarrhea can result in failure to thrive during the 1st years of life. The growth failure may be exacerbated by the effects of hypoglycosylation on the function and stability of components of the GH/IGF cascade. The mortality rate in CDG-Ia is apparently 20% in the 1st years of life. Patients die of severe infections or liver, cardiac, or renal failure. With increasing age, the clinical condition stabilizes and loss of acquired developmental skills is unusual.

Diagnosis Primary diagnostics in CDG-Ia are conducted by isoelectric focusing of serum transferrin, which reveals the characteristic CDG type I pattern due to the loss of complete N-glycan chains that lead to an increased amount of di- and asialotransferrin at the expense of tetrasialotransferrin (Figure 25-3). In the next step, phosphomannomutase activity is determined in an in vitro assay by using extracts from patient-derived fibroblasts or leukocytes. In case of reduced enzyme activity, genetic analysis of the *PMM2* gene is performed. In some cases, CDG-Ia patients, even with severe clinical phenotype, presented with only intermediately reduced phosphomannomutase activities (11). In any case of suspected CDG-Ia with an abnormal CDG-I transferrin pattern and only moderately reduced phosphomannomutase activity, genetic analysis of the *PMM2* gene should be performed. Mutation analysis is also the only reliable method for prenatal diagnostics of CDG-Ia (16) (Table 25-2).

Treatment Although it has been shown in cultured fibroblasts from CDG-Ia patients that supplementation with mannose (17) as

TABLE 25-2	CDG-Ia: Laboratory Findings
Decreased	**Increased**
AT III	disialotransferrin
thyroxine-binding globulin	asialotransferrin
cholesterol levels	liver transaminases
cholinesterase levels	serum transaminases
tetrasialotransferrin	
factor XI	
protein C	

well as glucose starvation (18) led to normalization in size of dolichol-linked oligosaccharides, mannose supplementation is not effective in vivo and no specific treatment of patients is so far available.

Treatment is complex; the possible multisystem manifestations must be considered, and treatment must be coordinated within an interdisciplinary team to monitor neurologic and cardiac function, onset of puberty, gonadal function, and growth.

CDG-Ib: PHOSPHOMANNOSE ISOMERASE DEFICIENCY

Etiology/Pathophysiology The molecular defect in CDG-Ib is caused by mutations in the MPI gene located on chromosome 15q22, which encodes phosphomannose isomerase, a cytosolic enzyme that catalyzes the conversion of fructose-6-phosphate to mannose-6-phosphate (Figure 25-1). As in CDG-Ia the reduced enzyme activity results in a decrease of GDP-mannose, the donor substrate in the assembly of dolichol-linked oligosaccharides outside and inside the endoplasmic reticulum, which leads in turn to loss of complete N-glycan chains linked to glycoproteins (19).

Clinical Presentation In contrast to CDG-Ia, patients with CDG-Ib do not have dysmorphic features, development delays, or neurologic manifestations. Rather the phenotype is characterized by gastrointestinal and hepatic disease. Approximately 25 patients are known to date. CDG-Ib presents with chronic diarrhea and recurrent vomiting, which start mostly in the 1st year of life and may lead to protein-losing enteropathy and failure to thrive. Duodenal biopsies showed in some cases a partial villus atrophy that might be misinterpreted as celiac disease. Hepatic fibrosis and hyperinsulinemic hypoglycemia have been reported. Complications of recurrent venous thrombosis may lead to life-threatening intestinal bleeding (19).

Diagnosis As described for CDG-Ia, primary diagnostics in CDG-Ib are conducted by isoelectric focusing of serum transferrin, which reveals a characteristic CDG type I pattern with an increased amount of di- and asialotransferrin at the expense of tetrasialotransferrin (Figure 25-3). Follow-up investigations include determination of phosphomannose isomerase activity in leukocytes or fibroblasts and mutation analysis of the MPI gene (19). In addition, albumin is low, liver transaminases are frequently raised, and the coagulopathy seen in CDG-Ib is indistinguishable from that of CDG-Ia, with

TABLE 25-3   CDG-Ib: Laboratory Findings

Decreased	Increased
AT III	disialotransferrin
thyroxine-binding globulin	asialotransferrin
tetrasialotransferrin	aminotransferases

low levels of factor XI, AT III, and protein C (Table 25-3).

Treatment Symptoms of CDG-Ib can be effectively treated by oral uptake of 1 g mannose/kg body weight/day divided into five portions. Due to the fact that mannose, which is directly taken up by the cell and phosphorylated by hexokinase, can bypass the defective phosphomannose isomerase (Figure 25-1), mannose supplementation leads to an increase in the depleted mannose-6-phosphate pool and thereby to normalization of protein glycosylation. Oral mannose treatment was reported to normalize hypoproteinemia and blood coagulation as well as protein-losing enteropathy and hypoglycemia (19).

CDG-Ic: DOLICHOL-P-Glc: Man₉GlcNAc₂-PP-DOLICHOL GLUCOSYLTRANSFERASE DEFICIENCY

Etiology/Pathophysiology Mutations in the human ortholog of the yeast *ALG6* gene (*hALG6*) located on chromosome 1p22, which encodes for dolichol-P-Glc: $Man_9GlcNAc_2$-PP-dolichol glucosyltransferase cause CDG-Ic, which was formerly termed CDGS type V (20,21). The enzyme is located inside the endoplasmic reticulum where it catalyzes the transfer of the first glucose residue from dolichol-phospate glucose onto $Man_9GlcNAc_2$-PP-dolichol (Figure 25-1). Due to reduced enzyme activity, $Man_9GlcNAc_2$-PP-dolichol accumulates. Because $Man_9GlcNAc_2$-PP-residues are not transferred onto newly synthesized proteins by the oligosaccharyltransferase complex, the amount of N-glycans is reduced due to unoccupied glycosylation sites on many glycoproteins, which leads to the appearance of di- and asialotransferrin.

Clinical Presentation The clinical phenotype of CDG-Ic patients is milder compared to CDG-Ia patients; CDG-Ic patients are not dysmorphic and have normal tendon reflexes and nerve conduction velocities. Cerebellar development may be mildly affected (Figures 25-6 and 25-7 (22)). In 40 known patients, psychomotor retardation, muscular hypotonia, ataxia, dystonic movements, recurrent seizures, and reduced coagulation factors were common.

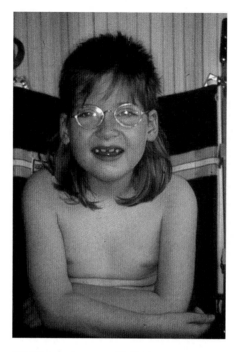

FIGURE 25-6. Seven-year-old girl with CDG-Ic (Dolichol-P-Glc:Man₉GlcNAc₂-PP-dolichol glucosyltransferase deficiency). Obvious features are muscular hypotonia, impaired coordination, and strabismus.

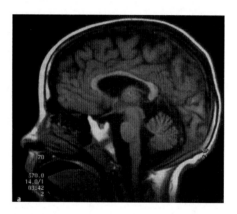

FIGURE 25-7. T1-weighted MRI in CDG-Ic. Sagittal view of mild cerebellar atrophy in a nearly 4.5-year-old CDG-Ic patient.

Diagnosis Primary diagnostic of CDG-Ic is made by isoelectric focusing of serum transferrin. The CDG type 1 pattern of serum transferrin by isoelectric focusing is characterized by an accumulation of di- and asialotransferrin resembles CDG-Ia and CDG-Ib, although in some cases the asialotransferrin band is weaker (Figure 25-3). Further analysis entails metabolic labeling of patients' fibroblasts with radioactive mannose, subsequent extraction of dolichol-linked oligosaccharides and high-performance liquid chromatography (HPLC) analysis of the oligosaccharide moiety. In case of a $Man_9GlcNAc_2$ accumulation, genetic analysis of the *hALG6* gene is performed (Table 25-4).

Treatment No specific treatment is available.

TABLE 25-4   CDG-Ic: Laboratory Findings

Decreased	Increased
AT III	disialotransferrin
factor XI	asialotransferrin
tetrasialotransferrin	dolichol-linked Man₉GlcNAc₂
	ammonia level

CDG-Id: DOLICHOL-P-Man Man₅GlcNAc₂-PP-DOLICHOL

Mannosyltransferase Deficiency

Etiology/Pathophysiology The molecular defect that leads to abnormal N-glycosylation in CDG-Id, formerly termed CDGS type IV, is caused by mutations in the dolichol-P-Man: $Man_5GlcNAc_2$-PP-dolichol mannosyltransferase gene, the human ortholog of the yeast *ALG3* gene (*hALG3*) located on chromosome 3q27 (23). The mannosyltransferase transfers mannose residues from dolichol-phosphate mannose onto $Man_5GlcNAc_2$-PP-dolichol in the endoplasmic reticulum (Figure 25-1). The defect leads to an accumulation of a $Man_5GlcNAc_2$-PP-dolichol intermediate, transfer of shortened oligosaccharides onto nascent glycoproteins, and incomplete usage of N-glycosylation sites in glycoproteins.

Clinical Presentation Three CDG-Id patients have been identified (3). The clinical phenotype comprises tetraspastic paresis, hypoplasia of the cerebellum, microcephaly, seizures, severe psychomotor retardation, and multiple dysmorphisms including abnormalities of the uvula, a high-arched palate, dysplastic ears, atrophy of the optic nerve, and coloboma of the iris.

Diagnosis Primary diagnostic evaluation in CDG-Id is made by isoelectric focusing of serum transferrin. In contrast to other CDG-I types, the asialotransferrin band is less pronounced. Further analysis is performed by metabolic labeling of patients' fibroblasts with radioactive mannose, subsequent extraction of dolichol-linked oligosaccharides, and HPLC analysis of the oligosaccharide moiety. In case of a $Man_5GlcNAc_2$ accumulation, genetic analysis of the *hALG3* gene is performed. In parallel, the dolichol-phosphate-mannose synthase-1 gene should be analyzed because its deficiency leads to a comparable $Man_5GlcNAc_2$ accumulation (see CDG-Ie) (Table 25-5).

Treatment No efficient treatment is available. Epilepsy may be reasonably controlled by valproic acid (23).

TABLE 25-5	CDG-Id: Laboratory Findings
Decreased	**Increased**
AT III	disialotransferrin
apolipoprotein B	asialotransferrin
tetrasialotransferrin	dolichol-linked $Man_5GlcNAc_2$

TABLE 25-6	CDG-Ie: Laboratory Findings
Decreased	**Increased**
factor XI	disialotransferrin
tetrasialotransferrin	creatine kinase
	transaminases
	dolichol-linked $Man_5GlcNAc_2$

$Man_5GlcNAc_2$ and $Man_9GlcNAc_2$ a genetic analysis of the MPDU1 gene is performed. (Table 25-7).

Treatment No specific treatment is available.

CDG-Ie: DOLICHOL-PHOSPHATE-MANNOSE SYNTHASE-1 DEFICIENCY

Etiology/Pathophysiology The molecular defect underlying CDG-Ie is due to mutations in the dolichol-phosphate-mannose synthase-1 gene (DPM1) located on chromosome 20q13 (24,25). It encodes the catalytic subunit of the dolichol-phosphate-mannose synthase complex, which catalyzes the biosynthesis of dolichol-phosphate mannose from dolichol-phosphate and GDP-mannose at the outer leaflet of the endoplasmic reticulum. Dolichol-phosphate mannose serves as the donor substrate for mannose residues during the elongation of $Man_5GlcNAc_2$-PP-dolichol to $Man_9GlcNAc_2$-PP-dolichol in the endoplasmic reticulum (Figure 25-1). Due to reduced activity of the dolichol-phosphate-mannose synthase complex, an accumulation of $Man_5GlcNAc_2$-PP-dolichol was detected in CDG-Ie patients similar to what has been observed in CDG-Id.

Clinical Presentation The four CDG-Ie patients identified so far presented in their first year of life with severe psychomotor retardation, dysmorphic features (hypertelorism, gothic palate, and small hands with dysplastic and knee contractures), muscular hypotonia, cortical blindness, and intractable seizures. Other manifestations that develop in early childhood include microcephaly, hepatosplenomegaly elevated liver transaminases, and coagulopathy. Magnetic resonance imaging (MRI) revealed cerebellar atrophy. Patients suffer from severe infections and fail to develop social contact.

Diagnosis Primary diagnostic in CDG-Ie is conducted by isoelectric focusing of serum transferrin. In contrast to other CDG-I types, the asialotransferrin band is less pronounced like in CDG-Id. Further analysis is performed by metabolic labeling of patients' fibroblasts with radioactive mannose, subsequent extraction of dolichol-linked oligosaccharides, and HPLC analysis of the oligosaccharide moiety. In case of a $Man_5GlcNAc_2$ accumulation an in vitro assay for dolichol-phosphate-mannose synthase and a genetic analysis of the DPM1 gene are performed. In parallel the hALG3 gene should be analyzed because

its deficiency leads to a comparable accumulation of $Man_5GlcNAc_2$ (see CDG-Id) (Table 25-6).

Treatment No efficient treatment is available.

CDG-If: DEFECTIVE DOLICHOL-P-MANNOSE AND DOLICHOL-P-GLUCOSSE UTILIZATION

Etiology/Pathophysiology CDG-If is linked to mutations in the MPDU1 gene localized on chromosome 17p13 (26,27). The MPDU1 gene product is an integral membrane protein of the endoplasmic reticulum, which plays a crucial role in the translocation of dolichol-linked mannose and dolichol-linked glucose into the lumen of the endoplasmic reticulum. Due to deficiency in the MPDU1 protein, $Man_5GlcNAc_2$-PP-dolichol and $Man_9GlcNAc_2$-PP-dolichol accumulate in fibroblasts of CDG-If patients.

Clinical Presentation The four patients identified with CDG-If presented with psychomotor retardation, muscular hypotonia, seizures, absence of speech development, failure to thrive, ichthyosis-like skin rash, and retinitis pigmentosa. AT III may be reduced but liver transaminases are normal.

Diagnosis Primary diagnosis in CDG-If is conducted by isoelectric focusing of serum transferrin, where a CDG-I pattern with an accumulation of di- and asialotransferrin was found. Further analysis is performed by metabolic labeling of patients' fibroblasts with radioactive mannose, subsequent extraction of dolichol-linked oligosaccharides, and HPLC analysis of the oligosaccharide moieties. In case of an accumulation of

TABLE 25-7	CDG-If: Laboratory Findings
Decreased	**Increased**
AT III	asialotransferrin
tetrasialotransferrin	disialotransferrin
	dolichol-linked $Man_5GlcNAc_2$
	dolichol-linked $Man_9GlcNAc_2$

CDG-Ig: DOLICHOL-P-Man: $Man_7GlcNAc_2$-PP-DOLICHOL MANNOSYLTRANSFERASE DEFICIENCY

Etiology/Pathophysiology Mutations in the Dolichol-P-Man:$Man_7GlcNAc_2$-PP-dolichol mannosyltransferase gene, the human ortholog of the yeast ALG12 gene (hALG12) that is located on chromosome 22q13 (28–30) cause CDG-Ig. The mannosyltransferase catalyzes the transfer of mannose residues from dolichol-phosphate mannose onto $Man_7GlcNAc_2$-PP-dolichol in the endoplasmic reticulum. Due to reduced enzyme activity the majority of dolichol-linked oligosaccharides accumulate as $Man_7GlcNAc_2$-PP-dolichol (Figure 25-1), which is further on transferred onto newly synthesized glycoproteins. The truncated oligosaccharides are apparently not sufficient to support complete glycoprotein biosynthesis.

Clinical Presentation The index patient with CDG-Ig presented with psychomotor retardation, supragluteal fat pads, dysplastic ears, and a short philtrum. Convulsions started in the 2nd year of life. As in other CDG-types, microcephaly and muscular hypotonia were observed. AT III and immunoglobulins (Ig)A, IgG, and IgM were low and partial thromboplastin time was prolonged.

Diagnosis Primary diagnostic in CDG-Ig is conducted by isoelectric focusing of serum transferrin. The isoelectric focusing pattern strongly resembles other CDG-I types, with an accumulation of di- and asialotransferrin (Figure 25-3). Further analysis is performed by metabolic labeling of patient's fibroblasts with radioactive mannose, subsequent extraction of dolichol-linked oligosaccharides, and HPLC analysis of the oligosaccharide moieties. In case of an accumulation of $Man_7GlcNAc_2$, genetic analysis of the hALG12 gene is performed (Table 25-8).

Treatment No specific treatment is available.

TABLE 25-8	CDG-Ig: Laboratory Findings
Decreased	**Increased**
AT III	partial thromboplastin time
IgA, IgG, IgM	disialotransferrin
tetrasialotransferrin	asialotransferrin
	dolichol-linked $Man_7GlcNAc_2$

CDG-Ih: DOLICHOL-P-GLUCOSE: $Glc_1Man_9GlcNAc_2$-PP-DOLICHOL-$\alpha 1,3$ GLUCOSYLTRANSFERASE DEFICIENCY

Etiology/Pathophysiology The underlying cause for CDG-Ih is due to mutations in dolichol-P-glucose:$Glc_1Man_9GlcNAc_2$-PP-dolichol-$\alpha 1,3$ glucosyltransferase, the human ortholog of the yeast *ALG8* gene, localized on chromosome 11p15 (31). The affected glucosyltransferase catalyzes the transfer of glucose residues from dolichol-phosphate glucose onto $Glc_1Man_9GlcNAc_2$-PP-dolichol in the endoplasmic reticulum (Figure 25-1). Surprisingly, $Man_9GlcNAc_2$-PP-dolichol accumulates in patients' fibroblasts instead of $Glc_1Man_9GlcNAc_2$-PP-dolichol as would have been expected. This is probably due to deglucosylation of $Glc_1Man_9GlcNAc_2$-PP-dolichol by the endoplasmic reticulum glucosidase II. In fact, accumulation of $Glc_1Man_9GlcNAc_2$-PP-dolichol became apparent only when patients' fibroblasts were pretreated with the glucosidase II inhibitor castanospermine (31).

Clinical Presentation The clinical phenotype of the CDG-Ih index patient resembles CDG-Ib. The patient presented at 4 months of age with edematoascitic syndrome due to severe hypoalbuminemia from protein-losing enteropathy. Other findings included severe diarrhea, moderate hepatomegaly, and coagulopathy. Neither dysmorphic features nor central nervous system involvement was present.

In addition to the index patient, three other infants afflicted with CDG-Ih have been described (32). One of these patients differed from the others, as he had dysmorphic features including an asymmetrical skull, large fontanel, hypertelorism, low-set and abnormally positioned ears, long philtrum, short neck, cryptorchidism, camptodactyly, and clubfeet. He also had pulmonary hypoplasia, cardiac defects, cholestasis, and diffuse renal microcysts.

Diagnosis Primary diagnostic evaluation of CDG-Ih is conducted by isoelectric focusing of serum transferrin. The isoelectric focusing pattern shows a typical CDG-I pattern with an accumulation of di- and asialotransferrin (Figure 25-3). Further analysis is performed by metabolic labeling of patients' fibroblasts with radioactive mannose in the presence of castanospermine, subsequent extraction of dolichol-linked oligosaccharides, and HPLC analysis of the oligosaccharide moieties. In case of $Glc_1Man_9GlcNAc_2$ accumulation genetic analysis of the *hALG8* gene is performed. Routine blood tests reveal severe hypoalbuminemia and disturbed coagulation

TABLE 25-9	CDG-Ih: Laboratory Findings
Decreased	**Increased**
AT III	asialotransferrin
factor XI	disialotransferrin
protein C	dolichol-linked $Man_9GlcNAc_2$
hypoalbuminia	
tetrasialotransferrin	

(decreased factor XI, protein C, and AT III). Laboratory examination of the CDG-Ih patient with dysmorphic features revealed anemia, severe thrombocytopenia, and primary hypothyroidism (Table 25-9).

Treatment A low-fat diet in combination with essential fatty acid supplementation resolved diarrhea and protein-losing enteropathy after 18 months of treatment. Nevertheless, mild hepatomegaly and coagulation anomalies persisted (31).

CDG-Ii: GDP-Man: $Man_1GlcNAc_2$-PP-DOLICHOL MANNOSYLTRANSFERASE DEFICIENCY

Etiology/Pathophysiology Mutations in GDP-Man:$Man_1GlcNAc_2$-PP-dolichol mannosyltransferase, the human ortholog of the yeast *ALG2* gene (*hALG2*), which is localized on chromosome 9q22 cause CDG-Ii (33). The mannosyltransferase catalyzes the transfer of the second and third mannosyl residue from GDP-mannose onto $Man_1GlcNAc_2$-PP-dolichol at the cytosolic site of the endoplasmic reticulum. Deficiency of the enzyme leads to accumulation of $Man_1GlcNAc_2$-PP-dolichol and $Man_2GlcNAc_2$-PP-dolichol (Figure 25-1).

Clinical Presentation The CDG-Ii index patient showed neither perinatal nor postnatal complications up to the age of 2 months when ophthalmologic examination revealed bilateral colobomas of the iris. From the age of 4 months seizures appeared with infantile spasms and hypsarrhythmia on electroencephalography tracings. At the age of 5 months, a cranial MRI showed severely delayed myelinization. A follow-up MRI at the age of 8 months showed that myelin formation had come to a standstill and that the volume of white matter was markedly reduced. Mental and motor development were both severely impaired; tendon reflexes were brisk without distinct spasticity. With the exception of a coccygeal dimple, a faint cardiac murmur, and borderline enlargement of the liver, the remainder of physical findings were unremarkable.

TABLE 25-10	CDG-Ii: Laboratory Findings
Decreased	**Increased**
factor XI	partial thromboplastin time
tetrasialotransferrin	disialotransferrin
	asialotransferrin
	dolichol-linked $Man_{1-2}GlcNAc_2$

Diagnosis Primary diagnostic evaluation in CDG-Ii is conducted by isoelectric focusing of serum transferrin. The isoelectric focusing pattern is indistinguishable from other CDG-I types with an accumulation of di- and asialotransferrin (Figure 25-3). Further analysis is performed by metabolic labeling of patients' fibroblasts with radioactive mannose, subsequent hydrophobic extraction of short dolichol-linked oligosaccharides by thin-layer chromatography, or HPLC analysis of the oligosaccharide moieties. In case of $Man_2GlcNAc_2$ and $Man_1GlcNAc_2$ accumulation genetic analysis of the *hALG2* gene is performed (Table 25-10).

Treatment No efficient treatment is available.

CDG-Ij: UDP-GlcNAc: DOLICHOL-PHOSPHATE N-ACETYLGLUCOSAMINE-1-PHOSPHATE TRANSFERASE DEFICIENCY

Etiology/Pathophysiology The molecular defect in CDG-Ij is caused by mutations in the UDP-GlcNAc:dolichol-phosphate N-acetylglucosamine-1-phosphate transferase gene (*DPAGT1*), which is localized on chromosome 11q23 (34). The affected enzyme catalyzes the transfer of the first N-acetylglucosamine residue from UDP-N-acetylglucosamine onto dolichol phosphate on the cytosolic side of the endoplasmic reticulum membrane (Figure 25-1). Due to reduced enzyme activity the amount of full-length lipid-linked oligosaccharides is decreased, causing hypoglycosylation of serum glycoproteins.

Clinical Presentation Only one CDG-Ij patient has been identified. The girl suffered from markedly delayed development, severe hypotonia, and medically intractable seizures. Microcephaly, arched palate, micrognathia, exotropia, fifth finger clinodactyly, single-flexion creases, and skin dimples on the upper thighs were present. At the age of 6 years she had minimal speech. Although brain MRI was normal, positron emission tomography scanning showed multifocal areas of decreased metabolic activity.

TABLE 25-11	CDG-Ij: Laboratory Findings
Decreased	**Increased**
AT III	disialotransferrin
tetrasialotransferrin	asialotransferrin
dolichol-linked Glc$_3$Man$_9$GlcNAc$_2$	

TABLE 25-12	CDG-Ik: Laboratory Findings
Decreased	**Increased**
circulating B cells	disialotransferrin
IgG	asialotransferrin
tetrasialotransferrin	dolichol-linked GlcNAc$_2$

TABLE 25-13	CDG-IL: Laboratory Findings
Decreased	**Increased**
tetrasialotransferrin	disialotransferrin
	asialotransferrin
	dolichol-linked Man$_6$GlcNAc$_2$
	dolichol-linked Man$_8$GlcNAc$_2$

Diagnosis Primary diagnostic evaluation of CDG-Ij is conducted by isoelectric focusing of serum transferrin, where a CDG-I pattern with an accumulation of di- and asialo-transferrin is found (Figure 25-3). Further analysis is conducted by metabolic labeling of patients' fibroblasts with radioactive mannose. In case of a decreased amount of full-length lipid-linked oligosaccharides, genetic analysis of the *DPAGT1* gene is performed (Table 25-11).

Treatment No efficient treatment is available.

CDG-Ik: GDP-Man: GlcNAc$_2$-PP-DOLICHOL MANNOSYLTRANSFERASE DEFICIENCY

Etiology/Pathophysiology The molecular defect of CDG-Ik is caused by mutations in the GDP-Man:GlcNAc$_2$-PP-dolichol mannosyl-transferase gene, the human ortholog of the yeast *ALG1* gene *(hALG1)*, which is localized on chromosome 16p13 (35–37). The mannosyltransferase catalyzes the transfer of the first mannosyl residue from GDP-mannose onto GlcNAc$_2$-PP-dolichol at the cytosolic site of the endoplasmic reticulum (Figure 25-1). Deficiency of the enzyme results in accumulation of GlcNAc$_2$-PP-dolichol and thereby to a decreased amount of full-length dolichol-linked oligosaccharides, which causes hypoglycosylation of glycoproteins.

Clinical Presentation Four CDG-Ik patients have been described. Three of the patients had a very severe clinical phenotype with death in early infancy (35,36). Fetal hydrops and hepatosplenomegaly were identified in the index patient by ultrasonography in the 30th week of pregnancy (35). At birth, hydrops, multiple dysmorphic features with large fontanelle, hypertelorism, micrognathia, hypogonadism, contractures, areflexia, cardiomyopathy, and multifocal epileptic activity were noted. The patient died at 2 weeks of age. Another CDG-Ik patient presented with an uncomplicated pregnancy and a milder clinical phenotype. Impaired psychomotor development, intractable seizures, muscular hypotonia, and blindness developed during infancy. Liver dysfunction and coagulation defects developed before 1 year of age.

Another patient presented with nephrotic syndrome and a severe decrease of B cells with a complete absence of serum IgG (36).

Diagnosis Primary diagnostic evaluation in CDG-Ik is conducted by isoelectric focusing of serum transferrin. The isoelectric focusing pattern is comparable to other CDG-I types with an accumulation of di- and asialo-transferrin (Figure 25-3). In two cases the total amount of transferrin was significantly reduced (35,36). Further investigations are performed by metabolic labeling of patients' fibroblasts with radioactive glucosamine, subsequent hydrophobic extraction of short dolichol-linked oligosaccharides, and thin layer chromatography analysis of the oligosaccharide moieties. In case of GlcNAc$_2$-PP-dolichol accumulation genetic analysis of the *hALG1* gene is performed (Table 25-12).

Treatment No efficient treatment is available.

CDG-IL: DOLICHOL-P-MANNOSE: ∝1,2 MANNOSYLTRANSFERASE DEFICIENCY

Etiology/Pathophysiology CDG-IL is caused by mutations in the dolichol-P-mannose:α1,2 mannosyltransferase gene, the human ortholog to the yeast *ALG9* gene *(hALG9)* located on chromosome 11q23 (38). This mannosyltransferase catalyzes the transfer of mannose residues from dolichol-phosphate mannose in α1,2 linkage onto Man$_6$GlcNAc$_2$-PP-dolichol and Man$_8$GlcNAc$_2$-PP-dolichol in the endoplasmic reticulum (Figure 25-1). The reduced enzyme activity leads to accumulation of Man$_6$GlcNAc$_2$-PP-dolichol and Man$_8$GlcNAc$_2$-PP-dolichol, which are further transferred onto newly synthesized glycoproteins. The truncated oligosaccharides are unable to support complete glycoprotein biosynthesis.

Clinical Presentation The clinical phenotype of CDG-IL presents with severe microcephaly, central hypotonia, seizures, hepatomegaly, developmental delay, and bronchial asthma.

Diagnosis Primary diagnostic evaluation in CDG-IL is conducted by isoelectric focusing of serum transferrin. The isoelectric focusing pattern resembles other CDG-I types

with accumulation of di- and asialotransferrin (Figure 25-3). Further investigations are conducted by metabolic labeling of patients' fibroblasts with radioactive mannose, extraction of dolichol-linked oligosaccharides, and HPLC analysis of oligosaccharide moieties. In case of Man$_6$GlcNAc$_2$-PP-dolichol and Man$_8$GlcNAc$_2$-PP-dolichol accumulation genetic analysis of the *hALG9* gene is performed (Table 25-13).

Treatment No efficient treatment is available.

CDG-IIa: GOLGI N-ACETYL-GLUCOSAMINYLTRANSFERASE II DEFICIENCY

Etiology/Pathophysiology The molecular defect in CDG-IIa is caused by mutations in the Golgi N-acetyl-glucosaminyltransferase II gene *(MGAT2)* (39,40), which is located on chromosome 14q21. The integral membrane protein catalyzes the transfer of the second N-acetylglucosamine residue to the nascent protein-linked GlcNAc$_2$Man$_3$GlcNAc$_1$ oligosaccharide during glycoprotein processing in the Golgi apparatus (Figure 25-1) and is therefore essential for the biosynthesis of complex N-linked glycans. The severe reduction of enzyme activity in CDG-IIa results in an accumulation of glycoproteins linked to monoantennary-oligosaccharides.

Clinical Presentation The four CDG-IIa patients described so far presented with psychomotor retardation more severe than in CDG-Ia. Vision, speech, sitting, and walking were all affected. Generalized hypotonia, limb weakness and a characteristic stereotypic handwashing-behavior as described for Rett syndrome were observed. MRI revealed cortical atrophy, focal white matter lesions, and delayed myelination. In contrast to CDG-Ia, neither peripheral neuropathy nor cerebellar hypoplasia were present. CDG-IIa patients show dysmorphic features such as hooked nose, large dysplastic ears, prognathia, proximal implantation of the thumbs, crowded toes, and widely spaced nipples. Chronic feeding problems with severe diarrhea, frequent infections of the upper airway, and coagulopathy have been observed.

TABLE 25-14	CDG-IIa: Laboratory Findings
Decreased	**Increased**
factor IX	AST disialotransferrin
factor XII	
AT III	
tetrasialotransferrin	

TABLE 25-15	CDG-IIb: Laboratory Findings
Increased
AST
tetrasaccharides in urine

TABLE 25-16	CDG-IIc: Laboratory Findings
Decreased	**Increased**
absence of ABO (Bombay phenotype),	white blood cells
lack of Sialyl-Lewis X on neutrophils	

Diagnosis Primary diagnostic evaluation in CDG-IIa is conducted by isoelectric focusing of serum transferrin. The isoelectric focusing pattern differs completely from all known CDG-I types with a strong accumulation of disialotransferrin and a nearly undetectable amount of tetrasialotransferrin (Figure 25-3). Because in vitro determination of Golgi N-acetyl-glucosaminyltransferase II activity is complicated due to restricted availability of the $GlcNAc_2Man_3GlcNAc_1$ acceptor substrate, further investigations should be performed by genetic analysis of the *MGAT2* gene. In addition, increased liver enzymes and decreased AT III, factor IX, and factor XII are present (Table 25-14).

Treatment No efficient treatment is available.

CDG-IIb: ENDOPLASMIC RETICULUM GLUCOSIDASE I DEFICIENCY

Etiology/Pathophysiology Mutations in the gene encoding endoplasmic reticulum glucosidase I (*GCS1*), which is located on chromosome 2p13, cause CDG-IIb (41). Glucosidase I is an enzyme in N-linked glycoprotein processing, which removes specifically distal -1,2-linked glucose residues from the $Glc_3Man_9GlcNAc_2$ precursor after its *en bloc* transfer from the dolichyl phosphate carrier onto newly synthesized glycoproteins in the endoplasmic reticulum (Figure 25-1).

Clinical Presentation The only patient with CDG-IIb presented neonatally with generalized hypotonia, hypomobility, and edema. Dysmorphic features included a prominent occiput, short palpebral fissures, long eyelashes, a broad nose, retrognathia, high-arched palate, hypoplastic genitalia, overlapping fingers, and thoracic scoliosis. The clinical course of the disease was progressive and characterized by hepatomegaly, hypoventilation, feeding problems, seizures, and fatal outcome at 74 days after birth (41).

Diagnosis In contrast to other CDG types the isoelectric focusing pattern of serum transferring was unremarkable in CDG-IIb, which has not been elucidated. Thin-layer chromatography screening for oligosaccharides in urine revealed the presence of an abnormal

Glc$_3$Man-tetrasaccharide, probably released from the unprocessed oligosaccharide by an endo-α1,2-mannosidase in the Golgi. Moreover, the activity of glucosidase I in cultured skin fibroblasts was severely reduced. The amount of glucosidase I in liver homogenates and fibroblasts was likewise strongly reduced, and molecular analysis revealed substitution mutations in the corresponding *GCS1* gene (Table 25-15).

Treatment No efficient treatment is available.

CDG-IIc: GOLGI GDP-FUCOSE TRANSPORTER DEFICIENCY

Etiology/Pathophysiology The molecular defect in CDG-IIc is due to mutations in the Golgi GDP-fucose transporter gene, which is located on chromosome 11p11 (42,43). This transporter imports GDP-fucose into the lumen of the Golgi apparatus and deports the corresponding nucleoside monophosphate into the cytosol (Figure 25-1). Mutations in the transporter protein lead to a general hypofucosylation of N- and O-glycosylated proteins.

Clinical Presentation CDG-IIc patients present with moderate-to-severe psychomotor retardation, dwarfism, and dysmorphic features including a broad and depressed nasal bridge, long eyelashes, and broad palms. Adhesion of leukocytes to endothelial cells and migration of neutrophiles to sites of infections are decreased because of the absence of fucosylated selectin ligands. Recurrent infections with neutrophilia are present in the newborn period.

Diagnosis A hint to diagnosis is the persistently elevated number of leukocytes combined with no detectable ABO blood group on their erythrocytes (Bombay phenotype) (44). Because the oligosaccharide moieties linked to transferrin do not contain fucose residues, isoelectric focusing is not suitable to identify CDG-IIc. Instead, laboratory investigations should include fluorescence-activated cell sorting analysis of the sialyl-Lewis X carbohydrate structure as well as the H-antigen at the surface of erythrocytes, which are both absent in CDG-IIc. Further investigations are performed by measuring the import of radioactive GDP-fucose into Golgi-enriched vesicles of patient-derived fibroblasts or lymphoblasts.

In case of reduced import of GDP-fucose, genetic analysis of the Golgi GDP-fucose transporter gene is performed (Table 25-16).

Treatment In two patients, CDG-IIc deficiency was treated by giving oral fucose starting at 25 mg/kg per dose five times a day (45). Single doses were slowly increased to a maximum dose of 492 mg/kg. Fucose is taken up into the cell and converted to GDP-fucose by fucose-1-kinase and GDP-L-fucose pyrophosphorylase. The effect of fucose supplementation is not completely understood but it is hypothesized that the increase of the GDP-fucose pool in the cytosol leads to a higher import of GDP-fucose into the Golgi, thereby normalizing the hypofucosylation of glycoproteins. Oral fucose supplementation leads to the reexpression of selectin ligands on neutrophils and to the correction of the core fucosylation of serum glycoproteins. Subsequently, the number of peripheral neutrophils was reduced to normal levels and infections or episodes of fever of unknown origin disappeared. The improvement of psychomotor capabilities and growth of the patients by fucose therapy remain unclear and the H-antigen could not be normalized on patient-derived erythrocytes by fucose treatment (45).

CDG-IId: GOLGI UDP-GALACTOSE: N-ACETYLGLUCOSAMINE-β-1,4-GALACTOSYLTRANSFERASE I

Etiology/Pathophysiology Deficiency of the Golgi enzyme UDP-galactose:N-acetylglucosamine-ß-1,4-galactosyltransferase I causes CDG-IId (46). The gene encoding this galactosyltransferase is located on chromosome 9p13. It transfers galactose from UDP-galactose onto terminal N-acetylglucosamine residues of complex-type oligosaccharides in newly synthesized glycoproteins in the Golgi (Figure 25-1). Reduced enzyme activity leads to shortened N-glycan side chains of glycoproteins due to the lack of galactose residues and the sialic acid residues linked to galactose.

Clinical Presentation The index patient with CDG-IId presented at birth with macrocephaly caused by Dandy–Walker malformation, coagulopathy, and extensive abdominal

TABLE 25-17	CDG-IId: Laboratory Findings
Decreased	**Increased**
factor XI	partial thromboplastin time
AT III	serum creatine kinase
fibrinogen	trisialotransferrin
cholinesterase	disialotransferrin
tetrasialotransferrin	monosialotransferrin

TABLE 25-18	CDG-IIe: Laboratory Findings
Decreased	**Increased**
tetrasialotransferrin	trisialotransferrin
	disialotransferrin
	monosialotransferrin
	asialotransferrin

bleeding caused by a rupture of the hepatic capsule. In the following months a transient cholestatic syndrome, elevated creatine kinase indicating myopathy, and a progressive shy-drocephalus due to compression of the aqueduct developed. Nonproportional muscular hypotonia with decreased muscle mass and poor head control with weak tendon reflexes were present. Ocular fixation and hearing were preserved as well as the other cranial nerve functions. At the age of 2 years, the patient was able to distinguish between familiar and unfamiliar people and spoke some words (47).

Diagnosis Primary diagnostic evaluation in CDG-IId is conducted by isoelectric focusing. In contrast to other CDG-II types, the levels of asialo-, mono-, di-, and trisialotransferrin were increased at the expense of tetrasialotransferrin, which was nearly not detectable (Figure 25-3). Further analysis is performed by determination of Golgi ß-1,4-galactosyltransferase I activity by metabolic labeling of patients' fibroblasts with radioactive galactose. In case of a reduced activity of this enzyme genetic analysis of the ß-1,4-galactosyltransferase I gene is performed (Table 25-17).

Treatment No specific treatment is available.

CDG-IIe

Etiology/Pathophysiology CDG-IIe is caused by mutations in the gene of subunit 7 of the conserved oligomeric complex (COG7), which is located on chromosome 16p12 (48). This complex comprises a group of at least eight protein subunits that are located at the cytosolic site of the Golgi apparatus. The task of COG is to keep glycosyltransferases and sugar nucleotide transporters in the right positions. Disruption of the complex as in CDG-IIe by COG7 deficiency affects the localization of the interacting enzymes and transporters (Figure 25-1) and results in hypoglycosylation of glycoproteins.

Clinical Presentation Only two siblings with CDG-IIe have been described. Both presented with perinatal asphyxia and dysmorphic features including low-set dysplastic ears, micrognathia, short neck, and loose, wrinkled skin. Shortly after birth, generalized hypotonia, hepatosplenomegaly, and progressive jaundice developed. Both patients developed severe epilepsy and died at 5 and 10 weeks of age, respectively, from recurrent infections and cardiac insufficiency.

Diagnosis Primary diagnosis for CDG-IIe is conducted by isoelectric focusing of serum transferrin. The isoelectric focusing pattern shows an accumulation of tri-, di-, mono-, and asialotransferrin at the expense of tetrasialotransferrin (Figure 25-3), which diverges from all known CDG types. Additional diagnostics may require isoelectric focusing of apolipoprotein C-III (49) to confirm deficient N- and O-glycosylation, thereby indicating a generalized glycosylation defect. Because no diagnostic markers for intracellular trafficking disorders exist, direct mutation analysis is indicated (Table 25-18).

Treatment No specific treatment is available.

REFERENCES

1. Jaeken J, Carchon H. Congenital disorders of glycosylation: a booming chapter of pediatrics. *Curr Opin Pediatr.* 2004;16:434–439.
2. Helenius A, Aebi M. Intracellular functions of N-linked glycans. *Science.* 2001;23:2364–2369.
3. Marquardt T, Denecke J. Congenital disorders of glycosylation: review of their molecular bases, clinical presentations and specific therapies. *Eur J Pediatr.* 2003;162:359–379.
4. Jaeken J. Komrower Lecture. Congenital disorders of glycosylation (CDG): it's all in it! *J Inherit Metab Dis.* 2003;26:99–118.
5. Fang J, Peters V, Körner C, et al. Improvement of CDG diagnosis by combined examinations of several glycoproteins. *J Inherit Metab Dis.* 2004;27:581–590.
6. Clayton P, Winchester B, Di Tomaso E, et al. Carbohydrate-deficient glycoprotein syndrome: normal glycosylation in the fetus. *Lancet.* 1993;34:956.
7. Participants "First International Workshop on CDGS". Carbohydrate-deficient glycoprotein syndromes become congenital disorders of glycosylation: an updated nomenclature for CDG. First International Workshop on CDGS. *Glycoconj J.* 1999;16:669–671.
8. Matthijs G, Schollen E, Pardon E, et al. Mutations in PMM2, a phosphomannomutase gene on chromosome 16p13, in carbohydrate-deficient glycoprotein type I syndrome (Jaeken syndrome). *Nat Genet.* 1997;16:88–92.
9. van Schaftingen E, Jaeken J. Phosphomannomutase deficiency is a cause of carbohydrate deficient glycoprotein syndrome type I. *FEBS Lett.* 1995;377:318–320.
10. Körner C, Lehle L, von Figura K, et al. Abnormal synthesis of mannose 1-phosphate derived carbohydrates in carbohydrate-deficient glycoprotein syndrome type I fibroblasts with phosphomannomutase deficiency. *Glycobiology.* 1998; 8:165–171.
11. Grünewald S, Schollen E, Van Schaftingen E, et al. High residual activity of PMM2 in patients' fibroblasts: Possible pitfall in the diagnosis of CDG-Ia (Phosphomannomutase deficiency). *Am J Hum Genet.* 2001;68:347–354.
12. Kristiansson B, Andersson M, Tonnby B, et al. Disialotransferrin developmental deficiency syndrome. *Arch Dis Child.* 1989;64:71–76.
13. Miller BS, Freeze HH. New disorders in carbohydrate metabolism: CDG and their impact on the endocrine system. *Rev Endocrin Metab Dis.* 2003;4:103–113.
14. deZegher F. Jackson J. Endocrinology of the carbohydrate-deficient glycoprotein syndrome type I from birth through adolescence. *Pediatr Res.* 1995;37:395–401.
15. Kristiansson B. Stibler H, Wide L. Gonadal function and glycoprotein hormones in the carbohydrate-deficient glycoprotein (CDG) syndrome. *Acta Paediatr.* 1995;84:655–659.
16. Matthijs G, Schollen E, van Schaftingen E, et al. The prenatal diagnosis of congenital disorders of glycosylation (CDG). *Prenat Diagn.* 2004;24:114–116.
17. Panneerselvam K, Freeze HH. Mannose corrects altered N-glycosylation in carbohydrate-deficient glycoprotein syndrome fibroblasts. *J Clin Invest.* 1996;97:1478–1487.
18. Körner C, Lehle L, von Figura K, et al. Carbohydrate-deficient glycoprotein syndrome type 1: correction of the glycosylation defect by deprivation of glucose or supplementation of mannose. *Glycoconj J.* 1998;15:499–505.
19. Niehues R, Hasilik M, Alton G, Carbohydrate deficient glycoprotein syndrome type Ib: phosphomannose Isomerase deficiency and mannose therapy. *J Clin Invest.* 1998;101:1414–1420.
20. Körner C, Knauer R, Holzbach U, et al. Carbohydrate deficient glycoprotein syndrome type V: deficiency of Dolichol-P-Glc: Man₉GlcNAc₂-PP-dolichol glucosyltransferase. *Proc Natl Acad Sci USA.* 1998; 95:13200–13205.
21. Imbach T, Burda P, Kuhner P, et al. A mutation in the human orthologue of the *Saccharomyces cerevisiae* ALG6 gene causes carbohydrate-deficient glycoprotein syndrome type-Ic. *Proc Natl Acad Sci USA.* 1999;96:6982–6987.
22. Hanefeld F, Körner C, Holzbach-Eberle U, et al. Congenital disorder of glycosylation-Ic: case report and genetic defect. *Neuropediatrics.* 2000;31:60–62.
23. Körner C, Knauer R, Stephani U, et al. Carbohydrate deficient glycoprotein syndrome type IV: deficiency of dolichol-P-Man: Man₅GlcNAc₂-PP-dolichol mannosyltransferase. *EMBO J.* 1999;18:6818–6822.
24. Imbach T, Schenk B, Schollen E, et al. Deficiency of dolichol-phosphate-mannose synthase-1 causes congenital disorder of

glycosylation type Ie. *J Clin Invest.* 2000;105:233–239.

25. Kim S, Westphal V, Srikrishna G, et al. Dolichol phosphate mannose synthase (DPM1) mutations define congenital disorder of glycosylation Ie (CDG-Ie). *J Clin Invest.* 2000;105:191–198.

26. Schenk B, Imbach T, Frank CG, et al. *MPDU1* mutations underlie a novel human congenital disorder of glycosylation, designated type If. *J Clin Invest.* 2001;108:1687–1695.

27. Kranz C, Denecke J, Lehrman MA, et al. A mutation in the human *MPDU1* gene causes congenital disorder of glycosylation type If (CDG–If). *J Clin Invest.* 2001;108:1613–1619.

28. Chantret I, Dupre T, Delenda C, et al. Congenital disorders of glycosylation type Ig is defined by a deficiency in dolichol-P-mannose:Man7GlcNAc2-PP-dolichol mannosyltransferase. *J Biol Chem.* 2002;12:25815–25822.

29. Grubenmann C, Frank C, Kjaergaard S, et al. ALG12 mannosyltransferase defect in congenital disorder of glycosylation type Ig. *Hum Mol Genet.* 2002;15:2331–2339.

30. Thiel C, Schwarz M, Hasilik M, et al. Congenital disorder of glycosylation-Ig is caused by deficiency of dolichol-P-Man:Man₇GlcNAc₂-PP-dolichol mannosyltransferase. *Biochem J.* 2002;367:195–201.

31. Chantret I, Dancourt J, Dupre T, et al. A deficiency in dolichol-P-glucose:Glc₁Man₉-GlcNAc₂-PP-dolichol-α1,3-glucosyltransferase defines a new subtype of congenital disorders of glycosylation (CDG). *J Biol Chem.* 2003;278:9962–9971.

32. Schollen E, Frank CG, Keldermans L, et al. Clinical and molecular features of three patients with congenital disorders of glycosylation type Ih (CDG-Ih) (ALG8 deficiency). *J Med Genet.* 2004;41:550–556.

33. Thiel C, Schwarz M, Peng J, et al. A new type of congenital disorders of glycosylation (CDG-Ii) provides new insights into the early steps of dolichol-linked oligosaccharide biosynthesis. *J Biol Chem.* 2003;278:22498–22505.

34. Wu X, Rush J, Karaoglu D, et al. Deficiency of UDP-GlcNAc:dolichol phosphate N-acetylglucosamine-1 phosphate transferase (DPAGT1) causes a novel congenital disorder of glycosylation type Ij. *Hum Mutat.* 2003;22:144–150.

35. Schwarz M, Thiel C, Lübbehusen J, et al. Deficiency of GDP-Man:GlcNAc₂-PP-dolichol mannosyltransferase causes congenital disorder of glycosylation type Ik. *Am J Hum Genet.* 2004;74:472–481.

36. Kranz C, Denecke J, Lehle L, et al. Congenital disorder of glycosylation type Ik (CDG-Ik): a defect of mannosyltransferase I. *Am J Hum Genet.* 2004;74:545–551.

37. Grubenmann CE, Frank CG, Hulsmeier AJ, et al. Deficiency of the first mannosylation step in the N-glycosylation pathway causes congenital disorder of glycosylation type Ik. *Hum Mol Genet.* 2004;13:535–542.

38. Frank C, Grubenmann C, Eyaid W, et al. Identification and functional analysis of a defect in the human ALG9 gene: definition of congenital disorder of glycosylation type IL. *Am J Hum Genet.* 2004;75:146–150.

39. Jaeken J, Schachter H, Carchon H, et al. Carbohydrate deficient glycoprotein syndrome type II: a deficiency in Golgi localised N-acetyl-glucosaminyltransferase II. *Arch Dis Child.* 1994;71:123–127.

40. Tan J, Dunn J, Jaeken J, et al. Mutations in the MGAT2 gene controlling complex N-glycan synthesis cause carbohydrate-deficient glycoprotein syndrome type II, an autosomal recessive disease with defective brain development. *Am J Hum Genet.* 1996;59:810–817.

41. de Praeter C, Gerwig G, Bause E, et al. A novel disorder caused by defective biosynthesis of N-linked oligosaccharides due to glucosidase I deficiency. *Am J Hum Genet.* 2000;66:1744–1756.

42. Lübke T, Marquardt T, Etzioni A, et al. Complementation cloning identifies CDG-IIc (LADII), a new type of congenital disorders of glycosylation, as a GDP-fucose transporter deficiency. *Nat Genet.* 2001;28:73–76.

43. Lühn K, Wild M, Eckhardt M, et al. The defective gene in leukocyte adhesion deficiency II codes for a putative GDP-fucose transporter. *Nat Genet.* 2001;28:69–72.

44. Marquardt T, Brune T, Lühn K, et al. Leukocyte adhesion deficiency II syndrome, a generalized defect in fucose metabolism. *J Pediatr.* 1999;134:681–688.

45. Marquardt T, Lühn K, Srikrishna G, et al. Correction of leukocyte adhesion deficiency type II with oral fucose. *Blood.* 2000;95:3641–3643.

46. Hansske B, Thiel C, Lübke T, et al. Deficiency of UDP-galactose:N-acetylglucosamine beta-1,4-galactosyltransferase leads to congenital disorder of glycosylation-IId (CDG-IId). *J Clin Invest.* 2002;109:725–733.

47. Peters V, Penzien JM, Reiter G, et al. Congenital disorder of glycosylation IId (CDG-IId) - a new entity: clinical presentation with Dandy-Walker malformation and myopathy. *Neuropediatrics.* 2002;33:27–32.

48. Wu X, Steet R, Bohorov O, et al. Mutation of the COG complex subunit gene COG7 causes a lethal congenital disorder. *Nat Med.* 2004;10:518–523.

49. Wopereis S, Grünewald S, Morava E, et al. Apolipoprotein C-III isofocusing in the diagnosis of genetic defects in O-glycan biosynthesis. *Clin Chem.* 2003;49:1839–1845.

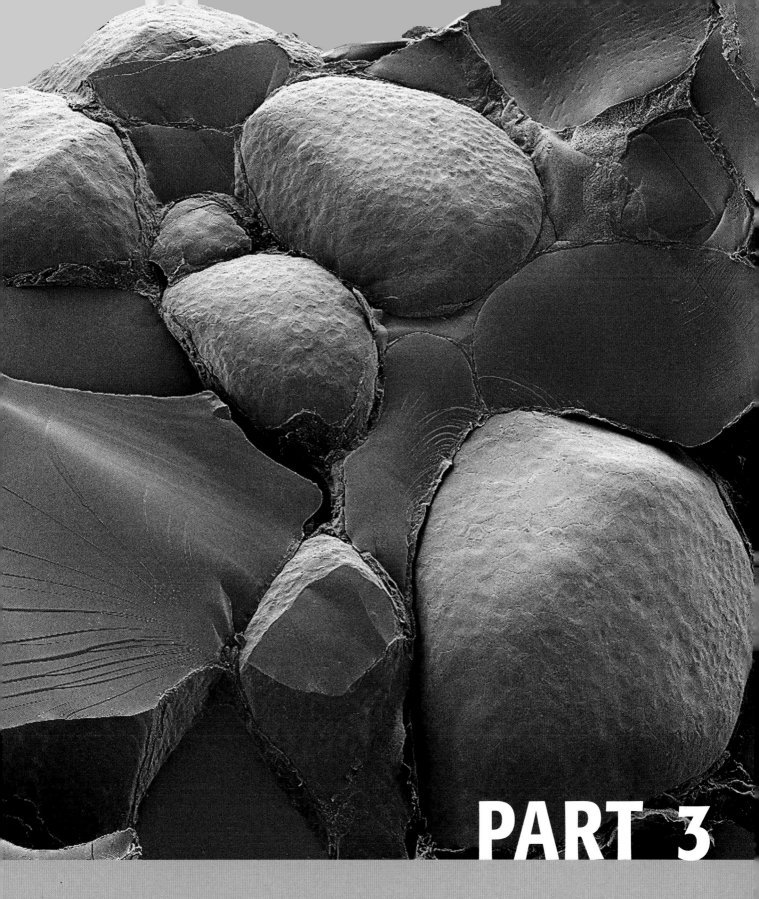

PART 3

Disorders of the Thyroid Gland

IN THIS PART

Previous page: Colored scanning electron micrograph (SEM) of a fracture through the thyroid gland revealing several follicles (orange and green). Between the follicles is connective tissue (red). A follicle consists of a layer of epithelial cells (green) around a central storage chamber. The cells produce the thyroid hormones triiodothyronin (T_3) and thyroxine (T_4) and secrete them into the central chamber where they are stored as the glycoprotein thyroid colloid (orange).

CHAPTER 26

Disorders of the Thyroid Gland

Michel Polak, MD, PhD
Guy Van Vliet, MD

NORMAL THYROID GLAND DEVELOPMENT AND FUNCTION

The thyroid gland is the first of the body's endocrine glands to develop (~24th day of gestation) and its maturation can be divided into two phases. The first phase involves embryogenesis of the thyroid gland and the hypothalamic-pituitary-thyroidal (HPT) axis. The second phase involves further development of the HPT axis including hormone production and regulation.

The thyroid gland originates from the median anlage and from two lateral anlagen. The single median anlage gives rise to the vast majority of the thyroxine-producing follicular cells: it evolves from an outpouching of the floor of the pharynx and at the tip of the foramen caecum at the base of the tongue (between the first and second branchial arches). As the thyroid gland develops it descends through the tissues of the neck, remaining connected to the foramen caecum by the thyroglossal duct, which generally solidifies and subsequently becomes entirely obliterated (during gestational weeks 7–10). Failure of subsequent closure and obliteration of the thyroglossal duct predisposes to thyroglossal cyst formation. The two lateral anlagen (one on each side of the neck) derive from the fourth branchial pouches and they eventually fuse with the median anlage. The lateral anlagen may give rise to a few thyroxine-producing cells but are the main source of the calcitonin-secreting cells (parafollicular or C cells). The calcitonin-producing cells are of neural crest origin and become dispersed between the thyroid follicles.

The thyroid follicular cells, which appear in the 9th to 10th week of gestation, are the major cellular component of the thyroid. They are organized in a structure made of a single layer of polarized cells surrounding a colloid-containing lumen, the thyroid follicle.

From the functional standpoint, the thyroid can be envisioned as a structure that extracts and concentrates the iodine that reaches the gland through the bloodstream to convert it

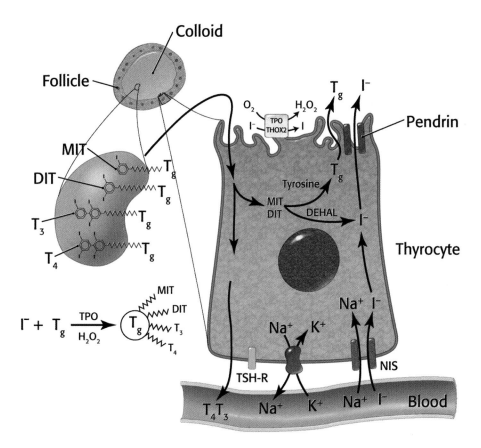

FIGURE 26-1. Steps in thyroid hormone synthesis. Iodine (I–) is taken up by the thyroid follicular cell via the NIS. Iodine is transported into the colloid lumen via the protein pendrin. Thyroperoxidase iodinates the tyrosines present on thyroglobulin (organification) and promotes synthesis of T_3 and T_4 from two iodotyrosines (coupling). H_2O_2 generation by THOX 2 is necessary for thyroperoxidase action.

into thyroxine (T_4) and triiodothyronine (T_3) (Figure 26-1). Briefly, iodide is taken up at the basal membrane of the follicular cells through a sodium-iodine symporter (NIS) and is transported to the apical membrane where thyroid hormone synthesis is initiated at the cell-colloid interface, through a protein complex consisting of iodide transporters (pendrin and possibly other proteins), a peroxidase (thyroid peroxidase, TPO), and a peroxide-generating system that includes thyroid oxidases, THOX1 or DUOX1 and THOX2 or DUOX2; peroxide (H_2O_2) generation is a limiting step in thy-

roid hormone biosynthesis. In addition to the oxidation of the iodine, TPO catalyzes the iodination of selected tyrosine residues within thyroglobulin (a process called organification of iodine) resulting in the formation of mono- and diiodotyrosines. Mono- and diiodotyrosines assemble (a process called coupling, which is also catalyzed by TPO) to make T_4 and T_3. Thyroglobulin is synthesized exclusively in the follicular cells of the thyroid gland and is found at a very high concentration in colloid. Iodinated thyroglobulin is next taken up by the follicular cell at its apical

Disorders of the Thyroid
AT A GLANCE

Normal development of the anatomic structures of the hypothalamic-pituitary-thyroid-target organ axis and of the physiologic interactions between the different levels of this axis are essential for brain development from before birth until the age of 3 years, for linear growth after birth, and for metabolism throughout life. Knowledge of both congenital and acquired disease processes that result in hypo- and hyperthyroidism are therefore essential for the practicing pediatric endocrinologist.

Hypothyroidism that remains unrecognized and untreated for several months after birth is by far the most dramatic example of the irreversible consequences that thyroid dysfunction can have on development. Indeed, the physical signs and symptoms of hypothyroidism at that age (jaundice, macroglossia, mottled skin, constipation, and hypotonia) are readily reversible with thyroxine replacement but brain damage is not. By contrast, hypothyroidism occurring after the age of 3 years does not lead to mental retardation but may affect growth and bone maturation so profoundly that the genetic height potential will not be reached (1). Severe iodine deficiency, which remains the most common cause of preventable mental and physical disability worldwide, exemplifies the impact of hypothyroidism throughout the lifespan (2).

Hyperthyroidism is less frequent but its impact on growth and development can be as dramatic. Exposure of the conceptus to excess thyroid hormone throughout gestation results in fetal loss and in decreased birth weight of the surviving newborns (3), severe congenital hyperthyroidism from activating mutations in the thyrotropin receptor gene occurring *de novo* in the fetus may lead to mental deficiency (4) and fetal hyperthyroidism from maternal Graves disease may lead to fetal death (5,6). Hyperthyroidism that develops during childhood and adolescence often results in a marked decrease in school performance due to a severe attention deficit.

The thyroid often becomes visible or palpable in euthyroid adolescents. If this is deemed to go beyond the normal growth of the thyroid at puberty, the possibility of low-grade Hashimoto thyroiditis, compensated defects of thyroid hormone biosynthesis, or mild iodine deficiency should be considered.

CAUSES	PATHOPHYSIOLOGIC FEATURES	PREVALENCE	OMIM
Permanent Congenital Hypothyroidism: Primary ($\downarrow T_4$, $\uparrow TSH$)		1:3500 newborns	
Thyroid dysgenesis	— Includes ectopy (~80%, female predominance), agenesis, hypoplasia, hemiagenesis (20%)	85% of permanent primary hypothyroidism, ectopy most common	#218700
	— $^{99m}TcO_4$ or ^{123}I scan may be diagnostic, ultrasound less sensitive		
	— Few known mutations:	Known mutations rare	
	• TTF-1: Hypotonia, choreoathetosis, respiratory distress		TTF-1: +600635
	• TTF-2: Cleft palate, kinky hair		TTF-2:*602617
	• PAX8: Autosomal dominant, thyroid hypoplasia, or apparent athyreosis		PAX8:*167415
	• TSH receptor: Autosomal recessive, thyroid hypoplasia, or apparent athyreosis		TSHR: #275200
Thyroid dyshormonogenesis	— Autosomal recessive mutations in thyroxine synthesis (NIS, PDS, THOX 2, TPO, Tg)	15% of permanent primary hypothyroidism, more common in inbred populations	NIS: *601843
	— Goiter that may not be immediately present at birth		PDS: *274600
	— TPO most common		THOX2: #607200
	— Deafness with Pendred syndrome		TPO: *606765
	— Perchlorate discharge test may help diagnose organification defects, but not usually performed (does not alter treatment)		Tg: *188450
Resistance to thyrotropin	— TSH receptor mutation: wide phenotypic spectrum with apparent athyreosis the most severe form	Rare	TSHR: #275200
	— Pseudohypoparathyroid (Gsα mutation): $\downarrow$Ca, $\uparrow$phos, $\uparrow$PTH		PHP: #103580
	— Others		

CAUSES	PATHOPHYSIOLOGIC FEATURES	PREVALENCE	OMIM
Permanent Congenital Hypothyroidism: Central ($\downarrow T_4$, $\downarrow$ or inappropriately normal TSH)		<1:50,000	
Developmental defects	— Pituitary or hypothalamic disorders; may have midline defects	Rare	Various
Inactivating mutations	— TRH receptor: isolated hypothyroidism — TSH ß-subunit: TSH levels low unless assay also measures mutant TSH — Pituitary transcription factors: multiple hormones deficient (HESX1, LHX3, LHX4, PROP1, PIT1)	Rare	TRHR: +188545 TSHß: *188540 HESX1: *601802 LHX3: *600577 LHX4: *602146 PROP1: +601538 PIT1: +173110
Permanent Congenital Hypothyroidism: Peripheral			
Abnormal thyroid hormone transport into the cell	— Mutations in MCT8; $\downarrow T_4$, $\downarrow rT_3$, $\uparrow T_3$, normal to slightly $\uparrow$TSH — Males more affected (X-linked), severe psychomotor and mental retardation	Rare	*300095
Thyroid hormone resistance	— Mutations in TRß most common (85%); $\uparrow T_4$, normal, or $\uparrow$TSH; goiter — Because of the distribution of α and ß thyroid hormone receptors, neurologic and cardiac effects can differ (i.e., mental retardation from central hypothyroidism but tachycardia)	Rare	+190160
Transient Congenital Hypothyroidism			
Severe iodine deficiency	— $\downarrow T_4$, $\uparrow$TSH, goiter; lack of iodine prevents thyroid hormone formation	Most common worldwide	NA
Acute iodine load	— Acute iodine overload from iodine-containing antiseptic	Rare	NA
Maternal antithyroid drug therapy	— $\downarrow T_4$, $\uparrow$TSH; transplacental passage of drug (usually propylthiouracil), clears 3–4 days after birth; hyperthyroidism may occur if TSIs are present	Most common cause in iodine-sufficient areas	NA
Transplacental transfer of TSH receptor-blocking antibodies	— $\downarrow T_4$, $\uparrow$TSH, scan may be negative; thyroglobulin present — Infant's TSH-stimulated thyroid hormone production blocked by maternal antibodies	~2% of congenital hypothyroidism	NA
Genetic causes	— Heterozygous mutation inactivating THOX2 (homozygous = permanent hypothyroidism)	Rare	#607200
Hypothyroxinemia of prematurity	— $\downarrow T_4$, $\downarrow T_3$, normal TSH; adaptation to prematurity rather than true central hypothyroidism	Common	NA
Childhood-Onset (Acquired) Hypothyroidism			
Hashimoto thyroiditis	— $\downarrow T_4$, $\uparrow$TSH; autoimmune—antithyroid peroxidase antibodies usually positive — Usually associated with a firm, pebbly goiter (2/3) but gland may be atrophic — Female preponderance; may be associated with other autoimmune diseases, Down syndrome, Turner syndrome — Pituitary enlargement (hyperplasia of thyrotrophs) reversible with thyroxine treatment	Most common cause of childhood-onset hypothyroidism in iodine-sufficient areas	%140300
Irradiation	— Radioiodine therapy for Graves disease usually leads to hypothyroidism — With external radiation therapy for tumors of the head and neck, antithyroid effects may occur early or late after exposure; may be primary or central (normal, $\downarrow$, or $\uparrow$ TSH)	Rare (but common after radiation)	NA
Thyroidectomy	— Usual reasons are cancer or, less commonly, treatment of hyperthyroidism	Rare	NA
Drug-induced	— Phenytoin and rifampin induce mixed function oxygenases — Interferon-α, amiodarone, and lithium	Rare	NA

CAUSES	PATHOPHYSIOLOGIC FEATURES	PREVALENCE	OMIM
Childhood-Onset (Acquired) Hypothyroidism			
Consumptive	— Overexpression of type 3 deiodinase by large liver or cutaneous hemangiomas — Suspect when a patient with hypothyroidism requires unusually high doses of thyroxine, especially in the first few months of life when hemangiomas are at maximum size	Rare	NA
Iodine deficiency	— Goiter	Common world wide	
Central tumors or infiltrative disease, developmental defects, growth hormone treatment	— Hypothalamic-pituitary axis disruption; $\downarrow T_4$, $\downarrow$ or inappropriately normal TSH — TRH stimulation test may help differentiate pituitary from hypothalamic disease — Usually other pituitary hormone deficiencies; slow growth, delayed bone age common	Rare	NA
Circulating thyroid stimulators			
Graves disease	— $\uparrow$ or normal T_4, $\uparrow T_3$, $\downarrow$ TSH; TSI detected in 90%, mimic TSH, stimulate growth and function of the thyroid gland — Increased preponderance in females, peak incidence around puberty, remission possible — Goiter present: symmetrical, smooth enlargement of the thyroid	2% of adult women, 0.25% of adult men, less common in children but can occur at any age	#275000
Neonatal Graves disease	— $\uparrow T_4$, $\uparrow T_3$, $\downarrow$ TSH; maternal TSI persist until up to 4 mo postnatally — Thyrotoxicosis may begin in utero if not controlled by maternal antithyroid therapy or TSH blocking antibodies, otherwise may begin 2-3 d postnatally after maternal antithyroid drug levels disappear	1:50,000 neonates	NA
Thyrotropin secreting tumor	— $\uparrow T_4$, $\uparrow T_3$, $\uparrow$ or normal TSH; pituitary adenoma	Very rare	NA
Thyroidal Autonomy ($\uparrow T_4$, $\uparrow T_3$, $\downarrow$ TSH)			
Toxic multinodular goiter	— Activating mutations in thyrotropin receptor or G proteins	Very rare	+603372
Toxic solitary adenoma	— Activating mutations in thyrotropin receptor or G proteins — Very rarely thyroid carcinomas can present as hyperfunctioning nodules in childhood	Very rare	+603372
Permanent congenital hyperthyroidism	— Autosomal dominant, variable severity, can present at birth or later; activating mutations in the thyrotropin receptor — No immune markers or eye signs, smooth goiter may become multinodular later in life	Very rare	+603372
McCune-Albright syndrome (MAS)	— Caused by an activating Gsα mutation; classic MAS clinical triad is fibrous dysplasia, precocious puberty, and café-au-lait spots; hyperthyroidism may or may not be present — Hyperthyroidism may be the initial sign in neonates with MAS or may appear later — Can be diffuse or can present as a toxic adenoma	Rare	174800
Iodine induced	— Children are rarely exposed to large iodine loads except for medical procedures — Excess iodine results in unregulated thyroid hormone production	Rare	NA

CAUSES	PATHOPHYSIOLOGIC FEATURES	PREVALENCE	OMIM
Destruction of Thyroid Follicles (Thyroiditis) ($\uparrow$ T$_4$, $\uparrow$ T$_3$, $\downarrow$ TSH)			
Hashitoxicosis	— Autoimmune with high titers of antithyroperoxidase antibodies	Uncommon	140300
	— Although hypothyroidism is more common, in the early phase damage to the gland can result in acute release of thyroid hormone		
	— Occasionally this can be accompanied by formation of lymphocytic nodules that may make it difficult to differentiate from a hyperfunctioning adenoma		
Subacute (de Quervain)	— Typically preceded by a viral infection; thyroid gland is tender	Very rare in children	NA
	— Generally self-limiting: thyrotoxic phase typically lasts 2–6 wk followed by euthyroid phase of variable duration, followed by recovery phase, which is associated with biochemical and possibly clinical features of hypothyroidism lasting 2–7 mo		
Amiodarone-induced	— Direct toxic drug effects, may induce hyper- or hypothyroidism	Uncommon	NA
Acute (infectious)	— Thyroid infection (bacterial, fungal, etc.) damages gland causes acute release of thyroxine	Very rare	NA
Exogenous Thyroid Hormone ($\uparrow$T$_4$, $\downarrow$ TSH)			
Iatrogenic	— Excess dosing of thyroid hormone	Rare	NA
Factitious	— Ingestion—accidental, Münchhausen syndrome by proxy, psychiatric or eating disorders	Rare	NA
	— To differentiate from Graves disease: low thyroglobulin level and low T$_3$/T$_4$ ratio (because most thyroid hormone preparations contain only T$_4$)		
Hamburger thyrotoxicosis	— Thyroid gland included in ground beef	Probably rare	NA

membrane through micro- and macropinocytosis and part of it is hydrolyzed in the lysosomes, whereupon T_4 and T_3 are released into the bloodstream, while the released mono- and diiodotyrosines are dehalogenated, allowing their iodine content to be recycled.

Fetal T_4 is detected by the 11th week of gestation and progressively increases throughout gestation. Placenta and pancreas produce thyrotropin-releasing hormone (TRH) early in the gestation and hypothalamic TRH synthesis is present at midgestation. Maternal TRH as well as iodine, maternal thiourea drugs, thyroid antibodies, and limited but significant amounts of thyroid hormones cross the placenta. Thyroid-stimulating hormone (TSH)-like activity by the human chorionic gonadotropin secreted by the placenta has minimal effect on the fetal HPT axis. Fetal TSH level starts progressively increasing at approximately 18 weeks of gestation to a peak value of 10 mU/L at term. At the same time T_4 levels begin to increase steadily until the end of gestation. Fetal serum T_3 remains low (<15 ng/dL) until the 30th week of gestation, and then slowly increases until birth.

TRH is a tripeptide secreted by the supraoptic and paraventricular nuclei of the hypothalamus and travels to the anterior pituitary through the hypophyseal portal venous system. Once at the anterior pituitary, TRH binds to TRH receptors that are coupled to intracellular G- proteins and through activation of adenylate cyclase and subsequent increase in cyclic adenosine monophosphate (cAMP) stimulates the synthesis and secretion of TSH-β subunit and prolactin. It appears that hypothalamic TRH controls TSH glycosylation, which is important for the biological activity of TSH. TRH production during cold is increased through peripheral and hypothalamic sensors.

TSH, through the same mechanism as TRH, after binding to the thyroid stimulating hormone receptor (TSHR) mediates through cAMP several effects on thyroid hormone metabolism, including among others iodide trapping, iodotyrosine synthesis, thyroglobulin synthesis, hormone release, and thyroid cell growth. TSH receptors are expressed in pituitary thyrotropes, which suggest that TSH may play a role in its own release. TSH is member of a family of heterodimeric glycoprotein hormones (follicle-stimulating hormone, luteinizing hormone, and human chorionic gonadotropin) that have a common α-subunit but differ in their hormone-specific β-subunit. TSH has a circadian rhythm with peak concentrations just prior to onset of sleep (10 PM to midnight). Antidiuretic hormone, norepinephrine, and adrenergic agonists stimulate TSH secretion, whereas dopamine and dopamine decrease TSH concentrations.

Growth hormone (GH) inhibits TSH secretion through increase in somatostatin levels, and glucocorticoids inhibit TSH release at the hypothalamic level.

Under normal circumstances, the thyroid secretes approximately 80% T_4 and 20% T_3 and also secretes thyroglobulin. Thyroid hormones are carried in the blood by three proteins; thyroxine binding globulin (TBG), transhyretin (TTR) and albumin. TBG has the highest affinity for T_4 and T_3, but is present in the lowest concentration. Despite its low concentration, TBG carries the majority of T_4 in serum (75%), followed by TTR (15%) and albumin (10%). Unlike TTR and albumin, TBG has a single binding site for T_4/T_3. Estrogen decrease clearance of TBG and increase its levels during pregnancy. Thyroid hormone synthesis is primarily regulated by the availability of iodine in the environment and by pituitary thyrotropin (TSH) that acts on its receptor (the TSHR) to stimulate the proliferation, differentiation, and function of the thyroid follicular cells. Negative feedback of the thyroid hormones on TSH secretion regulates thyroid hormone production and serum concentration, that is, the higher the serum levels of these hormones, the lower TSH release and vice versa. The negative feedback occurs at the pituitary anterior lobe and at the hypothalamus, principally, through T_4 taken from the circulation and converted into T_3 by outer-ring deiodinases (Figure 26-2). The major effects of

the thyroid hormones are mediated through the nuclear T_3 receptors, with T_3 having the highest affinity. The functions of thyroid hormone are reviewed in Table 26-1. Both T_4 and T_3 can exert a negative feedback on TRH and this action is mediated through thyroid receptor-β (TRβ).

The prohormone T_4 can be metabolized into the active T_3 by deiodinase type I and type II (DIO1 and DIO2) or into the inactive reverse T_3 (rT_3) by the inner-ring deiodinase type III. The deiodinases are a family of selenoproteins with each subtype having specific tissue distribution and regulation. A review of these is beyond the scope of this chapter. Two aspects of the deiodinase system, however, deserve to be highlighted. 1) The fact that the placenta expresses high levels of type III deiodinase explains why the fetal circulation is characterized by very low T_3 and very high rT_3; this can be seen as the mechanism responsible for the maintenance of a low level of in utero thermogenesis. 2) The fetal brain expresses type II deiodinase, which is upregulated in hypothyroidism; this, together with some transplacental transfer of T_4 (7), protects the fetal brain to a great extent when fetal thyroid hormone production is deficient. T_4 and T_3 are taken up into different tissues at very different rates probably through the existence of thyroid transporters that are selectively expressed in different tissues. Of particular importance is the monocarboxylate transporter 8 (MCT-8), which is essential

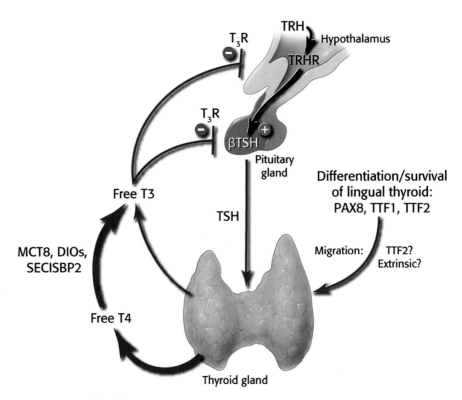

FIGURE 26-2. Regulation of the HPT axis.

TABLE 26-1   Actions of Thyroid Hormones

Increase Oxidative Metabolism

- ↑ oxygen consumption by increasing the activity of Na^+,K^+-ATPase (Na pump); this causes an increase in the basal metabolic rate and leads to heat production
- ↑ glucose metabolism by making glucose available (↑ gluconeogenesis and glycogenolysis) and promoting insulin-stimulated glucose uptake
- ↑ fat metabolism by stimulating fatty acid mobilization from adipose tissue and fatty acid oxidation

Promote Growth and Development

- essential for normal growth in childhood (direct effects as well as permissive effects on GH action)
- sustain normal muscle growth by enhancing protein synthesis
- amplify insulin-like growth factor-I actions on bone

Influence Nervous System Development and Function

- essential for normal myelination and development of the central nervous system in the first few years of life
- influence mental activity in older children and adults (↓ levels lead to mental sluggishness, ↑ levels lead to restlessness and anxiety)

Augment Cardiac Function

- ↑ heart rate, cardiac contractility, and cardiac output
- promote vasodilation to enhance blood flow to organs

Allow Normal Reproductive Function

- normal levels needed for normal reproductive function
- ↓ levels associated with delayed puberty in children and infertility in adults

---

for T_3 uptake in central neurons during development.

Immediately after birth, exposure to a cold environment triggers a surge in plasma TSH that peaks during the first 24 hours of life. This TSH surge is followed by a rise in plasma T_4, which peaks during the 2nd day of life. TSH levels remain elevated for 3 to 5 days after birth and elevated T_4 and T_3 levels gradually decline over the first 4 to 5 weeks of life. Both the TSH and T_4 surges are seen in premature and term neonates, although they are of lower amplitude in the former. The disappearance of the placenta with its abundant type III deiodinase activity results in a rise in plasma T_3 and a fall in plasma rT_3. Because iodine is no longer supplied by the mother, the neonate also becomes dependent on its own stores of iodine. Premature neonates have a low intrathyroidal iodine content and this explains in part their susceptibility to acute iodine overload and resultant inhibition of iodide organification and hypothyroidism (Wolff–Chaikoff effect), through exposure to iodine-containing antiseptic solutions or radiographic contrast solutions.

CONGENITAL HYPOTHYROIDISM

The clinical importance of permanent primary congenital hypothyroidism stems from its being the leading cause of preventable mental retardation and the most common congenital endocrine disorder. Congenital hypothyroidism has a birth prevalence of 1:3,500 newborns (1). As such, it is the major focus of this section. In approximately 85% of affected newborns, permanent primary congenital hypothyroidism is due to thyroid dysgenesis. Approximately 15% of cases of permanent primary congenital hypothyroidism are due to defects in thyroid hormone biosynthesis (thyroid dyshormonogenesis), which, because of the trophic action of thyrotropin, eventually lead to thyroid enlargement. This thyroid enlargement is very often not detected clinically at birth.

Thyroid dysgenesis includes defects in the differentiation or survival of thyroid follicular cells, resulting in thyroid agenesis or athyreosis (~20 % of cases of thyroid dysgenesis) or in the downward migration of the median thyroid anlage during embryonic development, resulting in ectopic thyroid (~80% of cases). Ectopic thyroid tissue has a round appearance because it lacks the lateral lobes typical of the orthotopic thyroid; it is located on the midline, anywhere between the foramen caecum of the tongue and the neck and is the only thyroid tissue present. Almost all individuals with ectopic thyroid are hypothyroid and this can be detected by biochemical screening at birth. Part of the spectrum of thyroid dysgenesis includes hypoplasia of a thyroid of normal shape and in the normal position (<5% of cases) and thyroid hemiagenesis, where one lobe, usually the left, and sometimes the isthmus, are missing (8). Thyroid hemiagenesis may be observed in as many as 1:500 euthyroid individuals but accounts for less than 1% of cases of congenital hypothyroidism. Ectopic thyroids are smaller than normal bilobed glands, and this likely explains why the patients are generally hypothyroid; the biochemical severity of the hypothyroidism is variable and more pronounced in girls (9).

Permanent central hypothyroidism, resulting from defects at the level of the hypothalamus or pituitary, is much rarer, occurring in fewer than 1:50,000 births. Transient alterations in thyroid function resulting from either primary (thyroidal) or secondary (hypothalamic or pituitary) causes are relatively frequent.

PATHOGENESIS OF PERMANENT CONGENITAL HYPOTHYROIDISM

Primary hypothyroidism

Thyroid Dysgenesis Thyroid dysgenesis was until recently considered a sporadic entity, although some familial cases had been reported. A systematic reevaluation of the heritability of thyroid dysgenesis in France revealed that 48 of 2,472 infants with thyroid dysgenesis (2%) had an affected relative; this is 15-fold higher than predicted by chance alone (10). Pedigree analysis was most compatible with dominant inheritance with variable penetrance, although there was genetic heterogeneity (11). Multigenic inheritance has also been proposed (12). In one study, subclinical abnormalities of thyroid development (mostly persistence of thyroglossal tract remnants) were identified by ultrasonography in 8% of euthyroid first-degree relatives of children with thyroid dysgenesis, compared with only 0.8% in a control population (13). On the other hand, a recent systematic survey of monozygotic twins revealed that discordance for thyroid dysgenesis was the rule, being observed in 12 of 13 reported twin pairs (92%) (14). Although it is not compatible with simple mendelian inheritance, thyroid dysgenesis (especially thyroid ectopy) has a marked female predominance (15).

Germline mutations in genes coding for transcription factors known to be involved in a hierarchical way in thyroid development (TTF-1, TTF-2, PAX8) and growth (TSHR) in mice (16) and in humans (17) may account for congenital hypothyroidism in patients with either isolated thyroid dysgenesis or thyroid dysgenesis with associated malformations of kidney, lung, forebrain, and palate. Thyroid transcription factor-1 (TITF-1) is expressed in the ventral forebrain and lung; TFF-2 in craniopharyngeal ectoderm (involved in palate formation) and the Rathke pouch; and paired-box 8 (PAX8) in the thyroglossal duct, central nervous system, and kidney, including the ureteric bud and the main collecting ducts (17). TTF-1, TTF-2 and PAX8 transcription factors are also involved in the regulation of the transcription of thyroglobulin, thyroid peroxidase (TPO), and NIS by binding to specific regulatory DNA sequences within their promoters. Overall mutations in TTF-1, TTF-2, PAX8, and TSHR have been identified in only approximately 50 of 500 patients with thyroid dysgenesis screened for mutations in these genes (18). This suggests that other genes may be involved in thyroid development (19). Although this is controversial (16), thyroid migration may be a passive phenomenon (20) and genes expressed by the surrounding mesenchyme may be involved in the extrinsic control of thyroid cell migration. A good example of an endocrine disorder caused by defective embryonic cell migration is X-linked Kallmann syndrome, which results from mutations not in genes expressed by the gonadotropin-releasing hormone-synthesizing neurons themselves but rather in genes coding for adhesion molecules involved in the extrinsic control of their migration (21). Unlike thyroid dysgenesis, Kallmann syndrome is a mendelian condition. Alternative mechanisms explaining the majority of cases of thyroid dysgenesis include epigenetic modifications (such as promoter methylation), somatic mutations occurring very early in embryogenesis in the parent thyroid follicular cell, or stochastic (random) developmental events. The lines of evidence in favor of mendelian and nonmendelian mechanisms of thyroid dysgenesis are depicted in Table 26-2 and are discussed in detail in references (1,22). The proportions of the different causes of congenital hypothyroidism differ somewhat between centers, probably in large part because of different scintigraphic techniques (23) but the overall prevalence of thyroid dysgenesis does not seem to vary substantially around the world. Suggestions of ethnic differences in prevalence of congenital hypothyroidism are based on small numbers (24) or on studies in which the distinction between dysgenesis and dyshormonogenesis was not made (25). The lack of consistent regional or seasonal variation in the frequency of thyroid dysgenesis and the discordance of twins argues against an important role of environmental factors (26).

Thyroid Dyshormonogenesis Thyroid dyshormonogenesis results from a defect in any one of the steps involved in the biosynthesis of thyroid hormone (Figure 26-1). Genetic mutations affecting the following steps of thyroid hormone synthesis have been defined.

1. Transport of iodide across the basolateral membrane of the thyroid follicular cell against a concentration gradient through the NIS: the human gene encoding NIS, mapped at chromosome 19p has been cloned. The severity of hypothyroidism is variable, goiter is not always present and individuals homozygous for NIS mutations but who have a high dietary iodine intake may remain euthyroid (27,28).

2. Transport of iodide from the cell into the colloid lumen through pendrin: Pendred syndrome is the most common cause (10%) of hereditary nonprogressive sensorineural deafness (29) and is associated with hypothyroidism of variable severity. The hypothyroidism is rarely diagnosed in the neonatal period (30). The thyroid disease usually presents as a multinodular or diffuse goiter of varying size, typically in the second decade of life. The gene for pendrin is the SLC26A4 gene on chromosome 7q and is expressed in both the cochlea and thyroid. Because mutations of SLC26A4 have not invariably been found in affected individuals, it is likely that Pendred syndrome is a heterogeneous disease.

3. Ca^{2+}/NADPH-dependent generation of H_2O_2 through the activity of thyroid oxidase 2 (THOX2), which is the rate-limiting step in thyroid hormonogenesis. The thyroid oxidase system is composed of at least two proteins, THOX1 and THOX2, and is responsible for generating hydrogen peroxide that oxidizes the iodide in the follicular cell. Thyroid peroxidase, the enzyme that catalyzes the oxidation of iodide, has no biologic activity in the absence of H_2O_2. Biallelic inactivating mutations in the THOX2 gene cause severe and permanent congenital hypothyroidism, while monoallelic mutations are associated with milder, transient hypothyroidism caused by insufficient thyroidal production of hydrogen peroxide, which prevents the synthesis of sufficient quantities of thyroid hormones to meet the large requirement for thyroid hormones at the beginning of life (31).

4. Iodide organification and iodotyrosine coupling via the thyroid peroxidase enzyme (TPO): this enzyme, which is located on the apical membrane of the thyroid follicular cell, is encoded by a gene that maps to chromosome 2p25. Mutations in this gene are the most prevalent cause of dyshormonogenesis (32) and are characterized by a complete or partial defect in iodide organification.

5. Synthesis of thyroglobulin: The two substrates needed for thyroid synthesis are iodide and tyrosine. Iodide is taken from the blood and tyrosine is part of the thyroglobulin molecule. The gene encoding thyroglobulin has been cloned and is located on chromosome 8q24. Thyroglobulin is synthesized in the follicular cell of the thyroid gland and is exported in the colloid to undergo iodination. Mutations of the thyroglobulin gene are associated with abnormal trafficking of thyroglobulin and moderate-to-severe congenital hypothyroidism, usually with low thyroglobulin concentrations (27).

Hormonogenesis defects are inherited as autosomal recessive traits, and they therefore occur at higher frequency in consanguineous families and in inbred populations. A goiter may be present in older individuals but not necessarily in newborns (33). Hypothyroidism is not necessarily present at birth. The perchlorate challenge test, if performed, shows excessive release of iodide from the thyroid gland, as perchlorate displaces intravenously infused radiolabeled iodide that accumulates in the thyrocyte due to abnormal hormonogenesis. Normally, discharge of unincorporated iodide is less than 10% 2 hours after administration of perchlorate but in disorders of dyshormonogenesis the unincorporated iodide discharge is greater than 15% and may be as high as 80%.

TABLE 26-2 Proposed Mechanisms of Thyroid Dysgenesis and Supporting Findings		
	Mechanisms	**Findings**
Mendelian inheritance	Autosomal dominant with variable penetrance; genetic heterogeneity; multigenic	2% of infants with thyroid dysgenesis have an affected relative (15-fold higher than chance); subclinical abnormalities of thyroid development in eight percent of first degree relatives of infants with thyroid dysgenesis (vs. 0.8% in a control population)
Non-Mendelian mechanisms	Epigenetic; early somatic mutations; stochastic events	Marked preponderance of females with ectopy (3 females to 1 male); 92% discordance among monozygotic twin pairs

Thyroid-Stimulating Hormone Resistance The TSHR is a G protein–coupled transmembrane receptor that mediates the effects of TSH in thyroid development, growth, and synthetic function. Autosomal recessive inheritance of TSH resistance caused by inactivating mutations in the TSHR was first described 10 years ago (34). The phenotypic spectrum of these recessively inherited TSHR mutations has now been shown to be very wide, ranging from asymptomatic elevations of TSH to severe hypothyroidism with apparent athyreosis. Patients with partial TSHR defects have elevated TSH levels, normal thyroid hormone levels, and a thyroid scintigraphy that is normal except for low uptake. Patients with severe impairment of the TSHR may present with profound thyroid hypoplasia, elevated TSH levels, low thyroid hormones, and low or absent ("apparent athyreosis") uptake on scintigraphy. Thyroglobulin levels are normal or high, probably due to leakage of thyroglobulin from the disorganized follicles (35–37). Dominant transmission of heterozygous TSHR mutations causing mild TSH resistance has also been described (38). In some pedigrees, the gene involved in mild TSH resistance remains unknown (39). In severe TSH resistance, the differential diagnosis includes true athyreosis, in which thyroglobulin is not measurable, TSHR antibodies passed in utero from the mother, and acute iodine overload. Patients with dominantly inherited pseudohypoparathyroidism type 1a and TSH resistance are occasionally identified because of a high TSH on neonatal screening.

Down Syndrome In newborns with trisomy 21, the whole distributions of T_4 and TSH at screening are shifted to the left and right, respectively (40), suggesting that, as a group, neonates with trisomy 21 have a subtle form of primary congenital hypothyroidism. One study suggests that treatment with thyroxine of infants with trisomy 21 may slightly reduce delayed motor development at 2 years (41). The molecular mechanisms underlying the TSH and T_4 shifts are unknown; there is no evidence that thyroid dysgenesis is more frequent (15) and there are only anecdotal reports of overt hypothyroidism from dyshormonogenesis (42). The skewed distribution of T_4 and TSH likely persists throughout life in trisomy 21, with true autoimmune hypothyroidism being more frequent in childhood (see section on acquired hypothyroidism).

Central (or Secondary) Hypothyroidism

Permanent central congenital hypothyroidism almost always occurs in conjunction with other pituitary hormone deficiencies and results from global structural or functional abnormalities in hypothalamic or pituitary development. Isolated central hypothyroidism caused by mutations of the gene for the β-subunit of TSH is very rare. These mutations result in the production of a TSH molecule with little or no biologic activity and the clinical and biochemical phenotype is therefore generally severe (43,44) A single patient with mild isolated central hypothyroidism from mutations in the thyrotropin-releasing hormone receptor has been reported (45). Hypothyroidism is seldom the presenting symptom of patients with mutations in the pituitary transcription factors HESX1, LHX3, LHX4, PROP1, and PIT1. These patients are usually identified because of growth failure. They are described in more detail in Chapters 30 and 32.

Peripheral Hypothyroidism

Abnormal transport of thyroid hormones in plasma, decreased conversion of the prohormone T_4 into the biologically active T_3 by deiodination, abnormal transfer across the cell membrane, and abnormal sensitivity of target cells could theoretically cause hypothyroidism. Only the latter two have been shown to lead to peripheral hypothyroidism (in which the cause of hypothyroidism does not originate from the thyroid or pituitary but rather at the target tissues). There is a recent report about a genetic disorder that affects deiodinase activity, which seems to be associated with abnormal biochemical values but no specific clinical manifestations (46).

Abnormal Transport of Thyroid Hormones in Blood Three proteins are involved in the transport of thyroid hormones in plasma: 1) thyroxine-binding globulin; 2) transthyretin (formerly named thyroxine-binding prealbumin); and, 3) albumin. Numerous mutations leading to either excess or deficiency of these hormones have been described. The circulating concentrations of free thyroid hormones are normal and patients bearing these abnormalities are therefore euthyroid. Because it is the measurement of free thyroxine that has now become routine in clinical biochemistry laboratories, these abnormalities are not as frequently identified as in the past. They will therefore not be discussed further in this chapter and the reader is referred elsewhere (27).

Abnormal Transport of Thyroid Hormones Across the Cell Membrane Thyroid hormone is essential for optimal brain development. T_3, the most active form of the thyroid hormone, can be transported across the cell membrane and exerts its biologic effects by binding to nuclear thyroid receptors. Recently, the membrane protein monocarboxylase transporter 8 (MCT8) has been identified as a specific thyroid hormone transporter. Furthermore, a syndrome of severe psychomotor retardation associated with very high plasma T_3, low reverse T_3 and T_4, and normal to mildly elevated TSH has recently been shown to be due to mutations in MCT8 (47,48). Consistent with the location of MCT8 on the X chromosome, hemizygous males are severely affected whereas heterozygous females have a milder thyroid phenotype and no neurologic deficits. The effects of MCT8 transporter defects on plasma thyroid hormone levels and on the function of different tissues remain to be defined.

Thyroid Hormone Resistance Since its initial description in 1967, the syndrome of resistance to thyroid hormone has been described in more than 200 families and is characterized by normal or increased TSH levels in the presence of increased levels of free T_4 and T_3 and variable refractoriness of the different tissues to the action of the thyroid hormone. Three clinical phenotypes of thyroid hormone resistance are often described, although the pathophysiologic validity of this classification is questionable (49): 1) generalized thyroid resistance; 2) predominant pituitary resistance, which may present as thyrotoxicosis; and, 3) peripheral thyroid resistance. It is generally due to missense mutations inactivating the β-type receptor for T_3 (TRβ1), although 15% of cases appear to be due to mutations in other as yet unidentified genes. TRβ1 mutations can occur *de novo* or be transmitted in an autosomal dominant fashion. There are two types of thyroid hormone receptors (TRα and TRβ), which have a tissue distribution that varies between organs and during development. Through alternative splicing of the TRα and TRβ mRNA, there are three isoforms of the TRα receptor and there are at least two isoforms of the TRβ (TRβ1, TRβ2). TRα receptors are widely distributed among tissues. TRβ1 receptor is distributed in brain, heart, kidney, and liver, whereas TRβ2 is found only in the pituitary and brain. Thyroid hormone receptors are hormone-activated transcription factors that modulate gene expression and contain a DNA-binding domain, a transactivation domain, a ligand-binding domain, and a dimerization domain. When thyroid hormone receptors bind DNA in the absence of hormone, transcriptional repression usually occurs, whereas hormone binding is associated with a conformational change in the receptor, resulting in transcriptional activation. The presence of multiple forms of the thyroid hormone receptor, with tissue and stage-dependent differences in their expression, suggests an extraordinary level of complexity in the physiologic effects of thyroid hormone. The mechanism for the dominant inheritance of the mutations is through a dominant negative effect of the mutant TRβ receptor on the normal TRβ receptor (presumably mediated by binding of the mutant TRβ receptor with the normal TRβ receptor, producing an inactive homodimer).

PATHOGENESIS OF TRANSIENT CONGENITAL HYPOTHYROIDISM

Iodine Deficiency or Excess, Maternal Factors

Most cases of transient primary congenital hypothyroidism stem from environmental, iatrogenic, or maternal causes. Severe iodine deficiency remains an important cause of transient hypothyroidism in newborns. In areas where the iodine intake of the population is moderately decreased, acute iodine overload from the application of iodine-containing antiseptic agents to newborns or to pregnant or lactating women may result in transient hypothyroidism, mostly in premature newborns whose thyroid iodine stores are particularly low (50). In iodine-sufficient areas, the most common cause of transient primary hypothyroidism is maternal therapy with antithyroid drugs (ATDs) (see section on hyperthyroidism in this chapter). Transplacental transfer of maternal antibodies that block the action of TSH is much rarer, causing only approximately 2% of cases of congenital hypothyroidism (51).

Genetic Causes of Transient Congenital Hypothyroidism

The first genetic cause of transient primary congenital hypothyroidism has been recently described. One patient bearing two mutated THOX2 alleles had permanent dyshormonogenesis; patients carrying only one mutated allele had transient congenital hypothyroidism (31). The frequency of this disorder remains to be determined.

Hypothyroxinemia of Prematurity

Although the early neonatal surges of TSH and T_4 are qualitatively similar in term and preterm newborns, the latter subsequently present with low plasma free T_4. Plasma TSH is generally not elevated in these premature infants and their biochemical profile therefore meets the definition of transient central hypothyroidism. Because a low free T_4 is an indicator of a poorer outcome in premature babies, thyroxine treatment has been evaluated in the last decade. In the largest, randomized, controlled trial to date, 200 babies born before 30 weeks of gestation were treated with either thyroxine or placebo. Overall, thyroxine did not

improve short- or long-term outcome (52). Post-hoc subgroup analyses of this trial, which are questionable from the methodologic standpoint, suggested possible benefit in very preterm newborns (<27 wk) but possible harm in the more mature newborns. The Cochrane review of this trial and of other data on this topic does not support the use of thyroid hormones in preterm infants to reduce neonatal mortality, improve neurodevelopmental outcome, or to reduce the severity of respiratory distress syndrome (53). Although future trials may be warranted in neonates born before 27 weeks, current evidence suggests that the hypothyroxinemia of prematurity represents an adaptation to the premature delivery rather than true central hypothyroidism.

Biochemical Screening for Congenital Hypothyroidism

Studies of children with congenital hypothyroidism performed in the 1970s had clearly shown that prevention of mental retardation required that treatment be started within the first few weeks of life, the period of maximal brain vulnerability to hypothyroidism. Methods for mass biochemical screening of newborns for congenital hypothyroidism have led to the eradication of mental retardation from this condition; however, continuous auditing of all steps of the neonatal screening process is essential. Cases missed by biochemical screening can occur (54).

Clinical Presentation of Congenital Hypothyroidism

Signs and symptoms of hypothyroidism are presented in Table 26-3. At birth, the clinical manifestations of hypothyroidism are relatively mild and the diagnosis is suspected clinically in only 1% to 4% of affected newborns (54). At recall after a positive screening test result, some of the clinical manifestations described in Table 26-3 may be noted. Very few infants

TABLE 26-3 Signs and Symptoms of Hypothyroidism
At Birth
• postmaturity
• macrosomia
• open posterior fontanel, large head circumference
• generalized delay in skeletal maturation (but normal or near-normal length)
During Early Infancy
• decreased muscle tone, lethargy, poor feeding
• hypothermia
• constipation
• prolonged jaundice
• abdominal distension, umbilical hernia
• dry and mottled skin
• macroglossia
• hoarse cry
• myxedematous appearance
In Childhood
• delayed linear growth
• puffy face (myxedema)
• fatigue
• constipation
• dry skin
• cold intolerance
• delayed bone age, stippling of epiphyses, delayed tooth eruption
• delayed central puberty
• pseudopuberty from follicle-stimulating hormone receptor stimulation by TSH
girls: ovarian cysts, vaginal bleeding, ↑estrogen levels, +/− breast development, no pubic hair
boys: adult-sized testes with unmeasurable testosterone, no pubic hair
• hypercholesterolemia
• goiter present in 2/3, but may have thyroid atrophy

Presenting Concerns

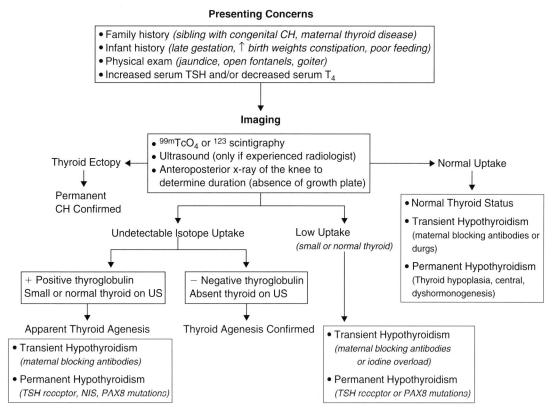

- Family history *(sibling with congenital CH, maternal thyroid disease)*
- Infant history *(late gestation, ↑ birth weights constipation, poor feeding)*
- Physical exam *(jaundice, open fontanels, goiter)*
- Increased serum TSH and/or decreased serum T₄

Imaging

- $^{99m}TcO_4$ or ^{123} scintigraphy
- Ultrasound (only if experienced radiologist)
- Anteroposterior x-ray of the knee to determine duration (absence of growth plate)

Thyroid Ectopy

Permanent CH Confirmed

Normal Uptake

- Normal Thyroid Status
- Transient Hypothyroidism *(maternal blocking antibodies or durgs)*
- Permanent Hypothyroidism *(Thyroid hypoplasia, central, dyshormonogenesis)*

Undetectable Isotope Uptake

Low Uptake *(small or normal thyroid)*

+ Positive thyroglobulin Small or normal thyroid on US

− Negative thyroglobulin Absent thyroid on US

Apparent Thyroid Agenesis

- Transient Hypothyroidism *(maternal blocking antibodies)*
- Permanent Hypothyroidism *(TSH receptor, NIS, PAX8 mutations)*

Thyroid Agenesis Confirmed

- Transient Hypothyroidism *(maternal blocking antibodies or iodine overload)*
- Permanent Hypothyroidism *(TSH receptor or PAX8 mutations)*

FIGURE 26-3. Algorithm for the diagnostic evaluation of an infant with suspected congenital hypothyroidism.

have a clinically detectable goiter, and goiters large enough to impede delivery or cause airway obstruction are even rarer. A clinical suspicion of hypothyroidism in a newborn or very young infant should always lead to the immediate measurement of plasma TSH and free T₄, regardless of the screening results.

When an infant is referred because of an abnormal screening result, a family history should be obtained, with focus on consanguinity and on the existence of even distant relatives with congenital hypothyroidism. A family history of thyroid disorders with onset in later life in distant relatives is usually irrelevant, but a maternal history of thyroid disease, treatment for thyroid disease, or recent exposure to iodine-rich compounds such as radiographic contrast agents may be relevant. The detection of a goiter usually requires that the infant's neck be hyperextended. The only extrathyroid malformations consistently associated with thyroid dysgenesis are defects in heart septation (11,15,55); these are usually mild and, in our experience, an audible murmur has never been discovered at the first endocrine visit.

The manifestations of central congenital hypothyroidism are in general milder than the clinical expression of the associated pituitary hormone deficiencies, which usually lead to the diagnosis (hypoglycemia due to corticotropin or GH deficiency, micropenis and cryptorchidism due to gonadotropin deficiency, or

cholestasis due to corticotropin deficiency). Midline malformations such as cleft lip or palate or optic nerve hypoplasia are occasionally associated with hypopituitarism.

Individuals with generalized thyroid resistance are commonly eumetabolic, have goiters, elevated plasma levels of total and free T₄ and T₃, normal thyroid hormone metabolism, and normal or slightly elevated TSH levels. A variable degree of delayed bone maturation, failure to thrive, mental retardation, learning disabilities, attention deficit/hyperactivity, tachycardia (through the effect of increased circulating thyroid hormone concentrations on the cardiac TRα receptor), and hearing defects have been reported. Because of the different concentration of TRα and TRβ receptors among the different tissues, patients may be hypothyroid in some tissues and hyperthyroid in others.

In the very rare instance of thyroid hormone resistance predominantly affecting the pituitary (predominant pituitary resistance), the patient may appear to have overt hyperthyroidism (27). Unlike in Graves disease, the TSH level is normal or slightly elevated. Finally, when an affected mother bears an unaffected fetus, there is a higher risk of miscarriage and of intrauterine growth retardation and blood TSH is suppressed in the neonate, demonstrating that excess thyroid hormone in the mother crosses the placenta and can cause fetal thyroxicosis (3).

Diagnostic Evaluation of Congenital Hypothyroidism

An algorithm for the diagnostic evaluation of an infant with suspected hypothyroidism is presented in Figure 26-3. Plasma TSH and free T₄ should be measured in all newborns recalled because of an abnormal screening result. The onset of hypothyroidism can be estimated from an anteroposterior X-ray of the knee: absence of both the femoral and tibial epiphyseal centers in a term newborn infant suggests hypothyroidism of prenatal onset, which has consistently been found to be a reliable predictor of greater risk of developmental delay, even in the screening era (56). Because the results of thyroid function testing do not distinguish among infants with athyreosis, ectopy, and dyshormonogenesis, scintigraphy is required to make an etiologic diagnosis. Pertechnetate ($^{99m}TcO_4$) is taken up by the thyroid like iodine. It is available daily in most nuclear medicine services and provides good anatomic detail in 15 to 30 minutes. Feeding the baby between the $^{99m}TcO_4$ injection and scanning will empty the salivary glands so that any uptake in the lingual area can be ascribed to thyroid tissue. Iodine-123 generally has to be ordered and imaging can only be done several hours after radioisotope administration. Some centers using ^{123}I, when a goiter is detected, perform a

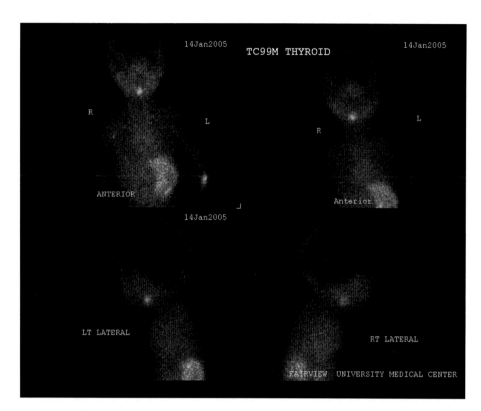

FIGURE 26-4. $^{99m}TcO_4$ scintigraphy of an ectopic thyroid gland in a 30-week gestational age girl with TSH 352 mU/L and free T_4 0.4 ng/dL (5.1 pmol/L). The robust increase in TSH shows that even premature babies can mount an appropriate pituitary response to primary thyroid insufficiency. Photo courtesy of Antoinette Moran.

perchlorate discharge test to identify iodine organification defects and orient molecular investigations. Detection of thyroid ectopy immediately establishes the permanent and predominantly (>90%) sporadic nature of the disorder (Figure 26-4). If there is no detectable isotope uptake, plasma thyroglobulin should be measured; if it is undetectable, true athyreosis is diagnosed; if it is normal or elevated (apparent athyreosis), the possibility of mutations inactivating the TSHR or the sodium-iodide symporter (NIS) or of transplacental transfer of TSHR-blocking antibodies should be considered (57).

If scintigraphy cannot be performed before treatment is started, it should be performed if hypothyroidism is confirmed at 3 years of age. At that time, thyroxine therapy can be safely discontinued for 1 month. If after 1 month plasma TSH increases to abnormally high values, scintigraphy is performed to identify the cause of congenital hypothyroidism. Infants with dyshormonogenesis do not require any further studies to determine the specific biosynthetic defect because a precise diagnosis has no impact on genetic counseling or on treatment. Thyroid ultrasonography is noninvasive but it is operator dependent and less sensitive than scintigraphy in identifying small amounts of ectopic thyroid tissue (58), even when color Doppler ultrasonography is used (59). Very experienced pediatric radiologists can distinguish normal thyroid lobes from the hyperechogenic structures that are found in the empty thyroid area in cases of ectopy or athyreosis (60), and this information can be used to start immediate treatment.

Given the low yield of the search for germline mutations discussed previously, molecular genetic analyses are only performed on a research basis and could probably be restricted to patients with positive family histories or suggestive phenotypes. Thus, unexplained respiratory distress, hypotonia and choreoathetosis suggest heterozygous TTF-1 mutations, which may appear *de novo* (61,62) or be inherited in a dominant fashion (63). Cleft palate and kinky hair, especially if there is parental consanguinity, suggest homozygosity for recessive TTF-2 mutations (64,65). In infants with isolated thyroid hypoplasia or apparent athyreosis, a family history suggesting dominant inheritance points to PAX8 mutations (66–69), whereas a history of autosomal recessive inheritance points to TSHR mutations (36).

Treatment and Outcome of Permanent Primary Congenital Hypothyroidism

Treatment should be started at recall, regardless of whether imaging has been obtained and without waiting for the results of the confirmatory tests. Every day of delay may result in loss of IQ points; the loss is likely greater soon after birth than later (70). Therefore, it is safer to start treatment in all newborns, even those with marginal screening values. Treatment should be stopped if the confirmatory tests show normal plasma TSH and free T_4 concentrations.

Medication

The treatment of choice is levothyroxine (Table 26-4). Tablets can be crushed and given in water with a spoon. For many years, we have instructed the parents to put the crushed whole tablet on the baby's tongue just before feeding without any problems: this ensures that the entire dose is swallowed. Conversely, the tablet should never be diluted in a bottle that the infant may not finish. Levothyroxine in solution for oral administration is available in some countries. Although bioavailability may be better and therefore the initial required dose may be less (71), levothyroxine is not as stable in solution as in tablet form. Soy formulas tend to decrease the absorption of thyroxine (72). Compared with infants with thyroid ectopy, infants with athyreosis generally need higher doses of levothyroxine, whereas those with thyroid dyshormonogenesis need lower doses (73,74); this further underlines the importance of trying to establish an etiological diagnosis by scintigraphy to individualize treatment.

During chronic oral therapy, a missed dose can be given later that day or two doses can be given the next day. Mental retardation, however, has been attributed to more infrequent (i.e., weekly) dosing in one case (75) and regular daily treatment is therefore recommended. The dose should be repeated if an infant or child vomits within an hour after taking levothyroxine. If needed, levothyroxine can be given as a daily intravenous injection; the dose should be approximately 75% of the oral dose. The addition of T_3 has no benefit (76).

In the first decade after screening was implemented, treatment was typically started at a mean age of 20 to 35 days with mean doses of levothyroxine of 5 to 6 μg/kg/day. Studies of outcome in infants and children treated at this age and with these doses revealed that bone maturation remained delayed until 3 years of age (77) and that those with more severe congenital hypothyroidism (defined on the basis of retarded bone maturation or low serum T_4 concentration at diagnosis) had a loss of 6 to 22 IQ points (78–81). Since 1990, term newborns have been treated with levothyroxine in doses of 10 to 15 μg/kg/day (in practice, 50 μg/d for a term infant of normal weight) at many centers (82). The effi-

TABLE 26-4   Treatment of Hypothyroidism, with Levothyroxine

Age	Approximate Dose*	Guidelines
Infants	10–15 μg/kg/d (50 μg/d for full-term, normal size infants)	• TSH should be normalized within 2 weeks (may require fT$_4$ levels as high as 65 pmol/L, (5 ng/dL) • Crush or give whole (do not dilute in bottle or some may be missed) • Infants with athyreosis require higher doses than those with thyroid ectopy, central hypothyroidism, or dyshormonogenesis • There is decreased absorption in the presence of soy formula • Daily dosing best, if a dose is missed give a double dose the next day • The intravenous dose is 75% of the oral dose • Assess thyroid function every 2–3 months
1–5 years	5 μg/kg/d	• There is decreased absorption in the presence of iron or calcium supplements • Assess thyroid function every 3–6 months
6–12 years	4 μg/kg/d	• Assess thyroid function every 6–12 months • Treatment may be associated with a decline in school performance or, rarely, with more serious effects including psychosis or benign intracranial hypertension
Adolescents	3 μg/kg/d	• Higher doses are needed if the patient is also taking an estrogen-containing oral or 100 μg/m^2/d contraceptive or is pregnant • Assess thyroid function every 6–12 months

*Exact dose must be determined by regular monitoring of thyroid hormone and TSH levels.

cacy of these doses was confirmed in a randomized study: only in the group randomized to 50 μg/day (corresponding to 16.5 μg/kg/d) was the mean plasma TSH concentration normalized within 2 weeks (83). Furthermore, developmental outcome at age 5 years was better in that group (84). On the other hand, observational studies strongly suggest that both initiation of treatment within 2 weeks after birth and a high initial dose are required for children with severe congenital hypothyroidism if they are to attain their full intellectual potential (85–87).

Biochemical targets of treatment

Targets in the Newborn There is considerable variation in the frequency at which treated infants are seen and in the biochemical targets of treatment. Reference intervals for plasma free T$_4$ and TSH are higher in infants than in older children and adults (88,89) but normative data for the 1st months of life are scarce and the different commercially available serum free T$_4$ assays are variably influenced by changes in plasma thyroid hormone–binding proteins (90). Based on the rule of thumb that four times the half-life of T$_4$ should elapse before steady state is achieved, it seems unnecessary to measure plasma free T$_4$ before infants are treated for 2 or 3 weeks. In terms of what the target plasma free T$_4$ value should be when the first follow-up sample is obtained, the study mentioned previously (83) suggests that a free T$_4$ as high as 65 pmol/L (5 ng/dL) after treat-

ment for 2 weeks may be needed to normalize plasma TSH.

Targets in the Older Infant and Child The required dose quickly declines from 10 to 15 μg/kg/day in very young infants to 4 μg/kg/day at age five years; this is due to the progressive decrease in the turnover rate of thyroxine with age. Conversely, the rate of weight gain decreases quickly in early infancy, so that an absolute starting dose of 50 μg/day will often remain unchanged for many months. Low plasma TSH concentrations indicate subclinical hyperthyroidism but in rapidly growing infants the same dose becomes in time more appropriate. Overt hyperthyroidism is rare, perhaps because plasma T$_3$ remains in the normal range even in infants with high free T$_4$ and low TSH (85), but should lead to a decrease in dose. An early report of temperamental difficulties in infants with high plasma T$_4$ (91) has not been confirmed (92). The finding of a high plasma TSH concentration should lead to inquiry about compliance, and if satisfactory, the dose of levothyroxine should be increased to maintain plasma TSH and free T$_4$ concentrations in the normal range for age, the normal plasma TSH being more important than the latter.

Frequency of Medical Visits

The frequency of follow-up visits varies considerably between clinics. Based on the rapid growth rates of infants, it seems reasonable to reassess thyroid function at intervals of no less than 3 months in the 1st year and of no

less than 6 months from age 1 to 3 years. After 3 years, because there is no irreversible effect of undertreatment on brain function, yearly assessments may be sufficient. Poor compliance with treatment is associated with poorer developmental outcome (87,93) and may justify more frequent visits.

Growth and Bone Maturation

If treatment is adequate, the mean heights and weights are similar to those of normal children, but the mean head circumference of infants with congenital hypothyroidism is approximately one standard deviation above the mean of normal infants. This increase is likely related to differential maturation of the cranial base and of the skull and has no impact on the size of the brain or cerebral ventricles (85). It may sometimes be so marked in an individual infant that it will lead to unnecessary imaging. Bone maturation at 3 years is normal even in infants with delayed bone maturation at diagnosis. The appropriate bone maturation for chronological age in treated children (94) suggests that the treatment regimen does not induce overt hyperthyroidism (95,96).

Developmental Outcome

Sensorineural hearing loss, a known consequence of congenital hypothyroidism, does not seem to occur in children treated within 2 weeks after birth (97,98). Through the initiation of an early, high-dose regimen, cognitive performance and mean behavioral indices up to school age are within normal limits and there is no specific cognitive or behavioral trait that can be ascribed to congenital hypothyroidism or its treatment in any individual child (94). Even infants with severe congenital hypothyroidism, if treated before 2 weeks of age, should have normal development.

Genetic and Prenatal Counseling

Because of the recent studies on the genetic component of thyroid dysgenesis (10,11), the risk of congenital hypothyroidism for subsequent siblings and for the offspring of the affected child is probably higher than 1:3,500. Particular attention should be given to the neonatal screening sample of subsequent siblings. Progress in fetal thyroid imaging by ultrasound may lead to the prenatal detection of thyroid dysgenesis. Because of the importance of euthyroidism in pregnant women from the beginning of gestation for the brain development of their offspring (99,100) girls with congenital hypothyroidism should have measurements of plasma TSH and free T_4 when they contemplate pregnancy and throughout their pregnancies, as the requirement of levothyroxine may increase during pregnancy (101).

ACQUIRED (CHILDHOOD-ONSET) HYPOTHYROIDISM

Essentially all chronic diseases in childhood will result in slowing of growth and physical maturation, but hypothyroidism is one of the conditions in which this is most pronounced. In utero, hypothyroidism delays skeletal maturation but does not decrease linear growth (i.e., even newborns with severe congenital hypothyroidism have normal birth length). Immediately after birth (102) and until epiphyseal fusion, longitudinal bone growth becomes exquisitely sensitive to thyroid hormone. Thus, slowing of linear growth in children is the most sensitive clinical indicator of incipient hypothyroidism. Development of hypothyroidism in children aged 3 years or older does not have the same impact on brain development as in the perinatal period

when delayed treatment causes irreversible brain damage. Initiation of treatment of severe hypothyroidism acquired during childhood and adolescence may transiently decrease learning ability and alter behavior, sometimes dramatically.

Pathogenesis of Childhood-Onset Hypothyroidism

One should be aware that some congenital causes may have a delayed mode of presentation: this appears to be more common for dyshormonogenesis (103,104) but has also been reported for ectopy (105). There are relatively few studies of the prevalence of acquired hypothyroidism in children. In a recent study of 103,500 people aged 0 to 22 years in Scotland, 140 patients (or one in 735) had received prescriptions for thyroxine on a regular basis (106). The male to female ratio was 1:2.8 and 75% of the patients had acquired hypothyroidism.

Autoimmune Hypothyroidism

The vast majority of cases of childhood-onset hypothyroidism are primary and are due to autoimmune thyroid disease. Comorbidities that are noted at a higher prevalence than in the general population include type 1 diabetes mellitus (3.5%), juvenile rheumatoid arthritis (2%), and Down syndrome (1.5%) (106). Geographic variations in the prevalence of hypothyroidism caused by autoimmune thyroid disease in humans and studies in animal models suggest that iodine deficiency may be protective (107). Indeed, Hashimoto thyroiditis is very common in iodine-replete North America and is much more rare in European countries with lower iodine intake such as France and Belgium (personal observations).

Radiation-Induced Hypothyroidism

Radiation-induced hypothyroidism is much less common than hypothyroidism because of autoimmune thyroid disease. It may occur as a result of external radiation therapy for tumors of the head and neck or after radioiodine therapy for hyperthyroidism (108).

Drug-Induced Hypothyroidism

Hypothyroidism due to drugs is also rare. Anticonvulsants such as phenytoin and the antituberculosis drug rifampicin induce hepatic mixed-function oxygenases, increasing thyroxine metabolism. This may lead to an increased need for thyroxine in treated children but generally has no significant effects in children with normal thyroid function. Interferon-α, amiodarone, and lithium may induce hypo- or hyperthyroidism. The mech-

anisms leading to thyroid dysfunction differ for each of these drugs. Excessive iodide ingestion paradoxically causes hypothyroidism due to inhibition of organic binding of iodine, which is called the Wolff–Chaikoff effect). The increased susceptibility of patients with preexisting autoimmune thyroiditis to drug-induced thyroid dysfunction remains poorly understood.

Hemangiomas

"Consumptive" hypothyroidism, resulting from the overexpression of type 3 deiodinase by large liver or cutaneous hemangiomas, has been recently described (109). Increased conversion of T_4 to rT_3 and T_3 to T_2 due to elevated levels of type 3 deiodinase in hemangiomas eventually resulted in low serum T_4 and T_3 and hypothyroisism. Some of these infants were already hypothyroid at birth (110) but most presented in the first few months of life, when hemangiomas are typically at their maximal size. Importantly, severe primary hypothyroidism requiring a very high dose of thyroxine was the presenting manifestation of occult multiple hepatic hemangiomas in one child, suggesting that a search for these tumors should be performed in any child with unexplained primary hypothyroidism who requires an unusually high dose of thyroxine (111).

Iodine Deficiency

Iodine deficiency remains an important cause of acquired hypothyroidism worldwide. Although overt hypothyroidism from iodine deficiency is very rare in industrialized countries, it has been infrequently reported in children whose diets are severely restricted in salt- and iodine-containing foods and rich in thiocyanate-containing goitrogens such as cabbage and broccoli (112).

Acquired Central Hypothyroidism Acquired central hypothyroidism is typically associated with other pituitary hormone deficiencies. It is rarely the first clinical manifestation of hypothalamic or pituitary disease due to tumors or infiltrative diseases such as histiocytosis (113).

Hypothyroidism in Children on GH Replacement Therapy

Some children with GH deficiency may develop central hypothyroidism during the course of GH treatment, and hypothyroidism is one reason for a poor therapeutic response to GH. This central hypothyroidism is generally due to evolving hypothalamic or pituitary disease. It should be distinguished from the decrease in free T_4 that has been observed during the first few

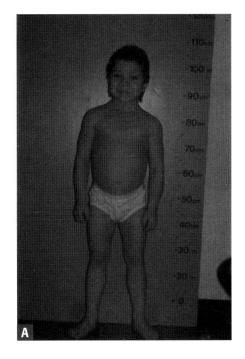

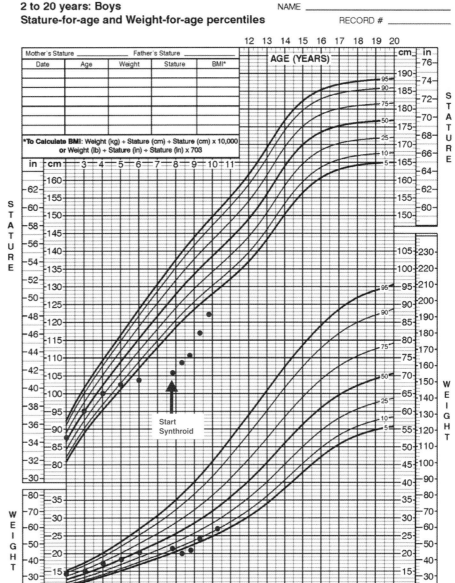

FIGURE 26-5. A 7.8-year-old boy who was diagnosed with hypothyroidism by a dermatologist who was seeing him for eczema. His only other complaint was constipation. TSH was 858 mU/L, total T₄ 1.2 mg/dL (15.4 nmol/L), and bone age 3.5 years. He had been measured but not plotted on a growth chart at his primary care clinic, where his 3-year lack of growth was not appreciated. Note the classic physical appearance (panel A), the growth chart showing cessation of growth with subsequent catch-up following thyroid hormone replacement (panel B), and the testicular enlargement in the face of low testosterone levels (testosterone = <10 ng/dL or <0.4 nmol/L) and absence of pubic hair (panel C). Photo courtesy of Antoinette Moran.

months of GH treatment in both GH-deficient (114) and GH-replete (115) children and which appears to be mainly due to increased conversion of T₄ into T₃. On the other hand, an increased hypothalamic somatostatin secretion during GH treatment may induce a fall in TSH concentrations and true central hypothyroidism (116). Thyroxine replacement therapy should be initiated in children who have a suboptimal response to GH therapy, symptoms and signs of hypothyroidism, and unequivocally low plasma free T₄ concentrations. This occurs mainly in children with organic hypo-

pituitarism (117). Thyroid replacement therapy of GH deficient children should not be taken lightly because overtreatment may result in acceleration of bone maturation and reduced final adult height (118).

Clinical Presentation of Childhood-Onset Hypothyroidism

Physical Signs and Symptoms The symptoms and signs of acquired hypothyroidism in children and adolescents depend on its severity and duration (Table 26-3). Some patients present with a relatively short history of fa-

tigue, constipation, dry skin, and cold intolerance, without growth deceleration or delay in bone maturation, reflecting a sudden onset of hypothyroidism. In the vast majority of patients, there is deceleration in height gain with increased and sometimes excessive weight gain. Thus, the patients present with short stature, weight gain, delayed bone age, and they may have puffy facies from subcutaneous myxoedema (Figure 26-5). The effect of hypothyroidism on bone maturation is even more pronounced than its effect on linear growth, so that the bone age is often younger than the "height age" (i.e., the age at which the child's height corresponds to the 50th percentile). Tooth eruption is also delayed. Other skeletal effects of hypothyroidism in children include stippling of the epiphyses and a slipped capital femoral epiphysis (119).

Longstanding hypothyroidism retards bone maturation and generally delays the onset of puberty; however, rare instances of sexual precocity have been reported in severe and longstanding primary hypothyroidism (120), which appears to result from chronic stimulation of the follicle-stimulating hormone receptor by very high plasma TSH concentrations. Accordingly, the most common changes in girls are functional ovarian cysts with vaginal bleeding, either with no other sign of puberty (121) or with breast development and galactorrhea but no pubic hair (120); plasma estradiol levels may be markedly elevated and there may be mild hyperprolactinemia. In boys, adult-size testes with undetectable plasma testosterone concentrations may be observed (122).

School-age children with severe longstanding hypothyroidism may require more time to accomplish the assigned tasks but are rarely held back academically. Quite often, school performance deteriorates after treatment is started (see later).

Of note, severe hypothyroidism has also been reported in otherwise asymptomatic children with hypercholesterolemia (123).

Appearance of the Thyroid Gland In all children with symptoms and signs of hypothyroidism, the volume of the thyroid should be determined. The World Health Organization's definition that a goiter is present when the thyroid lobes are larger than the distal phalanx of the thumb of the child may seem rather crude, but it is useful in children given their greatly varying size (124). In iodine-replete areas, the most common cause of goiter associated with hypothyroidism is Hashimoto thyroiditis, in which both lobes of the thyroid are in general moderately enlarged but are firm and sometimes irregular ("pebbly"). Nodules greater than 1 cm in diameter are rare, but a "Delphian node" is frequent (a lymph node sometimes as small as a grain of rice that can be palpated above the isthmus, close to the midline). A family history of autoimmune thyroid disease is very often present. Although a goiter is present at the time of diagnosis in approximately two thirds of pediatric patients with Hashimoto thyroiditis (125), the gland will usually atrophy over the years. Thyroid atrophy may also be present at diagnosis at any age but this appears to be more common in infants with autoimmune thyroiditis (126).

Pituitary Enlargement Imaging of the pituitary is often performed in children with growth failure. Children and adolescents, as well as adults, with longstanding primary hypothyroidism can have pituitary enlargement, caused by hypertrophy and hyperplasia of the thyrotrophs. The pituitary enlargement that may mimic a pituitary tumor is reversed after a few months of T_4 therapy (127). This pituitary pseudotumor may be responsible for the rare occurrence of transient GH deficiency, presumably from compression of the somatotrophs, during the 1st years of thyroxine therapy in children with primary hypothyroidism (128).

Diagnostic Evaluation of Childhood-Onset Hypothyroidism Primary Hypothyroidism

A clinical suspicion of hypothyroidism should always be confirmed by the measurement of plasma TSH and free T_4. On the other hand, the serendipitous discovery of a high plasma TSH in a normally growing child or adolescent without any symptoms and signs of hypothyroidism needs to be verified before embarking on long-term treatment, because episodes of transient hypothyroidism may occur in autoimmune thyroiditis. If primary hypothyroidism is confirmed, the next step is to determine its cause: in infants, a radionuclide scan should be done to rule out either congenital hypothyroidism that may have been missed on neonatal screening or late-onset congenital hypothyroidism, most likely due to thyroid dyshormonogenesis (103,104). Ectopic thyroid tissue was the cause of severe hypothyroidism in a 3-year-old boy with normal blood-spot TSH and T_4 values at neonatal screening (105). Intense radionuclide uptake by a normal-sized or enlarged thyroid in an infant with acquired hypothyroidism may suggest the presence of consumptive hypothyroidism (111).

In older infants, children, and adolescents, serum antithyroid peroxidase antibodies should be measured. These are more often elevated than antithyroglobulin antibodies (125). Elevated thyroid antibodies confirm the diagnosis of chronic autoimmune thyroiditis, whether the patient has a goiter or not. On radionuclide imaging studies, the size of the thyroid may vary from small to large, and the heterogeneous pattern of uptake often seen in adults, which probably results from areas of fibrosis, is rarely seen in children (125). On ultrasonography, heterogeneous echogenicity is usually present (129). In fact, neither scintigraphy nor ultrasonography is necessary to establish the diagnosis of chronic autoimmune thyroiditis and imaging should be re-

stricted to those children with a palpable thyroid nodule.

The child's growth trajectory should be carefully reconstructed and analyzed. A bone age should be obtained at diagnosis in to estimate the duration of hypothyroidism by the degree of retardation of bone maturation, particularly if previous growth data are not available.

Chronic autoimmune thyroiditis is prevalent in children with type 1 diabetes, in children with chromosomal disorders, principally aneuploidies (trisomy 21) (130) and Turner syndrome (131); the evidence for an association with Klinefelter syndrome is less clear (132). Although hypothyroidism may occur in association with other autoimmune endocrinopathies, it is seldom the presenting feature of the polyglandular autoimmune syndromes.

CENTRAL HYPOTHYROIDISM

Central hypothyroidism in children and adolescents is much less common and has a more subtle onset than primary hypothyroidism. Presenting symptoms include growth deceleration and delayed bone maturation (45). Central hypothyroidism is characterized by low plasma free T_4 and a low or normal TSH (which is inappropriate for the degree of hypothyroxinemia). Once the diagnosis is established, other pituitary functions should be evaluated. Magnetic resonance imaging of the pituitary with gadolinium should be performed to rule out space-occupying lesions, infiltrative processes of the hypothalamic pituitary area, or interruption of the pituitary stalk. Most patients with central hypothyroidism have other pituitary hormone deficiencies, especially GH deficiency.

TRH Stimulation Testing Whether a TRH stimulation test should be performed before treatment remains controversial (133) and currently, as of 2008, TRH is not commercially available in the United States. In children and adolescents with untreated central hypothyroidism, a TRH injection typically induces an ample and sustained plasma TSH response, with a peak concentration at 60 minutes or later. This response suggests that the pituitary thyrotrophs are not only present but also store TSH because of lack of stimulation from endogenous TRH (134). The TSH produced in these patients has low bioactivity (135). Imaging studies usually reveal an interrupted pituitary stalk, often associated with other developmental defects such as an ectopic posterior pituitary (136).

In the rare cases of central hypothyroidism resulting from pituitary transcription factor mutations, the plasma TSH response to TRH is generally blunted or absent, and the pituitary stalk is normal on imaging (137).

Treatment and Outcome of Childhood-Onset Hypothyroidism

As in adults, the treatment of choice for children and adolescents with either primary or central hypothyroidism is daily oral administration of thyroxine (Table 26-4). A full replacement dose of approximately 100 $\mu g/m^2$/day (138) may be prescribed from the outset in children and adolescents. There is substantial variation in the effect of thyroxine in different patients, so these estimates are a rough guide for the dose likely to be needed for an individual patient.

In primary hypothyroidism, the dose should be adjusted so that the patient's plasma TSH concentration is normal. Even though absorption may be better if thyroxine is administered 30 minutes or more before meals, this is seldom of clinical importance. Iron and calcium supplements should not be taken at the same time, as this may decrease thyroxine absorption (139,140).

The dose of thyroxine required in central hypothyroidism cannot be titrated against plasma TSH in the same way as in primary hypothyroidism; however, in the majority of patients with central hypothyroidism who have a measurable plasma TSH before treatment, a TSH that becomes undetectable suggests overtreatment even if serum free T_4 and T_3 are in the normal range. This should be avoided because it may lead to undue bone maturation, and the dose should be the lowest possible for optimal growth and maturation.

Response to therapy

Behavioral and Neurologic Response The initiation of treatment may occasionally initiate acute (and transient) psychosis in a few adolescents even after gradual dose escalation (141). Another rare side effect in the early phase of thyroxine therapy in children is benign intracranial hypertension, even with a gradual dose escalation (142). Thus, parents should be warned that dramatic behavioral changes may occur after therapy initiation, and that if severe headache develops, a prompt funduscopic examination is necessary.

Growth and Puberty After initiation of therapy, the appearance of children with severe longstanding hypothyroidism changes dramatically. Weight loss and a decrease in height of up to 0.5 cm may be seen, likely a reflection of the loss of myxoedema of the scalp. Subsequently, catch-up growth in height with proportionate weight gain occurs. Plasma TSH should not be measured earlier than 6 weeks after therapy is started or changed. Once the patient's plasma TSH

concentration is normal and catch-up growth is complete, height, weight, pubertal development, and plasma TSH can be monitored only once a year. Prepubertal children with severe longstanding hypothyroidism should be monitored closely to ensure that pubertal development and the associated acceleration of bone maturation are not too rapid. Administration of a gonadotropin-releasing hormone agonist to treat early puberty may be considered, although the impact of combined thyroxine and agonist therapy on adult height is uncertain (143). Ideally, hypothyroidism should be diagnosed before it has had an important impact on growth, and this can be achieved with yearly height and weight monitoring of all children.

Remission In most patients, and specifically those who have chronic autoimmune thyroiditis, hypothyroidism will be permanent. Although as in many other autoimmune diseases, there may be periods of remission. In particular, thyroid function may fluctuate, sometimes widely (144) (Figure 26-6) and it may therefore be appropriate to withdraw thyroxine for 6 to 8 weeks every several years or at the end of growth. This is not necessary in patients who have plasma TSH concentrations above the normal range while taking thyroxine or in those who had severe hypothyroidism with thyroid atrophy at the time of diagnosis.

Lipid Metabolism In both genders, the importance of maintaining lifelong euthyroidism for lipid metabolism should be stressed. This is especially true in primary hypothyroidism because the impact of thyroxine treatment on lipid profiles in central hypothyroidism is less clear (145).

Contraception and Pregnancy

Because estrogens increase plasma thyroxine-binding globulin, the dose of thyroxine may need to be increased in adolescent girls if they are taking an estrogen-containing oral contraceptive, although currently used oral contraceptives have only a minimal influence on thyroid function (146). More important, adolescent girls with congenital or acquired hypothyroidism should be advised that the adequacy of treatment should be determined before and as soon as possible after they become pregnant, because most pregnant women with hypothyroidism need a higher dose of thyroxine (101).

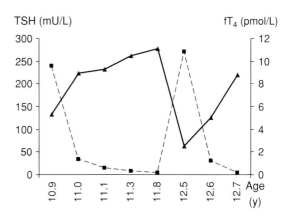

FIGURE 26-6. Serial plasma TSH (dotted line) and free T_4 (fT_4, solid line) between ages 10.9 and 12.7 years of a girl who had her initial blood work done because of headaches. When referred to the endocrinology clinic, she was growing normally and had neither symptoms nor signs of hypothyroidism and she had no goiter. The serum titer of antithyroid peroxidase antibodies was weakly positive (1:100, increasing to 1:400 after 2 months). The episode of biochemical hypothyroidism resolved spontaneously, as did the one that occurred 2 years later. The thyroid became firm in consistency but never increased in size. Now aged 20 years, the patient has remained euthyroid. This case, although rare, illustrates the need to confirm a diagnosis of acquired hypothyroidism when it is made by chance in an asymptomatic child before embarking on long-term treatment. This contrasts with the situation in congenital hypothyroidism, in which treatment is started on the basis of the screening test alone. (The upper limit of the normal range for TSH in this age group is 4.4 mU/L and the lower limit for free T_4 is 7.6 pmol/L or 0.6 ng/dL (88)).

When the patient's hypothyroidism is due to chronic autoimmune thyroiditis, plasma TSHR-blocking antibodies may be present but rarely in sufficient quantities to affect fetal thyroid function (51).

CONGENITAL HYPERTHYROIDISM

Fetal and neonatal hyperthyroidism have mostly been described in the context of maternal Graves disease (Table 26-5). It has been estimated that approximately 0.2% of pregnant women have Graves disease; however, only 1% of children born to these women have hyperthyroidism. Thus, transient neonatal hyperthyroidism due to maternal Graves disease is rare, affecting 1:50,000 neonates.

Persistent congenital hyperthyroidism, mostly with a dominant pattern of inheritance, has been described and can now be explained by molecular abnormalities of the thyrotropin receptor.

Pathogenesis of Congenital Hyperthyroidism

Transfer of Maternal Antibodies: Transient Congenital Hyperthy-roidism In most cases, the disease is due to thyroid-stimulating immunoglobulins (TSIs), which are transferred from the maternal into the fetal compartment, leading to stimulation of the fetal thyroid by

TABLE 26-5   Fetal and Neonatal Hyperthyroidism

Causes

- Most common cause is maternal Graves disease
- Other (rare) causes:
  - Activating TSHR mutation
  - MAS

Epidemiology of neonatal Graves disease

- Prevalence of Graves disease in pregnant women = 0.1%–0.4 %
- Prevalence of hyperthyroidism in offspring of women with Graves disease = 0.6%–1%
- Definition of women at risk:
  - Hyperthyroidism diagnosed for the first time during pregnancy
  - Women with known Graves disease on ATD therapy during pregnancy
  - Patient in remission after ATD therapy
  - History of ablation therapy (^{131}I, surgery)

Mechanism

- Transfer of TSHR antibodies from mother to fetus

activation of the TSHR (Table 26-5). This leads to an increase in thyroid hormone secretion, and as a consequence, to thyrotoxicosis, first in utero, and then postnatally until the maternal antibodies have disappeared from the infant's circulation (147), which occurs at the latest by 4 months of life. The fetal thyroid gland starts secreting thyroid hormone at approximately 10 weeks of gestation; the TSHR starts responding to the stimulation of TSH and therefore to the stimulation by TSI during the second trimester of gestation. The fetal concentration of immunoglobulin G-type immunoglobulin, in particular TSI, is low at approximately the 15th week of gestation, and increases progressively to reach the maternal level at approximately the 30th week of gestation. As there is a correlation between the elevated level of transmitted antibodies and the appearance of thyrotoxicosis, fetal hyperthyroidism develops during the second half of gestation mostly in fetuses of women with high levels of TSI (147).

TSHR-blocking antibodies may also be present in pregnant women with Graves disease. Their transplacental passage has been demonstrated (51), and the clinical symptoms in the fetus are the result of the balance between the stimulating action of the TSI and the inhibitory action of the TSHR-blocking antibodies.

Constitutive Activation of TSH Receptor Signaling: Persistent Congenital Hyperthyroidism

An even rarer type of neonatal hyperthyroidism was initially described as dominantly transmitted Graves disease with persistence of hyperthyroidism years after a neonatal onset (148). It was subsequently realized that markers of autoimmunity were generally lacking in these cases (149). Another decade later, dominantly inherited mutations resulting in an increase in the constitutive activity of the TSHR were shown to be responsible for this phenotype (150). Subsequently, the same mechanism occurring *de novo* was identified in neonates with severe persistent nonautoimmune hyperthyroidism (4,151). Neonatal hyperthyroidism has also been reported in McCune–Albright syndrome (MAS) due to activating mutations in GNAS, the gene encoding the α-subunit of the stimulatory G proteins (152,153), which have a central role in TSHR signal transduction.

In five kindreds with familial congenital nonautoimmune hyperthyroidism due to germline activating mutations of the TSHR, Leclère et al. found that 49 of 120 patients were hyperthyroid and that women were more frequently affected (32 women vs 17 men). The onset of thyrotoxicosis was generally early, but varied from 1 to 23 years, depending on the family. Interestingly, a systematic screening of the families identified two children with suppressed TSH but no signs of hyperthyroidism, emphasizing the possibility of detecting affected children before the development of symptoms with their potential deleterious consequences. The goiters were homogeneous in children but tended to become multinodular later in life. No ophthalmopathy or circulating antithyroid antibodies, including anti-TSHR antibodies, were detected in these patients. Recurrence after ATD therapy, non-ablative radioiodine treatment or partial thyroidectomy was frequent. Pathologic examination of the thyroid glands of patients with activating TSHR mutations showed no mononuclear cell infiltration, which is a characteristic finding in the thyroid glands of patients with Graves disease (154). Sporadic congenital nonautoimmune hyperthyroidism with thyroid hyperplasia due to *de novo* mutations of the TSHR gene have also been described (4,151). Interestingly, the mutations found in these cases are also found in toxic adenomas in adults, whereas those found in familial cases are private. This may suggest a historical bias due to the fact that these private mutations are milder and would not significantly decrease reproductive fitness (155). By contrast, the sporadic cases are so severe that they probably did not survive before the advent of modern treatments for neonatal thyrotoxicosis. These severe cases who have developmental delay also emphasize the potentially deleterious effect of suboptimal treatment of fetal hyperthyroidism, independently of the presence of craniosynostosis and/or microcephaly, (4,149,151). Finally, a somatic activating mutation in the extracellular TSH-binding domain of the TSHR has been reported in a male infant with congenital hyperthyroidism due to a toxic adenoma (156).

In conclusion, constitutive activation of TSH signaling due to mutations in TSHR or GNAS is a rare cause of persistent nonautoimmune neonatal hyperthyroidism, which may develop in utero. It should be suspected in the absence of maternal thyroid antibodies. The decision as to when definitive treatment (near total thyroidectomy in the very young, ablative radioiodine in older children) should be initiated depends on the severity of the disease and on tolerance and compliance to chronic treatment with ATDs.

CLINICAL PRESENTATION OF CONGENITAL HYPERTHYROIDISM

Fetal hyperthyroidism may be suspected because of intrauterine growth retardation and fetal tachycardia. Premature birth is frequent. In contrast to Graves disease in older children, the neonatal form affects both sexes equally. The clinical signs of hyperthyroidism generally appear several days after birth. This is due to the ATDs given to the mother, which are transferred across the placenta and control the fetal hyperthyroidism. As soon as the ATD from the mother disappears in the newborn (which takes only a few days), the newborn thyroid is no longer blocked, and the TSIs, which have a longer half-life than the ATDs, lead to an increase in thyroid hormone production and therefore to overt clinical hyperthyroidism. As during fetal life, if both TSHR-blocking antibodies and TSIs are present in the neonate, euthyroidism may ensue.

The clinical signs vary in severity (Table 26-6) and it is likely that some neonates born to mothers with autoimmune hyperthyroidism have transient hyperthyroidism that is not detected. Hyperexcitability, increased appetite with poor weight gain, vomiting or diarrhea, fever, diaphoresis, and erythema have been described. The fontanels are small and bone maturation is often advanced, as a consequence of increased thyroid hormone action on fetal bone.

Tachypnea is sometimes noticed in the context of heart failure or pulmonary arterial hypertension, which can be documented by echocardiography. Sinus tachycardia is frequent, sometimes associated with cardiac arrhythmia and rarely with high blood pressure. Heart failure is one of the major risks in the neonate. Early diagnosis and treatment are required for a good prognosis. A congenital or neonatal infection should be excluded in the presence of hepatomegaly, splenomegaly, polyadenopathy, jaundice, cholestasis, and thrombocytopenia, all of which have been described in thyrotoxicosis. Abnormalities of liver function tests can occur even in the absence of cardiac insufficiency. A goiter is

TABLE 26-6	Clinical Signs Present at Diagnosis in 10 Neonates with Hyperthyroidism (Nine Autoimmune Cases and One Case Due to a Neomutation in the TSHR)*	
Tachycardia (can lead to heart failure)		10/10
Goiter		7/10
Hyperexcitability		7/10
Poor weight gain (despite ↑ appetite)		5/10
Hepatomegaly and/or splenomegaly		5/10
Stare and/or eyelid retraction		5/10
Bilateral gynecomastia		2/10
Cardiac insufficiency		1/10

Intrauterine growth retardation, premature birth, vomiting, diarrhea, fever, tachypnea, jaundice, thrombocytopenia, and advanced skeletal maturation have been described in other infants.

* = reference 144.

present in approximately 50% of the cases but rarely is large enough to lead to compression of the airway. Thyroid volume is best evaluated by thyroid ultrasound. Traditionally, stare and eyelid retraction have been linked to thyrotoxicosis per se and exophthalmia to the autoimmune process. Exophthalmia can also occur in nonautoimmune neonatal hyperthyroidism (151).

Diagnosis of Congenital Hyperthyroidism

In newborns who have signs suggestive of congenital hyperthyroidism, the diagnosis should be confirmed by the determination of the plasma levels of free T_4, T_3, and TSH. Even if these are normal, they should be repeated 3 to 7 days later because of the possibility of the delayed appearance of hyperthyroidism, especially in the autoimmune cases in which the ATD is cleared from the newborn circulation whereas thyroid-stimulating antibodies are still present due to a longer half life (157). They should be interpreted taking into account the peculiarities of the reference ranges for thyroid hormone levels in the neonatal period. The presence of TSIs in cord blood may be predictive of the occurrence of neonatal thyrotoxicosis (5,158). Once neonatal hyperthyroidism is confirmed, its autoimmune origin should be established by determining the levels of TSI. In practice, these are measured by inhibition of the binding of TSH to thyroid membranes in a radioreceptor assay.

Treatment and Outcome of Congenital Hyperthyroidism

Treatment of the Neonate Immediate treatment of overt neonatal hyperthyroidism is essential for a good prognosis (157) (Table 26-7). Propylthiouracil (PTU) should be administered orally at a dose of 5 to 10 mg/kg/day di-

vided in three doses. Compared with methimazole (MMI) or carbimazole (CMZ), it has the advantage that, in addition to blocking thyroid hormone secretion, it decreases the conversion of T_4 to T_3 through its action on deiodinase type I. A saturated solution of potassium iodide (SSKI) (1 drop/d) or Lugol's solution (1–3 drops/d) may be added in severe cases to decrease thyroglobulin proteolysis and thyroid hormone secretion. Propranolol promptly restores a normal heart rate. Other drugs, such as sodium iopanoate (iopanoic acid 500 mg orally once every 3rd day) and glucocorticoids, are seldom used to decrease thyroid hormone production and to inhibit T_4 to T_3 conversion (159). Additional supportive measures, including high fluid and caloric intake, are essential. Infants with neonatal Graves disease should be monitored clinically and biochemically at frequent intervals, initially weekly. Tapering of the antithyroid medication and β-blockers can be initiated as serum free T_4 and T_3 fall in the lower half of the normal range for the age. Serum TSH can be suppressed even after euthyroid stage is achieved and routine measurement may not be useful.

In the immune-mediated form, treatment should be only maintained as long as the TSIs are detectable (usually between 3 and 12 weeks). It is often convenient to apply the "block and replace" approach: a fixed dose of ATD is given, and thyroxine is added when plasma thyroxine reaches the hypothy-

roid range. On average, treatment is required for 1 month (5). Even though it is transient, symptomatic neonatal hyperthyroidism should be treated to avoid both short-term (heart failure) and long-term morbidity (craniosynostosis, intellectual impairment).

Treatment of the Fetus for Hyper- or Hypothyroidism

A few cases of fetal hyperthyroidism related to maternal TSHR antibodies have been described (5). In the absence of maternal treatment with ATDs, hyperthyroidism develops in the fetus during the second half of pregnancy. Fetal tachycardia is a useful alarm signal but occurs later than fetal goiter. Therefore, fetal goiter on the sonogram is the earliest sign of fetal thyroid dysfunction. Normative data on the size of the fetal thyroid gland according to gestational age have been reported (160). Accelerated bone maturation may already be detected by neonatal ultrasound. Treatment of the fetus by administering ATD to the mother has been shown to improve fetal and neonatal prognosis. In pregnant women, PTU is preferred over MMI because of reports that MMI may be associated with aplasia cutis congenita and other malformations (161).

Because ATDs cross the placenta, hypothyroidism can develop in fetuses borne by women on ATD therapy for Graves disease. The diagnosis can be suggested by ultrasound visualization of fetal goiter and confirmed by tests on fetal blood samples. Because thyroid hormones play a crucial role in fetal brain development, fetal hypothyroidism can cause permanent intellectual impairment. Although ATD dosage reduction should restore normal fetal thyroid function, use of intraamniotic thyroxine injection has also been tried. Fetal

TABLE 26-7	Take Home Messages on Perinatal Graves Disease

- High risk of fetal and neonatal thyroid dysfunction (either hyper or hypo) when mother is positive for TSI and/or takes ATDs during the last trimester
- Prenatal treatment is effective in improving fetal/neonatal thyroid function and prognosis. The following are used to routinely evaluate the at-risk fetus:
  - Fetal growth
  - Fetal heart rate
  - Bone maturation (distal femoral center at 32 weeks gestation)
  - Size of thyroid gland (ultrasound perimeter and circumference)
- When a fetal goiter is found, one can distinguish between fetal hypo- or hyperthyroidism using the following factors:
  - Maternal factors: level of TSI, administration of 3rd trimester antithyroid drug
  - Fetal factors: heart rate, bone maturation, Doppler
- Fetal blood sampling should be reserved for those at risk of severe fetal hypothyroidism and when intraamniotic thyroxine injection is planned.
- Cord blood thyroid hormone concentration does not predict postnatal hyperthyroidism but an elevated titer of anti-TSHR antibodies does.

blood sampling should be reserved for those cases in which intraamniotic thyroxine injection is considered or when the thyroid status is in doubt in a fetus whose mother has positive TSIs and takes ATD therapy. Thus, fetuses of mothers on ATD therapy can develop either hypo- or hyperthyroidism. Early diagnosis and treatment of fetal hyperthyroidism are crucial to prevent premature delivery, death in utero, or permanent neurologic impairment.

In pregnant women with current or a history of Graves disease, TSI should be assayed routinely at the beginning of pregnancy. In pregnant women who are taking ATD therapy and/or have positive TSIs, monthly ultrasounds after 20 weeks of gestation to detect the development of goiter and/or other evidence of thyroid dysfunction in the fetus may be justified (6). It should also be remembered that fetal hyperthyroidism can occur in fetuses borne by women who are on thyroxine replacement after radioiodine treatment for Graves disease, because elevated levels of TSIs may persist in such women. In pregnant women with a history for Graves disease but negative TSI and no ATD treatment, routine prenatal care suffices.

Long-Term Outcome of Congenital Hyperthyroidism

Since the historical descriptions of craniosynostosis and developmental delay after recovery from transient neonatal hyperthyroidism (95), there have been very few studies of long-term developmental outcome of these patients. In one study, no difference in growth or psychomotor development was found at age 7 to 8 years between children with neonatal Graves born to mothers with treated hyperthyroidism and children born to euthyroid mothers (162). Neuropsychologic sequelae may be difficult to disentangle from those of prematurity per se (163). With this caveat, it seems that an optimistic long-term prognosis can be given to the parents of neonates with Graves disease.

Acquired Hyperthyroidism

Graves disease is the most common cause of childhood thyrotoxicosis and is characterized by diffuse goiter, hyperthyroidism, and occasionally, ophthalmopathy (164,165).

Pathogenesis of Graves Disease

Graves disease is an autoimmune disorder characterized by antibodies directed against the TSHR. These antibodies are detected in more than 90% of the patients and mimic the effects of pituitary TSH, thereby stimulating thyroid growth and function. Whether the disease is triggered by abnormal clones of autoreactive T cells, or by abnormal antigen presentation by thyroid follicular cells, either independently or in response to cytokines released by infiltrating T cells, is uncertain. The cause of Graves ophthalmopathy and dermatopathy is also unknown, but a strong candidate is cross-reactivity of circulating antibodies against thyroidal antigens, such as the TSHR, with antigens in orbital and extraorbital tissues (especially preadipocyte fibroblasts (154,155). A concordance rate of only 20% in monozygotic twins indicates that environmental factors trigger the development of Graves disease in genetically susceptible individuals. These factors include life stresses, sex steroids, smoking, a high dietary iodine intake, and immune modulators such as interferon-α.

Clinical Presentation and Diagnostic Evaluation

Because Graves disease is uncommon in childhood, hyperthyroidism is often discovered when the child or adolescent is evaluated for nonspecific complaints after having been symptomatic for months. A large female preponderance has been described for Graves disease and the peak incidence is around puberty (164,165). One of the most distressing symptoms is the inability to concentrate, causing deterioration of school performance as Graves disease develops. Other symptoms include an almost constant tachycardia, palpitations with heart rate providing the best index of the hyperthyroid state. The patient may be thin and complain of fatigue, decreased exercise tolerance, increased frequency of bowel movements and nocturia (Table 26-8). Skin is often moist and warm but pretibial myxoedema is extremely rare in children with Graves disease.

Graves disease is often associated with eye findings, but these are less dramatic in children than in adults. Stare due to eyelid retraction should be differentiated from true exophthalmos. Protrusion of the eyes should be measured by an ophthalmologist. Proptosis may be present along with fullness of the eyelids and redness of the conjunctivae. Occasionally, eye disease may antedate the development of overt hyperthyroidism. The thyroid gland is usually symmetrically enlarged and smooth and either firm or soft in consistency. Care should be taken to determine if an isolated thyroid nodule is present because autonomously functioning nodules may produce hyperthyroidism. Thyroid storm is extremely rare in children, except in neonates. It may manifest as high fever, tachycardia, and encephalopathy with seizures. In some cases withdrawal of ATD therapy for too long before radioiodine treatment has been implicated (166).

Diagnostic Evaluation

Biochemically, the cardinal feature of hyperthyroidism is a suppressed TSH level. Free T_4 and T_3 levels are generally elevated, but in some cases only T_3 is elevated (T_3 toxicosis). If free T_4 and T_3 levels are high but TSH levels are not suppressed, resistance to thyroid hormones (27) or a TSH-producing pituitary adenoma (167) should be considered. Clinical and laboratory findings may be more severe in younger children, and patients of African origin are more likely to have an earlier onset of disease in childhood (<6 years of age) (168,169). Thyroid scanning is usually not necessary for the diagnosis of Graves disease; a thyroid ultrasound may be useful to eliminate a toxic nodule, especially if the goiter is small.

TABLE 26-8   Clinical Signs of Graves Disease*

	Children, Adolescents (%)	Adults (%)
Tachycardia	85	88
Loss of weight	50	79
Polyphagia	60	13
Shaking	52	41
Irritability/Emotivity	82	53
Thermophobia	30	62
Accelerated growth		
Prepubertal	80	Not applicable
Ongoing puberty	24	
Advanced bone age		
Prepubertal	70	Not applicable
Ongoing puberty	24	

Other common symptoms include declining school performance, palpitations, increased frequency of bowel movements, nocturia, fatigue, decreased exercise tolerance, eyelid retraction, and stare. * = reference 179.

Treatment and Outcome of Graves Disease

Because Graves disease rarely resolves spontaneously within a short period, treatment of hyperthyroidism is essential. Current treatment approaches include ATDs, radioiodine therapy, and surgery. The risks and benefits of each approach must be considered by the physician and patient in developing a treatment strategy (Table 26-9). There is no consensus regarding the first-line treatment and the results of ongoing prospective studies will impact on our current recommendations.

Antithyroid Drug Therapy

Treatment with ATDs remains the first-line therapy for children with Graves disease in many centers, especially in Europe. Available drugs include the thionamide derivatives PTU and MMI or CMZ. MMI is 10-fold more potent than PTU and has a longer half-life. Recommended doses for initial therapy are 5 to 10 mg/kg/day for PTU and 0.5 to 0.8 mg/kg/day for MMI or CMZ; however, lower doses may be effective for induction or maintenance therapy with fewer side effects.

To control the hyperthyroid state, PTU is typically given every 8 hours and CMZ or MMI every 12 hours. Once a day dosing of CMZ or MMI, however, may bring remission as rapidly as divided doses and is especially well suited for maintenance therapy. Because of the dosing schedule and the smaller size of MMI and CMZ pills (5 or 10 mg) than PTU tablets (50 mg), MMI, or CMZ are easier to take than PTU. Another advantage of MMI or CMZ is the much lower risk of severe hepatitis than with PTU use.

Although MMI or CMZ and PTU promptly inhibit hormone formation, they do not inhibit thyroid hormone release. Thus, the levels of circulating thyroid hormones may remain elevated for several weeks after initiation of treatment as stored hormone is released. Until normalization of circulating levels of thyroid hormones occurs, the signs and symptoms of hyperthyroidism can be controlled with β-blockers such as propranolol (0.5–2 mg/kg/d in divided doses) or atenolol (25 or 50 mg, one or twice daily).

Clinical responses to treatment with PTU or MMI or CMZ are seen in 4 to 6 weeks. The dose of ATD can be reduced or levothyroxine can be added if hypothyroidism develops, usually 2 to 3 months later. The latter solution ("block and replace") does not improve the rate of remission but is very convenient and probably allows for fewer blood tests once euthyroidism has been reached.

In certain series, more than 25% of children treated with ATDs develop minor complications and up to 1% of children serious complications (Table 26-9). Common side effects include a pruritic rash and painful joints. A switch to another ATD may be tried but allergic reactions often recur. Agranulocytosis is rare, seldom fatal, and usually reversible when the drug is stopped. Severe hepatitis, however, may not be reversible and may progress to end-stage liver disease requiring transplantation. In children as in adults, deaths due to PTU-induced liver failure have been reported.

Remission rates in children, after several years of drug therapy, are usually lower than 30%. Some have suggested that remission rates in children are 25% after 2 years of treatment and that 4 years of drug therapy are needed to achieve remission in 50% of cases (170). Prospective, ongoing, long-term studies will provide more accurate figures (169). When responses to medical therapy are compared between prepubertal and pubertal children, remission rates appear to be lower in prepubertal children (17%) than in pubertal children (30%) (171). Thus, prepubertal children have a lower chance of spontaneous remission. Children with the greatest chance of going into and staying in remission after medical treatment of Graves disease are those with small thyroid glands and levels of TSIs in the normal range.

Radioiodine Therapy

In comparison with other forms of treatment, radioiodine therapy is the simplest and most cost-effective treatment of Graves disease (Table 26-7), but reports of its routine used in pediatric centers were few until 5 years ago (108). Treatment is achieved when ^{131}I is trapped in thyroid cells, which leads to thyroid cell destruction by internal radiation. In comparison with the gland of adults, the thyroid gland in children and adolescents is more sensitive to the destructive effects of radioiodine. Whereas 200 Gy of absorbed radioactivity results in hypothyroidism in 44% of adults with Graves disease, 100 Gy achieves hypothyroidism in 50% of pediatric patients, 200 Gy results in hypothyroidism in 70%, and hypothyroidism generally develops if doses higher than 270 Gy (300 μCi/g of thyroid tissue) are used (172). Hypothyroidism usually occurs within 2 to 6 months of treatment. If hyperthyroidism persists, additional courses of ^{131}I are indicated. After repeated treatments, 6 to 12 months may elapse before hypothyroidism develops. ATDs may need to be resumed after ^{131}I, until the thyroid is destroyed. The calculation of the dose of ^{131}I requires that the weight of the gland be estimated, which is traditionally done by clinical examination. Determining thyroid volume by ultrasonography may be more precise but whether it will result in a higher rate of ablation after only one treatment remains to be determined. When deciding the dose in children that will achieve the desired outcome, the age of the patient should be taken into consideration because total-body radiation doses after ^{131}I administration varies with age. The same absolute dose of ^{131}I will result in more radiation exposure in a young child than in an adolescent or adult. There is very little published experience of treatment with ^{131}I in children younger than 6 years of age (173,174).

Studies show that the risk for thyroid cancer or leukemia is not increased in children treated with doses of radioiodine high enough to destroy the gland (175). On the other hand, if low doses of radioiodine are given, the risk of thyroid neoplasia is increased in the residual irradiated thyroid tissue. At present, no data are available to assess actual lifetime cancer risks for children treated with ^{131}I or medication for Graves disease. Among adults with hyperthyroidism treated with ^{131}I in the original Cooperative Thyrotoxicosis Therapy Follow-up Study cohort, the total number of cancer deaths was close to that expected based on mortality rates in the general population (2,950 vs. 2,857). On the other hand, increased cancer mortality was seen among patients treated exclusively with ATDs. Radioiodine therapy was not linked to total cancer deaths or to any specific cancer, with the exception of thyroid cancer, the occurrence of which was very small in absolute numbers. In these cases, the underlying thyroid disease, rather than ^{131}I therapy, was concluded to play a role in the pathogenesis of malignancy (176). Large-scale studies involving individuals treated as children and adolescents have not been performed to assess long-term outcome in relation to age, treatment modality, dose, and residual thyroid tissue (175). One should note that some centers routinely give the same dose of ^{131}I to all children irrespective of thyroid size and report good outcomes. Adjusting the dose based on thyroid uptake and size allows lower doses of ^{131}I to be used and reduces whole-body radiation exposure. Importantly, responses to ^{131}I therapy are much less favorable in patients with large goiters and surgery may be preferable in these patients.

Discussions have focused on the association between ^{131}I therapy for Graves disease and the development or progression of ophthalmopathy in adult patients. In contrast to adults, children rarely develop severe ophthalmopathy, and proptosis is generally mild. Of 87 children treated with ^{131}I for Graves disease at one center, eye signs improved in 90% of children, did not change in 7.5%, and worsened in 3%; these did not

TABLE 26-9 Comparison of the Various Treatments in Graves Disease in the Pediatric Patient*

Treatment	Advantages	Disadvantages	Complications (incidence)	Comments
ATDs	• Noninvasive • Less initial cost • Low risk of permanent hypothyroidism • Possible remission	• Low cure rate • Drug compliance	• Mild increase in liver enzymes (28%) • Mild leukopenia (25%) • Skin rash [a] (9%) • Granulcytopenia [b] (5%) • Arthritis [b] (2%) • Nausea [a] (1%) • Reversible granulocytosis [b] (0.4%) • Potentially irreversible hepatitis [b] (0.4%) *[a]May try substituting another thioamide drug* *[b]Discontinue all thioamide drugs*	• First-line treatment in children and adolescents in many European centers • Mandatory before surgery
Radioactive ¹³¹I	• Cure of hyperthyroidism • Most cost effective	• Permanent hypothyroidism almost inevitable • Pregnancy and breastfeeding must be deferred for 6-12 mo • Small potential risk of exacerbation of hyperthyroidism	• Worsening of eye disease (3%-5%) • Transient thyroid pain (5%) • Nausea (rare) • Thyroid storm (rare) • Transient hypocalcemia (rare) • Hyperparathyroidism (rare)	• No evidence for infertility, birth defects, or leukemia or thyroid cancer • First-line treatment for adolescents in some North American centers
Surgery	• Rapid • Effective, especially in patients with large goiters	• Most invasive • Most costly • Permanent hypothyroidism • Scar	• Pain (100%) • Transient hypocalcemia (1-7 d) (10%) • Keloid (3%) • Permanent hypoparathyroidism (2%) • Vocal cord paralysis (1%) • Transient hoarseness (1%) • Temporary tracheostomy (1%) • Hemorrhage/hematoma (0.2%) • Death (0.1%)	• Potential in pregnancy if major side effects from ATDs • Useful when coexisting suspicious nodule present • Ovption for patients who refuse radioiodine • Few surgeons, especially pediatric ones, with enough experience

* = reference 162, 171, 180.

differ from the results for the drug-treatment group (174).

Thyroidectomy

If surgery is performed, near-total thyroidectomy is now recommended to reduce the risk of recurrent hyperthyroidism (Table 26-9). In preparation for surgery, the child should be rendered euthyroid or hypothyroid. This is typically done with PTU, MMI, or CMZ. One week before the procedure, stable iodine in the form of 5% Lugol's solution (7 drops three times a day orally in an adolescent) may be added to cause the gland to become firmer and less vascular, which facilitates surgery. It also decreases thyroglobulin proteolysis and therefore thyroid hormone production.

Complication rates are comparable after subtotal and near-total thyroidectomy. Reported in-hospital mortality rates are 0.5% for adults and 0.08% for children. The most frequent complications include pain and transient hypocalcemia. Less common problems (1%–4%) include hemorrhage, permanent hypoparathyroidism, and vocal cord paralysis.

Surgery is especially useful for patients with very large thyroid glands and individuals who have not gone into remission with drug therapy and do not desire radioiodine treatment. Yet, because of the increasing use of radioiodine, fewer thyroid surgeries are now performed and fewer pediatric surgeons can develop and maintain their skills than in the past. Only surgeons with expertise in performing thyroidectomy in children should perform surgery; if such an individual is not available, a surgeon expert in adult thyroid should cooperate with a pediatric surgeon.

Treatment of Hyperthyroidism During Pregnancy

The goal of treatment of pregnant women is to give ATDs at the lowest dose that can maintain the woman's thyroxine level in the upper range of normal and decrease the risk of ATD-induced fetal hypothyroidism. PTU is preferred over MMI and CMZ during organogenesis because this drug does not seem to be teratogenic. By contrast, CMZ-related malformations have been reported (161). Initial reports were of an increased incidence of scalp defects in the infants of treated mothers, but many other anomalies have now been described. Choanal atresia, gastrointestinal anomalies—particularly esophageal atresia, atelia/hypothelia, developmental delay, hearing loss, and dysmorphic facial features—have all been reported (158). Careful follow up of the fetus, especially with thyroid ultrasound, is mandatory to avoid ATD-induced fetal hypothyroidism or to treat it if present (5).

Uncommon Causes of Childhood Thyrotoxicosis

Hashimoto Thyroiditis Rarely, Hashimoto thyroiditis in children can lead to thyrotoxicosis, the so-called "Hashitoxicosis," in its first phase of evolution. This is linked to the lymphocytic infiltration of thyroid tissue, which leads to a certain degree of destruction of the gland and therefore to acute release of thyroid hormone. Occasionally, this entity can be accompanied by the formation of thyroid lymphocytic nodules, in which case Hashitoxicosis needs to be clinically differentiated from a hyperfunctioning adenoma. The diagnosis is based the presence of high titers of antithyroperoxidase or antithyroglobulin antibodies, but clinical features may overlap with those of Graves disease (177). No thyroid scintigraphy is necessary unless the diagnosis is uncertain. Hashitoxicosis can be associated with other autoimmune disorders, such as diabetes mellitus type 1. β-blockers may be used transiently to treat the signs of thyrotoxicosis, which is short-lived.

Subacute Thyroiditis

Subacute (or de Quervain's) thyroiditis (SAT) occurs only rarely in childhood. The disease is typically preceded by a viral illness, with the manifestations of sore throat, fever, neck pain, and a tender thyroid gland. Some children may have minimal symptoms and signs, rendering SAT difficult to differentiate clinically from Hashitoxicosis. Although children are frequently exposed to and infected with viruses, SAT is surprisingly rare in childhood. Early in the course of SAT, the erythrocyte sedimentation rate is elevated, as are the $\alpha 2$ and γ-globulin levels. The clinical course of SAT can be generally divided into three phases: 1) an acute thyrotoxic phase, lasting 2 to 6 weeks, 2) a euthyroid phase of variable duration, and 3) a recovery phase, which is associated with biochemical and possibly clinical features of hypothyroidism, usually lasting 2 to 7 months and that should be treated. Typically, thyroid function returns to normal after the third phase, although permanent hypothyroidism may develop in some patients. Because SAT is generally self-limiting, only symptomatic therapy with β-blockers is advised. Additionally, nonsteroidal antiinflammatory drugs are given for the alleviation of local pain/discomfort. Aspirin is to be avoided in younger children. Rarely, prednisone (0.5 mg/kg/d) can be used if nonsteroidal antiinflammatory drugs are ineffective or contraindicated.

Toxic Adenoma

Hyperfunctioning adenomas are rare in childhood and adolescence. In the early part of the natural history of toxic adenomas (i.e., when they are small in size), they cause only mild hyperthyroidism sometimes with tachycardia as the only symptom. On the other hand, most adenomas larger than 3.5 cm in diameter will present with overt thyrotoxicosis. Occasionally, plasma free T_4 is normal but T_3 is always elevated (T_3 toxicosis). Surgery is the therapy of choice because the adenomas are encapsulated and their removal with a partial lobectomy is usually not associated with increased perioperative risk. Radioiodine therapy for hyperfunctioning adenomas is to be avoided in children because the radioiodine doses required for their ablation can be quite high (600–1,500 μCi/g [22.2–55.5 MBq/g] of adenomatous tissue). This is a rather significant exposure to radiation and can lead to sublethal radiation of peritumoral normal thyroid tissue, with an obvious increase in the lifelong risk of developing nodules (both benign and malignant).

Toxic adenomas can also develop in the context of MAS. These nodules are typically benign. The optimal management of MAS-associated hyperthyroidism in childhood and adolescence is a highly debatable subject because these children typically relapse even after long-term ATD therapy and surgery should then be performed.

Cancer

Very rarely, thyroid carcinomas in children can be hyperfunctioning, leading to excessive secretion of thyroid hormone by the tumor. Considering that most hyperfunctioning thyroid carcinomas in adults are follicular carcinomas, the preponderance of papillary over follicular thyroid carcinomas in children and adolescents, and the rarity of thyroid cancer in general, pediatric cases of hyperfunctioning thyroid cancer causing hyperthyroidism are extremely rare (178).

Iodine-Induced Hyperthyroidism

Iodine-induced hyperthyroidism is quite rare in children because they are rarely exposed to acute, large iodine loads, except in the context of medical procedures that involve iodinated radiographic contrast administration. Occasionally, iodine-induced hyperthyroidism can develop after amiodarone administration for arrhythmia control in children. Patients treated with amiodarone may manifest altered thyroid hormone profile without thyroid dysfunction or they present with clinically significant amiodarone-induced hypothyroidism due to the blockade of thyroglobulin proteolysis or amiodarone-induced thyrotoxicosis due to iodine overload (179). Amiodarone administration to euthyroid patients results almost immediately in a decrease in serum T_3 levels and an increase in serum T_4, free T_4, rT_3, and TSH levels (176). After 3 months of therapy, a steady state is reached, with some hormonal changes persisting indefinitely. Serum levels of total and free T_4 and rT_3 remain at the upper end of normal or slightly elevated, and serum T_3 levels remain low (usually in the low normal range). In contrast, serum TSH levels return to normal after 12 weeks of therapy.

TSH-Producing Pituitary Adenoma

TSH-producing pituitary adenomas are very rare in children. These tumors induce a state of TSH-dependent hyperthyroidism in which the plasma TSH level is inappropriately normal or elevated in the context of increased thyroid hormone levels (167,180). Their diagnosis is made on the basis of biochemical tests including measurement of plasma pituitary glycoprotein hormone α-subunit level, the α-subunit/TSH ratio, and TRH dynamic testing showing the absence of TSH increase; magnetic resonance imaging of the pituitary is also performed. Given the rarity of these tumors, the diagnosis of a TSH-producing adenoma justifies prompt referral to a tertiary pituitary neurosurgery center with excellent pediatric endocrinology support.

Thyrotoxicosis Factitia

In contrast to the underlying causes of this entity in adults, hyperthyroidism due to exogenous ingestion of thyroid hormone preparations in children and adolescents is primarily the result of accidents or Münchhausen syndrome by proxy. The latter, of course, represents a potentially serious form of child abuse. Nevertheless, intentional intake of thyroid hormone does occur in pediatric patients, primarily in adolescents with either psychiatric disease or eating disorders (i.e., bulimia or anorexia nervosa). Due to its rarity, this diagnosis tends to be missed, leading to the erroneous assumption that the hyperthyroid state is due to either Graves disease or thyrotoxic thyroiditis. Excessive thyroid hormone ingestion leads to a pathognomonic constellation of biochemical findings, which, in addition to those of hyperthyroidism, include an undetectable or inappropriately low plasma thyroglobulin level and an inappropriately low T_3/T_4 ratio (because most thyroid hormone preparations contain only T_4).

Thyroid Hormone Suppression Therapy

Although thyroid hormone suppression therapy (THST) is used by some for the suppression of goiter and nodules in adults, THST has been very rarely used for the treatment of simple (usually diffuse) euthyroid goiter in children. Most children with simple euthyroid goiter have Hashimoto thyroiditis, compensated defects of thyroid hormone biosynthesis (including Pendred syndrome), or iodine deficiency. The effect of THST on goiter size in euthyroid children with Hashimoto thyroiditis is controversial (181,182). THST is typically used in the long-term management of children with thyroid carcinoma after their initial therapy. Although the aim of TSHT in these children should be to maintain TSH levels below the normal range, they do not become clinically thyrotoxic.

REFERENCES

1. Van Vliet G. Hypothyroidism in infants and children. In: Braverman LE, Utiger RD, eds. *The Thyroid: A Fundamental and Clinical Text*. 9th ed. New York: Lippincott Williams & Wilkins; 2005:1029–1047.
2. Delange F, de Benoist B, Pretell E, et al. Iodine deficiency in the world: where do we stand at the turn of the century? *Thyroid*. 2001;11(5):437–447.
3. Anselmo J, Cao D, Karrison T, et al. Fetal loss associated with excess thyroid hormone exposure. *JAMA*. 2004;292(6):691–695.
4. Kopp P, Van Sande J, Parma J, et al. Brief report: congenital hyperthyroidism caused by a mutation in the thyrotropin-receptor gene. *N Engl J Med*. 1995;332(3):150–154.
5. Polak M, Le G, I, Vuillard E, et al. Fetal and neonatal thyroid function in relation to maternal Graves' disease. *Best Pract Res Clin Endocrinol Metab*. 2004;18(2):289–302.
6. Luton D, Le GI, Vuillard E, et al. Management of Graves' disease during pregnancy: the key role of fetal thyroid gland monitoring. *J Clin Endocrinol Metab*. 2005;90(11):6093–6098.
7. Vulsma T, Gons MH, de Vijlder JJ. Maternal-fetal transfer of thyroxine in congenital hypothyroidism due to a total organification defect of thyroid agenesis. *N Engl J Med*. 1989;321:13–16.
8. Castanet M, Leenhardt L, Leger J, et al. Thyroid hemiagenesis is a rare variant of thyroid dysgenesis with a familial component but without Pax8 mutations in a cohort of 22 cases. *Pediatr Res*. 2005; 57(6):908–913.
9. Eugene D, Djemli A, Van Vliet G. Sexual dimorphism of thyroid function in newborns with congenital hypothyroidism. *J Clin Endocrinol Metab*. 2005;90(5):2696–2700.
10. Castanet M, Lyonnet S, Bonaiti-Pellie C, et al. Familial forms of thyroid dysgenesis among infants with congenital hypothyroidism. *N Engl J Med*. 2000;343(6):441–442.
11. Castanet M, Polak M, Bonaiti-Pellie C, et al. Nineteen years of national screening for congenital hypothyroidism: familial cases with thyroid dysgenesis suggest the involvement of genetic factors. *J Clin Endocrinol Metab*. 2001;86(5):2009–2014.
12. De Felice M, Di Lauro R. Thyroid development and its disorders: genetics and molecular mechanisms. *Endocr Rev*. 2004;25(5):722–746.
13. Leger J, Marinovic D, Garel C, et al. Thyroid developmental anomalies in first degree relatives of children with congenital hypothyroidism. *J Clin Endocrinol Metab*. 2002;87(2):575–580.
14. Perry R, Heinrichs C, Bourdoux P, et al. Discordance of monozygotic twins for thyroid dysgenesis: implications for screening and for molecular pathophysiology. *J Clin Endocrinol Metab*. 2002;87(9):4072–4077.
15. Devos H, Rodd C, Gagne N, et al. A search for the possible molecular mechanisms of thyroid dysgenesis: sex ratios and associated malformations. *J Clin Endocrinol Metab*. 1999;84(7):2502–2506.
16. Parlato R, Rosica A, Rodriguez-Mallon A, et al. An integrated regulatory network controlling survival and migration in thyroid organogenesis. *Dev Biol*. 2004;276(2):464–475.
17. Trueba SS, Auge J, Mattei G, et al. PAX8, TITF1, and FOXE1 gene expression patterns during human development: new insights into human thyroid development and thyroid dysgenesis-associated malformations. *J Clin Endocrinol Metab*. 2005;90(1):455–462.
18. Van Vliet G. Development of the thyroid gland: lessons from congenitally hypothyroid mice and men. *Clin Genet*. 2003;63(6):445–455.
19. Castanet M, Sura-Trueba S, Chauty A, et al. Linkage and mutational analysis of familial thyroid dysgenesis demonstrate genetic heterogeneity implicating novel genes. *Eur J Hum Genet*. 2005;13(2):232–239.
20. Fagman H, Grande M, Edsbagge J, et al. Expression of classical cadherins in thyroid development: maintenance of an epithelial phenotype throughout organogenesis. *Endocrinology*. 2003;144(8):3618–3624.
21. Legouis R, Hardelin JP, Levilliers J, et al. The candidate gene for the X-linked Kallmann syndrome encodes a protein related to adhesion molecules. *Cell*. 1991;67(2):423–435.
22. Polak M, Sura-Trueba S, Chauty A, et al. Molecular mechanisms of thyroid dysgenesis. *Horm Res*. 2004;62 Suppl 3:14–21.
23. Schoen EJ, Clapp W, To TT, et al. The key role of newborn thyroid scintigraphy with isotopic iodide (123I) in defining and managing congenital hypothyroidism. *Pediatrics*. 2004;114(6):e683–e688.
24. Rosenthal M, Addison GM, Price DA. Congenital hypothyroidism: increased incidence in Asian families. *Arch Dis Child*.1988;63(7):790–793.
25. Brown AL, Fernhoff PM, Milner J, et al. Racial differences in the incidence of congenital hypothyroidism. *J Pediatr*. 1981;99(6):934–936.
26. Toublanc JE. Comparison of epidemiological data on congenital hypothyroidism in Europe with those of other parts in the world. *Horm Res*. 1992;38(5-6):230–235.
27. Refetoff S, Dumont J, Vassart G. Thyroid disorders. In: Scriver CR, Beaudet AL, Sly WS, Valle D, eds. *The Metabolic and Molecular Basis of Inherited Disease*. 8th ed. New York: McGraw-Hill; 2001:4029–4076.

28. Szinnai G, Kosugi S, Derrien C, et al. Extending the clinical heterogeneity of iodide transport defect (ITD): a novel mutation R124H of the sodium/iodide symporter (NIS) gene and review of genotype-phenotype correlations in ITD. *J Clin Endocrinol Metab.* 2006; 91(4): 1199–1204.

29. Everett LA, Glaser B, Beck JC, et al. Pendred syndrome is caused by mutations in a putative sulphate transporter gene (PDS). *Nat Genet.*1997;17(4):411–422.

30. Gaudino R, Garel C, Czernichow P, et al. Proportion of various types of thyroid disorders among newborns with congenital hypothyroidism and normally located gland: a regional cohort study. *Clin Endocrinol* (Oxf). 2005;62(4):444–448.

31. Moreno JC, Bikker H, Kempers MJ, et al. Inactivating mutations in the gene for thyroid oxidase 2 (THOX2) and congenital hypothyroidism. *N Engl J Med.* 2002;347(2):95–102.

32. Ambrugger P, Stoeva I, Biebermann H, et al. Novel mutations of the thyroid peroxidase gene in patients with permanent congenital hypothyroidism. *Eur J Endocrinol.* 2001;145(1):19–24.

33. Kosugi S, Bhayana S, Dean HJ. A novel mutation in the sodium/iodide symporter gene in the largest family with iodide transport defect. *J Clin Endocrinol Metab.* 1999;84(9):3248–3253.

34. Sunthornthepvarakui T, Gottschalk ME, Hayashi Y, et al. Brief report: resistance to thyrotropin caused by mutations in the thyrotropin-receptor gene. *N Engl J Med.* 1995;332(3):155–160.

35. de Roux N, Misrahi M, Brauner R, et al. Four families with loss of function mutations of the thyrotropin receptor. *J Clin Endocrinol Metab.* 1996;81(12):4229–4235.

36. Abramowicz MJ, Duprez L, Parma J, et al. Familial congenital hypothyroidism due to inactivating mutation of the thyrotropin receptor causing profound hypoplasia of the thyroid gland. *J Clin Invest.* 1997;99(12):3018–3024.

37. Gagne N, Parma J, Deal C, et al. Apparent congenital athyreosis contrasting with normal plasma thyroglobulin levels and associated with inactivating mutations in the thyrotropin receptor gene: are athyreosis and ectopic thyroid distinct entities? *J Clin Endocrinol Metab.* 1998;83(5):1771–1775.

38. Alberti L, Proverbio MC, Costagliola S, et al. Germline mutations of TSH receptor gene as cause of nonautoimmune subclinical hypothyroidism. *J Clin Endocrinol Metab.* 2002;87(6):2549–2555.

39. Grasberger H, Mimouni-Bloch A, Vantyghem MC, et al. Autosomal dominant resistance to thyrotropin as a distinct entity in five multigenerational kindreds: clinical characterization and exclusion of candidate loci. *J Clin Endocrinol Metab.* 2005;90(7):4025–4034.

40. van Trotsenburg AS, Vulsma T, Van Santen HM, et al. Lower neonatal screening thyroxine concentrations in down syndrome newborns. *J Clin Endocrinol Metab.* 2003;88(4):1512–1515.

41. van Trotsenburg AS, Vulsma T, Rozenburg-Marres SL, et al. The effect of thyroxine treatment started in the neonatal period on development and growth of two-year-old Down syndrome children: a randomized clinical trial. *J Clin Endocrinol Metab.* 2005;90(6):3304–3311.

42. Hardy O, Worley G, Lee MM, et al. Hypothyroidism in Down syndrome: screening guidelines and testing methodology. *Am J Med Genet.* 2004;124A(4):436–437.

43. Brumm H, Pfeufer A, Biebermann H, et al. Congenital central hypothyroidism due to homozygous thyrotropin beta 313 Delta T mutation is caused by a Founder effect. *J Clin Endocrinol Metab.* 2002;87(10):4811–4816.

44. Deladoey J, Vuissoz JM, Domene HM, et al. Congenital secondary hypothyroidism due to a mutation C105Vfs114X thyrotropin-beta mutation: genetic study of five unrelated families from Switzerland and Argentina. *Thyroid.* 2003;13(6):553–559.

45. Collu R, Tang J, Castagne J, et al. A novel mechanism for isolated central hypothyroidism: inactivating mutations in the thyrotropin-releasing hormone receptor gene. *J Clin Endocrinol Metab.* 1997;82(5):1561–5.

46. Dumitrescu AM, Liao XH, Abdullah MS, et al. Mutations in SECISBP2 result in abnormal thyroid hormone metabolism. *Nat Genet.* 2005;37(11):1247–1252.

47. Dumitrescu AM, Liao XH, Best TB, et al. A novel syndrome combining thyroid and neurological abnormalities is associated with mutations in a monocarboxylate transporter gene. *Am J Hum Genet.* 2004;74(1):168–175.

48. Friesema EC, Grueters A, Biebermann H, et al. Association between mutations in a thyroid hormone transporter and severe X-linked psychomotor retardation. *Lancet.* 2004;364(9443):1435–1437.

49. Weiss RE, Refetoff S. Treatment of resistance to thyroid hormone—primum non nocere. *J Clin Endocrinol Metab.* 1999;84(2):401–404.

50. Chanoine JP, Pardou A, Bourdoux P, et al. Withdrawal of iodinated disinfectants at delivery decreases the recall rate at neonatal screening for congenital hypothyroidism. *Arch Dis Child.* 1988; 63(10):1297–1298.

51. Brown RS, Bellisario RL, Botero D, et al. Incidence of transient congenital hypothyroidism due to maternal thyrotropin receptor-blocking antibodies in over one million babies. *J Clin Endocrinol Metab.* 1996;81(3):1147–1151.

52. van Wassenaer AG, Kok JH, de Vijlder JJ, et al. Effects of thyroxine supplementation on neurologic development in infants born at less than 30 weeks' gestation. *N Engl J Med.* 1997;336:21–26.

53. Osborn DA. Thyroid hormones for preventing neurodevelopmental impairment in preterm infants. *Cochrane Database Syst Rev.* 2001;(4):CD001070.

54. Van Vliet G, Czernichow P. Screening for neonatal endocrinopathies: rationale, methods and results. *Semin Neonatol.* 2004;9(1):75–85.

55. Olivieri A, Stazi MA, Mastroiacovo P, et al. A population-based study on the frequency of additional congenital malformations in infants with congenital hypothyroidism: data from the Italian Registry for Congenital Hypothyroidism (1991-1998). *J Clin Endocrinol Metab.* 2002;87(2):557–562.

56. Wasniewska M, De Luca F, Cassio A, et al. In congenital hypothyroidism bone maturation at birth may be a predictive factor of psychomotor development during the first Year of life irrespective of other variables related to treatment. *Eur J Endocrinol.* 2003;149(1):1–6.

57. Djemli A, Fillion M, Belgoudi J, et al. Twenty years later: a reevaluation of the contribution of plasma thyroglobulin to the diagnosis of thyroid dysgenesis in infants with congenital hypothyroidism. *Clin Biochem.* 2004;37(9):818–822.

58. Bubuteishvili L, Garel C, Czernichow P, et al. Thyroid abnormalities by ultrasonography in neonates with congenital hypothyroidism. *J Pediatr.* 2003;143(6):759–764.

59. Ohnishi H, Sato H, Noda H, et al. Color Doppler ultrasonography: diagnosis of ectopic thyroid gland in patients with congenital hypothyroidism caused by thyroid dysgenesis. *J Clin Endocrinol Metab.* 2003;88(11):5145–5149.

60. Chanoine JP, Toppet V, Body JJ, et al. Contribution of thyroid ultrasound and serum calcitonin to the diagnosis of congenital hypothyroidism. *J Endocrinol Invest.* 1990;13(2):103–9.

61. Pohlenz J, Dumitrescu A, Zundel D, et al. Partial deficiency of thyroid transcription factor 1 produces predominantly neurological defects in humans and mice. *J Clin Invest.* 2002;109(4):469–473.

62. Krude H, Schutz B, Biebermann H, et al. Choreoathetosis, hypothyroidism, and pulmonary alterations due to human NKX2-1 haploinsufficiency. *J Clin Invest.* 2002;109(4):475–480.

63. Doyle DA, Gonzalez I, Thomas B, et al. Autosomal dominant transmission of congenital hypothyroidism, neonatal respiratory distress, and ataxia caused by a mutation of NKX2-1. *J Pediatr.* 2004;145(2):190–193.

64. Clifton-Bligh RJ, Wentworth JM, Heinz P, et al. Mutation of the gene encoding human TTF-2 associated with thyroid agenesis, cleft palate and choanal atresia. *Nat Genet.* 1998;19:399.

65. Castanet M, Park SM, Smith A, et al. A novel loss-of-function mutation in TTF-2 is associated with congenital hypothyroidism, thyroid agenesis and cleft palate. *Hum Mol Genet.* 2002;11(17):2051–2059.

66. Macchia PE, Lapi P, Krude H, et al. PAX8 mutations associated with congenital hypothyroidism caused by thyroid dysgenesis. *Nat Genet.* 1998;19(1):83–86.

67. Vilain C, Rydlewski C, Duprez L, et al. Autosomal dominant transmission of congenital thyroid hypoplasia due to loss-of-function mutation of PAX8. *J Clin Endocrinol Metab.* 2001;86(1):234–238.

68. Congdon T, Nguyen LQ, Nogueira CR, et al. A novel mutation (Q40P) in PAX8 associated with congenital hypothyroidism and thyroid hypoplasia: evidence for phenotypic variability in mother and child. *J Clin Endocrinol Metab.* 2001;86(8):3962–3967.

69. Komatsu M, Takahashi T, Takahashi I, et al. Thyroid dysgenesis caused by PAX8 mutation: the hypermutability with CpG dinucleotides at codon 31. *J Pediatr.* 2001;139(4): 597–599.

70. Fisher DA. The importance of early management in optimizing IQ in infants with congenital hypothyroidism. *J Pediatr.* 2000;136(3):273–274.

71. Touati G, Leger J, Toublanc JE, et al. A thyroxine dosage of 8 micrograms/kg per day is appropriate for the initial treatment of the majority of infants with congenital hypothyroidism. *Eur J Pediatr.* 1997;156(2):94–98.

72. Conrad SC, Chiu H, Silverman BL. Soy formula complicates management of congenital hypothyroidism. *Arch Dis Child.* 2004;89(1):37–40.

73. Germak JA, Foley TP Jr. Longitudinal assessment of L-thyroxine therapy for congenital hypothyroidism. *J Pediatr.* 1990;117 (2 Pt 1):211–219.

74. Hanukoglu A, Perlman K, Shamis I, et al. Relationship of etiology to treatment in congenital hypothyroidism. *J Clin Endocrinol Metab.* 2001;86(1):186–191.

75. Rivkees SA, Hardin DS. Cretinism after weekly dosing with levothyroxine for treatment of congenital hypothyroidism. *J Pediatr.* 1994;125(1):147–149.

76. Cassio A, Cacciari E, Cicognani A, et al. Treatment for congenital hypothyroidism: thyroxine alone or thyroxine plus triiodothyronine? *Pediatrics.* 2003;111(5 Pt 1): 1055–1060.

77. Van Vliet G, Barboni Th, Klees M, et al. Treatment strategy and long term follow up of congenital hypothyroidism. In: Delange F, Fisher DA, Glinoer D, eds. *Research in Congenital Hypothyroidism.* New York: Plenum Press; 1989:245–252.

78. Glorieux J, Dussault J, Van Vliet G. Intellectual development at age 12 years of children with congenital hypothyroidism diagnosed by neonatal screening. *J Pediatr.* 1992;121(4):581–584.

79. Derksen-Lubsen G, Verkerk PH. Neuropsychologic development in early treated congenital hypothyroidism: analysis of literature data. *Pediatr Res.* 1996;39(3):561–566.

80. Oerbeck B, Sundet K, Kase BF, et al. Congenital hypothyroidism: influence of disease severity and L-thyroxine treatment on intellectual, motor, and school-associated outcomes in young adults. *Pediatrics.* 2003; 112(4):923–930.

81. Rovet JF. Children with congenital hypothyroidism and their siblings: do they really differ? *Pediatrics.* 2005;115(1):e52–e57.

82. Fisher DA, Foley BL. Early treatment of congenital hypothyroidism. *Pediatrics.* 1989;83(5):785–789.

83. Selva KA, Mandel SH, Rien L, et al. Initial treatment dose of L-thyroxine in congenital hypothyroidism. *J Pediatr.* 2002;141(6):786–792.

84. Selva KA, Harper A, Downs A, et al. Neurodevelopmental outcomes in congenital hypothyroidism: comparison of initial T4 dose and time to reach target T4 and TSH. *J Pediatr.* 2005;147(6):775–780.

85. Dubuis JM, Glorieux J, Richer F, et al. Outcome of severe congenital hypothyroidism: closing the developmental gap with early high dose levothyroxine treatment. *J Clin Endocrinol Metab.* 1996;81(1):222–227.

86. Bongers-Schokking JJ, Koot HM, Wiersma D, et al. Influence of timing and dose of thyroid hormone replacement on development in infants with congenital hypothyroidism. *J Pediatr.* 2000;136(3):292–297.

87. Leger J, Larroque B, Norton J. Influence of severity of congenital hypothyroidism and adequacy of treatment on school achievement in young adolescents: a population-based cohort study. *Acta Paediatr.* 2001;90(11):1249–1256.

88. Zurakowski D, Di Canzio J, Majzoub JA. Pediatric reference intervals for serum thyroxine, triiodothyronine, thyrotropin, and free thyroxine. *Clin Chem.* 1999;45: 1087–1091.

89. Djemli A, Van Vliet G, Belgoudi J, et al. Reference intervals for free thyroxine, total triiodothyronine, thyrotropin and thyroglobulin for Quebec newborns, children and teenagers. *Clin Biochem.* 2004;37(4):328–330.

90. Bongers-Schokking JJ, de Muinck Keizer-Schrama SM, Docter R. Pitfalls in serum free thyroxine measurements in infants with and without congenital hypothyroidism. *Horm Res.* 1999; 51[suppl 2]:17. (Abstract)

91. Rovet JF, Ehrlich RM, Sorbara DL. Effect of thyroid hormone level on temperament in infants with congenital hypothyroidism detected by screening of neonates. *J Pediatr.* 1989;114(1):63–68.

92. Oerbeck B, Sundet K, Kase BF, et al. Congenital hypothyroidism: no adverse effects of high dose thyroxine treatment on adult memory, attention, and behaviour. *Arch Dis Child.* 2005;90(2):132–137.

93. New England Congenital Hypothyroidism Collaborative. Effects of neonatal screening for hypothyroidism: prevention of mental retardation by treatment before clinical manifestations. *Lancet.* 1981;2(8255): 1095–1098.

94. Simoneau-Roy J, Marti S, Deal C, et al. Cognition and behavior at school entry in children with congenital hypothyroidism treated early with high-dose levothyroxine. *J Pediatr.* 2004;144(6):747–752.

95. Daneman D, Howard NJ. Neonatal thyrotoxicosis: intellectual impairment and craniosynostosis in later years. *J Pediatr.* 1980;97(2):257–259.

96. Penfold JL, Simpson DA. Premature craniosynostosis-a complication of thyroid replacement therapy. *J Pediatr.* 1975;86(3): 360–363.

97. Francois M, Bonfils P, Leger J, et al. Role of congenital hypothyroidism in hearing loss in children. *J Pediatr.* 1994;124(3):444–446.

98. Rovet J, Walker W, Bliss B, et al. Long-term sequelae of hearing impairment in congenital hypothyroidism. *J Pediatr.* 1996;128(6):776–783.

99. Haddow JE, Palomaki GE, Allan WC, et al. Maternal thyroid deficiency during pregnancy and subsequent neuropsychological development of the child. *N Engl J Med.* 1999;341:549–555.

100. Lavado-Autric R, Auso E, Garcia-Velasco JV, et al. Early maternal hypothyroxinemia alters histogenesis and cerebral cortex cytoarchitecture of the progeny. *J Clin Invest.* 2003;111(7):1073–1082.

101. Alexander EK, Marqusee E, Lawrence J, et al. Timing and magnitude of increases in levothyroxine requirements during pregnancy in women with hypothyroidism. *N Engl J Med.* 2004;351(3):241–249.

102. Leger J, Czernichow P. Congenital hypothyroidism: decreased growth velocity in the first weeks of life. *Biol Neonate.* 1989;55(4-5):218–223.

103. de Zegher F, Vanderschueren-Lodeweyckx M, Heinrichs C, et al. Thyroid dyshormonogenesis: severe hypothyroidism after normal neonatal thyroid stimulating hormone screening. *Acta Paediatr.* 1992;81(3):274–276.

104. Vincent MA, Rodd C, Dussault JH, et al. Very low birth weight newborns do not need repeat screening for congenital hypothyroidism. *J Pediatr.* 2002;140(3):311–314.

105. Rochiccioli P, Dutau G, Augier D. [Thyroid ectopia, a cause of error in neonatal screening for hypothyroidism]. *Arch Fr Pediatr.* 1983;40(5):405–406.

106. Hunter I, Greene SA, MacDonald TM, et al. Prevalence and aetiology of hypothyroidism in the young. *Arch Dis Child.* 2000;83(3):207–210.

107. Pearce EN, Farwell AP, Braverman LE. Thyroiditis. *N Engl J Med.* 2003;348(26):2646–2655.

108. Ward L, Huot C, Lambert R, et al. Outcome of pediatric Graves' disease after treatment with antithyroid medication and radioiodine. *Clin Invest Med.* 1999;22(4):132–139.

109. Huang SA, Tu HM, Harney JW, et al. Severe hypothyroidism caused by type 3 iodothyronine deiodinase in infantile hemangiomas. *N Engl J Med.* 2000;343(3):185–189.

110. Ayling RM, Davenport M, Hadzic N, et al. Hepatic hemangioendothelioma associated with production of humoral thyrotropin-like factor. *J Pediatr.* 2001;138(6):932–935.

111. Konrad D, Ellis G, Perlman K. Spontaneous regression of severe acquired infantile hypothyroidism associated with multiple liver hemangiomas. *Pediatrics.* 2003;112(6):1424–1426.

112. Pacaud D, Van Vliet G, Delvin E, et al. A Third World endocrine disease in a 6-year-old North American boy. *J Clin Endocrinol Metab.* 1995;80(9):2574–2576.

113. Donadieu J, Rolon MA, Thomas C, et al. Endocrine involvement in pediatric-onset Langerhans' cell histiocytosis: a population-based study. *J Pediatr.* 2004;144(3):344–350.

114. Jorgensen JO, Pedersen SA, Laurberg P, et al. Effects of growth hormone therapy on thyroid function of growth hormone-deficient adults with and without concomitant thyroxine-substituted central hypothyroidism. *J Clin Endocrinol Metab.* 1989;69(6):1127–1132.

115. Grunfeld C, Sherman BM, Cavalieri RR. The acute effects of human growth hormone administration on thyroid function in normal men. *J Clin Endocrinol Metab.* 1988;67(5):1111–1114.

116. Lippe BM, Van Herle AJ, Lafranchi SH, et al. Reversible hypothyroidism in growth

hormone-deficient children treated with human growth hormone. *J Clin Endocrinol Metab.* 1975;40(4):612–618.

117. Giavoli G, Porretti S, Ferrante E, et al. Recombinant hGH replacement therapy and the hypothalamus-pituitary-thyroid axis in children with GH deficiency: when should we be concerned about the occurrence of central hypothroidism? *Clin Endocrinol* (Oxf). 2003;59:806–810.

118. Van den Brande JL, Van Wyk JJ, French FS, et al. Advancement of skeletal age of hypopituitary children treated with thyroid hormone plus cortisone. *J Pediatr.* 1973;82(1):22–27.

119. Burrow SR, Alman B, Wright JG. Short stature as a screening test for endocrinopathy in slipped capital femoral epiphysis. *J Bone Joint Surg (Br).* 2001;83(2):263–268.

120. Van Wyk JJ, Grumbach MM. Syndrome of precocious mentruation and galactorrhea in juvenile hypothyroidism: an example of hormonal overlap in pituitary feedback. *J Pediatr.* 1960;57:416–435.

121. Gordon CM, Austin DJ, Radovick S, et al. Primary hypothyroidism presenting as severe vaginal bleeding in a prepubertal girl. *J Pediatr Adolesc Gynecol.* 1997;10(1):35–38.

122. Bruder JM, Samuels MH, Bremner WJ, et al. Hypothyroidism-induced macroorchidism: use of a gonadotropin-releasing hormone agonist to understand its mechanism and augment adult stature. *J Clin Endocrinol Metab.* 1995;80(1):11–16.

123. Lavin A, Nauss AH. Hypothyroidism in otherwise healthy hypercholesterolemic children. *Pediatrics.* 1991;88(2):332–334.

124. Van Vliet G, Delange F. Goiter and thyroiditis. In: Bertrand J, Rappaport R, Sizonenko PC, eds. *Pediatric Endocrinology: Physiology, Pathophysiology, and Clinical Aspects.* 2nd ed. Baltimore: Williams & Wilkins; 1993:270–276.

125. Alos N, Huot C, Lambert R, et al. Thyroid scintigraphy in children and adolescents with Hashimoto disease. *J Pediatr.* 1995;127(6):951–953.

126. Foley TP, Jr., Abbassi V, et al. Brief report: hypothyroidism caused by chronic autoimmune thyroiditis in very young infants. *N Engl J Med.* 1994;330(7):466–468.

127. Papakonstantinou O, Bitsori M, Mamoulakis D, et al. MR imaging of pituitary hyperplasia in a child with growth arrest and primary hypothyroidism. *Eur Radiol.* 2000;10(3):516–518.

128. Dahlem ST, Furlanetto RW, Moshang T, et al. Transient growth hormone deficiency after treatment of primary hypothyroidism. *J Pediatr.* 1987;111(2):256–258.

129. Set PA, Oleszczuk-Raschke K, von Lengerke JH, et al. Sonographic features of Hashimoto thyroiditis in childhood. *Clin Radiol.* 1996;51(3):167–169.

130. Noble SE, Leyland K, Findlay CA, et al. School based screening for hypothyroidism in Down's syndrome by dried blood spot TSH measurement. *Arch Dis Child.* 2000;82(1):27–31.

131. Radetti G, Mazzanti L, Paganini C, et al. Frequency, clinical and laboratory features of thyroiditis in girls with Turner's syndrome. The Italian Study Group for Turner's Syndrome. *Acta Paediatr.* 1995;84(8):909–912.

132. Kondo T. Klinefelter syndrome associated with juvenile hypothyroidism due to chronic thyroiditis. *Eur J Pediatr.* 1993;152(6):540.

133. Mehta A, Hindmarsh PC, Stanhope RG, et al. Is the thyrotropin-releasing hormone test necessary in the diagnosis of central hypothyroidism in children. *J Clin Endocrinol Metab.* 2003;88(12):5696–5703.

134. Suter SN, Kaplan SL, Aubert ML, et al. Plasma prolactin and thyrotropin and the response to thyrotropin-releasing factor in children with primary and hypothalamic hypothyroidism. *J Clin Endocrinol Metab.* 1978;47(5):1015–1020.

135. Beck-Peccoz P, Amr S, Menezes-Ferreira MM, et al. Decreased receptor binding of biologically inactive thyrotropin in central hypothyroidism. Effect of treatment with thyrotropin-releasing hormone. *N Engl J Med.* 1985;312(17):1085–1090.

136. Hamilton J, Blaser S, Daneman D. MR imaging in idiopathic growth hormone deficiency. *AJNR Am J Neuroradiol.* 1998;19:1609–1615.

137. Ward L, Chavez M, Huot C, et al. Severe congenital hypopituitarism with low prolactin levels and age-dependent anterior pituitary hypoplasia: a clue to a PIT-1 mutation. *J Pediatr.* 1998;132:1036–1038.

138. Guyda HJ. Treatment of congenital hypothyroidism. In: Dussault JH, Walker P, eds. *Congenital Hypothyroidism.* New York: Marcel Dekker; 1983:385–396.

139. Sherman SI, Malecha SE. Absorption and malabsorption of levothyroxine sodium. *Am J Ther.* 1995 Oct;2(10):814–8.

140. Schneyer CR. Calcium carbonate and reduction of levothyroxine efficacy. *JAMA* 1998;279(10):750.

141. Rovet JF, Daneman D, Bailey JD. Psychologic and psychoeducational consequences of thyroxine therapy for juvenile acquired hypothyroidism. *J Pediatr.* 1993;122(4):543–549.

142. Van Dop C, Conte FA, Koch TK, et al. Pseudotumor cerebri associated with initiation of levothyroxine therapy for juvenile hypothyroidism. *N Engl J Med.* 1983;308(18):1076–1080.

143. Teng L, Bui H, Bachrach L, et al. Catch-up growth in severe juvenile hypothyroidism: treatment with a GnRH analog. *J Pediatr Endocrinol Metab.* 2004;17(3):345–354.

144. Maenpaa J, Raatikka M, Rasanen J, et al. Natural course of juvenile autoimmune thyroiditis. *J Pediatr.* 1985;107(6):898–904.

145. Alexopoulou O, Beguin C, De Nayer P, et al. Clinical and hormonal characteristics of central hypothyroidism at diagnosis and during follow-up in adult patients. *Eur J Endocrinol.* 2004;150(1):1–8.

146. Wiegratz I, Kutschera E, Lee JH, et al. Effect of four oral contraceptives on thyroid hormones, adrenal and blood pressure parameters. *Contraception.* 2003;67(5):361–366.

147. Zakarija M, McKenzie JM. Pregnancy-associated changes in the thyroid-stimulating antibody of Graves' disease and the relationship to neonatal hyperthyroidism. *J Clin Endocrinol Metab.* 1983;57(5):1036–1040.

148. Hollingsworth DR, Mabry CC, Eckerd JM. Hereditary aspects of Graves' disease in infancy and childhood. *J Pediatr.* 1972;81(3):446–459.

149. Thomas JS, Leclere J, Hartemann P, et al. Familial hyperthyroidism without evidence of autoimmunity. *Acta Endocrinol.* (Copenh) 1982;100(4):512–518.

150. Duprez L, Parma J, Van Sande J, et al. Germline mutations in the thyrotropin receptor gene cause non-autoimmune autosomal dominant hyperthyroidism. *Nat Genet.* 1994;7(3):396–401.

151. de Roux N, Polak M, Couet J, et al. A neomutation of the thyroid-stimulating hormone receptor in a severe neonatal hyperthyroidism. *J Clin Endocrinol Metab.* 1996;81(6):2023–2026.

152. Yoshimoto M, Nakayama M, Baba T, et al. A case of neonatal McCune-Albright syndrome with Cushing syndrome and hyperthyroidism. *Acta Paediatr Scand.* 1991;80(10):984–987.

153. Shenker A, Weinstein LS, Moran A, et al. Severe endocrine and nonendocrine manifestations of the McCune-Albright syndrome associated with activating mutations of stimulatory G protein GS. *J Pediatr.* 1993;123(4):509–518.

154. Leclere J, Bene MC, Aubert V, et al. Clinical consequences of activating germline mutations of TSH receptor, the concept of toxic hyperplasia. *Horm Res.* 1997;47(4-6):158–162.

155. Duprez L, Parma J, Van Sande J, et al. Pathology of the TSH receptor. *J Pediatr Endocrinol Metab.* 1999,12 Suppl 1.295–302.

156. Kopp P, Muirhead S, Jourdain N, et al. Congenital hyperthyroidism caused by a solitary toxic adenoma harboring a novel somatic mutation (serine281—>isoleucine) in the extracellular domain of the thyrotropin receptor. *J Clin Invest.* 1997;100(6):1634–1639.

157. Polak M. Hyperthyroidism in early infancy: pathogenesis, clinical features and diagnosis with a focus on neonatal hyperthyroidism. *Thyroid.* 1998 Dec;8(12):1171–1177.

158. Skuza KA, Sills IN, Stene M, et al. Prediction of neonatal hyperthyroidism in infants born to mothers with Graves disease. *J Pediatr.* 1996;128(2):264–268.

159. Transue D, Chan J, Kaplan M. Management of neonatal Graves disease with iopanoic acid. *J Pediatr.* 1992;121(3):472–474.

160. Ranzini AC, Ananth CV, Smulian JC, et al. Ultrasonography of the fetal thyroid: nomograms based on biparietal diameter and gestational age. *J Ultrasound Med.* 2001;20(6):613–617.

161. Foulds N, Walpole I, Elmslie F, et al. Carbimazole embryopathy: An emerging phenotype. *Am J Med Genet.* 2004 Dec 2.

162. Messer PM, Hauffa BP, Olbricht T, et al. Antithyroid drug treatment of Graves' disease in pregnancy: long-term effects on somatic growth, intellectual development and thyroid function of the offspring. *Acta Endocrinol.* (Copenh) 1990; 123(3):311–316.

163. Smith C, Thomsett M, Choong C, et al. Congenital thyrotoxicosis in premature

infants. *Clin Endocrinol.* (Oxf) 2001;54(3):371–376.

164. Weetman AP. Graves' disease. *N Engl J Med.* 2000;343(17):1236–1248.

165. Cooper DS. Hyperthyroidism. *Lancet.* 2003;362(9382):459–468.

166. Kadmon PM, Noto RB, Boney CM, et al. Thyroid storm in a child following radioactive iodine (RAI) therapy: a consequence of RAI versus withdrawal of antithyroid medication. *J Clin Endocrinol Metab.* 2001;86(5):1865–1867.

167. Polak M, Bertherat J, Li JY, et al. A human TSH-secreting adenoma: endocrine, biochemical and morphological studies. Evidence of somatostatin receptors by using quantitative autoradiography. Clinical and biological improvement by SMS 201-995 treatment. *Acta Endocrinol.* (Copenh) 1991;124(4):479–486.

168. Lazar L, Kalter-Leibovici O, Pertzelan A, et al. Thyrotoxicosis in prepubertal children compared with pubertal and postpubertal patients. *J Clin Endocrinol Metab.* 2000;85(10):3678–3682.

169. Guitteny MA, Castanet M, Alberti C, et al. Graves' disease in children: ethnic difference of the age at presentation in France. *Horm Res.* 2003;60 [Suppl 2]:102. (Abstract)

170. Glaser NS, Styne DM. Predictors of early remission of hyperthyroidism in children. *J Clin Endocrinol Metab.* 1997;82(6):1719–1726.

171. Shulman DI, Muhar I, Jorgensen EV, et al. Autoimmune hyperthyroidism in prepubertal children and adolescents: comparison of clinical and biochemical features at diagnosis and responses to medical therapy. *Thyroid.* 1997;7(5):755–760.

172. Rivkees SA, Cornelius EA. Influence of iodine-131 dose on the outcome of hyperthyroidism in children. *Pediatrics.* 2003;111(4 Pt 1):745–749.

173. Rahman MA, Birrell G, Stewart H, et al. Successful radioiodine treatment in a 3 year old child with Graves' disease following antithyroid medication induced neutropenia. *Arch Dis Child.* 2003;88(2):158–159.

174. Safa AM, Schumacher OP, Rodriguez-Antunez A. Long-term follow-up results in children and adolescents treated with radioactive iodine (131I) for hyperthyroidism. *N Engl J Med.* 1975;292(4):167–171.

175. Read CH, Jr., Tansey MJ, et al. A 36-year retrospective analysis of the efficacy and safety of radioactive iodine in treating young Graves' patients. *J Clin Endocrinol Metab.* 2004;89(9):4229–4233.

176. Ron E, Doody MM, Becker DV, et al. Cancer mortality following treatment for adult hyperthyroidism. Cooperative Thyrotoxicosis Therapy Follow-up Study Group. *JAMA.* 1998;280(4):347–355.

177. Nabhan ZM, Kreher NC, Eugster EA. Hashitoxicosis in children: clinical features and natural history. *J Pediatr.* 2005;146(4):533–536.

178. Mircescu H, Parma J, Huot C, et al. Hyperfunctioning malignant thyroid nodule in an 11-year-old girl: pathologic and molecular studies. *J Pediatr.* 2000;137(4):585–587.

179. Loh KC. Amiodarone-induced thyroid disorders: a clinical review. *Postgrad Med J.* 2000;76(893):133–140.

180. Brucker-Davis F, Oldfield EH, Skarulis MC, et al. Thyrotropin-secreting pituitary tumors: diagnostic criteria, thyroid hormone sensitivity, and treatment outcome in 25 patients followed at the National Institutes of Health. *J Clin Endocrinol Metab.* 1999;84(2):476–486.

181. Rother KI, Zimmerman D, Schwenk WF. Effect of thyroid hormone treatment on thyromegaly in children and adolescents with Hashimoto disease. *J Pediatr.* 1994;124(4):599–601.

182. Svensson J, Ericsson UB, Nilsson P, et al. Levothyroxine treatment reduces thyroid size in children and adolescents with chronic autoimmune thyroiditis. *J Clin Endocrinol Metab.* 2006;91(5):1729–1734.

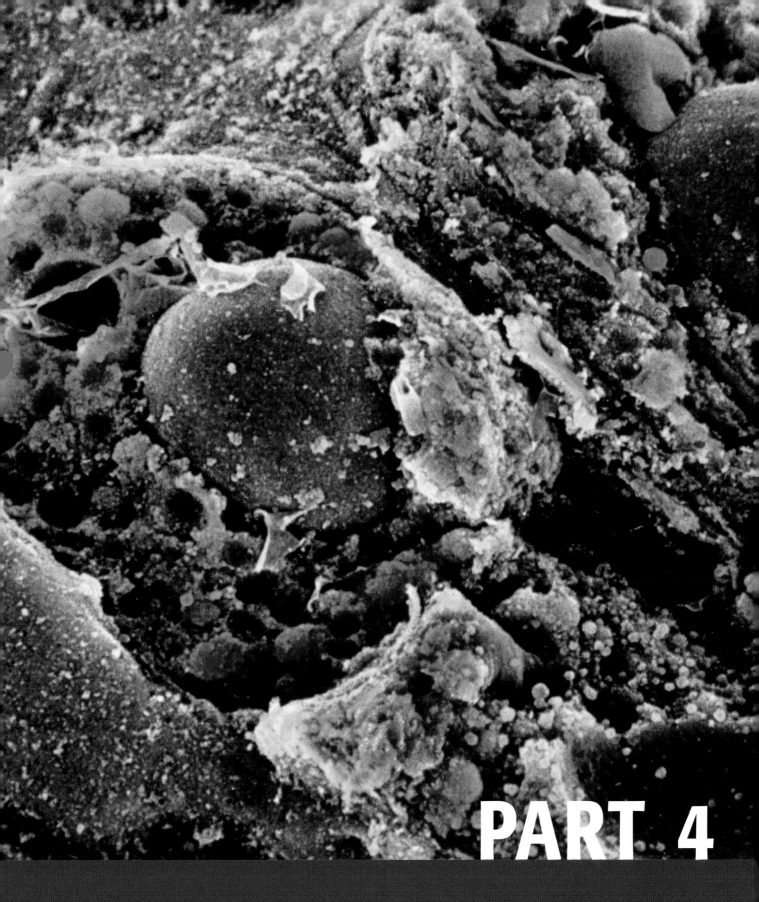

PART 4

Disorders of the Adrenals

IN THIS PART

Previous page: Colored Scanning Electron Micrograph (SEM) of secretory cells of the zona fasciculata region of the adrenal gland. Three cells are seen, sectioned by cell fracture to show internal anatomy. There is a large rounded nucleus (brown) in two of the cells. The cell cytoplasm is filled with lipid droplets (pink); larger mitochondria (pink) are seen at upper right; the cell membrane is colored blue.

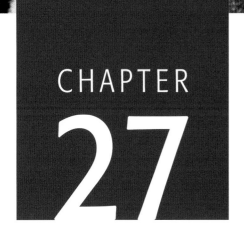

CHAPTER 27

Congenital Adrenal Hyperplasia

Kyriakie Sarafoglou, MD
Kathryn D. Harrington, MD
Walter O. Bockting, PhD

ADRENALS

Anatomy

Each adrenal gland (weighing approximately 4 g) is located above the upper pole of each kidney and consists of the adrenal cortex and adrenal medulla. The adrenal cortex (which forms about 90% of the adrenal gland's total mass) consists of three anatomical zones: the outer zona glomerulosa (approximately 15% of the cortex), the intermediate zona fasciculata (75%), and the inner zona reticularis (10%). These zones are where the three main types of hormones are produced, respectively: glucocorticoids (e.g., cortisol and corticosterone), mineralocorticoids (e.g., aldosterone and 11-deoxycorticosterone), and sex steroids (mainly androgen precursors dehydroepiandrosterone and androstenedione). Lying next to the zona reticularis is the adrenal medulla, which comprises approximately 10% of the adrenal gland's mass and secretes catecholamines.

Embryology

The adrenal cortex and medulla develop independently, with the cortex deriving from mesodermal cells and the medulla from neuroectoderm. Mesodermal cells also play a role in the developing gonad; both the adrenals and gonads have common enzymes involved in steroidogenesis. At approximately 5–6 weeks of gestation, the gonadal ridge develops into separate steroidogenic cells of the gonads and adrenal cortex; specifically, mesothelial cells migrate into the underlying mesenchyme (close to the developing gonad) and become the fetal zone of the adrenal cortex. A second migration of mesothelial cells forms the adult (definitive) zone. Neural crest cells migrate toward the coelomic cavity wall and form the adrenal medulla. In later stages of embryonic development, the cortex engulfs and ultimately encapsulates the entire medulla. By 9–12 weeks of gestation, the fetal zone is capable of steroidogenesis.

The fetal adrenals consists histologically of the following zones: 1) the large fetal zone, which is functionally similar to the adult zona reticularis, 2) the transitional zone, which is thought to give rise to zona fasciculata because this zone expresses both 17α-hydroxylase and 3β-hydroxysteroid dehydrogenase II (3β-HSD-II), allowing production of cortisol, and 3) the outer zone, or definite zone, which is later considered to evolve to the adult zona glomerulosa because it expresses only enzymes needed for the production of aldosterone.

STEROIDOGENESIS

Cholesterol

Cholesterol is an essential component of many cellular and developmental processes and is the precursor for all adrenal and gonadal steroid hormones, bile acids, and neurosteroids. The cholesterol molecule (27 carbons) is synthesized from lanosterol through a series of approximately 30 enzymatic reactions. (For a discussion of cholesterol biosynthesis and associated disorders, see Chapter 23).

Adrenals can synthesize cholesterol *de novo* from acetate and coenzyme A, but most cholesterol is of dietary origin, provided by plasma low-density lipoproteins (LDLs). Two families of enzymes play a leading role in the conversion of cholesterol to adrenal steroid hormones: cytochrome P450s and hydroxysteroid dehydrogenases.

Steroidogenic Enzymes

Cytochrome P450s and Hydroxysteroid Dehydrogenases Most of the enzymes involved in the synthesis of adrenal steroids belong to the cytochrome P450 enzyme family, which are membrane-bound proteins associated with either mitochondria or the endoplasmic reticulum (microsomal). P450 enzymes function as monooxygenases using reduced nicotinamide adenine dinucleotide phosphate (NADPH) as the electron donor for the reduction of the molecular oxygen (1).

The mitochondrial P450scc enzyme and P450c11 isozymes, P450c11β and P450c11AS, respectively, receive electrons from the NADPH through a sequential electron shuttle transfer involving two proteins, adrenodoxin reductase (a flavoprotein) (2) and adrenodoxin (a nonheme iron–sulfur protein) (3). The microsomal P450c17, P450c21, P450arom enzymes, receive electrons from the reduced form of NADPH using only one membrane-bound flavoprotein, P450 oxidoreductase (POR), to transfer the electrons from NADPH to POR to P450 enzymes.

The hydroxysteroid dehydrogenases, which include 3β-HSD and 17β-HSD isozymes, are involved in the reduction and oxidation of adrenal and gonadal steroids in the presence of $NAD^+/NADP^+$ or their reducing equivalents as cofactors (Table 27-1).

Conversion of Cholesterol into Adrenal Steroids (Figure 27-1)

CYP11A (P450scc) After uptake of cholesterol by the mitochondrion, the first and rate-limiting step in adrenal steroidogenesis is conversion of cholesterol to pregnenolone by the P450scc (cholesterol side-chain cleavage) enzyme, which is encoded by the CYP11A. P450scc is a single enzyme that catalyzes three chemical reactions (20α-hydroxylation, 22-hydroxylation, and cleavage of the cholesterol side-chain bond at position 20–22).

HSD3B1 (3β-HSD-I) and HSD3B2 (3β-HSD-II) There are two 3β-hydroxysteroid dehydrogenase isozymes (3β-HSD-I and 3β-HSD-II) encoded by two different genes, HSD3B1 and HSD3B2, respectively, and expressed in different tissues; 3β-HSD-II enzyme is expressed exclusively in the adrenals and the gonads, and 3β-HSD-I enzyme is expressed in placenta, breast, and skin.

Both 3β-HSD-I and 3β-HSD-II isozymes, through two sequential enzymatic steps, convert Δ^5-3β-hydroxysteroids, pregnenolone, 17α-hydroxypregnenolone, and dehydroepiandrosterone (DHEA) to Δ^4-3β-hydroxysteroids,

Congenital Adrenal Hyperplasia

AT-A-GLANCE

Congenital adrenal hyperplasia (CAH) refers to histological alterations of adrenal cortical tissue secondary to chronic overstimulation by elevated ACTH levels due to impaired cortisol synthesis. CAH is the most common monogenic endocrinopathy and the leading cause of ambiguous genitalia in the newborn. Replacing deficient cortisol in order to suppress ACTH and the subsequent elevation of adrenal steroid precursors is the goal of treatment. Mineralocorticoid, glucocorticoid, and/or sex steroid replacement may be necessary depending on the enzymatic defect.

TYPES OF CAH	OCCURRENCE	GENE	LOCUS	OMIM
21α-Hydroxylase deficiency	90%	CYP21A2	6p21.3	201910
11β-Hydroxylase deficiency	5%	CYP11B1	8q21	202010
3β-Hydroxysteroid dehydrogenase II deficiency	Rare	HSD3B2	1p13.1	201810
17α-Hydroxylase/17,20-lyase deficiency	Rare	CYP17	10q24.3	202110, 609300
Congenital lipoid adrenal hyperplasia	Very rare	StAR, CYP11A	8p11.2	201710, 60617, 118485
P450 oxidoreductase deficiency	Very rare	POR	7q11.2	201750

FORM	FINDINGS		CLINICAL PRESENTATION BIRTH	CHILDHOOD & ADOLESCENCE
21-OHD (classical) Salt wasting	↑ K ↓ Na ↑ PRA ↓ Aldo	↑ 17-OHP ↑ Androgens ↓ F	Females: Always present at birth with ambiguous genitalia; virilization of external genitalia from clitoromegaly to phallic urethra	Males with salt-wasting CAH present at 2–3 weeks of life in salt-wasting crisis
Simple virilizing	=↑ PRA = Lytes = Aldo	↑ 17-OHP ↑ Androgens ↓ F	Males: Normal external genitalia with hyperpigmentation of scrotum and postnatal virilization	Males with simple virilizing typically present in infancy or early childhood with growth acceleration and virilization
21-OHD (nonclassical)	= PRA = Lytes = Aldo	↑ 17-OHP ↑ Androgens = F	Normal genitalia in both sexes	May present with premature adrenarche, growth acceleration, bone advancement, PCO, irregular menses, acne, hirsutism, infertility
11β-OHlase deficiency	↓ K ↑ Na ↓ PRA ↓ Aldo	↑ DOC ↑ S ↑ 17-OHP ↑ Androgens ↓ F	Females: Virilization of external genitalia ranging from clitoromegaly to phallic urethra Males: Normal external genitalia with hyperpigmentation of scrotum and postnatal virilization; hypertension may be present	Milder defects (nonclassical) may manifest later as premature adrenarche, growth acceleration, bone advancement, PCO, irregular menses, acne, hirsutism, and infertility
3β-HSD-II deficiency	↑ K ↓ Na ↑ PRA ↓ Aldo	↑ 17-OH Preg ↑ DHEA ↓ Δ4A ↓ T, ↓ F ↑ LH, ↑ FSH	Females: Near normal to clitoromegaly Males: Micropenis and severe hypospadias to near-normal female genitalia	Milder defects (nonclassical) manifest as premature adrenarche, growth acceleration, bone advancement, PCO, irregular menses, acne, hirsutism; Δ5:Δ4 ratio mildly elevated after ACTH stimulation
17α-OHlase/17, 20 lyase deficiency	↓ K ↑ Na ↓ PRA ↓ Aldo	↑ Preg, ↑ Prog ↑ DOC, ↑ B ↓ F ↓ Sex steroids ↑ LH, ↑ FSH	Females: Normal external genitalia Males: Ambiguous genitalia with most presenting as phenotypic females Hypertension present in 85–90% of patients	Primary amenorrhea and lack of secondary sex characteristics 46,XY males may present as phenotypic females with hernia or inguinal mass
Lipoid CAH (StAR, P450scc)	↓ K, ↑ Na ↑ PRA ↓ Aldo	Steroids absent ↓ F ↑ LH, ↑ FSH	Females: Normal genitalia Males: Phenotypic female external genitalia	High mortality in infancy
POR deficiency	=↓ K =↑ Na =↓ PRA =↓ Aldo	↑ 17-OHP ↑ 17-OHPreg =↑ DOC =↓ Androgens =↓ F	Females have ambiguous genitalia, and males are undervirilized; no progression of virilization in females after birth; mothers may experience virilization during pregnancy, which resolves after birh	Skeletal malformations similar to Antley–Bixler (midface hypoplasia, choanal stenosis craniosynostosis, clinodactyly, radiohumeral or radiulnar synostosis, and arachnodactyly)

K = potassium; Na = sodium; aldo = aldosterone; PRA = renin; Prog = progesterone; 17-OHP = 17α-hydroxyprogesterone; Preg = pregnenolone; 17-OHpreg = 17α-pregnenolone; B = corticosterone; F = cortisol; DOC = 11-deoxycorticosterone; S = 11-deoxycortisol; T = testosterone; DHEA = dihydroepiandrosterone; Δ4A = androstenedione; PCO = polycystic ovarian disease.

TABLE 27-1 Steroidogenic Enzymes

Cytochrome P450

Enzyme	Gene	Locus	Cellular Site	Electron Transfer/ Target Tissue	Coenzymes	Enzymatic Activity
P450scc	CYP11A1	15q23-q24	Mitochondrial	Adrenal cortex, placenta, testes, ovaries	Adrenodoxin/adrenodoxin reductase/NADPH/O_2	Converts cholesterol to pregnenolone via 20α-hydroxylation, 22-hydroxylation, and cleavage of the cholesterol chain bond at position 20–22.
P450c11β	CYP11B1	8q21	Mitochondrial	Zona fasciculata and reticularis	Adrenodoxin/adrenodoxin reductase/NADPH/O_2	Converts 11-deoxycortisol (S) to cortisol in the zona fasciculata and 11-deoxycorticosterone (DOC) to corticosterone (B) in the zona glomerulosa via 11β-hydroxylase activity
P450c11AS	CYP11B2	8q21-q22	Mitochondrial	Zona glomerulosa	Adrenodoxin/adrenodoxin reductase/NADPH/O_2	Through three sequential enzymatic steps converts DOC to B via 11β-hydroxylase activity, B to 18-OHB through 18-hydroxylase or corticosterone methyl oxidase I (CMOI) activity, and 18-OHDOC to aldosterone through 18-oxidase (CMOII) activity.
P450c17	CYP17	10q24.3	Microsomal	Leydig and theca cells, zonae fasciculata and reticularis	P450 oxidoreductase/b_5 cytochrome/NADPH/O_2	Through two subsequent enzymatic steps converts pregnenolone to 17α-hydroxypregnenolone and progesterone to 17α-hydroxyprogesterone (17-OHP) through 17α-hydroxylase activity; 17-hydroxyperegnenolone, and, to a lesser degree, 17-(OHP) are converted to DHEA and Δ_4A, respectively, through 17,20-lyase activity.
P450arom	CYP19	15q21.1	Microsomal	Leydig and granulosa cells, placenta, bone, fat	P450 oxidoreductase/NADPH/O_2	Converts testosterone to estradiol (E_2) and Δ_4A to estrone (E_1)
P450c21	CYP21B	6p21.3	Microsomal	Adrenal cortex	P450 oxidoreductase/NADPH/O_2	Converts progesterone to DOC in zona glomerulosa and 17-OHP to 11-deoxycortisol (S) in zona fasciculata

3β-Hydroxysteroid dehydrogenase

Enzyme	Gene	Locus	Cellular Site	Target Tissue	Coenzymes	Enzymatic Activity
3β-HSD-I	HSD3B1	1p13.1	Mitochondrial and microsomal	Placenta, skin, breast	NAD^+/NADH	Both convert Δ_5-3β-hydroxysteroids (pregnenolone, 17α-pregnenolone, and DHEA) to Δ_4-3β-hydroxysteroids (progesterone, 17α-OHP, and Δ_4A), respectively.
3β-HSD-II	HSD3B2	1p13.1	Mitochondrial and microsomal	Leyding, theca, and granulosa cells, adrenal cortex		

17β-Hydroxysteroid dehydrogenase

Enzyme	Gene	Locus	Cellular Site	Target Tissue	Coenzymes	Enzymatic Activity
17β-HSD-1	HSD17B1	17q11-q21	Cytoplasm	Granulosa cells, placenta	NADPH	Converts E_1 to E_2
17β-HSD-3	HSD17B3	9q22	Microsomal	Testes	NADPH	Converts Δ_4A to testosterone
17β-HSD-7	HSD17B7	1q23	Microsomal	Corpus luteum	NADPH	Converts E_1 to E_2

progesterone, 17α-hydroxyprogesterone (17-OHP), and androstenedione (Δ_4A). The first enzymatic step requires NAD^+ coenzyme and through dehydrogenation converts the Δ^5-3β-hydroxysteroids into Δ^5-3β-ketosteroids and NAD^+ to NADH. The second enzymatic step is activated by NADH and through isomerization converts the Δ^5-3β-ketosteroids to Δ^4-3β-ketosteroids.

CYP17 (P450c17) The P450c17 enzyme is encoded by CYP17 gene and has both 17α-hydroxylase and 17,20-lyase activities; the first reaction involves 17α-hydroxylation of pregnenolone and progesterone to 17α-hydroxypregnenolone and 17-OHP; subsequently, 17,20-lyase activity of the P450c17 enzyme cleaves the C17,20 bond of these two 17α-hydroxylated steroids, converting mostly 17α-hydroxypregnenolone to DHEA and, at a smaller rate, 17-OHP to Δ_4A. The P450c17 enzyme has a key role in regulation of the three classes of adrenal steroids. For example, in the zona glomerulosa, where there is no expression of the P450c17 enzyme, pregnenolone is converted to mineralocorticoids, whereas in the zona fasciculata, where 17α-hydroxylation predominates, pregnenolone is converted to cortisol. In the zona reticularis, where both activities of the enzyme are present, precursors of sex steroids are produced (DHEA and Δ_4A).

Mechanisms that favor 17,20-lyase activity of the P450c17 enzyme include a high molar ratio of POR to P450c17 or factors that facilitate the transfer of electrons to P450c17, such

Normal Adrenal Steroidogenesis

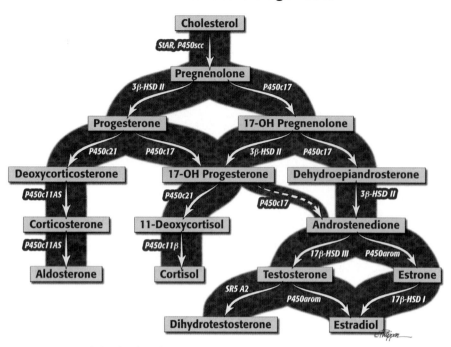

FIGURE 27-1. Normal adrenal and gonadal steroidogenesis showing the conversion of cholesterol into steroid hormones.

as cytochrome β_5 (4) and serine phosphorylation of P450c17 (5,6).

CYP21B (P450c21) The P450c21 enzyme, through 21α-hydroxylation, converts progesterone to 11-deoxycorticosterone (DOC) in the zona glomerulosa and 17-OHP to 11-deoxycortisol in the zona fasciculata. The P450c21 enzyme, encoded by the CYP21B gene, is expressed exclusively in the adrenal cortex and is essential for the synthesis of glucocorticoids such as cortisol and corticosterone and mineralocorticoids such as DOC and aldosterone.

CYP11B1 (P450c11β) and CYP11B2 (P450c-11AS) The two P450c11 isozymes, P450c-11β and P450c11AS, catalyze the final steps in the synthesis of cortisol and aldosterone and are encoded by the CYP11B1 and CYP11B2 genes, respectively. The P450c11β isozyme (11β-hydroxylase) is highly expressed in the zona fasciculata and converts 11-deoxycortisol (S) to cortisol and DOC to corticosterone (B). The P450c11AS isozyme is expressed only in the zona glomerulosa and catalyzes three sequential reactions: 11β-hydroxylase, 18-hydroxylase or corticosterone methyl oxidase I (CMO-I), and 18-oxidase or CMO-II activity. The synthesis of cortisol and production of of P450c11β isozyme are regulated by adrenocorticotropic hormone (ACTH), whereas the synthesis of aldosterone and P450c11AS isozyme is regulated primarily by angiotensin II and potassium.

Peripheral Conversion and Metabolism of Adrenal Steroids

The synthesis of active androgens and estrogens from the adrenal inactive androgen precursors DHEA and Δ_4A involves several enzymes, including the 17β-HSD superfamily and P450 aromatase enzyme.

17β-Hydroxysteroid Dehydrogenases The enzymes of the 17β-HSD gene family are responsible for the interconversion of DHEA and androstenediol, Δ_4A and testosterone, and estrone (E_1) and estradiol (E_2) in the gonads and several peripheral target tissues. The 17β-HSD enzymes are required for the synthesis of all active androgen and estrogen, as well as for their inactivation. Other names for 17β-HSDs are 17-oxoreductases or 17-ketosteroid reductases when they are used to reflect the direction of the reaction being studied (7). Overall, the enzymatic activity catalyzed by each type of 17β-HSD enzyme is almost exclusively unidirectional. Three 17β-HSD isoforms, types 1, 3, and 7, are involved in the synthesis of sex steroids in the gonads and are described briefly below.

HSD17B1 (17β-HSD-1), HSD17B3 (17β-HSD-3), HSD17B7 (17βHSD-7) 17β-HSD-1 enzyme catalyses the conversion of E_1 into estradiol E_2 using NADPH as a cofactor and is expressed in the placenta, breast, and granulosa cells of the ovary. 17β-HSD-7 catalyzes the conversion of E_1 into E_2 using NADPH as a cofactor in the corpus luteum during the luteal phase of the ovarian cycle. 17β-HSD-3 is expressed only in testes, converting Δ_4A to testosterone. Deficiency of 17-ketosteroid reductase due to mutations in the 17β-HSD-3 gene impairs the formation of testosterone in the fetal testis from Δ_4A, resulting in undervirilized genetic males with normal male Wolffian duct structures (8).

CYP19 or P450aro P450 aromatase enzyme converts androgens Δ_4A and testosterone to estrogens, E_1, and E_2, respectively. The tissue-specific expression of the aromatase enzyme is determined at least in part by alternative use of tissue-specific promoters, which give rise to unique transcripts of the CYP19 gene. The enzyme is found in the gonadal tissues but also extragonadal tissues such as muscle, liver, hair follicles, adipose tissue, and brain (9). Aromatization of fetal adrenal androgens and their desulfation are essential for production of estrogen in vivo by the human placenta. Placental aromatase deficiency appears to cause maternal virilization during pregnancy and virilization of the female fetus (see Chapter 35).

Fetal Adrenal Steroidogenesis

Through most of gestation, the production of cortisol and aldosterone by the fetal adrenal gland is low due to the very low expression of the 3β-HSD-II enzyme. Production of DHEA and DHEA-S is increased due to very high expression of 17,20-lyase, particularly in the large fetal zone (10). The large fetal adrenal zone has increased sulfotransferase (SULT2A1) activity in comparison with sulfatase favoring the production of DHEA-S over DHEA. The DHEA-S can be either 16α-hydroxylated in the liver and subsequently converted to estriol (E_3) by the placental enzymes 3β-HSD-I, 17β-HSD-1, and aromatase enzyme. Alternatively, it can be converted to DHEA by sulfatase and then to Δ_4A by placental 3β-HSD-I; Δ_4A then can be aromatized to E_1 by aromatase and then converted to E_2 by 17β-HSD-1. Estriol during pregnancy is a marker of function of the fetoplacental unit. Fetal adrenal steroids account for 90% of the E_3 and 50% of the E_1 and E_2 in the maternal circulation.

Placental aromatase increases throughout the pregnancy, preventing female fetuses and their mothers from getting virilized by the large amounts of DHEA-S secreted by the fetal adrenal cortex (11). Placental aromatase also protects female fetuses from virilization when their mothers have elevated testosterone levels due to uncontrolled congenital adrenal hyperplasia (CAH) due to 21–hydroxylase deficiency (12). Another factor that has been suggested to prevent virilization in female fetuses is the robust capacity of fetal adrenals to secrete ACTH-responsive cortisol early in gestation, with cortisol secretion peaking at weeks 8–9 of gestation; after the 9th week of gestation, cortisol secretion declines to almost undetectable levels until later in pregnancy when it is required for lung maturation. It is believed that the high levels of cortisol during this critical period for sexual differentiation suppress the fetal hypothalamic–pituitary–adrenal axis (HPA), keeping DHEA-S levels low and therefore preventing virilization of female fetuses (13) during this period when aromatase has not reached high levels.

Maternal cortisol cannot normally reach the fetus because it is oxidized to cortisone by the placental 11β-hydroxysteroid dehydrogenase type 2 enzyme (11β-HSD-2); cortisone is an inactive steroid. However, dexamethasone is not metabolized by 11β-HSD-2 and can cross the placenta, suppressing the fetal HPA axis, when administered to the mother. For this reason, dexamethasone is used for prenatal treatment of CAH before the 8th week of gestation, when the gonads, internal sex ducts, and external genitalia are bipotential.

Cortisol Metabolism The main function of cortisol at normal physiological concentrations is regulation of carbohydrate metabolism by decreasing insulin-stimulated glucose cellular uptake and stimulating hepatic gluconeogenesis (14). Glucocorticoids stimulate adipocyte differentiation and induce catabolic changes in muscle, skin, and connective tissue. Cortisol enhances vasoconstrictor response to catecholamines and increases water clearance (15,16). Effects of cortisol on endocrine systems include direct suppression of thyroid-stimulating hormone (TSH), decrease in growth hormone (GH) secretion, most likely through an increase in somatostatinergic tone and inhibition of the gonadotropin-releasing hormone (GnRH) pulsatility, as well as the luteinizing hormone (LH) and follicle-stimulating hormone (FSH) release. Cortisol can alter the immunological response to inflammation and autoimmune disorders by direct actions on both T- and B-cell lymphocytes functions (17). Elevated cortisol levels, both lsupraphysiologic and physiological, are associated with a decrease in some cytokines, such as interferon-γ (IFN-γ), tumor necrosis factor α (TNF-α), interleukin 1α (IL-1α), and IL-12 (18). This decrease in cytokines is part of the immune suppression seen with high-dose steroid therapy.

Circulating cortisol is bound with high affinity to the α_2-globulin, cortisol-binding globulin (CBG or transcortin), which is synthesized in the liver; only 10% of cortisol is in the free, active form. Glucocorticoids, cirrhosis, nephrotic syndrome, and hyperthyroidism reduce CBG levels. Increased estrogen levels during pregnancy are associated with an increase in CBG and total cortisol levels, whereas the free cortisol level remains stable.

The circulating half-life of cortisol varies between 70 and 120 minutes. The major routes of cortisol (F) metabolism include 1) interconversion of cortisol (F) to cortisone (E) through the activity of 11β-HSD isozymes and 2) reduction of the C_{4-5} double bond by either 5β-reductase or 5α-reductase to yield 5β-tetrahydrocortisol (THF) or 5α-THF (allo-THF).

The interconversion of cortisol to cortisone is the most important metabolic pathway of cortisol. There are two distinct 11β-HSD isozymes: 11β-HSD-2, which is coexpressed with the mineralocorticoid receptor (MR) in the kidney, colon, and salivary gland, and 11β-HSD-1, which is a bidirectional enzyme expressed mainly in liver and adipose tissues. The 11β-HSD-2 isozyme favors inactivation of cortisol by converting cortisol to cortisone and thus enabling aldosterone to bind to the MR, whereas the 11β-HSD-1 isozyme favors the conversion of cortisone to cortisol in the liver and adipose tissue. The latter results in enhanced glucocorticoid-dependent hepatic gluconeogenesis and glucose output, as well as adipocyte differentiation (19,20). Homozygous inactivating mutations of the 11β-HSD-2 isozyme result in cortisol-mediated hypertension or apparent mineralocorticoid excess (AME) (21,22). In this disorder, cortisol due to 11β-HSD-2 deficiency is not inactivated to cortisone and is free to bind and activate the mineralocorticoid receptor. Affected children have severe hypertension with suppressed renin and aldosterone levels, hypokalemia, and an increased urinary ratio of cortisol to cortisone metabolites. Spironolactone or amiloride at high doses can be used therapeutically.

Elevated thyroid hormone levels and GH/insulin-like growth factor 1 (IGF-1) levels increase cortisol clearance mainly by inhibiting the hepatic 11β-HSD-1 conversion of cortisone to cortisol (23,24).

REGULATION OF ADRENAL STEROIDOGENESIS

Hypothalamic–Pituitary–Adrenal (HPA) Axis

Cortisol and androgen secretion are under the control of ACTH, whereas aldosterone secretion is regulated mainly through the renin–angiotensin system. ACTH is secreted by the corticotropes of the anterior pituitary, has 39 amino acids, and is derived from pro-opiomelanocortin (POMC), a large 241-amino-acids precursor. POMC is cleaved into several active biological peptides such as N-terminal glycopeptide, corticotrophin-like intermediate-lobe peptide (CLIP), α- and β-melanocyte-stimulating hormone (MSH), β-endorphin, and β-lipoprotein. The first 20–24 amino acids

constitute the biologically active part of the ACTH molecule; synthetic ACTH, which is used for diagnostic purposes, consists of these 24 amino acids. Hypothalamic control of ACTH secretion is exerted primarily by corticotropin-releasing hormone (CRH), a 41-amino-acid peptide, and to a lesser degree by antidiuretic hormone (ADH). Both hormones are produced by parvocellular neurons of the paraventricular nucleus, secreted into the hypophyseal–portal system, and have a synergistic effect on ACTH release. Stress conditions such as major surgery, blood loss, high fever, severe illness, hypoglycemia, and psychological stress increase adrenal secretion of cortisol via increase in CRH and ACTH output.

ACTH stimulates adrenal cortisol production via the melanocortin-2 receptor (MC2R), also known as the ACTH receptor (ACTHR), a member of the G protein–coupled receptor family. Acute response of the adrenals to ACTH occurs within seconds to minutes through cyclic adenosine monophosphate (cAMP) activation and is mediated through the steroidogenic acute regulatory protein (StAR), which facilitates rapid flux of cholesterol into the mitochondrion. The chronic phase occurs within hours to days and involves increased transcription of the adrenal steroidogenic enzymes.

Cortisol, through a negative-feedback system, regulates the resting activity of the HPA axis; increased cortisol levels exert negative feedback at both the hypothalamus and pituitary, causing a decrease in ACTH and CRH release and thus a decrease in adrenal cortisol production. Conversely, a decrease in cortisol levels increases both CRH and ACTH release, resulting in increased adrenal cortisol secretion (Figure 27-2).

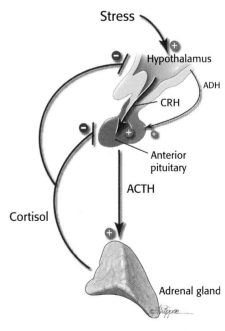

FIGURE 27-2. Regulation through cortisol-mediated negative feedback of the hypothalamic–pituitary–adrenal (HPA) axis.

ACTH and cortisol have a pulsatile secretion every 30–120 minutes. ACTH levels peak at 4 to 6 a.m., and cortisol levels peak around 8 a.m. because the frequency and amplitude of ACTH and cortisol pulses are much greater in the morning. The nadir of ACTH and cortisol secretion is 1 hour after going to sleep at night. In infants, the diurnal rhythm of ACTH and cortisol is not established during the first 6–12 months of life and may remain irregular for up to 3 years of life (25). The adrenal cortisol secretion rate under basal conditions is 6–9 mg/m^2/day in children and adults (15,16). In normal individuals, the highest plasma cortisol and ACTH levels are in the morning between 6 and 8 a.m. and the lowest at about midnight.

Unlike cortisol, aldosterone is less ACTH-dependent, and the major controlling factor in its secretion is the renin–angiotensin system. An acute bolus of ACTH will increase aldosterone secretion by no more than 10% to 20% above baseline, and chronic ACTH stimulation has either no effect or an inhibitory effect on aldosterone production.

Renin is an enzyme produced by the juxtaglomerular cells of the kidney whose secretion is increased in response to decreased low-perfusion pressure and/or low tubular sodium content, as seen in dehydration, hemorrhage, renal artery stenosis, and salt wasting. Hypokalemia increases renin secretion, whereas hyperkalemia has a negative effect; changes in potassium concentration of only 0.1–0.5 mEq/L may produce marked changes in alodsterone concentrations (26).

Renin cleaves angiotensinogen to form angiotensin I, a precursor for the formation of angiotensin II; angiotensin II is a potent vasoconstrictor that together with its metabolite, angiotensin III, acts on G-coupled protein mineralocorticoid receptor, inducing the synthesis and secretion of aldosterone.

Cortisol also can stimulate the mineralocorticoid receptor, but inactivation of cortisol to cortisone by the 11β-HSD-2 isozyme protects the mineralocorticoid receptor from being stimulated by cortisol, which is secreted at quantities 100-fold more than aldosterone.

CONGENITAL ADRENAL HYPERPLASIA

Etiology/Pathophysiology The congenital adrenal hyperplasias (CAHs) are a group of adrenal disorders characterized by histological alterations of adrenal cortical tissue secondary to chronic overstimulation by elevated levels of ACTH due to a defect in the pathway that converts cholesterol into cortisol. In most forms of CAH, the enzymatic defect blocks cortisol synthesis, impairing cortisol-

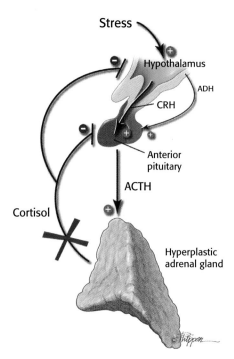

FIGURE 27-3. Impaired cortisol-mediated negative feedback due to congenital adrenal hyperplasia on the hypothalamic–pituitary–adrenal (HPA) axis.

mediated negative-feedback control of ACTH secretion (Figure 27-3). Consequently, oversecretion of ACTH ensues, stimulating excessive synthesis of the adrenal steroids from those pathways unimpaired by an enzyme deficiency and causing an accumulation of precursor molecules in pathways blocked by the enzyme deficiency. The constant unsuccessful ACTH stimulation of the adrenals to produce cortisol causes the adrenals to increase in size (see Figure 27-3). The range and severity of the phenotypes found in CAH depend on the degree of the defect (partial or complete), the location of the defect in the pathway, and which precursors become elevated as a result of the defect.

Sex Differentiation of Affected Females with CAH

Prior to sexual differentiation (the bipotential gonad stage), both male and female embryos have two pairs of genital ducts (Wolffian and Müllerian). In males, through expression of SRY (the testis-determining gene on the Y chromosome), the gonad, during sexual differentiation, becomes the testis and secretes anti-Müllerian hormone (AMH) and testosterone. In turn, testosterone promotes the differentiation of the Wolffian duct into the male reproductive tract through the formation of the epididymides, vas deferans, and seminal vesicles, whereas AMH eliminates the Müllerian duct. During the sexual differentiation of females, the bipotential gonad becomes the ovary, and the Müllerian ducts differentiate into the fallopian tubes, the uterus, and the upper two-thirds of the vagina. In the absence of testosterone, the Wolffian duct regresses, and the vesicovaginal septum forms along with creation of two separate openings, urethral and vaginal, in the perineum (Figure 27-4). (For a more detailed discussion of sex differentiation, see Chapter 35.) Similarly, in the absence of dihydrotestosterone (DHT), which is the hormone that masculinizes external genita-

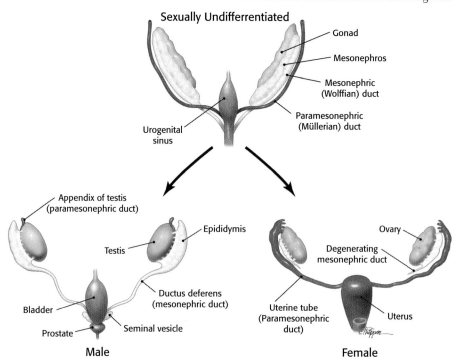

FIGURE 27-4. Sex differentiation of internal genital ducts (Müllerian and Wolffian ducts) from the undifferentiated stage in male and female embryos.

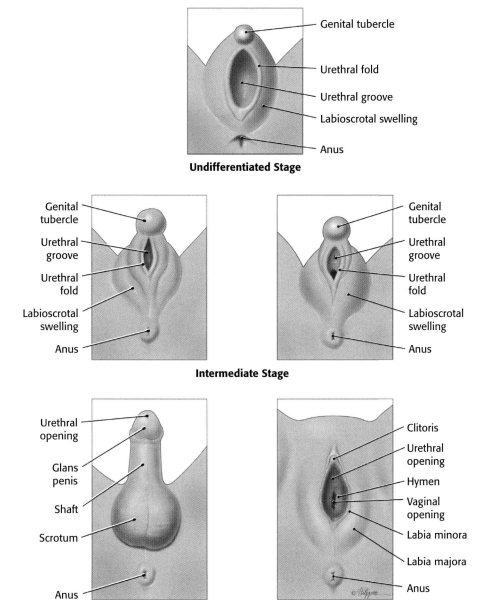

Genital tubercle

Urethral fold

Urethral groove

Labioscrotal swelling

Anus

Undifferentiated Stage

Genital tubercle

Urethral groove

Urethral fold

Labioscrotal swelling

Anus

Genital tubercle

Urethral groove

Urethral fold

Labioscrotal swelling

Anus

Intermediate Stage

Urethral opening

Glans penis

Shaft

Scrotum

Anus

Clitoris

Urethral opening

Hymen

Vaginal opening

Labia minora

Labia majora

Anus

Male   Final stage   Female

FIGURE 27-5. Sex differentiation of external genitalia from the undifferentiated stage in male and female embryos.

lia in males, the genital tubercle becomes a clitoris, the urethral folds form the labia majora, and the urogenital sinus becomes the urethra and lower third of the vagina (Figure 27-5).

Females affected with classical CAH (due to either 21α-hydroxylase or 11β-hydroxylase deficiency) are exposed in utero to elevated adrenal androgens during the critical period of sex differentiation (8–10 weeks). While the exposure to elevated androgens does not affect the development of the internal genitalia (ovaries or uterus), these patients do have masculinization of the external genitalia and inhibition of vesicovaginal septum formation, resulting in a urogenital sinus and a single opening. Depending on the severity of the enzymatic defect, genital masculinization can range from clitoral enlargement, mild posterior labial fusion and normal urethral and vag-

inal openings, to a markedly enlarged phallus with a penile urethra. Typing of the degree of virilization of the external genitalia in females can be done using the Prader classification (27), a five-point classification (Figure 27-6) in which stage I is minimal clitoral enlargement, stage II describes partial labioscrotal fusion, stage III is characterized by a funnel-shaped urogenital sinus at the posterior end of the vulva, stage IV demonstrates a small urogenital sinus at the base of an enlarged phallus, and stage V indicates a penile urethra.

CAH DUE TO 21α-HYDROXYLASE DEFICIENCY

Etiology/Pathophysiology Of the six main enzymes involved in the synthesis of cholesterol into glucocorticoid (cortisol), min-

eralocorticoid (aldosterone), and sex steroid hormones, deficiency of 21α-hydroxylase enzyme (P450c21) is the most frequent cause of CAH (found in more than 90% of cases). 21α-hydroxylase (21α-OHlase) a cytochrome P450 enzyme, is located on the endoplasmic reticulum and catalyzes two reactions involving the synthesis of aldosterone and cortisol. In the aldosterone pathway, 21α-OHlase is important in the conversion of progesterone to DOC and in the cortisol pathway, it catalyzes the conversion of 17-OHP to 11-deoxycortisol (Figure 27-7).

There are two 21-OHlase genes, one active and one nonfunctional (pseudogene). The active CYP21 gene (CYP21, CYP21A2, or CYP21B) and the pseudogene (CYP21A, CYP21A1P, or CYP21P) are located on chromosome 6p21.3 in the human histocompatability leukocyte antigen (HLA) complex and alternate with the C4B and C4A genes that encode the fourth component of serum complement (28). The pseudogene is located 30 kb from CYP21, has almost identical nucleotide sequences, but expresses no active enzyme because it carries deleterious mutations and eight missense mutations. The three main deleterious mutations present in the pseudogene include an Δ8-bp deletion in exon 3 (G110Δ8nt), a nonsense mutation in exon 8 (Q318X), and a nucleotide insertion in exon 7 (V281L). Several of the missense mutations carried by the pseudogene have been described in patients with CAH due to 21α-OHlase deficiency (21-OHD) (29,30). About 90% of the mutant alleles in CAH are generated by recombinations between the active gene and pseudogene (31,32) (Figure 27-8) either by transferring the deleterious mutations that are normally present in the pseudogene to the active gene (gene conversion) or by misalignment and unequal crossover during meiosis, resulting in large-scale deletion of the active gene (usually the deletion also includes the C4B gene).

Depending on the type of mutation and degree of enzyme deficiency, patients are categorized in three clinical phenotypes of 21-OHD: classical salt wasting, classical simple virilizing, and nonclassical CAH. About 75% of patients with classical CAH due to 21-OHD have the salt-wasting phenotype, in which synthesis of both cortisol and aldosterone is severely impaired secondary to CYP21 gene deletions or nonsense mutations that completely obliterate enzyme activity. As a result of the decreased adrenal cortisol production and impaired negative feedback, excessive secretion of CRH and ACTH occurs. Deficient aldosterone synthesis results in severe hyponatremic dehydration, hyperkalemia, hypotension, and shock.

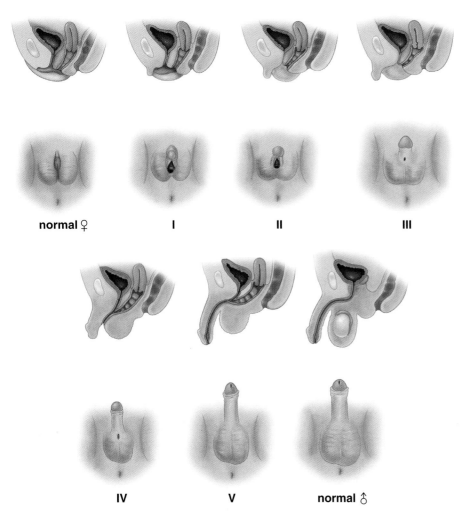

FIGURE 27-6. Prader classification depicting the increasing degrees of virilization of the female internal and external genitalia, flanked on the upper left side by a normal female schematic and on the lower right side by a normal male. Stage I: clitoral enlargement; Stage II: clitoral enlargement, partial labioscrotal fusion, and a funnel-shaped urogenital sinus: Stage III: increased phallus size with complete labioscrotal fusion forming a urogenital sinus at the base of the penis; Stage IV: further increased phallus size and further elongated urogenital sinus; Stage V: female with normal male-appearing penile urethra.

The remaining 25% of patients with classical CAH have the simple virilizing phenotype, in which cortisol synthesis is impaired, but there is enough aldosterone production to maintain normal sodium balance because these patients still have some activity of the 21α-OHlase enzyme (as little as 1% enzymatic activity of the 21α-OHlase enzyme allows sufficient aldosterone synthesis to prevent salt wasting). Predominant clinical manifestations include virilization and adrenal crises when stressed.

The least severe clinical manifestations of CAH secondary to 21-OHD are caused by the nonclassical phenotype, in which aldosterone production is normal and ACTH-stimulated cortisol levels are near normal or slightly subnormal. CYP21 gene mutations associated with the nonclassical CAH phenotype allow the 21α-OHlase enzyme to maintain 20% to 50% of its enzymatic activity. Affected patients can be either asymptomatic or have symptoms associated with mild androgen excess.

The worldwide incidence of 21-OHD has been estimated at 1 in 15,000 live births for homozygous patients and 1 in 60 for heterozygous patients (33). The incidence varies according to ethnicity and geographical areas, with the highest incidence found in Yupic Eskimos of Alaska (1 in 280) and on the French island of La Reunion (1 in 2100) (33,34). The incidence in the United States is 1 in 15,500 in Caucasians and 1 in 42,000 in African Americans (35). The incidence of nonclassical CAH has not been determined for the following reasons: 1) Newborn screening does not accurately detect nonclassical CAH because the cutoff levels for 17-OHP are set high to decrease false-positive results, and nonclassical CAH patients have only mildly elevated 17-OHP, and 2) the diagnosis of nonclassical CAH may be missed in patients who develop only the most mild symptoms of androgen excess or because their mild clinical manifestations may be attributed to other hyperandrogenemic conditions such as polycystic

ovarian disease or exaggerated adrenarche in childhood. However, the incidence of nonclassical CAH is more common than classical CAH, with a prevalence estimated to be 3.7% in Ashkenazi Jews, 1.9% in Hispanics, 1.6% in Yugoslavs, 0.3% in Italians, and 0.1% in the diverse Caucasian population (36).

Presentation

Classical CAH (Salt Wasting and Simple Virilizing) Clinical phenotype will vary based on the differences in 21α-OHDase activity, as outlined earlier. Affected male newborns with classical CAH may not be diagnosed clinically at birth because they do not have genital ambiguity except for scrotal hyperpigmentation and phallic enlargement. Affected male newborns with the salt-wasting phenotype usually are undiagnosed at birth, and they present 2–3 weeks later, or earlier if stressed, in salt-wasting adrenal crisis.

Affected males with the simple virilizing phenotype, if not diagnosed at birth, will present at 2 years of age or older with early development of pubic, axilliary, and facial hair, penile enlargement (Figure 27-9), body odor, and growth acceleration with bone age advancement. Virilization in boys due to CAH is distinguished from true precocious puberty by the testicular size, which is prepubertal (<3 mL) in boys affected with CAH. Untreated or poorly controlled boys with classical CAH have early epiphyseal closure, compromised final adult height, small testes, and infertility. Elevated estrogens through aromatization of adrenal androgens during childhood and the pubertal years may affect spermatogenesis directly or due to gonadotropin suppression through negative feedback of the hypothalamic–pituitary–gonadal (HPG) axis. In addition, elevated ACTH levels in poorly controlled men may stimulate enlargement of adrenal rests in the testes (some adrenal cells migrate along with gonadal cells during adrenal and gonadal development). Adrenal rests futher compromise spermatogenesis by a pressure effect on the testicular parenchyma and by production of steroid hormones that further elevate intratesticular estrogen concentration.

Females with classical CAH due to salt wasting or simple virilizing forms will have virilized genitalia at birth, ranging from clitoral enlargement, rugated labioscrotal folds (with or without posterior fusion), to complete fusion of labioscrotal folds, urogenital sinus, and a single opening (Figure 27-10). The presence of a single opening and penile urethra in severe virilized females instead of separate urethral and vaginal openings is the result of inhibition of vesicovaginal septum formation by the elevated adrenal

Steroidogenesis in 21α-hydroxylase Deficiency (P450c21)

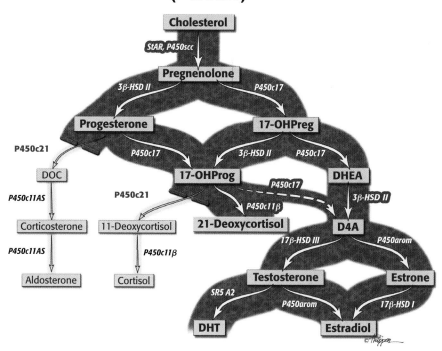

FIGURE 27-7. Congenital adrenal hyperplasia due to 21α-hydroxylase deficiency. Impaired enzymatic activity blocks the results the conversion of 17-hydroxyprogesterone (17-OHP) to 11-deoxycortisol (S), a precursor of cortisol, and the conversion of progesterone to 11-deoxycorticosterone (DOC), a precursor of aldosterone. Through increased ACTH secretion in an effort to promote adrenal cortisol synthesis, there is an overproduction of cortisol precursors, which are diverted to the pathway of androgen synthesis.

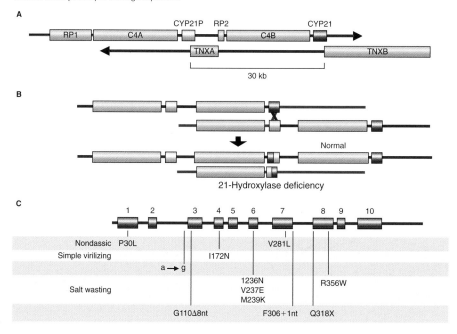

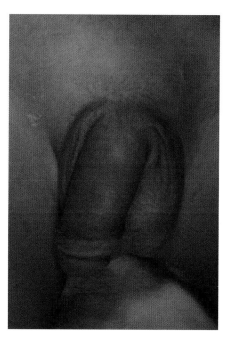

FIGURE 27-9. A 4-year-old boy with simple virilizing CAH due to 21-OHD presenting with penile enlargement, pubic hair, and early puberty.

androgens. In both sexes, if treatment for CAH is started late, a decrease in adrenal androgens and adrenal estrogens removes the chronic inhibition of the sex steroids on the HPG axis and may result in true precocious puberty. This can have a further negative impact on final adult height. Short stature also may occur with overtreatment because excess glucocorticoid inhibits the growth axis.

Untreated females or those in poor control may develop further clitoral enlargement, hirsutism, acne, and a clinical picture similar to polycystic ovarian syndrome, including ovarian cysts, anovulation, irregular bleeding, and insulin resistance. Breast development also is often suboptimal, menarche often occurs late, and infertility may be encountered.

Presentations in salt-wasting CAH may include poor appetite, vomiting, lethargy, failure to thrive, and shock. The latter is secondary to the combination of aldosterone deficiency (causing hyponatremia and hyperkalemia), cortisol deficiency (causing poor

FIGURE 27-8. The chromosomal region of 6p21.3 containing the 21-hydroxylase genes (A), 21-hydroxylase genes undergoing an unequal crossover during meiosis **(B)**, and mutations in steroid 21-hydroxylase causing congenital adrenal hyperplasia **(C)**. **A.** CYP21P and CYP21 are the steroid 21-hydroxylase pseudogene and active gene, respectively. C4A and C4B encode the fourth component of serum complement. RP1 encodes a nuclear protein of unknown function, and RP2 is the corresponding truncated pseudogene. On the opposite chromosomal strand, TNXB encodes tenascin-X, and TNXA is the corresponding truncated pseudogene. A bar delineates the 30-kb region that is deleted in approximately 20% of 21-hydroxylase deficiency chromosomes. **B.** 21-Hydroxylase genes undergo an unequal crossover during meiosis, and the resulting daughter chromosomes possess either three CYP21 alleles or one nonfunctional CYP21 gene as a result of a large deletion. **C.** The positions of mutations normally found in CYP21P; any of these can be transferred to CYP21 in gene-conversion events. Recombinant enzymes carrying each missense mutation have been expressed in cultured cells. Numbered boxes represent exons. The percentage of normal activity seen in each mutant hnzyme is denoted by the position of each mutation on a vertical scale; the mutations that affect activity most severely, causing salt-wasting disease, are at the bottom of the figure. The mutations are as follows: P30L, Pro30Leu; a→g, mutation in intron 2 activating a cryptic splice site; G110Δ8nt, deletion of eight nucleotides; I172N, Ile172Asn; I236N, V237E, and M239K are a cluster of three mutations almost invariably inherited together (Ile236Asn, Val237Glu, and Met239Lys, respectively); V281L, Val281Leu; F306+1nt, the insertion of a single nucleotide; Q318X, a nonsense mutation of Gln318; R356W, Arg356Trp; and P453S, Pro453Ser. (From Speiser PW, White PC. Congenital adrenal hyperplasia. *N Engl J Med.* 2003;349:776–788, with permission.)

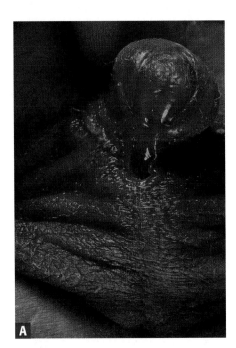

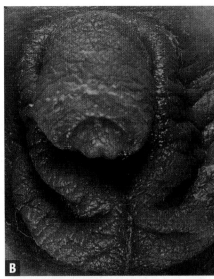

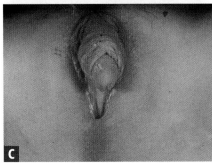

FIGURE 27-10. Females with the salt wasting and simple virilizing forms of CAH due to 21OHD can present with virilized genitalia at birth ranging from clitoral enlargement, rugated labioscrotal folds (with or without posterior fusion) to complete fusion of labioscrotal folds, urogenital sinus, and a single opening. **A, B.** An infant with rugated labioscrotal folds with posterior fusion and a single urogenital sinus. **C.** A female child with clitoromegaly.

cardiac function and poor vascular response to catecholamines), and catecholamine deficiency (caused by failure of adrenal medulla to develop fully), ultimately leading to hyponatremic dehydration and shock.

Nonclassical CAH Patients with nonclassical CAH do not have symptoms at birth. Clinical presentation during childhood may include early pubic hair development, growth acceleration, and bone age advancement. Hirsutism is the most common symptom (60%), followed by irregular menses (54%) and acne (33%) in adosescent or adult women with nonclassical CAH. Thus the presentation of nonclassical CAH and polycystic ovarian syndrome are similar, and at the time of diagnosis, both disorders may coexist. Infertility appears to be the presenting symptom in only 13% of nonclassical CAH females (37). It should be noted that some patients with nonclassical CAH may never develop any symptomatology of androgen excess. Carriers for 21-OHD are not at increased risk for developing symptoms of hyperandrogenism (38).

Adrenal Rests, Male Reproductive Function, and the Role of Estrogen Male CAH patients, as early as 3 years of age, can develop ectopic testicular adrenal rests, which may become hypertropic under chronic ACTH stimula-

tion and further impair gonadal function (39). Besides the mechanical pressure on the testicular parenchyma, another cause may contribute to decreased reproductive function in CAH males; increased estrogen levels aromatized from the increased androgen levels.

Within the reproductive system, estrogen plays a role in the regulation of fluid resorption from the efferent ducts and appears to be important in the structural and functional development of the Wolffian–excurrent duct system, as well as that of the prostate (40,41). Inappropriately low or high estrogen exposure during development can cause permanent changes to these tissues, which may lead to disorders of spermatogenesis and infertility (42,43).

More than in any other tissue, the highest concentrations of estrogen receptors (ER-α and ER-β) are found in Sertoli, Leydig, and germ cells, male reproductive tract ducts, and accessory sex organs, which signifies the importance of estrogen for regulation of these tissues (44). The widespread distribution of aromatase suggests that many of the effects of estrogens in the male might stem from its local production and action and, furthermore, that the balance in action between androgens and estrogens might be of central importance at many estrogen target sites, particularly the reproductive system. Elevated estrogens af-

fect testicular steroidogenesis by suppressing pituitary gonadotropins and affecting testicular steroidogenesis at the Leydig cells, which is LH-driven. An interesting study in which the effects of administration of an aromatase inhibitor were compared in normal versus GnRH-treated hypogonadotropic-hypogonadal men demonstrated that estrogen acts at the hypothalamus to decrease GnRH pulse frequency and at the pituitary to decrease responsiveness to GnRH (45).

In a study of 30 adult males with CAH in which 16 were tested for fertility, 9 were found to have decreased spermatogenesis and low testosterone (46). Adrenal rests were found in 7 of these 9 patients. Of the other 14 CAH male patients (those who did not have semen analysis), 7 had low testosterone (normal range 20 ± 6.6 nmol/L). However, only 1 of the 7 patients with low testosterone had adrenal rests, which supports the idea that adrenal rests are not the only cause of testicular dysfunction. In another study (47) of 17 male CAH patients, 16 had adrenal rests, and 12 had decreased testicular volume (<13 mL). In females, the prevalence of ovarian adrenal rests is rare (48–50).

Diagnosis Elevated random serum 17-OHP (>10,000 ng/dL or 300 nmol/L versus 100 ng/dL or 3 nmol/L for normal) is characteristic of classical CAH due to 21-OHD. Patients with nonclassical CAH may have normal baseline 17-OHP levels. However, a baseline, 8 a.m., 17-OHP level greater than 100ng/dL in children and adolescents with clinical symptoms of hyperandrogenemia should be followed by an ACTH stimulation test to rule out nonclassical CAH (in females, the 17-OHP level should be drawn at the early follicular phase of the menstrual cycle). A study of 220 patients with nonclassical CAH showed that 10% of the patients had a baseline 17-OHP level of less than 200 ng/mL. Adolescent patients had higher baseline values than children and older adult women (37).

A corticotropin (cosyntropin or ACTH) stimulation test is the "gold standard" for the diagnosis of CAH due to 21-OHD and, furthermor, can help to distinguish 21-OHD from other enzyme defects. An ACTH stimulation test should be performed in all infants with an elevated 17-OHP level or in whom clinical suspicion of CAH is high. The test is performed by injecting a bolus of cosyntropin (0.25 mg) and measuring baseline and stimulated 17-OHP levels at 60 minutes. The highest elevations after stimulation (up to 100,000 ng/dL) are indicative of salt-wasting CAH. Patients with simple virilizing CAH usually have 17-OHP levels that are somewhat elevated (10,000–30,000 ng/dL). Genetic testing in patients with classical CAH often can further delineate the form of CAH, simple virilization CAH versus salt-wasting CAH, because there is a good correlation between genotype and clinical phenotype. Stimulated 17-OHP values above 30.3 nmol/L or 1000 ng/dL (range 1000–10.000 ng/dL) are considered diagnostic of nonclassical CAH, although heterozygous CAH patients with 17-OHP values above 30.3 nmol/L have been reported (38,51). Figure 27-11 illustrates the diagnostic workup of infants with positive CAH newborn screens.

Baseline and stimulated adrenal androgens are elevated in CAH due to 21-OHD. Cortisol baseline and stimulated levels are low or absent in patients with classical 21-OHD, whereas patients with nonclassical CAH usually have a normal cortisol response to the ACTH stimulation test.

The majority of carriers of 21-OHD have an exaggerated 17-OHP response to the ACTH stimulation test, with levels usually less than 30.3 nmol/L or 1000 ng/dL (38). However, there is a significant overlap between the heterozygotes and the control population; a normal 17-OHP response does not exlude heterozygosity for 21-OHD, and a 17-OHP stimulated level above 30.3 nmol/L does not always indicate nonclassical CAH (51). Molecular studies in families with CAH therefore are important to distinguish between normal controls and heterozygotes. Genetic sequencing should be offered as part of the diagnostic evaluation of patients with clinical signs of hyperandrogenism and heterozygosity for one of the most common CAH tested mutations if the ACTH-stimulated 17-OHP values are above 30.3 nmol/L; nonclassical CAH unidentified alleles are at a higher frequency than classical CAH alleles in several population studies.

Increased plasma renin activity, decreased aldosterone levels, hyponatremia, hyperkalemia, elevated urinary sodium excretion, and increased potassium reabsorption are characteristic findings in salt-wasting CAH. Patients with simple virilizing CAH and nonclassical CAH have normal electrolytes.

A retrograde genitogram in virilized females affected with classical CAH would anatomically define the urogenital sinus by localizing the position and entrance of the urethra and the vagina into the sinus.

Genetic Testing and Counseling Correlations between the CYP21 genotype and phenotype have been studied in various ethnic populations (52–56). Several CYP21 mutations have been described and can be grouped into three categories (57): 1) deletions or nonsense mutations that totally ablate enzyme activity and are associated most often with salt-wasting disease, 2) mutations that allow 1% to 2% of enzyme

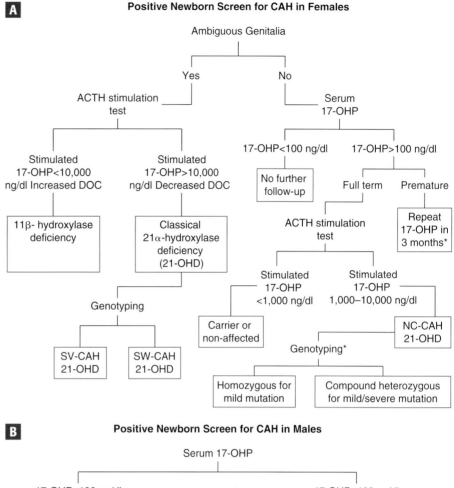

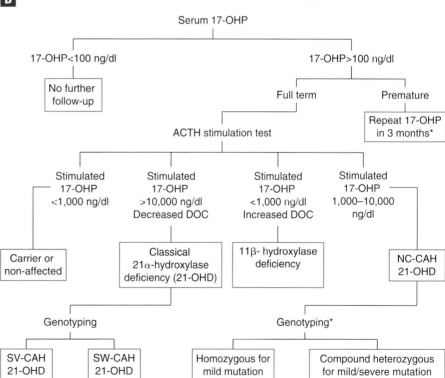

FIGURE 27-11. Diagnostic algorithms of male and female infants with a positive newborn screen for CAH.

activity and therefore permit adequate aldosterone synthesis, causing simple virilizing CAH (one such mutation is the I172N mutation, a missense mutation and the most common

mutation causing simple virilizing CAH) (58), and 3) mutations such as as V281L and P30L that produce enzymes retaining 20% to 60% of normal activity (these are the most frequent mutations associated with the nonclassical CAH) (59).

Compound heterozygotes for two different CYP21 mutations usually have a phenotype compatible with the presence of the milder of the gene defects. A source of phenotype–genotype variability can be the leakiness of splice mutations (60). For example, the intron 2 splice mutation that consists of an A-to-G transition in the splice acceptor site at the 3' end of intron 2 comprises 25% of all classical 21-OHD alleles and usually results in abnormally spliced mRNA transcripts, but with a small amount of the mRNA being normally spliced. If the amount of normal mRNA is enough to allow 1% to 2% of normal 21-OHlase enzyme activity, the patient's phenotype can change from salt- wasting to simple virilizing disease. More than half of nonclassical CAH females are compound heterozygotes, carrying a severe mutation of the CYP21 gene, and may give birth to a fetus affected with classical CAH if the father is also a carrier of a severe CYP21 mutation (61).

Genetic testing includes screening for the most common mutations (see Figure 29-8) that cause CAH due to 21-OHD, followed by genetic sequencing in patients who are heterozygotes for one of the screened mutations but their biochemical and clinical symptoms suggest CAH due to 21-OHD.

Treatment Patients with classical CAH due to 21-OHD require long-term treatment with glucocorticoids. Replacement with glucocorticoids may be indicated for symptomatic patients with nonclassical disease. Glucocorticoid therapy suppresses excessive secretion of CRH and ACTH by the hypothalamus and pituitary gland and subsequently decreases adrenal androgen secretion. Since physiological secretion of cortisol is 6–7 mg/m^2/day (62–64), the preferred maintenance dose of hydrocortisone should be in the range of 8–12 mg/m^2/day divided into two to three doses and should not exceed 15 mg/m^2/day. In the neonatal period, during the first weeks of treatment, higher doses of glucocorticoids may be used (up to 25 mg/m^2/day) in order to suppress the elevated ACTH levels and the HPA axis. Measurement of 17-OHP and Δ_4A levels, renin, and electrolytes, as well as weight and length, every 2 weeks until the hydrocortisone dose is reduced to 8–12 mg/m^2/day is recommended.

Hydrocortisone, a short-acting glucocorticoid, is the drug of choice during childhood to minimize the growth-suppressive effects of longer-acting glucocorticoids such as prednisone, prednisolone, and dexamethasone. Treatment efficacy is monitored by measurement of 17-OHP and Δ_4A and a yearly bone age to assess bone age advancement. One should keep in mind that elevated adrenal androgens, due to aromatization to estrogens, induce bone age advancement and premature epiphyseal closeure, whereas excess glucocorticoids suppress growth. Therefore, the treatment aim, especially in children, should be to keep 17-OHP levels between 100 and 1000 ng/dL, allowing for normal growth and bone age maturation. Weight gain, hypertension, growth failure in children, and osteopenia are indicative of glucorticoid overtreatment. Prednisone (5–7.5 mg/day in two divided doses) or dexamethasone (0.25–0.5 mg/day divided into one or two doses) are acceptable alternative treatments in older adolescents and adults.

Adrenal Crisis and "Stress" Dosing Glucocorticoid "stress" dosing is also necessary in patients with classical CAH during febrile illnesses or surgery because these patients are unable to produce the normal burst of endogenous adrenal secretions during these periods. The goal is to administer the typical physiological dose, but common practice is to err on the side of overtreatment. Patients often are told to double or triple their hydrocortisone doses during febrile illnesses. If children are unable to take an oral dose, intramuscular hydrocortisone sodium succinate (Solu-Cortef) can be used. For surgeries, hydrocortisone 100 mg/m^2 should be given intramuscularly on call to the operating room, followed by intravenous hydrocortisone (100 mg/m^2/day during the procedure). Postoperatively 100 mg/m^2 of hydrocortisone can be given over the next 24 hours divided in four doses and tapered by half each day until maintenance dose is achieved as long as the patient is stable clinically. Hydrocortisone can be administered orally as soon as the patient can take oral intake. If after surgery a patient needs to stay on high doses of steroids longer than 5 days, tapering should be considered over several days until daily maintenance doses are achieved. There is no evidence that higher doses are needed in times of mental or emotional stress. Patients with classical CAH may be at risk for hypoglycemia during stress because adrenomedullary function may be impaired (65). For emergency treatment of adrenal crisis, see Chapter 1.

Mineralocorticoid Replacement Therapy Patients with salt wasting require mineralocorticoid replacement in addition to glucocorticoid replacement, as outlined earlier. Mineralocorticoid often is given in the form of fludrocortisone (0.1–0.2 mg/day). Infants during the first 6–12 months of life require sodium chloride replacement (17–34 mEq/day or 1–2 g/day of sodium) because breast milk and formula do not provide sufficient supplementation. Measuring plasma renin activity, blood pressure, and electrolyte levels monitors treatment efficacy. Decreased renin levels, hypertension, growth suppression, and increased weight gain suggest overtreatment with glucocorticoids.

Other Treatment Issues Many of the same issues involving glucocorticoid therapy and control of excess androgens that troubled physicians 20 years ago (e.g., correct dose and measuring control) still plague physicians today. Ideally, the production of adrenal androgens is normalized in CAH patients by glucocorticoid replacement therapy. However, because glucocorticoids lack the close temporal relationship to ACTH pulses, increased adrenal activity will continue despite glucocorticoid treatment, resulting in greater than normal androgen production. Higher treatment doses needed to achieve satisfactory androgen suppression can expose children to the negative effects of excessive glucocorticoids (66–73). It also has been shown that glucocorticoids have a dose-dependent negative effect on linear growth and that the negative effect is age-dependent (74,75). A study in the Netherlands further pinpointed the negative effects of glucocorticoids on linear growth as being worse between the ages of 6 and 12 months, 8 and 10 years, and 12 and 14 years (76).

Further complicating the clinical management equation is the lack of a single test that accurately reflects and monitors the control of a CAH patient from the previous visit. Measuring plasma levels of cortisol precursors, such as 17-OHP, is limited by the circadian rhythm of adrenal steroid secretion, making a single morning plasma sample not a perfectly reliable marker of the metabolic status of CAH children over a 24-hour period (77,78). This is why in patients with CAH, the balancing of glucocorticoid replacement therapy dose and assessment of control are governed by clinical parameters (i.e., bone age, growth acceleration, and pubertal stage), together with biochemical data. However, even with close follow-up, certain problems still can arise because even "well controlled" CAH patients still may manifest early puberty, compromised final height, polycystic ovarian disease, and male infertility (46,79–83).

Patients with nonclassical CAH do not need treatment unless they develop symptoms of androgen excess, such as growth acceleration and bone age advancement in children or irregular menses, hirsutism, acne, and infertility in adolescents and adult women. They do not require "stress" dose coverage unless they are on glucocorticoid therapy.

Surgical Intervention Surgical intervention of affected females born with virilized genitalia is complex and controversial. Surgical correction of ambiguous genitalia traditionally is undertaken early, at 2–6 months, in a single-stage procedure involving vaginal reconstruction and clitoroplasty because it is technically easier than at later stages. However, long-term outcomes and patient satisfaction with the early-age approach are still being investigated. Previous surgical techniques generally have yielded unsatisfactory results, often requiring revisions for sexual function and cosmesis (84). The appropriateness of procedures that are solely cosmetic is a topic of much debate (85,86). Arguments for early surgery include reducing potential social stigma associated with genital ambiguity and the superior healing and tissue remodeling potential of children as compared with adults (87). Arguments against early surgery include a potential negative impact on sexual functioning and, in some cases, uncertainty about the child's future gender identity (87,88). A multidisciplinary team including specialists in pediatric endocrinology, psychology, pediatric urology, and surgery can discuss early surgery as well as the option of not doing surgery so that the patient can decide at an older age and participate fully in an informed-consent process (89).

Bilateral adrenalectomy, a controversial intervention, has been proposed as a surgical treatment for severe classical CAH that is unresponsive to high doses of glucocorticoid treatment (90). Following this procedure, patients must adhere to strict hormone replacement. A minimum dose of 11 mg/m^2/day of hydrocortisone is required to prevent hyperpigmentation due to Nelson syndrome (ACTH-secreting pituitary macroadenoma), as well as activation of adrenal rests.

During pregnancy, women affected with classical CAH are optimally managed with hydrocortisone or prednisone because they both do not cross the placenta; the dose usually is increased during pregnancy due to pregnancy-induced altered clearance and steroid metabolism (91,92). Dexamethasone during pregnancy is used only for prenatal treatment. Unaffected female infants born to mothers with classical CAH have no signs of virilization even in the presence of elevated maternal androgens during pregnancy (91).

Newborn Screening CAH is well suited for neonatal screening because it is common and easily diagnosed and early treatment can lead to a greatly improved outcome. Newborn screening for CAH due to 21-OHD began in 1997 and is now commonplace in many countries worldwide. A heel stick is performed on babies in the first week of life, and 17-OHP concentrations are analyzed. Babies with increased 17-OHP concentrations are at risk of having CAH secondary to 21-OHD. It is important to note that collecting samples before 36 hours of life results in a higher

false-positive rate (93). Additionally, because the current newborn screens test only for elevation of 17-OHP, they are limited to the detection of CAH secondary to 21-OH deficiency only. Therefore, a negative newborn screen for CAH in a virilized infant does not rule out all forms of CAH.

Multiple laboratory techniques are available to measure 17-OHP concentrations. Radioimmunoassay (RIA) is the least expensive and most widely used technique (94), but enzyme-linked immunosorbent assay (ELISA) and time-resolved fluoroimmunoassay also have been used (93). Fluoroimmunoassays measure significantly higher concentrations of 17-OHP than RIAs. Additionally, fluoroimmunoassays may overestimate levels on 17-OHP in infants weighing less than 1500 g (95).

A screening test is considered positive when the 17-OHP level is greater than the 99th percentile of the mean level in healthy newborns. Cutoffs for normal 17-OHP concentrations vary across testing centers based on technique accounting for differences in antibodies and reagents and the ethnic makeup of the reference newborns. Preterm infants, especially those less than 30 weeks gestation, will have higher 17-OHP concentrations due to decreased 11β-OHlase activity (96). Therefore, many testing centers have varying cutoff levels based on birth weight or gestation. Other factors that could contribute to falsely elevated 17-OHP levels and subsequent false-positive results are severe illness or dehydration and crossreactions with immunoassay antibodies or reagents.

When a 17-OHP level is found to be elevated, some centers will initiate a second screen with liquid chromatography tandem mass spectrometry (LC-MS/MS), measuring Δ$_4$A and cortisol levels in addition to 17-OHP to ensure that the level is truly elevated and not a false-positive result (see Chapter 2). False-negative results are rare but may occur when an infant is tested before 3 days of life or with corticosteroid use in pregnancy or the neonatal period (93). Maternal glucocorticoid therapy for preterm labor may suppress adrenocorticol function transiently in the newborn, leading to low 17-OHP levels and false-negative newborn screening tests (97). For diagnostic algorithms on patients who receive a positive newborn screen, see Figure 27-11.

Prenatal Diagnosis and Treatment Genetic testing can be used for prenatal diagnosis in women who have previously had children affected with salt-wasting or simple virilizing CAH due to 21-OHD or when both parents are known carriers of a classical (severe) mutation. In the past, prenatal diagnosis was made by measuring amniotic fluid concentrations of 17-OHP, Δ$_4$A, and 11-deoxycortisol and

HLA typing becauses the different forms of CAH can be associated with characteristic HLA haplotypes (genetic disequilibrium). For example, the nonclassical CAH phenotype has been associated with the HLA-B14, DR1 haplotype, particularly in the eastern European population; the simple virilizing form has been associated with the B5(w51) haplotype, and the salt-wasting phenotype with the HLA-A3, Bw47, DR7 haplotype in the northern European population (98).

Prenatal treatment with dexamethasone has been used since 1984 to prevent virilization of the external genitalia of affected female fetuses. However, the safety of this treatment has not been fully established through rigorously controlled trials, and many advocate that it remain experimental (103). The aim is to increase fetal glucocorticoid concentration (because dexamethasone crosses the placenta and is not inactivated by placental 11β-HSD-2 enzyme) and through negative feedback to suppress the elevated ACTH that drives fetal adrenal androgen production in affected fetuses. Generally, treatment must be initiated before 8 weeks' gestation. Currently, if both parents are known CAH carriers, dexamethasone therapy (20 μg/kg/day in three divided doses based on prepregnancy weight) can be initiated before the eighth week of gestation. Chorionic villus sampling can be performed and provide information about sex and CYP21 genotype. If the child is a male, dexamethasone treatment can be stopped regardless of genotype. If the child is a female and affected with CAH, dexamethasone therapy is continued throughout the pregnancy. Prenatal dexamethasone treatment appears to decrease the degree of virilization in affected females, but long-term treatment effects are largely unknown.

One of the drawbacks of the prenatal therapy is that a fetus at risk for 21OHD will receive at least 6 weeks of dexamethasone treatment before a diagnosis is made. CAH is an autosomal recessive disease, and only one in four treated fetuses will be affected, and half of these fetuses will be males. As a result, only one in eight of the affected fetuses will be female and therefore will have a theoretical chance to be helped by prenatal therapy. Seven of the eight fetuses will receive therapy needlessly for at least 6 weeks. Long-term follow-up studies are in need not only of the affected female fetuses, whose mothers were treated with dexamethasone throughout pregnancy, but also of the seven of eight fetuses whose mothers received dexamethasone treatment at least for 6 weeks before it was determined that they were not affected or that they were affected but males. Of note, 20 μg/kg of dexamethasone exposes the fetus to cortisol levels 10 times higher than they are normally exposed to in utero (99).

Treatment of rats with 20 μg/kg of dexamethasone throughout pregnancy resulted in reduced birth weight and elevated blood pressure at 6 months of age, which is equivalent to 35 years of age in humans (100). Long-term follow-up, including carbohydrate metabolism, blood pressure, and cognitive evaluation, should extend beyond childhood to adulthood (92).

The minimum dose of steroid required to achieve sufficient fetal adrenal suppression is yet to be determined. The dose generally recommended for prenatal treatment is based on the dose needed to suppress 17-OHP concentrations in the amniotic fluid at midterm and may be higher than the required dose to suppress the fetal HPA axis. A recent study showed that adrenal explants from 8 weeks postconception (wpc) fetuses have a robust capacity to secrete cortisol that is ACTH-responsive and that cortisol secretion decreases after 10 wpc, rising rapidly again toward term (13). This study indicates 1) that high dose of dexamethasone should be used during the time that cortisol levels are normally high (8 wpc until perhaps 16 wpc) (101) and 2) that reduced doses of dexamethasone for the remainder of the pregnancy may be effective in preventing female virilization and reducing adverse maternal side effects (102).

Psychological Support Psychological support and counseling should be provided for children born with CAH of any type and their families. Parents may experience a range of emotions when they learn about their child's condition, from initial shock and confusion, shame and anxiety, to anger and sadness. Out of concern, parents also may become overprotective of their child with CAH, sometimes causing other children in the family to be neglected. Addressing these feelings will facilitate the acceptance necessary to act in the child's best interest. Health providers can provide reassurance by expressing empathy, normalizing these reactions, and emphasizing that children with CAH are no less likely than other children to become well-adjusted, productive members of society (104,105). Parents will have questions about the child's future, including issues of gender identity and role, sexual orientation, and sexual and reproductive functioning. At birth, parents should be informed completely about their child's condition and counseled in order to make a fully informed decision regarding sex assignment and the available medical interventions (e.g., hormone therapy, genital reconstructive surgery, and their timing). Such counseling is best provided by a mental health professional who is part of a multidisciplinary team that specializes in the clinical

management of CAH and other disorders of sex development (106). These teams are not always readily available, and parents are not always amenable to seeing a psychologist or psychiatrist (107). The treating physician can help by explaining that counseling is a regular part of the assessment and treatment process. Peer support organizations are another potential resource.

Affected patients are best served by accurate information about their condition and prognosis. However, information needs to be paced and provided in a sensitive, age-appropriate manner (108), and preferably by the parents (88), although this is easier said than done. Many parents have great difficulty talking about sex, gender, and sexuality, especially to children. Above all, parents, counselor, and treating physicians should agree on what information to provide and when. Information and emotional support will help most children and adolescents to accept and adapt to their CAH condition. Children and adolescents who are ridiculed by their peers for being different may need additional assistance in the form of psychological and school-based interventions (e.g., a private locker room). Teasing by peers appears to be an important contributor to mental health problems of patients with an intersex condition (109).

All patients with CAH are likely, at one time or another, to struggle with shame as a result of the stigma associated with their condition. In an analysis of the life histories of adults with CAH and other disorders of sex development, their adaptation to being different was likened to the "coming out" process for gay and lesbian individuals (110). Contact with similar others enabled participants to "own" their condition, create greater visibility to combat isolation, and shape their treatment. CAH patients may encounter challenges associated with their condition at any point in their lives. These may stem from gender identity or body image concerns (111,112), sexual functioning or infertility concerns (113), or social difficulties. Almost all patients with 46,XX CAH develop a female gender identity (114), but in terms of gender role, girls with CAH have been shown to be more masculine (115,116). Body image concerns may relate to genital appearance, precocious puberty, or height. Patients with CAH may avoid dating and sexual relations (117) because of shame and fear of rejection. They may experience grief associated with infertility. In all situations, providers should be prepared to offer knowledgeable and sensitive care and provide appropriate referrals to mental health professionals, specialists in gender and sexual health, and peer support.

CAH DUE TO 17α-HYDROXYLASE/17,20-LYASE (P450c17) DEFICIENCY

Etiology/Pathophysiology CAH due to 17α-hydroxylase/17,20-lyase deficiency (P450c17) is a rare autosomal recessive disorder causing decreased production of cortisol and sex steroids and increased synthesis of mineralocorticoid precursors due to a defect of the CYP17 gene that encodes the P450c17 microsomal enzyme. This enzyme has two distinct activities: 1) 17α-hydroxylase (17α-OHlase) which catalyzes the 17α-hydroxylation of the C_{21} steroids (pregnenolone and progesterone) and is necessary for cortisol synthesis, and 2) 17,20-lyase, which catalyzes the scission of the C_{17-20} bond, converting C_{21} compounds to C_{19} steroids and yielding DHEA and to a lesser extent Δ_4A. These adrenal steroids do not bind to the androgen receptor but exert either estrogenic or androgenic action after their conversion into active estrogens and/or androgens in target tissues. These two enzymatic activities are differentially regulated in a tissue- and time-dependent manner. The CYP17 gene is mapped to chromosome 10q24.3 and is expressed in the zonae fasciculata and reticularis of the adrenals, Leydig cells of the testis, and theca cells of the ovary (118–120).

The P450c17 enzyme, like the P450c21 enzyme, receives electrons from flavoprotein P450 oxidoreductase (POR). Both enzymes compete for the electrons provided by POR. Decreased electron availability or mutations that disrupt electron transfer result in decreased 17,20-lyase activity. On the other hand, factors that facilitate electron transfer, such as high concentrations of POR or cytochrome b5 (4) and serine phosphorylation of P450c17 (5,6), favor 17,20-lyase activity and DHEA and Δ_4A formation. Expression studies in patients with isolated 17,20-lyase activity showed that mutant P450c17 enzymes retained 17α-OHlase activity but had minimal 17,20-lyase activity due to 1) diminished ability to interact with POR or 2) decreased phosphorylation of P450c17, resulting in loss of the electron transfer or diversion to uncoupling reactions (121).

In 17α-OHlase/17,20-lyase deficiency, increased ACTH stimulation of the zona fasciculata results in increased production of DOC a steroid with mineralocorticoid activity, and corticosterone (B), a steroid with glucocorticoid activity through the 17-deoxy pathway that does not require 17α-hydroxylation (122), resulting in sodium retention, hypertension, and hypokalemia (Figure 27-12). The sodium retention and subsequent plasma volume expansion suppress plasma renin activity (PRA) and inhibit aldosterone synthesis in the zona

Steroidogenesis in 17α-hydroxylase/ 17, 20 lyase Deficiency (P450c17)

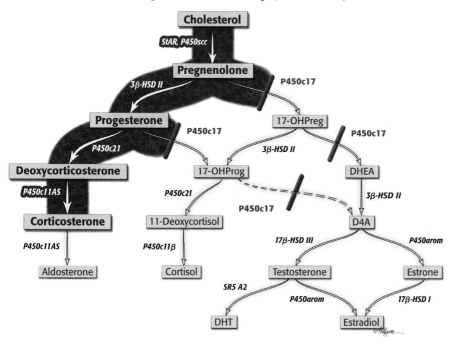

FIGURE 27-12. Congenital adrenal hyperplasia due to 17α-hydroxylase/17,20-lyase deficiency. This is a rare autosomal recessive disorder causing decreased production of cortisol and sex steroids and increased synthesis of mineralocorticoid precursors due to a defect of the CYP17 gene that encodes the P450c17 microsomal enzyme. This enzyme has two distinct activities: 1) 17α-hydroxylase, which catalyzes the 17α-hydroxylation of the C_{21} steroids (pregnenolone and progesterone) and is necessary for the cortisol synthesis, and 2) 17,20-lyase, which catalyzes the scission of the C_{17-20} bond, converting C_{21} compounds to C_{19} steroids, yielding DHEA and to a lesser extent Δ_4A.

glomerulosa through the renin–angiotensin–aldosterone axis. A distinguishing characteristic in these patients is that while they are cortisol-deficient, they do not experience adrenal crisis. Corticosterone has some glucocorticoid activity and thus at elevated levels (50–100 times normal) prevents adrenal insufficiency.

Clinical Presentation Patients with P450c17 deficiency (partial or complete) have reduced or absent levels of both gonadal and adrenal sex hormones, resulting in sexual infantilism in 46,XX females and genital ambiguity in 46,XY males ranging from phenotypic female (complete 46,XY sex reversal) to undervirilized male genitalia. In sex-reversed affected males, there is no Wolffian duct development due to absence of testoterone synthesis in utero. However, since the Sertoli cells produce anti-Müllerian hormone (AMH), these patients present with a blind vaginal pouch and absence of Müllerian structures (123–126).

Sex-reversed 46,XY males or 46, XX affected females may go undetected until puberty, at which time they present as an apparent female patient with a hernia or inguinal mass, primary amenorrhea, hypertension, and lack of secondary sex development (including pubic and axillary hair). Patients may be tall, with

eunuchoid proportions due to lack of sex steroids. Histology of the testes reveals atrophic tubules and Sertoli cells, Leydig cell hyperplasia, and little evidence of spermatogenesis. Ovaries of the affected 46,XX females often have multiple cysts and few ova and follicles.

Some degree of hypokalemia and hypertension is present in 85% to 90% of patients due to the mineralocorticoid properties of DOC and corticosterone.

Partial combined 17α-OHlase/17,20-lyase deficiency may present with irregular menses and, subsequently, amenorrhea, hypertension, hypokalemia with metabolic alkalosis, hypoplastic or absent breast development, and no axilliary or pubic hair. Hyperplasia of the adrenals and uterine hypoplasia and atrophy of the ovaries may be present (127–129).

A very mild P450c17 deficiency has been described in a female, homozygous for the Y201N mutation, who presented with low-renin hypertension, history of irregular menses, infertility, and sparse pubic and axillary hair. She was normocalemic and had significant elevation of B along with mildly elevated DOC (130).

Affected 46,XY patients with isolated 17, 20-lyase deficiency may present with undervirilization at birth, such as penoscrotal hypospadias, bifid scrotum, micropenis, blind

vaginal pouch, incomplete virilization during pubertal years, and gynecomastia (121,123).

Diagnosis Biochemical evaluation of patients with combined 17α-OHlase/17,20-lyase deficiencies shows that all steroids requiring P450c17 enzymatic activity (17-hydroxypregnenolone, 17-OHP, 11-deoxycortisol, cortisol, DHEA, Δ_4A, and testosterone) are decreased or absent. Baseline and ACTH-stimulated progesterone levels are significantly elevated, ranging from 0.7–14 ng/mL (124), which along with low 17-OHP and 11-deoxycortisol and the absence of virilized phenotype, differentiates CAH due to P450c17 deficiency from CAH due to 21-OHD or 11-OHD. Aldosterone levels are decreased due to elevated DOC (>100 ng/dL) and B (50–100 times higher than the reference range). Renin levels can be low or normal in the presence of hypertension. LH and FSH levels are elevated secondary to low sex steroid levels (androgens and estrogens). Decreased baseline cortisol and adrenal androgens (DHEA and Δ_4A) do not rise after ACTH stimulation. There is no increase in sex steroids (testosterone, DHT, and E_2) in response to human chorionic gonadotropin (β-hCG) stimulation tests. The decreased testosterone levels and subnormal response to β-hCG stimulation differentiate affected 46,XY patients from patients with complete or partial testicular feminization, who also can present at birth with sex reversal or undervirilization.

Patients with isolated 17,20-lyase deficiency show no significant testosterone response to the β-hCG stimulation test but can show an increase or even an exaggerated 17-OHP response. LH and FSH levels are elevated secondary to low sex steroid levels. The ACTH stimulation test shows normal cortisol response, a significant rise in progesterone levels, and no rise in DHEA and Δ_4A levels.

Genetic Testing Several mutations have been identified, with most of them eliminating both activities of the P450c17 enzyme, whereas some others reduce both activities partially or cause selective deficiency of the 17,20-lyase activity. Two mutations, R358Q and R347H, have been shown to cause isolated 17,20-lyase deficiency. When expressed in COS-1 cells, the mutant proteins retained 17α-OHlase activity but had minimal 17,20-lyase activity because their ability to interact with redox partners was diminished. Heterozygotes may have exaggerated responses to ACTH stimulation. Most mutations are random and spontaneous. Prenatal diagnosis is possible by measuring amniotic fluid concentrations of adrenal steroids. A PHE53/54DEL mutation with high prevalence in the Japanese population is associated with well-preserved gonadal function in young-adult patients but may cause early reduction of gonadal function with increasing age (129).

Treatment Patients with P450c17 deficiency usually require a smaller dose of glucocorticoid replacement than the standard dose used in treating other CAH disorders. The goal of treatment is to suppress ACTH secretion, decrease DOC and B accumulation, and normalize serum potassium and blood pressure. Patients who remain hypertensive on glucocorticoid replacement therapy require the addition of a mineralocorticoid antagonist (e.g., spironolactone or eplerenone) or calcium channel blocker. Dietary control of sodium intake is recommended.

Patients with severe hypertension at presentation should be monitored closely at the start of treatment. Glucocorticoid therapy suppresses ACTH-driven DOC production through the zona fasciculata and may lead to acute sodium loss and volume depletion until the suppressed renin–angiotensin–aldosterone axis recovers (recovery of the axis is variable and can take months to years).

Sex steroid replacement therapy appropriate for the phenotypic sex is started at the expected time of puberty to induce secondary sexual characteristic development and bone mass accrual (for details, see Chapter 36).

46,XX females require both estrogen and progestin every month to prevent endometrial hyperplasia from unopposed estrogen. However, 46,XY sex-reversed males, because they are phenotypic females but lack Müllerian structures, are treated with estrogen alone.

Measuring renin, DOC, B, electrolytes, weight gain, growth rate, and blood pressure monitors adequacy of treatment. Infants and young children should be evaluated every 3 months. A bone age determination should be obtained yearly to evaluate skeletal maturation. Unlike other forms of CAH, accelerated growth is not a concern. However, a decreased growth rate and delayed bone age may indicate a supraphysiological glucocorticoid dose that needs to be decreased. Alternatively, dexamethasone (0.25–0.5 mg/day) may be used as treatment in adults.

Surgical Treatment Affected 46,XY patients with sex reversal require gonadectomy to prevent malignant degeneration of their gonads. Preferably this is performed before 8–10 years of age.

CAH DUE TO 3β-HYDROXYSTEROID DEHYDROGENASE TYPE-II (3β-HSD-II) DEFICIENCY

Etiology/Pathophysiology CAH due to 3β-hydroxysteroid dehydrogenase type-II (3β-HSD-II) deficiency is a rare autosomal re-

Steroidogenesis in 3β-Hydroxysteroid Dehydrogenase Deficiency (3β-HSD II)

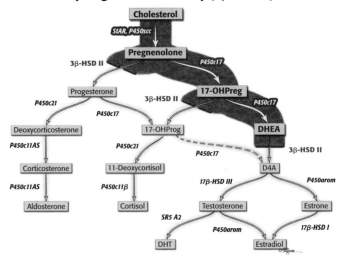

FIGURE 27-13. Congenital adrenal hyperplasia due to 3β-hydroxysteroid dehydrogenase type II (3β-HSD-II) deficiency. Impaired enzymatic activity affects the catalyzation of the 3β-dehydrogenation and isomerization of the Δ_5-3β-hydroxysteroids to Δ_4-β-ketosteroids, which convert pregnenolone to progesterone (mineralocorticoid pathway), 17α-hydroxypregnenolone to 17α-hydroxyprogesterone (glucocorticoid pathway), and dehydroepiandrosterone (DHEA) to androstenedione (sex steroid pathway in both adrenals and gonads).

cessive disorder that accounts for 1% of all cases of CAH and is characterized by impaired synthesis of all adrenal and gonadal steroids. The 3β-HSD isozymes catalyzes the 3β-dehydrogenation and isomerization of the Δ_5-3β-hydroxysteroids to Δ_4-β-ketosteroids, converting pregnenolone to progesterone (mineralocorticoid pathway), 17α-hydroxypregnenolone to 17-OHP (glucocorticoid pathway), and DHEA to Δ_4A (sex steroid pathway in both adrenals and gonads). Decreased cortisol synthesis results in increased ACTH stimulation and accumulation of steroids prior to enzymatic block, including pregnenolone, 17α-hydroxypregnenolone, and DHEA (Figure 27-13). There are two isozymes of 3β-HSD that are 93.5% homologous in their amino acid sequences and are encoded by two different genes, HSD3B1 and HSD3B2. Both genes have been localized to chromosome 1p11-13 and consist of four exons and three introns (131,132).

The 3β-HSD-I enzyme is expressed in the placenta and peripheral tissues such as liver, skin, and mammary glands, whereas the 3β-HSD-II enzyme is expressed in the adrenals and the gonads. Although 3β-HSD-I is detected at very low levels in normal gonads, its affinity is 10-fold higher than the 3β-HSD-II isozyme. No patients have been described with CAH due to mutations of the HSD3B1 gene (133).

Clinical Presentation Severe deficiency of the 3β-HSD-II enzyme presents in early infancy with adrenal insufficiency and salt wasting in both sexes. 46,XY infants present

with varying degrees of undervirilization ranging from hypospadias and micropenis to penoscrotal hypospadias with bifid scrotum due to decreased synthesis of androgens; the peripheral conversion of adrenal and testicular DHEA by the 3β-HSD-I enzyme to active androgens and the residual activity, if there is any, of the 3β-HSD-II enzyme are insufficient to allow normal male genital development. Conversely, 46,XX infants may present with normal genitalia or mild to moderate clitoromegaly and/or partial labial fusion due to peripheral conversion of elevated DHEA to testosterone by the isozyme 3β-HSD-I.

Affected males with partial or complete 3β-HSD-II deficiency, like affected males with 5α-reductase type 2 deficiency and 17β-HSD-III deficiency, have intact Wolffian duct structures, including the vas deferens. The salt-wasting form of classic 3β-HSD-II deficiency usually is diagnosed during the first few months of life due to decreased aldosterone synthesis.

In contrast, the non-salt-wasting form of 3β-HSD-II deficiency can be diagnosed either early in infancy in the presence of perineal hypospadias in males and mild clitoromegaly in female newborns, especially in the presence of other factors such as family history of death in early infancy, or at a later age when patients can present with premature adrenarche, growth acceleration, and bone advancement.

Increased LH levels during puberty secondary to low testosterone levels stimulate 3β-HSD-I activity in affected patients, resulting in increased conversion of Δ_5 to Δ_4 steroids.

As a result, affected 46,XY patients who present with or without salt wasting and undervirilized genitalia at birth may develop premature adrenarche and undergo normal to incomplete masculinization with gynecomastia during puberty. Similarly, affected females who present with or without salt wasting and normal to mild virilized external genitalia at birth may have premature adrenarche, usually spontaneous pubertal maturation and menarche, and irregular menses due to partial ovarian 3β-HSD-II deficiency (133–138); lack of pubertal development in affected females as well as males has been described (133,139). Spermatogenesis may be adequate (133) or impaired (azoospermia) with coexistence of adrenal rests in the testes.

A milder, late-onset form of 3β-HSD-II deficiency may present in affected females during childhood and adolescence with premature adrenarche and advanced linear and skeletal growth (140). Delayed diagnosis of CAH with salt wasting due to 3β-HSD-II deficiency also has be described (141).

Diagnosis The basal plasma levels of Δ_5 steroids such as pregnenolone, 17α-hydroxypregnenolone, and DHEA are elevated in affected individuals, and the ratio of Δ_5 to Δ_4 steroids is also elevated. However, females with hyperandrogenism and insulin-resistant PCO syndrome or children with exaggerated adrenarche and no mutations of the 3β-HSD-II gene may appear with a hormonal phenotype suggesting dysfunction of the 3β-HSD-II enzyme (142).

The validity of hormonal criteria used in the past for diagnosing mild 3β-HSD-II deficiency in a substantial number of women with hyperandrogenism or children with exaggerated premature adrenarche have been questioned because the diagnosis of mild 3β-HSD-II deficiency in these patients was based solely on elevations (greater than or equal to 2 SD) of Δ_5 steroids and Δ_5:Δ_4 ratios, and later studies found no mutations of the 3β-HSD-II gene in these patients (143).

Hormonal evaluation in patients with mutations of the HSD-II gene have shown that ACTH-stimulated 17-hydroxypregnenolone determination is more accurate in diagnosing 3β-HSD-II deficiency than baseline and ACTH-stimulated levels of DHEA: Δ_4A ratios. Patients with genotypical proof of 3β-HSD-II deficiency have been described to have ACTH-stimulated 17α-hydroxypregnenolone levels greater than 378 nmol/L in neonates, 165 nmol/L in prepubertal children with ambiguous genitalia, 294 nmol/L in affected children presenting with premature pubarche, and 289 nmol/L

in adult affected males (144). Overall, a 17-hydroxyprenenolone level greater than 147 nmol/L after ACTH stimulation is considered consistent with 3β-HSD-II deficiency (134,140,144–146).

Carriers of 3β-HSD-II gene mutations have normal enzymatic activity and baseline stimulated ACTH values of 17-hydroxypregnenolone, and the ratio of Δ_5 to Δ_4 steroids does not differ significantly from that of age-matched normal females and males (147).

Baseline 17-OHP levels in patients with 3β-HSD-II deficiency and salt wasting may be elevated as a result of normal 3β-HSD-I activity in the peripheral tissues, leading to erroneous diagnosis of CAH due to 21-OH deficiency. However, the discordance between the elevated 17-OHP levels and the clinical phenotype (salt wasting in the presence of normal or mild virilized genitalia in females and salt wasting in undervirilized males) should suggest the possibility of CAH due to 3β-HSD-II deficiency.

In males, the response to β-hCG is usually poor in infancy but may be substantial in pubertal boys seconday to increased activity of 3β-HSD-I, ranging from subnormal to normal.

Genetic Testing

Multiple mutations have been identified; missense mutations usually cause only partial deficiency of the enzyme (148).

Treatment Glucocorticoid replacement and mineralocorticoid therapy are indicated in patients with the salt-wasting form. Sex steroid replacement therapy appropriate for the phenotypic sex is started in patients who fail to develop secondary sex characterisitics (mean age for the appearance of secondary sexual characteristics in the general population is 11.5–12.0 years for males and 10.5 years for females). For detailed sex replacement therapy see Chapter 36.

Adequacy of treatment is monitored by measuring renin, electrolytes, Δ_5 steroids (i.e., DHEA/DHEA-S, pregnenolone, and progesterone), weight gain, and growth rate. Infants and young children should be evaluated every 3 months. A bone age should be obtained yearly to evaluate skeletal maturation. A decreased growth rate and delayed bone age may indicate that the glucocorticoid dose is supraphysiological and needs to be decreased.

In the milder, late-onset form of 3β-HSD deficiency, glucocorticoid replacement therapy is initiated in females to treat sequelae of androgen excess (i.e., hirsutism, acne, and menstrual irregularities).

CAH DUE TO 11β-HYDROXYLASE (P450C11) DEFICIENCY

Etiology/Pathophysiology CAH due to 11β-hydroxylase (P450c11) deficiency is the second most common defect causing CAH (5% to 8% of cases) and results in decreased production of cortisol with accumulation of mineralocorticoid precursors in the zona fasciculata and increased synthesis of adrenal androgens in the zona reticularis. An increased relative frequency of 11β-hydroxylase deficiency (11-OHD) has been noted in Jews from Morocco and Iran, as well in Saudi Arabians (149–151). The CYP11B1 gene that encodes 11β-hydroxylase enzyme is 93% identical with the CYP11B2 gene that encodes P450c11AS (aldosterone synthase); both genes are localized to chromosome 8q24.3 (152,153). P450c11 isozyme is responsible for synthesis of cortisol and corticosterone in the zona fasciculata, and P450c11AS is responsible for aldosterone synthesis in the zona glomerulosa. As with other P450 isozymes, the transfer of electrons from NADPH is achieved through adrenodoxin reductase and adrenodoxin.

Cortisol is synthesized in the zona fasciculata through five enzymatic conversions, including cholesterol side-chain cleavage, 17α-hydroxylation, 3β-dehydrogenation, and successive hydroxylations at the 21β and 11β positions. A 17-deoxy pathway is also active in the zona fasciculata, in which 17-hydroxylation does not occur, and the final product is normally corticosterone (B) (154).

The isozyme, under the regulation of ACTH, converts 1) 11-deoxycortisol (S) to cortisol and 2) DOC to corticosterone (B) in the zona fasciculata. Blockage of the production of cortisol leads to ACTH-stimulated adrenal hyperplasia and subsequent accumulation of steroid precursors, which are diverted toward the androgen synthesis pathway (Figure 27-14). The 17-deoxy pathway in the zona fasciculata, with B as the end product, is similar to the pathway in the zona glomerulosa, in which aldosterone is the final product. The zona fasciculata production of DOC, through the 17-deoxy pathway, increases in patients with P450c11 deficiency secondary to elevated ACTH levels. The accumulation of DOC increases sodium absorption with subsequent volume expansion and results in the suppression of plasma renin and decreased production of aldosterone in the zona glomerulosa.

The P450c11AS isozyme, or aldosterone synthase, is expressed only in the zona glomerulosa and mediates all three steps necessary for aldosterone synthesis (11β-hydroxylation, 18-hydroxylation, and 18-oxidation). It is regulated

Steroidogenesis in 11β-hydroxylase Deficiency
(P450c11β)

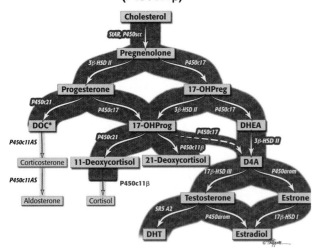

FIGURE 27-14. Congenital adrenal hyperplasia due to 11β-hydroxylase deficiency. Impaired enzymatic activity affects the CYP11B1 isozyme, which converts 1) 11-deoxycortisol (S) to cortisol and 2) 11-deoxycorticosterone (DOC) to corticosterone (B) in the zona fasciculata, resulting in decreased production of cortisol with accumulation of mineralocorticoid precursors in the zona fasciculata and increased synthesis of adrenal androgens in the zona reticularis. *Of note, there is an ACTH-stimulated 7-deoxy pathway in the zona fasciculata, with B as the end product, and it is similar to the pathway in the zona glomerulosa, in which aldosterone is the final product. In patients with CYP11B1 deficiency, DOC's conversion to B in the zona fasciculata through the 17-deoxy pathway is blocked, resulting in increased DOC levels secondary to elevated ACTH levels. The accumulation of DOC increases sodium absorption with subsequent volume expansion and results in suppression of plasma renin and decreased production of aldosterone in the zona glomerulosa.

by the renin–angiotensin system. A deficiency of P450c11AS causes isolated aldosterone deficiency with salt wasting and is not associated with CAH (for details, see Chapter 29).

Clinical Presentation In the newborn period, affected 46,XX patients typically present with ambiguous external genitalia ranging from clitoromegaly to phallic urethra with fused labial-scrotal folds. Affected 46,XY patients present with hyperpigmentation of the scrotum, and they usually are diagnosed in early childhood when they present with increased virilization.

Both sexes have normal internal genitalia and experience postnatal virilization (i.e., growth acceleration, advanced bone age, and early development of secondary sexual characteristics). Hypertension of various degrees of severity is present in 75% of patients of both sexes and is the distinguishing feature of 11-OHD that differentiates it from CAH due to 21-OHD (particularly the simple virilizing form). There is usually no correlation between the severity of the cardiovascular manifestations and the degree of virilization (150). Some of the cardiovascular manifestations include left ventricular hypertrophy and retinopathy; deaths from cerebrovascular accidents also have been reported. Although excess of DOC may contribute to hypertension, it is not the sole factor because DOC excess does not correlate with the degree of severity of hypertension. Few patients have been reported to present in salt-wasting crisis,

precipitated by glucocorticoid therapy; it has been suggested that suppression of the ACTH-stimulated excessive secretion of DOC from zona fasciculata with the initiation of therapy and the absence of an immediate increase in aldosterone secretion from the zona glomerulosa are responsible for the salt wasting (155–157). However, some patients developed salt-wasting crises before initiation of treatment, and the mechanism is not clear (155).

A mild form of nonclassical 11-OHD is rare and may present with menstrual irregularities and hirsutism in adolescent or adult women (158). Elevated DOC levels and/or hypertension distinguishes 11-OHD deficiency from 21-OHD.

Diagnosis Characteristic biochemical abnormalities include high basal or ACTH-stimulated levels of S and DOC, although some patients have been described with selective elevation of either DOC or S (155). A 24-hour urine collection shows elevated excretion of the tetrahydrometabolites of DOC and S, as well as of 17-ketosteroids. The diagnosis should be suspected in patients who have ACTH-stimulated levels of S and DOC that are more than five times the 95th percentile for age (158,159) and impaired cortisol response. Renin usually is suppressed, and aldosterone is low due to volume expansion secondary to the mineralocorticoid effect of elevated DOC. Hypokalemia is present in a minority of patients. Heterozygous carriers have no consistent bio-

chemical abnormalities at baseline after the ACTH stimulation test. The diagnosis of 11-OHD may be missed in neonates, who often lack the diagnostic features of hypertension and suppressed renin. An erroneous diagnosis of CAH due to 21-OHD can be made in patients with mild to moderate elevations of 17-OHP (17-OHP is often elevated in patients with 11-OHD), in whom DOC and S levels have not been measured.

Genetic Testing

Several mutations have been described (160,161), with the R448H being more prevalent in Moroccan Jews. Prenatal diagnosis is feasible in families in which the mutation has been identified.

Treatment Patients with CAH secondary to 11β-OH deficiency require glucocorticoid replacement (usually in the form of hydrocortisone 8–10 mg/m²/day) to replace deficient cortisol and suppress ACTH secretion. Glucocorticoid replacement prevents further virilization and ameliorates hypertension by suppressing the excess production of mineralocorticoid agonists stimulated by ACTH. At times, it is necessary to use antihypertensives, such as potassium-sparing diuretics or calcium channel blockers, in patients who are still hypertensive on glucocorticoid therapy or have had long-standing high blood pressure before diagnosis. Generally, angiotensin-converting enzymes inhibitors or β-adrenergic receptor blockers are not effective in the treatment of low-renin hypertension. The approach to females with ambiguous genitalia is similar to that for virilized females due to 21-OH deficiency.

Monitoring of the adequacy of glucocorticoid replacement dose includes measurement of renin, DOC and S, adrenal androgens, and growth rate and weight gain during each visit, every 3–4 months. Pubic hair development or progression or signs of early puberty should be monitored carefully. Bone age should be checked once a year. A decreased growth rate, weight gain, or delay in bone age suggests overtreatment, even in the presence of hypertension and normal DOC and S levels.

GLUCOCORTICOID-SUPPRESSIBLE HYPERALDOSTERONISM (GSH)

Etiology/Pathophysiology Although not a form of CAH, glucocorticoid suppressible hyperaldosteronism (GSH), known as *dexamethasone-suppressible hyperaldosteronism*, is an autosomal dominant disorder. It is characterized by inappropriate expression of aldosterone synthase activity in the zona fasciculata that results in low-renin hypertension, ACTH-stimulated hyperaldosteronism, and increased production of two "hybrid" steroids, 18-hydroxycortisol (18-OHF) and 18-oxocortisol (18-OXOF). GSH is rare, accounting for 1% of cases of primary hyperaldosteronism. As the name implies, all symptoms are normalized by glucocorticoid therapy.

The genetic defect in GSH is the formation of a hybrid gene from unequal crossover of genetic material at meiosis between the CYP11B1 (11β-hydroxylase) gene, which encodes the enzyme that catalyzes the last step of cortisol biosynthesis in the zona fasciculata, and the CYP11B2 (aldosterone synthase) gene, which encodes the enzyme that catalyzes the conversion of DOC to aldosterone in the zona glomerulosa (162,163).

Specifically, the chimeric gene represents a fusion of the 5'-adrenocorticotropin-responsive regulatory region of the CYP11B1 gene (the ACTH-responsive promoter) and the 3' coding sequence of the CYP11B2 gene, thereby causing ectopic expression of aldosterone synthase in the cortisol-producing zona fasciculata under the strong direction of ACTH (164). Normally, aldosterone is affected only indirectly by ACTH stimulation, with the main regulators being angiotensin II and potassium.

Another characteristic of GSH is the increased production (20–30 times normal levels) of "hybrid" steroids 18-OHF and 18-OXOF, which are the 17α-hydroxylated analogues of 18-hydroxycorticosterone and aldosterone, respectively. The markedly elevated levels of these steroids are the best indication of the overproduction of aldosterone in the zona fasciculata because the 17α-hydroxylase enzyme is expressed only in the zona fasciculata. Interestingly, since the chimeric gene is ACTH-regulated, aldosterone production of affected patients does not increase after stimulation with angiotensin II or in response to upright posture after overnight recumbency (165). From a pathophysiological point of view, it is the ACTH regulation of aldosterone production that explains the effectiveness of glucocorticoid therapy in controlling the manifestations of GSH. The mechanism of this effectiveness could be the following: because this is an autosomal dominant disorder, there is the chimeric gene and copies of the normal CYP11B1 and CYP11B2 genes. Cortisol production is slightly decreased (166) but continues through the CYP11B1 gene expression in the zona fasciculata. However, to maintain normal cortisol levels, there is an increase in ACTH production, which increases cortisol synthesis to appropriate levels but also increases the synthesis of aldosterone and the "hybrid" steroids 18-OHF and 18-OXOF through the chimeric gene.

Clinical Presentation Patients present with moderate to severe hypertension before age 20 and with the typical complications associated with hypertension (i.e., left ventricular hypertrophy and retinopathy). Patients are at risk for early stroke (<45 years of age) due to intracerebral hemorrhage. Females seem to have milder hypertension than males (165).

Diagnosis Aldosterone levels may be moderately elevated or normal. Potassium may be normal to low (approximately 50% of patients have hypokalemia). Renin levels are always low. The aldosterone:renin ratio is always elevated (>30) (167). Patients with GSH have elevated urinary levels of hybrid steroids such as 18-OHF and 18-OXOF; 18-OXOF levels seem to correlate with the severity of hypertension (165,168). A dexamethasone suppression test administered as 0.5 mg every 6 hours for 2 days is suggestive of GSH if it results in an aldosterone level of less than 4 ng/dL (166). However, some patients with aldosterone-producing adenomas may have similarly suppressed aldosterone levels in response to dexamethasone. Aldosterone-secreting adenomas are rare causes of hyperaldosteronism in children. Genetic testing is available and confirms the diagnosis of GSH.

Treatment In patients with GSH, treatment with glucocorticoids suppresses ACTH secretion and thus hybrid gene expression, resulting in amelioration of hyperaldosteronism and hypertension. In accordance with a recent study (169), lower doses of steroids can be used for control of hypertension, such as an initial dose of 0.125 mg dexamethasone and a maintenance dose that should be the minimum to maintain normotension and normal left ventricular mass index (LVMI) on echocardiography and should not exceed 0.25 mg dexamethasone in adults; dexamethasone should be administered in the evening in order to cover the ACTH peak during the morning period and optimally suppress the activity of the hybrid gene. In children, because of growth concerns, hydrocortisone twice a day instead of dexamethasone should be administered instead, with the higher dose of hydrocortisone given in the evening. Normalization of urinary 18-OXOF and elevation of renin levels to the upper end of normal may indicate that the steroid dose needs to be decreased.

CONGENITAL LIPOID ADRENAL HYPERPLASIA (StAR DEFICIENCY)

Etiology/Pathophysiology Congenital lipoid adrenal hyperplasia (lipoid CAH) is the most severe form of CAH, in which adrenal and gonadal steroidogenic cells are unable to convert cholesterol to pregnenolone, affecting the synthesis of virtually all adrenal and gonadal steroids (Figure 27-15). The defect in lipoid CAH is primarily in the steroidogenic acute regulatory protein (StAR), which is encoded by the StAR gene, which has been mapped to chromosomal 8p11.2 region. StAR protein shuttles cholesterol into the mitochondria, where the P450scc enzyme catalyzes the conversion of cholesterol to pregnenolone. Few patients so far have been reported with lipoid CAH due to homozygous or compound heterozygous disruptive mutations of the CYP11A1 gene that result in P450scc enzyme deficiency (170–172).

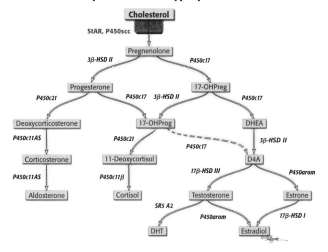

FIGURE 27-15. Congenital lipoid adrenal hyperplasia (lipoid CAH). In congenital lipoid adrenal hyperplasia (lipoid CAH), adrenal and gonadal steroidogenic cells are unable to convert cholesterol to pregnenolone due to a defect primarily in the steroidogenic acute regulatory protein (StAR), which shuttles cholesterol into the mitochondria, thereby affecting the synthesis of virtually all adrenal and gonadal steroids.

One patient was born prematurely (170) and had 46,XY reversal and severe adrenal insufficiency. The other patients presented in late infancy (171,172). No patients with defects of adrenodoxin reductase and adrenodoxin enzymes of the P450scc complex have been found.

StAR gene transcription increases in response to ACTH or LH stimulation, resulting in increased cholesterol transport to the P450scc enzyme and a surge of the stimulated steroids. Transfection of COS-1 cells with the P450scc complex has shown independent of StAR conversion of cholesterol to pregnenolone, particularly in tissues such as the brain and placenta, where there is no StAR expression (173), but following transfection of COS-1 cells with StAR. the conversion rate increased 4–20 times. The StAR independent steroidogenesis and the profound effect of StAR defiency in the active steroidoigenic tissues such as fetal testes and adrenals, with the fetal dormant ovaries being spared, suggest that the lipoid CAH phenotype is the result of two separate events (two-hit model). The first hit involves a genetic defect of the StAR gene, affecting StAR-dependent steroidogenesis in both adrenals and gonads. In response to decreased adrenal and gonadal steroids, ACTH and gonadotropin levels increase, causing accumulation of cholesterol esters in the adrenal cortex and gonads. The second hit is the subsequent loss of StAR-independent steroidogenesis due to cellular damage from accumulated cholesterol esters. Since fetal adrenals and testes are active in utero, producing large amounts of steroids, they are the first to lose both dependent and indepent StAR steroidogenesis in affected patients; 46,XY affected males have profound testosterone deficiency because they fail to develop male genitalia (complete sex reversal at birth) or to go through spontaneous puberty. In contrast, fetal ovaries are dormant until puberty, and ovarian cells are spared from damage (no cholesterol accumulation), maintaining the StAR-independent steroidogenesis and allowing some 46,XX patients to undergo feminization and have menses. Lipoid CAH is more common among the Japanese, Korean, and Palestinian Arab populations but is rare elsewhere.

Clinical Presentation The majority of affected patients with lipoid CAH present during the first month of life with salt wasting and adrenal crisis and female phenotype irrespective of gonadal sex (174,175). 46,XY patients have testes, a blind vaginal pouch, and no Müllerian structures (because Sertoli cells remain undamaged, producing AMH). Wolffian duct derivates may be present because some testosterone produc-

tion may occur early in fetal life through independent of StAR steroidogenesis. Testes can be in the abdomen, inguinal canal, or labia. Most affected patients present with hypoglycemia and generalized pigmentation at birth due to intrauterine glucorticoid deficiency that results in elevated ACTH levels; however, delayed presentations have been reported. Affected 46,XX patients, unlike the 46,XY patients, may experience spontaneous puberty, menarche, premature menopause, and anovulatory menses because their ovaries are able to produce estrogen through StAR-independent pathways (174,176,177). XX females with lipoid CAH also may possess multiple cysts in their ovaries, possibly from anovulation.

Recently, a nonclassical form of lipoid CAH has been reported, in which affected 46,XY patients presented in adrenal crisis during the first 2 years of life with normal male genitalia (178).

Diagnosis Characteristic hormonal abnormalities include elevated ACTH, elevated LH, and decreased or absent adrenal and gonadal steroids, including their precursors, such as pregnenolone and progesterone. Urinary 17-ketosteroids (17-KS) and 17-hydroxycorticosteroids (17-OHCS) are also low. Adrenal and gonadal steroids do not rise with ACTH or β-hCG stimulation. A karyotype should be done on all patients, and an abdominal ultrasound should be done to assess reproductive organs and adrenal gland size. Mothers pregnant with an affected fetus with lipoid CAH have low estriol levels.

The most difficult diagnosis is between affected 46,XY or 46,XX patients with lipoid adrenal hyperplasia and those with congenital adrenal hypoplasia. Small adrenals in 46,XX patients or sex-reversed 46,XY patients with adrenal insufficiency suggest congenital adrenal hypoplasia because patients with lipoid CAH usually have massively enlarged adrenals. Genetic testing for StAR and SFI or DAX-1 genes may be needed to establish an unambiguous diagnosis.

In 46,XX females, estrogen levels vary, LH levels are elevated, and progesterone levels may be undetectable (anovulatory cycles). The ovaries may be polycystic, but in contrast to patients with PCO, females with lipoid CAH have untedectable levels of Δ_4A and testosterone.

Low DOC levels, hyperkalemia, and absence of hypertension in 46,XY males with lipoid CAH differentiate them from 46,XY males with 17α-OHlase/17,20-lyase deficiency because both disorders are characterized by low 17OHP levels and 46,XY sex reversal.

Low 17α-hydroxypregenenolone and low DHEA levels in affected 46,XY or 46,XX patients with lipoid CAH differentiate them from affected 46,XY patients with CAH due

to 3β-HSD-II deficiency because both disorders are characterized by glucocorticoid and mineralcorticoid deficiency, including deficient testosterone synthesis; however, females with 3β-HSD-II deficiency usually are virilized due to elevated DHEA levels.

Genetics

Genetic analysis of patients with lipoid CAH has revealed several mutations of the StAR gene. The mutation Q258X has been found in 80% of affected alleles from Japanese and Korean patients, whereas an R182L mutation has been found in 78% of affected alleles from Palestinian patients (175).

Treatment Patients with lipoid CAH require glucocorticoid and mineralocorticoid replacement therapy similar to patients with salt-wasting CAH due to 21-OHD. Measuring plasma renin activity, blood pressure, and electrolyte levels monitors treatment efficacy for mineralocorticoid replacement. Decreased growth rate or weight gain suggests overtreatment with glucocorticoid.

46,XY sex-reversed males should have their undescended testicles removed to reduce the risk of malignant transformation and require estrogen therapy for development of sex characteristics and subsequently estrogen-replacement therapy without progesterone (because they lack Müllerian structures) (for more details on estrogen-replacement therapy, see Chapter 36). 46,XX patients may experience spontaneous puberty and anovulatory cycles. When ovarian steroidogenesis fails in 46,XX females with lipoid CAH, they are replaced with both estrogen and progestin every month to prevent endometrial hyperplasia from unopposed estrogen.

P450 OXIDOREDUCATASE DEFICIENCY (POR)

Etiology/Pathophysiology CAH due to P450 oxidoreductase deficiency is characterized by apparent combined 21α-OHlase and 17α-OHlase/lyase deficiency with a biochemical phenotype consisting of elevated 17-OHP level (although not as high as in 21-OHD), low adrenal androgens, and no aldosterone deficiency. POR is a single flavoprotein that transfers electrons from nicotinamide adenine dinucleotide phosphate (NADPH) to P450 microsomal enzymes, including P450c21, P450c17, and P450arom. Disruption of the POR gene in knockout mice results in early embryonic death. So far, all patients affected with POR deficiency are either homozygotes for partially inactivating POR mutations or compound heterozygotes for major loss-of-function mutations. The majority of patients described with recessive mutations of the POR gene presented with skeletal abnormalities characteristic of Antley–Bixler syndrome (ABS) and had genital abnormalities; patients with relatively milder mutations of the POR gene had abnormal steroidogenesis but did not have ABS (179–181).

The mechanism by which POR mutations cause skeletal malformations has not been elucidated but may be connected to disorders of cholesterol biosynthesis, particularly of the POR-dependent 14α-demethylase CYP51A1 (182,183).

It has been shown that individuals with an ABS phenotype, autosomal dominant inheritance, and normal steroidogenesis have FGFR mutations, whereas those who have ABS phenotype, autosomal recessive inheritance, ambiguous genitalia and abnormal steroidogenesis have mutations in the POR gene (181).

Clinical Presentation Affected girls are born with ambiguous genitalia (Prader stages III–V) indicating intrauterine androgen excess, but in contrast to what is occurring in 21-OHD or 11-OHD, there is no progression of virilization because circulating adrenal androgens after birth are low or normal. In order to explain the antenatal androgen excess and postnatal androgen deficiency in patients with P450 oxidoreductase deficiency, an alternative pathway in androgen synthesis that is present only during fetal life and ceases after birth has been proposed, as well as an impairment of placental aromatase activity. Conversely, affected boys are born undervirilized, with degrees varying from micropenis to penoscrotal hypospadias due to impairment of P450c17 enzyme in the testes. Most patients also have the characteristic skeletal malformations of the ABS such as craniofacial malformations, including midface hypoplasia, pear-shaped nose, choanal stenosis or atresia, stenotic external auditory ear canals, dysplastic ears, various degrees of craniosynostosis, clinodactyly, radiohumeral or radioulnar synostosis, arachnodactyly, joint contractures, and femoral bowing. Poor masculinization has been reported in some affected males, as well as decreased spermatogenesis (180). Primary amenorrhea has been described in one female (179) and ovarian cysts in at least five affected females (179,180,182). A few patients with hypertension and elevated DOC levels have been described (179,182).

Pregnant mothers of fetuses affected with POR deficiency have low estriol (E_3) concentrations and develop signs of virilization (e.g., acne and hirsutism) that resolve rapidly after birth (182). Maternal virilization also has been observed in mothers carrying fetuses with mutations in CYP19 gene, encoding

P450 aromatase. In normal physiology, Δ_4A and testosterone are aromatized to E_1 and E_2 in the placenta, but in patients with aromatase deficiency, these androgens are converted downstream to 5α-dihydrotestosterone and, on entering the maternal bloodstream, lead to maternal virilization. However, the characteristic metabolites associated with aromatase deficiency, urinary 16-hydroxyandrosterone and 16-hydroxyetiocholanolone (metabolites of the estriol precursor 16α-hydroxyandrostenedione), have not been seen in the urine of mothers carrying affected fetuses with POR deficiency.

Diagnosis Characterisitc steroid abnormalities in patients with POR deficiency, which reflect the combined deficiencies of P450c21 and P450c17 enzymes, include 1) normal or decreased adrenal androgens (DHEA and Δ_4A) before and/or after ACTH stimulation testing (0.25 mg), 2) testosterone levels that may be low and unresponsive to ACTH or β-hCG, 3) elevated progesterone, pregnenolone, 17-OHP, and 17α-hydroxypregnenolone levels at baseline and/or after ACTH stimulation, 4) cortisol levels that may be normal at baseline but may not increase after ACTH strimulation, 5) DOC level that may be elevated in some patients with hypertension, and 6) urinary metabolites that show increased concentrations of pregnediol (pregnenolone metabolites) and pregnanediol (progesterone metabolites).

Genetic Testing

Genetic testing is available on a clinical basis.

Treatment Depending on the degree of 21α-OHlase and of 17α-OHlase/17,20-lyase deficiencies, treatment can include 1) glucocorticoid replacement therapy in patients with low ACTH-stimulated cortisol levels, 2) testosterone treatment in infancy in males with micropenis at birth, and 3) sex steroid replacement for induction of secondary sex characteristics in individuals with decreased 17α-OHlase/17,20-lyase activity.

Treatment of craniosynostosis should be performed at an early age for better cognitive outcome. Joint contractures improve with age and with physical therapy. Airway management is a primary concern, and nasal stents or tracheotomy may be required because patients with ABS phenotype may have choanal atresia, a narrow trachea, and/or shortening of the larynx.

Surgical correction of clitoromegaly and/or vaginal reconstruction should be discussed with the family in the presence of a multidisciplinary team.

REFERENCES

1. Payne AH, Hales DB. Overview of steroidogenic enzymes in the pathway from cholesterol to active steroid hormones. *Endocr Rev.* 2004;25:947–970.
2. Lin D, Shi YF, Miller WL. Cloning and sequence of the human adrenodoxin reductase gene. *Proc Natl Acad Sci USA.* 1990;87:8516–8520.
3. Chang CY, Wu DA, Lai CC, et al. Cloning and structure of the human adrenodoxin gene. *DNA.* 1988;7:609–615.
4. Auchus RJ, Lee TC, Miller WL. Cytochrome b5 augments the 17,20-lyase activity of human P450c17 without direct electron transfer. *J Biol Chem.* 1998;273:3158–3165.
5. Zhang LH, Rodriguez H, Ohno S, et al. Serine phosphorylation of human P450c17 increases 17,20-lyase activity: Implications for adrenarche and the polycystic ovary syndrome. *Proc Natl Acad Sci USA.* 1995;92:10619–10623.
6. Pandey AV, Miller WL. Regulation of 17,20 lyase activity by cytochrome b5 and by serine phosphorylation of P450c17. *J Biol Chem.* 2005;280:13265–13271.
7. Labrie F, Luu-The V, Lin SX, et al. Intracrinology: Role of the family of 17β-hydroxysteroid dehydrogenases in human physiology and disease. *J Mol Endocrinol.* 2000;25:1–16.
8. Geissler WM, Davis DL, Wu L, et al. Male pseudohermaphroditism caused by mutations of testicular 17β-hydroxysteroid dehydrogenase 3. *Nat Genet.* 1994;7:34–39.
9. Jones ME, Boon WC, McInnes K, et al. Recognizing rare disorders: Aromatase deficiency. *Nat Clin Pract Endocrinol Metab.* 2007;3:414–421.
10. Rainey WE, Rehman KS, Carr BR. The human fetal adrenal: Making adrenal androgens for placental estrogens. *Semin Reprod Med.* 2004;22:327–336.
11. Kitawaki J, Inoue S, Tamura T, et al. Increasing aromatase cytochrome P450 level in human placenta during pregnancy: Studied by immunohistochemistry and enzyme-linked immunosorbent assay. *Endocrinology.* 1992;130:2751–2757.
12. Lo JC, Schwitzgebel VM, Tyrrell JB, et al. Normal female infants born of mothers with classic congenital adrenal hyperplasia due to 21-hydroxylase deficiency. *J Clin Endocrinol Metab.* 1999;84:930–936.
13. Goto M, Piper HK, Marcos J, et al. In humans, early cortisol biosynthesis provides a mechanism to safeguard female sexual development. *J Clin Invest.* 2006;116:953–960.
14. Arlt W, Walker EA, Draper N, et al. Congenital adrenal hyperplasia caused by mutant P450 oxidoreductase and human androgen synthesis: Analytical study. *Lancet.* 2004;363:2128–2135.
15. Yang S, Zhang L. Glucocorticoids and vascular reactivity. *Curr Vasc Pharmacol.* 2004;2:1–12.
16. Raff H. Glucocorticoid inhibition of neurohypophysial vasopressin secretion. *Am J Physiol.* 1987;252:R635–644.
17. McKay LI, Cidlowski JA. Molecular control of immune/inflammatory responses:

Interactions between nuclear factor-κβ and steroid receptor-signaling pathways. *Endocr Rev.* 1999;20:435–459.

18. Petrovsky N, McNair P, Harrison LC. Diurnal rhythms of pro-inflammatory cytokines: Regulation by plasma cortisol and therapeutic implications. *Cytokine.* 1998;10:307–312.

19. Bujalska IJ, Kumar S, Stewart PM. Does central obesity reflect "Cushing's disease of the omentum"? *Lancet.* 1997;349:1210–1213.

20. Kotelevtsev Y, Holmes MC, Burchell A, et al. 11β-Hydroxysteroid dehydrogenase type 1 knockout mice show attenuated glucocorticoid-inducible responses and resist hyperglycemia on obesity or stress. *Proc Natl Acad Sci USA.* 1997;94:14924–14929.

21. Stewart PM, Krozowski ZS, Gupta A, et al. Hypertension in the syndrome of apparent mineralocorticoid excess due to mutation of the 11β-hydroxysteroid dehydrogenase type 2 gene. *Lancet.* 1996;347:88–91.

22. Mune T, Rogerson FM, Nikkila H, et al. Human hypertension caused by mutations in the kidney isozyme of 11β-hydroxysteroid dehydrogenase. *Nat Genet.* 1995;10:394–399.

23. Zumoff B, Bradlow HL, Levin J, et al. Influence of thyroid function on the in vivo cortisol in equilibrium cortisone equilibrium in man. *J Steroid Biochem.* 1983;18:437–440.

24. Moore JS, Monson JP, Kaltsas G, et al. Modulation of 11β-hydroxysteroid dehydrogenase isozymes by growth hormone and insulin-like growth factor: In vivo and in vitro studies. *J Clin Endocrinol Metab.* 1999;84:4172–4177.

25. Onishi S, Miyazawa G, Nishimura Y, et al. Postnatal development of circadian rhythm in serum cortisol levels in children. *Pediatrics.* 1983;72:399–404.

26. Dluhy RG, Axelrod L, Underwood RH, et al. Studies of the control of plasma aldosterone concentration in normal man: II. Effect of dietary potassium and acute potassium infusion. *J Clin Invest.* 1972;51:1950–1957.

27. Prader A. [Genital findings in the female pseudo-hermaphroditism of the congenital adrenogenital syndrome: Morphology, frequency, development and heredity of the different genital forms.] *Helv Paediatr Acta.* 1954;9:231–248.

28. Levine LS, Zachmann M, New MI, et al. Genetic mapping of the 21-hydroxylase- deficiency gene within the HLA linkage group. *N Engl J Med* 1978;299:911–915.

29. Higashi Y, Yoshioka H, Yamane M, et al. Complete nucleotide sequence of two steroid 21-OH genes tandemly arranged in the human chromosome: A pseudogene and a genuine gene. *Proc Natl Acad Sci USA.* 1986;83:2841–2845.

30. White PC, New MI, Dupont B. Structure of human steroid 21-hydroxylase genes. *Proc Natl Acad Sci USA* 1986;835111–5115.

31. Tajima T, Fujieda K, Nakayama K, et al. Molecular analysis of patient and carrier genes with congenital steroid 21-hydroxylase deficiency by using polymerase chain reaction and single strand conformation polymorphism. *J Clin Invest.* 1993;92:2182–2190.

32. White PC, Tusie-Luna MT, New MI, et al. Mutations in steroid 21-hydroxylase (CYP21). *Hum Mutat.* 1994;3(4):373–378.

33. Pang SY, Wallace MA, Hofman L, et al. Worldwide experience in newborn screening for classical congenital adrenal hyperplasia due to 21-hydroxylase deficiency. *Pediatrics.* 1988;81:866–874.

34. Pang S, Murphey W, Levine LS, et al. A pilot newborn screening for congenital adrenal hyperplasia in Alaska. *J Clin Endocrinol Metab.* 1982;55:413–420.

35. Therrell BL Jr, Berenbaum SA, Manter-Kapanke V, et al. Results of screening 1.9 million Texas newborns for 21-hydroxylase-deficient congenital adrenal hyperplasia. *Pediatrics.* 1998;101:583–590.

36. Speiser PW, Dupont B, Rubinstein P, et al. New MI: High frequency of nonclassical steroid 21-hydroxylase deficiency. *Am J Hum Genet.* 1985;37:650–667.

37. Moran C, Azziz R, Carmina E, et al. 21-Hydroxylase-deficient nonclassic adrenal hyperplasia is a progressive disorder: A multicenter study. *Am J Obstet Gynecol.* 2000;183:1468–1474.

38. Knochenhauer ES, Cortet-Rudelli C, Cunnigham RD, et al. Carriers of 21-hydroxylase deficiency are not at increased risk for hyperandrogenism. *J Clin Endocrinol Metab.* 1997;82:479–485.

39. Kirkland RT, Kirkland JL, Keenan BS, et al. Bilateral testicular tumors in congenital adrenal hyperplasia. *J Clin Endocrinol Metab.* 1977;44:369–378.

40. Hess RA, Bunick D, Lee KH, et al. A role for oestrogens in the male reproductive system. *Nature,* 1997;390:509–512.

41. Eddy EM, Washburn TF, Bunch DO, et al. Targeted disruption of the estrogen receptor gene in male mice causes alteration of spermatogenesis and infertility. *Endocrinology.* 1996;137:4796–4805.

42. Luconi M, Bonaccorsi L, Forti G, et al. Effects of estrogenic compounds on human spermatozoa: Evidence for interaction with a nongenomic receptor for estrogen on human sperm membrane. *Mol Cell Endocrinol.* 2001;178:39–45.

43. Toyama Y, Ohkawa M, Oku R, et al. Neonatally administered diethylstilbestrol retards the development of the blood-testis barrier in the rat. *J Androl.* 2001;22:413–423.

44. Inkster S, Yue W, Brodie A. Human testicular aromatase: Immunocytochemical and biochemical studies. *J Clin Endocrinol Metab.* 1995;80:1941–1947.

45. Hayes FJ, Seminara SB, Decruz S, et al. Aromatase inhibition in the human male reveals a hypothalamic site of estrogen feedback. *J Clin Endocrinol Metab.* 2000;85:3027–3035.

46. Cabrera MS, Vogiatzi MG, New MI. Long term outcome in adult males with classic congenital adrenal hyperplasia. *J Clin Endocrinol Metab.* 2001;86:3070–3078.

47. Stikkelbroeck NM, Otten BJ, Pasic A, et al. High prevalence of testicular adrenal rest tumors, impaired spermatogenesis, and Leydig cell failure in adolescent and adult males with congenital adrenal hyperplasia. *J Clin Endocrinol Metab.* 2001;86:5721–5728.

48. Stikkelbroeck NM, Hermus AR, Schouten D, et al. Prevalence of ovarian adrenal rest tumours and polycystic ovaries in females with congenital adrenal hyperplasia: results of ultrasonography and MR imaging. *Eur Radiol.* 2004;14:1802–1806.

49. Russo G, Paesano P, Taccagni G, et al. Ovarian adrenal-like tissue in congenital adrenal hyperplasia. *N Engl J Med.* 1998;339:853–854.

50. Al Ahmadie HA, Stanek J, Liu J, et al. Ovarian "tumor" of the adrenogenital syndrome: The first reported case. *Am J Surg Pathol.* 2001;25:1443–1450.

51. Bachega TA, Brenlha EM, Billerbeck AE, et al. Variable ACTH-stimulated 17-hydroxy-progesterone values in 21-hydroxylase deficiency carriers are not related to the different CYP21 gene mutations. *J Clin Endocrinol Metab.* 2002;87:786–790.

52. Baumgartner-Parzer SM, Schulze E, Waldhausl W, et al. Mutational spectrum of the steroid 21-hydroxylase gene in Austria: Identification of a novel missense mutation. *J Clin Endocrinol Metab.* 2001;86:4771–4775.

53. Jaaskelainen J, Levo A, Voutilainen R, et al. Population-wide evaluation of disease manifestation in relation to molecular genotype in steroid 21-hydroxylase (CYP21) deficiency: Good correlation in a well defined population. *J Clin Endocrinol Metab.* 1997;82:3293–3297.

54. Stikkelbroeck NM, Hoefsloot LH, de Wijs IJ, et al. CYP21 gene mutation analysis in 198 patients with 21-hydroxylase deficiency in The Netherlands: Six novel mutations and a specific cluster of four mutations. *J Clin Endocrinol Metab.* 2003;88:3852–3859.

55. Speiser PW, New MI, Tannin GM, et al. Genotype of Yupik Eskimos with congenital adrenal hyperplasia due to 21-hydroxylase deficiency. *Hum Genet.* 1992;88:647–648.

56. Wedell A, Thilen A, Ritzen EM, et al. Mutational spectrum of the steroid 21-hydroxylase gene in Sweden: Implications for genetic diagnosis and association with disease manifestation. *J Clin Endocrinol Metab.* 1994;78:1145–1152.

57. Speiser PW, White PC. Congenital adrenal hyperplasia. *N Engl J Med* 2003;349(8):776–788.

58. Amor M, Parker KL, Globerman H, et al. Mutation in the CYP21B gene (Ile-172nAsn) causes steroid 21-hydroxylase deficiency. *Proc Natl Acad Sci USA.* 1988;85:1600–1604.

59. Tusie-Luna MT, Speiser PW, Dumic M, et al. A mutation (Pro-30 to Leu) in CYP21 represents a potential nonclassic steroid 21-hydroxylase deficiency allele. *Mol Endocrinol.* 1991;5:685–692.

60. Witchel SF, Bhamidipati DK, Hoffman EP, et al. Phenotypic heterogeneity associated with the splicing mutation in congenital adrenal hyperplasia due to 21-hydroxylase deficiency. *J Clin Endocrinol Metab.* 1996;81:4081–4088.

61. Deneux C, Tardy V, Dib A, et al. Phenotype–genotype correlation in 56 women with nonclassical congenital adrenal hyperplasia

due to 21-hydroxylase deficiency. *J Clin Endocrinol Metab* 2001;86:207–213.

62. Kerrigan JR, Veldhuis JD, Leyo SA, et al. Estimation of daily cortisol production and clearance rates in normal pubertal males by deconvolution analysis. *J Clin Endocrinol Metab.* 1993;76:1505–1510.

63. Linder BL, Esteban NV, Yergey AL, et al. Cortisol production rate in childhood and adolescence. *J Pediatr.* 1990;117:892–896.

64. Metzger DL, Wright NM, Veldhuis JD, et al. Characterization of pulsatile secretion and clearance of plasma cortisol in premature and term neonates using deconvolution analysis. *J Clin Endocrinol Metab.* 1993;77:458–463.

65. Merke DP, Chrousos GP, Eisenhofer G, et al. Adrenomedullary dysplasia and hypofunction in patients with classic 21-hydroxylase deficiency. *N Engl J Med.* 2000;343:1362–1368.

66. Silva IN, Kater CE, Cunha CF, et al. Randomised controlled trial of growth effect of hydrocortisone in congenital adrenal hyperplasia. *Arch Dis Child.* 1997;77:214–218.

67. Hughes IA. Management of congenital adrenal hyperplasia. *Arch Dis Child* 1988;63:1399–1404.

68. Miller WL. Clinical review 54: Genetics, diagnosis, and management of 21-hydroxylase deficiency. *J Clin Endocrinol Metab.* 1994; 78:241–246.

69. van der Kamp HJ, Otten BJ, Buitenweg N, et al. Longitudinal analysis of growth and puberty in 21-hydroxylase deficiency patients. *Arch Dis Child.* 2002;87:139–144.

70. Hargitai G, Solyom J, Battelino T, et al. Growth patterns and final height in congenital adrenal hyperplasia due to classical 21-hydroxylase deficiency: Results of a multicenter study. *Horm Res.* 2001;55:161–171.

71. Eugster EA, Dimeglio LA, Wright JC, et al. Height outcome in congenital adrenal hyperplasia caused by 21-hydroxylase deficiency: A meta-analysis. *J Pediatr.* 2001;138:26–32.

72. Cutler GB Jr, Laue L. Congenital adrenal hyperplasia due to 21-hydroxylase deficiency. *N Engl J Med.* 1990;323:1806–1813.

73. Merke DP, Cutler GB Jr. New approaches to the treatment of congenital adrenal hyperplasia. *JAMA.* 1997;277:1073–1076.

74. Jaaskelainen J, Voutilainen R. Growth of patients with 21-hydroxylase deficiency: An analysis of the factors influencing adult height. *Pediatr Res.* 1997;41:30–33.

75. Manoli I, Kanaka-Gantenbein C, Voutetakis A, et al. Early growth, pubertal development, body mass index and final height of patients with congenital adrenal hyperplasia: factors influencing the outcome. *Clin Endocrinol (Oxf).* 2002;57:669–676.

76. Stikkelbroeck NM, Hof-Grootenboer BA, Hermus AR, et al. Growth inhibition by glucocorticoid treatment in salt wasting 21-hydroxylase deficiency: In early infancy and (pre)puberty. *J Clin Endocrinol Metab.* 2003;88:3525–3530.

77. Atherden SM, Barnes ND, Grant DB. Circadian variation in plasma 17-hydroxy-progesterone in patients with congenital adrenal hyperplasia. *Arch Dis Child.* 1972; 47:602–604.

78. Frisch H, Parth K, Schober E, et al. Circadian patterns of plasma cortisol, 17-hydroxyprogesterone, and testosterone in congenital adrenal hyperplasia. *Arch Dis Child.* 1981;56:208–213.

79. Muirhead S, Sellers EA, Guyda H. Indicators of adult height outcome in classical 21-hydroxylase deficiency congenital adrenal hyperplasia. *J Pediatr.* 2002;141:247–252.

80. Dimartino-Nardi J, Stoner E, O'Connell A, et al. The effect of treatment of final height in classical congenital adrenal hyperplasia (CAH). *Acta Endocrinol Suppl (Copenh).* 1986;279:305–314.

81. Urban MD, Lee PA, Migeon CJ. Adult height and fertility in men with congenital virilizing adrenal hyperplasia. *N Engl J Med.* 1978;299:1392–1396.

82. Kirkland RT, Kirkland JL, Keenan BS, et al. Bilateral testicular tumors in congenital adrenal hyperplasia. *J Clin Endocrinol Metab.* 1977;44:369–378.

83. Jaaskelainen J, Tiitinen A, Voutilainen R. Sexual function and fertility in adult females and males with congenital adrenal hyperplasia. *Horm Res.* 2001;56:73–80.

84. Ogilvie CM, Crouch NS, Rumsby G, et al. Congenital adrenal hyperplasia in adults: A review of medical, surgical and psychological issues. *Clin Endocrinol (Oxf).* 2006;64:2–11.

85. Diamond M, Sigmundson HK. Management of intersexuality: Guidelines for dealing with persons with ambiguous genitalia. *Arch Pediatr Adolesc Med.* 1997;151:1046–1050.

86. Minto CL, Liao LM, Woodhouse CR, et al. The effect of clitoral surgery on sexual outcome in individuals who have intersex conditions with ambiguous gen- italia: A cross-sectional study. *Lancet.* 2003; 361:1252–1257.

87. Bockting WO, Fung LCT. Genital reconstruction and gender identity disorders. In: Sarwer D, ed. *The Psychological Aspects of Cosmetic and Reconstructive Plastic Surgery.* Philadelphia: Lippincott Williams & Wilkins; 2005:207–229.

88. Cohen-Kettenis PT. *Transgenderism and Intersexuality in Childhood and Adolescence: Making Choices.* Sage; Thousand Oaks, London 2003.

89. Houk CP, Hughes IA, Ahmed SF, et al. Summary of consensus statement on intersex disorders and their management. International Intersex Consensus Conference. *Pediatrics.* 2006;118:753–757.

90. Van Wyk JJ, Ritzen EM. The role of bilateral adrenalectomy in the treatment of congenital adrenal hyperplasia. *J Clin Endocrinol Metab.* 2003;88:2993–2998.

91. Lo JC, Schwitzgebel VM, Tyrrell JB, et al. Normal female infants born of mothers with classic congenital adrenal hyperplasia due to 21-hydroxylase deficiency. *J Clin Endocrinol Metab.* 1999;84:930–936.

92. Miller WL. Congenital adrenal hyperplasia in the adult patient. *Adv Intern Med.* 1999;44:155–173.

93. van der Kamp HJ, Wit JM. Neonatal screening for congenital adrenal hyperplasia. *Eur J Endocrinol* 2004;1513:U71–U75.

94. Therrell BL. Newborn screening for congenital adrenal hyperplasia. *Endocrinol Metab Clin North Am.* 2001;30:15–30.

95. al Saedi S, Dean H, Dent W, et al. Screening for congenital adrenal hyperplasia: The Delfia screening test overestimates serum 17-hydroxyprogesterone in preterm infants. *Pediatrics.* 1996;97:100–102.

96. Hingre RV, Gross SJ, Hingre KS, et al. Adrenal steroidogenesis in very low birth weight preterm infants. *J Clin Endocrinol Metab.* 1994;78:266–270.

97. Ng PC, Wong GW, Lam CW, et al. Effect of multiple courses of antenatal corticosteroids on pituitary–adrenal function in preterm infants. *Arch Dis Child Fetal Neonatal Ed.* 1999;80:F213–F216.

98. Holler W, Scholz S, Knorr D, et al. Genetic differences between the salt-wasting, simple virilizing, and nonclassical types of congenital adrenal hyperplasia. *J Clin Endocrinol Metab.* 1985;60:757–763.

99. Kari MA, Raivio KO, Stenman UH, et al. Serum cortisol, dehydroepiandrosterone sulfate, and steroid-binding globulins in preterm neonates: Effect of gestational age and dexamethasone therapy. *Pediatr Res.* 1996;40:319–324.

100. Benediktsson R, Lindsay RS, Noble J, et al. Glucocorticoid exposure in utero: New model for adult hypertension. *Lancet* 1993;341:339–341.

101. White PC. Ontogeny of adrenal steroid biosynthesis: Why girls will be girls. *J Clin Invest.* 2006;116:872–874.

102. Coleman MA, Honour JW. Reduced maternal dexamethasone dosage for the prenatal treatment of congenital adrenal hyperplasia. *Br J Obstet Gynaecol.* 2004; 111:176–178.

103. Seckl JR, Miller WL. How safe is long-term prenatal glucocorticoid treatment? *JAMA.* 1997;277:1077–1079.

104. Hurtig AL, Radhakrishnan J, Reyes HM, et al. Psychological evaluation of treated females with virilizing congenital adrenal hyperplasia. *J Pediatr Surg.* 1983;18:887–893.

105. Kuhnle U, Bullinger M, Schwarz HP. The quality of life in adult female patients with congenital adrenal hyperplasia: A comprehensive study of the impact of genital malformations and chronic disease on female patients life. *Eur J Pediatr.* 1995;154:708–716.

106. Lee PA, Houk CP, Ahmed SF, et al. Consensus statement on management of intersex disorders. International Consensus Conference on Intersex. *Pediatrics.* 2006; 118:e488–e500.

107. Eugster EA. Reality vs recommendations in the care of infants with intersex conditions. *Arch Pediatr Adolesc Med.* 2004; 158:428–429.

108. Alderson J, Madill A, Balen A. Fear of devaluation: Understanding the experience of intersexed women with androgen insensitivity syndrome. *Br J Health Psychol.* 2004;9:81–100.

109. Rickert VI, Hassed SJ, Hendon AE, et al. The effects of peer ridicule on depression

and self-image among adolescent females with Turner syndrome. *J Adolesc Health.* 1996;19:34–38.

110. Preves SE. For the sake of the children: Destigmatizing intersexuality. *J Clin Ethics.* 1998;9:411–420.

111. Krege S, Walz KH, Hauffa BP, et al. Long-term follow-up of female patients with congenital adrenal hyperplasia from 21-hydroxylase deficiency, with special emphasis on the results of vaginoplasty. *Br J Urol Int.* 2000;86:253–258.

112. Kuhnle U, Bullinger M. Outcome of congenital adrenal hyperplasia. *Pediatr Surg Int.* 1997;12:511–515.

113. Minto CL, Liao KL, Conway GS, et al. Sexual function in women with complete androgen insensitivity syndrome. *Fertil Steril.* 2003;80:157–164.

114. Dessens AB, Slijper FM, Drop SL. Gender dysphoria and gender change in chromosomal females with congenital adrenal hyperplasia. *Arch Sex Behav.* 2005;34:389–397.

115. Berenbaum SA. Effects of early androgens on sex-typed activities and interests in adolescents with congenital adrenal hyperplasia. *Horm Behav.* 1999;35:102–110.

116. Meyer-Bahlburg HF, Dolezal C, Baker SW, et al. New MI: Prenatal androgenization affects gender-related behavior but not gender identity in 5–12-year-old girls with congenital adrenal hyperplasia. *Arch Sex Behav.* 2004;33:97–104.

117. Hurtig AL, Rosenthal IM. Psychological findings in early treated cases of female pseudohermaphroditism caused by virilizing congenital adrenal hyperplasia. *Arch Sex Behav.* 1987;16:209–223.

118. Matteson KJ, Picado-Leonard J, Chung BC, et al. Assignment of the gene for adrenal P450c17 (steroid 17α-hydroxylase/17,20-lyase) to human chromosome 10. *J Clin Endocrinol Metab.* 1986;63:789–791.

119. Chung BC, Picado-Leonard J, Haniu M, et al. Cytochrome P450c17 (steroid 17α-hydroxylase/17,20-lyase): Cloning of human adrenal and testis cDNAs indicates the same gene is expressed in both tissues. *Proc Natl Acad Sci USA.* 1987;84:407–411.

120. Sparkes RS, Klisak I, Miller WL. Regional mapping of genes encoding human steroidogenic enzymes: P450scc to 15q23-q24, adrenodoxin to 11q22; adrenodoxin reductase to 17q24-q25; and P450c17 to 10q24-q25. *DNA Cell Biol.* 1991;10:359–365.

121. Geller DH, Auchus RJ, Mendonca BB, et al. The genetic and functional basis of isolated 17,20-lyase deficiency. *Nat Genet.* 1997;17:201–205.

122. White PC. Genetic diseases of steroid metabolism. *Vitam Horm.* 1994;49:131–195.

123. Van Den Akker EL, Koper JW, Boehmer AL, et al. Differential inhibition of 17α-hydroxylase and 17,20-lyase activities by three novel missense CYP17 mutations identified in patients with P450c17 deficiency. *J Clin Endocrinol Metab.* 2002;87:5714–5721.

124. Martin RM, Lin CJ, Costa EM, et al. P450c17 deficiency in Brazilian patients: Biochemical diagnosis through progesterone levels confirmed by CYP17 genotyping. *J Clin Endocrinol Metab.* 2003;88:5739–5746.

125. Costa-Santos M, Kater CE, Auchus RJ. Two prevalent CYP17 mutations and genotype–phenotype correlations in 24 Brazilian patients with 17-hydroxylase deficiency. *J Clin Endocrinol Metab.* 2004;89:49–60.

126. Scaroni C, Biason A, Carpene G, et al. 17α-Hydroxylase deficiency in three siblings: Short- and long-term studies. *J Endocrinol Invest.* 1991;14:99–108.

127. Yanase T, Kagimoto M, Suzuki S, et al. Deletion of a phenylalanine in the N-terminal region of human cytochrome P-450(17α) results in partial combined 17α-hydroxylase/17,20-lyase deficiency. *J Biol Chem.* 1989;264:18076–18082.

128. Matsuzaki S, Yanase T, Murakami T, et al. Induction of endometrial cycles and ovulation in a woman with combined 17α-hydroxylase/17,20-lyase deficiency due to compound heterozygous mutations on the p45017α gene. *Fertil Steril.* 2000;73:1183–1186.

129. Miura K, Yasuda K, Yanase T, et al. Mutation of cytochrome P45017α gene (CYP17) in a Japanese patient previously reported as having glucocorticoid-responsive hyperaldosteronism: With a review of Japanese patients with mutations of CYP17. *J Clin Endocrinol Metab.* 1996;81:3797–3801.

130. Taniyama M, Tanabe M, Saito H, et al. Subtle 17α-hydroxylase/17,20-lyase deficiency with homozygous Y201N mutation in an infertile woman. *J Clin Endocrinol Metab.* 2005;90:2508–2511.

131. Berube D, Luu T, Lachance Y, et al. Assignment of the human 3β-hydroxysteroid dehydrogenase gene (HSD-β3) to the p13 band of chromosome 1. *Cytogenet Cell Genet.* 1989;52:199–200.

132. Morissette J, Rheaume E, Leblanc JF, et al. Genetic linkage mapping of HSD3B1 and HSD3B2 encoding human types I and II 3β-hydroxysteroid dehydrogenase/Δ₅-Δ₄-isomerase close to D1S514 and the centromeric D1Z5 locus. *Cytogenet Cell Genet.* 1995;69:59–62.

133. Rheaume E, Simard J, Morel Y, et al. Congenital adrenal hyperplasia due to point mutations in the type II 3β-hydroxysteroid dehydrogenase gene. *Nat Genet.* 1992;1:239–245.

134. Rheaume E, Sanchez R, Simard J, et al. Molecular basis of congenital adrenal hyperplasia in two siblings with classical non-salt-losing 3β-hydroxysteroid dehydrogenase deficiency. *J Clin Endocrinol Metab.* 1994;79:1012–1018.

135. Mendonca BB, Bloise W, Arnhold IJ, et al. Male pseudohermaphroditism due to non-salt-losing 3β-hydroxysteroid dehydrogenase deficiency: Gender role change and absence of gynecomastia at puberty. *J Steroid Biochem.* 1987;28:669–675.

136. Chang YT, Kulin HE, Garibaldi L, et al. Hypothalamic–pituitary–gonadal axis function in pubertal male and female siblings with glucocorticoid-treated non-salt-wasting 3β-hydroxysteroid dehydrogenase deficiency congenital adrenal hyperplasia. *J Clin Endocrinol Metab.* 1993;77:1251–1257.

137. Marui S, Torrealba IM, Russell AJ, et al. A novel homozygous nonsense mutations E135* in the type II 3β-hydroxysteroid dehydrogenase gene in a girl with salt-losing congenital adrenal hyperplasia. Mutations in brief no. 168. Online. *Hum Mutat,* 1998;12:139.

138. Alos N, Moisan AM, Ward L, et al. A novel A10E homozygous mutation in the HSD3B2 gene causing severe salt-wasting 3β-hydroxysteroid dehydrogenase deficiency in 46,XX and 46,XY French-Canadians: Evaluation of gonadal function after puberty. *J Clin Endocrinol Metab.* 2000;85:1968–1974.

139. Zachmann M, Forest MG, de Peretti E. 3β-Hydroxysteroid dehydrogenase deficiency: Follow-up study in a girl with pubertal bone age. *Horm Res.* 1979;11:292–302.

140. Marui S, Castro M, Latronico AC, et al. Mutations in the type II 3β-hydroxysteroid dehydrogenase (HSD3B2) gene can cause premature pubarche in girls. *Clin Endocrinol (Oxf).* 2000;52:67–75.

141. Johannsen TH, Mallet D, Dige-Petersen H, et al. Delayed diagnosis of congenital adrenal hyperplasia with salt wasting due to type II 3β-hydroxysteroid dehydrogenase deficiency. *J Clin Endocrinol Metab.* 2005;90:2076–2080.

142. Carbunaru G, Prasad P, Scoccia B, et al. The hormonal phenotype of nonclassic 3β-hydroxysteroid dehydrogenase (HSD3B) deficiency in hyperandrogenic females is associated with insulin-resistant polycystic ovary syndrome and is not a variant of inherited HSD3B2 deficiency. *J Clin Endocrinol Metab.* 2004;89:783–794.

143. Sakkal-Alkaddour H, Zhang L, Yang X, et al. Studies of 3β-hydroxysteroid dehydrogenase genes in infants and children manifesting premature pubarche and increased adrenocorticotropin-stimulated Δ₅-steroid levels. *J Clin Endocrinol Metab.* 1996;81:3961–3965.

144. Lutfallah C, Wang W, Mason JI, et al. Newly proposed hormonal criteria via genotypic proof for type II 3β-hydroxysteroid dehydrogenase deficiency. *J Clin Endocrinol Metab.* 2002;87:2611–2622.

145. Moisan AM, Ricketts ML, Tardy V, et al. New insight into the molecular basis of 3β-hydroxysteroid dehydrogenase deficiency: Identification of eight mutations in the HSD3B2 gene of eleven patients from seven new families and comparison of the functional properties of twenty-five mutant enzymes. *J Clin Endocrinol Metab.* 1999;84:4410–4425.

146. Mermejo LM, Elias LL, Marui S, et al. Refining hormonal diagnosis of type II 3β-hydroxysteroid dehydrogenase deficiency in patients with premature pubarche and hirsutism based on HSD3B2 genotyping. *J Clin Endocrinol Metab.* 2005;90:1287–1293.

147. Pang S, Carbunaru G, Haider A, et al. Carriers for type II 3β-hydroxysteroid dehydrogenase (HSD3B2) deficiency can only be identified by HSD3B2 genotype study and not by hormone test. *Clin Endocrinol (Oxf).* 2003;58:323–331.

148. Simard J, Moisan AM, Morel Y. Congenital adrenal hyperplasia due to 3β-hydroxysteroid dehydrogenase/Δ₅-Δ₄ isomerase deficiency. *Semin Reprod Med.* 2002;20:255–276.

149. Hochberg Z, Schechter J, Benderly A, et al. Growth and pubertal development in patients with congenital adrenal hyperplasia due to 11β-hydroxylase deficiency. *Am J Dis Child.* 1985;139:771–776.

150. Rosler A, Leiberman E, Cohen T. High frequency of congenital adrenal hyperplasia (classic 11β-hydroxylase deficiency) among Jews from Morocco. *Am J Med Genet*. 1992;42:827–834.

151. Al Jurayyan NA. Congenital adrenal hyperplasia due to 11β-hydroxylase deficiency in Saudi Arabia: Clinical and biochemical characteristics. *Acta Paediatr*. 1995;84:651–654.

152. Mornet E, Dupont J, Vitek A, et al. Characterization of two genes encoding human steroid 11β-hydroxylase (P-450(11)β). *J Biol Chem*. 1989;264:20961–20967.

153. Taymans SE, Pack S, Pak E, et al. Human CYP11B2 (aldosterone synthase) maps to chromosome 8q24.3. *J Clin Endocrinol Metab*. 1998;83:1033–1036.

154. White PC, Curnow KM, Pascoe L. Disorders of steroid 11β-hydroxylase isozymes. *Endocr Rev*. 1994;15:421–438.

155. Zachmann M, Tassinari D, Prader A. Clinical and biochemical variability of congenital adrenal hyperplasia due to 11β-hydroxylase deficiency: A study of 25 patients. *J Clin Endocrinol Metab*. 1983;56:222–229.

156. Hochberg Z, Benderly A, Zadik Z. Salt loss in congenital adrenal hyperplasia due to 11β-hydroxylase deficiency. *Arch Dis Child*. 1984;59:1092–1094.

157. Liel Y. Acute adrenal crisis complicating hypertensive congenital adrenal hyperplasia due to 11β-hydroxylase deficiency. *Clin Genet*. 1993;43:92–93.

158. Joehrer K, Geley S, Strasser-Wozak EM, et al. CYP11B1 mutations causing non-classic adrenal hyperplasia due to 11β-hydroxylase deficiency. *Hum Mol Genet*. 1997;6:1829–1834.

159. Lashansky G, Saenger P, Dimartino-Nardi J, et al. Normative data for the steroidogenic response of mineralocorticoids and their precursors to adrenocorticotropin in a healthy pediatric population. *J Clin Endocrinol Metab*. 1992;75:1491–1496.

160. Curnow KM, Slutsker L, Vitek J, et al. Mutations in the CYP11B1 gene causing congenital adrenal hyperplasia and hypertension cluster in exons 6, 7, and 8. *Proc Natl Acad Sci USA*. 1993;90:4552–4556.

161. Geley S, Kapelari K, Johrer K, et al. CYP11B1 mutations causing congenital adrenal hyperplasia due to 11β-hydroxylase deficiency. *J Clin Endocrinol Metab*. 1996;81:2896–2901.

162. Pascoe L, Curnow KM, Slutsker L, et al. Glucocorticoid-suppressible hyperaldosteronism results from hybrid genes created by unequal crossovers between CYP11B1 and CYP11B2. *Proc Natl Acad Sci USA*. 1992;89:8327–8331.

163. Lifton RP, Dluhy RG, Powers M, et al. A chimaeric 11β-hydroxylase/aldosterone synthase gene causes glucocorticoid-remediable aldosteronism and human hypertension. *Nature*. 1992;355:262–265.

164. Pascoe L, Jeunemaitre X, Lebrethon MC, et al. Glucocorticoid-suppressible hyperaldosteronism and adrenal tumors occurring in a single French pedigree. *J Clin Invest*. 1995;96:2236–2246.

165. Stowasser M, Bachmann AW, Huggard PR, et al. Severity of hypertension in familial hyperaldosteronism type I: Relationship to gender and degree of biochemical disturbance. *J Clin Endocrinol Metab*. 2000;85:2160–2166.

166. Ganguly A, Weinberger MH, Guthrie GP, et al. Adrenal steroid responses to ACTH in glucocorticoid-suppressible aldosteronism. *Hypertension*. 1984;6:563–567.

167. Dluhy RG, Lifton RP. Glucocorticoid-remediable aldosteronism. *J Clin Endocrinol Metab*. 1999;84:4341–4344.

168. Mulatero P, di Cella SM, Williams TA, et al. Glucocorticoid remediable aldosteronism: Low morbidity and mortality in a four-generation italian pedigree. *J Clin Endocrinol Metab*. 2002;87:3187–3191.

169. Stowasser M, Bachmann AW, Huggard PR, et al. Treatment of familial hyperaldosteronism type I: Only partial suppression of adrenocorticotropin required to correct hypertension. *J Clin Endocrinol Metab*. 2000;85:3313–3318.

170. Hiort O, Holterhus PM, Werner R, et al. Homozygous disruption of P450 side-chain cleavage (CYP11A1) is associated with prematurity, complete 46,XY sex reversal, and severe adrenal failure. *J Clin Endocrinol Metab*. 2005;90:538–541.

171. Katsumata N, Ohtake M, Hojo T, et al. Compound heterozygous mutations in the cholesterol side-chain cleavage enzyme gene (CYP11A) cause congenital adrenal insufficiency in humans. *J Clin Endocrinol Metab*. 2002;87:3808–3813.

172. al Kandari H, Katsumata N, Alexander S, et al. Homozygous mutation of P450 side-chain cleavage enzyme gene (CYP11A1) in 46,XY patient with adrenal insufficiency, complete sex reversal, and agenesis of corpus callosum. *J Clin Endocrinol Metab*. 2006;91:2821–2826.

173. Sugawara T, Holt JA, Driscoll D, et al. Human steroidogenic acute regulatory protein: functional activity in COS-1 cells, tissue-specific expression, and mapping of the structural gene to 8p11.2 and a pseudogene to chromosome 13. *Proc Natl Acad Sci USA*. 1995;92:4778–4782.

174. Bose HS, Sato S, Aisenberg J, et al. Mutations in the steroidogenic acute regulatory protein (StAR) in six patients with congenital lipoid adrenal hyperplasia. *J Clin Endocrinol Metab*. 2000;85:3636–3639.

175. Bose HS, Sugawara T, Strauss JF III, et al. The pathophysiology and genetics of congenital lipoid adrenal hyperplasia. International Congenital Lipoid Adrenal Hyperplasia Consortium. *N Engl J Med*. 1996;335:1870–1878.

176. Nakae J, Tajima T, Sugawara T, et al. Analysis of the steroidogenic acute regulatory protein (StAR) gene in Japanese patients with congenital lipoid adrenal hyperplasia. *Hum Mol Genet*. 1997;6:571–576.

177. Fujieda K, Tajima T, Nakae J, et al. Spontaneous puberty in 46,XX subjects with congenital lipoid adrenal hyperplasia: Ovarian steroidogenesis is spared to some extent despite inactivating mutations in the steroidogenic acute regulatory protein (StAR) gene. *J Clin Invest*. 1997;99:1265–1271.

178. Baker BY, Lin L, Kim CJ, et al. Nonclassic congenital lipoid adrenal hyperplasia: A new disorder of the steroidogenic acute regulatory protein with very late presentation and normal male genitalia. *J Clin Endocrinol Metab*. 2006; 91:4781–4785.

179. Fluck CE, Tajima T, Pandey AV, et al. Mutant P450 oxidoreductase causes disordered steroidogenesis with and without Antley–Bixler syndrome. *Nat Genet*. 2004;36:228–230.

180. Fukami M, Horikawa R, Nagai T, et al. Cytochrome P450 oxidoreductase gene mutations and Antley–Bixler syndrome with abnormal genitalia and/or impaired steroidogenesis: Molecular and clinical studies in 10 patients. *J Clin Endocrinol Metab*. 2005;90:414–426.

181. Huang N, Pandey AV, Agrawal V, et al. Diversity and function of mutations in p450 oxidoreductase in patients with Antley–Bixler syndrome and disordered steroidogenesis. *Am J Hum Genet*. 2005;76:729–749.

182. Arlt W, Walker EA, Draper N, et al. Congenital adrenal hyperplasia caused by mutant P450 oxidoreductase and human androgen synthesis: analytical study. *Lancet*. 2004;363:2128–2135.

183. Miller WL, Huang N, Pandey AV, et al. P450 oxidoreductase deficiency: A new disorder of steroidogenesis. *Ann NY Acad Sci*. 2005;1061:100–108.

CHAPTER 28

Cushing Syndrome in Children and Adolescents

Maria Alexandra Magiakou, MD

Kyriakie Sarafoglou, MD

Constantine A. Stratakis, MD, D. Med. Sci.

George P. Chrousos, MD, FAAP, MACP, MACE, FRCP

Etiology/Pathophysiology Dr. Harvey Cushing first described the syndrome that carries his name in 1912. Cushing syndrome is a term used to describe the manifestations resulting from prolonged exposure of the organism to high levels of glucocorticoids. Cushing disease, on the other hand, solely describes adrenocorticotropic hormone (ACTH)-secreting pituitary corticotroph adenomas or corticotroph hyperplasia.

The cause of Cushing syndrome can be exogenous, resulting from the administration of glucocorticoids or ACTH, or endogenous, secondary to increased secretion of cortisol, ACTH, or corticotropin-releasing hormone (CRH) (1,2). Exogenous administration of glucocorticoids (iatrogenic) accounts for the majority of cases of Cushing syndrome in children and adolescents because supraphysiologic doses of glucocorticoids are frequently prescribed for a wide range of nonendocrine diseases (3).

Endogenous glucocorticoid excess, a rare condition among the general population (incidence is 2–5 new cases per million per year, with a female to male preponderance of 9 : 1) with only 10% of all cases presenting in childhood and adolescence, is divided in two categories: ACTH dependent, which accounts for 85% of endogenous cases, and ACTH independent, which accounts for the rest. The classification of endogenous Cushing syndrome and rate of occurrence for ages younger than 7 years are summarized in the At-a-Glance section. For a discussion of the physiology of the hypothalamic-pituitary-adrenal axis (HPA), please see Chapter 27.

ACTH-Dependent Cushing

ACTH-dependent Cushing syndrome results from ACTH excess, originating either from the pituitary (Cushing disease) secondary to microadenomas or macroadenomas (80%), or from ectopic production of ACTH- or CRH-secreting tumors, such as bronchial, thymic, and pancreatic carcinoids (20%) (4,5). A very small number of patients with chronic Cushing disease go on to develop adrenal macroadenomas, autonomously secreting cortisol (6), which is called a

"transitional state." The molecular pathophysiology of ACTH-secreting tumors, either in the pituitary or ectopically, remains elusive.

ACTH-Independent Cushing

ACTH-independent Cushing occurs from autonomous secretion of cortisol by primary adrenal disease (i.e., cortisol-secreting adrenal tumors, primary pigmented micronodular adrenal disease (PPNAD), macronodular adrenal hyperplasia) (7–11,12). In children younger than 7 years of age ACTH-independent causes—primarily bilateral adrenal hyperplasias and carcinoma—are more frequently seen than ACTH-dependent ones (2,7).

Adrenal carcinomas in children can be associated with hemihypertrophy, Beckwith–Wiedemann syndrome, and Li Fraumeni syndrome. Adrenal adenomas and carcinomas are monoclonal in origin. Aberrant or 'illicit' expression of membrane receptors (mainly G-protein–coupled receptors) has been observed in adrenal adenomas and ACTH-independent macronodular bilateral adrenal hyperplasia, but never in children (12,13).

PPNAD is a rare hereditary cause of adrenal Cushing, characterized by multiple, microscopic (<6 mm), pigmented bilateral, cortisol-secreting nodules and small adrenals due to suppression of pituitary ACTH secretion by the elevated cortisol levels. This condition is frequently part of the Carney complex, an autosomal dominant disorder presenting with multiple spotty pigmentation of the skin and mucosae, cardiac, and skin myxomas and other endocrine tumors (14).

Cushing syndrome can be part of the McCune–Albright syndrome due to the autonomous cortisol production by the hyperplastic adrenal nodules that carry the activating mutation in the GNAS gene. This form of Cushing syndrome is usually seen in infancy and it is often self-limited.

Clinical Presentation The clinical manifestations of the syndrome are due to glucocorticoid excess; the adrenal cortisol secretion rate under basal conditions is 6 to 9 mg/m2/day in

children and adults (15,16) combined with mineralocorticoid and/or adrenal androgen excess. One of the earliest signs in almost all patients with Cushing syndrome is obesity, mostly truncal, which is characterized by facial rounding (moon facies), plethora, and fat collections in the nuchal (buffalo hump), supraclavicular, and visceral areas. The spectrum of clinical manifestations is quite broad, particularly in children, where the characteristic centripetal fat distribution may be more generalized and not been seen at time of presentation. Although patients may exhibit some of the features at the time of diagnosis, few, if any, will have all of them. Pictures of the patient taken over a period of years are particularly helpful in the clinical evaluation (2,7).

The effects of Cushing syndrome on growth are profound (see Figures 28-1 and 28-2), causing growth deceleration or arrest, and all children presenting with weight gain and growth failure should be evaluated for Cushing's syndrome, if their thyroid function tests are normal (17). The somatotropic axis is negatively

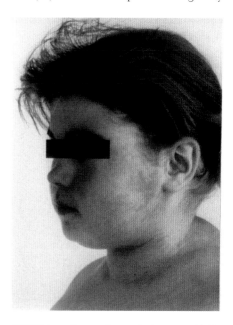

FIGURE 28-1. Close-up photograph of a 15-year-old girl with Cushing disease. Note the facial rounding, the facial hirsutism, and the filling in of the supraclavicular fossae.

Cushing Syndrome

AT-A-GLANCE

Cushing syndrome is a term used describe the manifestations associated with glucocorticoid excess. Cushing disease, on the other hand, solely describes adrenocorticotropic hormone (ACTH)-secreting pituitary corticotroph adenomas or corticotroph hyperplasia. The most common cause of glucocorticoid excess in children and adolescents is iatrogenic. Endogenous Cushing syndrome, a rare condition among the general population with only 10% of all cases presenting in childhood and adolescence, can be either ACTH dependent (Cushing disease) or ACTH independent (Cushing syndrome).

CLASSIFICATION OF ENDOGENOUS CUSHING SYNDROME AND RATE OF OCCURRENCE* (IN AGES OLDER THAN 7 YEARS)

ACTH-dependent	85%	ACTH-independent	15%
Pituitary (disease)	80%	Adrenal adenoma	30%
Ectopic ACTH	20%	Adrenal carcinoma	70%
Ectopic CRH	Rare	Micronodular adrenal disease (Carney complex, PPNAD)	Rare
		Macronodular adrenal hyperplasia	Rare
		McCune–Albright syndrome	Rare
		MEN Type I	Rare

PRESENTATION OF ENDOGENOUS (SYMPTOM AND FREQUENCY)

SYMPTOM	%	SYMPTOM	%	SYMPTOM	%	SYMPTOM	%
Weight gain	90	Violaceous skin striae	61	Mental changes	19	Sleep disturbances	8
Growth retardation	83	Acne	47	Hyperpigmentation	14	Hypercalcemia	7
Menstrual irregularities	78	Hypertension	47	Muscle weakness	12	Hypokalemic alkalosis	7
Hirsutism	78	Fatigue or weakness	44	Acanthosis nigricans	12	Delayed puberty	3
Osteoporosis/osteopenia	75	Premature sexual devel.	38	Bone age delayed	11	Slipped femoral capital epi	2
Obesity (BMI > 85th %)	75	Bruising	25	Bone age accelerated	8		

	CUSHING DISEASE	ECTOPIC ACTH	ADRENAL TUMORS	NODULAR ADRENAL HYPERPLASIA
Plasma ACTH	↑	↑	↓	↓
LDDST	Suppression	No suppression	No suppression	No suppression
HDDST	Suppression	No suppression	No suppression	No suppression
CRH Stimulation	↑ ACTH, ↑ Cortisol	No response	No response	No response
MRI Pituitary	Tumor (60%)	Normal	Normal	Normal
BIPSS	Gradient	No gradient	n/a	n/a

LDDST = low-dose dexamethasone suppression test; HDDST = high-dose DST; CRH = corticotropin-releasing hormone; MRI = magnetic resonance imaging; BIPSS = bilateral inferior petrosal sinus sampling; ACTH = adrenocorticotropic hormone.

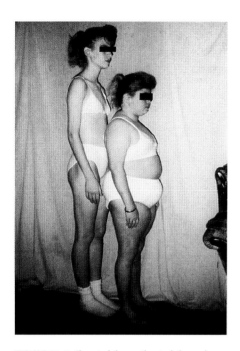

FIGURE 28-2. Characteristic growth retardation and obesity in a 15-year-old patient with Cushing disease in comparison to her healthy identical twin sister.

affected by hypercortisolism through suppression of the spontaneous secretion of (GH) and peripheral resistance of tissues to insulin-like growth factor–1 and other growth factors (18,19,20,63,64).

Young children may have premature sexual development, acne, and accelerated epiphyseal maturation as a result of increased adrenal androgen secretion. Older children and adolescents may develop delayed puberty, irregular menses, and amenorrhea, as a result of glucocorticoid-induced hypogonadotropic hypogonadism, which is further worsened by ACTH-induced hyperandrogenism. Hirsutism and occasionally virilization are the consequences of hyperandrogenemia.

Fatigue due to proximal muscle weakness, easy bruising, and typical purple skin striae due to inhibition of collagen synthesis by glucocorticoids and spontaneous fractures of ribs and vertebrae may also be encountered. Hypercortisolism in children, through the effects of glucocorticoids on bone and calcium metabolism, may lead to reduction in peak bone mass, osteopenia, or osteoporosis. Although the exact mechanisms have not been elucidated, it is generally thought that glucocorticoids cause loss of cortical osteo-

- In general, rapidly progressing and very severe Cushing syndrome with hypertension and hypokalemic alkalosis points toward the ectopic ACTH syndrome, whereas rapid and severe virilization is frequently due to adrenocortical carcinoma.

cytes; prevent bone repair; decrease bone collagenous matrix synthesis and osteoblast formation; inhibit calcium absorption from the intestine independently of vitamin D; and inhibit calcium reabsorption by the renal tubule. In addition, the effects of glucocorticoids on GH secretion and gonadotropins may further decrease BMD (17).

Manifestations of metabolic syndrome X (hypertension, carbohydrate intolerance, visceral adiposity, dyslipidemia, acanthosis nigricans, and/or diabetes mellitus type II) may develop as a direct or indirect consequence of hypercortisolism.

Mental changes such as emotional lability, irritability, or depression, as well as muscle weakness and sleep disturbances are rare in children in comparison to adults with Cushing syndrome; however hypercortisolic children have been reported to exhibit obsessive-compulsive behavior (21).

Hypercortisolism may cause subtle changes in thyroid function tests probably through inhibition of thyroxine-releasing hormone and thyroid-stimulating hormone secretion and suppression of the 5′-deiodinase enzyme that converts T_4 into active T_3. Free thyroxine levels are usually normal (22); however, these changes are not associated with clinical symptoms. Once the Cushing syndrome is cured, the values return to normal. Cushing patients are no more prone to thyroid disease than other individuals.

DIAGNOSIS OF CUSHING SYNDROME

The investigation of suspected Cushing syndrome is a three-step process. The first step, which must be completed before imple-

menting the tests in step two or three, is to establish hypercortisolism. First-line screening tests for Cushing syndrome are based on history, clinical evaluation, and, most importantly, biochemical documentation of hypercortisolism (23,24). These tests can be performed in the outpatient setting. Once confirmed, the second-line screening tests distinguish mild Cushing syndrome from pseudo-Cushing (Figure 28-3). The third step is to determine the cause of Cushing syndrome (Figure 28-4).

First-Line Screening Tests

Twenty four–hour urinary free cortisol excretion The 24-hour urinary free cortisol (UFC) provides a measurement of integrated cortisol secretion over 24 hours (25,26,27,28). To ensure a complete 24-hour collection, urinary creatine should be measured, and the UFC values should be corrected for body surface area. Because of the variability of cortisol secretion, possible errors in collecting samples, and to rule out the possibility of intermittent hypercortisolism (found in 5%–10% of patients with Cushing of any etiology), it is recommended to collect 24-hour urine for at least 3 consecutive days. Overall, there are very few false-negative results. The reference range for UFC depends on the assay used, with high-performance liquid chromatography or gas chromatography coupled with mass spectrometry being the most specific for measurement of UFC (26). Cortisol values fourfold greater than the upper limit of normal are diagnostic of Cushing syndrome. Milder elevations of urinary cortisol may be obtained in several non-Cushing hypercortisolemic states (i.e., chronic anxiety,

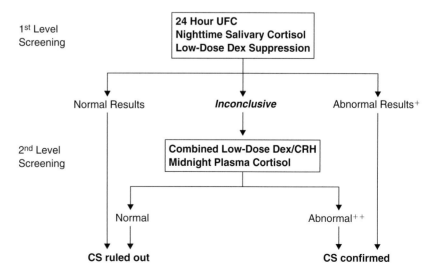

FIGURE 28-3. Establishing hypercortisolism and confirming Cushing states through first-level screening tests. + = Abnormal results of >4-fold upper normal limits for 24 hour UFC, >.27 mcg/dl for salivary cortisol, and cortisol 1.8 mcg/dl for low-dose dex. + + = Combined low-dose Dex/CRH: a simulated cortisol value > 1.4 mcg/dl after 15 minutes; Midnight plasma cortisol above 1.8 mcg/dl indicates loss of diurnal rhythm and the presence of Cushing's disease. CRH = corticotropin-releasing hormone; Dex = dexamethasone; UFC = urinary free cortisol.

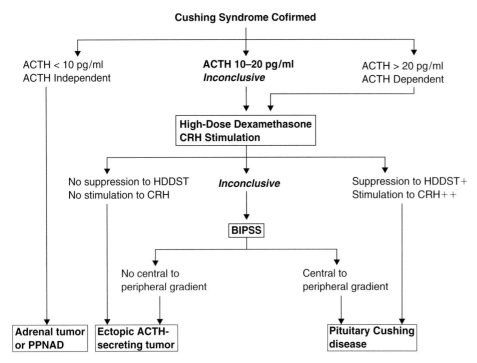

FIGURE 28-4. Identifying the etiology of Cushing syndrome. Once Cushing syndrome is confirmed, ACTH measurement, high-dose dexamethasone and CRH stimulation tests followed by BIPSS for inconclusive test results are used to identify the cause of Cushing syndrome. + = High-dose dex: plasma cortisol 50–80% suppression from baseline. ++ = CRH stimulation: ACTH increase above baseline 35–50% and cortisol increase over baseline 14–20%. PPNAD = Primary pigmented nodular adrenocortical disease; HDDST = High dose dexamethasone stimulation test; CRH = corticotropin-releasing hormone; BIPSS = bilateral inferior petrosal sinus sampling; ACTH = adrenocorticotropic hormone.

alcoholism, depression, and obesity), which are however rare in children. Patients with periodic and/or cyclical Cushing syndrome may also have UFCs in the mid- or upper-normal range; this form of Cushing syndrome is often caused by bilateral adrenocortical hyperplasias (27,28).

Nighttime salivary cortisol sampling Regardless of the etiology, derangement in cortisol's diurnal rhythm from mild changes to complete disruption is the hallmark of Cushing syndrome (30). Although the peak morning value of cortisol may be within the normal range, the evening cortisol level in patients with Cushing syndrome does not reach its nadir and stays elevated. A sleeping, unstressed midnight cortisol level if elevated is the earliest and most sensitive marker for Cushing syndrome.

Measurement of salivary cortisol at bedtime or midnight has been recently proposed as a simple, accurate way to screen for hypercortisolism in children. Salivary cortisol values higher than 1 μg/dL at bedtime and higher than 0.27 μg/dL at midnight establish the diagnosis of Cushing syndrome in nearly all cases (30,31,32).

Overnight low-dose dexamethasone suppression test In unaffected individuals, administration of 1 mg dexamethasone (in children 15 μg/kg body weight) will result in suppression of ACTH and subsequently, cortisol secretion.

In Cushing syndrome, of any cause, there is a failure to suppress cortisol in response to the low-dose dexamethasone test, which has a 3% false-negative rate and a 15% to 20% incidence of false-positive results. The classical 2 day test, where the patient takes 0.5 mg Dexamethasone orally every 6 hours is used as a first line screening test in some centers. Suppression of serum cortisol level to less than 1.8 μg/dL excludes Cushing syndrome (26,28).

In first-line screening tests, Cushing syndrome is generally excluded if the 24-hour UFC, nighttime salivary cortisol sampling, and the response to a single-dose dexamethasone suppression test are normal (26,28,30,31).

Patients receiving drugs such as phenytoin, phenobarbital, and primidone, which stimulate enzymatic activity in the liver and increase dexamethasone metabolism may fail to suppress cortisol levels after low-dose dexamethasone (32). Similarly, patients with psychiatric disorders (i.e., depression, anxiety, and posttraumatic stress) may also fail to suppress cortisol levels during the test.

Second-Line Screening Tests

The clinical and biochemical presentation of hypercortisolism in mild Cushing syndrome is often difficult to distinguish from pseudo-Cushing states and the following tests may be used to differentiate between the two.

Midnight plasma cortisol The principle behind the timing of the test is similar to the salivary nighttime cortisol test. This test requires a 2-day admission, with the 1st night to allow for acclimation of the patients to the hospital setting. During the 2nd night, a single cortisol sample is drawn during sleep at midnight. A cortisol level above 1.8 μg/dL indicates loss of diurnal rhythm and the presence of Cushing syndrome (33,34).

Combined low-dose 2-day dexamethasone and CRH test Combination of the low-dose 2-day dexamethasone test (0.5 mg every 6 h for 2 d) with the CRH test (1 μg/kg) has been shown to be highly accurate in distinguishing Cushing syndrome from pseudo-Cushing states. In patients with pseudo-Cushing the pituitary is appropriately suppressed by dexamethasone and does not respond to CRH, whereas patients with Cushing syndrome have a stimulated cortisol value greater than 1.4 μg/dL 15 minutes after the CRH test (35,36).

Third-Level Tests (Establishing the cause of Cushing Syndrome)

Once the diagnosis of endogenous Cushing syndrome has been established, testing should be undertaken to clarify the specific cause. The tests include biochemical evaluation of the HPA axis (when patient is hypercortisolemic), several imaging techniques are used to examine the size and shape of the pituitary and adrenal glands or to detect and evaluate tumors, and catheterization studies to localize ACTH-secreting tumors in the pituitary versus a peripheral site.

Adrenocorticotropic hormone measurement Determination of plasma ACTH simultaneously with plasma cortisol is the first step in distinguishing ACTH-dependent from ACTH-independent Cushing syndrome. It is recommended that a two-site immunoradiometric assay should be used for measurement of ACTH as it has sensitivity of 10 pg/mL or less.

In ACTH-independent causes of Cushing syndrome, autonomous cortisol production by adrenal cortisol-secreting tumors and micro- and macronodular adrenal disease are often associated with suppressed levels of plasma ACTH (<10 pg/mL) at 9:00 AM) through the negative feedback of cortisol at the hypothalamus (which decreases CRH release) and at the pituitary (which decreases ACTH release). ACTH levels may not be fully suppressed in patients with macronodular adrenal hyperplasia or small adrenal tumors because of intermittent or relatively low secretion of cortisol.

ACTH-dependent Cushing disease and the ectopic ACTH syndrome are associated with normal or elevated plasma ACTH concentrations (>20 pg/mL) as both pituitary and nonpituitary ACTH-secreting tumors have some degree of sensitivity to the negative feedback of cortisol. The magnitude of elevation of plasma ACTH may have differential diagnostic value because often patients with the ectopic ACTH syndrome have greater plasma ACTH levels than those with Cushing disease. The overlap in ACTH values is such that ACTH values alone rarely distinguish between the two conditions (1,2,7,28).

For values between 10 and 20 pg/dL, in order to differentiate between ACTH-dependent and ACTH-independent Cushing syndrome, a CRH stimulation test (explained later) is usually required.

High-Dose Dexamethasone Suppression Test

This test, originally described by Liddle and used to differentiate between Cushing disease and ectopic ACTH syndrome, is based on the theory that the negative feedback control of ACTH resets itself to an elevated threshold in response to higher levels of glucocorticoids in Cushing disease. Under this paradigm, cortisol levels that are not suppressed under low-dose dexamethasone, are suppressed under high dose (40).

In patients with Cushing disease the abnormal corticotrophs are sensitive to glucocorticoid inhibition only at high doses of dexamethasone. The standard high-dose dexamethasone test is 2 mg every 6 hours for 2 days (corrected for weight in children). Approximately 85% of patients with Cushing disease demonstrate a decrease in UFC excretion and plasma cortisol to values, respectively, less than 64% and 90% of the baseline values on day 2 of the test, whereas less than 10% of patients with the ectopic ACTH syndrome or ACTH-independent Cushing syndrome respond in this manner (40,41). There are several versions of the high-dose dexamethasone suppression test, including the 8-mg overnight oral, and the intravenous 4- to 7-mg tests, both corrected for weight in children (28).

Corticotropin-releasing hormone stimulation test

Approximately 85% of patients with Cushing disease respond to CRH with increases in ACTH and cortisol levels. In contrast, patients with ectopic ACTH production (over 95%) or with ACTH-independent Cushing syndrome show little or no cortisol/ACTH response to CRH (37,38,39). The CRH test should be performed when the patient is hypercortisolemic by intravenous injection of 1 μg/kg or 100 μg synthetic ovine or human CRH. In normal individuals, CRH produces a 15% to 20% rise in ACTH and cortisol, but in Cushing disease the response is more dramatic with a typical rise in ACTH greater than 50% and cortisol greater than 20%. The diagnostic power of the Liddle dexamethasone suppression test and the CRH test is enhanced when both tests are performed. Negative results from both tests rule out the diagnosis of Cushing disease with a diagnostic accuracy of more than 98% (38,40).

Imaging Evaluation

Pituitary More than 95% of pituitary ACTH-secreting tumors are microadenomas with a diameter less than 7 mm. Gadolinium-enhanced magnetic resonance imaging (MRI) of the pituitary will reveal an adenoma in up to 60% of patients with Cushing disease, but less frequently in children (27,42). Most pituitary microadenomas do not enhance with gadolinium contrast medium and appear as foci of reduced signal intensity. Because 5% of pituitary microadenomas uptake gadolinium and become isodense with the pituitary, MRI before the gadolinium administration should be performed.

Adrenals Computed tomography (CT) or MRI of the adrenal glands is useful in distinguishing between Cushing disease and a cortisol-secreting adrenal adenoma or carcinoma. The adrenal CT or MRI in patients with Cushing disease will demonstrate bilateral cortical hyperplasia, diffuse or nodular, and a relatively normal overall glandular configuration in approximately 60% of the patients, making it difficult to distinguish radiographically from ACTH-independent forms of bilateral adrenal hyperplasia. In 30% of patients with proven Cushing disease the adrenal glands are not hyperplastic. Both adrenal carcinomas and adenomas are clearly detectable with CT scanning or MRI of the adrenal glands (43).

The iodocholesterol scan, although not frequently used in diagnosing patients with adrenal Cushing, may help define whether there is unilateral or bilateral autonomous steroidosynthetic tissue when adrenal masses are seen bilaterally on CT or MRI studies. Also, it may help with the localization of adrenal rests or adrenal remnants after adrenalectomy (44).

Ectopic ACTH tumors CT and MRI studies of the chest, abdomen, and pelvis should be performed if biochemical diagnostic testing is suggestive of an ectopic ACTH source. In some cases scanning with radiolabeled osteotride may detect occult carcinoid tumor.

Catheterization studies Simultaneous bilateral inferior petrosal sinus sampling (BIPSS) and peripheral vein catheterization is one of the most specific tests to localize the source of ACTH production, before and after CRH stimulation, and to distinguish between Cushing disease and ectopic ACTH syndrome as both pituitary microadenomas and ectopic ACTH-secreting tumors may be radiologically occult (45,46,47,48,49). The test takes advantage by which ACTH and other hormones of the anterior pituitary reach systemic circulation. Venous blood from the anterior pituitary drains into the cavernous sinus and subsequently into the inferior petrosal sinuses. Samples for measurement of plasma ACTH are collected simultaneously from each inferior petrosal sinus and a peripheral vein at baseline and at 3, 5, and 10 minutes after injection of 1 μg/kg (or 100 μg) of CRH. Generally, patients with the ectopic ACTH syndrome have no ACTH concentration gradient between either inferior petrosal sinus and the peripheral sample before or after CRH. On the other hand, an increased baseline or stimulated gradient (>2 and >3, respectively) of plasma ACTH between any or both of the inferior petrosal sinuses and the peripheral sample is highly suggestive of Cushing disease. Basal gradients distinguish 95% of patients with Cushing disease from those with ectopic. Stimulated gradients separate up to 98% (Figure 28-3).

In addition, if a microadenoma cannot be identified at surgery, the only data on which the surgeon can base the decision to perform hemihypophysectomy are the results of BIPSS (47). The overall diagnostic value of the BIPSS depends on its being performed while the patient is hypercortisolemic, and this should always be ensured prior to performing the test (47,48). The use of BIPSS for localization of pituitary microadenoma to the right or left side of the pituitary is controversial (28,50). Lienhardt et al, in a small series of patients found BIPSS be more accurate than other imaging studies (46).

TREATMENT OF CUSHING SYNDROME

The treatment of choice depends on the specific cause of the hypercortisolism, which must be established unequivocally. Optimal treatment is the correction of hypercortisolism without permanent dependence on hormone replacement. Patients with ectopic tumors and primary adrenal disease are treated with tumor excision and bilateral or unilateral (in the case of adrenal adenomas or carcinomas) adrenalectomy, respectively. Currently, the following therapeutic modalities are available for the treatment of pituitary ACTH-secreting tumors: transsphenoidal removal of the adenoma, "Gamma Knife" and linear accelerator-assisted radiosurgery, pituitary irradiation with concomitant therapy with mitotane, combinations of other pharmacologic agents, and bilateral adrenalectomy (49,50).

Transsphenoidal adenomectomy is the treatment of choice for most cases of Cushing syndrome caused by pituitary microadenomas (51–53). In most specialized centers the success rate of initial transsphenoidal surgery varies from 66% to 80%. If BIPSS has lateralized the microadenoma and the surgeon cannot identify it at surgery, 75% to 80% of patients can be cured by ipsilateral hemihypophysectomy. Successful surgery leads to cure of hypercortisolism with no need for permanent glucocorticoid replacement. The success rate of repeated transsphenoidal surgery is considerably lower in patients with recurrent Cushing disease (54).

Transient diabetes insipidus and, less frequently, inappropriate antidiuretic hormone secretion may occur during the first weeks postsurgery. Central hypothyroidism, GH deficiency, hypogonadism, and permanent hypocortisolism may also occur. Successful cure of hypercortisolism may unmask a preexisting primary autoimmune thyroid disease. Permanent diabetes insipidus, hemorrage, cerebrospinal fluid rhinorrhea, injury of the internal carotid artery, cranial nerve palsy, and meningitis are uncommon complications but may occur more frequently in patients who undergo repeated transsphenoidal surgery. The perioperative mortality rate of transsphenoidal surgery is probably less than 1%, lower than that of bilateral adrenalectomy (~3%). After a successful transsphenoidal operation in Cushing disease, a period of adrenal insufficiency ensues in most of patients cured, during which glucocorticoids must be replaced (see postoperative glucocorticoid replacement) (52–54).

Gamma Knife and linear accelerator-assisted radiosurgery have been proposed as an alternative in the treatment of functioning pituitary adenomas with good results, but the long-term effects are not yet known (55,56).

Combined pituitary X-irradiation and mitotane is a reasonable alternative treatment after failure of transsphenoidal surgery, presence of cavernous sinus wall invasion by the tumor, or as the first line of treatment in patients judged unsuitable for surgery (57). The recommended dosage of pituitary irradiation is 4,500 to 5,000 rad total. High-voltage, conventional X-radiation is given in 180- to 200-rad fractions over a period of 6 weeks. Biochemical and clinical amelioration of Cushing syndrome is delayed by several months (6–18 mo). Full effect can take years to occur. Progressive anterior hypopituitarism, including GH deficiency, hypothyroidism, and hypogonadism, occurs in approximately 40% of patients receiving radiotherapy. These complications may occur several years after radiotherapy and children should be followed closely both clinically and biochemically even through adulthood. Combined pituitary radiation and mitotane improves the success rate of either modality given alone, curing approximately two thirds of the patients (57,58).

Heavy particle-beam irradiation and Bragg peak proton irradiation therapy appear to be as effective as conventional irradiation but experience is limited.

Drug therapy alone is rarely used to treat Cushing disease except temporarily, prior to definitive treatment. Mitotane is the only available pharmacologic agent that both inhibits biosynthesis of corticosteroids and destroys adrenocortical cells secreting cortisol, thus producing a long-lasting effect. Therapy with mitotane alone can be successful in 30% to 40% of patients with Cushing disease. Adrenal enzyme inhibitors—aminoglutethimide, metyrapone, trilostane, and ketoconazole—have been used alone or in combination with mitotane or each other to control some of the symptoms and metabolic abnormalities associated with the hypercortisolemia of Cushing disease (50).

Bilateral adrenalectomy should be considered for patients in whom selective pituitary adenomectomy or hemihypophysectomy, radiation or both failed have. When performed properly, it cures hypercortisolism. The major disadvantages of bilateral adrenalectomy are lifelong daily cortisol and fludrocortisone replacements; failure to attack the cause underlying the hypersecretion of ACTH; relapses, although uncommon, may occur as a result of growth of adrenal rest tissue or an adrenal remnant; perioperative mortality approximately three times higher than that of transsphenoidal surgery; and the risk of developing Nelson syndrome (large pituitary macroadenomas secreting large amounts of ACTH) in 10% to 15% of patients months or years after bilateral adrenalectomy (59,60). The younger the patient, the higher is the risk for developing Nelson syndrome.

FOLLOW UP AFTER TREATMENT

When to Consider the Patient Cured There is still no widespread agreement regarding the definition of apparent cure, and the remission rates after surgery vary according to the criteria used and the time of assessment. The definition of cure and the prognostic effect of subtle or unrecognized residual hypercortisolism have a major clinical impact on the follow up and therapeutic decisions in these patients. Success after surgery is defined as a drop in serum cortisol or UFC to an undetectable level in the immediate postoperative period. Patients are considered in remission if urinary cortisol values are less than 10 μg /24 hours and morning plasma cortisol values are less than 1 μg/dL the 3rd day after surgery. Definition of remission is based on the physiological principle that high cortisol levels will suppress normal corticotroph function such that complete removal of a corticotroph adenoma will render the patient ACTH deficient, with low or undetectable cortisol levels. (53,54).

Most series from major centers quote remission rates of approximately 80%, defining remission as a series of normal postoperative cortisol levels, either as mean serial serum cortisol measurements, obtained throughout the day, of 5.4 to 10.8 μg/dL, or as a UFC in the normal range and disappearance of signs and symptoms of Cushing syndrome (51–57). Serum cortisol below 1.8 μg/dL at 9:00 AM within 2 weeks after surgery is probably the best index of remission (52,53,54). Long-term follow up of patients with Cushing disease shows a significant incidence of recurrence (~25% or more at 10 years).

Postoperative Glucocorticoid Replacement

After a successful transsphenoidal operation in Cushing disease, a period of adrenal insufficiency ensues in most of patients cured, during which glucocorticoids are replaced. Adrenal insufficiency may persist for a 1 year or longer, and rarely can be permanent (52,53,62). Intraoperatively, and during the first 2 postoperative days, 75 to 150 mg/m^2/day of hydrocortisone or its equivalent is given intravenously. Once the patient has recovered from the surgical procedure, oral replacement doses of hydrocortisone, 20 to 30 mg/day (12–15 mg/m^2/d), are started. Patients often complain of weakness, lack of energy, and irritability at these doses. This is a sign of successful surgery and the symptoms can be alleviated with pharmacologic doses of glucocorticoids. The replacement dose of hydrocortisone is maintained for 3 months and adrenocortical function is evaluated at that time with a rapid Cortrosyn test (250 μg ACTH 1–24 intravenous bolus, with plasma cortisol measured at 0, 30, and 60 min). If the test is normal (cortisol >18 and >20 μg/dL at 30 and 60 min, respectively), glucocorticoid replacement is discontinued. If the response is subnormal, the patient is reevaluated at 3-month intervals. Seventy percent to 80% of the patients will have a normal test at 6 months postoperatively. Patients should be given extra glucocorticoids during stress (twice replacement for minor stress, such as febrile illness or dental surgery, and 8–10 times replacement for major stress, such as major trauma or surgery).

Postoperative Evaluation For Probable Complications In Patients With Cushing Disease

Monitoring The HPA axis should be monitored for probable recurrence (repeated measurements of UFC excretion every 3 months during the first postoperative year, and every 6 months during the second). After the end of the second postoperative year close monitoring for clinical signs and symptoms of recurrence is recommended.

The hypothalamic-pituitary-thyroid axis should be assessed every 3 months.

Central hypothyroidism usually persists for at least 3 months after surgical cure of hypercortisolism. The time course of recovery of the hypothalamo-pituitary-thyroid axis is not well known. Patients with persistently subnormal free T_4 values should receive T_4 replacement therapy, using free T_4 and not thyroid stimulating hormone plasma levels as the therapeutic end point. Of note, successful cure of hypercortisolism may unmask a pre-existing primary autoimmune thyroid disease, which may present either as hypothyroidism or transient hyperthyroidism (22).

The hypothalamic-pituitary-growth axis in growing patients should be carefully monitored, every 6 months in terms of linear growth. GH hyposecretion continues for at least a year after convalescence, in spite of significant increases in the growth rate of all growing patients. GH secretion recovers approximately 18 months after surgery (22). Catch-up growth is not usually achieved in children with Cushing syndrome even after successful surgical treatment resulting in compromised final adult height (63). These findings underscore the significance of early diagnosis and treatment. Thus, after becoming eucortisolemic, children with a decreased growth rate should be evaluated for GH deficiency; if GH deficient, GH therapy should be initiated. Gonadotropin-releasing hormone analog may be used in patients already in puberty (66).

In successfully treated children and adolescents, loss of weight, a decrease of body mass index, and an increase of bone mineral density into the normal range invariably take place. A residual effect on the body composition of these patients, such as decreased muscle mass and an increase in total body or visceral fat mass may increase their risk for development of metabolic syndrome, or syndrome X. Some patients may exhibit anxiety, melancholic symptoms irritability, deterioration in school performance in the first postoperative year or even longer and may require treatment (64, 65).

REFERENCES

1. Orth DN. Cushing's syndrome. N Engl J Med. 1995;332:791–803.
2. Kamilaris T, Chrousos GP. Adrenal diseases. In: Moore WT, Eastman R, eds. Diagnostic Endocrinology. Toronto: B.C. Decker; 1989:79–109.
3. Magiakou MA, Chrousos GP. Corticosteroid therapy, nonendocrine disease and corticosteroid withdrawal. In Bardin CW, ed. Current Therapy in Endocrinology and Metabolism. 5th ed. St. Louis: Mosby Year Book; 1994:120–124.
4. Carey RM, Varma SK, Drake CR, et al. Ectopic secretion of corticotropin-releasing factor as a cause of Cushing's syndrome. N Engl J Med. 1984;311:13–20.
5. Auchus RJ, Mastorakos G, Friedman TC, et al. Corticotropin-releasing hormone production by a small cell carcinoma in a patient with ACTH-dependent Cushing syndrome. J Endocrinol Invest. 1994;17:447–452.
6. Malchoff CD, Rosa J, DeBold CR. Adrenocorticotropin-independent bilateral macronodular adrenal hyperplasia: an unusual cause of Cushing's syndrome. J Clin Endocrinol Metab. 1989;68:855–860.
7. Magiakou MA, Chrousos GP. Diagnosis and treatment of Cushing disease. In: Imura H, ed. The Pituitary Gland. 2nd ed. New York:Raven Press; 1994:491–508.
8. Doppman JL, Travis WD, Nieman L, et al. Cushing syndrome due to primary pigmented nodular adrenocortical disease: findings at CT and MR imaging. Radiology. 1989;172:415–420.
9. Doppman JL, Nieman LK, Travis WD, et al. CT and MR imaging of massive macronodular adrenocortical disease: a rare cause of autonomous primary adrenal hypercortisolism. J Comput Assist Tomogr. 1991;15:773–779.
10. Lacroix A, Bolté E, Tremblay J, et al. Gastric inhibitory polypeptide–dependent cortisol hypersecretion—a new cause of Cushing's syndrome. N Engl J Med. 1992;327:974–980.
11. Boscaro M, Barzon L, Fallo F, et al. Cushing's syndrome. Lancet. 2001;357:783–791.
12. Stratakis CA, Kirschner LS. Clinical and genetic analysis of primary bilateral adrenal diseases (micro- and macronodular disease) leading to Cushing syndrome. Horm Metab Res. 1998;30:456–463.
13. Bertagna X, Groussin L, Luton JP, et al. Aberrant receptor-mediated Cushing's syndrome. Horm Res. 2003;59 (Suppl. 1):99–103.
14. Sandrini F, Stratakis C. Clinical and molecular genetics of Carney complex. Mol Genet Metab 2003;78:83–92.
15. Linder BL, Esteban NV, Yergey AL, et al. Cortisol production rate in childhood and adolescence. J Pediatr. 1990;117:892–896.
16. Kerrigan JR, Veldhuis JD, Leyo SA, et al. Estimation of daily cortisol production and clearance rates in normal pubertal males by deconvolution analysis. J Clin Endocrinol Metab. 1993;76(6):1505–1510.
17. Leong GM, Mercado-Asis LB, Reynolds JC, et al. The effect of Cushing disease on bone mineral density, body composition, growth and puberty: a report of an identical adolescent twin pair. J Clin Endocrinol Metab. 1996;81:1905–1911.
18. Magiakou MA, Mastorakos G, Gomez MT, et al. Suppressed spontaneous and stimulated growth hormone secretion in patients with Cushing's disease before and after surgical cure. J Clin Endocrinol Metab. 1994;78:131–137.
19. Hughes NR, Lissett CA, Shalet SM. Growth hormone status following treatment for Cushing's syndrome. Clin Endocrinol (Oxf). 1999;51:61–66.
20. Savage MO, Storr HL, Grossman AB, et al. Growth and growth hormone secretion in paediatric Cushing's disease. Hormones (Athens). 2003;2:93–97.
21. Magiakou MA, Mastorakos G, Oldfield EH, et al. Cushing syndrome in children and adolescents: presentation, diagnosis and therapy. N Engl J Med. 1994;331:629–636.
22. Stratakis C, Magiakou MA, Mastorakos G, et al. Thyroid function in children with Cushing disease before and after transsphenoidal surgery. J Pediatr. 1997;131:905–909.
23. Magiakou MA, Chousos GP. Cushing's syndrome in children and adolescents: current diagnostic and therapeutic strategies. J Endocrinol Invest. 2002;25:181–194.
24. Schuff KG. Issues in the diagnosis of Cushing's syndrome for the primary care physician. Prim Care. 2003;30:791–799.
25. Murphy BEP. Urinary free cortisol determinations: what they measure. The Endocrinologist. 2002;12:143–150.
26. Findling JW, Raff H. Newer diagnostic techniques and problems in Cushing's disease. Endocrinol Metab Clin North Am. 1999;28:191.
27. Boscaro M, Barzon L, Sonino N. The diagnosis of Cushing's syndrome: atypical presentations and laboratory shortcomings. Arch Intern Med. 2000;160:3045–3053.
28. Newell-Price J, Trainer P, Besser M, et al. The diagnosis and differential diagnosis of Cushing's syndrome and pseudo-Cushing's states. Endocr Rev.1998;19:647–672.
29. Bierwolf C, Kern W, Molle M, et al. Rhythms of pituitary-adrenal activity during sleep in patients with Cushing's disease. Exp Clin Endocrinol Diabetes. 2000;108:470–479.
30. Gafni RI, Papanicolaou DA, Nieman LK. Nighttime salivary cortisol measurement as a simple, noninvasive, outpatient screening test for Cushing's syndrome in children and adolescents. J Pediatr. 2000;137: 30–35.
31. Papanicolaou DA, Mullen N, Kyrou I, et al. Nighttime salivary cortisol: a useful midnight serum cortisol measurement distinguishes Cushing's syndrome from pseudo-Cushing states. J Clin Endocrinol Metab. 1998;83:1163.
32. Jubiz W, Meikle AW, Levinson RA, et al. Effect of diphenylhydantoin on the metabolism of dexamethasone. N Engl J Med. 1970;283:11–14.
33. Yaneva M, Mosnier-Pudar H, Dugue MA, et al. Midnight salivary cortisol for the initial diagnosis of Cushing's syndrome of various causes. J Clin Endocrinol Metab. 2004;89:3345–3351.
34. Papanicolaou DA, Yanovski JA, Cutler GB Jr, et al. A Single midnight serum cortisol measurement distinguishes Cushing's syndrome from pseudo-Cushing's syndrome. J Clin Endocrinol Metab. 1998;83:1163–1167.

35. Morris DG, Grossman AB. Dynamic tests in the diagnosis and differential diagnosis of Cushing's syndrome. *J Endocrinol Invest.* 2003;26:64–73.

36. Yanovski JA, Cutler GB Jr, Chrousos GP, et al. Corticotropin-releasing hormone stimulation following low-dose dexamethasone administration. A new test to distinguish Cushing's syndrome from pseudo-Cushing's states. JAMA. 1993;269:2232–2238.

37. Chrousos GP, Schulte HM, Oldfield EH, et al. The corticotropin releasing factor stimulation test: an aid in the evaluation of patients with Cushing's syndrome. *N Engl J Med.* 1984;310:622–626.

38. Newell-Price J, Morris DG, Drake WM, et al. Optimal response criteria for the human CRH test in the differential diagnosis of ACTH-dependent Cushing's syndrome. *J Clin Endocrinol Metab.* 2002;87:1640–1645.

39. Reimondo G, Paccotti P, Minetto M, et al. The corticotrophin-releasing hormone test is the most reliable noninvasive method to differentiate pituitary from ectopic ACTH secretion in Cushing's syndrome. *Clin Endocrinol* (Oxf). 2003;58:718–724.

40. Liddle GW. Tests of pituitary-adrenal suppressibility in the diagnosis of Cushing's syndrome. *J Clin Endocrinol Metab.* 1960;20:1539–1560.

41. Nieman LK, Chrousos GP, Oldfield EH, et al. The ovine CRH test and the dexamethasone suppression test in the differential diagnosis of Cushing's syndrome. *Ann Intern Med.* 1986;105: 862–867.

42. Doppman JL, Frank JA, Dwyer AJ, et al. Gadolinium DPTA enhanced MR imaging of ACTH-secreting microadenomas of the pituitary gland. *J Comp Assist Tomogr.* 1988;12:728–735.

43. Rockall AG, Babar SA, Sohaib SA, et al. CT and MR imaging of the adrenal glands in ACTH-independent Cushing syndrome. *Radiographics.* 2004;24:435–452.

44. Lumachi F, Zucchetta P, Marzola MC, et al. Usefulness of CT scan, MRI and radiocholesterol scintigraphy for adrenal imaging in Cushing's syndrome. *Nucl Med Commun.* 2002;23:469–473.

45. Oldfield EH, Doppman L, Nieman LK. et al. Petrosal sinus sampling with and without corticotropin releasing hormone in patients with Cushing's syndrome. N Engl J Med. 1991;325:897–905.

46. Lienhardt A, Grossman AB, Dacie JE, et al. Relative contributions of inferior petrosal sinus sampling and pituitary imaging in the investigation of children and adolescents with ACTH-dependent Cushing's syndrome. *J Clin Endocrinol Metab.* 2001;86:5711–5714.

47. Lefournier V, Martinie M, Vasdev A, et al. Accuracy of bilateral inferior petrosal or cavernous sinuses sampling in predicting the lateralization of Cushing's disease pituitary microadenoma: influence of catheter position and anatomy of venous drainage. *J Clin Endocrinol Metab.* 2003;88:196–203.

48. Findling JW. Inferior petrosal sinus sampling: pros and cons; when and where. *J Endocrinol Invest.* 2000;23:193–195.

49. Diez JJ, Iglesias P. Complications of inferior petrosal sinus sampling for the etiological diagnosis of Cushing's syndrome. *J Endocrinol Invest.* 2002;25:195–196.

50. Arnaldi G, Angeli A, Atkinson AB, et al. Diagnosis and complications of Cushing's syndrome: a consensus statement. *J Clin Endocrinol Metab.* 2003;88:5593–5602.

51. Malpalam TJ, Tyrrell JB, Wilson CB. Transsphenoidal microsurgery for Cushing disease: a report of 216 cases. *Ann Intern Med.* 1988;109:487–493.

52. Rees DA, Hanna FW, Davies JS, et al. Long term follow-up results of transsphenoidal surgery for Cushing's disease in a single centre using strict criteria for remission. *Clin Endocrinol* (Oxf). 2002;56:541–551.

53. Hoybye C, Grenback E, Thorén M, et al. Transsphenoidal surgery in Cushing disease: 10 years of experience in 34 consecutive cases. *J Neurosurg.* 2004;100:634–638.

54. Friedman RB, Oldfield EH, Nieman LK, et al. Repeat transsphenoidal surgery in Cushing's disease. *J Neurosurg.* 1989;71:520–527.

55. Kobayashi T, Kida Y, Mori Y. Gamma knife radiosurgery in the treatment of Cushing disease: long-term results. *J Neurosurg.* 2002;97: 422–428.

56. Hentschel SJ, McCutcheon IE. Stereotactic radiosurgery for Cushing disease. *Neurosurg Focus.* 2004; 16:E5.

57. Mahmoud -Ahmed AS, Suh JH. Radiation therapy for Cushing's disease: a review. *Pituitary.* 2002;5:175–180.

58. Storr HL, Plowman PN, Carroll PV, et al. Clinical and endocrine responces to pituitary radiotherapy in pediatric Cushing's disease: an effective second-line treatment. *J Clin Endocrinol Metab.* 2003;88:34–37.

59. Moore TJ, Dluhy RG, Williams GH, et al. Nelson's syndrome: frequency, prognosis, and effect of prior pituitary irradiation. *Ann Intern Med.* 1976;85:731–734.

60. Vella A, Thompson GB, Grant CS, et al. Laparoscopic adrenalectomy for adrenocorticotropin-dependent Cushing's syndrome. *J Clin Endocrinol Metab.* 2001;86:1596–1599.

61. Miller KA, Albanese C, Harrison M, et al. Experience with laparoscopic adrenalectomy in pediatric patients. *J Pediatr Surg.* 2002;37:979–982.

62. Gomez MT, Magiakou MA, Mastorakos G, et al. The pituitary corticotroph is not the rate limiting step in the postoperative recovery of the hypothalamic-pituitary-adrenal axis in patients with Cushing syndrome. *J Clin Endocrinol Metab.* 1993;77:173–177.

63. Rollin GA, Ferreira NP, Junges M, et al. Dynamics of serum cortisol levels after transsfenoidal surgery in a cohort of patients with Cushing's disease. *J Clin Endocrinol Metab.* 2004;89:1131–1139.

64. Magiakou MA, Mastorakos G, Chrousos GP. Final stature in patients with endogenous Cushing's syndrome. *J Clin Endocrinol Metab.* 1994;79:1082–1085.

65. Dorn LD, Burgess ES, Friedman TC, et al. The longitudinal course of psychopathology in Cushing syndrome after correction of hypercortisolism. J Clin Endocrinol Metab. 1997;82:912–919.

66. Sonino N, Fava GA. Psychiatric disorders associated with Cushing's syndrome. Epidemiology, pathophysiology and treatment. CNS Drugs.2001;15:361–373.

CHAPTER 29

Adrenal Insufficiency

Lynda E. Polgreen, MD
Kyriakie Sarafoglou, MD
Anna Petryk, MD

Adrenal insufficiency describes a condition of deficient production of adrenal cortical hormones caused by diseases affecting the adrenal gland (primary), the pituitary and the secretion of adrenocorticotropic hormone (ACTH) (secondary) or the hypothalamus and the secretion of corticotropic-releasing hormone (CRH) (tertiary). The severity of illness depends on the relative deficiency in the production of adrenal hormones both at a basal rate and in response to stressors. In primary adrenal insufficiency, usually all three zones of the adrenal cortex are involved, and therefore, secretion of all adrenal steroids is impaired. In secondary adrenal insufficiency, only the zona fasciculata and zona reticularis are affected; the zona glomerulosa remains intact for normal mineralocorticoid production.

The relative frequencies of the causes of adrenal insufficiency vary with age. In infancy, the most common cause is congenital adrenal hyperplasia (see Chapter 27). In children, adrenal hemorrhage secondary to anoxia or sepsis is most common, and during adolescence, the predominant cause is autoimmune adrenalitis (1).

PRESENTATION OF PRIMARY AND SECONDARY ADRENAL INSUFFICIENCY

The presentation of adrenal insufficiency can range from subtle and nonspecific to severe shock depending on the degree of insufficiency and level of stress. Infants with acute primary adrenal insufficiency during the first weeks of life present with acute dehydration, failure to regain birth weight, hypotension, hypoglycemia, and lethargy. Infants with a gradual onset of primary adrenal insufficiency may present with failure to thrive, hyperpigmentation, and fasting hypoglycemia. Charactcristic biochemical abnormalities consist of hyponatremia, hyperkalemia, elevated renin and low or absent aldosterone. The most common cause of adrenal insufficiency in the first 2–3 weeks of life is the salt-wasting form of congenital adrenal hyperplasia (CAH) due to 21α-hydroxylase deficiency (21OHD).

In the older child and adolescent, symptoms may include salt craving, fasting hypoglycemia, decline in linear growth rate, weight loss due to anorexia, vomiting and diarrhea, abdominal pain, generalized fatigue, muscle and joint pain, postural hypotension, and hyperpigmentation (see Figure 29-1). Hyperpigmentation seen in primary adrenal insufficiency (PAI) is due to increased melanocortin-stimulating hormone (MSH) secretion and

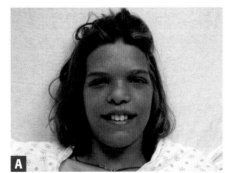
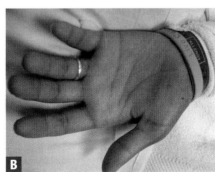
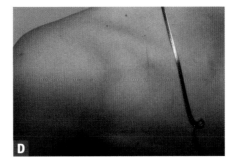

involves skin creases, axillae, groin, buccal, gingival, and vaginal mucosa, scars, and moles. Corticotropin and melanocyte-stimulating hormone (MSH) are both components of the same progenitor hormone. When corticotropin is cleaved from the prohormone, MSH is concurrently released. Hyperpigmentation of body areas unexposed to sun is characteristic of PAI (Figure 29-1). If PAI is associated with vitiligo, alopecia, autoimmune thyroiditis, diabetes, celiac disease, and/or mucocutaneous candidiasis, the possibility of autoimmune polyendocrinopathies should be explored.

The clinical manifestations of patients with secondary, or tertiary adrenal insufficiency are similar to those of patients with PAI but less severe and without salt wasting because aldosterone is regulated mainly via the

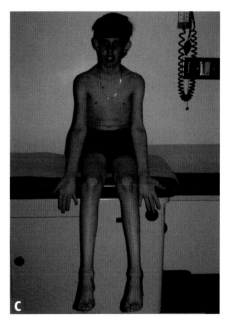

FIGURE 29-1. Hyperpigmentation Associated with Addison Disease. **A.** Notice the hyperpigmentation of the lips and mouth creases. **B.** Hyperpigmentation in the hand creases. **C.** Diffuse hyperpigmentation and thin appearance. **D.** Hyperpigmentation caused from an electrocardiograph lead placed on the patient for only a few hours 2 days earlier.

Adrenal Insufficiency

AT-A-GLANCE

Adrenal insufficiency describes a condition of deficient production of adrenal cortical hormones. The etiology is either inadequate production of cortical hormones by the adrenal glands (primary adrenal insufficiency [PAI]) or hypothalamic/pituitary dysfunction (secondary adrenal insufficiency [SAI]). Adrenal insufficiency is quite rare in pediatric patients. It is caused by a variety of both congenital and acquired disorders. Replacement of both glucocorticoid and mineralocorticoid with the least amount of cushingoid side effects is the goal of treatment.

TYPES OF PAI	GENE	LOCUS	OMIM
Congenital adrenal hypoplasia (AHC)	DAX1, SF1	Xp21.3-p21.2, 9q33	300473, 184757
Adrenoleukodystrophy (ALD)	ABCD1	Xq28	300371
Neonatal ALD	PEX1, PEX5, PEX10, PEX13, PEX26	7q21-q22, 12p13.3, Chr 1, 2p15, 22q11.21	602136, 600414, 602859, 601789, 608666
Familial glucocorticoid deficiency type 1 (FGD1)	ACTHR(MC2R)	18p11.2	607397
Familial glucocorticoid deficiency type 2 (FGD2)	FGD2	18q11.2-q13.2	607398
Triple A or Allgrove syndrome (AAA)	AAAS	12q13	605378
Wolman disease (WD)	LIPA	10q24-q25	278000
Kearns-Sayre syndrome (KSS)	mtDNA deletions		530000
Smith-Lemli-Opitz syndrome (SLO)	DHCR7	11q12-q13	602858
Isolated autoimmune adrenalitis	Multiple HLA	6p21.3	
Autoimmune polyglandular syndrome (APS 1)	AIRE1	21q22.3	607358
Autoimmune polyglandular syndrome (APS 2)	CTLA-4 HLA-B8	2q33 6p21.3	123890 142830
Glucocorticoid resistance	GCR	5q31	138040
Infections (HIV, turberculosis, CMV, meningococcemia, etc).	N/A	N/A	N/A
Adrenal hemorrhage	N/A	N/A	N/A

TYPES OF SECONDARY/TERTIARY AI SAI	GENE	LOCUS	OMIM
Isolated ACTH deficiency	TBX19, POMC, CRH	1q23-24, 2p23.3, 8q13	604614, #609734, 122560
CPHD	PROP1	5q	601538
PCSK1 deficiency	PCSK1	5q15-q21	#600955

TYPES OF HYPOALDOSTERONISM	GENE	LOCUS	OMIM
18-Hydroxylase deficiency (or CMO1)	CYP11B2	8q21	203400
FHHA1 (or CMO2)	CYP11B2	8q21	124080
FHHA2	Unknown	NA	606984
PHA1	SCNN1A, SCNN1B, SCNN1G	16p13-p12, 16p13-p12, 12p13	264350
PHA2	WNK1, WNK4	12p13, 17q21-q22	605232, 601844

FORM	FINDINGS	CLINICAL PRESENTATION	
		INFANCY	CHILDHOOD & ADOLESCENCE
AHC due to DAX-1/ SF-1defects *DAX1(X-linked recessive)*	↑K, ↓Na, ↑PRA, ↓Aldo, ↑ACTH, ↓Cortisol	Severe salt wasting; adrenal crisis; hypoglycemia	Males with DAX1 mutations may present later with failure to thrive, hypoglycemia, hyperpigmentation, adrenal crisis, growth failure, hypogonadotropic hypogonadism and impaired spermatogenesis. Duchenne muscular dystrophy suggests contiguous gene deletions. Females carriers for DAX-1 mutations do not develop adrenal insufficiency and may present with delayed puberty.
SF-1(AR or AD)		46,XY infants homozygous for the R92Q mutation or heterozygous for the G35E mutation of the SF1 gene present with 46,XY complete GD and adrenal insufficiency; 46,XY heterozygous patients for the 8-bp or 18delC deletion and C16X, V15M, M78I, G91S, L437Q missence mutations of the SF1 gene, present with various degrees of GD and normal adrenal function.	46, XX heterozygous females with the R255L mutation present with isolated adrenal failure, whereas 46, XX heterozygous for the M78I, G91S and R92Q mutations are not affected. 46,XY heterozygous for the L437Q mutation develop hypogonadotropic hypogonadism.
ALD	↑K, ↓Na, ↑PRA, ↓aldo, ↑ACTH, ↓cortisol	NA	*Females:* asymptomatic carriers; they may occasionally have subnormal cortisol response; rarely develop adrenal insufficiency. *Males:* behavioral/neurologic symptoms; adrenal insufficiency, which may precede neurological symptoms; auditory and visual deficits
Neonatal ALD	↑ pipecolic, ↑ plasmalogen, ↑ VLCFA, ↑ ACTH, ↓ cortisol	Hypotonia; seizures; FTT; facial dysmorphism; retinal leopard spot pigmentation; deafness; hepatomegaly; no chondrodysplasia punctuata	Developmental delay; ataxia; optic atrophy; hearing loss; CNS abnormalities such as heteropias, micropachygyrias; adrenal atrophy with or without a adrenal insufficiency; affected patients typically die before 7 years of age; liver disease may develop
FGD (FGD1 and FGD2)	Nl Na, K, Nl aldo, Nl PRA, ↑ ACTH, ↓ cortisol	Hyperpigmentation; jaundice; hypotonia; hypoglycemia	FTT; hypoglycemia; hypoglycemic seizures; hyperpigmentation; tall stature in FGD1
AAA	Nl Na, K, Nl aldo, Nl PRA (Nl in 10–15%), ↑ ACTH, ↓ cortisol	NA	Alacrima, achalasia and adrenal insufficiency; hypoglycemia; FTT; papillary and cranial nerve abnormalities; amyotrophy, dystonia and chorea; hyperkeratosis, fissured palms, and cutis anserine; developmental delay
WD	Nl Na, K, Nl aldo, Nl PRA, ↑ ACTH, ↓ cortisol	Hepatomegaly; splenomegaly; anemia; foam cells in bone marrow; adrenal calcifications adrenal crisis; steatorrhea; FTT; fatal by 1 year of age, if untreated	Milder, later onset form is CESD presenting with hepatomegaly, hyperlipidemia, adrenal calcifications, short stature, and foam cells
KSS	Rarely: ↑ ACTH, ↓ cortisol	NA	Pigmentary retinopathy; progressive external ophthalmoplegia; cardiac conduction defects; hearing loss; short stature; gonadal failure; type 1 diabetes mellitus; thyroid disease; hypoparathyroidism; adrenal insufficiency rare
SLO	Rarely: ↑ ACTH, ↓ cortisol	Multiple congenital abnormalities	Growth retardation; FTT; developmental delay; adrenal insufficiency rare
AAD	↑K, ↓Na, ↑PRA, ↓aldo, ↑ACTH, ↓cortisol	NA	Female to male ration is 0.8; mean age of onset of adrenal insufficiency is 30 years

FORM	FINDINGS	CLINICAL PRESENTATION	
		INFANCY	CHILDHOOD & ADOLESCENCE
APS 1	↑K, ↓Na, ↑PRA, ↓aldo, ↑ACTH, ↓cortisol	NA	Adrenal insufficiency; hypoparathyroidism; mucocutaneous candidiasis, chronic active hepatitis, ovarian failure; type I diabetes; alopecia; vitiligo may also develop
APS 2	↑K, ↓Na, ↑PRA, ↓aldo, ↑ACTH, ↓cortisol	NA	Adrenal insufficiency; Graves disease or Hashimoto thyroiditis; type 1 diabetes mellitus
APS 3	↑K, ↓Na, ↑PRA, ↓aldo, ↑ACTH, ↓cortisol	NA	Graves disease or Hashimoto thyroiditis plus other autoimmune disease; no adrenal insufficiency
APS 4	↑K, ↓Na, ↑PRA, ↓aldo, ↑ACTH, ↓cortisol	NA	Adrenal insufficiency plus other autoimmune disease excluding the major components of APS 1 or APS 2
Glucocorticoid resistance	Nl or ↓K, Nl or ↑Na, Nl or ↓aldo, Nl or ↓PRA, Nl or ↑ACTH, ↑cortisol, ↑adrenal androgen ↑DOC, ↑B, ↑24 hr urine for 17 OHCS and 17-KS	NA	Ranges from asymptomatic to severe hyper-androgenism and/or mineralocorticoid excess and mild cortisol deficiency; symptoms may include low renin hypertension, androgen excess with acne, hirsutism, infertility, fatigue and in one case ambiguous genitalia
IAD			
18-hydroxylase deficiency (CMO 1)	↑K, ↓Na↓, ↑PRA, ↓18-OHB/aldo, absent aldo	Dehydration; FTT	Salt wasting; intermittent fevers; vomiting; FTT; recurrent dehydration, hypotension and metabolic acidosis; electrolytes normalize by 4 years of age; adults are asymptomatic but may be sensitive to severe salt loss
FHHA 1 (CMO 2)	↑K, ↓Na, ↑PRA, ↑18-OHB/aldo, ↓ or Nl aldo	Dehydration; FTT	Similar as in CMO1
FHHA 2	↑K, ↓Na, ↑PRA, ↓ or Nl aldo	Dehydration; FTT	Similar as in CMO1 and CMO2; no mutation in CYP11B2
PHA 1	↑K, ↓Na, ↑PRA, ↑aldo	Salt wasting; dehydration; FTT	Salt wasting, recurrent dehydration and FTT in both AR and AD forms of PHA1; patients with AR form may present with CF-like clinical picture; improves with age in the AD form
PHA 2	↑K, ↓Na, ↓PRA, Nl aldo	NA	FTT; hypertension
ACTH deficiency	Nl Na, K, Nl aldo, Nl PRA, ↓ACTH, ↓cortisol	Adrenal crisis; hypoglycemia	FTT; hypoglycemia; adrenal insufficiency; hyperphagia, obesity, and red hair in patients homozygous for mutations in the POMC gene
CPHD	Nl Na, K, Nl aldo, Nl PRA, ↓ACTH, ↓cortisol, ↓GH, ↓free T$_4$, ↓LH, ↓FSH, ↓PRL	Hypoglycemia; hypothyroidism; growth failure	Hypoglycemia; short stature; hypothyroidism; late adrenal insufficiency

IAD = isolated aldosterone deficiency; NA = not applicable; Nl = normal; K = potassium; Na = sodium; Cl = chloride; Ur Ca = urinary calcium; PRA = renin; ACTH = adreno-corticotropin; CMO 1 = corticosterone methyloxidase deficiency type 1; CMO 2 = corticosterone methyloxidase deficiency type 2; FHHA 1 = familial hyperreninemic hypoaldosteronism type 1; FHHA 2 = familial hyperreninemic hypoaldosteronism type 2; PHA 1 = pseudohypoaldosteronism type 1; PHA 2 = pseudohypoaldosteronism type 2; GH = growth hormone; TSH = thyroid-stimulating hormone; LH = luteinizing hormone; FSH = follicle-stimulating hormone; PRL = prolactin; FTT = failure to thrive; APS = autoimmune polyglandular syndrome; HIV = human immunodeficiency virus; CMV = cytomegalovirus; FTT = failure to thrive; VCLFA = very long chain fatty acids; MI = mineralocorticoid insufficiency; CESD = cholesterol ester storage disease; Aldo = aldosterone; DOC = deoxycorticosterone; GD = gonadal dysgenesis.

renin-aldosterone system and is only partially dependent on ACTH. Skin hyperpigmentation is not present, and ACTH deficiency often is associated with other anterior pituitary hormone deficiencies. The usual chronologic sequence of the development of anterior pituitary hormone deficiencies begins with growth hormone (GH) deficiency and is followed by gonadotropin deficiency, thyroid-stimulating hormone (TSH) deficiency, and lastly, ACTH deficiency. Thyroid hormone supplementation in patients with anterior pituitary deficiencies including ACTH may precipitate an acute adrenal crisis because thyroxine increases cortisol metabolism. For this reason, cortisol replacement should precede thyroid hormone replacement.

Secondary adrenal insufficiency is relatively common compared to the primary form as prolonged exogenous steroid use frequently leads to suppression of the hypothalamic-pituitary axis. Recovery of the hypothalamic-pituitary-adrenal axis in patients who have been on pharmacologic doses of glucocorticoids may take weeks to months and is related to duration of pharmacological glucocorticoid exposure. These patients are at risk for developing acute adrenal insufficiency because they are unable to mount an appropriate cortisol response to stress due to chronic suppression of corticotropin-releasing hormone (CRH) and ACTH by exogenous glucocorticoids.

Acute adrenal crisis is a medical emergency and can result in cardiovascular collapse and death. Other clinical scenarios where adrenal insufficiency should be considered include newborns with sepsis, disseminated intravascular coagulopathy, meningococcemia, severe bilateral hemorrhages, and anticoagulant therapy and patients known to have adrenal insufficiency who fail to absorb or receive proper oral doses of glucocorticoids.

DIAGNOSIS OF PRIMARY AND SECONDARY ADRENAL INSUFFICIENCY

First-Level Tests

First-level screening laboratory evaluation includes basal morning (8 A.M.) plasma ACTH, cortisol, aldosterone, renin, adrenal androgens [i.e., dehydroepiandrosterone (DHEA), dexydroepiandrosterone-sulfate (DHEA-S) and androstenedione (D4A)], and electrolytes. A basal morning cortisol level greater than 20 μg/dL excludes adrenal insufficiency. Cortisol levels less than 3 μg/dL associated with elevated ACTH levels (>100 pg/mL) are consistent with PAI, and a cortisol level of less than 3 μg/dL associated with low or normal levels of ACTH is diagnostic of SAI. Cortisol levels between 4 and 19 μg/dL are equivocal (2).

Since secretion of cortisol and ACTH is episodic with a diurnal rhythm, 24-hour urine collection of free cortisol, 17-hydroxycorticosteroids, and 17-ketosteroids provides an integrated excretion of adrenal metabolites and is a useful additional tool in the assessment of adrenocortical function in equivocal cases (adrenal insufficiency is unlikely if their excretion is at the upper limit of normal for the assay). Overall, baseline urinary measurements are not recommended for the diagnosis of adrenal insufficiency. Low aldosterone, increased renin, decreased sodium and chloride, increased potassium levels and an elevated ratio of blood urea nitrogen to creatinine (prerenal azotemia) suggest mineralocorticoid deficiency.

Second-Level Tests

The screening tests may be sufficient to establish the diagnosis of overt primary adrenal insufficiency. Detection of more subtle adrenocortical dysfunction and differentiation between PAI and SAI may require dynamic testing, including a cosyntropin stimulation test, a CRH or metyrapone test (see Chapter 43) (2). The cosyntropin stimulation test uses either 1 μg (low-dose test) or 250 μg (high-dose test) of synthetic ACTH 1–24, and the rise in cortisol is measured at 30 and 60 minutes. A normal response to a cosyntropin stimulation test is a peak plasma cortisol level of 18 to 20 μg/dL (500 to 550 nmol/L) or greater (3). A low-dose ACTH stimulation test is preferred in patients suspected of early SAI/tertiary because these patients may respond normally to a high-dose cosyntropin stimulation test unless atrophy of the adrenal gland has occurred due to prolonged lack of adrenal stimulation by ACTH.

The metyrapone stimulation test evaluates the function of the entire hypothalamic-pituitary-adrenal axis (4). Physiologically, metyrapone blocks 11β-hydroxylation, resulting in decreased cortisol secretion and a compensatory rise in ACTH and 11-deoxycortisol(S) levels. Lack of increase in ACTH and 11-deoxycortisol levels after metyrapone administration is diagnostic of ACTH hyposecretion. When the diagnosis of ACTH hyposecretion is made, it is important to rule out other pituitary hormone deficiencies because isolated ACTH hyposecretion is rare. Finally, a CRH stimulation test is helpful in distinguishing between a hypothalamic and pituitary cause of adrenal insufficiency, secondary vs. tertiary; in both conditions cortisol levels are low at baseline and remain low after CRH. In patients with secondary adrenal insufficiency, there is little or no ACTH response, whereas in patients with tertiary disease there is an exag-

gerated and prolonged response of ACTH to CRH stimulation, which is not followed by an appropriate cortisol response.

Abdominal computed tomographic (CT) scanning or even plain radiographs may reveal adrenal calcification in the case of adrenal hemorrhage, Wolman disease, or tuberculosis of the adrenal glands. Magnetic resonance imaging (MRI) of the head with gadolinium enhancement is used to evaluate the hypothalamus and pituitary, when SAI/tertiary is suspected.

Additional Tests for Differentiation of Primary Adrenal Insufficiency

Further diagnostic evaluation for determination of the different causes of adrenal insufficiency is determined based on associated findings and presentation. If the presentation is in the early neonatal period and is associated with ambiguous genitalia, an elevated 17α-hydroxyprogesterone (17-OHP) level would suggest the diagnosis of congenital adrenal hyperplasia (CAH) due to 21OHD and rarely of 3β-hydroxysteroid dehydrogenase type II (3β-HSDII). A low 17-OHP level in the presence of enlarged adrenals would suggest 1) either lipoid CAH due to StAR deficiency and rarely due to inactivating mutations of the CYP11A gene encoding the P450scc enzyme (the first enzyme in adrenal steroidogenesis), or 2) mutations or deletions of P450 oxidoreductase, resulting in combined deficiencies of 17-hydroxylase/17,20 lyase and, 21-hydroxylase, enzymes. A low 17-OHP level and hypoplastic adrenals suggest congenital adrenal hypoplasia due to SF-1 or DAX-1 mutations. Karyotype is suggested even in the absence of ambiguous genitalia; patients with congenital lipoid CAH or congenital adrenal hypoplasia due to SF-1 mutations may have 46, XY sex reversal.

The presence of autoimmune endocrinopathies or autoimmune disease in the patient or other family members including hypocalcemia, or mucocutaneous candidiasis suggests autoimmune polyglandular syndromes (APSs). The presence of adrenal antibodies, including antibodies to 21α-hydroxylase, suggests adrenalitis, either isolated or as part of an APS.

If antibodies are negative, particularly in boys presenting with PAI, fasting very long-chain fatty acids (VLCFAs) should be measured in order to rule out adrenoleukodystrophy. Possible adrenal hemorrhage, or infiltrative processes to the adrenal gland should be sought as well. The presence of lactic acidosis, myopathy, or sensorineural deafness suggests mitochondrial disease such as Kearns–Sayre syndrome.

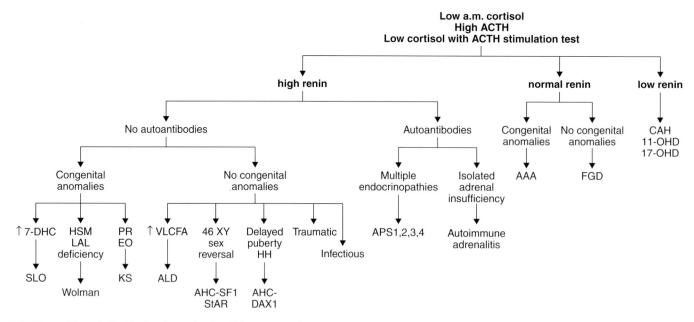

FIGURE 29-2. Diagnostic Algorithm for Primary Adrenal Insufficiency. AHC = adrenal hypoplasia congenita, APS = autoimmune polyglandular syndromes, ALD = adrenoleukodystrophy, FGD = familial glucocorticoid deficiency, KS = Kearns-Sayre syndrome, SLO = Smith-Lemli-Opitz syndrome, PR = pigmentary retinopathy, EO = external ophthalmoplegia, HH = hypogonadotropic hypogonadism, LAL= lysosomal acid lipase, 7-DHC = 7-dehydrocholesterol, HSM = hepatosplenomegaly, StAR = steroidogenic acute regulatory protein.

If physical findings suggest Allgrove syndrome, Wolman disease, or Smith–Lemli–Opitz syndrome, specific biochemical and genetic tests are recommended. Sequence analysis of the AAAS gene in Allgrove syndrome, enzyme analysis for lysosomal acid lipase activity in Wolman disease, genetic testing and enzymatic tests for Smith–Lemli–Opitz are clinically available.

Emergency Tests

Since diagnosis of adrenal insufficiency may be a lengthy process, treatment for presumed acute adrenal insufficiency is often necessary in the absence of any diagnostic certainty. To assist in future diagnosis, a critical blood sample for cortisol, ACTH, aldosterone, and renin should be obtained in critically ill patients before treatment begins. A recent study of adrenal insufficiency in septic shock suggests using a cutoff of a random cortisol level greater than 34 μg/dL to diagnose a sufficienct adrenal response; a cortisol level less than 15 μg/dL to suggest adrenal insufficiency; and a rise of cortisol level greater than 9 ug/dL above baseline response to high-dose (250 μg) cosyntropin stimulation suggests an appropriate adrenal response (5). However, in the setting of shock or severe illness, cortisol levels are extremely variable, and no standard has been set for diagnosing adrenal insufficiency.

Newborn Screening

Newborn screening for CAH is mandatory in all but five states (U.S. National Screening Status Report, 2006).

Prenatal Diagnosis Prenatal diagnosis is available for some of the heritable causes of adrenal insufficiency. If a familial mutation is known, such as in CAH, familial glucocorticoid deficiency (FGD), or Allgrove syndrome, prenatal genetic testing could be performed. Adrenoleukodystrophy (ALD) can be diagnosed by measurement of VLCFA levels in cultured amniocytes and chorion villus cells. Screening for Smith–Lemli–Opitz (SLO) syndrome can be done by prenatal ultrasound or by genetic or enzymatic analysis. Eighty percent of congenital anomalies associated with SLO syndrome are diagnosed by ultrasound. A prenatal ultrasound that shows nonvascular intrauterine growth retardation plus another congenital anomaly should raise the suspicion of SLO syndrome (9). Low sterol levels in maternal plasma (included in the prenatal triple screen), chorionic villi, or amniotic fluid will confirm the diagnosis of SLO syndrome. Figures 29-2 and 29-3 present diagnostic algorithms.

TREATMENT

Standard Treatment Regimen Maintenance therapy for PAI requires both glucocorticoid and mineralocorticoid replacement. Dosing of glucocorticoid is based on the physiologic cortisol secretion rate (5–7 mg/m2/day) (7). Taking into account incomplete intestinal absorption and drug metabolism, the suggested

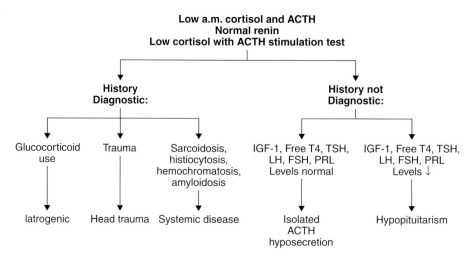

FIGURE 29-3. Diagnostic Algorithm for Secondary Adrenal Insufficiency. ACTH = adrenocorticotropin hormone, IGF-1 = insulin-like growth factor-1, TSH = thyroid stimulating hormone, LH = luteinizing hormone, FSH = follicle stimulating hormone, PRL= prolactin.

physiologic replacement dose of hydrocortisone in pediatric patients is usually 8–10 mg/m^2/day divided in two or three doses. In patients with ACTH deficiency, doses closer to 8 mg/m^2/day administered twice daily may be sufficient. The relative potency must be considered when treating with glucocorticoids other than hydrocortisone. Dosage adjustments are clinically based and titrated to a minimum needed to control the symptoms.

In PAI, mineralocorticoid replacement is also required. Fludrocortisone is currently the only mineralocorticoid available, and it is given at a dose of 0.05–0.1 mg/day orally. Treatment with fludrocortisone is effective only if adequate salt is ingested (1–2 g/day or 17–34 mEq of sodium) (1). This is not difficult to achieve in children on a regular adult diet, but most infant formulas are low in salt and need supplementation either added to the formula or given separately due to the noxious effect of salt on the taste of formula. The necessary minimum salt intake increases during hot weather and exercise.

In patients with multiple hormonal deficiencies, it is exceedingly important to initiate cortisol replacement at least 1 week prior to replacement of thyroid hormone because thyroid hormone accelerates the metabolism of glucocorticoids and mineralocorticoids and may precipitate adrenal crisis.

GH also has been shown to affect the metabolism of cortisol in adult patients with ACTH deficiency (8). The main mechanism is through the inhibition of hepatic 11β-hydroxysteroid dehydrogenase type 1 (11β-HSD-1), which catalyzes the conversion of cortisone to active cortisol (9). As a result, circulating cortisol levels are reduced. Therefore, adjustment of the hydrocortisone dose may be required once GH replacement is commenced.

Patients with adrenal insufficiency need to double or triple their daily cortisol dose during times of stress, such as during a febrile illness. If the patient is vomiting and is unable to take the dose orally, he or she should be given intramuscular hydrocortisone succinate (Solucortef) 50–100 mg/m^2/24 h or methylprednisolone acetate (Depo-Medrol) 15–20 mg/m^2/24 h as a single dose (10). All patients on cortisol replacement therapy have to be instructed on administration of intramuscular hydrocortisone and need a home supply as well as a supply at school.

Immediate/Emergency In adrenal crisis, immediate treatment consists of stress doses of corticosteroids, fluid for blood volume expansion, and electrolyte replacement. An initial loading dose of hydrocortisone of 100 mg/m^2 is given intravenously or intramuscularly if intravenous access is not possible immediately, followed by 100 mg/m^2/24 h of hydrocortisone given intravenously by continuous drip or divided every 6 hours. Prednisone and cortisone should be avoided in hypotensive patients because they both need to be metabolized in the liver to become active, a process that may be delayed in hypotensive patients. Hydrocortisone in large doses has sufficient mineralocorticoid activity to make fludrocortisone administration unnecessary during acute treatment. However, if hyperkalemia develops, fludrocortisone (0.05–0.2 mg/24 h) could be added or the dose of hydrocortisone increased. Patients should be monitored closely for hyperkalemia and hypoglycemia and treated appropriately.

Adjustment of the daily cortisol replacement regimen is required for surgical procedures. The usual dose of fludrocortisone should be given with 15 mL of water 4–6 hours before scheduled surgery. On the day of surgery, before initiation of anesthesia, the patient is given an intravenous bolus of hydrocortisone of 50–100 mg/m^2 and then started on a continuous infusion of hydrocortisone at 100 mg/m^2/24 h during the procedure, followed by 100 mg/m^2/24 h divided into four doses. This regimen should be continued as long as the patient is unable to take the medication by mouth (11).

Post–Critical Care Once the patient takes fluids by mouth, hydrocortisone should be given by mouth at 50–75 mg/m^2/24 h in three doses (every 8 hours). Once stress is over, hydrocortisone dose should be tapered to the maintenance dose over the next few days.

Treatment Monitoring The effectiveness of treatment should be monitored clinically (e.g., blood pressure, growth velocity, weight, and skin pigmentation) and by laboratory testing (e.g., ACTH, renin, serum, electrolytes, and fasting serum glucose).

LONG-TERM CONCERNS AND FOLLOW-UP MANAGEMENT

There are many potential side effects of glucocorticoid treatment, including hypertension, hyperglycemia, weight gain, osteoporosis, and gastric ulcers. In children on long-term glucocorticoid replacement, growth suppression is a concern. Long-acting synthetic glucocorticoids (e.g., prednisone and prednisolone) have been shown to have negative effects on growth (12) and are not recommended in growing children. When growth velocity decreases, the glucocorticoid dose may need to be lowered.

Bone mineral density should be followed annually by bone densitometry in children older than 5 years of age. Dietary intake of calcium and vitamin D should be assessed and supplemented if needed.

All patients with adrenal insufficiency should keep a glucocorticoid injection kit at home and at school. They also should wear a medical alert bracelet or necklace or carry a medical alert card.

Controversial Issues The use of DHEA in children has been controversial. DHEA has gained popularity over the last 10 years as a dietary supplement purported to decrease the risk of common adult diseases such as cardiovascular disease, osteoporosis, breast cancer, and impaired memory. Since DHEA is sold as an over-the-counter supplement, its use is entirely unregulated at this time.

A double-blind, placebo-controlled crossover study on the use of DHEA in adult women with adrenal insufficiency found a significant decrease in total and high-density lipoprotein (HDL) cholesterol levels, depression, and anxiety and improved sexuality (13).

PRIMARY ADRENAL INSUFFICIENCY

Etiology/Pathophysiology Primary adrenal insufficiency (PAI) results from destruction or dysfunction of the adrenal cortex; the adrenal medulla is typically preserved. Recent studies estimate the prevalence of PAI to be approximately 1 in 8000 in Western countries and 1 in 10.000, when an iatrogenic cause is excluded (14).

The etiologies of PAI are broken down into congenital and acquired.

Congenital Adrenal Hypoplasia

Etiology/Pathophysiology Congenital adrenal hypoplasia (AHC) is a rare cause of adrenal insufficiency with an estimated incidence of 1 per 12,500 live births (15). AHC is usually an X-linked recessive disease but it may also be autosomal recessive. The autosomal recessive form is due to certain defects of the gene that encodes for steroidogenic factor 1 (SF-1) or due to defects of an unidentified gene.

X-linked recessive AHC results from a deletion or point mutation in the dosage-sensitive sex reversal–adrenal hypoplasia congenital gene on the X chromosome, gene 1 (DAX1 or NR0B1) (16). The genetic locus for X-linked AHC was mapped to Xp21 through studies of male patients whose adrenal insufficiency were part of contiguous gene deletion syndromes (17). This region of the X chromosome is also the location of the dosage-sensitive sex reversal (DSS) locus important in sex determination; duplications of this area result in XY sex reversal. The DAX1 gene, also called NR0B1, encodes an orphan nuclear receptor that is required early in embryologic development of the hypothalamus, adrenal glands, and gonads (18). The DAX1 nuclear receptor has been shown to suppress SF-1-mediated transactivation (19) and is required for normal gonadal development in boys but not girls (20).

The adrenal cortices in X-linked AHC are structurally abnormal, lacking the individual zones of the normal adrenal cortex. The adrenal gland is hypoplastic, with characteristic "cytomegalic" adrenal cells. In the autosomal recessive form of AHC, the adrenal glands are hypoplastic, and the adrenal cortex consists almost exclusively of permanent cortex (miniature adult type). Hypoplasia of the adrenal gland results in an inability to produce glucocorticoids, mineralocorticoids, and sex steroids. Patients with AHC due to DAX1 defects develop hypogonadism, as well as impaired spermatogenesis.

It appears that DAX1 mutations have a direct effect on Sertoli cell function and spermatogenesis because neither gonadotropin-releasing hormone (GnRH) nor pituitary gonadotropin administration has been successful in stimulating spermatogenesis (21).

Clinical Presentation The majority of boys with AHC due to a DAX1 defect present with adrenal insufficiency—that is, adrenal crisis with salt wasting, hypoglycemia, lethargy, even shock—within the first 2 months of life (22). Some boys may present later in childhood with failure to thrive, vomiting, hypoglycemia, and hyperpigmentation. Growth failure with subsequent short stature is common.

AHC due to a contiguous gene deletion including the DAX1 gene can be associated with infantile glycerol kinase deficiency (GKD) or Duchenne muscular dystrophy (DMD). Patients with infantile GKD have elevated serum and urine glycerol levels and severe developmental delays. DMD is a progressive muscular dystrophy characterized by pseudohypertrophy of the calves.

Hypogonadotropic hypogonadism invariably has been associated with AHC due to DAX1 mutations and has both pituitary and hypothalamic components. However, the hypothalamic-pituitary-testicular axis can be active during infancy with the expected rise in gonadotropins and testosterone during the first 3 months of life. Chronic excessive ACTH levels due to adrenal insufficiency may stimulate Leydig cells and lead to gonadotropin-independent precocious puberty in some boys with DAX1 gene mutations (23). Boys with X-linked AHC frequently fail to enter puberty or have arrest of pubertal progression due to hypogonadotropic hypogonadism. Spermatogenesis typically is impaired. Female carriers of DAX1 mutations do not develop adrenal insufficiency but may present with delayed puberty (24).

Very few cases of autosomal recessive AHC associated with other pituitary hormone abnormalities due to unidentified genes have been described.

AHC can be part of the very rare IMAGe syndrome. IMAGe syndrome is defined by intrauterine growth retardation, metaphyseal dysplasia, AHC, and genital anomalies. No mutation in the DAX1 or SF-1 genes was identified in patients with IMAGe syndrome (25).

Diagnosis AHC should be considered in boys presenting with severe adrenal insufficiency in the newborn period or childhood and/or delayed puberty. Boys with isolated X-linked AHC will have signs of PAI: elevated ACTH, low cortisol, high renin, and low aldosterone (i.e., hyperkalemia or hyponatremia). Luteinizing hormone (LH) and follicle-stimulating hormone (FSH) levels may be normal at birth but low during pubertal years. The response to human chorionic gonadotropin (hCG) during adolescence is normal.

Genetic testing is available; the mutation detection rate with a positive family history of X-linked AHC is nearly 100% and with no family history is 50% to 70% (26). Testing for contiguous gene deletions in the DAX1 gene, which are associated with GKD and DMD, are detected by fluorescent in situ hybridization (FISH). The mutation detection rate in patients with X-linked AHC and GKD is 100% (26). Genetic testing or FISH for contiguous gene deletions can be used for prenatal diagnosis.

Childhood X-linked AHC resembles early adrenoleukodystrophy (ALD). The treatment and prognosis are quite different for ALD compared with AHC, and therefore, ALD needs to be excluded in these children through measurement of VLCFAs.

Treatment Adrenal insufficiency is treated with standard glucocorticoid and mineralocorticoid treatment. Hypogonadotropic hypogonadism in males secondary to DAX1 mutations is treated with hCG 1500–2000 IU two to three times weekly and human FSH 75 IU two to three times weekly to stimulate testosterone production and spermatogenesis (22); results vary however, and no effect on fertility was shown in small case series (22,24). Delayed puberty due to the hypogonadotropic hypogonadism in AHC can be treated with gradually increasing doses of testosterone (see Chapter 37).

Congenital Adrenal Insufficiency due to SF-1 Defects

Etiology/Pathophysiology SF-1 (NR5A1) gene defects may cause adrenal failure and/or XY sex reversal or isolated adrenal failure in

females (27–33). SF-1 is an orphan nuclear receptor that is critical for the development and function of the adrenal glands, gonads, pituitary gonadotropes, ventromedial nucleus of the hypothalamus, and male sexual differentiation.

Clinical Presentation 46,XY males heterozygous for the G35E mutation and homozygous for the R92Q in the SF-1 gene may present with gonadal dysgenesis (46,XY sex reversal), along with adrenal insufficiency (27–28). The presence of uterus differentiates 46, XY sex reversed patients due to SF-1 mutations from 46,XY sex reversed patients due to lipoid CAH. In lipoid CAH the Sertoli cells are intact and secretion of Antimullerian hormone inhibits the formation of uterus and fallopian tubes. 46,XY heterozygotes with 8-bp deletion and 18delC deletion and C16X, V15M, M78I, G91S, and L437Q missence mutations of the SF1 gene, have been associated with normal adrenal function and isolated gonadal impairment ranging from subnormal testicular structure with normal seminiferous tubules, to testes with very few germ cells, to testicular agenesis (29–32). SF-1 has a crucial role in adrenal gland formation in both sexes but is probably not necessary for female gonadal development. A 46,XX female heterozygous for missence R255L SF-1 mutation was diagnosed at 14 months of age with adrenal insufficiency but had normal ovarian function (33). Of note, 46,XX heterozygous for the recessive R92Q mutation (28), and the M78I and G91S sex-limited dominant mutations (32) have normal adrenal function. Experiments in mice suggest that heterozygotes for SF-1 mutations may have subclinical adrenal insufficiency with normal adrenal levels under basal conditions due to compensatory mechanisms such as cellular hypertrophy and increased expression of the rate-limiting steroidogenic protein StAR but inadequate adrenal stress response (34). The long term risk of adrenal dysfunction in 46,XY heterozygous individuals with isolated gonadal dysgenesis needs to be determined.

Diagnosis Affected patients have elevated ACTH, low cortisol, high renin and low aldosterone. In males, baseline gonadotropins can be normal to elevated during the first months of life. During late childhood and adolescence, pituitary gonadotropins may be low with an absent LH response to GnRH indicating a partial form of hypogonadotropic hypogonadism in addition to primary testicular defect (32). β-hCG stimulation test shows abnormal testosterone response. Genetic testing is available only on a research basis.

Treatment Comprehensive management of XY sex reversal is discussed in Chapter 36.

Adrenoleukodystrophy

Etiology/Pathophysiology

X-Linked Adrenoleukodystrophy X-ALD is an X-linked recessive peroxisomal disorder affecting the nervous system white matter and the adrenal cortex with an incidence of approximately 1 in 21,000 in the U.S. male population (35). X-ALD is characterized by accumulation of VLCFAs (>24 carbons, particularly C_{26}), primarily in the adrenal cortex, myelin of the central nervous system (CNS), and the Leydig cells of the testes. The genetic defect in X-ALD is in the adenosine triphosphate (ATP)–binding cassette, subfamily D, member 1 (ABCD1) gene on chromosome Xq28a (36). The ABCD1 gene codes for a peroxisomal membrane protein, ALDP, that is a member of the ABC transporter superfamily. The mechanism through which ABCD1 regulates the transport of VLCFAs into the peroxisome has not yet been clearly defined.

Neonatal Autosomal Recessive Adrenoleukodystrophy Neonatal ALD (NALD) is a peroxisomal biogenesis disorder similar to Zellweger syndrome that presents in the newborn period. It is characterized by a defect in peroxisome assembly and a generalized loss of peroxisomal function resulting in multiple enzyme abnormalities and accumulation of VLCFAs in the plasma, adrenal glands, CNS, and fibroblasts. The inheritance is autosomal recessive, and it affects males and females equally. NALD is distinct from Zellweger syndrome in that the clinical course is less severe, likely due to differences in peroxisomal enzyme activity (37).

Presentation

X-ALD Adrenal insufficiency in young males should prompt consideration of X-ALD as the underlying abnormality. Adrenal insufficiency has been documented in 70% to 90% of boys with X-ALD. The secretion of both cortisol and aldosterone is diminished. Adrenal insufficiency can precede neurological symptoms by several years in X-ALD and may in fact be the only manifestation in one form of the disorder.

The presentation and disease progression are variable and may range from a rapidly progressive childhood and adolescent ALD, characterized by neurological impairment and adrenal insufficiency, to the milder adrenomyeloneuropathy (AMN) in adults with and without adrenal disease, to isolated adrenal insufficiency (38).

Childhood- and adolescent-onset X-ALD is characterized by progressive neurological impairment and adrenal insufficiency. Adrenal insufficiency may be the presenting symptom, but symptoms of attention-deficit/hyperactivity

disorder with declining school function or auditory and visual processing deficits may be the first signs as well (39). Rapid neurological deterioration over 2 to 3 years is typical.

Isolated adrenal insufficiency occurs in about 14% to 20% of patients, presenting between 2 years of age and adulthood (most commonly by 7½ years of age) without evidence of neurological abnormality. However, most of these patients eventually develop AMN or cerebral disease. In asymptomatic boys with X-ALD, up to 80% have biochemical evidence of subclinical adrenal insufficiency (40).

NALD NALD is a peroxisomal biogenesis disorder, together with the Zellweger syndrome and infantile Refsum disease, are often referred to as Zellweger spectrum disorders (ZSDs). In ZSDs, peroxisome biogenesis is fully defective as caused by mutations in a number of different so-called PEX genes, which encode peroxins, the proteins required for normal peroxisomal assembly (for details see Chapter 24). Mutations of PEX5, PEX1, PEX10, PEX13 and PEX26 have been associated with NALD. Affected patients with NALD present in the newborn period with mild craniofacial abnormalities, hypotonia, progressive visual and hearing loss, global developmental delays, leopard spot retinal pigmentation, seizures, and liver disease. During autopsy of the brain cerebral abnormalities included heteropias and micropachygyria; autopsy of the adrenals has shown adrenal atrophy, especially of the zonae fasciculata and reticularis. Despite the severe adrenal atrophy clinical signs of adrenal insufficiency were not always present (41). Although there is clinical and biochemical overlap between NALD and Zellweger syndrome, the presence of moderate to severe dysmorphism, chondrodysplasia punctuata, renal cortical cysts, and the absence of adrenal atrophy suggest Zellweger syndrome (41). Children with NALD typically die before the age of 7 years.

Diagnosis

X-ALD All patients with X-ALD need to have a complete adrenal evaluation with baseline cortisol, ACTH, and low-dose cosyntropin-stimulated cortisol level determinations. Random cortisol levels may be within the normal range. Female carriers (heterozygotes) may have a subnormal cortisol response and decreased mineralocorticoid activity, although they rarely develop complete adrenal insufficiency (42).

High plasma levels of VLCFAs and elevated ratios of C_{26} and C_{22} VLCFAs are diagnostic of ALD and can be elevated even on the day of birth (43). The plasma concentration of VLCFAs is elevated in more than 99% of

males with X-ALD of all ages regardless of the presence or absence of symptoms. This assay is extremely specialized and therefore is performed only in a few laboratories worldwide. The assay has a sensitivity of approximately 85% in female carriers. Genetic testing for mutations in the ABCD1 gene is clinically available. If the disease-causing ABCD1 mutation has been identified in the family, genetic testing should be offered to females with normal VLCFA concentration because 20% of carriers register normal VLCFA concentrations.

Prenatal genetic testing can be offered to pregnant women who are carriers of a 46,XY fetus when a pathogenic mutation has been identified in the family. VLCFA can be measured in cultured amniocytes or cultured chorionic villus cells when genetic testing is not possible.

NALD In contrast to other forms of ALD, in NALD, abnormal concentrations of metabolites suggesting peroxisomal dysfunction are seen, such as decreased plasmalogen and elevated bile acids and serum pipecolic acid, in addition to the elevation in VLCFAs. Complementation analysis with cultured skin fibroblasts to determine affected PEX gene precedes genetic testing. Genetic testing is clinically available. Prenatal genetic testing can be offered if a mutation in the family has been identified (see Chapter 24).

Treatment

X-ALD Adrenal insufficiency in X-ALD is treated with standard glucocorticoid and mineralocorticoid treatment. Multiple therapies have been attempted in X-ALD. Hematopoietic cell transplantation (HCT) is effective in preventing the neurological deterioration in select patients with early brain involvement (11). Dietary therapy with glyceryl trierucate and trioleate oil (Lorenzo's oil) lowers VLCFAs; however, lowering VLCFA levels has not been effective in preventing disease progression in patients with symptomatic cerebral ALD. New therapies being investigated include lovastatin, phenylbutyrate, arginine butyrate, gene therapy, and therapies that increase ABCD2 expression (39).

NALD Adrenal insufficiency in NALD is treated with standard glucocorticoid and mineralocorticoid treatment. Treatment is aimed at the specific comorbidities with a multidisciplinary approach.

Familial Glucocorticoid Deficiency

Etiology/Pathophysiology Familial glucocorticoid deficiency (FGD) is a rare, genetically heterogeneous, autosomal recessive form of adrenal insufficiency. Fewer than 100 cases have been reported. FGD is caused by adrenal gland insensitivity to ACTH (45). Previously, FGD was divided into two forms based on the presence (FGD1) or absence (FGD2) of ACTH receptor mutations. Recently, however, with the identification of mutations at new genetic loci, FGD has been divided into three categories: FGD1, which is always characterized by mutations in the ACTH (MC2R gene) receptor (46); FGD2, in which patients have mutations in the melanocortin 2 receptor accessory protein (MRAP) gene; and FGD3, which includes those patients with mutations in chromosome 8q (47,48). All forms of FGD are indistinguishable clinically.

The ACTH receptor is a transmembrane protein involved in activation of adenyl cyclase and belongs to the melanocortin receptor family (MC-R). It is classified as melanocortin receptor 2 (MC2-R). Mutations in the MC2R gene account for approximately 25% of cases of FGD.

Histologically, the adrenal zona fasciculata and zona reticularis are significantly atrophied. The zona glomerulosa is preserved. This is true for all forms of FGD.

Clinical Presentation Clinically, FGD presents similarly to other congenital adrenal insufficiency disorders, with infant feeding problems resulting in failure to thrive, hypoglycemia, hypoglycemic seizures, and hyperpigmentation (49). The hyperpigmentation is secondary to ACTH stimulation of MC1R in melanocytes. Multiple episodes of hypoglycemia can result in developmental delays. The most common cause of death results from undiagnosed adrenal insufficiency. With early diagnosis and glucocorticoid treatment, patients with FGD live into adulthood. Tall stature with normal GH secretion is associated with FGD1. The etiology of the tall stature is unknown, but it has been hypothesized to be related to a stimulatory effect of ACTH because growth decelerates after treatment with glucocorticoids (50).

Diagnosis Plasma ACTH levels are very high, and cortisol is low. Due to preservation of the zona glomerulosa, mineralocorticoid activity is normal, with normal sodium, potassium, renin, and aldosterone levels and a normal response to dietary salt changes.

Genetic testing is clinically available for FGD1 by sequence analysis of the MC2R gene. FGD2 and FGD3 are diagnosed based on clinical findings and exclusion of a mutation in MC2R. Mutational analysis for FGD2 and FGD3 is currently only available on a research basis.

Treatment The treatment for all forms of FGD is standard glucocorticoid replacement.

Triple A Syndrome (Allgrove Syndrome)

Etiology/Pathophysiology Triple A or Allgrove syndrome is a rare (fewer than 100 described cases), autosomal recessive disorder characterized by alacrima, achalasia, and adrenal insufficiency. Triple A syndrome is caused by mutations in the achalasia–addisonianism–alacrima syndrome (AAAS) gene, which maps to chromosome 12q13 (51). This gene codes for a protein called aladin (alacrima-achalasia-adrenal insufficiency neurologic disorder) and is expressed in both neuroendocrine and cerebral structures (52). Although the exact mechanism of disease is not known at this time, mutations in the AAAS gene disrupt the nuclear localization process of aladin; it is hypothesized that this disruption results in abnormal development of certain tissues resulting in the clinical findings of triple A syndrome (53). Varying degrees of dysfunction could explain the phenotypic heterogeneity (54).

Clinical Presentation Triple A syndrome typically presents in the first decade of life with severe hypoglycemia similar to FGD. Distinct from FGD, aldosterone deficiency is present in 10% to 15% of patients (55). Adrenal insufficiency is frequently the presenting feature of Allgrove syndrome. Achalasia may lead to failure to thrive in infants. The neurological features include papillary and cranial nerve abnormalities, autonomic dysfunction, distal motor neuropathy, amyotrophy, dystonia, and chorea. Dermatologic complications include hyperkeratosis, fissured palms, and cutis anserine ("goose bumps"). Developmental delay is common in this syndrome; it is likely intrinsic to the disorder and compounded by multiple episodes of hypoglycemia.

Diagnosis Diagnosis of triple A syndrome is made by identification of two components of the diagnostic triad. Adrenal insufficiency is diagnosed by elevated ACTH with low cortisol levels or insufficient cortisol response to cosyntropin stimulation. Mineralocorticoid activity is impaired only in 15% of patients and is associated with high renin, low aldosterone levels, hyperkalemia and hyponatremia. Diagnosis of achalasia is made by barium esophagography or motility test. The Schirmer test is used in the diagnosis of alacrima.

Sequence analysis of the AAAS gene is clinically available. Prenatal genetic testing is offered as well. Since the presentation of triple A syndrome is similar to that of ALD—adrenal insufficiency and neurological findings—VLCFAs should be measured to exclude ALD.

Treatment Treatment is symptomatic. Adrenal insufficiency is treated with standard glucocorticoid and mineralocorticoid (when indicated) treatment. Ophthalmological, gastroenterological, and neurological consults are indicated to manage comorbidities.

Wolman Disease

Etiology/Pathophysiology Wolman disease is a rare autosomal recessive disorder with an incidence of fewer than 1 in 100,000 live births. The disease is caused by a deficiency in lysosomal acid lipase (LAL, LIPA) that is involved in cholesterol esters and triglycerides metabolism (56). LAL deficiency results in the intracellular accumulation of cholesterol esters and triglycerides, most notably in the liver, gastrointestinal tract, and adrenal glands. Foam cells are found in bone marrow and vacuolated lymphocytes in peripheral blood. LAL is encoded by a gene (LIPA) on chromosome 10 (57). Two major disorders, the severe infantile-onset Wolman disease and the milder late-onset cholesteryl ester storage disease (CESD), are seemingly caused by mutations in different parts of the LIPA gene.

Clinical Presentation Affected infants with of Wolman disease present in the first month of life. Accumulation of cholesterol esters and triglycerides in the liver and spleen results in hepatomegaly and splenomegaly, in the zona reticularis of the adrenal glands leads to adrenal insufficiency and adrenal calcifications, and in the villi of the small intestine contributes to diarrhea and steatorrhea. Other symptoms include failure to thrive, anemia, vomiting, and jaundice. Hepatomegaly can be the only clinical sign of CESD, and unlike Wolman disease, which is typically fatal by 1 year of age, CESD may go undiagnosed until adulthood. Splenomegaly, adrenal calcifications, short stature have been described.

Diagnosis Diagnosis is suspected by the clinical picture and confirmed by LAL enzyme testing in cultured fibroblasts or peripheral lymphocytes. Enzyme and genetic testing are available clinically and can by done prenatally as well. A plain x-ray of the abdomen typically reveals calcification of the adrenal glands. Intestinal wall thickening has been seen by ultrasound and CT scan as well (58).

Treatment Successful hematopoietic cell transplantation (HCT) of a patient with Wolman disease was reported by Krivit et al. (59). Normalization of peripheral leukocyte LAL activity was achieved and persisted at 3-year follow-up; however, HCT was not as successful for children who were already severely affected by Wolman disease. Therefore, early diagnosis is particularly important if HCT is to be considered. Enzyme supplementation and gene transfer were tested and proven successful in animal models (60,61). Human studies have not yet been completed.

Adrenal insufficiency is treated with standard glucocorticoid and mineralocorticoid treatment.

Kearns–Sayre Syndrome

Etiology/Pathophysiology Kearns–Sayre syndrome (KSS) is a complex multisystem disorder that is part of a continuum of disorders (Pearson syndrome and progressive external ophthalmoplegia) resulting from mitochondrial deletions.

Clinical Presentation The characteristic features of the syndrome are onset before 20 years of age, pigmentary retinopathy, and progressive external ophthalmoplegia (PEO). Other clinical features include hearing loss, ataxia, myopathy, hyperpigmented skin, and pernicious anemia. Multiple endocrinopathies are associated with KSS including adrenal insufficiency (rare), growth hormone deficiency, gonadal failure, diabetes mellitus, thyroid disease, and hypoparathyroidism (62).

Diagnosis Diagnosis of KSS is made by both clinical and laboratory assessments. Two of three of the following clinical criteria must be present for the diagnosis of KSS: onset before 20 years of age, pigmentary retinopathy, and PEO. In addition, one of the following abnormalities is required for diagnosis: cardiac conduction defects, cerebrospinal (CSF) fluid protein level greater than 100 mg/dL, and cerebral ataxia (63).

Muscle biopsy shows characteristic "ragged-red fibers" with modified Gomori trichrome stain. Approximately 90% of patients with KSS have a large mitochondrial deletion.

Treatment Treatment is symptomatic. Adrenal insufficiency is treated with standard glucocorticoid and mineralocorticoid treatment.

Smith–Lemli–Opitz Syndrome

Etiology/Pathophysiology Smith–Lemli–Opitz (SLO) syndrome is due to 7-dehydrocholesterol reductase (DHCR) deficiency, DHCR catalyzes the conversion of 7-dehydrocholesterol to cholesterol and is required for the *de novo* synthesis of cholesterol from acetate. Cholesterol is crucial in embryogenesis as well as in production of steroid hormones. However, the majority of cholesterol used in adrenal steroid production is derived from plasma low-density lipoproteins and does not depend on DHCR. Only *de novo* cholesterol production, which also occurs in the adrenal glands, starts with acetate and requires DHCR in the final step of conversion from 7-dehydrocholesterol to cholesterol. This may explain the rarity of chronic adrenal insufficiency in patients with SLO syndrome.

Clinical Presentation Characteristic features include microcephaly, anteverted nares, two/three toe syndactyly, polydactyly, broad alveolar ridges, and genital anomalies such as hypospadias. Postnatal growth retardation, severe feeding disorder, global developmental delay, and rarely, adrenal insufficiency are part of the clinical course.

Diagnosis The diagnosis of SLO syndrome is suspected based on physical findings. Confirmation is obtained by elevated levels of 7-dehydrocholesterol and the ratio of 7-dehydrocholesterol to cholesterol. Genetic testing is also clinically available and detects a mutation in more than 80 percent of SLO patients.

Treatment Adrenal insufficiency, if present, is treated with standard glucocorticoid and mineralocorticoid treatment. Cholesterol supplementation and simvastatin therapy are currently being evaluated as possible treatments for SLO syndrome (64,65).

Glucocorticoid Resistance

Etiology/Pathophysiology Glucocorticoid resistance (GR) is a rare disorder, characterized by partial end-organ insensitivity to glucocorticoids. Affected patients usually have adequate compensatory elevations in circulating cortisol and ACTH without clinical manifestations of hypo or hypercortisolism; however, the excess ACTH secretion often results in increased adrenal androgen and mineralocorticoid steroid production; in addition increased cortisol levels further stimulate the mineralocorticoid receptor. Inheritance can be either autosomal recessive or dominant. Sporadic cases also have been described. Multiple mutations have been found in patients with GR that group into at least two clusters (66). One cluster is in the glucocorticoid receptor (GCCR/NR3C1; 5q11-13), and the other is in the glucocorticoid receptor ligand (GRL; 5q31-32) (67,68). The glucocorticoid receptor has two isoforms, named GRα and GRβ. GRα is a ligand-dependent transcription factor (69). GRβ is transcriptionally inactive and inhibits GRα by competing for binding sites (70). Mutations in the GCCR or the GRL result in varying levels of inhibition of glucocorticoid signaling at target tissues (71). In the dominant form of GR, the heterozygous state tends to have a milder phenotype, indicating a gene dose effect (72). Complete glucocorticoid resistance is incompatible with life.

Because partial sensitivity to glucocorticoids is preserved in GR, the diurnal variation of cortisol is present, with a higher baseline set point and appropriate response to stress.

Clinical Presentation The phenotype ranges from asymptomatic to severe hyperandrogenism and/or mineralocorticoid excess, depending on the degree of receptor and receptor-ligand dysfunction; rarely some patients may have some degree of cortisol deficiency, presenting with prolonged fatigue. ACTH stimulated adrenal steroids including androgen and estrogen through aromatization of adrenal androgen may result in acne, hirsutism, oligoanovulation, and oligospermia. Similarly, ACTH stimulated deoxycorticosterone (DOC) and corticosterone (B) as well as cortisol cause low renin hypertension, with or without hypokalemic alkalosis. Homozygous mutations in the GR has been reported in a female presenting with ambiguous genitalia and severe hypokalemia (73).

Diagnosis A high serum cortisol level without signs or symptoms of hypercortisolemia is diagnostic of GR. Serum cortisol, urinary free cortisol, and 24 urine of 17-hydroxycorticosteroid urinary excretion are elevated. ACTH typically is elevated but can be normal. Adrenal androgens, DOC, and B are elevated. In contrast to Cushing disease, 17OHP levels can be elevated and can lead to an erroneous diagnosis of classical CAH due to 21OHD; however 17OHP elevations are not as high as in the classical forms of CAH (73) and a significant rise in serum cortisol is elicited following hypoglycemic stress. Affected patients nay have low renin hypertension associated with hypokalemia.

Genetic testing is available only on a research basis.

Treatment Asymptomatic patients, without hypertension or significant hyperandrogenism, do not require treatment. If a patient is symptomatic, treatment with high-dose dexamethasone (as HPA axis is resistant to dexamethasone suppression) can correct the hypertension and hypokalemic alkalosis by suppression of ACTH and decrease hyperandrogenemia (74). Dexamethasone can be titrated to keep the morning cortisol in the normal range (75).

Isolated Autoimmune Adrenalitis

Etiology/Pathophysiology Following CAH, isolated autoimmune adrenalitis, or Addison disease (76), is the most common cause of primary adrenal insufficiency in children (77). The prevalence of isolated autoimmune adrenalitis in children is reported to be 8 of 100 diagnosed cases of primary adrenal insufficiency (77). The exact pathogenesis of destruction of the adrenal gland in autoimmune adrenalitis has not been

TABLE 29-1   Comorbidities of the Autoimmune Polyglandular Syndromes

APS-1	APS-2	APS-3	APS-4
Adrenal insufficiency	Adrenal insufficiency	Thyroid autoimmune disease	Combination of endocrinologic
Hypoparathyroidism	Graves disease or	No adrenal insufficiency	organ- specific autoimmunity not
Mucocutaneus candidiasis	Hashimoto thyroiditis	or hypoparathyroidism	included in previous categories
Hypothyroidism	Type 1 diabetes mellitus	Celiac disease	
Gonadal failure	Pernicious anemia	Sarcoidosis	
Type 1 diabetes mellitus	Vitiligo	Atrophic gastritis	
Alopecia	Gonadal failure	Pernicious anemia	
Pernicious anemia	Celiac disease		
Vitiligo	Myasthenia gravis		
Chronic hepatitis	Primary biliary cirrhosis		
	Sjögren's syndrome		
	Lupus erythematosus		

determined, but antibodies against 21α-hydroxylase, 17α-hydroxylase, side-chain cleavage enzyme (P450scc), and adrenal cortex antibodies (ACAs) are markers of this destruction (78).

In children with another autoimmune disease and with antibodies to 21-hydroxylase and ACAs, progression to adrenal insufficiency develops frequently (90%) with a mean onset of 2.7 years (79). Time interval to overt disease in children with only adrenal antibodies and no other autoimmune disease is not known. Although a specific gene has not been identified in autoimmune adrenalitis, polymorphism in the CTLA-4 gene has been found in certain populations (80), and HLA haplotypes DR3–DQ2/DR4–DQ8 are associated with an increased risk of disease (81).

Clinical Presentation Isolated autoimmune adrenalitis presents with acute adrenal insufficiency and, in children, frequently with hypoglycemic seizures. Unlike autoimmune adrenalitis that is part of polyglandular syndromes, the isolated form is more common in males than in females (female : male ratio = 0.8), and the mean age of onset is 30 years (81).

Diagnosis Diagnosis of isolated adrenalitis is made by laboratory evaluation consistent with PAI (i.e., low serum cortisol, high ACTH, and insufficient response to a cosyntropin stimulation test) in the presence of antibodies against 21α-hydroxylase, 17α-hydroxylase, side-chain cleavage enzyme (P450scc), and/or ACAs.

Since isolated autoimmune adrenalitis can be the presenting feature of an autoimmune polyglandular syndrome (APS), patients should be followed closely for the development of other autoimmune endocrinopathies. In addition to clinical monitoring, APS antibodies could be checked every 2–3 years to help anticipate future endocrine abnormalities.

Treatment Adrenal insufficiency is treated with standard glucocorticoid and mineralocorticoid treatment.

Acquired PAI due to Autoimmune Polyglandular Syndromes

Etiology/Pathophysiology The autoimmune polyglandular syndromes (APSs) are divided into two main categories, APS-1 and APS-2. Some classifications recognize APS-3 and APS-4 as separate entities rather than subtypes of APS-2. APS-1 consists of adrenal insufficiency, hypoparathyroidism, and mucocutaneous candidiasis. APS-2 is a constellation of adrenal insufficiency, Graves disease or Hashimoto thyroiditis, and type 1 diabetes mellitus. Both may have multiple comorbidities (Table 29-1). APS-3 is a combination of thyroid autoimmune disease and other autoimmune diseases (e.g., atrophic gastritis and pernicious anemia) but not adrenal insufficiency and therefore will not be discussed in this chapter. APS-4 refers to a combination of adrenal insufficiency and other autoimmune diseases excluding the major components of APS-1 or APS-2.

Patients with APS-associated adrenal insufficiency can have positive antibodies years before developing signs or symptoms of adrenal insufficiency. In fact, overt adrenal insufficiency develops when 80% to 90% of adrenal cortices are destroyed. Usually the first sign of impending adrenal failure is an increase in renin activity, followed by increased ACTH level and subsequently blunted cortisol response to ACTH stimulation (82). Pathologically, there is a lymphocytic infiltration of the adrenal cortex.

APS-1 is caused by mutations in a transcription factor called *autoimmune regulator* (AIRE) on chromosome 21q22.3 (83). The specific mechanism by which these mutations result in the syndrome of APS-1 is unknown.

The inheritance is autosomal recessive; sporadic mutations have been documented. APS-1 is more common among people of Finnish, Sardinian, and Iranian Jewish ancestry. APS-2 does not result from a mutation in a single gene but is a complex genetic disorder associated with a certain HLA genotype DR3–DQ2/DR4–DQ8 (84). Patients with adrenal insufficiency have an additional association with MHC class I chain-related A (MICA-A5.1) allele (85).

Clinical Presentation APS-1 is also called *autoimmune polyendocrine–candidiasis–ectodermal dystrophy* (APECED). The prevalence varies significantly among populations, ranging from 1 in 9000 in Iranian Jews to 1 in 80,000 in Norway (82). At least two of the three components of the syndrome (i.e., mucocutaneous candidiasis, hypoparathyroidism, and adrenal insufficiency) need to be present for the diagnosis of APS-1. Candidiasis is usually the first manifestation (86). It is typically found in the diaper region early on and then in the vulvovaginal area at puberty. Colonization of the gut can lead to intermittent abdominal pain and diarrhea. Retrosternal pain results from esophageal candidiasis. It is important to consider APS-1 in children with a primary diagnosis of chronic mucocutaneous candidiasis because nearly half of these children may have an associated endocrine disorder, most commonly Addison's disease (87).

Candidiasis is followed by hypoparathyroidism, which usually develops before the age of 10 years, and when ACAs are present, 70% go on to develop adrenal insufficiency within 4 years (82). Hypoparathyroidism is diagnosed commonly only after severe hypocalcemia results in carpopedal spasms, muscle twitching, laryngospasm, or seizures. The symptoms of hypoparathyroidism can be masked by adrenal insufficiency, in which the calcium level typically is increased due to reduced renal excretion of calcium and increased proximal tubular reabsorption (88).

Chronic, active, autoimmune hepatitis is found in 5% to 31% of patients with APS-1 and is the leading cause of death in these patients. Multiple other comorbidities are associated with APS-1: hypothyroidism, gonadal failure, type 1 diabetes mellitus, celiac disease, chronic atrophic gastritis, pernicious anemia, cholelithiasis, alopecia areata and totalis, autoimmune skin disease (vitiligo), ectodermal dystrophy (keratoconjunctivitis and hypoplasia of dental enamel and nails), Sjögren syndrome (autoimmune exocrinopathy), acquired asplenism, and vasculitis (82). Primary gonadal failure is more common in females with APS-1 than in males. By age 13 in girls and age 16 in boys, one study found gonadal failure in 60% and 14%, respectively (86). Gastric parietal cell autoimmunity leads to atrophic gastritis with resulting achlorhydria and intrinsic factor deficiency. Consequently, iron-deficiency anemia or vitamin B12–deficient pernicious anemia can develop. Alopecia usually occurs before puberty.

APS-2 consists of adrenal insufficiency, thyroid autoimmunity, and type 1 diabetes mellitus (89). It is the most common polyendocrinopathy, with a prevalence of 1.4–2.0 per 100,000 (82). Unlike APS-1, presentation of APS-2 is typically in the third and fourth decades with adrenal failure and is rare in children (90).

APS-2 is also known as *Schmidt syndrome* when the thyroid gland is involved and *Carpenter syndrome* when type 1 diabetes mellitus is present. APS-2 is about three times more common in females than in males. Other associated diseases include chronic atrophic gastritis and pernicious anemia, vitiligo, hypergonadotropic hypogonadism, celiac disease, and Graves ophthalmopathy (89).

APS-4 is characterized by adrenal insufficiency with another autoimmune disorder, excluding the diagnostic comorbidities of APS-1 or APS-2 described earlier. It is the least common of the autoimmune polyendocine syndromes. A small study of patients with APS-4 found a female predominance (3.3:1), and all patients presented as adults with a mean age of onset, with adrenal insufficiency, of 36 years (82).

Diagnosis In patients with PAI, identification of serum 21α-hydroxylase or ACAs confirms the diagnosis of autoimmune adrenal insufficiency. Clinical context will distinguish APS-1 in that the mucocutaneous candidiasis and hypoparathyroidism typically precede adrenal insufficiency. APS-2 is confirmed by the presence of thyroid antibodies or type 1 diabetes mellitus. APS-4 is diagnosed in the presence of autoimmune adrenal insufficiency with one other autoimmune disease, excluding

mucocutaneous candidiasis, hypoparathyroidism, thyroiditis, and type 1 diabetes mellitus.

Treatment In APS-1, aggressive treatment of candidiasis is necessary because candidiasis can lead to carcinoma of the oral mucosa with a high mortality rate. If asplenism is present, prophylactic antibiotics need to be prescribed. Adrenal insufficiency is treated with standard glucocorticoid and mineralocorticoid supplementation.

Monitoring In APS-1 without adrenal insufficiency, yearly ACA, 21-hydroxylase autoantibody, and serum renin determinations as well as cosyntropin stimulation test should be performed. If adrenal autoantibodies are present, then continuation with yearly low dose cosyntropin stimulation tests and serum renin determinations is recommended (91). In APS-1 without hypoparathyroidism, yearly calcium and phosphorous measurements are recommended, and if they are abnormal, an intact parathyroid hormone level should be determined. Gonadal evaluation, including determination of LH, FSH, testosterone or estradiol, and 3β-HSD autoantibody levels when available, should be performed near the time of puberty. Since chronic active hepatitis is the leading cause of death in these patients, frequent liver function tests, and annually measurement of mitochondrial and smooth muscle autoantibodies is recommended.

In patients with APS-2, if adrenal insufficiency and type 1 diabetes mellitus are present, then yearly screening for thyroid disease is indicated (TSH and free thyroxine). Thyroid autoantibodies (thyroperoxidase, thyroglobulin and thyroid-stimulating and thyrotropin-binding inhibitory immunoglobulins) can be checked as well. If the diagnosis is made by the presence of adrenal insufficiency and Graves disease, then yearly fasting glucose tests and clinical assessment for signs and symptoms of diabetes mellitus should be done, as well as islet cell, insulin, and glutamic acid decarboxylase (GAD) autoantibody determinations. Gonadal evaluation is the same as in APS-1.

Patients with APS-4 should be screened for islet cell, insulin, and GAD antibodies, as well as the thyroid antibodies. Any of these positive antibodies would change the diagnosis to APS-2. Yearly calcium and phosphorous evaluations are indicated, and if they are abnormal, they would change the diagnosis to APS-1.

All patients with an APS should have yearly celiac screening with transglutaminase antibody (celiac disease is typically asymptomatic) and a hemoglobin to check for anemia. Yearly physical examinations will detect some

of the other comorbidities, such as alopecia areata and totalis, autoimmune skin disease (vitiligo), ectodermal dystrophy (keratoconjunctivitis and hypoplasia of dental enamel and nails), Sjögren syndrome, and Graves ophthalmopathy.

If chronic lymphocytic gastritis or pernicious anemia is suspected, gastric parietal cell and intrinsic factor blocking autoantibodies can be measured. If vitiligo is found on physical examination, determination of melanocyte or tyrosinase autoantibodies can confirm an autoimmune etiology.

An important component of monitoring is patient education. Patients should be educated about the symptoms of other autoimmune diseases for which they are at risk.

Infectious Adrenal Insufficiency

Etiology/Pathophysiology Multiple infectious agents—mycobacterial, bacterial, fungal, and viral—can cause destruction of the adrenal gland leading to acquired PAI (92). In areas such as Southeast Asia and Africa, adrenal insufficiency due to tuberculosis has been found to account for up to 34% of patients with acute PAI (93), and in patients with active tuberculosis, adrenal involvement is found in approximately 6% (94). The mechanism of damage to the adrenal glands is frequently adrenal hemorrhage, referred to as *Waterhouse-Friderichsen syndrome* in the case of meningococcemia (95). Adrenal hemorrhage also may occur in nonmeningococcal infections, such as group A *Streptococcus* (96). Adrenal necrosis due to vascular changes with endotoxin release and hypotension may contribute as well. Hypotension can result in damage to the pituitary, causing a secondary adrenal insufficiency with decreased ACTH, and cytokine release inhibits ACTH stimulation of the adrenal gland (97).

Up to 20% of patients with human immunodeficiency virus (HIV) disease have an abnormal response to the cosyntropin stimulation test (98,99). Some of the causes of adrenal insufficiency in acquired immune-deficiency disease (AIDS) patients include opportunistic infections and medications used in the treatment of HIV (e.g., ketoconazole, fluconazole, rifampin, and megestrol acetate). Cytomegalovirus (CMV) is the most common cause of adrenal insufficiency in this patient population (100).

Clinical Presentation Presentation is typically of acute adrenal insufficiency. Infectious adrenal insufficiency should be suspected in any patient with active tuberculosis or HIV infection. In patients with septic shock, the signs and symptoms of acute adrenal insufficiency may be difficult to distinguish from those of septic shock.

Diagnosis Diagnosis of the etiology in infectious adrenal insufficiency typically is done after acute crisis management. A random cortisol determination during sepsis of greater than 34 μg/dL suggests normal ad-renal response, less than 15 μg/dL suggests adrenal insufficiency, and a cortisol rise to a low dose cosyntropin stimulation of greater than 9 μg/dL above baseline suggests appropriate adrenal response (6). However, cortisol resistance may be present, and this area is still quite controversial, so these values should be considered within the clinical context. Adrenal hemorrhage can be seen on ultrasound or CT scan. The adrenal glands typically are enlarged bilaterally.

Treatment Treatment of adrenal insufficiency during septic shock has been controversial. Early studies showed an increased mortality in patients treated with high-dose glucocorticoids during septic shock, but more recent studies showed that in patients with vasopressor-dependent shock, when physiologic doses of hydrocortisone given with a 5- to 7-day taper have a survival benefit (101).

Adrenal Hemorrhage

Etiology/Pathophysiology In the newborn, the most common cause of primary acquired adrenal insufficiency is adrenal hemorrhage associated with a prolonged labor or traumatic delivery (102). The incidence of adrenal hemorrhage in full-term babies is 1 in 400, with 70% right-sided and 5% to 10% bilateral (103). The bleeding occurs in a network of small vessels between the capsule and the cortex.

Clinical Presentation If the hemorrhage is severe and bilateral, patients may present in acute shock secondary to both the adrenal insufficiency and blood loss into the adrenal gland. A mass in the flank may be palpable, and the kidney is displaced downward on ultrasound.

Diagnosis Diagnosis is made by ultrasound— by the appearance of a cystic mass. The natural history of these hemorrhages by ultrasound, is of continual decrease in size with initial cystic transformation and disappearance or calcification by up to 1 year (104). All newborns with adrenal hemorrhage need to be tested with a low dose cosyntropin stimulation test when stable to determine the need for replacement therapy.

Treatment Adrenal insufficiency is treated with standard glucocorticoid and mineralcorticoid treatment.

SECONDARY ADRENAL INSUFFICIENCY

Secondary adrenal insufficiency (SAI) describes a condition of deficient production of adrenal cortical hormones due to hypothalamic-pituitary dysfunction. SAI may be caused by any disease which affects the anterior pituitary and decreases ACTH secretion; ACTH deficiency may be isolated or occur in association with other pituitary hormone deficiencies. Tertiary adrenal insufficiency may be caused by any process that involves the hypothalamus and decreases CRH secretion.

Deficiency in CRH or ACTH leads to atrophy of the adrenal cortex and adrenal insufficiency. The causes of secondary adrenal insufficiency can be congenital or acquired, while the most common cause of tertiary adrenal insufficiency is iatrogenic as in abrupt discontinuation without tapering of prolonged high dose glucocorticoid therapy. Deficiency of ACTH as part of multiple pituitary hormone deficiencies is discussed in detail in Chapter 32.

Isolated ACTH Deficiency

Etiology/Pathophysiology Isolated ACTH deficiency (IAD) is a rare disorder that is clinically and genetically heterogeneous. Mutations of the following genes have been associated with IAD presenting in the neonatal period: (1) T-Box19 (TBX19), a gene that encodes a transcription factor called TPIT, required for the expression of proopiomelanocortin (POMC) and differentiation of the pituitary, (2) POMC, a gene that encodes POMC, the precursor of ACTH, MSH, endorphin, and lipotropin, and (3) CRH, the gene for corticotropin-releasing hormone (105–107).

Clinical Presentation The clinical spectrum of IAD is variable, and presentation typically is in the newborn period. However, it can occur in childhood as well. Mutations in TBX19 have been described in neonatal-onset IAD (108) but seem to not be associated with onset later than 5 years of age (109). Patients with mutations in the POMC gene may present in the newborn period with hyperphagia leading to obesity and red hair; hepatic failure due to severe neonatal cholestasis and IAD has also been described. (106,110).

IAD typically has not been associated with a syndrome. Recently, however, a 7-year-old boy was found to have multiple malformations including micrognathia, cleft palate, hypospadias, an atrial septal defect, mental retardation, and isolated ACTH deficiency (111).

Diagnosis Diagnosis of IAD is made by confirming the absence of any other pituitary hormone deficiency in the presence of secondary adrenal insufficiency. Mutational analysis of the TBX19, POMC, or CRH gene is not available at this time.

Treatment Adrenal insufficiency is treated with standard glucocorticoid replacement.

Exogenous (Iatrogenic) Glucocorticod Exposure

Etiology/Pathophysiology IAD resulting from glucocorticoid therapy is the most common cause of SAI (112). Administration of exogenous glucocorticoids for longer than a week in pharmacological doses for the treatment of illnesses (e.g., asthma, nephrotic syndrome, hematologic neoplasms, rheumatoid arthritis, etc.) may result in adrenal insufficiency. Suppression of the hypothalamic-pituitary-adrenal (HPA) axis by exogenous glucocorticoids results in atrophy of the adrenal cortex and corticotrophic cells of the pituitary gland.

Clinical Presentation Prolonged use of high-dose topical steroids, particularly on inflamed skin (113), and high-dose (>500 μg/d) inhaled steroids (such as fluticasone propionate) has been reported to impair adrenal function, although less frequently than oral or intravenous steroids (114,115).

Weight gain and growth failure may precede symptoms of adrenal insufficiency, such as weakness, hypoglycemia, and orthostatic hypotension. The onset of adrenal insufficiency is gradual, with the vague signs and symptoms of chronic adrenal failure. Recovery of the HPA axis may take up to 9 months depending on the dose and duration of treatment (112).

Diagnosis For children who require prolonged high-dose inhaled steroids, routine monitoring of the morning plasma cortisol level should be done. One method of monitoring is by assessment of morning plasma cortisol. If the morning cortisol level is greater than 10 μg/dL normal adrenal function should be confirmed by a low-dose ACTH stimulation test (115).

Treatment Until full recovery of the HPA axis, glucorticorticoid replacement therapy is required. Depending on the degree of HPA axis suppression, daily and/or stress-dose steroids may be necessary.

Prenatal Glucocorticoid Exposure

Etiology/Pathophysiology Prenatal exposure to glucocorticoids that cross the fetoplacental barrier may cause some degree of adrenal insufficiency due to suppression of HPA axis. Placental 11β-HSD type 2 (11β-HSD2) converts cortisol to its biologically inactive metabolite cortisone and thus limits transplacental passage of maternal endogenous cortisol (116). As a result, the majority of active cortisol in the fetal circulation originates from the fetal adrenals. This mechanism provides some protection to the fetus against maternal endogenous and exogenous glucocorticoids, (cortisol, prednisone, prednisolone) as these are substrates for 11β-HSD2. However, dexamethasone and betamethasone, which are given to mothers at risk for premature labor, are poorly metabolized by 11β-HSD2 and readily cross the placenta. Therefore, HPA suppression is possible with prenatal exposure to dexamethasone or betamethasone and needs to be considered in these infants. A recent study did not find a difference in plasma ACTH levels between preterm infants whose mothers were and were not treated with prenatal glucocorticoids, but serum cortisol levels were significantly lower in the group treated with one or two doses of prenatal glucocorticoids (117).

Clinical Presentation Presentation of adrenal insufficiency in the preterm newborn is with acute adrenal crisis, characterized by hypotension not responsive to volume expansion or inotropes usually within the first 12 hours of life. Adrenal insufficiency caused by prenatal exposure to glucocorticoids may last several weeks postnatally depending on the amount and duration of prenatal steroid administration.

Diagnosis Multiple factors can affect the HPA axis perinatally: prenatal glucocorticoid exposure, mode of delivery, perinatal stress and maternal condition, gestational age and birth weight, respiratory compromise, and mode of mechanical ventilation. Reference ranges following CRH stimulation testing for the first few weeks of life have been published for very-low-birth-weight infants (117). It also has been suggested that a post–stimulated cortisol level less than 9 μg/dL on day 7 of life is diagnostic of adrenal insufficiency (118).

Treatment Treatment of adrenal crisis is with intravenous glucocorticoid replacement. Dosing is not yet standardized in preterm infants, but published data for stress-dose glucocorticoid treatment suggest a dose ranging from 1 mg/kg every 8 hours for 5 days of intravenous hydrocortisone, to 1 mg/kg every 4 hours for 5 days, to a single intravenous dose of dexamethasone 0.5 mg/kg (119,120). Glucocorticoid replacement then is tapered to physiological doses until recovery of the HPA axis.

Miscellaneous Causes of SAI

Secondary, late adrenal insufficiency as part of hypopituitarism has been described in patients with mutations of the PROP1 gene (Chapter 32); patients with a defect in Proprotein convertase-1 (PCSK1), a neuroendocrine convertase, which process large precursor proteins into mature bioactive products, can also develop secondary adrenal insufficiency due to impaired processing of POMC to ACTH. Two patients, compound heterozygotes for PCSK1 mutations have been described with extreme childhood obesity, severe refractory neonatal diarrhea, abnormal glucose homeostasis, hypogonadotropic hypogonadism and hypocorticosolism; these patients had elevated plasma proinsulin and POMC with very low insulin levels, low to normal ACTH levels and low cortisol levels due to defective prohormone processing (121). Significant trauma to the head, brain tumors, and hemorrhage may disrupt the HPA axis. Cranial irradiation can damage the pituitary and hypothalamus, resulting in SAI (121). A threshold dose of irradiation to the brain has not yet been identified as damaging to the hypothalamus or pituitary. However, a positive relationship has been found between increasing fractionated irradiation dose and HPA dysfunction (122).

Similar to iatrogenic adrenal insufficiency from exogenous glucocorticoid treatment, a cortisol-secreting adrenal tumor can cause suppression of the HPA axis and subsequent atrophy of the adrenal glands. Patients with a cortisol-secreting tumor will present with Cushing syndrome. Stress-dose steroids are used during removal of cortisol-secreting tumors and then are tapered as with iatrogenic adrenal insufficiency to avoid an adrenal crisis.

Systemic disorders such as hemochromatosis, sarcoidosis, and Langerhans cell histiocytosis may infiltrate and disrupt any part of the HPA axis. SAI is a rare sequela of meningitis and encephalitis.

ALDOSTERONE DEFICIENCY

Aldosterone is produced in the zona glomerulosa, the only part of the adrenal cortex where aldosterone synthase is present. Aldosterone it is the most potent mineralocorticoid and regulates intravascular volume and electrolyte balance by increasing reabsorption of sodium and excretion of potassium in the distal convoluted tubules. By increasing sodium reabsorption, water is also reabsorbed, and blood volume increases.

Synthesis of aldosterone begins, as with all adrenal steroids, with cholesterol. Cholesterol conversion to aldosterone involves P450scc, 3β-HSDII, P450c21, and P450c11AS or aldosterone synthase (AS) enzymes. Aldosterone synthase is encoded by the CYP11B2 gene and facilitates all three enzymatic reactions needed to convert DOC to aldosterone: 11β-hydroxylation, which converts DOC to corticosterone (B); 18-hydroxylation, which converts B to 18-hydroxycorticosterone (18-

OHB); and finally, 18-oxidation, which converts 18-OHB to aldosterone (123). Of note the isozyme of AS, 11β-hydroxylase, hydroxylates 11-deoxycortisol to cortisol in zona fasciculata and can also convert 11-deoxycorticosterone to either corticosterone (the predominant product) or 18-hydroxy, 11-deoxycorticosterone; however, it 18-hydroxylates corticosterone poorly and cannot convert deoxycorticosterone into aldosterone.

Production and secretion are regulated predominantly by the renin-angiotensin system and potassium levels, with ACTH having only a short-term effect. Aldosterone is exquisitely sensitive to changes in serum sodium and potassium and intravascular volume via sensors in the kidneys. Decreased blood flow to the kidneys, decreased afferent arteriolar pressure to the kidneys, and increased delivery of potassium and decreased delivery of sodium to the macula densa cells in the distal convoluted tubules of the kidneys all result in increased production of aldosterone. This is accomplished by a cascade of events beginning with the release of renin from the juxtaglomerular cells of the kidneys in response to these changes. Renin then cleaves angiotensinogen and releases angiotensin I. Angiotensin I then is cleaved by angiotensin-converting enzyme (ACE), which is produced in the lungs and plasma, to angiotensin II. Angiotensin II stimulates the production and secretion of aldosterone from the adrenal gland. In addition, angiotensin II acts on vascular smooth muscle to cause contraction.

The most common inherited disorder of aldosterone synthesis is CAH due to 21OHD (see Chapter 27). Aldosterone deficiency with otherwise normal adrenal steroid synthesis is rare. Two forms of AS deficiency due to CYP11B2 gene defects are recognized and are termed *corticosterone methyloxidase deficiency type 1* and *type 2* (CMO1 and CMO2). Another form of isolated aldosterone deficiency has been described in which no mutations in the CYP11B2 gene have been identified and is called *familial hyperreninemic hypoaldosteronism type 2* (FHHA2). The two forms of AS deficiency (CMO1 and CMO2) are classified under the term *familial hyperreninemic hypoaldosteronism type 1* (FHHA1).

Patients with pseudohypoaldosteronism also present clinically with isolated aldosterone deficiency due to impaired response of target organs to aldosterone.

Corticosterone Methyloxidase Deficiency Types 1 and 2

Etiology/Pathophysiology These two clinical forms of aldosterone synthase deficiency have identical clinical features but differ in profiles of secreted steroids. Patients with CMO1 have mutations of the CYP11B2 gene that impair both the 18-hydroxylase and 18-oxidase activities of aldosterone synthase, whereas patients with CMO2 have CYP11B2 gene mutations that selectively impair the 18-oxidase activity of the enzyme (124). The biochemical distinction between CMO1 and CMO2 is not always clear. Patients with mutations that completely inactivate the enzyme and therefore should have undetectable serum aldosterone and low to normal 18-OHB levels, the biochemical phenotype of CMO1, may present with low to normal serum aldosterone and elevated 18-OHB levels, the biochemical phenotype of CMO2 (125) or vice versa (126).

Clinical Presentation Presentation of both CMO1 and CMO2 typically is in infancy, with recurrent dehydration, hyponatremia, and hyperkalemia. Failure to thrive, intermittent fevers, and vomiting may be the presenting signs in early childhood. CMO1 and CMO2 are indistinguishable clinically.

Although electrolyte abnormalities usually normalize by 4 years of age (even with a low-sodium diet), growth retardation may persist throughout childhood. Morbidity of AS deficiency is usually not as severe as in the salt-wasting form of CAH propably due to normal synthesis of deoxycorticosterone (DOC), corticosterone and cortisol in aldosterone synthase deficiency, which ameliorates the development of hyponatremia and shock. Adults are usually asymptomatic but may have decreased tolerance to severe salt loss compared to unaffected individuals.

Diagnosis CMO1 and CMO2 are characterized by hyperkalemia, hyponatremia, elevated renin, decreased aldosterone, and normal 24 hour urinary excretion of 17-ketosteroids, and 17-hydroxycorticosteroids (126). Electrolytes may be normal in untreated children older than 3–4 years of age; plasma rennin, although markedly elevated (up to 100 times normal) in infants and children, may be normal in adults. Serum DOC is elevated in both CMO1 and CMO2, as well as urinary corticosterone (B) metabolites relative to excretion of cortisol metabolites. CMO1 may be distinguished from CMO2 by undetectable serum aldosterone and mildly decreased 18-hydroxycorticosterone, whereas serum aldosterone typically is normal (particularly in older children and adults) and 18-hydroxycorticosterone is elevated in CMO2 (127). The elevated ratio of 18-hydroxycorticosterone to aldosterone (typically 100-fold) in either urine or serum is useful in diagnosing CMO2; the ratio does not vary with age and may be the sole biochemichal abnormality in adults.

Genetic, enzymatic, protein, and prenatal testing are available for both CMO1 and CMO2 and are needed to distinguish between these disorders.

Treatment Standard treatment is with mineralocorticoid replacement (fludrocortisone of 0.1–0.3 mg/d orally) and sodium chloride supplementation to ensure 1–2 g daily or 17–34 mEq of sodium (127). Sodium supplementation is stopped after plasma renin has decreased to a normal level; plasma renin activity and levels of steroid precursors may not return to normal for several months. Because infant formula is low in sodium, infants may need continued supplementation until transitioned to solid foods. Mineralocorticoid therapy is maintained through childhood. Sodium balance should be checked before discontinuing therapy.

Familial Hyperreninemic Hypoaldosteronism Type 2

Etiology/Pathophysiology Isolated hypoaldosteronism presenting in infancy similar to FHHA, but without a mutation in CYP11B2, was described in five Iranian Jewish patients (128) and named *familial hyperreninemic hypoaldosteronism type 2* (FHHA2). The etiology of this disorder is currently unknown.

Clinical Presentation Presentation of FHHA2 is in infancy with the usual signs and symptoms of hypoaldosteronism: vomiting, hyponatremia, hyperkalemia, dehydration, and failure to thrive.

Diagnosis Renin is elevated and aldosterone is low or normal even during dehydration (128). Genetic and enzymatic testing is not available.

Treatment Treatment is the same as for CMO1 and CMO2.

Pseudohypoaldosteronism

Etiology/Pathophysiology Pseudohypoaldosteronism (PHA) can be indistinguishable clinically from true hypoaldosteronism. PHA results when the kidney is unable to recognize and respond to aldosterone or when there is an abnormality of the epithelial sodium channel. There are two forms of PHA— type 1 and type 2. PHA1 is further divided into an autosomal recessive and autosomal dominant forms (129).

Autosomal Recessive PHA1 Autosomal recessive PHA1 results from mutations in the α, β, or γ subunit of the epithelial sodium channel (130). Since epithelial sodium channels are present in the colon, lungs, and sweat and salivary glands, disruption of the epithelial sodium channel in autosomal recessive PHA1 is associated with salt wasting from the colon and sweat and salivary glands, as well as pul-

monary involvement resulting in an inability to resorb lung water (131). Mutations in the α subunit are associated with more severe pulmonary involvement (132).

Autosomal Dominant PHA1 Autosomal dominant PHA1 results from mutations in the mineralocorticoid receptor (132,133). Unlike the epithelial sodium channel, disruption of the mineralocorticoid receptor only affects mineralocorticoid activity at the kidney.

Pseudohypoaldosteronism Type 2 Pseudohypoaldosteronism type 2 (also known as Gordon hyperkalemia–hypertension syndrome) is characterized by hyperkalemia, low renin, low to normal aldosterone, normal renal function, and hypertension. Mild hyperchloremia and metabolic acidosis are variable associated findings. Mutations in WNK1 and WNK4 have been identified in patients with PHA2. WNK1 and WNK4 are kinases involved in the mineralocorticoid pathway (135) whose defects seem to affect predominantly potassium balance at the kidney level. The inheritance is autosomal dominant with variable penetrance (136).

Clinical Presentation PHA1 presents similarly to true hypoaldosteronism with vomiting, failure to thrive, dehydration, hyponatremia, and hyperkalemia. All forms of PHA typically present in infancy. Autosomal recessive PHA1 presents with severe salt-wasting crisis in infancy, and salt wasting does not improve with age. In the autosomal dominant form, the salt loss is less severe, is restricted to the kidneys, and usually improves with age. Due to variable penetrance of the autosomal dominant mutation causing PHA1, some affected family members are asymptomatic and may be identified during family studies only after salt restriction (134).

Infants with autosomal recessive PHA1 frequently have pulmonary symptoms (e.g., cough, wheezing , and pneumonia) due to increased volume of airway surface liquid (131) and may be misdiagnosed with cystic fibrosis due to an elevated sweat chloride level (137). Infants with PHA1, in contrast to those with cystic fibrosis, do not develop chronic lung disease or bronchiectasis, and pulmonary symptoms resolve by around 6 years of age (131,132).

Hyperkalemia and hypertension are characteristic of PHA2. Onset has been described in childhood with hyperkalemia, but the onset of hypertension more typically is in adulthood. Mild hyperchloremia and metabolic acidosis also may be present.

Diagnosis In contrast to true hypoaldosteronism, in PHA1, both aldosterone and renin levels are elevated. In PHA2, case reports describe normal aldosterone levels but low in relation to potassium levels, low renin, and hyperkalemia that is resistant to exogenous mineralocorticoid administration.

For PHA1, clinical testing by sequence analysis for mutations in the epithelial sodium channel or the mineralocorticoid receptor is available. Prenatal testing is offered as well. Genetic testing for PHA2 is not currently available.

Treatment PHA1 is treated with sodium chloride supplementation to ensure 1–2 g daily or 17–34 mEq of sodium. In autosomal recessive PHA1 potassium-binding resins (kayexalate 1 g/kg orally every 4–6 hours) for treatment of severe hyperkalemia may be required (134). If hyperkalemia persists, hydrochlorothiazide (2 mg/kg/day orally every 12 or 24 hours) should be added (138).

Hydrochlorothizide is the first-line treatment for PHA2 (135).

TRANSIENT PSEUDOHYPOALDOSTERONISM

Obstructive uropathy, sickle cell disease, and urinary tract infections may be associated with a reversible or transient form of mineralocorticoid resistance presenting with hyperkalemia and high aldosterone and renin levels.

REFERENCES

1. Ten S, New M, Maclaren N. Clinical review 130: Addison's disease 2001. *J Clin Endocrinol Metab.* 2001;86:2909–2922.
2. Nieman LK. Dynamic evaluation of adrenal hypofunction. *J Endocrinol Invest.* 2003;26:74–82.
3. May ME, Carey RM. Rapid adrenocorticotropic hormone test in practice: Retrospective review. *Am J Med.* 1985;79:679–684.
4. Fiad TM, Kirby JM, Cunningham SK, et al. The overnight single-dose metyrapone test is a simple and reliable index of the hypothalamic-pituitary-adrenal axis. *Clin Endocrinol (Oxf).* 1994;40:603–609.
5. Gonzalez H, Nardi O, Annane D. Relative adrenal failure in the ICU: An identifiable problem requiring treatment. *Crit Care Clin.* 2006;22:105–118, vii.
6. Goldenberg A, Wolf C, Chevy F, et al. Antenatal manifestations of Smith-Lemli-Opitz (RSH) syndrome: A retrospective survey of 30 cases. *Am J Med Genet [A].* 2004;124:423–426.
7. Kenny FM, Preeyasombat C, Migeon CJ. Cortisol production rate: II. Normal infants, children, and adults. *Pediatrics.* 1966;37:34–42.
8. Swords FM, Carroll PV, Kisalu J, et al. The effects of growth hormone deficiency and replacement on glucocorticoid exposure in hypopituitary patients on cortisone acetate and hydrocortisone replacement. *Clin Endocrinol (Oxf).* 2003;59:613–620.
9. Gelding SV, Taylor NF, Wood PJ, et al. The effect of growth hormone replacement therapy on cortisol-cortisone interconversion in hypopituitary adults: Evidence for growth hormone modulation of extrarenal 11β-hydroxysteroid dehydrogenase activity. *Clin Endocrinol (Oxf).* 1998;48:153–162.
10. Urban MD, Kogut MD. Adrenocortical insufficiency in the child. In: Bardin CW, ed. *Current Therapy in Endocrinology and Metabolism,* 6th ed. St. Louis: Mosby-Year Book; 1997:147–151.
11. Migeon CJ, Lanes R. Adrenal cortex: hypo- and hyperfunction. In: Lifshitz F, ed. *Pediatric Endocrinology,* 4th ed. New York: Marcel Dekker; 2003:147–173.
12. Punthakee Z, Legault L, Polychronakos C. Prednisolone in the treatment of adrenal insufficiency: A re-evaluation of relative potency. *J Pediatr.* 2003;143:402–405.
13. Arlt W, Callies F, van Vlijmen JC, et al. Dehydroepiandrosterone replacement in women with adrenal insufficiency. *N Engl J Med.* 1999;341:1013–1020.
14. Lovas K, Husebye ES. High prevalence and increasing incidence of Addison's disease in western Norway. *Clin Endocrinol (Oxf).* 2002;56:787–791.
15. McCabe E. Adrenal hypoplasias and aplasias. In: Scriver CR, Valle D, Sly WS, et al., eds. *The Metabolic and Molecular Bases of Inherited Disease,* 8th ed. New York: McGraw-Hill; 2001:4263–4274.
16. Muscatelli F, Strom TM, Walker AP, et al. Mutations in the DAX-1 gene give rise to both X-linked adrenal hypoplasia congenita and hypogonadotropic hypogonadism. *Nature.* 1994;372:672–676.
17. Wise JE, Matalon R, Morgan AM, et al. Phenotypic features of patients with congenital adrenal hypoplasia and glycerol kinase deficiency. *Am J Dis Child.* 1987;141:744–747.
18. Swain A, Zanaria E, Hacker A, et al. Mouse Dax1 expression is consistent with a role in sex determination as well as in adrenal and hypothalamus function. *Nat Genet.* 1996;12:404–409.
19. Ito M, Yu R, Jameson JL. DAX-1 inhibits SF-1-mediated transactivation via a carboxy-terminal domain that is deleted in adrenal hypoplasia congenita. *Mol Cell Biol.* 1997;17:1476–1483.
20. Yu RN, Ito M, Saunders TL, et al. Role of Ahch in gonadal development and gametogenesis. *Nat Genet.* 1998;20:353–357.
21. Mantovani G, De Menis E, Borretta G, et al. DAX1 and X-linked adrenal hypoplasia congenita: Clinical and molecular analysis in five patients. *Eur J Endocrinol.* 2006;154:685–689.
22. Binder G, Wollmann H, Schwarze CP, et al. X-linked congenital adrenal hypoplasia: New mutations and long-term follow-up in three patients. *Clin Endocrinol (Oxf).* 2000;53:249–255.
23. Domenice S, Latronico AC, Brito VN, et al. Adrenocorticotropin-dependent precocious puberty of testicular origin in a boy with X-linked adrenal hypoplasia congenita due to a novel mutation in the DAX1 gene. J Clin Endocrinol Metab. 2001;86:4068–4071.
24. Seminara SB, Achermann JC, Genel M, et al. X linked adrenal hypoplasia congenita: A mutation in DAX1 expands the phenotypic spectrum in males and females. *J Clin Endocrinol Metab.* 1999;84:4501–4509.
25. Vilain E, Le Merrer M, Lecointre C, et al. IMAGe, a new clinical association of intrauterine growth retardation, metaphyseal dysplasia, adrenal hypoplasia congenita, and genital anomalies. *J Clin Endocrinol Metab.* 1999;84:4335–4340.
26. Vilain E. X-linked adrenal hypoplasia congenita. In: *GeneReviews.* Seattle: University of Washington; November 20, 2001.
27. Achermann JC, Ito M, Ito M, et al. A mutation in the gene encoding steroidogenic factor-1 causes XY sex reversal and adrenal failure in humans. *Nat Genet.* 1999;22:125–126.
28. Achermann JC, Ozisik G, Ito M, et al. Gonadal determination and adrenal development are regulated by the orphan nuclear receptor steroidogenic factor-1 in a dose-dependent manner. *J Clin Endocrinol Metab.* 2002;87:1829–1833.
29. Mallet D, Bretones P, Michel-Calemard L, et al. Gonadal dysgenesis without adrenal insufficiency in a 46,XY patient heterozygous for the nonsense C16X mutation: A case of SF1 haploinsufficiency. *J Clin Endocrinol Metab.* 2004;89:4829–4832.
30. Hasegawa T, Fukami M, Sato N, et al. Testicular dysgenesis without adrenal insufficiency in a 46,XY patient with a heterozygous inactive mutation of steroidogenic factor-1. J Clin Endocrinol Metab. 2004;89:5930–5935.
31. Correa RV, Domenice S, Bingham NC, et al. A microdeletion in the ligand binding domain of human steroidogenic factor 1 causes XY sex reversal without adrenal insufficiency. *J Clin Endocr Metab.* 2004; 89: 1767–1772.
32. Lin L, Philibert P, Ferraz-de-Souza B, et al. Heterozygous missense mutations in steroidogenic factor 1 (SF1/Ad4BP, NR5A1) are associated with 46,XY disorders of sex development with normal adrenal function. *J. Clin. Endocr. Metab.* 2007;92: 991–999.
33. Biason-Lauber A, Schoenle EJ. Apparently normal ovarian differentiation in a prepubertal girl with transcriptionally inactive steroidogenic factor 1 (NR5A1/SF-1) and adrenocortical insufficiency. *Am J Hum Genet.* 2000;67:1563–1568.
34. Bland ML, Fowkes RC, Ingraham HA. Differential requirement for steroidogenic factor-1 gene dosage in adrenal development versus endocrine function. *Mol Endocrinol.* 2004;18:941–952.
35. Bezman L, Moser AB, Raymond GV, et al. Adrenoleukodystrophy: Incidence, new mutation rate, and results of extended family screening. *Ann Neurol.* 2001;49:512–517.
36. Mosser J, Douar AM, Sarde CO, et al. Putative X-linked adrenoleukodystrophy gene shares unexpected homology with ABC transporters. *Nature.* 1993;361:726–730.
37. Chen WW, Watkins PA, Osumi T, et al. Peroxisomal beta-oxidation enzyme proteins in adrenoleukodystrophy: Distinction between X-linked adrenoleukodystrophy and neonatal adrenoleukodystrophy. *Proc Natl Acad Sci USA.* 1987;84:1425–1428.
38. Moser HW. Adrenoleukodystrophy. *Curr Opin Neurol.* 1995;8:221 226.
39. Moser HW. Therapy of X-linked adrenoleukodystrophy. *NeuroRx.* 2006;3:246–253.
40. Dubey P, Raymond GV, Moser AB, et al. Adrenal insufficiency in asymptomatic adrenoleukodystrophy patients identified by very long-chain fatty acid screening. *J Pediatr.* 2005;146:528–532.

41. Kelley RI, Datta NS, Dobyns WB, et al. Neonatal adrenoleukodystrophy: New cases, biochemical studies, and differentiation from Zellweger and related peroxisomal polydystrophy syndromes. *Am J Med Genet.* 1986;23:869–901.

42. el-Deiry SS, Naidu S, Blevins LS, et al. Assessment of adrenal function in women heterozygous for adrenoleukodystrophy. *J Clin Endocrinol Metab.* 1997;82:856–860.

43. Moser AB, Kreiter N, Bezman L, et al. Plasma very long chain fatty acids in 3000 peroxisome disease patients and 29,000 controls. *Ann Neurol.* 1999;45:100–110.

44. Peters C, Charnas LR, Tan Y, et al. Cerebral X-linked adrenoleukodystrophy: The international hematopoietic cell transplantation experience from 1982 to 1999. *Blood.* 2004;104:881–888.

45. Clark AJ, Weber A. Adrenocorticotropin insensitivity syndromes. *Endocr Rev.* 1998;19:828–843.

46. Penhoat A, Naville D, El Mourabit H, et al. Functional relationships between three novel homozygous mutations in the ACTH receptor gene and familial glucocorticoid deficiency. *J Mol Med.* 2002;80:406–411.

47. Metherell LA, Chapple JP, Cooray S, et al. Mutations in MRAP, encoding a new interacting partner of the ACTH receptor, cause familial glucocorticoid deficiency type 2. *Nat Genet.* 2005;37:166–170.

48. Genin E, Huebner A, Jaillard C, et al. Linkage of one gene for familial glucocorticoid deficiency type 2 (FGD2) to chromosome 8q and further evidence of heterogeneity. *Hum Genet.* 2002;111:428–434.

49. Migeon CJ, Kenny EM, Kowarski A, et al. The syndrome of congenital adrenocortical unresponsiveness to ACTH: Report of six cases. *Pediatr Res.* 1968;2:501–513.

50. Elias LL, Huebner A, Pullinger GD, et al. Functional characterization of naturally occurring mutations of the human adrenocorticotropin receptor: Poor correlation of phenotype and genotype. *J Clin Endocrinol Metab.* 1999;84:2766–2770.

51. Weber A, Wienker TF, Jung M, et al. Linkage of the gene for the triple A syndrome to chromosome 12q13 near the type II keratin gene cluster. *Hum Mol Genet.* 1996;5:2061–2066.

52. Tullio-Pelet A, Salomon R, Hadj-Rabia S, et al. Mutant WD-repeat protein in triple-A syndrome. *Nat Genet.* 2000;26:332–335.

53. Cronshaw JM, Matunis MJ. The nuclear pore complex protein ALADIN is mislocalized in triple A syndrome. *Proc Natl Acad Sci USA.* 2003;100:5823–5827.

54. Huebner A, Kaindl AM, Braun R, et al. New insights into the molecular basis of the triple A syndrome. *Endocr Res.* 2002;28:733–739.

55. Allgrove J, Clayden GS, Grant DB, et al. Familial glucocorticoid deficiency with achalasia of the cardia and deficient tear production. *Lancet.* 1978;1:1284–1286.

56 Anderson RA, Rao N, Byrum RS, et al. In situ localization of the genetic locus encoding the lysosomal acid lipase/cholesteryl esterase (LIPA) deficient in Wolman disease to chromosome 10q23.2-q23.3. *Genomics.* 1993;15:245–247.

57. Anderson RA, Bryson GM, Parks JS. Lysosomal acid lipase mutations that determine phenotype in Wolman and cholesterol ester storage disease. *Mol Genet Metab.* 1999;68:333–345.

58. Ozmen MN, Aygun N, Kilic I, et al. Wolman's disease: ultrasonographic and computed tomographic findings. *Pediatr Radiol.* 1992;22:541–542.

59. Krivit W, Peters C, Dusenbery K, et al. Wolman disease successfully treated by bone marrow transplantation. *Bone Marrow Transplant.* 2000;26:567–570.

60. Du H, Schiavi S, Levine M, et al. Enzyme therapy for lysosomal acid lipase deficiency in the mouse. *Hum Mol Genet.* 2001;10:1639–1648.

61. Du H, Heur M, Witte DP, et al. Lysosomal acid lipase deficiency: Correction of lipid storage by adenovirus-mediated gene transfer in mice. *Hum Gene Ther.* 2002;13:1361–1372.

62. Artuch R, Pavia C, Playan A, et al. Multiple endocrine involvement in two pediatric patients with Kearns-Sayre syndrome. *Horm Res.* 1998;50:99–104.

63. DiMauro, Salvatore, Hirano, et al. Mitochondrial DNA deletion syndromes GeneReviews. University of Washington, February 8, 2006.

64. Starck L, Lovgren-Sandblom A, Bjorkhem I. Cholesterol treatment forever? The first Scandinavian trial of cholesterol supplementation in the cholesterol-synthesis defect Smith-Lemli-Opitz syndrome. *J Intern Med.* 2002;252:314–321.

65. Correa-Cerro LS, Wassif CA, Kratz L, et al. Development and characterization of a hypomorphic Smith-Lemli-Opitz syndrome mouse model and efficacy of simvastatin therapy. *Hum Mol Genet.* 2006;15:839–851.

66. Bray PJ, Cotton RG. Variations of the human glucocorticoid receptor gene (NR3C1): Pathological and in vitro mutations and polymorphisms. *Hum Mutat.* 2003;21:557–568.

67. Weinberger C, Evans R, Rosenfeld MG, et al. Assignment of the human gene encoding the glucocorticoid receptor to the q11-q13 region on chromosome 5. *Cytogenet Cell Genet.* 1985;40:776.

68. Francke U, Foellmer BE. The glucocorticoid receptor gene is in 5q31-q32 [corrected]. *Genomics.* 1989;4:610–612.

69. Carson-Jurica MA, Schrader WT, O'Malley BW. Steroid receptor family: structure and functions. *Endocr Rev.* 1990;11:201–220.

70. Bamberger CM, Bamberger AM, de Castro M, et al. Glucocorticoid receptor beta, a potential endogenous inhibitor of glucocorticoid action in humans. *J Clin Invest.* 1995;95:2435–2441.

71. Schaaf MJ, Cidlowski JA. Molecular mechanisms of glucocorticoid action and resistance. *J Steroid Biochem Mol Biol.* 2002;83:37–48.

72. Chrousos GP, Vingerhoeds AC, Loriaux DL, et al. Primary cortisol resistance: A family study. *J Clin Endocrinol Metab.* 1983;56:1243–1245.

73. Mendonca BB, Leite MV, de Castro M, et al. Female pseudohermaphroditism caused by a novel homozygous missense mutation of the GR gene. *J Clin Endocrinol Metab.* 2002;87:1805–1809.

74. Charmandari E, Kino T, Chrousos GP. Familial/sporadic glucocorticoid resistance: Clinical phenotype and molecular mechanisms. *Ann NY Acad Sci.* 2004;1024:168–181.

75. Malchoff CD, Malchoff DM. Glucocorticoid resistance and hypersensitivity. *Endocrinol Metab Clin North Am.* 2005;34:315–326, viii.

76. Addison T. On the constitutional and local effects of disease of the supra-renal capsules 1855.

77. Perry R, Kecha O, Paquette J, et al. Primary adrenal insufficiency in children: Twenty years experience at the Sainte-Justine Hospital, Montreal. *J Clin Endocrinol Metab.* 2005;90:3243–3250.

78. Winqvist O, Karlsson FA, Kampe O. 21-Hydroxylase, a major autoantigen in idiopathic Addison's disease. *Lancet.* 1992;339:1559–1562.

79. Betterle C, Volpato M, Rees Smith B, et al. Adrenal cortex and steroid 21-hydroxylase autoantibodies in children with organ-specific autoimmune diseases: Markers of high progression to clinical Addison's disease. *J Clin Endocrinol Metab.* 1997;82:939–942.

80. Blomhoff A, Lie BA, Myhre AG, et al. Polymorphisms in the cytotoxic T lymphocyte antigen-4 gene region confer susceptibility to Addison's disease. *J Clin Endocrinol Metab.* 2004;89:3474–3476.

81. Lovas K, Husebye ES. Addison's disease. *Lancet.* 2005;365:2058–2061.

82. Betterle C, Dal Pra C, Mantero F, et al. Autoimmune adrenal insufficiency and autoimmune polyendocrine syndromes: autoantibodies, autoantigens, and their applicability in diagnosis and disease prediction. *Endocr Rev.* 2002;23:327–364.

83. Aaltonen J, Bjorses P, Sandkuijl L, et al. An autosomal locus causing autoimmune disease: Autoimmune polyglandular disease type I assigned to chromosome 21. *Nat Genet.* 1994;8:83–87.

84. Robles DT, Fain PR, Gottlieb PA, et al. The genetics of autoimmune polyendocrine syndrome type II. *Endocrinol Metab Clin North Am.* 2002;31:353–368, vi–vii.

85. Park YS, Sanjeevi CB, Robles D, et al. Additional association of intra-MHC genes, MICA and D6S273, with Addison's disease. *Tissue Antigens.* 2002;60:155–163.

86. Ahonen P, Myllarniemi S, Sipila I, et al. Clinical variation of autoimmune polyendocrinopathy-candidiasis-ectodermal dystrophy (APECED) in a series of 68 patients. *N Engl J Med.* 1990;322:1829–1836.

87. Herrod HG. Chronic mucocutaneous candidiasis in childhood and complications of non-*Candida* infection: A report of the Pediatric Immunodeficiency Collaborative Study Group. *J Pediatr.* 1990;116:377–382.

88. Vasikaran SD, Tallis GA, Braund WJ. Secondary hypoadrenalism presenting with hypercalcaemia. *Clin Endocrinol (Oxf).* 1994;41:261–264.

89. Falorni A, Laureti S, Santeusanio F. Autoantibodies in autoimmune polyendocrine syndrome type II. *Endocrinol Metab Clin North Am.* 2002;31:369–389, vii.

90. Betterle C, Volpato M, Greggio AN, et al. Type 2 polyglandular autoimmune disease (Schmidt's syndrome). *J Pediatr Endocrinol Metab.* 1996;9:113–123.

91. Eisenbarth GS, Gottlieb PA. Autoimmune polyendocrine syndromes. *N Engl J Med.* 2004;350:2068–2079.

92. Alevritis EM, Sarubbi FA, Jordan RM, et al. Infectious causes of adrenal insufficiency. *South Med J.* 2003;96:888–890.

93. Soule S. Addison's disease in Africa: A teaching hospital experience. *Clin Endocrinol (Oxf).* 1999;50:115–120.

94. Lam KY, Lo CY. A critical examination of adrenal tuberculosis and a 28-year autopsy experience of active tuberculosis. *Clin Endocrinol (Oxf).* 2001;54:633–639.

95. Agraharkar M, Fahlen M, Siddiqui M, et al. Waterhouse-Friderichsen syndrome and bilateral renal cortical necrosis in meningococcal sepsis. *Am J Kidney Dis.* 2000;36:396–400.

96. Hamilton D, Harris MD, Foweraker J, et al. Waterhouse-Friderichsen syndrome as a result of nonmeningococcal infection. *J Clin Pathol.* 2004;57:208–209.

97. Prigent H, Maxime V, Annane D. Science review: Mechanisms of impaired adrenal function in sepsis and molecular actions of glucocorticoids. *Crit Care.* 2004;8:243–252.

98. Gonzalez-Gonzalez JG, de la Garza-Hernandez NE, Garza-Moran RA, et al. Prevalence of abnormal adrenocortical function in human immunodeficiency virus infection by low-dose cosyntropin test. *Int J STD AIDS.* 2001;12:804–810.

99. Wolff FH, Nhuch C, Cadore LP, et al. Low-dose adrenocorticotropin test in patients with the acquired immunodeficiency syndrome. *Braz J Infect Dis.* 2001;5:53–59.

100. Seel K, Guschmann M, van Landeghem F, et al. Addison-disease: An unusual clinical manifestation of CMV end-organ disease in pediatric AIDS. *Eur J Med Res.* 2000;5:247–250.

101. Minneci PC, Deans KJ, Banks SM, et al. Meta-analysis: the effect of steroids on survival and shock during sepsis depends on the dose. *Ann Intern Med.* 2004;141:47–56.

102. Velaphi SC, Perlman JM. Neonatal adrenal hemorrhage: Clinical and abdominal sonographic findings. *Clin Pediatr (Phila).* 2001;40:545–548.

103. Goodman SN. Neuroblastoma screening data: An epidemiologic analysis. *Am J Dis Child.* 1991;145:1415–1422.

104. Deeg KH, Bettendorf U, Hofmann V. Differential diagnosis of neonatal adrenal haemorrhage and congenital neuroblastoma by colour coded Doppler sonography and power Doppler sonography. *Eur J Pediatr.* 1998;157:294–297.

105. Pulichino AM, Vallette-Kasic S, Couture C, et al. Human and mouse TPIT gene mutations cause early onset pituitary ACTH deficiency. *Genes Dev.* 2003;17:711–716.

106. Krude H, Biebermann H, Luck W, et al. Severe early-onset obesity, adrenal insufficiency and red hair pigmentation caused by POMC mutations in humans. *Nat Genet.* 1998;19:155–157.

107. Kyllo JH, Collins MM, Vetter KL, et al. Linkage of congenital isolated adrenocorticotropic hormone deficiency to the corticotropin-releasing hormone locus using simple sequence repeat polymorphisms. *Am J Med Genet.* 1996;62:262–267.

108. Atasay B, Aycan Z, Evliyaoglu O, et al. Congenital early onset isolated adrenocorticotropin deficiency associated with a TPIT gene mutation. *J Pediatr Endocrinol Metab.* 2004;17:1017–1020.

109. Metherell LA, Savage MO, Dattani M, et al. TPIT mutations are associated with early-onset, but not late-onset isolated ACTH deficiency. *Eur J Endocrinol.* 2004;151:463–465.

110. Krude H, Biebermann H, Schnabel D, et al. Obesity due to proopiomelanocortin deficiency: Three new cases and treatment trials with thyroid hormone and ACTH4–10. *J Clin Endocrinol Metab.* 2003;88:4633–4540.

111. Kajantie E, Otonkoski T, Kivirikko S, et al. A syndrome with multiple malformations, mental retardation, and ACTH deficiency. *Am J Med Genet [A].* 2004;126:313–318.

112. Krasner AS. Glucocorticoid-induced adrenal insufficiency. *JAMA.* 1999;282:671–676.

113. Woo WK, McKenna KE. Iatrogenic adrenal gland suppression from use of a potent topical steroid. *Clin Exp Dermatol.* 2003;28:672–673.

114. Todd GR, Acerini CL, Buck JJ, et al. Acute adrenal crisis in asthmatics treated with high-dose fluticasone propionate. *Eur Respir J.* 2002;19:1207–1209.

115. Allen DB. Inhaled steroids for children: Effects on growth, bone, and adrenal function. *Endocrinol Metab Clin North Am.* 2005;34:555–564, viii.

116. Murphy BE, Clark SJ, Donald IR, et al. Conversion of maternal cortisol to cortisone during placental transfer to the human fetus. *Am J Obstet Gynecol.* 1974;118:538–541.

117. Ng PC, Lam CW, Lee CH, et al. Reference ranges and factors affecting the human corticotropin-releasing hormone test in preterm, very low birth weight infants. *J Clin Endocrinol Metab.* 2002;87:4621–4628.

118. Watterberg KL, Scott SM. Evidence of early adrenal insufficiency in babies who develop bronchopulmonary dysplasia. *Pediatrics.* 1995;95:120–125.

119. Ng PC, Lam CW, Fok TF, et al. Refractory hypotension in preterm infants with adrenocortical insufficiency. *Arch Dis Child Fetal Neonatal Educ.* 2001;84:F122–124.

120. Ng PC, Lee CH, Bnur FL, et al. A double-blind, randomized, controlled study of a "stress dose" of hydrocortisone for rescue treatment of refractory hypotension in preterm infants. *Pediatrics.* 2006;117:367–375.

121. Jackson RS, Creemers JWM, Farooqi IS, et al. Small-intestinal dysfunction accompanies the complex endocrinopathy of human proprotein convertase 1 deficiency. *J. Clin. Invest.* 2003;112: 1550–1560.

122. Schmiegelow M, Feldt-Rasmussen U, Rasmussen AK, et al. Assessment of the hypothalamo-pituitary-adrenal axis in patients treated with radiotherapy and chemotherapy for childhood brain tumor. *J Clin Endocrinol Metab.* 2003;88:3149–3154.

123. Curnow KM, Tusie-Luna MT, Pascoe L, et al. The product of the CYP11B2 gene is required for aldosterone biosynthesis in the human adrenal cortex. *Mol Endocrinol.* 1991;5:1513–1522.

124. Pascoe L, Curnow KM, Slutsker L, et al. Mutations in the human CYP11B2 (aldosterone synthase) gene causing corticosterone methyloxidase II deficiency. *Proc Natl Acad Sci USA.* 1992;89:4996–5000.

125. Zhang G, Rodriguez H, Fardella CE, et al: Mutation T318M in the CYP11B2 gene encoding P450c11AS (aldosterone synthase) causes corticosterone methyl oxidase II deficiency. *Am J Hum Genet.* 1995;57:1037–1043.

126. Portrat-Doyen S, Tourniaire J, Richard O, et al. Isolated aldosterone synthase deficiency caused by simultaneous E198D and V386A mutations in the CYP11B2 gene. *J Clin Endocrinol Metab.* 1998;83:4156–4161.

127. White PC. Aldosterone synthase deficiency and related disorders. *Mol Cell Endocrinol.* 2004;217:81–87.

128. Kayes-Wandover KM, Tannin GM, Shulman D, et al. Congenital hyperreninemic hypoaldosteronism unlinked to the aldosterone synthase (CYP11B2) gene. *J Clin Endocrinol Metab.* 2001;86:5379–5382.

129. Hanukoglu A. Type I pseudohypoaldosteronism includes two clinically and genetically distinct entities with either renal or multiple target organ defects. *J Clin Endocrinol Metab.* 1991;73:936–944.

130. Chang SS, Grunder S, Hanukoglu A, et al. Mutations in subunits of the epithelial sodium channel cause salt wasting with hyperkalaemic acidosis, pseudohypoaldosteronism type 1. *Nat Genet.* 1996;12:248–253.

131. Kerem E, Bistritzer T, Hanukoglu A, et al. Pulmonary epithelial sodium-channel dysfunction and excess airway liquid in pseudohypoaldosteronism. *N Engl J Med* 1999;341:156–162.

132. Schaedel C, Marthinsen L, Kristoffersson AC, et al. Lung symptoms in pseudohypoaldosteronism type 1 are associated with deficiency of the alpha-subunit of the epithelial sodium channel. *J Pediatr.* 1999;135:739–745.

133. Geller DS, Rodriguez-Soriano J, Vallo Boado A, et al. Mutations in the mineralocorticoid receptor gene cause autosomal dominant pseudohypoaldosteronism type I. *Nat Genet.* 1998;19:279–281.

134. Riepe FG, Krone N, Morlot M, et al. Autosomal-dominant pseudohypoaldosteronism type 1 in a Turkish family is associated with a novel nonsense mutation in the human mineralocorticoid receptor gene. *J Clin Endocrinol Metab.* 2004;89:2150–2152.

135. Geller DS. Mineralocorticoid resistance. *Clin Endocrinol (Oxf).* 2005;62:513–520.

136. Mansfield TA, Simon DB, Farfel Z, et al. Multilocus linkage of familial hyperkalaemia and hypertension, pseudohypoaldosteronism type II, to chromosomes 1q31-42 and 17p11-q21. *Nat Genet.* 1997;16:202–205.

137. Prince LS, Launspach JL, Geller DS, et al. Absence of amiloride-sensitive sodium absorption in the airway of an infant with pseudohypoaldosteronism. *J Pediatr.* 1999;135:786–789.

138. Stone RC, Vale P, Rosa FC. Effect of hydrochlorothiazide in pseudohypoaldosteronism with hypercalciuria and severe hyperkalemia. *Pediatr Nephrol.* 1996;10:501–503.

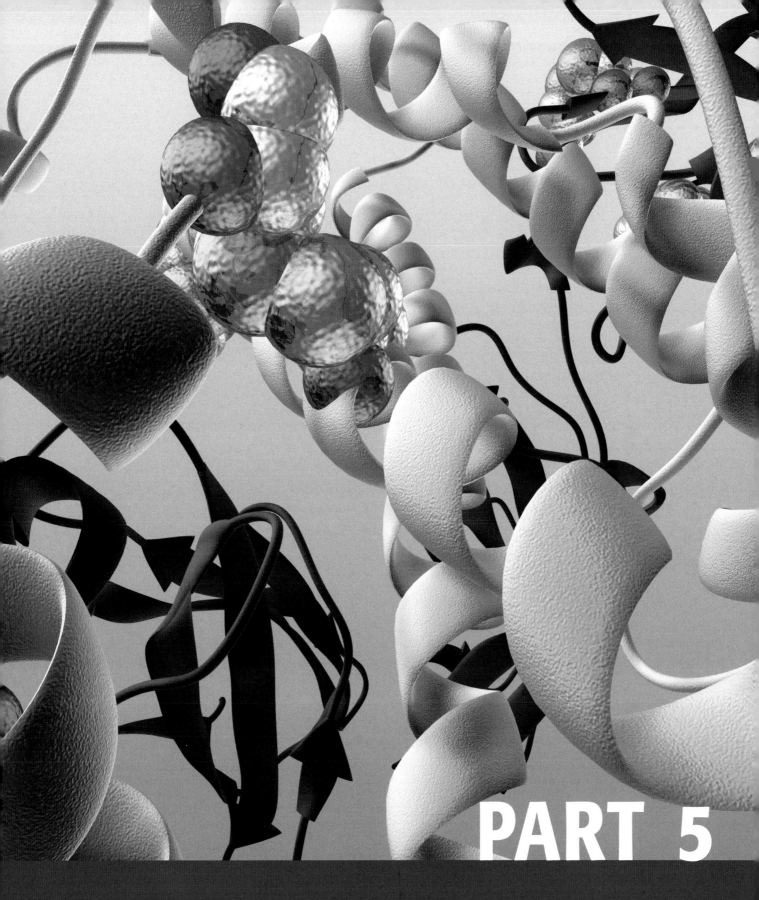

PART 5

Disorders of Growth and Puberty

IN THIS PART

Previous page: Image of human growth hormone (GH) produced from x-ray crystallographic data. GH (orange ribbons in foreground) is shown bound to its receptor (dark brown ribbons in background). A disulfide bond, formed by two cysteine amino acids (spheres) is shown in foreground. Disulfide bonds crosslink and stabilize the internal structure of proteins.

CHAPTER 30

Disorders of Growth

Stephen F. Kemp, MD, PhD
J. Paul Frindik, MD, CDE, FACE

NORMAL GROWTH: IN UTERO THROUGH PUBERTY

Human growth is characterized by a wide range of normals for height, weight, and growth velocity, with each stage of life having a characteristic growth pattern and tempo, such as 1) dramatic fetal growth (the most rapid phase of human growth), 2) deceleration of growth immediately after birth, 3) a prolonged childhood phase, 4) prepubertal deceleration, and 4) a pronounced adolescent growth spurt (1). Adult height results from the degree to which genetic potential is realized, which depends on adequate nutrition and integration of hormonal and environmental factors.

Growth charts for height and weight are available from the U.S. National Center for Health Statistics (NCHS) for ages birth to 36 months (Figures 30-1 and 30-2) and from ages 2–20 years (Figures 30-3 and 30-4) for both males and females. The growth charts were derived originally from a large cross-sectional sampling of children from North America and tend to flatten out the pubertal growth spurts. Children from other racial, ethnic, or geographical backgrounds may appear to grow differently from the NCHS curves.

The North American growth charts developed by Tanner are derived from longitudinal data and are more useful for tracking pubertal development than are the NCHS growth curves (2). The Tanner growth charts include growth curves for early and late pubertal developers; spaces for tracking breast, pubic hair, and testicular development; and growth velocity standards.

In addition, a number of specialty growth curves are available for various syndromes, such as Turner syndrome, and conditions such as achondroplasia.

Fetal (Intrauterine) Growth

Intrauterine growth is regulated by a number of extrinsic and intrinsic factors (3). Fetal insulin probably is the single most important hormone affecting fetal size, along with maternal insulin-like growth factor 1 (IGF-1) and placental growth hormone (PGH). Fetal pituitary-derived growth hormone (pitGH) and fetal thyroid hormone are not particularly important in fetal growth, in marked contrast to their paramount roles in later life. Other growth factors that regulate intrauterine growth include fetal IGF-1 and IGF-2, IGF-binding protein 3, epidermal growth factor (EGF), fibroblast growth factor (FGF), and nerve growth factor (NGF), among others. Leptin, produced by adipocytes and synytiotrophoblast cells, also may contribute to the control of fetal growth. The major non-hormonal, nongenetic factor determining birth size is *maternal constraint*, the term applied to a series of ill-defined processes by which maternal size and uteroplacental factors act to limit fetal growth.

The vast majority of births are appropriate for gestational age (AGA); that is, birth weight and length are within 2 standard deviations (2 SD) of the mean for gestational age. The newborn is said to be small for gestational age (SGA) if either birth length or weight is less than or equal to 2 SD below mean for age, and an SGA baby with intrauterine growth retardation is called *IUGR*. Intrauterine growth deficits can have lasting consequences on later growth, particularly if growth insults or deficits occur early in gestation.

Infancy

Growth in infancy is rapid and highly variable. The average growth rate during the first 12 months of age is about 24.5 cm/year and declines normally thereafter to an average of 10 cm/year by 24 months of life and 8 cm/year during the third year. Unless permanent intrauterine insults occur, growing children normally may cross growth percentiles (increase or decrease) during the first 2 years of life as maternal constraint and other prenatal effects on birth size begin to wane, and postnatal factors (i.e., hormones, nutrition, environment, and genetics) become increasingly important.

Children born SGA or to small-weight mothers may grow more rapidly and increase growth percentiles, whereas infants born large for gestational age (LGA) may grow more slowly and decrease growth percentiles (1). Thus growth percentiles may not stabilize until after 24 months of age, making it very difficult to access growth during this time.

Childhood

By 2–3 years of age, the vast majority of children have established stable, genetically predetermined growth patterns (1). Linear growth is remarkably consistent from this time until puberty, and the normal average growth rate during childhood is about 5–6 cm/year. Any deviation, increase or decrease, from previously established growth percentiles during childhood should be easy to detect and be cause for investigation. However, both early detection of abnormal growth and confirmation of normal growth require accurate measuring and consistent plotting of growth curves, neither of which may be done routinely in busy primary-care settings (4).

Puberty

In the normal child, prepubertal growth accounts for about 85% and pubertal growth for about 15% of total final adult height. Pubertal growth is influenced by the interactions of androgen, estrogen, and growth hormone and varies by age of onset, rapidity, and duration. The Tanner North American growth velocity curves are particularly helpful in tracking normal and detecting abnormal growth trends during this time (2). However, there are also ethnic differences in pubertal tempo, and the caveat must remain that standards of normal growth and pubertal development for one population do not necessarily apply to other populations (5).

Growth rates slow after the pubertal spurt, and linear growth ceases following epiphyseal growth plate fusion. In general, the average chronological age for epiphyseal fusion is

Disorders of Growth

AT-A-GLANCE

The growth of an individual is a complicated process influenced by many factors including endocrine, genetic, nutritional, illnesses and medications. Disorders of growth may be caused by one or a combination of any of these factors and are categorized according to their underlying cause.

GROWTH DISORDER	GENE	LOCUS	INHERITANCE	OMIM	AVERAGE ADULT HEIGHT (UNTREATED)
POU1F1 deficiency	POU1F1 (PIT-1)	3q	Recessive	173110	No available data but probably as in isolated GH deficiency
PROP-1 deficiency	PROP-1	5q	Recessive	601538	No available data but probably as in isolated GH deficiency
Septo-optic dysplasia	HESX1	3p21.2-p21.1	Recessive	182230	Variable but probably as in isolated GH deficiency
GH deficiency type IA	GH	17q22-q24	Recessive	262400	~143 cm (male) ~129 cm (female)
GH deficiency type IB	GH	17q22-q24	Recessive	262400	~143 cm (male) ~129 cm (female)
GH deficiency type II	GH	17q22-q24	Dominant	262400	No available data but probably as in isolated GH deficiency
GH deficiency type III	GH	17q22-q24	X-linked	262400	No available data but probably as in isolated GH deficiency
Isolated GH deficiency	N/A	N/A	N/A	139250	~143 cm (male) ~129 cm (female)
Organic GH deficiency	N/A	N/A	N/A	N/A	Variable
Biologically inactive GH	GH	17q22-q24	Recessive	262400	No available data
GH insensitivity syndrome	GH receptor	5p13-p12	Recessive	600946	108–142 cm
STAT5b deficiency	STAT5b	17q11.2	Recessive	245590	Near-adult height: 117.8–130.5 cm in female patients
IGF-1 deficiency	IGF-1	12q22-q24.1	Recessive	608747	Predicted adult height: 132.3 cm in a male patient
IGF-I receptor deficiency	IGF-I receptor	15q25-q26	Recessive	147370	No reported data
ALS deficiency	ALS	16p13.3	Recessive	601489	Predicted adult height: 168.8 cm in a male patient
Small for gestational age (SGA)	N/A	N/A	N/A	N/A	Variable
Idiopathic short stature	N/A	N/A	N/A	N/A	Variable, about −2.2 SD, which is ~160 cm (males) ~149 cm (females)
Leri–Weill dyschondrosteosis	SHOX	Ypter-p11.2, Xpter-p22.32	Dominant	127300	Variable, from 135 cm to normal

Turner syndrome	SHOX	Xpterp22.32	Dominant	312865	139–147 cm
Noonan syndrome	N.D.	12q24.1	N. D.	163950	~162.5 cm (males) ~152.7 cm (females)
Silver–Russell syndrome	N. D.	11p15.5, 7p11.2	N. D.	180860	~151.2 cm (males) ~139.9 cm (females)
Prader–Willi syndrome	N. D.	15q12, 15q11-q13, 15q11	N. D.	176270	~147.7 cm (males) ~141.2 cm (females)
Achondroplasia	FGFR3	4p16.3	Dominant	100800	131 ± 5.6 cm (males) 124 ± 5.9 cm (females)
Hypochondroplasia	FGFR3	4p16.3	~Dominant	146000	Not as severely short as achondroplasia

| GROWTH DISORDER | BASELINE | | | GH PROVOCATIVE | IGF GENERATION |
	GH	IGF-1	IGFBP3		
POU1F1 deficiency	↓	↓	↓	<10	=
PROP-1 deficiency	↓	↓	↓	<10	=
Septo-optic dysplasia	↓	↓	↓	<10	=
GH deficiency type IA	↓	↓	↓	<10	=
GH deficiency type IB	↓	↓	↓	<10	=
GH deficiency type II	↓	↓	↓	<10	=
GH deficiency type III	↓	↓	↓	<10	=
Isolated GH deficiency	↓	↓	↓	<10	=
Organic GH deficiency	↓	↓	↓	<10	=
Biologically inactive GH	= to ↑	↓	↓	>10	=
GH insensitivity	↑	↓	↓	>10	↓
STAT5b deficiency	= to ↑	↓	↓	>10	↓
IGF-1 deficiency	↑	↓	=	>10	↓
IGF-1 receptor deficiency	↑	↑	=	>10	=
ALS deficiency	↑	↓	↓	>10	↓
Small for gestational age (SGA)	=	= or ↓	=	>10	=
Idiopathic short stature	=	= or ↓	=	>10	=
Leri–Weill dyschondrosteosis	=	=	=	>10	=
Turner syndrome	=	=	=	>10	=
Noonan syndrome	=	=	=	>10	=
Silver–Russell syndrome	=	=	=	>10	=
Prader–Willi syndrome	=	=	=	>10 or <10	=
Achondroplasia	=	=	=	>10	=
Hypochondroplasia	=	=	=	>10	=

SYNDROME (INCIDENCE)	GENETICS	CLINICAL PRESENTATION: BIRTH	CLINICAL PRESENTATION: CHILDHOOD AND ADOLESCENCE
Turner (50:100,000 live births)	Most frequent karyotype is monosomy of X chromosome (45,X); deletion of portions of an X chromosome and chromosomal mosaicism with or without occult Y chromosome sequences also occur	Lymphedema of the hands and feet; redundant skin ("webbing") on the back of the neck; cardiovascular anomalies (coarctation of the aorta, bicuspid aortic valves, hypertension); renal anomalies (single "horseshoe" kidney)	Short stature (often associated with short fingers and toes and irregular rotations of the wrists and elbows); ovarian failure (delayed puberty/absent secondary sexual characteristics); short neck with redundant skin, low hairline, low-set ears, upturned nails; multiple pigmented nevi
Noonan (1:1000–2500 live births)	Mutations of the PTPN11 (protein tyrosine phosphatase, nonreceptor type 11) gene present in 40% to 50% of Noonan syndrome; however, contributions of PTPN11 mutations to the Noonan phenotype are unclear, and some patients may have only partial or even no correlation between PTPN11 genotype and phenotype	Usually normal size at birth; congenital anomalies include facial dysmorphia (including hypertelorism and down-slanted eyes, low-set and posteriorly rotated ears, high arched palate, small jaw); cardiovascular anomalies (in about two-thirds of patients, valvular pulmonic stenosis, atrial septal defects, and hypertrophic cardiomyopathy); webbed neck; chest deformities (pectus carinatum/pectus excavatum, broad barrel- or square-shaped chest); and cryptorchidism	Short stature and slow growth: mean height of males and females progresses along the 3rd height percentile; pubertal onset delayed about 2 years; mild mental retardation may be present, but average to even superior intelligence also seen; bleeding diathesis in about 20%
Silver–Russell (1:3000–100,000 live births)	Usually sporadic; anomalies of chromosomes 7 (7p and 7q regions) and 17 (17q23.3-q25 and 17q24.1) reported; maternal uniparental disomy for chromosome 7 (mUPD(7)) in 7% to 10%; mutations involving chromosomes 8, 15, and 18 also have been associated with either Silver–Russell syndrome or phenotypically similar cases	Low birth weight (secondary to prenatal, intrauterine growth retardation and ususally below or equal to − 2 SD below mean); fifth finger clinodactyly, skeletal asymmetry (hemihypertrophy), and genital anomalies (hypospadias and inguinal hernia in affected males)	Characteristic small, triangular face (with relative macrocephaly); short stature; slow postnatal growth and loss of height percentiles during the first 3 years of life; growth generally paralleling the 3rd percentile; limited pubertal growth; marked heterogeneity
Prader–Willi (1:10,000–16,000 live births)	Majority due to a sporadic deletion of chromosomal material on the paternally donated chromosome 15; about 5% of PWS have abnormalities of gene expression rather than deletion of the paternally donated chromosome 15; more rarely can result from maternal uniparental disomy of the same region	Profound hypotonia, poor feeding due to poor suck reflex and poor swallowing, cryptorchidism	Poor linear growth: mean adolescent height is − 2 SD and decreases below −2 SD thereafter; developmental delay, excessive appetite, obesity, learning disability, and behavioral problems, including moderate to severe obsessive–compulsive symptoms; delayed sexual development; sleep and respiratory dificulties (excessive daytime sleepiness, obstructive sleep apnea, hypoventilation, abnormal central [hypothalamic] ventilatory responses to hypoxia and hypercapnia, respiratory muscle insufficiency)

Note: All disorders besides Prader Willi present with normal GH, IGF-1 and IGFBP3 levels. Prader Willi have high GH levels and low IGF-1.

Disorders of Tall Stature

SYNDROME (INCIDENCE)	GENETICS	CLINICAL PRESENTATION: BIRTH	CLINICAL PRESENTATION: CHILDHOOD AND ADOLESCENCE
Familial (3:100 live births)	Tall parents	May or may not be tall at birth	Tall stature throughout childhood with bone age that is normal for age
Klinefelter (1:500 live births)	47,XXY	May have relatively small penis and testes	Tall stature throughout childhood; may start into puberty and then not continue; may have gynecomastia
Marfan (1:10,000– 1:3000–5000 live births)	Abnormality in the fibrillin-1 gene at 15q21.1; usually autosomal dominant; 25% from new mutations	May be diagnosed at birth	Tall stature with long, thin limbs; arachnodactyly; subluxation of the lens of the eye; dilatation (possibly with dissecting aneurism) of the ascending aorta; inguinal and/or femoral hernias
Homocystinuria (1:344,000 live births)	Autosomal recessive; decreased activity of the enzyme cystathionine synthase	Described in as young a child as 6 months	Tall stature; developmental delay in about 50%; arachnodactyly, pectus excavatum or carinatum, genu valgum, pes cavus, osteoporosis; medial degeneration of aorta and elastic arteries; both arterial and venous thromboses are common; subluxation of the lens of the eye
Cerebral gigantism (Sotos) (rare)	Sporatic; associated with 5q35	Large birth size with large span and large hands and feet; macrocephaly with mild dilation of the cerebral ventricles; prominent forehead (dolichocephaly); prognathism with narrow anterior mandible; high, narrow palate with prominent lateral palatine ridges	Tall stature; large head circumference; advanced bone age
Beckwith–Wiedemann (1:15,000 live births)	Probable autosomal dominance with variable penetrance; associate with contiguous duplication at 11p15.5; there is imprinting– associated with absence of maternally derived gene	Large size (macrosomia), large tongue, omphalocele; large kidneys; pancreatic hyperplasia associated with hypoglycemia	The growth rate is slower after the first several years; growth of the mouth may accommodate tongue

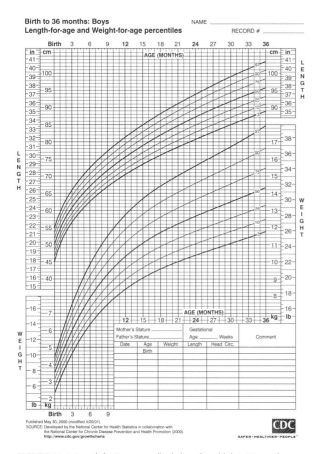

FIGURE 30-1. Length for Age percentiles in boys from birth to 36 months (from CDC website, www.cdc.gov/growthcharts).

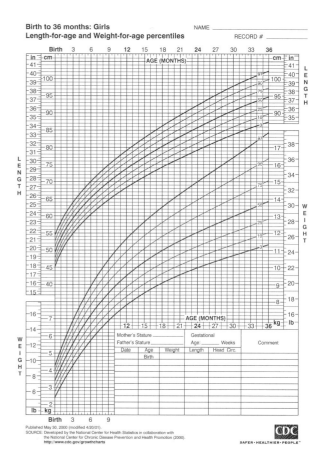

FIGURE 30-2. Length for Age percentiles in girls from birth to 36 months (from CDC website, www.cdc.gov/growthcharts).

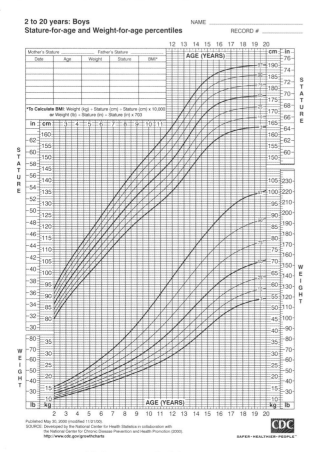

FIGURE 30-3. Height for age percentiles in boys from 2 to 20 years (from CDC website, www.cdc.gov/growthcharts).

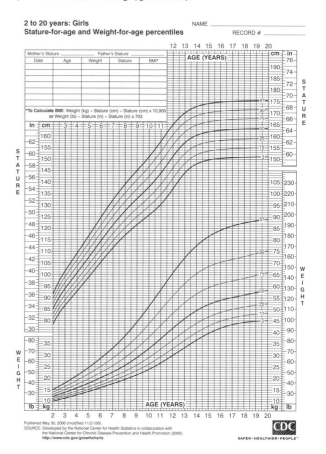

FIGURE 30-4. Height for age percentiles in boys from 2 to 20 years (from CDC website, www.cdc.gov/growthcharts).

17–18 years for males and 15 years for females. Depending on pubertal tempo, bone maturity (*bone age*) may differ from chronological age, and hand/wrist radiographs should be obtained to evaluate the epiphyseal growth plate status when there is concern about abnormal growth or question regarding remaining growth potential.

Secular Trends

Adult height has been increasing since the 19th century (6). In northern Europe, this trend is about 1 cm per decade, whereas in southern and eastern Europe, it is as much as 3 cm per decade. The effect is more apparent in childhood; because pubertal maturation also has been earlier, adult height is less affected. Menarchal age appears to have stabilized at 12–12.5 years (5). The recent secular trend has been increasing body fat and obesity. This is most apparent in the United States but also has been observed in Europe and the rest of the world.

PHYSIOLOGY OF GROWTH

Normal growth is a complex, multifactorial process that involves both endocrine and nonendocrine processes. Factors contributing to the growth process include genetic factors, endocrine factors (e.g., growth hormone and the nonpeptide hormones thyroxine, androgens, estrogens, and glucocorticoids), as well as environmental factors, such as nutrition, stress, and sleep (3).

Embryonic Development of the Pituitary Somatotrophs

The anterior pituitary develops in an orderly sequence of events (7). The pituitary, which derives from both stomodeal ectoderm and neural ectoderm, develops in close proximity to the hypothalamus and the optic chiasm. At about day 8.5 in the mouse, an invagination of the oral ectoderm occurs that forms a region known as *Rathke's pouch*. Rathke's pouch is the source of the cells that proliferate, migrate, and differentiate to become the anterior pituitary. These processes are controlled by opposing gradients of factors; several of these are in a class of bone morphogenetic proteins (BMPs), and another is one of the fibroblast growth factors (FGFs). BMP-4 appears to be necessary for the first stage of development, which is commitment of tissue to become the pituitary gland. The second stage of development is determination of the various cell types in the pituitary, and this appears to be accomplished through a dorsal-to-ventral gradient of FGF-8 and a ventral-to-dorsal gradient of BMP-2. The anterior pituitary has three distinct lobes—the

TABLE 30-1	FDA-Approved Uses of Growth Hormone	
Indication		**Year**
Childhood GH deficiency		1985
Childhood GH deficiency, pubertal dosing		2000
Adult GH deficiency		1996
Chronic renal insufficiency		1993
Turner syndrome		1996
AIDS wasting syndrome		1996
Prader–Willi syndrome		2000
Small for gestational age (SGA)		2001
Idiopathic short stature		2003
Short gut syndrome		2004
Noonan syndrome		2007

pars distalis, the pars intermedia, and the *pars tuberalis.* There are five distinct cell types in the anterior pituitary: somatotrophs, lactotrophs, thyrotrophs, gonadotrophs, and corticotrophs. It is in the pars distalis that the somatotrophs (or growth hormone–producing cells) reside.

Five pituitary-specific homeodomain transcription factors have been identified that contribute to development and differentiation of the pituitary gland and, ultimately, to cell-specific expression of anterior pituitary hormones, including growth hormone (Table 30-1). Two factors essential for development of the pituitary gland are POU1F1 (homologous to the mouse gene Pit-1) and PROP1, so named because it was recognized to be related to POU1F1 (*Prophet of Pit-1*). POU1F1 is important for development of somatotrophs, lactotrophs, and thyrotrophs. POU1F1 was the first pituitary transcription factor shown to be associated with combined pituitary hormone deficiency syndromes. POU1F1 mutations have been shown to impair DNA binding, resulting in an inability to activate promoters for growth hormone, prolactin, and the thyroid-stimulating hormone (TSH) subunit, and most commonly result in growth hormone deficiency and secondary hypothyroidism. The most common mutation reported is an arginine-to-tryptophan mutation at codon 271, which also was the first reported mutation (7). The mutations are mostly autosomal recessive, indicating that one functioning factor is sufficient for normal development, although there have been reports of autosomal dominant mutations, some of which do not appear to impair DNA binding. While it is clear that POU1F1 is involved in recruiting a number of nuclear cofactors (both coactivators and corepressors) that then act on the DNA to affect

development, the specific factors involved and the exact mechanisms of action are an area of current research interest.

The gene for PROP1 is located on human chromosome 5q and encodes a protein of 225 amino acids that resembles other "paired-like" transcript factors (7). The transcription factor encoded by PROP1 is necessary for expression of POU1F1. There have been cases of PROP-1 mutations reported since the first reported case in 1998. PROP1 contributes to early determination and differentiation of multiple anterior pituitary cell forms before emergence of four of the five anterior pituitary hormones (growth hormone [GH], prolactin, TSH, luteinizing hormone [LH], follicle-stimulating hormone [FSH]). Because it is required for POU1F1 expression, mutations of PROP-1 are also associated with deficiencies of GH, prolactin, and TSH. Children with mutations in PROP-1 often have delayed or absent pubertal development, suggesting that PROP-1 may be important in human gonadotroph development. As in the case of POU1F1, most of the PROP-1 mutations impair DNA binding and tend to be autosomal recessive. However, a 2-bp deletion (delA031, G302) of the PROP-1 gene has been described, resulting in a frameshift and termination of PROP-1 transcription factor synthesis. Patients with PROP-1 mutations usually have pituitary glands that are small or normal in size (as seen by magnetic resonance imaging [MRI]). However, some have had enlarged pituitaries, which appear to regress over time.

The HESX1 gene is similar in structure to PROP-1, but it is a transcriptional repressor. Mutations of HESX1 gene result in septo-optic dysplasia (also called *de Morsier syndrome*), which is characterized by optic nerve hypoplasia, absence of the septum pallucidum, and varying degrees of hypopituitarism. Inheritance of HESX1 mutations is autosomal recessive, although there have been reports of autosomal dominant inheritance. The exact role of HESX1 in pituitary development is not well understood. It has been hypothesized that HESX1 may block PROP-1 action until the appropriate moment in pituitary development. If this is the case, it would predict that a mutation that leads to an overactive HESX1 protein also should result in hypopituitarism; indeed, such a case has been reported.

Mutations in several other transcription factors have been associated with congenital GH deficiency. These situations have not been as well described as those associated with POU1F1, PROP-1, or HESX1. LHX3 transcription factor seems to be necessary for the proper development of all anterior pituitary cell types, except corticotropes. Mutations in the LHX3 transcription factor have been associated with combined pituitary hormone deficiency and rigid cervical spine. Finally, the homeobox gene REIG is implicated in development of the eye, and absence of this transcription factor gene has been associated with Reiger syndrome (Axenfield's posterior embryotoxon–juvenile glaucoma), which may include hypoplasia of the anterior stroma of the iris with glaucoma, oligodontia or microdontia, short stature, myotonic dystrophy, malformations of the hand, and developmental delay.

GH Gene, GH Protein

There are two GH genes, located on chromosome 17 in the human, GH-1 and GH-2. The GH-1 (or GH-N) gene is expressed in the pituitary and encodes for GH. It is part of a cluster of five genes on human chromosome 17q22-24. The genes in this region from 5′ to 3′ are GH-1, chorionic somatomammotropin-like (CS-L), CS-A, GH-2, and CS-B. The GH-2 gene product is a variant (GH-V) that is not expressed in the pituitary and differs from GH-1 by 13 amino acids. It is not usually active in terms of producing a GH product, except that it is known to be the gene that codes for a GH secreted by the placenta during the second half of pregnancy and results in suppression of the maternal pituitary GH-1 gene.

The gene for GH consists of five exons separated by four introns (8). GH (somatotropin) is synthesized by the somatotrophs in the anterior pituitary gland, where it is stored in secretory granules. GH is actually the most abundant hormone of the pituitary gland. GH is a single-chain α-helical nonglycosylated polypeptide consisting of 191 amino acids with two intramolecular disulfide bonds between amino acids 52–165 and 282–189. Through alternative splicing, different forms of GH exist, with the most common form of GH being the one with a molecular weight of 22 kDa (accounts for about 75% of the GH produced in the pituitary gland). Alternative splicing of the second codon results in a 20-kDa form that make up about 5% to 10% of the total GH. Other forms include an N-acetylated form and oligomers. There is structural homology between the GH molecule and prolactin and human placental lactogen (i.e., human chorionic somatotropin), suggesting that they all may have descended from a common ancestral gene (9).

Pattern and Regulation of GH Secretion

The GH–IGF axis is shown in Figure 30-5. Three peptides, two from the hypothalamus and one from the gastrointestinal tract regulate GH pulsatile release. These peptides are GH-releasing hormone (GHRH), somatostatin (SRIF), and ghrelin. GH is secreted in discrete bursts and remains in the circulation for about 20 minutes.

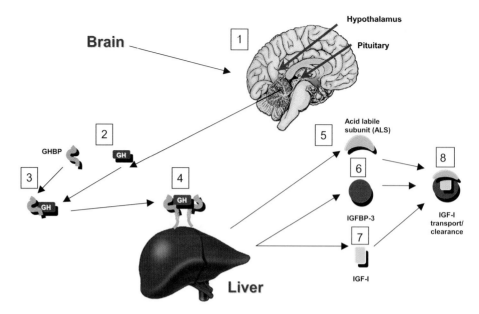

FIGURE 30-5. The Growth Hormone-IGF-Axis. 1. Growth hormone (GH) is secreted from the pituitary gland under the influence of somatostatin (−) or GHRH (+). 2. GH is secreted, and GHBP circulates as the cleaved extracellular portion of the GH receptor. 3. GH circulates bound to GHBP. 4. Growth hormone binds to its receptors. ALS (5) IGFBP3 (6) and IGF-I (7) are produced by the liver as a result of GH binding. 8. IGF-I circulates as part of a 140,000 kd complex.

GH secretion increases at night, particularly during stage 4 sleep, where increasing deep sleep triggers a proportional increase in GH secretion. At other times, GH secretion is stimulated by exercise or hypoglycemia. It also can be induced by a number of pharmacological agents. Since GHRH secretion is under control of dopaminergic pathways, dopaminergic agents such as L-dopa or clonidine will stimulate GH secretion. Also, GHRH secretion can be stimulated by glucagon.

Growth Hormone–Releasing Hormone (GHRH)

GHRH is a 44-amino-acid protein with homology to the vasoactive intestinal polypeptide/glucagons family of peptides; it was the most recent pituitary-releasing hormone to be characterized (10). It is produced by the hypothalamus and travels through the hypothalamic hypophyseal portal system to act on the somatotrophs in the anterior pituitary.

GHRH Receptor

The GHRH receptor is a G protein–coupled receptor. It has seven transmembrane domains with three extracellular and three cytoplasmic loops (11). When GHRH binds its receptor, there is an increase in intracellular Ca, leading to activation of protein kinase A, which phosphorylates and activates cyclic adenosine monophosphate (cAMP) response element–binding protein, which binds to cAMP response elements in the GH promoter, which, in turn, enhance GH-1 gene transcription.

Somatostatin

Somatostatin (12) is a small hypothalamic polypeptide hormone (14 amino acids) whose receptor (sstr, subtype 2) activates a Gi-coupled protein, resulting in decrease of cAMP and Ca influx with subsequent inhibition of GH secretion. Ultimately, somatostatin regulates the pulse frequency of GH.

GH-Releasing Peptides

GH-releasing peptides (GHRPs) are synthesized compounds shown to stimulate GH release (13), but they do not act through the GHRH or the somatostatin receptor. The structure of GHRP-6 (the first reported GHRP) is His-D-Trp-Ala-Trp-D-Phe-Llys-NH2. The GHRPs stimulate GH secretion and increase the GH response to GHRH. This observation suggested that there must be a unique receptor for the GHRPs, and indeed, one was discovered and cloned. This receptor is a seven transmembrane G protein–coupled receptor that acts through protein kinase C activation (14). Subsequently, a natural ligand was discovered and was named *ghrelin* (15). Ghrelin is produced predominantly in the stomach. It is distinct from other peptides in that it is the first peptide isolated from natural sources in which one of the serine residues is acylated by *n*-octanoic acid. The human gene for ghrelin is located on chromosome 3p26-25. The role of ghrelin in normal physiological regulation of GH secretion is not yet entirely clear.

Leptin (16) is a cytokine-like hormone secreted by fat cells that affects satiety, energy expenditure, and body weight. Leptin does stimulate GH secretion both by stimulating spontaneous secretion and by potentiating the effect of GHRH. The receptor for leptin is part of the type 1 cytokine family of receptors.

GH Receptor/Signaling

The GH receptor actually is a member of the cytokine family of receptors. The gene for the human GH receptor is located on chromosome 5p13.1-p12. It spans a region that is greater than 87 kb. The receptor consists of 620 amino acids (molecular weight 70 kDa before glycosylation). It is highly homologous with the prolactin receptor, as well as receptors for interleukins 2, 3, 4, 6, and 7; erythropoietin; granulocyte–macrophage colony-stimulating factor; and interferon. The GH receptor has extracellular, transmembrane, and intracellular domains, but it lacks intrinsic tyrosine kinase activity. The GH receptor is encoded by nine exons (numbered 2–10), with exons 3–7 encoding the extracellular GH-binding domain. Similar to other members of the cytokine family of receptors, it uses the JAK-STAT pathway for signal transduction. Initially, GH binds one GH receptor and then recruits a second GH receptor (Figure 30-6). This dimerization is followed by a conformational shift that initiates the JAK-STAT cascade (Figure 30-7). Janus kinase (JAK2) is activated (it is a receptor-associated kinase that both autophosphorylates and phosphorylates the GH receptor). Once phosphorylated, these sites act as docking sites for molecules that undergo phosphorylation by JAK2, resulting in activation of STAT1, STAT3, and STAT5 (STAT stands for signal *trans*ducers and *a*ctivators of *t*ranscription proteins). Once phosphorylated, cytoplasmic proteins form homodimers and heterodimers, travel to the nucleus, and bind specific DNA sequences that activate gene transcription.

Growth Hormone–Binding Protein (GHBP)

GH circulates at least 50% bound to its binding protein, GHBP (17). In the human, the circulating GHBP actually is the extracellular domain of the GH receptor. It binds specifically with high affinity and low capacity. It is thought that GHBP is shed or cleaved from intact receptors. The site of cleavage appears to be related to three residues close to the transmembrane domain, and the enzyme responsible for cleavage is most

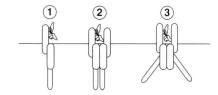

FIGURE 30-6. Growth hormone binding takes place in three phases. 1. GH binds a GH receptor. 2. A second GH receptor is recruited, which results in dimerization of the receptors, and 3. a conformation change takes place in the bound GH receptors, which results in phosphorylation of the receptors and activation of the JAK-STAT signaling system.

likely metalloprotease tumor necrosis factor α–converting enzyme (TACE). The physiological significance of GH binding by GHBP is not understood. It may act to prolong the half-life of GH in the serum, or it may compete with the GH receptor for binding.

GH Action

IGF Genes (IGF-1, IGF-2) In 1957, Salmon and Daughaday (18) described a "sulfation factor" to explain the observation that while normal rat serum stimulated sulfate incorporation into cartilage tissue (a marker for synthesis of glycosaminoglycan, a component of cartilage), this effect was reduced when serum from hypophysectomized (i.e., GH-deficient) rats was used and could not be restored by treating cartilage directly with GH. Sulfation factor was renamed *somatomedin* and became the basis of the classical somatomedin hypothesis (17), namely, that most of the actions of GH are carried out by factors originally named *somatomedins*. At the same time, others were studying a compound in the serum that they called *nonsuppressible insulin-like activity* (NSILA), whose insulin-like action persisted even after removing insulin by the addition of anti-insulin antibodies. Rinderknecht and Humbel (19,20) identified and sequenced two proteins, NSILA-I and NSILA-II, that were structurally similar to proinsulin. In the early 1980s, it became apparent that NSILA-I and somatomedin C were identical, which led to the renaming of NSILA-I and NSILA-II to the insulin-like growth factors (IGFs) IGF-1 and IGF-2. Of these two proteins, IGF-1 is the most GH-dependent. It is also now apparent that there are distinct cell membrane receptors for insulin, IGF-1, and IGF-2.

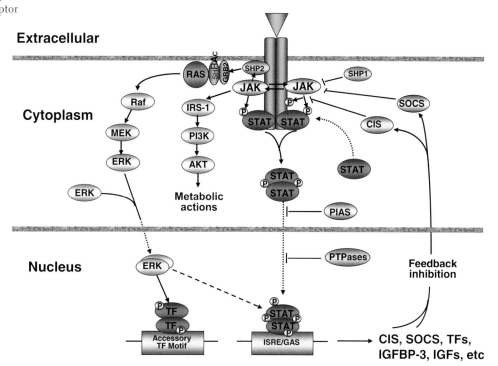

FIGURE 30-7. The JAK-STAT signaling system represents a series of reactions that take place when a hormone binds a receptor that uses this system. While the hormone binds the receptor on the outside of the cell surface, these reactions take place on the inside of the cell. Earlier steps take place in the cytoplasm, while the final steps take place in the nucleus. Receptors that use the JAK-STAT system include growth hormone and the cytokines. Abbreviations: JAK = janus kinase; STAT = signal transducer and activator of transcription; MEK = MAP kinase and ERK activator kinase; ERK = extracellular-signal regulated kinase; TF = transcription factors; CIS = cytokine inducible SH2-containing protein; PIAS = protein inhibitor of activated STAT; GRB2 = growth factor receptor-bound protein-2; IRS-1 = insulin receptor substrate-1; ISRE/GAS = interferon-stimulated response element/ IFN gamma activation site; SHP = Src-homology-2 containing protein tyrosine phosphatase-1 & -2; SOCS = suppressor of cytokine signaling; IGFBP-3 = insulin-like growth factor binding protein-3; PTPases = protein tyrosine phosphatases; PI3K = phosphoinositide 3-kinase.

IGF Proteins There are three peptide hormones in the IGF family—insulin, IGF-1, and IGF-2 (17). Insulin-like growth factors (IGF-1 and IGF-2) are small peptide hormones (~7.5 kDa) that share a high degree of homology with proinsulin. As with insulin, the IGFs have A and B chains connected by disulfide bonds and a C-peptide region that bears no homology with that of proinsulin. IGF-1 and IGF-2 have a C-terminal extension of variable amino acid lengths. Almost ubiquitously produced, compared with insulin, which circulates at picomolar concentrations and has a half-life of minutes, IGF-1 and IGF-2 circulate at much higher (i.e., nanomolar) concentrations in serum and have much longer half-lives primarily because they are part of a complex with IGF-binding proteins. Beyond their insulin-like effects, these growth-promoting peptides influence cellular proliferation and differentiation in numerous tissues. For IGFs to exert their effects at the cell surface, they first must bind specific, high-affinity cell-surface receptors, principally the type 1 IGF receptor. The interaction of IGFs with cell-surface receptors, however, is tightly regulated by at least six distinct high-affinity carrier proteins, the IGF-binding proteins (IGFBPs), and possibly by several low-affinity IGFBP-like molecules. IGFBPs 1–6, which are present in serum and many biological fluids, have similar or higher affinities for IGF-1 and IGF-2 than does the type 1 IGF receptor. Therefore, the interaction of IGFs with IGFBPs can prevent untoward IGF effects, such as uncontrolled cellular proliferation or hypoglycemia. Conversely, disruption of the IGF-IGFBP complex is probably a prerequisite for IGFs to exert their mitogenic and metabolic effects through the type 1 IGF receptor. It is probably binding of unbound IGF-1 to receptors on chondrocytes in the epiphyseal growth plate that stimulates linear growth. IGF-1 is the IGF most directly under GH control. It circulates in serum as part of a 140-kDa complex consisting of IGF-1, IGFBP-3, and a third 85-KDa factor named *acid-labile subunit* (ALS). Production of IGF-1, IGFBP-3, and ALS is stimulated by GH. The mechanism of IGF-2 regulation by the liver is not understood.

Pattern and Regulation of IGF Secretion

Regulated functioning of the IGF system has been shown to be an important component of numerous biological systems and processes, including reproductive physiology, gastrointestinal physiology, renal growth and hemodynamics, the development of malignancy, and the process of wound healing or tissue regeneration, in addition to bone growth and development (17). IGF-1, IGFBP-3, and ALS all appear to be regulated by GH because they are all low in GH deficiency and are restored with GH treatment. About 80% of circulating IGF-1 is produced in the liver (IGF-1 and ALS are produced by hepatocytes, whereas ALS is produced by Kupffer cells and sinusoidal endothelial cells). Several studies provided evidence of local production of IGF-1, including bone, suggesting, that the circulating form of IGF-1 might not be required for longitudinal bone growth and that hormones other than GH might affect IGF-1 expression at the autocrine/paracrine level. Experiments using the Cre/lox P–induced conditional knockout system generated a mouse that did not produced IGF-1 from the liver, and eventually it was shown that the effect of IGF-1 on the growth plate appears to be directly influenced by hepatic-derived circulating IGF-1. It is not clear whether GH regulates all components of the 140-kDa complex directly, or whether one of the components may be regulated by GH, which, in turn, regulates synthesis of the others. Transcription of the rat ALS gene and ALS promoter activity have been shown to be stimulated by GH. Patients with GH insensitivity syndrome (GHIS) are unresponsive to GH and have high circulating levels of GH and low circulating levels of IGF-1 and IGFBP-3, whereas patients with IGF-1 gene deletion (21) have circulating levels of GH and low circulating levels of IGF-1 but normal circulating levels of IGFBP-3, suggesting that GH regulates IGF-1 and IGFBP-3 synthesis.

IGF Receptors The IGF-1 receptor is similar in molecular structure to the insulin receptor (17); in fact, it has approximately 60% homology in amino acid composition. There are two membrane-spanning α-subunits connected by disulfide bonds, which form a pocket that mediates binding of IGF-1. There are two intracellular β-subunits that contain a transmembrane domain, an adenosine triphosphate (ATP)–binding site, and a tyrosine kinase domain that accounts for the presumed signal-transduction mechanism for the receptor. The type 1 IGF receptor binds IGF-1, IGF-2, and insulin with high affinity and mediates the actions of IGF on all tissue-specific cell types. IGF-2 also binds to a second receptor, the mannose-6-phosphate receptor, that has neither an intrinsic tyrosine kinase domain nor a known signal-transduction mechanism. Since this receptor also binds mannose-6-phosphate–containing lysomal enzymes at binding sites distinct from that of IGF-2, transporting them between intracellular compartments, it may serve as a biological sink that would remove IGF-2 as well as enzymes such as cathepsin and urokinase from the cellular environment.

IGFBPs IGFs circulate bound with high affinity to one of six IGF binding proteins (IGFBPs). Although the primary site of synthesis of IGF binding proteins is the liver, it has been shown that most tissues produce IGFBPs locally. They may act as part of paracrine and autocrine functions of the IGFs. The IGFBPs tend to temper the activity of the IGFs by restricting the bioavailability of the free IGF-1 to the IGF-1 receptor. Functions that the IGFBPs may perform include 1) increasing the half-life of IGF-1 in serum, 2) decreasing binding of IGF-1 with the insulin receptor, reducing the risk of IGF-induced hypoglycemia, 3) being involved in the transport of IGF-1 between the intravascular and extravascular spaces, 4) blocking the local effects of IGF-1, 5) enhancing IGF-1 action by keeping the IGF-1 in a slowly-releasing pool, and 6) modulating cellular proliferation and apoptosis through interaction with receptors other than the IGF-1 receptor.

There is some evidence that indicates that the IGFBPs have bioactivity other than the binding of IGFs. They have been shown both to stimulate and inhibit growth of certain cell types. They may induce apoptosis or modulate the effects of other non-IGF growth factors.

GROWTH ASSESSMENT

Evaluation of growth is at the heart of pediatrics. A child who is growing well is generally healthy. Assessment of growth involves three processes: 1) assessment of present size with comparison with population standards, 2) follow-up over time to evaluate growth velocity, and 3) predicting future growth from present size and our body of knowledge (22).

Measurement

The measurement of growth is called *anthropometry* (i.e., "measurement of man") (22). From birth until about age 2–3 years, the child is measured lying down. This measurement is referred to as *length*. As soon as the child is able to stand, the measurement is *height*; height tends to be shorter than length. Other anthropometric assessments include weight, head circumference, waist circumference, and skinfold thickness.

Length is best assessed using a device in which the infant may be placed with a movable piece that is put against the infant. It generally takes two people (an observer and an assistant) to obtain good length measurements. Height is best measured using a stadiometer. It is important that the child is standing erect with head, shoulders, and buttocks touching the wall and with shoes off. The child is instructed to take a breath, and the height measurement is taken. For precision, it is advisable use the mean of at least three height or length measurements.

To be considered short, a child's height must be 2 standard deviations (SD) or more below the mean and unlikely to reach normal adult height, based on a determination of height velocity (or growth rate), which is the amount a child grows during a given period, usually expressed as centimeters per year. To determine growth velocity accurately, a sufficient number of height measurements must be taken over a period of time that allows a reasonable amount of growth; usually this is a minimum of two height determinations at least 3 months apart.

Stage of puberty is assessed by the method of Tanner (23). Modest patients may perform their own self-assessment of puberty (24), although self-assessment may introduce some bias (25).

Growth Charts

The most useful tool for assessment of growth is the growth chart, where length, height, or weight-for-age are plotted. Examples are shown in Figures 30-1 through 30-4, and the charts are available from the Centers for Disease Control and Prevention (http://www.cdc.gov/growthcharts). A child who is growing normally should follow his or her own growth line, which is parallel to the lines on the chart after the first few years of life (i.e., "track" along centile lines). During the first year of life, it is not uncommon for a child to move somewhat across the centile lines. The highest and lowest lines on these growth charts are the 97th and the 3rd centiles, which are roughly equivalent to 2 SD above and below the mean. After the first year of life, if a child grows fast or slowly, he or she is demonstrating "catch-up" or "catch-down" growth, which may raise suspicion of a pathological situation. Also, it is important to know the birth weight and (if possible) the birth length of the child to evaluate the possibility that the child was small for gestational age (SGA) (see below).

Body Proportions

Measurements of body proportions are helpful, particularly when evaluating children with either tall or short stature. The most useful measurements are arm span (fingertip to fingertip) and upper-to-lower-segment ratios. Armspan normally is close to height. Upper-to-lower-segment ratio is determined by measuring from the top of the symphysis pubis (lower segment) and then subtracting this number from the height to determine the upper segment. The upper-to-lower-segment ratio begins at about 1.73 at birth and drops gradually as the child's extremities grow in

relation to the trunk. It reaches 1.0 at about age 10 years, where it remains for the rest of the individual's life. Published tables for interpretation of upper-to-lower-segment ratio are available (26). In thyroid hormone deficiency, growth is slow, and the maturation of the upper-to-lower-segment ratio is delayed. In Klinefelter syndrome, the upper-to-lower-segment ratio is less than 1.0 because the tall stature is caused largely by increased leg length. Also, in a child with a skeletal dysplasia, the upper-to-lower-segment ratio may be greater than 1 if the legs are dysproportionally short, and in children with irradiation of the spine, the upper-to-lower-segment ratio may be less than 1 because of failure of growth of the spine.

Predicting Adult Height Based on Parental Target Height

In examining a child with short stature, an effort should be made to predict as accurately as possible the child's expected adult height. The child's parents' heights are key factors in making this prediction. The relationship between a child's expected adult height and the parents' heights is represented as a bell-shaped distribution curve with the peak of the distribution at the midparental height. When the adult heights are separated by gender, two distribution curves result, with the peaks separated by 12.7 cm (5 in). A boy's most likely adult height is the midparental height + 5 cm (2.5 in); a girl's is the midparental adult height −5 cm (2.5 in). This value represents the sex-adjusted midparental height, commonly referred to as the target height (27).

Skeletal Maturation

One way to refine height predictions is to include an estimation of skeletal maturation, or bone age. In addition to aiding in the estimation of growth potential, the skeletal age also assists in identifying any pathology that likely may explain the etiology of a growth disorder. A radiograph of the left hand and wrist can be used to determine bone age after the age of 3 years; readings then can be compared with the published standards of Greulich and Pyle (28). Two other methods that involve a scoring system for individual indicators (parts of specific bones) also could be used (29,30). A locally read bone age normally will suffice for a clinical evaluation. While prevailing wisdom suggests that for situations in which precise bone age readings are important (e.g., clinical studies), it is desirable to have all bone ages determined by a single reader, there actually is a very good correlation between

centrally read bone ages and bone ages read by many different readers (31).

Several caveats must be considered in using bone age as a predictor of height. First, the left hand, while representative of the skeleton, does not contribute to growth. Although there is a strong correlation of bone age determined by a radiograph of the wrist with bone ages determined by a radiograph of the knee (31), there are occasional children in whom a significant discrepancy between the wrist and the knee exists. Second, the Greulich and Pyle standards were developed in the 1950s using data from American white children only. Third, all standards have been developed using data from normally growing children and may not apply to children with growth disorders.

The simplest method for estimating growth potential from bone age is to plot the height on the growth chart using the bone age rather than the chronological age. In an attempt to increase the accuracy of these predictions, a number of refinements have been developed, including the addition of other variables and the application of statistical methods.

Three different methods may be employed to use bone age to predict height: the Bayley–Pinneau (BP) method (variables include bone age and gender) (32), the Tanner–Whitehouse (TW) method (variables include bone age, gender, and pubertal status) (29), and the Roche–Wainer–Thissen (RWT) method (variables include weight, bone age, gender, and parental heights) (33). Unfortunately, all these methods—with the possible exception of the TW method—as well as the methods for calculating bone ages have been established with normally growing children, so whether these methods can predict adult height in children with growth disorders remains unclear.

Bramswig and colleagues (34) compared the reliability of height prediction by each of these three methods with others and with the target height in children with short stature and constitutional delay in growth and maturation. The most accurate method for boys was RWT, which underestimated adult height by −0.6 cm, whereas the TW–Mark 1 method (TWMI) and its refinement, TW–Mark II (TWMII), which used larger numbers of normal children and included children who were tall, short, and growth-delayed, underestimated adult height by −7.3 and −4.2 cm, respectively. The BP method, the one used most commonly, overestimated adult heights in boys by 3.1 cm. For girls, the mean prediction error was −0.8, −2.1, and −1.8 cm for BP, TWMI, and TWMII, respectively. RWT overpredicted height by 2.3 cm. Target height overpredicted adult height in boys by 1.7 cm and in girls by 1.2 cm.

EVALUATION OF SHORT STATURE

History, Physical Examination, and Clinical Findings

There are several issues in the history that help in the evaluation of short stature. The first is parents' heights. Next, it is important to know the birth weight and, if known, the birth length. If the child was SGA, it might explain why the child is now short because about 10% of children with SGA do not catch up in terms of height. The other very important data in the history include previous growth points. When plotted on a growth chart, these points can give an idea of the child's growth pattern, and a growth velocity can be determined. A history of hypoglycemia, particularly in infancy, or micropenis increases the suspicion of GH deficiency. It is also important to assess the child for other issues that may affect growth, such as nutritional status or symptoms of a chronic disease (e.g., renal failure, inflammatory bowel disease, or celiac disease).

On physical examination, it is important to obtain an accurate weight and height. If disproportionality is suspected, it is helpful to determine arm span and upper-to-lower-segment ratio. The physical examination also should include looking for signs of Turner syndrome, Russell–Silver syndrome, Noonan syndrome, Laron syndrome, and midfacial anomalies such as a single central maxillary incisor.

Biochemical Evaluation

If a child has a slow growth velocity, is short (>2.5 SD below the mean, for example), or is short compared with parents' heights, initial laboratory investigation should include thyroid functions (T_4 or free T_4 and TSH), electrolytes (to rule out renal tubular acidosis), bone age, and IGF-1 and IGFBP-3 levels. If there is a suspicion of Turner syndrome, a karyotype should be obtained; some endocrinologists believe that all short girls should have a karyotype because abnormalities of the X chromosome or various degrees of XO mosaicism may present with Turner syndrome without having frank signs on physical examination. If there is suspicion of a chronic disease, such as inflammatory bowel disease, an erythrocyte sedimentation rate should be done. IGF-1 and IGFBP-3 serum levels vary with age, making it important to compare levels in a patient with normal values at that child's age. Further, it may be more relevant to compare them with the child's bone age. Since there is overlap between the high GH-deficient range and the low-normal range, values in the lowest quartile of the normal range are suspicious for GH deficiency. A

stimulation test of the GH–hypothalamic axis using an agent such as insulin, arginine, glucagon, or clonidine may confirm the suspicion of GH deficiency. However, there is the recognition that these GH stimulation tests have difficulties in interpretation, and a growing number of endocrinologists prefer not to perform them, relying solely on the clinical picture and IGF-1 and IGFBP-3 levels for their diagnosis of GH deficiency.

In the past, a skull radiograph was part of the evaluation of patients with short stature to determine whether there was evidence of a central nervous system (CNS) tumor. The development of computed tomographic (CT) scanning and especially MRI allows evaluation of the pituitary anatomy in greater detail. In a study designed to identify common practice in a short-stature evaluation by pediatric endocrinologists, only 5% of patients undergoing evaluation for short stature had an MRI performed (35). Reports of abnormalities on MRI in children diagnosed with GH deficiency have ranged between 12% and 96% (36). Explanations for this wide variation include the heterogeneity of the GH-deficient population, inconsistency in the use of contrast-enhanced MRI (for delineation of the pituitary stalk), and variability in interpretation. The likelihood of finding an abnormality appears to increase with the severity of GH deficiency, with ectopic neurohypophysis mostly associated with GH deficiency. Failure to visualize the pituitary stalk is associated with more severe deficiency of GH, as well as multiple pituitary hormone deficiencies. In general, it appears useful to perform an MRI on any child who is diagnosed with severe GH deficiency. In patients with suspected or partial GH deficiency, MRI may aid in the diagnosis. When MRI is performed, the use of gadolinium contrast material is recommended for better delineation of the pituitary stalk. The Update of Guidelines for the Use of Growth Hormone in Children (37) suggests that GH therapy for GH deficiency be initiated only after an MRI or a CT scan has excluded an intracranial mass lesion.

NORMAL-VARIANT SHORT STATURE

There are two recognized short-stature normal variants—genetic or familial short stature and constitutional delay in growth and maturation. They are both characterized by short stature in a healthy child who is growing at a normal-height growth velocity (growth rate).

Genetic or Familial Short Stature

Familial short stature is characterized by short stature (height > 2 SD below the mean) in an otherwise healthy child with a normal-

height growth velocity (growth rate), a normal bone age, and short parents. It had been sufficient not to pursue a workup in such children; however, now some people raise the issue that there may be a reason that such parents are short, and therefore, it is appropriate to pursue such a workup. In 2003, the Food and Drug Administration (FDA) approved GH therapy for the indication "idiopathic short stature" (ISS). To qualify for this indication, the child should have 1) a height more than 2.25 SD below the mean and 2) a height velocity that would not permit attainment of a normal height (within 2 SD of the mean), open epiphyses, and no other explanation for the short stature that would better be treated by observation or some other means. Many children with familial short stature thus would qualify for GH therapy as described as ISS. It is hoped that as our understanding of the details of the physiology of growth increases, more etiologies for short stature and growth failure will be elucidated, likely causing the pool of children identified with ISS to become smaller.

Constitutional Delay in Growth and Maturation

This is the term applied to the second normal variant of short stature. It is actually the most common cause of short stature and delayed puberty. It is a diagnosis that actually can be made only after adult height is achieved; however, it is possible to describe a growth pattern in a growing child that is consistent with a diagnosis of constitutional delay. Children with constitutional delay are short, have a normal-height growth velocity (growth rate), have parents with normal heights, have a bone age that is delayed (often about 2 years behind chronological age), and may have either a history of something such as a serious illness (which explains why growth was delayed originally) or a constitutional delay in one of the parents. The typical pattern is that the child is born with a normal birth length and birth weight. During the first few years of life, the gain in height slows, causing the child's height to drop to below the 5th centile. Horner and colleagues (38) examined growth velocities in children with the diagnosis of constitutional delay and demonstrated that as a group, these children had a slowing of their growth velocity during the first year of life, with the slowest velocity at 6 months of age. This slowing results in a downward crossing of growth centiles that may continue until 2–3 years of age. At that time, height velocity resumes its normal rate, and these children grow along the lower growth centiles or below the curve but parallel to it for the remainder of the prepubertal years. Consistent with bone age delay, the onset of puberty is also delayed, which allows the child to continue to grow at the prepubertal height velocity while others at that age are having their pubertal growth spurt and closing their epiphyses. The child with constitutional delay then has a pubertal growth spurt and ends up with an adult height in the normal range and near the Tanner target height. In a recent study, Han and colleagues (39) have shown that boys with constitutional delay have higher rates of energy expenditure compared with age- and size-matched controls, suggesting that the increased metabolism may explain their lower tempo of growth.

In children with constitutional delay, their heights drift further from the growth curve because of the delay in the onset of the pubertal growth spurt; while peers are experiencing their pubertal growth spurt, the child with constitutional delay is still decelerating his or her growth velocity, as is typical just before puberty. Constitutional delay may contribute to psychological difficulties, as much related to the pubertal delay as to the short stature (40), which can be improved with treatment. It is not clear whether constitutional delay is more common in boys, but there appear to be twice as many boys as girls with constitutional delay who are referred for short stature. The preponderance of boys probably reflects a societal bias of greater concern for short boys than for short girls.

Treatment Treatment for children with constitutional delay in growth and maturation is first to offer assurance that they eventually will end up at a normal height if left untreated. Boys may be offered the option for testosterone therapy as long as the bone age is at least 11.5 years (testosterone given earlier than this bone age may result in loss of adult height because of early epiphyseal fusion). A typical scheme is to give 200 mg testosterone enanthate in oil as an intramuscular injection in three injections spaced 3 weeks apart (40). Studies have shown that if given at a bone age of at least 11.5 years, there is no difference in adult height compared with an untreated control group (41,42).

GROWTH FAILURE DUE TO DEFECTS IN THE GH–IGF–I AXIS

The etiology of familial GH deficiency was elucidated when technology allowed determination of GH gene deletions. Because GH gene deletions are rare and are transmitted in an autosomal recessive fashion, deletions in the GH gene are discovered more commonly in patients with consanguineous families (43). These gene deletions result in up to four forms of isolated GH deficiency, named type IA, type IB, type II, and type III.

Familial GH Deficiency Type IA

Etiology/Pathophysiology First described in 1971 in a consanguineous family (44), idiopathic GH deficiency type IA (IGHD-IA) was determined to be the result of absence of the GH gene (45). Transmission was autosomal recessive. Other similar patients have been described (11), and the extent of the GH gene deletions varies among the reported cases. Most cases (70% to 80%) have reported a 6.7-kb deletion in the GH gene, whereas others had a 7.6- or a 7.0-kb deletion. The GH-1 gene is at risk for such deletions because it is situated in an area that has long stretches of highly homologous DNA (46).

Clinical Presentation Children with type IA have the severest form of GH deficiency (11). At birth, they are short and somewhat obese with a small head circumference. Boys have micropenis. Hypoglycemia is present in infancy. These children grow very slowly, and their stature is usually more than 2 SD below the mean in height. They also have delay in skeletal and motor development. Etiology of the delay in motor development is not clear; there is no report of hypotonia. These children have a protruding forehead and a saddle nose and sparse hair.

Diagnosis Diagnosis is made by a failure to produce adequate GH in response to two provocative stimuli. Baseline IGF-1 level is low but rises in response to an IGF-1 generation test (IGF-1 is produced in response to 4–8 days of GH administration at 2.5 mg/day). DNA analysis will demonstrate a deletion in the GH gene.

Treatment What is particularly characteristic of children with type I GH deficiency is that many of the patients produce antibodies against GH when they are treated. The antibodies have been shown to appear even when the starting dose of GH was 1/10 the usual dose. These antibody titers may become quite high—high enough to attenuate their growth response to treatment (11). Interestingly, there are patients with type I GH deficiency in whom these antibodies do not develop (11), and treatment with GH at standard replacement doses can be effective. Several patients with high (growth-attenuating) antibody titers to GH have been treated with IGF-1 at doses of 80–240 µg/kg/day (47,48).

Familial GH Deficiency Type IB

Type IB GH deficiency (IGHD-IB) is not as well defined as type IA (49). It appears to be autosomal recessive with low but measurable GH levels in respose to GH stimulation tests. It was first described in two Saudi Arabian patients in whom a first-base transition of intron 4 ($+1G \rightarrow C$) resulted in activation of a cryptic splice site in exon 4, with the result that amino acids 103–126 in exon 4 were deleted, along with a frameshift in exon 5. A subsequent report (50) described a $G \rightarrow C$ transversion at base 5 of intron 4 that resulted in the same splice abnormality reported earlier by Cogan (51). These mutations reduce the stability and the biological activity of the mutant GH, which may disrupt the movement of the GH into secretory granules.

Clinical Presentation The consanguineous Bedouin kindred from Israel were very short (−3.6 to −5.2 SD). In some families the phenotype resembles IGHD-IA, whereas in others there may be relatively normal growth during infancy, with growth failure detected only in midchildhood.

Diagnosis Many of the children with IGHD-IB have little or no GH response to pharmacological stimuli. Initial IGF-1 and IGFBP-3 levels are low (in the GH-deficient range).

Treatment Patients with type IB familial GH deficiency respond to treatment with GH at usual replacement doses (0.3 mg/kg/week).

Familial GH Deficiency Type II

Type II familial GH deficiency (IGHD-II) is similar to type IB, except that it is autosomal dominant (49). There have been reports of transitions in intron 3 that inactivate the donor splice site and result in a deletion of exon 3. A missense transition mutation G6664A has been described in four families that replaces arginine with histidine at position 183 (Arg183His-R183H) in exon 5 of GH-1. All had heights of at least −3.5 SD. IGHD-II has the same phenotype as IGHD-IB; there is also variability (similar to type IB) depending on the exact nature of the gene deletion. Patients with type II familial GH deficiency are not as short as those with type IA, and they do respond to treatment with GH at usual replacement doses (11).

Familial GH Deficiency Type III

Type III familial GH deficiency has X-linked inheritance and is associated with deletions at the Xp22.3 region or microduplications of Xq13.3-q21.2 region. Patients have been reported to have hypogammaglobulinemia, which suggests a contiguous Xq21.2-Xq22 deletion (49) or a microdeletion of contiguous genes in the midportion of the long arm of the X chromosome (11) because the long arm of the X chromosome appears to have a locus necessary for immunoglobulin production and a second locus necessary for GH expression. Agammaglobulinemia is diagnosed in patients who have a susceptibility to certain bacterial infections. A typical history might include recurrent pneumonia and otitis media, for instance (52). X-linked agammaglobulinemia usually is diagnosed in the first few years of life. Patients present with growth failure at a later age and are discovered to have GH deficiency. Children with IGHD-III respond well to treatment with GH at usual replacement doses.

Isolated GH Deficiency

GH deficiency may be associated with other pituitary hormone deficiencies or may be the only pituitary hormone deficiency (isolated). Idiopathic isolated GH deficiency is the most common form of GH deficiency, accounting for as many as 44% of patients treated with GH (53). The incidence of GH deficiency, although difficult to determine accurately, has been estimated to be from 1 in 10,000 in the United Kingdom (54,55) to 1 in 3500 in the United States (56). Most cases of idiopathic isolated GH deficiency presumably result from inadequate signaling of the pituitary by GHRH.

Clinical Presentation The most characteristic feature of GH deficiency is a slow growth velocity. Patients may be short (i.e., height > 2 SD below the mean) at the time of presentation, or they may have a height that is decreasing in its centile on a growth chart. Birth weight should be considered because children with GH deficiency usually are not SGA. There may be a history of hypoglycemia in infancy. GH-deficient children may have increased body fat (which makes them appear younger than their ages; they have been described as looking like cherubs painted by Rubens). They may have midline abnormalities, which can be a cleft lip or, even more associated with GH deficiency, a single maxillary incisor (Figure 30-8). The most likely times that they are brought to the endocrinologist are at

the time of kindergarten (when they are first noticed to be shorter than their peers) or at the time of puberty (when they suddenly seem shorter than their peers because of a delay in the pubertal growth spurt coupled with their already short stature). It is important to rule out other possible causes of growth failure, such as chronic disease, renal tubular acidosis, hypothyroidism, and (in girls) Turner syndrome.

Diagnosis Laboratory studies should include thyroid functions (free T_4 and TSH), serum electrolytes, and serum levels of IGF-1 and IGFBP-3. If other studies are normal and the IGF-1 and IGFBP-3 levels are below normal or in the low-normal range, most endocrinologists would further evaluate the GH axis with a provocative test, although some now argue that this testing is unreliable and not helpful in making the diagnosis of GH deficiency as there is an overlap in the GH response between normal and GH-deficient patients. It is difficult to know exactly where to draw the line between normal and GH deficiency. The distinction between the GH-deficient, partially GH-deficient, and non-GH-deficient child with short stature largely has been drawn by payors during the 1990s, who arbitrarily considered a short child as GH-deficient if the peak GH response was less than 10 ng/mL to provocative stimuli. Unfortunately, provocative tests of GH secretion have been shown to be rather unreliable, which makes it even more difficult to establish a diagnosis of isolated GH deficiency unless there is virtually no GH secretion coupled with a slow growth velocity and perhaps an abnormal finding in the pituitary on an MRI. Current consensus guidelines indicate that a diagnosis of GH deficiency requires integration of auxological criteria, medical history, laboratory tests, and radiological assessments (37). Consequently, primary-care physicians can expedite the evaluation and treatment of children with growth disorders by regularly performing accurate height measurements and carefully recording growth data on the appropriate CDC growth charts. Because studies indicate that adult height outcomes improve with early diagnosis, larger recombinant human (rh)GH doses, and continuous therapy, early referral of children with declining height percentiles or those who show significant disparity between projected height and expected midparental height is recommended (57).

Treatment The treatment for isolated GH deficiency is replacement GH at a dose of 0.3 mg/kg/week divided into six to seven daily doses per week. The adult height outcomes for patients treated with GH for GH deficiency have continued to improve as we

have had more GH available, with adult heights approximating −1.0 SD (58). Data from the National Cooperative Growth Study have demonstrated an increase from heights of −2.7 SD at entry to near-adult heights of −1.4 SD (59). Similar data from the KIGS database demonstrated an increase in heights of Caucasians from −2.4 SD (males) and −2.6 SD (females) at entry to near-adult heights of −0.8 SD (males) and −1.0 SD (females). Japanese children had height increases from −2.9 SD (males) and −3.3 SD (females) to near-adult heights of −1.6 SD (males) and −2.4 SD (females) (60). Similarly, patients in France with idiopathic GH deficiency have demonstrated increases from −2.6 SD (males) and −2.8 SD (females) before treatment to near-adult heights of −1.6 SD (61). Standard GH replacement for GH deficiency usually is initiated at a dose of 0.3 mg/kg/week divided into daily (i.e., six or seven times per week) doses. The usual first-year response is about 9–10 cm of growth, followed by a waning over the next 2 years, with subsequent growth continuing at about 5–6 cm/year. The FDA has approved increasing the dose of GH during puberty to as much as 0.7 mg/kg/week (divided into daily doses). While this is an option, most endocrinologists reserve it for patients who are in puberty and have not yet achieved adequate catch-up growth. It is now recommended that IGF-1 levels be followed annually in order to ensure that they do not exceed 2 SD above the mean. There have been recent reports of success in adjusting doses of GH based on IGF-1 levels to achieve a maximal growth response. Some patients required very high GH doses to raise their IGF-1 levels to the upper quartiles of the normal range. IGFBP-3 levels do not tend to be helpful in following GH therapy. It was customary in the past to measure thyroid function annually, and it is still done in some practices. However, it is unusual for these patients to develop hypothyroidism, and if they do, it is usually apparent because of a poor growth response to GH therapy. Therefore, annual determination of thyroid function is considered optional. It also was customary in the past to obtain bone ages annually; however, many endocrinologists believe that the data from annual bone age determinations do not have an impact on therapeutic decision making. It is probably necessary to determine the bone age at the beginning of therapy and when there is concern about continued growth potential. A recent study has suggested that short children with a deletion of exon 3 (a common polymorphism) of the GH receptor may be more responsive to treatment with GH (62); however, it is argued in another study that the presence of these sequence changes in

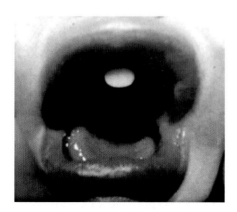

FIGURE 30-8. A child with a single maxillary incisor, a finding which is highly correlated with growth hormone deficiency.

the control subjects as well as in normal stature family members of children with ISS, indicates that these changes represent a simple polymorphism of the GHR without any functional importance (63).

An analysis of patients who received human-derived GH from the National Hormone and Pituitary Program (64) has shown that the death rate in this population is four times the expected rate. One risk was Jacob–Creutzfeld disease (CJD; there have been 26 cases in the United States in recipients of human-derived GH); however, hypoglycemia and adrenal insufficiency accounted for many more deaths. The epidemic of CJD related to contaminated pituitary-derived GH (65) prompted the establishment of patient registries that allow long-term safety monitoring in a large number of patients. Data from the largest of these registries, the National Cooperative Growth Study, indicate that long-term use of GH is not associated with an increased risk of primary leukemia or other malignancies in patients without risk factors or tumor recurrence (66). GH can reduce insulin sensitivity, but frank diabetes mellitus is rare. Other events that are reported rarely in association with rhGH treatment include benign intracranial hypertension, slipped capital femoral epiphysis, scoliosis, pancreatitis, and adrenal insufficiency. Benign intracranial hypertension is thought to be related to GH therapy. It presents with severe headaches (often associated with vomiting, especially on awakening). Papilledema may be present. It is a rare finding; there were 15 reported cases in a database of 20,000 children being treated with GH. Benign intracranial hypertension usually resolves with discontinuation of the GH. On resolution, GH usually may be restarted at about one-quarter the previous starting dose, and the dose can be increased over several weeks to the standard starting dose without a relapse of the headache. Slipped capital femoral epiphysis (SCFE), which is a fracture of the femoral growth plate in the hip, actually does not occur in idiopathic isolated GH deficiency at an increased rate compared with the general population; it does, however, appear to be increased in patients who have GH deficiency after an intracranial tumor or those who are being treated with GH for other conditions. SCFE presents with hip or knee pain and often with a history of having fallen on the hip. It is diagnosed radiographically and may require pinning of the fracture. GH therapy may be continued during the period of healing. Scoliosis is related to GH in that growth of the spine will exacerbate already existing scoliosis; therefore, while GH itself does not cause scoliosis, successful treatment with GH may worsen existing scoliosis. Scoliosis may require the attention of an orthopedist; it does not require changes in GH therapy. The report of pancreatitis is thought not to be related to GH because GH-treated patients who were found to have pancreatitis all were taking other medications known to be associated with pancreatitis. The association with adrenal insufficiency is thought to be related to GH. GH is known to inhibit 11β-hydroxysteroid dehydrogenase 1 activity in the liver, resulting in decreased conversion of inactive cortisone to active cortisol. Patients with known adrenal insufficiency not completely replaced with cortisol may experience adrenal insufficiency with initiation of GH therapy. This situation does not require a change in GH therapy; it requires ensuring that glucocorticoid function or replacement is appropriate in all patients before initiating GH therapy. Patients with adrenal insufficiency should be receiving the equivalent of 8–12 mg hydrocortisone per m^2 per day to be adequately treated. In general, these events represent heightened sensitivity to the physiological effects of GH (e.g., sodium and water retention and growth rate acceleration) or underlying patient conditions that are also treated. Importantly, correction of GH deficiency may unmask underlying central hypothyroidism and/or adrenal insufficiency, necessitating careful monitoring of hormone levels and clinical status in patients at risk. Preliminary results from a recent survey of rhGH prescribing practices in the United States indicate that the benefits of rhGH outweigh the risks, a finding surely supported by the existence of databases that monitor the outcomes of long-term rhGH administration. Patients with GH deficiency usually are treated until they have reached a height that is acceptable to them or until they experience epiphyseal fusion and are no longer able to respond to GH with linear growth. The time for discontinuing GH because of completed epiphyseal fusion is usually a growth velocity of less than 2.5 cm (1 in) per year in a patient who is known to be compliant with the GH injections. Some studies have suggested that it may be possible to extend the time for responding to GH with the use of luteinizing hormone–releasing hormone (LHRH) analogues or with aromatase inhibitors. LHRH analogues prevent progression of puberty, which may extend the time for a GH response. However, the amount of extra growth, while probably statistically significant, is small, and the child who is already behind his or her peers in terms of pubertal maturation may not feel that the tradeoff is worthwhile. Recently, there have been studies using aromatase inhibitors, which block conversion of testosterone to estradiol (which is known to be the hormone that matures the epiphysis). With aromatase inhibitors, there is no stopping of puberty (puberty actually may progress faster because of a buildup of testosterone when its conversion to estradiol is blocked). The results of these studies are just becoming available, and it is too soon to know whether this medication actually is effective.

It is now recognized that some GH-deficient children will not make sufficient GH as adults to meet metabolic needs. Features of adult GH deficiency include central (intra-abdominal) obesity, high cholesterol (particularly low-density lipoprotein [LDL] cholesterol), low bone mineral densitiy, and fatigue. The fatigue often is treated as depression. Only a minority (<10%) of patients treated for childhood GH deficiency will need GH as an adult. Those at particularly high risk are patients with familial GH deficiency, those with multiple pituitary hormone deficiencies, those with anatomical abnormalities of the pituitary gland or other organic GH deficiency, and those who had particularly low (<3–5 ng/mL) GH responses to provocative testing. It is a good practice to have patients who have completed GH therapy as children return in 6 months to 1 year to evaluate for signs of adult GH deficiency. It has been our practice to measure IGF-1 and cholesterol levels at that time. If there are indications of adult GH deficiency or a high cholesterol or low IGF-1, GH stimulation testing is recommended. Patients with multiple pituitary hormone deficiencies or anatomical abnormalities involving the pituitary gland may not require retesting as adults.

Organic GH Deficiency

Organic GH deficiency is a term that describes a group of children with structural or other insults to the CNS that affect GH production. This group includes septo-optic dysplasia or other CNS malformations, such as holoprosencephaly, or craniopharyngioma or other CNS tumors (e.g., medulloblastoma, dysgerminoma, and astrocytoma), trauma, infection, and radiation to the brain. This group makes up about 14% of children treated for GH deficiency (53) and includes both congenital and acquired conditions. A recent report demonstrated that treatment for most of these groups resulted in adult heights near the target height predicted by Tanner except for patients with septo-optic dysplasia and those who had received radiation, in whom adult heights were within the normal range but still below the Tanner target heights (67). Similarly, adult height in children with medulloblastoma averaged −1.9 SD (68); the poor growth response was attributed to craniospinal radiation. Not only does cranial radiation result in GH deficiency, irradiation of the skeleton may result in it being resistant to the growth-promoting effects of GH. In order to have optimal adult height, this group of patients needs to be diagnosed early with GH deficiency and treated with adequate GH doses.

Clinical Presentation Presentation of organic GH deficiency depends on the specific etiology. If the condition was present from birth (e.g., septo-optic dysplasia), the initial presentation may include hypoglycemia and micropenis, as well as other pituitary deficiencies. Growth failure may not be apparent until the end of the first year of life. If the condition was acquired (e.g., a craniopharyngioma that was treated by surgery), GH deficiency may be apparent because of decreasing growth velocity causing a downward crossing of a centile on the child's height chart.

Diagnosis Diagnosis of organic GH deficiency is based on low serum IGF-1 and IGFBP-3 levels and usually a failure to respond to provocative stimuli with appropriate GH levels. Because the likelihood of GH deficiency increases with increasing numbers of other pituitary hormone deficiencies, if there are three or more other pituitary hormone deficiencies, it may not be necessary to do provocative GH testing; GH deficiency may be presumed in these patients if there is growth deceleration and a low IGF-1 level. If the pituitary–hypothalamic axis has been irradiated or has suffered another traumatic insult (e.g., surgery for an intracranial tumor), there is the possibility of other pituitary deficiencies appearing with time. Therefore, with most situations where there is acquired GH deficiency, it is wise to recheck thyroid and adrenal function every few years.

Treatment GH is replaced using the standard replacement dose of 0.3 mg/kg/week divided into six to seven daily doses per week. Patients with organic GH deficiency often have other pituitary hormone deficiencies and are at risk for complications such as adrenal crisis (64). GH has been known to influence cortisol metabolism, particularly by increasing the activity of the 11β-HSD-1 enzyme (11β-HSD-1 metabolizes cortisol to its inactive form, cortisone). Thus patients with adrenal insufficiency on suboptimal glucocorticoid replacement therapy may develop adrenal crisis when GH therapy is initiated because GH increases cortisol clearance (69).

Children with organic GH deficiency are at high risk for having continuing GH needs into adulthood. If it is not certain that the child will have adult GH deficiency, GH administration should be discontinued for 1 month when height growth is complete, and then the GH stimulation test should be repeated. If there is no GH response greater than 5 ng/mL, the child is diagnosed with adult GH deficiency, and GH should be restarted at a low dose (0.2 mg/kg/week divided daily) and increased every 2–4 weeks until IGF-1 levels are in the normal range. If the child has multiple pituitary hormone deficiencies, it may be assumed that the child also will require GH replacement as an adult. At the time of finishing height growth, the GH replacement dose may be decreased to half the present dose and decreased further by titrating the dose every 4 weeks to achieve an IGF-1 level that is in the normal range for age.

Biologically Inactive GH

Mutations of the human GH gene result in severe short stature (−3.5 height SD or less) due to decreased biological activity of GH caused by either defective homodimerization of the receptor or increased binding but decreased GH signal transduction (70). Further, the mutant GH did not stimulate phosphorylation of the tyrosine of the GH receptor and acted to inhibit tyrosine phosphorylation by wild-type GH.

Clinical Presentation Patients reported with biologically inactive GH have been quite short (−3.7 and −6.1 SD). The patients reported with this abnormal GH also had high foreheads but otherwise appeared similar to GH-deficient patients.

Diagnosis Patients with biologically inactive GH produce immunoreactive GH robustly in response to provocative stimuli (from about 10 to about 35 ng/mL) but have low IGF-1 (7–14 μg/mL) levels.

As a result of genetic testing, two mutations of the GH gene have been described: substitution of glycine for aspartic acid at position 112 and substitution of a cystine for an arginine at position 77 (70). The first mutation interferes with receptor binding, with the mutant GH affecting homodimerization of the GH receptor, and the second mutation increases binding affinity of GH to GHBP by six times the normal affinity but decreases GH signal transduction.

Treatment Treatment with GH (0.3 mg/kg/week divided daily) resulted in increasing the IGF-1 level by about threefold. However, in one case, the first-year growth was 11 cm; in the other, growth responded to GH for only a short time. It has been suggested these patients should respond to treatment with IGF-1 (11).

GH Resistance/Insensitivity

Although previously referred to as *Laron syndrome* (because the syndrome was first described by Laron in 1966), the preferred terminology for this condition is now *complete GH insensitivity syndrome* (GHIS). Patients resembled those with IGHD, except that they had high circulating levels of GH with very low serum IGF-1 levels. They did not respond to GH administration either by increasing IGF-1 levels or by increasing growth velocity. The actual defect in these patients is an abnormal GH receptor. The largest concentration of patients with this condition is in Ecuador (71). Because these patients do not have GH receptors, they are also missing the serum GH-binding protein, which can be assayed easily in serum. Many of the patients reported with this condition are from families with consanguineous marriages (11); however, the patients in Ecuador are clustered in villages located in a 120-km region in the Andes of southern Ecuador (Figure 30-9). Since they have the same GH receptor mutation described in patients from Israel, it has been postulated that this mutation may have been introduced into the Ecuadorian population by a *converso* (a Spanish Jew who converted to Catholocism during the Spanish Inquisition and fled to South America). The mutation present in the Ecuadorian population is an A→G substitution that results in shortening the mRNA for the receptor by 24 nucleotides. It is assumed that this deletion results in intracellular degradation of the receptor. To date, there have been over 60 distinct mutations of the GH receptor (72), with the overwhelming majority of them affecting the extracellular domain. Two transmembrane region (exon 8) mutations have been reported. These mutations differ from typical GHIS in that the circulation levels of GHBP are normal or high. In addition, two splice mutations also have been reported that have resulted in loss of the intracellular domain of the GH receptor, causing the extracellular domain to circulate freely in serum. As a result, the levels of GHBP are high, but the GH receptor is not functional, resulting in a clinical picture of GHIS. There also have been six reports of mutations in the intracellular domain of the GH receptor that resulted in loss of function of the receptor (72). These mutated receptors may bind GH without causing activation of the JAK-STAT system.

Clinical Presentation The clinical phenotype in patients with GHIS is dominated by their short stature (71). They usually have a normal birth weight, but the growth velocity is about half normal. They have a bone age that is delayed but not as delayed as their height age. Body proportions are normal for bone age in children, but adults have a reduced upper-to-lower-segment ratio and arm span. In addition, patients with GHIS have craniofacial abnormalities consisting of sparse hair before age 7, frontal temporal hairline recession (all ages), a prominent forehead, a hypoplastic nasal bridge, retrognathic maxilla and mandible, and a sculpted chin. The head size is normal but appears disproportionately large because of the small stature. Many patients younger than 10 years of age (25%) show a

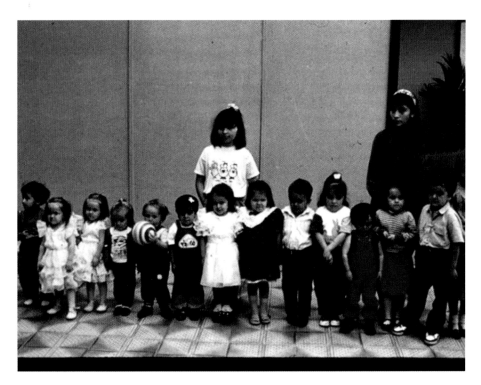

FIGURE 30-9. Patients with Laron syndrome who live in Ecuador. This photograph was kindly supplied by Dr. Ron Rosenfeld.

"setting sun" sign. There is prolonged retention of primary dentition with crowded permanent teeth. Unilateral ptosis and facial asymmetry are present in 15% of patients. Patients with GHIS have hypotonia, which gives rise to a delay in walking. They tend to have avascular necrosis of the femoral head (25%). All the children and 90% of adults have high-pitched voices. Their skin is thin and ages prematurely. Most of the children are underweight for height; most adults are overweight. They are prone to developing osteopenia. There is a propensity to have hypoglycemia, increased cholesterol (particularly LDL cholesterol), and decreased sweating. Males have a micropenis in childhood with normal penile growth in puberty. Both sexes have delayed puberty, but they have normal reproductive function.

Diagnosis Diagnosis of GHIS is made in a child who has the features of GH deficiency but has high baseline levels of GH with low serum IGF-1 and IGFBP-3 levels. An IGF-1 generation test may be performed. In this test, GH (~0.05 mg/kg/dose) is administered daily for 4–9 days. In GHIS, the serum IGF-1 does not respond to the GH administration. GHBP is also low in patients in whom there is a defect in the extracellular domain of the GH receptor. A normal or high GHBP suggests a defect in the transmembrane, intracellular, or postreceptor region of the GH receptor.

Treatment There have been a number of studies using IGF-1 to treat GHIS. Most `trials of IGF-1 treatment of GHIS began in the late 1980s and involved twice-daily dosing of IGF-1 (73). Doses of 40–150 μg/kg/day have resulted in increases in linear growth. From reports of trials from 1993 to 1997, growth velocity increased from 3.6 cm/year (range 2.9–4.7 cm/year) to a mean of 8.4 cm/year (range 7.2–9.3 cm/year) during the first year of treatment. Ranke (74–76) and Backeljauw (47,77) reported treatment of a European cohort of 17 patients with GHIS and demonstrated sustained catch-up growth, with a change in mean height SD from −6.2 to −4.2, and maintenance of the mean growth velocity at 6.3 cm/year. Some patients reached the 3rd centile.

Treatment of GHIS with IGF-1 has resulted in mild to moderate adverse events. Most commonly reported events have been pain at the injection site and headaches. The European study reported that these events seem to occur during the first month of treatment and then improve. Other adverse events have included lipohypertrophy at the injection site, papilledema related to increased intracranial hypertension (78), and facial nerve paralysis. Most of these adverse events resolved after interrupting treatment and restarting with a lower dose, usually dropping the dose from 120 to 80 μg/kg (74). A further concern has been hypoglycemia, which occurred in some of the patients receiving IGF-1 but only rarely resulted in seizures (74). Risk of hypoglycemia is reduced by giving the IGF-1 dose with meals; it is usually a problem during an intercurrent illness resulting in loss of appetite. Hypoglyce-

mia was dose-dependent; it hardly ever occurred in patients receiving less than 80 μg/kg. Another effect of IGF-1 therapy is lymphoid tissue enlargement, in particular, splenic and tonsillar hypertrophy. Renal size also increased, but renal function remained normal (74). There were changes in facial appearance (i.e., coarsening of features and an increase in hair growth) that were most noticeable during puberty.

Treatment of GHIS with IGF-1 has been reviewed recently (79). There are presently two IGF-1 compounds available for treatment of severe GHIS. One, mecasermin, which is rhIGF-1 alone (Increlex, Tercica, Inc., Brisbane, CA), received approval from the FDA for treatment of severe GH resistance in August 2005. The second compound is mecasermin rinfabate (iPlex, Insmed, Richmond, VA), which received FDA approval in December 2005. Formerly called SomatoKine, iPlex is a complex of equimolar amounts of rhIGF-1 and its most abundant binding protein insulin-like growth factor I–binding protein 3 (rhIGFBP). Ideally, administration of IGF-1 should raise IGF-1 levels into the normal range. In addition, it should result in an increase in growth velocity similar to what is seen with GH administration. Children should be monitored on physical examination for an increase in lymphoid tissue (particularly tonsils) and papilledema (by funduscopic examination at regular visits).

Partial GH Insensitivity

Definition Partial GH insensitivity (PGHIS) is a mild form of complete GHIS. It has been considered to be the cause in some cases of ISS and SGA.

Etiology/ Pathopysiology PGHIS is thought to be caused by a mutation in the GH receptor that does not completely inactivate the receptor but does cause lower GH binding or decreases the response to GH binding.

Clinical Presentation Patients with PGHIS are similar to patients with IGHD. They appear otherwise healthy, but have a slow growth velocity.

Biochemical Findings In order to determine whether partial GH insensitivity was responsible for growth failure in children who were not GH-deficient, data were analyzed from 773 children who were being treated with GH and were enrolled in a postmarketing surveillance project, the National Cooperative Growth Study (NCGS) (80). Patients enrolled in this study had levels of IGF-1 and GHBP determined. In addition, these patients had been evaluated for GH deficiency by response to provocative stimuli. Patients who had a GH response to provocative stimuli of greater than 10 ng/mL were classified as having ISS. Children with ISS had GHBP levels more than 2 SD below those of normal control patients, IGF-1 levels lower than those of controls (108–120 versus 217–308 μg/L) but higher than those of GH-deficiency patients (84–99 μg/L) and a mean 12-hour GH concentration similar to that of controls (2.2 versus 2.1–2.7 μg/L) but lower than that of GH-deficiency patients (1.2–1.4 μg/L). A subset of 14 of these patients (height more than 2.5 SD below the mean, normal GH secretion, IGF-1 levels more than 2.0 SD below the mean, and serum concentrations of GHBP more than 2 SD below the mean) were studied further (81). Four of the 14 patients had mutations in the GH receptor (but none of the 24 contol subjects). One of these patients was a compound heterozygote with respect to the GH receptor.

Postreceptor Defects in GH Action

Etiology/Pathophysiology In 2003, a patient was described who was very short but not GH-deficient who was shown to have a mutation in STAT5b, a postreceptor factor that is necessary for one of the steps that occurs after GH binds its receptor (72) (see the "Physiology of Growth" above).

Clinical Presentation The patient was born at 33 weeks' gestation to consanguineous parents of normal height. Birth weight was 1400 g (3rd centile). The patient had growth failure during the first 3 years of life. He had a prominent forehead, a saddle nose, and a high-pitched voice. At 7 years, his height was 97 cm, and his weight was 14 kg, both significantly below the 3rd centile. He was treated with GH for 1 year with no response in terms of height velocity. At age 16.5 years, his height was 117.8 cm, again well below the 3rd centile. The GH level was 9.4 ng/mL at baseline and rose to 53.8 ng/mL with insulin-induced hypoglycemia. Nonetheless, IGF-1, IGFBP-3, and ALS levels all were markedly low, with a poor response to 7 days of GH therapy (0.05 mg/kg/day). This patient was determined to have a mutation in the postreceptor factor STAT5b. A second patient with STAT5b deficiency has been reported (72) (see Figure 30-10). In addition to short stature, the patients identified with STAT5b deficiencies have histories of infections, consistent with STAT5b being a part of other cytokine receptor systems.

Treatment These patients do not respond to GH administration but should respond to IGF-1 in much the same way as GHIS patients. There has not yet been a report of IGF-1 treatment of a child with STAT5b deficiency.

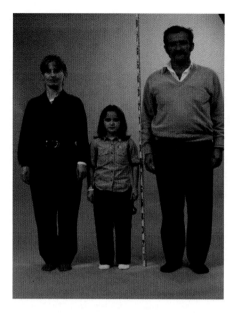

FIGURE 30-10. A patient with a deficiency of STAT5b with her parents. This picture was kindly supplied by Dr. Ron Rosenfeld.

IGF-1 Deficiency

There has been one case reported of an IGF-1 gene deletion (72).

Clinical Presentation The child was born by cesarean section at 37 weeks' gestation and had significant intrauterine growth failure (birth weight 1.4 kg, or −3.9 SD; birth length 37.8 cm, or −5.4 SD; head circumference 27 cm, or −4.9 SD) with continued postnatal growth failure. At age 15¾ years, height was −6.9 SD. This patient also had microcephaly, severe developmental delay, sensorineural deafness, and delayed puberty. This patient had no history of hypoglycemia or other metabolic disorder but was evaluated for GHIS. There was no family history of growth failure or IUGR; however, thes parents were first cousins once removed. This patient has been treated with IGF-1 with a response in the growth velocity. Unlike patients with GHIS, the patient had only a deficiency in IGF-1, not GH-binding proteins or ALS. Thus, when he was given a dose of IGF-1, it had a longer half-life than in patients with GHIS (82). He did develop antibodies to IGF-1 that have continued to increase over time.

A 55-year-old man with a very similar phenotype has been reported, in whom there are striking elevations of IGF-1 (83). The patient had a birth length of −4.3 SD and an adult height of −8.5 SD. His IGF-1 was found to have a missense mutation with the substitution of a methionine for a valine at position 44. The IGF-1 that resulted bound the IGFBPs, but with a decreased affinity to the IGF-1 receptor. It was poorly effective in stimulating the receptor to become phosphorylated and

stimulate DNA synthesis. In this case, conventional immunoassay detected the mutant IGF-1; it could be differentiated from normal IGF-1 only by bioassay.

IGF-1 Receptor Defect or IGF-1 Resistance

Definition IGF-1 resistance is characterized by short stature, IUGR, and elevated GH and IGF-1 (84).

Clinical Presentation The first patient identified after screening 42 patients with unexplained IUGR was a compound heterozygote for IGF-1 receptor defects, carrying two point mutations in exon 2. Her birth weight was 1.4 kg (3.5 SD below the mean for gestational age). She was taking 124 kcal/kg/ body weight but did not have catch-up linear growth. She got her first tooth at 14 month (normal is 6–8 months). At age 4½ years, her bone age was 3 years. The second patient had a nonsense mutation (Arg59stop) that reduced the number of IGF-1 receptors on the patient's fibroblasts and was identified after screening a second cohort of 50 children who had short stature and elevated IGF-1 levels. This patient had a birth weight of 2000 g and a birth length of 40 cm. He did not have catch-up linear growth despite normal caloric intake. At 14 months, his height was 3.8 SD below the mean. At 5 years, physical examination showed severe short stature, a receding hairline, bushy eyebrows, a broad nasal bridge, a broad and rounded nasal tip, a long and smooth philtrum, a thin upper lip, and a broad, everted, and fleshy lower lip. He had short fingers (especially thumbs), widely set nipples, and pectus excavatum. Bone age was delayed by 1–1.5 years. Both patients not only had IUGR but also demonstrated poor postnatal growth.

Diagnosis Patient 1 had a robust GH response of 51 ng/mL to clonidine. Pretreatment IGF-1 concentration was 63 ng/mL (normal for age). Patient 2 had a GH response of 6.0 ng/mL to arginine and 5.7 ng/mL to insulin-induced hypoglycemia. IGF-1 levels ranged from 121–222 μg/L (1.1–2.3 SD above the mean for age). The normal to high circulating levels of IGF-1 and GH indicated that these patients had IGF-1 resistance.

Treatment Patient 1 was treated with GH at 0.375 mg/kg/week divided into three doses per week. Her first-year growth rate increased from 5.2 to 7.2 cm/year. At age 6 years, GH was discontinued for 2 years to redetermine her baseline growth velocity, which was 3.6 cm/year. GH therapy was resumed at the same dose with an increase in growth velocity to 6.5 cm/year. At age 15, she remained well more than 2 SD below the mean for height. Patient 2 was not treated.

ALS Deficiency

ALS deficiency is characterized by moderate short stature and reduced levels of circulating IGF-1 presumably because of the failure to circulate as part of the usual 140,000-kDa complex, resulting in a more rapid clearing of IGF-1 from the circulation. To date, there have been two reports of mutations in the gene for ALS (85,86).

Clinical Presentation Both patients were characterized by modest short stature, with heights in the range of −2.5 SD. In addition, if it is indeed the case that ALS is not required for growth at the growth plate, these patients provide strong evidence that circulating IGF-1 is critical for normal human growth. The first patient was referred for short stature and pubertal delay at age 14½ years. His height was near the 3rd centile. Physical examination showed only mild micrognathia and truncal obesity. Bone age was 12½ years.

Diagnosis Routine laboratory tests ruled out liver, renal, and hematological disease. Thyroid function was normal. Brain MRI was normal. GH responses to arginine and clonidine were normal. IGF-1 was low (31 ng/mL, which is 5.3 SD below the mean for age). IGFBP-3 also was low (0.22 μg/mL, which is 9.7 SD below the mean for age). ALS serum measurement led to the diagnosis of ALS deficiency. Patient 2 had a similar workup but also had an IGF-1 generation test (0.033 mg/kg/day of GH for 7 days) that showed no measurable increase in IGF-1 or IGFBP-3.

Treatment Patient 1 was treated with GH (0.17 mg/kg/week) for 6 months without an increase in growth velocity. Patient 2 has not been treated.

GROWTH FAILURE DUE TO POSSIBLE DEFECTS IN THE GH–IGF-1 AXIS

Small for Gestational Age (SGA)

Adequate growth in a normal fetus depends on the ability of mother to provide nutrients, the ability of placenta to deliver nutrients, and the ability of fetus to use nutrients (87). SGA is defined as having either a birth length or a birth weight that is more than 2 SD below the mean for gestational age (88). Growth charts are available that allow easy determination of birth length and birth weight for gestational age (89). Of all newborns, 2.4% are short only, 1.6% are underweight only, and 1.5% are both short and underweight (90). In 40% of SGA births, there is no identified underlying pathology (91), whereas 50% of cases are due to maternal influences (91). About 5% of cases are due to chromosomal abnormalities (87),

and a small proportion of cases are related to placental factors (92), including placental insufficiency, infarction, abruption, or vascular abnormalities (87). Other factors associated with low-birth-weight infants include hormonal factors (e.g., insulin and IGFs), chromosomal abnormalities, congenital anomalies, and infections. Most children who are born SGA (approximately 90%) catch up their growth (i.e., have heights greater than −2 SD below the mean) by age 2 years (93). In children who do catch up, accelerated growth occurs in the first 3 months postpartum. Average weight and length increase to the 10th to the 25th percentile at 6 months (94). A predictor of catch-up growth is birth length; there is no association with gestational age, multiple birth, or gender (95). If catch-up growth does not occur by 2 years of age, it is unlikely that it will occur (except in the very premature infant). SGA children who have not experienced catch-up growth by age 2 years have an abnormal rhythm of bone maturation throughout childhood. Spontaneous acceleration of bone maturation and decreased height standard deviations occur from ages 6–12 years in untreated short children born SGA. Prediction of final height in untreated short children born SGA is not reliable and results in overprediction of final height in most.

It has been recognized that some children who are born SGA have early puberty, which may limit the time that GH may be administered successfully and thus may limit the potential for achievement of maximal adult height. Other problems seen in children born SGA are a tendency to obesity, insulin resistance, and polycystic ovarian syndrome (i.e., metabolic syndrome). The etiologies of these issues are not well understood; it has been suggested that these children may have had altered metabolism in utero that results in these metabolic changes that continue throughout life. There had been concern that GH therapy may exacerbate these metabolic changes; however, there has been no unusual advancement of bone age in SGA children treated with GH. Further, although SGA children receiving GH therapy may exhibit some insulin resistance, as evidenced by higher insulin levels and an increase in fasting blood sugar concentrations (9 mg/dL above controls), there appears to be no clinical significance, and the insulin resistance is reversible on discontinuing GH therapy.

Diagnosis Compared with normal neonates, serum GH hormone levels were significantly increased and IGF-1 and IGFBP-3 levels were significantly decreased in IUGR neonates (96). All parameters were within normal limits at 1 month of age and remained

normal thereafter. Low serum IGF-1 and IGFBP-3 levels at birth were related to fetal malnutrition and did not predict later growth. Boguszewski and colleagues (97) demonstrated that short children born SGA had lower GH secretion than normal short children or children of normal stature. In addition, the levels of IGF-1 and IGFBP-3 tended to be in the lower part of the normal range.

Treatment GH, particularly at high doses (0.48–0.72 mg/kg/week), has been shown to increase the growth velocity of children born SGA (98). This increase in growth velocity has been shown to persist for at least 2 years and even as long as 6 years (99), with a dose–response curve over 0.24–0.48 mg/kg/week. Based on these data, in 2003, the FDA approved the use of GH at a dose of 0.48 mg/kg/week for treating children who were born SGA and who had not brought up their height into the normal range by age 2 years.

Idiopathic Short Stature (ISS)

ISS has been used to describe short stature in children who do not have GH deficiency, in whom all recognizable causes of short stature (i.e., IUGR, genetic or syndromic causes of short stature, and psychosocial deprivation) have been ruled out, and in whom the etiology of the short stature is not understood (100). Other terms have been used in the past to describe these children, and some of the following terms overlap with those now described as having ISS: *familial short stature, constituitional delay of growth and maturation, normal-variant short stature, growth hormone neurosecretory dysfunction, idiopathic growth failure, non-GH-deficient short stature,* and *nonendocrine short stature.* As a group, children with ISS do not achieve their adult height predictions, and many have adult heights that are quite short.

Etiology/Pathophysiology Some patients with ISS may have partial GH insensitivity due to mutations in the GH receptor gene, as described earlier.

Treatment Children with ISS treated with GH are as short at the beginning of GH therapy as children with chronic renal insufficiency, idiopathic GH deficiency, Turner syndrome, or those born SGA; that is, their heights before treatment range from −2.6 to −2.9 SD (53). In this group of children, IGF-1 levels often are normal, but in about 25% they are low, suggesting that some in this group may have GH insensitivity. Many of the published studies of GH therapy in children with ISS have involved small sample sizes and did not have control groups. A meta-analysis of these studies (101) suggested that the overall height gain may have been an increase from −2.5 to −3.0 SD to −1.5 to −1.8 SD with GH therapy, which is a height increase of 3.6–4.6 cm. In studies with a control group, it appeared that the control group increased its height as well (consistent with previous reports of spontaneous growth in children with ISS) (102), but the treated group exceeded the control group by about 0.78 SD. Subsequent to this meta-analysis, results of a placebo-controlled study to adult height (103) demonstrated a height increase of 3.7–5.0 cm with GH therapy despite a low dose of GH (0.22 mg/kg/week) and an injection schedule of three times per week. A subsequent study evaluating two treatment protocols (104) demonstrated a dose effect, with a dose of 0.37 mg/kg/week resulting in an increase in adult height of 7.2 cm compared with 5.4 cm in the group receiving only 0.24 mg/kg/week. An analysis of children with ISS treated with GH followed in the National Cooperative Growth Study (NCGS) showed an increase in adult height from about −3.0 SD to about −1.5 SD (105). These studies, as well as an evaluation of over 8000 ISS patients followed in the NCGS (105), have shown that there are no safety issues in GH therapy different from what is seen with treatment of GH deficiency. Based on these studies, the FDA in 2003 approved the use of GH for the treatment of children with ISS, defined by a height that is at least −2.25 SD and associated with a growth rate that is unlikely to permit attainment of an adult height within the normal range of children whose epiphyses are not closed and for whom the diagnostic evaluation excludes other causes of short stature that should be observed or treated by other means.

It is interesting that children with ISS have been treated with GH at least since the inception of the NCGS in 1985, accounting for about 20% of all patients treated with GH (106). Nonetheless, it has been difficult to demonstrate that an increase in height also results in an increased quality of life. This is a particularly relevant question because GH therapy is quite expensive—perhaps as much as $52,634 per inch (107). A recent review of this issue (108) has concluded that parents and children retrospectively perceive the GH therapy to be positive; however, there are not good studies from which we can conclude evidence-based positive effects. A recent study has demonstrated a 5.9-cm increase in predicted adult height in boys with ISS using an inhibitor of aromatase (letrozole) for 24 months (109). Although this report appears quite promising, further studies in which subjects are followed to adult height are needed to determine whether this approach is viable.

SYNDROMES/CHROMOSOMAL ABNORMALITIES ASSOCIATED WITH GROWTH FAILURE

SHOX Gene

Growth and final adult height are determined by a number of intrinsic (i.e., hormonal and genetic) and extrinsic (i.e., environmental) factors. One of the most interesting and recently described gene mutations associated with short stature is the SHOX, or short stature homeobox-containing, gene. The SHOX gene exists on the distal part of the short-arm pseudoautosomal region (PAR1) of the sex chromosomes and is expressed from normal Y chromosomes and from both active and inactive X chromosomes, suggesting that SHOX escapes X inactivation. SHOX is also strongly expressed in bone-marrow fibroblasts, implying a positive role in bone growth and development (110).

SHOX haploinsufficiency can be caused by intragenic mutations, pseudoautosomal submicroscopic deletions, and cytogenetically recognizable Xp deletions (110) and was recognized originally as one of the genetic causes of "idiopathic" short stature (111). SHOX haploinsufficiency since has been shown to result not only in short stature but also in a number of phenotypic features associated with Turner syndrome, including cubitus valgus, short metacarpals, Madelung deformity, Leri–Weill dyschondrosteosis, high arched palate, and short neck (110). Clinically, any child presenting with short stature combined with short limbs, wrist changes, and tibial bowing is likely to have SHOX haploinsufficiency (112).

Turner Syndrome

Presentation, Diagnosis, and Genetics Phenotypic presentation of girls with Turner syndrome can vary, although short stature and ovarian failure are the most common and consistent clinical features. The short stature often is associated with short fingers and toes and irregular rotations of the wrists and elbows. Other features and associated conditions that may be seen include a characteristic appearance thought to be the result of fetal lymphatic system obstruction (i.e., short "webbed" neck, low hairline, low-set ears, edematous hands and feet at birth, and upturned nails), multiple pigmented nevi, cardiovascular anomalies (i.e., coarctation of the aorta, bicuspid aortic valves, and hypertension), renal anomalies (single "horseshoe" kidney), thyroiditis, and type 2 diabetes (113) (Figure 30-11). Girls with Turner syndrome have normal intelligence but may have difficulty with tasks requiring visual-spatial coordination.

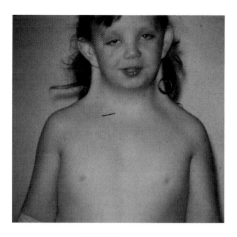

FIGURE 30-11. A child with Turner Syndrome. Photo courtesy of Robert Gorlin, D.D.S., M.S., D.Sc.

Turner syndrome may present at any age, although the predominant presenting complaints will vary. Turner syndrome in the neonatal period can present with lymphedema of the hands and feet as well as redundant skin ("webbing") on the back of the neck. Thereafter, the child with Turner syndrome may present with a chief complaint of short stature. Characteristic phenotypic findings are extremely variable and may be missing in some children; thus Turner syndrome should be considered in any female with apparent "idiopathic" short stature. The adolescent-age girl may present with short stature, delayed puberty (i.e., absence of female secondary sex characteristics), and/or absence of menses. Neck webbing, when present at any age, correlates positively with the existence of congenital cardiovascular defects (114).

Turner syndrome, the most common sex chromosome abnormality in girls, occurs in about 50 per 100,000 live births and is due to abnormalities of the X chromosome: either the absence of an X chromosome (complete deletion), deletion of portions of an X chromosome, or chromosomal mosaicism (113). The most frequent karyotype associated with Turner syndrome is monosomy of the X chromosome (45,X), found in 63.3% of patients in one review; other karyotypes in descending order of frequency are isochromosome Xq (46,XisoXq), 16.7%; mosaic (46,XX/45,X), 6.7%; deletion of Xp (46,XdelXp), 6.7%; deletion of Xq (46,XdelXq), 3.3%; and ring Xp (46,XX/46,XringXp), 3.3% (115). Occult Y chromosome sequences also may occur (116). SHOX haploinsufficiency has been shown recently to be responsible for many of the phenotypic features of Turner syndrome (110). See also SHOX gene discussion above.

Management/Treatment Initial diagnosis generally is suspected based on physical characteristics and history and should be confirmed by karyotype analysis and a probe for Y chromosome material. Girls with Turner syndrome generally do quite well but may have a variety of associated endocrine, renal, and cardiovascular anomalies (113), all of which can affect growth. See following sections for discussions of growth, puberty, and associated anomalies (117).

Growth and Puberty The spontaneous final height of untreated adults with Turner syndrome ranges between 139 and 147 cm, which is equivalent to an adult height as much as 20 cm less than that of the general female population (118). GH therapy increases adult height of girls with Turner syndrome and is given at a dose of 0.375 mg/kg/week. Growth is monitored on therapy every 3–6 months, and GH dose is adjusted as the child grows to maintain 0.375 mg/kg/week. Older girls likely also will be receiving oral conjugated estrogen to help with pubertal development and growth. Finally, a combination therapy consisting of GH plus an anabolic steroid (e.g., oxandrolone 0.05–0.1 mg/kg/day) is recommended by some pediatric endocrinologists, particularly when the diagnosis of Turner syndrome is made relatively late during adolescence, for further height enhancement (119).

In one review, treatment with GH for 3.2 ± 2.0 years resulted in an increase in height of 1.2 ± 0.8 SD compared with Turner syndrome standards (120). With more prolonged GH therapy of 6–7 years, there was a cumulative increase of +2.0 SD in mean height. In another review, mean adult height after 5.0 ± 2.2 years of GH plus estrogen was 149.9 ± 6.1 cm, or 8.5 cm above projected height (121). The most important predictors of adult height outcome are age at initiation of GH treatment and length of treatment (121). Thus potential strategies to improve growth should be presented and discussed with the patient and/or family soon after diagnosis to allow early initiation, if desired, of GH therapy. Although linear growth can be improved with GH, there should be an understanding of treatment costs, long-term safety uncertainties, and the lack of demonstrable positive correlates between improved adult height and psychosocial outcome (121).

About 20% of girls with Turner syndrome will have spontaneous pubertal development of varying degrees, whereas the remaining 80% show no puberty and will require estrogen replacement. For example, in 704 girls followed from 1986–1997 in one study, 10% had spontaneous puberty, and 13% had spontaneous pubertal advancement after the addition of low-dose secondary estrogen. The remaining 77% of girls had no pubertal signs at a mean age 15.0 ± 1.9 years and required pubertal inducement with estrogen treatment (121). The beginning of estrogen therapy should be individualized, but therapy may be started with low-dose oral premarin at 0.3 mg/day between the ages of 13 and 14 years or with small doses of transdermal estradiol (0.0125 mg/day); earlier initiation of oral conjugated estrogen, particularly before age 12 years, may compromise adult height (119). The addition of very-low-dose parenteral estradiol (depot estradiol at an initial dose of 0.2 mg/month intramuscularly) to GH therapy in girls as young as 12.0–12.9 years has been advocated recently as improving growth, allowing relatively age-appropriate feminization, and having no negative effects on GH therapy or height outcomes (122). Finally, the majority of adults with Turner syndrome will need continued long-term estrogen-replacement treatment to maintain feminization and prevent osteoporosis.

Other Endocrine Disorders in Turner Syndrome
Autoimmune thyroid dysfunction occurs commonly in girls with Turner syndrome. In one review, hypothyroidism was found in 24% of girls with Turner syndrome and hyperthyroidism in 2.5%. Elevated levels of thyroid autoantibodies were found in 42% of these girls and were predictive of the development of thyroid dysfunction (123). Autoimmune hypothyroidism is also common in adults with Turner syndrome with an annual incidence of 3.2% (124). Thus children and adults should have periodic screening for thyroid autoantibodies and thyroid function tests.

Impaired glucose tolerance may occur in Turner syndrome. Although type 1 diabetes has been reported in some girls with Turner syndrome, carbohydrate intolerance, when present, usually is seen more in conjunction with insulin resistance (i.e., elevated plasma glucose, insulin, C-peptide, and proinsulin response during an oral glucose tolerance test [OGTT]) (125). Since impaired glucose tolerance does not correlate with obesity, it has been suggested that haploinsufficiency for X chromosome gene(s) may directly impair β-cell function and predispose to diabetes mellitus in Turner syndrome (126). Fortunately, GH therapy of children with Turner syndrome has no adverse effect on glucose levels. Higher levels of serum insulin are found while receiving GH, indicating relative insulin resistance. However, insulin values decrease to baseline levels once GH treatment is discontinued (127).

Noonan Syndrome

Presentation, Diagnosis, and Genetics
Noonan syndrome (NS) is a cardiofacial syndrome characterized by short stature, facial dysmorphia (including hypertelorism and down-slanted eyes, low-set and posteriorly rotated ears, high arched palate, and small jaw), cardiovascular anomalies in about two-thirds of patients (e.g., valvular pulmonic stenosis, atrial septal defects, and hypertrophic cardiomyopathy), webbed neck, chest deformities (e.g., pectus carinatum/pectus excavatum and broad barrel- or square-shaped chest), and cryptorchidism (Figures 30-12A to 30-12E). NS individuals may have mild mental retardation, but average to even superior intelligence also occurs. A bleeding diathesis is found in about 20% of patients.

NS occurs with an estimated incidence of 1 in 1000–2500 live births and often appears to be sporadic, although autosomal dominant inheritance has been documented in many families. Clinical presentation can be extremely variable. Although the NS population is genetically heterogeneous, about 40% to 50% of NS patients are now known to have gain-of-function mutations of the PTPN11 (protein tyrosine phosphatase, nonreceptor type 11) gene located on the long arm of chromosome 12 (128). Both deletion and missense mutations of PTPN11 have been described. The PTPN11 gene encodes the protein tyrosine phosphatase SHP-2 and can interfere with multiple hormonal signaling pathways, including those for GH and IGF-1 (129,130). However, the exact contributions of the PTPN11 mutation genotype to the NS phenotype are unclear. For example, one review found no differences in growth patterns or birth lengths between PTPN11 mutation–positive and PTPN11 mutation–negative patients (131). Conversely and in the same group of patients, both hematological and cardiovascular abnormalities did vary depending on the mutation status. Bleeding diathesis and juvenile myelomonocytic leukemia were found only in PTPN11 mutation–positive patients. Pulmonary valve stenosis and atrial septal defects were more frequent in mutation-positive patients, whereas hypertrophic cardiomyopathy was present only in mutation-negative patients (131).

Short Stature and GH Treatment in NS
Short stature and slow growth are prominent features of NS. Size is usually said to be normal at birth (132), although one recent review noted a smaller mean birth length of −1.2 SD in some NS patients (129). During childhood, the mean height of both males and females typically progresses along the 3rd centile. Pubertal onset is delayed an average of about 2 years, and final mean adult height is 162.5 cm for males and 152.7 cm for females (132). GH has been used in attempts to improve growth and adult height in NS with variable results. Auxological measurements

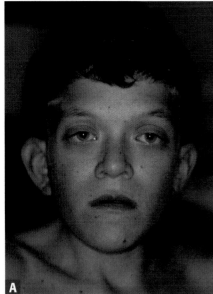
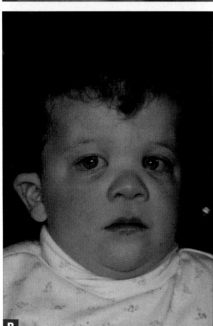
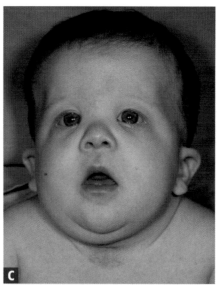
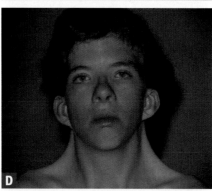
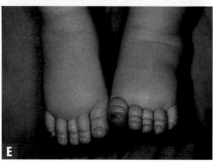

FIGURE 30-12 A to **E.** Children and adolescents with Noonan Syndrome. Note the low set posterior rotated ears and thick helices, low nasal bridge with wide based nose and bulbous tip, epicanthal folds, downslanting palpebral fissures, hypertelorism, webbing of the neck. Photos courtesy of Robert Gorlin, D.D.S, M.S., D.Sc.

status is important in interpreting response to GH treatment in NS because it is now known that PTPN11 mutation–positive NS patients do not respond as well to GH treatment, having both lesser IGF-1 levels and poorer growth following GH treatment (47 μg/kg/day) than do PTPN11 mutation–negative NS patients (130).

There have been no reports of negative effects of GH administration in NS. Specifically, GH treatment does not have clinically significant adverse effects on left ventricular size in children with NS (136). NS was added to the list of FDA-approved indications for GH treatment in 2007.

Silver Russell Syndrome

Presentation, Diagnosis, and Genetics The major clinical features of Silver Russell (SR) syndrome are low birth weight (secondary to prenatal or intrauterine growth retardation), short stature (secondary to postnatal growth retardation), and a characteristic small, triangular face. SR syndrome is accompanied frequently by other dysmorphic features, including relative macrocephaly, fifth-finger clinodactyly, skeletal asymmetry, and genital anomalies (e.g., hypospadias and inguinal hernia in affected males) (137) (Figures 30-13A to 30-13G). SR syndrome is a clinically and genetically heterogeneous congenital disorder, the diagnosis of which depends on clinical criteria. The presence of the three major characteristics (i.e., low birth weight, short stature, and triangular facies) plus one or more of the minor characteristics (i.e., relative macrocephaly, fifth-finger clinodactyly, skeletal asymmetry, hypospadias, or inguinal hernia) is usually required for a diagnosis. However, the major criteria may not be present in all patients, and diagnosis thus can be somewhat subjective (137).

Mutations involving chromosomes 7, 8, 15, 17, and 18 all have been associated with either SR syndrome or phenotypically similar patients. However, if the strictest clinical criteria are used for the diagnosis of SR syndrome, anomalies of chromosomes 7 (7p and 7q regions) and 17 (17q23.3-q25 and 17q24.1) become the most likely candidates (137,138). Maternal uniparental disomy for chromosome 7 (mUPD(7)) has been found in about 10% of SR syndrome patients (138).

Short Stature and GH Treatment in SR Syndrome In a review of 386 patients (163 girls and 223 boys) with SR syndrome, the mean (±SD) birth weight for full-term infants was 1940 ± 353 g in boys and 1897 ± 325 g in girls; mean birth length was 43.1 ± 3.7 cm (both males and females). There was poor growth and loss of height centiles during the first 3 years of life, with growth thereafter

should be performed before, at initiation of, and at least every 6 months during GH therapy to evaluate the effectiveness of therapy. Thus there is no standard GH dosage for the treatment of short stature and NS, and different researchers have chosen varying doses. Initially, GH treatment (0.15 U/kg/day given by daily injection) increases height velocity and height standard deviations in NS, comparable with the increases seen in GH treatment of Turner syndrome (133). More prolonged GH treatment (33 or 66 μg/kg/day) can improve final height outcomes in some NS patients, one study reporting a mean gain of 1.7 SD and final mean heights close to

midparental heights (134). Others report much more modest gains in height, such as changes in mean height standard deviations scores from −2.9 pretreatment to −2.6 after 1 year and −2.3 after 5 years of GH therapy and a mean incremental final height increase of only 3.1 cm (range −1.1 to 6.5 cm) (135). Only one patient in this study achieved a final adult height after GH treatment that was greater than the mean height for untreated NS patients (135); however, this result should be interpreted with caution given the small number of patients (n = 10) who achieved final adult height and the uncertain PTPN11 mutation status of this group. Knowledge of genetic

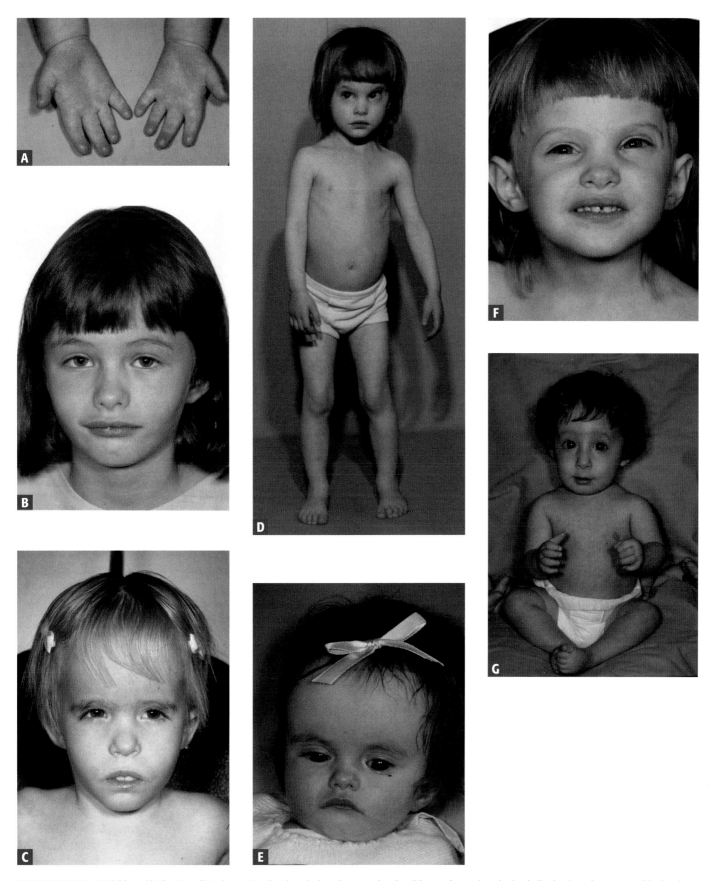

FIGURE 30-13 A to **G.** Children with Silver Russell Syndrome. Note the triangular face, downturned angles of the mouth, prominent forehead, clinodactaly, and asymmetry of the face, legs and hands. Photos courtesy of Robert Gorlin, D.D.S, M.S., D.Sc., and Susan Berry, M.D., University of Minnesota Medical School.

(ages 4–10 years) generally paralleling the 3rd centile. Pubertal growth was reduced, and mean final adult height was 151.2 ± 7.8 cm in males and 139.9 ± 9.0 cm in females (139).

Children with IUGR and/or born SGA may have poor growth throughout childhood and short stature as adults. Although these children usually are not GH-deficient, GH treatment (in doses ranging from 14 IU/m²/week to 0.3 mg/kg/week) has been shown to improve growth velocity and height SD scores significantly in children with SR syndrome, SGA, and unclassified IUGR (140–142). Furthermore, GH treatment of short children born SGA (33 μg/kg or 0.1 U/kg daily) can improve final height above the pretreatment predicted height, allowing many SGA individuals to achieve target heights (143). Early pubertal development or spontaneous acceleration of bone maturation with subsequent decreased height standard deviations may be seen in some children with SR syndrome, IUGR, or SGA and potentially could limit the effects of GH therapy on height. Whether or not attempts to slow skeletal maturation or delay puberty would be beneficial on final height is unknown because there are no published studies on the use of GnRH agonists or aromatase inhibitors in these specific populations. See "Growth Failure Due to Possible Defects in the GH–IGF-1 Axis" above for further discussion of SGA and GH treatment of SGA.

Prader–Willi Syndrome (PWS)

PWS Presentation, Diagnosis, and Genetics PWS is a genetic disorder characterized by short stature, infantile hypotonia, hypogonadism, learning disabilities, behavioral abnormalities, dysmorphic features, excessive appetite, and progressive obesity (144) (see Figure 30-14A to 30-14H). Presentation of PWS varies by age. Infants present most frequently with hypotonia, cryptorchidism, low birth weight, failure to thrive, and a poor suck reflex. Growth retardation, developmental delay, excessive appetite, small hands and feet, obesity, and behavioral problems become increasingly prominent in older children and adolescents. Adolescents also have delayed sexual development.

The characteristic behavioral phenotype of PWS includes hyperphagia and intense preoccupation with food. Moderate to severe obsessive–compulsive symptoms are seen in up to 60% of PWS patients, and over 50% of patients in one study met clinical criteria for obsessive–compulsive disorder (OCD) (145). Learning disabilities, including dyslexia and difficulties with mathematics and writing, may be profound and greater than would be expected on the basis of IQ. Average full-scale

IQ in a group of 18 PWS children was 73.7 ± 8.9 (1 SD below normal), whereas performance on various cognitive and visuospatial tasks ranged from 2.1–7.0 SD below the expected means (146).

PWS patients often suffer from a variety of sleep- and ventilation-related disturbances, including excessive daytime sleepiness, obstructive sleep apnea, sleep-related alveolar hypoventilation, and abnormal central (hypothalamic) ventilatory responses to hypoxia and hypercapnia (147). Respiratory muscle insufficiency, pharyngeal narrowness, and obesity all contribute to frequent and severe respiratory difficulties among PWS children (148). Other long-term multisytem complications of PWS include osteoporosis, type 2 diabetes, and cardiorespiratory failure (149). Sudden, unexpected death can occur in PWS (148).

PWS has an estimated incidence of 1 in 10,000–16,000 live births, suggesting that about 60 of every 1 million people are affected (144). Fluorescence in situ hybridization (FISH) and methylation studies have made it possible to confirm a diagnosis of PWS genetically in a majority of cases; the syndrome is due to a sporadic deletion of chromosomal material in the region 15q11-q13. In PWS, the deletion is always found on the paternally donated chromosome 15. About 5% of PWS patients have abnormalities of gene expression, rather than deletion, in the 15q11-q13 region of the paternally donated chromosome. More rarely, PWS also can result from maternal uniparental disomy (UPD) of the same region, a situation in which the affected individual inherits two maternal copies of the affected region with no paternal contribution (145). Genetic material on chromosome 15 may affect various GABAnergic, serotonergic, or other neurotransmitters or receptors responsible for feeding regulation, and thus alterations in this chromosomal region could provide a genetic basis for PWS phenotypical behavior (150).

Growth and GH Treatment in PWS From birth until about 2 years of age, weights of both boys and girls with PWS are below average. From about 2–4 years of age and older, PWS children develop the prominent features of PWS with progressive weight gain, poor linear growth, and short stature. The mean height of PWS children by the time of adolescence is −2 SD and decreases below −2 SD thereafter, presumably due to lack of the pubertal growth spurt. In one review, mean spontaneous final adult height in PWS was 141.2 ± 4.8 cm for females and 147.7 ± 7.7 cm for males, or about 15.8 cm (for females) and 21.9 cm (for males) below the mean height of unaffected adults (151).

Certain clinical features of PWS resemble those seen in many patients with GH deficiency. These GH deficiency–like symptoms include poor linear growth despite increasing obesity, decreased lean body mass, decreased IGF-1 and insulin levels, and a positive growth response to GH treatment (149). In addition, many PWS patients have decreased GH secretory capacity and hypogonadotropic hypogonadism, further suggesting hypothalamic–pituitary dysfunction (144).

PWS children treated with GH (1 mg/m²/day) have accelerated linear growth, decreased percentage of body fat, and increased fat oxidation (152). Respiratory muscle tone can improve (152) or may, more rarely, worsen with GH treatment (153). GH therapy improves overall muscle tone, physical strength, and agility, although some positive effects of GH in PWS may wane over time (149). Carbohydrate metabolism is not adversely affected by up to 3 years of GH therapy (8 mg/m²/week or 0.037 mg/kg/day) in PWS (154), and longer-term GH therapy (0.5 IU/kg/week for up to 5 years) can improve final adult height (155). Auxological measurements should be performed before, at initiation of, and at least every 6 months during GH therapy. Polysomnographic studies have been recommended before and during administration of GH, although the frequency of such monitoring has not been established (see below).

Sex steroid replacement will be needed in adolescent or older patients with PWS and hypogonadism. PWS patients with bone ages greater than 12 years may be started on low-dose testosterone (50 mg intramuscularly montly) in males and low-dose oral estrogens (0.3 mg premarin daily) in females.

Following the advent of GH therapy for PWS, there have been worldwide reports of sudden death in multiple PWS patients receiving GH (148), raising concerns of a possible causal relationship between GH administration and PWS sudden death. To date, there have been at least 17 PWS patients worldwide who have died suddenly while being treated with GH. Of these, 13 have been described by Eiholzer (148). An additional 2 patients were reported previously from the Genentech National Cooperative Growth Study database, and 2 additional patients were included in a recent abstract (the third patient in this abstract was already included in the Eiholzer report) (156). While the exact cause of sudden death is unknown, apnea due to respiratory compromise probably is a major contributing factor. Another possible explanation is that GH therapy increases basal metabolic rate and oxygen consumption, leading to increased ventilatory demands in patients who already have a compromised

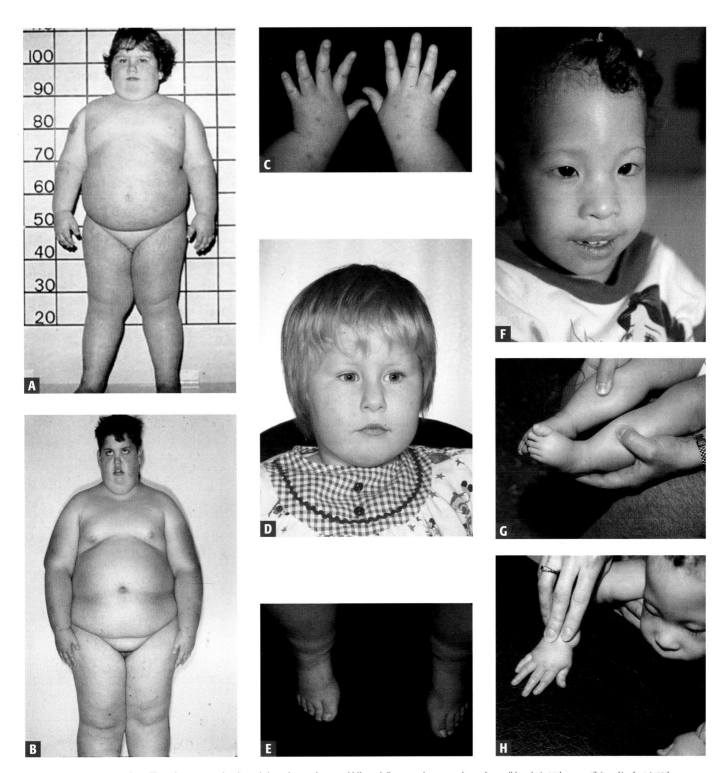

FIGURE 30-14 A to **H.** Prader Willi Syndrome. Note the almond shaped eyes, decreased bifrontal diameter, downturned mouth, small hands (<25th percentile) and/or feet (<10th percentile) for height age. Photos B–H courtesy of Robert Gorlin, D.D.S, M.S., D.Sc., and Susan Berry, M.D., University of Minnesota Medical School.

respiratory status. Possibly supporting this theory, there has been at least one documented case of respiratory deterioration on GH therapy that improved after GH therapy was stopped (153). Worsening apnea and/or hypoxia in other GH-treated PWS patients have been associated with upper respiratory infections, tonsillar hypertrophy, and elevated IGF-1 levels (157). However, deaths in PWS children have been reported among both GH-treated and GH-untreated patients (148), and the relationship, if any, of GH therapy to PWS sudden death is unclear. Nonetheless, in 2003, a voluntary label change was made to the package insert of GH intended for the long-term treatment of PWS, the insert now stating that GH therapy is contraindicated in PWS patients with severe obesity or severe respiratory impairment. The GH manufacturer suggests evaluation and monitoring of sleep apnea, weight control, and aggressive treatment of respiratory infections in PWS patients.

A recent prospective study examined the acute respiratory effects of GH therapy in 25 PWS patients. All patients (children and adults) had abnormal baseline polysomnographic studies prior to GH treatment. After 6 weeks of GH therapy, 19 (76%) patients actually had improvement, whereas 6 (24%) had worsening of their apnea/hypoxia index. The authors recommended that polysomnographic studies should be performed on all PWS children prior to initiation of GH therapy and 6 weeks thereafter, that an otorhinolaryngolical evaluation be obtained if sleep apnea or snoring occurred, and that IGF-1 levels be maintained near normal (157). Whether or not these recommendations will have an impact on the incidence of sudden death in PWS remains to be determined. It also should be noted that at least one death has been reported in a PWS patient after more prolonged (7 months) GH therapy who had never had respiratory difficulties (156).

Skeletal Dysplasias

Presentation, Diagnosis, and Genetics The skeletal dysplasias are a heterogeneous group of genetic skeletal malformation syndromes characterized by abnormal endochondral but normal periosteal ossification. The skeletal dysplasias can be classified on the basis of clinical presentation, radiographic features, and molecular pathogenesis and may be broadly divided into three related groups: achondroplasia, hypochondroplasia, and thanatophoric dysplasia (158).

Achondroplasia is the most common inherited cause of disproportionate (i.e., short-limbed) short stature. Affected patients have short trunk and limbs, bowing of the legs, kyphosis, a decreased anteroposterior chest diameter, and maxillar hypoplasia. In contrast to the relatively small jaw, head circumference usually is greater than the 97th percentile, and frontal bossing may be prominent. Neurological complications are frequent in achondroplasia and include hydrocephalus, subdural hematomas, spinal stenosis (secondary to abnormal vertebral endochondral ossification), and nerve root compression in the foramen magnum (secondary to periosteal overgrowth with foraminal obstruction). Cervical medullary compression can present with pain, ataxia, incontinence, apnea, or progressive quadriparesis. Both shunting for hydrocephalus and decompression of the small foramen magnum may be required (159). Other frequent complications include restrictive and obstructive lung disease and otitis media. Achondroplasia may be diagnosed prenatally with ultrasound in the third and sometimes the second trimesters (158), as well as via prenatal genetic testing.

Hypochondroplasia is a relatively common, milder form of skeletal dysplasia, and clinical manifestations can vary within and between families. Hypochondroplasia usually

lacks the neurological complications seen in achondroplasia, and accurate prenatal ultrasonographic diagnosis is rare (158). Thanatophoric dysplasia is the most severe and lethal dysplasia and is characterized by distinct features (i.e., short tubular bones and short ribs with platyspondyly) that allow accurate prenatal ultrasonographic diagnosis (158).

Achondroplasia occurs in between 1 in 15,000 and 1 in 40,000 live births (160). Most cases (>90%) are sporadic, and there is usually an increased paternal age at the time of conception (160). At least 97% of achondroplasia cases are due to a Gly380Arg mutation in the transmembrane domain of the fibroblast growth factor receptor 3 (FGFR3) gene (160). Mutations in the FGFR3 gene on chromosome 4p result not only in achondroplasia but also in hypochondroplasia, thanatophoric dysplasia, the recently described achondroplasia variant SADDAN (severe achondroplasia with developmental delay and acanthosis nigricans), and two craniosynostosis disorders (160).

Growth and GH Treatment in Skeletal Dysplasias Standard growth curves for achondroplasia are available and were constructed from height, growth velocity, upper and lower segment, and head circumference measurements in 400 patients with achondroplasia. Mean height for adult males with achondroplasia is just over 130 cm and for adult females is approximately 125 cm.

GH treatment (0.3 mg/kg/week divided into daily injections) has had only modest, if any, effects on growth in children with achondroplasia in some trials (161), whereas others report significant improvements (162,163). Height-velocity improvement in one limited study of 6 patients ranged from no effect to an increase of 1.1–2.6 cm/year compared with baseline after 12 months of GH therapy (0.1 IU/kg/day) (164). GH treatment (1 IU/kg/week) improved height velocity a mean of 3.7 cm/year after 1 year and 3.1 cm/year after 2 years in another group of 15 children (165). Achondroplasia children with the lowest pre–GH treatment growth velocities had better responses to GH therapy in these smaller groups (161,165). Emphasizing the variable response of achondroplasia to GH treatment, other studies with larger numbers of children ($n = 35$, GH dose of median 30 U/m^2/week [range 15.8–40 U/m^2/week], and $n = 145$, GH dose of either 0.5 or 1.0 IU/kg/ week) demonstrated significant improvements in height velocity and height SD scores with up to 6 years of GH therapy (162,163). Younger age at onset of GH therapy and higher GH doses (1.0 IU/kg/week versus 0.5 IU/kg/week) produced better growth responses in these later groups. Auxological measurements

should be performed before, at initiation of, and at least every 6 months during GH therapy.

Perhaps not surprisingly, children with relatively milder hypochondroplasia respond better to GH than do those with achondroplasia. In a direct comparison of GH effects on hypochondroplasia versus achondroplasia, 3 years of GH therapy improved mean height SD in hypochondroplasia from 1.2 SD to 2.6 SD but only from −0.2 SD to 0.1 SD in achondroplasia (166). This differential response to GH may be due in part to the greater quantitative decrease in endochondral ossification that occurs in achondroplasia than in hypochondroplasia (158).

Few adverse effects have been seen with GH treatment in the majority of these clinical trails. GH at a dose of 0.1 IU/kg/day does not, for example, seem to adversely stimulate periosteal bone growth at the foramen magnum (164). However, prolonged GH therapy (median dose of 30 U/m^2/week [range 15.8–40 U/m^2/week] or 0.06 mg/kg/day [range 0.04–0.08 mg/kg/day]) can accelerate spinal growth to a greater extent than long bone growth, actually accentuating the disproportionate short stature in some achondroplasic children (163). Other long-term effects and final adult outcomes of GH therapy in skeletal dysplasia remain to be determined, and GH use in these conditions must be considered investigational.

CHRONIC ILLNESS AS ETIOLOGY OF GROWTH FAILURE

Chronic disease can affect physical growth and the timing of puberty as well as psychosocial development. Growth failure may be the initial presentation of an undiagnosed chronic disease or may develop slowly secondary to disease progress or treatment. The prevalence of childhood chronic disease as well as disease-associated growth failure is difficult to ascertain. However, school-based self-administered surveys suggest that about 10% of adolescents suffer from some type of chronic illness (167). Growth retardation in these children and adolescents has multiple mechanisms that may include side effects of treatment (particularly chemotherapy, radiation therapy, or glucocorticoids), inadequate nutrition (either from poor intake or excessive demands and overconsumption of available energy substrates), inefficient management of body components (increased proteolysis), and alterations in the GH–IGF-1 system.

Prolonged use of glucocorticoids is especially common and problematic in children with chronic diseases. Long-term exposure to pharmacological glucocorticoids is associated with a variety of negative effects: insulin resistance (resulting in excessive weight gain or impaired glucose tolerance); generalized antianabolic and catabolic activity on protein, cartilage, and bone (poor wound healing, poor linear growth, and osteoporosis); and decreased GH release and action (suppressed linear growth) (168,169). In fact, glucocorticoids have so many profound antagonistic effects on the GH–IGF-1 axis at the hypothalamic, pituitary, and target-organ levels that a state of "functional" GH deficiency can be said to exist in many children receiving chronic pharmacological glucocorticoids (169). This later observation, plus experimental data demonstrating that exogenous GH can counteract some of the negative effects of glucocorticoids, has led to studies of GH use in children receiving chronic prednisone therapy for cystic fibrosis, chronic renal failure, juvenile rheumatoid arthritis, and inflammatory bowel disease. Preliminary data indicate that exogenous GH can improve lean body mass, increase linear growth, and increase bone calcium accretion (169), but longer-term studies are needed to better define the safety and efficacy of GH therapy in children with chronic diseases.

Iatrogenic growth retardation should be suspected in any child with linear growth failure receiving prolonged steroid therapy. The adverse growth effects of glucocorticoids may be minimized by using the lowest possible effective dose and alternate-day therapy and normalizing calcium balance (170). In addition, the use of nasal and inhaled glucocorticoids, when applicable, generally will produce fewer systemic effects at recommended doses, but adrenal suppression and short-term growth suppression also can occur with these glucocorticoid preparations.

One particular chronic disease that has been treated with GH is chronic renal insufficiency. In chronic kidney disease, there is a progressive decline in glomerular filtration that requires hemodialysis or peritoneal dialysis and then eventually renal transplantation. Growth failure is a frequent result of this process. In 1993, the FDA authorized the use of GH to treat children who had growth failure as a result of chronic kidney disease but who had not yet had a renal transplant. The usual dose is 0.35 mg/kg/week (divided into daily doses), a dose that is just a bit higher than replacement doses for GH deficiency. It is clear that GH replacement therapy significantly improves growth outcomes in children with GH deficiency, particularly when treatment is begun early and adequate doses are administered. At the time that the FDA approved this indication, it was assumed that once the patient received a renal transplant, he or she would no longer need GH therapy. As it

turns out, there is also an issue of growth failure related in part to the medications that are necessary to preserve the function of the transplanted kidney. There were early reports that GH may hasten rejection of the transplanted kidney, but these observations have not been borne out by subsequent studies. At present, there is no FDA approval to treat after transplantation, and it is still not clear whether this should be undertaken. However, it appears that GH may be helpful for the transplant patient in terms of reaching a normal adult height.

ENDOCRINE ETIOLOGIES OF GROWTH FAILURE (OTHER THAN GH)

Other endocrinopathies, besides GH deficiency, can adversely affect growth. Deficiencies of thyroid hormone or gonadotropins and androgens/estrogens can cause decreased linear growth and delayed puberty. Conversely, excess exposure to glucocorticoids, either from increased endogenous production or from prolonged exogenous administration, also can cause growth failure. Lastly, early puberty or excess androgen production or exposure can result in rapid growth during childhood but with accompanying bone age advancement, which, if untreated, results in early epiphyseal closure and adult short stature. This section will focus primarily on the linear growth failure associated with the following conditions.

Multiple Pituitary Hormone Deficiency (MPHD)

Etiology Children or adolescents with GH deficiency may have either isolated (i.e., idiopathic) GH deficiency (IGHD) or a combination of GH plus other pituitary hormone deficiencies. Patients with multiple pituitary hormone deficiency (MPHD) often have associated congenital or acquired CNS anomalies (36). Such patients with CNS structural anomalies or lesions often are said to have *organic GH deficiency* (OGHD). MPHD also may occur in association with chromosomal mutations (171). CNS malformations, trauma, and tumors are relatively uncommon causes of GH deficiency in the pediatric population, comprising only about 14% of all GH-reated patients in one large national database (53).

Clinical Presentation Children with MPHD may present in one of several ways: 1) MPHD may be discovered during the initial evaluation of short stature (e.g., a child with growth failure may be found to have both GH and ACTH or both GH and TSH deficiencies at

presentation); 2) MPHD may develop in a patient being treated with GH for "isolated" GH deficiency; in one review, hypothyroidism became evident during the course of GH treatment in as many as 50% of GH-deficient patients with organic but not idiopathic GH deficiency (172). Hypothyroidism in these OGHD patients was felt to be due to either the effects of GH administration on thyroid hormone metabolism and/or the "unmasking" of previously hidden, i.e., subclinical, hypothyroidism; 3) MPHD may be suspected or diagnosed in a neonate or infant with hypoglycemia, congenital nystagmus, or other midline structural anomalies such as microphallus; and, 4) patients with known histories of CNS trauma, CNS tumor, or craniospinal radiation therapy are at risk for MPHD. Finally, the presence of CNS structural anomalies involving the pituitary–hypothalamic region on an MRI study should alert the pediatric endocrinologist to investigate for MPHD regardless of the presenting symptoms (36).

Diagnostic Evaluation In general, the diagnostic evaluation of suspected MPHD is identical to that used when investigating possible GH deficiency, as described under "Evaluation of Short Stature" above. Indeed, the diagnosis of isolated or idiopathic GH deficiency is one of exclusion and is made only after all other pituitary hormones are shown to be intact. During the biochemical evaluation of short stature, all hormones that potentially affect growth are tested, either at initial presentation or during subsequent stimulation testing. During the initial screening process, free T_4 and TSH values are obtained to rule out hypothyroidism; LH, FSH, and testosterone/estrogen values are checked in adolescent patients with short stature and delayed puberty. Random ACTH and cortisol levels are obtained if there is a history suggesting adrenal insufficiency, such as weight loss, fatigue, or frequent infectious illnesses, followed by a low dose ACTH stimulation test if random levels are equivocal. Electrolytes, glucose, serum osmolarity, urine osmolarity, and urine specific gravity all are determined if a history of polyuria, polydipsia, excessive thirst, or excessive drinking is elicited to rule out diabetes. If insulin-induced hypoglycemia is used as part of the GH stimulation process, the HPA axis is tested by obtaining cortisol levels prior to and during induced hypoglycemia. When the HPA is intact, serum cortisol levels should increase two- to threefold during hypoglycemia. If insulin-induced hypoglycemia is not used, or if serum cortisol response to hypoglycemia is equivocal, a low-dose

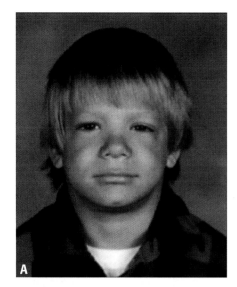

A

ACTH stimulation test may be used to evaluate adrenal function. One microgram of ACTH is given as an IV push; again, an adequate HPA is demonstrated by a rise in cortisol levels two- to three-fold above baseline.

Treatment/Management Management of children with MPHD is complex and requires a continual balancing of hormonal replacement to achieve optimal growth. Treatment must be individualized, with replacement of deficient hormone(s). In addition to GH replacement, adolescents with gonadotropin deficiency will need sex steroid replacement for pubertal growth and development. Serum T_4 must be maintained within normal limits in hypothyroidism; and the smallest dose of hydrocortisone (8–10 mg/m^2/day divided into three doses) should be used to avoid glucocorticoid growth suppression when treating ACTH/cortisol insufficiency. Poor growth in a GH-deficient child who is already receiving adequate GH treatment and has normal IGF-1 levels may indicate developing hypothyroidism that requires investigation and treatment (172). In patients with multiple defects at initial diagnosis, the usual sequence of replacement therapy is to first treat ACTH/cortisol deficiency to avoid adrenal crisis, then levothyroxine therapy to normalize serum T_4, and lastly GH replacement. Finally, adults with a history of pediatric-onset MPHD will require lifelong hormone replacement.

Hypothyroidism and Growth Failure

Newborns with congenital hypothyroidism (CH) typically are within population norms for birth length and weight. Short stature and growth failure usually are not presenting symptoms in CH, although CH certainly can

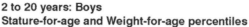

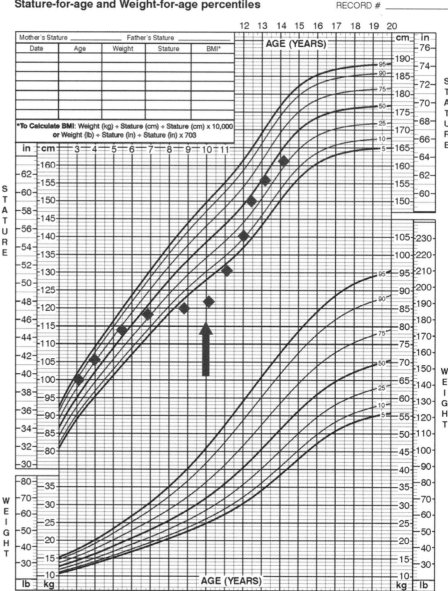

B

FIGURE 30-15 A and **B.** A child with hypothyroidism. (A) This child presented because of short stature. (B) The arrow on the growth chart represents the time of diagnosis and treatment.

result in growth failure if undiagnosed and untreated (see Figure 30-15A to 30-15B). Conversely, linear growth and pubertal tempo generally are normal in properly treated CH, and target heights, day of start of treatment, and compliance with therapy are the main prognostic factors for adult height in children with CH (173).

Growth failure occurs in untreated, acquired hypothyroidism but can be expected to improve once L-thyroxine therapy is instituted. However, severe height deficits secondary to prolonged untreated hypothyroidism can persist despite proper L-thyroxine replacement therapy.

Cushing/Glucocorticoid Excess

Etiology Hypercortisolism results from either increased endogenous production of cortisol or excessive exogenous administration. Endogenous hypercortisolism can arise from an ACTH-producing pituitary adenoma (Cushing disease) or a cortisol-producing adrenal tumor (Cushing syndrome). Both Cushing disease and Cushing syndrome are rare in infants and children but may be seen with a somewhat increased frequency in adolescents. By far the more common cause of hypercortisolism in the pediatric population is prolonged exposure to supraphysiologic (i.e., pharmacological) doses of exogenous glucocorticoids (see Chapter 28).

To understand which patients are at risk for this iatrogenic hypercortisolism, an appreciation of normal physiological production and replacement therapy is required. Cortisol production rates in humans had been estimated via radiotracer methodology to be about 12–15 mg/m²/day. Recent studies have questioned the validity of this value, and newer techniques, such as high-pressure liquid chromatography–mass spectrometry, have shown that physiological cortisol production is actually lower. Daily cortisol production in healthy children and adolescents in one study was found to be 6.8 ± 1.9 mg/m²/day (mean ± SD) with no variation for gender or pubertal stage (174). Similar cortisol production rates were demonstrated in early (Tanner I–II) pubertal males of about 16.8 ± 1.3 μmol/m²/day (6.1 ± 0.4 mg/m²/day) and for Tanner IV–V males of 14.8 ± 1.4 μmol/m²/day (5.3 ± 0.5 mg/m²/day) (175). Cortisol production is higher in the mornings and also correlates with body size, being greater in obese than in nonobese patients.

When glucocorticoids are used in replacement therapy, such as for adrenal insufficiency, congenital adrenal hyperplasia, or hypopituitarism, the treatment goal is to mimic physiological production. Hydrocortisone (cortisol) is the preferred drug in infants and children; more potent compounds such as prednisone are not recommended due to difficulty titrating dose in rapidly growing children and the potential for greater growth suppression. Bioavailability of hydrocortisone varies by route of administration, preparation, diet, and gastric motility and acidity. Daily intramuscular or intravenous doses of hydrocortisone, when given for replacement therapy, should approximate the daily physiological secretion rates, whereas oral doses should be double because only about one-half of oral hydrocortisone is absorbed (176). Pediatric patients receiving carefully monitored and adjusted physiological replacement doses of exogenous glucocorticoids should not be at risk for hypercortisolism. Conversely, chronic administration of glucocorticoid doses in excess of physiological production rates places patients at risk for iatrogenic hypercortisolism.

Glucocorticoid Excess and Growth Failure

Short stature and increased body weight (particularly centripetal obesity) are typical complaints in endogenous or exogenous glucocorticoid excess during childhood (177,178). Other common presenting signs include hirsutism (53%), striae (53%), and hypertension (47%) (177). A major clinical difference between the adult and pediatric forms of Cushing disease, regardless of the etiology, is that growth failure is often a predominant feature of pediatric hypercortisolism. However, short stature may not always be an initial complaint; one review noted that growth failure was a presenting feature in just slightly over two-thirds (71%) of pediatric patients with Cushing disease (177). Accumulation of dorsocervical fat, or a "buffalo hump," is not pathognomonic for hypercortisolism and is instead found in many conditions associated with hyperinsulinemia, including obesity and human immunodeficiency virus (HIV)–associated lipodystrophy, as well as Cushing disease (179). Successful treatment of Cushing disease may require both transsphenoidal adenomectomy and pituitary radiotherapy. Long-term clinical and biochemical remission can result, but GH therapy with or without GnRH analogue may be required to achieve final adult heights within expected ranges (180–182). Body mass index (BMI) also improves following successful treatment, but in some patients, BMI remains greater than population norms (182).

Exogenous Hypercortisolism Symptom severity tends to vary as a function of dose and duration of pharmacological steroid use. However sensitivity to the effects of exogenous glucocorticoids varies among individuals (183), and it is worth remembering that growth suppression and weight gain may be seen with chronic administration of all forms of glucocorticoids, including nasal, inhaled, ocular (184,185), and topical preparations. Management of iatrogenic hypercortisolism is difficult because the adverse effects of therapy must be balanced against the therapeutic needs of the patient. Growth suppression and weight gain may be lessened by using the lowest possible effective dose and alternate-day therapy. See also "Chronic Illness as Etiology of Growth Failure" above for a further discussion of the effects and management of chronic glucocorticoid administration.

Androgen Excess and Growth Failure

At puberty, gonadal steroids are secreted that result in a growth spurt but, ultimately, in closure of the epiphyses. The steroid most important for epiphyseal closure appears to be estrogen, which was verified by the discovery of an estrogen-resistant man who had a homozygous mutation in his estrogen receptor (186). This individual was quite tall and had not fused his epiphyses at age 27, although he had experienced all the androgen aspects of puberty. In males, androgen is converted to estrogen by the action of the enzyme aroma-tase. Androgen excess in the pediatric population that can potentially cause growth failure is seen most commonly in either undiagnosed or untreated 1) inborn errors of adrenal biosynthesis, that is, congenital adrenal hyperplasia (CAH), or 2) disorders in the timing of pubertal onset, that is, gonadotropin-dependent central precocious puberty (CPP). Rarer causes of androgen excess are gonadotropin-independent precocious puberty, β-human chorionic gonadotropin (β-hCG)–secreting germ cell tumors, virilizing tumors, and ingestion of or exposure to anabolic steroids. In all these conditions, excess androgen production or exposure during infancy or childhood initially causes increased, rather than decreased, linear growth. However, this rapid growth is accompanied by bone age advancement that, if untreated, results in early epiphyseal closure and, ultimately, short adult stature. Management options to prevent growth failure are aimed at suppressing or removing the source of excess androgens and vary depending on the etiology. Abnormalities of androgen biosynthesis, such as premature adrenarche and polycystic ovarian syndrome, usually are milder or occur in adolescence (or later) and are not associated with growth failure.

Congenital Adrenal Hyperplasia

Treatment and Growth Outcomes Early diagnosis and treatment of CAH, good compliance and careful adjustment of glucocorticoid suppression therapy are important variables in achieving optimal height outcomes (187). Depending on the specific defect involved, mineralcorticoid replacement with 9α-fludrocortisone will be required to prevent salt wasting and assist in maintaining normal blood pressure, but the effects of mineralcorticoid replacement on growth are minimal. The mainstay of therapy for most forms of CAH and the therapeutic modality that will have the most effect on stature is glucocorticoid administration (see Chapter 27). Exogenous glucocorticoids are given for physiological cortisol replacement therapy (to prevent adrenal crises) and to suppress ACTH-driven excess production of adrenal steroid precursors and androgens. Inadequate cortisol therapy results in continued growth acceleration due to a lack of ACTH suppression. Conversely (and to be expected), excessive glucocorticoid administration results in growth suppression, weight gain, and other effects of hypercortisolism. See also "Cushing/Glucocorticoid Excess" and "Chronic Illness as Etiology of Growth Failure" above for further discussions on physiological replacement, as well as adverse effects of glucocorticoids.

There are variable reports of adult height outcomes in patients with CAH and glucocorticoid suppression therapy. In one meta-analysis of 18 studies, many patients were found to have adult height within 1 SD of target height with a mean adult height SD minus target height SD for 65 patients of −1.03 (187). Nonethess, final adult height may be compromised in some patients wth CAH, and one recent clinical trail found that GH plus a GnRH analogue added to glucocorticoid therapy could improve adult heights in patients with CAH (188).

Central Precocious Puberty

Treatment and Growth Outcomes The current treatment choice for central precocious puberty (CPP) is GnRH agonist therapy, and such treatment should be considered only after evaluating pubertal progression, bone age, and final height prognosis (189). Children with CPP can be grouped into two broad categories on the basis of rapidity of pubertal development: accelerated and slowly progressive (190). Treatment of CPP with GnRH agonists such as leuprolide or nafarelin is indicated in accelerated pubertal progression, that is, in children with continual, rapid increase in pubertal maturation and abnormal height potential. Such children have a significantly advanced bone age for chronological age and thus are at risk for early epiphyseal closure and adult short stature. GnRH agonist therapy usually is not indicated in the slowly progressive group, that is, in those with minimal to moderate puberty, slow advancement, and normal bone age. Age also may be a factor in patient selection because GnRH therapy has not been shown to have a significant effect on adult height in most girls who have had onset of puberty between 6 and 8 years of age (191). However, GnRH therapy must be individualized and also may be indicated in children with coexisting GH deficiency, CAH, hypothyroidism, or pyschosocial issues.

With careful patient selection and treatment, height prognosis in CPP generally is good. Patients with slowly progressive early puberty tend to have normal height outcomes without therapy. In children with accelerated pubertal progression, advanced bone maturity and poor predicted heights, GnRH agonist therapy suppresses gonadotropins, decreases height velocity, and slows bone maturation, resulting in significant improvement in final height compare with initial predicated adult height (190).

Type 1 Diabetes and Growth Failure

Insulin has an important role in the GH–IGF-1 axis, and insulin deficiency potentially can lead to growth disturbances. GH resistance

has been described in some type 1 diabetes. Two children with Mauriac syndrome, a rare combination of poorly controlled diabetes, profound growth retardation, and hepatomegaly, had normal hypothalamic–pituitary function, GHBP, IGF-1 generation, and IGFBPs but no response to GH therapy, suggesting impaired IGF-1 receptor function (192). A growth pattern has been described in some diabetic children consisting of taller stature at diabetes onset, followed by growth deceleration after diagnosis and subsequent "rebound" to normal adult heights (193).

While growth failure certainly can be seen in poorly controlled diabetes, it should be emphasized that most adolescents with type 1 diabetes have normal pubertal onset, normal sexual maturation, and final heights within the normal centiles (194) despite varying degrees of control or mean hemoglobin A1c values. A recent review of a large number of children with type 1 diabetes (7598 growth data points collected over 25 years in 587 subjects, 317 males and 270 females) confirmed this lack of correlation between diabetes control (hemoglobin A1c values) and height outcomes (193). Thus poor growth in the diabetic should not be blamed automatically on poor glucose metabolism. Any child with type 1 diabetes and growth failure deserves an investigation for other causes of growth decline, particularly autoimmune endocrinopathies such as hypothyroidism and adrenal insufficiency, that can occur in conjunction with type 1 diabetes. Celiac disease is also found in type 1 diabetes and should be screened for. Finally, GH deficiency also has been described in type 1 diabetes and should be considered in any child with diabetes and poor growth, particularly when accompanied by unexplained hypoglycemia.

TALL STATURE

Tall stature is defined as a height that is more than 2 SD above the mean for age. Some of the causes are normal variants of growth (e.g., familial or constitutional tall stature). Non-endocrine causes of tall stature include cerebral gigantism (Sotos syndrome), Klinefelter syndrome, XYY males, Marfan syndrome, and homocystinuria. There are several endocrine causes of excessive growth, such as excessive secretion of GH and hypogonadism. Also, precocious puberty can cause a growth spurt, although, if untreated, it usually results in early fusion of the epiphyses and short stature as an adult.

Familial Tall Stature

It is now unusual to encounter children whose parents are seeking treatment for tall

statue. In the few instances where this has occurred in our practice, it has been girls who have been concerned because they perceive that they will have excessive adult height.

Diagnosis In familial tall stature, calculation of the Tanner target height will show that the child is growing as would be expected considering parents heights. A determination of a bone age will estimate the predicted adult height.

Growth markers such as IGF-1 and IgFBP3, if tested, will be normal.

Treatment Girls who are tall and have not yet had epiphyseal fusion may be given an estrogen parparation. One example would be ethinyl estradiol 0.25 mg/day given until epiphyseal fusion occurs. Boys may be given 750–1000 mg of depo-testosterone monthly, usually divided into three or four injections (195). In general, it takes 1–2 years for these therapies to result in epiphyseal fusion.

Pituitary Gigantism

Pituitary gigantism is caused by an excess of GH, usually from a GH-secreting pituitary tumor. It is extremely rare in children; the incidence of all pituitary tumors in children is approximately 0.1 in 1 million.

Clinical Presentation The usual presentation consists of tall stature with an abnormally fast growth velocity. Since this condition is acquired, a good growth chart demonstrates an acceleration in growth velocity.

Diagnosis The best screening test is an IGF-1 determination. If it is elevated (compared with age- and puberty-matched standards), it is highly suspicious for a GH-secreting pituitary tumor. IGFBP-3 also will be elevated. Also diagnostic is the failure to suppress GH levels with an OGTT.

Treatment Ideal treatment consists of removing the tumor. Medical treatment to inhibit GH secretion may include bromocriptine (a dopamine agonist), octreotide (an analogue of somatostatin), or pegvisomant (a GH receptor antagonist) (for details, see Chapter 46).

Cerebral Gigantism (Sotos Syndrome)

Clinical Presentation This syndrome was first described in 1964 (196). It usually presents with a large birth size (birth length averages almost 22 in). In addition to tall stature, other findings include macrocephaly, downslanting palpebral fissures, hypertelorism, prognathism with narrow anterior mandible, a high narrow palate with prominent lateral palatine ridges, and coarse-looking facies (Figure 30-16). The bone age is advanced, and along with advanced skeletal maturation, there is premature eruption of dentition. Because of the advanced skeletal maturation, children with this syndrome have early puberty and, ultimately, have normal adult stature.

Diagnosis Diagnosis is largely based on clinical findings.

Treatment Treatment consists reassurance because these children achieve normal adult stature.

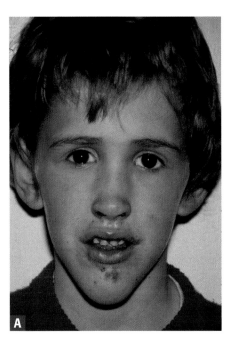

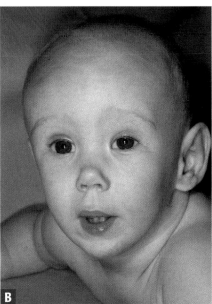

Klinefelter Syndrome

Clinical Presentation This disorder was first described by Klinefelter in 1942 and was discovered subsequently to be caused by one or more extra X chromosomes. Today, it may present prenatally because of a prenatal karyotype. It may present as a child with a small penis and testes. It may present during puberty if puberty is not completed after starting. It is characteristic to have tall stature because of long legs with a rather normal trunk (or sitting height). Arms also tend to be long. Gynecomastia beginning at the time of puberty occurs in about 40% of patients. The average IQ tends to be 10–15 points below that of normal siblings. The presence of an extra Y chromosome (XYY) also predisposes to tall stature. The incidence is thought to be between 1 in 500 and 1 in 1000 live births. When this karyotype is discovered in an infant, it does not predict the child's future behavior or development. Most individuals with this karyotype are tall normal men who likely had a karyotype obtained for unrelated reasons. The diagnosis is made by karyotype; the most common karyotype is 47,XXY, although it is also possible to have additional X chromosomes. After puberty, serum testosterone levels often are low (i.e., half the normal adult value). Patients often are infertile with hyalinization and fibrosis of the seminiferous tubules secondary to excess gonadotropin.

If there is hypogonadism, testosterone replacement will allow normal pubertal development. A usual beginning dose is 200 mg testosterone enanthate in oil per month as

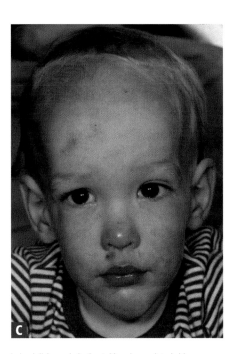

one or two injections per month. Another alternative is a testosterone patch or testosterone gel at usual adult replacement doses (for details, see Chapter 37).

Marfan Syndrome

Clinical Presentation Marfan syndrome usually presents as tall stature with long digits. Features are predominantly in three systems: the skeleton, the eyes, and the cardiovasular system. A common ocular feature is subluxation of the lens; occasionally, there may be retinal detachment. Problems with the vascular system include mitral valve prolapse, mitral regurgitation, dilatation of the aortic root, and aortic regurgitation. There is also the possibility of aortic aneurysm and aortic dissection, which are life-threatening. This syndrome is caused by a mutation in the fibrillin 1 gene, which is located on chromosome 15. Marfan syndrome is inherited as an autosomal dominant trait. It is caused by mutations in a gene located on chromosome 15 (15q21.1), which codes for a glycoprotein called *fibrillin*. Fibrillin is a part of microfibrils, which are part of structural components, such as the suspensory ligaments of the lens of the eye and elastin in the aorta and other connective tissues. Marfan syndrome affects about 1 in 10,000 individuals. Diagnostic criteria for Marfan syndrome were established in 1995. Known as the *Ghent criteria*, this system divides findings into major and minor criteria. Major criteria include family history and biochemical findings (i.e., evidence for a fibrillin mutation). If family history and genetic histories do not provide a diagnosis, it is possible to make the diagnosis from physical findings. There are major and minor findings in a number of organ systems; for a diagnosis, there should be major findings in at least two organ systems with minor findings in a third. Major skeletal findings include severe pectus excavatum, disproportionately long limbs, arachnodactyly, significant scoliosis, reduced extension of the elbows, medial displacement of the medial malleolus, and intrapelvic protrusion of the acetabulum. Minor criteria include mild pectus excavatum, mild scoliosis, thoracic lordosis, joint hypermobility, high arched palate, dental crowding, and typical facies. A major eye finding is subluxation of the lens. Minor eye findings include a flat cornea, increased length of the globe (on ultrasound), a cataract or glaucoma in a patient younger than 50 years of age, hypoplastic iris, myopia, and retinal detachment. Major cardiovascular findings include aortic root dilatation or dissection; minor criteria include mitral valve prolapse, dilatation of the proximal main pulmonary artery in the absence of peripheral pulmonic stenosis, calcification of

FIGURE 30-16 A to **C.** Children with Sotos. Note the macrocephaly, dolichocephaly, frontal bossing, pointed chin, downslanting palpebral fissures. Photos courtesy of Robert Gorlin, D.D.S, M.S., D.Sc.

a mitral annulus, or dilatation of the abdominal or descending thoracic aorta. There are minor criteria for the pulmonary system and for the skin that include a spontaneous pneumothorax or atypical blebs on a chest x-ray, striae, or recurrent or excisional hernia.

Treatment is aimed at preventing progression of aortic expansion and includes β-blockers. There is no agreement as to the age at which this therapy should be started. If there are problems with a heart valve, it may require replacement, followed by anticoagulant therapy and antibiotic prophylaxis for certain procedures, such as dental work. It is possible in the prepubertal child to treat with androgen or estrogen to cause early epiphyseal fusion. The estrogen dose for girls is 0.3–0.5 mg of ethinyl estradiol and the androgen dose for boys is 200 mg of testosterone enanthate in oil per month as one or two injections per month (195). In either case, the patient should be treated until epiphyseal fusion occurs.

Homocystinuria

Clinical Presentation Homocystinuria is an autosomal recessive disorder caused by a deficiency of cystathionine synthetase, an enzyme involved in methionine metabolism. In addition to tall, Marfanoid stature, there are other problems involving connective tissue, including subluxation of the lens (usually downward) and medial degeration of the aorta. There is also a characteristic rash consisting of red papules or erythematous blotches. More than half of those with homocystinuria have developmental delay. The incidence of homocystinuria is about 1 in 344,000 births.

Treatment Treatment is mainly dietary, supplemented with pyridoxine in high doses and/or folic acid (in pharmacological doses), betaine, or cyanocobalamin (for more details, see Chapter 16).

Beckwith–Wiedemann Syndrome

Clinical Presentation The usual presentation is in the immediate newborn period and consists of macrosomia with an omphalocele, macroglossia, and ear creases. In the newborn period, there is usually hypoglycemia due to hyperinsulinism. Hepatomegaly and large kidneys are seen commonly. The incidence is approximately 1 in 15,000 births.

Diagnosis is based largely on clinical findings. It is known that in some cases there is disrupted imprinting of one or more genes. The sex of the transmitting parent determines the pattern and risk of transmission in familial cases. Typically, individuals with this syndrome who survive infancy tend to be healthy adults. Many of the features of this disorder

are thought to result from elevated levels of IGF-2. Since IGF-2 is most important for fetal growth, the theory that IGF-2 is involved would be consistent with the observation that those with this syndrome who survive infancy do not have problems in later childhood or adulthood.

Treatment Treatment consists of observing blood glucose levels and treating hypoglycemia. It is also important to screen for Wilms tumor with ultrasound. It has been recommended to screen at 3-month intervals for the first 3 years and 6-month intervals thereafter.

REFERENCES

1. Rosenfield RL. Essentials of growth diagnosis. *Endocrinol Metab Clin North Am.* 1996;25:743–758.
2. Tanner JM, Davies PS. Clinical longitudinal standards for height and height velocity for North American children. *J Pediatr.* 1985;107:317–329.
3. Rosenfeld RG. Insulin-like growth factors and the basis of growth. *N Engl J Med.* 2003;349:2184–2186.
4. Frindik JP, Kemp SF, Kearns FS, et al. Growth screening: A positive medical experience. *Clin Pediatr.* 1992;31:497–500.
5. Herman-Giddens ME, Slora EJ, Wasserman RC. Secondary sexual characteristics and menses in young girls seen in office practice. *Pediatrics.* 1997;99:505–512.
6. Cole TJ. Secular trends in growth. *Proc Nutr Soc.* 2000;59:317–324.
7. Cohen RN. Update on genetic regulation of pituitary development. *Pediatr Endocrinol Rev.* 2006;3:312–317.
8. Parks JS, Nielsen PV, Sexton LA, et al. An effect of gene dosage on production of human chorionic somatomammotropin. *J Clin Endocrinol Metab.* 1985;50:994–997.
9. Cooke NE, Ray J, Watson MA, et al. Human growth hormone gene and the highly homologous growth hormone variant gene display different splicing patterns. *J. Clin Invest* 1988;82:270–275.
10. Campbell RM, Scanes CG. Evolution of the growth hormone–releasing factor (GHRF) family of peptides. *Growth Reg.* 1992;2:175–191.
11. Laron Z. Biologic and clinical aspects of molecular defects along the growth hormone–insulin-like growth factor I axis. In: Pescovitz OH, Eugster EA, eds. *Pediatric Endocrinology: Mechanisms, Manifestations, and Management.* Philadelphia: Lippincott Williams & Wilkins; 2004:129–130.
12. Botero D, Evliyaoglu O, Cohen LE. Hypopituitarism. In: Radovick S, MacGillivray MH, eds. *Pediatric Endocrinology: A Practical Clinical Guide.* Totowa, NJ: Humana Press; 2003:4–5.
13. Bowers CY, Momany F, Reynolds GA, et al. On the in vitro and in vivo activity of a new synthetic hexapeptide that acts on the pituitary to specifically release growth hormone. *Endocrinology.* 1984;114:1537.
14. Howard AD, Feighner SD, Cully DF. A receptor in pituitary and hypothalamus that functions in growth hormone release. *Science.* 1996;273:972–977.
15. Kojima M, Hosoda H, Date Y, et al. Ghrelin is a growth hormone–releasing acylated peptide from the stomach. *Nature.* 1999;402:656.
16. Lustig RH, Preeyasombat C, Velasquez-Mieyer PA. Childhood obesity. In: Pescovitz OH, Eugster EA, eds. *Pediatric Endocrinology: Mechanisms, Manifestations, and Management.* Philadelphia: Lippincott Williams & Wilkins; 2004:682–714.
17. Rosenfeld RG. The IGF system: New developments relevant to pediatric practice. *Endocr Dev.* 2005;9:1–10.
18. Salmon WD, Daughaday WH. A hormonally controlled serum factor which stimulates sulfate incorporation by cartilage in vitro. *J Lab Clin Med.* 1957;49:825–836.
19. Rinderknecht E, Humbel RE. Primary structure of human insulin-like growth factor II. *FEBS Lett.* 1978;89:283–286.
20. Rinderknecht E, Humbel RE. The amino acid sequence of human insulin-like growth factor I and its structural homology with proinsulin. *J Biol Chem.* 1978;253:2769–2776.
21. Woods KA, Camacho-Hubner C, Savage MO, et al. Intrauterine growth retardation and postnatal growth failure associated with deletion of the insulin-like growth factor I gene. *N Engl J Med.* 1996;335:1363–1367.
22. Cole TJ. Assessment of growth. *Best Pract Res Clin Endocrinol Metab.* 2002;16:383–398.
23. Tanner JM. *Growth at Adolescence.* Oxford, UK: Blackwell; 1962.
24. Duke PM, Whincup PH, Gross RT. Adolescents' self-assessment of sexual maturation. *Pediatrics.* 1980;66:918–920.
25. Hick KM, Katzman DK. Self-assessment of sexual maturation in adolescent females with anorexia nervosa. *J Adolesc Health.* 1999;24:206–211.
26. Robertson J, Shilkofski N. *The Harriet Lane Handbook: A Manual for Pediatric House Officers,* 17th ed. St. Louis: Mosby; 2005.
27. Tanner JM, Goldstein H, Whitehouse RH. Standards for children's height at ages 2–9 years allowing for heights of parents. *Arch Dis Child.* 1970;45:755–762.
28. Greulich WW, Pyle SI. *Radiographic Atlas of Skeletal Development of the Hand and Wrist,* 2nd ed. Stanford, CA: Stanford University Press; 1959.
29. Tanner JM, Whitehouse RH, Marshall WA, et al. *Assessment of Skeletal Maturity and Prediction of Adult Height (TW2 Method).* New York: Academic Press; 1975.
30. Roche AF, Chumlea WC, Thissen D. *Assening the Skeletal Maturity of the Hand-Wrist.* Springfield, IL: Charles C. Thomas; 1988.
31. Kemp SF. Analysis of bone age data from National Cooperative Growth Study Substudy VII. *Pediatrics.* 1999;104:1031–1036.
32. Bayley N, Pineau SR. Tables for predicting adult height from skeletal age: Revised for use with the Greulich–Pyle hand standards. *J Pediatr.* 1952;40:423–441.

33. Roche AF, Wainer H, Thissen D. The RWT method for the prediction of adult stature. *Pediatrics.* 1975;56:1027–1033.

34. Bramswig JH, Fasse M, Holthoff ML, et al. Adult height in boys and girls with untreated short stature and constitutional delay of growth and puberty: Accuracy of five different methods of height predicition. *J Pediatr.* 1990;117:886–891.

35. Kemp SF, Alter C, Dana K, et al. Use of magnetic resonance imaging in short stature: Data from the National Cooperative Growth Study (NCGS) Substudy 8. *J Pediatr Endocrinol Metab.* 2002;15:675–679.

36. Frindik JP. Pituitary morphologic anomalies and magnetic resonance imaging in pediatric growth hormone deficiency. *Endocrinologist* 2001;11:289–295.

37. Wilson TA, Rose SR, Cohen P, et al. Update of guidelines for the use of growth hormone in children: The Lawson Wilkins Pediatric Endocrinology Society Drug and Therapeutics Committee. *J Pediatr.* 2003;143:415–421.

38. Horner JM, Thorsson AV, Hintz RL. Grwoth deceleration patterns in children with constitutional short stature: An aid to diagnosis. *Pediatrics.* 1978;62:529–534.

39. Han JC, Balagopal P, Sweeten S, et al. Evidence for hypermetabolism in boys with constitutional delay of growth and maturation. *J Clin Endocrinol Metab.* 2006;91:2081–2086.

40. Rosenfeld RG, Northcraft GB, Hintz RL. A prospective, randomized study of testosterone treatment of constitutional delay of growth and development in male adolescents. *Pediatrics.* 1982;69:681–187.

41. Blethen SL, Gaines S, Weldon V. Comparison of predicted and adult heights in short boys: Effect of androgen therapy. *Pediatr Res.* 1984;18:467–469.

42. Zachmann M, Studer S, Prader A. Short-term testosterone treatment at bone age of 12–13 years does not reduce adult height in boys with constitutional delay in growth and adolescence. *Helv Paediatr Acta.* 1987;42:21–28.

43. Moseley CT, Orenstein MD, Phillips JA 3rd. GH gene deletions and IGHD type IA. *Rev Endocr Metab Disord.* 2002;3:339–346.

44. Illig R, Prader A, Ferrandez M, et al. Hereditary prenatal growth hormone deficiency with increased tendency to growth hormone antibody formation: A type of isolated growth hormone deficiency. *Acta Paediatr Scand.* 1971;60:607.

45. Phillips JA 3rd, Hjelle B, Seeburg PH, et al. Molecular basis for familial isolated growth hormone deficiency. *Proc Natl Acad Sci USA.* 1981;78:6372–6375.

46. Vnencak-Jones CL, Phillips JA 3rd, Chen EY, et al. Molecular basis of human growth hormone gene deletion. *Proc Natl Acad Sci USA.* 1988;85:5615–5619.

47. Backeljauw PF, Underwood LE. Prolonged treatment with recombinant insulin-like growth factor-I in children with growth hormone insensitivity syndrome: A clinical research center study. *J Clin Endocrinol Metab.* 1996;81:3312–3317.

48. Arnhold IJ, Oliveira SB, Osorio MG, et al. Insulin-like growth factor-I treatment in two children with growth hormone gene deletions. *J Pediatr Endocrinol Metab.* 1999;12:499–506.

49. Mullis PE. Genetic control of growth. *Eur J Endocrinol.* 2005;152:11–31.

50. Abjul-Latif HE, Leiberman HE, et al. Growth hormone deficiency type IB caused by cryptic splicing of the GH-1 gene. *J Pediatr Endocrinol Metab.* 2000;13:21–38.

51. Cogan JD, Phillips JA 3rd, Schenkman SS, et al. Familial growth hormone deficiency: A model of dominant and recessive mutations affecting a monometric protein. *J Clin Endocrinol Metab.* 199479: 1261–1265.

52. Sitz KB, Burks AW, Williams LW, et al. Confirmation of X-linked hypogammaglobulinemia with isolated growth hormone as a disease entity. *J Pediatr.* 1990;116:292–294.

53. Root AW, Kemp SF, Rundle AC, et al. Effect of long-term recombinant growth hormone therapy in children. National Cooperative Growth Study, 1985–1994. *J Pediatr Endocrinol Metab.* 1998;11:403–412.

54. Rona RJ, Tanner JM. Aetiology of idiopathic growth hormone deficiency in England and Wales. *Arch Dis Child.* 1997;52:197–208.

55. Lacey KA, Parkin JM. Causes of short stature: A community study of children in Newcastle-upon-Tyne. *Lancet.* 1974;1:42–45.

56. Lindsay R, Feldkamp M, Harris D, et al. Utah growth study: Growth standards and the prevalence of growth homrone deficiency. *J Pediatr* 1994;125:29–35.

57. Lipman TH, Hench KD, Benyi T, et al. A multicentre randomized, controlled trial of an intervention to improve the accuracy of linear growth measurement. *Arch Dis Child.* 2004;89:342–346.

58. Bramswig JH, Schlosser H, Kiese K. Final height in children with growth hormone deficiency. *Horm Res.* 1995;43:126–128.

59. Frindik JP, Kemp SF. Near adult heights after growth hormone treatment in patients with idiopathic short stature or idiopathic growth hormone deficiency. *J Pediatr Endocrinol Metab.* 2003;16:607–612.

60. Reiter EO, Price DA, Wilton P, et al. Effect of growth hormone (GH) treatment on final height of 1258 patients with idiopathic GH deficiency: Analysis of a large international database. *J Clin Endocrinol Metab.* 2006;91:2047–2054.

61. Carel JC, Ecosse E, Nicolino M, et al. Adult height after long term treatment with recombinant growth hormone for idiopathic isolated growth hormone deficiency: Observational follow up study of the French population based registry. *Br Med J.* 2002;325:70–76.

62. Dos Santos C, Essioux L, Teinturier C, et al. A common polymorphism of the growth hormone receptor is associated with increased responsiveness to growth hormone. *Nat Genet.* 2004;36:720–724.

63. Hujeirat Y, Hess O, Shalev S, et al. Growth hormone receptor sequence changes do not play a role in determining height in children with idiopathic short stature. *Horm Res.* 2006;65:210–216.

64. Mills JL, Schonberger LB, Wysowski DK, et al. Long-term mortality in the United States cohort of pituitary-derived growth hormone recipients. *J Pediatr.* 2004;144:430–436.

65. Brown P. Human growth hormone therapy and Creutzfeldt–Jacob disease: A drama in three acts. *Pediatrics.* 1988;81:85–92.

66. Maneatis T, Baptista J, Connelly K, et al. Growth hormone safety update from the National Cooperative Growth Study. *J Pediatr Endocrinol Metab.* 2000;13: 1035–1044.

67. Frindik JP, Morales A, Shulman D, et al. Near-adult hieght in 1448 growth hormone (GH)–treated patients with organic GH deficiency from the National Cooperative Growth Study (NCGS). *Pediatr Acad Soc.* 2006;4330–4331.

68. Ranke MB, Price DA, Lindberg A, et al. Final height in children with medulloblastoma treated with growth hormone. *Horm Res.* 2005;64:28–34.

69. Swords FM, Carroll PV, Kisalu J, et al. The effects of growth hormone deficiency and replacement on glucocorticoid exposure in hypopituitary patients on cortisone acetate and hydrocortisone replacement. *Clin Endocrinol (Oxf).* 2003;59:613–620.

70. Takahashi Y, Chihara K. Short stature by mutant growth hormone. *Growth Horm IGF Res.* 1999;9:37–41.

71. Rosenbloom AL, Guevara-Aguirre J, Rosenfeld RG, et al. Growth hormone receptor deficiency in Ecuador. *J Clin Endocrinol Metab.* 1999;84: 4436–4443.

72. Rosenfeld RG. Molecular mechanisms of IGF-I deficiency. *Horm Res.* 2006;65:15–20.

73. Savage MO, Camacho-Hubner C, Dunger DB. Therapeutic applications of the insulin-like growth factors. *Growth Horm IGF Res.* 2004;14:301–308.

74. Ranke MB, Wollmann HA, Savage MO. Experience with insulin-like growth factor I (IGF-I) treatment of growth hormone insensitivity syndrome (GHIS). *J Pediatr Endocrinol Metab.* 1999;12:259–266.

75. Ranke MB, Savage MO, Chatelain P. Insulin-like growth factor (IGF) I improves height in growth hormone insensitivity: Two year's results. *Horm Res.* 1995;44:253–264.

76. Azcona C, Preece M, Rose SJ, et al. Growth response to rhIGF-I 80 μg/kg twice daily in children with growth hormone insensitivity syndrome: Relationship to severity of phenotype. *Clin Endocrinol.* 1999;51:787–792.

77. Backeljauw PF, Underwood LE, Group TGC. Therapy for 6.5–7.5 years with recombinant insulin-like growth factor I in children with growth hormone insensitivity syndrome: A clinical research center study. *J Clin Endocrinol Metab.* 2001;86: 1510–1514.

78. Guevara-Aguirre J, Vasconez O, Martinez V, et al. A randomized, double-blinded, placebo-controlled trial on safety and efficacy of recombinant human insulin-like growth factor-I in children with growth hormone deficiency. *J Clin Endocrinol Metab.* 1995;80:1393–1398.

79. Kemp SF, Thrailkill KM. Investigational agents for the treatment of growth hormone–insensitivity syndrome. *Exp Opin Invest Drugs.* 2006;15:409–415.

80. Attie KM, Carlsson LM, Chen Rundle A, et al. Evidence for partial growth hormone insensitivity among patients with idiopathic short stature. *J Pediatr.* 1995;127:244–250.

81. Goddard AD, Covello R, Luoh S-M, et al. Mutations of the growth hormone receptor in children with idiopathic short stature. *N Engl J Med.* 1995;333:1093–1098.

82. Camacho-Hubner C, Woods KA, Miraki-Moud F, et al. Effects of recombinant human insulin-like growth factor-I (IGF-I) therapy on the growth hormone-IGF system of a patient with a partial IGF-gene deletion. *J Clin Endocrinol Metab.* 1999;84:1611–1616.

83. Walenkamp MJE, Karperien M, Pereira AM, et al. Homozygous and heterozygous expression of a novel insulin-like growth factor-I mutation. *J Clin Endocrinol Metab.* 2005;90:2855–2864.

84. Abuzzahab MJ, Schneider A, Goddard A, et al. IGF-I receptor mutations resulting in intrauterine and postnatal growth retardation. *N Engl J Med.* 2003;349:2211–2222.

85. Hwa V, Hausler G, Pratt KL, et al. Total absence of functional acit labile subunit, resulting in severe insulin-like growth factor deficiency and moderate growth failure. *J Clin Endocrinol Metab.* 2006;91:1826–1831.

86. Domene HM, Bengolea SV, Martinez AS, et al. Deficiency of the circulating insulin-like growth factor system associated with inactivation of the acid-labile subunit. *N Engl J Med.* 2004;350:570–577.

87. Neerhof MG. Causes of intrauterine growth restriction. *Clin Perinatol.* 1995;22:375–385.

88. Alkalay AL, Graham JM, Pomerance JJ. Evaluation of neonates born with intrauterine growth retardation: Review and practice guidelines. *J Perinatol.* 1998;18:142–151.

89. Usher R, McLean F. Intrauterine growth of live-born Caucasian infants at sea level: Standards obtained from measurements in 7 dimensions of infants born between 25 and 44 weeks of gestation. *J Pediatr.* 1969;74:901–910.

90. Albertsson-Wikland K, Karlberg J. Natural growth in children born small for gestational age with and without catch-up growth. *Acta Paediatr.* 1994;399:64–70.

91. Wollmann HA. Intrauterine growth restriction: Definition and etiology. *Horm Res.* 1998;49:1–6.

92. Pollack RN, Divon MY. Intrauterine growth retardation: Definition, classification, and etiology. *Clin Obstet Gynecol.* 1992;35:99–107.

93. Leger J, Limoni C, Collin D, et al. Prediction factors in the determination of final height in subjects born small for gestational age. *Pediatr Res.* 1998;43:808–812.

94. Hediger ML, Overpeck MD, Maurer KR, et al. Growth of infants and young children born small or large for gestational age: Findings from the Third National Health and Nutrition Examination Survey. *Arch Pediatr Adolesc Med.* 1998;152:1225–1231.

95. Karlberg J, Albertsson-Wikland K. Growth in full-term small-for-gestational-age infants: From birth to final height. *Pediatr Res* 1996;39:175.

96. Leger J, Oury JF, Noel M, et al. Growth factors and intrauterine growth retardation: I. Serum growth hormone, insulin-like growth factor (IGF)-I, IGF-II and IGF binding protein 3 levels in normally grown and growth-retarded human fetuses during the second half of gestation. *Pediatr Res* 1996;40:94–100.

97. Boguszewski M, Bjarnason R, Jansson C, et al. Hormonal status of short children born small for gestational age. *Acta Paediatr* 1997;423:189–192.

98. de Zegher F, Maes M, Gargasky SE, et al. High-dose growth hormone treatment of short children born small for gestational age. *J Clin Endocrinol Metab.* 1996; 81:1887–1892.

99. De Zegher F, Du Caju MV, Heinrichs C, et al. Early, discontinuous, high dose growth hormone treatment to normalize height and weight of short children born small for gestational age: Results over 6 years. *J Clin Endocrinol Metab.* 1999;84:1558–1561.

100. Lee MM. Idiopathic short stature. *N Engl J Med.* 2006;354:2576–2582.

101. Finkelstein BS, Imperiale TF, Speroff T, et al. Effect of growth hormone therapy on height in children with idiopathic short stature: A meta-analysis. *Arch Pediatr Adolesc Med.* 2002;156:230–240.

102. Rekers-Mombarg LT, Witt JM, Massa GG, et al. Spontaneous growth in idiopathic short stature. European Study Group. *Arch Dis Child.* 1996;75:175–180.

103. Leshek EW, Rose SR, Yanovski JA, et al. Effect of growth hormone treatment on adult height in peripubertal children with idiopathic short statue: A randomized, double-blind, placebo-controlled trial. *J Clin Endocrinol Metab.* 2004;89:3140–3148.

104. Witt JM, Rekers-Mombarg LTM, Cutler GB Jr, et al. Growth hormone (GH) treatment to final height in children with idopathic short stature: Evidence for a dose effect. *J Pediatr.* 2005;146:45–53.

105. Kemp SF, Kuntze J, Attie KM, et al. Efficacy and safety results of long-term growth hormone treatment of idiopathic short stature. *J Clin Endocrinol Metab.* 2005;90:5247–5253.

106. Kemp SF. Growth hormone treatment of idiopathic short stature: History and demographic data from the NCGS. *Growth Horm IGF Res.* 2005;15:S9–12.

107. Lee JM, Davis MM, Clark SJ, et al. Estimated cost-effectiveness of growth hormone therapy for idiopathic short stature. *Arch Pediatr Adolesc Med.* 2006;160:263–269.

108. Visser-van Balen H, Sinnema G, Geenen R. Growing up with idiopathic short stature: psycholsocial development and hormone treatment: A critical review. *Arch Dis Child.* 2006;91:433–439.

109. Hero M, Norjavaara E, Dunkel L. Inhibition of estrogen biosynthesis with a potent aromatase inhibitor increases predicted adult height in boys with idiopathic short stature: A randomized, controlled trial. *J Clin Endocrinol Metab.* 2005;90:6396–6402.

110. Ogata T. SHOX haploinsufficiency and its modifying factors. *J Pediatr Endocrinol Metab.* 2002;15:1289–1294.

111. Blaschke RJ, Roppold GA. SHOX in short stature syndromes. *Horm Res.* 2001;55:21–23.

112. Ross JL, Kowal K, Quigley CA, et al. The phenotype of short stature homeobox gene (SHOX) deficiency in childhood: contrasting children wtih Leri–Weill dyschondrosteosis and Turner syndrome. *J Pediatr.* 2005;147:499–507.

113. Gravholt CH. Epidemiological, endocrine and metabolic features in Turner syndrome. *Eur J Endocrinol.* 2004;151:657–687.

114. Loscalzo ML, Van PL, Ho VB, et al. Association between fetal lymphedema and congenital cardiovascular defects in Turner syndrome. *Pediatrics.* 2005;115:732–735.

115. Catovic A. Cytogenetics findings at Turner syndrome and their correlation with clinical findings. *Bosnian J Basic Med Sci.* 2005;5:54–58.

116. Meng H, Hager K, Rivkees SA, et al. Detection of Turner syndrome using high-throughput quantitative genotyping. *J Pediatr Endocrinol Metab.* 2005;90:3419–3422.

117. Frias JL, Davenport ML, Endocrinology Committee on Genetics and Section on Endocrinology. Health supervision for children with Turner syndrome. *Pediatrics.* 2003;111:692–702.

118. Parvin M, Roche E, Costigan C, et al. Treatment outcome in Turner syndrome. *Irish Med J.* 2004;97:14–15.

119. Guarneri MP, Abusrewil SA, Bernasconi S, et al. International workshop on management of puberty for optimum auxological results: Turner syndrome. *J Pediatr Endocrinol Metab.* 2001;14:959–965.

120. Plotnick L, Attie KM, Blethen SL, et al. Growth hormone treatment of girls with Turner syndrome: The National Cooperative Growth Study experience. *Pediatrics.* 1998;102:479–481.

121. Soriano-Guillen L, Coste J, Ecosse E, et al. Adult height and pubertal growth in Turner syndrome after treatment with recombinant growth hormone. *J Pediatr Endocrinol Metab.* 2005;90:5197–5204.

122. Rosenfield RL, Devine N, Hunold JJ, et al. Salutary effects of combining early very low-dose systemic estradiol with growth hormone therapy in girls with Turner syndrome. *J Clin Endocrinol Metab.* 2005;90:6424–6430.

123. Livadas S, Xekouki P, Fouka F, et al. Prevalence of thyroid dysfunction in Turner's syndrome: A long-term follow-up and brief literature review. *Thyroid.* 2005;15:1061–1066.

124. El-Mansoury M, Bryman I, Berntorp K, et al. Hypothyroidism is common in Turner syndrome: Results of a five-year follow-up. *J Clin Endocrinol Metab.* 2005;90:2131–2135.

125. Choi IK, Kim DH, Kim HS. The abnormalities of carbohydrate metabolism in Turner syndrome: Analysis of risk factors associated with impaired glucose tolerance. *Eur J Paediatr.* 2005;164:442–447.

126. Bakalov VK, Cooley MM, Quon MJ, et al. Impaired insulin secretion in the Turner metabolic syndrome. *J Clin Endocrinol Metab.* 2004;89:3516–3520.

127. Sas T, de Muinck Keizer-Schrama S, Aanstoot HJ, et al. Carbohydrate metabolism during growth hormone treatment and after discontinuation of growth hormone treatment in girls iwth Turner syndrome treated with once or twice daily growth hormone injections. *Clini Endocrinol.* 2000;52:741–747.

128. Tartaglia M, Gelb BD. Noonan syndrome and related disorders: Genetics and pathogenesis. *Annu Rev Genom Hum Genet.* 2005;6:45–68.

129. Limal JM, Parfait B, Cabrol S, et al. Noonan syndrome: Relationships between genotype, growth, and growth factors. *J Clin Endocrinol Metab.* 2006;91:300–306.

130. Ferreira LV, Souza SA, Arnhold IJ, et al. PTPN11 (protein tyrosine phosphatase, nonreceptor type 11) mutations and response to growth hormone therapy in children with Noonan syndrome. *J Clin Endocrinol Metab.* 2005;90:5156–5160.

131. Yoshida R, Hasegawa T, Hasegawa Y, et al. Protein-tyrosine phosphatase, nonreceptor type 11 mutation analysis and clinical assessment in 45 patients with Noonan syndrome. *J Clin Endocrinol Metab.* 2004;89:3359–3364.

132. Ranke MB, Heidemann P, Knupfer C, et al. Noonan syndrome: Growth and clinical manifestations in 144 cases. *Eur J Paediatr.* 1988;148:220–227.

133. de Schipper J, Otten BJ, Francois I, et al. Growth hormone therapy in pre-pubertal children with Noonan syndrome: First year growth response and comparison with Turner syndrome. *Acta Paediatr.* 1997;86:943–946.

134. Osio D, Dahlgren J, Wikland KA, et al. Improved final height with long-term growth hormone treatment in Noonan syndrome. *Acta Paediatr.* 2005;94:1232–1237.

135. Kirk JM, Betts PR, Butler GE, et al. Short stature in Noonan syndrome: Response to growth hormone therapy. *Arch Dis Child.* 2001;84:440–443.

136. Noordam C, Draaisma JM, van den Nieuwenhof J, et al. Effects of growth hormone treatment on left ventricular dimensions in children with Noonan's syndrome. *Horm Res.* 2001;56:110–113.

137. Preece M. The genetics of the Silver–Russell syndrome. *Rev Endocr Metab Disord.* 2002;3:369–379.

138. Hitchens MP, Stanier P, Preece M, et al. Silver–Russell syndrome: A dissection of the genetic aetiology and candidate chromosomal regions. *J Med Genet.* 2001;38:810–819.

139. Wollmann HA, Kirchner T, Enders H, et al. Growth and symptoms in Silver–Russell syndrome: Review on the basis of 386 patients. *Eur J Paediatr.* 1995;154:958–968.

140. Chernausek SD, Breen TJ, Frank GR. Linear growth in response to growth hormone treatment in children with short stature associated with intrauterine growth retardation: The National Cooperative Growth Study experience. *J Pediatr.* 1996;128:S22–27.

141. Rakover Y, Dietsch S, Ambler GR, et al. Growth hormone therapy in Silver Russell syndrome: 5 years experience of the Australian and New Zealand Growth database (OZGROW). *Eur J Paediatr.* 1996;155:851–857.

142. Albanese A, Stanhope R. GH treatment induces sustained catch-up growth in children with intrauterine growth retardation: 7-year results. *Horm Res.* 1997;48:173–177.

143. Dahlgren J, Wieland KA, Treatment TSS-GfGH. Final height in short children born small for gestational age treated with growth hormone. *Pediatr Res.* 2005;57:216–222.

144. Burman P, Ritzen EM, Lindgren AC. Endocrine dysfunction in Prader–Willi syndrome: A review with special reference to GH. *Endocr Rev.* 2001;22:787–799.

145. State MW, Dykens EM. Genetics of childhood disorders: XV. Prader–Willi s;syndrome: Genes, brain, and behavior. *J Am Acad Child Adolesc Psychiatry.* 2000;39:797–800.

146. Gross-Tsur V, Landau YE, Benarroch F, et al. Cognition, attention, and behavior in Prader–Willi syndrome. *J Child Neurol.* 2001;16:288–290.

147. Nixon GM, Brouillette RT. Sleep and breathing in Prader–Willi syndrome. *Pediatr Pulmonol.* 2002;34:209–217.

148. Eiholzer U. Deaths in children with Prader–Willi syndrome: A contribution to the debate about the safety of growth hormone treatment in children with PWS. *Horm Res.* 2005;63:33–39.

149. Allen DB, Carrel AL. Growth hormone therapy for Prader–Willi syndrome: A critical appraisal. *J Pediatr Endocrinol Metab.* 2004;17:1297–1306.

150. Dimitropoulos A, Feurer ID, Roof E, et al. Appetitive behavior, compulsivity, and neurochemistry in Prader–Willi syndrome. *Ment Retard Dev Disabil Res Rev.* 2000;66:125–130.

151. Nagai T, Matsuo N, Kayanuma Y, et al. Standard growth curves for Japanese patients with Prader–Willi syndrome. *Am J Med Genet.* 2000;95:130–134.

152. Carrel AL, Myers SE, Whitman BY, et al. Growth hormone improves body composition, fat utilization, physical strength and agility, and growth in Prader–Willi syndrome: A controlled study. *J Pediatr.* 1999;134:215–221.

153. Wilson SS, Cotterill AM, Harris MA. Growth hormone and respiratory compromise in Prader–Willi syndrome. *Arch Dis Child* 2006;81:349–350.

154. l'Allemand D, Eiholzer U, Schlumpf M, et al. Carbohydrate metabolism is not impaired after 3 years of growth hormone therapy in children with Prader–Willi syndrome. *Horm Res.* 2003;59:239–248.

155. Obata K, Sakazume S, Yoshino A, et al. Effects of 5 years growth hormone treatment in patients with Prader–Willi syndrome. *J Pediatr Endocrinol Metab.* 2003;16:155–162.

156. Sacco M, Di Giorgio G. Sudden death in Prader–Willi syndrome during growth hormone therapy. Horm Res. 2005; 63:29–32.

157. Miller J, Silverstein J, Shuster J, et al. Short–term effects of growth hormone on sleep abnormalities in Prader–Willi syndrome. *J Clin Endocrinol Metab.* 2006;91:413–417.

158. Lemyre E, Azouz EM, Teebi AS, et al. Bone dysplasia series: Achondroplasia, hyopchondroplasia and thanatophoric dysplasia: Review and upate. *Can Assoc Radiol J.* 1999;50:185–197.

159. Gordon N. The neurological complications of achondroplasia. *Brain Dev.* 2000;22:3–7.

160. Vajo Z, Francomano CA, Wilkin DJ. The molecular and genetic basis of fibroblast growth factor receptor 3 disorders: The achondroplasia family of skeletal dysplasias, Muenke craniosynostosis, and Crouzon syndrome with acanthosis nigricans. *Endocr Rev.* 2000;21:23–29.

161. Horton WA, Hecht JT, Hood OJ, et al. Growth hormone therapy in achondroplasia. *Am J Med Genet.* 1992;42:667–670.

162. Seino Y, Yamanaka Y, Shinohara M, et al. Growth hormone therapy in achondroplasia. *Horm Res.* 2000;53:53–56.

163. Ramaswami U, Rumsby G, Spoudeas HA, et al. Treatment of achondroplasia with growth hormone: Six years of experience. *Pediatr Res.* 1999;46:435–439.

164. Weber G, Prinster C, Meneghel M, et al. Human growth hormone treatment in prepubertal children with achondroplasia. *Am J Med Genet.* 1996;61:396–400.

165. Stamoyannou L, Karachaliou F, Neou P, et al. Growth and growth hormone therapy in children with achondroplasia: A two-year experience. *Am J Med Genet.* 1997;72:1.

166. Tanaka N, Katsumata N, Horikawa R, et al. The comparison of the effects of short-term growth hormone treatment in patients with achondroplasia and with hypochondroplasia. *Endocr J.* 2003; 50:69–75.

167. Suris JC, Michaud PA, Viner R. The adolescent child with a chronic condition: I. Developmental issues. *Arch Dis Child.* 2004;89:938–942.

168. Ward LM. Osteoporosis due to glucocorticoid use in children with chronic illness. *Horm Res.* 2005;64:209–221.

169. Mauras N. Growth hormone therapy in the glucocorticiosteroid-dependent child: Metabolic and linear growth effects. *Horm Res.* 2001;56:13–18.

170. Hochberg Z. Mechanisms of steroid impairment of growth. *Horm Res.* 2002;58:33–38.

171. Tiulpakov A, Zdravkovic V, Hamilton J, et al. Novel mutations within the POU1F1 gene associated with variable combined pituitary hormone deficiency. *J Clin Endocrinol Metab.* 2005;90:4762–4770.

172. Giavoli C, Porretti S, Ferrante E, et al. Recombinant hGH replacement therapy and the hypothalamus–pituitary–thyroid axis in children with GH deficiency: When should we be concerned about the occurrence of central hypothyroidism? *Clin Endocrinol.* 2003;59:806–810.

173. Bain P, Toublanc JE. Adult height in congenital hypothyroidism: Prognostic factors and the importance of compliance with treatment. *Horm Res.* 2002;58:136–142.

174. Linder BL, Esteban NV, Yergey AL, et al. Cortisol production rate in childhood and adolescence. *J Pediatr*. 1990;117:892–896.

175. Kerrigan JR, Veldhuis JD, Leyo SA, et al. Estimation of daily corticol production and clearance rates in normal pubertal males by deconvolution analysis. *J Clin Endocrinol Metab*. 1993;76:1505–1510.

176. Miller WL. The adrenal cortex. In: Sperling MA, ed. *Pediatric Endocrinology*, 2nd ed. Philadelphia: Saunders; 2002:385–438.

177. Savage MO, Leinhardt A, Lebrethon MC, et al. Cushing's disease in childhood: Presentation, investigation, treatment and long-term outcome. *Horm Res*. 2001;55:24–30.

178. Cirak B, Palaoglu S, Akalan N. Clinical and therapeutic properties of Cushing's disease in childhood. *Pediatr Neurosurg*. 1999;31:12–15.

179. Mallon PW, Law M, Miller J, et al. Buffalo hump seen in HIV-associated lipodystrophy is associated with hyperinsulinemia but not dyslipidemia. *J AIDS*. 2005;38:156–162.

180. Lebrethon MC, Grossman AB, Afshar F, et al. Linear growth and final height after treatment for Cushing's disease in childhood. *J Clin Endocrinol Metab*. 2000;85:3262–3265.

181. Johnston LB, Grossman AB, Plowman PN, et al. Normal final height and apparent cure after pituitary irradiation for Cushing's disease in childhood: Long-term follow-up of anterior pituitary function. *Clin Endocrinol*. 1998;48:663–667.

182. Davies JH, Storr HL, Davies K, et al. Final adult height and body mass index after cure of paediatric Cushing's disease. *Clin Endocrinol*. 2005;62:466–472.

183. Stevens A, Ray DW, Zeggini E, et al. Glucocorticoid sensitivity is determined by a specific glucocorticoid receptor haplotype. *J Clin Endocrinol Metab*. 2004;89:892–897.

184. Steelman J, Kappy M. Adrenal suppresion and growth retardation from ocular corticosteroids. *J Pediatr Ophthalmol Strabis*. 2001;38:177–178.

185. Afandi B, Toumeh MS, Saadi HF. Cushing's syndrome caused by unsupervised use of ocular glucocorticoids. *Endocr Pract*. 2003;9:526–529.

186. Smith EP, Boyd J, Frank GR, et al. Estrogen resistance caused by a mutation in the estrogen-receptor gene in a man. *N Engl J Med*. 1994;331:1056–1061.

187. Eugster EA, Dimeglio LA, Wright JC, et al. Height outcome in congenital adrenal hyperplasia caused by 21-hydroxylase deficiency: A meta-analysis. *J Pediatr*. 2001;138:26–32.

188. Lin-Su K, Vogiatzi MG, Marshall I, et al. Treatment with growth hormone and luteinizing hormone releasing hormone analog improves final adult height in children with congenital adrenal hyperplasia. *J Clin Endocrinol Metab*. 2005;90:3318–3325.

189. Heger S, Sippell WG, Partsch CJ. Gonadotropin-releasing hormone analogue treatment for precocious puberty: Twenty years of experience. *Endocr Dev*. 2005;8

190. Lanes R, Soros A, Jakubowicz S. Accelerated versus slowly progressive forms of puberty in girls with precocious and early puberty: Gondotropin suppressive efffect and final height obtained with two different analogs. *J Pediatr Endocrinol Metab*. 2004;17:759–766.

191. Kaplowitz PB, Oberfield SE. Reexamination of the age limit for defining when puberty is precocious in girls in the United States: Implication and treatment. Drug and Therapeutics and Executive Committees of the Lawson Wilkins Pediatric Endocrine Society. *Pediatrics*. 1999;104:936–941.

192. Mauras N, Merimee T, Rogol AD. Function of the growth hormone-insulin-like growth factor I axis in the profoundly growth-retarded diabetic child: Evidence for defective targe organ responsiveness in the Mauriac syndrome. *Metab Clin Exp*. 1991;40:1106–1111.

193. Lebl J, Schober E, Zidek T, et al. Growth data in large series of 587 children and adolescents with type 1 diabetes mellitus. *Endocr Reg*. 2003;37:153–161.

194. Salerno M, Argenziano A, Di Maio S, et al. Pubertal growth, sexual maturation, and final height in children with IDDM: Effects of age at onset and metabolic control. *Diabetes Care*. 1997;20:721–724.

195. Kemp SF, Elders MJ, Fiser RH Jr, Butenandt O. Disorders of growth. In: Eichenwald HF, Stroder J, Ginsburg CM, eds. *Pediatric Therapy*, 3rd ed. St. Louis: Mosby; 1993:230–233.

196. Sotos JF, Dodge PR, D M, et al. Cerebral gigantism in childhood: A syndrome of excessively rapid growth with acromegalic features and a nonprogressive neurologic disorder. *N Engl J Med*. 1964;271:109.

CHAPTER 31

Turner Syndrome

Constantine A. Stratakis, MD, D(Med)Sci
Kyriakie Sarafoglou, MD
Bradley S. Miller, MD, PhD, FAAP

ETIOLOGY OF TURNER SYNDROME

Turner syndrome (TS) is the most common genetic disorder affecting only women. The criteria of diagnosis are complete or partial absence of the second sex chromosome (with or without cell line mosaicism) and the presence of phenotypic TS features. The genotype in TS is most commonly 45,X. Besides the X chromosome monosomy (45,X), other karyotype abnormalities in TS patients include 45,X/46,XX (the most frequent mosaicism usually resulting in a milder clinical phenotype), 45,X/46,XY (resulting in partial or mixed gonadal dysgenesis), and structural abnormalities of the X chromosome such as deletions, rings, translocations, or isochromosomes (an abnormal X chromosome with equal arms caused by a transverse division of the centromere during cell division instead of normal longitudinal division). Overall, mosaicism was found in approximately 80% of patients with 45,X when two tissues (lymphocytes and fibroblasts) were examined (1).

The frequency of TS at conception is approximately 3%; however, 99% of these fetuses are aborted spontaneously, and the disorder affects only 1 in 1800 to 5000 live-born females in different populations (2). The prevalence of the syndrome (at birth) has been estimated in the white population at 25–55 cases per 100,000 females (3). However, we are also beginning to see a significant difference both in prevalence and in incidence of X chromosome anomalies between prospective studies and the analysis of case series and cohorts of patients presenting to endocrine/genetics clinics. In a 13-year prospective study of 17,038 girls born in Denmark who had karyotype testing, the incidence of TS was 1 in 1893 live female births, with only 1 of the 9 detected cases having a 45,X karyotype and the remaining cases being mosaic and having a variety of X abnormalities (4). This differs from the case series and cohort studies where X chromosome complete monosomy is responsible for TS in approximately half of

patients (5). Thus ascertainment bias likely plays a significant role in the clinical detection of TS.

The phenotypic characteristics of TS reflect the haploinsufficiency of specific genes located mainly in the pseudoautosomal region (PAR) of the X chromosome (Xp11.2-p22.1). Normally in females, one X chromosome is randomly inactivated, except in PAR, which retain two allelic pairs. One of these genes, the SHOX gene (short stature homeobox-containing gene) is located in the pseudoautosomal region of the X chromosome and is considered the gene responsible for most of the skeletal abnormalities in TS, such as short stature, short neck, cubitus valgus (increased carrying angle), genu valgum, and short fourth metacarpals (6). SHOX expression in primary fibroblasts and chondrocytes leads to cell cycle arrest and apoptosis, suggesting that the protein plays a direct role in regulating the differentiation of these cells in the growth plate (7). Besides TS, mutations in SHOX have been associated with Léri–Weill dyschondrosteosis, characterized by dorsal subluxation of the distal end of the ulna (Madelung deformity) and mesomelic short stature (8).

Many of the other phenotypic features found in a minority of patients (most notably webbed neck) are deformations secondary to the intrauterine lymphedema that results from an as yet unidentified lymphogenic gene in a non-pseudoautosomal region of the X chromosome (9). Abnormalities in two other regions on the X chromosome, POF1 and POF2, are considered important in the development of premature ovarian failure. However, the genes involved within these regions have not been delineated.

Studies have shown the presence of Y chromosome material in patients with TS (5,10–14) with a frequency of between 4% and 5%, as detected in the peripheral blood G-banding karyotype of TS patients; an additional 3% to 5% of TS patients who have an unidentifiable marker may have chromosomal material derived from the Y chromosome

that may be identified by fluorescent in situ hybridization (FISH) (5,10–16). In addition, molecular analysis by DNA amplification of Y chromosome–located genes (or microsatellite repeats) identifies an additional 2% to 4% of TS patients with presumably Y chromosome–negative karyotypes (12–14). Thus the true incidence of Y chromosome material among TS patients may be as high as 10% to 15% (5,10–14). While Y chromosome material in a small percentage of patients and some degree of virilization in an even smaller percent are compatible with TS when the internal genitalia are female and the phenotype is otherwise compatible with monosomy of genes on the X chromosome (short stature and other features of TS), intersex disorders with similar chromosomal karyotypes need to be differentiated from Turner syndrome (17–19). Similarly, phenotypic characteristics such as webbed neck and short stature can be found in both males and females who do not have TS (no X monosomy) but who have other genetic disorders, such as Noonan syndrome. These phenotypic characteristics of Noonan syndrome have been found to be due to heterozygosity of an activating mutation of PTPN11 in approximately 50% of cases (20–21); other Noonan syndrome genes have recently been identified as well.

Clinical Presentation The age at diagnosis of TS is related to the phenotypic features present in that individual (1). Some phenotypic characteristics are shown in Figure 31-1 and are listed on the At-A-Glance page.

During the prenatal period, ultrasonography and amniocentesis performed due to abnormal fetal screening and advanced maternal age commonly lead to the diagnosis of TS. Cardiovascular and lymphatic abnormalities are the most likely reasons for diagnosis by prenatal ultrasound and in the newborn period. In the toddler and prepubertal child, failure to thrive/short stature, otologic abnormalities, and school difficulties are common reasons for diagnosis. In the young

Turner Syndrome

AT-A-GLANCE

Turner syndrome (TS) is a rare chromosomal disorder of females characterized by short stature and the lack of sexual development at puberty. Patients with TS have an abnormal karyotype involving the X chromosome. More than 50% of girls with TS have the 45,X karyotype, whereas others have 46,XX with one of the X chromosomes being abnormal; a wide range of X abnormalities exists, including gene deletions, ring chromosomes, and isochromosomes.

Between 20% and 35% of TS patients have mosaic karyotypes such as 45,X/46,XX, and between 5% and 10% of patients have a cell line with Y chromosome material present. The 45,X karyotype generally is the most severely affected. The clinical presentation is quite variable depending on the amount of normal X or Y chromosome material present. Almost 99% of conceptions with the 45,X karyotype result in miscarriage, and thus the true prevalence of TS is consider-

ably higher than the birth prevalence of about 1 in 2000. Patients with TS require a multidisciplinary approach throughout their lives as clinical and molecular investigations examine a cascade of issues–from those associated with the TS-related phenotype (i.e., short stature, bone density and skeletal defects, cardiovascular, fertility, and other anomalies) and from those associated with post–growth hormone and post-estrogen replacement effects.

PRESENTATION

Frequent (>50%)

Growth deficiency
Gonadal dysgenesis
Lymphedema of hands and feet as newborn
Deep-set, hyperconvex nails
Unusual shape and rotation of ears
Narrow maxilla and dental crowding
Micrognathia
Low posterior hairline
Broad chest (with inverted or hypoplastic nipples)
Cubitus valgus
Short fourth metacarpals
Tibial exostosis
Tendency to obesity
Recurrent otitis media
Feeding difficulties in newborn period

Less Frequent (<50%)

Hearing loss
Pigmented nevi
Webbed neck
Renal abnormalities
Cardiovascular anomalies
Hypertension
Hypothyroidism
Glucose intolerance
Hyperlipidemia
Gonadoblastoma (<5%)
Juvenile rheumatoid arthritis (<5%)
Scoliosis, kyphosis, Madelung deformity (<5%)
Gastrointestinal–celiac, inflammatory bowel disease (IBD) (<5%)
Elevated liver function tests
Eye–strabismus, ptosis, epicanthal folds

HEALTH SUPERVISION GUIDELINES FOR CHILDREN WITH TURNER'S SYNDROME

System	Procedure/Evaluation	Monitoring
Eyes	Strabismus	Objectively from 4 months; at least one evaluation by ophthalmologist
Ears	Hearing	Audiologist at birth/diagnosis and every 3–5 years.
Mouth	Malocclusion	Starting at 2 years; at least one evaluation by orthodontist
Genetics	Counseling	Diagnosis (parents) and late adolescence or early adulthood (patient)
Heart	Echocardiography Fasting lipid profile	At diagnosis; repeat every 3–5 years beginning at 12 years; consider MRI; annual screening starting at time of puberty
Kidney	Sonography	At diagnosis
Gastrointestinal	Celiac and IBD screen	At regular intervals after 3 years of age
Skeletal	Hip dysplasia Scoliosis/kyphosis	Every visit from birth to 9 months Start screening yearly at 5 years of age
Stature	Growth chart	At every visit from birth; consider growth hormone therapy early
Thyroid	Function tests	Start screening from 4 years
Ovary	Puberty/ovarian failure	Start evaluations from 5 years
Psychosocial	Development, behavior, learning disabilities, socialization	At every visit from birth

Modified from ref. 1.

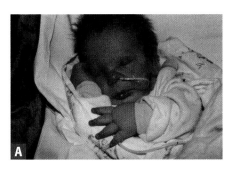

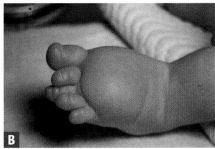

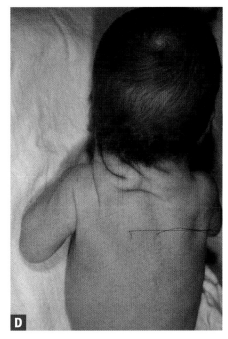

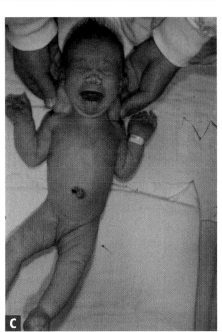

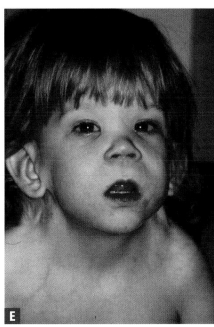

FIGURE 31-1. A to **E.** Spectrum of phenotypic characteristics in Turner's syndrome (edema of the dorsum of hands (A) and feet (B), webbing of the neck (C,D,E), low hairline (D), epicanthal folds (E), downward droop of outer corner of eyes (E), low-set ears and micrognathia (C,E). (Courtesy of Robert Gorlin, D.D.S., M.S., D.Sc., and Susan Berry, M.D., University of Minnesota Medical School.)

adolescent woman, short stature and delay of pubertal development are common reasons for suspecting TS. In adulthood, secondary amenorrhea is a common reason for diagnosis of TS. The major categories of phenotypic features are described below.

Short Stature

Short stature is the most common clinical characteristic of TS. Without intervention, TS patients attain a mean adult height of 143 cm (20 cm below that of the control female population). In 1995, a comprehensive report on almost 200 adults with TS showed that the final height of these women (age >18 years) was 146.7 ± 6.6 cm, whereas the subset that had been treated with some growth-promoting agent (9 patients) had a final height of 149.1 ± 6 cm (22). Growth in children with TS is characterized by a slight intrauterine growth retardation (−1 standard deviation [SD]), slow growth during infancy and childhood, and lack of the pubertal growth spurt. More than

half the girls with TS have fallen below the fifth percentile by 2 years of age (23).

Primary Ovarian Failure

Primary ovarian failure resulting in pubertal delay is a common phenotypic feature of TS. At 14–18 weeks' gestation, the ovaries of the 45,X fetus appear to be completely normal. After this, however, there is rapid loss of oocytes and stromal fibrosis so that in the majority of girls with TS, complete or near-complete follicular atresia has occurred prenatally or within the first several months or years of postnatal life. The genetic mechanism for this follicular atresia is as yet unknown. However, some pubertal development may occur in up to 30% of children with TS: 12% experience spontaneous menses, some go through complete puberty, and spontaneous pregnancies have been reported in 2% to 5% of the patients (24,25). Spontaneous menses may occur in as many as 47% of patients with a mosaic karyotype (24). The variability in pubertal development is the likely reason that a recent study found that about 10% of individuals with TS are not diagnosed until adulthood (24).

Plasma gonadotropins are elevated as early as 5 days of life in patients in whom the ovarian failure is present at birth (26). At 2 years of age, the elevated gonadotropin levels decline, but with mean concentrations that are still higher than in normal children. Between the ages 4 and 10–11 years, a trough in gonadotropin levels similar to that which occurs in gonadally normal females is noted, followed by a gradual rise of gonadotropin levels in normal children and a more rapid and exaggerated rise in TS patients with gonadal failure.

Congenital Cardiovascular Defects

Congenital cardiovascular defects (CCVDs) including most commonly bicuspid aortic valve (BV) and coarctation of the aorta (COA) are well-known features of TS (27–29). Aortic root dilatation is present in 3% to 8% of TS girls and may be progressive, leading to dissecting aneurysm, rupture, and death. Other less common cardiovascular defects in patients with TS are mitral valve prolapse, partial anomalous pulmonary venous return, and hypoplastic left heart syndrome. The prevalence of cardiovascular abnormalities is higher in TS patients with X chromosome monosomy. On the basis of these observations, the American Academy of Pediatrics (AAP) recommends that all patients with TS have a careful cardiac evaluation as part of their initial workup (1). In addition to physical examination, the evaluation may consist of echocardiography (ECHO) and magnetic resonance imaging (MRI). The MRI can detect dilatation missed by ECHO, provide accurate measurements of the aortic root dilatation, and assess the possibility of aortic dissection. The periodicity of cardiac evaluations will be determined by the cardiologist, but some have advocated repetition of all imaging every 3 years (1,27,30,31). Patients with a normal cardiac evaluation during childhood should have their blood pressure, peripheral pulses, and heart sounds for possible murmur monitored by their pediatrician. Up to 40% of TS patients develop hypertension, which in most cases is idiopathic and should be treated vigorously. A follow-up evaluation by a cardiologist during adolescence has been proposed to identify aortic root dilatation and late-presenting COA. Women with TS considering assisted fertility also should have an echocardiogram. Prophylactic administration of antibiotics in patients with cardiac malformations before dental or surgical procedures is essential because of increased susceptibility to endocarditis.

It is unknown if cardiac defects in TS are due to haploinsufficiency for X chromosome gene(s) involved in cardiovascular development or secondary to other features of the syndrome, such as massive fetal lymphedema impinging on heart and major vessel formation. This latter possibility was suggested by observations of an apparent increased prevalence of CCVDs in individuals with TS and neck webbing and supported by further epidemiological observations in studies of infants with neck webbing and 45,X embryos ascertained because of cystic hygromas and similar anomalies (9,32–34). These studies were retrospective and had a likely bias toward the most severely affected individuals. In a recent prospective study from the National Institutes of Health (NIH) of 134 volunteers with TS who were not selected for cardiovascular disease and who underwent physical examination and evaluation by MRI and ECHO, the association between cardiovascular defects and lymphedema was confirmed; however, unlike previous studies, it was suggested that haploinsufficiency for an X chromosome gene independently causes fetal lymphedema (webbed neck) and congenital heart defects (35).

Hearing Loss

Hearing loss is a major cause of disability and discomfort for TS patients (36). At NIH, it has been found that up to 90% of the TS population has some degree of hearing impairment. It is predominantly sensorineural hearing loss (sensorineural dip in the 1.5- to 2-kHz region) and less commonly mixed (conductive and sensorineural) (36). Pure conductive hearing loss is rare in TS (37). The etiology of this condition is unclear and, given the large sensorineural component, can be explained only in part by the numerous episodes of otitis during childhood. This said, otitis media is still a serious problem in children with TS, and in fact, some children with short stature have been diagnosed with TS as a result of recurrent otitis media. The increased incidence of otitis media is due to short and abnormally positioned eustachian tubes, resulting in poor drainage and poor aeration of the middle ear space. Colds, flues, allergies, and other sources that could lead to chronic middle ear problems should be treated immediately to prevent future sequelae, including cholesteatoma formation. It also should be noted that the onset of hearing loss is quite insidious, and if screening is not performed periodically, then patients may have communication problems without realizing that they have hearing impairment. Otologic impairment in adults with TS can have a major negative impact on perceived quality of life (38). AAP guidelines recommend hearing testing as soon as the diagnosis of TS is made (1).

Cognitive Defects

Certain cognitive deficits characterize patients with TS (1,39). However, there has been controversy regarding the degree to which these deficits are due to the genetic or hormonal deficiencies. Indeed, some of these defects (e.g., memory, reaction time, and speeded motor function) are at least partially reversed with estrogen replacement (40,41). In contrast, other areas of cognitive function (e.g., visual-spatial/perceptual skills) are present in both children and adults with TS and are not responsive to estrogen therapy (42). There is converging functional and structural neuroimaging evidence that TS-associated limitations in certain cognitive domains are secondary to perturbations of neural development involving specific cortical areas. TS females have significantly smaller structures in several subcortical areas, including the cerebellum and pons, the thalamus, and nuclei in both limbic (hippocampus) and striatal (caudate, lenticular nuclei) systems (43). Reductions also have been observed in cortical neuroanatomy, particularly in parieto-occipital areas bilaterally and the white matter tracts that connect these areas (genu of the corpus callosum), and the right temporal lobe (44). The extent of some of these structural differences appears related, at least in part, to the degree of monosomy X; TS individuals with a mosaic karyotype had relatively fewer anomalies than the those with the nonmosaic 45,X karyotype (45,46). A recent study that compared the cognitive phenotypes of women with premature ovarian failure (POF) and normal controls with those of women with TS found no difference between normal controls and women with POF. However, both groups were distinctly different from women with TS, indicating that prior estrogen deficiency does not have a major impact on cognitive function in adult females. The study concluded that the genetic deficiencies of women with TS most likely accounted for their specific cognitive phenotype (42).

Hypothyroidism

Hypothyroidism is more prevalent in TS than in the general population and is the most prevalent autoimmune disorder in TS (47). Antithyroid antibodies are present in up to 50% of individuals with TS regardless of karyotype (12,48). However, even higher rates of positive antithyroid antibodies (>80%) have been reported in those with isochromosome [46,Xi(Xq)] karyotype (12). The presence of antithyroid antibodies may predict future development of hypothyroidism. However, hypothyroidism also can develop in the absence of detectable antithyroid antibodies or overt clinical symptoms. The onset of hypothyroidism in TS rarely occurs before 4 years of age, and the incidence increases with age (47,49). Therefore, we recommend screening for hypothyroidism in TS annually after 4 years of age by measuring thyroperoxidase antibodies, thyroid-stimulating hormone (TSH), and thyroxine (free or total). Once thyroperoxidase antibodies are positive, determinations do not need to be repeated. Hypothyroidism in TS should be treated with appropriate L-thyroxine replacement therapy (1).

Congenital Developmental Dysplasia of the Hip

Congenital developmental dysplasia of the hip occurs more frequently in TS. Individuals with TS are also at risk for scoliosis and kyphosis, which can progress during growth hormone administration.

Strabismus

Strabismus develops between the ages of 6 months and 7 years in a third of TS individuals (50). Anterior chamber abnormalities are more common in TS and may present as congenital glaucoma. Approximately 10% of TS individuals are red-green color blind. An eye examination should be part of every clinic visit, and a formal evaluation by an ophthalmologist should be done at around 2 years of age. Children with strabismus after 3 months of age should be referred sooner for ophthalmologic evaluation (1).

Urinary Tract Abnormalities

Urinary tract abnormalities have been reported in 20% to 30% of children with TS (51–53). The incidence may be higher depending on the karyotype, with an increased incidence in 45,X individuals compared with those with mosaicism (51,52). The most common abnormality is horseshoe kidney, followed by duplicated collecting systems (53). Therefore, a renal ultrasound should be completed at diagnosis. Hypertension is a frequent problem in adults with TS (12,22,24,27). Renovascular disease, in addition to preexisting cardiovascular abnormalities, is a major contributing factor (22).

Metabolic Abnormalities

Metabolic abnormalities occur in most patients with TS and are first detectable around the time of adolescence. An increased prevalence of both type 1 and type 2 diabetes mellitus is also reported in TS (54). A number of studies have reported impaired glucose homeostasis in children (55,56) as well as adults (57–59). Women with TS tend to have increased adiposity compared with age-matched controls, and their hypogonadism and/or hormone-replacement therapy may have confounded studies of glucose homeostasis (58,59). However, all these studies lacked proper controls. A recent study that compared glucose homeostasis in women with TS with age- and body mass index (BMI)–matched women with POF and normal healthy female controls showed that insulin sensitivity was higher in women with TS compared with both control groups. Thus glucose intolerance in TS is most likely not due to obesity or hypogonadism but is caused by haploinsufficiency for specific X chromosome gene(s) (60). The same group, when investigating the parents of these TS individuals (79 adults and 32 children with TS), did not find a higher prevalence of diabetes among parents of TS individuals (61). These data did not support earlier evidence that had suggested that diabetes (and other autoimmune disorders) may contribute to the generation of offspring with X chromosomal aneuploidy (4,62) and further strengthened the notion that diabetes or glucose intolerance in TS patients is not classic type 2 diabetes but due to X chromosome–located gene(s) (60). Young, nonobese women with TS have been shown to exhibit an atherogenic lipid profile compared with 46,XX women of the same age and body composition with POF (63,64), confirming earlier data suggesting dyslipidemia in this condition (65). As part of routine care, individuals with TS should have fasting blood glucose, insulin, and lipid profile measured annually starting in the adolescent years.

Bone Mineral Density (BMD)

BMD in individuals with TS is relatively decreased, but it remains unclear whether this is due to an intrinsic bone defect or the lack of gonadal steroids. It has been said that many girls with TS have radiographic osteopenia and a coarse trabecular bone pattern even in the prepubertal years (66), but the supporting evidence is weak due to the difficulties in assessing bone mass and comparing it with appropriate age- and other dimension-matched controls. Recently, at the NIH, individuals with TS were shown to have a selective reduction of cortical BMD at the radius, as measured by dual X-ray absorptiometry (DXA) also known as dual energy X-ray absorptiometry (DEXA), that was independent of hypogonadism and hormone-replacement therapy (66,67). It was noted that a subset of women who had been treated with recombinant growth hormone (rGH) showed lower cortical BMD than those who had not been treated. GH administration to TS individuals in some studies has been associated with improvements in BMD (68,69) and in other studies had no effect (70,71) or suggested a decrease in BMD related to rGH treatment (67,72). The prevalence of osteoporosis and bone fractures is not increased significantly in women with TS who are treated with standard estrogen therapy (73,74).

It is very important to consider that women less than 150 cm in height are likely to be misdiagnosed with osteoporosis when a real bone density is measured unless adjustments for body size are made. The incidence of fractures in girls with TS probably is not increased significantly overall, other than in a particular location, the wrist, despite references in the literature in support of the opposite (73–79). During preteen years, adequate calcium intake should be ensured (1000 mg of elemental calcium daily), and after 11 years of age, 1200–1500 mg/day should be administered. Adequate vitamin D intake (at least 400 IU/day) also should be encouraged.

Gastrointestinal Disorders

Gastrointestinal (GI) disorders are more common in TS individuals. Inflammatory bowel disease (IBD) is two to three times more common in TS individuals than in the general population, with Crohn's disease more frequent than ulcerative colitis (22,80). Celiac disease, intestinal telangiectasia and resulting GI bleeding, hepatic abnormalities, and polyps also may be more common in TS individuals than in the general population (22,81–83).

Liver Enzyme Abnormalities

Liver enzyme abnormalities are also quite common and probably affect as many as 20% to 25% of the population of women with TS. Abnormal liver function tests raise questions and are troublesome for patients and health care providers (84–86). Few studies have been done to determine the pathophysiology of the "transaminitis." Concepts vary between autoimmune etiology, steatohepatitis, and possible X chromosome gene haploinsufficiency. Liver enzyme values fluctuate, and in one series, levels improved with estrogen replacement (89). Our initial observations suggest that this is not an autoimmune process but rather is related to simple steatosis or a nonalcoholic steatohepatitis-like picture.

Autoimmune Diseases

Autoimmune diseases such as hypothyroidism, celiac disease, IBD, and juvenile rheumatoid arthritis are increased in individuals with TS (47,83,88,89). Screening for these conditions ranges from awareness of the association and directed clinical history to routine laboratory evaluation. Due to the rate of asymptomatic hypothyroidism and celiac disease, routine laboratory screening is recommended at diagnosis and periodically thereafter.

Neoplasia

Neoplasia is not significantly more common in adult patients with TS save for gonadoblastoma, colon cancer, and gynecologic cancer (90). Whether the gynecologic cancers are related to estrogen replacement, favored by a defective genetic background, is a hypothesis that remains to be investigated (12,24,36). Since the data regarding the incidence of colon cancer predate therapy of TS individuals with rGH, long-term follow-up of these individuals will be necessary to address this issue. The incidence of gonadoblastoma in TS individuals and what to do to detect it, however, are a matter of debate. The overall prevalence of this tumor among individuals with any TS-causing karyotype does not seem to exceed 12% (10). Among patients with G-banding-detected Y chromosome material, the incidence of gonadoblastoma may be as high as 25%. There is no evidence that the presence of the SRY gene confers risk for gonadoblastoma; deletion analysis of patients' chromosomes and their tumors showed that the putative gonadoblastoma gene (GBY) is in fact near the Y chromosome centromere, not on distal Yp (where SRY is located) (14).

Diagnosis

Prenatal Diagnosis Most concepti with a 45,X karyotype abort spontaneously. Most, if not all, of those who survive to birth are suspected to have mosaicism for a normal cell line. TS may be diagnosed prenatally by amniocentesis or chorionic villus sampling. A karyotype should be obtained by one of these methods if ultrasonography of a fetus shows a nuchal cystic hygroma, horseshoe kidney, left-sided cardiac anomalies, or nonimmune fetal hydrops. A postnatal karyotype may be performed instead of amniocentesis or chorionic villus sampling, and it is also recommended if the human chorionic gonadotropin, estradiol, or alpha-fetoprotein is elevated during pregnancy.

When a prenatal diagnosis of TS is made by ultrasonography (91), prenatal biochemical screening (92), or amniocentesis performed for other reasons, counseling needs to be provided to the family (1). However, the phenotype cannot be predicted from the karyotype alone, even in nonmosaic TS, and the AAP recommends that careful sonographic investigation of the fetus be performed to define phenotypic abnormalities "as accurately as possible" and the gender of the fetus (in cases of Y chromosome mosaicism). For the latter, determination of amniotic fluid testosterone levels may be helpful (93). If a prenatal diagnosis is made, then the ultrasound is the best predictor of phenotype. Since many of the "malformations" of TS are, in fact, deformations secondary to edema (e.g., neck webbing, low hairline, rotated ears, upturned nails, etc.), if no edema is detected, these malformations are unlikely or are not going to be present, and the risk for COA is significantly lower.

Postnatal Diagnosis

In females, pedal edema in the neonate, growth failure at any age, or pubertal delay should warrant a diagnostic evaluation for TS. Other phenotypic features also may lead to suspicion of TS (1). A high-resolution karyotype should be performed with a sufficient number of cells to exclude low-level mosaicism.

At present, the AAP does not recommend "routine use of polymerase chain reaction (PCR) [techniques] to identify cryptic material," although it emphasizes that "girls with TS should have an adequate cytogenetic examination for covert Y chromosome mosaicism, including FISH" (1). This is perhaps the most prudent path given three factors: (1) lack of evidence that all patient with Y chromosome material develop gonadoblastoma and the need for more research to define the exact region of Y associated with this tumor, (2) the possibility of unnecessary operations and associated risks (e.g., in a previously quoted study of seven patients with Y material detected by PCR alone, three went on to have

ovariectomies that did not reveal tumors, and all the others, more than 50 years of age, had detailed imaging studies that failed to show any tumors), and (3) gonadoblastoma is not a malignant tumor per se. Gonadoblastoma is a gonadal tumor that consists of normal components of the ovary, granulosa–Sertoli type and Leydig–thecal type cells. It is only the germ cell component that may acquire a malignant potential and invade the ovarian stroma, where it forms a malignant germinoma or a seminoma; only rarely, a more aggressive tumor such as embryonal carcinoma or choriocarcinoma may develop within a gonadoblastoma.

Screening for Y chromosome material by molecular techniques should be done in all patients with (1) evidence for the presence of a marker chromosome (approximately 3% of all TS patients) because most markers are indeed derived from the Y chromosome (94) and (2) if any signs of masculinization exist at birth or develop later in life because many of the Y-containing tissues may lead to androgen (or even estrogen sometimes) production (1).

GENETIC COUNSELING

The molecular investigation of patients with a karyotype associated with TS is significant for two reasons: (1) for counseling reasons because there is an association of a mosaicism containing a second X or a Y with higher chances for fetal survival (when the karyotype information is obtained as part of prenatal screening) and (2) for medical care because patients with Y chromosome material are at risk for the development of gonadoblastoma.

The presence of X chromosome monosomy (or other X chromosome abnormalities) in association with Down syndrome also has been reported with an incidence that appears to be greater than that due to chance alone (95). This is not surprising because different chromosomal anomalies can coexist presumably due to the same deficient molecular mechanism that would have to do with dysregulation of chromosome separation or duplication; for example, Klinefelter syndrome also occurs with trisomy 21 at a frequency greater than expected by chance alone.

Disposition of a TS-associated chromosomal defect is not clear. Overall, there is no increased risk for recurrence of such chromosomal defects among TS families. However, carriers of X chromosome–involved translocations, as well as families with other chromosomal defects, including Down syndrome, are at increased risk (96). Advanced paternal age is a factor for the X,i(Xq) karyotype (97); twin sisters of patients with both the 45,X and the X,i(Xq) karyotype also may be at increased risk (98). Although earlier studies had shown no association of the chance

for a 45,X karyotype with advanced maternal age (99,100), newer observations suggest that such correlation in fact may exist, albeit weakly (66). There is an inverse correlation between maternal age and X chromosome abnormalities in a spontaneously aborted fetus (101), reflecting perhaps the increasing incidence of other chromosomal anomalies in spontaneous abortions of older mothers. Environmental factors, autoimmunity (in the mother or the family), seasonality of conception and birth, or the birth date or year do not seem to play a role.

TREATMENT AND MANAGEMENT

The results of baseline screening for anatomical abnormalities of the renal and cardiovascular systems and the presence of Y chromosome material, otolaryngological problems, learning disabilities, and associated autoimmune conditions such as thyroiditis, celiac disease, and IBD will determine the initial management and subsequent monitoring of children and adults with TS. After baseline screening, it is important to monitor individuals with TS for the development of associated conditions (1,102). During childhood and adolescence, most of the active treatment of TS is directed at correcting the somatic abnormalities, augmenting the short stature, and inducing secondary sexual development.

Growth-Promoting Therapy

Growth-promoting therapy regimen selection often is based on the age at diagnosis. Recombinant growth harmone (rGH), at doses up to 0.375 mg/kg per week, has been approved for use and is now considered the standard care for a child with TS (1). It is usually not started until the child's height falls below the 5th percentile for healthy girls of the same age. However, a recent study has shown that earlier rGH treatment of young TS patients can abrogate the height loss compared with their peers (103). Final height gains may be as high as 8 to 10 cm with or without delaying estrogen-replacement therapy (104–107). Higher doses of rGH may be associated with increased height gain (108), although the potential for adverse late effects has not been evaluated adequately. There are no current data on the utility of monitoring insulin-like growth factor type 1 (IGF-1) levels during rGH therapy in TS. rGH dose appears to be the most important predictor of height velocity in the first year of rGH therapy, whereas for height gain in years 2–4 of therapy, the velocity during the previous year is the most important predictor.

When given in conjunction with rGH, low-dose nonaromatizable anabolic steroids (such as 0.0625 mg/kg/d oxandrolone) may or may not have a beneficial effect on final height (104,109–113); when used alone, anabolic steroids lead to increased short-term height velocity, which again most likely does not lead to improvements in final height (111). Oxandrolone therapy should be considered in individuals with TS who are of pubertal age and are unlikely to attain a satisfactory adult height.

Standard estrogen feminization therapy has been felt to have a negative impact on growth. The near-adult height has been shown to increase with the number of estrogen-free years of rGH therapy (114). These data suggest that estrogen should not be used as a growth-promoting agent and should be reserved for feminization when the child has reached an appropriate height. The use of low-dose estrogen (as low as 25 ng/kg/d) leads to short-term increases in growth velocity but also may accelerate bone maturation (especially in younger patients with bone ages before 11 years), which may or may not compromise final height (115,116). However, early parenteral administration of low-dose estrogen (0.2 mg estradiol cypionate monthly) did not interfere with the effect of GH on height enhancement (117). Transdermal estrogen therapy, as a patch or cream applied daily or intermittently, would be expected to deliver similar levels of estradiol to parenteral injection without the negative effect on IGF-1 production seen with oral estrogens. Therefore, low-dose estrogen therapy, either parenteral or transdermal, may be an option for early feminization. Further studies of the impact of transdermal patch and cream delivery methods of low-dose estrogen therapy on final adult height, feminization, uterine growth, and pregnancy success are needed.

Stature versus Maturation Earlier diagnosis and initiation of GH treatment in children with TS should help patients to attain heights near the normal range at a younger age. Better growth, in turn, leads to the earlier introduction of estrogen therapy, allowing feminization to occur at a time closer to that of the child's peers. According to the 2006 Turner Syndrome Consensus Study Group, puberty should not be delayed to promote statural growth because this approach undervalues the psychosocial importance of age-appropriate pubertal maturation (126). In addition, the earlier initiation of estrogen would be expected to improve uterine growth, which may reduce the risk of miscarriage in adult women with TS seeking assisted pregnancy.

In children diagnosed with TS after 11 years of age, giving at least 1 year of GH prior to initiating estrogen therapy improved final adult height in a fashion similar to initiating standard estrogen therapy at 12 years of age (104).

Feminization

Feminization regimens for girls with TS should follow a protocol of slow introduction of sex steroids with the ultimate goals of cycling and achieving near-normal serum estradiol levels (39). A common practice involves initiation of estrogen therapy at a bone age greater than 12 years and not later than a chronological age of 15 years. The timing of this therapy should be discussed with the child and her parents as it relates to their height target. The common feminization regimen uses oral estrogen beginning with 0.3 mg of conjugated estrogens (Premarin) daily for 6 months, followed by 0.625 mg Premarin daily for another 6 months. After the first year of estrogen alone therapy, the Premarin dose is increased to 1.25, and cycling starts with the addition of 10 mg medroxyprogesterone acetate (Provera). The increased dose is recommended to start on the first of the month; 1.25 mg Premarin is received on days 1–23 of the month, and 10 mg Provera is received on days 10–23; no medication is given on days 23–30/31, when withdrawal menses usually occur. Many other feminization regimens exist, including transdermal and parenteral forms of estrogen and different progestins. Current guidelines (126) suggest waiting 2 years after starting estrogen or until breakthrough bleeding occurs before initiating progestin to improve breast and uterine development. One published transdermal feminization regimen involves initiation of 0.0125 mg transdermal 17β-estradiol. The transdermal 17β-estradiol is increased by 0.0125 mg every 6 months until the adult target dose (0.1 mg) is reached (102). Delaying estrogen therapy is likely to have a negative impact on uterine growth. This may become relevant when women with TS consider assisted fertility. Small uterine size can be a limiting factor in the ability to carry a pregnancy resulting from donated ova and in vitro fertilization to term. Normal gynecological care is provided for all cycling TS girls.

Pregnancy

Pregnancy in TS was addressed by a recent review (118). Some women with TS are able to conceive and have children of their own (24,25,118). The majority have the option of receiving a donated ovum with a success rate of 40% per treatment cycle and a 50% chance for each pregnancy to achieve a live birth (24,25). A hypoplastic or bicornuate uterus has been associated with a high rate of miscarriage once fertilization and implantation occur (119). The trophic response of the uterus to estrogen diminishes with age. Therefore, earlier initiation of estrogen therapy is likely to allow uterine growth to achieve proportions similar to those of adult 46,XX females (120,121). More recently, oocytes were found in adolescents with TS who did not have ovarian function clinically (122). This raises the possibility of cryopreservation and later reimplantation of ovarian tissue for adult women with TS, which previously has led to pregnancy in a woman following chemotherapy (123). Transplantation of ovarian tissue also may be a future pregnancy option (124). It is unclear whether either of these options will be viable in TS individuals.

The safety of pregnancy in women with TS should be considered carefully due to the risk of aortic root rupture and other cardiovascular implications. All patients with TS need to undergo careful cardiovascular assessment prior to pregnancy. When a pregnancy occurs, cephalopelvic disproportion is common, and caesarean section is the most likely mode of delivery (24).

Adult women with TS require ongoing health care management and screening. Many of the conditions associated with TS develop or progress over time. The adult care provider needs to be aware of the complex medical needs of TS individuals. A smooth transition process from the care of pediatricians to adult care providers may be facilitated by a "transition passport"(125). This transition passport is designed to be a summary of previous health issues as well as an educational tool for the patient and provider regarding adult health care guidelines for TS (12,125).

Information and educational materials for families, patients, and health care providers are available from the Turner's Syndrome Society of the United States (www.turner-syndrome-us.org). Links to regional, national, and international societies are available through this website. The Turner Syndrome International Registry (www.tsregistry.org) houses a confidential patient database and a public provider database. The registry's goals are to connect patients with providers knowledgeable about TS and to connect researchers with patients willing to participate in surveys and clinical trials with the ultimate goal of advancing health care of individuals with TS.

REFERENCES

1. Frias JL, Davenport ML. Health supervision for children with Turner syndrome. *Pediatrics.* 2003;692–702.
2. Lippe B. Turner syndrome. *Endocrinol Metab Clin North Am.* 1991;20.121–152.
3. Gravholt GH, Juul S, Naera RW, et al. Prenatal and postnatal prevalence of Turner

syndrome: A registry study. *Br Med J.* 1996;312:16–21.

4. Nielsen J, Wohlert M. Sex chromosome abnormalities found among 34,910 newborn children: Results from a 13-year incidence study in Arhus, Denmark. *Birth Defects.* 1990;26:209–223.

5. Alvarez-Nava F, Soto M, Sanchez MA, et al. Molecular analysis in Turner syndrome. *J Pediatr.* 2003;142:336–340.

6. Kosho T, Muroya K, Nagai T, et al. Skeletal features and growth patterns in 14 patients with haploinsufficiency of SHOX: Implications for the development of Turner syndrome. *J Clin Endocrinol Metab* 1999;84:4613–4621.

7. Marchini A, Marttila T, Winter A, et al. The short stature homeodomain protein SHOX induces cellular growth arrest and apoptosis and is expressed in human growth plate chondrocytes. *J Biol Chem* 2004;279:37103–37114.

8. Shears DJ, Vassal HJ, Goodman FR, et al. Mutation and deletion of the pseudoautosomal gene SHOX cause Leri-Weill dyschondrosteosis. *Nat Genet.* 1998;19:70–73.

9. Boucher CA, Sargent CA, Ogata T, et al. Breakpoint analysis of Turner patients with partial Xp deletions: Implications for the lymphoedema gene location. *J Med Genet.* 2001;38:591–598.

10. Gravholt CH, Fedder J, Naeraa RW, et al. Occurrence of gonadoblastoma in females with Turner syndrome and Y chromosome material: A population study. *J Clin Endocrinol Metab.* 2000;85:3199–3202.

11. Chu CE, Connor JM, Donaldson MD, et al. Detection of Y mosaicism in patients with Turner's syndrome. *J Med Genet.* 1995;32:578–580.

12. Elsheikh M, Dunger DB, Conway GS, et al. Turner's syndrome in adulthood. *Endocr Rev.* 2002;23:120–140.

13. Robinson DO, Dalton P, Jacobs PA, et al. A molecular and FISH analysis of structurally abnormal Y chromosomes in patients with Turner's syndrome. *J Med Genet.* 1999;36:279–284.

14. Page DC. Y chromosome sequences in Turner syndrome and risk of gonadoblastoma or virilization. *Lancet.* 1994;343:240–242.

15. Coto E, Toral JF, Menendez MJ, et al. PCR-based study of the presence of Y-chromosome sequences in patients with Ullrich-Turner syndrome. *Am J Med Genet.* 1995;57:393–396.

16. Monroy N, Lopez M, Cervantes A, et al. Microsatellite analysis in Turner syndrome: Parental origin of X chromosomes and possible mechanism of formation of abnormal chromosomes. *Am J Med Genet.* 2002;107:181–189.

17. Salo P, Ignatius J, Simola KO, et al. Clinical features of nine males with molecularly defined deletions of the Y chromosome long arm. *J Med Genet.* 1995;32:711–715.

18. Tzancheva M, Kaneva R, Kumanov P, et al. Two male patients with ring Y: Definition of an interval in Yq contributing to Turner syndrome. *J Med Genet.* 1999;36:549–553.

19. Barbaux S, Vilain E, Raoul O, et al. Proximal deletions of the long arm of the Y chromosome suggest a critical region associated with a specific subset of characteristic Turner stigmata. *Hum Mol Genet.* 1995;4:1565–1568.

20. Binder G, Neuer K, Ranke MB, et al. PTPN11 mutations are associated with mild growth hormone resistance in individuals with Noonan syndrome. *J Clin Endocrinol Metab.* 2005;90:5377–5381.

21. Tartaglia M, Mehler EL, Goldberg R, et al. Mutations in PTPN11, encoding the protein tyrosine phosphatase SHP-2, cause Noonan syndrome. *Nat Genet.* 2001;29:465–468.

22. Sybert V. The adult patient with Turner syndrome. In: Albertsson-Winkland K, Ranke M, eds. *Turner Syndrome in a Life-Span Perspective.* New York: Elsevier Science; 1995:205–218.

23. Davenport M, et al: Growth failure in early life: An important manifestation of Turner syndrome *Horm Res.* 2002;57:157–164.

24. Ostberg JE. Conway GS. Adulthood in women with Turner syndrome. *Horm Res.* 2003;59:211–221.

25. Conway GS. The impact and management of Turner syndrome in adult life. *Best Pract Res Clin Endocrinol Metab.* 2002;16:243–261.

26. Conte FA, et al. A diphasic pattern of gonadotropin secretion in patients with the syndrome of gonadal dysgenesis. *J Clin Endocrinol Metab.* 1975;40:670–674.

27. Sybert VP. Cardiovascular malformations and complications in Turner syndrome. *Pediatrics.* 1998;101:e11.

28. Gotzsche CO, Krag-Olsen B, Nielsen J, et al. Prevalence of cardiovascular malformations and association with karyotypes in Turner's syndrome. *Arch Dis Child* 1994;71:433–436.

29. Mazzanti L, Cacciari E. Congenital heart disease in patients with Turner's syndrome. Italian Study Group for Turner Syndrome (ISGTS). *J Pediatr.* 1998;133:688–692.

30. Lin AE, Lippe B, Rosenfeld RG. Further delineation of aortic dilation, dissection, and rupture in patients with Turner syndrome. *Pediatrics* 1998;102:e12.

31. Ho VB, Bakalov VK, Cooley M, et al. Major vascular anomalies in Turner syndrome: Prevalence and magnetic resonance angiographic features. *Circulation* 2004;110:1694–1700.

32. Berdahl LD, Wenstrom KD, Hanson JW. Web neck anomaly and its association with congenital heart disease. *Am J Med Genet.* 1985;56:304–307.

33. Brady A, Patton M. Web-neck anomaly and its association with congenital heart disease. *Am J Med Genet.* 1996;64:605–606.

34. Clark EB. Neck web and congenital heart defects: A pathogenic association in 45, X-O Turner syndrome. *Teratology.* 1984;29:355–361.

35. Lozcalzo ML, Van PL, HoVB, et al. Association between fetal lymphedema and congenital cardiac and renal anomalies in Turner syndrome pediatrics. 2005;115(3):732–735.

36. Hultcrantz M. Ear and hearing problems in Turner syndrome. *Acta Otolaryngol.* 2003;123:253–257.

37. Barrenas M-L, Landin-Wilhelmsen K, Hanson C. Ear and hearing in relation to genotype and growth in Turner syndrome. *Hear Res.* 2000;144:21–28.

38. Carel JC, Ecosse E, Bastie-Sigeac I, et al. Quality of life determinants in young women with Turner's syndrome after growth hormone treatment: Results of the StaTur

39. Stratakis CA, Rennert OM. Turner syndrome: *An update. Endocrinologist.* 2005;15:27–36.

40. Ross JL, Roeltgen D, Feuillan P, et al. Use of estrogen in young girls with Turner syndrome: Effects on memory. *Neurology.* 2000;54:164–170.

41. Ross JL, Roeltgen D, Feuillan P, et al. Effects of estrogen on nonverbal processing speed and motor function in girls with Turner's syndrome. *J Clin Endocrinol Metab.* 1998;83:3198–204.

42. Ross JL, Stefanatos GA, Kushner H, et al. The effect of genetic differences and ovarian failure: Intact cognitive function in adult women with premature ovarian failure versus turner syndrome. *J Clin Endocrinol Metab.* 2004;89:1817–1822.

43. Murphy DG, DeCarli C, Daly E, et al. X-chromosome effects on female brain: A magnetic resonance imaging study of Turner's syndrome. *Lancet.* 1993;342:1197–1200.

44. Reiss AL, Mazzocco MM, Greenlaw R, et al. Neurodevelopmental effects of X monosomy: A volumetric imaging study. *Ann Neurol.* 1995;38:731–738.

45. Murphy DG, Mentis MJ, Pietrini P, et al. A PET study of Turner's syndrome: Effects of sex steroids and the X chromosome on brain. *Biol Psychiatry.* 1997;41:285–298.

46. Lawrence K, Kuntsi J, Coleman M, et al. Face and emotion recognition deficits in Turner syndrome: A possible role for X-linked genes in amygdala development. *Neuropsychology.* 2003;17:39–49.

47. Radetti G, Mazzanti L, Paganini C, et al. Frequency, clinical and laboratory features of thyroiditis in girls with Turner's syndrome. The Italian Study Group for Turner's Syndrome. *Acta Paediatr.* 1995;84:909–912.

48. El-Mansoury M, Bryman I, Berntorp K, et al. Hypothyroidism is common in Turner syndrome: Results of a five-year follow-up. *J Clin Endocrinol Metab.* 2005;90:2131–2135.

49. Medeiros CC, et al. Turner's syndrome and thyroid disease: A transverse study of pediatric patients in Brazil. *J Pediatr Endocrinol Metab.* 2000;13:357–362.

50. Chrousos GA, Ross JL, Chrousos G, et al. Ocular findings in Turner syndrome: A prospective study. *Ophthalmology.* 1984;91:926–928.

51. Mazzanti L, Bergamaschi R, Scarano E, et al. Renal malformations in patients with Turner's syndrome. *Horm Res.* 1999;51:59.

52. Flynn MT, Ekstrom L, De Arce M, et al. Prevalence of renal malformation in Turner syndrome. *Pediatr Nephrol.* 1996;10:498–500.

53. Parker KL, Wyatt DT, Blethen SL, et al. Screening girls with Turner syndrome: The National Cooperative Growth Study experience. *Journal of Pediatrics.* 2003;143:133–135.

54. Polychronakos C, Letarte J, Collu R, et al. Carbohydrate intolerance in children and adolescents with Turner syndrome. *J Pediatr.* 1980;96:1009–1014.

55. Cicognani A, Mazzanti L, Tassinari D, et al. Differences in carbohydrate tolerance in Turner syndrome depending on age and karyotype. *Eur J Pediatr.* 1988;148:64–68.

56. Gravholt CH, Naeraa RW, Nyholm B, et al. Glucose metabolism, lipid metabolism, and

cardiovascular risk factors in adult Turner's syndrome: The impact of sex hormone replacement. *Diabetes Care*. 1998;21:1062–1070.

57. Caprio S, Boulware S, Diamond M, et al. Insulin resistance: An early metabolic defect of Turner's syndrome. *J Clin Endocrinol Metab*. 1991;72:832–836.

58. Gravholt CH, Naeraa RW. Reference values for body proportions and body composition in adult women with Ullrich-Turner syndrome. *Am J Med Genet*. 1997;72:403–408.

59. Landin-Wilhelmsen K, Bryman I, Wilhelmsen L. Cardiac malformations and hypertension, but not metabolic risk factors, are common in Turner syndrome. *J Clin Endocrinol Metab*. 2001;86:4166–4170.

60. Bakalov VK, Cooley MM, Quon MJ, et al. Impaired insulin secretion in the Turner metabolic syndrome. *J Clin Endocrinol Metab*. 2004;89:3516–3520.

61. Bakalov VK, Cooley MM, Troendle J, et al. The prevalence of diabetes mellitus in the parents of women with Turner's syndrome. *Clin Endocrinol (Oxf)*. 2004;60:272.

62. Forbes AP, Engel E. The high incidence of diabetes mellitus in 41 patients with gonadal dysgenesis and their close relatives. *Metabolism*. 1963;12:428–439.

63. Cooley M, Bakalov V, Bondy CA. Lipid profiles in women with 45,X vs 46,XX primary ovarian failure. *JAMA*. 2003;290:2127–2128.

64. Taylor SH. Genetic vs hormonal factors in lipid metabolism in women. *JAMA*. 2004;291:424–425.

65. Elsheikh M, Conway GS. The impact of obesity on cardiovascular risk factors in Turner's syndrome. *Clin Endocrinol (Oxf)*. 1998;49:447–450.

66. Hanton L, Axelrod L, Bakalov V, et al. The importance of estrogen replacement in young women with Turner syndrome. *J Womens Health (Larchmt)*. 2003;12:971–977.

67. Bakalov VK, Axelrod L, Baron J, et al. Selective reduction in cortical bone mineral density in Turner syndrome independent of ovarian hormone deficiency. *J Clin Endocrinol Metab*. 2003;88:5717–5722.

68. Sas TC, de Muinck Keizer-Schrama SM, Stijnen T, et al. Bone mineral density assessed by phalangeal radiographic absorptiometry before and during long-term growth hormone treatment in girls with Turner's syndrome participating in a randomized dose-response study. *Pediatr Res*. 2001;50:417–422.

69. Neely EK, Marcus R, Rosenfeld RG, et al. Turner syndrome adolescents receiving growth hormone are not osteopenic. *J Clin Endocrinol Metab*. 1993;76:861–866.

70. Shaw NJ, Rehan VK, Husain S, et al. Bone mineral density in Turner's syndrome: A longitudinal study. *Clin Endocrinol (Oxf)*. 1997;47:367–370.

71. Carrascosa A, Gussinye M, Terradas P, et al. Spontaneous, but not induced, puberty permits adequate bone mass acquisition in adolescent Turner syndrome patients. *J Bone Miner Res*. 2000;15:2005–2010.

72. Suganuma N, Furuhashi M, Hirooka T, et al. Bone mineral density in adult patients with Turner's syndrome: Analyses of the effectiveness of GH and ovarian steroid hormone replacement therapies. *Endocr J*. 2003;50:263–269.

73. Shaw NJ, Rehan VK, Husain S, et al. Bone mineral density in Turner's syndrome: A longitudinal study. *Clin Endocrinol (Oxf)*. 1997;47:367–370.

74. Bakalov VK, Chen ML, Baron J, et al. Bone mineral density and fractures in Turner syndrome. *Am J Med*. 2003;115:259–264.

75. Davies MC, Gulekli B, Jacobs HS. Osteoporosis in Turner's syndrome and other forms of primary amenorrhoea. *Clin Endocrinol (Oxf)*. 1995;43:741–746.

76. Sylven L, Hagenfeldt K, Ringertz H. Bone mineral density in middle-aged women with Turner's syndrome. *Eur J Endocrinol*. 1995;132:47–52.

77. Landin-Wilhelmsen K, Bryman I, Windh M, et al. Osteoporosis and fractures in Turner syndrome: Importance of growth promoting and oestrogen therapy. *Clin Endocrinol (Oxf)*. 1999;51:497–502.

78. Ross JL, Long LM, Feuillan P, et al. Normal bone density of the wrist and spine and increased wrist fractures in girls with Turner's syndrome. *J Clin Endocrinol Metab*. 1991;73:355–359.

79. Smith MA, Wilson J, Price WH. Bone demineralization in patients with Turner's syndrome. *J Med Genet*. 1982;19:100–103.

80. Hayward PA, Satsangi J, Jewell DP. Inflammatory bowel disease and the X chromosome. *Q J Med*. 1996;89:713–718.

81. Garavelli L, Donadio A, Banchini G, et al. Liver abnormalities and portal hypertension in Ullrich-Turner syndrome. *Am J Med Genet*. 1998;80:180–182.

82. Wardi J, Knobel B, Shahmurov M, et al. Chronic cholestasis associated with Turner's syndrome: 12 years of clinical and histopathological follow-up. *Digestion*. 2003;67:96–99.

83. Bonamico M, Pasquino AM, Mariani P, et al. and the Italian Society of Pediatric Gastroenterology Hepatology (SIGEP) and the Italian Study Group for Turner Syndrome (ISGTS). Prevalence and clinical picture of celiac disease in Turner syndrome. *J Clin Endocrinol Metab*. 2002;87:5495–5498.

84. Salerno M, Di Maio S, Gasparini N, et al. Liver abnormalities in Turner syndrome. *Eur J Pediatr*. 1999;158:618–623.

85. Larizza D, Locatelli M, Vitali L, et al. Serum liver enzymes in Turner syndrome. *Eur J Pediatr*. 2000;159:143–148.

86. Roulot D, Degott C, Chazouilleres O, et al. Vascular involvement of the liver in Turner's syndrome. *Hepatology*. 2004;39:239–247.

87. Elsheikh M, Hodgson HJ, Wass JA, et al. Hormone replacement therapy may improve hepatic function in women with Turner's syndrome. *Clin Endocrinol (Oxf)*. 2001;55:227–231.

88. Zulian F, Schumacher HR, Calore A, et al. Juvenile arthritis in Turner's syndrome: A multicenter study. *Clin Exp Rheumatol*. 1998;16:489–494.

89. Scarpa R, Lubrano E, Castiglione F, et al. Juvenile rheumatoid arthritis, Crohn's disease and Turner's syndrome: A novel association. *Clinical & Experimental Rheumatology*. 1996;14:449–451.

90. Hasle H, Olsen JH, Nielsen J, et al. Occurrence of cancer in women with Turner syndrome. *Br J Cancer*. 1996;73:1156–1159.

91. Bronshtein M, Zimmer EZ, Blazer S. A characteristic cluster of fetal sonographic markers that are predictive of fetal Turner syndrome in early pregnancy. *Am J Obstet Gynecol*. 2003;188:1016–1020.

92. Wenstrom KD, Williamson RA, Grant SS. Detection of fetal Turner syndrome with multiple-marker screening. *Am J Obstet Gynecol*. 1994;170:570–573.

93. Koeberl DD, McGillivray B, Sybert VP. Prenatal diagnosis of 45,X/46,XX mosaicism and 45,X: Implications for postnatal outcome. *Am J Hum Genet*. 1995;57:661–666.

94. Patsalis PC, Sismani C, Hadjimarcou MI, et al. Detection and incidence of cryptic Y chromosome sequences in Turner syndrome patients. *Clin Genet*. 1998;53:249–257.

95. Villaverde MM, Da Silva JA. Turner-mongolism polysyndrome: Review of the first eight known cases. *JAMA*. 1975;234:844–847.

96. Massa G, Vanderschueren-Lodeweyckx M, Fryns JP. Deletion of the short arm of the X chromosome: A hereditary form of Turner syndrome. *Eur J Pediatr*. 1992;151:893–894.

97. Carothers AD, Frackiewicz A, De Mey R, et al. A collaborative study of the aetiology of Turner syndrome. *Ann Hum Genet*. 1980;43:355–368.

98. Pescia G, Ferrier PE, Wyss-Hutin D, et al. 45,X Turner's syndrome in monozygotic twin sisters. *J Med Genet*. 1975;12:390–396.

99. Hassold T, Pettay D, Robinson A, et al. Molecular studies of parental origin and mosaicism in 45,X conceptuses. *Hum Genet*. 1992;89:647–652.

100. Mathur A, Stekol L, Schatz D, et al. The parental origin of the single X chromosome in Turner syndrome: Lack of correlation with parental age or clinical phenotype. *Am J Hum Genet*. 1991;48:682–686.

101. Kajii T, Ohama K. Inverse maternal age effect in monosomy X. *Hum Genet*. 1979;51:147–151.

102. Davenport ML, et al. Turner syndrome. In: Pescovitz OH, Eugster EA, eds. *Pediatric Endocrinology: Mechanisms, Manifestations, and Management*. Philadelphia: Lippincott Williams & Wilkins; 2004:203–223.

103. Davenport ML. Evidence for early initiation of growth hormone and transdermal estradiol therapies in girls with Turner syndrome. *Growth Horm IGF Res*. 2006;16:91–97.

104. Chernausek SD, Attie KM, Cara JF, et al. Growth hormone therapy of Turner syndrome: The impact of age of estrogen replacement on final height. Genentech, Inc., Collaborative Study Group. *J Clin Endocrinol Metab*. 2000;85:2439–2445.

105. Saenger P. Growth-promoting strategies in Turner syndrome. *J Clin Endocrinol Metab*. 1999;84:4345–4348.

106. van Pareren YK, de Muinck Keizer-Schrama SM, Stijnen T, et al. Final height in girls with turner syndrome after long-term growth hormone treatment in three dosages and low dose estrogens. *J Clin Endocrinol Metab*. 2003;88:1119–1125.

107. Plotnick L, Attie KM, Blethen SL, et al. Growth hormone treatment of girls with Turner syndrome: The National Cooperative Growth Study experience. *Pediatrics*. 1998;102:479–481.

108. Ranke MB, Lindberg A, Chatelain P, et al. and KIGS International Board. Kabi International Growth Study. Prediction of long-term response to recombinant human growth hormone in Turner syndrome: Development and validation of mathematical models. KIGS International Board. Kabi International Growth Study. *J Clin Endocrinol Metab*. 2000;85:4212–4218.

109. Haeusler G, Schmitt K, Blumel P, et al. Growth hormone in combination with anabolic steroids in patients with Turner syndrome: Effect on bone maturation and final height. *Acta Paediatr*. 1996;85:1408–1414.

110. Stahnke N, Keller E, Landy H and the Serono Study Group. Favorable final height outcome in girls with Ullrich-Turner syndrome treated with low-dose growth hormone together with oxandrolone despite starting treatment after 10 years of age. *J Pediatr Endocrinol Metab*. 2002;15:129–138.

111. Sybert VP. Adult height in Turner syndrome with and without androgen therapy. *J Pediatr*. 1984;104:365.

112. Rosenfeld RG, Hintz RL, Johanson AJ, et al. Methionyl human growth hormone and oxandrolone in Turner syndrome: Preliminary results of a prospective randomized trial. *J Pediatr*. 1986;109:936–943.

113. Rosenfeld RG, Attie KM, Frane J, et al. Growth hormone therapy of Turner's syndrome: Beneficial effect on adult height. *J Pediatr*. 1998;132:319–324.

114. Reiter EO, et al. Early initiation of growth hormone treatment allows age-appropriate estrogen use in Turner's syndrome. *J Clin Endocrinol Metab*. 2001;86:1936–1941.

115. Vanderschueren-Lodeweyckx M, Massa G, Maes M, et al. Growth-promoting effect of growth hormone and low dose ethinyl estradiol in girls with Turner's syndrome. *J Clin Endocrinol Metab*. 1990;70:122–126.

116. Naeraa RW, Nielsen J, Kastrup KW. Growth hormone treatment and 17β-estradiol treatment of Turner girls: 2-year results. *Eur J Pediatr*. 1994;153:72.

117. Rosenfield RL, Devine N, Hunold JJ, et al. Salutary effects of combining early very low-dose systemic estradiol with growth hormone therapy in girls with Turner syndrome. *J Clin Endocrinol Metab*. 2005;90:6424–630.

118. Tarani L, Lampariello S, Raguso G, et al. Pregnancy in patients with Turner's syndrome: Six new cases and review of literature. *Gynecol Endocrinol*. 1998;12:83–87.

119. Khastgir G, Abdalla1 H, Thomas A, et al. Oocyte donation in Turner's syndrome: An analysis of the factors affecting the outcome. *Hum Reprod*. 1997;12:279–285.

120. McDonnell CM, Lee Coleman L, Zacharin MR. A 3-year prospective study to assess uterine growth in girls with Turner's syndrome by pelvic ultrasound. *ClinEndocr*. 2003;58:446–450.

121. Paterson WF, Hollman AS, Donaldson MDC. Poor uterine development in Turner syndrome with oral oestrogen therapy. *Clin Endocr*. 2002;56:359–365.

122. Hreinsson JG, Otala M, Fridstrom M, et al. Follicles are found in the ovaries of adolescent girls with Turner's syndrome. *J Clin Endocrinol Metab*. 2002;87:3618–3623.

123. Meirow D, Levron J, Eldar-Geva T, et al. Pregnancy after transplantation of cryopreserved ovarian tissue in a patient with ovarian failure after chemotherapy. *N Engl J Med*. 2005;353:318–321.

124. Silber SJ, Lenahan KM, Levine DJ, et al. Ovarian transplantation between monozygotic twins discordant for premature ovarian failure. *N Engl J Med*. 2005;353:58–63.

125. Rubin K. Transitioning the patient with Turner's syndrome from pediatric to adult care. *J Pediatr Endocrinol Metab*. 2003;16:651–659.

126. Bondy CA. Care of girls and women with Turner syndrome: A guideline of the Turner syndrome study group. *J Clin Endocrinol Metab*. 2007;92:10–25.

CHAPTER 32

Developmental Disorders of the Anterior Pituitary

Brigitte Frohnert, MD, PhD, FAAP
Bradley S. Miller, MD, PhD, FAAP

INTRODUCTION

The pituitary plays a vital role in orchestrating complex functions of the body including growth, metabolism, homeostasis, reproduction, lactation, and the stress response. The anterior pituitary gland consists of five distinct cell types that are responsible for the synthesis, storage, and release of six hormones: growth hormone (GH), luteinizing hormone (LH), follicle-stimulating hormone (FSH), thyroid-stimulating hormone (TSH), prolactin (PRL), and adrenocorticotropin hormone (ACTH). Under the influence of the hypothalamus and regulated through feedback loops, all anterior pituitary hormones are secreted in a pulsatile fashion and follow a diurnal pattern. When deficiencies of either isolated or multiple pituitary hormones occur they do so through both congenital and acquired mechanisms.

Gene mutations that impact anterior pituitary function can affect either the hypothalamic-releasing hormone receptors, the pituitary hormones themselves, or regulatory transcription factors, which are critical to the normal anatomic development and cellular differentiation of the pituitary gland. Mutations in the genes encoding regulatory transcription factors cause a disruption of normal pituitary development, resulting in pituitary hormone deficiencies. The advent of molecular biology, genomics, and animal models has allowed for greater insight into these genetic causes of abnormal pituitary development.

PITUITARY DEVELOPMENT

The pituitary develops through a time- and position-dependent interaction of an invagination of the oral ectoderm (Rathke's pouch) with the brain neuroectoderm originating from the base of the diencephalon. The oral ectoderm of Rathke's pouch eventually evolves into the anterior pituitary and the posterior pituitary is derived from the neuroectoderm of the ventral diencephalon. Many steps and multiple transcriptions factors (Figures 32-1 and 32-2) contribute to the differentiation of the ectoderm of Rathke's pouch into the five mature cell types: somatotrophs (50% of total cell mass), lactotrophs (15%–20%), gonadotrophs (10%), and thyrotrophs and corticotrophs (15%). This cascade of differentiation

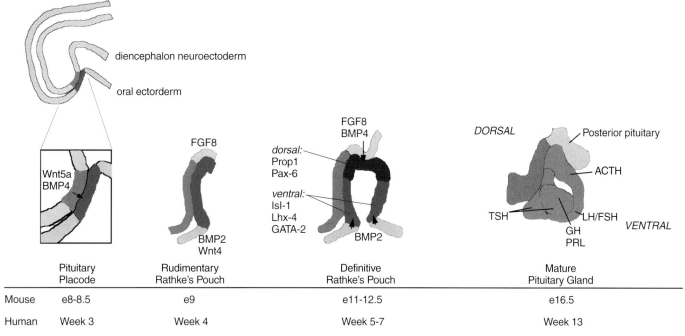

FIGURE 32-1. Stages of anterior pituitary development and key signaling molecules. Anterior pituitary development can be described as involving four stages: 1) pituitary placode, which forms as a thickening of the oral ectoderm when in contact with the neuroectoderm of the diencephalon; 2) rudimentary Rathke's pouch, formed by an invagination of the oral ectoderm; 3) definitive Rathke's pouch, formed by further development of this tissue; and finally 4) mature pituitary gland, formed by the final differentiation into the five major cell lines (somatotrophs, lactotrophs, corticotrophs, gonadotrophs, and thyrotrophs). Multiple signaling molecules and transcription factors are involved in this process. Time in embryonic development for both mouse (embryonic day) and human (embryonic week) indicated below each stage. Arrows denote signaling. Adapted from Mullis (39).

Developmental Disorders of the Anterior Pituitary

AT-A-GLANCE

Developmental disorders of the anterior pituitary involve a complex cascade of transcription factors that orchestrate the growth and differentiation of the five major cell types. These cells are responsible for the synthesis, storage, and release of the six anterior pituitary hormones: growth hormone (GH), luteinizing hormone (LH), follicle-stimulating hormone (FSH), thyroid-stimulating hormone (TSH), prolactin (PRL), and adrenocorticotropin (ACTH). Thus far, mutations in five important transcription factors have been identified that cause either isolated or combined pituitary hormone deficiency. There are two additional genes that have been associated with the pituitary hormone deficiencies in combination with the clinical syndromes of Septo-Optic Dysplasia and Rieger Syndrome.

DISORDERS	OCCURRENCE	GENE	INHERITANCE	LOCUS	OMIM
Congenital Isolated Adrenocorticotrophin Deficiency	Rare	TPIT	AR/AD	1q23-24	604614
Combined Pituitary Hormone Deficiency (CPHD)	1:8,000	LHX3	AR	9q34.3	600577
		LHX4	AD	1q25	602146
		PROP1	AR	5q	601538
		PIT1	AR/AD	3p11	173110
Septo-Optic Dysplasia	Rare	HESX1	AD/AR	3p21.2-p21.1	601802
Rieger Syndrome	Rare	PITX2	AD	4q25-q26	601542
		RIEG			180500

AR = autosomal recessive; AD = autosomal dominant

GENE	ENDOCRINE DISORDERS	MRI FINDINGS	CLINICAL PRESENTATION
TPIT	Isolated ACTH deficiency	Normal or hypoplastic pituitary	Profound neonatal hypoglycemia, may present with seizures; prolonged cholestatic jaundice; +/− hepatomegaly; family history of neonatal death
LHX3	CPHD (GH, TSH, PRL, LH, FSH)	Pituitary hypoplasia; enlarged anterior pituitary; possible pituitary microadenoma	Limitation of neck rotation; short cervical spine; short stature; pubertal delay
LHX4	CPHD (GH, TSH, ACTH)	Ectopic posterior pituitary; small sella turcica; small anterior pituitary; abnormal cerebellar tonsils; persistent craniopharyngeal canal	Short stature; adrenal insufficiency
PROP1	CPHD (GH, TSH, PRL; evolving LH/FSH and ACTH)	Small anterior pituitary; intrasellar or suprasellar mass	Hypoglycemia in infancy; short stature; evolving adrenal insufficiency; pubertal delay; infertility; no GHD re-evaluation necessary in adulthood
PIT1 (POU1F1)	CPHD (GH, TSH, PRL)	Small anterior pituitary	Congenital hypothyroidism; hypoglycemia in infancy; short stature
HESX1 (RPX)	IGHD or CPHD (GH, TSH, FSH, LH, PRL)	Ectopic posterior pituitary; small anterior pituitary; empty sella	Septo-optic dysplasia (eye abnormalities, midline brain deformities); short stature; spectrum of pubertal abnormalities from precocious to delayed
PITX2 (RIEG)	IGHD	Empty sella	Rieger Syndrome (eye, dental or umbilical abnormalities); short stature
Unknown	IGHD	Normal or small anterior pituitary; normal location of posterior pituitary; normal pituitary stalk	Short stature; delayed bone age

IGHD = Isolated growth hormone deficiency.

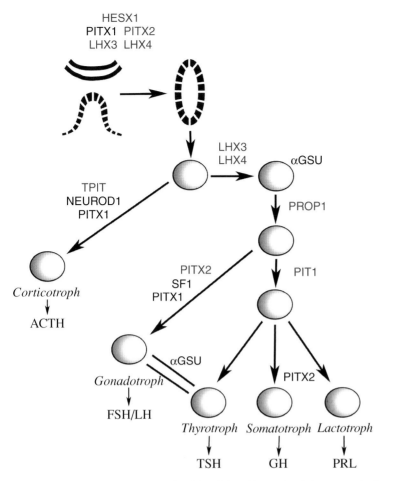

FIGURE 32-2. Cascade of transcription factors involved in differentiation of the anterior pituitary. Factors implicated in human disease are shown in red.

has been chiefly elucidated by studies in the mouse and other mammals. Signaling factors involved in the process of pituitary development are summarized in Table 32-1.

There are four steps in the development of the anterior pituitary. The initial step involves the thickening of the oral ectoderm into the pituitary placode. During the middle of the 4th week of human development, the oral ectoderm invaginates, forming the rudimentary Rathke's pouch. At the same time the neuroectoderm of the ventral diencephalon evaginates, maintaining contact with Rathke's pouch. This portion of neuroectoderm eventually develops into the posterior pituitary (Figure 32-1). In the third step, during weeks 5 through 7 of human embryonic development, there is further development of the oral ectoderm into the definitive Rathke's pouch. Finally, the various cell types within the mature pituitary gland differentiate into the five major cell types noted above, which is completed in the human by developmental week 13 (1,2).

The apposition of the two tissues, oral ectoderm and neuroectoderm, through-out the process of development allows for signaling interaction between these tissues. Initially, signaling factors, including BMP4 (bone morphogenetic protein 4), Wnt5A (wingless-type MMTV integration site family, member 5A), and FGF8 (fibroblast growth factor 8) (see Table 32-2), are released from the embryonic neuroectoderm, which induces invagination of the oral ectoderm and activation of early transcription factors in the maturing Rathke's pouch (Figure 32-1) including Pitx1 (Paired-like homeodomain transcription factor 1), Pitx2, Lhx3 (LIM homeobox gene 3), Lhx4, and HesX1/Rpx (homeobox gene expressed in ES cells/Rathke's pouch homeobox). The rudimentary Rathke's pouch produces the signaling proteins BMP2 and Wnt4 (3). During this time, the pouch expands via proliferation of cells producing Pitx1, Pitx2, Lhx3, Lhx4, and HesX1 and begins to separate from the oral ectoderm, becoming the mature Rathke's pouch.

From the early stages of the rudimentary Rathke's pouch, there is an orientation of transcription factor expression along the dorsal–ventral axis. The transcription factors

Prop1 (prophet of Pit1) and Pax6 (paired box gene 6) are chiefly found in the dorsal area of Rathke's pouch where the somatolactotrophs and thyrotrophs will eventually reside. Prop1 is thought to be a commitment factor. Other transcription factors, including Lhx4, Isl-1 (islet 1), and GATA-2 (GATA-binding protein 2) are more ventrally expressed; however there is no cognate commitment factor for the ventrally occurring gonadotrophs or corticotrophs. The spatial and temporal cascade of transcription factors results in the eventual development of the terminal cell types in a spatially oriented pattern. Corticotrophs develop on the dorsal side toward the rostral tip. Somatotrophs and lactotrophs are also found in the dorsal region. Thyrotrophs develop in the central region, and gonadotrophs are found in the ventral region (1). Although this distribution of cell types is found during development, the mature human pituitary does not show the same degree of organization.

One of the earliest branch points is the differentiation in the ventral region of Rathke's pouch of the corticotroph lineage, which produces pro-opiomelanocortin (POMC) and its product ACTH (Figure 32-2). This differentiation relies on the interaction of Pitx1 with the transcriptional activators Tpit (T-box factor, pituitary) and NeuroD1 (Neurogenic differentiation 1). These specifically activate POMC gene transcription (3).

The transcription factor, Prop1, which is present in the dorsal region, seems to play a significant role in commitment of progenitor cells into the somatolactotroph, thyrotroph, and gonadotroph lineages. Prop1, in addition to the upstream factor Lhx4, is required for expression of *Pit1* (pituitary-specific transcription factor 1), also known as POU1F1 (POU domain, class 1, transcription factor 1) (4). Pit1 continues the process of differentiation of the somatolactotroph and thyrotroph lineages. Additionally, low levels of GATA-2 dorsally are thought to allow expression of Pit-1. Another transcription factor, Pax6, plays a role in defining the boundary between thyrotroph and gonadotroph cell lineages.

High levels of GATA-2, in the ventral region, indirectly down regulate Pit-1 expression and allow the induction of gonadotroph factors such as Isl-1 and the orphan nuclear receptor, steroidogenic factor-1 (SF-1). SF-1 is specific to the gonadotroph lineage.

Although many transcription factors have been identified, in addition to those mentioned here, mutations of most of them have not been described in humans. This review will focus on the group of transcription factors associated with clinical disease. These transcription factors and their endocrine phenotypes are summarized in the At-A-Glance table. It is likely that this list will

TABLE 32-1	Pituitary Transcription Factors		
Protein	**Full Name**	**OMIM**	**Other Information**
T-Box Transcription Factor Family			
Tpit	T-Box factor, Pituitary	604614	Requires cooperation with Pitx1; T-box is N-terminal DNA-binding domain; family members play critical roles in human embryonic development
LIM Homeobox Gene Family			
Lhx3	LIM homeobox gene 3	600577	Large gene family; unique cysteine-rich zinc-binding LIM domain composed of
Lhx4	LIM homeobox gene 4	602146	50 to 60 amino acid residues; LIM homeobox genes are well conserved in evolution;
Isl-1	Islet 1	600366	play important roles as transcriptional regulators of embryonic development in vertebrates
Paired-Like Homeodomain Transcription Factor Family			
Pitx1	Paired-like homeodomain transcription factor 1	602149	Play role in development of anterior structures; bind to specific DNA sites, referred to as bicoid sites
Pitx2	Paired-like homeodomain transcription factor 2	180500/ 601542	
HesX1 (Rpx)	Homeobox gene expressed in ES cells (Rathke's pouch homeobox)	601802	
Paired Box Gene Family			
Pax6	Paired box gene 6	607108	Contain conserved paired domains; the helix-turn-helix structure of their carboxy-terminal portion suggests that these proteins are capable of DNA binding
GATA Family			
GATA-2	GATA-binding protein 2	137295	Zinc fingers in DNA-binding domain
bHLH (Basic Helix-Loop-Helix) Transcription Factor Family			
NeuroD1	Neurogenic differentiation 1	601724	Group of eukaryotic transcription factors important in development; highly conserved bHLH domain mediates dimerization of transcription factors
Nuclear Hormone Receptor Transcription Factor Family			
SF-1	Steroidogenic factor-1	184757	Orphan nuclear hormone receptor
Miscellaneous Transcription Factors			
Prop1	Prophet of Pit1	601538	Both DNA-binding and transcriptional activation ability
Pit1	Pituitary-specific transcription factor 1	173110	Exclusively expressed in the anterior pituitary
(POU1F1)	(POU domain, class 1, transcription factor 1)	173110	Significant similarity at its C terminus to the homeodomains encoded by Drosophila developmental genes

continue to expand significantly in the future as our understanding of pituitary development improves.

CONGENITAL ISOLATED ADRENOCORTICOTROPIN DEFICIENCY

TPIT

Etiology/Pathophysiology TPIT is a T-box transcription factor that is specific to the terminal differentiation of corticotrophs from the other anterior pituitary cell lineages. TPIT acts in synergy with PITX1 to activate the POMC gene. This protein contains an N-terminal element, the T-box, which is responsible for DNA binding. Many of the clinically important mutations of *TPIT* are found in this region; however, there are also a few other mutations thought to result in defective, poorly transcribed, or truncated proteins.

Clinical Presentation Congenital isolated adrenocorticotropin deficiency (IAD) is a genetically heterogeneous disorder. Individuals with IAD have either low or absent cortisol production due to low levels of plasma ACTH. All other pituitary hormones are present at normal levels. Administration of exogenous corticotrophin-releasing hormone rarely elicits a response in ACTH levels. Interestingly, patients with IAD demonstrate no structural pituitary defects (5). Onset of IAD has been noted to occur in two time periods, either in neonates (<1 y of age) or during later childhood (>5 y of age). Individuals with *TPIT* mutations express only the phenotype of neonatal onset IAD. Before identification of the role of the *TPIT* gene, IAD was an underestimated cause of neonatal death (6).

Presentation of infants with neonatal IAD includes severe hypoglycemia often associated with seizures. In one study, the major factor leading to diagnosis of these infants was failure to thrive, despite normal food intake (6). Other clinical features included prolonged cholestatic jaundice, sometimes associated with hepatomegaly. Plasma ACTH and cortisol levels were noted to be very low (mean 6.8 pg/mL and 24 nmol/L, respectively). A family history of unexplained neonatal death may also be present.

Magnetic resonance imaging (MRI) showed normal pituitary morphology in most patients with *TPIT* mutations; however, one patient was noted to have a hypoplastic pituitary (6). All had normal pituitary stalk and no evidence of posterior pituitary ectopia.

TABLE 32-2	Signaling proteins		
Protein	**Full Name**	**OMIM**	**Other Information**
WNT Family of Protooncogenes			
Wnt4	Wingless-type MMTV integration site family, member 4	603490	The WNT gene family consists of structurally related genes that encode cysteine-rich secreted glycoproteins that act as extracellular signaling factors; developmentally regulated in a precise temporal and spatial manner; 1 of the 3 major families of signaling molecules in the mouse
Wnt5A	Wingless-type MMTV integration site family, member 5A	164975	
Fibroblast Growth Factor Family			
FGF8	Fibroblast growth factor 8	600483	Secreted proteins that interact with the FGF receptor tyrosine kinases to mediate growth and development; the FGF gene family is also 1 of the 3 major families of signaling molecules in the mouse
Transforming Growth Factor-Beta Family			
BMP2	Bone morphogenetic protein 2	112261	Member of the transforming growth factor-beta (TGFβ) superfamily, one of 3 major families of signaling molecules in the mouse
Other Growth Factors			
BMP4	Bone morphogenetic protein 4	112262	Functions throughout development in mesoderm induction, tooth development, limb formation, bone induction, and fracture repair; unlike BMP2, is not member of TGFβ superfamily

Ten different human *TPIT* loss-of-function mutations have been identified. These mutations include nonsense, missense, point, and genomic deletions with both autosomal dominant and recessive inheritance patterns (7).

COMBINED PITUITARY HORMONE DEFICIENCIES (CPHD)

Combined pituitary hormone deficiency (CPHD) is defined as deficiency of growth hormone (GH) in combination with a decrease in one or more other pituitary hormones. The incidence of CPHD is approximately 1 in 8,000 live births (8). Mutations in transcription factors involved in early pituitary development have been identified that cause CPHD, including LHX3, LHX4, PROP1, and PIT1.

LHX3

Etiology/Pathophysiology In mice, the deletion of *Lhx3* is associated with the failure of Rathke's pouch to grow and differentiate. There is, however, a relative sparing of the corticotroph lineage, which differentiates, but does not proliferate. This observation led Netchine et al. to identify *LHX3* mutations in members of two separate consanguineous families with CPHD with sparing of ACTH function. (9)

Clinical Presentation The first four individuals who have been identified to have CPHD due to *LHX3* mutations all presented with severe growth failure. A more recently identi-

fied infant with homozygous *LHX3* mutation presented on day 1 of life with poor feeding, persistent jaundice, cyanosis, and micropenis (10). Further evaluation showed deficits of all anterior pituitary hormones except ACTH, which was detected at normal levels. Other phenotypic features noted include elevated and anteverted shoulders along with severe restriction of rotation of the cervical spine. X-rays of the neck did not show any malformation of the vertebra, but MRI of the neck demonstrated an abnormal steepness of the cervical spine in one patient. This unusual neck conformation did not appear to be muscular in origin, as MRI showed normal soft tissue structures without fibrosis or atrophy. In two patients, electromyograms of the sternocleidomastoid and brachioradial muscles did not show evidence of denervation or myopathy (9). Another patient showed normal nerve conduction studies, but moderate fasciculation potentials and occasional fibrillation potentials of the deltoid muscle, suggestive of dysfunction at the anterior horn cell (10). Interestingly, *LHX3* is focally expressed in ventral motor neurons and likely plays a role in the development and enervation of the neck musculature (11). Only one of the five described individuals with *LHX3* mutations has been noted to have delay in speech development (10).

In the members of one family with an identified *LHX3* point missense mutation, MRI of the brain showed severe hypoplasia of the anterior pituitary. An individual with a 23-bp deletion in *LHX3* causing a frame shift and premature termination had an enlarged

anterior pituitary at the age of 19 years, which had not been seen by computed tomography scans 10 years previously. The mechanism of this enlargement is not known. The frame shift deletion results in a severely truncated protein lacking significant functional regions. A third individual with a single base pair deletion in exon II was noted to have a hypointense lesion in the anterior pituitary, consistent with a microadenoma and leading to the appearance of an enlarged pituitary (10). All three mutations identified in the humans are thought to result in loss of function of this transcription factor (9,10).

LHX4

Etiology/Pathophysiology LHX4 is a LIM-transcription factor that works in conjunction with LHX3 during early steps of anterior pituitary development (Figure 32-2). The gene for LHX4 is on human chromosome 1. Interestingly it occurs in a region that is syntenic to the region of mouse chromosome 1, which contains the mouse ortholog *Lhx4* (12). The mouse and human amino acid sequences are 99% identical for these proteins. In humans, studies have shown that expression of *LHX4* is specific to the central nervous system, including fetal brain, spinal cord, and cerebral cortex. (13) The expression of *LHX4* is transient and it is found in the developing pituitary gland at 5 and 6 weeks of development, during the period of Rathke's pouch formation. (14)

Using mutation analysis, individuals with combined pituitary hormone deficiency were screened for defects in the *LHX4* gene. One family was identified with an intronic point mutation involving a splice acceptor site. This mutation resulted in two mutant splice variants, one with an in-frame deletion of four conserved amino acids and one with a premature termination of the protein. The affected individuals were heterozygous for this dominant mutation.

Clinical Presentation Individuals with LHX4 deficiency had a common phenotype including deficiency of GH, TSH, and ACTH. Because the patients studied were prepubertal, gonadotropins were not studied. Although the development of lactotroph cell lineage is downstream of LHX4 activity, interestingly, patients with *LHX4* mutations have thus far not shown deficiencies of PRL (4). As would be expected with GH deficiency, the four identified carriers of the *LHX4* mutation had short stature (12).

In addition to hormonal abnormalities, head MRI showed a small sella turcica, hypoplastic anterior pituitary, persistent craniopharyngeal canal, deformation of the cerebellar tonsils into pointed configuration (the Chiari I malformation), and an ectopic posterior pituitary. The ectopic posterior pituitary tissue was found in a variety of locations, including near the optic chiasm and in the middle of the pituitary stalk; however in some patients, the posterior pituitary was also found in its normal position (12).

PROP1

Etiology/Pathophysiology PROP1 is a paired-like homeodomain transcription factor in the same class as HESX1. It is thought to function chiefly as a transcription activator (15). As would be expected by its prominent role early in the differentiation of anterior pituitary cell lineages, *PROP1* mutations have been associated with CPHD. At least 14 mutations have been identified in *PROP1*, all of which act in an autosomal recessive manner. A hot spot of gene mutation was located in a series of three tandem repeats of the dinucleotides GA at location 296–302 (16). *PROP1* mutations have been noted to be a common cause of CPHD in patients from nine countries (17,18). The exception to this trend was a study in Australian children, which showed no *PROP1* mutations in a group of 33 CPHD children.

Clinical Presentation The phenotype of human *PROP1* mutations includes deficiencies of GH, TSH, PRL, FSH, and LH. This results in the phenotype of short stature, hypothyroidism, delayed or absent puberty, and infertility.

The severity of the phenotype, age of onset, and size of the pituitary gland can vary greatly, even among members of the same family (16). Many affected individuals are first noted to have growth failure during infancy or early childhood, ranging from 9 months to 8 years of age. Secondary sexual development can be absent or delayed. Some women undergo menarche, but may require later hormone replacement. Males often are noted to have micropenis and small testes. Incomplete secondary sexual development in both genders is associated with infertility. Hypothyroidism is generally mild and does not typically present until later infancy or childhood. ACTH deficiency is variable, and when it is noted, occurs in adolescence or adulthood. MRI of the pituitary can show either a small anterior pituitary gland or intrapituitary mass, but the mechanism of this finding is unknown.

PIT1 (POU1F1)

Etiology/Pathophysiology *PIT1* (*POU1F1*) is specifically expressed quite late in the anterior pituitary differentiation cascade. It is found in somatotrophs, lactotrophs, and thyrotrophs. Target genes regulated by PIT1 include the genes encoding GH, PRL and the β-subunit of TSH as well as the gene for PIT1 itself. Mutations in *PIT1* are some of the most commonly identified causes of CPHD.

Clinical Presentation Patients with *PIT1* mutations display a phenotype that includes short stature caused by GH deficiency, PRL deficiency, and variable central hypothyroidism. Patients may present in the newborn period with severe congenital hypothyroidism (19,20). Because corticotroph and gonadotroph cell lineages differentiate at an earlier stage of the developmental cascade, ACTH, FSH, and LH are not affected in *PIT1* mutants. Pituitary hypoplasia is commonly seen on MRI. Both dominant and recessive mutant alleles of *PIT1* exist and at least 14 distinct mutations have been described (19,21–23).

SYNDROMIC HYPOPITUITARISM

Septo-Optic Dysplasia (HESX1)

Etiology/Pathophysiology HESX1 (also called Rpx) is a paired-like homeodomain transcription factor that plays an important role in early pituitary development (15). HESX1 contains a repression domain that can inhibit expression of target genes. Down-regulation of *HESX1* correlates with differentiation of anterior pituitary cells (24). Interestingly, HESX1 is closely related to another pituitary transcription factor, PROP1, which acts as an activator of transcription. Both factors bind

to the same DNA response elements. The sequential function of these factors results in the temporal regulation of down-stream genes. The importance of HESX1 in development is supported by the high degree of conservation among the human, mouse, and *Xenopus* genes (25).

Clinical Presentation Mutations of *HESX1* have been associated with septo-optic dysplasia (SOD) and varying degrees of panhypopituitarism (25). SOD is a constellation of abnormalities including varying degrees of panhypopituitarism, pituitary hypoplasia, optic nerve hypoplasia, and midline abnormalities, such as absence of the septum pellucidum and corpus callosum (26). The endocrine abnormalities range from partial idiopathic GH deficiency (IGHD) to CPHD. In one study 36% of children with SOD had associated posterior pituitary dysfunction in the form of antidiuretic hormone deficiency (27). In addition, these children can have pubertal development along the entire spectrum from precocious, rapidly progressive puberty to severely delayed or absent pubertal development (28). The SOD phenotype can vary widely, and only approximately 30% of individuals express the full phenotype (22). MRI findings varied from small or absent anterior pituitary with an ectopic posterior pituitary. Children with SOD were noted in one study to present at an earlier age than children with other forms of CPHD, and maternal age was significantly lower, with a mean age of 21, compared with a mean age of 27 for mothers of children with other forms of CPHD (27). This age discrepancy could support an environmental exposure contributing to SOD, and although SOD is usually sporadic, it has been associated with exposure to teratogens including cocaine and alcohol (29,30). Overall, SOD is relatively rare, occurring in approximately 1 in 50,000 births (22).

There have been seven separate mutations of *HESX1* identified, which include both dominant and recessive alleles (22,25,26,31–33). Four of these mutant alleles are associated with SOD. All have some element of pituitary hypoplasia, but not all mutant alleles confer panhypopituitarism. The milder alleles show only isolated GH deficiency. In one mutation, the affected individual with features of SOD was initially noted to have a small anterior pituitary gland, but no hormone abnormalities at age 3. Over the subsequent 2 years he began to show decreased growth velocity, GH deficiency, and borderline TSH (31). Other mutations have also shown evolving pituitary hormone deficiencies including GH, TSH, FSH, LH, and PRL (32); therefore, these individuals require ongoing surveillance and hormone testing.

Rieger Syndrome (PITX2, RIEG)

Etiology/Pathophysiology PITX2 is a bicoidlike homeodomain transcription factor that is expressed in Rathke's pouch as well as in the adult pituitary, which implies that it plays a role in both the early differentiation and more terminal pituitary development (34). Experiments have shown that the mouse homolog, *Pitx2*, is expressed in many tissues, including the first branchial arch, eye, brain, mandible, heart, and limbs. In the pituitary, PITX2 acts in the early development of Rathke pouch in conjunction with HESX1 and LHX3 (35). In a later stage of pituitary development, *PITX2* is expressed in gonadotroph, thyrotroph, and somatolactotroph cell lineages and has been shown to play a role in the activation of hormone genes (35). The promoters for the αGSU, αLH, αFSH, αTSH, GH, PRL, and POMC genes all contain a binding site for PITX2 (and the related protein PITX1), indicating an ongoing role for this transcription factor in the mature pituitary.

Clinical Presentation Rieger syndrome is an autosomal dominant disorder consisting of a heterogeneous group of abnormalities. It is part of the Axenfeld–Rieger group of anomalies, which are thought to be related disorders that represent a continuum of defects. The first member of the group is the Axenfeld anomaly, which consists of defects of the peripheral anterior segment and iris of the eye. These include a prominent, anteriorly displaced Schwalbe line (the posterior embryotoxon) to which iris strands adhere, reaching the angle of the anterior chamber. The next member of the group, Rieger's anomaly, includes the Axenfeld anomaly in addition to hypoplasia of the iris stroma. There may be other associated findings such as abnormally situated pupils (corectopia), slit pupils, or multiple pupils (polycoria). It is associated with glaucoma in approximately half of affected patients. The final member of this group is Rieger syndrome, which is characterized by the eye abnormalities included in the Rieger anomaly in addition to other developmental defects.

There are multiple nonocular findings associated with Rieger syndrome with variable presentations. One common finding is dental hypoplasia, which can present as missing, small, or malformed teeth. Umbilical stump abnormalities are another nonocular component of Rieger syndrome. These are thought to represent a failure of the involution of the periumbilical skin, and can include umbilical hernias as well as an elongated, protuberant umbilicus. A third class of associated features includes mild craniofacial dysmorphism.

This consists of a broad nasal root, telecanthus, maxillary hypoplasia, and a protruding lower lip associated with mild prognathism.

Endocrine findings associated with Rieger's syndrome include pituitary disorders such as GH deficiency and empty sella syndrome (36). Rieger syndrome represents a family of genetic disorders and has been associated with abnormalities on several chromosomes. One subset of this syndrome, Rieger syndrome type 1 (RIEG 1), has been associated with multiple mutations of *PITX2*. Thus far, all *PITX2* mutations have a dominant phenotype. The varied phenotype of Rieger syndrome correlates with the expression pattern of *PITX2* in tissues that lead to formation of the eye, brain, mandible, and pituitary. Despite the role of PITX2 in pituitary development, it is interesting to note that only a subset of Rieger syndrome patients manifest the pituitary-related phenotype of GH deficiency. This has been hypothesized to be either the result of a differential gene dosage effect, that is, one normal copy is enough for pituitary development, whereas other tissues are affected differently. The pituitary phenotype is perhaps also more or less penetrant depending on the genetic milieu of other important transcription factors (36).

Diagnosis Initial identification of patients with developmental disorders of the anterior pituitary generally occurs when the signs or symptoms of a specific hormone deficiency are noted. The presence of a family member with similar hormone deficiencies or the presence of dysmorphic features can both be clues to a genetic etiology.

MRI findings in a child with pituitary hormone deficiencies can be helpful in further delineating possible genetic etiologies. In children with GH deficiency, MRI can reveal abnormal pituitary morphology that may be associated with mutations in genes encoding transcription factors important in pituitary development. Children with an ectopic posterior pituitary are unlikely to have *PIT1*, *PROP1*, or *LHX3* mutations. An ectopic posterior pituitary is a specific marker of permanent GH deficiency and may be associated with *HESX1* or *LHX4* mutations (37). In the cases of combined pituitary hormone deficiency, the presence of multiple findings on MRI may indicate *PIT1*, *PROP1*, *HESX1*, or *LHX3* mutations. These MRI findings include normal or small anterior pituitary gland, enlarged empty sella, pituitary hyperplasia, and intrasellar or suprasellar mass. Neck stiffness and Chiari I malformations may be associated with *LHX3* or *LHX4* mutations (37).

Children who present with central hypothyroidism in infancy, whether detected by

newborn screen or by clinical suspicion, should also be evaluated for hypoglycemia and linear growth as a marker for GH deficiency after thyroid hormone replacement. Furthermore, evaluation for both GH and ACTH deficiency should be considered as these children are at risk for severe hypoglycemia and its related morbidity (21).

The majority of children with IGHD or CPHD do not have identified mutations. This implies that these children have unidentified mutations of the previously identified genes or mutations in other unknown or unstudied genes. It is likely that there will be many more candidates identified in the future. Despite this, it is suggested that patients with IGHD or CPHD associated with abnormalities of pituitary development undergo genetic testing, as the identification of known mutations can help with understanding likely evolution of the hormone deficiencies and can assist with genetic counseling (38). At this time, the *PROP-1*, *POU1F1*, *LHX3*, *LHX4*, *HESX1*, and Rieger syndrome (*PITX2*) genes have testing available for clinical use; however, the spectrum of genetic testing opportunities is constantly evolving. The web site www.genetests.org is a useful, regularly updated resource to find laboratories that perform genetic testing on a clinical basis for multiple conditions. These laboratories are either US-CLIA certified or are clinical laboratories outside the USA. In some cases, genetic testing of individuals may be coordinated with the specific research laboratories involved in the initial characterization of the human diseases described.

At this point, the molecular diagnosis of pituitary hormone deficiencies is still in its infancy. Both greater access to genomic data and further studies on the development of the mammalian pituitary will almost certainly lead to an ever-increasing list of candidate genes.

Treatment The treatment of these disorders of congenital pituitary development should focus on the replacement of deficient hormones. Screening for other hormonal deficiencies should be based on the known role of a particular genetic mutation in the ontogeny of the pituitary cells involved in the hormone production. Because of the rarity of these conditions and the lack of extensive studies, no general screening paradigm can be endorsed other than persistent clinical vigilance. In addition, subsequent MRI may be indicated in individuals with *LHX3* and *PROP1* mutations to screen for abnormalities of the pituitary. The natural history and clinical relevance of these lesions has not been established. Other conditions associated with these disorders, including precocious puberty in individuals with *HESX1* mutations, neck abnormalities in individuals with *LHX4* mutations, and ophthalmologic abnormalities in individuals with *PITX2* mutations should be managed by appropriate specialists.

REFERENCES

1. Savage JJ, Yaden BC, Kiratipranon P, et al. Transcriptional control during mammalian anterior pituitary development. *Gene.* 2003;319:1–19.

2. Tran PV, Savage JJ, Ingraham HA, et al. Molecular genetics of hypothalamic-pituitary axis development. In: Pediatric endocrinology: mechanisms and management. Pescovitz O, Eugster E, eds. Philadelphia, PA: Lippincott, Williams & Wilkins, 2004, p. 63–79.

3. Reynaud R, Saveanu A, Barlier A, et al. Pituitary hormone deficiencies due to transcription factor gene alterations. *Growth Horm IGF Res.* 2004;14:442–448.

4. Machinis K, Amselem S. Functional relationship between LHX4 and POU1F1 in light of the LHX4 mutation identified in patients with pituitary defects. *J Clin Endocrinol Metab.* 2005;90:5456–5462.

5. Metherell LA, Savage MO, Dattani M, et al. TPIT mutations are associated with early-onset, but not late-onset isolated ACTH deficiency. *Eur J Endocrinol.* 2004; 151:463–465.

6. Vallette-Kasic S, Brue T, Pulichino AM, et al. Congenital isolated adrenocorticotropin deficiency: an underestimated cause of neonatal death, explained by TPIT gene mutations. *J Clin Endocrinol Metab.* 2005;90:1323–1331.

7. Pulichino AM, Vallette-Kasic S, Couture C, et al. Human and mouse TPIT gene mutations cause early onset pituitary ACTH deficiency. *Genes Dev.* 2003;17(6):711–716.

8. Dattani MT, Robinson IC. HESX1 and septo-optic dysplasia. *Rev Endocr Metab Disord.* 2002;3:289–300.

9. Netchine I, Sobrier ML, Krude H, et al. Mutations in LHX3 result in a new syndrome revealed by combined pituitary hormone deficiency. *Nat Genet.* 2000;25:182–186.

10. Bhangoo AP, Hunter CS, Savage JJ, et al. Clinical case seminar: a novel LHX3 mutation presenting as combined pituitary hormonal deficiency. *J Clin Endocrinol Metab.* 2006;91/747–753.

11. Sharma K, Sheng HZ, Lettieri K, et al. LIM homeodomain factors Lhx3 and Lhx4 assign subtype identities for motor neurons. *Cell.* 1998;95:817–828.

12. Machinis K, Pantel J, Netchine I, et al. Syndromic short stature in patients with a germline mutation in the LIM homeobox LHX4. *Am J Hum Genet.* 2001;69:961–968.

13. Liu Y, Fan M, Yu S, et al. cDNA cloning, chromosomal localization and expression pattern analysis of human LIM-homeobox gene LHX4. *Brain Res.* 2002;928: 147–155.

14. Sobrier ML, Attie-Bitach T, Netchine I, et al. Pathophysiology of syndromic combined pituitary hormone deficiency due to a LHX3 defect in light of LHX3 and LHX4 expression during early human development. *Gene Expr Patterns.* 2004;5:279–284.

15. Cushman LJ, Showalter AD, Rhodes SJ. Genetic defects in the development and function of the anterior pituitary gland. *Ann Med.* 2002;34:179–191.

16. Deladoey J, Fluck C, Buyukgebiz A, et al. "Hot spot" in the PROP1 gene responsible for combined pituitary hormone deficiency. *J Clin Endocrinol Metab.* 1999;84:1645–1650.

17. Vallette-Kasic S, Barlier A, Teinturier C, et al. PROP1 gene screening in patients with multiple pituitary hormone deficiency reveals two sites of hypermutability and a high incidence of corticotroph deficiency. *J Clin Endocrinol Metab.* 2001;86:4529–4535.

18. Cogan JD, Wu W, Phillips JA 3rd, et al. The PROP1 2-base pair deletion is a common cause of combined pituitary hormone deficiency. *J Clin Endocrinol Metab.* 1998;83:3346–3349.

19. Hendriks-Stegeman BI, Augustijn KD, Bakker B, et al. Combined pituitary hormone deficiency caused by compound heterozygosity for two novel mutations in the POU domain of the Pit1/POU1F1 gene. *J Clin Endocrinol Metab.* 2001;86:1545–1550.

20. Blankenstein O, Muhlenberg R, Kim C, et al. A new C-terminal located mutation (V272ter. in the PIT-1 gene manifesting with severe congenital hypothyroidism. Possible functionality of the PIT-1 C-terminus. *Horm Res.* 2001;56:81–86.

21. Malvagia S, Poggi GM, Pasquini E, et al. The de novo Q167K mutation in the POU1F1 gene leads to combined pituitary hormone deficiency in an Italian patient. *Pediatr Res.* 2003;54:635–640.

22. Dattani MT, Robinson IC. The molecular basis for developmental disorders of the pituitary gland in man. *Clin Genet.* 2000; 57:337–346.

23. Salemi S, Besson A, Eble A, et al. New N-terminal located mutation (Q4ter) within the POU1F1-gene (PIT-1) causes recessive combined pituitary hormone deficiency and variable phenotype. *Growth Horm IGF Res.* 2003;13:264–268.

24. Cohen RN, Cohen LE, Botero D, et al. Enhanced repression by HESX1 as a cause of hypopituitarism and septooptic dysplasia. *J Clin Endocrinol Metab.* 2003;88: 4832–4839.

25. Dattani MT, Martinez-Barbera JP, Thomas PQ, et al. Mutations in the homeobox gene HESX1/Hesx1 associated with septo-optic dysplasia in human and mouse. *Nat Genet.* 1998;19:125–133.

26. Brickman JM, Clements M, Tyrell R, et al. Molecular effects of novel mutations in Hesx1/HESX1 associated with human pituitary disorders. *Development.* 2001;128:5189–5199.

27. Rainbow LA, Rees SA, Shaikh MG, et al. Mutation analysis of POUF-1, PROP-1 and HESX-1 show low frequency of mutations in children with sporadic forms of combined pituitary hormone deficiency and septo-optic dysplasia. *Clin Endocrinol.* (Oxf) 2005;62:163–168.

28. Hanna CE, Mandel SH, LaFranchi SH. Puberty in the syndrome of septo-optic dysplasia. *Am J Dis Child.* 1989;143:186–189.

29. Dominguez R, Aguirre Vila-Coro A, Slopis JM, et al. Brain and ocular abnormalities in infants with in utero exposure to cocaine and other street drugs. *Am J Dis Child.* 1991;145:688–695.

30. Coulter CL, Leech RW, Schaefer GB, et al. Scheithauer BW, Brumback RA. Midline cerebral dysgenesis, dysfunction of the hypothalamic-pituitary axis, and fetal alcohol effects. *Arch Neurol.* 1993;50:771–775.

31. Cohen LE, Radovick S. Molecular basis of combined pituitary hormone deficiencies. *Endocr Rev.* 2002 Aug;23:431–442.

32. Carvalho LR, Woods KS, Mendonca BB, et al. A homozygous mutation in HESX1 is associated with evolving hypopituitarism due to impaired repressor-corepressor interaction. *J Clin Invest.* 2003;112:1192–1201.

33. Thomas PQ, Dattani MT, Brickman JM, et al. Heterozygous HESX1 mutations associated with isolated congenital pituitary hypoplasia and septo-optic dysplasia. *Hum Mol Genet.* 2001;10:39–45.

34. Drouin J, Lamolet B, Lamonerie T, et al. The PTX family of homeodomain transcription factors during pituitary developments. *Mol Cell Endocrinol.* 1998;140:31–36.

35. Quentien MH, Pitoia F, Gunz G, et al. Regulation of prolactin, GH, and Pit-1 gene expression in anterior pituitary by Pitx2: An approach using Pitx2 mutants. *Endocrinology.* 2002;143:2839–2851.

36. Amendt BA, Semina EV, Alward WL. Rieger syndrome: a clinical, molecular, and biochemical analysis. *Cell Mol Life Sci.* 2000;57:1652–1666.

37. Maghnie M, Ghirardello S, Genovese E. Magnetic resonance imaging of the hypothalamus-pituitary unit in children suspected of hypopituitarism: who, how and when to investigate. *J Endocrinol Invest.* 2004;27:496–509.

38. Dattani MT. DNA testing in patients with GH deficiency at the time of transition. *Growth Horm IGF Res.* 2003;13 Suppl A:S122–9.

39. Mullis PE. Genetic control of growth. *Eur J Endocrinol.* 2005;152:11–31.

CHAPTER 33

Precocious Puberty

Melena Bellin, MD
Kyriakie Sarafoglou, MD
Brandon Nathan, MD

INTRODUCTION

Normal pubertal development is dependent on a change in the activity of the hypothalamic-pituitary-gonadal (HPG) axis from a period of relative quiescence during childhood to its re-activation during puberty. Any disruption to the normal inhibition of this axis during childhood results in central precocious puberty. Alternatively, secretion of or exposure to sex steroids independent of this axis can result in a peripheral form of precocious puberty. The challenge to the practitioner is to identify children with pathologic forms of precocious puberty and determine whether the etiology is central (gonadotropin-releasing hormone [GnRH]-dependent) or peripheral (GnRH-independent) in order to initiate appropriate therapy.

NORMAL PUBERTAL DEVELOPMENT

The HPG Axis

Pubertal onset is heralded by the increased secretion of hypothalamic GnRH, which enters the hypothalamic–pituitary portal circulation and stimulates the anterior pituitary to secrete luteinizing hormone (LH) and follicle-stimulating hormone (FSH). LH and FSH enter the systemic circulation and stimulate the ovaries and testis to produce the sex steroids, estrogen and testosterone, respectively. Sex steroids, along with the peptides inhibin (primarily secreted from gonads with a direct inhibitory effect on FSH release) and follistatin (produced in multiple tissues exerting inhibitory effects by inhibiting activin) exert selective negative feedback inhibition on hypothalamic GnRH and pituitary gonadotropin release. Estradiol (during the midcycle surge in females) and another peptide, activin, present in the gonads and multiple other tissues, have stimulatory roles (Figure 33-1) [reviewed in (1,2)].

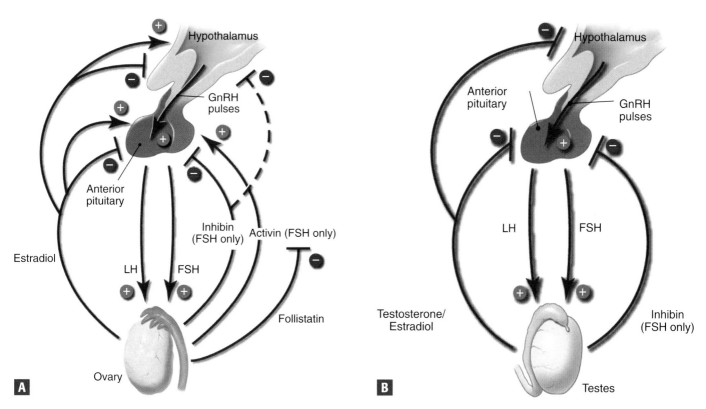

FIGURE 33-1. A. Hypothalamic-Pituitary-Ovarian Axis. In the presence of a GnRH pulse, the pituitary and ovarian hormones exert mutual control over the circulating levels of one another in a complex interaction involving positive and negative feedback that serves to sustain the perpetual monthly menstruation cycle. **B.** Hypothalamic-Pituitary-Testicular Axis. Negative feedback regulation of gonadotropin synthesis and release. Gonadotropin release from the pituitary is controlled by GnRH and the negative feedback of gonadal steroids is exerted at the pituitary and hypothalamic level. Inhibin is produced from Sertoli cells through FSH stimulation and its main function is to regulate, through negative feedback, the secretion of FSH from the pituitary.

Precocious Puberty

AT-A-GLANCE

Precocious puberty refers to the onset of pubertal changes at an age that is earlier than expected for the normal population. Boys are considered to have precocious puberty with pubertal changes at younger than 9 years of age. Girls are traditionally considered to have precocious puberty with development of secondary sexual characteristics at younger than 8 years old, although newer guidelines suggest lowering the age limit to 7 years for white girls and 6 years for black girls. Precocious puberty is classified as either central precocious puberty (CPP), involving premature activation of the hypothalamic-pituitary-gonadal (HPG) axis, or peripheral precocious puberty (PPP) due to increased sex steroid exposure in the absence of increased gonadotropin secretion. Treatment in CPP is directed at suppression of HPG axis after evaluation for central nervous system (CNS) lesions affecting the hypothalamus and/or pituitary gland. Treatment in PPP is directed at the underlying etiology.

	PRESENTATION	LAB FINDINGS	TREATMENT
CPP			
Idiopathic CPP	Breast and pubic hair development in girls. Testicular and penile enlargement, pubic hair in boys. Increased growth velocity. Puberty progresses in expected sequence but may occur more rapidly than normal	• Elevated basal LH • Elevated peak LH with GnRH agonist (leuprolide) stimulation • Elevated estradiol or testosterone • Advanced bone age	• GnRH agonist
CPP due to CNS lesion	Similar to idiopathic CPP but may experience symptoms of headaches, diplopia, other neurologic symptoms. May have history of CNS insult	Same as above, plus • MRI or CT evidence of underlying CNS tumor or lesion	• Directed at underlying lesion for CNS tumors • GnRH agonists for hypothalamic harmatoma or irreversible CNS insult
PPP			
General comments	Isosexual or contrasexual development without evidence for hypothalamic-pituitary–driven gonadarche	• Prepubertal response to GnRH agonist stimulation • Low basal LH	
hCG-secreting tumors	Mainly in males, rarely in females. Boys have testicular enlargement, penile enlargement, and pubic hair. Breast development and pubic hair in girls	• Elevated β-hCG • Elevated estradiol or testosterone • Imaging evidence of tumor	• Combination of resection, chemotherapy, +/−radiation
Gonadal tumors: – **Leydig cell (LC)** – **Granulosa cell (GC)**	LC tumor in males associated with rapid onset penile growth and pubic hair; asymmetric testes. GC tumor in girls associated with rapid onset breast development, menstruation.	• Elevated testosterone or estradiol • Ultrasound or CT evidence of tumor	• Resection
Adrenocortical tumors	Virilization in boys and girls. Boys have prepubertal testes.	• Elevated adrenal androgens- DHEA, DHEA-S, androstenedione • Ultrasound or CT evidence of tumor	• Resection • Adjuvant chemotherapy with malignant lesions
Congenital Adrenal Hyperplasia	Premature pubarche in girls and boys; ambiguous genitalia, small testes in boys, prepubertal ovaries in girls; hypertension or hypotension with classic forms of CAH	• Elevated 17-OH-progesterone, 17-OH-pregnenelone, or 11-deoxycortisol, DHEA, DHEAS in response to ACTH stimulation.	• Glucocorticoid replacement
McCune-Albright Syndrome	Precocious puberty, irregular café-au-lait spots, polyostotic fibrous dysplasia, other endocrinopathies	• Elevated estradiol • Asymmetric, multicystic ovaries on ultrasound	• Tamoxifen or testolactone /aromatase inhibition
Male-Limited Precocious Puberty	Precocious puberty in males only enlarged testicles and virilization in first years of life.	• Elevated testosterone. • Suppressed baseline and stimulated LH and FSH	• Spironolactone and aromatase inhibitor +/− ketoconazole
Unknown Mechanism of PP			
Hypothyroidism	Breast development and menstruation in girls, macroorchidism in boys	• Elevated TSH, low free T_4 • Bone age normal or delayed	• Levothyroxine

Hypothalamic GnRH secretion is active by the end of the first trimester. At birth, plasma FSH and LH are low due to the inhibitory effect of placenta-derived steroids (particularly estrogen). Within the first few minutes of life, a surge of LH secretion accompanied by a rise in testosterone levels can be seen in males, lasting for approximately 12 hours (3, 4). A similar surge of LH is not observed in females. As placenta-derived steroids dissipate, reactivation of the HPG axis occurs within 2 weeks of age ("mini-puberty") resulting in an increase in FSH and LH levels and gonadal sex steroid levels (5). During this period, gonadotropin levels peak between 4 and 10 weeks (LH-predominate response in males whereas FSH levels predominate in females), followed by a gradual decline until a nadir is reached at approximately 6 months in males. Females may retain minimal, variable GnRH activity for the first several years of life (5–7).

Approximately 2 years prior to the appearance of physical changes of puberty, there is an increase in nocturnal pulsatile release of GnRH leading to an increase in LH secretion at night. Both genders experience similar overnight LH values; however, girls have increased FSH release (8). As the onset of puberty progresses, nocturnal LH pulses increase in amplitude and frequency eventually occurring during the daytime. Testosterone concentrations rise quickly during central puberty. In males, a circadian rhythm is established in which there are significantly higher testosterone levels in the early morning compared with the rest of the day. Estradiol levels in females tend to be more episodic than testosterone levels in boys but do increase with Tanner stage and tend to peak in the morning as well (9).

Pubertal Physical Characteristics

The increase in both adrenal androgens and GnRH-driven sex steroids leads to the development of secondary sexual characteristics. The first visible sign of central puberty in boys is testicular enlargement (4 mL testicular volume and 2.5 cm length) and puberty in girls is most often characterized by breast development although pubic hair may precede breast budding in one-third of girls. Progression of sexual characteristics can be described clinically by Tanner staging or the sexual maturation scale (see Chapter 34).

The growth spurt that occurs at puberty is driven largely by the gradual increasing secretion of gonadal sex steroids. Rising growth hormone (GH) levels also contribute to this growth acceleration as a physiologic correlation exists between the

amount of gonadal steroids produced and the amount of GH produced with a doubling of GH production occurring in puberty (10). Attainment of higher sex steroid levels ultimately results in termination of linear growth. It is now well established that the peak growth velocity, maturation of the epiphyseal plates, and accrual of bone mineral density during puberty are estrogen-dependent processes (11–13). Deficiencies in aromatase, the enzyme responsible for the conversion of androgen to estrogen, and resistance to the effects of estrogen caused by a mutations in the receptor for estrogen have highlighted the importance of pubertal estrogen to growth and bone mineral accrual in males (14–17). Growth plate senescence, referring to the estrogen-dependent, gradual decline of proliferative cells in the resting zone of the growth plate, has also emerged as an important factor in epiphyseal fusion (18,19).

Normal Pubertal Timing

The timing of pubertal onset is dependent on both genetic and environmental factors. An estimated 50% to 80% of the variation in pubertal timing is determined by genetic factors as evidenced by the correlation within families, monozygotic twins, and different ethnic groups (20–24) On average, black girls enter puberty earlier than other girls of other racial backgrounds, followed by Mexican-American and then white girls (20). Pubertal timing is also likely influenced by environmental factors such as nutrition, which is illustrated by the association between obesity and earlier pubertal onset in girls (25–27). Recent reports of environmental industrial compounds causing breast development in girls highlights the potential for other environmental influences on the HPG axis (28,29).

Historically, the standards for the normal ranges of pubertal timing came from the observational studies of British children from the 1960s by Tanner and Marshall (30,31). Their findings demonstrated that 95% of males started puberty (as assessed by an increase in testicular volume) between 9.5 and 13.5 years, with a mean age of 11.6 years. The duration from pubertal onset to full maturity of external genitalia took an average of 3 years. Among girls, 95% experienced breast development between 8.5 to 13 years, with an average age of 11.2 years and the duration from breast development to menarche was 2.3 years. Based on these studies, the traditional cut-offs for precocious puberty were development of secondary sex characteristics prior to the age of 9 years in boys and 8 years in girls.

Defining Precocious Puberty

Precocious puberty is defined as the onset of puberty at a younger age than would be expected for the normal population (i.e., 2 standard deviations (SDs) earlier than the population mean). Classically, pubertal signs occurring prior to 8 years for girls or 9 years for boys have been considered precocious. However, recent data based on a cross-sectional observational study of over 17,000 girls from the Pediatric Research in Office Settings (PROS) network suggested that puberty may be occurring earlier than previously thought. In this study, white girls experienced thelarche at a mean age of 9.96 ± 1.82 years and black girls at a mean age of 8.87 ± 1.93. Furthermore, 6.7% of white and 27.2% of black girls from this study would have been characterized as having precocious puberty when using the historic cutoff of 8 years (32).

Based on this study, the Drug and Therapeutics and Executive Committees of the Lawson Wilkins Pediatric Endocrine Society recommended lowering the age cut-off for precocious puberty to younger than 7 years in white girls and younger than 6 years in black girls. Pubertal onset occurring between 7 and 8 years in white girls and 6 and 8 years in black girls should be evaluated if there is unusually rapid pubertal progression resulting in bone age advancement by more than 2 years and a predicted height that is less than 150 cm or 2 SDs below genetic target height; signs or symptoms of a central nervous system (CNS) lesion; or behavior-based factors suggesting a child's emotional state is adversely affected by early puberty and potential early menses (33).

These new guidelines have not been universally accepted by endocrinologists and several have questioned the validity of the data from the PROS study. Concerns about ascertainment bias, accuracy of physical examination data, and a lack of change in the timing of menarche have all been raised as potential confounders (34–37). Perhaps most important, girls in this study were not evaluated for pathologic causes of precocious puberty or followed to determine the outcome of early puberty, prompting concerns about whether the new guidelines would fail to identify pathology. Supporting this concern were the findings in one patient population where 12% of girls evaluated solely for precocious puberty at age 6 to 8 years old had a treatable pathology (38).

There has not been similar controversy surrounding the normal age range of pubertal timing in boys. A recent analysis of the National Health and Nutritional Examination Survey III data found an earlier onset of testicular enlargement (Tanner genital stage 2) compared with traditional norms (39). Perhaps due to concerns about the criteria used for genital staging in this study and a lack of corroborating data, there have been no alterations to the accepted cut-off for precocity in boys (33,40).

Defining the correct cut-off for diagnosing precocious puberty ultimately rests on a consensus determination of the normal age range among different ethnic groups as well as an accurate background rate of pathologic cases among 6 to 8 year olds (24). At a minimum, sexual development in girls younger than 8 years and boys younger than 9 years warrants a thorough history and clinical examination, close longitudinal follow up, and a bone age.

VARIATIONS OF NORMAL PUBERTAL DEVELOPMENT

Premature Adrenarche

Adrenarche refers to the maturation of the adrenal cortex that leads to increased production of androgens responsible for many secondary sexual characteristics such as pubic hair, body odor, and acne. Adrenarche is a gradual process, occurring independent of the HPG axis (41). Most often, adrenarche precedes the onset of central puberty, typically around the age of 8 years. The etiology for premature adrenal androgen secretion is not well understood. Because the physical signs of adrenarche may indicate an underlying disorder of puberty, children with adrenarchal characteristics occurring at a young age should be evaluated for disorders of either central or peripheral precocious puberty. Benign premature adrenarche can be distinguished from pathologic forms of precocity due to a lack of significant bone age advancement (usually <2 years advanced or equivalent to height age), a lack of linear growth acceleration, absence of breast development in girls or testicular enlargement in boys, and a moderate increase in the concentrations of adrenal androgens, dehydroepiandrosterone (DHEA), DHEA-S, or androstenedione, which are usually consistent with Tanner stage of pubic hair development. Such children should be monitored clinically to ensure the tempo of further pubertal maturation is normal. Premature adrenarche generally occurs with increasing frequency between the ages of 3 and 8 years, although it may present as early as the 1st year of life. Girls are much more frequently affected than boys, with a ratio of almost 10:1 (42).

Although generally considered a benign variation in maturation, girls with premature adrenarche are at increased risk for developing insulin resistance and polycystic ovary syndrome (42). Evidence for an association between infants born small for gestational age and premature adrenarche has emerged as well (43).

Premature Thelarche

Premature thelarche refers to the isolated development of breast tissue in girls within the first 2 years of life. Breast tissue in premature thelarche is self-limited and is most often characterized by Tanner stage 2 or 3 development. Unlike precocious puberty, there is no accompanying linear growth acceleration or bone age advancement. Although the cause for premature thelarche remains unclear, girls with premature thelarche have increased estradiol levels compared with matched controls (44) and may have FSH-driven follicular maturation (45). Girls with intermittent or exaggerated thelarche have also been described. A subset of these girls may have mutations in the α subunit of the Gs protein, representing a nonclassic form of McCune–Albright syndrome (MAS) (46).

No therapy is required in cases of premature thelarche with the exception of close clinical follow up to ensure there is no evidence for clinical progression. Although rare, premature thelarche can represent early HPG axis activation (47) that may progress to true central precocious puberty (CPP) (48).

CENTRAL PRECOCIOUS PUBERTY

Etiology/Pathophysiology CPP results from the premature reactivation of the HPG axis. The increase in pulsatile LH secretion, increase in sex steroids, and progression of pubertal stages in CPP mimics that of normal puberty (49). The approximate incidence of CPP is 1:5,000 to 10,000 persons (50) and is more common in girls than boys, occurring at a ratio of approximately 10:1. When CPP occurs in boys it is more likely to be the result of a demonstrable CNS lesion. Approximately 20% of boys with CPP have an underlying CNS lesion compared with a rate of approximately 5% for girls (51,52). Idiopathic CPP is the most common cause in girls, accounting for approximately 85% of cases of CPP (52). Idiopathic CPP is more common among children adopted from developing nations, possibly due to nutritional factors, ethnicity, psychosocial factors, and inaccuracies in age (26,53,54). There also appears to be a familial tendency toward CPP in a subset of patients. Recent evidence suggests an autosomal dominant inheritance pattern with incomplete penetrance and sex-limited expression within this population (55).

Idiopathic CPP is a diagnosis of exclusion. CNS mass lesions or malformations should first be considered in the differential diagnosis of CPP. Risk factors for a CNS etiology include a young age and male gender. The most common CNS lesion associated with CPP is the hypothalamic hamartoma, a congenital, nonneoplastic, heterotopic collection of neural tissue located at the floor of the third ventricle. Hamartomas contain neurosecretory neurons composed of LH-releasing hormone (LHRH) or tumor necrosis factor-α (a stimulus for LHRH release), which likely function as an "ectopic GnRH-pulse generator" and are responsible for initiating the premature release of pulsatile gonadotropins (56,57). Several other CNS suprasellar and pineal tumors may cause CPP including optic gliomas, astrocytomas, and ependymomas. Congenital and acquired malformations and illnesses including empty sella syndrome, Arnold-Chiari malformation, subarachnoid cyst, neurofibromatosis type I, hydrocephalus, cranial irradiation, head trauma, and meningitis or encephalitis may also predispose to the development of CPP (24,49,58–60).

Clinical Presentation Children with CPP exhibit isosexual pubertal development at an early age. In girls, breast development and estrogenization of the vaginal mucosa precede the development of pubic and maxillary hair. Onset of menstruation follows in untreated girls. In boys, testicular enlargement is followed by penile enlargement, development of pubic hair, increased muscle mass, and deepening of the voice. Penile or breast development may be signs of both central and peripheral onset of puberty; however, ovarian follicle maturation and/or menarche and testicular enlargement usually result from central activation of the HPG axis. Boys and girls exhibit an increased growth velocity typical of the pubertal growth spurt. Bone age is significantly advanced compared with chronologic age. Slowly progressive or incomplete forms of progressive puberty have also been reported. In these cases, pubertal duration is longer and is associated with a less advanced bone age and better adult height prognosis (61,62).

Headaches, seizures, or other neurologic signs and symptoms should raise suspicion for an underlying CNS tumor. Patients with hypothalamic hamartoma have early precocious puberty, usually before 4 years of age and often at younger than 2 years of age. Approximately 50% of girls with hypothalamic hamartoma undergo menarche by the age of 4 years (58). Seizure disorders are common with intrahypothalamic as opposed to parahypothalamic hamartoma (63). Gelastic seizures, which manifest as laughing spells, are characteristic of hypothalamic hamartomas and are often resistant to anticonvulsant medications (64–66).

Diagnosis Classic laboratory findings in CPP include elevated estradiol (>20 pg/mL) or testosterone levels (>50 ng/dL), detectable, elevated basal LH levels higher than 0.3 IU/L (although these cutoffs may be dependent on the sensitivity of the assay used), and a pubertal response to GnRH agonist stimulation testing. Historically, GnRH stimulation testing has been the single most important diagnostic test to distinguish CPP from peripheral precocious puberty (PPP). GnRH stimulation is performed by giving a 100-μg intravenous or subcutaneous GnRH bolus and serially sampling serum LH and FSH for 60 to 90 minutes (67,68). Peak LH values are used to distinguish between pubertal and prepubertal activity of the HPG axis. Patients with CPP will demonstrate an LH-dominant pubertal response with an LH rise commonly greater than 8 to 10 IU/L. Prepubertal patients or those with PPP have little to no response or may have a FSH-predominant response (69,70). Significant overlap exists in GnRH-stimulated FSH responses between pubertal and prepubertal children. FSH measurements, therefore, have little value in the diagnosis of CPP except in determining the LH:FSH ratio.

Recently, GnRH has become commercially unavailable, making other means of diagnostic testing necessary. Older radioimmunoassays for LH and FSH lack sensitivity and specificity at lower gonadotropin levels, previously making basal LH and FSH levels unreliable. Newer immunofluorometric assays and immunochemiluminometric assays (ICMAs) improve accuracy with sensitivity down to 0.01 IU/L (70,71). A morning or basal LH level greater than 0.3 IU/L when using an ICMA has been demonstrated to correlate strongly with elevated peak LH levels on GnRH stimulation testing with a specificity of 100% for CPP (72). Basal LH will be elevated in approximately 66% of patients with CPP diagnosed by GnRH stimulation testing, making it a useful screening tool (72,73). A basal LH:FSH ratio above 1 may be sufficient for the diagnosis of CPP without GnRH stimulation (49). Many centers have now adopted the GnRH agonist stimulation test as an alternative to the historic GnRH [Factrel® (gonadorelin)] test. A commonly used protocol includes the administration of aqueous leuprolide acetate given subcutaneously at a dose of 20 μg/kg (maximum dose 500 μg). LH and FSH levels are measured at time 0, 60, 120, and 180 minutes post leuprolide administration

along with a testosterone or estradiol measurement at 24 hours. An LH-predominant response with an LH peak greater than 8 IU/L (67) and estradiol levels higher than 100 pg/mL or testosterone >50 ng/mL are suggestive of centrally mediated puberty. Other agents that have been used for this purpose include depot leuprolide (73), nafarelin (74), and triptorelin (75) but each of these may be limited by duration of effect, cost, and/or availability. Twenty-four-hour urinary gonadotropin values lack reliability and have no role in diagnosis (69).

Elevation of estradiol by ultrasensitive assay in females (76) and elevation of testosterone in males are also seen in CPP. Similar elevations in estradiol may be seen in benign premature thelarche (44), but this condition can be distinguished from true CPP based on a nonprogressive course, lack of bone age advancement, and prepubertal basal and GnRH-stimulated gonadotropin levels. Estradiol or testosterone at the upper limits of normal may be consistent with CPP but should also prompt consideration of gonadotropin-independent puberty.

Radiographs of the left wrist for bone age are indicated in all cases of precocious puberty. Bone age is advanced for chronologic age in cases of progressive precocious puberty. Although not routinely performed, the most reliable indicator of CPP on pelvic ultrasound is enlarged ovarian volume (>2SDs for age), although uterine length and volume and ovarian morphology may also support the diagnosis (77) (Figure 33-2). Due to the potential risk of CNS pathology, magnetic resonance imaging (MRI) of the brain should be performed in all children with a diagnosis of CPP (78).

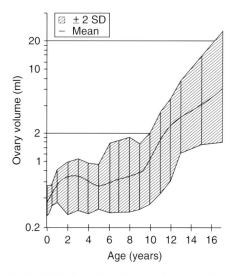

FIGURE 33-2. Ovary Volume Normal Values. Mean value of right and left ovarian volumes in relation to age. Ranges are expressed as mean and ± 2 SD. Figure used by permission (Ranke MB. *Diagnostics of Endocrine Function in Children and Adolescents.* London: Karger; 2003).

Outcomes of Untreated (Central) Precocious Puberty Because epiphyseal maturation is an estrogen-dependent process, a primary deleterious outcome of premature sex steroid exposure is rapid growth with advancement in bone age that ultimately leads to adult short stature (Figure 33-3). Children with earlier and more rapid pubertal progression and significant advancement in bone age present the greatest risk for loss of potential adult height (79,80). Patients with slowly progressive or unsustained CPP can achieve normal adult height without intervention (61,62,81).

Girls with precocious puberty may also be at an increased risk for behavioral difficulties, impaired peer relations, and psychologic problems. Children with precocious puberty often appear older than their chronologic age, leading adults to place greater responsibilities and have higher expectations than appropriate for their developmental level (82). Girls with precocious puberty may be moody, depressed, socially withdrawn, and aggressive (83,84). In one study with long-term follow up, adolescents and young adult females with a history of CPP exhibited an increased frequency of psychosomatic complaints compared with a control population (82). Despite these tendencies, there was not an increased rate of psychiatric diagnosis in women with a history of CPP nor were there significant differences in perception of attractiveness, satisfaction with appearance, or self-regard.

Treatment Treatment of CPP should be aimed at the underlying cause. Children with invasive tumors such as gliomas or astrocytomas should undergo appropriate neurosurgical and oncologic evaluation and intervention, if necessary. Most CNS tumors are surgically treated with the exception of hypothalamic hamartomas for which resection is not necessary unless the tumor is pedunculated or the tumor size poses additional risks to surrounding neural tissue. Primary treatment for hypothalamic hamartoma is directed at suppression of CPP with GnRH agonists.

Treatment is generally indicated in cases of idiopathic CPP in girls younger than 6 years of age and boys younger than 9 years of age. The decision about whether to treat CPP is more difficult with girls in the 6 to 8 year old age range. Most common indications for therapy include bone age advancement greater than 2 years beyond chronologic age, predicted adult height greater than 2 SDs below target height or less than 150 cm, rapid advancement of pubertal development, or psychosocial or behavioral concerns. Girls with unsustained or slowly progressive CPP who are not treated need close follow up, with clinical evaluation of

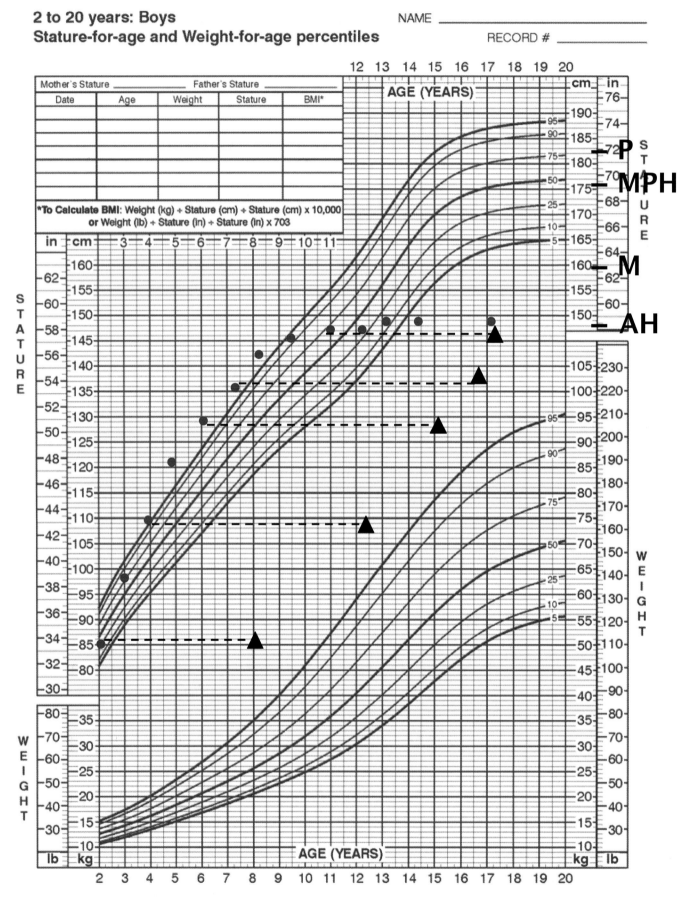

2 to 20 years: Boys
Stature-for-age and Weight-for-age percentiles

NAME _____

RECORD # _____

FIGURE 33-3. Growth Pattern Example of Male with Undiagnosed Precocious Puberty. Red circles represent individual height measurements. Black triangles represent theoretical bone ages. P: Paternal height; M: Maternal height; MPH: Midparental height; AH: Adult Height. Note accelerated growth rate earlier in childhood prior to premature epiphyseal fusion and slowing of growth velocity in early adolescence.

pubertal development and growth every 6 months (81,85).

Chronic administration of a synthetic GnRH agonist is the treatment of choice for CPP. After an initial stimulatory effect, chronic exposure to a GnRH agonist suppresses the HPG axis through continuous stimulation of pituitary GnRH receptors, rendering these receptors insensitive to the effect of endogenous pulsatile GnRH. Multiple formulations of GnRH agonists are available. Frequency of administration is daily with subcutaneous or intranasal formulations or monthly with intramuscular or subcutaneous injection of depot formulations. A 3-month depot form has been used primarily in Europe (86,87) and may soon be available in the United States as well, although concerns about its effectiveness compared with standard 4-week depot forms remain (86,88). Most recently, an implantable GnRH analog, Histrelin, has become available with preliminary evidence for effective HPG axis suppression over a one-year period (89). In the United States, leuprolide depot formulation is most commonly used at a starting dose of 7.5 mg every 4 weeks. Adequacy of suppression can be assessed by performing repeated GnRH stimulation testing or by monitoring gonadotropin levels shortly after routine monthly depot injection (73,90). An LH level of 3 IU/L or less 30 to 60 minutes, or 6 IU/L or less 2 hours after a depot injection have been proposed for defining therapeutic response. If suppression is inadequate, the GnRH agonist dose or frequency of depot administration can be increased.

Suppression of the HPG axis with GnRH agonists leads to regression of secondary sexual characteristics, slowing of growth velocity, and decreased bone age advancement. Withdrawal bleeding may occur in the first few weeks secondary to a transient stimulatory effect of therapy but is followed by cessation of menses. LH response to GnRH decreases to prepubertal level within 2 to 4 weeks and sex steroid levels are suppressed to prepubertal levels within 4 to 12 weeks of beginning treatment. Ovarian and uterine volumes decrease in girls and testicular volume decreases in boys. Following completion of therapy, LH, FSH, and sex steroid levels should return to pretreatment levels within 6 months. Pubertal development resumes with onset of menstruation typically 1 to 1.5 years after cessation of treatment (91–93). Time to menses may be shorter for patients with a history of menstruation prior to GnRH analog therapy compared with those with no menstrual history (94).

In idiopathic CPP, the purpose of treatment is to preserve adult height potential and prevent psychosocial problems associated with early puberty. Multiple clinical trials have confirmed improved adult height outcomes with GnRH agonist therapy (reviewed in (50, 79)). Approximately three-fourths of patients treated with GnRH agonists will reach their genetic target height range and 90% will have a height of more than 150 cm. Height gains are dependent on several factors but the greatest gains in adult height or predicted adult height are seen with early initiation of treatment prior to the age 6 years in girls and in those with lower predicted height at onset of treatment (85,95,96). Additional factors that may influence final height outcomes include pretreatment bone age, duration of treatment, bone age advancement and height at the end of treatment, target height, chronologic age at the end of treatment, and posttreatment growth spurt (50,79,92,97–99). To maximize adult height, GnRH analog treatment should be discontinued in girls at a chronological age of 11 years or a bone age of 12 to 12.5 years, and in boys at a bone age of 13 years. Continuing treatment beyond 11 years of age in girls might be detrimental to adult height by compromising a posttreatment growth spurt (97). Girls with an older age at onset of CPP, less advancement in bone age, and better predicted adult height may demonstrate adequate height gains without treatment.

Patients should be aware of rare yet potential side effects of GnRH agonists. Perimenopausal symptoms including hot flashes, irritability, and insomnia have been reported at the onset of treatment. Potential local reactions at the injection site include erythema, induration, muscle pain, and wheal formation. Sterile abscesses may occur with depot formulations (100). BMD is typically increased for chronologic age prior to treatment in CPP. Conflicting studies have shown either stable (101–103) or decreased BMD (104,105) following treatment with GnRH agonists. Any potential decreases in BMD may be prevented or reversed with calcium supplementation during treatment (106). Body mass index tends to be higher than normal in CPP girls both before and after treatment with GnRH analogs. Treatment itself does not appear to have any significant long-term effect on body mass index (92,107). Polycystic ovaries have been observed in females after treatment but the incidence appears to be no greater than in asymptomatic women in the general population (108). Fertility has not been formally studied, although pregnancies have occurred in women treated with GnRH analogs. Urinary hormone levels followed in menstruating patients who had received treatment for idiopathic CPP in childhood suggest these patients have normal ovulatory cycles (94). More recent evidence suggests that no differences exist in adult menstrual patterns or function of the pituitary–gonadal axis between women with a history of CPP treated with a GnRH agonist and two control populations (107).

Prior to the availability of GnRH agonists for treatment of CPP, medroxyprogesterone acetate or cyproterone acetate were the primary treatment modalities. Cyproterone acetate and medroxyprogesterone acetate inhibit gonadotropin release, leading to the suppression of menstruation and some arrest of secondary sexual characteristics development; however, the effect on adult height preservation was minimal (109,110). Although infrequently used, these agents may remain useful as an adjunct treatment during initiation of GnRH agonist therapy to oppose the initial stimulatory effects of GnRH agonists (109).

PERIPHERAL PRECOCIOUS PUBERTY

PPP, or gonadotropin-independent precocious puberty, refers to the development of secondary sex characteristics without activation of the HPG axis. Pubertal development may be virilizing or feminizing depending on the underlying disorder. Excess sex steroids may originate from the adrenal glands, gonads, or exogenous sources. The differential diagnosis for this set of disorders is vast and includes McCune–Albright syndrome (MAS), familial or sporadic male-limited precocious puberty, gonadal tumors, adrenal tumors, congenital adrenal hyper-plasia (CAH), β-human chorionic gonadotropin (hCG)-secreting tumors, hypothyroidism, ovarian cysts, and exogenous exposure to sex steroids. MAS and male-limited precocious puberty (MLPP) represent a unique category of gonadotropin-independent precocious puberty in which genetic mutations lead to autonomous production of sex steroids by the gonads in absence of pubertal gonadotropin stimulation.

Distinguishing CPP from peripheral forms of precocious puberty is important for therapeutic considerations but can be quite challenging. Both forms of precocity are associated with development of secondary sexual characteristics, bone age advancement, and linear growth acceleration. Unlike in central precocity, disorders of peripheral precocity do not cause significant gonadal maturation (i.e., testicular or ovarian growth) although mild degrees may be seen in MAS and MLPP. Gonadotropin levels and response to GnRH stimulation testing are prepubertal in PPP; however, transition from PPP to CPP has been reported with most etiologies of PPP including MAS, MLPP, CAH, gonadal tumors, and adrenal tumors (111,112). The mechanism for this phenomenon is not well understood but may be related to the direct effects of increased sex steroids on the maturation of the HPG axis. The subsequent treatment and decrease in sex steroids may then lead to decreased negative feedback inhibition at the level of the hypothalamus and pituitary gland. Alternatively, skeletal maturation may provide feedback to the CNS regarding developmental status resulting in CPP.

A proposed guide for the diagnostic evaluation of both boys and girls with precocious puberty is illustrated in Figures 33-4 through 33-8. These figures should be used only as a source to guide preliminary diagnostic decision making and should not be seen as absolute because exceptions to the proposed decision-making tree for individual presentations and/or diagnoses may occur.

McCUNE–ALBRIGHT SYNDROME

Etiology and Pathophysiology MAS is characterized by café-au-lait skin lesions, precocious puberty, and polyostotic fibrous dysplasia of bone. These features result from a gain-of-function mutation in the *GNAS1* gene for the α-subunit of the stimulatory G protein (Gsα) (113). Ligand binding to the normal receptor induces Gsα to exchange guanine diphosphate (GDP) for guanine triphosphate (GTP). The GTP-bound α-subunit dissociates from the receptor and stimulates adenylate cyclase to increase intracellular cyclic adenosine monophosphate concentration activating second messenger pathways (PKA and PKC) important in gene expression and cellular regulation. Under normal circumstances, intrinsic GTPase of Gsα activity converts GTP to GDP, inactivating the Gsα subunit. In individuals with MAS, this intrinsic GTPase activity is deficient, resulting in persistent activation of the signaling pathway in the absence of an external signal.

Stimulatory G proteins interact with a variety of transmembrane receptors including FSH and LH receptors. Thus, LH receptors of individuals with MAS are tonically activated, resulting in pubertal levels of estradiol or testosterone despite prepubertal levels of circulating gonadotropins. Additional endocrinopathies, including hyperthyroidism, Cushing syndrome, and acromegaly similarly may result from constitutive activation of stimulatory G protein within the thyroid gland, adrenal gland, and pituitary gland, respectively. Hypophosphatemic rickets or osteopenia can occur due to decreased renal tubular phosphate reabsorption, possibly from altered renal adenylate cyclase activity or a phosphaturic substance produced by dysplastic bone lesions (114,115).

Mutations in MAS occur in multiple tissues from all three germ layers—endoderm, mesoderm, ectoderm—but are not present in all tissues, suggesting a postzygotic somatic mutation occurring early in embryologic development prior to the formation of the trilaminar disk (113,116). This variation in tissue mosaicism accounts for the variety of clinical manifestations seen in MAS. Germ line mutations likely represent a lethal mutation (117). The *GNAS1* gene on chromosome 21 encodes the α-subunit of G-stimulatory protein. The genetic etiology of MAS appears to be a point mutation in the *GNAS1* gene, which leads to the constitutive activation of Gsα. Two mutations were identified in exon 8 of Gsα at position 201, resulting in substitution of cysteine or histidine for arginine (113,116). Similar isolated mutations of Gsα at codon 201 and 227 have been described in GH-secreting pituitary tumors and thyroid tumors (116).

Clinical Presentation MAS does not appear to follow a classic inheritance pattern and females are affected more often than males. Diagnosis is based on the presence of the classic triad of café-au-lait spots, precocious puberty, and polyostotic fibrous dysplasia (Figures 33-9 to 33-11). Disease is considered nonclassic when only two components of the triad are present (118–120).

Precocious puberty occurs in more than 90% of females with MAS but less frequently in males. Signs of precocious puberty in girls may be present as early as the 1st year of life and increase with age thereafter. Estradiol production by autonomously functioning ovarian cysts can lead to rapid breast development and/or menstruation. Onset of menses may also precede breast development. Pubic hair is seen less frequently. Progression of pubertal signs may slow and spontaneous regression of secondary sex characteristics is common. Potential for autonomous ovarian hyperfunction persists even after the onset

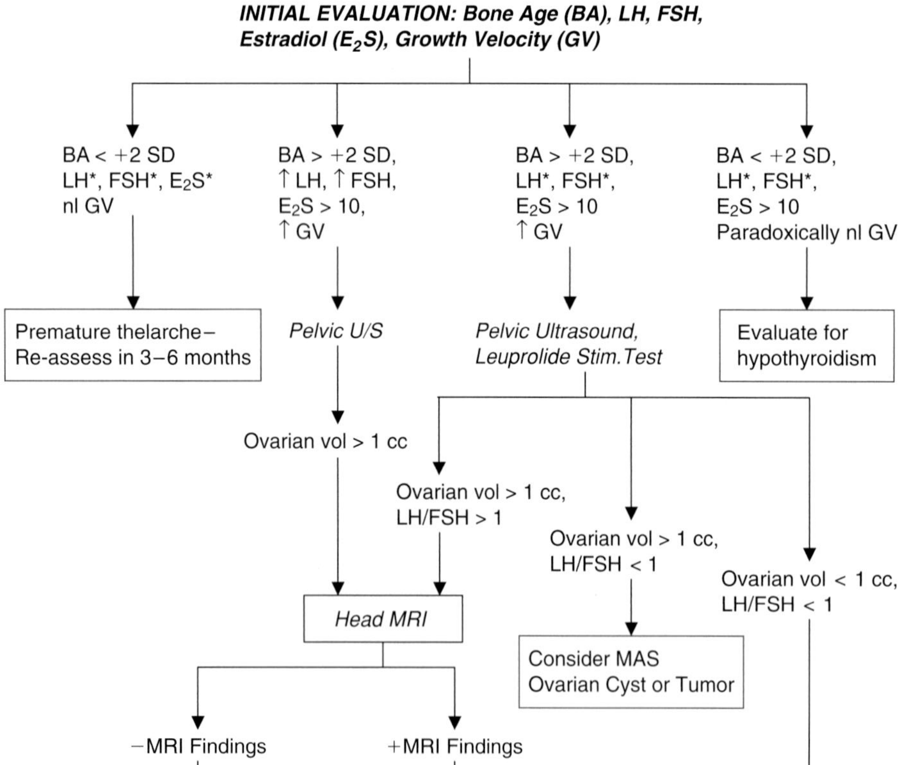

INITIAL EVALUATION: Bone Age (BA), LH, FSH, Estradiol (E₂S), Growth Velocity (GV)

FIGURE 33-4. Precocious Puberty Evaluation–Females with Isolated Breast Development.
*Normal prepubertal values.
LH–Luteinizing hormone; FSH–Follicle-stimulating hormone; GnRH–Gonadotropin-releasing hormone; MAS–McCune Albright Syndrome.

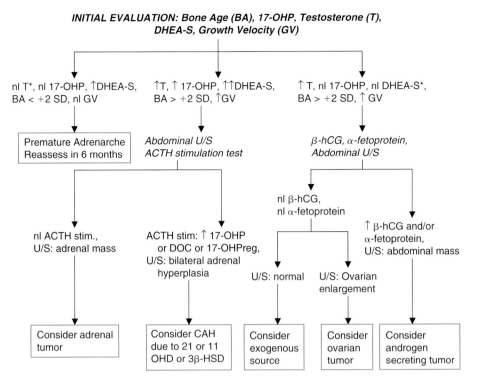

FIGURE 33-5. Precocious Pubarche Evaluation–Females with Increased Virilization and No Breast Development.
*Appropriate for age or adrenarche.
LH–Luteinizing hormone; FSH–Follicle-stimulating hormone; 17-OHP–17α-hydroxyprogesterone; 17-OHPreg–17α-hydroxypregnenolone; DHEA-S–Dehydroepiandrosterone sulfate; DOC–Deoxycorticosterone; GnRH–Gonadotropin-releasing hormone; β-hCG–β-human chorionic gonadotropn; ACTH–Adrenal corticotropin stimulating hormone; U/S–Ultrasound; SD–Standard deviation; 21-OHD–21-hydroxylase deficiency; 11-OHD–11β-hydroxylase deficiency; 3 β-HSD–3β-hydroxysteroid dehydrogenase deficiency.

of central puberty (121). Precocious puberty in males generally occurs later, most often between the ages of 4 to 9 years. In males, precocious puberty is characterized by testicular enlargement, androgenization of external genitalia, and, less often, pubic hair development. Adrenarche typically occurs appropriately for chronologic age.

Café-au-lait macules are pigmented skin lesions with well-demarcated irregular borders occurring in more than 90% of patients with MAS. Café-au-lait macules are usually present at birth and do not typically increase in size or number with age. Café-au-lait spots are few in number and often occur near the midline. They may be bilateral or unilateral and the trunk, limbs, or face may be affected.

Polyostotic fibrous dysplasia occurs in more than 60% of patients, most commonly involving the long bones and base of the skull. In fibrous dysplasia, cysticlike areas of bone reabsorption are replaced by fibrous spindle cells and weakened, poorly formed, bony trabeculae. Signs and symptoms include pain, pathologic fractures of long bones, and deformity. Cranial fibrous dysplasia may cause facial asymmetry and compression of the optic or auditory nerves leading to visual or hearing impairment (118,122).

Additional endocrinopathies and systemic involvement of the liver, kidneys, thymus,

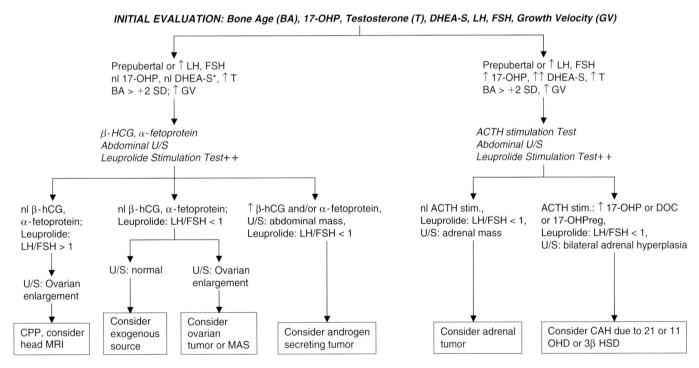

FIGURE 33-6. Precocious Puberty Evaluation–Females with Breast and Pubic Hair Development.
LH–Luteinizing hormone; FSH–Follicle-stimulating hormone; 17-OHP–17α-hydroxyprogesterone; 17-OHPreg–17α-hydroxypregnenolone; DHEA-S–Dehydroepiandrosterone sulfate; DOC–Deoxycorticosterone; GnRH–Gonadotropin-releasing hormone; β-hCG–β-human chorionic gonadotropn; ACTH–Adrenal corticotropin stimulating hormone; U/S–Ultrasound; SD–Standard deviation; 21 OHD 21 hydroxylase deficiency; 11-OHD–11β-hydroxylase deficiency; 3β-HSD–3β-hydroxysteroid dehydrogenase deficiency. MAS–McCune Albright Syndrome.
*Appropriate for age and adrenarche.
**Leuprolide stimulation test for patients with prepubertal gonadotropins.

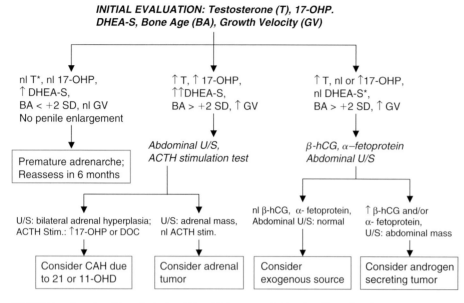

INITIAL EVALUATION: Testosterone (T), 17-OHP. DHEA-S, Bone Age (BA), Growth Velocity (GV)

nl T*, nl 17-OHP, ↑ DHEA-S, BA < +2 SD, nl GV, No penile enlargement → Premature adrenarche; Reassess in 6 months

↑ T, ↑ 17-OHP, ↑↑DHEA-S, BA > +2 SD, ↑ GV → *Abdominal U/S, ACTH stimulation test*
- U/S: bilateral adrenal hyperplasia; ACTH Stim.: ↑17-OHP or DOC → Consider CAH due to 21 or 11-OHD
- U/S: adrenal mass, nl ACTH stim. → Consider adrenal tumor

↑ T, nl or ↑17-OHP, nl DHEA-S*, BA > +2 SD, ↑ GV → *β-hCG, α–fetoprotein Abdominal U/S*
- nl β-hCG, α- fetoprotein, Abdominal U/S: normal → Consider exogenous source
- ↑ β-hCG and/or α- fetoprotein, U/S: abdominal mass → Consider androgen secreting tumor

FIGURE 33-7. Precocious Puberty Evaluation–Males with Testes ≤3cc, Pubic Hair, and/or Penile Enlargement. *Appropriate for age and/or adrenarche.

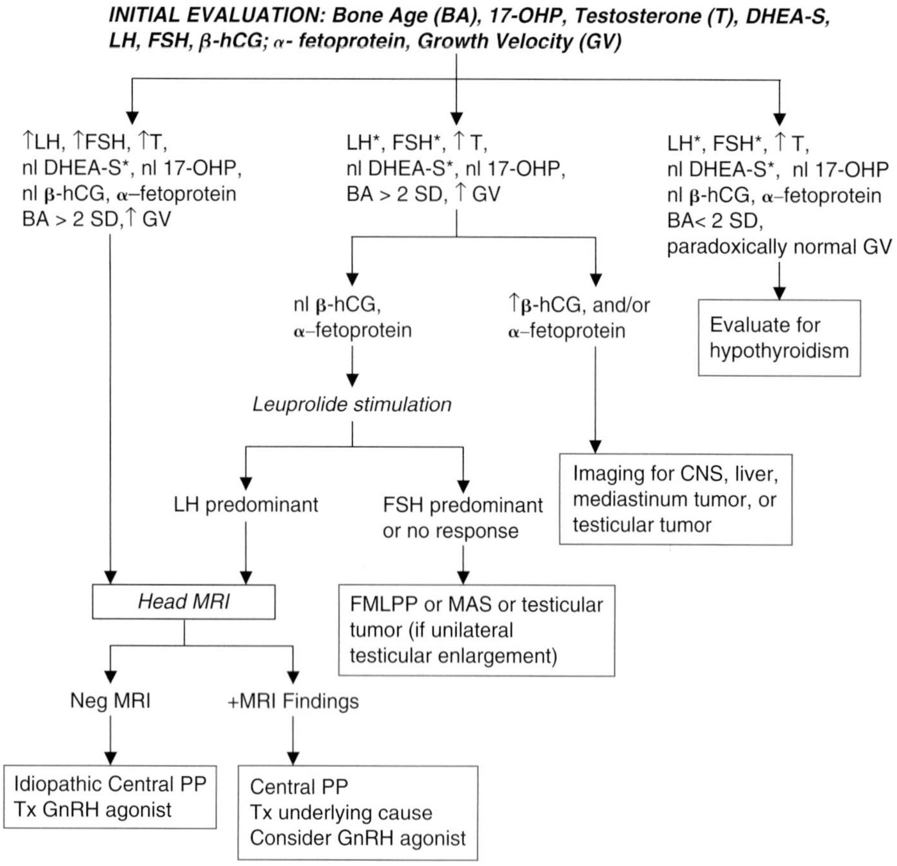

INITIAL EVALUATION: Bone Age (BA), 17-OHP, Testosterone (T), DHEA-S, LH, FSH, β-hCG; α- fetoprotein, Growth Velocity (GV)

↑LH, ↑FSH, ↑T, nl DHEA-S*, nl 17-OHP, nl β-hCG, α–fetoprotein BA > 2 SD,↑ GV

LH*, FSH*, ↑ T, nl DHEA-S*, nl 17-OHP, BA > 2 SD, ↑ GV
- nl β-hCG, α–fetoprotein → *Leuprolide stimulation*
  - LH predominant → *Head MRI*
  - FSH predominant or no response → FMLPP or MAS or testicular tumor (if unilateral testicular enlargement)
- ↑β-hCG, and/or α–fetoprotein → Imaging for CNS, liver, mediastinum tumor, or testicular tumor

LH*, FSH*, ↑ T, nl DHEA-S*, nl 17-OHP nl β-hCG, α–fetoprotein BA< 2 SD, paradoxically normal GV → Evaluate for hypothyroidism

Head MRI
- Neg MRI → Idiopathic Central PP Tx GnRH agonist
- +MRI Findings → Central PP Tx underlying cause Consider GnRH agonist

FIGURE 33-8. Precocious Puberty Evaluation–Males with Testes ≥3 cc, Pubic Hair, and/or Penile Enlargement. Gonadotropins and testosterone samples should be drawn in a.m.
*Appropriate for age.
**Prepubertal.
LH–Luteinizing hormone; FSH–Follicle-stimulating hormone; 17-OHP–17α-hydroxyprogesterone; 17-OHPreg–17α-hydroxypregnenolone; DHEA-S–Dehydroepiandrosterone sulfate; DOC–Deoxycorticosterone; GnRH–Gonadotropin-releasing hormone; β-hCG–β-human chorionic gonadotropn; ACTH–Adrenal corticotropin stimulating hormone; U/S–Ultrasound; SD-Standard deviation; 21-OHD–21-hydroxylase deficiency; 11-OHD–11β-hydroxylase deficiency; 3β-HSD–3β-hydroxysteroid dehydrogenase deficiency. MAS–McCune Albright Syndrome; FMLPP–Familiar male–limited precocious puberty.

gastrointestinal tract, and heart have been described in MAS (117,118,122–124). Hyperthyroidism occurs in 20% of patients and is the second most common endocrine manifestation in MAS. Other reported endocrinopathies include acromegaly due to GH hypersecretion and Cushing syndrome. GH hypersecretion is associated with hyperprolactinemia in 80% to 90% of cases. Additional nonendocrine manifestations include hepatocellular disease with direct hyperbilirubinemia in infancy, renal tubular phosphate wasting, electrolyte imbalances, thymic hyperplasia, adenomatous gastrointestinal polyps, acute pancreatitis, cardiomegaly, and cardiac arrest.

Diagnosis Diagnosis of MAS is made clinically based on the presence of the classic triad. Precocious puberty is associated with elevated levels of estradiol in girls and testosterone in boys, prepubertal basal and stimulated LH and FSH levels, and an advanced bone age. Pelvic ultrasound may demonstrate asymmetric ovaries and ovarian cysts. Fibrous dysplasia of bone lesions is often evident on radiographs, but milder lesions may be detected on a bone scan. Lesions are typically radiolucent and cysticlike on plain radiographs, although skull lesions are often sclerotic. In individuals with hyperthyroidism, thyroid autoantibodies and thyroid-stimulating immunoglobulins are negative. Pituitary adenomas are present in 40% of patients with GH excess. In patients with Cushing features, ACTH is low and cortisol levels cannot be suppressed with dexamethasone. In hypophosphatemia, serum phosphorus levels are low but serum calcium, vitamin D, and parathyroid hormone levels are normal.

GNAS1 mutations can be identified in affected tissue samples although genetic diagnosis is not always necessary when clinical features are prominent. Because individuals with MAS are mosaic for the GNAS1 mutation, DNA analysis of peripheral blood leukocytes is often negative for the mutation.

Treatment Multiple medication regimens have been used to treat precocious puberty in MAS. Older regimens included the use of medroxyprogesterone acetate, a progesterone with antiestrogen effects, and cyproterone acetate, an antiandrogen with inherent progestin and antiestrogen activity. Both medroxyprogesterone and cyproterone acetate decrease breast development and menstrual bleeding but have had little effect on adult height (reviewed in (125)). Ketoconazole has been used for its inhibitory effects on the CYP-450 enzymes 17, 20-desmolase and 11-, 17-, and 18-hydroxylase involved in gonadal steroidogenesis. Patients receiving ketoconazole have reduced estradiol levels, cessation

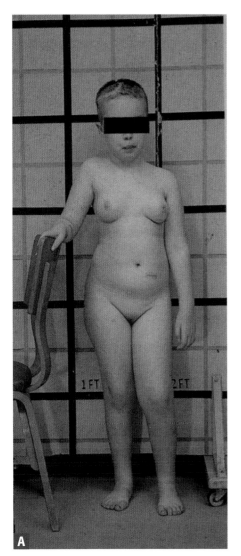

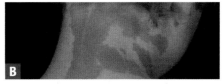

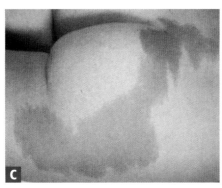

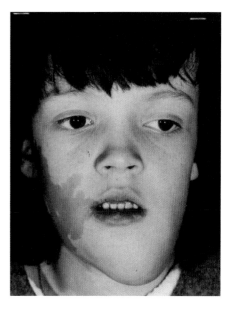

FIGURE 33-10. McCune–Albright. Patient has enlarged and extended jaw, secondary to fibrous dysplasia, and café-au-lait spots on the face (which is rare). Photo provided by Dr. Robert Gorlin.

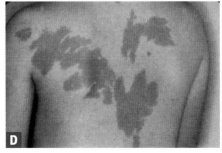

FIGURE 33-9. A to D. McCune–Albright Café-au-Lait spots. Female patient with characteristic, well-defined, irregular cutaneous light brown pigmented areas (café-au-lait spots in an irregular outline known as the "coast of Maine") and precocious puberty. Photos provided by Dr. Robert Gorlin.

of menses, and regression of pubertal signs. The main disadvantages of ketoconazole are its multiple side effects including idiopathic hepatotoxicity in 0.01% (126).

More recently, testolactone and tamoxifen have become the treatments of choice for precocious puberty in MAS. Normally, ovarian thecal cells produce androgens that are converted to estrogens in ovarian granulosa cells by the enzyme aromatase (127). Testolactone, an aromatase inhibitor, inhibits the enzymatic conversion of androgens to estrogens, thereby decreasing ovarian estrogen production, decreasing frequency of menses, and slowing the rates of bone maturation in patients with MAS (128,129). Estradiol levels may not be decreased to prepubertal levels and intermittent menses can occur (130). Adverse effects of testolactone include transient abdominal pain, headaches, diarrhea, and

elevated liver enzymes. More specific aromatase inhibitors such as anastrozole, a third generation aromatase inhibitor, have shown promise in decreasing bone age progression and improving predicted adult height in one patient with MAS (131). It has the advantage of fewer side effects and more convenient once-a-day dosing. In contrast, another selective aromatase inhibitor, fadrozole, had limited benefit in slowing pubertal progression in 16 girls with MAS (132).

Tamoxifen, a nonsteroidal antiestrogen, has shown recent promise in the treatment of precocious puberty in MAS. Tamoxifen use results in a slowing of pubertal progression and linear growth velocity, decreased rate of skeletal maturation, and decreased frequency of menstruation (133). Estradiol levels remain elevated on tamoxifen, and persistent enlargement of the ovaries and increased

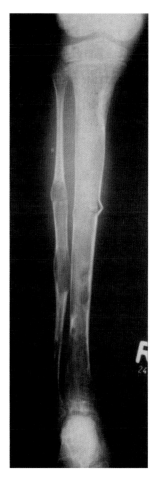

FIGURE 33-11. McCune–Albright: Thickening and pseudocystic involvement of tibia and fibula. Photo provided by Dr. Robert Gorlin.

uterine volumes have been observed (133). Periodic pelvic ultrasounds are thus advised while on tamoxifen to follow uterine volumes (117). Surgical ovarian cyst removal is generally not recommended in MAS as the recurrence rate is high but may be successful in select cases with unilateral ovarian involvement (134). GnRH analogs are effective only if central precocious puberty develops. Hyperthyroidism, when present, is treated by surgical or radioiodine ablation (118). Treatment of fibrous dysplasia with pamidronate, a bisphosphonate, may decrease pain and fracture risk (135–137). A commonly used regimen of pamidronate has been administered at a dose of 1 mg/kg/day for 3 days every 3 to 6 months (119,137). Surgical treatment of fibrous dysplasia is reserved for cases involving cranial nerve compression with loss of function, progressive deformity, or uncontrolled pain.

MALE-LIMITED PRECOCIOUS PUBERTY

Etiology/Pathophysiology Sporadic and familial MLPP, also known as familial testotoxicosis, is an autosomal dominant disorder with greater than 90% penetrance; it is characterized by precocious pubertal development in males. In MLPP, an activating mutation of the LH receptor in Leydig cells results in autonomous testosterone production (138). Expression of the LH receptor mutation is gender limited as females are asymptomatic carriers (139). Twelve missense mutations in the LH receptor, located on chromosome 2 have been identified, typically in the fifth or sixth transmembrane spanning region or third cytoplasmic loop (140). More recently, mutations have been identified in the first transmembrane loop in select ethnic backgrounds (141). Mutations result in the persistent activation of the LH receptor, thereby activating the G protein pathway and increasing cyclic adenosine monophosphate concentrations in the absence of gonadotropin stimulation (122,142).

Clinical Presentation Boys with MLPP have onset of precocious puberty early in life, typically between 1–4 years of age (139). Increased androgen levels result in penile growth, development of axillary and pubic hair, and acne. A significant increase in linear growth velocity and bone age advancement can occur that may result in compromised final adult height (122,125). A mild degree of testicular enlargement is observed but is less than would be typical for the stage of pubertal development (125,130).

Diagnosis Pubertal testosterone levels in the face of prepubertal basal and stimulated gonadotropin levels are encountered. Bone age is advanced. Testicular ultrasound should be performed to exclude a testosterone-producing tumor. Testicular biopsy is not indicated for diagnostic work up but when performed shows Leydig cell maturation or hyperplasia and varying degrees of spermatogenesis in affected males. Family history should reveal other male members with precocious puberty, although a minority of MLPP index cases may be sporadic. Genetic testing for the LH receptor mutations by polymerase chain reaction–based gene sequencing is commercially available.

Treatment Similar to MAS, treatments for MLPP in the past included agents that inhibit androgen biosynthesis such as cyproterone acetate, medroxyprogesterone acetate, or ketoconazole. Medroxyprogesterone and cyproterone acetate have efficacy in decreasing testosterone levels and height velocity (143,144). Treatment with ketoconazole is associated with a rapid decrease in testosterone levels, decreased growth velocity, and slowing of bone age advancement. Adult height achieved with ketoconazole treatment has been reported to exceed pretreatment predicted adult height (145).

Testolactone, an aromatase inhibitor, and spironolactone, an androgen receptor blocker, are alternative forms of therapy for MLPP. Neither testolactone nor spironolactone alone have demonstrated satisfactory control of precocious puberty, but when used in combination, treatment result in slowed bone age advancement, decreased growth velocity, lower frequency of spontaneous erections, and decreased aggressive behavior (146,147). Predicted adult height increased from 160.7 cm to 173.6 cm in 10 boys treated with testolactone and spironolactone in one study (147). Although generally well-tolerated, testolactone may cause gastrointestinal upset potentially limiting adherence to the regimen. Recently, the third generation aromatase inhibitor, anastrazole, administered in combination with antiandrogen therapy was shown to slow growth velocity, skeletal maturation, and progression of secondary sexual characteristics in 2 boys with FMLPP. Anastrazole has several advantages over testolactone, including more complete inhibition of the P450 aromatase and the convenience of once daily dosing (148).

Following initiation of treatment, some boys may develop CPP, characterized by a pubertal LH response to GnRH stimulation testing. If GnRH stimulation indicates development of CPP, a GnRH analog should be added to the treatment regimen to suppress the HPG axis (147,149). GnRH analogs have no efficacy in the treatment of MLPP in the absence of secondary CPP.

GONADAL TUMORS

Etiology/Pathophysiology Stromal cell tumors of the gonad are rare causes of PPP in both genders. Leydig cell tumors are the most common sex steroid–secreting testicular tumor in males, accounting for 6% of testicular tumors in prepubertal boys (150). Somatic mutations of the LH receptor have been identified in a subset of Leydig cell tumors activating the LH receptor and G protein pathway implicated in MLPP (151). Granulosa cell is the most common ovarian tumor type in girls presenting with PPP (152). Other less frequently encountered tumor types include Sertoli cell, theca cell, Sertoli–Leydig cell, and granulosa–thecal cell tumors (152).

Clinical Presentation Precocious pubertal development may be feminizing or virilizing depending on the tumor type. Boys with Leydig cell tumors exhibit penile growth and development of pubic hair. Spontaneous erections and penile emissions can occur. Testes are asymmetric in size, with one enlarged tumor-containing testis and one prepubertal unaffected testis (153). Granulosa cell tumors present with precocious puberty in 70% of affected girls. Initially, areolar pigmentation and breast development occurs, followed by the onset of menstruation and growth of pubic hair. The onset of precocious puberty can be particularly rapid. Less common presenting signs include abdominal pain, fever, irritability, and ascites (152). Granulosa cell tumors can present at any age but most often occur in the first decade of life, frequently before the age of 4 years. Sertoli–Leydig cell tumors occur rarely in girls and can be associated with symptoms of androgen and less often, estrogen excess (154).

Diagnosis In Leydig cell tumors, testosterone and, rarely, androstenedione, levels are elevated (153). Granulosa cell tumors are associated with increased estradiol levels (152,155). Inhibin levels may be elevated with granulosa or Sertoli–Leydig cell tumors and may serve as a useful tumor marker (154). Response to GnRH stimulation testing is prepubertal, although CPP with a pubertal response to GnRH stimulation can develop after treatment (156). Testicular tumors are typically diagnosed by ultrasound, although MRI may have some utility in determining tumor type (157). Ovarian tumors can be diagnosed by ultrasound, computed tomography (CT) scan, or MRI (158).

Treatment Treatment of gonadal tumors involves a multidisciplinary approach. The overall prognosis is good for both ovarian and testicular stromal cell tumors (159,160). Resection is usually curative and leads to regression of pubertal signs. Among all prepubertal boys younger than the age of 12 with testicular stromal cell tumors in one tumor registry, only one patient (with an undifferentiated stromal cell tumor) had metastatic disease, which was characterized by local invasion (159). No patient with a Leydig cell tumor experienced metastatic disease. Resection is typically the sole treatment modality for testicular stromal cell tumors, with either orchiectomy or a testis-sparing approach.

Advanced disease is slightly more common in ovarian stromal cell tumors but overall survival is still high (160,161). Among 72 pediatric patients in a German tumor registry, the 10-year event free survival rate for children with ovarian stromal cell tumors was 88%. The most important predictors of relapse and metastatic disease were the clinical stage of disease and mitotic activity on histopathology (160). Most juvenile granulosa and thecal cell tumors presenting with precocious puberty are localized at diagnosis and have a good prognosis (152,154). The primary treatment modality is resection, usually by oophorectomy or salpingo-oophorectomy, with adjuvant chemotherapy required in rare cases (160). If secondary CPP occurs, GnRH analogs should be used (154).

ADRENAL TUMORS

Etiology/Pathophysiology Adrenocortical neoplasms, including benign adenomas and malignant carcinomas, comprise only 0.5% of all pediatric neoplasms (162) and represent an exceedingly rare cause of PPP in children. In functional adrenocortical neoplasms, supraphysiologic amounts of adrenocortical steroids (glucocorticoids or androgens) are produced in the absence of ACTH stimulation. Feminization from adrenal tumors may occur rarely and is likely associated with tumor expression of aromatase causing conversion of androgens to estrogens (163). Adrenocortical tumors in children have been associated with several genetic syndromes, including Beckwith–Wiedemann and Li–Fraumeni syndromes (162,164).

Clinical Presentation Childhood adrenocortical tumors most commonly present in the first decade of life, at a mean age of 4 years (162,165). Females are two to four times more likely than males to be affected and there is a higher incidence among children from southern Brazil (166). Unlike in adults, most adrenocortical tumors in children are hormonally active. The predominant manifestations of hormonally active adrenocortical tumors are precocious puberty and Cushing syndrome (167). Precocious development of pubic hair, increased penile size or clitoromegaly, deep-

ening voice, increased muscle mass, and an increased linear growth are signs of increased secretion of androgens. Abdominal distention or a palpable mass may be present on examination. Postpubertal females may have amenorrhea or oligomenorrhea secondary to hyperandrogenism. In males testes are usually prepubertal in size, although mild testicular enlargement has been reported, possibly due to androgen's effect on seminiferous tubular growth (167). Rare feminizing adrenocortical tumors lead to breast development and menstruation in girls (163). Physical examination shows features of Cushing syndrome, including weight gain with centripetal fat pattern, hypertension, acne, striae, hirsutism, and linear growth deceleration. Hypertension, hypokalemia, and pseudoparalysis from hyperaldosteronism have been reported (164).

Diagnosis Elevations in hormones of the adrenocortical/androgen biosynthetic pathways such as DHEA and its sulfated counterpart, DHEA-S, androstenedione, testosterone, and/or cortisol are present. Basal gonadotropin levels and response to GnRH stimulation are prepubertal. Adrenal steroid precursors including 11-deoxycorticosterone, 17-hydroxypregnenolone, and 17-hydroxyprogesterone may also be elevated. Imaging studies including ultrasonography, CT, or MRI of the abdomen are essential to diagnosis. CT is superior to ultrasound for identifying small lesions (0.5–1 cm) and can help delineate regional spread and vascular invasion (164). MRI may further differentiate adrenal tumor from surrounding tissue (164).

Treatment Resection is the mainstay of treatment for adrenocortical adenoma and carcinoma. Corticosteroids at stress doses should be given perioperatively as cortisol overexpression by tumor tissue may lead to suppression of the unaffected adrenal gland. Adjuvant chemotherapy is often given with metastatic or invasive disease. No optimal chemotherapy regimen exists but commonly used agents include mitotane and cisplatin (168,169). Radiation has not been found to be beneficial (170).

Overall survival rates for children with adrenocortical tumors are high, reported at 50% to 85% (162). Presence of vascular and capsular invasion on histopathological examination is considered predictive of poor outcome, although tumor size is more important than the histological features in predicting prognosis (170). Tumor size is a strong predictor of malignancy, with tumors larger than 500 g and/or more than 10 cm likely to be malignant (164,170). Factors conferring good prognosis include small tumor size (<5 cm), a young age (<2 y), and a functional status of the neoplasm (162,164,168).

In adrenocortical carcinoma, metastatic disease occurs by contiguous spread into the kidney or hematogenous metastasis to the liver, lungs, and regional lymph nodes (167). For carcinoma, rapid diagnosis and early age at diagnosis are crucial as the long-term survival rate is much greater for children younger than 2 years and with symptom duration less than 6 months (168).

CONGENITAL ADRENAL HYPERPLASIA

Etiology/Pathophysiology The CAHs are a heterogenous group of autosomal recessive genetic disorders characterized by enzyme defects in adrenal steroidogenesis that result in adrenal hyperplasia, variable deficiencies in cortisol and aldosterone synthesis, and increased androgen production (CAHs are further detailed in Chapter 27). Loss of function in several different enzymes in the steroidogenesis pathway can result in CAH, but the most common are deficiencies in 21-hydroxylase(21-OHD), 11-hydroxylase(11-OHD), and 3-β-hydroxysteroid dehydrogenase (3β-HSD).

Newborn females with classical CAH have varying degrees of virilization. Both boys and girls may present in adrenal crisis with symptoms of shock (hypotension, hypoglycemia). In addition, dehydration, hyponatremia and/or hyperkalemia due to mineralocorticoid deficiency can be seen in 21-OHD and 3β-HSD deficiencies. Other features may include hypertension in 11-OHD deficiency due to excess production of the aldosterone precursor, deoxycorticosterone.

Boys and girls without a salt-wasting defect can present at an older age with signs of increased androgen exposure including pubic hair development, acne, axillary hair, and body odor. Increased growth velocity and advanced bone age are usually present. Virilization may occur in girls, causing clitoromegaly and deepening of the voice. Boys may have penile enlargement with prepubertal testes.

Nonclassic CAH patients may present during childhood with findings of hyperandrogenism such as premature pubarche, bone advancement, and growth acceleration. Adolescents may present with acne in both sexes, and hirsutism, oligomenorrhea, polycystic ovarian disease, and infertility in females. Milder forms of 3β-HSD may also be encountered among girls with premature pubarche (174,175).

Diagnosis Diagnosis is based on identifying elevated precursors of adrenal steroidogenesis. ACTH stimulation testing with 250 μg of cosyntropin in older children or 10 to 15 μg/kg in infants can accentuate steroid precursor levels and aid in diagnosis (172,173). Classically, 17-hydroxyprogesterone is elevated in 21-OHD, 17-hydroxypregnenolone is elevated with 3β-HSD deficiency, and 11-deoxycortisol and deoxycorticosterone are is elevated in 11-hydroxylase deficiency. For complete detail about the diagnosis of all forms of CAH, please see Chapter 27, are also elevated.

Treatment Hydrocortisone is the treatment of choice for classic CAH in younger children. Mineralocorticoids (fludrocortisone) should be used for children who have accompanying salt wasting. GH in combination with a GnRH agonist has shown recent promise in augmenting adult height outcomes in children with CAH and precocious puberty (176). Aromatase inhibitor therapy is also emerging as a potential therapeutic option in CAH as a means of preserving growth velocity and adult height potential while using a lower dose of glucocorticoids (177). Future studies incorporating such therapies are ongoing and may help clarify their respective roles in CAH treatment.

Treatment is generally not indicated for asymptomatic nonclassic disease. In cases of rapid progression of pubarche, significantly advanced bone age, excessive virilization, or persistent oligomenorrhea, a trial of glucocorticoids may be considered.

β-hCG-SECRETING TUMORS

Etiology/Pathophysiology β-hCG-secreting tumors are rare causes of precocious puberty in children. Precocity results from the effects of unregulated hCG secretion on the LH receptor. LH, FSH, TSH, and β-hCG are all composed of an α- and a β-subunit. The a subunits for each hormone are derived from a single gene and exhibit 95% homology whereas the β subunits confer specificity for each hormone. The β subunits of LH and β-hCG are 82% homologous, which may lead to an overlap in their function and an ability of β-hCG to bind and stimulate the LH receptor. Because β-hCG acts specifically on the LH receptor and in females, estrogen production requires both LH and FSH action, precocious puberty from β-hCG-secreting tumors occurs primarily in boys. Precocious puberty in girls has been reported (178), possibly related to aromatase expression by tumor tissue or a limited effect of high levels of β-hCG on FSH receptors as well.

β-hCG-producing tumors are a heterogeneous group of tissue types and include immature teratomas, germinomas, choriocarcinoma, embryonal carcinoma, hepatoma, and chorioepithelioma. β-hCG secreting tumors are most frequently identified in the CNS, commonly located in suprasellar or pineal gland location.

Clinical Presentation Boys present with androgen-specific effects including penile enlargement, the appearance of pubic hair, and testicular enlargement. In rare cases of affected girls, pubertal development is characterized by breast development and pubic hair. Other signs or symptoms of a CNS mass lesion may be present such as headaches or other neurologic symptoms.

Diagnosis The findings of precocious puberty with elevated β-hCG levels are highly suspicious for a β-hCG tumor. Elevated α-fetoprotein levels may also be present with certain tumor types, including immature teratomas and embryonal carcinomas. Testosterone or estradiol levels are elevated. FSH and LH basal levels are low and response to GnRH stimulation testing is prepubertal. An MRI evaluation of the head is imperative in determining the presence, location, and extent of tumor.

Treatment Treatment involves a multidisciplinary approach, typically consisting of a combination of surgery, cisplatin-based chemotherapy, and radiation. Successful treatment results in regression of secondary sexual characteristics. Because there are several tumor types that may produce β-hCG and they are all rare, long-term survival rates are difficult to determine. Marked neurologic symptoms at diagnosis, suprasellar tumor location, and tumor hemorrhage are poor prognostic factors in children with intracranial disease (179,180).

HYPOTHYROIDISM

Etiology/Pathophysiology The association between severe and prolonged hypothyroidism and precocious pubertal development, also referred to as the Van Wyk–Grumbach syndrome was first described in the early 1900s (181). The mechanism for sexual precocity in this entity remains unknown but several theories exist. High TRH levels associated with primary hypothyroidism may act nonspecifically on gonadotropin receptors of the pituitary gland, resulting in an increased secretion of FSH, the α-subunit, and prolactin (182–185). This theory is supported by the mild elevations in serum FSH and prolactin that are commonly observed in such patients (182,184,186,187). Moreover, in males, there is a linear correlation between FSH and testicular enlargement (184). Another prevailing theory is that elevated serum TSH acts on the FSH and, to a lesser extent, LH receptor. This theory is supported by the observation that the degree of TSH elevation correlates with the onset of sexual precocity (182). In addition, TSH stimulation of the FSH receptor has been demonstrated *in vitro* (183). Other theories regarding the mechanism of sexual precocity in hypothyroidism include hyperprolactinemia resulting in either increased production of estrogens or secretion of gonadotropins, increased ovarian sensitivity to gonadotropins, and decreased sex steroid metabolism.

Clinical Presentation Classic signs and symptoms of hypothyroidism (see Chapter 26) are present. Characteristics of pubertal development are specific to FSH-dependent effects, with girls exhibiting breast development and menstruation and boys displaying macroorchidism without significant virilization. Galactorrhea is rare, but also may occur in cases associated with elevated prolactin levels. Unlike other forms of precocious puberty, these children are often quite short for chronologic age and display a slowed rather than rapid growth velocity.

Diagnosis Elevated TSH and low free thyroxine are diagnostic of hypothyroidism. Elevations in FSH, α-subunit, prolactin, and possibly LH may be present (182,186,187). Despite elevated basal gonadotropins, response to GnRH stimulation testing is blunted, without significant increases in FSH and LH levels (184,185). Perhaps related to predominant FSH effect, estradiol levels may be elevated in girls, but in boys, testosterone levels are prepubertal. Ovaries may have a multicystic appearance if pelvic ultrasound is performed (186). In contrast to other etiologies of precocious puberty, bone age is typically delayed.

Treatment Treatment with levothyroxine results in regression of breast development, suppression of menses, and normalization of estradiol and gonadotropin levels. Testicular volume decreases in boys following treatment, but may remain greater than expected for the degree of sexual maturation and even after full pubertal development is attained in well-treated males (184). Height prognosis may be particularly poor in such cases as children with prolonged, severe hypothyroidism may fail to manifest sufficient catch-up growth (188). GnRH agonist therapy with or without GH administration has shown little to no benefit in a limited number of such cases associated with precocious puberty (189), but additional study is still needed to assess its full potential for augmenting final height in these children.

REFERENCES

1. de Kretser DM, Hedger MP, Loveland KL, et al. Inhibins, activins and follistatin in reproduction. *Hum Reprod Update.* 2002;8:529–541.

2. Kaplan SL, Grumbach MM. Clinical review 14: Pathophysiology and treatment of sexual precocity. *J Clin Endocrinol Metab.* 1990;71:785–789.

3. Corbier P, Dehennin L, Castanier M, et al. Sex differences in serum luteinizing hormone and testosterone in the human neonate during the first few hours after birth. *J Clin Endocrinol Metab.* 1990;71:1344–1348.

4. de Zegher F, Devlieger H, Veldhuis JD. Pulsatile and sexually dimorphic secretion of luteinizing hormone in the human infant on the day of birth. *Pediatr Res.* 1992;32:605–607.

5. Schmidt H, Schwarz HP. Serum concentrations of LH and FSH in the healthy newborn. *Eur J Endocrinol/Eur Fed Endocr Soc.* 2000;143:213–215.

6. Apter D, Butzow TL, Laughlin GA, et al. Gonadotropin-releasing hormone pulse generator activity during pubertal transition in girls: pulsatile and diurnal patterns of circulating gonadotropins. *J Clin Endocrinol Metab.* 1993;76:940–949.

7. Penny R, Olambiwonnu NO, Frasier SD. Serum gonadotropin concentrations during the first four years of life. *J Clin Endocrinol Metab.* 1974;38:320–321.

8. Manasco PK, Umbach DM, Muly SM, et al. Ontogeny of gonadotrophin and inhibin secretion in normal girls through puberty based on overnight serial sampling and a comparison with normal boys. Hum Reprod 1997;12:2108–2114.

9. Norjavaara E, Ankarberg C, Albertsson-Wikland K. Diurnal rhythm of 17 beta-estradiol secretion throughout pubertal development in healthy girls: evaluation by a sensitive radioimmunoassay. *J Clin Endocrinol Metab.* 1996;81:4095–4102.

10. Martha PM Jr, Rogol AD, Veldhuis JD, et al. Alterations in the pulsatile properties of circulating growth hormone concentrations during puberty in boys. *J Clin Endocrinol Metab.* 1989;69:563–570.

11. Caruso-Nicoletti M, Cassorla F, Skerda M, et al. Short term, low dose estradiol accelerates ulnar growth in boys. *J Clin Endocrinol Metab.* 1985;61:896–898.

12. Cutler GB Jr. The role of estrogen in bone growth and maturation during childhood and adolescence. *J Steroid Biochem Mol Biol.* 1997;61:141–144.

13. Grumbach MM, Auchus RJ. Estrogen: consequences and implications of human mutations in synthesis and action. *J Clin Endocrinol Metab.* 1999;84:4677–4694.

14. Morishima A, Grumbach MM, Simpson ER, et al. Aromatase deficiency in male and female siblings caused by a novel mutation and the physiological role of estrogens. *J Clin Endocrinol Metab.* 1995;80:3689–3698.

15. Carani C, Qin K, Simoni M, et al. Effect of testosterone and estradiol in a man with aromatase deficiency. *N Engl J Med.* 1997;337:91–95.

16. Bilezikian JP, Morishima A, Bell J, et al. Increased bone mass as a result of estrogen therapy in a man with aromatase deficiency. *N Engl J Med.* 1998;339:599–603.

17. Smith EP, Boyd J, Frank GR, et al. Estrogen resistance caused by a mutation in the estrogen-receptor gene in a man. *N Engl J Med.* 1994;331:1056–1061.

18. Weise M, De-Levi S, Barnes KM, et al. Effects of estrogen on growth plate senescence and epiphyseal fusion. *Proc Natl Acad Sci USA.* 2001;98:6871–6876.

19. Weise M, Flor A, Barnes KM, et al. Determinants of growth during gonadotropin-releasing hormone analog therapy for precocious puberty. *J Clin Endocrinol Metab.* 2004;89:103–107.

20. Wu T, Mendola P, Buck GM. Ethnic differences in the presence of secondary sex characteristics and menarche among US girls: the Third National Health and Nutrition Examination Survey, 1988–1994. *Pediatrics.* 2002;110:752–757.

21. Palmert MR, Boepple PA. Variation in the timing of puberty: clinical spectrum and genetic investigation. *J Clin Endocrinol Metab.* 2001;86:2364–2368.

22. Nathan BM, Palmert MR. Regulation and disorders of pubertal timing. *Endocrinol Metab Clin North Am.* 2005;34:617–641, ix.

23. Plant TM, Barker-Gibb ML. Neurobiological mechanisms of puberty in higher primates. *Hum Reprod Update.* 2004;10:67–77.

24. Parent AS, Teilmann G, Juul A, et al. The timing of normal puberty and the age limits of sexual precocity: variations around the world, secular trends, and changes after migration. *Endocr Rev.* 2003;24:668–693.

25. Kaplowitz PB, Slora EJ, Wasserman RC, et al. Earlier onset of puberty in girls: relation to increased body mass index and race. *Pediatrics.* 2001;108:347–353.

26. Biro FM, McMahon RP, Striegel-Moore R, et al. Impact of timing of pubertal maturation on growth in black and white female adolescents: The National Heart, Lung, and Blood Institute Growth and Health Study. *J Pediatr.* 2001;138:636–643.

27. Wang Y. Is obesity associated with early sexual maturation? A comparison of the association in American boys versus girls. *Pediatrics.* 2002;110:903–910.

28. Colon I, Caro D, Bourdony CJ, et al. Identification of phthalate esters in the serum of young Puerto Rican girls with premature breast development. *Environ Health Perspect.* 2000;108:895–900.

29. Parent AS, Rasier G, Gerard A, et al. Early onset of puberty: tracking genetic and environmental factors. *Horm Res.* 2005;64 Suppl 2:41–47.

30. Marshall WA, Tanner JM. Variations in the pattern of pubertal changes in boys. *Arch Dis Child.* 1970;45:13–23.

31. Marshall WA, Tanner JM. Variations in pattern of pubertal changes in girls. *Arch Dis Child.* 1969;44:291–303.

32. Herman-Giddens ME, Slora EJ, Wasserman RC, et al. Secondary sexual characteristics and menses in young girls seen in office practice: a study from the Pediatric Research in Office Settings network. *Pediatrics.* 1997;99:505–512.

33. Kaplowitz PB, Oberfield SE. Reexamination of the age limit for defining when puberty is precocious in girls in the United States: implications for evaluation and treatment. Drug and Therapeutics and Executive Committees of the Lawson Wilkins Pediatric Endocrine Society. *Pediatrics.* 1999;104:936–941.

34. Rosenfield RL, Bachrach LK, Chernausek SD, et al. Current age of onset of puberty. *Pediatrics.* 2000;106:622–623.

35. Reiter EO, Lee PA. Have the onset and tempo of puberty changed? *Arch Pediatr Adolesc Med.* 2001;155:988–989.

36. Lee PA, Kulin HE, Guo SS. Age of puberty among girls and the diagnosis of precocious puberty. *Pediatrics.* 2001;107:1493.

37. Pathomvanich A, Merke DP, Chrousos GP. Early puberty: a cautionary tale. *Pediatrics.* 2000;105:115–116.

38. Midyett LK, Moore WV, Jacobson JD. Are pubertal changes in girls before age 8 benign? *Pediatrics.* 2003;111:47–51.

39. Herman-Giddens ME, Wang L, Koch G. Secondary sexual characteristics in boys: estimates from the national health and nutrition examination survey III, 1988-1994. *Arch Pediatr Adolesc Med.* 2001;155:1022–1028.

40. Lee PA, Guo SS, Kulin HE. Age of puberty: data from the United States of America. *Apmis.* 2001;109:81–88.

41. Palmert MR, Hayden DL, Mansfield MJ, et al. The longitudinal study of adrenal maturation during gonadal suppression: evidence that adrenarche is a gradual process. *J Clin Endocrinol Metab.* 2001;86:4536–4542.

42. Ibanez L, Dimartino-Nardi J, Potau N, et al. Premature adrenarche—normal variant or forerunner of adult disease? *Endocr Rev.* 2000;21:671–696.

43. Ong KK, Potau N, Petry CJ, et al. Opposing influences of prenatal and postnatal weight gain on adrenarche in normal boys and girls. *J Clin Endocrinol Metab.* 2004;89:2647–2651.

44. Klein KO, Mericq V, Brown-Dawson JM, et al. Estrogen levels in girls with premature thelarche compared with normal prepubertal girls as determined by an ultrasensitive recombinant cell bioassay. *J Pediatr.* 1999;134:190–192.

45. Crofton PM, Evans NE, Wardhaugh B, et al. Evidence for increased ovarian follicular activity in girls with premature thelarche. *Clin Endocrinol.* (Oxf) 2005;62:205–209.

46. Roman R, Johnson MC, Codner E, et al. Activating GNAS1 gene mutations in patients with premature thelarche. *J Pediatr.* 2004;145:218–222.

47. Pescovitz OH, Hench KD, Barnes KM, et al. Premature thelarche and central precocious puberty: the relationship between clinical presentation and the gonadotropin response to luteinizing hormone-releasing hormone. *J Clin Endocrinol Metab.* 1988;67:474–479.

48. Pasquino AM, Pucarelli I, Passeri F, et al. Progression of premature thelarche to central precocious puberty [see comments]. *J Pediatr.* 1995;126:11–14.

49. Lee PA. Central precocious puberty. An overview of diagnosis, treatment, and outcome. *Endocrinol Metab Clin North Am.* 1999;28:901–918, xi.

50. Partsch CJ, Heger S, Sippell WG. Management and outcome of central precocious puberty. *Clin Endocrinol. (Oxf)* 2002; 56:129–148.

51. De Sanctis V, Corrias A, Rizzo V, et al. Etiology of central precocious puberty in males: the results of the Italian Study Group for Physiopathology of Puberty. *J Pediatr Endocrinol Metab.* 2000;13 Suppl 1:687–693.

52. Cisternino M, Arrigo T, Pasquino AM, et al. Etiology and age incidence of precocious puberty in girls: a multicentric study. *J Pediatr Endocrinol Metab.* 2000;13 Suppl 1:695–701.

53. Virdis R, Street ME, Zampolli M, et al. Precocious puberty in girls adopted from developing countries. *Arch Dis Child.* 1998;78:152–154.

54. Bona G, Marinello D. Precocious puberty in immigrant children: indications for treatment. *J Pediatr Endocrinol Metab.* 2000;13 Suppl 1:831–834.

55. de Vries L, Kauschansky A, Shohat M, et al. Familial central precocious puberty suggests autosomal dominant inheritance. *J Clin Endocrinol Metab.* 2004;89:1794–1800.

56. Jung H, Carmel P, Schwartz MS, et al. Some hypothalamic hamartomas contain transforming growth factor alpha, a puberty-inducing growth factor, but not luteinizing hormone-releasing hormone neurons. *J Clin Endocrinol Metab.* 1999;84:4695–4701.

57. Judge DM, Kulin HE, Page R, et al. Hypothalamic hamartoma: a source of luteinizing-hormone-releasing factor in precocious puberty. *N Engl J Med.* 1977;296:7–10.

58. Cassio A, Cacciari E, Zucchini S, et al. Central precocious puberty: clinical and imaging aspects. *J Pediatr Endocrinol Metab.* 2000;13 Suppl 1:703–708.

59. Virdis R, Sigorini M, Laiolo A, et al. Neurofibromatosis type 1 and precocious puberty. *J Pediatr Endocrinol Metab.* 2000;13 Suppl 1:841–844.

60. Rivarola MA BA, Mendilaharzu H, et al. Precocious puberty in children with tumors of the suprasellar and pineal areas: organic central precocious puberty. *Acta Pediatri.* 2001;90:751–756.

61. Palmert MR, Malin HV, Boepple PA. Unsustained or slowly progressive puberty in young girls: initial presentation and long-term follow-up of 20 untreated patients. *J Clin Endocrinol Metab.* 1999;84:415–423.

62. Fontoura M, Brauner R, Prevot C, et al. Precocious puberty in girls: early diagnosis of a slowly progressing variant. *Arch Dis Child.* 1989;64:1170–1176.

63. Jung H, Neumaier Probst E, Hauffa BP, et al. Association of morphological characteristics with precocious puberty and/or gelastic seizures in hypothalamic hamartoma. *J Clin Endocrinol Metab.* 2003;88:4590–4595.

64. Breningstall GN. Gelastic seizures, precocious puberty, and hypothalamic hamartoma. *Neurology.* 1985;35:1180–1183.

65. Kuzniecky R, Guthrie B, Mountz J, et al. Intrinsic epileptogenesis of hypothalamic hamartomas in gelastic epilepsy. *Ann Neurol.* 1997;42:60-67.

66. Brandberg G, Raininko R, Eeg-Olofsson O. Hypothalamic hamartoma with gelastic seizures in Swedish children and adolescents. *Eur J Paediatr Neurol.* 2004;8:35–44.

67. Ibanez L, Potau N, Zampolli M, et al. Use of leuprolide acetate response patterns in the early diagnosis of pubertal disorders: comparison with the gonadotropin-releasing hormone test. *J Clin Endocrinol Metab.* 1994;78:30–35.

68. Eckert KL, Wilson DM, Bachrach LK, et al. A single-sample, subcutaneous gonadotropin-releasing hormone test for central precocious puberty. *Pediatrics.* 1996;97:517–519.

69. Iughetti L, Predieri B, Ferrari M, et al. Diagnosis of central precocious puberty: endocrine assessment. *J Pediatr Endocrinol Metab.* 2000;13 Suppl 1:709–715.

70. Neely EK, Hintz RL, Wilson DM, et al. Normal ranges for immunochemiluminometric gonadotropin assays. *J Pediatr.* 1995;127:40–46.

71. Wu FC, Butler GE, Kelnar CJ, et al. Ontogeny of pulsatile gonadotropin releasing hormone secretion from midchildhood, through puberty, to adulthood in the human male: a study using deconvolution analysis and an ultrasensitive immunofluorometric assay. *J Clin Endocrinol Metab.* 1996;81:1798–1805.

72. Neely EK, Wilson DM, Lee PA, et al. Spontaneous serum gonadotropin concentrations in the evaluation of precocious puberty. *J Pediatr.* 1995;127:47–52.

73. Brito VN, Latronico AC, Arnhold IJ, et al. A single luteinizing hormone determination 2 hours after depot leuprolide is useful for therapy monitoring of gonadotropin-dependent precocious puberty in girls. *J Clin Endocrinol Metab.* 2004;89:4338–4342.

74. Rosenfield RL, Garibaldi LR, Moll GW Jr, et al. The rapid ovarian secretory response to pituitary stimulation by the gonadotropin-releasing hormone agonist nafarelin in sexual precocity. *J Clin Endocrinol Metab.* 1986;63:1386–1389.

75. Salerno M, Di Maio S, Gasparini N, et al. Central precocious puberty: a single blood sample after gonadotropin-releasing hormone agonist administration in monitoring treatment. *Horm Res.* 1998;50:205–211.

76. Ikegami S, Moriwake T, Tanaka H, et al. An ultrasensitive assay revealed age-related changes in serum oestradiol at low concentrations in both sexes from infancy to puberty. *Clin Endocrinol. (Oxf)* 2001; 55:789–795.

77. Herter LD, Golendziner E, Flores JA, et al. Ovarian and uterine findings in pelvic sonography: comparison between prepubertal girls, girls with isolated thelarche, and girls with central precocious puberty. *J Ultrasound Med.* 2002;21:1237–1246.

78. Ng SM, Kumar Y, Cody D, et al. Cranial MRI scans are indicated in all girls with central precocious puberty. *Arch Dis Child.* 2003;88:414–418.

79. Carel JC LN, Roger M, Chaussain JL. Precocious puberty and statural growth. *Hum Reprod Update.* 2004;10:135–147.

80. Kletter GB, Kelch RP. Clinical review 60: Effects of gonadotropin-releasing hormone analog therapy on adult stature in precocious puberty. *J Clin Endocrinol Metab.* 1994;79:331–334.

81. Klein KO. Precocious puberty: who has it? Who should be treated? [editorial; comment]. *J Clin Endocrinol Metab.* 1999;84:411–414.

82. Ehrhardt AA, Meyer-Bahlburg HF, Bell JJ, et al. Idiopathic precocious puberty in girls: psychiatric follow-up in adolescence. *J Am Acad Child Psychiatry.* 1984;23:23–33.

83. Sonis WA, Comite F, Blue J, et al. Behavior problems and social competence in girls with true precocious puberty. *J Pediatr.* 1985;106:156–160.

84. Graber JA, Seeley JR, Brooks-Gunn J, et al. Is pubertal timing associated with psychopathology in young adulthood? *J Am Acad Child Adolesc Psychiatry.* 2004;43:718–726.

85. Brauner R, Adan L, Malandry F, et al. Adult height in girls with idiopathic true precocious puberty. *J Clin Endocrinol Metab.* 1994;79:415–420.

86. Schroeter M, Baus I, Sippell WG, et al. Long-term suppression of pituitary-gonadal function with three-month depot of leuprorelin acetate in a girl with central precocious puberty. *Horm Res.* 2002;58:292–296.

87. Carel JC, Lahlou N, Jaramillo O, et al. Treatment of central precocious puberty by subcutaneous injections of leuprorelin 3-month depot (11.25 mg). *J Clin Endocrinol Metab.* 2002;87:4111–4116.

88. Badaru A, Wilson DM, Bachrach LK, et al. Sequential comparisons of one-month and three-month depot leuprolide regimens in central precocious puberty. *J Clin Endocrinol Metab.* 2006;91:1862–1867.

89. Eugster SA, Clarke W, Kletter GB, et al. Efficacy and safety of histrelin subdermal implant in children with central precocious puberty: A multicenter trial. *J Clin Endocrinol Metab.* 2007;92(5)1697–1704.

90. Bhatia S, Neely EK, Wilson DM. Serum luteinizing hormone rises within minutes after depot leuprolide injection: implications for monitoring therapy. *Pediatrics.* 2002;109:E30.

91. Jay N, Mansfield MJ, Blizzard RM, et al. Ovulation and menstrual function of adolescent girls with central precocious puberty after therapy with gonadotropin-releasing hormone agonists. *J Clin Endocrinol Metab.* 1992;75:890–894.

92. Heger S, Partsch CJ, Sippell WG. Long-term outcome after depot gonadotropin-releasing hormone agonist treatment of central precocious puberty: final height, body proportions, body composition, bone mineral density, and reproductive function. *J Clin Endocrinol Metab.* 1999;84:4583–4590.

93. Paterson WF, McNeill E, Young D, et al. Auxological outcome and time to menarche following long-acting goserelin therapy in girls with central precocious or early puberty. *Clin Endocrinol. (Oxf)* 2004;61:626–634.

94. Tanaka T, Niimi H, Matsuo N, et al. Results of long-term follow-up after treatment of central precocious puberty with leuprorelin acetate: evaluation of effectiveness of treatment and recovery of gonadal function. The TAP-144-SR Japanese Study Group on Central Precocious Puberty. *J Clin Endocrinol Metab.* 2005;90:1371–1376.

95. Paul D, Conte FA, Grumbach MM, et al. Long-term effect of gonadotropin-releasing hormone agonist therapy on final and near-final height in 26 children with true precocious puberty treated at a median age of less than 5 years. *J Clin Endocrinol Metab.* 1995;80:546–551.

96. Partsch CJ, Heger S, Sippell WG. Treatment of central precocious puberty: lessons from a 15 years prospective trial. German Decapeptyl Study Group. *J Pediatr Endocrinol Metab.* 2000;13 Suppl 1:747–758.

97. Carel JC, Roger M, Ispas S, et al. Final height after long-term treatment with triptorelin slow release for central precocious puberty: importance of statural growth after interruption of treatment. French study group of Decapeptyl in Precocious Puberty. *J Clin Endocrinol Metab.* 1999;84:1973–1978.

98. Oerter KE, Manasco P, Barnes KM, et al. Adult height in precocious puberty after long-term treatment with deslorelin. *J Clin Endocrinol Metab.* 1991;73:1235–1240.

99. Cacciari E, Cassio A, Balsamo A, et al. Long-term follow-up and final height in girls with central precocious puberty treated with luteinizing hormone-releasing hormone analogue nasal spray. *Arch Pediatr Adolesc Med.* 1994;148:1194–1199.

100. Tonini G, Lazzerini M. Side effects of GnRH analogue treatment in childhood. *J Pediatr Endocrinol Metab.* 2000;13 Suppl 1:795–803.

101. Unal O, Berberoglu M, Evliyaoglu O, et al. Effects on bone mineral density of gonadotropin releasing hormone analogs used in the treatment of central precocious puberty. *J Pediatr Endocrinol Metab.* 2003;16:407–411.

102. Neely EK, Bachrach LK, Hintz RL, et al. Bone mineral density during treatment of central precocious puberty. *J Pediatr.* 1995;127:819–822.

103. Boot AM, De Muinck Keizer-Schrama S, Pols HA, et al. Bone mineral density and body composition before and during treatment with gonadotropin-releasing hormone agonist in children with central precocious and early puberty. *J Clin Endocrinol Metab.* 1998;83:370–373.

104. Saggese G, Bertelloni S, Baroncelli GI, et al. Reduction of bone density: an effect of gonadotropin releasing hormone analogue treatment in central precocious puberty. *Eur J Pediatr.* 1993;152:717–720.

105. Antoniazzi F, Bertoldo F, Zamboni G, et al. Bone mineral metabolism in girls with precocious puberty during gonadotrophin-releasing hormone agonist treatment. *Eur J Endocrinol.* 1995;133:412–417.

106. Antoniazzi F, Zamboni G, Bertoldo F, et al. Bone mass at final height in precocious puberty after gonadotropin-releasing hormone agonist with and without calcium supplementation. *J Clin Endocrinol Metab.* 2003;88:1096–1101.

107. Cassio A, Bal MO, Orsini LF, et al. Reproductive outcome in patients treated and not treated for idiopathic early puberty: Long-term results of a randomized trial in adults. *J Pediatr.* 2006;149:532–536.

108. Heger S, Muller M, Ranke M, et al. Long-term GnRH agonist treatment for female central precocious puberty does not impair reproductive function. *Mol Cell Endocrinol.* 2006;254-255:217–220.

109. Laron Z, Kauli R. Experience with cyproterone acetate in the treatment of precocious puberty. *J Pediatr Endocrinol Metab.* 2000;13 Suppl 1:805–810.

110. Lee P. Medroxyprogesterone therapy for sexual precocity in girls. *Am J Dis Child.* 1981;135:443–445.

111. Pescovitz OH, Comite F, Cassorla F, et al. True precocious puberty complicating congenital adrenal hyperplasia: treatment with a luteinizing hormone-releasing hormone analog. *J Clin Endocrinol Metab.* 1984;58: 857–861.

112. Pescovitz OH, Hench K, Green O, et al. Central precocious puberty complicating a virilizing adrenal tumor: treatment with a long-acting LHRH analog. *J Pediatr.* 1985;106:612–614.

113. Weinstein LS, Shenker A, Gejman PV, et al. Activating mutations of the stimulatory G protein in the McCune-Albright syndrome. *N Engl J Med.* 1991;325:1688–1695.

114. Chattopadhyay A, Bhansali A, Mohanty SK, et al. Hypophosphatemic rickets and osteomalacia in polyostotic fibrous dysplasia. *J Pediatr Endocrinol Metab.* 2003;16:893–896.

115. Collins MT, Chebli C, Jones J, et al. Renal phosphate wasting in fibrous dysplasia of bone is part of a generalized renal tubular dysfunction similar to that seen in tumor-induced osteomalacia. *J Bone Miner Res.* 2001;16:806–813.

116. Schwindinger WF, Francomano CA, Levine MA. Identification of a mutation in the gene encoding the alpha subunit of the stimulatory G protein of adenylyl cyclase in McCune-Albright syndrome. *Proc Natl Acad Sci USA.* 1992;89:5152–5156.

117. Saenger P, Rincon M. Precocious puberty: McCune-Albright syndrome and beyond. *J Pediatr.* 2003;143:9–10.

118. Lee PA, Van Dop C, Migeon CJ. McCune-Albright syndrome. Long-term follow-up. *JAMA.* 1986;256:2980–2984.

119. Albers N, Jorgens S, Deiss D, et al. McCune-Albright syndrome—the German experience. *J Pediatr Endocrinol Metab.* 2002;15 Suppl 3:897–901.

120. De Sanctis L, Romagnolo D, Olivero M, et al. Molecular analysis of the GNAS1 gene for the correct diagnosis of Albright hereditary osteodystrophy and pseudohypoparathyroidism. *Pediatr Res.* 2003;53:749–755.

121. Boepple PA, Frisch LS, Wierman ME, et al. The natural history of autonomous gonadal function, adrenarche, and central puberty in gonadotropin-independent precocious puberty. *J Clin Endocrinol Metab.* 1992;75:1550–1555.

122. DiMeglio LA, Pescovitz OH. Disorders of puberty: inactivating and activating molecular mutations. *J Pediatr.* 1997;131:S8–12.

123. de Sanctis C, Lala R, Matarazzo P, et al. McCune-Albright syndrome: a longitudinal clinical study of 32 patients. *J Pediatr Endocrinol Metab.* 1999;12:817–826.

124. Shenker A, Weinstein LS, Moran A, et al. Severe endocrine and nonendocrine manifestations of the McCune-Albright syndrome associated with activating mutations of stimulatory G protein GS. *J Pediatr.* 1993;123: 509–518.

125. Holland FJ. Gonadotropin-independent precocious puberty. *Endocrinol Metab Clin North Am.* 1991;20:191–210.

126. Syed FA, Chalew SA. Ketoconazole treatment of gonadotropin independent precocious puberty in girls with McCune-Albright syndrome: a preliminary report. *J Pediatr Endocrinol Metab.* 1999;12:81–83.

127. Lupo VR NC Endocrinology of female reproduction. In: CB N ed. *Endocrine Pathophysiology.* 1st ed. Madison, CT: Fence Creek Publishing; 1998:185–209.

128. Feuillan PP, Foster CM, Pescovitz OH, et al. Treatment of precocious puberty in the McCune-Albright syndrome with the aromatase inhibitor testolactone. *N Engl J Med.* 1986;315:1115–1119.

129. Feuillan PP, Jones J, Cutler GB Jr. Long-term testolactone therapy for precocious puberty in girls with the McCune-Albright syndrome. *J Clin Endocrinol Metab.* 1993;77:647–651.

130. Low LC, Wang Q. Gonadotropin independent precocious puberty. *J Pediatr Endocrinol Metab.* 1998;11:497–507.

131. Roth C, Freiberg C, Zappel H, et al. Effective aromatase inhibition by anastrozole in a patient with gonadotropin-independent precocious puberty in McCune-Albright syndrome. *J Pediatr Endocrinol Metab.* 2002;15 Suppl 3:945–948.

132. Nunez SB, Calis K, Cutler GB Jr, et al. Lack of efficacy of fadrozole in treating precocious puberty in girls with the McCune-Albright syndrome. *J Clin Endocrinol Metab.* 2003;88:5730–5733.

133. Eugster EA, Rubin SD, Reiter EO, et al. Tamoxifen treatment for precocious puberty in McCune-Albright syndrome: a multicenter trial. *J Pediatr.* 2003;143:60–66.

134. Laven JS, Lumbroso S, Sultan C, et al. Management of infertility in a patient presenting with ovarian dysfunction and McCune-Albright syndrome. *J Clin Endocrinol Metab.* 2004;89:1076–1078.

135. Lala R, Matarazzo P, Bertelloni S, et al. Pamidronate treatment of bone fibrous dysplasia in nine children with McCune-Albright syndrome. *Acta Paediatr.* 2000;89:188–193.

136. Lala R, Matarazzo P, Andreo M, et al. Bisphosphonate treatment of bone fibrous dysplasia in McCune-Albright syndrome. *J Pediatr Endocrinol Metab.* 2006;19 Suppl 2:583–593.

137. Zacharin M, O'Sullivan M. Intravenous pamidronate treatment of polyostotic fibrous dysplasia associated with the McCune Albright syndrome. *J Pediatr.* 2000;137:403–409.

138. Shenker A, Laue L, Kosugi S, et al. A constitutively activating mutation of the luteinizing hormone receptor in familial male precocious puberty. *Nature.* 1993;365:652–654

139. Egli CA, Rosenthal SM, Grumbach MM, et al. Pituitary gonadotropin-independent male-limited autosomal dominant sexual precocity in nine generations: familial testotoxicosis. *J Pediatr.* 1985;106:33–40.

140. Laue L, Chan WY, Hsueh AJ, et al. Genetic heterogeneity of constitutively activating mutations of the human luteinizing hormone receptor in familial male-limited precocious puberty. *Proc Natl Acad Sci USA.* 1995;92:1906–1910.

141. Latronico AC, Shinozaki H, Guerra G Jr. Gonadotropin-independent precocious puberty due to luteinizing hormone receptor mutations in Brazilian boys: a novel constitutively activating mutation in the first transmembrane helix. *J Clin Endocrinol Metab.* 2000;85:4799–4805.

142. Kremer H, Martens JW, van Reen M, et al. A limited repertoire of mutations of the

luteinizing hormone (LH) receptor gene in familial and sporadic patients with male LH-independent precocious puberty. *J Clin Endocrinol Metab.* 1999;84:1136–1140.

143. Rosenthal SM, Grumbach MM, Kaplan SL. Gonadotropin-independent familial sexual precocity with premature Leydig and germinal cell maturation (familial testotoxicosis): effects of a potent luteinizing hormone-releasing factor agonist and medroxyprogesterone acetate therapy in four cases. *J Clin Endocrinol Metab.* 1983;57:571–579.

144. Itoh K, Nakada T, Kubota Y, et al. Testotoxicosis proved by immunohistochemical analysis and successfully treated with cyproterone acetate. *Urolog Intl.* 1996;57:199–202.

145. Soriano-Guillen L, Lahlou N, Chauvet G, et al. Adult height after ketoconazole treatment in patients with familial male-limited precocious puberty. *J Clin Endocrinol Metab.* 2005;90:147–151.

146. Laue L, Kenigsberg D, Pescovitz OH, et al. Treatment of familial male precocious puberty with spironolactone and testolactone. *N Engl J Med.* 1989;320:496–502.

147. Leschek EW, Jones J, Barnes KM, et al. Six-year results of spironolactone and testolactone treatment of familial male-limited precocious puberty with addition of deslorelin after central puberty onset. *J Clin Endocrinol Metab.* 1999;84:175–178.

148. Kreher NC, Pescovitz OH, Delameter P, et al. Treatment of familial male-limited precocious puberty with bicalutamide and anastrzole. *J Pediatr.* 2006;149:416–420.

149. Holland FJ, Kirsch SE, Selby R. Gonadotropin-independent precocious puberty ("testotoxicosis"): influence of maturational status on response to ketoconazole. *J Clin Endocrinol Metab.* 1987;64:328–333.

150. Castleberry RP KD, Joseph DB, et.al. ed. Gonadal and extragonadal germ cell tumors. St. Louis: Mosby Year Book; 1991.

151. Hirakawa T, Ascoli M. A constitutively active somatic mutation of the human lutropin receptor found in Leydig cell tumors activates the same families of G proteins as germ line mutations associated with Leydig cell hyperplasia. *Endocrinology.* 2003;144:3872–3878.

152. Cronje HS, Niemand I, Bam RH, et al. Granulosa and theca cell tumors in children: a report of 17 cases and literature review. *Obstet Gynecol Surv.* 1998;53:240–247.

153. Urban MD, Lee PA, Plotnick LP, et al. The diagnosis of Leydig cell tumors in childhood. *Am J Dis Child.* 1978;132:494–497.

154. Choong CS, Fuller PJ, Chu S, et al. Sertoli-Leydig cell tumor of the ovary, a rare cause of precocious puberty in a 12-month-old infant. *J Clin Endocrinol Metab.* 2002; 87:49–56.

155. Isguven P, Yoruk A, Adal E, et al. Adult type granulosa cell tumor causing precocious pseudopuberty in a 6 year-old girl. *J Pediatr Endocrinol Metab.* 2003;16:571–573.

156. Ghazi AA, Rahimi F, Ahadi MM, et al. Development of true precocious puberty following treatment of a Leydig cell tumor of the testis. *J Pediatr Endocrinol Metab.* 2001;14:1679–1681.

157. Fernandez CG TF, Rivas C. MRI in the diagnosis of testicular leydig cell tumor. *Br J Radiol.* 77:521–524. 2004;

158. Outwater EK, Marchetto B, Wagner BJ. Virilizing tumors of the ovary: imaging features. *Ultrasound Obstet Gynecol.* 2000;15:365–371.

159. Ross JH, Rybicki L, Kay R. Clinical behavior and a contemporary management algorithm for prepubertal testis tumors: a summary of the Prepubertal Testis Tumor Registry. *J Urol.* 2002;168:1675–1678.

160. Schneider DT, Janig U, Calaminus G, et al. Ovarian sex cord-stromal tumors—a clinicopathological study of 72 cases from the Kiel Pediatric Tumor Registry. *Virchows Arch.* 2003;443:549–560.

161. Vassal G, Flamant F, Caillaud JM, et al. Juvenile granulosa cell tumor of the ovary in children: a clinical study of 15 cases. *J Clin Oncol.* 1988;6:990–995.

162. Patil KK RP, McCullagh M, et al. Functioning adrenocrotical neoplasms in children. *BJU Intl.* 2002;89:562–565.

163. Phornphutkul C, Okubo T, Wu K, et al. Aromatase p450 expression in a feminizing adrenal adenoma presenting as isosexual precocious puberty. *J Clin Endocrinol Metab.* 2001;86:649–652.

164. Narasimhan KL, Samujh R, Bhansali A, et al. Adrenocortical tumors in childhood. *Pediatr Surg Intl.* 2003;19:432–435.

165. Rodriguez-Galindo C, Figueiredo BC, Zambetti GP, et al. Biology, clinical characteristics, and management of adrenocortical tumors in children. Pediatr Blood Cancer 2005;45:265–273.

166. Figueiredo BC, Cavalli LR, Pianovski MA, et al. Amplification of the steroidogenic factor 1 gene in childhood adrenocortical tumors. *J Clin Endocrinol Metab.* 2005;90:615–619.

167. Lee PD, Winter RJ, Green OC. Virilizing adrenocortical tumors in childhood: eight cases and a review of the literature. *Pediatrics.* 1985;76:437–444.

168. Albaugh G, Chen M. 2001; Adrenocortical carcinoma in two female children. *Pediatr Surg Intl.* 17:71–74

169. Zancanella P, Pianovski MA, Oliveira BH, et al. Mitotane associated with cisplatin, etoposide, and doxorubicin in advanced childhood adrenocortical carcinoma: mitotane monitoring and tumor regression. *J Pediatr Hematol Oncol.* 2006;28:513–524.

170. Wolthers OD, Cameron FJ, Scheimberg I, et al. Androgen secreting adrenocortical tumours. *Arch Dis Child.* 1999;80:46–50.

171. Hawkins LA, Chasalow FI, Blethen SL. The role of adrenocorticotropin testing in evaluating girls with premature adrenarche and hirsutism/oligomenorrhea. *J Clin Endocrinol Metab.* 1992;74:248–253.

172. New MI, Lorenzen F, Lerner AJ, et al. Genotyping steroid 21-hydroxylase deficiency: hormonal reference data. *J Clin Endocrinol Metab.* 1983;57:320–326.

173. Speiser PW, White PC. Congenital adrenal hyperplasia. *N Engl J Med.* 2003;349:776–788.

174. Marui S, Castro M, Latronico AC, et al. Mutations in the type II 3beta-hydroxysteroid dehydrogenase (HSD3B2) gene can cause premature pubarche in girls. *Clin Endocrinol.* (Oxf) 2000;52:67–75.

175. Mermejo LM, Elias LL, Marui S, et al. 2005 Refining hormonal diagnosis of type II 3beta-hydroxysteroid dehydrogenase deficiency in patients with premature pubarche and hirsutism based on HSD3B2 genotyping. *J Clin Endocrinol Metab.* 90:1287–1293.

176. Lin-Su K, Vogiatzi MG, Marshall I, et al. 2005 Treatment with growth hormone and luteinizing hormone releasing hormone analog improves final adult height in children with congenital adrenal hyperplasia. *J Clin Endocrinol Metab.* 90:3318–3325.

177. Merke DP, Keil MF, Jones JV, et al. 2000 Flutamide, testolactone, and reduced hydrocortisone dose maintain normal growth velocity and bone maturation despite elevated androgen levels in children with congenital adrenal hyperplasia. *J Clin Endocrinol Metab.* 85:1114–1120.

178. Starzyk J, Starzyk B, Bartnik-Mikuta A, et al. 2001 Gonadotropin releasing hormone-independent precocious puberty in a 5 year-old girl with suprasellar germ cell tumor secreting beta-hCG and alpha-fetoprotein. *J Pediatr Endocrinol Metab.* 14:789–796.

179. Calaminus G, Bamberg M, Harms D, et al. 2005 AFP/beta-HCG secreting CNS germ cell tumors: long-term outcome with respect to initial symptoms and primary tumor resection. Results of the cooperative trial MAKEI 89. Neuropediatrics 36:71–77.

180. Shinoda J, Sakai N, Yano H, et al. 2004 Prognostic factors and therapeutic problems of primary intracranial choriocarcinoma/germ-cell tumors with high levels of HCG. Journal of neuro-oncology 66:225–240.

181. Kendle V 1905 Case of precocious puberty in a female cretin. British Medical Journal 1:246.

182. Niedziela M, Korman E 2001 Severe hypothyroidism due to autoimmune atrophic thyroiditis—predicted target height and a plausible mechanism for sexual precocity. *J Pediatr Endocrinol Metab.* 14:901–907.

183. Anasti JN, Flack MR, Froehlich J, et al. 1995 A potential novel mechanism for precocious puberty in juvenile hypothyroidism. *J Clin Endocrinol Metab.* 80:276–279.

184. Castro-Magana M, Angulo M, Canas A, et al. 1988 Hypothalamic-pituitary gonadal axis in boys with primary hypothyroidism and macroorchidism. *J Pediatr.* 112:397–402.

185. Bruder JM, Samuels MH, Bremner WJ, et al. 1995 Hypothyroidism-induced macroorchidism: use of a gonadotropin-releasing hormone agonist to understand its mechanism and augment adult stature. *J Clin Endocrinol Metab.* 80:11–16.

186. Lindsay AN, Voorhess ML, MacGillivray MH 1980 Multicystic ovaries detected by sonography. Am J Dis Child. 134:588–592.

187. Buchanan CR, Stanhope R, Adlard P, et al. 1988 Gonadotrophin, growth hormone and prolactin secretion in children with primary hypothyroidism. *Clin Endocrinol.* (Oxf) 29:427–436.

188. Rivkees SA, Bode HH, Crawford JD 1988 Long-term growth in juvenile acquired hypothyroidism: the failure to achieve normal adult stature. *N Engl J Med.* 318:599–602.

189. Miyazaki R, Yanagawa N, Higashino H, et al. LHRH analogue and growth hormone did not improve the final height of a patient with juvenile hypothyroidism accompanied by precocious puberty. *Arch Dis Child.* 83:87.

CHAPTER 34

Variants of Pubertal Progression

Betsey Schwartz, MD
Kyriakie Sarafoglou, MD
Christopher P. Houk, MD, FAAP
Peter A. Lee, MD, PhD

CONSTITUTIONAL DELAY OF GROWTH AND PUBERTY

A delayed pubertal onset is defined as the failure to develop secondary sexual characteristics by an age 2 standard deviations (SDs) beyond the mean age of onset for that population. Constitutional delay of growth and puberty (CDGP) is the term used to characterize a normal variant of growth seen in healthy, and often short, children who manifest a pubertal delay alongside a delayed bone age. CDGP is more common in boys. Although a single definition may not apply to all populations, a practical definition for girls is the lack of breast development by age 13 years and for boys, a testicular volume of less than 4 mL by 14 years (1,2). Based on the expected distribution of the age of pubertal onset, delayed puberty is expected in at least 2.3% of children. Although the age of onset for female puberty is approximately normally distributed, the onset of male puberty does not follow a normal distribution.

Etiology/Pathophysiology CDGP accounts for approximately 60% of pubertal delay in boys and approximately 30% in girls (3). Although CDGP is particularly common in boys, there may also be a referral bias for males because of an expressed or perceived greater psychologic pressure on small and sexually immature boys (4,5). Because CDGP presents with both short stature and pubertal delay, medical attention may be sought before the onset of puberty because of concerns about height (1). In early life, CDGP presents with a growth pattern marked by a fall in growth centiles in the first 2 years of life followed by a normal childhood growth velocity that is followed by a pubertal delay. Typically, after an initial growth deceleration, the interval growth rate is normal, paralleling the normal growth curve. During childhood, both the height and growth velocity of children with CDGP are more typical of biologic age as estimated by skeletal age x-ray than of chronologic age (6,7). The extent of delay of

onset of puberty also correlates more closely with bone age than chronologic age. (8) Puberty generally begins at a skeletal age approximating 10.5 years in girls and 12.5 years in boys. In CDGP, the regulation of gonadarche, the hypothalamic-pituitary-gonadal axis, and the onset of adrenarche are linked to the biologic maturity as reflected by skeletal age; consequently it will occur at a later than average chronologic age (6), consistent with biologic maturity reflected by skeletal age. A family history of delayed puberty is frequently associated with CDGP in both sexes, often a delay in the same sex parent.

Available evidence (7,9) suggests that gonadotropin and sex steroid levels typify a normal pubertal pattern as bone age progresses and that once underway shows a normal pubertal duration. Once the initial signs of puberty spontaneously develop, children with GDGP should progress normally to sexual maturity.

In males with CDGP, skeletal age is typically delayed by 2 to 3 years with similar delay in the spontaneous onset of puberty. In more severe delay, spontaneous puberty may occur by 18 years of age; in rare circumstances pubertal onset may be delayed into the third decade of life (10). Hence, without intervention, sexual maturity may not be reached until boys are well into their twenties. In girls with CDGP, the average pubertal delay is also typically 2 to 3 years and the mean age of menarche has been reported to be 15.6 years (5) compared with the normal mean of 12.5 years (11).

Although it has been assumed that adult height in those with CDGP is normal, this has not been consistently verified. Reports of adult heights are: 1) within genetic potential (1,9,12,13); 2) less than genetic potential (5,15); and 3) less than midparental height or the height predicted at the time of delayed puberty (15–18). Adult height differences may relate to duration of delay, diminished growth hormone (GH) secretion, or treatment with exogenous sex steroids (7,13,17,19). Of note, the magnitude of provoked GH peaks does

not correlate with subsequent adult height in boys with CDGP (18).

Prolonged delay of puberty may be associated with altered body proportions such as relatively longer arms and legs, resulting from a greater growth of long bones relative to spinal growth during the prolonged prepubertal period. The resultant decreased spine to leg length ratio is a common feature of pubertal delay, with an increase in adult height developing from the disproportionate gains in the lower body segment (19). Conversely, relatively less spinal growth during puberty may account for failure to reach predicted height (7). In children with familial short stature, pubertal onset occurs at the expected chronologic age; however, many children being evaluated for short stature have both CDGP and familial short stature. This may be the explanation of reduced adult stature in a significant subset of the population (7,13).

Differential Diagnosis The primary goal of the evaluation of pubertal delay is to identify children with an underlying pathology (Figure 34-1). Pathology is expected in a larger percentage of girls than boys, with CDGP accounting for only 30% of the cases of pubertal delay in girls. The differential diagnosis of pubertal delay is subdivided into two major categories: 1) those with low plasma gonadotropin levels (also called hypogonadotropic hypogonadism) that may be temporary or permanent; and 2) those with elevated gonadotropin levels (also called hypergonadotropic hypogonadism) that indicate gonadal failure (except in cases of transient gonadal failure seen during chemotherapy or radiation) (20).

Deficient gonadotropin secretion (hypogonadotropic hypogonadism) occurs with hypothalamic or pituitary disorders, chronic diseases, and CDGP. A thorough physical examination and family history may distinguish between transient and permanent hypogonadotropism. Permanent hypogonadotropism may be suggested by a history of micropenis, cryptorchidism, and/or anosmia.

Variants of Pubertal Progression

AT-A-GLANCE

Variations of pubertal progression may occur in otherwise healthy children and include constitutional delay of growth and puberty, pubertal gynecomastia, premature thelarche, and premature adrenarche. These conditions are usually benign and often require no treatment other than reassurance. It is, however, important to differentiate these conditions from pathologic causes of pubertal delay or precocity.

CONDITION	CLINICAL PRESENTATION	FINDINGS	TREATMENT
Constitutional Delay of Growth and Puberty	Testicular volume <4 mL at 14 years in males; absent breast development at 13 years in females; CDGP more common in boys; associated with family history of pubertal delay and short stature for chronologic age	Bone age delayed; prepubertal testosterone, estrogen, FSH, and LH levels; prior to physical changes of puberty, gonadotropin and gonadal steroid level may be measured within the pubertal range; DHEA-S low for chronologic age, appropriate for bone age	Reassurance and observation; testosterone enanthate 50 mg IM given monthly for 3–6 months or Oxandrolone 0.0625 mg/kg oral daily for same period in males; low-dose estrogen therapy in females
Pubertal Gynecomastia	Breast tissue >5 cm; typically resolves within 2 years; testes are pubertal	Normal pubertal levels of testosterone, estradiol, FSH, LH, DHEA-S, androstenedione, and DHT; ratio of serum estradiol to testosterone may be elevated	Treatment with aromatase inhibitor or estrogen antagonist may be beneficial if started early; resection is definitive
Premature Thelarche	Female breast development before 8 years of age without other signs of sexual maturation; majority of cases occur before 2 years of age and regress; growth velocity is normal; pubertal onset and progression are usually normal	Bone age within range for chronologic age; estradiol normal or slightly elevated; gonadotropin levels usually prepubertal; response to leuprolide shows FSH predominance; pelvic ultrasound shows normal prepubertal uterus and ovaries; ovarian microcysts may occur	No treatment necessary; routine follow up indicated to ensure normal pubertal progression
Premature Adrenarche	Pubic hair development before the age of 8 years in girls and 9 years in boys; axillary hair, body odor, and mild acne may occur; no signs of gonadal development or virilization; more common in girls; growth velocity may be increased; normal pubertal onset and progression	Bone age often advanced by 1–2 years; DHEA, DHEA-S, 17OHP, androstenedione, and testosterone may be elevated for chronologic age but normal for the Tanner stage of pubic hair development	No treatment necessary; follow up important because of increased risk for later functional ovarian hyperandrogenism and insulin resistance

DHEA-S = dehydroepiandrosterine sulfate; FSH = follicular stimulating hormone; LH = luteinizing hormone; 17OHP = 17α-hydroxyprogesterone; DHT = dihydrotestosterone.

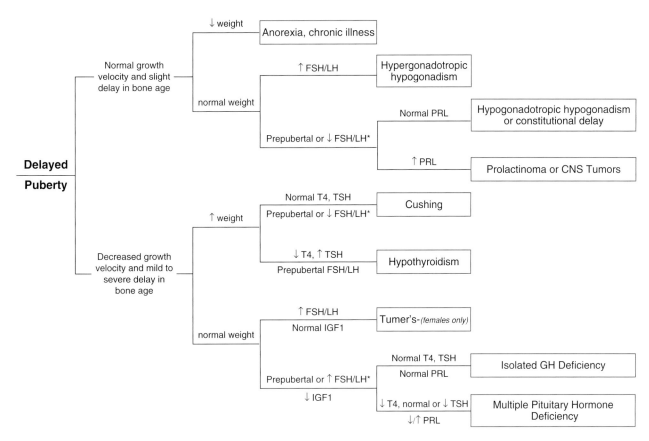

FIGURE 34-1. Diagnostic algorithm for boys and girls presenting with delayed puberty. * = Decreased gonadotropin response to GNRH agonist (LHRH, Leuprolide).

Chronic diseases, such as inflammatory bowel disease, celiac disease, asthma, chronic renal failure, cardiac disease, endocrine disorders such as hypothyroidism and diabetes mellitus, chronic therapy with glucocorticoids (3) may delay both linear growth and puberty and may be associated with disproportionate weight for height. Inadequate nutritional intake when associated with psychiatric disorders such as anorexia nervosa, or excessive energy utilization such as vigorous exercise in athletes or ballet dancers may result in pubertal delay. Successful intervention in such situations can be followed by catch-up growth and pubertal progression (6).

Pubertal delay associated with high gonadotropin levels always indicates gonadal failure as seen in Turner syndrome, disorders of sex differentiation and gonadal steroidogenesis, autoimmune gonadal destruction, and as a consequence of gonadotoxic chemotherapeutic regimens. An exception may be in the oncology patient who during chemotherapy has elevated gonadotropin levels but subsequently the gonadotropin levels decrease as he/she may have varying degrees of recovery. Of special note, although Klinefelter syndrome is a type of hypergonadotropic hypogonadism, males with this condition commonly present with unusually small testes or infertility rather than pubertal delay.

The frequency of the disorders responsible for pubertal delay is not well documented; however, a retrospective study of 232 children referred to an academic center for evaluation of pubertal delay reported that 53% had CDGP (63% of males and 30% of females) (21). Of the 158 males, 63% had CDGP, 20% had a delay because of an underlying condition, 9% had hypogonadotropic hypogonadism (Kallmann syndrome and craniopharyngioma being the most common), and 7% had hypergonadotropism (primary testicular failure). In the 74 females evaluated, 30% had CDGP, 19% were delayed because of an underlying condition, 15% had permanent hypogonadotropic hypogonadism, and 26% had hypergonadotropism (Turner syndrome and chemotherapy/gonadal radiation were the most common entities).

Evaluation An evaluation for pubertal delay should be initiated if pubertal onset does not occur by age 14 to 15 years in boys and age 12 to 13 in girls, or the lack of menarche by age 15 to 16 years. Because a hypogonadotropic state characterizes the prepubertal years, it is usually not possible to distinguish between transient CDGP and other pathologic permanent causes of hypogonadotropic hypogonadism including partial gonadotropin deficiency(9). Thus, at least annual reassessment should occur, even after sex steroid therapy has been instituted, until hormonal evidence

verifies endogenous puberty or permanent hypogonadotropism.

Lack of attainment of pubertal milestones within the expected intervals, including lack of attainment of testes larger than 15 mL in boys and lack of menarche in girls within 5 years of pubertal onset should be evaluated (7).

Initial Evaluation An initial evaluation of pubertal delay involves a careful history and physical examination. The focus of the history should be toward identifying chronic symptoms suggestive of illnesses or malnutrition, documenting birth history, subsequent growth and development, history of anosmia, hyposmia, and family history of pubertal delay, age of menarche, infertility, and consanguinity (7,11).

Using available data, a growth chart should be plotted. Height, weight, and body proportions should be determined. Compared with previous data, height and weight can be used to calculate annual growth rates preferable based on a 12-month interval, intervals less than 4 to 6 months being inadequate. Upper-to-lower segment ratio can be determined by measuring sitting height or lower segment (from top of pubic symphysis to floor) and compared with normal for age: ratio decrease with age to 1.0 or more depending on racial group. Arm span, (finger tip to finger tip) should be within 5 cm of the standing height.

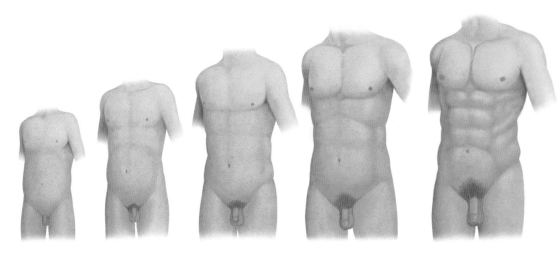

Figure 34-2. Tanner stages 1 to 5 of pubertal development in males.

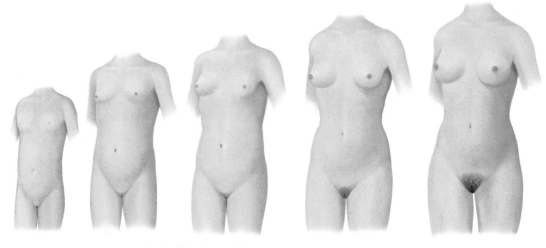

FIGURE 34-3. Tanner stages 1 to 5 of pubertal development in females.

Turner syndrome (22). A complete neurologic evaluation should include examination of the optic discs and visual fields testing to look for evidence of optic nerve damage from a CNS abnormality (7,11). Olfaction should also be tested because anosmia is part of some forms of Kallmann syndrome (7,11).

First Level of Tests Consideration for initial laboratory testing should include serum gonadotropins, free thyroxine, thyroid stimulating hormone (TSH), dehydroepiandrosterone sulfate (DHEAS), and prolactin levels, an electrolyte panel, complete blood count, erythrocyte sedimentation rate, and urinalysis to screen for chronic disease and endocrine disorders that may hinder growth (9). A bone age radiograph should also be obtained to assess the degree of bone maturity (biologic age). Serum sex steroid levels should be a part of the initial evaluation only if there is any physical evidence of pubertal changes (sex steroid levels are expected to be low in the absence of any pubertal development). If puberty has begun, transient nocturnal increases in luteinizing hormone (LH) secretion, which is characteristic of early puberty, may result in early morning detectable sex steroid levels. A daytime plasma testosterone greater than 45 ng/dL in boys and plasma estradiol level over 9 pg/ml in girls is associated with the onset of puberty. Measurement of gonadotropins allows the differentiation of hypergonadotropic hypogonadism from hypogonadotropic hypogonadism and CDGP (for further details and differentiation of the different causes of hypergonadotropic hypogonadism in both males and females, please see Chapters 35, 36 and 37). DHEAS levels may document adrenarche; hypogonadotropic patients usually undergo adrenarche at a normal age, although adrenarche is often delayed in CDGP (7). Other testing to be considered should include magnetic resonance imaging (MRI) of the brain if findings suggest a neurologic abnormality, and

The physical examination should concentrate on identifying markers of chronic disease, malnutrition, neurologic abnormalities, thyroid disease, or other endocrinopathies/syndromes. In boys, in addition to determining height, weight, and skeletal proportions, documentation should include stretched penile length, position of urethral opening, and whether both testes are present in a normal developed scrotum. Cryptorchidism, bifid scrotum, micropenis and/or perineoscrotal hypospadias may indicate defects in gonadal steroidogenesis, testicular disorders of sex development including, congenital anorchia (see Chapter 37), defects along the hypothalamus or pituitary and rare forms of congenital adrenal hyperplasia (CAH) such as 17α-hydroxylase/17,20 lyase, partial 17,20 lyase deficiencies or lipoid CAH. Small testes, eunuchoid habitus, and gynecomastia are suggestive of the Klinefelter syndrome. Obesity

and delayed puberty, in both boys and girls may suggest defects in prohormone convertase 1 (PC1), or in leptin and leptin receptor. When obesity is associated with delayed puberty and dysmorphic features it is suggestive of Prader-Willi, Bardet-Biedl or other genetic syndromes (see Chapter 21).

Tanner stage for pubic hair and breast development in girls should be carefully assessed, as should Tanner stage for public hair and testicular volume in boys (7,11) (see Figures 34-2 and 34-3; Tables 34-1 and 34-2). Children with CDGP typically have delay of both gonadarche no breast develpoment or ovarian volune increase in girls; no increase in testicular volume in boys and adrenarche (sexual hair, body odor, and oily skin). Signs of adrenarche in the absence of testicular or breast development, however, may occur in patients with gonadotropin deficiency, such as Kallmann syndrome or gonadal dysgenesis, including

TABLE 34-1   Pubertal Characteristics Correlated with Tanner Staging–Males

Stage	Growth Rate	Genital–Pubic Hair	Other Changes
1	5-6 cm/year	Penis size prepubertal: no coarse or pigmented pubic hair; testes < 4 ml volume; long axis <2.5 cm	
2	5-6 cm/year	Early penile and scrotum growth; minimal coarse and pigmented pubic hair at base of penis; testes 4–8 ml volume; length 2.5–3.3 cm	Scrotal thinning/reddening; early voice changes
3	Accelerates to 7.8 cm/year	Increase in penile length and width; coarse, dark curly pubic hair over pubis; testes 10-15 ml volume; length 3.4 – 4.0	Voice breaks; light hair on upper lip; acne; muscle mass increases
4	Peaks at 10 cm/year	Increase in penile length and width; scrotum pigmenting adult quality of pubic hair but more sparse distribution; testes 15–20 ml volume; 4.1–4.5 cm in length	Axillary hair; voice change; early sideburns
5	No further growth after epiphyseal closure	Adult size and shape penis; adult distribution of pubic hair (spread to medial thighs); testes > 20 ml volume; > 4.5 cm in length	Beard growth; mature male physique

TABLE 34-2   Pubertal Characteristics Correlated with Tanner Staging–Females

Stage	Growth Rate	Breast	Pubic Hair
1	5-6 cm/year	Papilla elevation	No pubic hair
2	7-8 cm/year	Palpable breast buds; areola enlargement	Sparse, pigmented hair mainly on labia
3	Peaks at 8 cm/year	Areola and breast enlargement; no projection of the areolae	Coarser and darker hair spread over mons pubis
4	7 cm/year	Projection of areola and papillla to form secondary mound	Adult type hair but not spreading to medial surface of the thighs
5	No further growth after epiphyseal closure	Mature with projection of papilla only	Adult type hair and distribution

a karyotype to diagnose Turner or other disorders of sex differentiation; Klinefelter syndrome rarely presents with lack of onset of puberty.

Second Level of Tests There are no tests that clearly distinguish between CDGP and hypogonadotropic hypogonadism at presentation with pubertal delay. Basal or stimulated serum gonadotropin levels in response to gonadotropin-releasing hormone (GnRH) analog testing greater than the prepubertal range (6,9,23) once the skeletal age is at the biologic age of puberty (11 y for girls and 13 y for boys) may distinguish these two entities; those with physiologic delay show serum gonadotropin levels within the pubertal response range with LH predominance.

Commonly monitoring the progression of puberty is recommended (6,7,9,11). If sex steroid therapy is given, it should be discontinued for intervals of 2 months and hormone levels measured. If by 18 years of age or bone age of 13 in girls or 15 in boys, there are no findings of pubertal maturation, levels of gonadotropins and sex steroids continue to be prepubertal, and the DHEAS level is normal for chronologic age, the diagnosis of gonadotropin deficiency can reasonably be made (7). Significantly increased testicular volume is indicative of pubertal gonadotropin secretion with or without interval androgen therapy in boys. Comparable monitoring in females involves imaging the ovaries with ultrasound (6).

Treatment Indications Patients and parents of children with a presumptive diagnosis of CDGP can be assured that their child most likely has a normal variant of puberty and reassured that sexual maturation will develop in time. Children with CDGP tend to have more behavioral problems and lower self-esteem than their peers and feel more vulnerable in social situations (24). Short-term therapy with sex steroids should be offered in the presence of psychosocial issues as there is no identified negative impact of treatment of delayed puberty. A retrospective study found that half of adult men and women with a history of CGDP reported that growth delay negatively impacted their social and academic success during adolescence and that they, in retrospect, would have liked to have had treatment to hasten their growth spurt (5,15).

Bone mineralization and future risk of osteoporosis is another consideration for treatment. There is inconsistent evidence of reduced spinal bone mineral density in both prepubertal children with CDGP and adult men with a history of CDGP (25,26). Because gonadal sex steroids have a significant impact on the peak bone mineral density attained during adolescence, normalizing the hormonal milieu earlier during adolescence in these children would be expected to improve adult bone mineralization (10).

Treatment Options Currently, low-dose testosterone is the therapy of choice for boys with CDGP. Testosterone increases growth velocity, advances bone age, induces appearance of sexual characteristics, and is safe in physiologic doses (13,27), without compromising final height (18,28–30). Depot testosterone preparations such as 50 to 100 mg per dose testosterone enanthate or cypionate can be given intramuscularly at 4-week intervals for a period of 6 months. Oral testosterone preparations have been used to promote growth but multiple daily doses and variable absorption from gastrointestinal tract make its use less predictable (11). There is sufficient experience with testosterone patches or gel preparations that these can also be used in pubertal delay if desired.

Oxandrolone, a non-aromatizable weak androgen, has limited efficacy in promoting growth in males and females with CDGP, except if used when bone age is peripubertal (6, 7, 10, 11, 31, 32) and in appropriate doses, 0.0625 mg/kg/day (8,13,33). Its utility is limited to stimulating linear growth with minimal androgen impact; hence, it does not stimulate puberty in males with CDGP.

In girls with CDGP, the mainstay of therapy is low-dose estrogen to stimulate growth and feminization without compromising adult height (7). Ethinyl estradiol is often provided orally at a dose of 2 to 4 μg (50–100 μg/kg/d) for 6 months or until spontaneous sexual development occurs (6,7,34).

The use of GH for these children remains controversial. Although GH enhances short-term growth, it does not appear to significantly improve adult height in children with CDGP (13). Furthermore, exogenous sex steroids eliminate the transient GH deficiency seen in CDGP (8,13).

Testosterone treatment in combination with aromatase inhibitors is a potentially promising therapy for treatment of short boys with CGDP. The rational is that testosterone therapy induces virilization and the aromatase inhibitor blocks the conversion of the administered testosterone to estrogen, thereby blocking the negative effects of increased estrogen on epiphyseal closure and adult height (34,34).

A reevaluation of linear growth, pubertal development, bone age, and sex hormone levels should follow 6 months of therapy (9). If signs of spontaneous puberty are absent or concentrations of sex steroids remain low, then treatment may be repeated (7). Only one or two courses are usually necessary and development of secondary sex characteristics starts once bone age reaches 12 to 13 years in boys or 11 to 12 years in girls (11). If pubertal development or sex steroid levels do not improve after the cessation of therapy, gonadotropin deficiency should be considered. Accordingly, it is important to follow these children carefully until puberty is complete.

PUBERTAL GYNECOMASTIA

Gynecomastia is defined as the development of glandular breast enlargement in males. Most commonly, gynecomastia is a transient condition that starts in early puberty and resolves within 1 to 2 years. Gynecomastia is common and as many as one half to two-thirds of all boys develop at least some degree of gynecomastia during puberty, with a peak incidence at 14 years of age (35). Although the vast majority of cases are benign, gynecomastia may signal an underlying disease or drug side effect. When gynecomastia develops in the prepubertal period, exceeds 5 cm, or fails to regress as sexual maturity is reached, additional evaluation should be undertaken.

Etiology/Pathophysiology More than half of all neonates will demonstrate breast enlargement of up to 2.0 cm caused by the action of maternal estrogens, placental estrogens, or both. The increased breast tissue usually disappears in a few weeks. This regression can be delayed in some infants, particularly those who are breastfed. Although the cause

of gynecomastia remains uncertain, a transient diagnostic alteration in serum estradiol to testosterone has been proposed (36–39). Because estrogens stimulate and androgens inhibit breast growth, gynecomastia is thought to occur when the male breast is exposed to unusually high ratios of estrogen/testosterone.

The balance of estrogen and testosterone may be altered during early puberty in boys because of diurnal variations in hormone secretion at this time. Testosterone is initially secreted by the testes only at night in response to nocturnal LH stimulation from the pituitary gland (40). As puberty progresses, LH and testosterone levels start to rise during the daytime as well (37). Circulating estrogens, however, rise both during the day and night during early puberty, leading to a relative estrogen dominance in the daytime, which may be exaggerated in boys with gynecomastia (40). Testosterone suppression of estrogen action on their breast tissue during the day may only become adequate in time as puberty ensues.

The literature evaluating the estrogen/androgen imbalance of pubertal gynecomastia offers various mechanisms to explain this phenomenon. Because the majority of circulating estrogens in males are derived from peripheral tissue aromatization of testosterone and adrenal androgens, it is likely that increased aromatase activity contributes to transient gynecomastia. This theory is supported by the finding of increased aromatase activity in pubic skin fibroblasts in individuals with gynecomastia (41). Also, decreased adrenal androgen levels in those with pubertal gynecomastia suggests that a greater conversion of adrenal androgens to estrogen may in part be responsible for this condition (42). In addition, boys with marked pubertal gynecomastia have a greater body mass index (43). Excess adipose tissue may provide some of these boys with increased peripheral aromatase activity, thereby increasing their estrogen/androgen ratio (44).

It is also possible that sex hormone binding globulin (SHBG), which binds more tightly to testosterone than estrogen, may also alter estrogen–androgen balance. An elevation of SHBG in pubertal boys with gynecomastia is associated with low free testosterone levels and a high estrogen/testosterone ratio when compared with controls (45). Other explanations for the pathogenesis of pubertal gynecomastia include elevated prolactin levels and increased sensitivity of receptors to circulating estrogen; however, a universally accepted theory does not yet exist (11).

Clinical Presentation Signs of male sexual development, such as testicular enlargement and the appearance of pubic hair, precede the

onset of gynecomastia for at least 6 months (37). Breast enlargement is bilateral in the majority of cases; however, approximately 25% of boys will present with unilateral gynecomastia, which is considered a stage in the development of bilateral gynecomastia (36,37). Glandular breast tissue usually measures less than 4 cm in diameter and resembles early female breast budding. Tissue extending 5 cm or more is referred to as pubertal macrogynecomastia and is unlikely to regress sufficiently after puberty (37).

Histopathology The histologic appearance of glandular breast tissue is related to the duration of gynecomastia. Initial changes include proliferation of ductal epithelium, periductal edema, and highly cellular fibroblastic stroma. After 1 year, the tissue matures to a "fibrous stage," which is characterized by dilation of the ducts and an almost acellular fibrous stroma (46). The inactive fibrotic tissue seen after longer durations of gynecomastia is unlikely to respond to medical therapy (47).

Differential Diagnosis Although pubertal gynecomastia is usually a benign and transient condition, gynecomastia may signify an underlying systemic disease, identifiable syndromes, or medication side effects. Prepubertal boys and boys with rapid or excessive breast development should be evaluated promptly. Although prepubertal gynecomastia, both unilateral and bilateral, seldom has an identifiable pathologic cause, except those with abrupt onset or progression. A study evaluating 60 boys referred to a pediatric endocrinology clinic for macrogynecomastia found a pathologic cause for gynecomastia in 25% of the patients. Of these, nearly half were diagnosed with a gynecomastia-associated syndrome, such as Klinefelter. The other half had a history of chronic illnesses, including diabetes mellitus and a variety of neurologic disorders (44). This study underscores the importance of a medical evaluation to rule out pathologic causes of gynecomastia.

Hypogonadism Hypogonadism caused by primary testicular failure or secondary to hypothalamic-pituitary disorders may lead to gynecomastia. Low androgen levels increase the estrogen/androgen ratio; high LH levels with primary hypogonadism seem to increase testicular estrogen synthesis production further altering the estrogen/androgen balance (48). The incidence of gynecomastia in Klinefelter syndrome is more than 50% (49). Defects in testosterone synthesis or action can lead to ambiguous genitalia at birth and gynecomastia with virilization in adolescence if the defect is partial. Congenital anorchia and postnatal causes of testicular damage such as viral orchitis, bilateral injury, or radiation may all predispose to gynecomastia. Ovarian and testicular activity in patients with 46, XX testicular DSD, 46, XY mixed or partial gonadal dysgenesis or ovotesticular DSD may result in a mixed pattern of virilization and feminization, including breast development during puberty (37).

Thyroid and Prolactin Disorders Gynecomastia occurs in 25% to 40% of boys with hyperthyroidism (49). An elevated estrogen/testosterone ratio is found in men with hyperthyroidism and is thought to result from an increase in serum SHBG concentration with preferential binding to testosterone (50). Also, hyperthyroidism is associated with increased peripheral conversion of androstenedione to estrogen (51,52). High prolactin levels, as seen with prolactinomas or hypothyroidism, may lead to galactorrhea and rarely gynecomastia, possibly by inducing secondary hypogonadism (53,54).

Tumors Tumors may cause gynecomastia by altering the hormonal milieu. More than in any other tissue, the highest concentrations of estrogen receptors (ER-α and ER-β) are found in Sertoli, Leydig, and germ cells, signifying the importance of estrogen for regulation of these tissues. Germ cell, Leydig cell, and some Sertoli cell tumors and adrenocortical neoplasms secrete estrogen, leading to testosterone/estrogen imbalance and gynecomastia (48). Testosterone is usually low due to the suppressive effects of estrogens on LH, which drives testicular androgen biosynthesis.

Breast tumors are an exceedingly rare cause of gynecomastia in boys, but should be considered if breast swelling is hard, unilateral, or fixed. Dimpling of the skin, nipple retraction, and axillary adenopathy are also suggestive of carcinoma (55). Although the risk of male breast cancer is increased 20-fold in Klinefelter syndrome, it is uncertain whether idiopathic gynecomastia, such as occurs in healthy boys, alone predisposes the breast to cancer (37).

Chronic Diseases A number of chronic diseases such as liver disease, renal failure, ulcerative colitis, cystic fibrosis, and AIDS may induce gynecomastia by various mechanisms. Liver disease may impair hepatic degradation of estrogens and chronic uremia of renal failure is damaging to the testes. Gynecomastia observed in malnutrition may be related to liver dysfunction. Decreased testicular function and gynecomastia may result from nervous system damage with paraplegia or herpes zoster infection (37).

Familial A heterogeneous group of cases of a familial form of gynecomastia have been described. These syndromes are inherited in an X-linked recessive or autosomal dominant manner and involve defective androgen receptor function or excess aromatase activity (56,57).

Drugs Gynecomastia can occur as an adverse reaction to drugs that inhibit testosterone action or enhance the effects of estrogen. Ketoconazole inhibits several of the enzymes required for testosterone synthesis and may lead to an increased estrogen/testosterone ratio. The combination of spironolactone and cimetidine inhibits testosterone synthesis and blocks the binding of androgens to their receptors and has been reported to cause gynecomastia. Cancer chemotherapeutic agents, particularly alkylating agents, may permanently impair testosterone synthesis through toxic effects on the testes (55).

Medications and substances that contain estrogen also may induce gynecomastia. Even exposure to estrogen-containing skin lotions, delousing powder, and embalming fluid can cause gynecomastia. Testosterone administration or human chorionic gonadotropin β-hCG injections in boys can cause gynecomastia from increased aromatization of testosterone to estrogens in the peripheral or gonadal tissues (37). Marijuana may cause gynecomastia and is associated with decreased testosterone levels. Alcohol also induces breast enlargement through toxic effects on the testes, increased clearance of testosterone by the liver, and enhanced conversion of testosterone to estrogen (56).

Clinical Assessment An evaluation should distinguish pubertal gynecomastia from pathologic causes. The duration and timing of breast enlargement should be established, particularly in relation to pubertal development. Breast enlargement before the onset of puberty or associated with precocious puberty may indicate an endocrine pathology (37). In the medical history it is important to identify any symptoms of hypogonadism or systemic diseases such as renal failure, liver disease, hyperthyroidism, and malnutrition. A history of medication or marijuana use and a family history of gynecomastia should also be sought. In addition, one should determine whether the breast enlargement is causing the patient psychologic distress or pain.

Physical examination A thorough physical examination should be performed to rule out signs of chronic illness. Glandular tissue of gynecomastia can be distinguished from fatty enlargement (pseudogynecomastia)

by grasping the breast between the thumb and forefinger and gently moving the two digits toward the nipple while the patient is supine. A firm or rubbery, mobile, disklike mound of tissue should arise from beneath the nipple and areolar region in true gynecomastia (48). The breast examination should determine whether glandular enlargement is unilateral or bilateral and if there is discharge or tenderness. It is also important to determine the stage of pubertal development, testicular size, and assess for ambiguous genitalia.

First Level of Tests The clinical picture will determine the laboratory tests needed for the evaluation of gynecomastia. Any boy who appears chronically ill or malnourished should undergo renal, hepatic, and thyroid function tests. Boys with signs of hypogonadism, precocious puberty, or macrogynecomastia are evaluated using serum levels of LH, follicle-stimulating hormone (FSH), prolactin, estradiol, testosterone, androstenedione, DHEA-S, dihydrotestosterone, and β-hCG levels. If the testicular size is small in relation to the stage of pubertal development, a karyotype will identify those with the Klinefelter syndrome.

Second Level of Tests A high estradiol level warrants testicular ultrasonography to rule out a germ cell, Leydig cell, or Sertoli cell tumor. If the testicular ultrasound is negative but the β-hCG level is elevated, a germ cell tumor should be sought with computed tomography and MRI studies of the brain, chest, and abdomen. If the β-hCG level is undetectable or adrenal androgens are markedly elevated, an adrenal tumor should be considered and abdominal computed tomography or MRI should be performed.

Treatment Idiopathic pubertal gynecomastia usually stabilizes within 18 months and resolves within 3 years without treatment, and as such requires no medical treatment other than reassurance. The traditional therapy is cosmetic surgical reduction, while more recently medical therapy has been tried and is often followed by reduction of breast volume but not total resolution.

Medical therapy is more effective if initiated when the breast tissue has been present less than 4 years (37). Although no medications are approved specifically for gynecomastia, many have been developed, studied, and are used in practice (49). These medications, in theory, reduce breast enlargement by decreasing the estrogen/androgen ratio. The medical therapies typically include estrogen antagonists and aromatase inhibitors. Tamoxifen, developed to treat breast cancer in women, competes for estrogen receptor binding in the breast. Studies in gynecomastia report partial regression of breast tissue when using a dose of 10 to 20 mg twice daily (58). Side effects occur in less than 5% of treated males and include mild nausea and abdominal discomfort (37). Theoretically, aromatase inhibitors would appear to be the best option because they decrease the peripheral aromatization of androgens to estrogens. Of these agents, testolactone has been studied and used the most at a dose of 150 mg three times daily. Recently, a third generation aromatase inhibitor (Arimidex) was found to improve the testosterone/estrogen ratio but did not show significant differences in the reduction of gynecomastia between the treated and placebo groups (59).

Surgery remains the therapy of choice for gynecomastia exceeding 6 cm breast tissue, for breast tissue that has been present for years, and tissue that does not respond to medical therapy. Various approaches are used to remove breast glandular tissue. The most satisfactory method involves periareolar excision of breast tissue combined with liposuction (59).

PREMATURE THELARCHE

Premature thelarche is a condition characterized by isolated breast development in girls younger than 8 years of age. This condition occurs in 20.8 per 100,000 patient-years and, according to one population-based study, 60% to 85% of cases occur by 2 years of age (60–62). When occurring at younger than 2 years of age, it is most likely a reflection of the increased ovarian activity characteristic of normal infancy. Premature thelarche may be bilateral or unilateral and regression occurs in the majority of cases over a period of 6 months to 6 years (61,63). Regression is less common for girls who show breast development after 2 years of age (62,63).

Etiology/Pathophysiology The etiology of premature thelarche is unknown. Elevated FSH levels and increased FSH response to GnRH stimulation have been found in girls with premature thelarche when compared with prepubertal controls (62,64). The exaggerated FSH production has been postulated to increase ovarian estrogen production and induce breast development. Prepubertal baseline and GnRH-stimulated LH levels distinguish girls with premature thelarche from girls with precocious puberty. Increased estradiol levels have been identified by some but not all investigators in girls with premature thelarche, although methods of estradiol quantification in these studies may lack sensitivity (62,64,66). Determination of estradiol levels by ultrasensitive recombinant cell bioassay has shown that estradiol

levels in girls with premature thelarche are significantly higher compared with prepubertal controls (65).

The source of excess estrogen in girls with premature thelarche is uncertain and debated in the literature. It is possible that increased FSH stimulation induces the development of ovarian follicular cysts, corresponding to changes seen in the follicular phase of a normal menstrual cycle (66). Ovaries of girls with premature thelarche have been found to contain cysts that enlarge or diminish in parallel to changes in breast size (66). Other studies have found no correlation between presence or absence of ovarian cysts in these girls with estradiol levels (67). This suggests that although ovarian cysts may not be the source of increased estradiol, it does not preclude the ovary as a source. An alternative nonovarian source of estradiol may be adrenal androgens. DHEA may serve as a precursor for peripheral conversion to estrogen; DHEA has been reported to be higher in girls with precocious thelarche in some studies but not others (66,67). In addition, an increased sensitivity of the breast to low levels of estrogen, perhaps related to estrogen receptor differences, may also play a role in premature thelarche, although this has not been demonstrated (66).

Clinical Presentation Most girls with premature thelarche are younger than 2 years old and the condition may be present at birth (62). Breast development is bilateral in one-half to three-quarters of cases and is usually at Tanner stage 2 or 3 (61,69). Commonly patients have fluctuation in breast size with a periodicity between 6 weeks and 2 months (68). Other than breast enlargement, these girls have no signs of estrogenization; their vaginal mucosa and labia appear prepubertal and they typically show no enlargement or elevation of the areolae (62,64,69). Linear growth velocity is normal and bone age corresponds with chronologic age (63,69). Signs of virilization, such as sexual hair or body odor, do not occur (69). Long-term follow up is consistent with normal menarche, normal fertility, and normal adult height (61,68).

A variant of premature thelarche, referred to as thelarche variant, exaggerated thelarche, nonprogressive precocious puberty or slowly progressive precocious puberty, has been described (63,69), occurring as frequently as in 30% of girls presenting with premature thelarche (63). Girls with such variants may have intermittent or moderate acceleration of growth velocity, skeletal maturity, and increase in uterine size most likely due to an intermittently increased estrogen secretion (70). Up to one-fifth of girls identified as having premature thelarche will

experience pubertal progression at an early age (63,64,71). Hence, careful follow up is indicated for girls with premature thelarche to monitor them for other signs of pubertal progression.

Differential Diagnosis A careful examination can usually distinguish a benign mass, such as a hemangioma, lipoma, lymphangioma, or a cyst from a breast bud. Breast cancer is extremely rare in children (72). Isolated premature thelarche should be differentiated from central or peripheral precocious puberty as premature breast development is often the presenting sign of precocious puberty.

Although later stages of central precocious puberty are characterized by an LH-predominant response to GnRH or GnRHa (leuprolide acetate), earlier stages are often indistinguishable from the FSH-predominant response of prepuberty or isolated premature thelarche (64,66,73,74). Ultrasound examination of the ovaries and uterus may or may not help to make this distinction (64,66,71,73,75).

Isolated breast development has been described in patients with exogenous estrogen exposure or juvenile hypothyroidism (76).

Clinical Assessment A thorough medical history should be obtained and the patient's growth and development should be reviewed. It is important to determine the onset and duration of breast development and to inquire about fluctuations in breast size. Other signs of puberty and exposure to exogenous hormones should be excluded. Pubertal history and growth patterns of parents and siblings should also be sought.

First Level of Tests Initial laboratory tests should include serum LH, FSH, and, if a sensitive assay is available, estradiol levels. Estradiol may be normal or slightly elevated and gonadotropin levels are usually prepubertal, with a typical prepubertal ratio of FSH/LH greater than 1. Thyroid function testing, bone age film, and pelvic ultrasound should also be obtained. Bone age is usually consistent with chronologic age, and pelvic ultrasound should reveal normal uterus and ovaries with prepubertal measurements. Although ovarian microcysts can occur with premature thelarche, unilateral enlargement or asymmetry found on ultrasound may indicate a tumor or cyst.

Second Level of Tests If signs of virilization are present, growth is accelerated, skeletal age is advanced, or pelvic ultrasound shows pubertal measurements, an evaluation for precocious puberty, early onset of ovarian hyperandrogenism, or adrenal androgen excess is indicated (see Chapter 33).

Treatment Premature thelarche is a benign condition that may regress. Follow up with appropriate work up or reassurance is indicated. Resection of breast tissue, even if a cyst is identified, is contraindicated because this may impair or preclude future breast development (7). As discussed previously, in some cases premature thelarche progresses into precocious puberty. Because these two entities can be difficult to distinguish, it is important to monitor all girls with premature thelarche for accelerated pubertal progression.

PREMATURE PUBARCHE/ ADRENARCHE

Premature adrenarche refers to an early increase in adrenal androgen production that usually results in the development of pubic hair (pubarche) before the age of 8 years in girls and 9 years in boys. Although axillary hair, body odor, and mild acne may be present, children with premature adrenarche lack other signs of sexual maturation or virilization. This condition occurs with increasing frequency between the ages of 3 and 8 years, although it may present as early as 6 months of age, and is much more common in girls than boys, at a ratio of almost 10 to 1 (77). Obesity, low birth weight, and family history of ovarian hyperandrogenemia all have been associated with an increased incidence of premature adrenarche (78). Although accelerated growth and advanced skeletal maturation are often seen on presentation, long-term data show that final height is normal. Girls with this condition also experience normal pubertal onset and progression (79,80). Early adrenarche is not associated with early pubertal changes of the hypothalamic-pituitary-gonadal axis as evidenced by a prepubertal response to gonadotropin stimulation (81–84). As in normal adrenarche, this condition occurs independently of hypothalamic-pituitary-gonadal maturation.

Premature adrenarche is generally considered a benign variant of puberty, but it may constitute a risk for the later development of ovarian hyperandrogenism and insulin resistance (85,86). Although the incidence is related to racial/ethnic differences, features of functional ovarian hyperandrogenism have been found in almost half of one series of postmenarchal girls with a history of premature adrenarche (87). Mild forms of adrenal androgen excess, as in nonclassic CAH due to 21α-hydroxylase deficiency, may present with early onset of sexual hair, acne, and oily skin in both boys and girls.

Etiology/Pathophysiology The clinical findings of premature adrenarche result from a mild-to-moderate over- secretion of adrenal androgens. Although adrenal androgens DHEA and DHEAS are relatively weak, they serve as a substrate for extraadrenal (peripheral) conversion to the potent androgen testosterone (79). Children with premature adrenarche have plasma concentrations of DHEA, DHEAS, androstenedione, and testosterone that are elevated for chronologic age, but fall within the expected range according to the pubertal stage of pubic hair; usually pubic hair development is at Tanner stages II to III of normal pubertal development (79,80,88–90).

An increase in the P450c17 enzymatic activity in the adrenal zona reticularis typically occurs between the ages of 6 and 8 years, leading to the initial rise in adrenal androgen levels characteristic of adrenarche (79). In premature adrenarche, this process is accelerated, leading to a greater rise in DHEA and its sulfated metabolite DHEA-S levels (80,87,91).

Clinical Presentation Girls with premature adrenarche usually present with dark, coarse, curly pubic hair along the labia majora and occasionally extending onto the mons pubis. In boys, pubic hair appears at the base of the penis. Children with premature adrenarche are otherwise prepubertal without any signs of breast development in girls or testicular enlargement in boys. Although axillary hair, body odor, and mild acne may occur, signs of androgen excess such as severe acne, hirsutism, clitoral or penile enlargement, and voice change are absent. Children with premature adrenarche are typically taller than average for their chronologic age with evidence of mildly increased growth velocity. Bone age is often advanced by 1 to 2 years and typically correlates with height age (79–81). An increased prevalence of premature adrenarche has been observed in children with severe central nervous system abnormalities (79,92). An increased incidence of behavioral problems has not been substantiated (93,94).

Differential Diagnosis Although isolated premature adrenarche is a benign variation of puberty, precocious pubic hair growth may also be the first sign of an underlying pathologic condition, particularly if accompanied by testicular or breast enlargement, and growth acceleration. If signs of virilization are present, rare androgen-secreting gonadal or adrenal tumors, nonclassic (NC) and simple virilizing (SV) CAH due to 21α-hydroxylase deficiency (and rarely CAH due to 3-β-dehydrogenase deficiency), and exogenous androgen medication may be responsible. Cushing syndrome may also lead to excessive androgen production and premature adrenarche; however, these children have impaired growth velocity, which distinguishes them from obese children with premature adrenarche.

Clinical Assessment The age of onset and subsequent progression of pubic hair development, presence or absence of associated axillary hair, acne, or body odor, testicular size in boys and breast development in girls should be determined. History should include a review of the patient's growth pattern and possible exposure to exogenous androgens. A family history of growth and pubertal patterns, including history of premature adrenarche and androgen excessive conditions, should be obtained.

First Level of Tests Initial laboratory tests should include serum levels of DHEA or DHEAS, 17α-hydroxyprogesterone (17OHP), androstenedione, testosterone, and a bone age. In premature adrenarche, adrenal androgens, particularly DHEAS, are expected to be high for chronologic age but within the normal range for Tanner stage of pubic hair development. Skeletal age is typically mildly advanced at 1 to 2 SDs.

Second Level of Tests A high dose adrenocorticotropin (ACTH) hormone stimulation test to rule out CAH due to 21-hydroxylase deficiency should be performed in the patient with signs of excessive virilization, elevated baseline serum 17OHP level above 100 ng/dL, or bone age advancement more than 2 SDs greater than chronologic age. If androgens are elevated and adrenal hyperplasia is ruled out, adrenal and ovarian imaging is indicated.

Treatment Premature adrenarche does not require treatment, but monitoring is pertinent. It is important to follow pubertal progression and growth every 3 to 6 months. In addition, because this condition is associated with the later development of insulin resistance and functional ovarian hyperandrogenism, careful follow up into adolescent and adult years is also recommended.

REFERENCES

1. Argente J. Diagnosis of late puberty. *Horm Res.* 1999;51:95–100.
2. Traggiai C, Stanhope R. Delayed puberty. *Best Pract Res Clin Endocrinol Metab.* 2002;16:139–151.
3. De Luca F, Argente J, Cavallo L, et al. Management of puberty in constitutional delay of growth and puberty. *J Pediatr Endocrinol Metab.* 2001;14:953–957.
4. Crowne EC, Shalet SM, Wallace WHB, et al. Final height in girls with untreated constitutional delay in growth and puberty. *Eur J Pediatr.* 1991;150:708–712.
5. Albanese A, Stanhope R. Investigation of delayed puberty. *Clin Endocrinol.* 1995;43:105–110.

6. Grumbach MM, Styne DM. Puberty: ontogeny, neuroendrocrinology, physiology, and disorders. In: Larsen PR, ed. *Williams Textbook of Endocrinology.* Philidelphia: WB Saunders; 1998:1509–1625.

7. Stanhope R, Preece MA. Management of constitutional delay of growth and puberty. *Arch Dis Child.* 1988;63:1104–1110.

8. Rosenfield RL. Diagnosis and management of delayed puberty. *J Clin Endocrinol Metab.* 1990; 70:559–562.

9. Kulin HE. Delayed puberty. *J Clin Endocrinol Metab.* 1996;81:3460–3464.

10. Styne DM. Disorders of sexual differentiation and puberty in the male. In: Sperling MA, ed. *Pediatric Endocrinology.* Philadelphia: WB Saunders, 2002:565–628.

11. Lee PA, Kulin HE, Guo SS. Age of puberty in girls and the diagnosis of precocious puberty. *Pediatrics.* 2001; 107:1493–1494.

12. Longas FA, Mayayo E, Valle A, et al. Constitutional delay in growth and puberty: a comparison of final height achieved between treated and untreated children. *J Pediatr Endocrinol Metab.*1996;9:345–357.

13. Volta C, Ghizzoni L, Buono T, et al. Final height in a group of untreated children with constitutional growth delay. *Helvet Paediatr Acta.* 1988;43:171–176.

14. Crowne EC, Shalet SM, Wallace WHB, et al. Final height in boys with untreated constitutional delay in growth and puberty. *Arch Dis Child.* 1990; 65:1109–1112.

15. Sperlich M, Butenandt O, Schwarz HP. Final height and predicted height in boys with untreated constitutional delay. *Eur J Pediatr.* 1995;154:627–632.

16. LaFranchi S, Hanna CE, Mandel SH. Constitutional delay of growth: expected versus final adult height. *Pediatrics.*1991;87:82–87.

17. Adan L, Souberbielle JC, Brauner R. Management of the short stature due to pubertal delay in boys. *J Clin Endocrinol Metab.* 1994;78:478–482.

18. Albanese A, Stanhope R. Predictive factors in the determination of final height in boys with constitutional delay of growth and puberty. *J Pediatr.*1995;126:545–550.

19. Bierich JR, Nolte K, Drews K, et al. Constitutional delay of growth and adolescence. Results of short-term and long-term treatment with GH. *Acta Endocrinol.* 1992;127:392–396.

20. Larsen EC, Muller J, Schmiegelow K, et al. Reduced ovarian function in long-term survivors of radiation- and chemotherapy-treated childhood cancer. *J Clin Endocrinol Metab.* 2003;88:5307–5314.

21. Sedlmeyer IL, Palmert MR. Delayed puberty: analysis of a large case series from an academic center. *J Clin Endocrinol Metab.* 2002;87:1613–1620.

22. Sklar CA, Kaplan SA, Grumbach MM. Evidence for dissociation between adrenarche and gonadarche: studies in patients with idiopathic precocious puberty, gonadal dysgenesis, isolated gonadotropin deficiency, and constitutionally delayed growth and adolescence. *J Clin Endocrinol Metab.* 1980;51:548–556.

23. Ghai K, Cara JF, Rosenfield RL. Gonadotropin releasing hormone agonist (Nafarelin) test to differentiate gonadotropin deficiency from constitutionally delayed puberty in teen-age boys - a clinical research center study. *J Clin Endocrinol Metab.* 1995;80:2980–2986.

24. Gordon M, Crouthamel C, Post EM, et al. Psychosocial aspects of constitutional short stature: Social competence, behavior problems, self-esteem, and family functioning. *J Pediatr.*1982;101:477–480.

25. Moreira MN, Canizo FJ, de la Cruz FJ, et al. Bone Mineral status in prepubertal children with constitutional delay of growth and puberty. *J Pediatr.* 1998;133:521–525.

26. Finkelstein JS, Klibanski A, Neer RM. A longitudinal evaluation of bone mineral density in adult men with histories of delayed puberty. *J Clin Endocrinol Metab.* 1996;81:1152–1155.

27. De Luca F, Argente J, Cavallo L, et al. Management of puberty in constitutional delay of growth and puberty. *J Pediatr Endocrinol Metab.*2001;14:953–957.

28. Kelly BP, Paterson WF, Donaldson MDC. Final height outcome and value of height prediction in boys with constitutional delay in growth and adolescence treated with intramuscular testosterone 125 mg per month for 3 months. *Clin Endocrinol.* 2003;58:267–272.

29. Arrigo T, Cisternino M, De Luca F, et al. Final height outcome in both untreated and testosterone-treated boys with constitutional delay of growth and puberty. *J Pediatr Endocrinol Metab.*1996;9:511–517.

30. Kulin HE, Finkelstein JW, D'Arcangelo MR, et al. Diversity of pubertal testosterone changes in boys with constitutional delay in growth and/or adolescence. *J Pediatr Endocrinol Metab.*1997;10:395–400.

31. Lampit M, Hochberg Z. Androgen therapy in constitutional delay of growth. *Horm Res.* 2003;59:270–275.

32. Wilson DM, McCauley E, Brown DR, et al. Oxandrolone therapy in constitutionally delayed growth and puberty. *Pediatrics.* 1995;96:1095–1100.

33. Traggiai C, Stanhope R. Disorders of pubertal development. *Best Pract Res Clin Obstet Gynaecol.* 2003;17:41–56.

34. Dunkel L, Wickman S. Novel treatment of delayed male puberty with aromatase inhibitors. *Horm Res.* 2002;57(S2):44–52.

35. Nydick M, Bustos J, Dale JH, et al. Gynecomastia in adolescent boys. *JAMA.* 1961; 178:449–454.

36. Mahoney CP. Adolescent gynecomastia: differential diagnosis and management. *Pediatr Clin No Am.* 1990;37:1389–1404.

37. Lee PA. The relationship of concentrations of serum hormones to pubertal gynecomastia. *J Pediatr.*1975;86:212–215.

38. LaFranchi S, Parlow AF, Lippe BM, et al. Pubertal gynecomastia and transient elevation of serum estradiol level. *Am J Dis Child.*1975;129:927–931.

39. Large DM, Anderson DC. Twenty-four hour profiles of circulating androgens and oestrogens in male puberty with and without gynecomastia. *Clin Endocrinol.*1979;11:505–521.

40. Judd HL, Parker DC, Siler TM, et al. The nocturnal rise of plasma testosterone in pubertal boys. *J Clin Endocrinol Metab.* 1974;38:710–713.

41. Bulard J, Mowszowicz I, Schaison G. Increased aromatase activity in pubic skin fibroblasts from patients with isolated gynecomastia. *J Clin Endocrinol Metab.* 1987;64:618–623.

42. Moore DC, Schlaepfer LV, Paunier L, et al. Hormonal Changes during puberty: V. transient pubertal gynecomastia: abnormal androgen-estrogen ratios. *J Clin Endocrinol Metab.* 1984;58:492–499.

43. Sher ES, Migeon CJ, Berkovitz GD. Evaluation of boys with marked breast development at puberty. *Clin Pediatr.* 1998;37:367–372.

44. Longcope C, Baker R, Johnston CC Jr. Androgen and estrogen metabolism: relationship to obesity. *Metabolism.* 1986;35:235–237.

45. Biro FM, Lucky AW, Huster GA, et al. Hormonal studies and physical maturation in adolescent gynecomastia. *J Pediatr.* 1990;116:450–455.

46. Bannayan GA, Hajdu SI. Gynecomastia: clinicopathologic study of 351 cases. *Am J Clin Pathol.* 1972;57:431–437.

47. Braunstein GD. Gynecomastia. *N Engl J Med.* 1993;328:490–495.

48. Lazala C, Saenger P. Pubertal gynecomastia. *J Pediatr Endocrinol Metab.*2002;15:553–560.

49. Salbenblatt JA, Bender BG, Puck MH, et al. Pituitary-gonadal function in Klinefelter syndrome before and during puberty. *Pediatr Res.* 1985;19:82–86.

50. Chopra IJ, Tulchinsky D. Status of estrogen-androgen balance in hyperthyroid men with Graves' disease. *J Clin Endocrinol Metab.* 1974;38:269–277.

51. Southren AL, Olivo J, Gordon GG, et al. The conversion of androgens to estrogens in hyperthyroidism. *J Clin Endocrinol Metab.* 1974;38:207–214.

52. Meikle AW. The interrelationships between thyroid dysfunction and hypogonadism in men and boys. *Thyroid.* 2004; 14 Suppl 1:S17–25.

53. Colao A, Loche S, Cappa M, et al. Prolactinomas in children and adolescents. Clinical presentation and long-term follow-up. *J Clin Endocrinol Metab.* 1998; 83:2777–2780.

54. Glass AR. Gynecomastia. *Endocrinol Metab Clin No Am.* 1994;23:825–837.

55. Mathur R, Braunstein GD. Gynecomastia: pathomechanisms and treatment strategies. *Horm Res.* 1997;48:95–102.

56. Grino PB, Griffin JE, Cushard WG Jr, et al. A Mutation of the androgen receptor associated with partial androgen resistance, familial gynecomastia, and fertility. *J Clin Endocrinol Metab.* 1988;66:754–761.

57. Stratakis CA, Vottero A, Brodie A, et al. The aromatase excess syndrome is associated with feminization of both sexes and autosomal dominant transmission of aberrant P450 aromatase gene transcription. *J Clin Endocrinol Metab.* 1998;83:1348–1357.

58. Gruntmanis U, Braunstein GD. Treatment of gynecomastia. *Curr Opin Invest Drugs.* 2001;2:643–649.

59. Plourde PV, Reiter EO, Jou HC, et al. Safety and efficacy of anastrozole for the treatment of pubertal gynecomastia: a randomized, double-blind, placebo-controlled trial. *J Clin Endocrinol Metab.* 2004;89:4428–4433.

60. Van Winter JT, Noller KL, Zimmerman D, et al. Natural history of premature thelarche in Olmsted County, Minnesota, 1940 to 1984. *J Pediatr.*1990;116:278–280.

61. Ilicki A, Lewin RP, Kauli R, et al. Premature thelarche - natural history and sex hormone secretion in 68 girls. *Acta Paediatr Scand.* 1984;73:756–762.

62. Volta C, Bernasconi S, Cisternino M, et al. Isolated premature thelarche and thelarche variant: clinical and auxological follow-up of 119 girls. *J Endocrinol Invest.* 1998; 21:180–183.

63. Verrotti A, Ferrari M, Morgese G, et al. Premature thelarche: a long-term follow-up. *Gynecol Endocrinol.* 1996;10:241–247.

64. Stanhope R, Abdulwahid NA, Adams J, et al. Studies of gonadotrophin pulsatility and pelvic ultrasound examinations distinguish between isolated and premature thelarche and central precocious puberty. *Eur J Pediatr.*1986;145:190–194.

65. Klein KO, Maricq V, Brown-Dawson JM, et al. Estrogen levels in girls with premature thelarche compared with normal prepubertal girls as determined by an ultrasensitive recombinant cell bioassay. *J Pediatr.*1999; 134:190–192.

66. Stanhope R, Adams J, Brook CGD. Fluctuation of breast size in isolated premature thelarche. *Acta Paediatr Scand.* 1985;74:454–455.

67. Dumic M, Tajic M, Mardesic D, et al. Premature thelarche: a possible adrenal disorder. *Arch Dis Child.* 1982;57:200–203.

68. Salardi A, Cacciari E, Mainetti B, et al. Outcome of premature thelarche: relation to puberty and final height. *Arch Dis Child.* 1998;79:173–174.

69. Stanhope R, Brook CCD. Thelarche variant: a new syndrome of precocious sexual maturation? *Acta Endocrinol.* 1990;123:481–486.

70. Garibaldi LR, Aceto T Jr, Weber C. The pattern of gonadotropin and estradiol secretion in exaggerated thelarche. *Acta Endocrinol.* 1993;128:345–350.

71. Pasquino AM, Pucarelli I, Passeri F, et al. Progression of premature thelarche to central precocious puberty. *J Pediatr.* 1995;126:11–14.

72. Simmons PS. Diagnostic considerations in breast disorders of children and adolescents. *Pediatr Adolesc Gynecol.* 1992;19:91–102.

73. Pescovitz OH, Hench KD, Barnes KM, et al. Premature thelarche and central precocious puberty: the relationship between clinical presentation and the gonadotropin response to luteinizing hormone-releasing hormone. *J Clin Endocrinol Metab.* 1988;67:474–479.

74. Haber HP, Wollmann HA, Ranke MB. Pelvic ultrasonography: early differentiation between isolated premature thelarche and central precocious puberty. *Eur J Pediatr.* 1995;154:182–186.

75. Buzi F, Pilotta A, Dordoni D, et al. Pelvic ultrasonography in normal girls and in girls with pubertal precocity. *Acta Paediatr.* 1998;87:1138–1145.

76. Barnes ND, Hayles AB, Ryan RJ. Sexual maturation in juvenile hypothyroidism. *Mayo Clin Proc.* 1973; 48:849–856.

77. Ibanez L, DiMartino-Nardi J, Potau N, et al. Premature adrenarche - normal variant or forerunner of adult disease? *Endocr Rev.* 2000;21:671–696.

78. Reiter EO, Saenger P. Premature adrenarche. *Endocrinologist.* 1997;7:85–88.

79. Ibanez L, Virdis R, Potau N, et al. Natural history of premature pubarche: an auxological study. *J Clin Endocrinol Metab.* 1992;74:254–257.

80. Ghizzoni L, Milani S. The Natural History of Premature Adrenarche. *J Pediatr Endocrinol Metab.*2000;13:1247–1251.

81. Pang S. Precocious thelarche and premature adrenarche. *Pediatr Ann.* 1981;10:29–34.

82. Lee PA, Gareis FJ. Gonadotropin and sex steroid response to luteinizing hormone-releasing hormone in patients with premature adrenarche. *J Clin Endocrinol Metab.* 1976;43:195–197.

83. Ibanez L, Virdis R, Potau N, et al. Natural History of Premature Pubarche: An Auxological Study. *J Clin Endocrinol Metab.* 1992; 74:254–257.

84. Ghizzoni L, Milani S. The Natural History of Premature Adrenarche. *J Pediatr Endocrinol Metab.*2000; 13:1247–1251.

85. DiMartino-Nardi J. Pre- and postpubertal findings in premature adrenarche. *J Pediatr Endocrinol Metab.* 2000;13:1265–1269.

86. Oppenheimer E, Linder B, DiMartino-Nardi J. Decreased insulin sensitivity in prepubertal girls with premature adrenarche and acanthosis nigricans. *J Clin Endocrinol Metab.* 1995;80:614–618.

87. Ibanez L, Potau N, Virdis R, et al. Postpubertal outcome in girls diagnosed of premature pubarche during childhood: increased frequency of functional ovarian hyperandrogenism. *J Clin Endocrinol Metab.* 1993;76:1599–1603.

88. Voutilainen R, Perheentupa J, Apter D. Benign premature adrenarche: clinical features and serum steroid levels. *Acta Paediatr Scand.* 1983;72:707–711.

89. Kaplowitz PB, Cockrell JL, Young RB. Premature adrenarche: clinical and diagnostic features. *Clin Pediatr.* 1986;25:28–34.

90. Riddick LM, Garibaldi LR, Wang ME, et al. 3?-Androstandediol glucuronide in premature and normal pubarche. *J Clin Endocrinol Metab.* 1991;72:46–50.

91. Ibanez L, Potau N, Zampolli M, et al. Girls diagnosed with premature pubarche show an exaggerated ovarian androgen synthesis from the early stages of puberty: evidence from gonadotropin-releasing hormone agonist testing. *Fertil Steril.* 1997; 67:849–855.

92. Liu N, Grumbach MM, deNapoli R, et al. Prevalence of electro-encephalographic abnormalities in idiopathic precocious puberty and premature pubarche: bearing on pathogenesis and neuroendocrine regulation of puberty. *J Clin Endocrinol Metab.* 1965;25:1296–1308.

93. Dorn LD, Hitt SF, Rotenstein D. Biopsychological and cognitive differences in children with premature vs on-time adrenarche. *Arch Pediatr Adolesc Med.* 1999;153:137–146.

94. Reiter EO, Kulin HE. Sexual maturation in the female: normal development and precocious puberty. *Pediatr Clin No Am.* 1972;19:581–603.

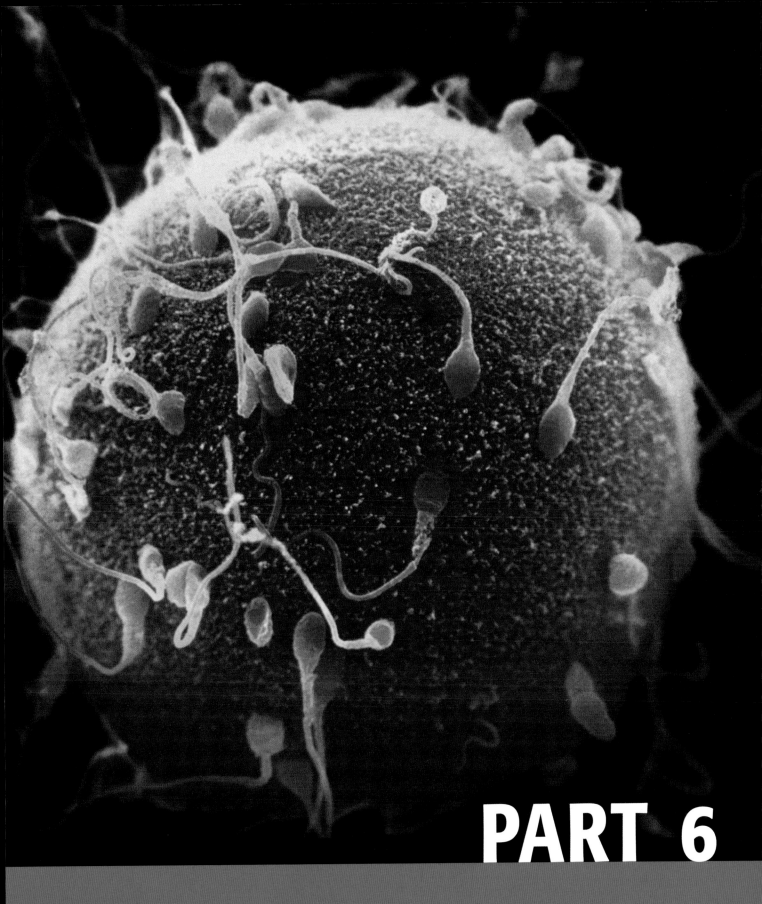

PART 6

Disorders of the Reproductive System

IN THIS PART

Previous page: Colored scanning electron micrograph (SEM) of sperm on the surface of a human egg (ovum) during fertilization.

Disorders of Sex Development

Eric Vilain, MD, PhD
Kyriakie Sarafoglou, MD
Nadir Yehya, MD

INTRODUCTION TO HUMAN SEX DEVELOPMENT

The field of sex development has been rapidly evolving in the past 15 years. From a biologic standpoint, the advances were considerable, with the identification of many genes and mutations responsible for a large number of disorders of sex development, allowing for rapid diagnosis, understanding of the pathophysiology and predicting functional outcomes. From a medical perspective, the management of individuals with ambiguous genitals has also considerably improved, with a better understanding of the needs of patients, and the involvement, in more and more centers (yet, not enough) of a multidisciplinary approach that recognizes the need for psychologic care for children and their parents. Surgical management, although still quite controversial in its indications and efficiency, has improved technically. Finally, it would be difficult not to mention in a chapter on disorders of sex development the broader social context in which these changes have occurred. The role of patient advocacy groups has been instrumental in forcing a dialogue between practitioners and their patients, and making physicians begin to understand the difficulties in defining normalcy and the ethical dilemma of acting medically on children before they reach an age of consent.

In October of 2005, 50 international experts were gathered under the auspices of the Lawson Wilkins Pediatric Endocrine Society (USA) and the European Society for Pediatric Endocrinology, and an international consensus conference was held in Chicago to review the management of disorders of sex development. The experts, as well as representatives of patients advocacy groups, were divided into six working groups (Genetics, Brain Programming, Medical Management, Surgical Management, Psychosocial Management, and Outcome Data) that eventually all agreed on a consensus statement published in *Pediatrics* (1). Our Genetics group was charged with implementing genetic advances in the care of intersex patients, which resulted in a much needed update to the nomenclature of intersexuality.

The significance of such a change goes far beyond the issues accompanying management of intersexuality. It symbolically brings together healthcare providers and patients on a very contentious medical matter. It prevents gender-labeling of patients and the use of classic terms such as "hermaphrodites" and "pseudohermaphrodites," all of which have been perceived as socially harmful. It is also a paradigm for the inclusion of new biologic concepts into long-established medical practice. We have endeavored in this chapter to use the new nomenclature. The term *disorders of sex development* (DSD) was proposed, as defined by "congenital conditions in which development of chromosomal, gonadal or anatomical sex is atypical." It is all-encompassing and should replace the word "intersex"—which has social connotations and reflects a concept of sexual identity—in the medical literature.

In this chapter, we have also avoided the use of "pseudohermaphroditism." Because it is widely used in the literature, we wish to argue why we believe the current nomenclature is vague, obsolete, potentially harmful, and should therefore be altered. The current classification is mainly based on the gonadal anatomy: male pseudohermaphroditism refers to individuals with testicular tissue who are not typically virilized, whereas female pseudohermaphroditism refers to individuals with ovaries who are masculinized. The first issue with this nomenclature is that it is scientifically questionable and ignores recent advances in endocrinology and genetics. Why emphasize the gonadal structure above all other parameters defining sex? In addition, the categories are broad and vague and do not allow for an accurate categorization of the patients, which in turn, prevents accurate outcome studies. The second issue is that the current nomenclature is not clinically adapted to the patients' situation and is potentially psychologically harmful. The example of complete androgen insensitivity syndrome is striking. These are women in many senses of the term and they identify as such; yet they are labeled "male pseudohermaphrodites." This classification is not clinically relevant (because the patients have female external genitalia, and mostly identify as women), and may be distressing to the patient (being labeled "male" while identifying as female).

SEX DETERMINATION AND DIFFERENTIATION

Development of the Bipotential Urogenital (Gonadal) Ridge

An overview of human sex determination and differentiation is depicted in Figure 35-1 and 35-2. The genetic sex of an infant is determined by which paternal sex chromosome, X or Y, was inherited (2–4). *Sex determination* refers to gonad differentiation that culminates with the developmental choice of the bipotential and undifferentiated gonad to become either testis or ovary. *Sex differentiation* refers to the developmental events that occur after the gonads have differentiated, for instance the formation of the penis or the clitoris.

The early stages of sex determination, equivalent in mammals to gonadal determination, begin when primordial germ cells migrate from the yolk sac to the undifferentiated urogenital ridge on the mesonephric bulge between the 6th and 7th weeks of gestation (between 4 and 5 wk postfertilization). The differentiation of these cells from the intermediate mesoderm is dependent on the transcriptional activity of several transcription factors whose roles remain poorly understood.

Disorders of Sex Development

AT-A-GLANCE

Sexual development is the process by which external and internal genitalia are formed and can be viewed as being composed of two processes: sex determination and sex differentiation. In sex determination disorders, there is abnormal development of the gonads, whereas in sex differentiation disorders the gonads develop normally, but the subsequent development of internal or external genitalia fails. Genital ambiguity occurs with an estimated frequency of 1%. Even with these developmental distinctions, defining sex is still an elusive task. As humans, we tend to dichotomize our worldview: male *or* female. As biologists, however, we cannot easily identify a simple characteristic that is necessary to qualify either a male or a female. Sex, indeed, is defined by a constellation of biologic parameters. *Genetic sex* generally refers to the chromosomal allotment of an individual (XX, XY, or mosaic) but may also refer to the presence of a particular sex-determining gene, such as SRY (Sex-determining Region on Y). *Gonadal sex* refers to the type of gonads present (testes, ovaries, ovotestes, or dysgenic streaks). An extension of gonadal sex is the pattern of gonadal hormone secretion (masculine or feminine). *Genital sex* refers to the architecture of external and internal genitalia. In the case of intersex individuals, the precise definition of what constitutes either a "penis" or a "clitoris" is often blurred. Despite a theoretically large spectrum of sexual variation, the legal definition offers no more than the two traditional choices.

SEX DETERMINATION DISORDERS	KARYOTYPE TO PHENOTYPE	GENE	LOCUS	OMIM
XY gonadal dysgenesis	Male to female	SRY	Yp11.3	480000
XX testicular DSD	Female to male	SOX9	17q24.3-q25.1	114290
Ovotesticular DSD		SF-1	9q33	184757
		WT-1	11p13	607102
		DAX-1	Xp21	300473
		WNT-4	1p35	603490
		DMRT1	9p24.3	154230
		XH2	Xq13.3	301040
		DHH	12q12-q13.1	605423

SEX DIFFERENTIATION DISORDERS	SEX REVERSAL	GENE	LOCUS	OMIM
Leydig cell hypoplasia	Male to female	LHCGR	2p21	152790
StAR deficiency, lipoid CAH	Male to female	StAR	8p11.2	201710
3β-HSD type II deficiency	Male to female	HSD3B2	1p13.1	201810
17α-hydroxylase/ 17,20-lyase deficiency	Male to female	CYP17	10q24.3	202110
P450 oxidoreductase deficiency	Male to female	POR	7q11.2	201750
17β-HSD type 3 deficiency	Male to female	HSD17B3	9q22	264300
21α-hydroxylase deficiency	Female to male	CYP21	6p21.3	201910
11β-hydroxylase deficiency	Female to male	CYP11B1	8q24.3	202010
P450 aromatase deficiency	Female to male	CYP19	15q21.1	107910
7-dehydrocholesterol reductase deficiency (Smith-Lemli-Opitz)	Male to female	DHCR7	11q12-q13	602858
5α-reductase type 2 deficiency	Male to female	SR5A2	2p23	264600
Androgen insensitivity syndrome	Male to female	AR	10q11-12	300068
Persistent Müllerian duct syndrome	Phenotypic males with uterus	AMH AMHR2	19p13.2-13.3 12q13	261550 600956

SYNDROME	FINDINGS	PHENOTYPE AT BIRTH	PHENOTYPE AT PUBERTY
XY female pure gonadal dysgenesis	↑ FSH, LH ↓↓ T, DHT, E2 ↓↓ AMH No ↑ with hCG	Normal female genitalia, uterus, and streak gonads	Sexual infantilism, pubertal delay, amenorrhea, gonadoblastoma
XY female partial/mixed gonadal dysgenesis	↑ FSH, LH ↓ T, DHT, E2 Nml to ↓ AMH No ↑ with β-hCG	Ambiguous genitalia with partial Müllerian structures; mixed gonadal dysgenesis may present with asymmetric genitalia	Pubertal delay, amenorrhea, or gonadoblastoma, similar to pure gonadal dysgenesis
XX testicular DSD	↑ FSH, LH ↓ T, DHT Nml AMH No ↑ with β-hCG	Usually with normal male genitalia; small minority (20%) may have evidence of mild androgen deficiency such as cryptorchidism or glandular hypospadias	Pubertal delay, gynecomastia, small testes, infertility
Ovotesticular DSD	Nml FSH,LH Nml T, DHT, E₂ Nml to ↓ AMH Nml to ↑ with β-hCG	Ambiguous external genitalia, mixed internal genitalia, ovotestes	Gynecomastia, cryptorchidism, pubertal delay, infertility in phenotypic males; amenorrhea, pubertal delay in females

DISORDER	FINDINGS	PHENOTYPE AT BIRTH	PHENOTYPE AT PUBERTY
Leydig cell hypoplasia (LCH)	↑ LH Nml FSH ↑ AMH ↓ T, DHT, E₂ ↓ β-hCG response Nml Δ4A/T ratio	XY variable feminized up to complete sex reversal with palpable inguinal/labial masses	XY females present with primary amenorrhea and sexual infantilism; XX females have amenorrhea and polycystic ovaries
Lipoid CAH (StAR, P45scc)	↑ Renin ↓ Aldo ↑ K ↓ Na ↓ All adrenal hormones	XX and XY appear as females; severe salt wasting, adrenal crisis, leading to death in infancy if not diagnosed.	XX females may experience spontaneous puberty, regular anovulatory menstruation, and polycystic ovaries
3β-HSD type II deficiency	↑ Renin ↓ Aldo, F ↑ K ↓ Na, ↑ Preg ↑ ratio of Δ⁵/Δ⁴ steroids ↓ Δ4A, T	XY frequently feminized; XX females rarely masculinized; may die prior to diagnosis; salt wasting and adrenal crisis	XY females may experience significant virilization and change gender; XX experience premature adrenarche/puberty and polycystic ovaries
17α-hydroxylase/ 17,20-lyase deficiency	↓ Renin ↓ Aldo, F ↑ Progesterone, DOC, B ↑ Na ↓ K ↓ DHEA-S, Δ4A, T	XX and XY appear as females; low-renin hypertension. In isolated 17,20-lyase deficiency, only sex steroids decreased	XX and XY have pubertal delay; XY females with mild defect may experience some virilization or testis descent
P450 oxido-reductase deficiency	↑ 17-OHP ↑ Progesterone ↓ F, DHEA-S ↓ Δ4A, T	XX and XY have ambiguous genitalia; virilization does not progress postnatally in XX; skeletal dysplasias reminiscent of Antley–Bixler	XX and XY have delayed puberty
17β-HSD type 3 deficiency	Nml to ↑ Δ4A ↑ ratio Δ4A/T (> 15) ↓ T, DHT	XX and XY appear as females	XX and XY have pubertal delay; XY females can be virilized at puberty and change gender
21α-hydroxylase deficiency	↑ Renin ↓ Aldo, DOC, F ↑ K ↓ Na ↑ 17-OHP ↑ DHEA-S, Δ4A, T	XX females have variable degrees of ambiguous genitalia; XY males are hyperpigmented; most common cause of CAH; may have septic-like presentation	XX females and XY males with nonclassic form may experience premature adrenarche; XX females may have virilization, polycystic ovaries
11β-hydroxylase deficiency	↓ Aldo, F, Renin ↑ DOC ↑ K ↓ Na ↑ 17-OHP ↑ DHEA-S, Δ4A, T	XX females have variable degrees of ambiguous genitalia; XY males are hyperpigmented; 2nd most common cause of CAH; low-renin hypertension	Hypertension in both XX and XY; XX females may become virilized during childhood or puberty

DISORDER	FINDINGS	PHENOTYPE AT BIRTH	PHENOTYPE AT PUBERTY
P450 aromatase deficiency	↑ 16OH-Δ4A (maternal) ↑ FSH, LH, Δ4A, T ↓ E_1, E_2	Maternal virilization; XX females virilized with ambiguous genitalia, normal adrenal function	XX females have amenorrhea, no breast development, polycystic ovaries, and virilization; XY males are sterile; both are tall, delayed bone age
Smith Lemli-Opitz (7DHCR)	↑↑↑ 7-DHC ↓ cholesterol	XY have ambiguous genitalia; XX and XY have classic facies, variable organ malformations, toe 2/3 syndactyly	XX and XY patients experience spontaneous puberty
5α-reductase type 2 deficiency	Nml FSH, LH Nml T, E_2 ↓ DHT ↑ ratio T/DHT (> 30)	XX appear as females; XY have variable degrees of sex reversal and may have palpable gonads	XY females have deep voice, increased muscle, amenorrhea and no gynecomastia (majority switch to female gender)
Androgen insensitivity syndrome (AIS)	Nml FSH, LH (PAIS) ↓ FSH, LH (CAIS) Nml to ↑ AMH Nml Δ4A, T, DHT ↑↑ β-hCG response	XY with complete reversal are females +/− palpable gonads; partial defect causes variable degrees of ambiguity	XY females with complete sex reversal have amenorrhea, blind vagina and are tall, with female secondary characteristics
Persistant Müllerian Duct syndrome (AMHR II)	Nml hormonal profile	Normal external genitalia; XY have cryptorchidism and inguinal hernia with Müllerian structures	May represent after an initial unsuccessful orchidopexy with inguinal hernia

LHCGR = luteinizing hormone-choriogonadotropin receptor; 3 β-HSD type II = 3 β-hydroxysteroid dehydrogenase type II; 17 β-HSD type 3 = 17 β-hydroxysteroid dehydrogenase type 3; 7DHCR = 7 dehydrocholesterol reductase; AR = androgen receptor; AMH = anti-Müllerian hormone; AMHR II = anti-Müllerian hormone receptor type II; β-hCG = β-human chorionic gonadotropin; Nml = normal; E_1 = estrone; E_2 = estradiol; K = potassium; Na = sodium; LH = luteinizing hormone; FSH = follicle-stimulating hormone; Aldo = aldosterone; Prog = progesterone; 17-OHP = 17α-hydroxyprogesterone; Preg = pregnenolone; 17-OHpreg = 17α-pregnenolone; F = cortisol; DOC = 11-deoxycorticosterone; B = corticosterone; T = testosterone; DHEA-S = dehydroepiandrosterone sulphate; Δ4A = androstenedione; DHT = dihydrotestosterone.

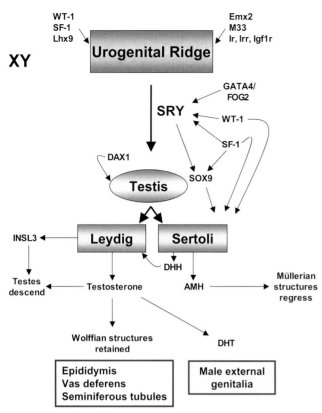

XY

FIGURE 35-1. Normal XY sex determination and differentiation. The male sex determination cascade has been elucidated through studies of human mutations and animal genetic models. The presence of SRY initiates the development of the bipotential urogenital ridge toward the formation of Sertoli cells, mature testicular cords, and Leydig cells. WT-1 = Wilm tumor 1; SF-1 = steroidogenic factor 1; Lhx9 = Lim homeobox 9; Emx2 = empty spiracles homolog 2; M33 = mouse homolog of chromobox homolog 2; Ir = insulin receptor; Irr = insulin-related receptor: Igf1r = insulin-like growth factor 1 receptor; FOG2 = friend of GATA 2; SRY = sex-determining region on Y; DAX1 = dosage-sensitive sex reversal (DSS) and adrenal hypoplasia congenita (AHC) on X; SOX9 = SRY-like homeobox 9; INSL3 = insulin-like growth factor 3; DHH = desert hedgehog; DHT = dihydrotestosterone.

Mouse genetic models have implicated several ubiquitously expressed homeobox genes (Lhx9, Emx2, M33), transcription factors (Sf1, GATA4), and growth factor signaling genes (Ir, Igf1r, Irr, Fgf9) in the development and maintenance of the urogenital ridge (5–7), largely by promoting cell proliferation and preventing apoptosis. Studies of human mutations have paralleled some of the mouse data. For instance, the transcription factors Wilms tumor 1 (WT-1) and steroidogenic factor 1 (SF-1) demonstrate high transcriptional activity in the bipotential gonadal ridge prior to gonadal differentiation, and inactivating mutations of the corresponding genes in humans affect the development of testes as well as other nearby structures.

The homeobox gene Lhx9 (LIM homeox gene 9) is also expressed on the bipotential gonadal ridge prior to divergence toward either a male or female pathway. Mice deficient in Lhx9 fail to develop gonads, and

show lower expression of Sf-1, suggesting an upstream role (8). Lhx9 remains the only candidate gene studied in mice that results in isolated gonadal agenesis in both males and females, without associated anomalies in other organs. No mutations in human LHX9 gene sequences have been detected in patients with gonadal maldevelopment, including bilateral gonadal agenesis (9). Nevertheless, Lhx9 and other genes identified in mouse studies remain promising targets for further investigation.

Testis Determination

In the presence of a Y chromosome with an intact SRY, the bipotential gonad diverges toward testes organogenesis (10–13) by week 8 of gestation. Mouse knockout studies suggest that in the bipotential gonad WT-1 and SF-1 interact with transcriptional factors GATA4 and its cofactor FOG2 (friend of GATA) and are necessary for proper SRY expression (14). SRY expression in the precursors to Sertoli cells, located in mesonephros, initiates testes determination. SRY activates downstream effectors SOX9 (SRY-related HMG-box 9) and SF-1. Under synergistic stimulation by SOX9 and SF-1, Sertoli precursors begin to proliferate and organize around germ cells into tubular cords and start secreting anti-Müllerian hormone (AMH). AMH expression in situ has been consistently detected by the 9th week of gestation (15,16). Peptide regulatory factors such as FGR9 (fibroblast growth factor 9) and FGFR2 (FGF receptor 2) are also requisite for Sertoli proliferation (17,18). A single copy of the orphan nuclear receptor DAX-1 also appears to be necessary for testes development and spermatogenesis, but two copies appear to suppress testes development and cause XY gonadal dysgenesis (GD) (19). DAX-1 illustrates the marked sensitivity to gene dosage underlying parts of the sex determination pathway.

Precursors to steroidogenic Leydig cells (under stimulation from placental human chorionic gonadotropin [β-hCG]) migrate into the developing testes in the 10th week,

while vascular endothelial cells from the mesonephros begin production of testosterone (T) and initiation of a testes-specific vasculature. Desert hedgehog (DHH) signaling positively regulates Leydig cell proliferation by up regulating SF-1 (20,21). Mature testes are morphologically recognizable at approximately 10 weeks gestational age.

Ovary Determination

Ovary determination is not default, as the absence of SRY in 46,XY and 45,X does not result in an ovary, but in a nonfunctional streak of fibrous tissue. In a 46,XX fetus without SRY, ovaries begin to develop in the 10th week with the proliferation of oogonia into oocytes. By approximately the 14th week, somatic granulosa cells encircle the oocytes and form primordial follicles consisting of a single somatic cell layer surrounding the oocyte. Oocytes are blocked at meiosis I at this stage until ovulation. In the absence of two functional X chromosomes, as in monosomy 45,X, oocytes develop initially, but begin to involute beginning at 13 weeks, and continue until loss of functional germ cells and associated stroma, with replacement of ovarian tissue by fibrous streaks. Germ cell survival therefore appears essential for proper ovarian development. At all stages of development the fetal ovary allows oocyte maturation, migration to the surface, and expulsion into the peritoneum. At 5 months of gestation, the fetal ovary contains 7 million oocytes, the maximum it will ever possess.

Ovary organogenesis is poorly understood, and relatively little is known about the role of "ovary-determining" genes. Initial studies in mice suggest that ovary development is a relatively gene-poor process compared with testes differentiation (22,23), although this may reflect differential timing of maximal transcriptional activity between developing testes and ovaries. Nevertheless, specific X chromosomal as well as autosomal genes such as WNT-4 (wingless-related MMTV integration site 4), and likely a downstream factor Follistatin (24), appear to be required for proper ovarian development.

Male Sexual Differentiation

The presence of a functional testis determines the internal and external genitalia, and thus governs *sexual differentiation*, a term that refers to the developmental events occurring after the gonads have differentiated. In 1953, Alfred Jost performed the critical and elegantly simple experiment that demonstrated that castration of an early male rabbit fetus results in feminine internal and external genitalia, and that the two testicular hormones, AMH and T, are required for

XX

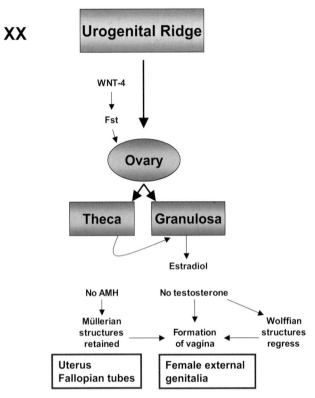

FIGURE 35-2. Normal XX sex determination and differentiation. Relative to male sex determination, the genetics of the female pathway are less well defined. Absence of SRY and expression of WNT-4 promote typical ovarian vasculature and the organization of oocytes and mesenchymal cells. The absence of testosterone and AMH allows for the development of female external and internal genitalia. WNT-4 = wingless-type integration factor 4; Fst = follistatin.

male genital development (25). This study established the current paradigm of sex determination and differentiation in placental mammals: genetic sex determines gonad development, and gonadal sex in turn governs anatomic sex.

Sertoli cells and testicular cords are the hallmark of a developed testis. AMH from the Sertoli cells induces regression of paramesonephric (Müllerian) ducts starting at gestational week 10; after week 12 the Müllerian ducts lose their responsiveness to AMH. T from Leydig cells promotes development of Wolffian structures (epididymis, vas deferens, and seminal vesicles). T, after conversion to the more potent androgen 5α-dihydrotestosterone (DHT), promotes fusion of the labioscrotal folds into a typical male scrotum, induces increased anogenital distance, and stimulates growth of the urogenital sinus during the 10th to 12th weeks of gestation. After week 14, male sexual differentiation is essentially complete; even very high doses of DHT will fail to mediate fusion of the labial folds, although androgen-sensitive phallic growth occurs during the third trimester.

Migration of the testes is also hormonally regulated. INSL3 (insulin-like 3) secreted by Leydig cells mediates the transabdominal descent of the testes from their initial location at the gonadal ridge to the internal inguinal ring between weeks 10 and 12 of gestation. T is responsible for the inguinoscrotal descent of the testes from weeks 30 to 32.

Female Sexual Differentiation

Unlike the determination of ovaries, the growth of female genitalia is the default process in sexual differentiation. In the absence of a testes or a functional gonad (i.e., streak), there is no AMH or T produced. Due to absence of AMH, Müllerian structures develop (fallopian tubes, uterus, and upper vagina), and Wolffian ducts regress at 12 weeks of gestation. Absence of T results in no further virilization of external genitalia: the anogenital distance does not increase, and the labioscrotal folds develop into the labia majora.

The origins of the vagina remain controversial. Traditionally, it has been thought that the upper vagina is a Müllerian derivative, whereas the lower is composed of an extension and subsequent canalization of cells derived from the urogenital sinus. Recently it has been suggested that a Wolffian and Müllerian origin for the lower vagina, postulating that in the absence of testicular androgens and AMH, both genital ducts continue on a caudal descent toward the urogenital sinus, fusing to form a Müllerian tubercle, from which the lower vagina is formed. The subsequent regression of the Wolffian ducts is thought to contribute to vaginal canalization and the formation of the vaginal os, including the hymen.

GENETICS OF SEX DETERMINATION AND ASSOCIATED SYNDROMES

Dozens of eponymous and otherwise recognized syndromes are associated with varying degrees of ambiguous genitalia. A subset of these syndromes that are linked with sex determination are presented in Table 35-1. Most of these conditions involve genes implicated in testes organogenesis and have helped us decipher the proposed sex determination pathway. Select syndromes that either positively or negatively influence the sex-determining pathway are discussed in further detail.

Denys-Drash and Frasier Syndromes

The WT1 gene encodes a zinc finger DNA-binding protein that acts as a transcriptional activator or tumor repressor depending on the cellular or chromosomal context. WT1 is required for normal development of the genitourinary system and mesothelial tissues and loss of WT1 function predisposes to Wilms tumor. Heterozygous mutations or deletions are associated with urogenital pathologies, including Denys Drash syndrome (DDS), Wilms tumor, aniridia, genitourinary malformations, and mental retardation (WAGR) syndrome, and Frasier syndrome (FS). The four major WT-1 isoforms are generated by alternative splicing of the WT-1 gene at two sites: splicing at exon 5 (26–29), results in either insertion or exclusion of 17 amino acids in the middle of the WT-1 protein, whereas splicing at exon 9 results in either insertion or exclusion of three amino acids (KTS) in between zinc fingers 3 and 4 of WT-1 protein (+KTS isoform is the one with the inserted three amino acids and −KTS isoform is the one without the three amino acids).

−KTS isoforms bind to the SRY promoter, inducing transcription of SRY (30) and synergize with SF1 promoting MIS expression (31). For reasons not currently understood, a precise ratio of +KTS/−KTS isoforms (~2:1) must exist for proper WT-1 gene function (32).

DDS is characterized by rapidly progressive diffuse mesangial sclerosis of the kidneys, Wilms tumor, and ambiguous genitalia in 46,XY males ranging from micropenis, penoscrotal hypospadias with cryptorchidism to 46,XY GD. The DDS phenotype is the result of dominant-negative mutations in WT-1, which render the protein incapable of binding DNA or synergizing with SF-1 (33). Mutant WT-1 is unable to initiate transcription of either SRY or AMH, leading to genital ambiguity or XY complete GD. In patients with DDS, development of Wilms tumor, which typically presents bilaterally at a mean age of 2 years, results from two independent events (the two-hit genetic model) that lead to loss of function of both alleles of the WT1 gene. DDS patients have a defective dominant-negative mutant WT-1 allele (first hit) and later a somatic mutation (second hit) or loss of heterozygosity in the second allele causes uncontrolled cell proliferation and Wilms tumor formation. WT-1 does not play a significant role in female gonadal development as gonadal defects are absent in 46,XX patients with DDS.

TABLE 35-1   Syndromes Associated with GD

Gene	Locus	Syndrome	Description	Genetics
SRY	Yp11.3	Swyer	GD, gonadoblastoma, primary amenorrhea, pubertal delay	Mutations and deletions responsible for 20% of 46,XY GD
		de la Chapelle	XX testicular DSD, small testes, infertile, under virilized, pubertal delay	Translocations to Xp responsible for 80% of 46,XX testicular DSD
WT-1	11p13	Denys-Drash	Diffuse mesangial sclerosis of kidneys in infancy, Wilms tumor, XY GD	Mutations affecting DNA binding of WT-1 cause DDS, including 46,XY GD
		Frasier	Focal segmental glomerulosclerosis in adolescence, gonadoblastoma, XY GD	Intron 9 mutations disrupt the +KTS/−KTS ratio, causing FS and XY GD
SF-1	9q33		XY GD, adrenal failure	Responsible for 10 cases of 46,XY GD, 2 with associated AHC
SOX9	17q24.3-q25.1	Campomelic dysplasia	Congenital bowing of long bones, hypoplastic scapulae, hypoplastic pedicles of thoracic vertebrae, variable genitalia	Mutations cause campomelic dysplasia and 46,XY GD in 75% of patients
				One case of SOX9 duplication in a 46,XX SRY-negative testicular DSD
DHH	12q12-13.1		XY GD with associated neuropathy	Four cases of mutations causing 46,XY GD; in one case there was also a minifasicular polyneuropathy
XH2	Xq13.3	X-linked alpha-thalassemia/mental retardation	Hemoglobin H inclusions, mental retardation, dysmorphic facies, genital abnormalities	Mutations cause ATR-X and related mental retardation syndromes; one case of XY GD
DMRT1	9p24.3		Isolated XY GD	Deletions of 9p24 result in 46,XY GD; the smallest defined deletion maps 30 kb adjacent to, but outside of, DMRT1
DAX-1	Xp21	Dosage-sensitive sex reversal	Isolated XY GD	Duplications of Xp21 cause DSS, possibly through suppression of SF-1 action
		AHC	Primary adrenal failure	Mutations cause AHC, hypogonadotropic hypogonadism, and a primary testes defect in XY males; ovaries are normal in XX females
WNT-4	1p35		Variable degrees of XY GD with associated anomalies	In 4 cases, duplications of 1p31-35 result in variable degrees of 46,XY GD
			Variant of MRKH syndrome	One case of a 46,XX virilized female lacking Müllerian structures with mutant WNT-4

Proteinuria may be evident during the first months of life, with end-stage renal failure usually appearing before the age of 4 years. Nephrotic syndrome is resistant to corticosteroids and immunosuppressive therapy.

By comparison, FS appears later in life (age 10–20 y) and is characterized by a nephrotic syndrome due to focal segmental glomerulosclerosis, GD, and an increased gonadoblastoma risk (27,32). FS is caused by a specific mutation at the intron 9 donor splice site of WT-1, leading to a deficiency of the usually more abundant +KTS isoform, and changing the +KTS/−KTS ratio from 2:1 to 1:2 (32). This aberrant ratio disrupts WT-1 regulation of SRY, causing GD. The gonadoblastoma risk is similar to that of other cases of 46,XY GD. In contrast to DDS, FS patients have one normal copy of WT1 and one that can only produce −KTS

isoform. The −KTS isoform has the same tumor suppressor effect as +KTS which may explain why FS patients do not develop Wilms tumor.

WAGR syndrome is due to homozygous deletions of band 11p13 and is characterized by urinary tract abnormalities without nephropathy, Wilms tumor, aniridia, genitourinary malformations, and mental retardation.

Dosage-Sensitive Gonadal Dysgenesis (Also Called Dosage-Sensitive Sex Reversal)

DAX-1 (Dosage Sensitive Sex reversal-Adrenal Hypoplasia Congenital critical region on the X chromosome, gene 1) belongs to the orphan nuclear receptor superfamily and lacks any known endogenous ligand. When mutated, DAX-1 (NR0B1) causes congenital ad-

renal hypoplasia (AHC) with associated hypogonadotropic hypogonadism, and when duplicated causes DSS in the presence of a normal SRY (34–38). DAX-1 is expressed in the developing adrenals, gonads, hypothalamus, and pituitary, an expression pattern that is intriguingly intertwined with another orphan nuclear receptor SF-1 (discussed further later); SF-1 upregulates DAX-1, while DAX-1 in turn represses virtually all known SF-1–mediated gene activations, including its own expression (38).

DAX-1 has also been theorized to be an "ovary-determining" gene in addition to its postulated "anti-testes" role. Subsequent studies have challenged this hypothesis, as the XX females with AHC show normal ovary development (39). Interestingly, a single copy of DAX-1 in 46,XY males appears to be necessary for proper testes development because

XY males with a DAX-1 mutation present with AHC, hypogonadotropic hypogonadism and infertility not correctable by gonadotropin or T treatment, implying a primary spermatogenic defect (39,40). It is postulated that duplication of DAX-1 in DSS results in an overwhelming inhibition of SF-1–mediated processes necessary for testes development, thereby causing XY GD (41,42). This underscores the exquisite sensitivity of the sex-determining pathway to gene dosage at multiple levels.

An intriguing new development is the discovery of a novel, shorter isoform of DAX-1 (called DAX-1α), generated by alternative splicing of intron 1 (43). Although the properties of this new isoform have yet to be completely elucidated, initial experiments suggest that DAX-1α does not antagonize SF-1 action.

XY Gonadal Dysgenesis and Adrenal Insufficiency

SF-1 is an orphan nuclear receptor (NR5A1) necessary for adrenal and testicular development. Interactions between SF-1 and the transcription factors GATA-4 and FOG2 appear to be necessary for SRY expression in developing testes (44,45). SF-1 also synergizes with SOX9 to upregulate AMH in developing Sertoli cells (2,44).

In ten reported cases, SF-1 mutations caused 46,XY GD (46–50). Two of the cases (46,47) were associated with failure of adrenal development (AHC). The mutations impaired SF-1 synergism with GATA-4 (45) and DNA binding (47), thereby rendering the mutant SF-1 incapable of activating SRY and AMH, leading to XY GD. The first heterozygous mutation described (G35E) lacked any transcriptional activity (46), and suggested that SF-1 haploinsufficiency was sufficient to cause both XY GD and AHC. The second mutation described (R92Q), exhibited partial DNA binding and transcriptional activity (47). The 46,XY affected infant was homozygous for the R92Q mutation and had both adrenal failure and severe gonadal dysgenesis. Both parents and his sister, who were carriers for the mutation, had normal adrenal and reproductive function.

Another mutation such as the nonsense C16X mutation (49) resulted in no demonstrably active protein while the heterozygous 8-bp deletion resulted in a dominant negative SF-1 isoform (49). The 46,XY patient with the C16X mutation presented at birth with perineal hypospadias, micropenis, hypoplastic scrotum, hypoplastic testes, low AMH, uterus and fallopian tubes as well as vas deferens and epididymis. The 46,XY patient with the 8-bp deletion presented with clitoromegaly, single perineal opening, Wolffian derivatives and testicular regression. Both mutations resulted

in normal adrenals. Overall, the data suggests that SF-1 haploinsufficiency is sufficient to disrupt testicular development, as shown by the three patients with varying phenotypic degrees of XY GD, but not sufficient enough to disrupt adrenal development, suggesting that other factors besides SF-1 have a role in modifying adrenal organogenesis (48,49,50). Recently four heterozygous missense mutations in the SF1 (V15M, M78I, G91S, L437Q) have been described; two of the mutations (V15, L437Q) appear to be *de novo*, and the other two mutations appear to be inherited in a sex-limited dominant manner (the mother was heterozygous for the mutation). All four patients had partial gonadal dysgenesis and impairment of Leydig cell steroidogenesis with normal adrenal function; their external genitalia phenotype ranged from clitoromegaly with single opening to penoscrotal hypospadias, well developed vasa diferrentia and epididymes, and no uterus or Müllerian ducts remnants (50). Postnatally, testicular architecture was relatively normal with more pronounced impairment in Leydig cell steroidogenesis; AMH levels were low even in the presence of Sertoli cells suggesting impaired SF1 transcription rather than a direct consequence of Sertoli cell dysfunction. Partial hypogonadotropic hypogonadism in late childhood and adolescence in addition to primary testicular defect developed in the patient with the L437Q mutation, who at birth presented with palpable testes, penoscrotal hypospadias and impaired androgen synthesis (50).

SF-1 appears not to be required for ovary development because a 46,XX phenotypic female with adrenal insufficiency and a heterozygous mutant SF-1 (R255L) possessed normal ovaries (51).

Campomelic Dysplasia

The SRY-type HMG box (SOX) proteins are a large family of transcription factors that play diverse roles in embryonic development of the central nervous system, the heart, and the gonads. The SOX9 gene product has roles in chondrogenesis and in testes differentiation. Although no direct targets immediately downstream of SRY have been identified to date, significant evidence in human and mouse models implicates SOX9 as the most probable candidate (2,52,53). Mutations in SOX9 result in campomelic dysplasia (CD), an autosomal dominant inherited disorder, characterized by bowing of the long bones and hypoplastic scapulae. No mutation in SOX9 has been so far associated with isolated sex reversal.

Interestingly, 75% of XY patients with CD display GD with female external genitalia, suggesting a role for SOX9 in male sex

determination. SOX9 activates SF-1, and in concert with SF-1, GATA-4, and WT-1, SOX9 upregulates AMH expression in Sertoli cells (52). The important role of SOX9 in testes determination and differentiation is supported by the report of a 46,XX testicular DSD (formerly known as XX maleness), SRY negative, who carried a 17q23-24 duplication including SOX9. This case suggests that extra dose of SOX9 is sufficient to initiate testis differentiation in the absence of SRY (54).

SOX9 is one of the genes that plays critical roles in male sexual differentiation. Recently, the pleiotropy of SOX9 mutations with respect to the presence or absence of XY GD was explained by the observation that the SOX9 protein binds the collagen gene promoters as a homodimer, but activates the gonadal SF-1 promoters as a monomer. A dimerization domain adjacent to the conserved HMG box of SOX-9 is required for the binding and transactivation activity of SOX-9 on the promoters of collagen, but not on the promoter of the sex determining gene SF1. Mutations in the SOX9 dimerization domain result in CD without GD, whereas mutations in the high mobility group (HMG) DNA-binding domain that affect DNA binding cause CD and XY GD (55).

In addition to bowing of the long bones and hypoplastic scapulae, other skeletal abnormalities include hypoplastic pedicles of thoracic vertebrae, small thoracic cage, narrow airways from defective tracheobronchial cartilages, talipes equinovarus deformities, and dislocated hips. Patients have flat facies with hypertelorism, Pierre Robin sequence, long philtrum, depressed nasal bridge, and relative macrocephaly. Renal and cardiac abnormalities, conductive hearing loss, and developmental delay may also present. The condition is generally lethal in infancy, but long-term survivors exist.

Although campomelia is one of the most common clinical features of this disorder and the feature that gives it its name, cases without campomelia (acampomelic CMPD) have also been reported (56).

Desert Hedgehog and XY Gonadal Dysgenesis

The hedgehog family of signaling proteins are involved in patterning and organogenesis. One of its members, desert hedgehog (DHH), has been implicated in human and mouse testes development. The majority of Dhh null XY mice have female external genitalia (20,57). Dhh is expressed in Sertoli cells immediately after Sry expression and is necessary for formation of seminiferous tubules. It is also implicated in Leydig cell proliferation via one of the hedgehog receptors Ptch1, which is expressed on interstitial cells of the testes (58). Dhh/Ptch1 signaling triggers Leydig differentiation by upregulating SF-1 (21). Dhh is also expressed in peripheral nerve Schwann cells (59).

The first human reported with a homozygous DHH mutation presented with partial GD and minifascicular polyneuropathy, consistent with the expression of DHH in developing testes and Schwann cells (60). The patient's heterozygous father was asymptomatic, consistent with the mouse studies that showed haploinsufficiency of Dhh did not disrupt nerve or testes development. Subsequently, investigation of six unrelated XY females with complete GD and normal SRY sequence demonstrated three cases of homozygous DHH mutations (61). All three patients had normal neurologic examinations and mentation. Although the investigators found mutations in three of six unexplained cases of XY females, the true prevalence of defective DHH as the etiology for XY GD is difficult to assess because of the rarity of this condition.

Distal 9p Deletion Syndrome and XY Gonadal Dysgenesis

Over 100 cases of 9p deletion syndrome have been reported. Associated dysmorphologies include midface hypoplasia, anteverted nares, hypertelorism, flat nasal bridge, microsomia, micrognathia, and trigonocephaly. The majority of 46,XY patients show some degree of genital ambiguity with GD, up to complete GD with female external genitalia, implying that haploinsufficiency of some gene product on 9p disrupts testes organogenesis (62,63). XX patients have reportedly experienced normal puberty with normal ovarian function (64). Cytogenetic investigations in humans with 9p deletion have localized the critical region for XY GD to 9p24.3, a region containing several genes associated with sexual development, DMRT1 (doublesex- and mab3-related transcription factor 1) and the related DMRT2 and DMRT3.

Humans possess at least seven related DM domain-containing genes, of which DMRT1, DMRT2, and DMRT3 are located at 9p24.3 (65, 66). Among adult human tissues, higher expression of DMRT1 is necessary for testicular differentiation, whereas lower expression is compatible with ovarian differentiation (65).

DMRT2 expression appears to be restricted to developing somites (67–69), and is necessary for somitogenesis. DMRT3 is also expressed more in developing testes than ovaries (69,70). Most reported 9p deletions with

XY GD involve all three DMRT genes, suggesting that haploinsufficiency of more than just one of these genes is necessary for disrupting testiculogenesis. The smallest interval associated with XY GD is a 700-kb deletion that maps to a region outside of, but immediately upstream to, DMRT1 (71), suggesting that loss of function of this gene may be most critical.

α-Thalassemia and Mental Retardation, X-Linked

The α-thalassemia/mental retardation syndrome (ATR-X) is a very rare X-linked condition, caused by mutations in XH2 (X chromosome helicase 2) gene and condition characterized by severe mental retardation and speech delay, genital anomalies and characteristic facial dysmorphism including carp-shaped mouth, anteverted nares, midface hypoplasia, hypotonic flat facies, congenital microcephaly and Hb H inclusions (72). XH2 protein localizes to the nucleus and associates with the short arm of acrocentric chromosomes during mitosis (73). It may also regulate transcription through effects on chromatin remodeling and methylation-dependent mechanisms (74). With the exception of the α-globin gene, no target genes have been identified.

Genital abnormalities in affected males range from mild hypospadias or cryptorchidism to ambiguous genitalia, and occasionally XY GD with female external genitalia (75, 76). The α-thalassemia is a common (but not constant) feature of this syndrome. Other associated anomalies include deafness, renal anomalies and mild skeletal defects. In familial cases, XX female relatives are usually unaffected, due to skewed X-inactivation; however, a carrier female with mental retardation and without a skewed X-inactivation pattern has been reported (77).

WNT-4 and Disorders of Sex Determination

The Wnts (Wingless-type integration factor) proteins are secreted glycoproteins that mediate various developmental and regulatory processes such as kidney and brain development. WNT-4, long associated with kidney development, is the first secreted signaling factor to be a candidate sex-determining gene. Duplication of 1p31-35 (including WNT-4) has resulted in various degrees of XY GD in four cases, similar to DSS (42,78). Molecular studies demonstrate that WNT-4 (1p35) inhibits migration of precursors to testicular (and adrenal) steroidogenic cells from the kidneys to the developing gonad (79), as well as directly represses hormone

synthesis by disrupting the SF-1/β-catenin synergy needed for transcription of steroidogenic enzymes. The immediate downstream targets of WNT signaling have yet to be identified. Duplications of WNT-4 are hypothesized to inhibit the normal SRY-induced cell migration necessary for testes organogenesis in normal XY individuals, resulting in GD.

Recently, an XX female was identified with extensive virilization, no Müllerian structures, and a mutation of the WNT-4 gene (E226G). The mutated gene was ineffective at repressing (79) steroidogenic gene activation when compared to wild-type WNT-4 (79,80), resulting in an increased production of androgens. The patient's gonads were identified as ovaries, but placed retroperitoneal above the iliac crest. A biopsy was not performed for the presence or absence of testicular tissue. The absence of Müllerian structures suggests the presence of some testicular tissue at some point in early genital development, suggesting that lack of appropriate WNT-4 signal in an XX individual is potentially sufficient to induce some testes development and prevent normal ovary development. To date, WNT-4 remains the only gene with a proven role in ovary determination.

APPROACH TO THE BABY WITH AMBIGUOUS GENITALIA

Genital ambiguity in a newborn can be an emotionally overwhelming experience for families. As with other birth defects, parental anger, guilt, and sociocultural background are important considerations when discussing their infant's condition. Due to the complex nature of these disorders, a multidisciplinary team approach is necessary to effectively help the parents during this time and guide a multifaceted support and treatment strategy.

Physical Examination

Physical examination of a newborn with ambiguous genitalia should include careful palpation of the scrotum, labia majora, and inguinal area. Inguinal hernias may contain gonadal tissue or Müllerian structures or both. Position of the testes in the scrotum or inguinal canal and their ability to be reduced should be documented. Palpated gonads below the inguinal ring in patients with feminized external genitalia are usually testes or ovotestes. Asymmetry of genital development may indicate ovotesticular DSD (formerly known as true hermaphroditism) or mixed GD. Measurements of the stretched phallus/clitoris should be recorded and adjusted for gestational age. Premature infants may appear to have relative clitoromegaly because of minimal labial fat, but a clitoris longer than 1 cm and width greater than 0.6 cm suggests abnormal virilization. The anogenital distance (anus to base of the labioscrotal structure) divided by the distance between the anus and the base of the phallus/clitoris is the *anogenital ratio*; a ratio greater than 0.5 is consistent with virilization and is independent of gestational age and body size. A single opening at the base of the phallus may be either penile urethra or urogenital sinus in Prader III-V virilized females.

Degree of "scrotalization" of the labia, presence or absence of chordee, and the position of the urethral meatus relative to the distal phallic tip (to evaluate degree of hypospadias) should be noted. Prader staging semiquantifies increasing degrees of virilization, from mild clitoromegaly in an otherwise normal female (stage I), clitoromegaly with labial fusion (II), intermediate phallus size with perineal hypospadias and bifid scrotum (III), normal-length penis with perineal hypospadias and empty scrotum (IV), to otherwise normal male with either normal meatal placement or only mild glandular hypospadias and empty scrotum (stage V). A detailed physical examination will eventually need to be reconciled to the preliminary laboratory work (particularly karyotype) and imaging studies.

The remainder of the physical examination is equally critical because some syndromes are associated with genital ambiguity or 46,XY GD (Smith-Lemli-Opitz, DDS, WAGR, campomelic dysplasia etc). Cleft lip and palate may also be associated with central nervous system midline defects, such as hypopituitarism and central gonadotropin deficiency. Flank masses may represent Wilms tumor in patients with ambiguous genitalia due to DDS or WAGR syndromes.

Along with the physical examination a detailed family history is also very important. History of consanguinity, infertility, short stature, or male infant death the first weeks of life during an acute illness may suggest the diagnosis of congenital adrenal hyperplasia (CAH). Medical history of the mother's pregnancy course should include medications used during pregnancy and any signs of virilization developed during pregnancy.

Initial Approach and Stabilization

Initial medical management of a newborn with ambiguous genitalia is relatively similar regardless of the underlying etiology and eventual diagnosis; the primary focus should be an immediate evaluation of medically concerning issues such as hypo-hypertension and electrolyte imbalances, which are some of the manifestations in CAH disorders. Electrolytes, however, may be normal during the first days of life unless there is significant perinatal stress. The flowcharts provided can be used as a framework for the decision-making process (Figures 35-3 to 35-4). If hyponatremia or hyperkalemia is present, particularly in a stressed newborn, stress dose glucocorticoids (hydrocortisone 25 mg intravenous bolus and then 100 mg/m²/d in 4 divided doses) should be initiated awaiting hormone evaluation tests results, while also starting a 5% dextrose of NS with the rate of NS and glucose administration depending on the presence of hypovolemia or hypoglycemia at the time of evaluation. A pelvic ultrasound for localization of gonads, evaluation of adrenals, and determination of presence and degree of Müllerian development would guide further evaluation and management. The presence of intraabdominal, inguinal, or labial gonads, absence of Müllerian structures and ambiguous genitalia varying from normal female external genitalia to under virilized male genitalia in a newborn with salt wasting and enlarged adrenals suggests 46,XY karyotype and CAH either due to lipoid CAH or 3β-dehydrogenase type II deficiency (3β-HSDII). Conversely, the presence of Müllerian structures, ovaries, and enlarged adrenals in a neonate with salt wasting and ambiguous genitalia varying from clitoromegaly, labial fusion urogenital sinus, to penile urethra is suggestive of a 46,XX karyotype and CAH due either to 21-hydroxylase (21OHD) deficiency in the majority of the cases or 3β-HSDII deficiency.

Laboratory Tests and Diagnostic Imaging

Karyotype is indicated in all cases of ambiguous genitalia (even when prenatal karyotype is available), accompanied by fluorescence in situ hybridization (FISH) using SRY-specific probes or screening for SRY by polymerize chain (PCR) reaction in cases in which the clinical examination and the pelvic ultrasound findings suggest ovotesticular DSD, mixed GD, or XX testicular DSD.

First-line hormone measurements should include assessment of adrenal and gonadal secretion, including measurement of 17α-hydroxyprogesterone (17-OHP), androstenedione (Δ4A), and T. These should be drawn alongside the initial electrolyte panel and prior to exogenous glucocorticoid administration. A basal T level quickly screens for the presence of Leydig cells and appropriate T synthesis.

The initial results of the karyotype, hormonal profile, and imaging should begin to elucidate an etiology and suggest second-line (usually subspecialty-assisted) testing. At this stage, more sophisticated imaging, such as magnetic resonance imaging of the pelvis, may be necessary to better define the internal anatomy. In addition a genitogram would assess the anatomy and size of the urogenital sinus and the entry of the vagina and the urethra. More than any other factor, the

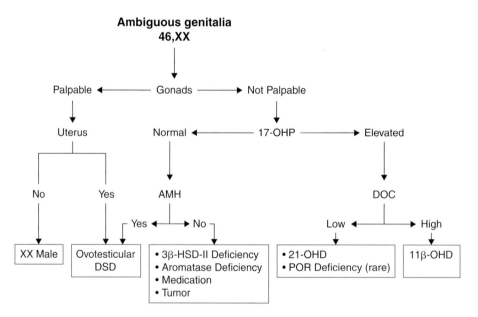

FIGURE 35-3. Diagnostic workup of ambiguous genitalia with XX karyotype. This algorithm for the diagnosis and laboratory and physical evaluation of infants with ambiguous genitalia is most useful for infants with 46,XX karyotype. 17OHP = 17α-hydroxyprogesterone; AMH = anti-Müllerian hormone; DOC = 11-deoxycorticosterone; 3β-HSD2 = 3β-hydroxysteroid dehydrogenase type II; 21-OHD = 21α-hydroxylase deficiency; POR = P450 oxidoreductase; 11β-OHD = 11β-hydroxylase deficiency.

Ambiguous genitalia
46,XY

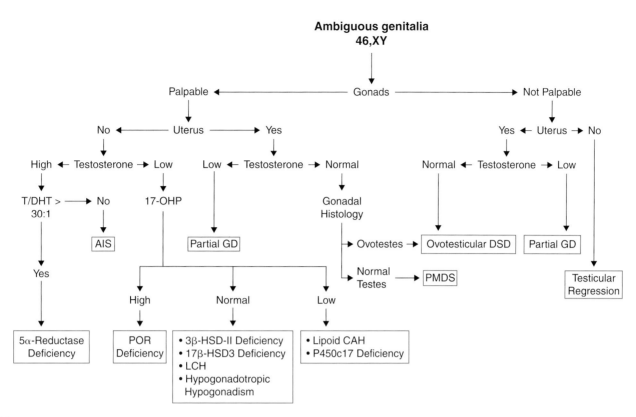

FIGURE 35-4. Diagnostic work up of ambiguous genitalia with XY karyotype. Algorithm for a 46,XY infant with ambiguous genitalia. T = testosterone; DHT = dihydrotestosterone; 17OHP = 17α-hydroxyprogesterone; AIS = androgen insensitivity syndrome; GD = gonadal dysgenesis; PMDS = persistent Müllerian duct syndrome; POR = P450 oxidoreductase; 3β-HSD2 = 3β-hydroxysteroid dehydrogenase type II; 17β-HSD3 = 17β-hydroxysteroid dehydrogenase type 3; LCH = Leydig cell hypoplasia; CAH = congenital adrenal hyperplasia; P450c17 = 17α-hydroxylase /17,20 lyase.

karyotype should direct subsequent hormonal testing. If 17-OHP is elevated, or electrolytes or vital signs suggest adrenal disorders, then further evaluation of the adrenal axis is warranted. Basal and ACTH-simulated (administer 0.25 mg synthetic ACTH and measure after 60 minutes, usually best in the morning) (17-OHP), 17α-hydroxy pregnenolone (17-OHPreg), progesterone, pregnenolone 11-deoxycorticosterone (DOC), corticosterone (B), androstenedione (Δ4A), dehydroepiandrosterone and dehydroepiandrosterone-sulfate (DHEA, DHEA-S, respectively), can be measured to differentiate between the various forms of CAH and other adrenal defects (81).

If the adrenal axis appears intact, and the patient has an XY karyotype, one should measure serum FSH, LH, T, DHT, Δ4A, to assess for pituitary or primary gonadal deficiencies. Sex steroid measurements may also require both pre- and post-β-hCG stimulation T levels, (a two- to threefold rise is normal). Several protocols exist for the β-hCG stimulation test; the most commonly used involves administration of β-hCG 1000 U/day for 3 days with steroids measured 24 hours after the last β-hCG administration. Alternatively, one can give a single dose of β-hCG 5000 U/m² and measure steroids after 72 hours.

Also, steroid ratios (DHT/T or T/Δ4A), both pre- and post-β-hCG stimulation, are frequently more diagnostic than are isolated values.

Patients with an XX karyotype and normal adrenal steroid levels also require measurement of basal and β-hCG-stimulated T and DHT to ascertain the presence of functional Leydig cells. Estradiol (E₂) should be measured alongside the androgenic steroids to evaluate for aromatase deficiency in an XX patient.

Additional tests that may be needed are measurement of serum inhibin B or AMH to evaluate for the presence of testicular tissue (specifically Sertoli cells), which is indicated to discriminate between XX testicular DSD syndrome (or ovotesticular DSD) and virilization secondary to androgen excess as in CAH. T stimulation (T heptylate 50 mg intramuscularly monthly for 3 months) and measurement of phallic growth to test for peripheral androgen responsiveness (>2.5 cm considered positive response) can be used if partial androgen insensitivity is suspected. A positive response to T heptylate may aid in sex assignment.

Initial studies should suggest a presumptive diagnosis, which can be further refined using molecular diagnostics or histologic analysis of a surgical specimen.

Sex Assignment and Surgical Management

An explanation of the basics of sex determination and genital virilization can assist parents with understanding how such a birth defect could happen. Counseling should involve a multidisciplinary approach, with specialists from endocrinology, genetics, psychiatry, social work, and (if necessary) pediatric urology or surgery. Comparisons can be made between genetic sex, hormonal sex, and external phenotype to empower parents in the decision-making process with respect to gender assignment. Although assigning sex is a priority, definitive surgery in infancy may not be. The role of early definitive surgery is controversial, and it is the opinion of the authors that the benefits of definitive surgery do not necessarily outweigh the risks.

The most common case of genital ambiguity at birth is an XX individual with CAH due to 21OHD. These patients possess ovaries and Müllerian structures and universally are reared as females. They can safely be declared "female," and any necessary surgical remodeling can likely proceed before a year of age without concern for future psychosocial impairment. Arguably, earlier surgery may improve child–parent bonding and provide a more comfortable environment of rearing. Long-term follow-up studies have demonstrated significant dissatisfaction with genital appearance and sexual ability, especially when clitoral surgery was performed (82,83). It may be preferable to defer decisions for cosmetic genital remodeling until later in life. "Moderate" clitoromegaly at birth may not appear quite as worrisome at 8 years of age.

A dilemma exists in the case of an XX female with CAH and a phallic urethra. Such patients show greater potential to identify as males, and a male gender identity may be preferred. One potential approach recommended by the authors is to allow these patients to be raised as males, but to defer any surgery until later in life, when the child can contribute to the decision.

In conditions such as XY gonadal dysgenesis, complete androgen insensitivity, and XX testicular DSD, sexual phenotype is opposite to chromosomal and gonadal sex, and patients almost universally identify with their apparent phenotypic gender. When the diagnosis of one of the above is certain, then early genital surgery may be preferred given the relatively unambiguous gender identity.

Delaying genital shaping until later childhood allows incorporation of the patient's views on their own gender identity, and does not demonstrably harm their psychosocial development, although parent and family expectations and relationships can potentially be compromised if a definitive procedure is not performed. Furthermore, conditions such as 17βHSD3- or 5α-reductase deficiency are associated with a switch in societal gender role at some point in childhood or adolescence (in some conditions, up to two-thirds of affected patients switch gender), and the harm represented by premature surgery may outweigh any possible benefits.

DISORDERS OF SEX DETERMINATION

Errors of sex determination are disorders of gonadal development leading to a phenotype opposite that predicted by the karyotype. This includes complete GD, XX testicular DSD (previously names XX maleness), and ovotesticular DSD (previously named true hermaphroditism). These conditions are uncommon and their etiologies are not completely understood. The phenotypic spectrum varies broadly with respect to genital appearance. The genetic basis for these disorders is similarly varied.

Turner syndrome results in GD and is covered in Chapter 31.

46,XY Gonadal Dysgenesis

Etiology and Pathophysiology of Pure/Complete Gonadal Dysgenesis XY GD occurs when fetal testes fail to differentiate normally. GD can be pure (or complete), partial, or mixed. Pure GD individuals lack any functional Sertoli or Leydig cells, and therefore produce no AMH or T. Instead of testes patients possess bilateral fibrous streaks usually located where ovaries are expected. Pure GD results in normal female external genitals with hypoplastic (but occasionally normal) Müllerian structures (previously referred to as Swyer syndrome).

Approximately 15% to 20% of all pure XY GD is caused by mutations in SRY (84–86), an unexpectedly low fraction given the role of SRY in human sex determination. The majority of mutations causing XY pure GD disrupt the high-mobility group (HMG) box, thereby either reducing DNA binding (86,87), interfering with DNA bending (87), or inhibiting nuclear import of the SRY protein (88). There are 50 known mutations of the SRY open reading frame (ORF). Deletions of Yp involving SRY have also been implicated in XY GD (84,85,89).

Mutations in genes necessary for testes organogenesis (XH2, SF-1, SOX9, WT-1, DHH) and duplications of putative "antitestes" genes (WNT-4) are responsible for a very small minority of all XY GD (30,41,78), but are usually associated with other syndromic features. Duplications of the DSS locus on Xp21, including DAX1, and mutations in DHH can cause isolated XY GD.

Presentation of Pure Gonadal Dysgenesis Pure XY GD presents as a phenotypic female with normal or tall stature, bilateral streak gonads, sexual infantilism, amenorrhea, small or normal Müllerian structures, and no Turner stigmata. Patients usually come to clinical attention in adolescence for pubertal delay and primary amenorrhea (please see Figure 35-5 for a diagnostic algorithm of disorders of sex determination and differentiation based on the phenotype at puberty). Rarely, patients can present with an abdominal or pelvic mass representing gonadoblastoma.

Occasionally, pure XY GD can be due to mutations in SF-1 gene, SXO9 or WT1 gene mutations or deletions.

Diagnosis of Pure Gonadal Dysgenesis Isolated 46,XY pure GD is considered in an adolescent with primary amenorrhea and sexual immaturity. FSH and LH levels are elevated and sex steroid levels are low or normal (relative to XX females). The adrenal axis is intact, and levels of steroid precursors such as 17-OHP, DHEA-S, D4A) are normal.

β-hCG stimulation results in minimal (or absent) increase in testosterone. Pelvic ultrasound demonstrates normal or hypoplastic uterus and streak gonads but atrophic gonads. Karyotype of peripheral lymphocytes shows 46,XY and FISH for SRY or for Yp rarely show complete or partial SRY deletion. The majority of patients are 46,XY SRY-positive. Sequencing of the SRY ORF for mutations is positive in only up to 20% of 46,XY GD. Certain isolated and syndromic forms of XY GD with large chromosomal duplications (DSS, 1p31-35) or deletions (del 9p24) will be detected with standard cytogenetics, but smaller rearrangements can be tested for with FISH or comparative genomic hybridization (CGH). SOX9 and WT-1 can be sequenced in patients with characteristic clinical findings (genetic testing is available). Mutations in SF-1 and DHH genes should be searched for as causes of pure 46,XY GD, even in the absence of adrenal failure or neuropathy; however, commercial sequencing is not widely available for these genes. Gonadal appearance and histology determined at gonadectomy differentiates between streak gonads due to pure 46,XY GD and normal testes due to 17-hydroxylase/lyase deficiency, isolated 17,20 lyase deficiency, or androgen resistance.

Etiology and Pathophysiology of 46,XY Partial and Mixed Gonadal Dysgenesis In a minority of cases, testes dysgenesis and sex reversal are not complete, resulting in a condition termed "partial" GD. These patients have varying degrees of Wolffian and Müllerian development and genital ambiguity correlating with the degree of testes dysgenesis. Mutations involving SRY have been implicated in partial 46,XYGD in three cases: a 3–7 kb deletion 2–3 kb 3' to the SRY polyadenylation site (90), and in two point mutations outside the HMG box in the 5' end of the gene (91,92). Notably, all three of these cases represent disruptions occurring outside of the HMG box, highlighting the significance of this highly conserved region. It is worth noting that although one of these mutations (Gln2Stop) resulted in a premature stop signal and complete absence of SRY protein, the resulting phenotype was one of a 46,XY female with only partial GD. Histology of the gonads in this patient showed incomplete dysgenesis and primitive tubules reminiscent of early testes development, which in the absence of SRY is inexplicable.

"Mixed" 46,XY GD refers to individuals with a completely dysgenic streak gonad on one side and a partially dysgenic (or even a normal-appearing) testis opposite. Mosaicism for 45,X/46,XY is the most frequent

Phenotype at Puberty

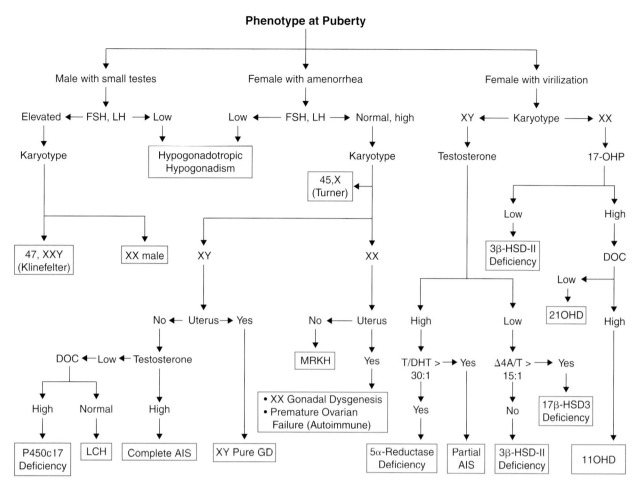

FIGURE 35-5. Diagnostic work up of disorders of sexual determination or differentiation presenting at puberty. This algorithm is designed for those disorders that may present at puberty, although premature virilization or adrenarche may prompt an earlier evaluation in childhood. FSH = follicle stimulating hormone; LH = luteinizing hormone; 17OHP = 17α-hydroxyprogesterone; 3β-HSD2 = 3β-hydroxysteroid dehydrogenase type II; 21α-OH = 21α-hydroxylase; DOC = 11-deoxycorticosterone; MRKH = Mayer-Rokitansky-Küster-Hauser syndrome; T = testosterone; DHT = dihydrotestosterone; Δ4A = androstenedione; P450c17 = 17α-hydroxylase/17,20 lyase; LCH = Leydig cell hypoplasia; AIS = androgen insensitivity syndrome; GD = gonadal dysgenesis; 17β-HSD3 = 17β-hydroxysteroid dehydrogenase type 3; 11OHD = 11β-hydroxylase deficiency.

cause of mixed GD, although a minority have a 46,Xi(Yq) karyotype (3). Mixed 46,XY GD is part of the phenotypic variation spectrum in an individual with 45,X/46,XY mosaicism. In one series of 10 45,X/46,XY patients, 3 presented as Turner females with bilateral streak gonads, 3 presented as mixed GD and genital ambiguity, and 4 as males possessing bilateral testes and varying degrees of under virilization (93). There is evidence that increasing proportion of gonadal Y chromosome material correlates with increasing testicular tissue and phenotypic maleness (94,96).

Although most cases are sporadic, familial cases of XY pure (86,96) and partial 46,XY GD (86,97,98) have been reported (98). Some intriguing cases involve SRY mutations detectable in the normal father and male relatives (96,98). Other reports of fathers who are mosaics for mutant and normal SRY transmitting the mutation to their XY female daughters (99,100) are less puzzling. Presumably, the normal father's mosaicism reflects a postzygotic mutation event.

These cases demonstrate the effect of genetic background on sex determination and may provide further clues for elucidating the molecular basis for gonad formation. This is especially relevant because the etiology of 80% of 46,XY with any degree of GD remains unknown.

Presentation of Partial and Mixed Gonadal Dysgenesis Partial and mixed 46,XY GD patients present in infancy or early childhood with varying degrees of ambiguous genitalia and Wolffian and Müllerian structures development. Although the streak gonad in mixed 46,XY GD is always abdominally located, dysgenic testes may be either abdominally or inguinally located, depending on the degree of testicular activity. If one of the testes is relatively normal, it can be present in the scrotum. Patients with partial 46,XY GD usually have female external genitalia with some degree of virilization, such as clitoromegaly or a bifid scrotum. Uterus and fallopian tubes are usually well formed, but occasionally may be hypoplastic. In

mixed 46,XY GD, the development of Wolffian and Müllerian structures as well as the virilization of external genitalia, correlates with the degree of development of the ipsilateral testis (Figure 35-6, 35-7), resulting in asymmetric virilization of the

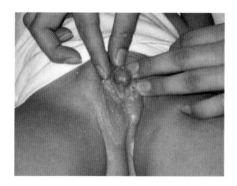

FIGURE 35-6. 45,X/46,XY mixed GD. This patient presented with genital ambiguity, with only one palpable testis on the right. The left scrotal skin shows fewer rogations and is more labial in appearance. The penis has hypospadias. Photograph courtesy of Dr. Gloria Queipo. Hospital General de Mexico.

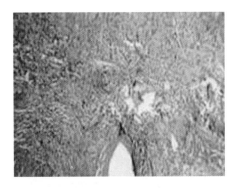

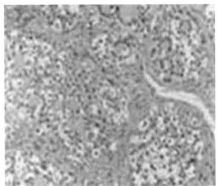

FIGURE 35-7. Gonadal histology of 45, X/46. XY mixed GD. A streak gonad with only fiber tissue is present on the top, and a dysgenetic testis on the bottom. Photograph courtesy of Dr. Gloria Queipo. Hospital General de Mexico.

external or internal genitalia and unilateral cryptorchidism. In rare cases, phenotypic female patients presented with premature adrenarche, reflecting a hormonally active gonadal tumor (101).

Diagnosis of Partial and Mixed Gonadal Dysgenesis As with all cases of GD, FSH and LH are elevated whereas E_2, T, and DHT levels are low to normal, and do not increase following β-hCG stimulation (less than twofold increase). Serum AMH or inhibin B levels are low to undetectable in partial GD, but may be normal in mixed. Steroid precursors such as 17-OHP, DHEA-S are normal. Pelvic ultrasound demonstrates a normal or hypoplastic uterus, but may show asymmetric Müllerian development in mixed GD, with fallopian tubes present only on the side ipsilateral to the streak gonad. Karyotype of peripheral lymphocytes usually shows 46,XY in partial GD, and mosaic 45,X/46,XY in mixed.

If FISH for SRY is positive, the gene can be sequenced. In the majority of the cases no mutations of the SRY are found, and the etiology remains uncertain. SRY mutations causing partial GD tend to be located outside of the highly conserved DNA-binding HMG box. After surgical removal, distinction between normal testes, dysgenic testes, streaks, and ovotestes is possible. Bilateral dysgenic

testes define partial GD, although the presence of at least one streak gonad is more consistent with mixed. If peripheral karyotype is 46,XY, and gonads' histology is asymmetric (e.g., streak gonad on one side, testis on the other), karyotyping of the gonads may reveal cryptic mosaicism.

If a mutation or translocation involving SRY is found, the father should be tested for a possible familial mutation because SRY mutations can result in a full spectrum of phenotypes, from 46,XY fertile males to 46,XY phenotypic females. The actual risk of recurrence of a GD phenotype in families is therefore difficult to predict.

Management of XY Gonadal Dysgenesis The primary concern governing treatment is the risk of gonadoblastoma, a mixed germ cell sex-cord tumor, which can undergo malignant transformation to germ cell neoplasms, including dysgerminomas. Patients with dysgenetic testes should undergo prophylactic or therapeutic gonadectomy soon after diagnosis, preferably in the first decade of life. Patients are followed with regular ultrasounds every 6 months starting at 2 years of age until gonadectomy can be performed. The use of laparoscopic gonadectomies is increasing, with good results reported (102).

In patients with XY pure GD, genitals are typically female and so is gender identity, however, issues of gender identity do arise in partial and mixed GD. Factors such as degree of genital ambiguity or the presence of a descended testis are indirect evidence for the degree of fetal androgen exposure, and may be used for initial gender assignment. Although it is advisable that a gender be assigned as soon as possible, decisions regarding definitive surgery may be postponed until the patient can contribute to the decision. Medically indicated surgery to correct urogenital malformations (e.g., fistula repair) should not be delayed.

Sex steroid replacement consistent with the chosen gender should be initiated at puberty for secondary sex development, growth spurt, and normal accrual of bone mineral density (for details please see Chapter 36 and 37). Height and weight should be monitored regularly, and a dual-energy X-ray absorptiometry (DEXA) scan for bone density should be performed prior to induction of puberty with exogenous hormone replacement, and yearly thereafter for the first 2 years. Once patients are on adult cyclic estrogen and progestin replacement doses, DEXA scans can be spaced to every 2 to 3 years as long as the initial DEXA scan was normal.

Hysterectomies are not routinely performed (because a functional uterus is pres-

ent) to preserve child-bearing potential with embryo-transfer techniques, although most patients do not carry successful pregnancies for unknown reasons (3).

Rare individuals with mixed GD and more virilized phenotypes are raised as males. These patients require testosterone replacement for life, most often via intramuscular injections or transdermal patches (please see Chapter 37).

Long-Term Concerns Gonadoblastomas are a common presentation for all forms of GD regardless of the phenotype of the genitals. Gonadoblastoma formation in patients with some form of XY GD increases with age and has been estimated to be as high as 30% by 30 years of age (85,89,102,103). The etiology remains unclear, but the vast majority of all patients possess some detectable Y chromosome material, leading some to postulate the presence of a gonadoblastoma locus on the Y chromosome (GBY locus), and a potential oncogenic role for mutant SRY (89,102–104). Although gonadoblastomas themselves have a low malignant potential, up to 50% of patients have an overgrowth of associated germinal or epithelial components, leading to tumors with higher malignant potential such as dysgerminomas and testicular intraepithelial neoplasms. Up to 10% of patients have overtly malignant disease (102).

XX testicular DSD

Etiology/Pathophysiology Phenotypic spectrum of individuals with XX testicular DSD can vary from males with immature testes and varying degrees of phenotypic genital ambiguity, to patients with ovotesticular DSD (who will be addressed more thoroughly in the following section).

The incidence of XX testicular DSD is estimated at 1:20,000. Approximately 85% of patients with XX testicular DSD have unambiguously masculine genitalia (106). Ninety percent of these males harbor an Xp:Yp translocation containing SRY. One-third of all recombination occurs at the PRKX locus hotspot on Xp22.3 and the Y-homolog PRKY (106).

Of the 15% of patients with XX testicular DSD and ambiguous genitals, only a minority carry SRY (107,108). Preferential inactivation of the Y-bearing X chromosome (105,107,109), and cryptic mosaicism with SRY expression confined to the testes (105,110) has been implicated in causing partial, rather than complete, sex-reversed phenotype. XX testicular DSD has also been associated with a 17q23-24 duplication including SOX9 (54). Familial cases of XX testicular DSD represent predominantly SRY-negative kindred, whose members can present with 46,XX partial or complete testicular DSD, or ovotesticular DSD (111).

Clinical Presentation
The majority of patients with XX testicular DSD (80%) have classic de la Chapelle syndrome with completely masculinized genitals, and present in adulthood as infertile males. The patients exhibit some similarities with Klinefelter (XXY), such as small testes, azoospermia, gynecomastia (37%), and sexual infantilism (109). Unlike Klinefelter individuals, patients with XX testicular DSD are short and have normal mentation. Phallus size varies from small to normal, and sexual function and ejaculation are normal.

Occasionally, patients will present in early childhood with undervirilized genitalia. There is some correlation between phenotype and genotype, as the presence of SRY is usually (but not always) associated with a more virilized appearance of the genitals. Less than 20% of cases have been reported prior to adolescence. Incidence of cryptorchidism has been estimated at 15%, and of hypospadias at 10% to 15% (112). Wolffian structures are normal, and Müllerian structures are absent.

Diagnosis
The diagnosis of most XX testicular DSD patients without genital ambiguity is often made during an investigation of infertility or delayed puberty. Patients have hypergonadotropic hypogonadism with elevated FSH and LH, decreased T, DHT, and a less than twofold increase in response to the β-hCG stimulation test. 17-OHP levels are normal. Serum AMH level greater than 75 nmol/L is unequivocal proof of functioning testicular tissue suggesting XX testicular DSD or ovotesticular DSD (113). An ultrasound shows absence of a uterus. Semen analysis demonstrates normal semen volume with azoospermia. FISH for SRY is positive in 90% of adults with XX testicular DSD who present without genital ambiguity. In patients with XX testicular DSD and negative SRY, further cytogenetic testing should include chromosome painting to determine the amount of Yp material present or FISH to detect SOX9 (17q24) microduplications.

In XX testicular DSD patients presenting with genital ambiguity, SRY is often not present.

If gonad biopsy is performed (for example, in work up of azoospermia), the histology of XX testicular DSD reveals hyalinized seminiferous tubules with Sertoli-cell-only appearance, absent germ cells, and Leydig hyperplasia. If ovotestes are found, the diagnosis is ovotesticular DSD.

Management
Medical management of adolescents and adults involves androgen replacement if indicated for virilization. Prosthetic testes can be used for cosmetic reasons. If gynecomastia is present and does not respond to androgens, it can be surgically corrected. Patients with XX testicular DSD, without genital ambiguity, although they are SRY-positive and possess dysgenic testes, are not at increased risk for gonadoblastomas because they lack a Y chromosome. It is not clear whether they are at an increased risk for breast cancer similar to those with Klinefelter syndrome. There is one reported case of a XX testicular DSD patient with breast cancer (114–116) and one case of a XX testicular DSD patient with M7 acute myelogenous leukemia (117).

Because the majority of individuals with XX testicular DSD carry the Xp:Yp translocation, paternal karyotype and FISH for SRY should also be performed to determine whether or not the father carries a balanced translocation, or if the translocation is de novo (germline). Fathers who carry the translocation can only produce offspring that are 46,XX SRY-positive testicular DSD or 46,XY SRY-negative complete gonadal dysgenesis offspring.

Ovotesticular DSD (formerly True Hermaphrodites)

Etiology and Pathophysiology
Ovotesticular DSD signifies the presence of both testicular (defined by seminiferous tubules) and ovarian (defined by follicles) tissues in one individual. This can take the following forms: ovotestis on one side with contralateral ovary or testis (50%); ovary and testis on opposite sides (30%); or bilateral ovotestes (20%). For unknown reasons, testicular tissue is more often located on the right and ovarian on the left (118).

The presence of both ovarian and testicular tissues in varying amounts leads to variable development of internal and external genitalia. The location of the individual gonad usually correlates with the predominant tissue type: gonads with ovarian predominance are most often abdominal and correctly positioned, whereas testes are usually scrotal (118). The degree of Müllerian and Wolffian structure correlates with the ipsilateral gonad; Wolffian structures generally develop only with a well-formed testis, confined to the same side. Müllerian structures develop in the presence of an ovary or an ovotestis. Gonadal hormone production and type of external genitalia depend on the predominant type of gonadal tissue (Figure 35-8).

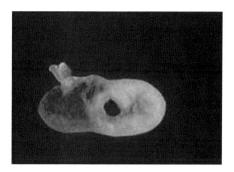

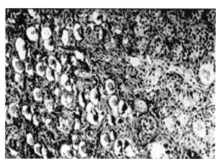

FIGURE 35-8. Microcopy (top) and gonadal histology (bottom) of ovotesticular DSD. An ovotestis possesses features of both testes and ovaries and is the most common gonadal type encountered among individuals with ovotesticular DSD. Testicular tissue with well-formed seminiferous tubules is evident on the right side of the histology slide. Ovarian tissue as defined by follicles is on the left. Photograph courtesy of Dr. Gloria Queipo. Hospital General de Mexico.

Approximately 60% of ovotesticular DSD have a 46,XX karyotype; 10% are SRY-positive (86,119–122), suggesting that these patients are part of the phenotypic spectrum that includes XX testicular DSD. This variability in presentation between XX testicular DSD and 46,XX ovotesticular DSD may be caused by preferential inactivation of the X chromosome with the Xp:Yp translocation (107,123), or by cryptic mosaicism for SRY (106,111,125), resulting in variable degrees of testes development leading to either ovotesticular DSD or XX testicular DSD.

Approximately 7% to 10% of ovotesticular DSD are 46,XY; in two cases a mutation was found in SRY (85,118,124). Between 30% and 33% of ovotesticular DSD are mosaics with at least one cell line containing Yp material (118,124). One-third of these mosaics are 46,XX/46,XY, although an unknown number of these are not actually mosaics but represent chimeras (125). At least five cases have been proven to be true tetragametic chimeras (126–130).

Clinical Presentation
Most patients with ovotesticular DSD present in infancy or early childhood with ambiguous genitalia. The phenotype of external genitalia and the

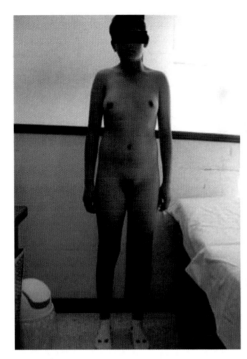

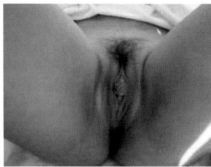

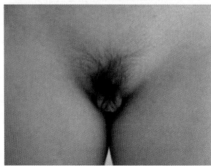

FIGURE 35-9. Patient with ovotesticular DSD. Moderately virilized external genitalia, with scrotalized labia and hooded clitoris. This patient with ovotesticular DSD has breast development. Photograph courtesy of Dr. Gloria Queipo. Hospital General de Mexico.

degree of development of internal genitalia reflect the hormonal status of the gonad (Figure 35-9). Unicornuate uterus is a common finding in all patients, whereas adnexa and vagina are generally better developed in phenotypic females. Approximately half of phenotypic females menstruate (119,122). Patients with a high degree of masculinization and male phenotype may have some uterine remnants, such as a prostatic utricle (prostatic vagina). Phenotypic males also tend to have bilateral palpable gonads, or at least one descended gonad. The undescended gonad may be an ovary and located intraabdominal or ovotestis and located at any point of the pathway of testicular descent. Sometimes the ovotestis along with the hypoplastic Müllerian structures may be present as inguinal hernia. Rarely, patients with relatively unambiguous genitalia may present later in adolescence or adulthood with delayed puberty, infertility, or with atypical secondary sex characteristics (e.g., gynecomastia in phenotypic males or clitoromegaly in females). In these cases, diagnosis may require gonadal biopsy demonstrating the presence of both ovarian and testicular tissue.

Diagnosis The diagnosis of ovotesticular DSD is made during the evaluation and work up of ambiguous genitalia. The combination of both male and female internal and external genitalia is suggestive, but final diagnosis requires gonadal tissue confirmation. Pelvic or transrectal ultrasound reveals asymmetry in the degree of Müllerian and Wolffian ducts development, depending on the gonadal make up of each side.

Unlike individuals with GD, the gonads of patients with ovotesticular DSD have some degree of function and therefore normal levels of FSH, LH, E_2, T, DHT, and Δ4A. Sex steroids also increase appropriately with β-hCG stimulation. The karyotype is most often 46,XX but can be XY or mosaic. As in patients with XX testicular DSD, AMH levels are usually normal (for males).

Initial evaluations are often unsatisfactory. When the karyotype conforms to the apparent phenotypic gender, it may erroneously be interpreted as "normal." FISH for SRY is positive in 10% of 46,XX patients. Sequencing of the SRY ORF can rarely reveal a mutation in 46,XY patients. At this time, fibroblasts can be collected from oral mucosa to test for hidden mosaicism.

Gonadal biopsies confirm the diagnosis of ovotesticular DSD. Histology of gonads reveals the ovarian follicles and seminiferous tubules in various combinations. Gonadal tissue can also be tested for karyotype, cryptic mosaicism, or SRY mutations because SRY-negative patients with ovotesticular DSD have been found to have SRY expression in the gonads (105,111,131). Patients with a mosaic karyotype (most commonly 46,XX/46,XY) should be tested as well as their parents with microsatellite markers to determine potential chimerism (especially in twin cases, or those conceived with in vitro fertilization).

Management Initial management consists of surgical correction of medically concerning issues, such as inguinal hernia repair, fistulas, and malignancies. Subsequent management will depend on the degree of masculinization or feminization of the external genitalia, which generally determines the initial gender assignment. In infants and young children, it may be advisable to defer any cosmetic surgery until the patient is capable of participating in the decision, allowing for the incorporation of the patients' own notion of their gender. During surgery, in addition to shaping of the external genitalia, internal genitalia inconsistent with the desired gender is often removed. The paradoxical portion of the gonad is also excised. Sex hormone replacement for the appropriate gender is initiated at puberty for secondary sex characteristics and bone density.

There is a 5% incidence of gonadal tumors in ovotesticular DSD (132,133), which likely represents an increased risk from abdominal gonads possessing testicular tissue, as well as the increased risk of gonadoblastomas in dysgenic gonads with Yp material. Breast cancer risks may also be increased, but this is less certain (115,116).

Fertility Ovotesticular DSD with adequate Müllerian structures possess ovarian follicles, and can become pregnant and carry to term (119). In 8 pregnancies, the patients' karyotype was 46,XX, supporting the widely held hypothesis that individuals with a Y chromosome cannot become naturally pregnant. There is one case report of a patient with ovotesticular DSD with karyotype of 20% 46,XX/80% 46,XY who carried a successful pregnancy (133).

Males are generally azoospermic, but there have been infrequent case of males with mature sperm (118,134), and even more rare cases of ovotesticular DSD who have fathered children (118). Theoretically, males with immotile but otherwise normal sperm could father a child with intracytoplasmic sperm injection techniques.

DISORDERS OF SEXUAL DIFFERENTIATION

In disorders of sexual differentiation, the gonads develop normally, but the subsequent development of internal or external genitalia fails. The etiology in XY patients with normal testes and sex differentiation disorders is either due to a defect in androgen biosynthesis or a defect in its receptor. In XX patients with normal ovaries, the etiology of the sex differentiation disorders stems from androgen excess (adrenal and exogenous). Prenatal development of external genitalia is bipotential, and is dependent on the presence of testosterone for development of Wolffian structures and inguinoscrotal testes descent, and on DHT for fusion of labial folds into a scrotum and phallic growth. The absence of androgens maintains the "typical" female anogenital distance and labial folds, and promotes development of the vaginal sinus. All conditions show autosomal recessive inheritance except for androgen receptor mutations, which are X-linked.

DEFECTS IN TESTOSTERONE PRODUCTION AND SYNTHESIS

Testosterone is essential for development of secondary sex characteristics in XY individuals including differentiation of Wolffian structures, inguinoscrotal testes descent, and masculinization of external genitalia after conversion to DHT. The inheritance pattern for all enzyme defects involved in testosterone production is autosomal recessive.

Leydig Cell Hypoplasia/Agenesis

Etiology and Pathophysiology Leydig cell hypoplasia (LCH) is an autosomal recessive disorder, caused by inactivating mutations of luteinizing hormone-choriogonadotropin receptor (LHCGR) gene and characterized by impaired Leydig cell differentiation and testosterone production. After the 10th week of gestation, when testes determination has occurred in XY individuals, male sexual differentiation is regulated by placental β-hCG stimulation of Leydig cells. Then, during the third trimester of gestation and the first 6 months after birth (mini puberty), fetal LH is predominantly responsible for Leydig development and testosterone production. Both β-hCG and LH activate the shared G protein–coupled LHCG receptor. Inactivating mutations of the LHCGR gene reduce the responsiveness of fetal Leydig cells to β-hCG and LH in utero causing a failure of male sexual differentiation termed Leydig cell hypoplasia (LCH). Over 20 inactivating mutations of LHCGR gene have been identified scattered throughout the gene (135,136), including missense, nonsense, deletions, and in-frame insertion mutations. These mutations are not localized in any particular region of the gene and cause variable degrees of loss of receptor activity. Mutations causing truncation or decreased surface expression and coupling efficiency of the receptor are usually associated with XY GD, whereas milder missense mutations result in XY males with micropenis or hypospadias (137). An intriguing mutation in LHCGR gene causing absence of exon 10 has been described in an 18-year-old male who pre-

sented with normal male phenotype, pubertal delay, small testicles, and delayed bone age (138). The highly elevated LH levels and low testosterone indicated decreased LHCGR response to LH, whereas the normal male sex differentiation in utero and the normal rise in testosterone in response to β-hCG stimulation test indicated that the LHCG receptor responded to β-hCG.

Clinical Presentation The phenotype of patients with LCH depends on the degree of residual LHCG receptor activity ranging from patients presenting at birth with micropenis, hypospadias and cryptorchidism to patients with completely female external genitalia and palpable labial or inguinal masses. Some patients may not be diagnosed until later in adolescence, when they present as phenotypic females with primary amenorrhea and lack of secondary sex characteristics such as breast development. Testes are only slightly smaller and histologic examination of the testes of patients with LCH show seminiferous tubules and absence of mature Leydig cells. LCH patients have a blind vagina and lack a uterus and fallopian tubes because of active Sertoli cells and AMH during sexual differentiation. Present epididymis and vas deferens, absent uterus and fallopian tubes, nearly normal male development, small testicles, and delayed puberty and bone age have been described in a male (138).

Homozygous inactivating mutations of LHCGR gene in XX females cause hypergonadotropic hypogonadism with primary amenorrhea or oligoamenorrhea, cystic ovaries, and infertility. (139–142). (Diagnosis and treatment of XX females with mutant LRH and amenorrhea is covered in Chapter 36).

Diagnosis The diagnosis of LCH is considered in an adolescent female with delayed puberty or in a male with varying degrees of genital ambiguity and hypergonadotropic hypogonadism. LH is universally elevated, and FSH is either elevated or normal. Inhibin B levels are normal to low. T, DHT, and E₂ are extremely low, and do not increase with β-hCG stimulation. Disorders of androgen biosynthesis are ruled out by the absence of abnormal step-up in testosterone biosynthesis precursors and by the normal baseline levels of the precursors Δ4A and DHEA-S. Although the presentation can be similar to 17HSD3 or 5α-reductase deficiency, LCH patients have significantly lower testosterone and DHT levels, are less responsive to β-hCG, and have a normal Δ4A/T ratio (<15:1) as well as a T/DHT ratio. Pelvic ultrasound shows absence of uterus and fallopian tubes. AMH is normal to high, which differentiates patients with LCH from patients with partial or complete

XY GD, where AMH is undetectable or low (113).

Gonadal biopsy reveals normal Sertoli cells, hyalinization of the seminiferous tubules, absence of mature Leydig cells and spermatogenesis. Rarely, immature Leydig cells are present. Mildly affected XY individuals may show some early spermatogenesis, with arrest prior to spermiation.

The LHCGR gene can be sequenced to detect small and large deletions, insertions, and point mutations.

Congenital Lipoid Adrenal Hyperplasia

Mutations of steroidogenic acute regulatory (StAR) protein, and rarely of cytochrome P450 side chain cleavage P450scc or CYP11A gene (143,144), affect the synthesis of virtually all adrenal and gonadal steroidogenesis, with progressive cholesterol accumulation in these organs (lipoid), CAH, and adrenal failure (145). StAR protein facilitates the transport of cholesterol across the mitochondrial membrane of the adrenal and gonadal steroidogenic cells (for details see Chapter 27).

Clinical Presentation Both sexes present with salt wasting and adrenal crisis at birth and with female phenotype irrespective of gonadal sex. 46,XY patients have testes, a blind vaginal pouch, no Müllerian structures, and absent Wolffian derivates due to absence of testosterone. Testes can be in the abdomen, inguinal canal, or labia. Partial defects are possible with various degrees of genital ambiguity and Wolffian duct development in males. The majority of affected patients have excess generalized pigmentation at birth due to intrauterine glucocorticoid deficiency that results in elevated ACTH levels. The condition is usually fatal if not diagnosed and treated within the first week of life, although delayed presentations have been reported. 46,XX patients with partial StAR deficiency may experience spontaneous puberty, menarche, and anovulatory menses because their ovaries are able to produce estrogen. Estrogen production by the ovaries is possible: 1) because ovaries are dormant until puberty, preventing accumulation of cholesterol and therefore sparing the ovarian cells from damage (146); 2) because of estrogen synthesis by StAR-independent pathways (145–147). XX females with lipoid CAH also possess multiple cysts in their ovaries, possibly from anovulation.

Diagnosis Characteristic biochemical abnormalities include elevated plasma renin, hyponatremia, hyperkalemia, absent adrenal steroids and their precursors (Δ4A, DHEA, DHEA-S, cortisol, aldosterone, 17OHP, DOC, etc.), and testicular steroids (T, DHT).

Urinary 17-ketosteroids (17-KS) and 17-hydroxycorticosteroids (17-OHCS) are also low. ACTH and gonadotropins are elevated, and adrenal and gonadal steroids do not rise with ACTH or β-hCG stimulation, respectively. Low DOC levels, hyperkalemia, and absence of hypertension differentiate 46,XY males with lipoid hyperplasia from patients with 17α-hydroxylase/17,20 lyase deficiency as both disorders are characterized by low 17-OHP levels.

3β-Hydroxysteroid Dehydrogenase Type II Deficiency

Defects in adrenal and gonadal 3β-hydroxysteroid dehydrogenase/Δ^5-Δ^4 isomerase type II (3βHSDII, HSD3B2 gene) affect cortisol, aldosterone, and testosterone synthesis in XX and XY individuals, leading to a rare variant of CAH that causes virilization of females due to elevated DHEA levels and undervirilization of XY patients due to decreased testosterone synthesis (for details see Chapter 27).

Clinical Presentation Both sexes present with variable degrees of salt wasting and genital ambiguity dependent upon the amount of residual enzyme activity. The decreased testosterone synthesis and overproduction of DHEA, a weak androgen, results in ambiguous genitalia in 46,XY patients such as micropenis, hypospadias, a blind vaginal pouch and cryptorchidism, whereas in 46,XX patients results in virilization of external genitalia such as posterior fusion of labia majora, clitoromegaly and urogenital sinus. In 46,XY males there are no Müllerian structures and there is various degrees of Wolffian duct development. During childhood peripheral conversion of elevated DHEA levels to androgen through the activity of the 3βHSD-I isoenzyme can result in premature adrenarche, growth acceleration, and excess virilization in both sexes, as well as polycystic ovaries in XX females (149,150). Undiagnosed XY individuals (or those who have not undergone gonadectomy) may experience phallic enlargement or labial/scrotal testis descent, leading to a change in gender role at puberty despite female sex of rearing (151). In addition 46,XY patients develop gynecomastia during puberty due to decreased testosterone levels and aromatization of androgens to estrogens. Gonadal function and fertility are variable and not well characterized in either XX or XY patients (152).

Diagnosis Baseline and ACTH-stimulated Δ^5/Δ^4 steroid ratios (17OH-Preg/17-OHP and DHEA/Δ4A ratios) are elevated and are a more useful diagnostic marker than serum levels alone (148). FSH and LH are elevated and spermatogenesis is impaired.

17α-Hydroxylase/17,20-Lyase Deficiency

Cytochrome P450 17α-hydroxylase/17,20-lyase (P450c17, CYP17 gene) catalyzes two distinct reactions in the adrenals and gonads: the hydroxylation of carbon-17 in C21 steroids (essential for glucocorticoid and sex hormone synthesis), and the lysis of the 17,20 carbon–carbon bond (necessary for sex steroids synthesis). The majority of reported mutations disrupt both actions (153), resulting in a rare variant of CAH characterized by decreased cortisol synthesis, low renin hypertension, and hypokalemia from excess mineralocorticoid precursor production in the zona fasciculata such as DOC and corticosterone (B). Occasional CYP17 mutations have been discovered which disrupt only 17,20-lyase activity (156), and thus affect only sex steroid synthesis (for details see Chapter 27).

Clinical Presentation 46,XX patients have normal genitalia at birth. 46,XY affected individuals with either 17α-hydroxylase/17,20-lyase or isolated 17,20 lyase deficiency have either female external genitalia and a blind vaginal pouch, or ambiguous genitalia if the defect is partial. Affected 46,XY patients have no Müllerian structures and the degree of Wolffian duct development depends on the degree of enzyme deficiency. Patients do not develop adrenal crisis because the elevated precursor B has glucocorticoid activity (155). Sexual development and puberty are delayed. Most often patients may not be diagnosed until pubertal years, when they present with primary amenorrhea, low renin hypertension, and hypokalemia (due to elevated mineralocorticoid precursors).

Diagnosis Patients have elevated levels of B and DOC, low renin, low aldosterone, hypokalemic alkalosis, and low levels of cortisol. Serum gonadotropins are elevated. In both 17α-hydroxylase/17,20-lyase and isolated 17,20 lyase baseline values of DHEA-S, Δ4A, testosterone, and E_2 are low and do not rise in response to β-hCG and ACTH stimulation testing. The 24-hour urinary collection of 17-ketosteroid metabolites are low. XY individuals with 17,20-lyase deficiency are variably feminized with low DHEA-S, Δ4A, and testosterone levels. Stimulation with β-hCG demonstrates a subnormal increase in these androgens.

P450 Oxidoreductase Deficiency

Cytochrome P450 oxidoreductase (POR) is a flavoprotein that donates electrons to all microsomal P450 enzymes, including the steroidogenic enzymes P450c17 and P450c21. A defect in POR is a rare cause of CAH due to

deficiencies of both P450c21 and P450c17 enzymes (157–159) (for details see Chapter 27).

Clinical Presentation As with P450c21 deficiencies, affected XX patients are virilized at birth, suggesting exposure to elevated androgen in utero. After birth, however, virilization does not progress as postnatal DHEA-S, Δ4A, and testosterone levels are low to normal. Affected 46,XY patients may have normal or ambiguous genitalia at birth. Bone malformations, resembling a pattern seen in patients with Antley–Bixler syndrome (ABS), may be seen in both males and females (see Chapter 23) The mechanism by which POR deficiency causes a skeletal disorder resembling ABS is unclear. Mothers of patients with POR deficiency experience virilization during pregnancy along with their XX offspring The suggested mechanism of increased androgen production by the fetoplacental is either decreased activity of POR-dependent aromatase or increased androgen synthesis through an alternative pathway not involving P450c17 enzyme activity and which is active only during fetal life (159). Increased androgen production by the aforementioned mechanisms in affected 46,XY patients may not fully compensate for defective P450c17 activity in utero and can result in ambiguous genitalia at birth.

Diagnosis The biochemical profile of affected infants may vary with cortisol levels being low to normal, 17-OHP elevated to normal and DHEA, Δ4A and testosterone levels being low to normal. Urinary excretion of 17-OHS in 24-hour urine may also vary from high to normal. Although the hormonal changes suggest different degrees of combined deficiencies of P450c21 and P450c17 hydroxylase enzymes, no mutations in the two genes (CYP21 and CYP17) have been identified. Recently, POR mutations have been reported as the etiology for ambiguous genitalia, disordered steroidogenesis, and/or ABS phenotype; individuals with ABS phenotype and normal steroidogenesis have FGFR2 mutations (mutations of FGFR2 cause ABS) (160).

17β-Hydroxysteroid Dehydrogenase Type 3 Deficiency (17-βHSD3)

The 17β-HSD type 3 enzyme (gene HSD 17B3) is mapped on chromosome 9q22 and is expressed primarily at the gonads. The enzyme catalyzes the conversion of Δ4A to testosterone and E_1 to E_2 and its deficiency causes impaired virilization of 46,XY males.

Clinical Presentation Depending on the degree of residual enzyme activity, 17β-HSD3 deficiency can cause a range of undervirilization of XY individuals at birth, from an empty bifid scrotum with perineoscrotal hypospadias to otherwise normal female genitalia with clitoromegaly and posterior labioscrotal fusion. Testes can be undescended or labial. Müllerian ducts are absent because of normal AMH production by Sertoli cells. Wolffian ducts are present ending blindly at a vaginal pouch. During puberty, 46,XY patients may experience progressive virilization, clitoral/phallic enlargement, muscle development, breast development, and testicular descent. (161,162). No affected 46,XX females have been reported.

Diagnosis Serum Δ4A and estrone E_1 are high and serum testosterone and E_2 are low at baseline. The diagnosis may require measurement of testosterone and Δ4A after β-hCG stimulation, and use of the Δ4A/T ratio (abnormal if ratio > 15:1) rather than isolated hormone levels (163). Serum FSH and LH are elevated due the absence of negative feedback inhibition. Histologic study of the testes show Leydig cell hypoplasia and decreased or absent sperm precursors in the seminiferous tubules.

17-βHSD3 deficiency may be difficult to recognize in infancy because XY individuals often appear with normal female external genitalia, and they have no significant clinical problems. Testosterone levels in infancy are near normal, thereby clouding the diagnosis (164), probably due to an excess of weakly androgenic DHEA and Δ4A and extraglandular testosterone production.

Management XY patients are usually raised female (161,163). In one study, up to 40% of affected XY individuals who were raised as females successfully switched gender roles at puberty (163). Surgical management appropriate to the chosen gender should be discussed. Patients with undescended testes throughout childhood are at increased risk for gonadoblastoma (161).

Management of Patients with LCH or Defective Steroid Metabolism Sex hormone replacement corresponding to the chosen gender is initiated between 12–14 years of age for development of secondary sex characteristics. Bone density should be measured prior to initiation of puberty with a DEXA scan, and yearly thereafter. Testosterone treatment slowly tapers up to adult doses (up to 300 mg q 3–4 wk) over 2 years (for details see Chapter 37). 46,XY patients with mild androgen synthesis defects can be fertile. Spermatogenesis may be impaired in patients with long-term cryptorchidism. Undescended testes can be corrected with orchidopexy, and patients should be moni-

tored because of tumor risk. Patients with isolated hypospadias should have surgical correction in the first year of life.

XY patients who are reared as females are treated with estrogens alone because they lack a uterus and are not at risk for endometrial hyperplasia from unopposed estrogens. Puberty can be initiated after age 12 with low-dose (0.2 mg/mo) ethinyl E_2 and a slow titration upward over 2 years, to the adult dose (for details see Chapter 36).

Gonadectomy in childhood may be performed in XY patients raised as females to remove a source of endogenous testosterone as well as to reduce risk of tumor from undescended testes. Many patients with 3β-HSD2 and especially 17β-HSD3 deficiency have successfully switched gender at puberty, when production of testicular androgens increase (152,163,162). Decisions involving gender assignment should not be rigid, and definitive surgeries can be delayed in deferment to societal roles and patient preferences.

Smith-Lemli-Opitz Syndrome

Etiology and Pathophysiology Smith-Lemli-Opitz syndrome (SLOS) is a congenital syndrome, variably associated with female external genitals in an XY patient, caused by defective cholesterol synthesis. Patients usually have low levels of cholesterol and steroid hormones, and marked elevations of cholesterol precursors due to defective 3β-hydroxysteroid-Δ7 reductase (*DHCR7*) activity, which catalyzes the hydration of 7-dehydrocholesterol (7-DHC) to cholesterol, the last step of cholesterol biosynthesis (165–168). Over 120 mutations in DHCR7 in SLOS patients have been reported to date (169).

The pathophysiology behind the dysmorphology and mental retardation in SLOS remains unclear. Because many of the affected organs in SLOS are dependent upon the hedgehog (Hh) proteins for embryonal patterning, disruption of Hh signaling due to intracellular cholesterol deficiency has been proposed as a possible etiology (170–172). In vivo and in vitro analyses of SLOS patients' gonads generally demonstrate adequate testosterone production and poor response to β-hCG (173). A combination of poor fetal response to β-hCG/LH and cholesterol deficiency with subsequently impaired androgen synthesis may explain the female phenotype in XY patients with severe SLOS. Additionally, there may be impairment of DHH signaling, which is required for testes organogenesis (for details see Chapter 23).

Clinical Presentation Phenotype depends on the severity of the enzymatic defect, from

variable presence of classic facial dysmorphisms (microcephaly, micrognathia, microglossia, cleft lip and palate, and anteverted nares) and major malformations (cardiac malformations, liver disease, and intestinal aganglionosis) to frank holoprosencephaly and intrauterine or neonatal death (174). One of the most consistent findings is syndactyly of toes 2 and 3, which has been reported to occur in up to 99% of biochemically diagnosed cases.

Genital ambiguity in XY infants with SLOS ranges from mild hypospadias to micropenis with perineoscrotal hypospadias (Prader III) and cryptorchidism to female genitals (rare) (175, 176). 46,XY SLOS patients who have female external genital are often severely affected, with poor survival. In females, hypoplastic labia minora and majora can occur, but usually the external genitalia are normal. Other abnormalities include renal and cardiac malformations, intestinal aganglionosis (Hirschsprung disease), intestinal or pyloric stenosis, or less well-defined functional dysmotility (178). Rarely, patients with severe SLOS may present with adrenal insufficiency at birth due to impaired adrenal steroidogenesis (175,177,179). SLOS patients surviving to adulthood had spontaneous puberty.

Diagnosis The diagnosis of SLOS requires measurement of serum cholesterol and the precursor 7-DHC by sensitive methods that can readily distinguish between different sterols, such as gas chromatography/mass spectrometry. Levels of the precursor 7-DHC are universally elevated (sometimes >1000 × normal), but only loosely correlate with the degree of clinical severity. Normal levels of 7-DHC are 0.1 ± 0.05 μg/mL in newborns; SLOS patients typically range between 50 and 300 μg/mL (168,180,181).

Treatment Treatment involves cholesterol supplementation (for more details see Chapter 23).

DEFECTS IN TESTOSTERONE METABOLISM AND ACTION

Defects in 5α-Reductase Type 2

Etiology and Pathophysiology Steroid 5α-reductase deficiency (SRD5A2) is a male-limited autosomal recessive disorder that results from a defect in the enzyme converting testosterone to DHT. DHT is responsible for the differentiation of male external genitalia, development and secretory function of the prostate and seminal vesicles, and development of secondary sex characteristics in males during puberty.

Peripheral conversion of testosterone to DHT is an irreversible reaction catalyzed by the two isoenzymes of 5α-reductase, SRD5A1 and SRD5A2. The genes encoding SRD5A1 and SRD5A2 have been mapped to chromosome 5(5p15) and chromosome 2 (2p23), respectively. The SRD5A1 isozyme is mainly expressed in skin during puberty, but recently has been shown to be expressed in genital fibroblasts (182). SRD5A2 isozyme is the only isozyme expressed during embryogenesis and is predominantly expressed in the genital skin tissue, male accessory sex organs, and prostate (183). The SRD5A2 enzyme levels decrease during childhood but increase during puberty. Defects in 5α-R2 (gene SR5A2) isozyme result in undervirilization of male external genitalia, differentiated Wolffian ducts, which terminate in a blind vaginal pouch, absent Müllerian structures, and a hypoplastic prostate (184–186). Testicular and adrenal androgen synthesis is unaffected.

Clinical Presentation Affected 46,XY infants present with various degree of under virilization and ambiguous genitalia, ranging from isolated glandular hypospadias to the most common presentation of perineal hypospadias with a blind perineal pouch (pseudovaginal perineoscrotal hypospadias), micropenis bound by chordee and bifid scrotum (187). 46,XY patients have complete Wolffian duct differentiation but absent uterus or other Müllerian derivatives (see Figure 35-10). At puberty, they develop male habitus, deepening of the voice, excellent muscular growth, and penile enlargement, yet they have a char-

acteristically scanty beard. They also have a rudimentary prostate and underdeveloped seminal vesicles. Semen is highly viscous, ejaculate volume is extremely low (<0.5–1 mL), but sperm counts may be normal. The ones who were not diagnosed at birth may present as phenotypic females with amenorrhea, complaints of deepening voice, increased musculature, and clitoromegaly. Unlike 17β-HSD3 deficiency and androgen insensitivity syndrome, they do not develop gynecomastia during puberty. 46,XX females with SRD5A2 deficiency have normal sexual differentiation, delayed puberty, sparse sexual hair, and normal fertility.

Diagnosis During early infancy and puberty testosterone levels increase and the diagnosis of SRD5A2 deficiency can be made based on an elevated ratio of testosterone to DHT (normal < 30:1), either with or without β-hCG stimulation (185,188). An β-hCG stimulation test may be required either during childhood, when the hypothalamic-pituitary-gonadal axis is inactive, or during adolescence to elicit the abnormally elevated DHT to testosterone ratio. DHT is low in infants but can reach near-normal levels during adolescence without treatment, presumably by peripheral SRD5A1 activity. Testosterone and estrogen levels are normal and explain the lack of gynecomastia. FSH and LH levels are normal. Urinary 5α steroid metabolites of both C21 and C19 (androgens) are low. Affected females although phenotypically normal have the same biochemical abnormalities as affected males.

Mutational analysis of the SR5A2 gene can be performed, and mutations have been reported in all five exons. To date, over 50 mutations in SR5A2 have been found, ranging from point mutations to deletions. There is poor genotype–phenotype correlation.

Treatment Most of XY patients with SR5A2 deficiency who were raised as females revert to male gender at puberty (189–191). It is not clear why there is such a high prevalence of change in gender identity in this disorder. Because this disorder has been described in consanguineous families in the Dominican Republic, Turkey, New Guinea, and Saudi Arabia, cultural and societal reasons may have an important role. Topical DHT cream application above the pubic area (25–50 mg daily), promotes phallic growth prior to puberty. Treatment can continue for several months until desired results are achieved. Facial and body hair may increase with topical DHT treatment. Corrective surgeries may include orchidopexy and external genitalia reconstruction to correspond with the chosen gender. Fertility is not possible without surgical correction because the sperm ducts end blindly in the vaginal pouch.

Complete and Partial Androgen Insensitivity Syndrome

Etiology and Pathophysiology Androgen insensitivity syndrome (AIS) is an X-linked disorder of male sexual differentiation caused by mutations affecting the androgen receptor (AR) gene resulting in decreased peripheral responsiveness to circulating androgens. AR is a member of the nuclear receptor superfamily of transcription factors and possesses distinct functional domains. AR is activated by testosterone and (preferentially) by DHT. Its function is essential for sexual differentiation and maintenance of normal spermatogenesis in males. Over 300 mutations have been identified worldwide (database at http://www.androgendb.mcgill.ca), which decrease the ligand-binding domain affinity for DHT, prevent homodimer formation, or disrupt the DNA-binding domain. The incidence of AIS is approximately 1:20,400 liveborn XY individuals.

AIS is characterized by various degrees of undervirilization of XY individuals. The least severe form, called minimal AIS (MAIS), is found in phenotypic XY males with the only manifestation being infertility, gynecomastia, or hypospadias (192,193). On the opposite end of the spectrum is complete AIS (CAIS), which refers to XY phenotypic females. Between these two extremes exists variable degrees of feminized or ambiguous XY genitalia, referred to as partial AIS (PAIS).

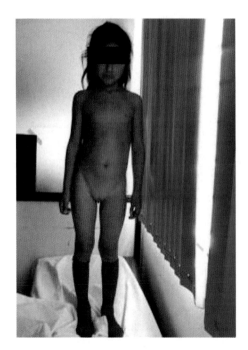
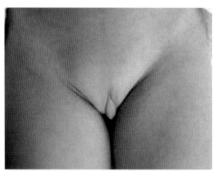
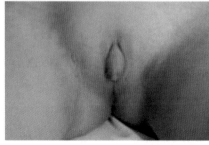

FIGURE 35-10. Patient with 5α reductase deficiency. Patient is prepubertal and was raised as a girl. Photograph courtesy of Dr. Gloria Queipo. Hospital General de Mexico.

All known forms of AIS are caused by disruption of the androgen receptor activity. There is little correlation between the level of residual AR activity and degree of AIS (194), but CAIS is generally associated with a complete absence of androgen binding and AR activation. This suggests that factors other than the AR mutations, such as genetic background and interactions of AR with coactivators or promoters, influence tissue response to androgens and the resultant phenotype.

Mutations causing AIS are equally spread throughout the AR ORF with not one defect particularly prevalent, although hotspots do exist (195). Of note, exon 1 rarely possesses a causative mutation (195). Single amino acid substitutions account for 90% of reported cases. The majority of cases are inherited, but 30% of all AIS cases are de novo mutations. The majority of de novo mutations originate in the mother in a single germ cell or as germ cell mosaicism and the recurrence risk seems to be very low.

In familial PAIS and in both familial and sporadic CAIS, mutations in AR exonic sequences are found in 85% to 90% of cases (195,196). In contrast, detectable mutations in AR account for only 10% to 15% of sporadic cases with hormonal profile and clinical presentation suggestive of PAIS (196). Although the genotypes causing CAIS are consistent in phenotypic presentation, in PAIS there is phenotypic variability among affected individuals carrying the same mutation.

Clinical Presentation The phenotype of patients with PAIS is extremely heterogenous. Patients present in infancy or childhood with variable degrees of virilization such as micropenis, cryptorchidism, and perineoscrotal hypospadias. Infants and children may present with unilateral or bilateral inguinal hernias. Wolffian derivative development is dependent on the degree of AR activity. Prostate is usually absent. Testes are present and functional, producing high levels of testosterone and AMH. Uterus and fallopian tubes are usually absent, but partial persistence of Müllerian structures has been reported (197). In patients presenting at puberty, breast development and sparse pubic hair are suggestive of PAIS, and help differentiate it from 5α-R2 deficiency.

CAIS presents at puberty with primary amenorrhea. Examination reveals a short, blind vagina and absent uterus. Inguinal or labial testes may be palpable. Wolffian derivatives and prostate are absent or vestigial because their development is testosterone dependent. Height, bone maturation, and breast development are normal, but pubic and axillary hair, an androgen-mediated feature, are absent or sparse. Patients' identity and behavior is feminine. Less commonly, CAIS may present in infancy with phenotypic female genitalia and inguinal or labial masses representing testes.

MAIS is considered in phenotypic XY males with infertility or gynecomastia, but normal male genitalia.

Diagnosis Postnatal testosterone and LH surge occurs in neonates with PAIS but is absent in those with CAIS, suggesting that postnatal testosterone rise requires the receptivity of the hypothalamo-pituitary axis to testosterone (198). Normal 17-OHP levels and normal androgen levels differentiates AIS from lipoid adrenal hyperplasia or CAH due to 17-hydroxylase/17,20 lyase or 3βHSD2 deficiency. In prepubertal children, basal LH and testosterone may be normal, but β-hCG stimulation elicits an exaggerated androgen response (a tripling instead of a doubling of testosterone and DHT). DHT and Δ4A levels should be measured in all patients in whom AIS is suspected to compare hormone ratios, and differentiate PAIS from defects in 17βHSD3 and 5α-R2 deficiencies. AMH levels are normal to elevated. Examination and pelvic ultrasound reveals absence of uterus and fallopian tubes, and abdominal testes.

Historically, residual AR function has been used to aid in the diagnosis of AIS; however, AR ligand-binding and saturation vary greatly between laboratories and between sites of skin biopsy. Fibroblasts obtained from nongenital skin show significantly different androgen binding and activation of AR when compared to perineoscrotal skin, limiting the usefulness of these assays (199).

PCR-based sequencing of AR exons 2 to 10 can be routinely performed, as well as sequencing of the much longer exon 1, and some intronic and promoter regions (199). Prenatal testing by mutation analysis is available for families in which the AIS-causing allele has been identified in an affected family member. Molecular genetic testing of the AR gene detects mutations in more than 95% of probands with CAIS.

Management PAIS patients present with issues similar to other XY patients with ambiguous genitalia. The relative prevalence and good characterization of AIS allows for some improved prognostic predictors for this condition, but wide variability exists. In PAIS and CAIS patients who choose to be raised as female, gonadectomy can be performed to reduce testicular tumor risk. Frequently, this gonadectomy occurs during repair of an inguinal hernia in a phenotypic female. This will, however, remove a source of endogenous estrogens, and XY female patients lacking testes must receive supplemental estrogens to promote female sexual development, normal bone maturation, and bone accrual. Rarely, mutation of the AR may occur at the postzygotic stage of the affected offspring, causing somatic mosaicism and increasing the chance of virilization during puberty due to coexistence of both a mutant and a wild-type AR (204).

In less severely affected PAIS patients, a male gender of rearing may be chosen. These patients generally show good response to androgen supplementation initiated at puberty. In infants, treatment with testosterone (intramuscular testosterone heptylate 50 mg monthly) for 3 months can be used therapeutically as well as diagnostically to assess degree of insensitivity. A positive response is increased penile length (>2.5 cm), scrotal development, or pubic hair formation (For a chart of penile lengths in normal males see Table 35-1). This does not rule out a milder degree of insensitivity, however. Orchidopexy should be performed for patients whose testes remain undescended to reduce tumor risk.

Approximately 70% of mothers carry the AR mutation, and should be counseled regarding their 50% chance of transmitting the trait to their XY offspring (195). Phenotype can vary within familial cases between PAIS and CAIS (195,197).

Other Conditions Associated with AR Mutations Exon 1 of AR contains a polymorphic number of CAG repeats. Fully fertile XY males possess 11 to 35 repeats, with an average among western males of 21 ± 2 repeats (195). There is an inverse correlation in vitro between number of CAG repeats and AR function. African Americans have an increased prevalence of alleles with few CAG repeats (<22), and are at higher risk for prostate cancer than are Asian males, where these alleles are less common (200). Also, increasing CAG repeats are associated with impaired rates of spermatogenesis reminiscent of MAIS patients (201–203), and patients possessing more than 28 repeats have a fourfold higher risk for impaired spermatogenesis (202).

The neurodegenerative condition spinal and bulbar muscular atrophy (also referred to as Kennedy's disease) often presents with gynecomastia and hypofertility in association with progressive muscle weakness and atrophy in the third through fifth decade of life (205–206). The condition maps to Xq12-21, and all reported patients possess an expanded AR exon 1 with 38 to 75 CAG repeats instead of the usual 11–35, with severity correlating with repeat number. Androgens are implicated in motor neuron development, but the relationship between spinal and bulbar muscular atrophy and increased AR CAG repeat numbers is unknown. AIS alone is not associated with neuron degeneration.

ADRENAL AND NONADRENAL VIRILIZING DISORDERS

Etiology and Presentation of Virilizing Disorders

Fetal external genitalia are bipotential, and XX fetuses will develop male external genitalia if exposed to excess intrauterine androgens or androgen precursors. The genitalia of virilized XX infants at birth include clitoromegaly, "scrotalization" of the labia, urogenital sinus and phallic urethra. Virilizing disorders of infancy can present with evidence of maternal androgen excess, and mothers may have variable degrees of hirsutism and acne as pregnancy progresses.

The most common cause of genital ambiguity in newborns is virilizing forms of CAH (81). Other causes of androgen excess leading to masculinization of XX individuals include P450 aromatase deficiency, maternal androgen intake, and androgenic tumors in pregnant mothers (e.g., luteoma).

Recent formulations of oral contraceptives no longer routinely use highly androgenic progestins (207–209), and maternal ingestion of androgens or progestins as a cause of XX virilization is rare. Luteomas and related tumors are also uncommon causes of maternal virilization and ambiguous genitalia in an XX baby (210). A bilateral cystic ovarian condition termed hyperreactio luteinalis is associated with virilization in 15% of cases (210), but overall is a very infrequent cause of XX masculinization. Despite the relative infrequency relative to CAH, iatrogenic and oncologic causes should always be considered in the differential diagnosis of maternal/fetal virilization.

Congenital Adrenal Hyperplasia

P450c21 (gene CYP21) deficiency accounts for over 90% of CAH, and represents the most common etiology of ambiguous genitalia in newborns. Mutations in 11β-hydroxylase (gene CYP11B1) account for another 5% of virilizing CAH. Defects in 3βHSD gene II is a rare cause of masculinization of XX infants and P450 oxidoreductase defects cause maternal and XX infant virilization that does not progress beyond infancy (for more details see Chapter 27).

P450 Aromatase Deficiency

Aromatase (gene CYP19A1), or estrogen synthetase, is a cytochrome P450 enzyme which catalyzes the formation of C18 estrogens from C19 androgens. Mutations in aromatase cause impairment of estrogen synthesis in both sexes. The initial manifestation of aromatase deficiency is placental, with maternal virilization

(211–213). Urine from these mothers has elevated levels of 16α-hydroxyandrostenedione (16OH-Δ4A) and its metabolites. XX fetuses are born with ambiguous genitalia, normal Müllerian structures, and normal ovaries. Serum FSH, LH, testosterone, and Δ4A levels are high, whereas E_1 and E_2 are low or undetectable. CAH due to 21OHD, 11OHD and 3-βHSDII is the major differential considered, and normal basal and ACTH-stimulated levels of adrenal hormones confirm a non-adrenal source of androgen excess.

At puberty, XX patients demonstrate amenorrhea, no breast development, progressive virilization, and polycystic ovaries (211,214–215). XY males experience normal puberty, but are sterile, reflecting the requirement of estrogen for spermatogenesis (213,216–217). Both XX and XY patients have linear growth throughout childhood and into adulthood (without a growth spurt) and are tall. Bone age is delayed and osteoporosis develops early (213,218). Patients often complain of bone pain (213).

Management of Virilized Patients with Aromatase Deficiency

In aromatase deficient XX individuals, virilization does not progress post-natally, but does recur during puberty (211,214–215). Estrogen replacement therapy starting at low doses, usually starting age 12–14 (see Chapter 36) promotes secondary sex characteristics and resolution of ovarian cysts. In both XX and XY patients, estrogen treatment promotes bone maturation and allows epiphyseal closure (211,213).

DISORDERS OF SEX ORGANS NOT OTHERWISE CLASSIFIED

Testicular Regression Syndrome

Failure of testes to develop properly leads to inadequate AMH and testosterone secretion and results in complete or partial GD, and variable degrees of feminization of both internal and external genitalia. Testicular regression syndrome (TRS), is a distinct but related entity occurring subsequent to initial testes development (219–221). Müllerian and Wolffian structures, and external genitalia, are variably developed depending on when the insult to the fetal testes occurred (219–220,222–223). Uncommonly, patients can present in adulthood as females with primary amenorrhea (222–223). Typically, however, TRS is characterized by primitive epididymis and spermatic cord in the absence of testicular tissue (220–221,224). The presence of spermatic cord structures, the absence of Müllerian derivatives, and normal male ex-

ternal phenotype suggest viable testes existed early in development, and imply a late-fetal early neonatal regression. This variant in the spectrum is sometimes known in the literature as "vanishing testes" (220).

The incidence of TRS has been estimated at 5% of males presenting with cryptorchidism (221), and as high as 12% of cryptorchid patients older than 1 year (221,225). Correct diagnosis is essential because of significant malignant potential of abdominal or dysgenic testes. Imaging including magnetic resonance, usually fails to detect any abdominal or inguinal structure consistent with a gonad. Laparoscopic exploration is frequently necessary and is the gold standard for diagnosis (226). Prior to surgery, measurement of basal and β-hCG-stimulated testosterone and DHT levels can be helpful in identifying functional Leydig cells. Serum AMH or inhibin B can similarly be used to identify Sertoli cells. During laparoscopy either a fibrous nodule is found (not a streak or dysgenetic gonad) at the end of the spermatic cord, or there is a complete absence of identifiable testis. Patients with TRS or "vanishing testes" are adequately virilized in utero, and appear and identify as male children.

Persistent Müllerian Duct Syndrome

Mutant AMH or AMH receptor type II in XY individuals cause a rare condition of mixed internal genitalia called persistent Müllerian duct syndrome (PMDS). Testicular AMH, a member of the transforming growth factor β (TGFβ) family of signaling proteins, causes the regression of Müllerian derivatives in the developing fetus between gestational weeks 10 and 12, after which the Müllerian ducts lose responsiveness to AMH signaling. TGFβ family members signal through two membrane-bound serine/threonine kinase receptors, designated I and II. The type II receptor binds the ligand on its own, and recruits the type I receptor. The AMH receptor type II is located on the mesenchyme of Müllerian ducts.

XY patients with PMDS have typical male external genitalia, but possess both uterus and fallopian tubes in addition to Wolffian derivatives. It is differentiated from mixed GD, which usually possesses a 45,X/46,XY karyotype with Müllerian structures ipsilateral to the streak gonad. Mutations in the AMH and AMHR2 have been implicated in 85% of PMDS cases in approximately equal proportions (227–228). Inheritance is autosomal recessive for both loci.

Boys present with cryptorchidism (20%) or with an inguinal hernia (229) containing Müllerian structures and normal virilization (227,230). Often the diagnosis of PMDS has been made incidentally during surgical exploration or imaging during evaluation of an abdominal mass (231). The incidence of testicular neoplasm in PMDS is 18%, mostly seminomas (232), corresponding to the increased tumor risk of abdominal testes.

Mayer-Rokitansky-Küster-Hauser Syndrome

The Mayer-Rokitansky-Küster-Hauser Syndrome (MRKHS) syndrome is characterized by congenital absence of the vagina, rudimentary uterus, normal ovaries, and fallopian tubes and normal female secondary sexual characteristics. The incidence is estimated at 1:5,000 females, and is thought to be the second most common cause of primary amenorrhea after ovarian dysgenesis (233). No mutations in either AMH or AMHR2 have been found in any reported cases and he etiology remains unknown (234–235). Most cases are sporadic, but familial aggregates have been reported (236–238), suggesting a genetic basis for MRKHS. The syndrome is variably associated with renal anomalies (unilateral renal aplasia, pelvic kidney, and horseshoe kidney) and spinal dysplasias (cervicothoracic somite dysplasia, scoliosis [237,239]). It has also been rarely associated with ovarian agenesis (240–245). The MURCS syndrome of Müllerian agenesis, renal aplasia, and skeletal anomalies occurs in approximately one-third of all MRKH patients (239). Affected females have normal FSH, LH levels, normal ovarian steroid production and ovulation.

46,XX Gonadal Dysgenesis

The majority of cases of ovarian dysgenesis involve abnormal complements of X chromosomes in phenotypic females (246). The most common of these is Turner syndrome (see Chapter 31) 46,XX GD, can occur as either an isolated entity or as part of a syndrome. Females possess normal female genitalia at birth, but remain sexually infantile and do not experience normal puberty. Ovarian failure with hypergonadotropic hypogonadism at puberty is highly suggestive of ovarian dysgenesis. Müllerian structures are normal, and gonadal histology reveals bilateral streaks. Patients present with amenorrhea and infertility and without the somatic stigmata characteristic of Turner syndrome.

Several studies in familial ovarian dysgenesis have noted the frequent reports of consanguinity, suggesting that isolated 46,XX GD is inherited as an autosomal recessive condition (247–250). Mutations in the gene for FSH receptor (gene FSHR, 2p16) have been implicated in some cases (249,251), but does not explain the phenotype in all populations studied (252–253). The molecular basis

TABLE 35-2	Stretched Penile Length (cm) in Normal Males		
		Mean ± SD	Mean −2.5 SD
Newborn: 25 wk		1.8 ± 0.4*	0.8
30 wk		2.5 ± 0.4**	1.5
34 wk		3.0 ± 0.4**	2.0
term		3.5 ± 0.4**,***	2.5;2.4
0–5 mo		3.9 ± 0.8	1.9
6–12 mo		4.3 ± 0.8	2.3
1–2 y		4.7 ± 0.8	2.6
2–3 y		5.1 ± 0.9	2.9
3–4 y		5.5 ± 0.9	3.3
4–5 y		5.7 ± 0.9	3.5
5–6 y		6.0 ± 0.9	3.8
6–7 y		6.1 ± 0.9	3.9
7–8 y		6.2 ± 1.0	3.7
8–9 y		6.3 ± 1.0	3.8
9–10 y		6.3 ± 1.0	3.8
10–11 y		6.4 ± 1.1	3.7
Adult		13.3 ± 1.6	9.3

*From Tuladhar R et al. 1998
**From Feldman and Smith, 1975
***From Flatau et al. 1975
Other data from Schonfeld and Beebe, 1942.

for 46,XX GD remains unknown for the majority of patients.

The blepharophimosis-ptosis-epicanthus inversus syndrome, caused by a mutation in the forkhead transcription factor gene FOXL2 (254–255), is the best characterized form of syndromic 46,XX GD. Molecular studies in mice implicate disruption of Foxl2 activity with failure of follicle maturation (256–257). Less understood forms of ovarian dysgenesis are associated with dwarfism and arachnodactyly (258), epibulbar dermoid (259), recurrent metabolic acidosis (260), and cerebellar ataxia and sensorineural deafness (261–264).

Aphallia and Cloacal Extrophy

Cloacal extrophy and aphallia, are extremely rare failures of urologic development that have historically resulted in female gender assignment to otherwise normal XY males with functional testes (265–266).

Cloacal extrophy represents a failure of proper midline structure formation and is considered a developmental field defect (267). The phenotype is bladder extrophy protruding into an anomalous cloacal structure located where genitalia and an anus would normally be expected. Other midline defects, such as omphalocele and imperforate anus are frequently associated. In XY males, a proper phallus does not form, but

the patient possess two hemipeniscs located laterally to the cloaca. There is no urethra, and the bladder empties via a vesicocutaneous or vesicorectal fistula (267). Traditionally, XX and XY patients underwent vaginal construction and were raised as females, with significant subsequent rejection by the XY individuals of their gender (266,268). The two "phallic" hemipenis structures are responsive to androgens, and can enlarge when treated with testosterone. Recently, there has been a move to raise these patients as males (269), and multistage operations to correct the deformity and construct a penis have been attempted in select XY males.

Aphallia is a very rare condition of congenital absence of the phallus and corporal tissue (265). XY patients possess functional bilateral testes and are otherwise normally virilized. The bladder empties via a very short urethra either anterior to, into, or posterior to the anal sphincter muscles via a vesicorectal fistula (265,270). Anteriorly displaced urethras are less associated with other urogenital anomalies, and these patients have the best mortality rates (265). Aphallic XY patients commonly undergo vaginoplasty and orchidectomy and are raised female. Recently, many have questioned the validity of assigning female gender to otherwise normal masculine patients (266,268,270), and such patients are increasingly being raised male, with genital reconstructions planned prepuberty.

REFERENCES

1. Lee PA, Houk CP, Ahmed SF, et al. International Consensus Conference on Intersex organized by the Lawson Wilkins Pediatric Endocrine Society and the European Society for Paediatric Endocrinology. Consensus statement on management of intersex disorders. *Pediatrics*. 2006;118(2):e488–500.

2. Cotinot C, Pailhoux E, Jaubert F, et al. Molecular genetics of sex determination. *Semin Reprod Med*. 2002;20:157–168.

3. Migeon CJ, Wisniewski AB. Human sex differentiation and its abnormalities. *Best Pract Res Clin Obstet Gynaecol*. 2003;17:1–18.

4. Fleming A, Vilain E. The endless quest for sex determination genes. *Clin Genet*. 2005;67: 15–25.

5. Yao HH, Tilmann C, Zhao GQ, et al. The battle of the sexes: opposing pathways in sex determination. *Novartis Found Symp*. 2002;244: 187–198, discussion 98–206, 53–57.

6. Guo JK, Hammes A, Chaboissier MC, et al. Early gonadal development: exploring Wt1 and Sox9 function. *Novartis Found Symp*. 2002;244: 23–31, discussion 42, 253–257.

7. Nef S, Verma-Kurvari S, Merenmies J, et al. Testis determination requires insulin receptor family function in mice. *Nature*. 2003;426:291–295.

8. Birk OS, Casiano DE, Wassif CA, et al. The LIM homeobox gene Lhx9 is essential for mouse gonad formation. *Nature*. 2000;403:909–913.

9. Ottolenghi C, Moreira-Filho C, Mendonca BB, et al. Absence of mutations involving the LIM homeobox domain gene LHX9 in 46,XY gonadal agenesis and dysgenesis. *J Clin Endocrinol Metab*. 2001;86: 2465–2469.

10. Koopman P, Munsterberg A, Capel B, et al. Expression of a candidate sex-determining gene during mouse testis differentiation. *Nature*. 1990;348: 450–452.

11. Sinclair AH, Berta P, Palmer MS, et al. A gene from the human sex-determining region encodes a protein with homology to a conserved DNA-binding motif. *Nature*. 1990;346.240–244.

12. Berta P, Hawkins JR, Sinclair AH, et al. Genetic evidence equating SRY and the testis-determining factor. *Nature*. 1990;348: 448–450.

13. Koopman P, Gubbay J, Vivian N, et al. Male development of chromosomally female mice transgenic for Sry. *Nature*. 1991;351:117–121.

14. Tevosian SG, Albrecht KH, Crispino JD, et al. Gonadal differentiation, sex determination and normal Sry expression in mice require direct interaction between transcription partners GATA4 and FOG2. *Development*. 2002;129:4627–4634.

15. Josso N, Lamarre I, Picard JY, et al. Anti-Müllerian hormone in early human development. *Early Hum Dev*. 1993;33:91–99.

16. Rajpert-De Meyts E, Jorgensen N, Graem N, et al. Expression of anti-Müllerian hormone during normal and pathological gonadal development: association with differentiation of Sertoli and granulosa cells. *J Clin Endocrinol Metab*. 1999;84:3836–3844.

17. Colvin JS, Green RP, Schmahl J, et al. Male-to-female sex reversal in mice lacking fibroblast growth factor 9. *Cell*. 2001;104:875–889.

18. Schmahl J, Kim Y, Colvin JS, et al. Fgf9 induces proliferation and nuclear localization of FGFR2 in Sertoli precursors during male sex determination. *Development*. 2004;131:3627–3636.

19. Muscatelli F, Strom TM, Walker AP, et al. Mutations in the DAX-1 gene give rise to both X-linked adrenal hypoplasia congenita and hypogonadotropic hypogonadism. *Nature*. 1994;372:672–676.

20. Clark AM, Garland KK, Russell LD. Desert hedgehog (Dhh) gene is required in the mouse testis for formation of adult-type Leydig cells and normal development of peritubular cells and seminiferous tubules. *Biol Reprod*. 2000;63:182518–38.

21. Yao HH, Whoriskey W, Capel B. Desert Hedgehog/Patched 1 signaling specifies fetal Leydig cell fate in testis organogenesis. *Genes Dev*. 2002;16:1433–1440.

22. McClive PJ, Hurley TM, Sarraj MA, et al. Subtractive hybridisation screen identifies sexually dimorphic gene expression in the embryonic mouse gonad. *Genesis*. 2003;37:84–90.

23. Menke DB, Page DC. Sexually dimorphic gene expression in the developing mouse gonad. *Gene Expr Patterns*. 2002;2:359–367.

24. Yao HH, Matzuk MM, Jorgez CJ, et al. Follistatin operates downstream of Wnt4 in mammalian ovary organogenesis. *Dev Dyn*. 2004;230:210–215.

25. Jost A. Problems of fetal endocrinology: the gonadal and hypophyseal hormones. *Recent Prog Horm Res*. 1953;8:379–418.

26. Haber DA, Sohn RL, Buckler AJ, et al. Alternative splicing and genomic structure of the Wilms tumor gene WT1. *Proc Natl Acad Sci USA*. 1991;88:9618–9624.

27. Barbaux S, Niaudet P, Gubler MC, et al. Donor splice-site mutations in WT1 are responsible for Frasier syndrome. *Nat Genet*. 1997;17:467–470.

28. Neri G, Opitz J. Syndromal (and nonsyndromal) forms of male pseudohermaphroditism. *Am J Med Genet*. 1999;89:201–209.

29. Saylam K, Simon P. WT1 gene mutation responsible for male sex reversal and renal failure: the Frasier syndrome. *Eur J Obstet Gynecol Reprod Biol*. 2003;110:111–113.

30. Hossain A, Saunders GF. The human sex-determining gene SRY is a direct target of WT1. *J Biol Chem*. 2001;276:16817–16823.

31. Hossain A, Saunders GF. Role of Wilms tumor 1 (WT1) in the transcriptional regulation of the Müllerian-inhibiting substance promoter. *Biol Reprod*. 2003;69:1808–1814.

32. Nachtigal MW, Hirokawa Y, Enyeart-VanHouten DL, et al. Wilms' tumor 1 and Dax-1 modulate the orphan nuclear receptor SF-1 in sex-specific gene expression. *Cell*. 1998;93:445–454.

33. Klamt B, Koziell A, Poulat F, et al. Frasier syndrome is caused by defective alternative splicing of WT1 leading to an altered ratio of WT1 1/-KTS splice isoforms. *Hum Mol Genet*. 1998;7:709–714.

34. Bardoni B, Zanaria E, Guioli S, et al. A dosage sensitive locus at chromosome Xp21 is involved in male to female sex reversal. *Nat Genet*. 1994;7:497–501.

35. Zanaria E, Bardoni B, Dabovic B, et al. Xp duplications and sex reversal. *Philos Trans R Soc Lond B Biol Sci*. 1995;350:291–296.

36. Dabovic B, Zanaria E, Bardoni B, et al. A family of rapidly evolving genes from the sex reversal critical region in Xp21. *Mamm Genome*. 1995;6:571–580.

37. Baumstark A, Barbi G, Djalali M, et al. Just W. Xp-duplications with and without sex reversal. *Hum Genet*. 1996;97:79–86.

38. Iyer AK, McCabe ER. Molecular mechanisms of DAX1 action. *Mol Genet Metab*. 2004;83:60–73.

39. Ozisik G, Mantovani G, Achermann JC, et al. An alternate translation initiation site circumvents an amino-terminal DAX1 nonsense mutation leading to a mild form of X-linked adrenal hypoplasia congenita. *J Clin Endocrinol Metab*. 2003;88:417–423.

40. Merke DP, Tajima T, Baron J, et al. Hypogonadotropic hypogonadism in a female caused by an X-linked recessive mutation in the DAX1 gene. *N Engl J Med*. 1999;340:1248–1252.

41. Capel B. Sex in the 90s: SRY and the switch to the male pathway. *Annu Rev Physiol*. 1998;60:497–523.

42. Jordan BK, Mohammed M, Ching ST, et al. Up-regulation of WNT-4 signaling and dosage-sensitive sex reversal in humans. *Am J Hum Genet*. 2001;68:1102–1109.

43. Hossain A, Li C, Saunders GF. Generation of two distinct functional isoforms of dosage-sensitive sex reversal-adrenal hypoplasia congenita-critical region on the X chromosome gene 1 (DAX-1) by alternative splicing. *Mol Endocrinol*. 2004;18:1428–1437.

44. Ozisik G, Achermann JC, Jameson JL. The role of SF1 in adrenal and reproductive function: insight from naturally occurring mutations in humans. *Mol Genet Metab*. 2002;76:85–91.

45. Tremblay JJ, Viger RS. A mutated form of steroidogenic factor 1 (SF-1 G35E) that causes sex reversal in humans fails to synergize with transcription factor GATA-4. *J Biol Chem*. 2003;278:42637–42642.

46. Achermann JC, Ito M, Hindmarsh PC, et al. A mutation in the gene encoding steroidogenic factor-1 causes XY sex reversal and adrenal failure in humans. *Nat Genet*. 1999;22:125–126.

47. Achermann JC, Ozisik G, Ito M, et al. Gonadal determination and adrenal development are regulated by the orphan nuclear receptor steroidogenic factor-1, in a dose-dependent manner. *J Clin Endocrinol Metab*. 2002;87:1829–1833.

48. Correa RV, Domenice S, Bingham NC, et al. A microdeletion in the ligand binding domain of human steroidogenic factor 1 causes XY sex reversal without adrenal insufficiency. *J Clin Endocrinol Metab*. 2004;89:1767–1772.

49. Mallet D, Bretones P, Michel-Calemard L, et al. Gonadal dysgenesis without adrenal

insufficiency in a 46,XY patient heterozygous for the nonsense C16X mutation: a case of SF1 haploinsufficiency. *J Clin Endocrinol Metab*. 2004;89:4829–4832.

50. Lin L, Philibert P, Ferraz-de-Souza B, et al. Heterozygous missense mutations in steroidogenic factor 1 (SF1/Ad4BP, NR5A1) are associated with 46,XY disorders of sex development with normal adrenal function. *J Clin Endocr Metab*. 2007;92: 991–999.

51. Biason-Lauber A, Schoenle EJ. Apparently normal ovarian differentiation in a prepubertal girl with transcriptionally inactive steroidogenic factor 1 (NR5A1/SF-1) and adrenocortical insufficiency. *Am J Hum Genet*. 2000);7:1563–1568.

52. Clarkson MJ, Harley VR. Sex with two SOX on: SRY and SOX9 in testis development. *Trends Endocrinol Metab*. 2002;13:106–111.

53. Harley VR, Clarkson MJ, Argentaro A. The molecular action and regulation of the testis-determining factors, SRY (sex-determining region on the Y chromosome) and SOX9 [SRY-related high-mobility group (HMG) box 9]. *Endocr Rev*. 2003;24:466–487.

54. Huang B, Wang S, Ning Y, et al. Autosomal XX sex reversal caused by duplication of SOX9. *Am J Med Genet*. 1999;87:349–353.

55. Bernard P, Tang P, Liu S, et al. Dimerization of SOX9 is required for chondrogenesis, but not for sex determination. *Hum Mol Genet*. 2003;12:1755–1765.

56. Moog U, Jansen NJ, Scherer G, et al. Acampomelic campomelic syndrome. *Am J Med Genet*. 2001;104: 239–245.

57. Pierucci-Alves F, Clark AM, Russell LD. A developmental study of the Desert hedgehog-null mouse testis. *Biol Reprod*. (2001) 65: 1392–402.

58. Bitgood MJ, Shen L, McMahon AP. Sertoli cell signaling by Desert hedgehog regulates the male germline. *Curr Biol*. 1996:6: 298–304.

59. Parmantier E, Lynn B, Lawson D, et al. Schwann cell-derived Desert hedgehog controls the development of peripheral nerve sheaths. *Neuron*. (1999) 23:713–24.

60. Umehara F, Tate G, Itoh K, et al. A novel mutation of desert hedgehog in a patient with 46,XY partial GD accompanied by minifascicular neuropathy. *Am J Hum Genet*. 2000;67:1302–1305.

61. Canto P, Soderlund D, Reyes E, et al. Mutations in the desert hedgehog (DHH) gene in patients with 46,XY complete pure gonadal dysgenesis. *J Clin Endocrinol Metab*. 2004;89: 4480–4483.

62. Veitia R, Nunes M, Brauner R, et al. Deletions of distal 9p associated with 46,XY male to female sex reversal: definition of the breakpoints at 9p23.3-p24.1. *Genomics*. 1997;41:271–274.

63. Muroya K, Okuyama T, Goishi K, et al. Sex-determining gene(s) on distal 9p: clinical and molecular studies in six cases. *J Clin Endocrinol Metab*. 2000;85:3094–3100.

64. Ounap K, Uibo O, Zordania R, et al. Three patients with 9p deletions including DMRT1 and DMRT2: a girl with XY complement, bilateral ovotestes, and extreme growth retardation, and two XX females

with normal pubertal development. *Am J Med Genet*. 2004;130:415–423.

65. Raymond CS, Shamu CE, Shen MM, et al. Evidence for evolutionary conservation of sex-determining genes. *Nature*. 1998;391:691–695.

66. Raymond CS, Parker ED, Kettlewell JR, et al. A region of human chromosome 9p required for testis development contains two genes related to known sexual regulators. *Hum Mol Genet*. 1999;8:989–996.

67. Meng A, Moore B, Tang H, et al. A Drosophila doublesex-related gene, terra, is involved in somitogenesis in vertebrates. *Development*. 1999;126:1259–1268.

68. Ottolenghi C, Veitia R, Barbieri M, et al. The human doublesex-related gene, DMRT2, is homologous to a gene involved in somitogenesis and encodes a potential bicistronic transcript. *Genomics*. 2000;64:179–186.

69. Kim S, Kettlewell JR, Anderson RC, et al. Sexually dimorphic expression of multiple doublesex-related genes in the embryonic mouse gonad. *Gene Expr Patterns*. 2003;3:77–82.

70. Smith CA, Hurley TM, McClive PJ, et al. Restricted expression of DMRT3 in chicken and mouse embryos. *Mech Dev*. 2002;119 Suppl 1:S73–76.

71. Calvari V, Bertini V, de Grandi A, et al. A new submicroscopic deletion that refines the 9p region for sex reversal. *Genomics*. 2000;65:203–212.

72. Gibbons RJ, Picketts DJ, Villard L, et al. Mutations in a putative global transcriptional regulator cause X-linked mental retardation with alpha-thalassemia (ATR-X syndrome). *Cell*. 1995;80:837–845.

73. McDowell TL, Gibbons RJ, Sutherland H, et al. Localization of a putative transcriptional regulator (ATRX) at pericentromeric heterochromatin and the short arms of acrocentric chromosomes. *Proc Natl Acad Sci USA*. 1999;96:13983–1398.

74. Cardoso C, Lutz Y, Mignon C, et al. ATR-X mutations cause impaired nuclear location and altered DNA binding properties of the XNP/ATR-X protein. *J Med Genet*. 2000;37:746–751.

75. Reardon W, Gibbons RJ, Winter RM, et al. Male pseudohermaphroditism in sibs with the alpha-thalassemia/mental retardation (ATR-X) syndrome. *Am J Med Genet*. 1995;55:285–287.

76. Ion A, Telvi L, Chaussain JL, et al. A novel mutation in the putative DNA helicase XH2 is responsible for male-to-female sex reversal associated with an atypical form of the ATR-X syndrome. *Am J Hum Genet*. 1996;58:1185–1191.

77. Wada T, Sugie H, Fukushima Y, et al. Non-skewed X-inactivation may cause mental retardation in a female carrier of X-linked alpha-thalassemia/mental retardation syndrome (ATR-X): X-inactivation study of nine female carriers of ATR-X. *Am J Med Genet*. 2005;138:18–20.

78. Domenice S, Correa RV, Costa EM, et al. Mutations in the SRY, DAX1, SF1 and WNT4 genes in Brazilian sex-reversed patients. *Braz J Med Biol Res*. 2004;37:145–150.

79. Biason-Lauber A, Konrad D, Navratil F, et al. A WNT4 mutation associated with Müllerian-duct regression and virilization in a 46,XX woman. *N Engl J Med*. 2004;351:792–798.

80. Jordan BK, Shen JH, Olaso R, et al. Wnt4 overexpression disrupts normal testicular vasculature and inhibits testosterone synthesis by repressing steroidogenic factor 1/beta-catenin synergy. *Proc Natl Acad Sci USA*. 2003;100:10866–10871.

81. New MI. Inborn errors of adrenal steroidogenesis. *Mol Cell Endocrinol*. 2003;211:75–83.

82. Creighton SM, Minto CL, Steele SJ. Objective cosmetic and anatomical outcomes at adolescence of feminising surgery for ambiguous genitalia done in childhood. *Lancet*. 2001;358:124–125.

83. Minto CL, Liao LM, Woodhouse CR, et al. The effect of clitoral surgery on sexual outcome in individuals who have intersex conditions with ambiguous genitalia: a cross-sectional study. *Lancet*. 2003;361:1252–1257.

84. McElreavey K, Vilain E, Abbas N, et al. XY sex reversal associated with a deletion 5′ to the SRY "HMG box" in the testis-determining region. *Proc Natl Acad Sci USA*. 1992;89:11016–11020.

85. Uehara S, Hashiyada M, Sato K, et al. Complete XY gonadal dysgenesis and aspects of the SRY genotype and gonadal tumor formation. *J Hum Genet*. 2002;47:279–284.

86. Assumpcao JG, Benedetti CE, Maciel-Guerra AT, et al. Novel mutations affecting SRY DNA-binding activity: the HMG box N65H associated with 46,XY pure gonadal dysgenesis and the familial non-HMG box R30I associated with variable phenotypes. *J Mol Med*. 2002;80:782–790.

87. Mitchell CL, Harley VR. Biochemical defects in eight SRY missense mutations causing XY gonadal dysgenesis. *Mol Genet Metab*. 2002;77:2172–25.

88. Li B, Zhang W, Chan G, et al. Human Sex Reversal Due to Impaired Nuclear Localization of SRY. *J Biol Chem*. 2001;276:46480–46484.

89. Uehara S, Funato T, Yaegashi N, et al. SRY mutation and tumor formation on the gonads of XY pure gonadal dysgenesis patients. *Cancer Genet Cytogenet*. 1999;113:78–84.

90. McElreavey K, Vilain E, Barbaux S, et al. Loss of sequences 3′ to the testis-determining gene, SRY, including the Y pseudoautosomal boundary associated with partial testicular determination. *Proc Natl Acad Sci USA*. 1996;93: 8590–85994.

91. Brown S, Yu C, Lanzano P, et al. A de novo mutation (Gln2Stop) at the 5′ end of the SRY gene leads to sex reversal with partial ovarian function. *Am J Hum Genet*. 1998;62:189–192.

92. Domenice S, Yumie Nishi M, Correia Billerbeck AE, et al. A novel missense mutation (S18N) in the 5′ non-HMG box region of the SRY gene in a patient with partial gonadal dysgenesis and his normal male relatives. *Hum Genet*. 1998;102:213–215.

93. Knudtzon J, Aarskog D. 45,X/46,XY mosaicism. A clinical review and report of ten cases. *Eur J Pediatr.* 1987; 146:266–271.

94. Reddy KS, Sulcova V. Pathogenetics of 45,X/46,XY gonadal mosaicism. *Cytogenet Cell Genet.* 1998;82:52–57.

95. Rosenberg C, Frota-Pessoa O, Vianna-Morgante AM, et al. Phenotypic spectrum of 45,X/46,XY individuals. *Am J Med Genet.* 1987;27:553–559.

96. Jordan BK, Jain M, Natarajan S, et al. Familial mutation in the testis-determining gene SRY shared by an XY female and her normal father. *J Clin Endocrinol Metab.* 2002;87:3428–3432.

97. Jawaheer D, Juo SH, Le Caignec C, et al. Mapping a gene for 46,XY gonadal dysgenesis by linkage analysis. *Clin Genet.* 2003;63:530–535.

98. Sarafoglou K, Ostrer H. Clinical review 111: familial sex reversal: a review. *J Clin Endocrinol Metab.* 2000;85:483–493.

99. Bilbao JR, Loridan L, Castano L. A novel postzygotic nonsense mutation in SRY in familial XY gonadal dysgenesis. *Hum Genet.* 1996;97:537–539.

100. Hines RS, Tho SP, Zhang YY, et al. Paternal somatic and germ-line mosaicism for a sex-determining region on Y (SRY) missense mutation leading to recurrent 46,XY sex reversal. *Fertil Steril.* 1997;67:675–679.

101. Iliev DI, Ranke MB, Wollmann HA. Mixed gonadal dysgenesis and precocious puberty. *Horm Res.* 2002;58:30–33.

102. Trobs RB, Hoepffner W, Buhligen U, et al. Video-assisted gonadectomy in children with Ullrich Turner syndrome or 46,XY gonadal dysgenesis. *Eur J Pediatr Surg.* 2004;14:1179–84.

103. Haddad NG, Walvoord EC, Cain MP, et al. Seminoma and a gonadoblastoma in an infant with mixed gonadal dysgenesis. *J Pediatr.* 2003;143:136.

104. Funato T, Uehara S, Takahashi M, et al. Kaku M. Microsatellite instability in gonadal tumors of XY pure gonadal dysgenesis patients. *Int J Gynecol Cancer.* 2002;12:192–197.

105. Queipo G, Zenteno JC, Pena R, et al. Molecular analysis in true hermaphroditism: demonstration of low-level hidden mosaicism for Y-derived sequences in 46,XX cases. *Hum Genet.* 2002;111:278–283.

106. Schiebel K, Winkelmann M, Mertz A, et al. Abnormal XY interchange between a novel isolated protein kinase gene, PRKY, and its homologue, PRKX, accounts for one third of all (Y+)XX males and (Y−)XY females. *Hum Mol Genet.* 1997;6:1985–1989.

107. Kusz K, Kotecki M, Wojda A, et al. Incomplete masculinisation of XX subjects carrying the SRY gene on an inactive X chromosome. *J Med Genet.* 1999;36:452–456.

108. Zenteno-Ruiz JC, Kofman-Alfaro S, Mendez JP. 46,XX sex reversal. *Arch Med Res.* 2001;32:559–566.

109. Bouayed Abdelmoula N, Portnoi MF, et al. Skewed X-chromosome inactivation pattern in SRY positiveness: a case report and review of literature. *Ann Genet.* 2003;46:11–18.

110. Jimenez AL, Kofman-Alfaro S, Berumen J, et al. Partially deleted SRY gene confined to testicular tissue in a 46,XX true hermaphrodite without SRY in leukocytic DNA. *Am J Med Genet.* 2000;93:417–420.

111. Jarrah N, El-Shanti H, Khier A, et al. Familial disorder of sex determination in seven individuals from three related sibships. *Eur J Pediatr.* 2000;159:912–918.

112. Li JH, Huang TH, Jiang XW, et al. 46,XX male sex reversal syndrome. *Asian J Androl.* 2004;6:165–167.

113. Rey RA, et al. Evaluation of gonadal function in 107 intersex patients by means of serum antiMüllerian hormone measurement. *J Clin Endocrinol Metab.* 1999;84:627–631.

114. Bernard-Gallon DJ, Dechelotte P, Vissac C, et al. BRCA1 and BRCA2 protein expressions in an ovotestis of a 46,XX true hermaphrodite. *Breast Cancer Res.* 2001;3:61–65.

115. Decker JP, Lerner HJ, Schwartz I. Breast carcinoma in a 46,XX true hermaphrodite. *Cancer.* 1982;49:1481–1484.

116. Hado HS, Helmy SW, Klemm K, et al. XX male: a rare cause of short stature, infertility, gynaecomastia and carcinoma of the breast. *Int J Clin Pract.* 2003;57:844–845.

117. Lau LC, Lim P, Lee LH, et al. Myelodysplastic syndrome with transformation to AML-M7 in a 46,XX male patient. *Cancer Genet Cytogenet.* 2002;136:153–154.

118. Krob G, Braun A, Kuhnle U. True hermaphroditism: geographical distribution, clinical findings, chromosomes and gonadal histology. *Eur J Pediatr.* 1994;153:2–10.

119. Boucekkine C, Toublanc JE, Abbas N, et al. Clinical and anatomical spectrum in XX sex reversed patients. Relationship to the presence of Y specific DNA-sequences. *Clin Endocrinol.* (Oxf) 1994;40:733–742.

120. McElreavey K, Rappaport R, Vilain E, et al. A minority of 46,XX true hermaphrodites are positive for the Y-DNA sequence including SRY. *Hum Genet.* 1992;90:121–125.

121. Berkovitz GD, Fechner PY, Marcantonio SM, et al. The role of the sex-determining region of the Y chromosome (SRY) in the etiology of 46,XX true hermaphroditism. *Hum Genet.* 1992;88:411–416.

122. Damiani D, Fellous M, McElreavey K, et al. True hermaphroditism: clinical aspects and molecular studies in 16 cases. *Eur J Endocrinol.* 1997;136:201–204.

123. Abbas N, McElreavey K, Leconiat M, et al. Familial case of 46,XX male and 46,XX true hermaphrodite associated with a paternal-derived SRY-bearing X chromosome. *C R Acad Sci III.* 1993;316:375–383.

124. Hadjiathanasiou CG, Brauner R, Lortat-Jacob S, et al. True hermaphroditism: genetic variants and clinical management. *J Pediatr.* 1994;125:738–744.

125. Niu DM, Pan CC, Lin CY, et al. Mosaic or chimera? Revisiting an old hypothesis about the cause of the 46,XX/46,XY hermaphrodite. *J Pediatr.* 2002;140: 732–5.

126. Cui Y, Zhu P, Ye X, et al. [The mechanism of tetragametic chimerism in a true hermaphroditism with 46,XX/46,XY]. *Zhonghua Nan Ke Xue* 2004;10:107–112.

127. Repas-Humpe LM, Humpe A, Lynen R, et al. A dispermic chimerism in a 2-year-old Caucasian boy. *Ann Hematol.* 1999;78:431–434.

128. Strain L, Dean JC, Hamilton MP, et al. A true hermaphrodite chimera resulting from embryo amalgamation after in vitro fertilization. *N Engl J Med.* 1998;338:166–169.

129. Uehara S, Nata M, Nagae M, et al. Molecular biologic analyses of tetragametic chimerism in a true hermaphrodite with 46,XX/46,XY. *Fertil Steril.* 1995;63:189–192.

130. Verp MS, Harrison HH, Ober C, et al. Chimerism as the etiology of a 46,XX/46,XY fertile true hermaphrodite. *Fertil Steril.* 1992;57:346–349.

131. Ortenberg J, Oddoux C, Craver R, et al. SRY gene expression in the ovotestes of XX true hermaphrodites. *J Urol.* 2002;167: 1828–1831.

132. Malavaud B, Mazerolles C, Bieth E, et al. Pure seminoma in a male phenotype 46,XX true hermaphrodite. *J Urol.* 2000;164:125–126.

133. Tanaka Y, Fujiwara K, Yamauchi H, et al. Pregnancy in a woman with a Y chromosome after removal of an ovarian dysgerminoma. *Gynecol Oncol.* 2000;79:519–521.

134. Jakubowski L, Jeziorowska A, Constantinou M, et al. Xp;Yp translocation inherited from the father in an SRY, RBM, and TSPY positive true hermaphrodite with oligozoospermia. *J Med Genet.* 2000;37:E28.

135. Richter-Unruh A, Martens JW, Verhoef-Post M, et al. Leydig cell hypoplasia: cases with new mutations, new polymorphisms and cases without mutations in the luteinizing hormone receptor gene. *Clin Endocrinol.* (Oxf) 2002;56:103–112.

136. Wu SM, Chan WY. Male pseudohermaphroditism due to inactivating luteinizing hormone receptor mutations. *Arch Med Res.* 1999;30:495–500.

137. Martens JW, Verhoef-Post M, Abelin N, et al. A homozygous mutation in the luteinizing hormone receptor causes partial Leydig cell hypoplasia: correlation between receptor activity and phenotype. *Mol Endocrinol.* 1998;12:775–784.

138. Gromoll J, Eiholzer U, Nieschlag E, et al. Male hypogonadism caused by homozygous deletion of exon 10 of the luteinizing hormone (LH) receptor: differential action of human chorionic gonadotropin and LH. *J Clin Endocrinol Metab.* 2000;85:2281–2286.

139. Latronico AC, Anasti J, Arnhold IJ, et al. Brief report: testicular and ovarian resistance to luteinizing hormone caused by inactivating mutations of the luteinizing hormone-receptor gene. *N Engl J Med.* 1996;334 507–512.

140. Toledo SP, Brunner HG, Kraaij R, et al. Post M, Dahia PL, Hayashida CY, Kremer HTAP. An inactivating mutation of the luteinizing hormone receptor causes amenorrhea in a 46,XX female. *J Clin Endocrinol Metab.* 1996;81:3850–3854.

141. Latronico AC, Chai Y, Arnhold IJ, et al. A homozygous microdeletion in helix 7 of the luteinizing hormone receptor associated with familial testicular and ovarian resistance is due to both decreased cell surface

expression and impaired effector activation by the cell surface receptor. *Mol Endocrinol*. 1998;12:442–450.

142. Stavrou SS, Zhu YS, Cai LQ, et al. A novel mutation of the human luteinizing hormone receptor in 46XY and 46XX sisters. *J Clin Endocrinol Metab*. 1998;83:2091–2098.

143. Tajima T, Fujieda K, Kouda N, et al. Heterozygous mutation in the cholesterol side chain cleavage enzyme (p450scc) gene in a patient with 46,XY sex reversal and adrenal insufficiency. *J Clin Endocrinol Metab*. 2001;86:3820–3825.

144. Katsumata N, Ohtake M, Hojo T, et al. Compound heterozygous mutations in the cholesterol side-chain cleavage enzyme gene (CYP11A) cause congenital adrenal insufficiency in humans. *J Clin Endocrinol Metab*. 2002;87:3808–3813.

145. Stocco DM. Clinical disorders associated with abnormal cholesterol transport: mutations in the steroidogenic acute regulatory protein. *Mol Cell Endocrinol*. 2002;191:19–25.

146. Fujieda K, Tajima T, Nakae J, et al. Spontaneous puberty in 46,XX subjects with congenital lipoid adrenal hyperplasia. Ovarian steroidogenesis is spared to some extent despite inactivating mutations in the steroidogenic acute regulatory protein (StAR) gene. *J Clin Invest*. 1997;99:1265–1271.

147. Fujieda K, Okuhara K, Abe S, et al. Molecular pathogenesis of lipoid adrenal hyperplasia and adrenal hypoplasia congenita. *J Steroid Biochem Mol Biol*. 2003;85:483–489.

148. Sakkal-Alkaddour H, Zhang L, Yang X, et al. Studies of 3 beta-hydroxysteroid dehydrogenase genes in infants and children manifesting premature pubarche and increased adrenocorticotropin-stimulated delta 5-steroid levels. *J Clin Endocrinol Metab*. 1996;81:3961–3965.

149. Mendonca BB, Russell AJ, Vasconcelos-Leite M, et al. Mutation in 3 beta-hydroxysteroid dehydrogenase type II associated with pseudohermaphroditism in males and premature pubarche or cryptic expression in females. *J Mol Endocrinol*. 1994;12:119–122.

150. Marui S, Castro M, Latronico AC, et al. Mutations in the type II 3beta-hydroxysteroid dehydrogenase (HSD3B2) gene can cause premature pubarche in girls. *Clin Endocrinol*. (Oxf) 2000;52:67–75.

151. Mendonca BB, Bloise W, Arnhold IJ, et al. Male pseudohermaphroditism due to non-salt-losing 3 beta-hydroxysteroid dehydrogenase deficiency: gender role change and absence of gynecomastia at puberty. *J Steroid Biochem*. 1987;28:669–675.

152. Alos N, Moisan AM, Ward L, et al. A novel A10E homozygous mutation in the HSD3B2 gene causing severe salt-wasting 3beta-hydroxysteroid dehydrogenase deficiency in 46,XX and 46,XY French-Canadians: evaluation of gonadal function after puberty. *J Clin Endocrinol Metab*. 2000;85:1968–1974.

153. Van Den Akker EL, Koper JW, Boehmer AL, et al. Differential inhibition of 17alpha-hydroxylase and 17,20-lyase activities by three novel missense CYP17 mutations identified in patients with P450c17 defi-

ciency. *J Clin Endocrinol Metab*. 2002;87:5714–57121.

154. Di Cerbo A, Biason-Lauber A, Savino M, et al. Combined 17alpha-Hydroxylase/17,20-lyase deficiency caused by Phe93Cys mutation in the CYP17 gene. *J Clin Endocrinol Metab*. 2002;87:898–905.

155. Scaroni C, Biason A, Carpene G, et al. 17-alpha-hydroxylase deficiency in three siblings: short- and long-term studies. *J Endocrinol Invest*. 1991;14:99–108.

156. Geller DH, Auchus RJ, Mendonca BB, et al. The genetic and functional basis of isolated 17,20-lyase deficiency. *Nat Genet*. 1997;17:201–205.

157. Peterson RE, Imperato-McGinley J, Gautier T, et al. Male pseudohermaphroditism due to multiple defects in steroid-biosynthetic microsomal mixed-function oxidases. A new variant of congenital adrenal hyperplasia. *N Engl J Med*. 1985;313:1182–1191.

158. Shackleton C, Marcos J, Arlt W, et al. Prenatal diagnosis of P450 oxidoreductase deficiency (ORD): a disorder causing low pregnancy estriol, maternal and fetal virilization, and the Antley-Bixler syndrome phenotype. *Am J Med Genet*. 2004;129A:105–112.

159. Arlt W, Walker EA, Draper N, et al. Congenital adrenal hyperplasia caused by mutant P450 oxidoreductase and human androgen synthesis: analytical study. *Lancet*. 2004;363:2128–2135.

160. Huang N, Pandey AV, Agrawal V, et al: Diversity and function of mutations in P450 oxidoreductase in patients with Antley-Bixler syndrome and disordered steroidogenesis. *Am J Hum Genet*. 2005;76:729–749.

161. Imperato-McGinley J, Peterson RE, Stoller R, et al. Male pseudohermaphroditism secondary to 17 beta-hydroxysteroid dehydrogenase deficiency: gender role change with puberty. *J Clin Endocrinol Metab*. 1979;49:391–395.

162. Mendonca BB, Inacio M, Arnhold IJ, et al. Male pseudohermaphroditism due to 17 beta-hydroxysteroid dehydrogenase 3 deficiency. Diagnosis, psychological evaluation, and management. *Medicine*. (Baltimore) 2000;79:299–309.

163. Bilbao JR, Loridan L, Audi L, et al. A novel missense (R80W) mutation in 17-beta-hydroxysteroid dehydrogenase type 3 gene associated with male pseudohermaphroditism. *Eur J Endocrinol*. 1998;139: 330–333.

164. Wilson JD. Androgens, androgen receptors, and male gender role behavior. *Horm Behav*. 2001;40:358–366.

165. Fitzky BU, Witsch-Baumgartner M, Erdel M, et al. Mutations in the Delta7-sterol reductase gene in patients with the Smith-Lemli-Opitz syndrome. *Proc Natl Acad Sci USA*. 1998;95:8181–8186.

166. Wassif CA, Maslen C, Kachilele-Linjewile S, et al. Mutations in the human sterol delta7-reductase gene at 11q12-13 cause Smith-Lemli-Opitz syndrome. *Am J Hum Genet*. 1998;63:55–62.

167. Waterham HR, Wijburg FA, Hennekam RC, et al. Smith-Lemli-Opitz syndrome is caused by mutations in the 7-dehydrocho-

lesterol reductase gene. *Am J Hum Genet*. 1998;63:329–338.

168. Tint GS, Irons M, Elias ER, et al. Defective cholesterol biosynthesis associated with the Smith-Lemli-Opitz syndrome. *N Engl J Med*. 1994;330:107–113.

169. Yu H, Patel SB. Recent insights into the Smith-Lemli-Opitz syndrome. *Clin Genet*. 2005;68:383–391.

170. Porter JA, Young KE, Beachy PA. Cholesterol modification of hedgehog signaling proteins in animal development. *Science*. 1996;274:255–259.

171. Cooper MK, Porter JA, Young KE, et al. Teratogen-mediated inhibition of target tissue response to Shh signaling. *Science*. 1998;280:1603–1607.

172. Cooper MK, Wassif CA, Krakowiak PA, et al. A defective response to Hedgehog signaling in disorders of cholesterol biosynthesis. *Nat Genet*. 2003;33:508–513.

173. Berensztein E, Torrado M, Belgorosky A, et al. Smith-Lemli-Opitz syndrome: in vivo and in vitro study of testicular function in a prepubertal patient with ambiguous genitalia. *Acta Paediatr*. 1999;88:1229–1232.

174. Cunniff C, Kratz LE, Moser A, et al. Clinical and biochemical spectrum of patients with RSH/Smith-Lemli-Opitz syndrome and abnormal cholesterol metabolism. *Am J Med Genet*. 1997;68:263–269.

175. Bialer MG, Penchaszadeh VB, Kahn E, et al. Female external genitalia and Müllerian duct derivatives in a 46,XY infant with the Smith-Lemli-Opitz syndrome. *Am J Med Genet*. 1987;28:723–731.

176. Fukazawa R, Nakahori Y, Kogo T, et al. Normal Y sequences in Smith-Lemli-Opitz syndrome with total failure of masculinization. *Acta Paediatr*. 1992;81:570–572.

177. Craigie RJ, Ba'ath M, Fryer A, et al. Surgical implications of the Smith-Lemli-Opitz syndrome. *Pediatr Surg Int*. 2005; 21:482–484.

178. Andersson HC, Frentz J, Martinez JE, et al. Adrenal insufficiency in Smith-Lemli-Opitz syndrome. *Am J Med Genet*. 1999; 82:382–384.

179. Nowaczyk MJ, Siu VM, Krakowiak PA, et al. Adrenal insufficiency and hypertension in a newborn infant with Smith-Lemli-Opitz syndrome. *Am J Med Genet*. 2001;103:223–225.

180. Chemaitilly W, Goldenberg A, Baujat G, et al. Adrenal insufficiency and abnormal genitalia in a 46XX female with Smith-Lemli-Opitz syndrome. *Horm Res*. 2003;59:254–256.

181. Tint GS, Salen G, Batta AK, et al. Correlation of severity and outcome with plasma sterol levels in variants of the Smith-Lemli-Opitz syndrome. *J Pediatr*. 1995;127:82–87.

182. Thiele S, Hoppe U, Holterhus PM, et al. Isoenzyme type 1 of 5alpha-reductase is abundantly transcribed in normal human genital skin fibroblasts and may play an important role in masculinization of 5alpha-reductase type 2 deficient males. *Eur J Endocrinol*. 2005;152:875–880.

183. Thigpen AE, Silver RI, Guileyardo JM, et al. Tissue distribution and ontogeny of

183. steroid 5 alpha-reductase isozyme expression. *J Clin Invest.* 1993;92:903–910.

184. Andersson S, Berman DM, Jenkins EP, et al. Deletion of steroid 5 alpha-reductase 2 gene in male pseudohermaphroditism. *Nature.* 1991;354:159–161.

185. Peterson RE, Imperato-McGinley J, Gautier T, et al. Male pseudohermaphroditism due to steroid 5-alpha-reductase deficiency. *Am J Med.* (1977) 62: 170–91.

186. Imperato-McGinley J, Gautier T, Zirinsky K, et al. Prostate visualization studies in males homozygous and heterozygous for 5 alpha-reductase deficiency. *J Clin Endocrinol Metab.* 1992;75:1022–1026.

187. Imperato-McGinley J. 5alpha-reductase-2 deficiency and complete androgen insensitivity: lessons from nature. *Adv Exp Med Biol.* 2002;511:121-131; discussion 31–34.

188. Saenger P, Goldman AS, Levine LS, et al. Prepubertal diagnosis of steroid 5 alpha-reductase deficiency. *J Clin Endocrinol Metab.* (1978) 46: 627–34.

189. Canto P, Vilchis F, Chavez B, et al. Mutations of the 5 alpha-reductase type 2 gene in eight Mexican patients from six different pedigrees with 5 alpha-reductase-2 deficiency. *Clin Endocrinol.* (Oxf) 1997;46:155–160.

190. Imperato-McGinley J, Peterson RE, Gautier T, et al. Androgens and the evolution of male-gender identity among male pseudohermaphrodites with 5alpha-reductase deficiency. *N Engl J Med.* 1979;300:1233–1237.

191. Mendonca BB, Inacio M, Costa EM, et al. Male pseudohermaphroditism due to steroid 5alpha-reductase 2 deficiency. Diagnosis, psychological evaluation, and management. *Medicine.* (Baltimore) 1996;75:64–76.

192. Galli-Tsinopoulou A, Hiort O, Schuster T, et al. A novel point mutation in the hormone binding domain of the androgen receptor associated with partial and minimal androgen insensitivity syndrome. *J Pediatr Endocrinol Metab.* 2003;16:149–154.

193. Pinsky L, Kaufman M, Killinger DW, et al. Human minimal androgen insensitivity with normal dihydrotestosterone-binding capacity in cultured genital skin fibroblasts: evidence for an androgen-selective qualitative abnormality of the receptor. *Am J Hum Genet.* 1984;36:965–978.

194. Bevan CL, Hughes IA, Patterson MN. Wide variation in androgen receptor dysfunction in complete androgen insensitivity syndrome. *J Steroid Biochem Mol Biol.* 1997;61:19–26.

195. Gottlieb B, Beitel LK, Wu JH, et al. The androgen receptor gene mutations database (ARDB): 2004 update. *Hum Mutat.* 2004;23:527–533.

196. Sultan C, Lumbroso S, Paris F, et al. Disorders of androgen action. *Semin Reprod Med.* 2002;20:217–228.

197. Rutgers JL, Scully RE. The androgen insensitivity syndrome (testicular feminization): a clinicopathologic study of 43 cases. *Int J Gynecol Pathol.* 1991;10:126–144.

198. Bouvattier C, Carel JC, Lecointre C, et al. Postnatal changes of T, LH, and FSH in 46,XY infants with mutations in the AR gene. *J Clin Endocrinol Metab.* 2002;87:29–32.

199. Brown TR, Migeon CJ. Cultured human skin fibroblasts: a model for the study of androgen action. *Mol Cell Biochem.* 1981;36:3–22.

200. Ris-Stalpers C, Hoogenboezem T, Sleddens HF, et al. A practical approach to the detection of androgen receptor gene mutations and pedigree analysis in families with x-linked androgen insensitivity. *Pediatr Res.* 1994;36:227–234.

201. Irvine RA, Yu MC, Ross RK, et al. The CAG and GGC microsatellites of the androgen receptor gene are in linkage disequilibrium in men with prostate cancer. *Cancer Res.* 1995;55:1937–1940.

202. Casella R, Maduro MR, Misfud A, et al. Androgen receptor gene polyglutamine length is associated with testicular histology in infertile patients. *J Urol.* 2003;169:224–227.

203. Tut TG, Ghadessy FJ, Trifiro MA, et al. Long polyglutamine tracts in the androgen receptor are associated with reduced transactivation, impaired sperm production, and male infertility. *J Clin Endocrinol Metab.* 1997;82:3777–3782.

204. Dowsing AT, Yong EL, Clark M, et al. Linkage between male infertility and trinucleotide repeat expansion in the androgen-receptor gene. *Lancet.* 1999;354:640–643.

205. Butler R, Leigh PN, McPhaul MJ, et al. Truncated forms of the androgen receptor are associated with polyglutamine expansion in X-linked spinal and bulbar muscular atrophy. *Hum Mol Genet.* 1998;7: 121–127.

206. Igarashi S, Tanno Y, Onodera O, et al. Strong correlation between the number of CAG repeats in androgen receptor genes and the clinical onset of features of spinal and bulbar muscular atrophy. *Neurology.* 1992;42:2300–2302.

206 Lumbroso S, Lobaccaro JM, Vial C, et al. Molecular analysis of the androgen receptor gene in Kennedy's disease. Report of two families and review of the literature. *Horm Res.* 1997;47:23–29.

207. Nelson KG, Goldenberg RL. Sex hormones and congenital malformations: a review. *J Med Assoc State Ala.* 1977;46:31.

208. Coenen CM, Thomas CM, Borm GF, et al. Comparative evaluation of the androgenicity of four low-dose, fixed-combination oral contraceptives. *Int J Fertil Menopausal Stud.* 1995;40 Suppl 2:92–97.

209. Ziaei S, Rajaei L, Faghihzadeh S, et al. Comparative study and evaluation of side effects of low-dose contraceptive pills administered by the oral and vaginal route. *Contraception.* 2002;65:329–31.

210. Joshi R, Dunaif A. Ovarian disorders of pregnancy. *Endocrinol Metab Clin North Am.* 1995;24:153–169.

211. Ito Y, Fisher CR, Conte FA, et al. Molecular basis of aromatase deficiency in an adult female with sexual infantilism and polycystic ovaries. *Proc Natl Acad Sci USA.* 1993;90:11673–1167.

212. Shozu M, Akasofu K, Harada T, et al. A new cause of female pseudohermaphroditism: placental aromatase deficiency. *J Clin Endocrinol Metab.* 1991;72:560–566.

213. Herrmann BL, Saller B, Janssen OE, et al. Impact of estrogen replacement therapy in a male with congenital aromatase deficiency caused by a novel mutation in the CYP19 gene. *J Clin Endocrinol Metab.* 2002;87:5476–5484.

214. Mullis PE, Yoshimura N, Kuhlmann B, et al. Aromatase deficiency in a female who is compound heterozygote for two new point mutations in the P450arom gene: impact of estrogens on hypergonadotropic hypogonadism, multicystic ovaries, and bone densitometry in childhood. *J Clin Endocrinol Metab.* 1997;82:1739–1745.

215. Conte FA, Grumbach MM, Ito Y, et al. A syndrome of female pseudohermaphrodism, hypergonadotropic hypogonadism, and multicystic ovaries associated with missense mutations in the gene encoding aromatase (P450arom). *J Clin Endocrinol Metab.* 1994;78:1287–1292.

216. Carreau S, Lambard S, Delalande C, et al. Aromatase expression and role of estrogens in male gonad: a review. *Reprod Biol Endocrinol.* 2003;1:35.

217. Rochira V, Balestrieri A, Madeo B, et al. Congenital estrogen deficiency in men: a new syndrome with different phenotypes; clinical and therapeutic implications in men. *Mol Cell Endocrinol.* 2002;193:19–28.

218. Belgorosky A, Pepe C, Marino R, et al. Hypothalamic-pituitary-ovarian axis during infancy, early and late prepuberty in an aromatase-deficient girl who is a compound heterocygote for two new point mutations of the CYP19 gene. *J Clin Endocrinol Metab.* 2003;88:5127–5131.

219. Edman CD, Winters AJ, Porter JC, et al. Embryonic testicular regression. A clinical spectrum of XY agonadal individuals. *Obstet Gynecol.* 1977;49:208–217.

220. Smith NM, Byard RW, Bourne AJ. Testicular regression syndrome—a pathological study of 77 cases. *Histopathology.* 1991;19:269–272.

221. Spires SE, Woolums CS, Pulito AR, et al. Testicular regression syndrome: a clinical and pathologic study of 11 cases. *Arch Pathol Lab Med.* 2000;124:694–698.

222. Corrado F, Stella NC, Triolo O. Testicular regression syndrome. A case report. *J Reprod Med.* 1991;36:549–550.

223. Rattanachaiyanont M, Phophong P, Techatraisak K, et al. Embryonic testicular regression syndrome: a case report. *J Med Assoc Thai.* 1999;82:506–510.

224. Coulam CB. Testicular regression syndrome. *Obstet Gynecol.* 1979;53:44–49.

225. Grady RW, Mitchell ME, Carr MC. Laparoscopic and histologic evaluation of the inguinal vanishing testis. *Urology.* 1998;52:866–869.

226. Radmayr C, Oswald J, Schwentner C, et al. Long-term outcome of laparoscopically managed nonpalpable testes. *J Urol.* 2003;170:2409–2411.

227. Josso N, Picard JY, Imbeaud S, et al. Clinical aspects and molecular genetics of the persistent Müllerian duct syndrome. *Clin Endocrinol.* (Oxf) 1997;47:137–144.

228. Josso N, Belville C, di Clemente N, et al. AMH and AMH receptor defects in persistent Müllerian duct syndrome. *Hum Reprod Update.* 2005;11:351–356.

229. Koksal S, Tokmak H, Tibet HB Olgun E. Persistent Müllerian duct syndrome. *Br J Clin Pract.* 1995;49:276–277.

230. Lang-Muritano M, Biason-Lauber A, Gitzelmann C, et al. A novel mutation in the anti-Müllerian hormone gene as cause of persistent Müllerian duct syndrome. *Eur J Pediatr.* 2001;160:652–654.

231. Beyribey S, Cetinkaya M, Adsan O, et al. Persistent Müllerian duct syndrome. *Scand J Urol Nephrol.* 1993;27:563–565.

232. Berkmen F. Persistent Müllerian duct syndrome with or without transverse testicular ectopia and testis tumours. *Br J Urol.* 1997;79:122–126.

233. Reindollar RH, Byrd JR, McDonough PG. Delayed sexual development: a study of 252 patients. *Am J Obstet Gynecol.* 1981;140:371–380.

234. Resendes BL, Sohn SH, Stelling JR, et al. Role for anti-Müllerian hormone in congenital absence of the uterus and vagina. *Am J Med Genet.* 2001;98:129–136.

235. Zenteno JC, Carranza-Lira S, Kofman-Alfaro S. Molecular analysis of the anti-Müllerian hormone, the anti-Müllerian hormone receptor, and galactose-1-phosphate uridyl transferase genes in patients with the Mayer-Rokitansky-Kuster-Hauser syndrome. *Arch Gynecol Obstet.* 2004;269:270–273.

236. Shokeir MH. Aplasia of the Müllerian system: evidence for probable sex-limited autosomal dominant inheritance. *Birth Defects Orig Artic Ser.* 1978;14:147–165.

237. Griffin JE, Edwards C, Madden JD, et al. Congenital absence of the vagina. The Mayer-Rokitansky-Kuster-Hauser syndrome. *Ann Intern Med.* 1976;85:224–236.

238. Carson SA, Simpson JL, Malinak LR, et al. Heritable aspects of uterine anomalies. II. Genetic analysis of Müllerian aplasia. *Fertil Steril.* 1983;40:86–90.

239. Oppelt P, Strissel PR, Kellermann A, et al. Clinical aspects of Mayer-Rokitansky-Kuester-Hauser syndrome: recommendations for clinical diagnosis and staging. *Hum Reprod.* 2006;21:792–797.

240. Levinson G, Zarate A, Guzman-Toledano R, et al. An XX female with sexual infantilism, absent gonads, and lack of Müllerian ducts. *J Med Genet.* 1976;13:68–69.

241. Guitron-Cantu A, Lopez-Vera E, Forsbach-Sanchez G, et al. Gonadal dysgenesis and Rokitansky syndrome. A case report. *J Reprod Med.* 1999;44:891–893.

242. Aydos S, Tukun A, Bokesoy I. Gonadal dysgenesis and the Mayer-Rokitansky-Kuster-Hauser syndrome in a girl with 46,X,del(X)(pter—>q22:). *Arch Gynecol Obstet.* 2003;267:173–174.

243. Marrakchi A, Gharbi M, Kadiri A. [Gonadal dysgenesis associated with Mayer-Rokitansky-Kuster-Hauser syndrome: a case report]. *Ann Endocrinol.* (Paris) 2004;65:466–468.

244. Gorgojo JJ, Almodovar F, Lopez E, et al. Gonadal agenesis 46,XX associated with the atypical form of Rokitansky syndrome. *Fertil Steril.* 2002;77:185–187.

245. Plevraki E, Kita M, Goulis DG, et al. Bilateral ovarian agenesis and the presence of the testis-specific protein 1-Y-linked gene: two new features of Mayer-Rokitansky-Kuster-Hauser syndrome. *Fertil Steril.* 2004;81:689–692.

246. Simpson JL, Rajkovic A. Ovarian differentiation and gonadal failure. *Am J Med Genet.* 1999;89:186–200.

247. Boczkowski K. Pure gonadal dysgenesis and ovarian dysplasia in sisters. *Am J Obstet Gynecol.* 1970;106:626–628.

248. Portuondo JA, Neyro JL, Benito JA, et al. Familial 46,XX gonadal dysgenesis. *Int J Fertil.* 1987;32:56–58.

249. Aittomaki K. The genetics of XX gonadal dysgenesis. *Am J Hum Genet.* 1994;54:844–851.

250. Namavar-Jahromi B, Mohit M, Kumar PV. Familial dysgerminoma associated with 46,XX pure gonadal dysgenesis. *Saudi Med J.* (2005) 26: 872–4.

251. Aittomaki K, Lucena JL, Pakarinen P, et al. Mutation in the follicle-stimulating hormone receptor gene causes hereditary hypergonadotropic ovarian failure. *Cell.* (1995) 82: 959–68.

252. De la Chesnaye E, Canto P, Ulloa-Aguirre A, et al. No evidence of mutations in the follicle-stimulating hormone receptor gene in Mexican women with 46,XX pure gonadal dysgenesis. *Am J Med Genet.* (2001) 98:125–8.

253. Layman LC, Amde S, Cohen DP, et al. The Finnish follicle-stimulating hormone receptor gene mutation is rare in North American women with 46,XX ovarian failure. *Fertil Steril.* 1998;69:300–302.

254. Crisponi L, Deiana M, Loi A, et al. The putative forkhead transcription factor FOXL2 is mutated in blepharophimosis/ptosis/epicanthus inversus syndrome. *Nat Genet.* 2001;27:159–166.

255. De Baere E, Dixon MJ, Small KW, et al. Spectrum of FOXL2 gene mutations in blepharophimosis-ptosisepicanthus inversus (BPES) families demonstrates a genotype—phenotype correlation. *Hum Mol Genet.* 2001;10:1591–1600.

256. Schmidt D, Ovitt CE, Anlag K, et al. The murine winged-helix transcription factor Foxl2 is required for granulosa cell differentiation and ovary maintenance. *Development.* 2004;131:933–942.

257. Uda M, Ottolenghi C, Crisponi L, et al. Foxl2 disruption causes mouse ovarian failure by pervasive blockage of follicle development. *Hum Mol Genet.* 2004;13:1171–1181.

258. Maximilian C, Ionescu B, Bucur A. [Two sisters with major gonadal dysgenesis, dwarfism, microcephaly, arachnodactyly, and normal karyotype 46,XX]. *J Genet Hum.* 1970;18:365–378.

259. Quayle SA, Copeland KC. 46,XX gonadal dysgenesis with epibulbar dermoid. *Am J Med Genet.* 1991;40:75–76.

260. Hisama FM, Zemel S, Cherniske EM, et al. 46,XX gonadal dysgenesis, short stature, and recurrent metabolic acidosis in two sisters. *Am J Med Genet.* 2001;98:121–124.

261. Amor DJ, Delatycki MB, Gardner RJ, et al. New variant of familial cerebellar ataxia with hypergonadotropic hypogonadism and sensorineural deafness. *Am J Med Genet.* 2001;99:29–33.

262. Arlazoroff A, Rosenberg T, Gadoth N, et al. Secondary amenorrhea in two sisters with hypogonadotropic hypogonadism and progressive cerebellar ataxia. *Brain Dev.* 1989;11:422–425.

263. Georgopoulos NA, Papapetropoulos S, Chroni E, et al. Spinocerebellar ataxia and hypergonadotropic hypogonadism associated with familial sensorineural hearing loss. *Gynecol Endocrinol.* 2004;19:105–110.

264. Skre H, Bassoe HH, Berg K, et al. Cerebellar ataxia and hypergonadotropic hypogonadism in two kindreds. Chance concurrence, pleiotropism or linkage? *Clin Genet.* 1976;9:234–244.

265. Skoog SJ, Belman AB. Aphallia: its classification and management. *J Urol.* 1989;141:589–592.

266. Reiner WG. Psychosexual development in genetic males assigned female: the cloacal exstrophy experience. *Child Adolesc Psychiatr Clin N Am.* 2004;13:657–674, ix.

267. Lund DP, Hendren WH. Cloacal exstrophy: a 25-year experience with 50 cases. *J Pediatr Surg.* 2001;36:68–75.

268. Reiner WG, Kropp BP. A 7-year experience of genetic males with severe phallic inadequacy assigned female. *J Urol.* 2004;172:2395–2398.

269. Reiner WG, Gearhart JP. Discordant sexual identity in some genetic males with cloacal exstrophy assigned to female sex at birth. *N Engl J Med.* 2004;350:333–341.

270. Threatt CB, Wiener JS. Aphallia with congenital urethrorectal fistula. *Urology.* 2003;61:458–459.

CHAPTER 36

Female Hypogonadism

Bala Bhagavath, MD
Bruce R. Carr, MD

NORMAL FUNCTION OF THE HYPOTHALAMIC-PITUITARY-OVARIAN AXIS

The hypothalamus secretes pulses of the oligopeptide gonadotropin-releasing hormone (GnRH), which is transported through the portal vessels to the pituitary. In childhood, GnRH pulse frequency is irregular and the amplitude is very low. As puberty approaches, there is initially a nocturnal increase in the frequency and amplitude of GnRH pulses, followed gradually by similar pulses during the daytime until an adult frequency of one pulse every 60 to 90 minutes is reached.

GnRH receptors (GNRHR) are G-protein–coupled receptors that are present on the cell membrane of the gonadotrope cells of the pituitary. GnRH acts on the GNRHR, activating adenylate cyclase. This results in an intracellular cascade of events culminating in the release of the stored glycoprotein hormones, follicle-stimulating hormone (FSH) or luteinizing hormone (LH). At the same time, further synthesis of these hormones within the gonadotropes is also activated.

Prior to puberty, FSH and LH levels are low but pulsatile secretion is nonetheless present with greater amplitude of FSH than LH pulses. As puberty progresses, LH pulses gradually predominate. Serum FSH levels rise approximately 2.5-fold over the course of puberty but LH levels increase approximately 25-fold. LH levels are similar between the sexes, whereas girls have higher FSH levels at all stages of puberty. FSH is preferentially released at a lower GnRH pulse frequency (1 pulse every 90 min) and LH is released at a higher frequency (1 pulse every 60 min). Thus, via alterations in GnRH pulse frequency, the hypothalamus can control the differential secretion of the gonadotropins at different stages of the menstrual cycle.

The normal menstrual cycle is described in detail in Chapter 38. Briefly, the cycle begins on day 1, the 1st day of menstruation, with the follicular phase. Low basal levels of LH act on ovarian theca cells to stimulate production of androgens. Theca cells lack aromatase and, therefore, steroidogenesis cannot proceed to estrogen formation. The androgens are transported to the adjacent granulosa cells where FSH, the predominant gonadotropin during the follicular phase, stimulates their conversion to estrogen. FSH acts on the granulosa cells surrounding the primordial follicles (oocytes surrounded by a single layer of cuboidal cells) to stimulate their growth to the preovulatory follicle stage (oocytes surrounded by many layers of granulosa cells and an outer layer of theca cells). During the midfollicular stage, a dominant follicle emerges that continues to grow while the other follicles that have developed beyond the primordial stage undergo atresia.

FSH also stimulates follicular synthesis of activin and inhibin B, members of the transforming growth factor—β family of peptides. Activin augments LH action on theca cells. Inhibin B is the most potent selective inhibitor of FSH synthesis and release. Rising levels of inhibin B and estradiol in the late follicular phase act on the pituitary to inhibit the secretion of FSH. This explains rising levels of FSH as follicle mass diminishes in perimenopausal women or women with partial follicular atresia (such as some Turner syndrome [TS] mosaics) despite normal levels of estradiol. In these women, a smaller primordial follicle pool results in decreased inhibin B and a consequent rise in the FSH level.

The increased level of estradiol during the late follicular phase stimulates a higher GnRH pulse frequency and release of LH from the pituitary. The surge in LH induces ovulation and the theca—granulosa cell complex, which had been part of the dominant follicle, becomes the corpus luteum. The corpus luteum synthesizes progesterone and estrogen for 2 weeks (luteal phase of the menstrual cycle), after which time it regresses unless it is supported by β-hCG from pregnancy. Estrogen and progesterone levels fall and there is sloughing of the endometrium and the onset of the next cycle. Menstrual irregularities are discussed in Chapter 38.

OVERVIEW OF OVARIAN FAILURE

Etiology/Pathophysiology Specific etiologies for hypergonadotropic and hypogonadotropic hypogonadism are discussed later. In general, pathology in the ovaries may be due to absence of the ovary, defective formation of the ovary, defective formation of the follicles, defective ovarian steroidogenesis or injury to the ovary by radiation, chemotherapy, infection, or autoimmune disease. A central pathology results in defective hormonal stimulation of the ovary. Pathology in the hypothalamus or the pituitary may result from defective migration of the neurons, absent gonadotropes, abnormal hormonal receptors, tumors and space-occupying lesions, or disturbance in the hormonal milieu due to psychogenic causes, illness, or lifestyle changes.

Clinical Presentation and Diagnostic Evaluation The most common presenting complaint of children with ovarian failure of any cause is delayed puberty or primary amenorrhea. In one large series of girls with delayed puberty who were referred to pediatric endocrinologists at an academic center, 30% had constitutional delay, 19% had functional hypogonadotropic hypogonadism, 20% had permanent hypogonadotropic hypogonadism, 26% had hypergonadotropic hypogonadism, and 4% had other causes (1). Girls given the diagnoses of "primary amenorrhea" have entered puberty but failed to progress to menarche. The most common causes for primary amenorrhea include ovarian failure (48.5%), anatomic defects (16.2%), GnRH deficiency (8.3%), and constitutional delay (6%) (2). The most common causes of secondary amenorrhea (amenorrhea with onset after menarche) are anovulation (28%), ovarian failure (10.5%), weight loss/anorexia (10%), and hypothalamic suppression (10%) (3). Please refer to Chapters 35 and 38 for discussion of menstrual cycle abnormalities and anatomic defects of the female genital tract. The discussion in this chapter will be limited to hypergonadotropic and hypogonadotropic hypogonadism.

Female Hypogonadism
AT-A-GLANCE

Normal ovarian function is characterized by spontaneous production of the sex hormones estrogen and progesterone and by ovulatory menstrual cycles. In childhood, the first physical sign of estrogen production, breast budding, usually begins between 9 and 11 years of age and the average age of menarche is 12.7 years. The median age of menopause is 51 years.

The term "premature ovarian failure" is conventionally used to describe women who develop ovarian failure before the age of 40. Delayed puberty in girls is defined as no secondary sex characteristics by age 13 (2 standard deviations above the mean), and primary amenorrhea as lack of menarche by age 16. Approximately 30% of girls with delayed puberty or primary amenorrhea have constitutional delay and will go on to experience normal, albeit late, pubertal development and ovarian function—this is a variation of normal growth. In many girls, however, either ovarian or central pathology is present. If the primary pathology is in the ovaries, serum gonadotropin levels become elevated and the conditions, which are generally permanent, are classified as "hypergonadotropic hypogonadism." If the primary pathology is in the hypothalamus or the pituitary and serum gonadotropins are low, then the conditions are classified as "hypogonadotropic hypogonadism." Hypogonadotropic hypogonadism can be functional (due to systemic illness, endocrinopathies, stress, excessive exercise, or undernutrition), or permanent.

HYPERGONADOTROPIC HYPOGONADISM IN PHENOTYPIC FEMALES

Type	Occurrence	(Gene) Locus	OMIM
Gonadal agenesis	rare	unknown	600171
Gonadal dysgenesis (Turner syndrome)	1:2000 live births	45,X most common, many forms abnormal X, mosaics	NA
Mixed gonadal dysgenesis	5-9% of Turner syndrome	Y genes present; mosaic 45,X/46XY or marker chromosome	NA
Pure gonadal dysgenesis			
Sex-determining region of Y (SRY)	25% of 46,XY pure gonadal dysgenesis	(SRY) Yp11.3	*480000
SOX9	rare	17q24.3-25.1	*608160, #114290
SF-1 (steroidogenic factor-1)	rare	(NR5A1) 19q33	+184757
DAX1	rare	(NR0B1) Xp21.2	*300473
Wilms tumor 1	rare	(WT1) 11p13	*607102
Bone morphogenetic protein 15	rare	(BMP15) Xp11.2	*300247
Perrault syndrome	rare	unknown	%233400
Gonadal steroid pathway enzyme defects			
Congenital lipoid hypoplasia (StAR)	rare	(StAR) 8p11.2	#201710
17α-hydroxylase/17,20-lyase deficiency	rare	(CYP17) 10q24.3	#202110
Aromatase deficiency	rare	(CYP19) 15q21.1	+107910
Genetic defects affecting gonadal function			
FSH receptor defects	Common only in Finland	2p21-p16	*136435
LH/β-hCG receptor defects	rare	2p21	+152790
Galactosemia	1:40,000-50,000	9p13	#230400
Fragile X premutation	1:6,000 females	(FMR1) Xq27.3	+309550
Multiple X syndromes	rare	47, XXX and 48,XXXX	NA
Blepharophimosis, ptosis, epicanthus, inversus syndrome (BPES)	rare	(FOXL2) 3q23	#110100
Diaphanous homolog 2	rare	Xq22	*300108
Eukaryotic initiation factor	rare	(EIF2B2) 14q24	*603162
		(EIF2B4) 2p23.3	*606687
		(EIF2B5) 3q27	*600495
Premature ovarian failure	1–2% of adult women		
Radiation/chemotherapy	common, lifetime risk	NA	NA
Autoimmune destruction	Present in 60% of APS-1, 4% of APS-2	APS type 1: (AIRE) 21q22.3 APS type 2: related to HLA-DR3-DQ2 and DR4-DQ8	# 240300 269200
Mumps oophoritis	5% of postpubertal females with mumps	NA	NA
Resistant ovaries	rare	unknown	NA

HYPERGONADOTROPIC HYPOGONADISM IN 46,XY AND 46,XX FEMALES

Form	Findings and Clinical Presentation
Gonadal agenesis	Both gonads absent, female external/internal genitalia when occurs prior to 6 wk fetal age, sexual infantilism
Gonadal dysgenesis (Turner syndrome)	Bilateral streak gonads; 45,X karyotype most common (>50%); short stature $+/-$ other characteristic physical features; most have sexual infantilism but 20-30% progress at least partially through puberty; mosaic karyotypes (gonadal dysgenesis variants) often less severely affected
Mixed gonadal dysgenesis	One streak gonad and one gonad with testicular tissue; Y chromosome structurally abnormal or present as mosaic; female phenotype, ambiguous genitalia or normal male depending on amount of Y present; $+/-$ short stature and features of Turner syndrome; risk of gonadal tumors
Pure gonadal dysgenesis (46,XX or 46,XY)	Bilateral streak gonads, female phenotype—difference between this and gonadal dysgenesis is normal stature; no Turner syndrome stigmata. Known gene defects causing pure gonadal dysgenesis in 46,XY: – SRY: complete 46,XY sex reversal (no testosterone or anti-Müllerian hormone) – SOX9; heterozygous loss-of-function mutations associated with campomelic dwarfism and phenotype ranging from complete 46,XY sex reversal with Müllerian structures present to ambiguous genitalia – SF-1: 46,XY complete sex reversal (no testosterone nor AMH) and/or adrenal failure; 46,XX have normal ovarian function with adrenal failure – DAX1: Duplication leads to variable 46,XY gonadal dysgenesis ranging from complete sex reversal with Müllerian structures to genital ambiguity – WT1: variable 46,XY gonadal dysgenesis ranging from complete sex reversal to ambiguity; 46,XX has normal external genitalia with normal or less impaired gonadal development; Frasier syndrome = 46,XY complete gonadal dysgenesis (+Müllerian structures), focal glomerular sclerosis and risk of gonadoblastoma; Denys-Drash syndrome = 46,XY gonadal dysgenesis with ambiguity, mesangial sclerosis and Wilms tumor Known gene defects causing gonadal dysgenesis in 46,XX: – BMP15, thought to be involved in oocyte maturation – Perrault syndrome: 46XX gonadal dysgenesis and sensorineural deafness; may have ataxia and cerebellar degeneration
Gonadal steroid pathway enzyme defects	Variable presentation depending on completeness and type of defect – StAR deficiency: lipoid congenital adrenal hyperplasia: early death from adrenal crisis if not detected; all patients present with female phenotype, 46,XY do not have Müllerian structures; 46,XX may undergo normal puberty – 17α-hydroxylase/17,20-lyase deficiency: no adrenal or salt wasting crisis (corticosterone (B) has glucocorticoid and 11-deoxycorticosterone (DOC) has mineralocorticoid activity.), hypokalemic, low renin hypertension ($\uparrow$ DOC); Severe defects: 46,XY-female phenotype but no Müllerian structures (+AMH); 46,XX no puberty (can't make sex hormones) – Aromatase deficiency: (no conversion of androgen to estrogen) in females result in virilization of the female fetus and ambiguous genitalia; at the age of puberty, affected females present with polycystic ovaries, amenorrhea, elevated gonadotropins, pubertal delay, progressive virilization and low estradiol and increased androgen levels
Genetic defects affecting gonadal function	Variable gonadal failure is associated with several genetic syndromes – FSH receptor defects: 46,XX delayed puberty, primary or secondary amenorrhea; 46,XY normal males (defects in spermatogenesis) – LH receptor defects: 46,XY phenotype ranges from ambiguous genitalia to normal female external genitalia, no Müllerian structures (+AMH); 46,XX normal genitalia and pubertal development, but amenorrhea and infertility – Galactosemia: ovarian failure soon after attaining puberty in majority, some before puberty – Fragile X premutation: 20% develop premature ovarian failure, mechanism unknown – Multiple X syndromes: 47,XXX is associated with ovarian failure; the association is less strong with 48,XXXX – DIAPH2: defect affecting actin-mediated morphogenetic processes, has been described in a family with premature menopause in a mother at age 32 and secondary amenorrhea in her 17-y-old daughter – FOXL2: blepharophimosis, ptosis, epicanthus inversus syndrome, type 1 associated with ovarian failure – Eukaryotic initiation factor defects result in childhood ataxia with central nervous system vanishing white matter disease leukodystrophy and premature ovarian failure
Premature ovarian failure	Normal menarche with subsequent oligomenorrhea/amenorrhea, risk of osteoporosis, infertility – Radiation/chemotherapy: lifelong risk (especially with alkylating agents); prepubertal girls are more resistant, perhaps simply because they have more primordial follicles; failure rates particularly high after bone marrow transplant (>40%) – Autoimmune: may be associated with the autoimmune polyglandular syndromes, no reliable serum antibody markers – Mumps oophoritis, doesn't necessarily impact fertility – Resistant ovaries: follicles arrested in preantral stage, may be transitional state in development of ovarian failure – Most cases in adults idiopathic, perhaps due to unidentified genetic defects; in contrast, an etiology is usually apparent in adolescents

HYPOGONADOTROPIC HYPOGONADISM IN 46,XX FEMALES

Type	Occurrence	Gene (Locus)	OMIM
Hypothalamic Defects			
Constitutional delay of growth and puberty	common	NA	NA
Functional defects	common	NA	NA
Hypothyroidism	relatively common	NA	NA
Genetic defects			
Kallmann syndrome	1:10,000 (M:F = 5:1)	X-linked = (KAL) Xp22.3	+308700
		AD = (FGFR1) 8p11.2	#147950
		AR = unknown	%244200
Leptin deficiency	rare	(LEP) 7q31.3	*164160
Leptin receptor defect	rare	(LEPR) 1p31	*601007
DAX1 (dosage sensitive sex reversal 1)	rare	(NR0B1) Xp21.2	*300473
G-protein coupled receptor 54 defect	rare	(GPR54) 19p13.3	*604161
Prader-Willi syndrome	1:10,000-25,000	(SNRPN and Necdin) 15q11-13	#176270
Bardet-Biedl syndrome	rare	Multiple loci	#209900
CHARGE syndrome	1:12,000	8q12.1	#214800
Physical insult to the hypothalamus	uncommon	NA	NA
Pituitary Defects			
Genetic defects			
GnRH receptor	20-50% of AR	(GNRHR) 4q21.2	*138850
FSHβ subunit	rare	11p13	*136530
HESX1	rare	3p21.2-p21.1	*601802
LHX3	rare	9q34.4	*600577
PROP1 (prophet of PIT1)	rare	5q	*601538
Prohormone convertase 1 defect	rare	(PCSK1) 5q15-q21	#600955
Physical insult to the hypothalamus	uncommon	NA	NA
Prolactinoma (isolated familial)	rare	unknown	600634
Prolactinoma with MEN1	42% of MEN1	11q13	+131100

AD=autosomal dominant; AR=autosomal recessive.

HYPOGONADOTROPIC HYPOGONADISM IN FEMALES

Type	Findings and Clinical Presentation

Hypothalamic Defects

Constitutional delay — Most common cause of delayed puberty, a variation of normal growth and development, slower tempo than usual

Functional defects — Chronic debilitating disease, anorexia nervosa, weight loss, stress or strenuous exercise can inhibit gonadotropin production, resulting in sexual infantilism in the prepubertal girl or amenorrhea in the sexually mature young woman

Hypothyroidism — Delayed puberty and growth in pre-pubertal children (or sometimes precocious puberty), menstrual irregularities post-puberty

Genetic defects
- Kallmann syndrome: anosmia, delayed puberty, normal growth but no pubertal growth spurt, eunuchoid proportions, synkinesis (mirror movements), midline facial defects, renal agenesis
- Leptin deficiency : hyperphagia, early childhood onset of morbid obesity; hypogonadotropic hypogonadism with impaired GnRH release; leptin infusion reverses obesity and hypogonadism
- Leptin receptor defect: similar to leptin deficiency, above, but leptin infusion has no effect
- NR0B1 (DAX1): listed in both Tables 1 and 2 because duplication leads to gonadal dysgenesis with 46,XY sex reversal. Loss-of-function mutations, however, lead to hypogonadotropic hypogonadism which may involve both the pituitary and the hypothalamus. Males but not females also have congenital adrenal hypoplasia and present with adrenal insufficiency. Involvement of adjacent genes can lead to glycerol kinase deficiency, Duchenne muscular dystrophy, ornithine transcarbam-ylase deficiency and mental retardation. Delayed puberty reported in female carriers of the DAX1 mutation.
- G-protein coupled receptor 54: autosomal recessive, described in two kindreds with boys and girls with hypogonadotropic hypogonadism; the ligand for this receptor is metastin, a peptide derived from the KISS1 protein which is expressed in the hypothalamus and placenta

Syndromes
- Prader-Willi syndrome: hypotonia in infancy, short stature, small hands and feet, hypothalamic obesity with an insatiable appetite, delayed puberty due to hypothalamic hypogonadism and mild mental retardation
- Bardet-Biedl syndrome: obesity, pigmentary retinopathy, polydactyly, mental retardation, and renal failure; hypogonadotropic hypogonadism variably present
- CHARGE syndrome: coloboma, heart disease, choanal atresia, retarded growth, genital hypoplasia in males, ear abnormalities +/− deafness; hypogonadism may be both hypothalamic and pituitary

Physical insult — May be due to tumor, infection, infiltrative processes, trauma, chemotherapy or radiation; may involve multiple pituitary hormones or non-endocrine hypothalamic sequelae (obesity, hyperphagia, temperature dysregulation, etc.)

Pituitary Defects

Genetic defects
- GnRH receptor: primary amenorrhea with absence or varying degrees of pubertal development
- FSHβ subunit gene: absent or delayed thelarche and primary amenorrhea with low levels of FSH and estradiol and high LH levels
- PROP1: heterogeneous clinical presentation with variable deficiencies of LH, FSH, GH, TSH, PRL, and ACTH
- HESX1: septo-optic dysplasia; hormone deficits range from isolated GH deficiency to panhypopituitarism
- LHX3: low gonadotropin levels, combined pituitary hormone deficiency and a rigid cervical spine
- Pro-hormone convertase 1: defect leads to inability to cleave POMC, proinsulin and proglucagon; characterized by severe childhood obesity, chronic gastro-intestinal disturbances, adrenal insufficiency and hypogonadotropic hypogonadism

Physical insult — May be due to tumor, infection, infiltrative processes, trauma, chemotherapy or radiation, autoimmune disease, degenerative disorders; usually involve multiple hormones; some specific causes listed below:
- Prolactinomas: delayed puberty or pubertal arrest, amenorrhea or oligomenorrhea and galactorrhea; normal TSH; if no lesion apparent on MRI consider drugs that can elevate prolactin levels
- Craniopharyngioma: headache, visual disturbance, poor growth; gonadotropin deficiency noted in up to 40%; calcified lesion on MRI
- Lymphocytic hypophysitis : usually associated with pregnancy; described in childhood in association with DI and panhypopituitarism; MRI reveals thickening of the sphenoid sinus mucosa, pituitary stalk enlargement, and tongue-shaped extension of the lesion along the basal hypothalamus; moderate elevation of prolactin
- Empty sella syndrome: extension of the subarachnoid space into the pituitary fossa due to tumor, surgery or radiotherapy; hyperprolactinemia, headaches, low bodyweight and short stature
- Sheehan's syndrome: postpartum pituitary necrosis; patients may present with fatigue, inability to lactate, amenorrhea, loss of axillary and pubic hair, severe hyponatremia and even coma; multiple pituitary hormones affected, most commonly growth hormone and gonadotropins

A thorough history with particular emphasis placed on family history of delayed puberty, early menopause, X-linked mental retardation or autoimmune disorders is essential. Family history of adrenal insufficiency and obesity may suggest defects in prohormone convertase 1 gene, whereas family history of X-linked adrenal insufficiency and hypogonadotropic hypogonadism in males may suggest that the female patient is a carrier of a DAX-1 mutation. Parental heights and calculated target height should be recorded. The girl's growth rate and weight gain as well as weight-to-height ratio throughout childhood and should be carefully evaluated; decreased growth rate, increased weight gain and predicted height below the target height suggest the following conditions: 1) existence of other pituitary hormone deficiencies either due to CNS structural lesions or pituitary transcription factors defects such as PROP-1, LHX3 and HESX1 (see Chapter 32); and, 2) primary hypothyroidism or Cushing syndrome.

History of early morbid obesity suggests leptin or leptin receptor defects. History of neonatal hypotonia, feeding difficulties, small feet and hands, cognitive delays, almond shape eyes and morbid obesity with short stature suggest Prader Willi whereas obesity associated with polydactyly, cognitive delays, pigmenatry retinopathy suggest Bardet-Biedl syndrome. Decreased weight-to- height ratio may indicate chronic disease or anorexia nervosa. History of lymphedema at birth, short stature, renal disease or cardiac disease suggest Turner syndrome. During physical examination, Tanner stage for breast development and pubic hair should be recorded and breasts should be examined for galactorrhea. Blood pressure should be also recorded. Hypertension in girls with primary amenorrhea suggest congenital adrenal hyperplaisa (CAH) due to 17α-hydroxylase/17,20 lyase (P450c17) deficiency. A complete neurologic evaluation should include examination of the optic discs and visual fields testing to rule out CNS CNS abnormality. The detailed systemic examination should also include evaluation of hearing (Perrault syndrome) and sense of smell as anosmia is part of some forms of Kallmann syndrome. Most anatomic defects causing primary amenorrhea can be diagnosed or at least suspected at the end of the physical examination. Attention must be paid to clinical evaluation of estrogen status during the examination of the breasts and the vaginal introitus.

After a thorough history and physical examination, laboratory evaluation should include the following: Serum FSH, LH, estradiol, prolactin levels, thyroid function tests, adrenal steroids such as 17α-hydroxyprogesterone(17-OHP), androstenedione, dehydroepiandrosterone-sulfate(DHEAS), progesterone and a testosterone level; testosterone level is particularly important to include if the patient has primary amenorrhea, normal breast development and absent pubic hair in order to rule out complete androgen insensitivity. General metabolic screening including electrolytes, CBC, ESR should be done to rule out systemic illness or inflammation.

If the serum gonadotropin levels are elevated, hypergonadotropic hypogonadism is the diagnosis; a pelvic ultrasound to evaluate uterus and ovaries should be obtained and a karyotype. A karyotype is suggested in order to differentiate between the following disorders associated with hypergonadotropic hypogonadism: 1) 46,XY sex reversal caused by gonadal dysgenesis, LHR defects or defects in testosterone biosynthesis or action; 2) Turner syndrome due to 45,XO or 45XO/46,XX or 46, XO/46,XY gonadal dysgenesis; 3) 46, XX gonadal dysgenesis or 46,XX ovarian failure due to LHR defects or defects in sex steroids production as in P450c17 deficiency; defect in estrogen synthesis as in aromatase deficiency or action as in estrogen receptor resistance should be suspected, especially if the patient has a history of ambiguous genitalia at birth, followed by pubertal failure and progressive virilization at the age of puberty, elevated gonadotropins, elevated androgens, low estradiol, and polycystic ovarian disease. If the serum gonadotropin levels are low or normal and the presence of a uterus is confirmed, constitutional delay is the most common diagnosis, followed by functional and permanent hypogonadotropic hypogonadism. Progression to spontaneous puberty confirms the diagnosis of constitutional delay (see Chapter 34).

If the diagnosis is not constitutional delay, functional hypogonadotropic hypogonadism is the second most likely diagnosis especially, in patients with anorexia nervosa, stress or strenous exercise in young athletes or dancers, or underlying chronic condition; chronic malnutrition and severe weight loss may suppress the hypothalamic-pituitary-gonadal axis resulting in low estradiol levels, pubertal failure and amenorrhea. If the patient has low to normal gonadotropins and evidence for estrogen secretion, chronic anovulation is most likely the cause of amenorrhea. If permanent causes of hypogonadotropic hypogonadism is suspected an MRI of the pituitary with gadolinium is recommended to evaluate to rule out space-occupying lesions even if the prolactin level is within the normal range. At any point during this algorithmic evaluation of delayed puberty or amenorrhea, it is appropriate to skip steps if a specific diagnosis is suspected based on history and physical examination. Laparoscopic ovarian biopsy is not necessary as ultrasound and FSH levels can reliably assess the ovary for the presence of antral follicles.

It is always important to consider the possibility of pregnancy when evaluating amenorrhea in a girl who has completed puberty. The test can be performed in the clinic and is inexpensive and rapid. Some patients with hypogonadism have renal abnormalities and it is prudent to perform a renal ultrasonographic examination if indicated.

Treatment of Female Hypogonadism

Hormone Replacement The goals of treatment of female hypogonadism with hormone replacement therapy are to induce sexual maturation at a gradual pace mimicking normal puberty, to augment growth without overly accelerating epiphyseal fusion, to maximize height potential, to promote accrual of bone mass, to maintain sexual health once development is complete, and, in adult women, to assist reproduction. With the exception of fertility therapy, treatment is the same regardless of whether the category of hypogonadism is hyper- or hypogonadotropic. Puberty should generally be initiated at approximately 12 years of age to allow normal psychosocial development and for bone health. Unopposed estrogen is essential for induction of breast development and is started at a low dose, which is gradually increased over a period of 2 to 4 years to mimic normal puberty. Progesterone is essential for converting the endometrium from the proliferative to the secretory phase, thereby preventing the development of endometrial hyperplasia and carcinoma. Cycling with progesterone is begun 2 to 2.5 years after initiation of low-dose estrogen therapy or sooner if breakthrough bleeding occurs. In girls who have spontaneously achieved some degree of pubertal development or in whom final adult height is not a concern, the initial estrogen dose can be higher and cycling can begin sooner. Suggested protocols including dosage of different preparations are summarized in (Tables 36-1 to 36-4).

A variety of natural estrogen and synthetic estrogen and progesterone preparations are available to initiate puberty and menstrual cycling. Of the various routes of administration available, the oral and transdermal routes are the most popular and convenient. A 2004 survey of Lawson Wilkins Pediatric Endocrine Society members indicated that 78% of pediatric endocrinologists in the US recommended the conjugated equine estrogen for puberty induction 10% favored oral ethinyl estradiol, and 8% transdermal 17-β estradiol (4). In contrast, European pediatric endocrinologists favored oral ethinyl estradiol (39%), oral 17-β estradiol (32%), and transdermal 17-β estradiol (10%), with only 12% selecting conjugated equine estrogen as their choice (5).

TABLE 36-1 General Protocols for Hormone Replacement

Aim	Timing	Principle	Method–Start With:
Induction of breast growth (skip this step if breast development has occurred to Tanner stage 4–5)	12–14 years, depending whether patient achieved satisfactory height	Unopposed estrogen for a 2–2.5 years (add progesterone if breakthrough bleeding occurs). Start with a low dose and increase to adult doses (see Table 6) gradually. Evaluate breast growth at least every 6 months	Typically start out with 1/8-1/4 of adult dose: Conjugated estrogen (equine, synthetic, or esterified) – 0.3 mg orally daily or every other day; may promote rapid epiphyseal fusion *Or* ethinyl estradiol 2-5 µg orally daily *Or* 17ß-estradiol 0.25 mg orally daily *Or* 17ß-estradiol transdermal patch starting with half or one quarter of a 0.025-mg patch weekly or twice weekly depending on the preparation
Hormone replacement to maintain sexual health and bone mass	2–2.5 years after starting unopposed estrogen therapy, sooner if breakthrough bleeding occurs	Cyclical progesterone for 7–10 days in a cycle to prevent development of endometrial cancer	*28-d cycles with hormone intake for 21 of these days and hormone free for 7 d; estrogen for 21 d; on d 15-21 of taking the estrogen, add*: Medroxyprogesterone 2.5 to 5 mg orally daily *Or* Norethindrone 0.5 to 1 mg orally daily *Or* Norethindrone 0.14- to 0.25-mg patch twice weekly (with estradiol as combination patch) *Or* Levonorgestrel 0.015-mg patch (with estradiol as combination patch) *Alternatively*, combined oral contraceptive pills may be used *Note:* Dose of conjugated estrogens can be increased to 1.25 mg daily when cyclical progesterone is added. Ethinyl Estradiol is not available as a single formulation in USA

TABLE 36-2 Common Estrogen-Only Drugs Used in Hormone Therapy to Induce and Maintain Puberty

Product Examples	Estrogen	Common Premenopausal Adult Dose	Available Doses (mg)
Premarin (Wyeth)	Oral equine conjugated estrogen	1.25 mg/d	0.3, 0.45, 0.625, 0.9, 1.25, 2.5 mg
Cenestin (Duramed) Enjuvia (Duramed)	Oral synthetic conjugated estrogen	1.25 mg/d	0.3, 0.45, 0.625, 0.9, 1.25 mg 0.625, 1.25 mg
Menetest (Monarch)	Oral esterified estrogen	1.25 mg/d	0.3, 0.625, 1.25, 2.5 mg
Ogen (Abbot)	Oral estropipate	1.25 mg/d	0.625, 1.25, 2.5 mg
Gynodiol (Novavax)	Oral 17β-estradiol	2.0 mg/d	0.5, 1.0, 2.0 mg
Estrace (Warner- Chilcott) Estradiol (Watson Labs)	Oral micronized 17β-estradiol	2.0 mg/d	0.5, 1.0, 2.0 mg
Alora (Watson) Esclim (Women First) Estraderm (Ciba-Geigy) Vivelle (Novartis) *Vivelle-Dot (Novartis)	Transdermal 17β-estradiol patch	0.1 mg, 2x/wk change patch	0.025, 0.05, 0.075, 0.1 mg 0.025, 0.0375, 0.05, 0.075, 0.1 mg 0.05, 0.1 mg 0.025, 0.0375, 0.05, 0.075, 0.1 mg 0.025, 0.05, 0.075, 0.10 mg
Climara (Berlex) FemPatch (Parke-Davis)		0.1 mg, 1x/wk change patch	0.025, 0.0375, 0.05, 0.06, 0.075, 0.1 mg 0.025 mg
EstroGel (Solvay)	Transdermal estradiol gel	0.1–1.5 mg/d	0.75 mg / pump unit dose (rub into arm)

*Vivelle-Dot may be particularly conducive to cutting into smaller pieces

**Transvaginal estrogen products are also available but are not usually considered practical in the pediatric population

TABLE 36-3 Common Progesterone-Only Drugs Used in Hormone Therapy to Induce and Maintain Puberty

Product Examples	Progesterone	Common Premenopausal Adult Dose	Available Doses (mg)
Prometrium (Solvay)	Micronized progesterone	200–300 mg 10–12 d/ cycle	100, 200 mg
Provera (Pharmacia-Upjohn)	Medroxyprogesterone acetate	5–10 mg daily 10–12 d/ cycle	2.5, 5, 10 mg
Aygestin (Barr)	Norethindrone acetate	5–10 mg daily 10–12 d/ cycle	5 mg

**Vaginal, intrauterine, and parenteral products are available but are not usually considered practical in the pediatric population

TABLE 36-4 Common Combination Products Used in Hormone Therapy

Oral Product	Estrogen	Progestin
Activella *(Novo Nordisk)*	17β-estradiol 1.0 mg	Norethindrone acetate 0.5 mg
Prefest *(Monarch)*	17β-estradiol 1.0 mg	Norgestimate 0.09 mg (3 d on and 3 d off)
Climara Pro *(Berlex)*	17β-estradiol 0.045 mg	Levonorgestrel 0.015 mg
FemHRT *(Pfizer)*	Ethinyl estradiol 0.05mg	Norethindrone acetate 1.0 mg
Premphase *(Wyeth)*	Conjugated equine estrogen 0.625 mg	Medroxy progesterone 5 mg (14-d/28-d cycle)
Prempro *(Wyeth)*	Conjugated equine estrogen 0.625 mg	Medroxy progesterone 2.5 mg or 5.0 mg
	Conjugated equine estrogen 0.45 or 0.3mg	Medroxy progesterone 1.5 mg
Oral contraceptive pills	Multiple formulations (usually 20-30 mg/ethinyl estradiol)	Multiple formulations
Transdermal product (2x/week)		
CombiPatch *(Novartis)*	17β-estradiol 0.05 mg	Norethindrone acetate 0.14 mg
	17β-estradiol 0.05 mg	Norethindrone acetate 0.25 mg

Generally, the initial estrogen dose for induction of puberty must be very low to maximize growth potential. Regimens using conjugated estrogen (Premarin 0.3 mg/d for 6–12 mo followed by 0.625 mg/d for 6–18 mo followed by addition of 10 mg medroxyprogesterone acetate 7–14 d/mo) may deliver too high a dose. The final height in girls with TS, was decreased when estrogen therapy was started at 12 years of age in comparison to the final height of TS patients starting estrogen therapy later at 15 years of age (6). Better results were also reported in TS girls treated with very low doses of intramuscular depot estradiol, 0.2 mg/month with gradual dose increases over a period of 2 years (4 7) or treated with 17-β estradiol starting at 5 μg/kg/day and increasing to a dose of 10 μg/kg/day over a period of 5 years (8). The authors acknowledge however that an intramuscular route is not practical for routine clinical application (4).

There is increasing evidence that the non-oral routes of estrogen administration offer important advantages in inducing puberty in hypogonadal girls. Transdermal 17-β estradiol patches with a matrix composition can be cut into pieces that deliver doses as small as one-eighth of a 0.025-mg dose. In one study, by gradually increasing the patch size, they were able to accurately mimic normal early and mid pubertal estrogen levels (9). Similarly, transdermal estrogen gel starting at a dose of 0.1 mg/day and increasing over 5 years to a dose of 1.5 mg was able to mimic levels found during normal puberty in girls with TS (10). Studies in adults suggest systemic advantages that may be pertinent in girls who are already at increased risk for the metabolic syndrome, such as those with TS. Compared with oral estrogens, transdermal estrogens reduce insulin resistance and have a more beneficial effect on body composition, lipid oxidation, and serum triglyceride levels (11,12). Insulin-like growth factor-I levels are greater with the transdermal route (13), which may have implications for achievement of adequate height.

In addition to the preparations listed in Tables 36-1 to 36-4, low-dose oral contraceptive pills may be used for combined hormone replacement. These are extremely convenient, but they provide a higher dose of estrogen than is physiologically necessary when birth control is not needed. Although it is clear that more studies need to be performed in the pediatric population to determine the optimum therapeutic regimen, it seems prudent to try to achieve near-physiologic estrogen/progesterone levels in adolescent girls (4).

Fertility Even though it is not an immediate problem, adolescent girls and their parents are extremely concerned about future fertility. Thus, it is important to inform them about currently available methods of assisted reproduction, along with the expectation that techniques will improve by the time the young woman is ready to contemplate pregnancy. Artificial reproductive techniques should be performed in a specialist center. In patients with hypogonadotropic hypogonadism, the method used for ovulation induction depends on the presence or absence of pituitary function. In the presence of pituitary function, pulsatile GnRH can be successfully used to induce ovulation. The advantage with this method is a lower rate of multiple pregnancies and ovarian hyperstimulation compared with induction of ovulation with gonadotropins. If pituitary function is absent, gonadotropins are used for ovulation induction. Microdose hCG or combined FSH and LH preparations are used to allow production of androgen precursors for aromatization to estrogens. Coitus, intrauterine insemination, or in vitro fertilization can then be performed to achieve conception. At present, the only option for hypergonado-tropic hypogonadism patients is donor oocyte and in vitro fertilization.

HYPERGONADOTROPIC HYPOGONADISM

Elevated gonadotropin levels are found when there is primary ovarian failure. Important management decisions depend on correctly diagnosing the cause of ovarian failure. For example, TS patients require special care involving multiple specialists while the pure gonadal dysgenesis patient does not require such rigorous medical attention. Individuals with a karyotype involving the Y chromosome have up to a 25% risk of developing gonadal malignancy, whereas gonadal tumors are rare in patients without Y chromosome in their karyotype. Tumors have been demonstrated in dysgenetic gonads in patients as young as 6 months old. In addition, there is a risk of virilization during puberty from androgen production, if testicular tissue is present in these gonads. Therefore, it is recommended that all women younger than 30 years of age with hypergonadotropic hypogonadism have their karyotype determined and prophylactic gonadectomy performed if Y chromosome material is present. An algorithm for the differential diagnosis of hypergonadotropic hypogonadism is presented in Figure 36-1.

Gonadal Agenesis

Gonadal agenesis refers to complete absence of both gonads. This generally manifests as sexual infantilism with female external genitalia (reflecting lack of functional testicular tissue from at least 6 wk fetal age) and is generally associated with a 46,XY karyotype, although rarely it can be associated with 46,XX (14). The diagnosis is usually made when laparoscopy is performed to remove the gonads in a 46,XY female. Thorough

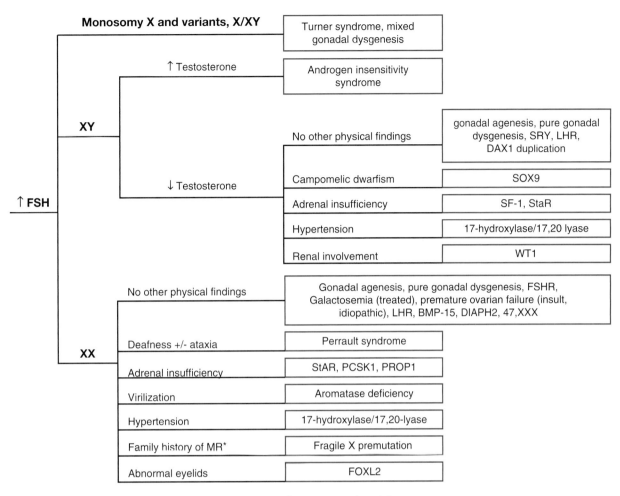

FIGURE 36-1. Algorithm for the differential diagnosis of hypergonadotropic hypogonadism; *MR = mental retardation.

examination of the inguinal canal must be performed to rule out undescended testes (see Chapter 35).

Gonadal Dysgenesis (Turner Syndrome)

Pathogenesis TS is discussed in detail in Chapter 31. Patients with TS have an abnormal karyotype involving the X chromosome. More than 50% of girls with TS have the 45,X karyotype, whereas others have 46,XX with one of the X chromosomes being abnormal; a wide range of X abnormalities exists, including gene deletions, ring chromosomes, and isochromosomes. Twenty percent to 35% of TS patients have mosaic karyotypes such as 45,X/46,XX (gonadal dysgenesis variants). Five percent to 10% of patients have a cell line with Y chromosome material present (mixed gonadal dysgenesis). The 45,X karyotype is generally associated with the most severely affected phenotype. The clinical presentation is quite variable with gonadal dysgenesis variants or mixed gonadal

dysgenesis, depending on the amount of normal X or Y chromosome material present. Almost 99% of conceptions with the 45,X karyotype result in miscarriage, and thus the true prevalence of TS is considerably higher than the birth prevalence of approximately 1:2000.

The phenotype of TS reflects the absence of specific genes. Normally in females one X chromosome is randomly inactivated except small regions called pseudoautosomal regions, which retain two alleles. The SHOX (short stature homeobox) gene is present in the pseudoautosomal regions on the X chromosome and absence of one of the allelic pair results in short stature. There is believed to be a lymphogenic gene on the X chromosome, absence of which leads to lymphedema. Abnormalities in two other regions on the X chromosome, POF1 & POF2, are considered important in the development of premature ovarian failure; however, the genes involved within these regions have not been delineated.

At 14 to 18 weeks gestation, the ovaries of the 45,X fetus appear to be completely nor-

mal. After this, there is rapid loss of oocytes and stromal fibrosis, so that in the majority of girls with TS, complete or near-complete follicular atresia has occurred prenatally or within the first several months or years of postnatal life. Some pubertal development may occur in up to 30% of TS patients and spontaneous pregnancies have been reported in 2% to 5% (15).

Clinical Presentation In the antenatal period, the diagnosis may be made incidentally upon karyotyping the fetus because of advanced maternal age. Left-sided cardiac anomalies, increased nuchal translucency or edema of the extremities noted during sonographic examination of the fetus should lead to karyotyping of the fetus even in a younger mother. In the newborn period, TS should be suspected if characteristic features are present such as edema of the hands and feet, low hairline, presence of a nuchal fold, or left-sided cardiac anomalies. Only approximately 20% to 30% of TS patients are diagnosed in the newborn period, however.

Short stature in childhood with declining growth velocity is the most frequent presentation of TS. Because other stigmata may be absent or subtle, the diagnosis is frequently overlooked initially by physicians (16,17). The average adult height of these patients if they are not treated with growth hormone is 147.3 ± 6.0 cm (16,18).

In adolescence, the common presenting complaint is delayed puberty. Although some girls spontaneously undergo puberty, the majority of girls with TS exhibit sexual infantilism with no breast development or evidence of estrogenization. Sparse pubic hair may be present in the pubertal-aged girl due to adrenal androgens. FSH levels are elevated during the first 2 years of life, decline normally to low levels during childhood, and rise again to castrate levels at the time of expected puberty. Estrogen levels are lower than normal even during the prepubertal years (19). A small percentage of women with TS may present with recurrent pregnancy loss or secondary amenorrhea.

Diagnosis and Treatment Karyotyping is usually performed on peripheral blood lymphocytes. Many laboratories will count only 20 cells. If TS is suspected and the karyotype is reported to be 46,XX, the number of cells counted must be increased to 100 or a fibroblast culture (skin biopsy) performed to rule out mosaicism. It has been shown that up to 67% of TS patients may have mosaicism if both lymphocyte and fibroblast cultures are performed (20). Up to 6% of patients may have a Y chromosome and up to 3% have a marker chromosome (a supernumerary chromosome that is structurally abnormal and cannot be classified as part of any of the normal chromosomes). In almost all these patients with a marker chromosome, a Y component is noted. Gonadectomy is indicated in patients with Y material in their karyotype.

Detailed guidelines for management of children with TS have been published by the American Academy of Pediatrics (21) and are discussed in the chapter on TS. Sex hormone replacement is essential in TS and has been shown to exert an anabolic effect on the skeleton of these patients (22). The timing of hormonal replacement is important because once estrogen therapy is started, there is a relatively short period of time (~24 mo) before the epiphyses close. In the girl who was started on growth hormone therapy at an early age and has achieved normal or acceptable stature, estrogen therapy can be stared at 12 years of age. In the very short girl with TS, however, many practitioners delay estrogen therapy until 15 years to allow time to gain increased height. Please see Table 36-1 for suggested sex hormone replacement protocols.

With increasing lifespan of TS patients and with advances in artificial reproductive technologies, reports of donor oocyte in vitro fertilization are beginning to emerge. Careful screening of organ systems must be performed before this is offered because a few cases of dissection of the aorta during pregnancy have been reported (23). It is important to note that the majority of TS patients becoming pregnant spontaneously or through assisted reproductive techniques do not suffer this complication (16,24).

Pure Gonadal Dysgenesis

Pure gonadal dysgenesis is a label used for individuals with 46,XX or 46,XY karyotype with streak gonads, sexual infantilism, and normal stature with no stigmata of TS. 46,XY sex reversal is sometimes called Swyer syndrome. Children with 46,XY gonadal dysgenesis have a uterus, as the dysgenetic gonads rarely produce anti-Müllerian hormone (AMH). Children with partial or mixed 46, XY gonadal dysgenesis may produce some AMH and testosterone, which may result in genital ambiguity (see Chapter 35). Notably, because key genes on the pseudoautosomal regions of the sex chromosomes are not affected, physical features of TS including short stature are absent. Other features may be present that point to specific chromosomal defects.

Several different etiologies are possible for pure gonadal dysgenesis. Patients with 46,XX gonadal dysgenesis and a female phenotype are likely to harbor mutations in one of the many autosomal and X-linked genes being enumerated as having a role in ovarian morphogenesis, such as BMP15, a gene on the short arm of the X chromosome that promotes folliculogenesis and granulosa cell growth and is thought to be involved in oocyte maturation (25). Several families with 46,XX gonadal dysgenesis and sensorineural deafness have been reported (Perrault syndrome) (26). Some of these patients may have ataxia and cerebellar degeneration. Up to 50% of women with 46,XX premature ovarian failure have some ovarian follicles remaining. Unpredictable intermittent ovulation can occur in these patients and pregnancies have been documented.

Sex-Determining Region of Y (SRY) Up to 25% of 46,XY gonadal dysgenesis patients have a mutation in SRY, a gene found on the Y chromosome that produces a transcription factor involved in differentiation of the bipotential gonad into testis. Depending on the specific mutation, disruption of SRY can result in complete 46,XY sex reversal with absence of Wolffian or Müllerian structures, true hermaphroditism, or ambiguous genitalia. Abnormalities in other genes are involved in the etiology of gonadal dysgenesis, because the majority of 46,XY females have normal

SRY (27). Although most of these mutations have yet to be determined, defects in the genes listed later have resulted in complete sex reversal in case reports in 46,XY individuals.

SOX9 SOX9 (an SRY homeobox gene) is involved in testis determination and may be a downstream target of SRY. Heterozygous loss-of-function mutations in 46,XY patients are associated with campomelic dwarfism and a phenotype ranging from complete sex reversal with the presence of Müllerian structures to ambiguous genitalia. Campomelic dysplasia usually leads to neonatal death from respiratory failure (see Chapter 35).

NR5A1 (Nuclear Receptor subfamily 5 type A member 1, or Steroidogenic Factor 1 or SF-1) SF-1 is a nuclear receptor involved in gene regulation of many aspects of the reproductive axis including gonadotrope function, male sexual differentiation, Müllerian regression, steroidogenesis, and testicular descent. Mutations in SF-1 have been reported to cause gonadal dysgenesis with complete XY sex reversal and/or adrenal failure. Affected 46,XY patients present with normal female external genitalia, streak gonads, and a hypoplastic uterus and respond to treatment with cyclical estrogen and progesterone resulting in pubertal maturation and regular menstruation (28). A female with an SF-1 deletion had adrenal hypoplasia but normal ovaries (29).

NR0B1 (nuclear receptor subfamily 0 type B member 1, or Dosage sensitive sex reversal Adrenal hypoplasia congenita X-linked gene 1, DAX1) Loss-of-function mutations in DAX1 are associated with both adrenal insufficiency (X-linked congenital adrenal hypoplasia) and hypogonadotropic hypogonadism only in males. Females carriers may present with delayed puberty. In contrast to deletions, duplication of the DAX1 locus leads to variable 46,XY gonadal dysgenesis ranging from complete sex reversal with Müllerian structures present to genital ambiguity (30) (see Chapter 35).

Wilms Tumor Suppressor Gene 1 (WT1) WT1, involved in both renal and gonadal differentiation, appears to function both as a transcription factor and a tumor suppressor. 46,XY individuals may have gonadal dysgenesis with normal female genitalia or, if less severely affected, may have ambiguous genitalia. 46,XX girls have normal external genitalia with normal or less impaired gonadal development. Different mutations result in various syndromes. Frasier syndrome is characterized by progressive focal glomerular sclerosis and streak gonads. Wilms tumor is rare but patients are at risk for gonadoblastoma. Patients with Denys-Drash syndrome have genitourinary abnormalities and Wilms tumor. Progressive renal failure with onset early in life is characterized by proteinuria and focal or diffuse mesangial sclerosis (see Chapter 35).

Gonadal Steroid Pathway Enzyme Deficiencies

Lipoid Congenital Adrenal Hyperplasia Lipoid congenital adrenal hyperplasia is mostly caused by a deficiency in the steroidogenic acute regulatory (StAR) protein. StAR is essential for the transport of cholesterol into mitochondria and a defect results in severe impairment of steroid synthesis in both adrenals and gonads. Cholesterol accumulates in the adrenal glands, leading to the enlarged, lipid-filled appearance. Absence of cortisol and aldosterone production leads to adrenal crisis with salt wasting in the newborn period, which is usually fatal.

All 46,XY patients with lipoid congenital adrenal hyperplasia present as phenotypic females because of absent of sex steroid production. These patients do not have a uterus because of normal Sertoli function and AMH production. Wolffian structures may be absent or hypoplastic. Some 46,XX individuals who survive to the teenage years have been noted to undergo normal puberty and attain menarche (31). Treatment includes glucocorticoid and mineralocorticoid replacement from birth and sex hormone replacement at puberty in 46,XY and perhaps 46,XX individuals (see Chapter 27).

17 α-Hydroxylase and 17, 20-Lyase Deficiencies The CYP17 gene codes for the P450c17 enzyme that exhibits both 17 α-hydroxylase and 17,20-lyase activities. Although both enzymes are usually affected together, specific mutations (amino acid positions 347 and 358) have been shown to interfere with the interaction of the enzyme with its redox partners, resulting in isolated deficiency of 17,20-lyase activity (32–34).

Conversion of pregnenolone and progesterone to 17-hydroxy steroids is blocked by 17 α-hydroxylase deficiency. This is a key step in human steroidogenesis. Formation of cortisol and sex steroids is blocked, and the mineralocorticoid pathway is unaffected. 11-Deoxycorticosterone (DOC) and corticosterone are formed in excess at the zona fasciculata secondary to stimulation by elevated ACTH levels. Elevation of DOC leads to low renin hypertension and hypokalemia. Although corticosterone is not as potent as cortisol, it possesses enough glucocorticoid activity that when it is present in excess it is able to prevent adrenal crisis and, thus, diagnosis of a CYP17 gene defect is not usually made until the time of puberty, when testosterone and estrogen deficiency become apparent.

Patients with complete enzyme defects present with female external genitalia, sexual infantilism, and elevated gonadotropin levels. 46,XX individuals have normal female internal sex structures and primary amenorrhea. 46,XY individuals, due to normal AMH secretion in utero, have a short vagina and absence of a uterus. If the defect is not complete and some testosterone production is possible, they may have hypoplastic Wolffian ducts and varying degrees of genital ambiguity. Laboratory findings include decreased serum levels of cortisol, dehydroepiandrosterone, androstenedione, renin, aldosterone and estrogens with increased levels of progesterone, DOC and corticosterone. Considerable heterogeneity in physical and laboratory findings have been described, depending on the severity of the defect (34).

Isolated 17,20 lyase deficiency presents with a unique phenotype of normal blood pressure, primary amenorrhea, and sexual infantilism. This condition is extremely rare (34). A recent case report described a 13-year-old girl presenting with large ovarian cysts elevated serum gonadotropins and 17-hydroxysteroids and low peripheral levels of androgens and estrogens. Female 46,XY sibling was found to harbor the same mutation (35).

Replacement with glucocorticoids (hydrocortisone in children, prednisone or dexamethasone in adults) normalizes the blood pressure by inhibiting adrenocorticotropin hormone secretion and its stimulation of the mineralocorticoid pathway. Estrogen replacement should be initiated as described earlier around the time of expected puberty (see Chapter 27).

Aromatase Deficiency The aromatase enzyme (P450arom) is coded by the CYP19 gene. Mutation in this gene results in absence of conversion of androgens to estrogen. Consequently, androgen levels are increased during fetal life, resulting in virilization of the female fetus. Depending on the severity of the defect, females present at birth with ambiguous genitalia, in childhood with ovarian cysts (36), or at the time of puberty with amenorrhea and polycystic ovaries (37–39). Hormone replacement as described in Table 36-1 leads to breast development, normalization of gonadotropin levels, resolution of ovarian cysts, and occurrence of menses. Aromatase deficiency was described in a male who had completely normal sexual development and function, tall stature, and incomplete fusion of the epiphyses, demonstrating that the primary role of estrogen in the male is to promote skeletal maturation (37).

Genetic Defects Affecting Gonadal Function

Follicle Stimulating Hormone Receptor Gene Mutations Females with homozygous inactivating mutations of the FSH receptor (FSHR) present with delayed puberty, primary amenorrhea, elevated FSH, elevated LH, and low estradiol levels The ovaries show arrest of follicular development. Very few FSHR mutations have been identified, with the first mutation (Ala189Val) described in Finnish women (40–42). The mode of transmission is autosomal recessive with a deleterious effect on fertility. Males have a normal male phenotype and undergo normal spontaneous puberty but may have defects in spermatogenesis.

The clinical presentation of females with compound heterozygous mutations in FSHR is variable, including normal pubertal development followed by primary or secondary amenorrhea. Sonographic examination reveals normal to slightly enlarged ovaries with several follicles arrested in the antral stage of development. Heterozygous carriers of inactivating mutations have normal pubertal development and fertility, suggesting that the presence of one wild-type FSHR allele is sufficient to permit normal reproductive function in humans. Treatment with FSH does not result in any steroid production by the ovary (43).

Luteinizing Hormone Receptor Gene (LHR) Mutations In males, inactivating mutations of the LHR gene lead to Leydig cell hypoplasia and inadequate secretion of testosterone. The 46,XY phenotype ranges from ambiguous genitalia to normal female external genitalia, depending on the severity of the defect. There are no Müllerian structures present because AMH secretion is normal (see Chapter 37).

Females are born with normal internal and external sex structures and undergo normal puberty. The LHR has an important role in follicular maturation and induction of ovulation, and patients with inactivating mutations in this gene have elevated FSH and LH levels with low-to-normal estradiol levels (44,45). The ovaries have many follicles in various stages of development. The phenotype may range from primary amenorrhea to dysfunctional uterine bleeding and infertility.

Galactosemia Galactosemia is a rare disorder with an estimated prevalence of 1:40,000 to 50,000 (46). Females with galactosemia due to complete deficiency of galactose-1-phosphate uridyl transferase invariably suffer from ovarian failure (47). Follicular depletion has been noted but the exact mechanism has not been elucidated (48). Ovarian failure is more likely if the mean galactose-1-phosphate level in the erythrocyte exceeds 3.5 mg/dL or if the patient has a homozygous Q188R mutation in the GALT gene (49). Variants of the classic disease present with varying levels of enzymatic activity (for other aspects of the disorder see Chapter 9). Most patients develop ovarian failure soon after puberty, but some develop it earlier (50). Prenatal identification and early treatment through newborn screening programs do not prevent the development of ovarian failure in patients with complete enzyme deficiency.

Fragile X Syndrome Premutation Fragile X syndrome is the most common cause of inherited mental retardation in humans with an incidence of 1:6,000 in females. There are less than 55 CGG repeats in the 5′ untranslated region of the FMR1 gene in normal individuals compared with 200 or more trinucleotide repeats in patients with fragile X syndrome. Those patients with CGG repeats between 55 and 199 in number are recognized to have a premutation, and their offspring have higher risk for developing the full mutation. Female patients with full mutations have normal ovarian function. Interestingly, approximately 20% of patients with premutation in FMR1 develop premature ovarian failure as opposed to 1% of the general population (51). The mechanism involved is unknown.

Multiple X chromosomes Trisomy for the X chromosome (47,XXX) is also associated with ovarian failure. In contrast, 48,XXXX women do not have a strong phenotypic association with premature ovarian failure (52), although a case has been reported in the literature (53).

DIAPH2 and FOXL2 Gene Defects Primary ovarian failure has been described with gene defects in DIAPH2 (54), FOXL2 and EIF2B (55,56). In particular, defects of the winged helix/forkhead transcription factor gene, (FOXL2) are associated with blepharophimosis/ptosis/epicanthus inversus syndrome and/or ovarian failure. Defects of the diaphanous drosophila homolog 2 (DIAPH2) gene are associated with premature ovarian failure. Eukaryotic initiation factor-2B (EIF2B) defects result in premature ovarian failure and childhood ataxia with central nervous system hypomyelination/vanishing white-matter leukodystrophy. The genetics of ovarian development has become a very complex field of study with the explosion in molecular genetic knowledge within the last decade. Genes at multiple levels are involved and the information is currently too fragmented to offer a coherent overview. Except for FSHR gene mutation testing in Finland, testing for these gene mutations is not offered for widespread clinical use yet.

Premature Ovarian Failure

Premature ovarian failure is conventionally used to describe patients who develop ovarian failure after menarche and before the age of 40. In adults, most cases of premature ovarian failure have no discernible etiology and are currently classified as idiopathic. Although karyotypes have generally been found to be normal (57), it is quite likely that many of these patients will eventually be assigned specific genetic causes in the future. In contrast

to adults, an etiology is usually apparent in children who have the capacity to achieve normal ovarian function but subsequently lose it. Many of these girls have TS. The following is a discussion of other conditions resulting in or leading to premature ovarian failure.

Injury to the Ovaries by Chemotherapy and Radiation Ovarian function in survivors of cancer remains a concern among the caregivers of young women. Cancer patients are usually subjected to chemotherapy, radiotherapy, or both. Among chemotherapeutic agents, the alkylating agents busulfan and cyclophosphamide are especially toxic to the ovaries. Following treatment with these agents, approximately 17% of women develop premature ovarian failure and 70% resume spontaneous menstrual cycles. The ovarian volume, mean number of antral follicles, and serum inhibin levels are significantly reduced in spontaneously menstruating survivors when compared with controls. Therefore, even individuals who spontaneously menstruate after chemotherapy have diminished ovarian reserve and are likely to suffer premature ovarian failure in the future (58–61). Increased age of the patient at the time of chemotherapy and/or irradiation increases the risk of premature ovarian failure (62). As a result, adolescents and young women are highly susceptible to the toxic effects of therapy, whereas prepubertal girls are more resistant, presumably due to a larger reserve pool of primordial follicles; however, those undergoing bone marrow transplantation may have ovarian failure rates of 43% or higher (63, 64). A longer duration of therapy also increases the likelihood of ovarian failure. Most bone mass accumulation in the hip and spine occurs between 14 and 18 years of age in women, and lack of estrogen during this time can result in decreased bone density. Rapid bone loss as measured by bone mineral density has been documented with chemotherapy-induced ovarian failure (65).

Fertility is always an emotional issue and the inability of the current state of medical technology to confidently preserve the fertility in girls and women undergoing chemotherapy is a frequent source of anguish to all parties involved. Many approaches have been tested to preserve ovarian function prior to chemotherapy or radiotherapy. The oldest and most effective is ovarian transposition in cases requiring pelvic irradiation. In fact, this is the only method proven to be effective in preserving ovarian function. Laparoscopic transposition of ovaries is as effective as the traditional approach via laparotomy and preservation rates as high as 88.6% have been noted in women undergoing pelvic radiation

(66). The use of oral contraceptives to preserve ovarian function in patients undergoing gonadotoxic chemotherapy appears to be ineffective (67). Use of GnRH analogs and antagonists remains controversial. The studies are small and poorly controlled (68–71). Recently published animal data are encouraging (72) but large, controlled, randomized studies in humans are needed before firm recommendations can be made. Cryopreservation of ovarian tissue and reimplantation after completion of therapy remains controversial and concerns have been raised about potential for transfer of malignant cells during this process (68). Recent case reports of success are encouraging, including a live birth from Belgium (73–76). Despite this success, cryopreservation and ovarian transplantation remains an option only in the realm of research and is not widely available in the mainstream. Live birth rate from cryopreservation of oocytes is dismal at less that 2% and is not currently available for routine use (69).

Autoimmune Ovarian Failure Autoimmune disease plays a minor role in the etiology of premature ovarian failure. No reliable serum antibody marker for premature ovarian failure exists and antibody testing has been recommended only within the context of clinical trials (77). Convincing evidence for the role of immune markers, antiovarian antibodies, antibodies blocking action of FSH to its receptor, antibodies to zona pellucida, and cell-mediated immunity in the etiology of premature ovarian failure is lacking (78).

Autoimmune ovarian failure may be associated with the autoimmune polyglandular syndromes (APS). In APS type I, adrenal failure, mucocutaneous candidiasis, and hypoparathyroidism are associated with premature ovarian failure in up to 60% of cases. Although the candidiasis generally presents in infancy, endocrine failure may occur gradually over a period of many years. APS type II is most common in adult women. Autoimmune adrenal failure, hypothyroidism, and type 1 diabetes mellitus are associated with premature ovarian failure in up to 4% of cases. Thus, it is reasonable to screen young women with idiopathic premature ovarian failure for these endocrine disorders.

Ovarian Injury due to Infection Mumps oophoritis is a well-documented but rare cause of premature ovarian failure (79–81). Only 5% of postpubertal females with mumps develop orchitis and there is no relationship to infertility. According to World Health Organization, the incidence of mumps remains high in Africa and southeast Asia but has declined in the last decade in the United States from 5,712 cases in 1989 to 231 cases in 2001 (82).

Resistant Ovaries This is a rare disorder marked by ovarian follicles arrested in the preantral stage of development. A recent case report describes the presentation in an 18-year-old girl with amenorrhea, sexual infantilism, elevated gonadotropin hormone levels, and a 46,XX karyotype (83). Although the diagnosis is made only by ovarian biopsy, biopsy in 46,XX patients is generally considered unnecessary as the management is not altered. Indeed, this may not even be a separate disease condition but may represent a transitional state or developing case of ovarian failure.

HYPOGONADOTROPIC HYPOGONADISM

Known causes of hypogonadotropic hypogonadism can be divided into those that originate in the hypothalamus and those that are primarily pituitary in origin. Despite the elucidation of a multitude of molecular mechanisms, we still do not know the etiology in the vast majority of patients with hypogonadotropic hypogonadism (84).

Hypothalamic Causes of Hypogonadotropic Hypogonadism

Constitutional Delay of Growth and Puberty
The most common cause of delayed puberty, constitutional delay, is not a pathological condition, but simply represents a variation of normal growth. These girls are "late-bloomers"—the tempo of growth and development is slower than usual, but ultimately they achieve a normal adult stature and normal sexual maturation. In general, bone age (skeletal maturation) is concordant with height age rather than with chronological age. If puberty has not started by a bone age of 13 years, one can be fairly certain that a pathologic cause of hypogonadotropic hypogonadism is present. Constitutional delay is discussed in detail in Chapter 34.

Functional Hypothalamic Amenorrhea
Functional hypothalamic amenorrhea is defined as amenorrhea with low levels of estrogens and low or normal levels of gonadotropins in the absence of organic hypothalamic disease. Strenuous exercise, weight loss, and eating disorders are the usual causes for functional hypothalamic amenorrhea (85). Chronic debilitating disease is also an etiology. Stress and strenuous exercise can induce menstrual irregularities and amenorrhea. In addition, strenuous exercise has been linked to eating disorders and bone loss. Both exercise and stress interfere with GnRH pulse frequency and decrease it from one pulse every hour to one every 3 hours (86). A critical body fat mass

has been proposed as necessary for maintenance of reproductive function. Low weight is hypothesized to result in low leptin levels (87), and a small study demonstrated improved hormonal milieu and follicular development and in some cases ovulation when underweight women were treated with recombinant leptin (88). The role of leptin in human reproduction remains to be clearly defined.

A combination of amenorrhea and body weight at 85% below the ideal body weight remains the *Diagnostic and Statistic Manual-IV* criteria for diagnosis of anorexia nervosa. Some of these patients may have associated bulimia (binge eating followed by induced vomiting). The disorder most commonly afflicts adolescent females and approximately 3.7% of women are estimated to have this condition at some point in their lifetime (89). The differential diagnosis for anorexia nervosa should include hyperthyroidism, inflammatory bowel disease, malignancy, CNS tumors, and depression.

Anorectic girls and women suffer significant health risks. Hypothermia, anemia, osteopenia, osteoporosis, hypokalemia, cardiac arrhythmia, hypotension, and obsessive–compulsive behavior are some of the complications that can ensue due to the eating disorder (Table 36-5). Management focuses on increasing body weight over the critical level of 85% of ideal weight. The aim is to achieve a weight gain of 1 lb/week in outpatient therapy. Cognitive psychotherapy is frequently required. Cure is difficult, and in one study up to 39% of patients had some form of eating disorder 6 years after completion of therapy, and 6% of patients were deceased, underscoring the seriousness of the condition (90). Death may result from cardiovascular complications (arrhythmias and hypotension) or suicide. A multidisciplinary team involving the primary care provider, psychiatrist, and dietician is frequently needed in the care of these patients.

Most patients with anorexia nervosa will resume menses within 6 months after reaching 90% of their ideal body weight (91). Estrogen therapy is indicated to prevent bone loss if the patient remains amenorrheic. Patients who recover from anorexia have normal fertility. Because amenorrheic anorexic patients can still become pregnant, contraception should be practiced if pregnancy is not desired. Female athletes in whom exercise is interfering with normal menses should be encouraged to decrease the intensity of exercise.

Evaluation of bone mineral density and aggressive management of osteopenia and osteoporosis is vital in these patients. The bone mineral density is much lower than predicted based on body weight, suggesting that endocrine abnormalities may independently and additively contribute to osteoporosis. There is marked improvement in bone during treatment of anorexia with some deterioration in the first 2 years after completion of therapy followed by steady improvement over the next 4 years (90). Even though recovery of bone mineral density is slow, the potential for recovery remains high for many years after menarche (92). Calcium 1500 mg/day with vitamin D 400 IU/day should be prescribed. The benefit from bisphosphonates is not proven.

Hypothyroidism Prepubertal children with central or primary hypothyroidism experience growth failure and, in general, delayed puberty (although precocious puberty may occur in primary hypothyroidism). After puberty, hypothyroidism leads to a wide variety of menstrual dysfunction. Changes in menstrual frequency range from absence of menses (amenorrhea) to shortened cycles with more frequent menses. Menstrual blood flow can be extremely light or menorrhagia (excessively heavy bleeding) may be present. Dysmenorrhea (menstrual discomfort) may be more severe in

TABLE 36-5	Features of Anorexia Nervosa (84)
Feature	**Anorexia Nervosa**
Patient characteristics	Most often adolescents; Caucasian; ballet dancers and athletes in sports requiring weight restriction
Weight	Severely underweight; wasting; reduced fat and lean body mass
Food intake	Starvation; avoidance of fatty and high-calorie food
Exercise	Hyperactivity in pursuit of athletic goals
Psychiatric	Preoccupation with and distorted attitudes about food; increased interest in exercise; negative and distorted body image (feeling fat despite wasting); cycles of binging and purging if bulimia nervosa present
Neuroendocrine	Neuroendocrine changes consistent with starvation
Other features	Osteopenia and osteoporosis common; hypercarotinemia; dry skin; lanugo-type hair; pedal edema; anemia, leukopenia, thrombocytopenia; low metabolic rate, cold intolerance, hypothermia; electrolyte imbalance (low sodium and potassium levels); bradycardia; hypotension; systolic murmur; dehydration

women with thyroid disease. Although hypothyroidism per se affects menstrual function, prolactin levels may be elevated in some women with hypothyroidism, further impairing the hypothalamic-pituitary-gonadal axis.

Genetic Defects and Syndromes

To date, no mutation in the GnRH gene has been described in humans, but multiple defects and syndromes have been described that affect GnRH secretion. Some of these are listed below, and other rare defects are listed in At-A-Glance, including mutations in prohormone-convertase-1 (93), DAX1 (30), and G protein–coupled receptor 54 (94, 95), This is an area where new knowledge of gene defects is rapidly being gained.

Kallmann Syndrome Kallmann syndrome is the most common form of isolated gonadotropin deficiency. It occurs when normal migration of GnRH and olfactory neurons from the olfactory placode to the basal forebrain does not occur during embryonic development. Three types of inheritance have been described: X-linked recessive, autosomal recessive, and autosomal dominant. The syndrome is five times more common in males than females.

- The gene involved in the X-linked form of the condition was the first found and is the best understood (96). It produces a protein called anosmin-1, which is an adhesion molccule essential for the migration of olfactory and GnRH neurons in embryologic development (97, 98).

- The gene involved in the autosomal dominant phenotype of Kallmann syndrome, FGFR1 (fibroblast growth factor receptor), is postulated to interact with anosmin-1 to effect its normal function (99).

- The autosomal recessive form of Kallmann syndrome is poorly characterized.

Kallmann syndrome patients have anosmia and low FSH/LH levels. The most common presentation is delayed puberty. Stature is normal, although there is absence of the pubertal growth spurt, and adolescent patients may develop eunuchoid proportions. Females have absent breast development. The history of anosmia has to be elicited in most cases by specific questioning and a smell test should be performed. Olfactory tract hypoplasia or aplasia can be demonstrated by magnetic resonance imaging (MRI). There is considerable heterogeneity in findings, even within the same family. Associated anomalies include midline facial defects, neurologic abnormalities including mirror movements of limbs (synkinesia), and renal anomalies (usually unilateral agenesis).

Leptin and leptin receptor genes Leptin is a protein produced by white adipose tissue that acts as a satiety signal to the hypothalamus. Mutation in the leptin gene or its receptor causes hyperphagia and early childhood onset of morbid obesity. Hypogonadotropic hypogonadism occurs with impaired GnRH release. Leptin infusion has been shown to successfully reverse obesity and hypogonadism in leptin-deficient patients but not in patients with mutations in the receptor gene (100).

Prader–Willi syndrome Prader–Willi syndrome is estimated to affect 1:10,000 to 25,000 live births and results from three different genetic mechanisms leading to lack of expression of paternally imprinted genes. The genes affected are SNRPN and Necdin. Over 70% of cases result from paternal deletion in 15q11-13. Approximately 25% are due to uniparental maternal disomy for 15q11-13. Approximately 5% result from abnormal methylation of DNA leading to a defect in the imprinting mechanism (101). Patients with Prader–Willi syndrome exhibit a constellation of symptoms including hypotonia in infancy, short stature, small hands and feet, hypothalamic obesity with an insatiable appetite, delayed puberty due to hypothalamic hypogonadism, and mild mental retardation (102). Only 39% of these patients attain menarche and if they do, they are likely to have irregular menses although the occasional patient may become pregnant (102,103). Estrogen status and bone mineral density must be monitored from their early teens and the need for hormone therapy determined on an individual basis (for other aspects of the disorder see Chapter 30).

Other syndromes Bardet–Biedl syndrome (formerly called Laurence-Moon-Biedl) is characterized by obesity, pigmentary retinopathy, polydactyly, mental retardation, and renal failure. Hypogonadotropic hypogonadism may be a feature of this syndrome, ranging from primary amenorrhea and sexual infantilism to menstrual irregularities, although female patients with normal gonadal function and several cases with normal fertility have been described. CHARGE syndrome (coloboma, heart disease, choanal atresia, retarded growth, genital hypoplasia in males, ear abnormalities +/- deafness) is associated with hypogonadal hypogonadism, which may involve both hypothalamic and pituitary dysfunction (104).

Physical Insult to the Hypothalamus

Central tumors, infiltrative processes such as Langerhans cell histiocytosis, tuberculosis, or sarcoidosis; infections such as encephalitis or meningitis; trauma; and cranial irradiation may cause hypogonadotropic hypogonadism and have to be considered when the history and/or clinical examination suggests the possibility of such a diagnosis. Examples of hypothalamic tumors include germinomas, hamartomas, and teratomas. Cranial irradiation can cause hypothalamic insufficiency, which may not become apparent until years after the initial insult (see Chapter 47).

Langerhans cell histiocytosis is characterized by granulomatous deposits in multiple sites throughout the body. Infiltration can lead to isolated thickening of the pituitary stalk or more diffuse pituitary and/or hypothalamic dysfunction including hypogonadotropic hypogonadism. Diabetes insipidus and multiple pituitary hormone deficiencies can occur along with hypothalamic defects including morbid obesity, sleeping disorders, defects in thermoregulation, and adipsia (105).

Pituitary Causes of Hypogonadotropic Hypogonadism

GnRH Receptor Mutations Multiple mutations in the GNRHR gene have been well documented and they may account for 7% to 40% of cases of autosomal recessive hypogonadotropic hypogonadism (106,107). Nineteen mutations have been described to date and they are predominantly compound heterozygous missense mutations. Two hotspots have been noted: Q106R and R262Q. The clinical presentation is variable. Female patients have been described as isolated cases and as part of kindred with male and female affected family members (108,109). Female patients present with primary amenorrhea with absence or varying degrees of pubertal development. Variable response to GnRH stimulation has been noted. Two patients with first trimester pregnancies have been documented. In one pregnancy there was a spontaneous conception and the other patient achieved three pregnancies through very high dose (250 ng/kg as opposed to normal dose of 75 ng/kg) exogenous pulsatile GnRH administration (110). All four pregnancies ended in first trimester miscarriages.

FSH β-subunit deficiency Compound heterozygous and homozygous mutations in the FSH-β gene cause absent or delayed thelarche and primary amenorrhea with low levels of FSH and estradiol and high LH levels (111). Exogenous administration of FSH has resulted in normal pregnancy in these patients. LH-β subunit defects have not been described in females to date.

Transcription Factor Mutations: PROP1, HESX1, LHX3 Mutations in genes involved in the development of the pituitary gland such as

HESX1, LHX3, and PROP1 result in hypogonadotropic hypogonadism as part of a general picture of hypopituitarism (see Chapter 32). PROP1 (prophet of PIT1) is involved in the development of pituitary gonadotropes, lactotropes, thyrotropes, and somatotropes. The clinical presentation of deficiency is heterogeneous with variable deficiencies of LH, FSH, growth hormone, thyroid-stimulating hormone, and prolactin (112, 113). HESX1 (homeobox genes expressed in ES cells) is involved in the initial determination of the anterior region of the developing embryo. Mutation is characterized by septo-optic dysplasia (absent septum pellucidum and optic nerve hypoplasia). Hormone deficits range from isolated growth hormone deficiency to panhypopituitarism (114,115). LHX3, LIM homeobox gene 3, is a transcription regulator involved in pituitary gland development. Individuals may have low gonadotropin levels, combined pituitary hormone deficiency, and a rigid cervical spine (116). Homozygous mutations in PCSK1 gene cause prohormone convertase-1 (PC-1) deficiency, characterized by morbid childhood obesity, chronic gastro-intestinal disturbances, adrenal insufficiency and hypogonadotropic hypogonadism. PC-1 is a neuroendocrine convertase that cleaves POMC, proinsulin and proglucagon (96). Other genetic factors not yet well characterized are likely to be important in gonadotropin secretion.

Physical Insult to the Pituitary Similar to the hypothalamus, the pituitary can be damaged by a variety of processes including infiltrative disease, infection, trauma, cranial irradiation, autoimmune disease, degenerative disorders, or tumors.

Prolactinoma Prolactinomas are the second most common tumors occurring in the region of the pituitary in childhood and are the most common pituitary tumors that cause amenorrhea or oligomenorrhea (117). Most prolactinomas arise from a single clone of acidophilic cells. These acidophilic cells are in turn derived from the same lineage as the somatotropes and thyrotropes. Reflecting their origin, prolactin-secreting adenomas may sometimes secrete growth hormone and thyroid-stimulating hormone.

Ninety-three percent of prolactinomas occur after the age of 12 in children (118). Delayed puberty or pubertal arrest, amenorrhea, and galactorrhea are common presenting symptoms (117,119). The diagnosis is established by elevated prolactin levels and by demonstration of a mass lesion on MRI of the pituitary fossa. An adenoma less than 1 cm is classified as a microadenoma and larger tumors as macroadenomas. If hyperprolac-

tinemia without any CNS tumor is encountered, drugs including metoclopramide, cimetidine, tricyclic antidepressants, phenothiazines, benzodiazepines, methyldopa, prostaglandins, and cocaine must be excluded as possible causes before starting dopamine agonist therapy.

Prolactin-secreting microadenomas are more common than macroadenomas and may be followed conservatively if the prolactin levels are only borderline high and if the patient does not have galactorrhea or menstrual disturbance (120). These tumors usually remain stable and rarely increase in size with time. In patients with amenorrhea and/or galactorrhea, treatment with dopamine agonists (bromocriptine, quinagolide, and cabergoline) results in quick resolution of symptoms. Cabergoline has the advantage of fewer side effects and once or twice weekly dosing (0.25–0.5 mg). The most common side effects are nausea and vomiting. Orthostatic hypotension is transient and occurs at the start of therapy. The side effects can be minimized with gradual increase in dose. With bromocriptine, the initial dose is 1.25 mg at night (to avoid orthostatic hypotension) with gradual increase to 2.5 mg twice daily over 2 weeks. Medical treatment usually results in swift resolution of symptoms. Even though there is no evidence for teratogenicity, if pregnancy occurs during therapy it is advisable to discontinue the medication and check visual fields regularly to assess for growth of the tumor during pregnancy.

Macroadenomas can also be treated conservatively but require referral to a specialist. The majority of macroadenomas are found in children and, although a higher percentage of them (compared with adults) are resistant to dopamine agonist therapy, most do respond with tumor shrinkage (121). Eighty percent to 90% of patients with visual field defects recover on medical therapy (122). There are no clear studies to assess the optimal duration of therapy. Discontinuation of treatment should be attempted with cautious tapering of the dose 1 to 2 years after normalization of prolactin levels. The possibility of a nonprolactin-producing adenoma causing hyperprolactinemia by compressing the stalk must be borne in mind if continued growth of the mass occurs.

Surgery is reserved for those patients in whom agonist therapy fails. Roughly one in five patients suffer a recurrence of the condition after surgery. Radiotherapy and stereotactic surgery are reserved for recurrent cases because hypopituitarism may occur in a large number of these patients.

Craniopharyngioma Craniopharyngioma is a rare tumor with an incidence of 0.13/100,000 person years, but it is the most common tumor (80%–90%) that arises in the region of the

pituitary during childhood (117). Squamous rest cells present in remnants of Rathke pouch (the diverticulum from the embryonic mouth that gives rise to the adenohypophysis) cause this tumor. Even though they are benign histologically, they can be locally invasive.

The usual age of presentation is between 5 and 14 years of age with symptoms of headache, visual disturbance, and poor growth. Up to 75% of patients have growth hormone deficiency and gonadotropin deficiency is noted in up to 40% of patients. Despite the large size of craniopharyngiomas, pituitary stalk compression leading to hyperprolactinemia occurs in only 20% of cases (117).

Surgery is the treatment of choice and this is usually followed with adjuvant radiotherapy. Unfortunately, endocrine dysfunction occurs postoperatively in a large group of patients and a substantial number have recurrence. If gonadotropin insufficiency occurs after surgery, hormone replacement should be instituted. These patients should be able to have children using artificial reproductive techniques.

Lymphocytic Hypophysitis Lymphocytic hypophysitis is a rare condition usually associated with pregnancy. It has been described in childhood in association with diabetes insipidus and panhypopituitarism (123). Plasma cells, macrophages, and lymphocytes infiltrate and enlarge the anterior pituitary gland resulting in impaired function. MRI reveals thickening of the sphenoid sinus mucosa, pituitary stalk enlargement, and tongue-shaped extension of the lesion along the basal hypothalamus. Moderate elevation of prolactin levels may occur presumably due to compression of the pituitary stalk by the enlarged gland. In the case of a macroadenoma presenting for the first time in pregnancy, it is worth considering this diagnosis because the mass may spontaneously resolve after pregnancy (124).

Empty Sella Syndrome Empty sella syndrome occurs due to a defect in the diaphragma sellae that allows the extension of the subarachnoid space into the pituitary fossa. The empty sella can also occur due to tumor, surgery or radiotherapy. Hyperprolactinemia occurs due to compression of the pituitary stalk. Although it is more common in adults, empty sella syndrome can present in the pediatric age group and the diagnosis must be actively entertained in children with headaches, low body weight increased fatigue, precocious or delayed puberty, and short stature (125). Suppression of nonadenomatous somatotropic cells leads to growth arrest and short stature in children with partial pituitary deficiency (118). Empty sella syndrome can also occur as a complication of Sheehan syndrome (126).

Sheehan Syndrome Sheehan syndrome occurs due to pituitary necrosis in the postpartum period secondary to postpartum hemorrhage leading to shock. Patients may present with fatigue, inability to lactate, amenorrhea, loss of axillary and pubic hair, severe hyponatremia, and even coma. The clinical picture depends on the hormones involved. Growth hormone and gonadotropins are the most commonly affected, followed by TSH and ACTH deficiency. Diabetes insipidus is reportedly rare. Treatment is by identification of the hormone deficiency and appropriate replacement (126,127).

REFERENCES

1. Sedlmeyer IL, Palmert MR. Delayed puberty: analysis of a large case series from an academic center. *J Clin Endocrinol Metab.* 2002;87(4):1613–1620.

2. Timmreck LS, Reindollar RH. Contemporary issues in primary amenorrhea. *Obstet Gynecol Clin North Am.* 2003;30(2): 287–302.

3. Reindollar RH, Novak M, Tho SP, et al. Adult-onset amenorrhea: a study of 262 patients. *Am J Obstet Gynecol.* 1986;155(3):531–543.

4. Drobac S, Rubin K, Rogol AD, et al. A workshop on pubertal hormone replacement options in the United States. *J Pediatr Endocrinol Metab.* 2006;19(1):55–64.

5. Kiess W, Conway G, Ritzen M, et al. Induction of puberty in the hypogonadal girl–practices and attitudes of pediatric endocrinologists in Europe. *Horm Res.* 2002;57(1-2):66–71.

6. Chernausek SD, Attie KM, Cara JF, et al. Growth hormone therapy of Turner syndrome: the impact of age of estrogen replacement on final height. Genentech, Inc., Collaborative Study Group. *J Clin Endocrinol Metab.* 2000;85(7):2439–24345.

7. Rosenfield RL, Perovic N, Devine N, et al. Optimizing estrogen replacement treatment in Turner syndrome. *Pediatrics.* 1998;102 (2 Pt 3):486–488.

8. van Pareren YK, de Muinck Keizer-Schrama SM, Stijnen T, et al. Final height in girls with Turner syndrome after long-term growth hormone treatment in three dosages and low dose estrogens. *J Clin Endocrinol Metab.* 2003;88(3):1119–1125.

9. Ankarberg Lindgren C, Elfving M, Wikland KA, et al. Nocturnal application of transdermal estradiol patches produces levels of estradiol that mimic those seen at the onset of spontaneous puberty in girls. *J Clin Endocrinol Metab.* 2001;86(7):3039–3044.

10. Piippo S, Lenko H, Kainulainen P, et al. Use of percutaneous estrogen gel for induction of puberty in girls with Turner syndrome. *J Clin Endocrinol Metab.* 2004;89(7):3241–3247.

11. O'Sullivan AJ, Crampton LJ, Freund J, et al. The route of estrogen replacement therapy confers divergent effects on substrate oxidation and body composition in postmenopausal women. *J Clin Invest.* 1998;102(5):1035–1040.

12. Godsland IF. Effects of postmenopausal hormone replacement therapy on lipid, lipoprotein, and apolipoprotein (a) concentrations: analysis of studies published from 1974–2000. *Fertil Steril.*2001;75(5):898–915.

13. Janssen YJ, Helmerhorst F, Frolich M, et al. A switch from oral (2 mg/day) to transdermal (50 microg/day) 17beta-estradiol therapy increases serum insulin-like growth factor-I levels in recombinant human growth hormone (GH)-substituted women with GH deficiency. *J Clin Endocrinol Metab.* 2000;85(1):464–467.

14. Sills ES, Harmon KE, Tucker MJ. First reported convergence of premature ovarian failure and cutis marmorata telangiectatica congenita. *Fertil Steril.* 2002;78(6): 1314–1316.

15. Hreinsson JG, Otala M, Fridstrom M, et al. Follicles are found in the ovaries of adolescent girls with Turner's syndrome. *J Clin Endocrinol Metab.* 2002;87(8):3618–3623.

16. Sybert VP, McCauley E. Turner's syndrome. *N Engl J Med.* 2004;351(12):1227–1238.

17. Massa G, Verlinde F, De Schepper J, et al. Trends in age at diagnosis of Turner syndrome. *Arch Dis Child.* 2005;90(3):267–268.

18. Lyon AJ, Preece MA, Grant DB. Growth curve for girls with Turner syndrome. *Arch Dis Child.* 1985;60(10):932–935.

19. Wilson CA, Heinrichs C, Larmore KA, et al. Estradiol levels in girls with Turner's syndrome compared to normal prepubertal girls as determined by an ultrasensitive assay. *J Pediatr Endocrinol Metab.* 2003;16(1):91–96.

20. Held KR, Kerber S, Kaminsky E, et al. Mosaicism in 45,X Turner syndrome: does survival in early pregnancy depend on the presence of two sex chromosomes? *Hum Genet.* 1992;88(3):288–294.

21. Frias JL, Davenport ML. Health supervision for children with Turner syndrome. *Pediatrics.* 2003;111(3):692–702.

22. Khastgir G, Studd JW, Fox SW, et al. A longitudinal study of the effect of subcutaneous estrogen replacement on bone in young women with Turner's syndrome. *J Bone Miner Res.* 2003;18(5):925–932.

23. Birdsall M, Kennedy S. The risk of aortic dissection in women with Turner syndrome. *Hum Reprod.* 1996;11(7):1587.

24. Karnis MF, Reindollar RH. Turner syndrome in adolescence. *Obstet Gynecol Clin North Am.* 2003;30(2):303–320.

25. Di Pasquale E, Beck-Peccoz P, Persani L. Hypergonadotropic ovarian failure associated with an inherited mutation of human bone morphogenetic protein-15 (BMP15) gene. *Am J Hum Genet.* 2004;75(1):106–111.

26. Nishi Y, Hamamoto K, Kajiyama M, et al. The Perrault syndrome: clinical report and review. *Am J Med Genet.*1988;31(3):623–629.

27. Dewing P, Bernard P, Vilain E. Disorders of gonadal development. *Semin Reprod Med.* 2002;20(3):189–198.

28. Achermann JC, Ito M, Hindmarsh PC, et al. A mutation in the gene encoding steroidogenic factor-1 causes XY sex reversal and adrenal failure in humans. *Nat Genet.* 1999;22(2):125–126.

29. Biason-Lauber A, Schoenle EJ. Apparently normal ovarian differentiation in a prepubertal girl with transcriptionally inactive steroidogenic factor 1 (NR5A1/SF-1) and adrenocortical insufficiency. *Am J Hum Genet.* 2000;67(6):1563–1568.

30. Merke DP, Tajima T, Baron J, et al. Hypogonadotropic hypogonadism in a female caused by an X-linked recessive mutation in the DAX1 gene. *N Engl J Med.* 1999;340(16):1248–1252.

31. Nakae J, Tajima T, Sugawara T, et al. Analysis of the steroidogenic acute regulatory protein (StAR) gene in Japanese patients with congenital lipoid adrenal hyperplasia. *Hum Mol Genet.* 1997;6(4):571–576.

32. Gupta MK, Geller DH, Auchus RJ. Pitfalls in characterizing P450c17 mutations associated with isolated 17,20-lyase deficiency. *J Clin Endocrinol Metab.* 2001;86(9):4416–4423.

33. Auchus RJ, Miller WL. Molecular modeling of human P450c17 (17alpha-hydroxylase/ 17,20-lyase): insights into reaction mechanisms and effects of mutations. *Mol Endocrinol.* 1999;13(7):1169–1182.

34. Auchus RJ. The genetics, pathophysiology, and management of human deficiencies of P450c17. *Endocrinol Metab Clin North Am.* 2001;30(1):101–19, vii.

35. ten Kate-Booij MJ, Cobbaert C, Koper JW, et al. Deficiency of 17,20-lyase causing giant ovarian cysts in a girl and a female phenotype in her 46,XY sister: case report. *Hum Reprod.* 2004;19(2):456–459.

36. Mullis PE, Yoshimura N, Kuhlmann B, et al. Aromatase deficiency in a female who is compound heterozygote for two new point mutations in the P450arom gene: impact of estrogens on hypergonadotropic hypogonadism, multicystic ovaries, and bone densitometry in childhood. *J Clin Endocrinol Metab.* 1997;82(6):1739–1745.

37. Morishima A, Grumbach MM, Simpson ER, et al. Aromatase deficiency in male and female siblings caused by a novel mutation and the physiological role of estrogens. *J Clin Endocrinol Metab.* 1995;80(12):3689–3698.

38. Conte FA, Grumbach MM, Ito Y, et al. A syndrome of female pseudohermaphrodism, hypergonadotropic hypogonadism, and multicystic ovaries associated with missense mutations in the gene encoding aromatase (P450arom). *J Clin Endocrinol Metab.* 1994;78(6): 1287–1292.

39. Ito Y, Fisher CR, Conte FA, et al. Molecular basis of aromatase deficiency in an adult female with sexual infantilism and polycystic ovaries. *Proc Natl Acad Sci USA.* 1993;90(24):11673–11677.

40. Aittomaki K, Lucena JL, Pakarinen P, et al. Mutation in the follicle-stimulating hormone receptor gene causes hereditary hypergonadotropic ovarian failure. *Cell.* 1995;82(6): 959–968.

41. Meduri G, Touraine P, Beau I, et al. Delayed puberty and primary amenorrhea associated with a novel mutation of the human follicle-stimulating hormone receptor: clinical, histological, and molecular studies. *J Clin Endocrinol Metab.* 2003;88(8):3491–3498.

42. Touraine P, Beau I, Gougeon A, et al. New natural inactivating mutations of the follicle-stimulating hormone receptor: correlations between receptor function and phenotype. *Mol Endocrinol.* 1999;13(11):1844–1854.

43. Vaskivuo TE, Aittomaki K, Anttonen M, et al. Effects of follicle-stimulating hormone (FSH) and human chorionic gonadotropin in individuals with an inactivating mutation of the FSH receptor. *Fertil Steril.* 2002;78(1):108–113.

44. Latronico AC, Anasti J, Arnhold IJ, et al. Brief report: testicular and ovarian resistance to luteinizing hormone caused by inactivating mutations of the luteinizing hormone-receptor gene. *N Engl J Med.*1996;334(8):507–512.

45. Toledo SP, Brunner HG, Kraaij R, et al. An inactivating mutation of the luteinizing hormone receptor causes amenorrhea in a 46,XX female. *J Clin Endocrinol Metab.* 1996;81(11):3850–3854.

46. Lambert C, Boneh A. The impact of galactosaemia on quality of life-A pilot study. *J Inherit Metab Dis.*2004;27(5):601–608.

47. Leslie ND. Insights into the pathogenesis of galactosemia. *Annu Rev Nutr.* 2003;23:59–80.

48. Laml T, Preyer O, Umek W, et al. Genetic disorders in premature ovarian failure. *Hum Reprod Update.* 2002;8(5):483–491.

49. Guerrero NV, Singh RH, Manatunga A, et al. Risk factors for premature ovarian failure in females with galactosemia. *J Pediatr.* 2000;137(6):833–841.

50. Waggoner DD, Buist NR, Donnell GN. Long-term prognosis in galactosaemia: results of a survey of 350 cases. *J Inherit Metab Dis.*1990;13(6):802–818.

51. Sherman SL. Premature ovarian failure in the fragile X syndrome. *Am J Med Genet.* 2000;97(3):189–194.

52. Rooman RP, Van Driessche K, Du Caju MV. Growth and ovarian function in girls with 48,XXXX karyotype–patient report and review of the literature. *J Pediatr Endocrinol Metab.* 2002;15(7):1051–1055.

53. Collen RJ, Falk RE, Lippe BM, et al. A 48,XXXX female with absence of ovaries. *Am J Med Genet.* 1980;6(4):275–278.

54. Bione S, Sala C, Manzini C, et al. A human homologue of the Drosophila melanogaster diaphanous gene is disrupted in a patient with premature ovarian failure: evidence for conserved function in oogenesis and implications for human sterility. *Am J Hum Genet.* 1998;62(3):533–541.

55. De Baere E, Dixon MJ, Small KW, et al. Spectrum of FOXL2 gene mutations in blepharophimosis-ptosis-epicanthus inversus (BPES) families demonstrates a genotype–phenotype correlation. *Hum Mol Genet.* 2001;10(15):1591–1600.

56. Fogli A, Rodriguez D, Eymard-Pierre E, et al. Ovarian failure related to eukaryotic initiation factor 2B mutations. *Am J Hum Genet.* 2003;72(6):1544–1550.

57. Davison RM, Quilter CR, Webb J, et al. A familial case of X chromosome deletion ascertained by cytogenetic screening of women with premature ovarian failure. *Hum Reprod.* 1998;13(11):3039–3041.

58. Larsen EC, Muller J, Schmiegelow K, et al. Reduced ovarian function in long-term survivors of radiation- and chemotherapy-treated childhood cancer. *J Clin Endocrinol Metab.* 2003;88(11):5307–5314.

59. Howell SJ, Shalet SM. Fertility preservation and management of gonadal failure associ-ated with lymphoma therapy. *Curr Oncol Rep.* 2002;4(5):443–452.

60. Blumenfeld Z. Gynaecologic concerns for young women exposed to gonadotoxic chemotherapy. *Curr Opin Obstet Gynecol.* 2003;15(5):359–370.

61. Cicognani A, Pasini A, Pession A, et al. Gonadal function and pubertal development after treatment of a childhood malignancy. *J Pediatr Endocrinol Metab.* 2003;16 Suppl 2:321–326.

62. Franchi-Rezgui P, Rousselot P, Espie M, et al. Fertility in young women after chemotherapy with alkylating agents for Hodgkin and non-Hodgkin lymphomas. *Hematol J.* 2003;4(2):116–120.

63. Sarafoglou K, Boulad F, Gillio A, et al. Gonadal function after bone marrow transplantation for acute leukemia during childhood. *J Pediatr.* 1997;130(2):210–216.

64. Thibaud E, Rodriguez-Macias K, Trivin C, et al. Ovarian function after bone marrow transplantation during childhood. *Bone Marrow Transplant.* 1998;21(3):287–290.

65. Shapiro CL, Manola J, Leboff M. Ovarian failure after adjuvant chemotherapy is associated with rapid bone loss in women with early-stage breast cancer. *J Clin Oncol.* 2001;19(14):3306–3311.

66. Bisharah M, Tulandi T. Laparoscopic preservation of ovarian function: an underused procedure. *Am J Obstet Gynecol.* 2003;188(2):367–370.

67. Longhi A, Pignotti E, Versari M, et al. Effect of oral contraceptive on ovarian function in young females undergoing neoadjuvant chemotherapy treatment for osteosarcoma. *Oncol Rep.* 2003;10(1): 151–155.

68. Posada MN, Kolp L, Garcia JE. Fertility options for female cancer patients: facts and fiction. *Fertil Steril.*2001;75(4):647–653.

69. Mardesic T, Snajderova M, Sramkova L, et al. Protocol combining GnRH agonists and GnRH antagonists for rapid suppression and prevention of gonadal damage during cytotoxic therapy. *Eur J Gynaecol Oncol.* 2004;25(1):90–92.

70. Revel A, Laufer N. Protecting female fertility from cancer therapy. *Mol Cell Endocrinol.* 2002;187(1-2):83–91.

71. Blumenfeld Z, Dann E, Avivi I, et al. Fertility after treatment for Hodgkin's disease. *Ann Oncol.* 2002;13 Suppl 1:138–147.

72. Meirow D, Assad G, Dor J, et al. The GnRH antagonist cetrorelix reduces cyclophosphamide-induced ovarian follicular destruction in mice. *Hum Reprod.* 2004;19(6):1294–1299.

73. Donnez PJ, Dolmans M, Demylle D, et al. Livebirth after orthotopic transplantation of cryopreserved ovarian tissue. *Lancet.* 2004;364(9443):1405–1410.

74. Kim SS. Ovarian tissue banking for cancer patients. To do or not to do? *Hum Reprod.* 2003;18(9):1759–1761.

75. Oktay K, Buyuk E. The potential of ovarian tissue transplant to preserve fertility. *Expert Opin Biol Ther.* 2002;2(4):361–370.

76. Radford JA, Lieberman BA, Brison DR, et al. Orthotopic reimplantation of cryopreserved ovarian cortical strips after high-dose chemotherapy for Hodgkin's lymphoma. *Lancet.* 2001;357(9263):1172–1175.

77. Wheatcroft NJ, Salt C, Milford-Ward A, et al. Identification of ovarian antibodies by immunofluorescence, enzyme-linked immunosorbent assay or immunoblotting in premature ovarian failure. *Hum Reprod.* 1997;12(12):2617–2622.

78. Bukulmez O, Arici A. Autoimmune premature ovarian failure. *Immunol Allergy Clin N Am.* 2002;22:455–470.

79. Sullivan KM, Halpin TJ, Kim-Farley R, et al. Mumps disease and its health impact: an outbreak-based report. *Pediatrics.* 1985;76(4):533–536.

80. Prinz W, Taubert HD. Mumps in pubescent females and its effect on later reproductive function. *Gynaecologia.* 1969;167(1):23–27.

81. Morrison JC, Givens JR, Wiser WL, et al. Mumps oophoritis: a cause of premature menopause. *Fertil Steril.*1975;26(7):655–659.

82. Mumps. In: *Epidemiology and Prevention of Vaccine-Preventable Diseases.* 8th ed. National Immunisation Program; 2004: 135–143.

83. Katz S, Marshall J, Khorram O. An unusual case of ovarian resistance syndrome. *Obstet Gynecol.* 2003;101(5 Pt 2):1078–1082.

84. Dode C, Hardelin JP. Kallmann syndrome: fibroblast growth factor signaling insufficiency? *J Mol Med.* 2004;82(11):725–734.

85. Ahima RS. Body fat, leptin, and hypothalamic amenorrhea. *N Engl J Med.* 2004;351(10):959–962.

86. Reame NE, Sauder SE, Case GD, et al. Pulsatile gonadotropin secretion in women with hypothalamic amenorrhea: evidence that reduced frequency of gonadotropin-releasing hormone secretion is the mechanism of persistent anovulation. *J Clin Endocrinol Metab.* 1985;61(5):851–858.

87. Miller KK, Grinspoon S, Gleysteen S, et al. Preservation of neuroendocrine control of reproductive function despite severe undernutrition. *J Clin Endocrinol Metab.* 2004;89(9):4434–4438.

88. Welt CK, Chan JL, Bullen J, et al. Recombinant human leptin in women with hypothalamic amenorrhea. *N Engl J Med.*2004;351(10):987–997.

89. Deering S. Eating disorders: recognition, evaluation, and implications for obstetrician/gynecologists. *Prim Care Update Ob Gyns.* 2001;8(1):31–35.

90. Fichter MM, Quadflieg N. Six-year course and outcome of anorexia nervosa. *Int J Eat Disord.* 1999;26(4):359–385.

91. Mehler PS. Diagnosis and care of patients with anorexia nervosa in primary care settings. *Ann Intern Med.* 2001;134(11): 1048–1059.

92. Valla A, Groenning IL, Syversen U, et al. Anorexia nervosa: slow regain of bone mass. *Osteoporos Int.* 2000;11(2):141–145.

93. Legouis R, Hardelin JP, Levilliers J, et al. The candidate gene for the X-linked Kallmann syndrome encodes a protein related to adhesion molecules. *Cell.* 1991;67(2):423–435.

94. Soussi-Yanicostas N, Hardelin JP, Arroyo-Jimenez MM, et al. Initial characterization of anosmin-1, a putative extracellular matrix protein synthesized by definite neuronal cell populations in the central nervous system. *J Cell Sci.* 1996;109 (Pt 7):1749–1757.

95. de Roux N, Genin E, Carel JC, et al. Hypogonadotropic hypogonadism due to loss of

function of the KiSS1-derived peptide receptor GPR54. *Proc Natl Acad Sci USA.* 2003;100(19):10972–10976.

96. O'Rahilly S, Gray H, Humphreys PJ, et al. Brief report: impaired processing of prohormones associated with abnormalities of glucose homeostasis and adrenal function. *N Engl J Med.* 1995; 333(21):1386–1390.

97. Soussi-Yanicostas N, Faivre-Sarrailh C, Hardelin JP, et al. Anosmin-1 underlying the X chromosome-linked Kallmann syndrome is an adhesion molecule that can modulate neurite growth in a cell-type specific manner. *J Cell Sci.* 1998;111 (Pt 19):2953–2965.

98. Seminara SB, Messager S, Chatzidaki EE, et al. The GPR54 gene as a regulator of puberty. *N Engl J Med.* 2003;349(17): 1614–1627.

99. Dode C, Levilliers J, Dupont JM, et al. Loss-of-function mutations in FGFR1 cause autosomal dominant Kallmann syndrome. *Nat Genet.* 2003;33(4):463–465.

100. Farooqi IS, Jebb SA, Langmack G, et al. Effects of recombinant leptin therapy in a child with congenital leptin deficiency. *N Engl J Med.* 1999;341(12):879–884.

101. Varela MC, Kok F, Setian N, et al. Impact of molecular mechanisms, including deletion size, on Prader-Willi syndrome phenotype: study of 75 patients. *Clin Genet.* 2005;67(1):47–52.

102. Holm VA, Cassidy SB, Butler MG, et al. Prader-Willi syndrome: consensus diagnostic criteria. *Pediatrics.* 1993;91(2):398–402.

103. Burman P, Ritzen EM, Lindgren AC. Endocrine dysfunction in Prader-Willi syndrome: a review with special reference to GH. *Endocr Rev.* 2001;22(6):787–799.

104. Wheeler PG, Quigley CA, Sadeghi-Nejad A, et al. Hypogonadism and CHARGE association. *Am J Med Genet.* 2000;94(3):228–31.

105. Kaltsas GA, Powles TB, Evanson J, et al. Hypothalamo-pituitary abnormalities in adult patients with Langerhans cell histiocytosis: clinical, endocrinological, and radiological features and response to treatment. *J Clin Endocrinol Metab.* 2000;85(4):1370–1376.

106. Bhagavath B, Ozata M, Ozdemir IC, et al. The prevalence of gonadotropin-releasing hormone receptor mutations in a large cohort of patients with hypogonadotropic hypogonadism. *Fertil Steril.* 2005;84(4):951–957.

107. Layman LC. Genetic causes of human infertility. *Endocrinol Metab Clin North Am.* 2003;32(3):549–572.

108. Meysing AU, Kanasaki H, Bedecarrats GY, et al. GNRHR mutations in a woman with idiopathic hypogonadotropic hypogonadism highlight the differential sensitivity of luteinizing hormone and follicle-stimulating hormone to gonadotropin-releasing hormone. *J Clin Endocrinol Metab.* 2004;89(7): 3189–3198.

109. Costa EM, Bedecarrats GY, Mendonca BB, et al. Two novel mutations in the gonadotropin-releasing hormone receptor gene in Brazilian patients with hypogonadotropic hypogonadism and normal olfaction. *J Clin Endocrinol Metab.* 2001;86(6):2680–2686.

110. Seminara SB, Beranova M, Oliveira LM, et al. Successful use of pulsatile gonadotropin-releasing hormone (GnRH) for ovulation induction and pregnancy in a patient with GnRH receptor mutations. *J Clin Endocrinol Metab.* 2000;85(2):556–562.

111. Matthews CH, Borgato S, Beck-Peccoz P, et al. Primary amenorrhoea and infertility due to a mutation in the beta-subunit of follicle-stimulating hormone. *Nat Genet.* 1993;5(1):83–86.

112. Deladoey J, Fluck C, Buyukgebiz A, et al. "Hot spot" in the PROP1 gene responsible for combined pituitary hormone deficiency. *J Clin Endocrinol Metab.* 1999;84(5): 1645–1650.

113. Fluck C, Deladoey J, Rutishauser K, et al. Phenotypic variability in familial combined pituitary hormone deficiency caused by a PROP1 gene mutation resulting in the substitution of Arg–>Cys at codon 120 (R120C). *J Clin Endocrinol Metab.* 1998;83(10): 3727–3734.

114. Dattani MT, Martinez-Barbera JP, Thomas PQ, et al. HESX1: a novel gene implicated in a familial form of septo-optic dysplasia. *Acta Paediatr Suppl.* 1999;88(433):49–54.

115. Thomas PQ, Dattani MT, Brickman JM, et al. Heterozygous HESX1 mutations associated with isolated congenital pituitary hypoplasia and septo-optic dysplasia. *Hum Mol Genet.* 2001;10(1):39–45.

116. Netchine I, Sobrier ML, Krude H, et al. Mutations in LHX3 result in a new syndrome revealed by combined pituitary hormone deficiency. *Nat Genet.* 2000;25(2):182–186.

117. Lafferty AR, Chrousos GP. Pituitary tumors in children and adolescents. *J Clin Endocrinol Metab.* 1999;84(12):4317–4323.

118. Mindermann T, Wilson CB. Pituitary adenomas in childhood and adolescence. *J Pediatr Endocrinol Metab.* 1995;8(2):79–83.

119. Pickett CA. Diagnosis and management of pituitary tumors: recent advances. *Prim Care.* 2003;30(4):765–789.

120. Schlechte J, Dolan K, Sherman B, et al. The natural history of untreated hyperprolactinemia: a prospective analysis. *J Clin Endocrinol Metab.* 1989;68(2):412–418.

121. Colao A, Loche S, Cappa M, et al. Prolactinomas in children and adolescents. Clinical presentation and long-term follow-up. *J Clin Endocrinol Metab.* 1998;83(8):2777–2780.

122. Molitch ME, Elton RL, Blackwell RE, et al. Bromocriptine as primary therapy for prolactin-secreting macroadenomas: results of a prospective multicenter study. *J Clin Endocrinol Metab.* 1985;60(4):698–705.

123. Bettendorf M, Fehn M, Grulich-Henn J, et al. Lymphocytic hypophysitis with central diabetes insipidus and consequent panhypopituitarism preceding a multifocal, intracranial germinoma in a prepubertal girl. *Eur J Pediatr.* 1999;158(4):288–292.

124. Levy A. Pituitary disease: presentation, diagnosis, and management. *J Neurol Neurosurg Psychiatry.* 2004;75 Suppl 3:iii47–52.

125. Ammar A, Al-Sultan A, Al Mulhim F, et al. Empty sella syndrome: does it exist in children? *J Neurosurg.* 1999;91(6):960–963.

126. Sert M, Tetiker T, Kirim S, et al. Clinical report of 28 patients with Sheehan's syndrome. *Endocr J.* 2003;50(3):297–301.

127. Kelestimur F. Sheehan's syndrome. *Pituitary.* 2003;6(4):181–188.

CHAPTER 37

Male Hypogonadism

Darius A. Paduch, MD, PhD
Peter N. Schlegel, MD

Acknowledgments

This work was supported by the Frederick J and Teresa Dow Wallace Fund of the New York Community Trust fellowship to Dr. Darius A. Paduch. The authors would like to thank our families for their patience and understanding during months spent preparing and writing this chapter.

FREQUENTLY USED ABBREVIATIONS

T	=	testosterone
LH	=	leutinizing hormone
FSH	=	follicle stimulating hormone
E_1	=	estrone
E_2	=	estradiol
β-hCG	=	human chorionic gonadotropin
MIS	=	Müllerian-inhibiting substance
GnRH	=	gonadotropin releasing hormone

ANATOMY, EMBRYOLOGY, AND DEVELOPMENT

Each testis is encapsulated in white fibrous membrane, the *tunica albuginea* with a large testicular artery located along the anterior surface of the gonad. The parenchyma of the testis consists of numerous tortuous tubules, the seminiferous tubules, which comprise 80% to 85% of the testicular mass, surrounded by the interstitial tissue containing Leydig cells. Lymphatic and blood vessels, macrophages and nerves are also contained in the interstitial tissue. The seminiferous tubuli loop around and eventually form straight tubules that are called *tubuli recti*. The *tubuli recti* then form a close anastomosing network, located in the hilum of the testis, called the *rete testis*. The *rete testis* tubules in turn join into three to five *ductuli efferentia*, which then join to form the duct of the epididymis. The seminiferous epithelium is the site of spermatogenesis and once spermatozoa are produced, they are released into the lumen of the seminiferous tubuli and are transported via the previously described network of tubules to the epididymis. From the epididymis the spermatozoa enter the vas deferens and then the ejaculatory ducts to enter the urethra.

The testis develops in the abdomen. Male differentiation of the primitive bipotential gonads depends on timely and spatially coordinated events that are triggered by the SRY gene (located on the short arm of chromosome Y) together with SOX-9, DAX-1, WT-1, and other genes and their products. These genes initiate the cascade of events necessary to commit the gonads to testicular development, the first step in normal male differentiation (1). Approximately 7 weeks after conception, primordial germ cells migrate from the yolk sac and populate the primitive cords of the gonad, where they evolve into prospermatogonia and spermatogonia. Gonadal mesenchymal stem cells differentiate into steroidogenic Leydig cells. Leydig cells are stimulated to produce testosterone (T) by maternal human chorionic gonadotropin (β-hCG) during the first half of pregnancy, and later, with the development and maturation of gonadotropin-producing cells in the fetal pituitary, by fetal luteinizing hormone (LH) (2).

The fetus initially has both male and female internal genital ducts. Persistence of the Wolffian ducts and differentiation into the male reproductive tract (epididymis, vas deferens, and seminal vesicles) depends on the presence of T (3). Precursors of Sertoli cells produce Müllerian-inhibiting substance (MIS) that causes regression of the female internal ducts. T is converted by 5-α reductase to dihydrotestosterone (DHT) in fibroblasts of the external genitalia and prostate; DHT affects male transformation of the external genitalia with fusion of the genital folds, development of the scrotum, and formation of the primordial phallus into a penis. Growth hormone (GH) acting in conjunction with insulin-like growth factors (IGFs) may modulate androgen action in these target tissues (4). This process is complete by the end of the first trimester.

Transabdominal migration of the fetal testes to a position at the internal inguinal ring occurs in the first trimester and may be more related to fetal growth than to actual migration. The testes remain in this location until approximately 7 months gestation, when they continue their descent into the scrotum. This entire process depends on normal abdominal wall development, lack of anatomic obstruction along the descent pathway, and an adequate endocrinologic milieu. Transabdominal descent is regulated by T, but transinguinal advancement of the testis is thought to be directed by relaxin and other autocrine substances. Abnormal descent results in cryptorchidism (undescended testis).

Just after birth. the Leydig cells increase in number and reach a peak at 2 to 3 months of age, contributing to a second surge in T levels (the first surge is in utero at 12–14 wk of gestation coinciding with an increase in Leydig cell number). After the postnatal peak, Leydig cells regress rapidly to a nadir by the end of the 1st year. Differentiation of the Leydig cells begins at 10 years of age and is complete by 13 years of age. During puberty the number of Leydig cells increases, reaching a maximum in early 20s.

There are also two phases of Sertoli proliferation, one immediately after birth and one later at puberty; both phases are characterized by elevated gonadotropin levels, LH, and follicle-stimulating hormone (FSH), both of which seem to be effective in stimulating Sertoli cell proliferation. The cessation of Sertoli cell proliferation and initiation of Sertoli cell maturation occur during early puberty and result in development of blood–testis barrier and initiation of spermatogenesis. Sertoli cells are the major determinant of testicular size, seminiferous tube development, and sperm count because each Sertoli cell supports a set number of germ cells. During puberty the dramatic increase in number

Male Hypogonadism

AT-A-GLANCE

Male hypogonadism is defined as endocrine or spermatogenic testicular dysfunction. The testis has two primary functions: (1) endocrine-producing and -releasing testosterone (T) and other endocrine hormones such as estradiol (E_2) and Müllerian-inhibiting substance (MIS), and (2) spermatogenic-producing sperm. Although both functions regulate and depend on each other, the endocrine function is especially important during fetal organogenesis, development of male external genitalia, and puberty.

Male hypogonadism may be anatomically classified as pretesticular (central deficits), testicular (i.e., Klinefelter syndrome, varicocele, cryptorchidism, or gonadal injury), and posttesticular (obstruction at the level of the epididymis, vas deferens, ejaculatory ducts; retrograde ejaculation, or erectile dysfunction).

NOTE: The At-A-Glance tables exclude disorders of gonadal development and sex differentiation which is covered in Chapter 35.

TYPE	OCCURRENCE	(GENE) LOCUS	OMIM
Pretesticular-Central Causes			
Injury to Pituitary/Hypothalamic area (Tumors, trauma, irradiation, infiltrative disease)	NA	NA	NA
Functional hypogonadotropic hypogonadism	NA	NA	NA
Idiopathic hypogonadotropic hypogonadism	rare	unknown	NA
Kallmann syndrome (KAL-1, KAL-2, KAL-3, KAL-4)	1:8,000	(KAL1) Xp22.3	+308700
		(FGFR1) 8p11.2	#147950
		(PROKR2) 20p13	#244200
		(PROK2) 3p21.1	*607002
Prader–Willi Syndrome	1:10,000–25,000	(Unknown) 15q12, 15q11-13	#176270
Gordon Holmes syndrome	rare	unknown	%212840
Leptin, deficiency	rare	(LFP) 7q31.3	*164160
Leptin receptor defect	rare	(LEPR) 1p31	*601007
CHARGE syndrome	rare	(CHD7, SEMA3E) 8q12.1, 7q21.1	#214800
Bardet–Biedl syndrome	rare	Multiple loci	#209900
Congenital adrenal hypoplasia	rare	(NR0B1) Xp21.q	*300473
Hyperprolactinemia*			
Drug effects	Relatively common	NA	NA
Sporadic prolactinoma	14:100,000	unknown	NA
Familial prolactinoma	Rare	unknown	600634
MEN1	320:100,000	(MEN1) 11q13	+131100
GnRH receptor defects	rare		
With LH and FSH deficiency		(GNRHR) 4q21.2	*138850
With isolated LH deficiency (fertile eunuch)			#228300
FSH receptor defect	rare	(FSHR) 2p21-p16	*136435
LHCG receptor defects	rare	(LHCGR) 2p21	+52790
FSHβ subunit defect	rare	(FSHB) 11p13	*136530
LHβ subunit defect	rare	(LHB) 19q13.32	+152780
Pituitary transcription factor defects	rare		
PROP1		(PROP1) 5q	*601538
HESX1		(HESX1) 3p21.2-21.1	*601802
LHX3		(LHX3) 9q34.3	*600577
Aromatase excess syndrome**	rare	(CYP19A1) 15q21.2	#139300

* Other endocrine causes of prolactinemia include GH tumors and hypothyroidism; **Common in obesity.

TYPE	OCCURRENCE	(GENE) LOCUS	OMIM
Testicular Causes			
Klinefelter syndrome	1:500–1,000	XXY	NA
Noonan Syndrome	1:2,000	(PTPN11) 12q24.1	#163950
		(SOS1) 2p22-p21	#610733
		(KRAS) 12p12.1	#609942
		(RAF1) 3p25	#611553
Anorchia	rare	unknown	273250
Cryptorchidism	1–3% newborn males	unknown, but may be 19p13.2, 13q13.1	#219050
Macroorchidism	rare	(FMR1) Xq27.3	+309550
Varicocele	common	NA	NA
Estrogen deficiency			
Aromatase deficiency	rare	(CYP19A1) 15q21.1	+107910
Estrogen receptor -1 defect	rare	(ESRA) 6q25.1	*133430
Genetic defects affecting spermatogenesis	rare		
AZF abnormities to AZF a, b, c, deletions		distal arm of Y chromosome	#400042
Posttesticular Causes			
Cystic fibrosis, CBAVD	1:2,500 live births	(CFTR) 7q31.2	*602421
			#277180
Immotile cilia syndrome	rare		
Primary ciliary dyskinesia (PCD1-7)		Multiple loci	#242650,
			%606763,
			#608644,
			%608646,
			%608647,
			#611884
Kartagener		(DNAI1, DNAH11, DNAH5) 9p21–p13, 7p21, 5p15-p14	#244400
Penile deformities			
Concealed penis	relatively common	NA	NA
Penile agenesis	extremely rare	unknown	NA
Phimosis and paraphimosis	very common in uncircumcised boys	NA	NA
Epispadias	1:117,000 male births	unknown	%600057
Hypospadias	1:300 male births, increasing	unknown, estrogen like pollutant	#146450

FORM	FINDINGS AND CLINICAL PRESENTATION
Pretesticular-Central Causes	
Physical damage to the hypothalamus or pituitary	Hypogonadism is seldom the only presenting symptom. Change in visual fields, new onset of blurred vision, or bilateral hemianopsia may reflect central tumors.
Functional hypogonadotropic hypogonadism	Depression of gonadotropin secretion due to chronic debilitating disease or eating disorders; no organic hypothalamic disease.
Idiopathic hypogonadotropic hypogonadism (IHH); Kallmann syndrome (KalS)	Both have delayed puberty, eunuchoid body habitus, gynecomastia; other pituitary hormone levels are normal; IHH is not associated with other phenotypic abnormalities; genetic cause(s) are unknown; KalS is associated with micropenis (60%), bilateral cryptorchism (25%–75%), hyposmia or anosmia (80%), synkinesia and renal aplasia (KAL-1), and cleft palate and dental agenesis (KAL-2); the extent of hypogonadotropic hypogonadism is variable.
Prader–Willi Syndrome	Hypotonia and feeding difficulties in infancy, hyperphagia and morbid obesity developing early in childhood, short stature, small hands and feet, mild mental retardation and behavioral problems; hypogonadotropic hypogonadism with bilateral cryptorchidism, micropenis (70%); appear to be infertile.
Gordon Holmes syndrome	Progressive neurologic deterioration with ataxia and hypogonadotropic that does not respond to GnRH therapy hypogonadism in mid-20s.
Leptin, leptin receptor deficiency	Hyperphagia, early onset obesity, and hypogonadotropic hypogonadism.

FORM	FINDINGS AND CLINICAL PRESENTATION
CHARGE syndrome	Coloboma, heart disease, choanal atresia, retarded growth, genital hypoplasia due to hypogonadotropic hypogonadism, ear anomalies
Bardet–Biedl, Laurence–Moon syndrome	Obesity, progressive retinal dystrophy and mental retardation; patients with Bardet–Biedl syndrome have hexadactyly while Laurence–Moon syndrome displays spastic paraplegia and ataxia
Congenital adrenal hypoplasia	Loss of function causes hypogonadotropic hypogonadism and adrenal insufficiency
Hyperprolactinemia	Patients present with impaired sexual function, rarely with galactorrhea, or with mass effect symptoms (panhypopituitarism, visual field deficits).
GnRH receptor mutations	The clinical picture is variable but in males it can range from delayed puberty to infertility; no response to GnRH; A variant of this is the fertile eunuch syndrome: isolated LH deficiency, normal FSH; normal sized testes with some degree of spermatogenesis, occasionally fertile, respond to β-hCG.
FSH receptor mutations	Normal puberty, decreased testicular volumes, variable degrees of spermatogenic failure but NOT azoospermia; high FSH, normal to elevated LH, normal T, and low inhibin.
LH receptor mutations	Leydig cell hypoplasia to agenesis; delayed puberty; phenotype varies from hypospadias and/or micropenis to complete 46,XY sex reversal; no pubertal gynecomastia; elevated LH, FSH, and low T.
FSHβ subunit defect	Mild pubertal delay or normal puberty; small testicles and spermatogenic failure, azoospermia; low FSH, elevated LH, and normal T.
LHβ subunit defect	Delayed puberty, normal sex development, small, soft testes, with arrested spermatogenesis, and absent Leydig cells; elevated LH, FSH, and low T. Normal T in response β-hCG stimulation test.
Pituitary Transcription Factor Defects	PROP1: variable deficiencies of LH, FSH, PRL, TSH and GH. HESX1: septo-optic dysplasia, isolated GH deficiency or panhypopituitarism. LHX3: low gonadotropin levels, combined pituitary hormone deficiency and a rigid cervical spine.
Aromatase excess syndrome	Excessive estrogen suppresses LH; aromatase inhibitors may be useful in men with high E_2:T ratios.
Anabolic steroid and other drug abuse	LH is suppressed by high androgen levels; small, soft testes, may lead to permanent sterility; acute and chronic alcohol intoxication in pubertal males is associated with a decrease in plasma T and lower LH and FSH; delayed puberty has been found in boys with chronic alcohol abuse.
Testicular Causes	High or Normal Gonadotropins, T May Be Normal or Low
Klinefelter syndrome	Broad phenotypic variation, eunuchoid body habitus, sparse facial and pubic hair, small, hard testicles, major intellectual impairment rare, mostly learning disability and auditory processing dysfunction; low T, high LH and FSH, and often elevated E_2; normal timing of puberty; T deficit may become worse with age; 47,XXY most common; those with more than two X chromosomes are usually more severely affected.
Noonan Syndrome	Similar to features of Turner syndrome in females, normal karyotype, short stature, triangular face, hypertelorism, refractive problems, amblyopia, low-set ears, high nasal bridge, short, webbed neck, scoliosis, pectus excavatum, cardiac abnormalities, coagulopathy, splenomegaly; undescended testes (>50%); normal LH, elevated FSH, normal or low T; fertility possible; risk of leukemia.
Anorchia	Present with bilateral testicular absence, otherwise phenotypically normal; no T response to β-hCG; no MIS; no increase in inhibin B level
Cryptorchidism	Especially common in premature infants; unilateral and right-sided most common; most resolve by 3 months corrected gestational age; boys with cryptorchidism generally undergo normal pubertal development; some syndromes (KalS, PWS) are associated with cryptorchism.
Macroorchidism	Unilateral: suspect testicular tumor or extratesticular mass, or compensatory hypertrophy after damage to the opposite testis; most common cause of bilateral is fragile X syndrome: mild to moderate mental retardation which may worsen with age; large ears, a prominent jaw, a high-pitched voice, flat feet and joint laxity; phenotypic expression is variable.

FORM	FINDINGS AND CLINICAL PRESENTATION
Testicular damage by trauma, infection, toxins, and drugs	Mumps orchitis after puberty, trauma to the testis, torsion or cryptorchidism can all affect spermatogenesis; hormonal function is usually intact unless bilateral severe atrophy is present; chemotherapy may not only affect sperm production but also increase slightly the risk of abnormal sperm; drugs like sulfasalazine and colchicines can cause transient spermatogenic arrest.
Varicocele	Dilation of the pampiniform plexus veins; the most common identifiable cause of male infertility; testicular atrophy, abnormal sperm, and poor T production in adulthood; first seen during puberty; timely diagnosis and treatment are essential to preserve fertility.
Estrogen deficiency	Lack of estrogen activity caused by resistance ER-1 defects or aromatase deficiency; boys go through puberty normally but the epiphyses do not close; adult men have tall stature, elevated FSH and LH, high E_2 (resistance) or low E_2 (aromatase def.), macroorchidism with abnormal sperm, osteoporosis, insulin resistance and impaired glucose tolerance, elevated lipid levels.
Genetic defects affecting spermatogenesis	These conditions are typically only discovered during work up for male infertility; microdeletions of AZFc on the long arm of Y may result in azoospermia or oligospermia with potential fertility (and passing on the genetic mutation to offspring); FSH may be elevated but T is normal; FSH receptor deficiency can cause defects in spermatogenesis in males.
Posttesticular	Normal Gonadotropin and T Levels
Mechanical obstruction	Bilateral inguinal hernia repair can result in obstruction of the vas deferens.
Retrograde ejaculation	Caused by retroperitoneal surgery, radiation, spina bifida, bladder neck reconstruction; α-blockers and serotonin reuptake inhibitors can cause retrograde ejaculation or anejaculation; 5 α-reductase inhibitors can decrease semen volume by 13%–20%.
Cystic fibrosis, CBAVD	Bilateral congenital absence of the vas deferens is the most common genetic cause of obstructive azoospermia; caused by mutations in the CFTR gene; when pulmonary and GI symptoms are present the diagnosis is cystic fibrosis; unilateral absence of the vas deferens is due to mesonephric duct malformation rather than CFTR and is associated with renal agenesis.
Immotile cilia syndrome	Abnormal tubular structure of sperm and cilia tail leading to motility problems (diagnosed by electron microscopy); when associated with situs inversus and bronchiectasis it is called Kartagener syndrome, otherwise primary ciliary dyskinesia.
Penile abnormalities	*Concealed penis:* An entirely normal penis appears small because it is hidden by the suprapubic fat pad (especially in obese children), or when the scrotal skin extends onto the ventrum of the penis ("webbed penis"); must be distinguished from micropenis. *Penile agenesis:* Failure of genital tubercle development; karyotype 46,XY; well-formed scrotum and descended testes; variable connection between the genitourinary and gastrointestinal tract, there are often associated renal abnormalities, which can be severe. *Phimosis:* the inability to retract the foreskin to see the glans; common and normal in uncircumcised boys. *Paraphimosis:* the retracted foreskin cannot be pulled back over the glans, causing constriction, pain, edema, and eventually may lead to necrosis—this is a urologic emergency; risk factors- poor hygiene, overly vigorous cleaning, inflammation, penis body piercing. *Epispadias:* urethral opening on the dorsal side of the penis; associated with varying degrees of dorsal chordee; degree of deformity and urinary incontinence varies depending on the location of the urethral meatus; the most severe type is associated with bladder exstrophy. *Hypospadias: urethral* opening on the ventral side of the penis; other malformations (esp. renal and urinary tract) present in about 15%.
Erectile dysfunction	Results from psychologic, neurologic, vascular, or mechanical problems; diabetes and smoking are risk factors.

of germ cells has a significant impact in determining ultimate testis size.

T levels in the newborn, which reach the level of an adult man by approximately 3 months of age, decrease to almost undetectable levels by age 6 months. This early infancy rise in T is necessary for normal penile development and growth (5). LH levels rise and fall in parallel with T, whereas FSH and inhibin B slowly decrease during the 1st year of life. The most reliable time to assess reproductive hormones in infancy is at the age of approximately 2 to 3 months. FSH should be between 0.9 and 2.93 IU/L, LH 0.9 and 2.64 IU/L, and T 75 and 240 mg/dL (1.8–11.9 nmol/L).

At approximately the age of 10 years, a higher frequency and amplitude of pulsatile LH discharge causes an increase in testicular volume (> 4 cc^3) and circulating T levels, all of which signal the onset of puberty. T acting via DHT stimulates growth of the penis, development of axillary, pubic and facial hair, and tertiary male sexual characteristics. T levels, testicular volumes, and penile length correlate better with Tanner stages of pubertal development than with chronologic age (Figure 37-1) because at the same age some boys may be just starting puberty whereas others have adult male body proportions and development. Normal mean stretched penile length and ranges, testicular volumes, and T levels are provided in Table 37-1. The occurrence of nocturnal emissions coincides with the start of normal spermatogenesis, when sperm can be found in the ejaculate and the morning urine of midpubertal boys. In distinction to females, men continue the process of spermatogenesis throughout their lifespan, although with age the quality and quantity of sperm production deteriorate.

TABLE 37-1 Testosterone Levels, Testicular Volume, and Penile Length in Different Developmental Groups (20,119–120)

Tanner Stage	Age years	Testicular Volume cc^3, mean (range)	Penile Length (cm) mean (95% CI)	Testosterone mg/dL (nmol/L) min		max	
T1	Birth	1	3.5 (2.5–4.5)	0	(0)	187	(6.5)
T1	3 mo	1	3.9 (2.7–4.9)	52	(1.8)	346	(12)
T1	18 mo	1	4.2 (3.1–5.3)	0	(0)	17	(0.6)
T1	36 mo	1	4.5 (3.3–5.8)	0	(0)	12	(0.4)
T1	5–11	1 (1–2)	6.2 (4.7–7.6)	0	(0)	12	(0.4)
T1	8–13	3 (2–3)	7.1 (4.7–11.3)	6	(0.2)	12	(0.4)
T2	9–14	4 (3–6)	9.8 (6.1–13.5)	12	(0.4)	29	(1.0)
T3	11–15	8 (8–12)	11.8 (9.1–14.8)	101	3.5	231	(8.0)
T4	13–17	15 (15–25)	12.5 (10.8–15.3)	176	6.1	433	(15)
T5	17–19	20 (15–25)	13.1 (10.8–15.5)	225	7.8	702	(24)

THE HYPOTHALAMIC-PITUITARY GONADAL AXIS

There are two types of hormones important in human reproduction, peptides (gonadotropin releasing-hormone [GnRH], LH, and FSH) and steroids (T, DHT, E$_2$). GnRH, a decapeptide, is produced by neurons in the hypothalamic preoptic and paraventricular nuclei and is transported via the hypothalamic portal blood to the anterior pituitary. GnRH binds to G protein–coupled receptors (GnRHR) on gonadotropes in the anterior pituitary and stimulates pulsatile release of the gonadotropins FSH and LH, which are both produced by the same cells in proportions determined at least in part, by the GnRH pulse frequency. Release of GnRH is regulated by many neuroendocrine factors and direct neuronal connections from the cortex and subcortical (hypothalamus and limbic system) regions (7) (Figure 37-2).

T inhibits the release of GnRH through negative feedback. This process depends on local conversion of T to estradiol (E$_2$) and DHT, each of which decreases release of GnRH from the hypothalamus. E$_2$ is produced from T through the activity of the aromatase enzyme in the brain, testis and the peripheral tissues, with 20% of the total circulating estrogens in males produced by the Leydig cells. In addition, GnRH effects on the pituitary are modulated by E$_2$, and high levels of circulating estrogens may dampen the response of the pituitary gland to GnRH stimulation. Pituitary release of FSH is inhibited by E$_2$ and is also regulated by the Sertoli cell–produced glycoproteins inhibin B (inhibitory) and activin (stimulatory). Prolactin decreases the responsiveness of gonadotrophs to GnRH and is a well-established cause of hypogonadism.

Pulsatile GnRH secretion is increased during the neonatal period and markedly decreased during childhood. The onset of puberty is characterized by a striking increase in the amplitude of the LH pulses, with less change in frequency during sleep. As puberty progresses gonadotropin secretion occurs throughout the day. In adult males pulsatile secretion of gonadotropins is characterized by one pulse every 2 hours. In testicular failure a further increase in pulsatile GnRH secretion increases the number of GnRHR resulting in elevated gonadotropin levels, whereas continuous GnRH treatment or GnRH deficiency results in decrease in the number of the GnRHRs and suppression of pituitary gonadotropin secretion.

GnRH neurons have been observed in the human hypothalamus by the 9th week of gestation; Gonadotropins LH, FSH are first detected in the fetus by the 12th to 14th weeks

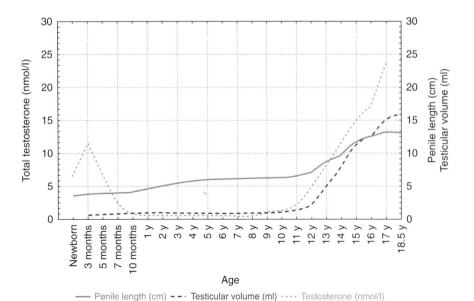

FIGURE 37-1. Total testosterone, penile length, and testicular volume changes in boys from 0 to 22 years of age (17,20,120–121).

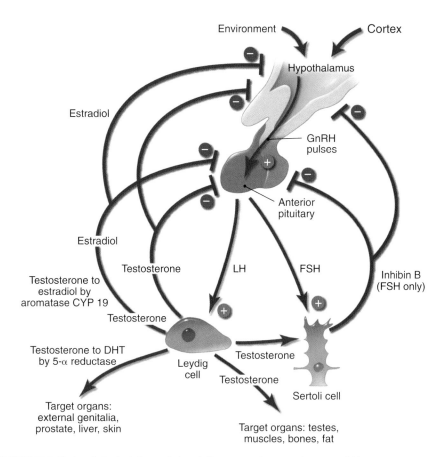

FIGURE 37-2. The hypothalamic-pituitary-testicular axis. Testosterone after conversion to estradiol by aromatase enzyme exerts negative feedback on GnRH release and on pituitary onadotropes, resulting in decreases of LH and FSH levels. LH stimulates the testes to secrete testosterone and FSH stimulates release of inhibin from the Sertoli cells and is necessary for spermatogenesis. FSH release is inhibited by inhibin B and follistatin and is stimulated by activin. Testosterone is converted to DHT by 5α-reductase enzyme.

of gestation. Anecenphalic fetuses that do not have hypothalamus secrete glucoprotein hormone α-subunit but do not produce LH or FSH. Gonadotropins are members of the glycoprotein family hormones, which includes thyroid-stimulating hormone (TSH) and β-hCG. All the glycoproteins of this family are heterodimers consisting of a common α-subunit and a unique β-subunit. The human α-subunit gene is on 6p21.1-23. The LH-β gene along with six CGB genes and pseudogenes is mapped on 19q13.3 and the FSH-β gene is on 11p13. After release from the pituitary to the blood stream, gonadotropins bind to G protein–coupled receptors. Both gonadotropin receptor genes are mapped on chromosome 2p21. LH and β-hCG are structurally similar so that they bind to the same receptor, LHCG receptor (LHCGR). In the early fetal period, placental β-hCG through the LHCGR stimulates Leydig cell steroidogenesis, which is essential for the male development of internal reproductive organs as fetal pituitary gonadotropin secretion does not begin until the end of the first trimester. FSH binds to FSHR on the Sertoli cell and LH binds to LHCGR on the Leydig

cell. LH binding to its receptor initiates a cyclic adenosine monophosphate second messenger system and production of T. The acute response of the Leydig cells to the LH stimulation is mediated through the steroidogenic acute regulatory protein (StAR), whereas the chronic response involves transcriptional activation of the genes encoding the steroidogenic enzymes of the T biosynthesis (P450scc, P450c17, 3β-HSD-II, and 17β-HSD3). Prolactin, growth hormone (GH), triiodothyronine (T_3), and inhibin B can also stimulate T synthesis directly, whereas glucocorticoids, E_2, activin, AVP and IL-1 may reduce T production by the Leydig cells. FSH receptor (FSHR) binding is necessary to initiate spermatogenesis during puberty. FSH is necessary for qualitative and quantitative normal spermatogenesis. Once spermatogenesis has been initiated, it can be sustained with β-hCG, which has implications for fertility in cases of gonadotropin deficiency.

In addition to the negative feedback of gonadal steroids at the hypothalamic–pituitary axis, peptides such as activin and follistatin, which are produced by the pituitary, and inhibin B produced by the Sertoli cells are

involved in gonadotropin regulation. In particular, FSH secretion is regulated through modulation of FSHβ gene expression through the actions of pituitary activin and follistatin and through the Sertoli cell-secreted inhibin B.

Inhibin belongs to a family of glucoprotein hormones and growth factors including transforming growth factor–β, Müllerian-inhibiting hormone, and activin. Inhibins are heterodimers consisting of an a-subunit and one of two β-subunits (βA and βB), which form inhibin A and inhibin B, respectively. In the testis, only the subunit βB is expressed and therefore testis make only inhibin B. Inhibin is produced and released from the Sertoli cells in response to FSH stimulation and exerts both paracrine and endocrine responses. The main function of inhibin is to suppress the secretion of FSH from the pituitary through a negative feedback mechanism.

Inhibin B levels rise during the neonatal period and again at puberty, which are also the developmental phases during which Sertoli cells number increases; circulating inhibin B levels reflect the number and function of Sertoli cells and is less dependent on FSH stimulation. As there is a correlation between inhibin B levels, sperm count, and testicular volume, inhibin B can be used as an index of spermatogenesis.

Activins are members of the same family of peptides as the inhibins and are homodimers or heterodimers of the β-subunit of the inhibins. Activin increases FSH release by stimulating FSHβ mRNA transcription and prolonging FSHβ mRNA half life. Activin's actions are antagonized by follistatin and by inhibin, which competes with activin for binding to the activin receptor.

Follistatin is a single chain gonadal protein that inhibits FSH release and binds to and antagonizes activin. There are three known isoforms of follistatin created by alternative splicing. Follistatin mRNA is expressed in nearly all tissues, with highest expression in adult ovary, pituitary, and kidney, and in fetal heart and liver. Activin, inhibin B, and follistatin may also act locally in the testis and may alter T production and gamete maturation.

SPERMATOGENESIS

Spermatogenesis involves a series of processes (mitosis, miosis, and spermiogenesis) that produce highly differentiated haploid spermatozoa from a limited population of stem (diploid) spermatogonia.

The epithelium of the seminiferous tubules consists of three types of germ cells, spermatogonia, spermatocytes, and spermatids and one somatic cell type, the Sertoli cell, which provide nutrients, growth factors, and support to the germ cells. The Sertoli cells lie on the basement membrane and extending to the lumen of the seminiferous tubules. The spermatogonia also lie on the basement membrane and are classified as stem cells or spermatogonia type A or differentiated spermatogonia or spermatogonia type B. Spermatogonia are mitotically active; division of the last generation of the spermatogonia B results in the production of the spermatocytes, which are the last diploid germ cells and compose the next layer of the seminiferous epithelium. Spermatocytes differentiate and through meioses I and II form the haploid spermatids, which comprise the layer of the epithelium adjacent to the tubular lumen. At the initial stage spermatids are round and undergo further maturational events to develop into spermatozoa, a process termed spermiogenesis. A spermatozoan, more commonly known as a sperm cell, is the haploid cell that is the male gamete. Both T and FSH are required for normal spermatogenesis. Increased FSH and low inhibin B levels are indicative of decreased spermatogenesis. Spermatozoa are produced continuously throughout the life of adult males.

Testosterone (T) Biology

Testosterone (T) is produced in the Leydig cells via four enzymatic steps. The first enzymatic step takes place in the mitochondrion, where cholesterol is converted to pregnenolone through the activity of the P450 cholesterol side cleavage enzyme (P450scc). Cholesterol transport into the mitochondrion is facilitated by the StAR protein. Subsequently, pregnenolone in the endocytoplasmic reticulum of the Leydig cell is converted to T through the activities of three enzymes: 3β-hydroxysteroid dehydrogenase type II (3βHSD-II), P450 17α-hydroxylase/lyase (P450c17) and 17β-hydroxysteroid dehydrogenase type 3 (17βHSD3).

T concentration in the testicular interstitium is 100 times higher than T levels found in serum. High local concentration of T within the testis is necessary for complete spermatogenesis. Extrinsic treatment with T suppresses LH release and thus ablates high intratesticular T levels, resulting in suppression of spermatogenesis and shrinkage of the testes. This is important information to provide to adolescent athletes because prolonged anabolic steroid abuse may irreversibly alter the hypothalamic-pituitary-gonadal (HPG) axis, leading to permanent sterility.

T produced in Leydig cells is washed out from the interstitium to the blood stream where it is bound to albumin and sex hormone–binding globulin (SHBG). Only approximately 2% of the total T in serum is free (not bound). In target tissues, T traverses cell membranes (mostly by diffusion but also through active transport) and after binding to its receptor, androgen receptor (AR) in the cytosol, the ligand-receptor complex travels to the nucleus where it binds to androgen response motifs of DNA. Although most of the T action occurs through activation of transcription, growing evidence supports the hypothesis that some of its action occurs directly through membrane bound steroid receptors (nongenomic action). Action of T is modulated by interaction with coactivators that enhance transcriptional activity of the AR complex. Coinhibitors may interfere with this action, and thus the circulating levels of T may not directly reflect cellular bioactivity of androgens. The net action of T on target tissues is a sum of its bioavailability, saturation of the AR, and the relative ratio of coinhibitors to coactivators in the transcriptional complex (8).

The AR gene is located on the long arm of the X chromosome (Xq11.2 to Xq12). It belongs to a class of proteins with a highly conserved sequence within the animal kingdom. There are at least four distinct regions in the AR: N-terminal transactivation domain, DNA-binding domain, hinge region, and hormone binding domain. The amino terminal section of the AR (referred to as the hypervariable region) contains a series of CAG repeats with a variable number of CAG nucleotides (usually 22–28) encoding glutamine. A longer length of CAG repeats causes allosteric changes in the AR and negatively affects AR-T transcriptional activation. The importance of long CAG sequences in causing male infertility and T resistance has been postulated but the evidence is inconclusive. Like many factors involved in T resistance, CAG repeats may modulate but not ablate AR action. Inactivating mutations in the AR may result in complete androgen insensitivity syndrome with a 46XY karyotype and a female phenotype, or in partial androgen insensitivity, which has a variable phenotype ranging from ambiguous genitalia to infertile male (see also Chapter 35).

T has important local and peripheral actions in males. It is responsible for the sexual imprinting of the brain, male type behavior, dimorphism of cognitive and spatial recognition functions of the brain, growth of bones and muscle, male type fat distribution, sexual drive, spermatogenesis, and indirectly it is involved in erectile function. Besides physical changes such as delayed puberty, infertility, and osteoporosis, T deficiency leads to changes in cognitive performance and emotional stability.

T is converted to estrogens through the action of aromatase CYP 19. Aromatase is expressed in the testis, brain, and fat tissue. E_2 plays an important role in the hormonal regulation of the hypothalamus-pituitary-testicular axis, spermatogenesis, bone maturation, and epiphyseal closure.

MALE HYPOGONADISM

Hypogonadism in a male refers to a decrease in one of the two major functions of the testes: sperm production or T production; or in rare cases, decreased response to T. Clinical presentation depends on timing of testicular deficiency during one's life and its extent.

Deficiency or defects in androgen production that occur during the first trimester may result in abnormal gonadal development and differentiation of Wolffian ducts with affected external genitalia. Presentation may range from ambiguous external genitalia to normal-appearing female external genitalia. Deficiency or defects in androgen production during the second and third trimesters can lead to micropenis, anorchism, or cryptorchism.

Deficiency or defects in androgen production in early childhood can result in pubertal delay and impairment of secondary sexual development. In adulthood, men typically present with infertility or sexual dysfunction.

Male hypogonadism may be anatomically classified in the following way:

Pretesticular: Acquired causes or genetic defects that negatively affect the HPG axis.

Testicular: Conditions that directly affect testicular function resulting from structural or chromosomal abnormalities (i.e., varicocele, cryptorchidism, gonadal injury, KS, XX male, and other disorders of gonadal development and sexual differentiation).

Posttesticular: Obstruction at the level of the epididymis, vas deferens, ejaculatory ducts; retrograde ejaculation, or erectile dysfunction.

Clinical Presentation and Diagnostic Evaluation

History The medical history should concentrate on two factors: development of the genitalia and pubertal progression. A family history of delayed puberty in otherwise normal adult relatives suggests constitutional delay. Change in visual fields, new onset of blurred vision, or bilateral hemianopsia should be taken seriously because they can indicate intracranial or pituitary tumors. Patients with Kallmann syndrome (KalS) may suffer from hyposmia or anosmia, as well as other midline craniofacial deformities. Hypotonia in infancy and hyperphagia and obesity starting in the toddler years suggests Prader–Willi syndrome (PWS). A history of unilateral cryptorchidism is rarely helpful in narrowing the differential diagnosis, but the presence of bilateral undescended testes and micropenis suggests potential hypogonadotropic hypogonadism.

Genitalia at Birth Normal T and DHT synthesis and action are necessary for genital formation during the first trimester, whereas growth of the phallus and testicular descent are dependent on androgen levels in the second half of pregnancy, when the testes are stimulated by fetal LH. Ambiguous genitalia suggests an early defect in androgen synthesis or action. In contrast, the presence of bilateral cryptorchidism or micropenis reflects androgen deficiency during the second half of gestation and suggests lack of central stimulation.

Pubertal History Timely onset and progression of puberty excludes major deficits in the hormonal axis and can direct further evaluation of testicular function. An increase in testicular volume to more than 4 cc heralds the onset of puberty and typically occurs between 9 and 14 years of age. Delayed puberty is present if there are no signs of testicular or genital development by the age of 14. Although delayed puberty is most commonly constitutional, it may also be the presenting sign in disorders causing hypergonadotropic or hypogonadotropic hypogonadism.

Sexual Drive and Semen Volume Sexual drive and performance depends on a complex interaction of hormonal, social, cultural, and psychologic factors that are often hard to quantify in an adolescent population. The literature, however, supports surprisingly uniform patterns and timing of sexual behavior development among boys from different cultural backgrounds. Frequency of sexual fantasies, masturbation, and timing of first coitus correlate well with T levels (9). The average age of first sexual fantasies is 12.0 years (10). Spermarche, assessed by microscopic examination of morning urine samples, occurs at a mean age of 13.4 years (11), and more than 90% of boys with Tanner 5 development will have sperm present in morning urine.

Change in sexual drive or low level of sexual interest can be seen in young males with hypogonadism. Decreased libido should be evaluated by measuring morning T levels. Low libido is not pathognomic for hypogonadism, and normal sexual performance does not exclude hypogonadism.

Seminal fluid is produced by the seminal vesicles and the prostate, and sperm contributes only 5% to the total seminal volume. Low semen volume can be a result of ejaculatory duct or seminal vesicle obstruction as well as hypogonadism. Hypogonadism may cause low semen volume because T is needed for normal prostate function. Antidepressants, especially serotonin reuptake inhibitors, can decrease seminal volume because they often cause retrograde ejaculation and anejaculation.

Damage to the Male Reproductive Tract Genital trauma or surgery, spinal damage or surgery,

testicular torsion, cryptorchidism, chemotherapy, irradiation, or previous mumps infection are all important risk factors to recognize in the medical history. A detailed history of medication and recreational drug use, smoking, alcohol abuse, and heat exposure is important because many drugs and environmental factors affect erectile function, libido, ejaculation, and spermatogenesis. Anabolic steroid abuse is common among adolescents and should be at least discussed with the patient.

Physical Examination

General Examination In children and adolescents, growth curves and body proportions play an important role in the evaluation of male hypogonadism. For example, both Klinefelter (KS) and hypogonadotropic hypogonadism (HH) are associated with eunuchoid body habitus (arm span exceeds body length, decreased upper-to-lower extremity ratio) and scarce facial, and pubic and auxiliary hair. There are several syndromes that have a characteristic phenotypic presentation. Patients with immotile cilia syndrome suffer from frequent respiratory tract infections and infertility. When this syndrome is associated with situs inversus and bronchiectasis, it is known as Kartagener syndrome.

Breasts Gynecomastia is often found in normal adolescents and should be distinguished from the lipomastia seen in obese males. With true gynecomastia one can feel distinct glandular breast tissue (Figure 37-3). Gynecomastia developing suddenly after puberty is complete, deserves a thorough evaluation of the breast, a scrotal ultrasound, and tumor markers (α-fetoprotein, β-hCG, LDH) because rapidly developing gynecomastia is seen in hormonally active testicular tumors. Leydig cell tumors can produce both E_2 and T and can cause precocious puberty in prepubertal males and gynecomastia in pubertal or adult males. T levels are initially elevated; however, in pubertal or adult males elevated E_2 levels may eventually suppress T production through LH suppression and alter E_2/T ratio leading to gynecomastia. Tumor markers a-fetoprotein and β-hCG are not elevated in Leydig cell tumors but are often elevated

in germ cell tumors of the testis. Only 10% of the Leydig cell tumors are malignant. Ninety-five percent of tumors that arise from testis are germ cell tumors and early diagnosis results in high cure rate. Gynecomastia is part of germ cell tumors presentation, such as choriocarcinoma because these tumors secrete β-hCG. (12). Men with KS have an increased risk of breast cancer (13).

Testes Testes descend into the scrotum during the last trimester of pregnancy. Cryptorchidism occurs in 1% to 3% of term newborns and is more common in preterm boys. Spontaneous testicular descent eventually occurs in most cases, with only a 1% frequency of cryptorchidism at 1 year of age. Bilateral cryptorchidism can be distinguished from bilateral anorchia by laparoscopy or β-hCG stimulation testing. Cryptorchidism associated with micropenis and hypoglycemia suggests panhypopituitarism. Prader V virilized female with congenital adrenal hyperplasia (CAH) due to 21α-hydroxylase (21-OHD) or 11β-hydroxylase deficiencies (11-OHD) can be mistakenly diagnosed as males with cryptorchidism. Other causes of cryptorchidism include KaLS, PWS and sometimes Noonan syndrome.

Testicular volume is measured by orchidometer (Prader beads) (Figure 37-4), ultrasound or calipers. Both testes should have similar size and consistency without any masses or localized tenderness. Testicular volumes are listed in Table 37-1; testicular volume at Tanner stage V of development is between 15 and 25 cc³.

To examine an infant or small child, the patient should be lying down in a frog leg position. The examiner should have warm hands and the child should be warm. With the examiner standing on the right side of the table, the left hand should be placed in the inguinal region to push the testis down toward the

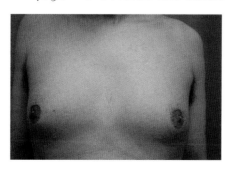
FIGURE 37-3. Gynecomastia in a 19-year-old man.

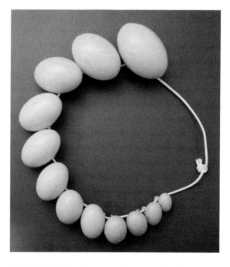
FIGURE 37-4. Orchidometer (Prader beads) with volumes from 1 to 25 mL.

scrotum, while at the same time the right hand is over the scrotal sac palpating and securing the testis.

In adolescent boys the examination is first done with the patient supine. The cord (upper part of the scrotum) is fixed between the thumb and the index finger of the left hand. One should feel a 2- to 3-mm thick vas deferens surrounded by veins and arteries. The testis is examined between the thumb and the opposing fingers and should be oval in shape and uniform in consistency. The epididymis should be less than 1 cm in width, positioned along the posterior aspect of the testis and the longitudinal axis. A tender, enlarged epididymis with irritative voiding symptoms is diagnostic of epididymitis and should be treated with antibiotics. Subsequently, the patient is asked to stand, while the physician is seated. The abdomen and external genitalia are examined. Normally the neck of the scrotum should be thinner than the lower portion. Any fullness in the scrotal neck should prompt an examination with a Valsalva maneuver to detect a varicocele.

Any suspicious testicular mass should be further evaluated by ultrasound. The presence of smooth epididymal masses is common and usually these are spermatoceles or epididymal cysts, which are benign lesions. Scrotal ultrasound confirms the cystic nature of the lesion and excludes the rare solid epididymal tumor.

Seventy percent of testicular volume is determined by the germinal epithelium. Small, hard testicles are typically found in end stage testicular failure and are most commonly seen in patients with KS. Small, soft testicles can be encountered in hypogonadotropic hypogonadism, anabolic androgen abuse, and spermatogenic failure after radiation or chemotherapy.

Varicocele Dilated veins of the pampiniform plexus are known as a varicocele (Figure 37-5). This lesion is described in detail later in "Testicular Causes of Male Hypogonadism." Varicocele most commonly occurs on the left side, and starts to be noticeable during puberty. The diagnosis can be established by physical examination. Timely diagnosis and treatment are essential because early on there may be a chance to preserve fertility (14).

Vas Deferens The vas deferens should be palpable on both sides. Bilateral congenital aplasia of the vas deferens (CBAVD) is the most common genetic cause of obstructive azoospermia. Cystic fibrosis (CF) gene mutations, cystic fibrosis transmembrane conductance regulator (CFTR) gene, are found in approximately 60% of men with CBAVD (15). Unilateral CBAVD can be either caused by a Cystic fibrosis transmembrane conductance

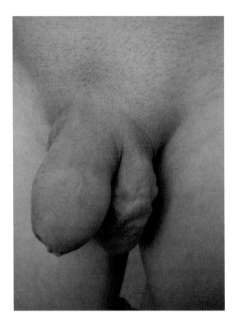

FIGURE 37-5. A grade III varicocele is easily seen as dilated veins in the scrotum. Photo courtesy of Dr. Jerzy Niedzielski.

regulator (CFTR) gene mutation or can be a result of mesonephric duct malformation. In the latter case, renal ultrasound should be performed to rule out associated renal abnormalities including agenesis (16).

Penis During the physical examination one should assess the Tanner stage of pubic hair, penile length, and localization and configuration of the meatus. In uncircumcised boys and young men the foreskin should be retracted to expose the urethral meatus. The penile size should be measured starting at the pubic symphysis and using a stretched penile length technique by applying mild traction at the glans. In an infant, one can place a tongue depressor at the pubic symphysis and stretch the penis along its ventral side, marking the point where the penis ends. Micropenis is defined as penile length that is 2.5 standard deviations (SDs) below the mean for age and ethnic population. For a full-term Caucasian male, the mean penile length at birth is 3.5 cm with an SD of 0.4 cm; thus, 2.5 cm is the lower limit of normal.

The meatus should be easily visible and present at the tip of the glans. Hypospadias is defined as transposition of the urethral meatus onto the ventral aspect of the penile shaft, whereas epispadias refers to transposition onto the dorsal shaft. Proximal hypospadias and midshaft hypospadias interfere with semen deposition and the defect is usually surgically repaired in early childhood in the majority of patients. Micropenis strongly suggests central hypogonadism, a defect in androgen production or action, or abnormal growth hormone function, and as such should be evaluated early.

Prostate and Seminal Vesicles The size of the prostate is directly related to androgenization. Hence, a very small prostate in a young adult male may suggest defects in androgen production or androgen action.

Laboratory and Imaging Studies of the Male Reproductive System

The Gonadotropins, LH and FSH LH and T are high the first day of birth, decrease during the first 2 weeks and then start to increase after the 2nd week postpartum; LH and T peak at approximately 2–3 months of age, and then decrease to low levels by age 6 months and remain low until the onset of puberty. Males infants have LH predominance in contrast to females who have FSH predominance. Early infancy provides a unique opportunity to detect and evaluate suspected hypogonadism, which may be isolated or may be part of multiple pituitary hormone deficiencies. Establishing the correct diagnosis in the newborn is less complex than evaluation starting during puberty, when it is often difficult to distinguish low LH and FSH levels secondary to constitutional delay from hypogonadotropic hypogonadism. Making the latter diagnosis in infancy avoids significant delay in initiation of hormone treatment at the time of puberty.

Baseline labs of gonadal function during the first week of life should include LH, FSH, T, inhibin B, and Müllerian-inhibiting substance (MIS). LH, FSH, and T should be repeated at the age of 4 to 12 weeks, allowing differentiation of hypogonadotropic versus hypergonadotropic hypogonadism.

After puberty is complete, males with normal spermatogenesis should have an FSH level below 7 IU/L (17). Elevated levels of FSH (especially greater than twice the upper limit of normal) are consistent with severe damage to the germinal epithelium and carry a poor prognostic value for natural fertility. Many laboratories report "normal" levels up to 12 to 15 IU/L because their reference population includes elderly males.

Testosterone T levels in boys are low after the end of mini puberty (~6 mo of age) and prior to the onset of puberty, but progressively increase during puberty and reach adult male levels at Tanner stage V of pubertal development. There is a diurnal rhythm for T, with the highest levels of T occurring during the early morning hours. Total T measured in the morning is a standard screening test to evaluate testicular function. Levels are approximately 25% lower when measured in the afternoon. A low-normal concentration requires measurement of free or bioavailable T. Free T is measured only if total T is below 300 mg/dL or the patient has low normal T in the presence of symptoms. Low free T is consistent with hypogonadism.

Estradiol (E₂) High E_2 levels can suppress release of LH and lower intratesticular levels of T, negatively affecting spermatogenesis. We routinely measure E_2 in patients with obesity (aromatase is expressed in adipose tissue), patients with low normal or low T levels, and patients with osteoporosis.

Sex Hormone Binding Globulin, Inhibin B, and Müllerian-Inhibiting Substance (MIS) High levels of SHBG are associated with obesity, hyperthyroidism, liver disease, androgen deficiency and estrogen excess. Male patients with hypogonadism may have high SHBG levels because of low T levels and increased E_2 production through intratesticular aromatization. Inhibin B and MIS reflect the integrity of Sertoli cells, and MIS has been used as a testis marker in the evaluation of suspected bilateral gonadal agenesis.

Semen Analysis Adolescents ejaculate on average 1 year after starting puberty (18). It takes 2 to 3 years from the time of first ejaculation for the seminal volume and sperm density and motility to be normal. A semen analysis, although commonly done in adults during evaluation of gonadal dysfunction, is seldom performed in adolescents, unless it is done prior to chemotherapy to preserve sperm (19).

Most andrology laboratories use World Health Organization standards. Recommended normal values are to some extent arbitrary, based more on consensus opinion than on rigorous scientific evidence. General principles of semen analysis include:

- Semen should be collected after 2 to 3 days of abstinence, and preferably on the premises of the laboratory to allow for prompt evaluation.

- The standard semen analysis includes sperm density (number of sperm per 1 mL of semen volume), total number of sperm, sperm motility, vitality, percentage of pathologic forms, total semen volume (normal is >2 mL) and pH of semen.

- The most common cause of low seminal volume is inadequate collection technique.

- Sperm density is one of the most important factors in semen analysis. Oligospermia refers to low sperm density, whereas azoospermia is complete absence of sperm.

- A high number of white blood cells may indicate genitourinary infection.

- Electron microscopy is useful if Kartagener syndrome is suspected as it allows one to confirm lack of central tubules in the tail of the sperm.

Genetic Testing Most syndromes that can be diagnosed by genetic testing have other associated signs and symptoms. CFTR gene screening should be considered in patients with suspected CF or those with bilateral or unilateral absence of vas deferens to establish the diagnosis and help with genetic counseling. Deletions of genes on the distal arm of the Y chromosome that are critical for spermatogenesis result in isolated azoospermia or severe oligospermia.

Scrotal Ultrasound Scrotal ultrasound is relatively inexpensive, easy to perform and safe for the patient. It allows measurement of the size of the testis and comparison between testicles. Color-enhanced Doppler assesses arterial perfusion of the testis—diminished or absent arterial perfusion is seen in testicular torsion. Ultrasound of the scrotum is invaluable in evaluating an intrascrotal mass. A solid mass on the ultrasound is a testicular cancer unless proven otherwise, and urological consultation is required because an orchiectomy needs to be anticipated in the majority of solid testicular masses. Cystic masses generally represent benign spermatoceles or epididymal cysts. One should also check the epididymis size and blood flow. An epididymal head diameter above 1 cm with increased perfusion is consistent with epididymitis. Ultrasound with color Doppler is often used in the evaluation of a varicocele.

Magnetic Resonance Imaging Imagining studies of the hypothalamus and pituitary gland should be ordered if an intracranial or pituitary tumor is anticipated. Magnetic resonance imaging (MRI) is helpful in the diagnosis of KalS if absence of the olfactory bulbs is noted. Elevated prolactin levels (especially if prolactin levels are >100 ng/dl) should also be evaluated by cranial MRI to exclude a prolactinoma, or a non prolactin producing pituitary tumor.

Testicular Biopsy and Scrotal Exploration Germinal cell function is usually assessed through FSH measurements. However, in pubertal males with azoospermia, normal FSH levels, and normal testicular size, a testicular biopsy and scrotal exploration should be considered to determine whether a germinal cell abnormality, an obstruction, or a congenital abnormality of the vasa is present.

Treatment of Male Hypogonadism The goal of therapy in patients with hypogonadism is geared toward support of normal progression of puberty, development of adequate masculinization, normal libido, and bone density. All of those goals can be achieved with T supplementation. Early diagnosis of hypogonadism and appropriate T replacement, gen-

erally started between the ages of 12 to14 years, allows for normal physical development and good social adjustment, even in boys with anorchia. In patients with HH due to pretesticular causes and with testes responsive to GnRH or gonadotropin treatment, replacement therapy is first initiated with T alone, with gonadotropins or GnRH therapy added later in life to induce spermatogenesis and achieve fertility. The penis may show disproportionate growth in these boys, with better improvement in length than girth (20).

Intramuscular T preparations are frequently used with T enanthate being one of the most common. It is inexpensive and can be delivered in small doses. It needs to be injected deep into the muscle to avoid abscess formation, and application may be painful. T enanthate is suspended in oil and once administered it is slowly absorbed from the muscle. Serum T levels peak 1 to 3 days after intramuscular administration and gradually decline to a trough after 2 to 3 weeks. The rate of absorption is not controllable and it is possible to achieve supraphysiological levels, which rarely might lead to priapism. Topical T may be a better choice because levels are more constant, without the extreme highs that are often seen after an intramuscular injection and the hypogonadal period that may occur before the next injection. Topical preparations allow for restoration of circadian rhythm with higher doses in the morning. Androgel pump is especially useful method of T replacement in pediatric endocrinology since it allows for easy age appropriate dosing from 1.25 mg to 10 mg a day. Common dosing regimens for intramuscular and other forms of T are presented in Table 37-2.

When inducing puberty in boys, one tries to mimic normal pubertal development as much as possible, with progression from Tanner I to Tanner V features gradually evolving over approximately 3 years. Thus, initial T doses are low and slowly increased at approximately 6-month intervals until an adult dosage is reached. For the boy who has already completed puberty and attained an adult stature at the time hypogonadism develops, adult replacement doses of T can immediately be instituted.

Patients with KalS or nonosmic HH (nIHH) often become concerned about their testicular size (particularly later in adolescence). β-hCG may be started to induce testicular growth and improve the patient's body image perception. Typical dosing is 1,000 to 2,500 U β-hCG intramuscularly or 100 to 250 μg of rhCG subcutaneously 2 to 3 times a week for 6 months followed by the addition of menotropins (75 IU LH and 75 IU FSH, Menopur or Repronex) three times a week subcutaneously for 1 year. Testicular size is measured

TABLE 37-2 Androgen Therapy in Hypogonadism

Indication	Dose	Clinical Implications
Micropenis	• *Standard:* 25 μg T enanthate or cypionate IM every 4 weeks × 3; (can give up to 6 injections) • Topical testosterone (oil preparation containing T propionate 25 mg and T enanthate 110 mg, equivalent to 100 mg of T–2 mg/kg/wk in twice daily application to the penis achieves similar serum T and penile growth to IM (but more likely to cause pubic hair) (121) • Androgel is an excellent choice for topical treatment (1.25 g, 1.25 mg T daily); side effects like skin irritation are very rare • DHT cream (Andractim 2.5 mg daily) is not available in the US but is under study in Europe with promising initial results (122) • Success with subcutaneous LH/FSH has been reported (123) • GH levels must be adequate for normal response—GH alone may increase penile length with isolated GH deficiency (124)	• 60%–70% of infants with micropenis respond to T therapy • Therapy should be started before age 3 months (but boys up to 8 years old have been treated) • The penis should increase by 0.9 cm after 3 months (if not, suggests androgen resistance) • Fathers, not mothers, should apply topical androgens because they are absorbed through the skin; should not wash the infant's skin for 6 hours to allow absorption • Concern from animal studies that high-dose T early in life might ↓ adult penis size has not been shown in humans (125) • T levels just before the injection or after 1 week of topical treatment should be 2–8 nmol/L • Pubic hair should resolve once the androgen is stopped; the dose should be reduced if erections lasting more than 2 h occur
Constitutional Delay	• IM: 40–50 mg/m^2/dose monthly (T cypionate or enanthate) for 6 mo; *OR,* 2.5 g Androgel daily or every other day for 6 mo	• Generally not given unless bone age is at least 11 years • Only 6 months of treatment to "tip" the patient into puberty
Adolescent Hypogonadism	• *Initiation:* 50 mg IM T cypionate or enanthate 1 × month for the first 6 months, then 100 mg IM for 6–12 months; *OR,* 2.5 gm topical androgens every other day for 6 months followed by 2.5 gm daily for 6–12 months, and 5 gm × 12 months. • *Terminal growth phase:* 100 mg IM T cypionate or enanthate monthly for about one year; *OR* 5 gm of topical Androgel daily for 1 year. • Alternative regimens include pellets for subcutaneous implantation 150–450 mg every 3–6 months; *OR* buccal androgen twice daily applied to the gum region above the incisor teeth • Then move to *adult dosing*	• Monitor therapy with clinical assessment and T levels; levels should be appropriate for Tanner stage • With IM, T should be checked a day prior to the 2nd injection; if topical, T can be check after 1 week • Should not shower or swim for 4–6 hours after Androgel • Testim leaves a white residue on the arms, which may be unacceptable to some adolescents; Androgel is better option • Measure liver function tests and hematocrit at baseline, after 3 months, and semiannually; measure lipids annually • IM tends to stimulate erythropoiesis more than topical testosterone; Androgel pump allows for convenient and physiological dosing
Adult Dosing, Hypogonadism	• IM T enanthate or cypionate in oil 50–400 mg every 2–4 wks (most common dose 200 mg every 2 weeks) • Androderm, 5–7.5 mg/day, nightly to clean, dry area on the back, abdomen, upper arms or thighs (do not apply to scrotum) • Androgel or Testim: 5–10 gm (delivers 50–100 mg T with 5–10 mg systemically absorbed), applied once daily (preferably in the morning) to clean, dry, intact skin on shoulders or upper arms; Androgel may also be applied to abdomen; do not apply to genitals	• Topical applications may be more physiologic because they can mimic normal diurnal variation better than IM • There have been reports of virilization of female partners of men using topical androgens • *In patients with cognitive impairment* where there is concern about inappropriate sexual behavior; using 1% Androgel pump at 1.25 to 2.5 mg dose may achieve T level in the low-normal range to provide the benefits of T therapy without as much concern about excessive masturbation or sexual aggression
Adult Dosing with HCG	• Stop testosterone therapy • 2,500 units IM hCG (or 250 μ rhCG) SQ 3× a week for 6 months, followed by adding menotropins (75 IU LH and 75 IU FSH, Menopur or Repronex) 3× a week SQ	• May induce testicular growth (to 8–10 cc over 1–2 years) in men with hypogonadotropic hypogonadism • Higher doses plus an aromatase inhibitor may be needed for fertility

before β-hCG and 3 and 6 months after starting therapy. If the testicular size is not increasing as expected, the dose of menotropins can be increased to 150 IU three times a week. This therapy is intended mainly to increase the size of the testes, but in some adolescents it will allow for induction of spermatogenesis. We aim to achieve T levels above 15 nmol/L. Because the maturation of spermatogonia to

sperm takes approximately 70 days, the first sperm does not appear in the ejaculate for at least 3 months after initiation of therapy and it may take 2 years for patients with congenital HH to respond to therapy and have sperm in the ejaculate. Testicular size increases in response to GnRH or gonadotropin therapy with final testicular size depending on the initial testicular volume. Patients with testicular

volumes more than 4 ml prior to initiation of therapy are considered partially gonadotropin resistant and respond better to stimulation therapy. Pulsatile GnRH therapy, through a portable minipump, can be used to induce spermatogenesis in patients with GnRH deficiency and normal pituitary function. The pump delivers a GnRH bolus every 120 minutes at a starting dose of 4 μg/pulse, with increases of 2 μg every 2 weeks, if LH secretion does not increase (maximum dose is 20 μg/pulse). Generally, after the initial 6 to 12 months of combination treatment qualitatively normal spermatogenesis can be sustained with β-hCG alone.

CAUSES OF MALE HYPOGONADISM

Pretesticular

Pretesticular causes of male hypogonadism include acquired or genetic defects of the hypothalamus and the pituitary affecting GnRH or pituitary gonadotropins secretion (hypogonadotropic hypogonadism), endocrine disorders that suppress the HPG axis such as estrogen excess, Cushing syndrome, and drugs that affect the HPG axis.

Hypogonadotropic Hypogonadism

HH is caused by defects in GnRH and/or gonadotropin secretion resulting in low/or inappropriate normal gonadotropin levels, low T/DHT levels, delayed or arrested puberty and decreased spermatogenesis in pubertal or adult males. HH can be congenital or acquired. Congenital anomalies leading to HH are rare and include isolated defects in GnRH secretion associated with or without anosmia, genetic defects of the GnRH receptor, pituitary transcription factors defects, leptin and leptin receptor defects, (see Chapter 21) DAX-1 defects (see Chapter 29) and complex genetic syndromes. Acquired causes of HH include destructive lesions such as tumors, trauma, inflammation, radiation, and vascular lesions of the hypothalamus and pituitary gland, which all cause secondary GnRH and/or LH/FSH deficiencies.

Acquired HH may also be caused by severe weight loss, intensive exercise, renal failure, malnutrition, and chronic disease. The effects of hypogonadism associated with chronic diseases of childhood, may not be seen until adolescence or early adulthood. Children with chronic renal failure have short stature, delayed puberty and bone age, but their levels of LH, FSH and T are similar to controls matched for pubertal stage. In contrast, chronic renal failure in adults is known to cause hypogonadism, which is usually reversed by renal transplantation. Type 1 diabetes may be associated with elevated LH and variably increased T with normal inhibin B and FSH levels in pubertal children compared with age-matched controls (21). Diabetes is one of leading causes of sexual and erectile dysfunction in younger men and smoking further increases this risk. This observation emphasizes the importance of discussing with adolescent patients the negative impact on sexual health of smoking or poor diabetic

control. Growth and puberty are often delayed in patients with thalassemias, and gonadal dysfunction has been found in 68% of patients (22).

Alcohol, illicit drugs, and use of anabolic steroids may also cause HH and are described later.

The postpubertal presentation of hypogonadism is less pronounced. Decreased libido, fatigue, impotence, decreased ejaculation volume, problems with concentration, decreased facial hair growth, thinning of pubic hair, fine wrinkles of the skin, and mild anemia are all symptoms and signs.

Congenital Hypogonadotropic Hypogonadism

Congenital HH is a very heterogeneous genetically disorder associated in some cases with anosmia/hyposmia (KalS) or in some other cases with normal sense of smell (normosmic IHH or nIHH).

KalS, a genetically heterogeneous disease, affects 1:8000. X-linked inheritance, autosomal dominant and autosomal recessive variants have been all described in the familial forms of KalS. More than 60% of the cases are sporadic. The anosmia in KalS is due to defective olfactory bulb formation and the hypogonadism due loss of GnRH function. In KalS, the GnRH neurons and usually the olfactory neurons do not migrate correctly and undergo apoptosis.

The link between the anosmia and the HH is due to GnRH-producing neuroendocrine cells migrating from the nasal placode to the forebrain along olfactory nerve fibers during embryogenesis. Loss-of-function mutations in KAL-1 gene, which encodes the anosmin-1, an extracellular matrix glucoprotein involved in cellular adhesion, result in the X-linked form of HH. Loss of function mutations of the fibroblast growth factor receptor 1 (FGFR1) underlie the autosomal dominant form of the disease (KAL2) (23). The FGFR1 protein is expressed in multiple embryonic tissues and organs such as skeletal tissues, inner ear and rostral forebrain and is required for initial olfactory bulb evagination. Mutations in these genes, however, only account for approximately 20% of all KalS with FGFR1 mutations accounting for 10% of KalS patients.

Other forms of autosomal KalS include KAL3 which is caused by mutation in the G protein-coupled prokineticin receptor-2 (PROKR2) gene, and KAL4 which is caused by mutation in the prokineticin-2 gene, encoding one of the ligands of PROKR2 receptor, accounting for an additional 10%. These findings reveal that insufficient prokineticin-signaling through PROKR2 leads to abnor-

mal development of the olfactory system and reproductive axis in man (24).

Clinical Presentation The phenotype of males affected with either KalS or nIHH include cryptorchidism and/or micropenis during infancy, delayed puberty, tall stature with disproportionately long limbs (eunuchoid body habitus), and gynecomastia. The extent of HH varies and phenotypc is not always complete. Most adolescent boys will have no signs of spontaneous pubertal development, their testes will be less than 2 cc in volume with normal consistency, and the majority will have a micropenis. The presence of anosmia or hyposmia and midline or other defects differentiates patients with KalS from those with IHH, who have an otherwise normal phenotype. Although KalS and nIHH are thought to represent two distinct entities, coexistence of both KalS and HH with normal olfaction (nIHH) have been reported in the same pedigree of patients having a loss-of function mutations in FGFR1. Females with KAL2 gene abnormalities may present with anosmia, primary amenorrhea, low gonadotropin and lack of response to LHRH.

Patients with the KAL1 gene abnormalities have hypogonadotropic hypogonadism, anosmia/hyposmia, mirror movements and renal abnormalities have been detected in 60% of patients with familial KalS and in only 10–15% of patients with sporadic KalS. Of note there has been no report of a patient with KAL1 mutations and normal smell; however, two males with normal gonadal function and impaired smell, whose brothers had typical KalS phenotype, have been reported.

The clinical spectrum in patients with KalS due to FGFR1 mutations ranges from typical KalS to apparently normal phenotype including anosmia only and dental agenesis phenotypes. Mirror hand movement and single kidney have been reported but in much less frequency than in KalS patients with KAL1 mutations. The higher prevalence of KalS in males suggests that these two proteins interact but the precise mechanism by which they interact is unknown.

Patients with KalS and mutations in PROK2 or PROKR2 had variable degrees of olfactory and reproductive dysfunction and do not seem to have any clinical anomalies such as mirror movements, renal agenesis, dental agenesis, and cleft lip or palate.

Diagnosis Before puberty the HPG axis is inactive and levels of T, LH, and FSH are naturally low and may be difficult to diagnose KalS. KalS should be suspected in children with bilaterally undescended testes (25%–75%), micropenis (60%), and midline facial defects. Careful history can reveal presence of bilateral or unilateral cryptorchidism, which normally would have been repaired within the first year of life. Boys with cryptorchidism without GnRH deficiency generally undergo normal pubertal development. Some boys with KalS may enter puberty with a modest increase in penile length and pubic hair development but eventually puberty fails to progress. The diagnosis may be made in early infancy by lack of the postnatal rise of LH and T (mini puberty) and a blunted response to LHRH and β-hCG stimulation. On physical examination one should record the body proportions, test smell with seven to eight different odors and consider evaluating hearing (25). Serum T, LH, and FSH are low in both KalS and IHH. Serum T levels should be measured in the morning because of the diurnal variation in T concentration. Patients with KalS have variable degrees of HH and may show poor or subnormal T response to β-hCG (26). Patients with KAL1 mutations have a pulsatile LH secretion (less than one LH peak in 24 h) whereas patients with autosomal KalS have some degree of GnRH secretion and low amplitude LH pulses during frequent LH sampling (27). Absent olfactory tracts on MRI help establish the diagnosis of KalS, but in 20% of cases the olfactory tract will be present. Identification of olfactory bulbs in first years of life is difficult and we defer MRI until a boy reaches 10 years.

Hypogonadotropic Hypogonadism due to GnRHR Mutations

The GnRHR is a G protein–coupled receptor, located on the cell surface of pituitary gonadotropes and mapped on 4q21.2 chromosomal area (28). GnRHR transduces signals from GnRH regulating the synthesis and secretion of pituitary gonadotropins and has a key role in the reproductive cascade in humans. Different GnRHR mutations may cause different degrees of decreased GnRH binding and/or activation of the mutant receptor resulting in variability of the clinical phenotype. At the mildest end lie the rare IHH patients with the so-called fertile eunuch syndrome who present with decreased virilization, eunuchoidal proportions, and hypogonadal T levels despite normal testicular size and preserved spermatogenesis. Typically, these patients achieve normal virilization and fertility with T or β-hCG therapy alone (29).

The other end of the clinical spectrum includes males with micropenis, cryptorchidism, complete lack of pubertal development, small, soft testes, and azoospermia. Plasma gonadotropins are very low and they do not rise in response to GnRH stimulation test or in response to GnRH pulsatile administration. Treatment with β-hCG 1,500 U twice a

week has been shown to normalize T levels and the addition of FSH at 150 U twice a week for 6 months induced spermatogenesis in azoospermic patients and an increase in testicular volume (30,31). It is estimated that 15% to 40% of patients with IHH and a normal sense of smell may have a GnRHR mutation (32). Whether therapy is initiated with T supplementation or FSH/LH injections to stimulate spermatogenesis is determined by the patient's age and reproductive goals.

Other Genetic Defects and Syndromes Affecting GnRH Secretion

Defects in the *leptin or the leptin receptor gene* cause hyperphagia, early onset childhood obesity, and hypogonadotropic hypogonadism. The response to exogenous GnRH or β-hCG may be normal (33). The Gordon Holmes or *ataxia hypogonadism syndrome* is characterized by progressive neurologic deterioration with hypogonadism developing in the mid-twenties (34). *Bardet-Biedl syndrome* (BBS), is a heterogeneous genetic disorder characterized by obesity, pigmentary retinopathy, polydactyly, mental retardation, male HH, and renal failure in some cases (35). The genetic mechanism that leads to BBS is still unclear. Recently, 12 (BBS1 to BBS12) that are responsible for the disease have been cloned. The syndrome is familial and inheritance is suggested to be "recessive inheritance with a modifier of penetrance" (36). In a 1999 survey of BBS patients, 60 of 62 patients had hypogonadism, 8 patients had maldescended testes, and 19 had delayed puberty (37). *CHARGE syndrome* is the constellation of coloboma, heart disease, choanal atresia, retarded growth, genital hypoplasia due to HH, and ear abnormalities (38).

Boys with adrenal hypoplacia congenita (AHC) usually present with adrenal insufficiency in childhood and subsequent HH as teenagers but some cases of men with HH and normal adrenal function have been reported (39). The response of patients with DAX-1 mutations to GnRH therapy is variable, suggesting a hypothalamic and/or combined pituitary defect. In addition failure of β-hCG to induce normal spermatogenesis implies an additional testicular defect. The diagnosis is usually established early in infancy. Treatment is similar to IHH and KalS. Patients with adrenal insufficiency must continue adrenal steroid replacement indefinitely (for details see Chapter 29).

Prader–Willi Syndrome

Pathophysiology PWS, also known as Prader-Labhart-Willi syndrome, is a complex devel-

opmental syndrome caused by deletion or disruption of genes on the proximal long arm of the paternal chromosome 15 (70% of cases), or by maternal uniparental disomy (20%–25% of cases). Several genes are located within the 15q11-13 region, but no single gene has been yet identified as critical for development of PWS. The region of interest encodes a group of proteins and possibly small RNAs essential for normal development of the CNS, especially the hypothalamus (40). Two of these are SNRPN, involved in RNA processing, and necdin, which is expressed by neurons and is involved in cellular growth and differentiation. The hypothalamus is involved in regulation of appetite, awareness, and reproductive functions; hence, children with PWS present with hyperphagia, somnolence, and HH.

Clinical Presentation PWS occurs in 1:10,000 to 1:25,000 live births and is characterized by diminished fetal activity, hypotonia, hypogonadism, characteristic facies, small hands and feet, and initial failure to thrive in infancy (41). They may require tube feeding in early childhood, but by 2 to 3 years of age hyperphagia becomes apparent with subsequent excessive weight gain. Strict control of caloric intake is difficult but manageable during the early childhood period. As they get older, PWS patients often become more difficult to control because of obsessive behavior and temper tantrums related to food restriction, and they develop severe obesity. Obesity may be one of the factors fundamental to development of type 2 diabetes in these patients.

PWS may be suspected during prenatal ultrasonography with signs of intrauterine growth arrest and decreased motor activity of the fetus. Postnatally, infants have central hypotonia, failure to thrive, cryptorchidism (bilateral in over 80%), and micropenis. A narrow face, almond-shaped eyes, fair eyes, skin and hair, small narrow hands, short stature, and morbid obesity are typical morphologic features in preadolescent and adolescent boys. Defects in speech articulation, sleep apnea, a high pain threshold, obsessive–compulsive behavior, violent temper tantrums, and skin picking reflect general neuropsychologic abnormalities (42) (for other aspects of the disorder see Chapter 30).

Adolescents present with delayed puberty and infantile external genitalia. A small penis may be confused with "concealed penis" (a normal size penis hidden because of the presence of a pubic fat pad, but 70% of boys with PWS have genuine micropenis with a stretched penile length below 2.5 SDs for age and pubertal stage and ethnic adjusted norms (Figure 37-6). Both T and GH deficiency may be responsible for infantile genitalia in

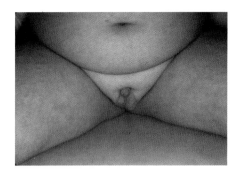

FIGURE 37-6. Micropenis in a child with PWS. Photo courtesy of Dr. Robert Gorlin.

boys with PWS. Testicular biopsy shows absent spermatogonia and spermatogenic arrest; however it is unknown if these changes are specific to PWS or reflective of changes secondary to cryptorchidism. Males with PWS are presumed to be infertile because paternity has not been reported. Osteoporosis and osteopenia are seen in men with PWS due to sex steroid insufficiency.

Diagnosis Endocrine evaluation demonstrates low T, LH, and FSH, consistent with HH, but stimulation with β-hCG results in a blunted T response, suggesting combined hypogonadism. PWS can be confirmed by genetic testing that includes fluorescence in situ hybridization for 15q deletion and methylation studies.

Treatment A multidisciplinary approach to management of boys with PWS appears to prolong the life span of affected individuals. Cardiovascular, pulmonary, and infectious complications of type 2 diabetes and morbid obesity contribute to a significantly lower life expectancy of adults with PWS. Hence, the treatment of these boys focuses on improving body weight and body composition. Children with PWS have high fat mass and low muscle mass compared with children with simple obesity with a similar body mass index (BMI). Because the low muscle mass correlates with basic energy expenditure, an increase in muscle mass should improve glycemic control, the lipid profile, and potentially prolong the life expectancy of PWS patients. Together with simple dietary control, two drugs have been used in children with PWS to alter body composition: GH and T.

The majority of boys with PWS have low GH levels and a blunted GH response to challenge tests. GH therapy for 1 to 2 years has been showed to slightly decrease BMI and to improve growth velocity, muscle mass, activity level, and the development of gross motor skills (43). T replacement has been shown to lower BMI in other hypogonadal patients and in boys with PWS. Treatment with T achieves normal progression of pu-

berty, lower BMI, increased muscle strength, and normalization of bone mineral density. Topical T may provide the benefits of androgen therapy with less risk of inappropriate sexual behavior in these patients with cognitive impairment (Table 37-2). Pharmacotherapy should be an adjunct to behavioral, vocational, and occupational therapy.

Defects in Pituitary Transcription Factors

HH as well as other features of hypopituitarism occur with deficiencies of transcription factors important in pituitary development.

PROP1 (prophet of PIT1) is involved in the differentiation and proliferation of gonadotropes, lactotropes, thyrotropes and somatotropes, and, thus, deficiency is associated with variable deficiencies of LH, FSH, prolactin, TSH, and GH (44).

Mutation in HESX1, a transcriptional repressor, is characterized by septo-optic dysplasia (absent septum pellucidum and optic nerve hypoplasia); patients may have isolated GH deficiency or panhypopituitarism (45). LHX3 (LIM homeobox gene 3) leads to low gonadotropin levels, combined pituitary hormone deficiency, and a rigid cervical spine (46) (see Chapter 32).

CENTRAL NERVOUS SYSTEM TUMORS
Prolactinoma

Pathogenesis Prolactin is secreted by the anterior pituitary and is regulated by the tonic inhibitory effects of hypothalamic dopamine, which acts on dopamine receptors (D_2 receptor) on the surface of lactotrophs. Hyperprolactinemia results from prolactinomas (benign prolactin-secreting tumors), CNS lesions interfering with dopamine inhibition of the pituitary, hypothyroidism, renal failure (47), or drugs such as metoclopramide, tricyclic antidepressants, cimetidine, ranitidine, famotidine, omeprazole, phenothiazines, benzodiazepines, reserpine, methyldopa, prostaglandins, and cocaine. Prolactinomas are usually sporadic, but familial prolactinomas do occur, in isolation or as part of the multiple endocrine neoplasia syndrome. Prolactinomas may occasionally also secrete growth hormone.

Clinical Presentation Although they appear to be equally common in males and females, prolactinomas tend to be larger in males (>10 mm in diameter), as the tumors are discovered later. Prolactin affects the testis directly and it seems that normal serum prolactin levels are required for normal testicu-

lar function and spermatogenesis. High levels of prolactin suppress GnRH secretion and decrease gonadotropin and T production. Most patients with elevated prolactin levels have low-normal levels of LH, T and DHT, low-frequency and low-amplitude LH secretion as well as a normal LH response to GnRH stimulation test. Prolactin levels are usually higher than 100 ng/dL and are proportional to the size of the tumor. In some cases hyperprolactinemia causes clinical hypogonadism in the presence of normal serum gonadotropins and T. Symptoms and signs of hypogonadism may not become obvious unless the tumor is large or hyperprolactinemia and gonadotropin deficiency become severe. The primary symptoms in adolescent boys are headaches, visual changes, and delayed puberty. Infertility, hypogonadism and erectile dysfunction are seen in adult men. With long-standing hypogonadism the testes are typically soft but of normal size and the semen analysis shows low semen volume, oligospermia, or azoospermia. Galactorrhea rarely occurs. Other pituitary hormone deficiencies or vision may be affected if the tumor is large enough to produce a mass effect. Gadolinium-enhanced MRI is the method of choice for detection of prolactinoma.

Treatment Treatment is either surgical removal of the adenoma or medical therapy with the dopamine D_2 receptor agonists cabergoline (Dostinex) or bromocriptine (Parlodel). Bromocriptine comes in 2.5 mg tablets and 5 mg capsules. The initial dose is half of a 2.5 mg tablet daily; this can be increased every 2 to 7 days up to a maximum of 10 mg/day. Cabergoline has largely replaced bromocriptine because of lower frequency of side effects (orthostatic hypotension, nausea, and vomiting) and easier dosing (once or twice weekly). It comes in 0.5 mg tablets. Therapy is started at half a tablet (0.25 mg) twice weekly for 1 month and increased by 0.25 mg increments each month, up to a maximum dose of 1 mg twice a week. It may take up to 8 weeks for the prolactin level to normalize after therapy is started, and therapy should be continued for 2 to 3 years in cases of large prolactinomas. Smaller tumors may respond to 1 year of therapy with Dostinex. Up to one third of patients appear to have remission after therapy is stopped (48). Surgery is generally only considered in patients in whom medical therapy fails because the rate of recurrence is high.

Growth Hormone–Secreting Tumors and Cushing Disease

Acromegaly is caused in 99% of cases by pituitary tumors secreting either GH or GH and prolactin and only in less than 1% of cases is caused by an ectopic tumor secreting GHRH. Hypogonadism is a known potential consequence of acromegaly encountered in more than 50% of patients with acromegaly. The mechanism underlying the pathogenesis of HH in patients with acromegaly is unclear. In patients without hypopituitarism from tumor mass effect, HH may be caused by the coexistent hyperprolactinemia due to stalk disruption or tumor secretion; however one third of the hypogonadal patients had normal prolactin levels indicating that GH excess may contribute to the development of hypogonadism (49). The symptoms of hypogonadism in men with acromegaly progress slowly and include oligospermia and decreased sperm motility. Restoration of gonadal function depends on whether the treatment of the tumor is successful and whether there is permanent damage to the pituitary-hypothalamic area secondary to the tumor or therapy.

Cushing disease is characterized by chronic glucocorticoid excess secondary to hypersecretion of ACTH from a pituitary corticotroph adenoma. Combined hypogonadism is common in hypercortisolic states such as Cushing disease or syndrome. The mechanisms by which elevated glucocorticoid levels affect T production include: 1) suppression of gonadotropin production decreasing gonadotropin levels by inhibitory effects at the hypothalamic and pituitary level; 2) glucocorticoid suppression of LH receptor signal transduction and Leydig cell steroidogenic activities; and, 3) induction of Leydig cell apoptosis directly suppressing testicular function (50,51). Adolescents on chronic glucosteroid therapy are at high risk for hypogonadism and osteoporosis. T replacement therapy, vitamine D3 and calcium should be instituted early to prevent osteoporosis.

Clinical manifestations of HH include loss of libido and oligospermia. Basal LH, FSH, and T levels are low and the response to GnRH is impaired. Successful treatment of hypercortisolism without permanent damage of the pituitary normalizes T and gonadotropin levels and improves hypogonadism symptoms (for more details see Chapter 28).

Nonpituitary Tumors

Intrasellar and parasellar tumors such as craniopharyngioma, Rathke cleft cyst, germinoma, Langerhans cell histiocytosis, and others may affect anterior pituitary and/or hypothalamic function and may present in children with growth failure, hypothyroidism, delayed or arrested puberty in pubertal males, and decreased gonadal function in adult males due to decreased gonadotropins and T levels.

Associated symptoms include visual impairment due to the effect of the tumor on the optic chiasm, headache, obesity, polyuria, and polydipsia due to tumor effect on the posterior pituitary (germinoma, Langerhans cell histiocytosis). As with the other tumors described previously, restoration of gonadal function depends on whether there is permanent damage to the hypothalamic-pituitary area and whether treatment of the tumor is successful.

Other causes of HH include head trauma, radiation to the head, and empty sella syndrome. Empty sella syndrome is a radiologic finding, in which cerebrospinal fluid is found within the space created for the pituitary. The cerebrospinal fluid pressure flattens the pituitary out within the sella. Generally, in this situation, pituitary function is normal, but a number of patients have headaches, mild hyperprolactinemia, galactorrhea, and hypogonadism.

Estrogen Excess

There is emerging interest in the role of E_2 in male development. Within the reproductive system, estrogens appear to be important in the structural and functional development of the Wolffian duct system and the prostate (52). Inappropriately low or high E_2 exposure during development can cause permanent changes to nucleosome and chromatin, thus changing expression profile of tissues which may lead to disorders of spermatogenesis and infertility.

Male reproductive system is highly sensitive to estrogens, although expression of estrogen receptors α and β is species specific. Humans don't express ERα in testis, although active estrogen response elements are found in the reproductive system including Sertoli, Leydig and germ cells, the reproductive tract ducts and the accessory sex organs, which signifies the importance of estrogen for regulation of these tissues. The widespread distribution of aromatase suggests that many of the effects of estrogens in the male might stem from its local production and action, and furthermore, that the balance in action between androgens and estrogens might be of central importance at many E_2 target sites, particularly the reproductive system.

Chronically elevated E_2 levels affect testicular morphology and steroidogenesis in the following ways: 1) suppression of pituitary gonadotropin secretion; 2) a direct adverse effect on the testes resulting in decreased T production; 3) decreased spermatogenesis due to lower intratesticular T levels; 4) a negative impact on Leydig, Sertoli and germ cell development; and 5) dysfunction of the efferent ductules and epididymis (53,54). Males with estrogen excess may have gynecomastia.

Aromatase gain of function mutations, which result in E_2 excess, have been reported but are rare (55). The most common reason for an elevated E_2 level in males is obesity, because of the aromatase activity of adipose tissue. Treatment with aromatase inhibitors has been shown to increase LH and T in both young and older patients, and in obese men (56,57).

Follicle-Stimulating Hormone-β and Luteinizing Hormone-β Subunit Defects

Disorders of FSHβ and LHβ subunits as well as FSH and LH receptor defects, although pretesticular causes of hypogonadism, mostly do not present with HH (low FSH, LH levels).

So far only one family has been reported with mutation of the LHβ gene. The proband, who was homozygous for Q54R missense mutation presented with delayed puberty at 17 years of age. He had a low serum T, elevated LH and FSH values and normal T response to β-hCG stimulation test. Biopsy of his testes showed arrested spermatogenesis and absent Leydig cells. He responded well to β-hCG treatment with increase in his testes size, normal development of secondary sex characteristics, and spermatogenesis. His parents were first cousins. All heterozygous women for the Q54R mutation including his mother were fertile. Some of the heterozygous family members had normal pubertal development but were infertile (58).

The very few males that have been reported with homozygous mutations of the FSHβ gene presented with azoospermia, low FSH levels, normal or elevated LH levels, normal T, small, soft testicles and mild pubertal delay to normal puberty. Testicular biopsy shows Leydig cell hyperplasia and sparse, small seminiferous tubules with germinal cell aplasia, peritubular fibrosis, and few Sertoli cells (59–61).

Follicle-Stimulating Hormone (FSH) and Lutropin-Choriogonadotropin Receptors Defects

Inactivating mutations of FSHR have been reported in homozygous brothers of women with hypergonadotropic hypogonadism. The affected males had normal puberty and secondary sex characteristics development, decreased testicular volumes, variable degree of spermatogenic failure, but, surprisingly, did not have azoospermia or absolute infertility as two of them fathered children. They had high FSH levels, low inhibin, normal or slightly elevated LH, and normal T levels (62).

In males the Lutropin-Choriogonadotropin (LHCG) receptor has an essential role in Leydig cell development and function, and subsequently, in the differentiation of internal and external genitalia, onset of puberty and spermatogenesis. The LHCG receptor belongs to a particular subgroup of G protein–coupled receptors that also includes the FSH and TSH receptors. They contain a seven-transmembrane domain characteristic of G protein-coupled receptors.

Loss-of-function mutations in the LHCGR gene in homozygous males result in Leydig cell hypoplasia and impaired testicular steroidogenesis. LHCGR gene mutations are not localized in any particular region of the gene and cause variable degrees of loss of receptor activity. Depending on the severity of the LHCGR gene defect the clinical manifestations may vary from hypospadias/micropenis to complete 46,XY sex reversal at birth and cryptorchidism (63,64) (for details see Chapter 36).

Phenotypic female 46,XY patients with complete LHCG receptor inactivation present with delayed puberty, elevated LH, FSH, low T, and no response β-hCG stimulation. These patients also have epididymis, vas deferens, and lack of Müllerian derivatives which indicates that a small amount of T is needed for normal development of vas and epididymis. Histologic examination of the testis shows seminiferous tubules and absence of mature Leydig cells (65). Although their clinical and biochemical phenotype resembles complete androgen insensitivity syndrome (CAI), they differ as they do not develop pubertal gynecomastia, which in CAI is explained by the increased aromatization of T to estrogen during puberty.

Adolescent Drug Abuse and Male Gonadal Function

Adolescent drug use may have a negative impact on gonadal function and also increases the risk of unsafe sexual and other behaviors, and thus creates a significant health care issue.

Anabolic Steroids Anabolic androgenic steroids (AAS) have been used for almost 40 years by competitive athletes to improve performance and strength. Strict enforcement of policies to detect exogenous androgens among international and national sport organizations has decreased the incidence of AAS use among professional athletes. Use of these drugs among amateur athletes and even non-athletes is much harder to estimate because obligatory testing programs do not exist.

There are several issues that are specific for adolescent AAS abuse. From the published literature it is estimated that 2% to 11% of late adolescents have used AAS (66). AAS in this age group are often used to improve physique rather than to gain muscle strength. Adolescents also use AAS as mood-enhancing drugs, often in association with other illicit drugs. The

high prevalence of AAS abuse and the poor knowledge of AAS-associated side effects among both health professionals and teenagers create significant health issues.

Supraphysiologic amounts of AAS can elevate liver transaminases and increase hematocrit and blood viscosity. Polycythemia is a risk factor for stroke (67). Adolescent acne may be exacerbated. Use of AAS during puberty may elevate E_2 levels, leading to gynecomastia and, if pubertal growth is not complete, decreased final height (premature closure of the epiphyses). High T levels suppress LH and FSH release, and thus cause transient oligospermia or sterility. Discontinuation of ASS does not always reverse altered control of the hypothalamic-pituitary-testicular axis and sterility may be permanent. In addition, a withdrawal syndrome from high AAS levels has been described among some adult athletes after prolonged use (68). The dependence is more psychologic than physical and can lead to depression and suicidal ideation.

Treatment of adolescent ASS abuse requires comprehensive care. Endocrinologically, clomiphene citrate or anastrozole may stimulate the pituitary to produce FSH and LH. In addition, a short course of β-hCG may allow for normal T production while the HPG axis is recovering. In our practice we use clomiphene 25 mg three times a week for 3 months plus a tapering dose of β-hCG (2500 IU IM 3 times weekly for the 1st month, 2000 IU IM 3 times weekly for the 2nd month, and 1500 IU IM 3 times weekly for the 3rd month). Unfortunately a significant number of men will continue to use AAS—this is evident by undetectable levels of FSH and LH despite normal T levels and treatment with clomiphene.

Alcohol and Illicit Drugs The effects of illicit drug use on testicular function are less well studied. Research data, with the exception of alcohol abuse, are primarily available for adult men rather than developing adolescents. Acute and chronic alcohol intoxication in pubertal males is associated with a decrease in plasma T, and lower LH and FSH and delayed puberty have been found in boys with chronic alcohol abuse (69).

There are no reports on effects of gamma-hydroxybutyrate or ketamine abuse on gonadal function. Marijuana use does not directly affect sex hormone levels or spermatogenesis (70). Crystal methamphetamine can cause apoptosis of Leydig cells in mice but data in humans are lacking (71). Chronic cocaine use may depress LH and T levels and limit spermatogenesis in rats, but the effects of chronic or acute cocaine use on the gonadal axis or spermatogenesis in man have not been adequately investigated (72).

TESTICULAR CAUSES OF MALE HYPOGONADISM

Klinefelter Syndrome

Pathogenesis KS is the most common chromosomal cause of male infertility, with an estimated frequency of 1:500 to 1:1,000 live births. KS is characterized by X chromosome polysomy, with X disomy being the most common variant (47,XXY). The risk factors for KS are poorly understood but advanced maternal or paternal age are associated with a higher incidence (73). Babies born from in vitro fertilization with intracytoplasmic sperm injection have a slightly higher risk of sex chromosomal aberrations.

Most cases of KS are sporadic and results from maternal or paternal nondisjunction of X chromosomes during meiosis I or II. In KS mosaic cases (~10%), the nondisjunction occurs during early embryo divisions. Tissue specific nondisjunction has also been reported but its prevalence is hard to assess.

Clinical Presentation KS is rarely diagnosed prior to puberty. It can be recognized in the neonatal period, but the signs of mild hypotonia and mildly delayed weight gain are nonspecific. Often T levels between 3 and 6 months of age are decreased in children with KS. There are no pathognomic features of KS in young children, but the phenotypic difference between boys with KS and their peers becomes more noticeable with the onset of puberty (74). The timing of puberty is usually normal in KS.

There is broad phenotypic variation, but classically boys with KS present with eunuchoid body proportions (long legs with an arm span greater than height), sparse facial and pubic hair, gynecomastia, small hard testicles (<5 mL), infertility, and learning disabilities including language deficits, neurodevelopmental lag, academic difficulties, and psychologic problems (Figure 37-7). Severe cognitive impairment is extremely rare. Most cognitive problems are secondary to difficulties in auditory processing and executive skills. Boys and men with more than two X chromosomes (48,XXXY; 49,XXXXY) tend to be more severely affected. Patients with mosaicism may have milder intellectual impairment (75). Patients with KS and gonadal mosaicism may present with a more subtle clinical phenotype.

KS patients have an increased risk for breast cancer, autoimmune diseases, and diabetes mellitus. Taurodontism, an enlargement of the pulp of the molar teeth, is frequently seen in KS, which predisposes them to early dental caries and tooth loss.

Diagnosis Adolescent patients may have low serum T, decreased free T because SHBG

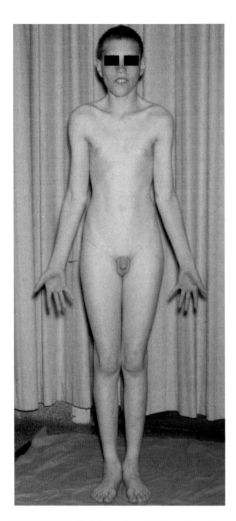

FIGURE 37-7. Klinefelter syndrome. Photo courtesy of Dr. Robert Gorlin.

levels are elevated, high LH and FSH levels, low inhibin and often elevated E_2. However, at the onset of puberty T levels may be relatively normal, with progressive deterioration over time (76). Likewise, prepubertal boys with KS typically have normal inhibin B and MIS levels which significantly decline during puberty, reflecting progressive damage to the Sertoli cells and spermatogenesis.

Testicular biopsy in adults with KS shows hyalinization of the seminiferous tubules and fibrosis. Testicular biopsies in prepubertal and pubertal boys show presence of spermatogenesis and deterioration of spermatogenesis most likely occurs during mid puberty.

The diagnosis of KS is established by peripheral blood karyotype, bearing in mind that low-level mosaicism may be missed. If there is high suspicion, testicular biopsy may show gonadal mosaicism and confirm the diagnosis. Genetic counseling is advisable because patients with KS have a higher risk of breast cancer and mediastinal germ cell tumors, and slightly decreased life expectancy (77).

Treatment There is no specific treatment for KS other than hormonal manipulation and cognitive, behavioral, and vocational therapy. Growing evidence suggests that early diagnosis and therapeutic intervention in boys and men with KS have a beneficial effect on their physical and intellectual development and health.

T therapy should be initiated in adolescence if T levels are low. Only topical T preparations like Androgel should be used since they allow for physiologic normalization of T level and avoid mood swings associated with high and low levels seen with the use of injectable T. The cognitive impairment in boys with KS may be at least in part related to low T because hypogonadism negatively affects brain development and is associated with decreased thickness of the left temporal lobe gray matter, global reduction in brain volume, and impairment in spatial recognition and executive skills (78). T replacement started in early adolescence can increase the thickness of the gray zone and improve the intellectual capabilities of these boys (79). Early T replacement may improve the shortened life expectancy for men with KS, which is mostly related to complications of cardiovascular disease. Twenty five percent of KS adult men are affected by osteoporosis, and early T replacement may prevent this complication. Men with KS are at higher risk to develop autoimmune diseases, with systemic lupus erythematosus being the most common (80). High E_2 levels and low T have been proposed as an underlying mechanism in systemic lupus erythematosus (81), and T replacement improves clinical and biochemical parameters. Low T levels can increase insulin resistance and may be one of the factors leading to development of diabetes mellitus in KS.

Unfortunately, only 10% of men affected by KS are diagnosed prior to adulthood, the time when treatment may be the most effective. Infertility in men with KS has been successfully treated by sperm extraction and in vitro fertilization (82). We and others found sperm in ejaculate in adolescents during early stages of puberty and semen analysis with potential cryopreservation is strongly advised in adolescents with KS.

Noonan Syndrome

Pathogenesis NS occurs in an estimated 1:2,000 live births. It is characterized by many of the same phenotypic features as Turner syndrome, except that NS affects both males and females and the affected patients have normal karyotypes,

Most of cases of NS are spontaneous mutations, but it can be transmitted in an autosomal dominant pattern with equal sex distribution. Advanced paternal age may be one of the risk factors (83). Germline missense mutations in the PTPN11 gene occur in 50% of patients with NS. The PTPN11 product, the ubiquitously expressed protein Shp2, is a tyrosine phosphatase which is essential for activation of the Ras-Erk cascade in receptor tyrosine kinase and cytokine receptor signaling pathways. NS is most likely due to gain of function mutations of Shp2 (84). Shp2 exhibits a negative regulatory effect on GH action, which may explain the short stature observed in these patients. PTPN11 mutations are also associated with myeloproliferative disease and acute leukemia, both of which occur more often in children with NS. An animal model of NS has been recently described (85). Other heterozygous mutations of SOS1, KRAS, and RAF1 can also cause NS.

Clinical Presentation Affected children suffer from typical facial and body dysmorphic features (86). Those features may not be easily noticeable in early childhood, and the diagnosis may escape the attention of skilled practitioners. Family history of mild mental retardation, congenital heart defects, short stature, or facial dysmorphic features may aid in the diagnosis. Adolescents have short stature, a triangular face, hypertelorism, refractive problems, amblyopia, low set ears, and a high nasal bridge. Short, webbed neck, scoliosis, and pectus excavatum represent typical torso findings. A dysplastic or stenotic pulmonary valve is the most common cardiac defect, but other abnormalities have been also described. Both hypertrophic cardiomyopathy (30%) and hepatosplenomegaly (25%) are common features of the syndrome. More than 50% of males have undescended testes (68). Some boys may start puberty spontaneously, but progression is often slow. Testicular histology in men shows persistence of fetal Leydig cells, immature Sertoli cells and spermatogenic arrest, and 80% have oligospermia or azoospermia. In one study, however, 4 of 11 men with NS fathered children (87). Endocrinologic evaluation reveals normal LH and normal-to-low T, and elevated FSH.

Diagnosis and Treatment The diagnosis of NS is made clinically due to the characteristic phenotypic features and can be confirmed by detection of mutations in the PTPN11 gene; however, the absence of mutation does not exclude the disease. Correction of cardiac defects usually takes priority over any other treatment. NS is associated with coagulation factor deficiencies (especially factor XI) and platelet dysfunction (88), so care needs to be taken to identify and correct any coagulopathy prior to invasive or surgical procedures. Cryptorchidism should be corrected within the 1st year of life, in an effort to preserve fertility. Delayed puberty or poor progression of puberty can be managed with T replacement. GH therapy has been evaluated in some studies with equivocal results.

DISORDERS OF SEX DETERMINATION, SEX DIFFERENTIATION, AND GONADAL DEVELOPMENT

Errors of sex determination and gonadal development such as XX male syndrome, 46,XX/XY gonadal dysgenesis, testicular and ovotesticular disorders of sex development, usually result in a male or under-virilized male phenotype and present with normal or elevated FSH and LH, ambiguous genitalia at birth, and some degree of testicular and spermatogenic failure. T levels may be low or normal.

Disorders of sex differentiation such as Leydig cell aplasia, partial androgen insensitivity (PAIS), 5α- reductase deficiency, CAH due to 17α-hydroxylase/17,20-lyase deficiency and 3β-hydroxysteroid dehydrogenase type II deficiency, and 17β-hydroxysteroid dehydrogenase type 3 deficiency, may present with undervirilized male phenotype, elevated FSH/LH levels and low-to-low normal T except for PAIS where T is elevated.

Patients with the classic forms of CAH due to 21α-hydroxylase(21-OHD) deficiency or 11β-hydroxylase (11-OHD) deficiency may also present with decreased testicular steroidogenesis and decreased spermatogenesis. Overtreatment with steroids or elevated adrenal androgen that are aromatized to estrogen in CAH patients with poor control may have a direct toxic effect on Sertoli or germ cells as well as an effect on the hypothalamic-pituitary axis by suppressing LH production and therefore T synthesis.

Adrenal rests, which arise from aberrant adrenal cells in the testes, are stimulated by ACTH and can also affect fertility directly by pressure effect or by the effect of adrenal rest steroids on the HPA axis. The preferred treatment for adrenal rests is dexamethasone 2 mg per day for 7 days and then replacement therapy with hydrocortisone at a dose to keep 17-OHP less than 1,000 ng/dL in growing adolescents, or with dexamethasone 0.25 to 0.5 mg daily in males who have completed growth. Surgical intervention is reserved for the cases that do not respond to glucocorticoid regimen (89). For more detail on the above disorders, please refer to Chapters 35 and 27.

Anorchia

Patients with congenital anorchia (also called vanishing testes or testicular regression syndrome) present with bilateral absence of the testes, and thus it is typically recognized early in life. Because they have normal external genitalia without ambiguity, it is believed that the testicular insult occurred sometime after the first trimester. The primary defect is unknown, but has been postulated to be related to vascular insult. Familial cases exist.

Anorchia must be distinguished from cryptorchidism. Boys with anorchia have a very low T level which does not respond to stimulation with intramuscular β-hCG.

Measurement of MIS in peripheral blood is recommended to confirm the diagnosis of bilateral anorchia: undetectable MIS is consistent with a lack of testicular tissue. Laparoscopy should be performed on boys believed to have congenital anorchia, although novel MRI protocols may change this recommendation (90). Blindly ending stumps of testicular arteries confirm the diagnosis. If any testicular tissue remains, it is usually laparoscopically removed because of concern about the risk of malignancy. These concerns are based on data from men with cryptorchidism, and some feel the risk of cancer in congenital anorchia may not be any higher than in the general population (91). T replacement is required to induce puberty, followed by life long T replacement to maintain normal male sexual health.

Acquired anorchia can be secondary to traumatic or iatrogenic orchiectomy. Once bilateral orchiectomy is performed, the chance for sperm production is lost. Hence, in cases of planned orchiectomy in a postpubertal patient (such as for a testicular cancer), semen collection and sperm cryopreservation should be discussed. Patients with acquired anorchia need to be placed on androgen replacement therapy at the time of puberty and thereafter.

Cryptorchidism

Pathogenesis Cryptorchidism, which refers to unilateral or bilateral undescended testes, is the most common urogenital disorder of childhood. The testes can be located anywhere along their embryologic path of descent, from the kidneys to just outside the scrotum. Rarely, they may be located in an ectopic position.

The etiology of cryptorchism is multifactorial and often unknown, but both hormonal and mechanical problems associated with testicular descent are involved. Adequate central gonadotropin secretion, testicular T production, sensitivity to T, normal development of the gubernaculum (the bandlike structure that directs intra-abdominal descent of the testes), and intra-abdominal pressure (because boys with abdominal wall defects have cryptorchidism) are all important for descent of the testes. Cryptorchidism is usually sporadic, but there is also a familial component because a male infant has approximately a 6% risk if a brother was affected. The incidence of cryptorchidism is rising and environmental factors such as endocrine disruptors have been postulated to play a role. Boys with KalS, KS, NS, PWS, and a number of other syndromes involving the urogenital system are all at risk of cryptorchidism.

Clinical Presentation Because the final descent of the testes does not occur until after 7 months gestation, 30% of premature infants have at least one undescended testis, whereas approximately 1% to 3% of term-delivered male newborns have cryptorchidism. In most cases the testes spontaneously descend after birth due to the postnatal surge in T, and by the age of 3 months the frequency drops to 0.5% to 1%. Cryptorchidism is usually unilateral with the right side affected more often than the left. Boys with cryptorchidism typically go through puberty normally and have normal sexual development and function. It is associated with a significant risk of infertility, although the earlier the surgical repair the less evident the impairment of fertility. A history of undescended testes increases the risk of testicular cancer 10-fold and this risk is not lowered by orchiopexy. Embryonal carcinoma is the most common testicular cancer seen in individuals who have had cryptorchidism repair, whereas seminoma is most common if there has not been surgical repair. If hypospadias is also present, intersex conditions need to be considered (and are discussed at length in Chapter 35).

Diagnosis and Treatment A phenotypically male newborn with bilateral nonpalpable testicles should be considered a severe virilized genetic female with CAH due to 21-OHD or 11-OHD until proven otherwise. An ultrasound of the abdomen to evaluate for the presence of an uterus/ovaries and enlarged adrenals, karyotype, measurement of serum electrolytes, T, 17-OHP level, DOC, MIS should be part of the work up to rule out CAH.

Bilateral cryptorchidism needs to be differentiated from bilateral anorchia. Elevation in LH and FSH, as well as the absence of detectable MIS and inhibin B suggest testicular absence due to bilateral anorchia. Imaging studies may help identify the location of a nonpalpable gonad; however, a negative study does not exclude the presence of testicles in the abdomen because they can be hard to visualize by current imaging techniques. An increase in T levels after β-hCG stimulation demonstrates the presence of functioning testicular tissue. Normal gonadotropin levels or detectable MIS levels warrant surgical exploration even with a negative β-hCG stimulation test.

In boys with low gonadotropin levels and low to normal MIS levels, measurements of thyroid hormone and cortisol should be included to rule out hypogonadism as part of panhypopituitarism, KalS or nIHH.

Cryptorchidism must be differentiated from the retractile testis. A retractile testis resides in the scrotum but frequently and temporarily enters the inguinal canal. Boys 6 month old or older have an active cremaster reflex resulting in retraction of the testis into the scrotum or external inguinaling, particularly if the boy is anxious, nervous, or cold.

The boy with bilaterally nonpalpable testes should undergo inguinal or laparoscopic abdominal exploration and have orchiopexy performed. Most pediatric urologists perform orchiopexy between 6 and 24 months of age based on the fact that spontaneous descent after 6 months of age is unlikely and repair before 2 years of age may have a better prognosis with respect to fertility (92). The main reason surgery for cryptorchidism is delayed is late referral, underscoring the need for early diagnosis and treatment (93).

Orchiopexy for adolescent and adult males is more controversial and the decision on how to proceed should be made by the patient and the urologist after discussing risks versus benefits of surgery. Options include orchiectomy, orchiopexy, or observation. Orchiectomy has been advocated by many because the cryptorchid testis is most likely nonfunctional and the patient has a significantly increased risk of developing testicular cancer (94). Orchiopexy is usually considered in young men because there might be potential for sufficient spermatogenesis for fertility, especially with new techniques of sperm extraction and in vitro fertilization using intracytoplasmic sperm injection (95).

β-hCG is used in Europe but is not often used in the United States, where it is thought to be useful only for a retractile testis. GnRH therapy combined with orchiopexy may have a positive effect on fertility (96).

The surgical procedure performed depends on the location of the testes. If they are palpable in the inguinal canal and can be brought down to the upper portion of the scrotum, then an open surgical inguinal orchiopexy is performed. Intraabdominal testicles may require a two-stage procedure for mobilization to the scrotum. Orchiopexy allows for easy examination of the testicle to monitor for malignancy; it may preserve hormonal function of the testicle and could potentially improve spermatogenesis.

Macroorchidism

Normal testicular size in adult men is 15 to 25 cc^3. The testes should generally be equal in size, and a single enlarged testis suggests tumor or an extratesticular mass such as hydrocele. If one testis has been damaged, however, such as by torsion or late cryptorchidism repair, compensatory hypertrophy of the other testis can occur (97).

The most common genetic cause of macroorchidism after puberty and sometimes in prepubertal boys is fragile X syndrome (98). Associated signs include mild-to-moderate mental retardation that may worsen with age, large ears, a prominent jaw, a high-pitched voice, flat feet, and joint laxity. Phenotypic expression is variable. The FMR1 (fragile-site mental retardation-1) gene is located on the X chromosome at a site where, in fragile X syndrome, expanded stretches of CGG repeats form an unstable region prone to breakage. Hypothyroidism can also cause macroorchidism, generally with low T levels, and macroorchidism has been described related to a Sertoli cell G protein mutation in an unusual case of McCune–Albright syndrome (99).

Damage to Normal Testes

Mumps orchitis after puberty, trauma to the testis, testicular torsion, and cryptorchidism and its repair can all affect spermatogenesis, although hormonal function is usually intact unless bilateral severe atrophy is present. Irradiation and/or chemotherapy can damage the testes; often the insult may not become apparent for several years. Cancer treatment also increases slightly the risk of abnormal sperm and chromatin structures (further discussion is found in Chapter 47).

Varicocele Varicocele is defined as a dilation of the pampiniform plexus veins and is the most common identifiable cause of male infertility. Although they are located exterior to the testis, they are included under testicular defects because they are associated with testicular atrophy, they can negatively affect sperm motility and morphology, and they may have deleterious effects on T production in adulthood. They are first seen during puberty. Timely diagnosis and treatment are essential because early on there may be a chance to preserve fertility (14).

The diagnosis can be established by physical examination. A varicocele felt only during a Valsalva maneuver is classified as grade I, a palpable varicocele in the standing position is grade II, and a grade III varicocele is visible as a prominent pampiniform plexus vein (Figure 37-5). Ultrasound is clinically useful in the evaluation. Dilated pampiniform plexus veins above 2 mm are consistent with the diagnosis. Varicoceles can be further confirmed by the presence of venous reflux (flow reversal) with the Valsalva maneuver, although this is not a consistent finding. A varicocele that does not change size in the supine position. or a large varicocele on the right side may indicate a retroperitoneal or renal fossa tumor.

A discrepancy in testicular volume of more than 2 mL in the presence of a palpable varicocele in adolescents is considered by many experts to be an indication for surgery (100). It is the authors' practice to repair varicoceles in patients with a grade III varicocele and abnormal semen analysis, or in adolescents with a large varicocele and decreased testicular volume.

Estrogen Deficiency

E_2 is necessary for closure of the epiphyses, normal mineral bone density, and normal spermatogenesis. Two rare genetic syndromes illustrate the effects of estrogen deficiency in males. A 28-year-old man with an estrogen receptor mutation had gone through puberty normally and was normally virilized, but he did not stop growing after puberty (101,102). He had tall stature (204 cm, 80 inches) and incomplete epiphyseal closure. E_2, E_1, FSH, and LH were all elevated, whereas T levels were normal. He had impaired glucose tolerance, insulin resistance with acanthosis nigricans, elevated lipid levels, early atherosclerosis and osteoporosis. Similarly, a man with aromatase deficiency had normal puberty and virilization, but was extremely tall with lack of epiphyseal fusion. He had undetectable E_2 levels, high LH and FSH, macroorchidism with abnormal sperm, and osteoporosis (103).

Genetic Defects Affecting Spermatogenesis

Spermatogenesis is regulated by many genes located on the Y and X chromosomes. The distal arm of the Y chromosome carries genes with a critical role in spermatogenesis called azoospermia factor (AZF). Deletion of one or more distinct regions known as AZF a, b, and c result in azoospermia or severe oligospermia. Sperm was never found in men with AZF a or AZF b deletion. Those regions are critical for normal spermatogenesis. Patients with AZF c deletions have a much less severe defect of spermatogenesis and produce sperm although sperm density is low in those patients (104). In this case (AZF c deletion), Y chromosome microdeletions will be transmitted to all male offspring and affected children are expected to have azoospermia or severe oligospermia.

FSH receptor deficiency may also cause defects in spermatogenesis in males, with otherwise normal virilization. The severity of the defect is variable, demonstrating that FSH is clearly more important for fertility in women than in men (105).

POSTTESTICULAR DEFECTS

Mechanical Obstruction and Retrograde Ejaculation

Bilateral inguinal hernia repair (especially done in the 1st year of life) can result in obstruction of the vas deferens. Bladder neck reconstruction, retroperitoneal surgery, trauma to the spine, or anterior approaches to spinal fusion can all damage the sympathetic chain–dependent bladder neck closure mechanism and contribute to retrograde ejaculation. α-blockers and serotonin reuptake inhibitors can cause retrograde ejaculation or anejaculation.

Cystic Fibrosis and Congenital Absence of the Vas Deferens

CBAVD is the most common genetic cause of obstructive azoospermia. Most males with CF have CBAVD, but only approximately 60% of men with CBAVD have CF (15). There are more than 800 mutations described in the responsible CF transmembrane conductance regulator gene (CFTR), with variable phenotype and penetrance.

CBAVD patients with renal malformations, especially renal agenesis, are likely not to have CF and instead have a mesonephric duct malformation. Confirmed renal agenesis makes detection of a CFTR mutation no more likely than in the general population (16). Any patient with CBAVD who does not have renal agenesis should have sweat chloride testing.

Immotile Cilia Syndrome, Kartagener Syndrome

Patients with immotile cilia syndrome suffer from frequent respiratory tract infections and infertility. When this syndrome is associated with situs inversus and bronchiectasis, it is known as Kartagener syndrome.

The normal sperm tail has 9+2 tubules involved in sperm movement. Patients with immotile cilia have abnormal sperm tails with 9+0 tubules, which do not allow the tail to move although the sperm are alive. The defect is uniform in all spermatozoa. This diagnosis can be confirmed by electron microscopy of the sperm tail or nasal cilia, showing a missing central pair of microtubules (106).

Penile Abnormalities

Concealed Penis A entirely normal penis may appear small or "inconspicuous" when it is hidden by the suprapubic fat pad, especially in obese children (Figure 37-8), or when the scrotal skin extends onto the ventrum of the penis ("webbed penis") (Figure 37-9). These

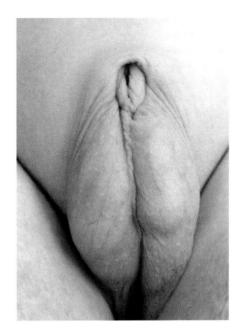

FIGURE 37-8. Concealed penis (a normal size penis hidden because of the presence of a pubic fat pad). Photo courtesy of Dr. Rosalia Misseri.

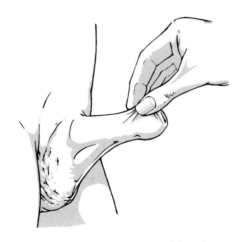

FIGURE 37-9. A webbed penis (a normal size penis concealed by scrotal skin extending onto the ventrum of the penis).

conditions, in which the penis is normal in size, must be distinguished from micropenis.

Phimosis and Paraphimosis Phimosis occurs in uncircumcised males, and refers to the inability to retract the foreskin to visualize any part of the glans (Figure 37-10). Congenital phimosis is entirely normal for uncircumcised young boys because the foreskin is always tight, nonretractable, and adherent to the glans at birth. During childhood, epithelial debris (smegma) accumulates, gradually separating the foreskin from the glans. In Japan, where males are generally not circumcised, congenital phimosis was present in approximately 90% of boys aged 1 to 3 months and in 35% of boys at

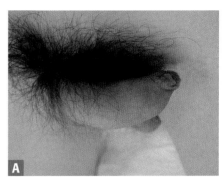
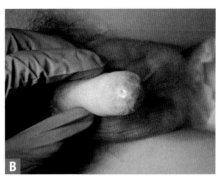
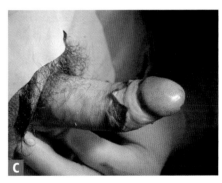

FIGURE 37-10. Phimosis in a 15-year-old boy before surgery (A and B) and after opening the foreskin (C). Photos courtesy of Dr. Leo Fung.

3 years. Only 40% of foreskins were fully retractable over the glans by 3 years of age (107). In Denmark, 6% of boys aged 8 to 11 years and 3% of boys aged 12 to 13 years were reported to still have congenital phimosis (108), and fully retractable foreskins were seen in only 20% of British boys aged 5 to 13 years (109). Thus, congenital phimosis is common throughout childhood. As long as it does not cause problems such as urinary obstruction, hematuria, or pain, it is not a concern. It usually disappears after puberty, although approximately 1% of males older than 16 years have phimosis.

Acquired phimosis can occur with inflammation or trauma, such as is seen with poor hygiene or with forceful retraction of a congenital phimosis (often by parents trying to clean the glans), which leads to scar formation with a fibrotic ring of tissue close to the opening of the prepuce. The patient should be referred to a urologist if the urinary stream decreases (obstruction) or if there is hematuria or pain. High potency steroids applied to the fibrotic band may be successful in treating acquired phimosis (110). Circumcision is therapeutic but is only performed when unavoidable in the older child or adolescent because it may be associated with decreased sexual sensation and the cosmetic results are not as good as when the procedure is done in infancy (111).

Paraphimosis is a true urologic emergency. It is present in uncircumcised or incorrectly circumcised males when one cannot move a retracted foreskin back over the glans into its naturally occurring position. This causes pain and edema of the glans, and eventually necrosis may occur secondary to arterial occlusion. The etiology includes poor hygiene, chronic inflammation, or a history of frequent catheterizations. On physical examination, it is important to rule out an encircling foreign body, such as hair, clothing, metallic objects, or rubber bands. With the rising incidence of body piercing, those obtaining penile rings are at increased risk of paraphimosis, especially if the newly placed ring causes enough discomfort to prevent the reduction of a retracted foreskin.

Penile Agenesis Penile agenesis is a rare condition that generally results from failure of genital tubercle development. The karyotype is 46,XY, and the appearance of the external genitalia is otherwise normal, with a well-formed scrotum and descended testes. The urethra may open into the rectum or the anus, but the connection between the genitourinary and gastrointestinal tract is variable and there are often associated renal abnormalities that can be severe. In the past, gender reassignment was routine because construction of a penis requires multiple surgeries throughout the lifetime of the individual and the cosmetic and functional results are poor. With greater understanding of the role of prenatal androgen exposure in the formation of gender identity, this is no longer considered standard. This dilemma was highlighted in the case of a child who lost his penis at several months of age following a botched circumcision (112). Because of the belief at that time that gender identity was plastic before the age of approximately 2 years, he was raised as a girl until adolescence, at which time he emphatically chose to reclaim his male identity, maintaining that he had always known he was not a girl. He eventually married and adopted children.

Epispadias Epispadias refers to a urethral opening on the dorsal side of the penis (113) (Figure 37-11). It occurs in 1:117,000 newborn boys. The degree of penile deformity

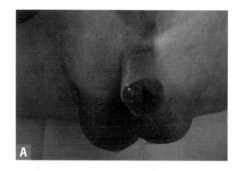
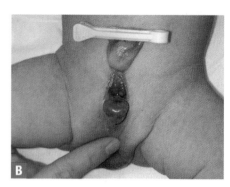
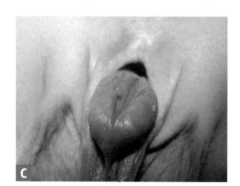
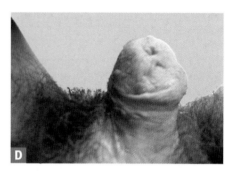

FIGURE 37-11. Epispadius. It ranges from mild (A) with almost normal appearance of the penis, to severe forms with variable exposure of the bladder neck mucosa (B,C). The reconstruction results in a functionally adequate penis, although the cosmetic results depend on the extent of the initial defect (D).

and of urinary incontinence varies depending on the location of the urethral meatus, which may be found on the glans (the mildest defect), the penile shaft, or the penopubic region (complete epispadius). The most severe type is associated with exstrophy of the bladder, where the entire penile urethra and bladder are open and the pubic symphysis is split. Urinary incontinence is not generally a problem with glandular epispadius, is seen in just over half of patients with penile epispadias, and is almost universal in those with the penopubic form. Epispadias is associated with varying degrees of dorsal chordae (upward curvature of the penis), and often the penis appears short and wide.

The cause of epispadias is unknown but may be related to abnormal development of the pubic symphysis. Surgical repair is required for all but the mildest forms to achieve urinary continence and to reconstruct a functional and cosmetically acceptable penis. Persistent urinary incontinence may be present in some patients even after multiple operations, and upper ureter and kidney damage as well as infertility may occur. Bladder exstrophy is associated with severe abnormalities that generally require multiple surgeries and have a less than optimal cosmetic and functional outcome.

Hypospadias Hypospadias is a common malformation in which the urethra opens on the ventral side of the penis, usually associated with ventral chordae (downward curvature of the penis) (Figure 37-12). It occurs in 3:1,000 male births. It is considered a complex disorder with both genetic and environmental factors involved in the pathogenesis (114). No specific gene defect is known, although defects in 5-a-reductase and, rarely, in the AR, are found in 30% of 118 severe forms of hypospadias (115).

Coronal or glandular hypospadias is considered mild and is present in approximately 80% to 85% of cases. Moderate hypospadias, located on the shaft of the penis, is present in 10% to 15% of cases. Only approximately 3% to 6% of patients have the most severe forms of hypospadias, penoscrotal or perineal. Other malformations are present in approximately 15% of infants with hypospadias, with renal and urinary tract abnormalities being most common. The recurrence risk for brothers is approximately 20% (116). The prevalence of hypospadias may be rising and has been postulated to be related to endocrine-disrupting chemicals in the environment (117).

Surgery (urethroplasty) is generally performed at an early age (8–12 mo), and most patients have an excellent outcome with normal appearance, normal urinary and sexual function, and normal fertility. Circumcision should never be done prior to hypospadias surgery because the foreskin may be used in the reconstruction. Hypospadias increases the risk of future testicular cancer.

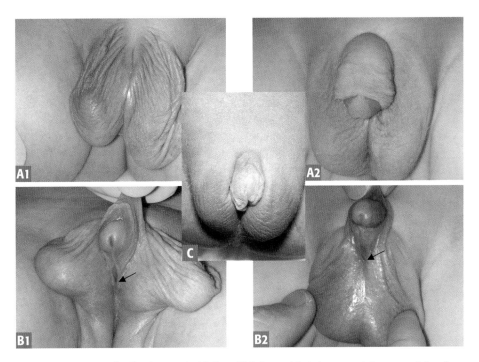

FIGURE 37-12. Hypospadias. The photos on the left (A1 and B1) show an infant who appears to have congenital penile agenesis, but careful examination reveals a scrotal penis with penoscrotal hypospadias. The boy on the right (A2 and B2) has severe penoscrotal hypospadias. The arrow points to the distal urethra. For comparison, the middle photo is a 46,XY boy with ambiguous genitalia.

Erectile Dysfunction

Pathogenesis Erectile dysfunction (ED) can be a result of psychologic, neurologic, vascular, or mechanical problems. Although not typically an endocrinologic or developmental problem, it may have its origin during childhood or adolescence, especially as a result of spinal cord or pelvic floor injury. Diabetes mellitus has been shown to be a risk factor for early erectile dysfunction. Young men with history of type 1 diabetes have higher rate of ED than men with type 2 diabetes (118). Smoking, so common among adolescents, further increases the risk of ED.

Normal erectile function requires an intact central and peripheral nervous system, peripheral vascular system, and penile anatomy. Tactile, auditory, and visual stimulation are carried via descending pathways to the erection center in the spinal cord at S2–S4. Parasympathetic fibers carry signals to the penis through the pelvic plexus via the *nervi cavernosi* along the pudendal artery. Sympathetic fibers that inhibit erections originate in the thoracolumbar region (T12–L2). Somatosensory innervation is carried through the dorsal penile nerve, which forms the pudendal nerve. During development of an erection, sympathetic discharge decreases with concurrent cavernosal nerve activity that stimulates cavernosal body relaxation and increased arterial inflow. Compression of the subtunical venous plexus and decreased outflow allows for adequate rigidity for penetration. T plays a role in erectile function.

Clinical Presentation, Diagnosis and Treatment A carefully performed history can facilitate the diagnosis and evaluation. Patients with spinal cord injury suffer from both ED and abnormal spermatogenesis, and occasionally hypogonadism. The presence of spontaneous erections in the morning or full rigidity during masturbation indicates normal physiologic function, and in this setting if ED is present it is likely psychogenic and hence should be evaluated by a sexual therapist. In adults and perhaps older adolescents, a history of type 1 diabetes, high blood pressure, elevated cholesterol, peripheral vascular disease, coronary artery disease, or smoking may be associated with vascular insufficiency and may prompt diagnostic vascular studies using penile Doppler ultrasound after injection of prostaglandin E1.

Oral 5-phosphodiesterase inhibitors are the first line of therapy for patients with) ED. They can help patients with psychologic dysfunction to avoid performance anxiety. They work well in patients with mild-to-moderate vascular insufficiency. There are other options for patients who cannot take such agents (sildenafil, vardenafil, and tadalafil) or who fail to respond to the medication. Vibratory stimulation or electroejaculation may be used to obtain semen for in vitro fertilization in patients with spinal cord injury.

REFERENCES

1. Koopman P. The genetics and biology of vertebrate sex determination. *Cell.* 2001;105:843–847.
2. Haider SG. Cell biology of Leydig cells in the testis. *Int Rev Cytol.* 2004;233:181–241.
3. Park SY, Jameson JL. Minireview: transcriptional regulation of gonadal development and differentiation. *Endocrinology.* 2005;146:1035–1042.
4. Laron Z, Klinger B. Effect of insulin-like growth factor-I treatment on serum androgens and testicular and penile size in males with Laron syndrome (primary growth hormone resistance). *Eur J Endocrinol.* 1998;138:176–180.
5. Boas M, Boisen KA, Virtanen HE, et al. Postnatal penile length and growth rate correlate to serum testosterone levels: a longitudinal study of 1962 normal boys. *Eur J Endocrinol.* 2006;154:125–129.
6. Andersson AM, Skakkebaek NE. Serum inhibin B levels during male childhood and puberty. *Mol Cell Endocrinol.* 2001;180:103–107.
7. Roth CL, Ojeda SR. Genes involved in the neuroendocrine control of normal puberty and abnormal puberty of central origin. *Pediatr Endocrinol Rev.* 2005;3:67–76.
8. Papaioannou M, Reeb C, Asim M, et al. Co-activator and co-repressor interplay on the human androgen receptor. *Andrologia.* 2005;37:211–212.
9. Halpern CT, Udry JR, Suchindran C. Monthly measures of salivary testosterone predict sexual activity in adolescent males. *Arch Sex Behav.* 1998;27:445–465.
10. Campbell BC, Prossinger H, Mbzivo M. Timing of pubertal maturation and the onset of sexual behavior among Zimbabwe school boys. *Arch Sex Behav.* 2005;34:505–516.
11. Nielsen CT, Skakkebaek NE, Richardson DW, et al. Onset of the release of spermatozoa (spermarche) in boys in relation to age, testicular growth, pubic hair, and height. *J Clin Endocrinol Metab.* 1986;62:532–535.
12. Daniels IR, Layer GT. Testicular tumours presenting as gynaecomastia. *Eur J Surg Oncol.* 2003;29:437–439.
13. Weiss JR, Moysich KB, Swede H. Epidemiology of male breast cancer. *Cancer Epidemiol Biomarkers Prev.* 2005;14:20–26.
14. Paduch DA, Skoog SJ. Diagnosis, evaluation and treatment of adolescent varicocele. *Sci World J.* 2004;4 Suppl 1:263–78.
15. Dohle GR, Veeze HJ, Overbeek SE, et al. The complex relationships between cystic fibrosis and congenital bilateral absence of the vas deferens: clinical, electrophysiological and genetic data. *Hum Reprod.* 1999;14:371–374.
16. Schlegel PN, Shin D, Goldstein M. Urogenital anomalies in men with congenital absence of the vas deferens. *J Urol.* 1996;155:1644–1648.
17. Sikaris K, McLachlan RI, Kazlauskas R, et al. Reproductive hormone reference intervals for healthy fertile young men: evaluation of automated platform assays. *J Clin Endocrinol Metab.* 2005;90:5928–5936.
18. Janczewski Z, Bablok L. Semen characteristics in pubertal boys. I. Semen quality after

first ejaculation. *Arch Androl.* 1985;
15:199–205.

19. Tournaye H, Goossens E, Verheyen G, et al.
Preserving the reproductive potential of men
and boys with cancer: current concepts and
future prospects. *Hum Reprod Update.*
2004;10:525–532.

20. Klugo RC, Cerny JC. Response of micropenis to topical testosterone and gonadotropin.
J Urol. 1978;119:667–668.

21. Salardi S, Zucchini S, Cicognani A, et al.
Inhibin B levels in adolescents and young
adults with type 1 diabetes. *Horm Res.*
2002;57:205–8.

22. De Sanctis V. Growth and puberty and its
management in thalassaemia. *Horm Res.*
2002;58 Suppl 1:72–79.

23. Dode C, Levilliers J, Dupont J-M, et al. Loss-of-function mutations in FGFR1 cause autosomal dominant Kallmann syndrome. *Nat
Genet.* 2003;33:463–465.

24. Dode C, Teixeira L, Levilliers J, et al.
Kallmann syndrome: mutations in the genes
encoding prokineticin-2 and prokineticin receptor-2. *PLoS Genet.* 2006;2:e175.

25. Coatesworth AP, Woodhead CJ. Conductive
hearing loss associated with Kallmann's syndrome. *J Laryngol Otol.* 2002;116:125–6.

26. Sato N, Katsumata N, Kagami M, et al.
Clinical assessment and mutation analysis
of Kallmann syndrome 1 (KAL1) and fibroblast growth factor receptor 1 (FGFR1, or
KAL2) in five families and 18 sporadic patients. *J Clin Endocrinol Metab.*
2004;89:1079–88.

27. Oliveira LMB, Seminara SB, Beranova M,
et al. The importance of autosomal genes in
Kallmann syndrome: genotype-phenotype correlations and neuroendocrine characteristics.
J Clin Endocrinol Metab. 2001;86:1532–1538.

28. Kakar SS, Neill JD. The human gonadotropin-releasing hormone receptor gene
(GNRHR) maps to chromosome band 4q13.
Cytogenet Cell Genet. 1995;70:211–214.

29. Pitteloud N, Boepple PA, DeCruz S, et al.
The fertile eunuch variant of idiopathic hypogonadotropic hypogonadism: spontaneous
reversal associated with a homozygous mutation in the gonadotropin-releasing hormone
receptor. *J Clin Endocrinol Metab.*
2001;86:2470–2475.

30. de Roux, N, Young, J, Misrahi, M, et al.
A family with hypogonadotropic hypogonadism and mutations in the gonadotropin-releasing hormone receptor. *N Engl J Med.*
1997;337: 1597–1602.

31. Roux N, Young J, Brailly-Tabard S, et al. The
same molecular defects of the gonadotropin-releasing hormone receptor determine a variable degree of hypogonadism in affected
kindred. *J Clin Endocrinol Metab.* 1999;84:
567–572.

32. Beranova M, Oliveira LM, Bedecarrats GY,
et al. Prevalence, phenotypic spectrum, and
modes of inheritance of gonadotropin-releasing hormone receptor mutations in
idiopathic hypogonadotropic hypogonadism. *J Clin Endocrinol Metab.*
2001;86:1580–1588.

33. Farooqi IS, Matarese G, Lord GM, et al.
Beneficial effects of leptin on obesity, T cell
hyporesponsiveness, and neuroendocrine/
metabolic dysfunction of human congenital

leptin deficiency. *J Clin Invest.* 2002;110:
1093–1103.

34. Seminara SB, Acierno JS Jr, Abdulwahid
NA, et al. Hypogonadotropic hypogonadism and cerebellar ataxia: detailed phenotypic characterization of a large, extended
kindred. *J Clin Endocrinol Metab.*
2002;87:1607–1612.

35. Moore SJ, Green JS, Fan Y, et al. Clinical
and genetic epidemiology of Bardet-Biedl
syndrome in Newfoundland: a 22-year prospective, population-based, cohort study.
Am J Med Genet. 2005;132:352–360.

36. Burghes AHM, Vaessin HEF, de la Chapelle
A. The land between mendelian and multifactorial inheritance. *Science.*
2001;293:2213–2214.

37. Beales PL, Elciouglu N, Woolf AS, et al.
New criteria for improved diagnosis of
Bardet-Biedl syndrome: results of a population survey. *J Med Genet.*1999;36:437–446.

38. Wheeler PG, Quigley CA, Sadeghi-Nejad A,
et al. Hypogonadism and CHARGE association. *Am J Med Genet.* 2000;94:228–31.

39. Peter M, Viemann M, Partsch CJ, et al. Congenital adrenal hypoplasia: clinical spectrum,
experience with hormonal diagnosis, and report on new point mutations of the DAX-1
gene. *J Clin Endocrinol Metab.*
1998;83:2666–2674.

40. Goldstone AP, Thomas EL, Brynes AE,
et al. Elevated fasting plasma ghrelin in
Prader-Willi syndrome adults is not solely
explained by their reduced visceral adiposity
and insulin resistance. *J Clin Endocrinol
Metab.* 2004;89:1718–1726.

41. Wigren M, Hansen S. Prader-Willi syndrome: clinical picture, psychosocial support
and current management. *Child Care
Health Dev.* 2003;29:449–56.

42. Holm VA, Cassidy SB, Butler MG, et al.
Prader-Willi syndrome: consensus diagnostic
criteria. *Pdeiatrics.* 1993;91:398–402.

43. Allen DB, Carrel AL. Growth hormone therapy for Prader-Willi syndrome: a critical appraisal. *J Pediatr Endocrinol Metab.* 2004;17
Suppl 4:1297–1306.

44. Deladoey J, Fluck C, Buyukgebiz A,
et al. "Hot spot" in the PROP1 gene
responsible for combined pituitary hormone deficiency. *J Clin Endocrinol Metab.*
1999;84:1645–1650.

45. Dattani MT, Robinson IC. HESX1 and
Septo-Optic Dysplasia. *Rev Endocr Metab
Disord.* 2002;3:289–300.

46. Netchine I, Sobrier ML, Krude H, et al.
Mutations in LHX3 result in a new syndrome
revealed by combined pituitary hormone
deficiency. *Nat Genet.* 2000;25:182–186.

47. Holley JL. The hypothalamic-pituitary axis
in men and women with chronic kidney
disease. *Adv Chronic Kidney Dis.* 2004;11:
337–341.

48. Biswas M, Smith J, Jadon D, et al. Long-term remission following withdrawal of
dopamine agonist therapy in subjects with
microprolactinomas. *Clin Endocrinol.* (Oxf)
2005;63:26–31.

49. L, Kleinberg D, Vance ML, et al.
Hypogonadism in patients with acromegaly:
data from the multicentre acromegaly registry pilot study. *Clin Endocrinol.*
2001;54:183–188.

50. Gao HB, Ming MH, Hu YQ, et al. Glucocorticoid induces apoptosis in rat Leydig
cells. *Endocrinology.* 2002;143:130–138.

51. Sankar BR, Maran RR, Sudha S, et al.
Chronic corticosterone treatment impairs
Leydig cell 11b-hydroxysteroid dehydrogenase activity and LH-stimulated testosterone
production. *Horm Metab Res.* 2000;
32:142–146.

52. Hess RA, Bunick D, Bahr J. Oestrogen, its
receptors and function in the male reproductive tract - a review. *Mol Cell Endocrinol.*
2001;178:29–38.

53. Wickman S, Dunkel L. Inhibition of P450
aromatase enhances gonadotropin secretion in early and midpubertal boys:
evidence for a pituitary site of action of
endogenous E. *J Clin Endocrinol Metab.*
2001;86:4887–94.

54. O'Donnell L, Robertson KM, Jones ME, et
al. Estrogen and spermatogenesis. *Endocr
Rev.* 2001; 22:289–318.

55. Shozu M, Sebastian S, Takayama K, et al.
Estrogen excess associated with novel
gain-of-function mutations affecting the
aromatase gene. *N Engl J Med.*
2003;348:1855–1865.

56. de Boer H, Verschoor L, Ruinemans-Koerts
J, et al. Letrozole normalizes serum testosterone in severely obese men with hypogonadotropic hypogonadism. *Diabetes Obes Metab.*
2005;7:211–215.

57. T'Sjoen GG, Giagulli VA, Delva H, et al.
Comparative assessment in young and elderly men of the gonadotropin response to
aromatase inhibition. *J Clin Endocrinol
Metab.* 2005;90:5717–5722.

58. Weiss J, Axelrod L, Whitcomb RW, et al.
Hypogonadism caused by a single amino
acid substitution in the beta subunit of luteinizing hormone. *N Engl J Med.*
1992;326:179–183.

59. Lindstedt G, Nystrom E, Matthews C, et al;
Follitropin (FSH) deficiency in an infertile
male due to FSHß gene mutation. A syndrome of normal puberty and virilization but
underdeveloped testicles with azoospermia,
low FSH but high lutropin and normal serum testosterone concentrations, *Clin Chem
Lab Med.* 1998;36:663–665.

60. Layman LC, Porto LAA, Xie J et al. FSHß
gene mutations in a female with partial
breast development and a male sibling with
normal puberty and azoospermia. *J Clin
Endocrinol Metab..* 2002;87(8):3702–3707.

61. Phillip M, Arbelle JE, Segev Y. Male
hypogonadism due to a mutation in the
gene for the beta-subunit of follicle-stimulating hormone. *N Engl J Med.*
1998;338(24):1729–1732.

62. Tapanainen JS, Aittomaki K, Min J, et al.
Men homozygous for an inactivating mutation of the follicle-stimulating hormone
(FSH) receptor gene present variable suppression of spermatogenesis and fertility. *Nat
Genet.* 1997;15:205–206.

63. Latronico A, Anasti J, Arnhold I, et al. Testicular and ovarian resistance to luteinizing
hormone caused by inactivating mutations
of the luteinizing hormone-receptor gene.
N Engl J Med. 1996;334:507–512.

64. Kremer H, Kraaij R, Toledo SP, et al. Male
pseudohermaphroditism due to a homozy-

gous missense mutation of the luteinizing hormone receptor gene. *Nat Genet.* 1995;9:160–164.

65. Misrahi M, Meduri G, Pissard S, et al. Comparison of immunocytochemical and molecular features with the phenotype in a case of incomplete male pseudohermaphroditism associated with a mutation of the luteinizing hormone receptor. *J Clin Endocrinol Metab.* 82: 2159–2165, 1997.

66. Tanner SM, Miller DW, Alongi C. Anabolic steroid use by adolescents: prevalence, motives, and knowledge of risks. *Clin J Sport Med.* 1995;5:108–115.

67. Palfi S, Ungurean A, Vecsei L. Basilar artery occlusion associated with anabolic steroid abuse in a 17-year-old bodybuilder. *Eur Neurol.* 1997;37:190–191.

68. Malone DA, Jr., Dimeff RJ. The use of fluoxetine in depression associated with anabolic steroid withdrawal. a case series. *J Clin Psychiatry.* 1992; 53:130–132.

69. Diamond F Jr, Ringenberg L, MacDonald D, et al. Effects of drug and alcohol abuse upon pituitary-testicular function in adolescent males. *J Adolesc Health Care.* 1986;7:28–33.

70. Block RI, Farinpour R, Schlechte JA. Effects of chronic marijuana use on testosterone, luteinizing hormone, follicle stimulating hormone, prolactin and cortisol in men and women. *Drug Alcohol Depend.* 1991;28:121–8.

71. Yamamoto Y, Yamamoto K, Hayase T, et al. Methamphetamine induces apoptosis in seminiferous tubules in male mice testis. *Toxicol Appl Pharmacol.* 2002;178:155–60.

72. Mendelson JH, Sholar MB, Mutschler NH, et al. Effects of intravenous cocaine and cigarette smoking on luteinizing hormone, testosterone, and prolactin in men. *J Pharmacol Exp Ther.* 2003;307:339–48.

73. Lowe X, Eskenazi B, Nelson DO, et al. Frequency of XY sperm increases with age in fathers of boys with Klinefelter syndrome. *Am J Hum Genet.* 2001;69:1046–1054.

74. Mandoki MW, Sumner GS, Hoffman RP, et al. A review of Klinefelter's syndrome in children and adolescents. *J Am Acad Child Adolesc Psychiatry.* 1991;30:167–72.

75. Bender BG, Linden MG, Robinson A. Neuropsychological impairment in 42 adolescents with sex chromosome abnormalities. *Am J Med Genet.* 1993;48:169–173.

76. Wikstrom AM, Raivio T, Hadziselimovic F, et al. Klinefelter syndrome in adolescence: onset of puberty is associated with accelerated germ cell depletion. *J Clin Endocrinol Metab.* 2004;89:2263–2270.

77. Hasle H, Mellemgaard A, Nielsen J, et al. Cancer incidence in men with Klinefelter syndrome. *Br J Cancer.* 1995;71:416–420.

78. Shen D, Liu D, Liu H, et al. Automated morphometric study of brain variation in XXY males. *Neuroimage.* 2004;23:648–653.

79. Patwardhan AJ, Eliez S, Bender B, et al. Brain morphology in Klinefelter syndrome: extra X chromosome and testosterone supplementation. *Neurology.* 2000: 54:2218–2223.

80. Gilliland WR, Stashower ME. Klinefelter's syndrome and systemic lupus erythematosus. *Clin Exp Rheumatol.* 2000; 18:107–109.

81. Lahita RG. Sex hormones and systemic lupus erythematosus. *Rheum Dis Clin North Am.* 2000;26:951–968.

82. Schiff JD, Palermo GD, Veeck LL, et al. Success of testicular sperm injection and intracytoplasmic sperm injection in men with Klinefelter syndrome. *J Clin Endocrinol Metab.* 2005;90:6263–6267.

83. Tartaglia M, Cordeddu V, Chang H, et al. Paternal germline origin and sex-ratio distortion in transmission of PTPN11 mutations in Noonan syndrome. *Am J Hum Genet.* 2004;75:492–497.

84. Tartaglia M, Kalidas K, Shaw A, et al. PTPN11 mutations in Noonan syndrome: molecular spectrum, genotype-phenotype correlation, and phenotypic heterogeneity. *Am J Hum Genet.* 2002;70:1555–1563.

85. Araki T, Mohi MG, Ismat FA, et al. Mouse model of Noonan syndrome reveals cell type- and gene dosage-dependent effects of Ptpn11 mutation. *Nat Med.* 2004;10: 849–857.

86. Jongmans M, Sistermans EA, Rikken A, et al. Genotypic and phenotypic characterization of Noonan syndrome: new data and review of the literature. *Am J Med Genet.* 2005;134:165–170.

87. Elsawi MM, Pryor JP, Klufio G, et al. Genital tract function in men with Noonan syndrome. *J Med Genet.* 1994; 31:468–470.

88. Bertola DR, Carneiro JD, D'Amico EA, et al. Hematological findings in Noonan syndrome. *Rev Hosp Clin Fac Med Sao Paulo.* 2003;58:5–8.

89. Stikkelbroeck NM, Otten BJ, Pasic A, et al. High prevalence of testicular adrenal rest tumors, impaired spermatogenesis, and Leydig cell failure in adolescent and adult males with congenital adrenal hyperplasia. *J Clin Endocrinol Metab.* 2001;86(12):5721–5728.

90. Yeung CK, Tam YH, Chan YL, et al. A new management algorithm for impalpable undescended testis with gadolinium enhanced magnetic resonance angiography. *J Urol.* 1999;162:998–1002.

91. Davenport M, Brain C, Vandenberg C, et al. The use of the hCG stimulation test in the endocrine evaluation of cryptorchidism. *Br J Urol.* 1995;76:790–794.

92. Engeler DS, Hosli PO, John H, et al. Early orchiopexy: prepubertal intratubular germ cell neoplasia and fertility outcome. *Urology* 2000; 56:144–8.

93. Brown JJ, Wacogne I, Fleckney S, et al. Achieving early surgery for undescended testes: quality improvement through a multifaceted approach to guideline implementation. *Child Care Health Dev.* 2004;30:97–102.

94. Oh J, Landman J, Evers A, et al. Management of the postpubertal patient with cryptorchidism: an updated analysis. *J Urol.* 2002;167:1329–33.

95. Raman JD, Schlegel PN. Testicular sperm extraction with intracytoplasmic sperm injection is successful for the treatment of nonobstructive azoospermia associated with cryptorchidism. *J Urol.* 2003; 170:1287–1290.

96. Schwentner C, Oswald J, Kreczy A, et al. Neoadjuvant gonadotropin-releasing hormone therapy before surgery may improve the fertility index in undescended testes: a prospective randomized trial. *J Urol.* 2005; 173:974–7.

97. Puri P, Barton D, O'Donnell B. Prepubertal testicular torsion: subsequent fertility. *J Pediatr Surg.* 1985; 20:598–601.

98. Vatta S, Cigui I, Demori E, et al. Fragile X syndrome, mental retardation and macroorchidism. *Clin Genet.* 1998;54:366–367.

99. Coutant R, Lumbroso S, Rey R, et al. Macroorchidism due to autonomous hyperfunction of Sertoli cells and G(s)alpha gene mutation: an unusual expression of McCune-Albright syndrome in a prepubertal boy. *J Clin Endocrinol Metab.* 2001;86:1778–1781.

100. Schiff J, Kelly C, Goldstein M, et al. Managing varicoceles in children: results with microsurgical varicocelectomy. *BJU Int* 2005;95:399–402.

101. Smith EP, Boyd J, Frank GR, et al. Estrogen resistance caused by a mutation in the estrogen-receptor gene in a man. *N Engl J Med.* 1994;331:1056–1061.

102. Sudhir K, Chou TM, Chatterjee K, et al. Premature coronary artery disease associated with a disruptive mutation in the estrogen receptor gene in a man. *Circulation.* 1997;96:3774–3777.

103. Morishima A, Grumbach M, Simpson E, et al. Aromatase deficiency in male and female siblings caused by a novel mutation and the physiological role of estrogens. *J Clin Endocrinol Metab.* 1995;80:3689–3698.

104. Hopps CV, Mielnik A, Goldstein M, et al. Detection of sperm in men with Y chromosome microdeletions of the AZFa, AZFb and AZFc regions. *Hum Reprod.* 2003;18:1660–1665.

105. Simoni M, Weinbauer GF, Gromoll J, et al. Role of FSH in male gonadal function. *Ann Endocrinol.* (Paris) 1999;60:102–106.

106. Afzelius BA. Genetics and pulmonary medicine. 6. Immotile cilia syndrome: past, present, and prospects for the future. *Thorax.* 1998;53:894–897.

107. Imamura E. Phimosis of infants and young children in Japan. *Acta Paediatr Jpn.* 1997; 39:403–405.

108. Oster J. Further fate of the foreskin. Incidence of preputial adhesions, phimosis, and smegma among Danish schoolboys. *Arch Dis Child.* 1968;43:200–203.

109. Gairdner D. The fate of the foreskin, a study of circumcision. *Br Med J.* 1949; 2: 1433–1437.

110. Zampieri N, Corroppolo M, Camoglio FS, et al. Phimosis: stretching methods with or without application of topical steroids? *J Pediatr.* 2005; 147:705–706.

111. Masood S, Patel HR, Himpson RC, et al. Penile sensitivity and sexual satisfaction after circumcision: are we informing men correctly? *Urol Int.* 2005;75:62–66.

112. Colapinto J. *As Nature Made Him: The Boy Who Was Raised as a Girl.* New York: HarperCollins Publishers; 2000:xvii.

113. Mitchell ME. Bladder exstrophy repair: complete primary repair of exstrophy. *Urology* 2005;65:5–8.

114. Utsch B, Albers N, Ludwig M. Genetic and molecular aspects of hypospadias. *Eur J Pediatr Surg.* 2004; 14:297–302.

115. Silver RI. Endocrine abnormalities in boys with hypospadias. *Adv Exp Med Biol.* 2004;545:45–72.

116. Stoll C, Alembik Y, Roth MP, et al. Genetic and environmental factors in hypospadias. *J Med Genet.* 1990; 27:559–563.

117. Dolk H. Rise in prevalence of hypospadias. *Lancet.* 1998;351:770.

118. Kubin M, Wagner G, Fugl-Meyer AR. Epidemiology of erectile dysfunction. *Int J Impot Res* 2003; 15:63–71.

119. Mori MM, Cedenho AP, Koifman S, et al. Sperm characteristics in a sample of healthy adolescents in Sao Paulo, Brazil. *Cad Saude Publica.* 2002;18:525–530.

120. Ankarberg-Lindgren C, Norjavaara E. Changes of diurnal rhythm and levels of total and free testerone secretion from pre to late puberty in boys: testis size of 3 ml is a transition stage to puberty. *Eur J Endocrinol.* 2004; 151:747–757.

121. Chalapathi G, Rao KL, Chowdhary SK, et al. Testosterone therapy in microphallic hypospadias: topical or parenteral? *J Pediatr Surg.* 2003;38:221–223.

122. Charmandari E, Dattani MT, Perry LA, et al. Kinetics and effect of percutaneous administration of dihydrotestosterone in children. *Horm Res.* 2001;56:177–181.

123. Main KM, Schmidt IM, Toppari J, et al. Early postnatal treatment of hypogonadotropic hypogonadism with recombinant human FSH and LH. *Eur J Endocrinol.* 2002;146:75–79.

124. Levy JB, Husmann DA. Micropenis secondary to growth hormone deficiency: does treatment with growth hormone alone result in adequate penile growth? *J Urol,* 1996;156:214–216.

125. Sutherland RS, Kogan BA, Baskin LS, et al. The effect of prepubertal androgen exposure on adult penile length. *J Urol.* 1996;156:783–787.

CHAPTER 38

Adolescent Menstrual Disorders

Hilary Smith, MD
Mitchell P. Rosen, MD
Marcelle I. Cedars, MD

NORMAL MENSTRUAL PHYSIOLOGY

Anatomy and Embryology of the Ovary

The main functions of mature ovaries are to generate a fertilizable ovum each month and to prepare the endometrium for implantation through the sequential release of estrogen and progesterone. The sexually mature ovary is approximately 3.3 cm³ in volume. It consists of three structurally distinct regions: 1) the outer cortex containing the surface germinal epithelium and follicles, 2) a central medulla consisting of stroma, and 3) a hilum around the area of attachment of the ovary to the mesovarium. The ovarian follicle, composed of the egg and surrounding granulosa and theca cells, is the fundamental functional unit of the ovary (Table 38-1).

By week 5 of gestation, premeiotic germ cells, which originate outside of the embryo proper, arrive at the genital ridge and are termed oogo-nia. Through three separate processes of mitosis, meiosis, and oogonial atresia, these oogonia gradually evolve to form primary oocytes. The number of primary oocytes reaches a peak of 5 to 7 million at approximately 5 months of gestation. Through the process of atresia, this number decreases to 1 to 2 million by birth and to approximately 500,000 by the first menses. The ovary is perhaps most unique for its continuous process of atresia. This process begins in utero and continues, without regeneration, until a woman reaches the point of menopause, around the fifth decade of life, when approximately 1,000 oocytes remain. Throughout life only 400 to 500 follicles, less than 1% of the total number, will ovulate.

Once formed, the primary oocyte will persist in the stage of prophase of the first meiotic division until the time of ovulation when meiosis is resumed. The primary oocyte then evolves into a secondary oo-cyte and the first polar body is formed and extruded. The change occurs just prior to ovulation but after the luteinizing hormone (LH) surge. At ovulation, the secondary oo-cyte and the surrounding granulosa cells (cumulus oophorus) are extruded from the ovary. If penetrated by a sperm, the secondary oocyte will undergo a second meiotic division after which the second polar body is extruded.

The Normal Menstrual Cycle

The menstrual cycle is divided into two main phases: the follicular (proliferative) phase and the luteal (secretory) phase. The follicular phase begins on day 1 of the cycle, with the onset of menses, and ends on the day of the LH surge. It is characterized by growth and maturation of the dominant follicle and by buildup of the uterine endometrium. The luteal phase begins on the day of the LH surge and ends at the onset of the next menses. Ovulation occurs at the beginning of this phase. The primary luteal phase hormone is progesterone. This is secreted by the corpus luteum, which is formed from the follicular cells remaining after release of the oocyte.

TABLE 38-1 Chapter Vocabulary

Amenorrhea–absence of menarche by age 16 or no menses for >3 cycles or >6 months in an individual who previously had cyclic menses

Atresia–the degeneration and resorption of one or more ovarian follicles

Corpus luteum–formed by luteinization of the remaining theca and granulosa cells of the dominant follicle after ovulation; produces progesterone and estrogen during the luteal phase

Chronic anovulation–repetitive *ovulation* failure, which differs from *ovarian* failure in that viable oocytes remain in the ovary

Dysfunctional uterine bleeding (DUB)–noncyclic, nonovulatory bleeding unrelated to anatomic lesions or systemic disease

Dysmenorrhea–a condition marked by painful menstruation

Hematocolpos–sequestration of blood in the vagina with imperforate hymen

Luteinization–the transformation of the mature ovarian follicle into a corpus luteum

Menometrorrhagia–prolonged (>7 days) or excessive (>80 cc) bleeding occurring *irregularly* at more frequent than normal intervals

Menorrhagia–prolonged (>7 days) or excessive (>80 cc) bleeding occurring at *regular intervals* (21–28 days)

Menstruation–the monthly discharge of blood from the uterus of nonpregnant women from puberty to menopause

Metrorrhagia (intermenstrual bleeding)–uterine bleeding between expected menstrual periods ("spotting," "breakthrough bleeding")

Oligomenorrhea–bleeding occurring at intervals of >35 days but <6 months

Polymenorrhea–bleeding occurring at intervals of <21 days

Progesterone withdrawal test–oral medroxyprogesterone acetate (Provera) is given as 10 mg daily for 7–10 days; withdrawal bleeding within 2 week of the last dose indicates an estrogenized endometrium

Adolescent Menstrual Disorders

AT-A-GLANCE

The normal menstrual cycle is a tightly regulated system of both inhibitory and stimulatory signals that function to select, mature, and release a single oocyte through the process of monthly ovulation. Menstrual disorders are among the most frequent gynecologic complaints of adolescents.

Most abnormal bleeding in adolescents is physiologic dysfunctional uterine bleeding (DUB) due to immaturity of the hypothalamic-pituitary-ovarian axis, leading to anovulatory cycles. This is especially common during the first 12 to 18 months after menarche, but anovulation can occur in 50% to 80% of girls 2 years after menarche, and in more than 20% of girls it can persist until 5 years after menarche. Anovulatory bleeding generally occurs irregularly and is not accompanied by typical premenstrual symptoms associated with ovulatory bleeding (breast tenderness, water weight gain, mood swings, and cramping). Exceptionally heavy bleeding may be a manifestation of severe DUB, but may also occur with clotting disorders.

Lack of menses by the age of 16 is defined as primary amenorrhea, whereas secondary amenorrhea is defined as the absence of menses for more than three cycles or 6 months in women who previously had menses. Disorders leading to amenorrhea, which are associated with delayed puberty or gonadal failure, are discussed in Chapter 36 and are not covered here. Other causes of amenorrhea or abnormal uterine bleeding in this age group include pregnancy, infection, the use of hormonal contraceptives, stress (psychogenic or exercised induced), eating disorders, endocrine disorders (hypothyroidism, hyperprolactinemia), and anatomic defects of the vagina or uterus. When accompanied by signs of hyperandrogenism, polycystic ovary syndrome (PCOS) is the most common cause.

CONDITION	OCCURRENCE	CAUSE
Adolescent Menstrual Complaints		
Dysfunctional Uterine Bleeding (DUB)	Extremely common in 2–5 years post menarche	Immaturity of the HPO axis, anovulation leading to unopposed estrogen
Menometrorrhagia	Rare	Severe DUB or bleeding disorder
Menorrhagia	Rare except for thyroid disease	Bleeding disorder, systemic disorder, thyroid disease, structural lesions
Metrorrhagia (intermenstrual bleeding)	Relatively common in adolescents on oral contraception	Problems with oral contraceptives (too low an estrogen dose, missed pills, irregular timing, drug interactions), progesterone only contraception, sexually transmitted disease, cervical lesions, foreign bodies (retained tampons)
Dysmenorrhea	60%–93% of adolescent females	Excess production of endometrial prostaglandins cause dysrhythmic uterine contraction, hypercontractility, increased uterine muscle tone, uterine ischemia and pain; secondary dysmenorrhea from pelvic pathology is more rare, includes endometriosis, pelvic inflammatory disease, ovarian cysts and tumors, congenital malformations of the reproductive tract, intrauterine contraceptive devices
Amenorrhea Without Androgen Excess		
Pregnancy	Common	Most common cause of amenorrhea in postpubertal girls
Functional amenorrhea	15%–35% of amenorrhea	Reduced GnRH pulse frequency and amplitude, leading to low or low-normal serum levels of FSH and LH and subsequent anovulation; related to stress, excessive exercise, or excessive weight loss
Amenorrhea in female athletes	Common in competitive athletes	The neuroendocrine abnormalities are similar to those of women with functional hypothalamic amenorrhea but may be more severe; severe suppression of GnRH, with low E_2
Eating disorders and malnutrition	0.1–3%	*Anorexia nervosa* characterized by relentless dieting in pursuit of a thin body habitus, severe reduction in GnRH pulsatility and FSH/LH secretion, anovulation, $\downarrow E_2$, $\uparrow$ACTH, and cortisol, $\downarrow$leptin, normal TSH and T_4 but $\downarrow T_3$ and $\uparrow$rT3, high mortality rate (6%–20%); *Bulimia* defined as binge eating followed by self-induced purging; weight is generally more normal, neuroendocrine abnormalities similar to but less severe than anorexia nervosa; *"Social thinness"* has less severe metabolic derangements, differs from classic eating disorders in that body image is positive, abnormally low body weight maintained for social reasons
Hyperprolactinemia	15–30% of amenorrhea	Causes, include pregnancy and breast-feeding, prolactinoma, other CNS lesions, hypothyroidism, renal failure, cirrhosis, chest wall injury/stimulation, seizure, idiopathic, and many drugs

CONDITION	OCCURRENCE	CAUSE
Thyroid disease	1%–2% of women	Both hypo- and hyperthyroid associated with altered LH surge, perhaps related to weight loss and psychologic disturbances; altered metabolic clearance of estradiol, estrone, testosterone, and dihydrotestosterone; primary hypothyroidism associated with ↑ prolactin in one-third of patients
Glucocorticoid excess	Exogenous—common	Whether endogenous or exogenous, it causes menstrual abnormalities by inhibiting GnRH secretion
Amenorrhea associated with obesity	common	Independent of the relation between obesity and PCOS, peripheral conversion of androgens to estrogen results in a hyperestrogenic state related to the degree of excess adiposity
Anatomic amenorrhea	15% of primary amenorrhea	Congenital absence or alteration in the uterus, endometrium, cervix, cervical os, or vagina; the most common are imperforate hymen, transverse vaginal septum, and vaginal agenesis
Amenorrhea With Androgen Excess		
Polycystic ovary syndrome (PCOS)	3%–7% of women of reproductive age	Hyperandrogenemia, anovulation, insulin resistance, and features of the metabolic syndrome are interrelated and it is difficult to determine which is primary
Nonclassic CAH due to 21-hydroxylase def.	1%–19% of women who appear to have PCOS	Autosomal recessive defects in adrenal cortisol synthesis lead to compensatory ACTH secretion and excessive androgen production
Tumor-related androgen excess	Rare	Ovarian androgen secreting tumors cause chronic anovulation and virilization; adrenal adenomas and carcinomas may cause anovulation via androgens but also related to glucocorticoid suppression of the hypothalamic-pituitary axis, they are rare in the adolescent or adult female; ACTH-secreting tumors stimulate both androgen and cortisol excess
Exogenous androgens	Becoming more common	Increasing usage of anabolic steroids for body building and athletic achievement; there are reports of virilization of family members in households where an adult male used testosterone gel

CONDITION	FINDINGS AND CLINICAL PRESENTATION	TREATMENT
Adolescent Menstrual Complaints		
Dysfunctional Uterine Bleeding (DUB)	Irregular, anovulatory cycles, most commonly within the first 2 years but occurring up to 5 years after menarche	Observation and reassurance; oral contraceptive pills
Menometrorrhagia	Heavy flow occurring at irregular intervals, anemia, or shock	Oral contraceptive pills, hospitalization, transfusion
Menorrhagia	Heavy menstrual flow occurring at regular intervals, anemia, or shock	Oral contraceptive pills, hospitalization, transfusion
Metrorrhagia (intermenstrual bleeding)	Irregular bleeding occurring between ovulatory cycles, "spotting" or "breakthrough bleeding"	Increase the estrogen content of oral contraceptives, encourage adherence, pelvic exam to assess for infection or cervical lesions
Dysmenorrhea	Painful lower abdominal cramping sensation often accompanied by sweating, tachycardia, headache, nausea, vomiting, diarrhea, and tremulousness in the absence of pelvic pathology; occurs just prior to the onset of menses and for 1–3 days	Nonsteroidal antiinflammatory agents (NSAIDS), oral contraceptive pills if resistant to NSAIDS
Amenorrhea Without Androgen Excess		
Pregnancy	Nausea, weight gain, urinary frequency, fatigue	Obstetrics/gynecology referral
Functional amenorrhea	Heterogeneous clinical presentation: luteal phase defects to anovulation with erratic bleeding to amenorrhea; FSH:LH ratio may be >1; E_2 may be low; rule out other cause (diagnosis of exclusion)	If no withdrawal bleeding after progesterone, start combined estrogen/progesterone therapy; if withdrawal bleeding occurs, progesterone alone is adequate; treat underlying condition

CONDITION	FINDINGS AND CLINICAL PRESENTATION	TREATMENT
Amenorrhea in female athletes	Competitive athlete with disordered eating, amenorrhea, and osteoporosis; muscular with low body fat (<10%)	As above for functional amenorrhea; evaluate bone mineral density
Eating disorders and malnutrition	—*Anorexia nervosa*: negative distorted body image, weight <85%, fear of weight gain, food preoccupation, hyperactive, obsessive-compulsive, depression, social withdrawal, inflexible, irritability, need for control; palpitations, weakness, dizziness, shortness of breath, constipation; exam will find hypothermia, bradycardia, lanugo, ↓ scalp hair, brittle nails, dry yellowish skin, after puberty at least 3 months of no menses	Multidisciplinary approach that includes nutritional counseling and psychotherapy, consider hospitalization, force-feeding or enteral/parenteral feeding may be necessary; hormone therapy either in the form of hormone replacement or combination contraceptive pills
	—*Bulimics:* may have normal weight, problems with impulse control, substance use, emotional lability and hypersexual activity; teeth may have decalcification due gastric acidic in vomit, amalgams may project above tooth surface	
	—*Social thinness*: may have same physical but not psychologic problems	
Hyperprolactinemia	Menstrual disturbances, galactorrhea, headaches, visual field defects, infertility, and osteopenia; prolactin level >20 ng/mL; may have lesion on MRI or visual field deficit; microadenoma unlikely to progress to macroadenoma (<7% chance)	Dopamine agonist treatment for at least 1 year; transsphenoidal surgery has high recurrence rate (microadenoma <30%, macroadenoma >60%); mild case consider oral contraceptives
Thyroid disease	Non reproductive symptoms described in Chapter 26. Both hypo- and hyperthyroid cause menstrual disorders including excessive bleeding, infertility, and spontaneous abortions; *Hypothyroid*: ↓SHBG, total E_2 and T; *Hyperthyroid*: ↑SHBG, total E_2 and T, but free levels normal in both states	Treatment of hypo- and hyperthyroidism normalizes reproductive abnormalities
Glucocorticoid excess	Amenorrhea or irregular menses along with other typical signs of ↑glucocorticoids	Treat underlying problem, discontinue or ↓ meds if possible, consider combination contraceptive pills
Amenorrhea associated with obesity	May have prolonged cycles of amenorrhea alternating with cycles of metrorrhagia or menometrorrhagia	Treat underlying problem, consider combination contraceptive pills
Anatomic amenorrhea	Primary amenorrhea in a sexually mature girl, cyclic pelvic pain and a perirectal mass resulting from sequestration of blood in the vagina (hematocolpos)	Can be corrected with surgery
	Amenorrhea With Androgen Excess	
Polycystic ovary syndrome	History of premature pubarche or small for gestational age birth; hirsutism, acne, anovulation with amenorrhea or irregular menses; may have hyperlipidemia, hypertension, type 2 diabetes; ovaries may appear polycystic on ultrasound, may have ↑LH:FSH ratio	Treat hyperandrogenism with oral contraceptive pills, may add Lupron or an antiandrogen such as spironolactone; insulin sensitizer such as metformin; cosmetic removal of excess body hair
Nonclassic CAH due to 21-hydroxylase def.	Nonclassic CAH commonly presents with normal female genitalia at birth. Early pubic hair development, bone age advancement, and acceleration of growth may be the presenting symptoms in childhood. In adolescence years clinical manifestations may include hirsutism, menstrual irregularities identical to PCO and infertility during reproductive years. A normal baseline 17-OHP level (<100 ng/dL [3.0 nmol/L]), especially if measured early in the morning (8 AM) and during the follicular phase in a menstruating patient can exclude a diagnosis of nonclassic CAH. A high-dose ACTH stimulation test should be performed for patients with a baseline 17-OHP level above >100 ng/dL (3.0 nmol/L).	Cortisol (only if symptomatic); oral contraceptives and antiandrogens may be useful and depending on the symptoms can alone be used.
Tumor-related androgen excess	Anovulation and virilization; imaging studies and tumor markers may be helpful in differentiating the various tumors; ACTH-secreting and adrenal tumors also have cortisol excess; adrenal tumors tend to have rapid onset of severe symptoms (male pattern baldness, deepening voice, clitoromegaly, and defeminization)	Surgical removal
Exogenous androgens	Virilization and menstrual abnormalities	Identify and remove the source

GnRH = gonadotropin releasing hormone; FSH = follicular stimulating hormone; LH = leutinizing hormone; TSH = thyrotropin stimulating hormone; E_2 = estradiol; T_4 = thyroxin; T_3 = triiodothyronine; rT_3 = reverse triiodothyronine; CAH = congenital adrenal hyperplasia; ACTH = adrenocorticotropic hormone; SHBG = sex hormone binding globulin; T = testosterone.

Menstrual bleeding occurs after the corpus luteum involutes and secretion of estrogen and progesterone tapers.

Menarche (the onset of menses) commences by the age of 16 in most females, with an average age of onset of 12.8 years. Girls have typically matured to a Tanner stage 4 of puberty at the time of menarche. Although some girls immediately establish regular cyclic menses, it is not uncommon for ovulation to be sporadic and menstrual cycles to be irregular for 2 or more years following menarche.

The average mature menstrual cycle is 28 days long, with a range of 24 to 35 days. Anything outside these parameters is considered to be abnormal bleeding. There are approximately 14 days in the follicular phase and 14 days in the luteal phase. Variation in the cycle length tends to be governed by changes in the number of days in the follicular phase, whereas the luteal phase tends to stay relatively constant at 12–15 days.

Menstruation typically occurs over 4 to 6 days and involves the disintegration and sloughing of the functionalis layer of the endometrium. The median blood loss during each menstrual cycle is 30 mL; the upper limit of normal is 60 to 80 mL. Usually, there are no more than 2 days of heavy flow. The average tampon holds 5 cc of blood whereas the average pad holds 5 to 15 cc.

Hormonal Control of the Menstrual Cycle

The three main organs orchestrating the menstrual cycle are the hypothalamus, the pituitary, and the ovary. Through a system of both positive and negative feedback, they work together to produce one follicle and egg targeted for monthly ovulation. The hypothalamic-pituitary-ovarian axis is discussed in detail in Chapter 36. Briefly, the hypothalamus secretes pulsatile gonadotropin-releasing hormone (GnRH), which stimulates the pituitary to release follicle-stimulating hormone (FSH) and LH. These gonadotropins then stimulate oocyte maturation and trigger the ovary to release an oocyte that is capable of fertilization. Concurrently, the ovary secretes hormones that act on the endometrial lining of the uterus to prepare for implantation. The ovarian hormones feed back to the hypothalamus and pituitary, regulating the secretion of gonadotropins during the phases of the menstrual cycle.

Early Follicular Phase

The 1st day of the menses marks the 1st day of the cycle and the start of the follicular phase. This is when the ovary is the least hormonally active and is shown to be quiescent by ultrasound. The inactivity of the ovary results in low levels of estradiol and progesterone, leading to decreased negative feedback inhibition of hypothalamic GnRH and a concomitant rise in pituitary FSH. The rise in FSH actually begins in the late luteal phase prompted by the fall in estradiol and progesterone from the failing corpus luteum. Increased FSH leads to the selection of follicles for this new cycle, one of which will become the dominant follicle and ultimately ovulate. There is also an increase in LH pulse frequency, from one pulse every 4 hours in the late luteal phase, to one pulse every 90 minutes in the early follicular phase.

Mid to Late Follicular Phase

During the midfollicular phase, FSH continues to stimulate estrogen production and progressive growth of the cohort of follicles selected for the cycle. Stromal tissue composed of connective tissue and interstitial cells of mesenchymal origin line the inside of the follicles. This tissue is composed of two main cell types. Theca cells make androgens, which are converted by granulosa cells to estrogens. LH/human chorionic gonadotropin (β-hCG) receptors are expressed primarily on theca cells, whereas FSH receptors are expressed on granulosa cells. LH promotes theca cell production of dehydroepiandrosterone, testosterone, and androstenedione. FSH activates granulosa cell aromatase, which converts the androgens to estrogens, of which estradiol is the most potent. FSH also stimulates granulosa cell production of progesterone from pregnenolone. Rising estrogen levels lead to negative feedback on the pituitary, suppressing production of LH.

Other peptides produced by ovarian granulosa cells under stimulation by FSH include, inhibin, activin, and follistatin. Inhibin and activin are members of the transforming growth factor–β superfamily. There are two forms of inhibin, A and B, which have identical α-subunits but different β-subunits. Both inhibins play a major role in the down-regulation of FSH through direct inhibitory effects on the pituitary. If pregnancy occurs, they are also important in embryonic and fetal development. Inhibin B is largely a product of the granulosa cells during the follicular phase and its levels are an indication of granulosa cell mass and total follicle reserve. Inhibin A is predominantly made by the corpus luteum during the luteal phase of the menstrual cycle. Activin acts in a manner opposite to the inhibins by exerting positive feedback on the pituitary to up-regulate FSH levels. Follistatin is a binding protein for activin and appears to regulate activin function, because the bound complex is not biologically active.

The continually enlarging follicles produce increasing amounts of estradiol and inhibin, which cause FSH levels to fall during the late follicular phase. During this process, a dominant follicle is selected as described below and proceeds to grow larger whereas the others stop developing and undergo a process of atresia.

Luteal Phase: Midcycle Surge and Ovulation

Rising estradiol levels reach a peak 1 day before ovulation. Suddenly there is a switch from an estrogen-exerted negative feedback to a positive feedback on pituitary production of LH leading to a 10-fold increase in LH levels. This phenomenon is referred to as the midcycle LH surge. The LH surge lasts approximately 48 to 50 hours. Thirty-six hours after onset of the LH surge, ovulation occurs.

Mid to Late Luteal Phase

Following the release of the oocyte during ovulation, the dominant follicle reorganizes to become the corpus luteum. The theca and granulosa cells inhabiting the corpus luteum are transformed by the process of luteinization. These cells continue to produce estradiol and progesterone in the late luteal phase.

If the egg becomes fertilized, trophoblast cells begin to make β-hCG, which maintains the corpus luteum. Without β-hCG stimulation, the corpus luteum deteriorates and progesterone and estradiol levels drop, leading to a loss of the endometrial blood supply, endometrial sloughing, and the onset of menses. The fully regressed corpus luteum is soon replaced by an avascular scar, referred to as the corpus albicans. This typically occurs 14 days from the onset of the LH surge.

OVARIAN AND ENDOMETRIAL CHANGES DURING THE MENSTRUAL CYCLE

Follicular Development

At the beginning of each menstrual cycle, approximately 15 to 20 primordial follicles develop into primary follicles. These begin to grow, but generally only one will emerge as the dominant graafian follicle destined for ovulation, and the others will undergo atresia. Early in the menstrual cycle, multiple, small follicles 3 to 8 mm in diameter are seen in the ovary. On approximately day 7, these primary follicles have grown to approximately 9 to 10 mm. By this point, the dominant follicle is enlarging at a rate of approximately 2 mm/day until it reaches its mature size of 20 to 26 mm.

The progression of each cycle to a single mature graafian follicle is a selection process. Rising estrogen levels in the follicular phase exert negative feedback on pituitary release of FSH. The decrease in FSH stimulation promotes follicular atresia. The dominant follicle escapes this effect and continues to grow despite decreasing levels of FSH because it accumulates a greater mass of granulosa cells with more FSH receptors. Simultaneously, increased vascularity of the theca cells allows preferential FSH delivery to the dominant follicle despite waning FSH levels.

Increased estrogen levels towards the end of the follicular phase facilitate FSH induction of LH receptors on the granulosa cells of the graafian follicle, allowing it to respond to the mid-cycle LH surge. The LH surge causes ovulation, whereby the oocyte in the follicle completes its first meiotic division and is subsequently released at the surface of the ovary. This occurs in a period approximately 36 hours from the start of the LH surge. The oocyte is taken up by the fallopian tube and travels down to the uterine cavity.

Uterine Changes

The endometrium consists of two regions. The innermost functionalis undergoes changes throughout the menstrual cycle and is shed during menstruation, whereas the basalis remains unchanged during the menstrual cycle and regenerates the functionalis each month.

Following menstruation, the endometrium is seen on ultrasound as a thin stripe. On approximately day 7 of the cycle, rising estradiol levels lead to proliferation of the functionalis from stem cells of the basalis, with an increase in the quantity of endometrial glands and the surrounding dense stroma. Spiral arteries elongate and span the length of the endometrium. As the follicular phase continues, rising levels of estradiol increase the quantity and fluidity of cervical mucus and the thickness of the endometrium, preparing them for the possibility of sperm penetration and implantation.

Under the influence of progesterone during the luteal phase, there is no further thickening of the endometrium, but its character changes. The endometrial glands become tortuous and have large lumens due to increased secretions. The spiral arteries extend into the superficial layer of the endometrium, which can be seen as an increase in echogenicity on ultrasound. This phase lasts 14 days, ending with either implantation of a fertilized ovum or menstruation.

In the absence of fertilization and resultant β-hCG stimulation, the corpus luteum begins to degenerate and, consequently, ovarian hormone levels decrease. As estrogen and pro-gesterone levels fall, the functionalis undergoes involution. The spiral arteries rupture secondary to vasoconstriction and ischemia, releasing blood into the uterus, and the apoptosed endometrium is sloughed off as the functionalis is completely shed. Menstrual flow contains arterial and venous blood and remnants of endometrial stroma and glands. Vasoconstriction of the spiral arteries is mediated by endothelin and thromboxin. The resulting ischemia may cause menstrual cramps.

ADOLESCENT MENSTRUAL COMPLAINTS

Dysfunctional Uterine Bleeding

Pathogenesis Noncyclic, nonovulatory endometrial bleeding, unrelated to anatomic lesions of the uterus or to systemic disease, is referred to as dysfunctional uterine bleeding (DUB). This is the most common cause of abnormal uterine bleeding in adolescents. In the absence of ovulation, there is no corpus luteum and, thus, no cyclical progesterone secretion. This results in continuous unopposed estradiol production, stimulating overgrowth and proliferation of the endometrium. The endometrium eventually outgrows its blood supply, leading to necrosis and irregular bleeding.

For ovulatory menstrual cycles to occur, the hypothalamic-pituitary-ovarian axis needs to mature, which occurs at different rates in individuals. Approximately 18% to 45% of teens will have ovulatory cycles by 2 years postmenarche, 45% to 70% by 2 to 4 years, and 80% by 4 to 5 years (1,2). This varies depending on the age of menarche; typically the earlier menarche occurs the quicker a girl will reach maturity (3). DUB generally resolves once maturation of the hypothalamic-pituitary-ovarian axis leads to establishment of regular ovulatory cycles (4).

Clinical Presentation DUB can be classified by the degree of bleeding as mild, moderate, or severe.

Mild dysfunctional bleeding is defined as long (>35 days) or short (<21 days) cycles for more than 2 months (5). Most adolescents with DUB fall into this group. Moderate DUB is characterized by prolonged (>7 days) or frequent (every 1–3 weeks) menses (5). Menstrual flow is moderate to heavy and mild anemia (hemoglobin 10–12g/dL) is often present, but without hemodynamic instability or signs of hypovolemia (6). Severe DUB with excessive menstrual flow is described later.

Diagnosis For most girls with mild DUB, a careful history and physical examination are sufficient to exclude a pathologic cause. For DUB, which is moderate or severe, coagulation defects should be considered, and pathological conditions should be excluded including hypo- or hyperthyroidism, exogenous hormone administration, sexually transmitted infections, or cervical anomalies. The diagnosis of DUB should only be used when other medical or structural causes for abnormal uterine bleeding have been ruled out.

Treatment Management of mild DUB consists of observation and reassurance. Keeping a menstrual calendar and following up in 3 to 6 months is recommended (7). With moderate DUB, treatment involves hormonal therapy to stabilize endometrial proliferation and shedding. Iron and folate supplementation should also be considered. Patients can be started on oral contraceptives, especially a combination pill of estrogen and progestin rather than a progestin-only preparation. The estrogen will provide acute hemostasis and stabilize the endometrium (5,8). Pills with a minimum of 30 μg of ethinyl estradiol should be given to ensure enough estrogen to prevent breakthrough bleeding.

For patients with active bleeding, the oral contraceptive pill is typically prescribed to be taken three times per day until the bleeding ceases (usually within 48 hours) (8). Following cessation of the bleeding, the pills are tapered to twice per day for 5 days, and then decreased to once per day to complete the rest of the 21 days of hormone therapy. An alternative is to give three packs of pills. All the placebo pills should be discarded. The first pack is taken as three pills per day, the second pack as two pills per day, and the last pack once daily. This will not only allow a longer bleed-free period but also decrease the amount of the ultimate bleed at the end of the three cycles. It is essential to maintain close follow up and be aware of side effects from high-dose estrogen including nausea, which may lead to noncompliance. (5) Prescriptions for antiemetics may be required to alleviate symptoms of nausea (5).

For all patients, close follow up is required. Prognosis will depend on the cause of the underlying problem (8). Girls with mild bleeding should undergo follow up in 3 to 6 months. With moderate or severe bleeding, follow up should be in 1 to 3 months (7).

Menorrhagia and Menometrorrhagia

Pathogenesis Menorrhagia is defined as heavy menstrual flow occurring at regular intervals, whereas menometrorrhagia is heavy flow occurring at irregular intervals. This may include a flow that is heavy in duration (>7 days) or in volume (>80 mL/cycle). Meno-metrorrhagia is seen with severe DUB. When bleeding occurs at regular intervals or occurs with menarche, it is often related to a bleeding diathesis or other pathology (9–14). Coagulation disorders among adolescents with menorrhagia include von Willebrand disease, Glanzmann thromboasthenia, idiopathic thrombocytopenic purpura, platelet dysfunction, and thrombocytopenia secondary to chemotherapy (9–12,15). Excessive bleeding, in adolescents, may also be related to the use of medications such as anticoagulants or platelet inhibitors or to liver disease.

Less common causes of menorrhagia and menometrorrhagia in adolescents include systemic illnesses, endocrine disorders, and structural lesions. Examples of systemic illnesses that can sometimes affect the ovary and lead to abnormalities in ovulation or coagulation include diabetes mellitus, systemic lupus erythematous, renal failure, malignancy, and myelodysplasia. Hypothyroidism and hyperthyroidism can also lead to heavy menses as well as anovulatory cycles, and decreased levels of factors VII, VIII, IX, and XI may be present with hypothyroidism (16), contributing to excessive bleeding. Structural lesions that cause menorrhagia include cervical polyps and uterine leiomyomas (fibroids); however, these are both rare in teenagers.

Clinical Presentation Menorrhagia and menometrorrhagia are characterized by disruptive normal menstrual cycles with heavy bleeding that causes a decrease in hemoglobin (<10 mg/dL) and may or may not cause hemodynamic instability (5,6). Other signs of bleeding disorders (bruising and petechiae), liver disease, or systemic disorders may be present.

Diagnosis Females who present with an extremely heavy first menses, with bleeding requiring blood transfusion, or with refractory menorrhagia and concomitant anemia, warrant a work up for bleeding dyscrasias. Work up should include a complete blood count with platelets and the examination of the peripheral blood smear to detect anemia or thrombocytopenia, and a coagulation assessment. If bleeding diathesis, thyroid disease, or other chronic or systemic illnesses have been excluded, a pelvic ultrasound should be done to rule out anatomic causes.

Treatment When considering treatment, decisions should be made depending on the degree to which the patient is bleeding. The main goals of treatment for excessive bleeding include: 1) establishment and/or maintenance of hemodynamic stability, 2) correc-

tion of acute or chronic anemia, 3) return to a normal menstrual cycle, 4) prevention of recurrence, and 5) prevention of long-term consequences of anovulation (4,5,17).

Hemodynamically unstable patients (hemoglobin <7 mg/dL or orthostatic changes, or heavy active bleeding and hemoglobin <10 mg/dL) should be hospitalized for stabilization of hemodynamic status, blood transfusion, pharmacologic therapy, and, rarely, surgical therapy (5). The need for blood transfusion is assessed on a case-by-case basis depending on hemoglobin, blood loss, orthostatic vital signs, and the ability to rapidly gain control of bleeding (5,6). When bleeding is this severe, a combination oral contraceptive pill (OCP) with high-dose estrogen, such as a monophasic combination with 50 μg of estradiol and 0.5 mg of norgestrel, is prescribed. The pills can be taken once every four hours until the bleeding subsides, then four times per day for four days, then three times per day for three days, followed by twice per day for two weeks. If bleeding recurs while tapering, then the dose of oral contraceptive pills should be increased to the lowest dose that controls bleeding (8). The regimen described above for DUB with 3 pill packs may also be given. Progestin-only pills are an alternative for patients in whom estrogen is contraindicated (5).

In patients with 1) atrophic bleeding or 2) endometrium progesterone breakthrough bleeding (i.e., patients on progesterone-only pill or long term use of OCP due to overall progesterogenic effect of OCP), or 3) prolonged hemorrhage that has resulted in minimal endometrial residual, estrogen therapy as conjugated estrogen 25 mg intravenously every 4 hours or oral conjugated estrogen 1.25 mg every 4 hours for 24 hours, then once daily for 7 to 10 days may work better. During intravenous estrogen administration, always premedicate for nausea. As soon as the bleeding slows down, OCP therapy is started with monophasic combination with 50 μg of estradiol and 0.5 mg of norgestrel, either as the regimen described above for DUB with three pill packs, or as two pills for 5 to 7 days until bleeding abates and then is continued as one pill per day for 2 weeks.

High-dose estrogen OCP may be continued for several months before decreasing to lower estrogen dose OCP. In patients with very atrophic endometrium lining, conjugated oral estrogen therapy 1.25 mg po daily 7 days along with OCP will rejuvenate the lining. The 7-day conjugated estrogen course may be repeated monthly as needed for up to 4 to 6 months. At that time if endometrium is still atrophic, revaluation is needed. Addition of the oral conjugated estrogen does not change efficacy of the contraception.

In cases of severe menorrhagia, unresponsive to 24 hours of hormonal therapy or in those with platelet dysfunction, nonhormonal hemostatic drugs may be used, including the antifibrinolytics, aminocaproic acid, and desmopressin (18,19). In the rare patient who continues to bleed heavily despite adequate hormonal therapy (20), a dilation and curettage (D&C) may be required as both a diagnostic and a treatment option. When performing the procedure, it is important that steps are taken to prevent Asherman syndrome (scarring of the endometrium) following the procedure (Table 38-2).

Metrorrhagia (Intermenstrual Bleeding)

Metrorrhagia is defined as irregular bleeding occurring between ovulatory cycles. It may also be called "spotting" or "breakthrough bleeding." The most common causes of intermenstrual bleeding include exogenous hormone administration and infections.

Breakthrough bleeding, when using oral or patch contraceptives, is a common cause of abnormal uterine bleeding in adolescents (21) and suggests that the doses of estrogen and progestin in the pill are inadequate for the patient. Most commonly, a relative estrogen deficiency leads to the breakthrough bleeding and thus an oral contraceptive pill with a higher estrogen content should be considered. It is important to keep in mind that breakthrough bleeding may indicate reduced birth control efficacy. Intermenstrual bleeding may also occur if oral contraceptive pills are not taken as prescribed, such as missed pills, varied ingestion times, or drug interactions. For example, phenobarbital, carbamazepine, some penicillins, tetracycline, trimethoprim-sulfamethoxazole may impact estrogen metabolism. Breakthrough bleeding is particularly common with progestin-only compounds for birth control, such as Depo-Provera or the Norplant system (surgically implanted levonorgestrel).

Cervicitis related to sexually transmitted disease is another common cause of acute vaginal bleeding unrelated to menses in sexually active adolescents or girls with a history of sexual abuse. Other less common causes of intramenstrual bleeding in adolescents include cervical polyps or ectropion, foreign bodies (most commonly retained tampons), trauma, and medications (anticoagulants).

Dysmenorrhea

Pathogenesis Dysmenorrhea occurs in 60% to 93% of all adolescent females, making it the most common gynecologic complaint among this age group (22–25). It generally

TABLE 38-2	Treatment of Excessive Uterine Bleeding
Mild	• Observation and reassurance, keep a menstrual calendar.
Moderate –hemoglobin 10–12 mg/dL –hemoglobin 7–10 mg/dL with hemodynamic stability and no active bleeding	• Start oral contraceptive pills with combination estrogen (minimum of 30 µg ethinyl estradiol) and progestin. — With active bleeding, take pill 3 times/day until the bleeding ceases (usually within 48 hours), then taper to 2 times/day for 5 days, then decrease to 1/day to complete the rest of the 21-day pill pack. — OR, give 3 packs of pills. Discard placebo pills. The first pack is taken as 3 pills/day, the second pack as 2 pills/day and the last pack, once daily. — Antiemetics may be necessary. • Provide iron and folate supplementation.

Severe
 	
–hemoglobin <7 mg/dL
–orthostatic changes or heavy active bleeding and hemoglobin <10 mg/dL
	• Hospitalize, transfuse if necessary.
	• Start a combination oral contraceptive pill with high-dose estrogen, such as a monophasic combination with 50 µg of estradiol and 0.5 mg of norgestrel.
	— The pills are taken once every 4 hours until the bleeding subsides, then 4 times/day for 4 days, then 3 times/day for 3 days, followed by 2/day for 2 weeks.
	— If bleeding recurs while tapering, then the dose of oral contraceptive pills should be increased to the lowest dose that controls bleeding.
	— OR, as above, give 3 packs of pills. Discard placebo pills. The first pack is taken as 3 pills/day, the second pack as 2 pills/day and the last pack, 1/day.
	• In patients with
	1) atrophic bleeding, OR
	2) endometrium progesterone breakthrough bleeding (i.e., patients on progesterone only pill or long term use of OCP due to overall progesterogenic effect of OCP), OR
	3) prolonged hemorrhage that has resulted in minimal endometrial residual:
	  –Estrogen therapy as conjugated estrogen 25 mg IV every 4 hours or
	  –Oral conjugated estrogen 1.25 mg every 4 hours for 24 hours, then once daily for 7–10 days may work better.
	• During IV estrogen administration, always pre-medicate for nausea. As soon as the bleeding slows down, OCP therapy is started with monophasic combination with 50 µg of estradiol and 0.5 mg of norgestrel, either as the regimen described above for DUB with 3 pill packs, or as 2 pills for 5–7 days until bleeding abates and then is continued as 1 pill/day for 2 weeks.
	• In cases of severe bleeding unresponsive to 24 hours of hormonal therapy or in patients with platelet dysfunction, nonhormonal hemostatic drugs may be used including the antifibrinolytics, aminocaproic acid, and desmopressin.
	• If patient continues to bleed heavily despite adequate hormonal therapy, a dilation and curettage may be required
	• Provide iron and folate supplementation.

does not occur until ovulatory menstrual cycles are established. It results from the excess production of endometrial prostaglandin F2α or an elevated PGF2α:PGE2 ratio. These compounds cause dysrhythmic uterine contraction, hypercontractility, and increased uterine muscle tone leading to uterine ischemia and pain. They also can stimulate the gastrointestinal tract leading to gastrointestinal symptoms. Factors associated with more severe episodes of dysmenorrhea include earlier age at menarche, long menstrual periods, heavy menstrual flow, smoking, and positive family history.

Secondary dysmenorrhea can result from pelvic pathology, including endometriosis, pelvic inflammatory disease, ovarian cysts and tumors, congenital malformations of the reproductive tract, or intrauterine contraceptive devices. Girls may report midcycle pelvic pain (mittelschmerz), which is related to ovulation.

Clinical Presentation Dysmenorrhea occurs as a painful cramping sensation in the lower abdomen, often accompanied by other symptoms such as sweating, tachycardia, headaches, nausea, vomiting, diarrhea, and tremulousness in the absence of pelvic pathology. Symptoms of dysmenorrhea occur prior to the onset of menses and continue for a period of 1 to 3 days.

Diagnosis When evaluating an adolescent female presenting with menstrual cramps, one begins with a complete medical and menstrual history followed by a thorough physical examination. The history should include age at menarche, duration of menstrual cycles, interval between, onset and duration of cramps, symptoms of nausea, vomiting, diarrhea and their severity; medications, and sexual history. The physical examination should include a pelvic examination and testing for sexually transmitted infections.

Treatment The first line of therapy for dysmenorrhea is nonsteroidal antiinflammatory drugs (NSAIDs) (26–28). The inhibitory effects these drugs have on the production of prostaglandins are often enough to alleviate the symptoms of primary dysmenorrhea and produce effective pain relief in 70% to 90% of patients (29–34). NSAIDs should be started at the onset of menses and continued for the first 1 or 2 days of the menstrual cycle or for the duration of the pain. If symptoms are severe, patients may take the NSAIDs a day or two prior to the onset of menses.

A second line of therapy is the use of OCPs. These are typically reserved for patients who do not respond to NSAIDs. OCPs act by suppressing ovulation, thereby decreasing the prostaglandin levels typically produced by the uterus within a normal menstrual cycle.

All patients should be followed closely for the first few months after treatment has started to evaluate the response to therapy. If treatment options fail, the patient has recurrent pain, or symptoms worsen, the patient should be re-evaluated for a possible secondary cause of dysmenorrhea such as endometriosis (28).

AMENORRHEA

Amenorrhea has been classified as primary or secondary depending on whether the individual experienced menses in the past. This classification may lead to misdiagnosis because most conditions that cause amenorrhea can present both before and after menarche. Each individual should be assessed by means of the history and clinical findings, including the presence or absence of secondary sexual characteristics. Amenorrhea per se does not cause harm, but in the absence of pregnancy it may be a sign of genetic, endocrine, and/or anatomic abnormalities. These aberrations can affect any level of control in the menstrual cycle and thus result in menstrual abnormalities.

The most common causes for primary amenorrhea are chromosomal abnormalities causing gonadal dysgenesis (50%), hypothalamic hypogonadism (20%), absence of the uterus, cervix, and/or vagina (15%), transverse vaginal septum or imperforate hymen (5%), or pituitary disease (5%). The remaining 5% of cases are due to a combination of disorders including androgen insensitivity, congenital adrenal hyperplasia (CAH), and polycystic ovary syndrome (35).

Secondary amenorrhea is defined as the absence of menses for more than three cycles or 6 months in women who previously had menses (20). Anovulation is the most common cause of secondary amenorrhea during the reproductive years. This differs from ovarian failure in that viable oocytes remain in the ovary. Secondary amenorrhea can result from dysfunction of the hypothalamus, pituitary, ovaries, uterus, or vagina. Pregnancy is the most common cause in postpubertal girls.

It is important in anyone who presents with secondary amenorrhea to first rule out pregnancy. This can be achieved through either serum or urine measurement of the β-hCG level. A thorough history includes questions covering recent stressors (functional hypogonadotropic hypogonadism), drugs (dopamine antagonists), development of acne or hirsutism (polycystic ovary syndrome), headaches and/or visual field defects (central nervous system tumor), galactorrhea (prolactinoma, pituitary mass), history of anorexia nervosa and fatigue (pituitary-hypothalamic disease including thyroid-stimulating hormone [TSH] and/or adreno-corticotropic hormone [ACTH] deficiency). Additional complaints in adult women that may occasionally be elicited by history in adolescents include hot flashes, vaginal dryness, poor sleep, decreased libido (ovarian failure), or a history of obstetric catastrophe (Asherman syndrome, Sheehan syndrome). The history should be followed by a physical examination including height and weight, an evaluation of any skin changes, and a pelvic examination. The minimal laboratory testing should include serum prolactin, thyrotropin, free T_4, LH and FSH levels; elevated TSH, low T_4 and normal/ or elevated prolactin suggests primary hypothyroidism, decreased TSH, low T_4, decreased gonadotropins, and normal/ or elevated prolactin suggest hypopituitarism or prolactinoma, where elevated LH and FSH suggest ovarian failure; normal thyroid studies, normal prolactin and decreased FSH, LH with an FSH/LH ratio >1 suggest functional hypothalamic amenorrhea or hypogonadotropic hypogonadism.

Disorders of hypothalamic GnRH or pituitary gonadotropin secretion (hypogonadotropic hypogonadism) and ovarian failure (hypergonadotropic hypogonadism) are covered in detail in Chapter 36. Disorders that play a particularly important role in adolescent menstrual dysfunction are described here in separate sections divided by the absence or presence of androgen excess.

AMENORRHEA AND ABNORMAL UTERINE BLEEDING NOT ASSOCIATED WITH ANDROGEN EXCESS

Functional Hypothalamic Amenorrhea

Pathogenesis Functional hypothalamic amenorrhea is one of the most common causes of amenorrhea, accounting for 15% to 35% of cases. It is an endocrine disorder, although the exact mechanism has not been definitively determined. It is characterized by reduced GnRH pulse frequency and amplitude, leading to low or low-normal serum levels of FSH and LH and subsequent anovulation. The ratio of serum FSH and LH in these patients is often equivalent to that of a prepubertal female with a relative FSH predominance. The cause of functional hypothalamic amenorrhea often remains unclear, but psychologic stress, strenuous exercise, and poor nutrition have all been implicated. Chronic medical conditions may also lead to this disorder.

The importance of stress or chronic strenuous exercise in functional hypogonadism is suggested by the slightly increased serum cortisol levels found in these women. The inciting event may be the excessive production of corticotropin-releasing hormone, which has been shown to decrease the pulse frequency of GnRH and increase cortisol levels in vivo. Patients with functional hypothalamic amenorrhea are often high achievers who have dysfunctional coping mechanisms when dealing with daily stress.

The relation between nutritional status and functional hypothalamic amenorrhea may be mediated by the adipocyte hormone leptin (36,37). Leptin is an important nutritional satiety factor, but it is also necessary for maturation of the reproductive system. The potential link to the reproductive system is thought to be through leptin receptors, which have been identified in the hypothalamus and on the gonadotropes. This is supported by the observation that leptin can stimulate GnRH pulsatility and gonadotropin secretion. Several studies suggest that women with functional hypothalamic amenorrhea have lower serum leptin levels in comparison with eumenorrheic controls. This relative deficiency may lead to dysfunctional release of GnRH. Leptin levels are related to body fat, and sufficient body fat (generally found in women who are at least 85% ideal body weight) is necessary for normal menstrual cycles.

Clinical Presentation Psychologic stress, strenuous exercise, and poor nutrition may act synergistically to suppress GnRH drive. The significant inter-patient variability in the degree of psychologic or metabolic stress required to induce menstrual disturbances explains the clinical heterogeneity, which range from luteal phase defects to anovulation with erratic bleeding to amenorrhea.

Diagnosis The diagnosis of functional hypothalamic amenorrhea can be made if the FSH:LH ratio is greater than 1 in the presence of hypoestrogenemia (38). A minor disturbance of hypothalamic function may be present in a young woman with normal laboratory results, a clinical history that coincides with "stress," and a negative evaluation for other causes of anovulation. Functional hypothalamic amenorrhea is frequently a diagnosis of exclusion. Interestingly, many of these patients, while hypoestrogenic, do not experience as hot flashes. Given the strong correlation between hypoestrogenemia and the development of osteoporosis, estrogen status should be evaluated by means of the progesterone withdrawal test or by measurement of the serum estradiol level, which should be greater than 50 pg/mL in a sexually mature young woman.

Treatment If there is no bleeding after progesterone withdrawal therapy (10 medroxyprogesterone orally daily for 10 days, the first 10 days of the month for 3 months), hormone replacement should be instituted. The various estrogen/progesterone regimens are discussed in Chapter 36. If withdrawal bleeding occurs, any cyclic progestin-containing therapy will be adequate to combat unopposed estrogen and the development of endometrial hyperplasia.

Functional hypothalamic amenorrhea is reversible. The factors that have best predicted the rate of recovery are body mass index and basal cortisol levels. When patients recover, ovulation is preceded by return of cortisol levels to baseline. Some experts have shown that cognitive behavioral therapy teaches the patient how to cope with stress and that nutritional consultation helps reverse this condition.

Amenorrhea in the Female Athlete

Pathogenesis The female athletic triad, as defined by the American College of Sports Medicine, is characterized by disordered eating, amenorrhea, and osteoporosis. The neuroendocrine abnormalities are similar to those of women with functional hypothalamic amenorrhea. There is evidence that a negative correlation between body fat and menstrual irregularities exists. In addition, there appears to be a critical body fat level that must be present to have a functioning reproductive system. Several studies have shown that amenorrheic athletes have significantly lower serum leptin levels, which further supports leptin's role as a mediator between nutritional status and the reproductive system. The strenuous exercise in which these athletes engage amplifies the effects of the associated nutritional deficiency. This synergism causes severe suppression of GnRH, leading to low estradiol levels.

Amenorrhea alone is not harmful; however, low serum estradiol, over a period of time, may lead to osteoporosis.

Clinical Presentation Competitive athletes in events such as gymnastics, ballet, marathon running, and diving can show menstrual irregularities ranging from luteal phase defects to amenorrhea. These patients have very low body fat, often below the 10th percentile.

Diagnosis and Treatment An analysis of estrogen status may be obtained with measurement of serum estradiol levels and with the progesterone withdrawal test. If estrogen is low, a bone mineral density scan should be performed. Patients diagnosed with female athletic triad need combination contraceptive therapy or hormone replacement.

Amenorrhea Associated with Eating Disorders and Malnutrition

Pathogenesis There is a continuum of disordered eating and nutritional deficiencies ranging from socially "fashionable" thinness to anorexia nervosa, and resulting in increasingly severe abnormalities in the reproductive system. The age at onset impacts the potential complications of these disorders. If these conditions occur prior to puberty, stunted growth and delayed development of secondary sexual characteristics may occur. If low estradiol levels are present before age 20, bone mineralization may be profoundly affected because this period is critical for accrual of peak bone mass. The prognosis for recovery is worse for patients with hypogonadotropic dysfunction due to nutritional disorders compared to that caused by excessive exercise.

Anorexia nervosa is a disorder characterized by relentless dieting in pursuit of a thin body habitus. These individuals have a negative and distorted body image, believing themselves to be "fat" despite emanciation. Approximately 95% of cases are females, with onset mainly in adolescence. Severe reduction in GnRH pulsatility leads to suppression of FSH and LH secretion, sometimes to undetectable levels, and results in anovulation and low serum estradiol levels. Given the severe psychologic and metabolic stress experienced by these individuals, the hypothalamic-pituitary-adrenal axis is affected. The circadian rhythm of adrenal secretion is maintained, but both cortisol production and plasma cortisol levels are persistently elevated secondary to increased pituitary secretion of ACTH. Serum leptin levels in these individuals are significantly lower than those of normal healthy controls and correlate with percentage of body fat and body weight. A rise in leptin levels in response to dietary treatment is associated with a subsequent rise in gonadotropin levels.

The self-induced starvation state associated with anorexia nervosa leads to additional endocrine abnormalities not observed in other causes of hypothalamic amenorrhea. Thyroid hormone metabolism is altered. TSH and T_4 levels are in the low-normal range, but T_3 levels are usually below normal. This is attributable to decreased peripheral conversion of T_4 to T_3 and increased conversion of T_4 to the metabolically inactive thyroid hormone, reverse T_3—a change that resembles other states of starvation. This may be a protective mechanism in that the relative hypothyroid state attempts to reduce basal metabolic function in response to a highly catabolic state.

Bulimia occurs in approximately half of anorectic patients and is defined as binge eating followed by self-induced purging (vomiting, laxative use, and enemas). Purging behaviors generally occur at least weekly. They also have a variety of neuroendocrine aberrations, albeit often to a lesser degree than those with anorexia, which lead to menstrual disturbances. Leptin levels are lower than in matched controls but not as low as in individuals with anorexia nervosa. They also have neurotransmitter abnormalities—notably low serotonin levels—which might help explain the often-coexisting psychologic difficulties.

"Social thinness" may also cause amenorrhea or oligomenorrhea. In contrast to patients with classic eating disorders, these young women have a positive body image, and maintain an abnormally low body weight for social reasons.

Clinical Presentation The clinical features of anorexia nervosa include extreme weight loss leading to a body weight less than 85% of normal for age and height, a distorted body image, and intense fear of gaining weight. These patients usually have a preoccupation with food and are hyperactive, with an obsessive–compulsive personality. Other characteristics of anorexia nervosa include depression, social withdrawal, inflexible thinking, irritability, and a need for control.

Patients may complain of palpitations, weakness, dizziness, shortness of breath, chest pain, constipation, or coldness of the extremities. On physical examination, in addition to severe underweight, hypothermia and bradycardia may be noted. The skin may develop lanugo, characterized by downy soft body hair on the face, forearms, and other surfaces of the body. This may be accompanied by a loss of scalp hair. Brittle nails and dry skin may be present with a yellowish discoloration, probably secondary to carotenemia. Furthermore, as part of the diagnostic criteria after puberty, patients must experience at least 3 months of no menses.

Not all bulimics have low body weight—in fact, normal-weight bulimic individuals are much more common. Compared with patients with isolated anorexia nervosa, these girls tend to have more problems with impulse control, substance use, emotional lability and hypersexual activity. Teeth in patients who engage in purging may have decalcification of the lingual, palatal, and posterior occlusal surfaces due to the effects of the acidic gastric contents of vomit. The amalgams, which are resistant to acid, may end up projecting above the surface of the teeth.

Diagnosis The diagnosis may often be made by history and physical examination, but other causes of malabsorption and malnutrition must be excluded, including celiac disease, inflammatory bowel disease, and cystic fibrosis.

Treatment Anorexia nervosa is a life-threatening illness with a significant mortality rate (6%–20% of deaths are from suicide or from complications of starvation and refeeding). Anorexic patients should be considered for inpatient therapy and management with a multidisciplinary approach that includes nutritional counseling and psychotherapy. Force-feeding may be necessary in some patients. If weight gain cannot be achieved with oral intake, meals may need to be supplemented by enteral or parenteral feeding.

Because anorexia nervosa is a hypoestrogenic state and there is a high potential for the development of osteoporosis, all patients should receive hormone therapy either in the form of hormone replacement or combination contraceptive pills. Evidence exists that when caloric intake is sufficient to match energy expenditure, patients will resume normal menstrual cycles (39,40).

Hyperprolactinemia

Pathogenesis Hyperprolactinemia is one of the most common causes of amenorrhea, accounting for 15% to 30% of cases. Although normal prolactin secretion is regulated by several stimulatory and inhibitory factors, it is primarily under tonic inhibition by dopamine. Any interference with dopamine synthesis or transport from the hypothalamus may result in elevated prolactin levels.

The mechanism by which hyperprolactinemia causes amenorrhea is not completely known. Studies have shown that prolactin can affect the reproductive system in several ways. Prolactin receptors have been identified on GnRH neurons and may directly suppress GnRH secretion (41). It has been postulated that elevated prolactin levels inhibit GnRH pulsatility indirectly by increasing other neuromodulators such as endogenous opioids. There is also evidence that GnRH receptors on the pituitary may be down regulated in the presence of excess prolactin. The best data now available suggest that hyperprolactinemia causes amenorrhea primarily by suppression of GnRH secretion.

Approximately half of patients with elevated prolactin levels have radiologic evidence of a pituitary tumor. The most common type is a prolactin-secreting tumor (prolactinoma). Prolactinomas are mainly composed of lactotrophs; rarely, however, these tumors may be mixed with other cell types present in the pituitary, most commonly secreting both growth hormone and prolactin. Prolactinomas are categorized into two groups based on their dimensions: microadenomas are those less than 10 mm in diameter and macroadenomas are 10 mm or larger. They are typically located in the lateral wings of the anterior pituitary. Rarely will a microadenoma infiltrate the surrounding tissue, including the dura, cavernous sinus, or adjacent skull base. A macroadenoma may expand farther and grow out of the sella to impinge on surrounding structures, including cranial nerve areas such as the optic chiasm, or may extend into the sphenoid sinus. As a result, macroadenomas are more frequently associated with severe headaches, visual field defects, and ophthalmoplegia. The incidence of a microadenoma regular lettering to a macroadenoma is relatively low, only 3% to 7%.

Other tumors of nonpituitary origin may also result in delayed puberty and amenorrhea. The most common of these is craniopharyngioma. Although they are most often located in the suprasellar region, anatomically these tumors originate from the anterior surface of the pituitary and they can distort the infundibulum of the pituitary. This tumor has not been shown to produce hormones, but because it may compress the infundibulum, it can interfere with the tonic inhibition of prolactin and result in mildly elevated prolactin levels.

Other causes of elevated prolactin are listed in Table 38-3. Hyperprolactinemia has been observed in several chronic diseases, including cirrhosis and renal disease. Furthermore, inflammatory diseases such as sarcoidosis and histiocytosis can infiltrate the hypothalamus or pituitary and result in hyperprolactinemia.

Persistently elevated prolactin levels may also be present in primary hypothyroidism. Approximately 40% of patients with primary hypothyroidism present with a minimal increase in prolactin (25–30 ng/mL), and 10% present with even higher serum levels. Individuals with primary hypothyroidism have an increase in hypothalamic thyrotroph-releasing hormone (TRH), which stimulates both TSH and prolactin release. Patients with long-standing primary hypothyroidism may eventually manifest profound pituitary enlargement due to hypertrophy of thyrotrophs. This mass effect with elevated prolactin levels mimics a prolactinoma.

Many different drugs increase prolactin levels. Prolactin elevation is a normal physiologic

TABLE 38-3 Causes of Hyperprolactinemia

PHYSIOLOGICAL	DRUGS
Pregnancy and breast-feeding	**Dopamine receptor antagonists**
In response to stress	phenothiazines
After a meal	butyrophenones
Chest wall or breast stimulation	thioxanthenes
	risperidone
PROLACTINOMA	metoclopramide
NONPROLACTINOMA CENTRAL TUMORS INTERFERING WITH DOPAMINE INHIBITION	sulpiride
	pimozide
OTHER HYPOTHALAMIC/CNS INSULT INTERFERING WITH DOPAMINE INHIBITION	**Dopamine-depleting agents**
	methyldopa
	reserpine
HYPOTHYROIDISM	**Other**
	antiandrogens
CHRONIC RENAL FAILURE	benzodiazepines
	cimetidine and other H2-blockers
CIRRHOSIS	cocaine and opiates
	danazol
SEIZURE	isoniazid
(during the postictal state)	marijuana
	methyldopa
IDIOPATHIC	monoamine antihypertensives
	neuroleptics
	oral contraceptives
	prostaglandins
	tricyclic antidepressants
	verapamil

response to pregnancy and breast feeding. During pregnancy, prolactin levels may be two to four times baseline. With postpartum breast-feeding, the prolactin level should be below 100 ng/mL after 7 days and below 50 ng/mL after 3 months. If a woman is not breast feeding, prolactin levels should return to baseline by 7 days postpartum.

Clinical Presentation In addition to menstrual disturbances, individuals with hyperprolactinemia may present with galactorrhea. Up to 80% of patients with both amenorrhea and galactorrhea have elevated prolactin levels. Other associated findings include headaches, visual field defects, infertility, and osteopenia.

Diagnosis A prolactin level greater than 20 ng/mL defines hyperprolactinemia though the limit of normal may vary between laboratories. Normal prolactin release follows a sleep circadian rhythm, but prolactin may also be secreted in response to stress, physical exercise, breast stimulation, or a meal. Therefore, prolactin should be measured in the mid morning hours and in the fasting state.

A careful clinical and pharmacologic history and physical examination should be performed to exclude other causes of hyperprolactinemia. Drugs most commonly associated with elevated prolactin include antipsychotics, some antiepileptics, and some antidepressants. All patients with hyperprolactinemia should have their thyroid function investigated to exclude hypothyroidism as the cause. If elevated prolactin levels persist or if any measurement is found to be above 100 ng/mL, MRI of the hypothalamic-pituitary region should be performed. If a thorough evaluation does not reveal a cause for the elevated prolactin, MRI should be considered for any persistent elevation of prolactin above the normal range due to the risk of a non-hormonal or a mixed (primarily GH) tumor. If a microadenoma is observed, the diagnosis of microprolactinoma can be made. If a macroadenoma is observed, other pituitary hormones should be measured to exclude other functioning adenomas or hypopituitarism. All patients diagnosed with macroadenoma should have a visual field examination.

Treatment The treatment of choice for prolactinoma is dopamine agonist therapy. These drugs (bromocriptine, cabergoline, pergolide, and quinagolide) are very effective at lowering prolactin levels, resolving symptoms, and stimulating tumor shrinkage. Bromocriptine was the first dopamine agonist on the market. Although it is still in use, it has a less than ideal side effect profile with nausea, postural hypotension, dizziness, headache, and constipation. Less common side effects include mild depression and occasional psychosis. New

agents with fewer side effects have been developed, including cabergoline and quiagolide. Both agents have a longer half-life and fewer side effects. Nonetheless, all three agents require low initial doses with gradual increases to minimize side effects. Treatment will result in a rapid reduction in prolactin levels and resumption of ovulatory menses within 6 weeks in 60% to 100% of cases, and galactorrhea disappears within 1 to 3 months after starting treatment. Reduction in tumor size is usually evident after 2 to 3 months of drug therapy, but may also occur within days after initiation of treatment. The extrasellar portion of the tumor appears to be particularly sensitive to drug therapy, which explains the improvement in symptoms such as visual impairment or ophthalmoplegia with drug therapy.

In patients with a microadenoma, in whom the only manifestation is a menstrual disturbance, observation should be considered. These individuals may be offered oral contraceptives to control the bleeding pattern or to protect bone from estrogen deficiency. Estrogen treatment is less expensive and has fewer side effects than dopamine agonists and will be generally effective in regulating menstrual cycles and protecting patients from bone loss. Only rarely tumor growth will occur. The long-term sequelae of persistently elevated prolactin levels are unknown.

If dopamine agonist treatment is initiated for a microadenoma, long-term therapy may be continued. If the tumor responds, the dose may be tapered and eventually stopped. A recent study evaluated withdrawal of cabergoline in patients treated for micro- or macroprolactinomas. At 2 to 5 years following withdrawal of medication, hyperprolactinemia recurred in 24% of patients with nontumoral hyperprolactinemia, 31% of patients with microprolactinomas, and 36% of patients with macroprolactinomas. Renewed tumor growth was not seen in any patient and only 22% demonstrated gonadal dysfunction (42). Treatment should be continued for at least 1 year prior to attempted withdrawal. All patients diagnosed with a prolactinoma should have follow-up imaging, determination of serum prolactin levels, and visual field examination.

An alternative to medical management of pituitary tumors is transsphenoidal surgery after which resolution of symptoms may be immediate; however, the success and recurrence rates vary and are dependent on the size of the tumor and the depth of invasion. The larger and more invasive the tumor is, the less chance there is for complete resection and the greater the chance for recurrence. In general, the success rate of surgery for a microadenoma may be up to 70% and for a macroadenoma less than 40%. Overall, the recurrence rate with surgery is approxi-

mately 50%. Surgery is a good alternative for resistant tumors or for patients intolerant of medical treatment, as well as for nonprolactin-secreting pituitary tumors, which tend to not respond well to medical therapy. The risks of surgery include infection, diabetes insipidus, and panhypopituitarism. Complete pituitary testing should be performed prior to surgery.

Thyroid Disease

The prevalence of overt thyroid dysfunction is 1% to 2% in women of reproductive age (43).

Pathogenesis Menstrual irregularities frequently occur in hyperthyroid and hypothyroid states and consist of changes in cycle length, amount of bleeding, including oligoamenorrhea, amenorrhea, polymenorrhea, or menorrhagia (44). The exact mechanism is unclear. Hyperthyroid patients may have normal FSH and LH responses to exogenous GnRH, but the LH surge may be impaired, perhaps related to the weight loss and psychologic disturbances associated with this disease. Peripherally, excess thyroid hormone stimulates hepatic production of SHBG. As a result, total serum estradiol, estrone, testosterone, and dihydrotestosterone are increased; yet free levels of these hormones remain within the normal range. The metabolic clearance pathways appear to be altered, which can be explained in part by the increased binding. The conversion rates of androstenedione to estrogen and testosterone are also increased. The significance of these alterations in sex steroid metabolism has not been determined.

The mechanism underlying menstrual abnormalities in hypothyroidism is also unclear. Because primary hypothyroidism is associated with elevated serum prolactin in up to one-third of patients, it is plausible that the hyperprolactinemia is a contributing factor; however, menstrual abnormalities are also observed in the absence of elevated prolactin. Midcycle LH surge like in hyperthyroidism seems to be impaired. Peripherally, inadequate thyroid levels decrease the production of SHBG. As a result, serum estradiol and testosterone concentrations are decreased, but free hormone levels remain within the normal range.

Clinical Presentation Hypothyroidism is a more common disorder than hyperthyroidism in women of reproductive age. Reproductive abnormalities associated with both hypo- and hyperthyroidism includes menstrual disorders, infertility, and spontaneous abortions. Excessive bleeding may result from estrogen breakthrough bleeding secondary to anovulation.

Menstrual or reproductive dysfunction may be the primary presenting symptoms of thyroid disease.

Diagnosis Measurement of free T$_4$, TSH as part of the initial work-up of menstrual irregularities will show low free T$_4$, increased or low to normal TSH in patients with primary or cental hypothyroidism; increased T$_4$ and suppressed TSH levels will be found in patients with hypwrthyroidism.

Treatment Successful treatment of thyroid disease resolves the associated menstrual and reproductive symptoms. Additionally, in cases of severe hypothyroidism with associated hyperprolactinemia, prolactin levels should return to normal as the TSH level normalizes (45).

Glucocorticoid Excess

Glucocorticoid excess, whether endogenous or exogenous, causes menstrual abnormalities by inhibiting GnRH secretion. Thus, it is common for menstrual dysfunction to occur in adolescent girls receiving high-dose glucocorticoid therapy, even if their primary disease condition does not affect the HPO axis. Endogenous glucocorticoid excess, whether caused by central or ectopic ACTH secretion or by primary adrenal lesions, is often accompanied by adrenal androgen excess as described below.

Amenorrhea Associated with Obesity

Obese women often experience amenorrhea of menstrual irregularities, even if they do not have PCO. Peripheral conversion of androgens to estrogen results in a hyperestrogenic state, correlating to the degree of excess adiposity. Patients may present with prolonged cycles of amenorrhea, alternating with cycles of metrorrhagia or menometrorrhagia.

Anatomic Amenorrhea

Menses cannot occur without an intact uterus, endometrium, cervix, cervical os, and vaginal conduit. The most common anatomic abnormalities seen include imperforate hymen, transverse vaginal septum, and vaginal agenesis. The most common presenting symptoms are pelvic or lower abdominal pain accompanied by primary amenorrhea.

An imperforate hymen is the simplest defect that results in primary amenorrhea. Classic symptoms are cyclic pelvic pain and a perirectal mass resulting from sequestration of blood in the vagina (hematocolpos). This can be easily corrected with surgery.

Transverse vaginal septum can occur at any level between the hymenal ring and the cervix. Presentation and treatment are very similar to an imperforate hymen although tissue grafting may be required.

Congenital absence of the vagina with variable uterine development is referred to as vaginal mullerian agenesis. This defect is a result of hypoplasia of the mullerian duct system. Typically, vaginal agenesis also results in some degree of cervical and uterine agenesis. Imaging studies (transvaginal ultrasound or MRI) help to make the diagnosis.

AMENORRHEA AND ABNORMAL UTERINE BLEEDING ASSOCIATED WITH ANDROGEN EXCESS

Menstrual irregularities including amenorrhea are common in the setting of androgen excess, and are often accompanied by acne and excessive sexual hair growth. There can also be temporal hairline recession and a deepening of the voice when androgen excess is present.

Polycystic Ovary Syndrome

Pathogenesis Polycystic ovary syndrome (PCOS) is the most common cause of chronic anovulation, occurring in 3% to 7% of women of reproductive age (46–48). The endocrine and metabolic abnormalities associated with this condition include hyperandrogenemia, anovulation, insulin resistance, and features of the metabolic syndrome (dyslipidemia, hypertension, type 2 diabetes, and cardiovascular disease) (49–52). These features are interrelated, and it is difficult to sort out which, if any, is the primary or the initiating factor. PCOS may be a common clinical manifestation of heterogeneous underlying ovarian, adrenal, and/or pituitary pathology.

Androgen excess is clearly a central feature of PCOS. It may precede the diagnosis of PCOS because young women with this condition frequently have a history of exaggerated or premature adrenarche during childhood. In these patients, adrenal androgens may be an important contributor to the disease state. Ovarian androgen excess may be related to an abnormally high LH:FSH ratio in some women with PCOS. Insulin resistance is also a cause of ovarian androgen excess, and women with PCOS are often profoundly insulin resistant, with decreased insulin-stimulated glucose utilization (peripheral resistance) and poor suppression of hepatic glucose production (hepatic resistance) (49). It is thought that insulin has a direct stimulatory effect on ovarian androgen production. This relationship is apparent in children born small for gestational age, who can be insulin resistant and have increased risk of premature pubarche with subsequent development of PCOS.

A prospective study demonstrated that PCOS patients have a 31.1% prevalence of impaired glucose tolerance and a 7.5% prevalence of undiagnosed type 2 diabetes mellitus (53). This risk of type 2 diabetes among PCOS patients may be as much as 5- to 10-fold higher than in the general population (54). VLDL and triglyceride levels are elevated, HDL levels are decreased, and blood pressure is increased (55–59). Insulin resistance and excessive androgens may have independent roles in the promotion of deleterious lipid profiles because antiandrogen medications reduce triglyceride and LDL levels in adolescent and adult women (60–62). Although metabolic syndrome abnormalities are present in both lean and obese PCOS patients, more than 50% of patients are obese, with a tendency toward excessive central adiposity. It is likely that obesity synergistically affects long-term sequelae of PCOS (63).

The anovulation and incomplete follicular development associated with PCOS lead to the characteristic "polycystic ovaries," although this feature is not uniformly present. There is an increased prevalence of both endometrial hyperplasia and carcinoma (64,65). This is thought to be a function of prolonged exposure to unopposed estrogen (primarily estrone). As a result of the anovulation, there is no luteal phase and no corpus luteum to produce progesterone. Without sufficient progesterone, proliferation of the endometrium is uninhibited and there is no differentiation to a secretory state. In addition, the predisposition to obesity and type 2 diabetes are features of PCOS that are known to be independent risk factors for endometrial cancer.

Clinical Presentation In most situations, the manifestations of PCOS emerge in the peripubertal years, revealed by premature pubarche and irregular cycles, which persist through much of reproductive life. A 1990 conference sponsored by the National Institutes of Health and the National Institute of Child Health and Human Development first standardized criteria for the diagnosis of PCOS, which they defined as the presence of: 1) chronic anovulation; 2) clinical hyperandrogenism (hirsutism, acne, androgenic alopecia) and/or hyperandrogenemia; and, 3) the exclusion of secondary causes such as hyperprolactinemia, thyroid dysfunction, and adrenal disorders (66). A consensus workshop held in Rotterdam in 2003 updated the diagnostic criteria to include the presence on ultrasound of polycystic-appearing ovaries. The conference further recognized that, although insulin resistance should not be used in the diagnosis of PCOS, patients with this syndrome were at increased risk for the development of insulin resistance, hyperinsulinemia, and type 2 diabetes mellitus in addition to other long-term sequelae such as obesity, infertility, cardiovascular risk, and endometrial carcinoma.

In addition to the metabolic consequences of PCOS, patients are often faced with reproductive issues as 75% of women who present for infertility with anovulation have PCOS (67). This is usually correctable with clomiphene citrate, metformin, or gonadotropins.

Diagnosis Diagnosis of PCOS may be challenging because normal adolescent girls commonly display irregular cycles during the 5 years after menarche. Evaluation should start with a careful history including birth history (i.e., small for gestational age), timing of development of pubertal changes and menarche, and cycle regularity. Clinically, patients should be examined for signs of androgen excess such as acne and hirsutism, and signs of insulin excess such as acanthosis nigricans (68).

Biochemical elevations in testosterone, free testosterone, or dehydroepiandrosterone sulfate may frequently be seen in PCOS patients; however, in the absence of clinical findings to suggest a tumor, the usefulness of these measurements is not clear. There are subsets of oligo- or amenorrheic patients, such as Asians, who are hyperandrogenemic without clinical manifestations, most likely as a result of relative insensitivity to circulating androgens. In these patients, assessing androgen levels may be of value in determining the cause of menstrual abnormalities.

Because of the association with the metabolic syndrome, evaluation for PCOS should include a fasting glucose and insulin level and/or an oral glucose tolerance test, a fasting lipid profile, and careful blood pressure measurement.

Ultrasonography may show the presence of polycystic ovaries; however many women with PCOS do not have polycystic appearing ovaries. Furthermore, the finding of polycystic ovaries is not unique to PCOS as it has been observed in late-onset congenital adrenal hyperplasia (CAH), human immunodeficiency virus, and epilepsy. In fact, polycystic ovaries occur in more than 20% of normal women.

Treatment Because PCOS may present with a variety of symptoms, treatment is targeting each problem independently. The typical individual abnormalities requiring treatment include: 1) hyperandrogenism, 2) insulin resistance and hyperinsulinemia, and 3) menstrual irregularities.

Hyperandrogenism The goal of treatment is to interrupt the steps leading to increased androgen production. Suppression of circulating ovarian androgens with low-dose oral contraceptives results in moderate improvement in hirsutism and acne, and these drugs continue to represent the first line approach to treatment. The mechanism of action is thought to be a combination of an increase in SHBG synthesis (and hence a decrease in free androgen), suppression of gonadotropin secretion, reduction of ovarian androgen secretion, inhibition of DHT receptor binding, and, in patients on antiandrogen drugs, enhancement of antiandrogen effectiveness (69,70). Gonadotropin agonist therapy, such as leuprolide acetate, has also been successful in improving hirsutism. Long-term use with this therapy requires the addition of estrogen and progesterone to prevent associated hypoestrogenism (71,72).

Spironolactone is the most commonly utilized antiandrogen in the United States. This drug is an anti-mineralocorticoid agent that inhibits androgen biosynthesis in the adrenal and ovary, inhibits 5α-reductase, and is a competitive inhibitor of the androgen receptor. Side effects are minimal and include diuresis in the first few days, dyspepsia, breast tenderness, and abnormal bleeding, which can be alleviated with concomitant use of oral contraceptives. Spironolactone is teratogenic to the male fetus, and should always be prescribed along with oral contraceptives to prevent pregnancy. The 5α-reductase inhibitors (e.g., finasteride) have been used for refractory cases with some success. These are also should be prescribed together with oral contraceptives.

Mechanical hair removal methods such as shaving, tweezing, waxing, depilatory creams, electrolysis, and laser therapy provide temporary improvement in hirsutism, but the combination of medical treatment and mechanical methods are needed for long-term improvement to remove and prevent new growth.

Insulin Resistance Insuline resistance represents the most serious long-term risk factor; treatment of insulin resistance usually improves androgen levels and menstrual irregularities.

All patients with PCOS should be counseled regarding lifestyle changes including aerobic and muscle building exercise and a healthy diet. Further data are necessary prior to widespread use of insulin-sensitizing medications to determine: 1) if these patients are indeed at risk for cardiovascular events, 2) if hyperinsulinemia is an independent risk factor for PCOS, and 3) whether long-term treatment with an insulin-sensitizing agent will decrease the potential sequelae. Currently available insulin sensitizers include metformin and the thiazolidinediones.

Metformin is used in the treatment of type 2 diabetes. It maintains glucose homeostasis primarily through suppression of hepatic glucose output. In PCOS, metformin leads to a decrease in serum insulin and androgen levels, as well as an improvement in ovulatory function (73). The metformin dose is 1,000 to 2,000 mg/day divided over one to two doses. Initially, to avoid side effects, a smaller dose is started. Renal and liver function should be evaluated before initiation of metformin.

Thiazolidinediones are another class of insulin sensitizers under investigation for the management of PCOS. These drugs are not approved for use in the pediatric population. They are selective ligands for PPARγ, a nuclear receptor that regulates the transcription of multiple insulin-responsive genes, crucial to the control of glucose and lipid metabolism. PPARγ plays a central role in the regulation of adipocyte gene expression and regulation (74–76). Early work with troglitazone, prior to its withdrawal from the market due to liver toxicity, found that this drug effectively decreased both insulin and free androgen levels in PCOS patients (77). Although pioglitazone (Actos) and rosiglitazone (Avandia) have been advocated for use in the treatment of PCOS, definitive studies have not yet been performed.

Menstrual Irregularities Menstrual irregularities in PCOS can be addressed by inducing endometrial shedding with progesterone. The recommended interval of use is no less than every 3 months. Medroxyprogesterone acetate (Provera) may be dosed at 10 mg/day for 14 days duration. If this does not result in control of the dysfunctional uterine bleeding often associated with PCOS, or if contol of ovarian hyperandrogenism is desired, oral contraceptive pills can be prescribed.

Nonclassic Congenital Adrenal Hyperplasia Due to 21 Hydroxylase Deficiency

Pathogenesis CAH due to 21-hydroxylase deficiency (21OHD) is an autosomal recessive defect that impairs adrenal cortisol synthesis and leads to compensatory ACTH secretion and excessive androgen production. This condition is discussed in detail in Chapter 27. The mildest form of CAH due to 21OHD is the nonclassic form.

Clinical Presentation Nonclassic CAH commonly presents with normal female genitalia at birth. Early pubic hair development, bone age advancement, and acceleration of growth may be the presenting symptoms in childhood. In adolescence years clinical manifestations may include hirsutism, menstrual irregularities identical to PCO, and infertility during reproductive years (79).

Diagnosis Nonclassic CAH may be difficult to distinguish from PCOS. Baseline elevation of dehydroepiandrosterone sulfate, androstenedione, and testosterone levels may be found in both conditions, and polycystic-appearing ovaries are not uncommon in patients with nonclassical CAH (80,81). Measurement of 17-hydroxyprogesterone (17-OHP) can differentiate these two conditions. A normal baseline 17-OHP level ($<$100 ng/dL [3.0 nmol/L]), especially if measured early in the morning (8 AM) and during the follicular phase in a menstruating patient can exclude a diagnosis of nonclassic CAH. A high dose ACTH stimulation test should be performed for patients with baseline 17OHP level above higher than 100 ng/dL (3.0 nmol/L). Poststimulation 17-OHP levels exceeding 1340 ng/dL (77) are suggestive of nonclassic CAH. Because there may be overlap between 17-OHP levels in heterozygotes and mild cases of nonclassic CAH, genotyping is recommended to confirm the diagnosis.

Treatment Treatment of nonclassic CAH in females is indicated only if symptomatic (for detailed treatment, please see Chapter 27).

Oral contraceptive pills may be a useful adjunct to control menstrual cycles and decrease hyperandrogenism. In fact, there is still some question regarding the need for glucocorticoid treatment in women with nonclassic CAH, given that frequently there is excellent response to contraceptive pills and antiandrogens without the added risk of adrenal suppression.

Tumor-Related Androgen Excess

Tumors of the ovary, adrenal, or ACTH-secreting tumors which stimulate the adrenal glands, may produce androgens.

In the presence of ovarian tumors, autonomous androgen production may result in chronic anovulation and virilization. The tumor types include hilus cell tumors, arrhenoblastomas (Sertoli–Leydig cell tumors), benign cystic teratomas, luteinized thecoma, gynandroblastoma (Leydig and granulosa cell elements), and ovarian sex cord tumors (granulosa and Sertoli cells). Tumor markers may be helpful in differentiating these various tumors. Inhibin, β-hCG, and anti-Müllerian hormone are markers for sex cord and germ cell tumors and, occasionally, for granulosa and Leydig cell tumors.

Adrenal adenomas and carcinomas are rare in the adolescent or adult female, but are the most common cause of Cushing syndrome in infants or children younger than the age of 7 years. These tumors are often virilizing. When present, they generally produce large amounts of 17-ketosteroids, such as dehydroepiandrosterone and androstenedione, as well as cortisol. Children with virilizing tumors have growth acceleration, advanced bone age and public hair development. Women with adrenal tumors tend to have a rapid onset of symptoms and often manifest with severe hyperandrogenism (frank virilization), which includes male pattern baldness, deepening voice, clitoromegaly, and defeminization.

ACTH-secreting tumors may be located in the pituitary or may be peripherally located, such as in the lungs. They stimulate the adrenal gland to produce excessive amounts of both corticol and androgens. Menstrual irregularities occur in over 80% of patients. Anovulation is related to glucocorticoid suppression of the hypothalamic-pituitary axis. Hyperandrogenism is present in 60% to 70% of women with Cushing syndrome and further contributes to anovulation.

In addition to blood tests, the work up for tumor-related androgen excess in suspected cases should include ultrasound, computed tomography and/or MRI. Further localization may necessitate the use of retrograde venous catheterization to clarify both location (ovary versus adrenal) and situs (left versus right) of the excess hormone production.

Exogenous Androgens

Exogenous androgens are occasionally the cause of virilization and menstrual abnormalities in children or young women. This has become a major concern in adolescents, including young women with the increasing usage of anabolic steroids for body building and athletic achievement. There have also been reports of virilization of family members in households where an adult male used testosterone gel.

REFERENCES

1. Hertweck SP. Dysfunctional uterine bleeding. *Obstet Gynecol Clin North Am.* 1992;19:129.
2. Lemarchand-Beraud T, Zufferey MM, Raymond M, et al. Maturation of the hypothalamic-pituitary-ovarian axis in adolescent girls. *J Clin Endocrinol Metab.* 2002;54:241–246.
3. Apter D, Vihko R. Early menarche, a risk for breast cancer indicates early onset of ovulatory cycles. *J Clin Endocrinol Metab.* 1983;57:82–86.
4. Lavin C. Dysfunctional uterine bleeding in adolescents. *Curr Opin Pediatr.* 1996;8:328–332.
5. Emans. Dysfunctional uterine bleeding. *Pediatric and Adolescent Gynecology.* Philadelphia: Lippincott Williams & Wilkins; 2003:270.
6. Mitan LA, Slap GB, et al. Dysfunctional uterine bleeding. *Adolescent Health Care: A Practical Guide.* 4th ed. Philadelphia; Lippincott Williams & Wilkins; 2003:966.
7. Bravender T, Emans SJ. Menstrual disorders. Dysfunctional uterine bleeding. *Pediatr Clin North Am.* 1999;46:545–553.
8. Rimsza ME. Dysfunctional uterine bleeding. *Pediatr Rev.* 2002;15:725–733.
9. Claessens EA, Cowell CA, et al. Acute adolescent menorrhagia. *Am J Obstet Gynecol.* 1981;139:277–280.
10. Bevan JA, Maloney KW, Hillery CA, et al. Bleeding disorders: A common cause of menorrhagia in adolescents. *J Pediatr.* 2001;138:856–861.
11. Smith YR, Quint EH, Hertzberg RB et al. Menorrhagia in adolescents requiring hospitalization. *J Pediatr Adolesc Gynecol.* 1998; 11:13–15.
12. Falcone T, Desjardins C, Bourque J, et al. Dysfunctional uterine bleeding in adolescents. *J Reprod Med.* 1994;39:761–764.
13. Kanbur NO, Derman O, Kutluk T, et al. Coagulation disorders as the cause of menorrhagia in adolescents. *Int J Adolesc Med Health.* 2004;16:183–185.
14. Oral E, Çagdas A, Gezer A, et al. Hematological abnormalities in adolescent menorrhagia. *Arch Gynecol Obstet.* 2002;266:77–84.
15. Minjarez DA. Abnormal bleeding in adolescents. *Semin Reprod Med.* 2003; 21:363–373.
16. Ansell JE. The blood in the hypothyroidism. In: Braverman L, Utiger R, eds. *Werner and Ingbar's the Thyroid, a Fundamental and Clinical Text.* Philadelphia: Lippincott Raven; 1996:821–825.
17. Cowan BD, Morrison JC. Management of abnormal genital bleeding in girls and women. *N Engl J Med.* 1991;324:1710–1715.
18. Mannucci PM. Hemostatic drugs. *N Engl J Med.* 1998;339:245–253.
19. Mannucci PM. Treatment of von Willebrand disease. *N Engl J Med.* 2004;351:683–694.
20. Slap GB. Menstrual disorders in adolescence. *Best Pract Res Clin Obstet Gynecol.* 2003;17:75–92.
21. Greydanus DE, Patel DR, Rimsza ME, et al. Contraception in the adolescent: an update. *Pediatrics.* 2001;107:562–573.
22. Campbell MA, McGrath PJ. Use of medication by adolescents for the management of menstrual discomfort. *Arch Pediatr Adolesc Med.* 1997;151:905–913.
23. Wilson CA, Keye WR Jr. A survey of adolescent dysmenorrhea and premenstrual symptom frequency. A model program for prevention, detection, and treatment. *J Adolesc Health Care.* 1989;10:317–322.
24. Klein JR, Litt IF. Epidemiology of adolescent dysmenorrhea. *Pediatrics.* 1981;68:661–664.
25. Johnson J. Level of knowledge among adolescent girls regarding effective treatment for dysmenorrhea. *J Adolesc Health Care.* 1988;9:398–402.
26. Proctor M, Farquhar C. Dysmenorrhea. *Clin Evid.* 2006;15:2429–2448.
27. Zhang WY, Li Wan A. Efficacy of minor analgesics in primary dysmenorrhoea: a systematic review. *Br J Obstet Gynaecol.* 1998;105(7):780–789.
28. French L. Dysmenorrhea. *Am Fam Physician.* 2005;71:285–291.
29. Smith RP. Primary dysmenorrhea and the adolescent patient. *Adolesc Pediatr Gynecol.* 1988;1:23–30.
30. Alvin PE, Litt IF. Current status of the etiology and management of dysmenorrhea in adolescence. *Pediatrics.* 1982;70:516–525.

31. Chan WY, Dawood MY, Fuchs F, et al. Prostaglandins in primary dysmenorrhea. Comparison of prophylactic and nonprophylactic treatment with ibuprofen and use of oral contraceptives. Am J Med. 1981;70:535–541.

32. Henzl MR, Buttram V, Segre EJ, et al. The treatment of dysmenorrhea with naproxen sodium: a report on two independent double-blind trials. Am J Obstet Gynecol. 1977;127:818.

33. Larkin RM, Van Orden DE, Poulson AN, et al. Dysmenorrhea: treatment with an antiprostaglandin. Obstet Gynecol. 1979;54:456–460.

34. Smith RP. Cyclic pelvic pain and dysmenorrhea. Obstet Gynecol Clin North Am. 1993;20:753–764.

35. Reindollar RH, Novak M, Tho SP, et al. Adult-onset amenorrhea: a study of 262 patients. Am J Obstet Gynecol. 1986;155:531–543.

36. Andrico, S, Gambera A, Specchia C, et al. Leptin in functional hypothalamic amenorrhea. Hum Reprod. 2002;17(8):2043–2048.

37. Chan JO, Mantzoros CS. Leptin and the hypothalamic-pituitary regulation of the gonadotropin-gonadal axis. Pituitary. 2001;4:87–92.

38. Santoro N, Filicori M, Crowley WF, et al. Hypogonadotropic disorders in men and women: diagnosis and therapy with pulsatile gonadotropin-releasing hormone. Endocr Rev. 1986;7:11–23.

39. Constantini NW, Warren MP. Menstrual dysfunction in swimmers: a distinct entity. J Clin Endocrinol Metab. 1995;80:2740–2744.

40. Warren MP. Amenorrhea in endurance runners. J Clin Endocrinol Metab. 1992;75:1393–1397.

41. Kooy A, de Greef WJ, Vreeburg JT, et al. Evidence for the involvement of corticotrophin-releasing factor in the inhibition of gonadotropin release induced by hyperprolactinemia. Neuroendocrinology. 1990;51(3):261–266.

42. Gillam MP, Molitch ME, Lombardi G, et al.: Advances in the treatment of prolactinomas. Endocr Rev. 2006;27(5):485–534.

43. Turnbridge WM, Evered DC, Hall R, et al. The spectrum of thyroid disease in a community: the Whickham survey. Clin Endocrinol. (Oxf) 1977;7:481–493.

44. Krassas GE, Pontikides N, Kaltsas T, et al. Disturbances of menstruation in hypothyroidism. Clin Endocrinol. (Oxf) 1999;50(5):655–659.

45. Krassas GE. Thyroid disease and female reproduction. Fertil Steril. 2000;74(6):1063–1070.

46. Knochenhauer ES, Key TJ, Kahsar-Miller M, et al. Prevalence of the polycystic ovary syndrome in unselected black and white women of the southeastern United States: a prospective study. J Clin Endocrinol Metab. 1998;83(9):3078–3082.

47. Diamanti-Kandarakis E, Kouli CR, Bergiele AT, et al. A survey of the polycystic ovary syndrome in the Greek island of Lesbos: hormonal and metabolic profile. J Clin Endocrinol Metab. 1999;84(11):4006–4011.

48. Michelmore KF, Balen AH, Dunger DB, et al. Polycystic ovaries and associated clinical and biochemical features in young women. Clin Endocrinol. (Oxf) 1999;51(6):779–786.

49. Dunaif A, Segal KR, Futterweit W, et al. Profound peripheral insulin resistance, independent of obesity, in polycystic ovary syndrome. Diabetes. 1989;38(9):1165–1174.

50. Conway GS, Agrawal R, Betteridge DJ, et al. Risk factors for coronary artery disease in lean and obese women with the polycystic ovary syndrome. Clin Endocrinol. (Oxf) 1992;37(2):119–125.

51. Talbott E, Guzick D, Clerisi A, et al. Coronary heart disease risk factors in women with polycystic ovary syndrome. Arterioscler Thromb Vasc Biol. 1995;15(7):821–826.

52. Taylor AE. Polycystic ovary syndrome. Endocrinol Metab Clin North Am. 1998;27(4):877–902, ix.

53. Legro RS, Kunselman AR, Dodson WC, et al. Prevalence and predictors of risk for type 2 diabetes mellitus and impaired glucose tolerance in polycystic ovary syndrome: a prospective, controlled study in 254 affected women. J Clin Endocrinol Metab. 1999;84(1):165–169.

54. Ovalle F, Azziz R. Insulin resistance, polycystic ovary syndrome, and type 2 diabetes mellitus. Fertil Steril. 2002;77(6):1095–1105.

55. Wild RA, Bartholomew MJ. The influence of body weight on lipoprotein lipids in patients with polycystic ovary syndrome. Am J Obstet Gynecol. 1988;159(2):423–427.

56. Slowinska-Srzednicka J, Zgliczynski S, Wierzbicki M, et al. The role of hyperinsulinemia in the development of lipid disturbances in nonobese and obese women with the polycystic ovary syndrome. J Endocrinol Invest. 1991;14(7):569–575.

57. Wild RA, Alaupovic P, Parker IJ, et al. Lipid and apolipoprotein abnormalities in hirsute women. I. The association with insulin resistance. Am J Obstet Gynecol. 1992;166(4):1191–1196;discussion 1196–1197.

58. Zimmermann S, Phillips RA, Dunaif A, et al. Polycystic ovary syndrome: lack of hypertension despite profound insulin resistance. J Clin Endocrinol Metab. 1992;75(2):508–513.

59. Elting MW, Korsen TJ, Bezemer PD, et al. Prevalence of diabetes mellitus, hypertension and cardiac complaints in a follow-up study of a Dutch PCOS population. Hum Reprod. 2003;16(3):556–560.

60. De Leo V, Lanzetta D, D'Antona D, et al. Hormonal effects of flutamide in young women with polycystic ovary syndrome. J Clin Endocrinol Metab. 1998;83(1):99–102.

61. Diamanti-Kandarakis E, Mitrakou A, Raptis S, et al. The effect of a pure antiandrogen receptor blocker, flutamide, on the lipid profile in the polycystic ovary syndrome. J Clin Endocrinol Metab. 1998;83(8):2699–2705.

62. Mather KJ, Kwan F, Corenblum B, et al. Hyperinsulinemia in polycystic ovary syndrome correlates with increased cardiovascular risk independent of obesity. Fertil Steril. 2000;73(1):150–156.

63. Wild RA. Polycystic ovary syndrome: a risk for coronary artery disease? Am J Obstet Gynecol. 2002;186(1):35–43.

64. Balen A. Polycystic ovary syndrome and cancer. Hum Reprod Update. 2001;7(6):522–525.

65. Hardiman P, Pillay OC, Atiomo W, et al. Polycystic ovary syndrome and endometrial carcinoma. Lancet. 2003;361(9371):1810–1812.

66. Zawadzki JK, Dunaif A. Diagnostic criteria for polycystic ovary syndrome: towards a rational approach. In: Merriam GR, ed. Polycystic Ovary Syndrome. Boston: Blackwell Scientific; 1992:377–384.

67. Homburg R. Management of infertility and prevention of ovarian hyperstimulation in women with polycystic ovary syndrome. Best Pract Res Clin Obstet Gynecol. 2004;18(5):773–788.

68. Hermanns-Le T, Scheen A, Pierard GE. Acanthosis nigricans associated with insulin resistance: pathophysiology and management. Am J Clin Dermatol. 2004;5(3):199–203.

69. Rittmaster RS. Hirsutism. Lancet. 1997;349(9046):191–195.

70. Eil C, Edelson SK. The use of human skin fibroblasts to obtain potency estimates of drug binding to androgen receptors. J Clin Endocrinol Metab. 1984;59(1):51–55.

71. Adashi EY, Potential utility of gonadotropin-releasing hormone agonists in the management of ovarian hyperandrogenism. Fertil Steril. 1990;53(5):765–779.

72. Rittmaster RS, Thompson DL. Effect of leuprolide and dexamethasone on hair growth and hormone levels in hirsute women: the relative importance of the ovary and the adrenal in the pathogenesis of hirsutism. J Clin Endocrinol Metab. 1990;70(4):1096–1102.

73. Seli E, Duleba AJ. Treatment of PCOS with metformin and other insulin-sensitizing agents. Curr Diab Rep. 2004;4(1):69–75.

74. Ibrahimi A, Teboul L, Gaillard D, et al. Evidence for a common mechanism of action for fatty acids and thiazolidinedione antidiabetic agents on gene expression in preadipose cells. Mol Pharmacol. 1994;46(6):1070–1076.

75. Brandes R, Arad R, Bara-Tana J, et al. Inducers of adipose conversion activate transcription promoted by a peroxisome proliferator's response element in 3T3-L1 cells. Biochem Pharmacol. 1995;50(11):1949–1951.

76. Kliewer SA, Lenhard JM, Wilson TM, et al. A prostaglandin J2 metabolite binds peroxisome proliferator-activated receptor gamma and promotes adipocyte differentiation. Cell. 1995;83(5):813–819.

77. Ehrmann DA, Schneider DJ, Sobel BE, et al. Troglitazone improves defects in insulin action, insulin secretion, ovarian steroidogenesis, and fibrinolysis in women with polycystic ovary syndrome. J Clin Endocrinol Metab. 1997;82(7):2108–2116.

78. Pang S. Congenital adrenal hyperplasia. Baillieres Clin Obstet Gynaecol. 1997;11(2):281–306.

79. Chrousos GP, Loriaux DL, Mann DL, et al. Late-onset 21-hydroxylase deficiency mimicking idiopathic hirsutism or polycystic ovarian disease. Ann Intern Med. 1982;96(2):143–148.

80. Hague WM, Adams J, Rodda C, et al. The prevalence of polycystic ovaries in patients with congenital adrenal hyperplasia and their close relatives. Clin Endocrinol. (Oxf) 1990;33(4):501–510.

81. Cobin RH, Futterweit W, Fiedler RP, et al. Adrenocorticotropic hormone testing in idiopathic hirsutism and polycystic ovarian disease: a test of limited usefulness. Fertil Steril. 1985;44(2):224–226.

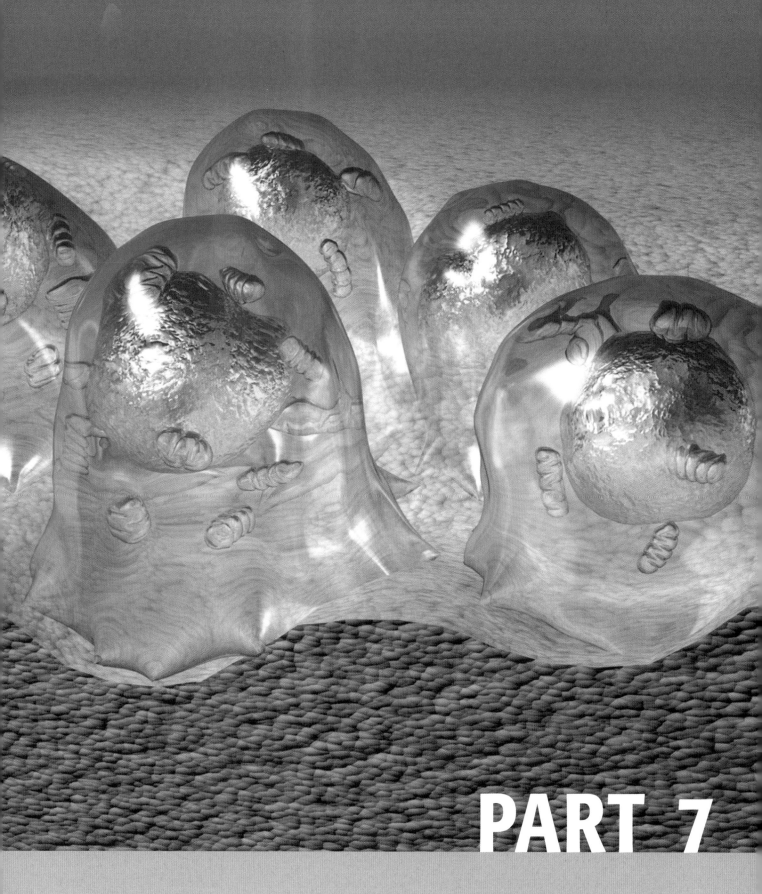

PART 7

Disorders of Bone and Mineral Metabolism

IN THIS PART

Previous page: Osteoblasts are active in the development and calcification of bony tissue.

CHAPTER 39

Disorders of Calcium, Phosphate, and Bone Metabolism

Karl S. Roth, MD
Robert J. Ward, MD
James C. M. Chan, MD
Kyriakie Sarafoglou, MD

PHYSIOLOGY OF BONE METABOLISM

The Skeleton

Bone is a calcium reservoir for many crucial body functions, such as activity of calcium-dependent ATPases in cellular metabolism, nerve transmission, and muscle contraction. The usual image of a reservoir is as a placid lake whose water level does not change appreciably from day to day. Yet it is possible for this reservoir to be supplying hundreds of thousands, if not millions, of gallons of water per day as long as the supply keeps pace. This is an analogy that amply illustrates the physiological concept of homeostasis, in which there is rapid turnover without appreciable change in quantity. Moreover, the health of the reservoir is maintained by a balance of ecological entities that live in harmony, each checking the growth rate of the others to preserve this balance. Thus it is with the skeleton, which is a highly vascularized and cellular tissue and an ion reservoir of calcium, phosphate, and (to a lesser extent) magnesium; the exquisitely orchestrated balance between building and destroying bone tissue maintains the contours and strength and enables corrective actions when necessary. Integrated with this activity is the ability to respond to external signaling in order to maintain calcium and phosphorus homeostasis. The complexity of the intimate and intricate interactions performed by the cellular elements of bone throughout the life of an individual is only recently becoming appreciated, and much about it remains to be elucidated.

Osteoblasts, Osteocytes, and Osteoclasts

The two fundamental concepts to keep in mind about bone during life are 1) modeling, which occurs during development and involves the shaping process of creation and destruction to move bone tissue with no net loss (indeed, in the end, there is a net gain because it is consonant with body growth), and 2) remodeling, which occurs throughout life and involves removal for homeostatic needs, in response to changes in physical stress, and for replacement with no net change. To accomplish these events, each of the cells has a specific role. The *osteoblast* provides matrix and initiates mineralization, the *osteocyte* is an osteoblast that has become entombed within the newly created bone, and the *osteoclast* plays the role of bone destruction (Figure 39-1). The osteoblast and osteoclast are both derived from embryonic progenitors within the bone marrow, but from distinctly different stem cell lines. Hence the initiating factors for differentiation of one or the other cell type, as well as cellular responsiveness to extracellular messengers, differ. Moreover, it appears that the osteoblast regulates osteoclastic activity through cell–cell interactions, thus coordinating the creative and destructive phenomena that result in the predictable shapes of specific bones of the skeleton.

Osteoblast The osteoblast originates from stromal multipotent mesenchymal stem cells within the bone marrow. The same stem cells also are precursors of adipocytes, chondrocytes, and myocytes (1–3). It is also possible that osteoblasts emerge from "stray" mesenchymal cells adhering to the vascular endothelium (4).

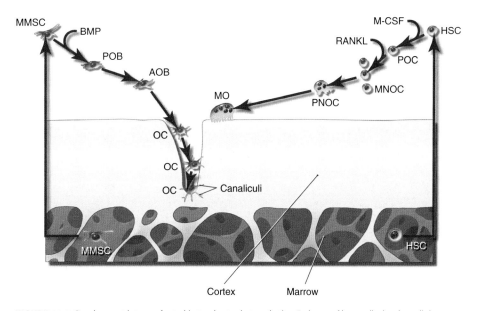

FIGURE 39-1. Developmental stages of osteoblast and osteoclast production. Each type of bone cell arises from distinct embryonic cell lines, which underscores the distinct nature of their functions. The *osteoblast* derives from bone marrow multipotent mesenchymal stem cells (MMSCs), acted on by a family of cytokines factors called *bone morphogenetic proteins* (BMPs) to become converted into a precursor osteoblast (POB). The mature, or active, osteoblast (O) migrates to the bone surface, where it secretes the bone matrix materials. With continued secretion and bone remodeling, some osteoblasts are trapped within the matrix and are entombed, becoming *osteocytes* (OCs) and communicating with the surface osteoblasts by means of syncitial processes extending through the canaliculi. The *osteoclast,* in contrast, emerges from the hematopoietic stem cell (HSC), a process initiated by macrophage colony-stimulating factor (M-CSF) as a precursor osteoclast (POC). Under the direction of many stimulating factors, especially RANK-L produced by the precursor osteoblast, the POC is converted to a mononuclear osteoclast (MNOC). These mononuclear cells then merge to form a polynuclear osteoclast (PNOC), which develops a ruffled border and then is considered to be a mature osteoclast (MO). The loose association of these mature cells at the bone surface comprises the basic multicellular unit (BMU) responsible for bone remodeling (see text).

Disorders of Calcium, Phosphate, and Bone Metabolism

AT-A-GLANCE

Bone contains approximately 99% of total-body calcium, whereas the remaining 900–1000 mg in the soluble fluids of the body are in constant flux. The normal human diet contains calcium, magnesium, and phosphorus in relatively large quantities, and although the renal tubule is remarkably efficient in conserving these elements, no biological system can achieve 100% efficiency, resulting in some loss. Bone formation and resorption, intestinal absorption, cellular uptake and exchange with serum, serum protein binding, and renal reabsorption and loss—all the mechanisms for maintenance of calcium, magnesium, and phosphate homeostasis—result in a highly cooperative and responsive homeostatic system.

Three hormones (PTH, calcitonin, and vitamin D $[1,25(OH)_2D_3]$) are mostly responsible for regulating the extracellular control of these minerals. A disturbance (genetic, nutritional, or intercurrent illness) at any level in this intricate regulatory network can lead to clinical disease.

TYPES	OCCURRENCE	LOCUS	OMIM
Hypoparathyroidism			
DiGeorge	12000–4,000	22q11.2	188400
HDR (Barakat)	Rare	10p15	146255
Kenny–Caffey	Rare	1q42-43	244460
HRD (Sanjad–Sakati)	Rare	1q42-43	241410
PTH gene defects	Rare	11p15.3-p15.1	168450, 146200
GCMB deletion	Rare	6p24.2	603716
Familial hypercalciuric hypocalcemia	Rare	3q13.3-q21	146200
Kearns–Sayre	Rare	mtDNA DEL	530000
Pearson marrow pancreas	Rare	mtDNA, ND4, ND5, A6-ND5, DEL	557000
APECED	Rare	21q22.3	240300
Pseudohypoparathyroidism			
Type 1a	Rare	20q13.2	103580
Type 1b	Rare	20q13.2	603233
Type 1c	Rare	20q13.2	103580
Type II	Rare	Unknown	203330
PPHP	Rare	20q13.2	103580
Hyperparathyroidism			
Primary hyperparathyroidism	Rare	N/A	145000-01
Neonatal, severe	Rare	3q13.3-q21	239200
MEN I	3–20:100,000	11q13	131100
MEN IIA	1:40,000	10q11.2	171400
Hyperparathyroidism–jaw-tumor	Rare	1q25-q31	145001
Familial isolated (FIHP)	Rare	1q25-q31, 11q13	145000
Familial hypocalciuric hypercalcemia	Rare	3q13.3-q21, 19q13, 19q13.3	145980, 600740, 145981
Jansen metaphyseal	Rare	3p22-p21.1	156400
Rickets			
Vitamin D–dependent rickets			
1α-Hydroxylase deficiency	Very rare	12q13.1-q13.3	264700
Calcitriol-resistant (VDR defect)	Rare	12q12-q14	277440
Hypophosphatemic rickets			
X-linked dominant	1:20,000	Xp22.2-p22.1	307800
Autosomal dominant	Rare	12p13.3	193100
Autosomal recessive	Rare	4q21	241520
Hypophosphatemic rickets with hypercalciuria			
HHRH, autosomal recessive	Rare	9q34	241530
HHRH, X-linked recessive	Rare	Xp11.22	300554
Fibrous dysplasia	Rare	20q13.2	174800

TYPES	OCCURRENCE	LOCUS	OMIM
Other bone disorders			
Hypophosphatasia			
Infantile	Rare	1p36.1-p34	241500
Childhood	Rare	1p36.1-p34	241510
Adult	Rare	1p36.1-p34	146300
Hyperphosphatasia	Rare	8q24	239000
Osteogenesis imperfecta			
Type I	1:30,000	17q21.31-q22, 7q22.1	166200
Type II	1:60,000	17q21.31-q22, 7q22.1, 3p22	166210, 610854
Type III	1:70,000	17q21.31-q22, 7q22.1	259420
Type IV	Very rare	17q21.31-q22	166220
Osteopetrosis			
Autosomal recessive	1:200,000–300,000	16p13, 11q13.4-q13.5, 6q21	259700
Autosomal dominant	1:100,000–500,000	11q13.4, 16p13	607634,166600
With RTA	Rare	8q22	259730

Hypoparathyroidism

FORM	FINDINGS	CLINICAL PRESENTATION
DiGeorge syndrome	↓ Ca; ↑ Pi; ↓ or absent intact PTH; ↓ 1,25(OH)$_2$D$_3$; nl alk. phosphatase; ±↓ IgA; ±↑ IgE; ↓ absolute lympocytes; ↓ 24-h urine for Ca/Cr	Neonatal hypocalcemia, seizures; dysmorphic facies, including bulbous nose, square nasal tip, cleft palate; short stature; mild to moderate learning difficulties; depression; hypothyroidism; thymic hypoplasia; T-cell deficiency; conotruncal cardiac defects
HDR (Barakat syndrome)		Asymptomatic neonatal hypocalcemia, seizures, tetany, bilateral sensorineural deafness, renal dysplasia
Kenny–Caffey	↓ Ca; ↑ Pi; ↓ or absent intact PTH; ↓ 1,25(OH)$_2$D$_3$; nl alk. phosphatase; ↓ 24-h urine for Ca/Cr	Hypocalcemia, cortical thickening, medullary stenosis of long bones, delayed fontanel closure, ± psychomotor delay, short stature
HRD (Sanjad–Sakati)		Low birth weight, deep-set eyes, microphthalmia, depressed nasal bridge, beaked nose, long philtrum, micrognathia, large earlobes, severe growth retardation, psychomotor retardation, microcephaly, delayed bone age, dental abnormalities, reduced T-cell subsets; susceptible to pneumococcal infections; found in patients of Arab origin
PTH gene defects		Familial isolated hypoparathyroidism, neonatal and childhood hypocalcemia
GCMB deletion		Familial isolated hypoparathyroidism, neonatal and childhood hypocalcemia
Familial hypercalciuric hypocalcemia	↓ Ca; ↑ Pi; normal intact PTH; ↓ or nl magnesium; ↑ 24-h urine for Ca/Cr	Usually asymptomatic
Kearns–Sayre	↓ Ca; ↑ Pi; ↓ or absent intact PTH; ↓ 1,25(OH)$_2$D$_3$; nl alk. phosphatase; ↓ 24-h urine for Ca/Cr	Does not generally appear in the neonatal period; progressive external opthalmoplegia; pigmentary degeneration of the retina; cardiomyopathy; generalized muscle weakness; increased CSF protein
Pearson marrow pancreas	↓ Ca; ↑ Pi; ↓ or absent intact PTH; ↓ 1,25(OH)$_2$D$_3$; nl alk. phosphatase; ↑ HbF ↓ 24-h urine for Ca/Cr; macrocytic anemia; neutropenia; thrombocytopenia	Congenital hypoplastic anemia, failure to thrive, pancreatic fibrosis with diabetes mellitus, neuromuscular dysfunction; believed to evolve into Kearns–Sayre syndrome with hypoparathyroidism
APECED	↓ Ca; ↑ Pi; ↓ or absent intact PTH; ↓ calcitriol; nl alk. phosphatase; ↓ 24-h urine for Ca/Cr	Hypoparathyroidism, Addison disease, chronic mucocutaneous candidiasis, malabsorption, juvenile pernicious anemia, gonadal failure, chronic active hepatitis; usually presents at 3–5 years or later in adolescence

Pseudohypoparathyroidism

FORM	FINDINGS	CLINICAL PRESENTATION
Type Ia	↓ Ca; ; ↑ Pi; ↑ intact PTH; ↓ U$_{cAMP}$; ↓ U$_{Pi}$ in response to hPTH infusion; ↓ 24-h urine for Ca/Cr; ↓ G$_s\alpha$ activity; ↓ IgF1; ↓ free T$_4$; ↑ TSH; ↑ LH/FSH	Hypocalcemia usually beginning at around 8 years of age and rarely before age 3; characteristic AHO phenotype consisting of short stature, round facies, obesity, brachydactyly, subcutaneous ossifications, dental defects, calcification of the basal ganglia; other endocrinapathies may include hypothyroidism, hypogonadism, GHRH resistance, testotoxicosis
Type 1b	↓ Ca; ; ↑ Pi; ↑ intact PTH; ↓ U$_{cAMP}$ and ↓ U$_{Pi}$ in response to hPTH infusion; nl G$_s\alpha$ activity; ↓ 24-h urine for Ca/Cr	Patients do not have the phenotypic features of Albright heridary osteodystrophy (AHO); they show renal resistance to PTH and may develop skeletal lesions similar to patients with hyperparathyroidism

FORM	FINDINGS	CLINICAL PRESENTATION
Type 1c	↓ Ca; ↑ Pi; ↑ intact PTH; ↓ U_{cAMP} and ↓ U_{Pi} in response to hPTH infusion; nl $G_s\alpha$ activity; ↓ 24-h urine for Ca/Cr	Patients have the AHO phenotype and resistance to multiple hormones
Type II	↓ Ca; ↑ Pi; ↑ intact PTH; nl U_{cAMP} and ↓ U_{Pi} in response to hPTH infusion; nl $G_s\alpha$ activity; ↓ 24-h urine for Ca/Cr	Patients do not have the AHO phenotype or resistance to other hormones
PPHP	No biochemical abnormalities; ↓ $G_s\alpha$ activity	AHO phenotype
	Hyperparathyroidism	
Primary hyperparathyroidism		Appears after adolescence; results from sporadic mutations causing isolated parathyroid adenoma
Neonatal, severe		Newborns can present with severe hypercalcemia and skeletal disease, anorexia, irritability, lethargy; may be rapidly fatal; caused by certain inactivating mutations of the CaSR in the homozygous state
MEN I	↑ Ca; ↓ Pi; ↑ intact PTH; ↑ 1,25(OH)$_2$D$_3$; ↓ or nl 25(OH)D$_3$; ↑ alk. phosphatase; ↑ 24-h urine for Ca/Cr; nl to ↑ U_{cAMP}	80% of patients present with hyperparathyroidism (multiglandular hyperplasia); can affect children under age 10 years; caused by mutations in the MENIN gene; autosomal dominant
MEN IIA		Autosomal dominant inheritance; caused by mutations in the RET proto-oncogene; 20% to 30% of patients develop hypoparathyroidism, typically in adulthood
Hyperparathyroidism jaw-tumor (HPT-JT)		Autosomal dominant inheritance; caused by mutations in the HPRT2; associated with hyperparathyroidism and malignant parathyroid tumors (15%), jaw-ossifying tumors, renal cysts, renal harmatomas, Wilm tumors, and uterine tumors
Familial isolated (FIHP)		Isolated hyperparathyroidism with adenomatous changes in the parathyroid gland; genetically heterogeneous; mutations of HPRT2 gene, MENIN, and CaSR have been identified in affected patients
Familial hypocalciuric hypercalcemia	↑ Ca; ↓ phosphorus; nl to ↑ intact PTH; ↑ magnesium; nl alk. phosphatase; spot Ca/Cr urine <0.01; ↓ 24 hour urine for Ca/Cr	Patients usually asymptomatic
Jansen metaphyseal dysplasia	↑ Ca; ↑ alk. phosphatase; ↓ intact PTH; ↑ U_{cAMP}	Hypercalcemia develops within the first few months of life; after puberty, calcium levels may improve but remain slightly elevated; dysmorphic facial features (micrognathia, prominent eyes, high skull vault, hypertelorism, wide-open cranial sutures, high arched palate), choanal atresia, markedly shorted limbs, short tubular bones with metaphyseal abnormalities, enlarged joints, limited mobility, flexion contractures of knees and hip, normal IQ, hearing loss, short stature
	Vitamin D–dependent rickets	
Vitamin D deficiency	↓ or nl Ca; ↓ or nl Pi; ↑ intact PTH; ↑ alk. phosphatase; ↓ 25(OH)D$_3$; ↓ or ↑ or nl 1,25(OH)$_2$D$_3$; ↑ or nl urinary Pi; ↓ urinary Ca	Bone pain, pseudofractures, reluctance to bear weight, seizures, poor growth, rachitic rosary, widening of the wrists, frontal bossing and craniotabes, delayed dentition, susceptibility to pneumonias
1α-Hydroxylase deficiency (VDDR I)	↓ Ca; nl or ↓ Pi; ↑ intact PTH; ↑ alk. phosphatase; nl 25(OH)D$_3$; ↓ 1,25(OH)$_2$D$_3$ ↑ urinary Pi; ↓ urinary Ca	Similar to nutritional rickets; in VDDR type II, alopecia may begin at the first year of life; the severity of alopecia may range from sparse hair to total alopecia without eyelashes
Calcitriol-resistant (VDDR II)	↓ Ca; ↓ Pi; ↑ intact PTH; ↑ alk. phosphatase; nl 25(OH)D$_3$; ↑ 1,25(OH)$_2$D$_3$ ↑ urinary Pi; ↓ urinary Ca	

Hypophosphatemic rickets

FORM	FINDINGS	CLINICAL PRESENTATION
X-linked dominant (XLH)	↓ Pi; nl Ca ; ↓ or nl 1,25(OH)$_2$D$_3$; nl 25(OH)D$_3$; nl PTH; nl uCa, ↑ urinary Pi;	Bone pain, progressive deformities (lower extremities) and stunted growth, delayed dentition, dental abscesses
Autosomal dominant (ADHR)	nl urinary PH, no proteinuria; ↑ serum FGF-23	*Infancy:* Rickets with with renal phosphate wasting. *Adolescence:* With renal wasting, bone pain, fatigue, weakness, pseudofractures, stress fractures. After giving birth, females may develop hypophosphatemia
Tumor-induced osteomalacia (TIO)		Bone pain, muscle weakness, fractures, osteomalacia or rickets; symptoms may be present for years before causal tumor is identified
Autosomal recessive (ARHR)		Bone pain, progressive deformities (lower extremities) and stunted growth, delayed dentition, dental abscesses; severe osteosclerosis combined with coarse and thickened calvaria, broad and undermodeled ribs, and clavicles has been described in older patients
Hypophosphatemia with hypercalciuria (HHRH)	↓ Pi; ↑ Ca; ↓ 1,25(OH)$_2$D$_3$; nl 25(OH)D$_3$; ↓ PTH; ↑ urinary Pi; ↑ urinary Ca; nl urinary PH; nl or ↓ FGF-23	Similar symptoms as with other forms of hypophosphatemic rickets; nephrocalcinosis secondary to hypercalciuria; obligate carriers may have borderline hypercalciuria but do not have hypophosphatemia or rickets
X-linked recessive with hypercalciuria (XRHR)	↓ Pi; ↑ Ca; ↓ PTH; ↑ 1,25(OH)$_2$D$_3$; nl 25(OH)D$_3$; ↑ urinary Pi; ↑ urinary Ca; glucosuria, ↑ aminoaciduria, proteinuria; nl urinary PH	Similar symptoms as with other forms of hypophosphatemic rickets; proteinuria, intermittent aminoaciduria, glucosuria, nephrocalcinosis secondary to hypercalciuria
Fibrous dysplasia	↓ Pi; nl Ca ; ↓ or nl 1,25(OH)$_2$D$_3$; nl 25(OH)D$_3$; nl PTH; nl urinary Ca; ↑ urinary Pi; nl urinary PH, no proteinuria; ↑ serum FGF-23	Facial asymmetry due to abnormal growth of the craniofacial bones and neurological symptoms due to bony encroachment on cranial nerves; also may have symptoms characteristic of associated endocrinopathies and of rickets secondary to hypophosphatemia
Fanconi syndrome	↓ Pi; nl Ca; nl or ↑ PTH; nl or ↓ 1,25(OH)$_2$D$_3$; nl 25(OH)D$_3$; ↑ urinary Pi; nl urinary Ca; glucosuria, aminoaciduria, proteinuria; ↑ urinary PH,	Rickets with renal tubular acidosis, glycosuria and generalized aminoaciduria; associated findings of underlying metabolic disorders may be present

Other bone disorders

FORM	FINDINGS	CLINICAL PRESENTATION
Hypophosphatasia	↓ alk. phosphatase; nl Ca; nl Pi; nl intact PTH; nl 25(OH)D$_3$; nl 1,25(OH)$_2$D$_3$; ↑ inorganic pyrophosphate; ↑ pyridoxal-5-phosphate; nl urinary Pi; nl urinary Ca; ↑ urinary phosphoethanolamine; ↑ urinary inorganic pyrophosphate; ↑ urinary pyridoxal-5-phosphate	*Perinatal form* manifests during gestation; skeletal hypomineralization; short, deformed limbs; most affected newborns survive only briefly *Infantile form:* Infant may appear normal at birth; by 6 months of age, poor feeding, failure to thrive, wide fontanels and hypotonia, hypercalcemia, hypercalciuria, recurrent vomiting, nephrocalcinosis; about 50% die within the year, and prognosis seems to improve if survival beyond infancy; chest bone deformity manifests with respiratory complications *Childhood form* presents with a history of delayed walking, waddling gait, bone pain, premature loss of dentition, frequent fractures *Adult form* shows pseudofractures and poor healing of stress fractures, especially at the metatarsus *Odontohypophosphatemic form:* Premature loss of the teeth is only finding
Hyperphosphatasia (juvenile Paget disease)	↑ alk. phosphatase; nl Ca; nl Pi; nl intact PTH; nl 25(OH)D$_3$; nl 1,25(OH)$_2$D$_3$; nl urinary Pi; nl urinary Ca	Normal at birth; progressive long bone deformities, fractures, vertebral collapse, skull enlargement due to massively thickened calvarium, deafness

Osteogenesis imperfecta

FORM	FINDINGS	CLINICAL PRESENTATION
OI type I		Most frequent form of OI, accounting for 60% to 80% of all OI; typically presents in infancy or early childhood with fractures, blue sclerae, hearing loss, dentinogenesis imperfecta; normal stature and little to no limb deformity
OI type II	Nl alk. phosphatase; nl Ca; nl Pi; nl intact PTH; nl 25(OH)D$_3$; nl 1,25(OH)$_2$D$_3$	Most severe form of OI; lethal during the perinatal period; extreme bone fragility with intrauterine fractures
OI type III		At birth present with triangular facies, frontal bossing, limb shortening; some with blue sclera; progressively deforming, with 50% of cases with intrauterine fragility, short staure
OI type IV		Mild to moderate limb deformities and fractures in infancy; short stature that may be responsive to GH therapy; dentinogenesis imperfect may be present; normal sclerae

Osteopetrosis

FORM	FINDINGS	CLINICAL PRESENTATION
Autosomal recessive		Present at birth or within the first year of life with brittle bones, pancytopenia, progressive blindness and deafness, facial palsy, difficulties with swallowing and feeding, nasal congestion; other clinical findings include hepatosplenomegaly, nystagmus, dental abnormalities, failure to thrive, macrocephaly, intercurrent infections, especially osteomyelitis and rickets
Autosomal dominant (ADO-I, ADO-II, ADO-III)	↑ TRAP in ADO-II and associated biochemical findings of RTA in osteopetrosis due to CAII gene defects	Half the patients with this variant of osteopetrosis are asymptomatic; this subform is characterized by diffuse osteosclerosis, more predominant in the cranial vault, and low fracture rate; affected patients have a normal height, proportion, intelligence, longevity; flattened forehead and elongation of the mandible may be seen during adolescent years
With RTA		Less severe form; RTA, short stature, developmental delay, cerebral calcifications, cranial nerve compressions, increased frequency of fractures, dental abnormalities; no hematological abnormalities

HDR (hypoparathyroidism, deafness, renal dysplasia syndrome); PTH (parathyroid hormone); APECED (autoimmune, polyendocinopath, candidiasis, and ectodermal dystrophy); VDR (vitamin D receptor); VDDR (vitamin D dependent rickets); HHRH (hereditary hypophosphatemic rickets with hypercalciuria); CaSR (calcium sensing receptor); Ca (calcium); Pi (phosphorus); Cr (creatinine); hPTH (human parathyroid hormone); TSH (thyrotropin stimulating hormone); FSH (follicle stimulating hormone); LH (luteinizing stimulating hormone); IgF1 (insuline like growth factor 1); $G_s a$ (a subunit of the stimulatory guanine nucleotide regulation protein); HbF (fetal hemoglobin); CSF (cerebrospinal fluid); ABO (Albright's osteodystrophy); U_{cAMP} (urinary cyclic adenosine monophosphate); U (urinary); HPRT2 (hypoxanthine phosphoribosyltransferase 2 gene); RTA (renal tubular acidosis); TRAP (tartrate–resistant acid phosphatase); FGF–23 (fibroblast growth factor 23)

The differentiation process that results in an osteoblast can be initiated only by a family of factors known as *bone morphogenetic proteins* (BMPs) (5). These proteins are numerous and comprise a subgroup of the class of cytokines responsible for cell–cell signaling and regulation of cell differentiation. The mature osteoblast secretes the proteins comprising bone matrix and contributes to mineralization of the matrix to form true bone. In the process, many osteoblasts become entombed in the mineralized matrix yet continue to communicate with the surface osteoblasts and each other by means of syncytial processes extending throughout a complex canicular system (6). Since the surface osteoblasts also communicate in a similar fashion with the vascular endothelium, the osteocyte appears to be capable of sending systemic signals (7) through what loosely resembles the ganglionic connections of the nervous system. It is thought possible that this system helps the osteocyte to "sense" mechanical stress and signal surface osteoblasts to deposit additional bone tissue as part of a remodeling to meet the stress.

Osteoclast In distinct contrast to the osteoblast, the osteoclast is derived from hematopoietic stem cells that also give rise to macrophages and monocytes (Figure 39-1). Initiation of the differentiation of an osteoclast is caused by macrophage colony-stimulating factor (M-CSF), and the process is carried to completion by many other factors, chief among which is the RANK ligand (RANKL) expressed at the surface of the primitive osteoblast. Together, these two osteoblast-produced molecules are acted on by many hormones to influence osteoclastic activity using the osteoblast as an intermediary. Other factors involved in controlling osteoclastic differentiation include interleukins (ILs), tumor necrosis factor β (TNF-β), and interferon γ (IFN-γ) (8). Emerging from the bone marrow, these cells reach the surface of bone via the circulation; they are large and multinucleated, with many mitochondria and lysosomes. Each osteoclast has a "ruffled border" that consists of many villus-like membrane projections that serve to increase surface area and facilitate resorption of the bone and bone matrix (9); the outer lamellar membrane surface, called the *clear zone*, is specialized to seal the undersurface of the cell to the bone (Figure 39-2). Within the clear zone, the osteoclast secretes H^+, generated by means of an ATPase in the ruffled border membrane, that solubilizes the mineral content of the bone surface directly below the osteoclast. Subsequently, the matrix protein is degraded by enzymes called *proteinases* that also are secreted by the osteoclast. The degradation products then are endocytosed. They traverse the cell until they reach the surface opposite the clear zone and are released (10,11).

Basic Multicellular Unit (BMU) All activity related to bone remodeling and homeostatic maintenance of extra- and intracellular calcium ionic balance derives from the association of osteoblast and osteoclast into the basic multicellular unit (BMU) (12). By virtue of this association alone, it should be apparent that all these activities are a result of coordinated, carefully directed processes that, if disrupted, can result in significant pathology. This is especially apparent when one realizes that in a healthy adult, the skeleton is completely turned over every 10 years. The BMU is a loose association of osteoblasts and osteoclasts clustered in a linear fashion about a blood and nerve supply; the unit is led by the osteoclasts, which resorb an area of bone and then either die or advance to the next site, followed by the osteoblasts. The latter cells lay down new bone in the resorbed area and, following completion of mineralization, flatten and become cells that line the bone surface over the site. The process repeats itself until the area of bone in need is replaced completely, at which point the unit comes to rest and terminates its activity. There is no clearly defined BMU during modeling, although it is self-evident that some degree of coordination is essential in formation and accretion of bone material in accordance with growth and shaping requirements.

The final destination for all cells is, of course, their death. In the case of the osteoblasts and osteoclasts, the chief cause of death is apoptosis. The lifespan of an osteoclast is approximately 2 weeks, whereas that of an osteoblast is much longer, up to 3 months. This is consistent with the differences between bone resorption time (~3 weeks) and complete mineralization of the matrix (~3 months). Osteoclasts, which have reached a specific depth of resorption in cancellous bone or a specific distance from the center in cortical bone, become apoptotic along with a majority of the osteoblasts at the site (13,14). Since approximately 60% of the osteoblasts in any given BMU are destined to undergo apoptosis, it is remarkable that osteocytes generally escape this fate, although some do undergo apoptosis as well. It is considered possible that the imminent death of an osteocyte signals the need for a BMU, thus acting as the reason for the time and site of arrival of the unit. Overall, endocrine-mediated "withdrawal" of materials from the massive bone reservoir depends on varying balances between the activities of the cellular components of the skeleton.

Role of Bone in Calcium–Phosphate Homeostasis

Simplistically described, the chief promoters of bone resorption and consequent systemic release of calcium and phosphate act by receptor binding to the osteoblast and exert minimal effects on the osteoclast. These include parathyroid hormone (PTH), 1,25-dihydroxycholecalciferol (vitamin D), interleukin-1 (IL-1), IL-6, and TNF-β, among many others, all of which act on the osteoblast to evoke a response through cell–cell interaction to dictate osteoclastic response. The single exception to this is calcitonin, for which the osteoclast membrane is richly

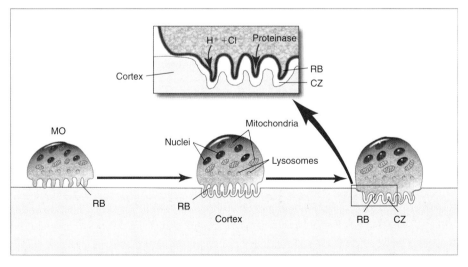

FIGURE 39-2. The mature osteoclast (MO). This is a large, multinucleated cell containing many mitochondria and lysosomes. It has a distinctive ruffled border (RB) consisting of villar projections that considerably increases the area of contact with the bone surface. The RB envelops the area of bone directly below it; within this area, the clear zone (CZ), which is a specialized area of the outer lamellar membrane, seals the area and secretes hydrogen ions and proteinases in order to solubilize and hydrolyze the bone matrix. The resulting products are endocytosed, traverse the cell, and are extruded at the opposite surface.

TABLE 39-1 Factors Affecting Bone Metabolism

	Effect on Bone	Effect on Kidney	Effect on Serum
Parathyroid hormone (PTH)	Binds to PTH receptor on osteoblast; osteoblast produces interleukin-6, which stimulates osteoclast activity and differentiation; calcium released from bone	Strongly inhibits tubule reabsorption of inorganic phosphate; stimulates activity of $25(OH)D_3$ 1α-hydroxylase in production of calcitriol	Raises serum Ca^{2+}; lowers serum P_i; ↑ calcitriol
Calcitriol	Stimulates monocytic precursors to differentiate to osteoclasts; stimulates osteoblast production of bone matrix proteins	Feedback inhibition of renal $25(OH)D_3$ 1α-hydroxylase; increases Ca^{2+} reabsorption	Normalizes serum calcium and P_i
Calcitonin	Inhibits bone resorption; acts directly on osteoclast via receptor binding	Decreases reabsorption of calcium, magnesium, and P_i	No measurable effect

endowed with receptors. The molecular mechanisms by which the deceptively complex anabolic–catabolic osteoblast–osteoclast pair is regulated are being investigated. Although the literature is rich with experimental results, many are contradictory or demand further study. For these reasons, our discussion here will follow the traditional mode regarding the major humoral factors regulating calcium–phosphate balance except where data exist that point clearly to a cellular basis for a given effect. Throughout, however, it will be important to keep in mind the concept that bone comprises a reservoir for calcium, phosphate, and, to a minor degree, magnesium that completes the homeostatic "loop." It is this complete loop that provides an enormous buffer against any losses compromising critical cell functions that otherwise might result in death.

Factors Affecting Bone Metabolism

There is a bewildering array of cell-surface factors and growth factors and a diversity of their interactions. This chapter will focus on the demonstrated and functional physiology, namely, the major regulatory factors of bone metabolism: parathyroid hormone, vitamin D, and to a lesser extent, calcitonin (Table 39-1).

Parathyroid Hormone (PTH) The primary effects of PTH are exerted on bone and the renal tubule; hence it provokes release of calcium and phosphate (as well as magnesium) from the reservoir, simultaneously inhibiting renal calcium and magnesium excretion while facilitating phosphate excretion. The net result is an increase in serum calcium that, in the absence of calcium and/or vitamin D intake, comes about at the ultimate expense of the skeletal stores. Therefore, in cases of dietary vitamin D or deficient calcium intake, homeostasis requires an elevation in PTH concentration for maintenance of normal serum calcium levels (see below). PTH is a polypeptide hormone produced by the chief cells of the parathyroid glands, where it is synthesized in a 115-amino-acid

sequence, cleaved to 90 amino acids as it leaves the endoplasmic reticulum, and finally, cleaved further to 84 residues (mature PTH) as it is stored in secretory vesicles within the cells. As well as providing a store of bioactive hormone, sequestration of PTH within the gland permits degradation intracellularly, an integral part of the mechanism controlling PTH secretion. The estimated half-life of PTH in the circulation is approximately 2 minutes; it is cleaved rapidly into fragments in the liver (~70%) and the kidney, in the latter by endocytosis of filtered hormone within the proximal tubule. Secretion and synthesis of PTH are controlled largely by the concentration of extracellular ionized calcium (Ca^{2+}_o). Lodged within the chief cell membrane is an integral membrane protein receptor called the *calcium-sensing receptor* (CaSR) that is a member of the G protein–coupled receptor group (15). Maintenance of an ionized calcium concentration range of 1.1–1.3 mM requires an extreme sensitivity of response; changes amounting to a few percent in ionized calcium concentration elicit a response. In the parathyroid chief cell, as Ca^{2+}_o increases, it binds to the extracellular domain of the CaSR, which triggers dissociation of a $G_{\alpha q}$ subunit from G protein complex. The $G_{\alpha q}$ subunit activates membrane-bound phospholipase C, which, in turn, causes generation of phosphoinositol trisphosphate and release of Ca^{2+} from the endoplasmic reticulum, thus inhibiting PTH secretion (16). A naturally occurring loss-of-function human mutation transmitted as an autosomal dominant trait known as *familial hypocalciuric hypercalcemia* (FHH) confirms the relationship of the CaSR to the set point at which Ca^{2+}_o inhibits parathyroid secretion of PTH (17). In addition, the increase of circulating PTH due to an elevated set point documents the physiological effects of PTH on renal calcium reabsorption addressed below. In contrast to FHH, an autosomal dominant form of familial hypoparathyroidism has been reported (18) in which the CaSR is exquisitely sensitive to very low Ca^{2+}_o so that PTH secretion is

largely and inappropriately suppressed. The consequences are hypocalcemia and hypercalciuria; such patients may be symptomatically hypocalcemic and develop tetany and seizures.

Many investigators (19–21) have reported the presence of CaSR expression in osteoblasts, a feature that may determine the osteoblastic attraction to the BMU by virtue of the increased local calcium concentration produced by osteoclastic activity. Teleologically, it makes sense for osteoblastic mineralization activity to be stimulated by release of calcium by osteoclasts. Viewed in this manner, one would expect the osteoclast to be reciprocally inhibited by high Ca^{2+}_o, as it actually is by virtue of CaSR expression on the osteoclast membrane as well (19,22). There are also reported data indicating that increased extracellular calcium increases the rate of osteoclastic cellular apoptosis (23). Thus the BMU exerts local control over its cellular elements through cellular communication via calcium concentration and, possibly phosphate as well.

As mentioned earlier, humoral control over the BMU generally is exerted on the osteoblast and is communicated selectively by that cell type to the osteoclast (24). The osteoblast membrane contains PTH receptor sites (25) and responds to binding of the receptor to PTH by secretion of IL-6 (26,27), which then stimulates osteoclastic activity (28,29) as well as osteoclastic differentiation (30,31). Production of IL-6, however, is not the only osteoblastic response to PTH-receptor binding; through stimulation of the α-chain of G protein, PTH increases the activity of adenyl cyclase and thus synthesis of cyclic adenosine monophosphate (cAMP). The cell also responds with production of a number of growth factors and expression of genes that contribute products involved with bone matrix degradation (32). Thus, by virtue of a CaSR sensitive to ambient Ca^{2+} concentration, the organism uses PTH secretion by the parathyroid gland as a message to the osteoblast, and the immediate response of the latter is to

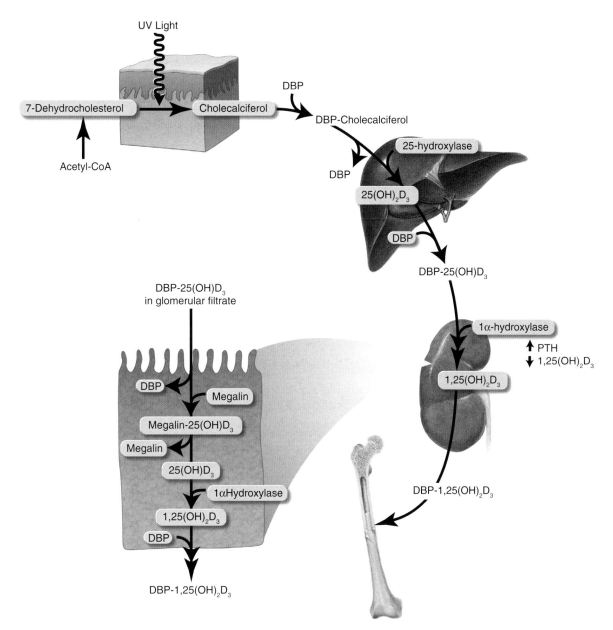

FIGURE 39-3. Synthesis of calcitriol. The dermal layer of the skin is capable of synthesizing 7-dehydrocholesterol (7-DH cholesterol); on ultraviolet (UV) light exposure, this compound is converted to cholecalciferol, or vitamin D_3. Cholecalciferol is avidly bound by vitamin D–binding protein (DBP) and transported in the circulation to the liver, where the DBP is released and the vitamin D_3 is rapidly taken up by the hepatocyte. Cholecalciferol is converted to biologically inactive 25-OH cholecalciferol or $25(OH)D_3$ by the action of a 25-hydroxylase that is a member of the cytochrome P450 family. On exit from the hepatocyte, 25-$(OH)D_3$ is bound tightly to DBP and transported to the kidney, where it is filtered at the glomerulus and taken up at the brush-border surface of the proximal tubule by endocytosis after binding to megalin. The DBP is degraded within the tubule cell, and the megalin–$25(OH)D_3$ complex is transported to the mitochondrion, where the megalin is released for degradation; within the mitochondrion, the free 25-OH cholecalciferol is acted on by a second P450 enzyme, 1α-hydroxylase, to form $1,25(OH)_2D_3$, or calcitriol. On release from the tubule cell across the antiluminal surface, the calcitriol is again bound to DBP, and the bulk circulates as the complex; only a very small fraction remains free in the circulation.

signal the osteoclast to differentiate and initiate activity to release calcium from bone. Simultaneously, PTH binding in the renal tubule directs the nephron to restrict calcium excretion, thus amplifying the net serum effect of the release of calcium from bone. There is also an offsetting effect of removal of calcium from bone by direct PTH stimulation of renal tubule production of active vitamin D, or calcitriol (see below).

Vitamin D Vitamin D is found in two forms: ergocalciferol (vitamin D_2), produced by ultraviolet exposure of ergosterol plants, and cholecalciferol (vitamin D_3), produced by animal tissues and by the action of ultraviolet light (UVB) on 7-dehydrocholesterol (7-DHC) in human skin (Figure 39-3). Cholecalciferol, or vitamin D_3, is among the most intriguing of all molecules in human biology and is not, strictly speaking, a vitamin at all. This is so because the oxidativly-metabolizing cells have the capacity to produce cholesterol from acetyl CoA in virtually unlimited quantities. Cholesterol in the skin can be converted to 7-DHC; with UVB and temperature exposure, this compound is converted to cholecalciferol (melanin competes with 7-DHC for UVB photons, reducing the production of vitamin D_3). Hence the ability to be produced *de novo* disqualifies vitamin D from the category of true vitamins. In addition, vitamin D exerts its biological actions through membrane-receptor binding; true vitamins are inactive cofactors for enzymes that often participate directly in the reaction being mediated through electron transfer or some other mechanism. Thus it is obvious that cholecalciferol meets more fully the criteria of a hormone than those of a vitamin, although cholecalciferol has no intrinsic biological activity and, like many vitamins, requires enzymatic "activation" to exert its effects. The major dietary source of vitamin D_3 is oily fish (e.g., salmon or mackerel) and fish liver oils.

The normal metabolism of cholecalciferol (vitamin D_3), a lipophilic compound that is poorly soluble in aqueous media, involves transport in blood to liver via binding to vitamin D–binding protein (DBP). This protein is present in serum at concentrations several times greater than vitamin D_3 plus all its metabolites; binding affinities for these are vitamin D_3 < $1,25(OH)_2D_3$ < $25(OH)D_3$ (33). This binding protein is critical to the production of active vitamin D, which requires that cholecalciferol undergo hydroxylation at the 25 position in the liver and subsequent 1α-hydroxylation in the kidney. On reaching the hepatocyte, vitamin D_3 is taken up avidly by the cells, where it is 25-hydroxylated (34); the 25-hydroxylase enzyme is a member of the cytochrome P450 family, specifically designated CYP2R1 (35). Activity of CYP2R1 is not tightly regulated because $25(OH)D_3$ concentration in blood is proportional to vitamin D_3 intake. Serum measurement of $25(OH)D_3$ reflects vitamin D stores, with low levels (<80 ng/liter) indicating vitamin D deficiency and high levels (>500 nmol/liter) indicating vitamin D toxicity. $25(OH)D_3$ has minimal, if any, biological activity and, when extracellular, is avidly bound by DBP (36). This bound $25(OH)D_3$ then is carried to the kidney, where it is filtered by the glomerulus (37). Subsequently the DBP–$25(OH)D_3$ complex binds to a receptor-associated protein called *megalin* along the brush border of the proximal tubule (37). The DBP–$25(OH)D_3$ complex then is endocytosed by the brush border, and the DBP is degraded. It was believed originally that transfer of the intracellular $25(OH)D_3$ to the mitochondria of the tubular epithelial cell occurred passively, but recent evidence has established at least two intracellular DBPs that attach to megalin and thus may subserve the need to direct the megalin–$25(OH)D_3$ complex to the mitochondria before the megalin is degraded (38). On entering the mitochondrion, free $25(OH)D_3$ is exposed to a second cytochrome P450–dependent enzyme, $25(OH)D_3$–1α-hydroxylase, which then results in the final biologically active form of vitamin D, $1,25(OH)_2D_3$, or calcitriol. Increases in $1,25(OH)_2D_3$ induce increases in megalin (39), thus enhancing uptake of $25(OH)D_3$ and resulting in a feed-forward system for active hormone production. Once freed from the renal tubular cell, the vast bulk of the newly synthesized $1,25(OH)_2D_3$ circulates in the blood bound again to DBP; only about 0.4% of the total is free in the circulation (40). An important aspect of $1,25(OH)_2D_3$ metabolism is its regulation because the biological potency of its effect is so great. As we have

seen, the 25-hydroxylation reaction is unregulated, and the amount of circulating DBP to carry it to the kidney is far in excess of available $25(OH)D_3$, providing unlimited substrate for the $25(OH)D_3$–1α-hydroxylase. This enzyme is stimulated by low circulating levels of calcitriol, elevated levels of PTH, and reduced serum concentrations of calcium and/or phosphate, thus essentially participating in a feedback loop. Two responses in the tubule cell guard against the generation of toxic levels of $1,25(OH)_2D_3$. The first is the feedback inhibition on the enzyme exerted by calcitriol (as well as other factors controlled by calcitriol, such as increased calcium and phosphate concentrations) (41). The second regulator is a separate enzyme system, the 24-hydroxylase, that is induced by elevated concentrations of calcitriol (33,40). This enzyme carries out a series of oxidative reactions that results in formation of $24,25(OH)_2D_3$, which has essentially no biological potency. Thus these two processes ensure against endogenous vitamin D intoxication, which was essential during evolution when sunlight exposure was virtually unlimited and photosynthetic precursor production unrestrained.

The bone-related actions of calcitriol depend, for the most part, on the presence of the vitamin D receptor (VDR). The VDR is a member of the nuclear receptor superfamily and interacts with the retinoic acid X receptor (RXR) to form a heterodimeric RXR–VDR complex that binds to specific DNA sequences called *vitamin D–response elements*. The VDR gene is located on chromosome 12q12-q14 (42).

Besides bone and kidneys, other tissues and cells in the body have VDRs, including activated T and B lymphocytes, gonads, prostate, brain, colon, and pancreas; the physiological action of calcitriol in these tissues is not clear. Some believe it to function as an intracellular messenger.

Acting through this receptor, calcitriol stimulates monocytic precursors to differentiate into osteoclasts by inducing the production by osteoblasts of a number of osteoclast-activating factors. In addition, there is osteoblast stimulation for the production of BMPs, as well as alkaline phosphatase, all of which indicate bone formation. In addition, expression of the PHEX gene, an essential component of phosphate homeostasis, is stimulated (43). Calcitriol is an essential component of the coordination between the constituents of the BMU in the process of bone remodeling (44). This effect is achieved through coordination of the expression of the RANK/RANKL–osteoprotegerin system that controls the interactions between osteoblasts and osteoclasts in the BMU (45,46). Reported data suggest that the PTH-directed effect on osteo-

clastogenesis depends on the calcitriol–VDR system, which facilitates osteoblastic expression of RANKL (47).

The parathyroid cell has VDRs and responds to calcitriol by decreasing PTH gene transcription and PTH synthesis and secretion. Calcitriol is the primary facilitator of calcium transfer across the intestinal epithelium and into blood (Figure 39-4). Once transferred into the intestinal epithelial cell, calcitriol binds to the nuclear VDR, the so-called AF2 domain undergoing a significant conformational change that initiates gene transcription of multiple factors involved in intestinal calcium uptake (48,49). A great deal is now understood of the mechanism(s) by which calcitriol exerts its nuclear effects to either enhance or down regulate calcium uptake (50), but these processes are far too complex to discuss here in detail. Suffice it to say that the major impact of the initiation of transcription is to increase the number of the two critical brush-border calcium channels, designated $ECaC_1$ and $ECaC_2$ (51). It is believed that one means of intestinal calcium absorption is by passive diffusion via paracellular channels, and this is, therefore, not rate-limited. A second pathway involves the specialized calcium channels under the control of calcitriol; by increasing the number of these calcium channels, the net effect of calcitriol on this initial step is to enhance the amount of calcium transferred per unit time (52). This impact on gene transcription has been verified in mice; normal mice show increased mRNA for both channel proteins (51), whereas VDR knockout mice are unresponsive to calcitriol (52).

The next step in the intestinal cell transfer of calcium is binding to an intracellular calcium-binding protein (CaBP) called *calbindin D*. Calbindin escorts the calcium to the basolateral cell surface; a secondary role of calbindin is to increase the accessibility of the lumen to the intracellular calcium gradient by reducing free intracellular calcium, thus enhancing the influx via the membrane channels (53). As demonstrated in mice genetically deficient in 1α-hydroxylase, in the absence of calcitriol, both the membrane calcium channels and the calbindin levels are low; both increase in response to increased luminal calcium and administered calcitriol (51). The final step in delivery of calcium across intestinal epithelium into the blood is transfer across the basolateral membrane, a process mediated by a calcium ATPase, designated PMCA1. It has been shown consistently that calcitriol upregulates PMCA gene expression (51,54) and increases mRNA stability and half-life (55). Thus it is apparent that $1,25(OH)_2D_3$ exerts control over and is a major determinant of calcium absorption in intestine, thereby facilitating increased calcium absorption.

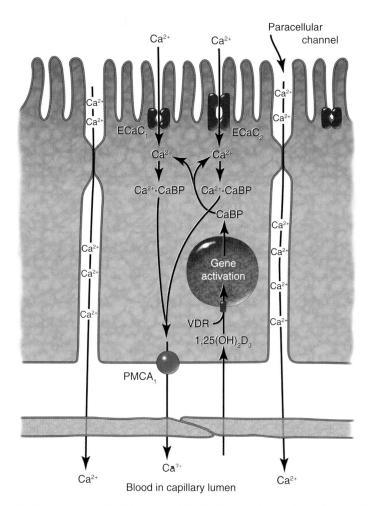

FIGURE 39-4. Intestinal calcium transport. Calcium transport in the intestine occurs by two pathways—the paracellular channel and two separate calcium channels (ECaC$_1$ and ECaC$_2$). Calcium flux through the paracellular channels is concentration-dependent, unsaturable, and unregulated. In contrast, active transport across the brush-border membrane is carried out under control of calcitriol. Calcitriol enhances gene transcription by binding to the nuclear vitamin D receptor (VDR), increasing mRNA for each of the two calcium channel proteins and increasing the number of channels available. After entry, the calcium binds to calbindin or calcium-binding protein (CaBP), which carries out transcellular carriage of the calcium to the inner antiluminal membrane. A secondary effect of the complexing of calcium with CaBP is to reduce the intracellular free calcium, thereby enhancing calcium entry through the calcium channels. Another effect of calcitriol is the up regulation of the antiluminal membrane calcium ATPase, PMCA1; this pump is responsible for transfer of calcium across the antiluminal membrane into blood.

Calcitonin (CT) Early in gestation, cells migrate from the neural crest to the developing thyroid gland, where they establish themselves as thyroid C cells. CT cells produce and secrete the 116-amino-acid proCT, which is cleaved to the active 32-amino-acid peptide hormone calcitonin. Control of the secretory process is independent of the follicular cells of the thyroid gland; the CT cell responds to serum Ca^{2+} concentration via the same calcium-sensing receptor (CaSR) as PTH (56). The clinical effect of calcitonin is, however, converse to that of PTH. The principal activity of calcitonin on bone is to inhibit resorption; among the three endocrine controls discussed here, only calcitonin affects osteoclasts directly. Osteoclasts possess many surface calcitonin receptor sites, and the calcitonin–receptor complex triggers an intracellular G protein–mediated response

that inhibits osteoclast activity (57). Interestingly, resistance to calcitonin's effect develops relatively quickly, apparently as a consequence of an accelerated decay of receptor mRNA concomitant with the formation of the calcitonin–receptor complex (58). Thus any serum calcium–lowering effect of calcitonin's action on osteoclasts is likely to be unmeasureable because such changes will be offset by other mechanisms.

CALCIUM–PHOSPHATE AND MAGNESIUM HOMEOSTASIS

Bone and teeth contain approximately 99% of total-body calcium, whereas the 900–1000 mg of calcium found in the soluble fluids and the 10 grams in soft tissue of the body are in constant flux. The normal human diet contains calcium, magnesium, and

phosphorus in relatively large quantities, and although the renal tubule is remarkably efficient in conserving these elements, no biological system can achieve 100% efficiency, thus resulting in some loss. Bone formation and resorption, intestinal absorption, cellular uptake and exchange with serum, serum protein binding, and renal reabsorption and loss—all the mechanisms for maintenance of calcium, magnesium, and phosphate homeostasis—result in a highly cooperative and responsive homeostatic system.

Calcium

This divalent ion is a crucial participant in many reactions in virtually every cell; it is intrinsic to muscle function (including cardiac muscle contraction and rhythm), neurotransmission, adenosine triphosphate (ATP) metabolism, and blood coagulation, among many other roles. In addition, as we saw earlier, calcium concentration in serum acts as a secretagogue binding to CaSR, thus initiating a series of G protein–mediated reactions and resulting in modulated release of hormones (e.g., calcitonin, PTH, PTH-related peptide [PTHrP], adrenocorticotropic hormone [ACTH], and growth hormone [GH]) involved in calcium homeostasis. It should be kept in mind that calcium is a highly reactive divalent cation, so *a priori* we might expect that it circulates *bound* in serum. Indeed, serum calcium normally is divided equally between bound and ionized forms; of the bound quantity, most is bound to serum proteins, whereas a smaller fraction is found in combination with the organic ions citrate and lactate, as well as the inorganic ions phosphate and sulfate. Although both citrate and lactate are metabolized, under conditions where these anions accumulate, the sole route for excretion is the kidney, resulting in calcium loss into urine. The same is true for phosphate and, in particular, sulfate, which are "fixed acids" and cannot be excreted by any other route but the kidney. Hence, in a simplified view, systemic acidosis will increase urinary calcium loss and require "bone buffering" for maintenance of serum calcium concentration. Clearly, only the ionized calcium fraction is biologically active and available for exchange with the intracellular milieu, as well as for binding to the CaSR.

Phosphate

The importance of phosphate to normal metabolism of bone and oxidative cells cannot be overstated. As a chemical component of hydroxyapatite, inorganic phosphate is integral to the crystal structure of normal bone tissue. As a chemical component of ATP, inorganic phosphate is a part of the most fundamental energy currency of oxidative metabolism. Inorganic phosphate is also associated with lipids as phospholipids, which are integral components of cell membranes and are found in the circulation, as well as phosphoproteins and nucleic acids. In the role of phosphate as an integral part of bone tissue, regulation of inorganic phosphate homeostasis is intimately intertwined with that of calcium. As was the case for calcium, the vast bulk of body inorganic phosphate is contained in bone. In the adult human, phosphate absorption occurs in the intestine in a manner similar to that described earlier for calcium, that is, by both passive and active means (59). Under most circumstances in the adult, except when the diet is severely restricted in phosphate content, passive diffusion through paracellular pathways is the major means of phosphate absorption in the intestine. The amount of phosphate lost in the urine is equivalent to the amount absorbed in the intestine minus the amount lost in pancreatic and intestinal secretions (thus the adult is normally in a zero phosphate balance) (60). This balance is regulated by absorption and excretion; the bulk of absorption occurs passively in the duodenum and jejunum, as well as by sodium cotransport via an ATPase under control of calcitriol. Phosphate excretion is more tightly regulated; from 85% to 90% of phosphate reabsorption takes place in the proximal tubule, the remainder being taken up in the distal convoluted tubule, so net urinary loss normally does not exceed 5% of the filtered total. In both locations, reabsorption is active and influenced by insulin, PTH, corticoids, and calcitriol.

Magnesium

Magnesium is the second most abundant intracellular cation, where it plays a crucial role in enzymatic reactions, and the fourth most abundant body cation, with the majority (60%) found in bone. The bone component of total-body magnesium is either firmly apatite-bound or absorbed to the surface of mineral crystals (61). Approximately 25% of the total is found in tissues with high metabolic rates, further attesting to magnesium's key role in metabolism. Approximately 75% of the magnesium delivered to the distal tubule (about 10% of total filtered by the glomerulus) is reabsorbed at that site. Consequently, the distal tubule plays a major role in control of urinary loss of magnesium. There is good evidence to suggest that reabsorption of magnesium by the distal tubule is at least partially under control of PTH (62). Interestingly, release of PTH from the parathyroid gland depends on normal magnesium concentration; PTH synthesis, however, is unaffected by magnesium fluctuations.

Fetal Skeletal Growth

Development of the fetal skeleton is utterly dependent on sufficient maternal supply of calcium, obviously requiring an increase in both maternal intake and absorption in order to prevent either hypocalcemia or osteoporosis or both in the mother. Consequently, during gestation, maximizing maternal intestinal calcium absorption and retention becomes of paramount importance, and the key to this are increases in maternal/fetal hormones that enhance this absorption. While maternal ionized calcium and PTH concentrations remain fairly undisturbed throughout gestation, the placenta and other fetal structures produce a substance called *PTH-related peptide* (PTHrP) that increases in maternal serum. In addition, maternal calcitriol levels increase to double the pregravid concentration due to a combination of increased maternal synthesis in the kidney and release from the placenta (63). Inasmuch as overall maternal bone mineral density (BMD) does not vary appreciably throughout a normal pregnancy, although there are regional alterations, it must be concluded that the combination of changes including increased calcitriol and PTHrP result in enhanced intestinal calcium absorption and minimal to no bone resorption (63,64).

Since the fetus is entirely dependent for bone mineralization on maternal supply, the fetoplacental unit actively removes calcium from the maternal circulation (65). During the first two trimesters, deposition of calcium in bone contributes primarily to the rapid rate of fetal linear growth rather than to BMD. The majority of the calcium demand occurs during the period of rapid bone mineralization (versus growth) in the third trimester, when an estimated 250 mg of calcium per day enters the fetal circulation from the mother. Since biological processes cannot rely wholly on increased supply in times of demand, it is not surprising that the evidence suggests that the fetal increment of calcium derives from increased intestinal absorption of dietary calcium in the mother, with a lesser increment derived from maternal bone resorption. Calcitriol facilitates increased calcium absorption in the gravid female for transfer to the growing fetus. Paradoxically, while maternal serum calcium levels fall and PTH/PTHrP levels rise, 24-hour urinary calcium excretion rises, along with creatinine clearance (66–68). The fall in serum calcium concentration is attributable to a simultaneous increase in circulating volume and a fall in serum albumin concentration; notably, the decreased serum albumin also enhances ionized calcium concentrations, compensated for by the hypercalciuria of pregnancy. However, measurement of fasting urine calcium excretion provides low to normal values; it is believed that this hypercalciuria is reflective of the increased intestinal absorption and is not representative of enhanced loss of bone calcium (69,70). It must be noted, however, that there is a steady increase in bone turnover throughout pregnancy, suggested by measurement of urinary collagen crosslinks, despite the stability of bone density parameters (71).

The active removal of calcium from the maternal circulation by the fetus establishes and maintains a significant, inwardly directed calcium gradient; fetal/maternal serum total calcium concentrations are approximately 1.4:1.0 (72,73). Data from work in animals suggest that fetal hypercalcemia is the result of concerted actions of PTHrP and PTH (among other potential factors). PTHrP and PTH have distinct roles and interlocking roles in relation to fetal skeletal development and mineralization. PTHrP acts on a unique placental receptor (different from the PTH/PTHrP-responsive receptor) and regulates placental calcium transfer (74,75). Experiments in mice have shown that PTHrP is produced locally at the growth plate, and its absence leads to abnormalities of chondrocyte differentiation and skeletal development. PTH, however, has a more dominant effect on calcium regulation than PTHrP and a critical role in maintaining skeletal mineral accretion (76).

In contrast to lower than maternal calcitriol concentration, fetal PTH is low in relation to maternal and postnatal levels, although PTH/PTHrP concentration is higher than corresponding maternal PTH concentration during gestation (77,78). While PTH remains low in relation to maternal levels, the fetal parathyroid gland has the capacity to produce and secrete PTH in response to hypocalcemia. Since the key effect of calcitriol is exerted on intestinal absorption, the fetus has little need for high concentrations of active vitamin D. Thus the increased maternal calcium absorption and the stimulation of transplacental transfer of calcium by PTHrP release with maintenance of a state of fetal hypercalcemia are sufficient for bone mineralization. Although the fetus is apparently capable of synthesizing calcitriol, fetal calcium metabolism appears to be relatively independent of vitamin D. Fetal calcitonin concentration is substantially higher than normal adult levels throughout gestation; although the reasons are not established, it is possible that high circulating calcitonin serves to inhibit fetal bone resorption. A substantial portion of the elevation in fetal total calcium is found in the ionized fraction. The physiological reasons for the maintenance of a state of hypercalcemia have not yet been elucidated.

Neonatal Changes in Calcium Metabolism

As mentioned earlier, fetal PTH concentrations are near undetectable at term, whereas serum calcium is increased, indicating that PTH secretion is suppressed by CaSR. This situation is immediately reversed at birth, when maternal calcium supply is interrupted; simultaneously, PTHrP synthesized by the feto-placental unit has diminished. Within 24 hours of life, the neonatal serum calcium (both total and ionized) and PTHrP have fallen to low-normal adult concentrations, whereas at the same time PTH and calcitriol concentrations slowly ascend into the low adult ranges (79). The PTH response of the neonate to declining serum calcium indicates the presence of functional parathyroid CaSR. Notably, as PTH increases, there is a slow decline in calcitonin, perhaps signaling the onset of bone remodeling.

Postnatally, the term infant slowly adapts to the interruption in maternal calcium supply, and as endogenous endocrine regulators of growth appear, linear growth resumes, usually within the first 1–2 weeks of life (80). Keeping in mind the many developmental/physical changes occurring in the first months of life, one would anticipate not simply increased BMD but bone remodeling as well. Recent data support this assumption, indicating that both bone formation and resorption increase in the first 3 days postnatally, coincident with the increases in PTH and calcitriol and the decrease in calcitonin (79,81). Specifically, there was an increase in the protein osteocalcin, which is made exclusively by osteoblasts and is believed to restrict bone formation without affecting mineralization (82); the C-terminal telopeptide of type I collagen also was increased, signifying bone resorption (81).

In order to support the calcium requirements for linear growth as well as adequate bone mineralization, the neonate requires assistance from the kidney. In addition to its role of 1α-hydroxylation in the production of active vitamin D (calcitriol), the postnatal kidney must assume the additional function of mineral conservation. In utero, any mineral losses in urine are either compensated by maternal supply or swallowed and reabsorbed, both sources obviously being lost at birth. Thus the consequences of birth on calcium metabolism include dependence on a continuing dietary source of calcium to support a skeletal accretion rate of 150 mg/day of cal-

cium, increased production of calcitriol to enhance intestinal absorption to meet this demand, and regulated renal conservation of calcium, phosphate, and magnesium for proper bone mineralization. The initial serum phosphate concentration in a term neonate is significantly above adult norms. The subsequent fall in serum phosphate is related to increased secretion of PTH.

Renal Calcium Handling By the Neonate

In response to the rapid fall in total and ionized calcium concentrations over the first 24–48 hours of life, there is a predictable and reciprocal increase in serum PTH. Acting through the calcium-sensitive receptor (CaSR), the falling ionized calcium triggers PTH secretion, which then enhances renal calcium reabsorption and activates the renal 1α-hydroxylase to increase production of calcitriol. Ontogentically, it is of interest that there are data suggesting that PTH responsiveness of the renal tubule increases with postnatal age (83,84). Functionally, the result is to provoke further PTH secretion due to persistently decreasing serum calcium levels and further induction of 1α-hydroxylase activity, resulting in increased intestinal absorption of calcium. As the renal tubule undergoes maturation, the effect of PTH in reducing calcium clearance becomes greater, and both PTH and calcitriol concentrations in the serum stabilize within the adult range by 3–4 days of postnatal life (79). Concurrently, calcium excretion, which is usually low at birth, increases slowly over the first 2 weeks of postnatal life, likely a result of increased glomerular perfusion as well as an increase in the filtered load consequent to the rise in serum concentration. It is worthy of mention that calcitonin, which remains above adult levels throughout this time frame, also has a calciuric effect; it also may moderate the reabsorptive impact of PTH on bone because PTH secretion drives production of calcitriol.

Neonatal Calcium Absorption

As indicated earlier, the initial rise in PTH activates renal 1α-hydroxylase and leads to an increased rate of synthesis of calcitriol. It is well established that calcium absorption in the intestine occurs by both passive and active means. Although we reviewed the active process earlier, it is important to note that passive absorption is directly proportional to intraluminal concentration, is unregulated, and occurs throughout the intestine. In the preterm infant, as well as in the early days of postnatal life in the term baby, passive absorption may be the predominant means of cal-

cium absorption as the active transport system undergoes maturation (85). Significantly, capacity for vitamin D absorption from the lumen is now recognized to undergo developmental changes, so oral vitamin D in the neonate may have little effect on absorption in comparison with the enhanced endogenous synthesis noted earlier (86).

Neonatal Phosphate Absorption

Again, as with calcium, the source of inorganic phosphate in fetal life is the maternal circulation. At birth, the neonate is required to absorb and conserve inorganic phosphate in order to keep pace with the needs of developing bone and the accumulation of calcium. The infant at term has accumulated approximately 50% of the adult inorganic phosphate load per kilogram of body weight, consistent with the relative densities of neonatal and adult human bone. The calcium/phosphorus ratio of human milk and most infant formulas is in the range of 2:1, yet the human infant is hyperphosphatemic as well as hypercalcemic in relation to the adult. A major contributor to the ability to maintain a positive phosphate balance, reflected in the higher serum phosphate concentration, is the enhanced intestinal absorption in the neonate, which can exceed 90% of the dietary intake of phosphate (85). In experimental animals, there appears to be enhanced expression of phosphate transporters throughout the neonatal gastrointestinal tract, thus increasing the contribution of active transport to overall phosphate balance (87).

Neonatal Renal Phosphate Handling

A second contributor to neonatal phosphate homeostasis is the kidney, where phosphate is filtered at the glomerulus and passes into the tubule. Neonates and children, in contrast to adults, have a positive phosphorus balance, which supports adequate bone mineralization and growth. How the developing kidney contributes to this balance is not entirely understood, but it has been accepted for some time that the threshold for inorganic phosphate (T_mPO_4) is substantially higher than the plasma phosphate concentration in the neonate (88). There is evidence that the tubule is less responsive to PTH in young rats than in adults, so the phosphaturic effect of high serum phosphate concentration is blunted (89,90). As a consequence, clearance of phosphate is lower than that in an adult; it also should be noted that glomerular filtration is reduced in the normal term neonate, which further contributes to a positive phosphate balance. Finally, the blunted PTH response and hyperphosphatemia increase

PTH secretion, which, in turn, further activates renal 1α-hydroxylase and results in greater calcitriol production. Calcitriol enhances the efficiency of phosphate absorption in the intestine and kidney, further contributing to maintenance of hyperphosphatemia until the renal tubule is competent to respond to PTH and produce phosphaturia.

Neonatal Magnesium Metabolism

During gestation, magnesium is transferred to the fetus across the placenta against a gradient by active transport (91). At birth, serum magnesium concentration is in the normal adult range and remains stable thereafter.

Summary

Overall, the developing fetus must accomplish two primarily important tasks: first, it must accumulate sufficient stores of calcium, phosphate, and magnesium to support both oxidative metabolism and rapid postnatal cellular replication; and second, it must establish an uninterrupted supply of calcium and phosphate to enable bone mineralization and growth in relation to gestational age. All three minerals are actively transported to the fetus across the placenta, and any intrauterine urinary losses are recovered from the amniotic fluid by swallowing. Maternal calcium uptake from the intestine is expedited by increased circulating calcitriol, produced as a consequence of placental/fetal production of PTHrP, which also expedites transfer of calcium across the placenta. Postnatally, the neonate must continue to engage in rapid mineral accumulation without benefit of recovered urinary losses. Neonatal intestinal calcium absorption is enhanced by a greater proportion of paracellular, nonsaturable, and gradient-dependent absorption than seen in the adult. Vitamin D absorption in the intestine develops with postnatal age, suggesting that oral supplements of vitamin D are not helpful in increasing neonatal calcium absorption. PTH levels increase in response to the initial fall in serum calcium concentration, having its primary effect on further calcitriol synthesis but also enhancing tubular reabsorption in the developing renal tubule. Phosphate transport is enhanced in the neonatal gut, and the renal threshold for phosphate is higher than in the older infant, permitting both increased phosphate absorption and retention. Magnesium is actively accumulated during gestation and is retained at the distal renal tubular level under the partial influence of the increased neonatal PTH levels. Consequently, the human neonate is well-equipped for sustained rapid growth and active oxidative metabolism as long as dietary supplies are adequate.

HYPOCALCEMIA

Hypocalcemia occurs in a wide range of disorders (Table 39-2) and results from an imbalance of calcium absorption, excretion, and/or distribution. Specifically, hypocalcemia is

---

TABLE 39-2 Causes of Hypocalcemia

Neonatal hypocalcemia	Childhood and adolescent hypocalcemia
Early neonatal (first 3 days of life)	Hypoparathyroidism
Maternal diabetes	Primary
Toxemia of pregnancy	DiGeorge syndrome (22q11.2 microdeletions)
Maternal hyperparathyroidism	Familial hypoparathyroidism (recessive, dominant, X-linked)
Congenital rubella	Partial deletion of GCMB
Sepsis	Kenny–Caffey syndrome
SGA, IUGR, prematurity	Hypoparathyroidism, retardation dysmorphism syndrome
Asphyxia	Kearns–Sayre mitochondropathy
Hypomagnesemia	Pearson mitochondropathy
Transfusion (citrated blood products/alkali)	PTH gene defects
Respiratory or metabolic alkalosis	CaSR-activating gene mutations
Late neonatal (from 4th to 10th day of life)	Pseudohypoparathyroidism
Excessive ingestion of evaporated/whole milk (increased phosphate load)	Secondary
Vitamin D deficiency	Autoimmune polyglandular syndrome type I (APS-I)
Nutritional	Radiation
Deficient 1α-hydroxylase activity	Surgery
VDR loss-of-function mutation	Infiltration (hemochromatosis, thalassemia, Wilson disease, etc.)
Nutritional calcium deficiency	Severe vitamin D deficiency (acquired PTH resistance)
Hypomagnesemia	Hypomagnesemia (acquired PTH resistance)
Acute/chronic renal insufficiency	Vitamin D deficiency
Hypoalbuminemia (e.g., nephrotic syndrome)	Nutritional
Transfusion (citrated blood products/alkali)	Deficient 1α-hydroxylase activity
Diuretics (furosemide)	VDR loss-of-function mutation
Organic acidemias	Nutritional calcium deficiency
Hypoparathyroidism, primary	Hypomagnesemia
DiGeorge syndrome (22q11.2 microdeletions)	Hyperphosphatemia
Familial hypoparathyroidism (recessive, dominant, X-linked)	Renal failure
Partial deletion of GCMB	Tumor lysis
Kenny–Caffey syndrome	Rhabdomyolysis (muscle injury, long-chain fatty acid oxidation disorders)
Hypoparathyroidism, retardation dysmorphism syndrome	Hypoalbuminemia (e.g., nephrotic syndrome)
Kearns–Sayre mitochondropathy	Drugs
Pearson mitochondropathy	Diuretics (furosemide)
PTH gene defects	Chemotherapy (cisplatin, asparaginase, doxorubicin, cytosine arabinoside)
CaSR-activating gene mutations	Transfusion (citrated blood products/alkali)
Pseudohypoparathyroidism	Organic acidemias (IVA, MMA, PPA)

defined as a total serum level of less than 7 mg/dL in preterm infants, less than 8 mg/dL in newborns, and less than 8.8 mg/dL in children. The organization of the discussion begins with the general pathophysiology of hypocalcemia, followed by neonatal hypocalcemia, the type encountered most frequently by the pediatrician, and concluding with hypoparathyroidism and miscellaneous causes of hypocalcemia. While Ca^{2+} has many functions that include a role in several critical enzymatic steps in oxidative metabolism, its most apparent role clinically is the one this cation plays in neuromuscular function. Keeping in mind that the myocyte converts biochemical to mechanical energy, any interference with this process is certain to manifest clinically. A brief review of this process is both instructive and serves to illustrate the reasons for the adverse neuromuscular implications of hypocalcemia.

Pathophysiology

In the normal course of events, transmission of the nerve impulse to the surface membrane of the myocyte initiates a depolarization phenomenon. The depolarization wave is conducted into the interior of the cell by the transverse (T) tubules, which are extensions of the surface membrane; the T-tubules form a specialized contact with the sarcoplasmic reticulum (SR) at the T–SR junction (Figure 39-5). The specialization unique to this junction is the presence of two key regulators of the excitation–contraction apparatus, the dihydropyridine (DHPR) and ryanodine (RyR) receptors (92,93). The DHPRs found in cardiac and skeletal muscle are distinct entities, coded differently, structurally distinct, and under separate regulatory constraints (94). It is also important to note that the DHPR is integral to the plasma membrane and T-tubules; it is thought to have bimodal functions as a voltage sensor and calcium channel (92,94). In contrast to the DHPR, the RyR is integral to the sarcomeric membrane, where it acts as a calcium channel, allowing brief but rapid efflux of stored Ca^{2+} under the tight control of the DHPR, especially in skeletal muscle (95). In this fashion, the phenomena of nerve transmission and myocyte response are tightly linked; in skeletal muscle, the DHPR acts primarily as a voltage sensor, monitoring the relatively slow calcium current and thereby controlling RyR-mediated release of stored calcium from the sarcomeric reticulum. The DHPR is far more critical to activation of RyR in cardiac muscle, where it plays a key role because of the rapid and substantial Ca^{2+} current (96).

The functional differences between skeletal and cardiac muscle is underscored by the seminal observation by Ringer in 1883 (97) that the latter muscle is nonfunctional in the absence of calcium, whereas skeletal muscle remains contractile for hours under similar conditions (98).

The distribution of Ca^{2+} across various cell boundaries is widely disparate. While extracellular ionized calcium generally is in the range of 1–1.5 mM, cytoplasmic calcium in the resting muscle cell is 20–50 nM, and SR contains 0.1–2.0 mM calcium. Within the various membrane structures, there are calcium pumps that are responsible for maintenance and/or restoration of these enormous gradients (99). It has been estimated that approximately 30% of total cardiac cell energy production at rest is devoted to maintenance of the homeostatic distribution of intracellular calcium (100). This relatively large fractional distribution is probably as related to protection of the critical enzymatic machinery for oxidative metabolism as it is to muscle contraction per se. Nonetheless, it serves to illustrate the importance of calcium to muscle cell function. At the cellular level, then, given the complexity of the regulatory and activation phenomena, as well as the enormous gradients of calcium to be maintained, the adverse effects of significant changes in extracellular calcium concentration are easy to envision.

At a macro level, the impact on cardiac muscle function of hypocalcemia is considerable. Approximately 10% of intracellular calcium contributing to the contractile phenomenon is derived from entry from the extracellular space (100).

It is this influx that is required for initiation of the release of calcium from the SR via the RyR. Thus significant alteration of the extracellular Ca^{2+} is likely to have a measurable effect on intracellular ionic shifts, depolarization phenomena, and cardiac muscle contractility. The first two are manifested in the electrocardiographic alterations mentioned earlier as signs of hypocalcemia. Changes in skeletal muscle are less likely to appear as early as those in cardiac muscle, but the underlying phenomena are similar; the DHPR in skeletal muscle is less of a factor in the RyR, so

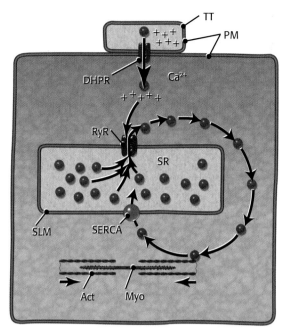

FIGURE 39-5. Role of calcium in muscle contraction. Following transmission of the neural impulse to the surface membrane, the depolarization wave is conducted along the T-tubule (TT), a specialized extension of the plasma membrane (PM). The figure shows the idealized structure of the myocyte at the T-SR junction, a specialized site at which the dihydropyridine (DHPR) and ryanodine (RyR) receptors are located. These receptors are key to regulation of the excitation–contraction process, in which each functions as a calcium channel but with distinct features. The DHPR is an integral structure of the PM and TT with voltage sensor and calcium channel properties; the RyR is located within the sarcolemmal membrane (SLM) and functions exclusively as a calcium channel. On activation, RyR permits rapid release of large amounts of calcium from the sarcoplasmic reticulum (SR); binding of calcium to the troponin C subunit (not shown) permits interaction of the actin (ACT) and myosin (MYO) filaments, which physically slide across each other to produce a contraction. The calcium released from the SR is returned to the SR by a high-capacity Ca^{2+}-ATPase (SERCA), and the actin–myosin complex relaxes by reversing the directions of the slide.

the transcytoplasmic membrane calcium gradient assumes a lower priority in determination of function.

Clinical Manifestations

In clinical practice, mild hypocalcemia is often seen in association with a variety of underlying disorders whose symptoms and signs may mask those of the hypocalcemia (Figure 39-6). However, clinically significant hypocalcemia eventually will manifest in physiologic changes, the severity of which can be striking. These include paresthesia, tetany, positive Chvostek and Trousseau signs, prolongation of the QT interval, QRS-complex and ST-segment changes, and in particularly acute circumstances, grand mal seizures and ventricular arrythmias. The important message in all this is that causes of hypocalcemia are both myriad and potentially devastating, and an etiological diagnosis always must be sought.

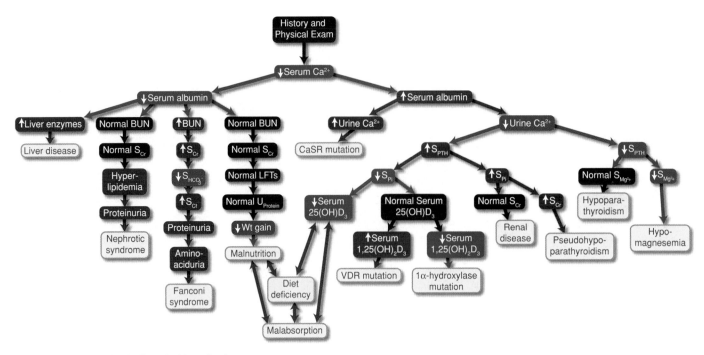

FIGURE 39-6. Algorithm for the diagnosis of hypocalcemia.

NEONATAL HYPOCALCEMIA

Neonatal hypocalcemia is defined as a serum concentration below 8 mg/dL in term infants and below 7 mg/dL in preterm infants. Depending on the time of onset, it can be classified as early or late neonatal hypocalcemia. Early neonatal hypocalcemia occurs during the first 3 days of life and is seen commonly in premature babies, infants of diabetic mothers (IDMs), and asphyxiated babies. Premature infants have a postnatal decrease in calcium levels that occurs earlier and is more exaggerated than in the term infants. The suggested mechanism behind the hypocalcemia of prematurity is a delayed response of the parathyroids to hypocalcemia as well as hyperphosphatemia due to delay in the phosphaturic action of PTH at the kidney. This is consistent with the earlier discussion regarding the blunted renal response of the neonatal kidney to hyperphosphatemia. The IDM shows changes in calcium levels similar to those in premature babies; hypocalcemia may be caused by decreased responsiveness of the parathyroid gland at birth (functional hypoparathyroidism) caused by hypomagnesemia (pregnant diabetic females have lower magnesium and PTH levels during pregnancy). Intrauterine growth-retarded (IUGR) infants, infants of preeclamptic mothers, and asphyxiated babies experience early hypocalcemia and tend to develop hypomagnesemia.

Late neonatal hypocalcemia presenting at between 5 and 10 days of life is more frequent in full-term neonates than in premature neonates and is not correlated with birth trauma or asphyxia. Causes of late hypocalcemia include hypophosphatemia, hypomagnesemia, and maternal hyperparathyroidism and vitamin D deficiency. Maternal use of anticonvulsants such as phenytoin and phenobarbital increases vitamin D clearance due to hepatic cytochrome P450 enzyme system induction and may result in low maternal vitamin D levels. Hyperphosphatemia is due to 1) inability of the immature kidney to excrete phosphate and 2) transient low PTH levels and high dietary phosphate load. Severe hypomagnesemia may occur in infants with intestinal malabsorption or renal tubular malabsorption. Hypocalcemia in infants born to mothers with hyperparathyroidism may occur within the first 3 weeks of life and as late as 1 year of age. Maternal hypercalcemia results in increased calcium delivery to the fetus and fetal hypercalcemia, which, in turn, inhibits parathyroid gland function and PTH production. In addition, maternal PTH cannot cross the placenta. Adverse fetal outcomes including abortion and stillbirth have been associated with maternal hyperparathyroidism. Similar suppression of fetal parathyroids occurs when the mother has hypercalcemia due to familial hypocalciuric hypercalcemia. At birth, these infants develop hypocalcemia due to oversuppressed parathyroid glands; therapy for the acute hypocalcemia may be required, but the disorder is usually self-limited.

Other causes of transient hypocalcemia in the newborn period may occur in infants receiving lipid infusions or citrated blood products; fatty acids or citrate forms complexes with ionized calcium and decreases serum ionized calcium. Respiratory distress and respiratory alkalosis also can cause hypocalcemia because alkalosis results in a shift of ionized calcium to the protein-bound compartment.

In most infants, hypocalcemia resolves after 2–4 weeks. If hypocalcemia and hyperphosphatemia persist beyond the 4 weeks, permanent causes of hypocalcemia should be sought, such as defects in vitamin D metabolism, isolated or syndromic hypoparathyroidism, and pseudohypoparathyroidism. Neonates with chronic renal failure from renal hypoplasia/dysplasia and obstructive nephropathy may develop hypocalcemia and hyperphosphatemia with elevated PTH levels, as well as increased blood urea nitrogen (BUN) and creatinine.

Diagnosis of Neonatal Hypocalcemia

The diagnostic evaluation of neonatal hypocalcemia should include serum total and ionized calcium, magnesium, phosphorus; spot urine for calcium-to-creatinine ratio; total protein and albumin; intact PTH; electrolytes, including BUN and creatinine; and vitamin D metabolites. In persistent hypocalcemia, if maternal hypoparathyroidism or vitamin D deficiency is suspected, maternal evaluation should include total and ionized serum calcium, magnesium, and phosphorus; intact PTH; $25(OH)D_3$ and $1,25(OH)_2D_3$; and spot urine for calcium-to-creatinine ratio. The diagnostic workup of a child with hypocalcemia is similar to that for the neonate.

Treatment of Neonatal Hypocalcemia

Acute Phase Asymptomatic hypocalcemic patients usually require no immediate intervention while a diagnostic investigation is undertaken. Therapy in neonatal hypocalcemia usually is recommended when total calcium level is less than 5–6 mg/dL in the premature infant and less than 6–7 mg/dL in the full-term infant. Rapid therapeutic intervention is warranted in any symptomatic neonate with hypocalcemia. A 10% calcium gluconate solution at a dose of 1–2 mL/kg (9 mg of elemental calcium/mL) is given slowly at a rate less than 1 mL/min over 5–10 minutes with constant electrocardiographic monitoring of the QT interval until symptoms disappear. If tetany or seizures recur, the dose can be repeated as necessary at 6- to 8-hour intervals (a dose of 1–3 mL of 10% calcium gluconate usually will stop seizures) until resolution of severe symptoms, or elemental calcium at 1–3 mg/kg/h can be started as a continuous infusion. An important caveat is that if the serum calcium concentration does not rise with such therapy, primary hypomagnesemia must be considered. If acute hypocalcemia is associated with hypomagnesemia, magnesium sulfate can be given intravenously at a dose of 0.1–0.2 mL/kg (50% solution) under cardiac monitoring or administered intramuscularly as an alternative. In the case of severe persistent hypocalcemia calcitriol at 20–100 ng/kg/day orally or intravenously may be used in addition to calcium supplementation.

Maintenance In infants that are not fed enterally, the resolution of symptomatic hypocalcemia should be followed by a continuous infusion at 1–3 mg/kg/h of elemenatal calcium to maintain the serum calcium level above 7.5–8.0 mg/dL while diagnostic investigation is in progress. Infants on parenteral nutrition may receive calcium supplementation as 50 mg elemental calcium per 100 mL until starting enteral feedings. Calcium gluconate and calcium chloride (10% preservative free solution) contain elemental calcium 9 mg/ml and 27.2 mg/ml, respectively. In asymptomatic infants with hypocalcemia, oral administration of 50–75 mg elemental Ca per kilogram per day in four to six divided doses is recommended. Oral suspension of calcium carbonate, 250 mg/ml, contains elemental calcium 100 mg/ml and chewable tablets contain elemental calcium 200 mg/500 calcium carbonate; oral suspension of calcium glubionate 360 mg/ml contain elemental calcium 27.2 mg/ml.

In infants with hyperphosphatemia, maintenance therapy of hypocalcemia with oral administration of calcium should include a low-phosphate formula such as PMK60/40 or breast milk and an overall calcium-to-phosphate ratio of 4:1. Infants with vitamin D–deficiency rickets due to maternal vitamin D deficiency respond well to 1000 U of daily oral vitamin D for 4 weeks and elemental calcium of at least 40–75 mg/kg/day. The duration of supplemental calcium therapy in early neonatal hypocalcemia is usually 2–3 days. Once the serum calcium level is normalized, the calcium supplementation can be reduced by half for 2 days and then discontinued. If higher doses and prolonged calcium supplementation are required, permanent causes of hypocalcemia are more likely (see sections on treatment of hypoparathyroidism, pseudo-hypoparathyroidism, and vitamin D metabolism defects).

Hypocalcemia Treatment in Children and Adolescents

The acute treatment of symptomatic hypocalcemia in children and adolescents, as well as maintenance therapy while investigating for the underlying cause, is the same as in neonatal hypocalcemia. Specific therapies depending on the cause are discussed in the related sections.

Monitoring of Hypocalcemia Laboratory evaluation during treatment includes studies to monitor the underlying cause of hypocalcemia as well the adequacy of calcium supplementation by measuring fasting, total, and ionized serum calcium; fasting serum phosphate; and spot urine for calcium-to-creatinine ratio.

HYPOPARATHYROIDISM

Etiology/Pathophysiology Hypoparathyroidism is a clinical disorder that can be due to 1) impaired synthesis or secretion of PTH, 2) target-organ PTH resistance, or 3) to inappropriate regulation due to constitutively activated or antibody-stimulated CaSR. In order to understand the basis for abnormalities of the parathyroid gland, it is crucial to have a grasp of the reciprocal relationships among PTH, vitamin D, and serum calcium, phosphate, and magnesium concentrations. These were discussed earlier in various contexts; the CaSR regulates PTH secretion, PTH activates renal 1α-hydroxylase to increase calcitriol production, and increased calcitriol and normalized serum calcium suppress PTH secretion. Phosphate is regulated chiefly by diet and the kidney; the latter responds to PTH by production of phosphaturia. Magnesium is essential to the normal secretory response of the parathyroids. Hence interruption in any arm of this loop will cause hypocalcemia; the *sine qua non* of hypoparathyroidism is hypocalcemia, hyperphosphatemia, and tetany. However, in seeking an etiology for hypocalcemia, differentiation between states of PTH deficiency and impaired PTH responsiveness can be very difficult in some cases.

PTH DEFICIENCY (CONGENITAL, ACQUIRED, TRANSIENT)

Abnormalities of branchial arch formation resulting in aplasia or hypoplasia of the parathyroid glands are the most common causes of hypoparathyroidism in infants and children; they can be part of complex congenital abnormalities such as DiGeorge, Bakarat, or HDR (hypoparathyroidism, nerve deafness, and renal dysplasia) syndrome; Kenny–Caffey syndrome (101); and HRD (hypoparathyroidism, retardation, and dysmorphism) syndrome (102) or isolated as in familial isolated hypoparathyroidism due to GCMB mutations or due to defects of an unknown developmental gene that result in agenesis of the parathyroid gland. The unknown gene is mapped to the Xq27 region and is transmitted through X-linked recessive inheritance. The SOX3 gene is located in the Xq27 region and is one of the candidate genes because SOX3 gene expression has been shown in the parathyroid glands (103).

Activating mutations of the CaSR gene are associated with chronic suppression of PTH secretion and autosomal dominant familial hypoparathyroidism, whereas magnesium deficiency (congenital or acquired) is associated with decreased PTH secretion as well as resistance to PTH action. Pearson syndrome and polyglandular autoimmune syndrome (APECED) are also associated with hypoparathyroidism (104).

Aquired causes of hypoparathyroidism include cervical irradiation with radioisotopic iodine (105) and surgical dissection for unrelated causes. Surgical thyroidectomy frequently results in inadvertent parathyroidectomy due to the anatomical relationships of the two endocrine glands. It is unclear why irradiation causes hypoparathyroidism. In addition, certain drugs, particularly anticonvulsants, may cause hypocalcemia (106). This effect is particularly common with use of drugs that induce hepatic cytochrome P450 because vitamin D catabolism is carried out by this family of enzymes, although the precise mechanism remains obscure. Administration of pamidronate also has been reported to cause hypocalcemia (107), probably because bone resorption is blocked.

Other miscellaneous causes for hypoparathyroidism include severe intrauterine or postnatally acquired infection (e.g., congenital rubella). The reasons for this are poorly understood, but the deficiency is usually transient. Infiltrative disorders, such as hemochromatosis and Wilson disease, may diminish parathyroid function over time.

By definition, all these conditions have in common a deficiency of PTH; the exception is the genetic defect in the PTH molecule, although even in this case PTH measured by the usual clinical methodologies is undetectable. Given the inverse relationship between serum ionized calcium concentration and PTH response, it also may be surmised that all have in common a degree of hypocalcemia. Approximately 10% of total calcium reabsorption in the kidney is under control of PTH at the distal tubule level, where it increases calcium reabsorption. Hence PTH deficiency will lead to enhanced urinary calcium loss. Moreover, the normal phosphaturic effect of PTH on the renal tubule is absent or diminished, so retention of phosphate will result in hyperphosphatemia. Since a major effect of PTH secretion is mobilization of bone calcium, PTH deficiency generally results in hypocalcemia and hyperphosphatemia without any change in the serum alkaline phosphatase.

CONGENITAL HYPOPARATHYROIDISM

DiGeorge Syndrome

One of the most common causes of this congenital endocrinopathy is the DiGeorge syndrome, in which the parathyroid glands are absent; DiGeorge syndrome is one of the phenotypes associated with 22q11 microdeletion syndrome and is caused by abnormal third and fourth branchial arch development, with various degrees of parathyroid and thymus glandular hypoplasia, cardiac maldevelopment, and facial abnormalities. Although the vast majority of patients are affected by the 22q11.2 defect, deletions have been identified at a second locus at 10p13, termed *DiGeorge locus type II* (DGSII) (108, 109).

The relationship of genotype to phenotype is loose at best, and the reasons for the wide clinical spectrum in these patients also remain problematic. However, hypoparathyroidism generally is associated only with the 22q microdeletion.

Clinical features of the classical DiGeorge syndrome include neonatal hypocalcemia and susceptibility to infection engendered by T-cell deficiency secondary to thymal hypoplasia. Across the rest of the clinical spectrum one frequently sees micrognathia, hypertelorism, short or hypoplastic philtrum, and cardiac defects, chiefly those of the outflow tract; tetralogy of Fallot, truncus arteriosus,

and right-sided aortic arch are common (Figure 39-7). Growth is slow, and learning difficulties are common in the older child.

Diagnosis in the classical presentation should be based on the manifestation of hypocalcemia, the frequent micrognathia, and a CD4 cell count to demonstrate T-cell deficiency. Measurement of very low to absent serum PTH concentration should provide the definitive diagnosis in such a patient, especially if outflow tract cardiac defects are also present. The major focus of management should be the PTH deficiency, which can be treated by the usual means outlined earlier. Immunocompetence tends to improve with age, although caution is advised in infancy with intercurrent infections. Clinically diagnosed infants should have echocardiography

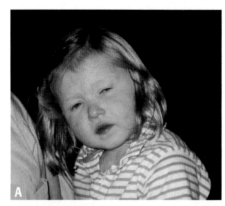

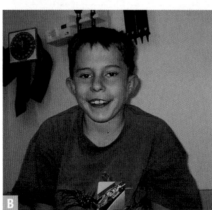

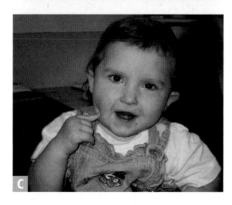

looking for cardiac defects. Hypocalcemia develops during the neonatal period and tends to resolve after the first year of life.

Hypoparathyroisism, Deafness, and Renal Dysplasia (HDR) or Barakat Syndrome

Barakat syndrome is a autosomal dominantly inherited disorder consisting of hypoparathyroidism, sensorineural deafness, and renal dysplasia that is caused by defects of the GATA3 gene. The GATA3 gene encodes the GATA3 transcription factor, which is expressed in the developing parathyroid glands, inner ears, kidneys, thymus, and central nervous system (CNS) and is mapped on 10p14-15, distal to Digeorge critical region II (110–112). Affected patients show wide phenotypic variability. Hypoparathyroidism manifestations range from asymptomatic neonatal hypocalcemia that resolves after the neonatal period to low PTH levels that persist to seizures and tetany between 1 month and 72 years of age. Sensorineural deafness is bilateral, whereas renal abnormalities usually are unilateral. Treatment for hypocalcemia is as

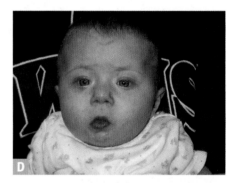

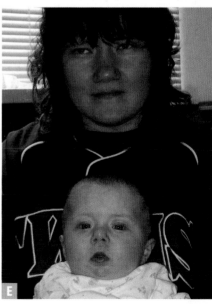

FIGURE 39-7. Spectrum of characteristics found in DiGeorge syndrome. **A–E.** Micrognathia; low set, posteriorly rotated ears; square nasal root and narrow alar base; smooth philtrum. **D, E.** Mother and infant share the same phenotypic features.

outlined earlier, and additional therapy is symptomatic.

Kenny–Caffey Syndrome

Kenny–Caffey syndrome is an extremely rare hereditary skeletal disorder characterized by thickening of the long bones, thin marrow cavities in the bones (medullary stenoses), abnormalities affecting the head and eyes, and short stature. Patients may have recurrent episodes of hypocalcemia due to insufficient PTH production. Two forms of inheritance, autosomal dominant (113) and autosomal recessive, have been described. The autosomal recessive form of the Kenny–Caffey is mapped at the same locus (1q43-44) as the Sanjad–Sakati syndrome, and both are caused by mutations of the TBCE gene (114,115). Mutations of the TBCE gene in both disorders affect synthesis of chaperone proteins that are necessary for normal folding of α,β-tubulins; and formation of α-β-tubulin heterodimers; abnormal tubulin formation adversely affects cellular organelles such as the Golgi apparatus and endosomes. Although the abnormalities in tubulin formation in association with PTH insufficiency suggests a physiologic relationship, this remains speculative.

Treatment for hypocalcemia is as outlined earlier, and additional therapy is symptomatic.

Hypoparathyroidism, Retardation, and Dysmorphism (HRD) or Sanjad–Sakati Syndrome

Hypoparathyroidism, retardation, and dysmorphism (HRD) syndrome, described in patients of Arab origin, consists of permanent hypoparathyroidism, severe prenatal and postnatal growth retardation, reduced T-cell subsets, and developmental delay (102,116). Both the HRD syndrome and the autosomal recessive form of Kenny–Caffey syndrome are believed to share a common founder mutation of the TBCE gene. The main dysmorphic features are microcephaly, microphthalmia, ear abnormalities, depressed nasal bridge, thin upper lip, hooked small nose, micrognathia, and small hands and feet. Early recognition and therapy of hypocalcemia are important, as is daily antibiotic prophylaxis against potential pneumococcal infections.

Isolated Hypoparathyroidism due to Mutations of the PTH Gene

Isolated hypoparathyroidism due to mutations of the PTH gene, which is located on chromosome 11p15.3-p15.1, has been described in a couple of families. The inheritance is autosomal recessive or autosomal dominant, and the reported mutations either impair the conversion of the pre-pro-PTH to pro-PTH, delete the entire exon 2 of the PTH gene, or result in inefficient processing of the mutated PTH peptide (117–119).

Familial Isolated Hypoparathyrodism and Partial Deletion of GCMB

Deletion of a large sequence in the GCM2 gene, which is mapped to chromosomal region 6p24.2 (120), was documented in a large pedigree by Ding et al., demonstrating an autsomal recessive transmission of this GCMB type of familial-isolated hypoparathyroidism (121). In a murine model, GCMB is the sole transcription factor, with its expression confined to the parathyroid; it is not known whether the same applies to humans. In the human pedigrees described thus far, the clinical picture is entirely consistent with a simple, uncomplicated PTH deficiency, so specific diagnosis requires heightened suspicion based on family history.

Familial Hypercalciuric Hypocalcemia (CaSR Mutation)

Familial hypercalciuric hypocalcemia is caused by activating mutations of the CaSR gene on chromosome 3q13.3-q21 that decrease the set point of parathyroid cells for calcium. The set point is defined as the calcium concentration in which PTH secretion is at 50% of maximum (122).

Most cases are familial, but a few are sporadic due to *de novo* mutations. A Ca^{2+}/Mg^{2+}-sensing reception has been demonstrated in the nephron, particularly in the loop of Henle, distal convoluted tubule, and medullary collecting duct (123). Structurally, this receptor closely resembles the one in the parathyroid gland and is involved in regulation of magnesium as well as calcium reabsorption. Depressed circulating PTH levels in CaSR mutations therefore lead to enhanced urinary magnesium loss and, eventually, to hypomagnesemia. In many patients, the degree of hypocalcemia and hypercalciuria may be mild and well tolerated without treatment.

Kearns–Sayre Mitochondropathy

Kearns–Sayre mitochondropathy is clearly a syndrome because various mitochondrial (mtDNA) deletions have been described in patients fitting the clinical criteria of ophthalmoplegia, retinal pigment degeneration, cardiomyopathy, and a variety of less prominent features, such as generalized muscle weakness and short stature. Endocrinopathies in general and hypoparathyroidism in particular are not uncommonly associated with these other findings (124). These patients experience significant morbidity because of the underlying features of their disease, and cardiomyopathy may be the cause of early demise.

The clinician should be alerted to this possibility in a child with short stature, ophthalmoplegia, and various findings such as facial muscle weakness, cardiomyopathy, etc. A pedigree that suggests maternal transmission should heighten suspicion still further, and mt DNA analysis will demonstrate the defect conclusively. Only symptomatic treatment is available other than that for hypocalcemia, as outlined earlier.

Pearson Mitochondropathy

Pearson marrow–pancreas syndrome presents in infancy as a combination of hematopoietic and exocrine pancreatic disease. Granulocytopenia, anemia, and hypocellular marrow are common features. The nature of the mtDNA deletion in Pearson syndrome is identical to that in Kearns–Sayre syndrome, which presents later (125). It is now believed that Pearson marrow–pancreas syndrome frequently will evolve into Kearns–Sayre syndrome, the distinction at the outset being a more restricted distribution of the mutated mtDNA. The stage at which hypoparathyroidism may become manifest is unpredictable and requires close follow-up. Treatment for hypocalcemia is as outlined earlier; all other treatment is symptomatic.

Autoimmune Hypoparathyroidism (Activating Antibodies to the Calcium-Sensing Receptor; Autoimmune Polyglandular Syndrome 1), APECED

The acronym APECED represents a complex of autoimmune polyendocrinopathy, candidiasis, and ectodermal dystrophy that is transmitted as an autosomal recessive trait. The disease typically presents in children 3–5 years of age or later in adolescence. Affected children present with a chronic fungal infection with subsequent development of hypoparathyroidism and adrenal failure. Malabsorption also may be a prominent feature of the disease, and chronic active hepatitis, juvenile pernicious anemia, and primary hypogonadism may be present. In a small population of Iranian Jews, the autoimmune hypoparathyroidism may appear as an isolated manifestation (126). The gene defect has been mapped to locus 21q22.3 (127), and the gene involved is called the *autoimmune regulator gene* (AIRE). Pathogenesis is based on autoimmunity, which may involve CaSR but is poorly understood.

The diagnosis should be suspected in young children with persistent fungal mucocutaneous disease, especially with accompanying alopecia. The major clinical threat to such a patient is the endocrinopathy, which demands investigation. Serum calcium, PTH, and thyroid function studies should be obtained. Hyponatremia should alert the physician to the potential for adrenocortical insufficiency. Treatment will depend on the manifestations in a given patient, but the tendency for additional manifestations to evolve with age always should be kept in mind.

ACQUIRED HYPOPARATHYROIDISM

Hypomagnesemia

It has been observed in patients with primary hypomagnesemia that both hypocalcemia and PTH deficiency are common and frequently quite severe. Inasmuch as the defect in this disease is genetically confined to magnesium absorption, calcium also becomes deficient because the parathyroid gland fails to respond to the situation in an appropriate manner. Infusion of calcium does little to alleviate the situation, the serum calcium falling rapidly to pretreatment levels. Infusion of magnesium, on the other hand, will both correct serum calcium and stimulate PTH secretion (128). There is a likelihood that magnesium deficiency also interferes with cAMP production in bone, creating PTH resistance as well (129).

Diagnosis of hypomagnesemia may be difficult clinically because of the frequent concurrence of hypocalcemia secondary to the hypoparathyroidism. The clinical findings are very similar and include tetany, generalized weakness, and anorexia. A distinguishing feature can be the frequent hypokalemia associated with hypomagnesemia; potassium handling in the loop of Henle and distal tubule is energy-dependent, and reduction of cellular magnesium may reduce ATP production, thereby permitting excessive potassium loss. Hypokalemia, of course, may cause exaggeration of the weakness perceived clinically. Correspondingly, overuse of thiazide and loop diuretics can inhibit magnesium reabsorption; malabsorption, severe diarrheal disease, and bowel bypass surgery also may cause hypomagnesemia.

Acute treatment of the tetanic patient with hypomagnesemia requires administration of up to 50 mEq of intravenous magnesium over an 8- to 24-hour period with electrocardiographic monitoring. The goal is raise the serum magnesium concentration to at least 1.0 mg/dL; for maintenance, the initial dose may be repeated as necessary. The asymptomatic hypomagnesemic patient should receive oral supplementation with either magnesium chloride or magnesium lactate preparations, each tablet of which delivers approximately 70 mg magnesium; up to 1 g total per day may be required. Abrupt correction of serum magnesium enhances urinary loss, and cellular repletion of magnesium requires a sustained serum correction, so monitoring is important to therapy.

PTH RESISTANCE: PSEUDOHYPOPARATHYROIDISM

Pseudohypoparathyroidism (PHP) describes a group of heterogeneous disorders that are characterized by hypocalcemia, hyperphosphatemia, decreased serum concentrations of $1,25(OH)_2D_3$, elevated PTH levels, and resistance of the target tisues to the biological actions of PTH. Since the time that Albright described the first patient, many patients affected with PHP of different clinical phenotypes of the disorder have been reported (130). PHP is divided in two types, PHP-I and PHP-II, based on the differences in renal cAMP production in response to PTH; patients with PHP-I have markedly reduced renal CAMP production after PTH stimulation, whereas patients with PHP-II show a normal cAMP urinary response but decreased phosphaturic response to PTH, indicating a signaling post cAMP defect. PHP-I is further subdivided into PTH-Ia, PHP-Ib, and PHP-Ic. Gene imprinting plays a significant role in the nature of the defect; the classical defect, as described originally by Albright (type Ia), is caused by mutations on the maternal allele of the GNAS gene, which is responsible for encoding the α-chain of the G_s stimulatory G protein. In patients with paternal allelic mutations, hormone resistance is unusual because the G_s paternal protein is obviated in many tissues by imprinting (131). These individuals are said to have *pseudopseudohypoparathyroidism* (PPHP).

Pathophysiology PTH exerts its biological action by binding to specific heptahelical (seven transmembrane helices) receptors on the target cells, which are called *PTH/PTHrP receptors* because they can bind with equivalent affinity both PTH and PTHrP. The PTH/PTHrP or type 1 PTH receptor is coupled by heterotrimeric guanine nucleotide–binding regulatory proteins (G proteins). G proteins transduce extracellular signals received by transmembrane receptors to effector proteins. Binding of PTH or PTHrP to the G-coupled PTH/PTHrP receptor results in the generation of second messengers such as cAMP via the activity of hormone-sensitive adenylate cyclase. Adenylate cyclase is regulated by at least two G proteins, one stimulatory (G_s) and one inhibitory (Gi). Each G protein is a heterotrimer composed of an α, a β, and a γ subunit. The molecular defect responsible for most types of PHP affects the α subunit of the stimulatory guanine nucleotide–binding protein ($G_s\alpha$), which is encoded by the GNAS1 gene (located on chromosome 20q13.3), a complex, imprinted gene with multiple transcriptional units. Heterozygous inactivating mutations of the GNAS1 gene have been found in PHP-Ia and PPHP and are distributed throughout the gene.

Patients with PTH-Ia, in addition to renal PTH resistance, have resistance to other hormones that act through $G_s\alpha$ activation via the cAMP–adenylate cyclase pathway, including thyroid-stimulating hormone (TSH) gonadotropins and growth hormone–releasing hormone (GHRH), as well as clinical abnormalities referred to as *Albright hereditary osteodystrophy* (AHO). The skeletal resistance to PTH in PHP-Ia is only partial, in contrast to the complete resistance of the proximal renal tubule. Radiological changes such as subperiostal resorption and/or cysts are rare; bone density is usually subnormal. The clinical manifestations of loss-of-function GNAS1 mutations depend on whether the mutated gene is transmitted by the mother or the father. In renal proximal tubules, pituitary, gonads, and thyroid, the $G_s\alpha$ protein encoded by GNAS1 is expressed from only the maternal allele, but in most other tissues it is expressed biallelically (from both parental alleles). Maternal transmission is associated with PHP-Ia for the following two reasons: 1) the $G_s\alpha$ activity is deficient at the kidney, where only the maternal alleles are expressed, leading to PTH resistance, and 2) the $G_s\alpha$ activity is impaired in the other tissues where the paternal alleles are imprinted, and the nonimprinted maternal alleles are mutated, leading to resistance to other hormones and the AHO phenotype. Paternal transmission of the same GNAS1 mutation is associated with PPHP because 1) the $G_s\alpha$ activity is normal in the kidney since the maternal alleles are not mutated or imprinted, thus resulting in normal action of PTH at the kidney, and 2) the $G_s\alpha$ activity is partially reduced in other tissues due to partial expression of the imprinted paternal alleles in a tissue-specific manner, leading to the AHO phenotype but no other hormone resistance (PPHP) (132–135). PHP-Ia and PPHP typically are present within the same kindred but are never present within the same sibship.

Patients with PHP-Ib have renal resistance to PTH without the accompanying AHO phenotype; the skeleton appears to respond normally to PTH, releasing calcium and phosphorus, which eventually may result in secondary hyperparathyroidism and skeletal disease. The majority of PHP-Ib cases are sporadic. Patients with familial or sporadic PHP-Ib have no mutations in the coding exons and splice junctions of the GNAS1 gene. Most individuals with the autosomal dominant form of PHP-Ib have loss of GNAS methylation at the exon A/B differentially methylated regions due to a maternally inherited deletion. The markedly decreased $G_s\alpha$ activity in the renal proximal tubules of patients with PHP-Ib due to silencing of both paternal and maternal alleles suggests that the inherited maternal deletion contains a cis-acting element required for imprinting of the GNAS1 gene in a tissue-specific manner (136–139).

PHP-Ic describes the phenotype of affected patients with normal erythrocyte N-protein activities, the AHO phenotype, and resistance to multiple hormones (133–135). Recent molecular studies suggest that these patients may have GNAS mutations that impair $G_s\alpha$ activity but not the response to the human PTH infusion test.

PHP-II is a very rare heterogeneous disorder characterized by a normal urinary cAMP response and decreased or absent phosphaturic response to PTH. The normal cAMP response to PTH and absence of other hormone resistance, as well as absence of the AHO phenotype, in these patients suggest normal $G_s\alpha$ activity and a post-$G_s\alpha$ defect of the signaling pathway. A similar clinical and biochemical phenotype is seen in patients with severe vitamin D deficiency.

Clinical Presentation Most patients with PHP-Ia do not develop hypocalcemia during the first several years of life. Hypocalcemia and hyperphospahatemia usually occur at an average of 8 years and rarely before the age of 3 years. Patients with PTH-Ia in addition to PTH resistance may have resistance to TSH and/or luteinizing hormone (LH)/follicle-stimulating hormone (FSH) and a characteristic AHO phenotype clinically, consisting of obesity, short stature, developmental delay, round facies, depressed nasal bridge, heterotopic ossifications, and brachydactyly (i.e., variable shortening of the metacarpals, metartasals, and phalanges) (Figure 39-8). Hand and foot abnormalities may not appear before the age of 4 years, and the AHO habitus may develop slowly during school years. Dental abnormalities are common, including enamel hypoplasia, enlarged pulps, root canals with open apices, delayed tooth eruption, and early tooth loss due to caries. Within a given kindred, affected patients may have PHP-Ia or the AHO phenotype alone, a variant termed PPHP. Among PHP-Ia and PPHP patients, AHO expression varies greatly, with brachydactyly reported in 70% of PHP patients (130).

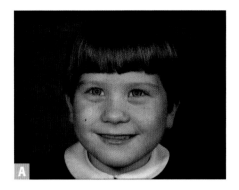
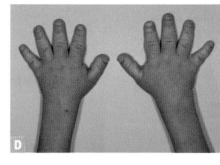
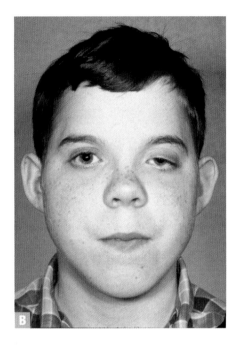
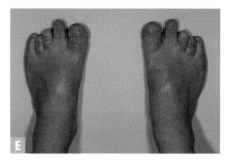
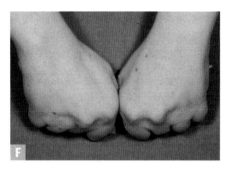
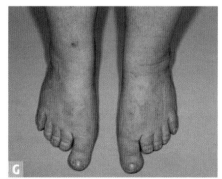
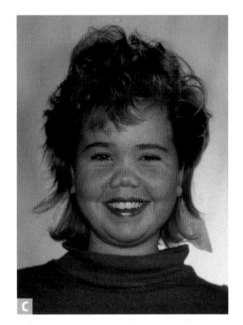
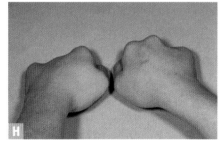

FIGURE 39-8. Spectrum of characteristics found in pseudohypoparathyroidism. Patients with pseudohypoparathyroidism have the characteristic Albright hereditary osteodystrophy (AHO) phenotype. **A–C.** *Craniofacial:* Round facies with full cheeks, short neck, depressed nasal bridge. **D–H.** *Musculoskeletal:* Short metacarpals and metatarsals, mainly of the fourth and fifth digits; absent knuckles when making fist; short distal thumb phalanx.

TABLE 39-3 PTH Stimulation Test

- Fast overnight; 4 hours for children younger than 3 months of age.
- Empty bladder at 7 a.m.; flush urine.
- Hydrate patient with 200–400 mL H_2O between 7 and 9 a.m.
- At 9 a.m.,
  - Collect 2-hour fasting urine sample by voluntary void for cAMP, phosphorus, and creatinine.
  - Collect 3 mL of blood for calcium, phosphate, creatinine, PTH and cAMP
  - (use an EDTA plasma tube: 0.2 g EDTA/mL of blood).
- Slowly (over 2 minutes) inject 3 U/kg (200 U maximum) human PTH [hPTH(1–34)] that has been dissolved in 10mL of normal saline.
- At 5 and 10 minutes after hPTH administration, collect 1 mL of blood in an EDTA tube to measure plasma cAMP levels.
- Obtain urine samples 30 and 60 minutes after hPTH administration to measure the following levels: cAMP, phosphate, creatinine.

Notes:

- Urinary cAMP is expressed as nmol cAMP/mg Cr.
- Percent tubular reabsorption of phosphate (%TRP) is calculated as

$$\%TRP = 100[1 - (Phos_u/Phos_s)(Cr_s/Cr_u)]$$

where u = urine and s = serum.
- hPTH should induce an increase in plasma cAMP levels of at least 50 nmol/L (median basal level approximately 17 nmol/L) and an increase in urinary cAMP of at least 40 nmol/mg Cr (median basal level approximately 8.4 nmol/mg Cr) and a variable decrease in the %TRP (0–11.4%; median value of 3.6%).
- Pseudohypoparathyroidism shows a markedly impaired increase in plasma cAMP (max increase: 27 nmol/L) and also in urinary cAMP (max increase: 21 nmol/mg Cr); the %TRP change is variable (0–6.9%; median 1.1%) and often overlaps the range of the appropriate response; thus it is less useful.

Brachydactyly involves shortening of the 3rd, 4th, and 5th metacarpals and 1st distal phalanx. In one study, evaluation of the metacarpophalangeal pattern profile in 14 genetically characterized PHP-Ia patients showed that shortening below the –2 standard deviation (SD) score was present in at least one bone in each subject, with a prevalence of 100%; however, great variability existed between subjects and between hand bone segments (143). Archibald's sign, which describes a characteristic shortening and widening of the 4th and 5th digits and dimpling over the knuckles of a clenched fist can be positive in PHP patients and in about 10% of normal individuals.

A GNAS1 mutation has been reported to cause PHP-Ia and testotoxicosis. The paradoxical coexistence of both activating and inactivating phenotypic features in the same patient was because the mutant $G_s\alpha$ protein was stable at the reduced temperature of the testes but was thermobile at 37°C, leading to reduced $G_s\alpha$ activity in other tissues and the AHO phenotype. Pituitary resistance to hypothalamic hormones acting via $G_s\alpha$-coupled receptors also may be present in patients with PHP-Ia, who may present with low IgF1 levels and growth failure due to GHRH resistance (131).

Other clinical features in patients with PHP-Ia may include nongoitrous hypothyroidism, which may be congenital; ovarian hypogonadism due to gonadotropin resistance; subcutaneous ossifications, which may be present at birth and years before hypocalcemia develops; and bone pain caused by cystic bone disease. Calcifications of the basal ganglia also may be present.

Patients with PHP-Ib have resistance to PTH only at the kidney and may present with short stature and normal appearance and development. However, because of elevated PTH levels (as in hyperparathyroidism) and the fact that the skeleton is not resistant to PTH, demineralization of the bones may develop. Symptomatic hypocalcemia may appear within the first 10 years of life, and occasionally, there is also resistance to TSH (134).

Diagnosis of the Different Forms of Hypoparathyroidism and Pseudohypoparathyroidism

The biochemical hallmarks of hypoparathyroidism are hypocalcemia and hyperphosphatemia in the presence of normal renal function. Laboratory evaluation of a patient suspected of hypoparathyroidism should include measurement of serum calcium, both total and ionized; phosphate; serum magnesium; alkaline phosphatase; and $25(OH)D_3$ and $1,25(OH)_2D_3$ levels and intact PTH levels; spot urine for the calcium-to-creatinine ratio also should be obtained. In hypoparathyroidism, total calcium and ionized levels are decreased (6–7 mg/dL and less than 4 mg/dL, respectively), phosphate levels are elevated (6–9 mg/dL), and magnesium and alkaline phosphatase levels are normal. Despite an increase in fractional excretion of calcium, the renal filtered load of calcium is decreased, and the 24-hour urinary calcium excretion is decreased for the following reasons: 1) decreased intestinal calcium absorption due to reduced calcitriol (the primary function of PTH is to stimulate calcitriol synthesis) and 2) diminished bone resorption. Renal tubular reabsorption of phosphate is increased.

The different types of PHP can be further differentiated depending whether resistance to other hormones or the AHO phenotype is present. Elevated gonadotropins with low testosterone in males and estradiol in females or growth failure with elevated GH and low IgF1 levels may be present in patients with PHP-Ia. Elevated TSH levels with low T_4 may be present in patients with PHP-Ia or PHP-Ib. Exogenous administration of hPTH(1–34) to patients with PHP-Ia or PHP-Ib, regardless of their serum calcium concentrations, results in a blunted urinary excretion of both cAMP and phosphate, whereas patients with PTH deficiency and normal controls show an increase in urinary cAMP excretion. Furthermore, this test can distinguish normocalcemic PHP patients from patients with PPHP (see Table 39-3 for a description of the hPTH infusion test). Measurement of G protein activity in fibroblasts and erythrocytes of PHP-Ia and PPHP patients shows a 50% decrease in expression or function of $G_s\alpha$ subunit. Of note, urinary cAMP and phosphate responses to PTH depend on the endogenous serum PTH and calcium levels; treatment with calcitriol to normalize calcium levels may normalize the phosphaturic response to PTH in patients with PHP-Ia or PHP-Ib, as well as calcium reabsorption from the renal tubule (144). Recent studies indicate that measurement of plasma cAMP or calcitriol levels may differentiate PHP-I from other causes of hypoparathyroidism (145,146). A diagnosis of PHP-Ib or PHP-II is suspected in patients with hypocalcemia, hyperphosphatemia, and elevated PTH and no clinical signs of the AHO phenotype. An infusion of hPTH(1–34) will show a normal cAMP and phosphorus response in patients with PHP-Ib, whereas an abnormal phosphaturic response will be seen in patients with PHP-II.

Chromosomal analysis in patients with the AHO phenotype may differentiate between patients with PPHP and patients with the AHO-like phenotype due to terminal deletions of 2q37. In addition, patients with proximal deletion of 15q, del(15)(q11q13), and classic features of PHP-Ia and Albright hereditary osteodystrophy have been reported (147).

If PTH is elevated in the presence of hypocalcemia, normal or low phosphorus, and elevated alkaline phosphatase, secondary causes of hyperparathyroidism should be sought such as vitamin D deficiency, low calcium or high phosphorus intake, chronic renal disease, malabsorption, and other causes of hypocalcemia or hyperphosphatemia.

Patients with PTH levels within the normal range but low for the degree of hypocalcemia, increased or inappropriate normal calcium excretion, hyperphosphatemia, and low or normal magnesium levels should be suspected of having autosomal dominant hypoparathyroidism caused by gain-of-function mutations of the CaSR gene.

If DiGeorge syndrome is suspected, evaluation of the immune system should include measurement of serum immunoglobulins; these are usually normal, although IgA may be low and IgE elevated. For these reasons, proper diagnosis rests on clinical recognition of the abnormal facies and likely hypocalcemia, followed by high-resolution chromosomal analysis and fluorescence in situ hybridization (FISH) for microdeletions of chromosome 22 in the region of 22q11.21-q11.23. A negative FISH result does not exclude the possibility of 22q abnormality, and in a patient with DiGeorge-like phenotype, testing for microdeletions of DiGeorge critical region II should be considered.

If candidiasis is present, polyglandular type I autoimmune syndrome should be suspected as the cause of hypoparathyroidism.

Of note, serum PTH and calcium concentrations will be severely reduced in primary hypomagnesemia because magnesium deficiency not only impairs normal release of PTH but also causes PTH resistance in target organs. Diagnostically, hypomagnesemic patients must be differentiated from individuals with Bartter and Gittelman syndromes.

Genetic Testing Genetic testing for most of the preceding causes of hypoparathyroidism is available clinically. For pseudohypoparathyroidism, GNAS mutational analysis for the diagnosis of PHP-Ia is available clinically; however, genetic testing for PHP-Ib is still a research test. Molecular studies to identify CaSR mutations are available on a research basis and recommended for cases of sporadic isolated hypoparathyroidism.

TREATMENT OF HYPOPARATHYROIDISM

Acute Phase

As in neonatal hypocalcemia (described earlier), treatment for tetany should be viewed as an emergeny. Keeping in mind that cardiac muscle is also affected in hypocalcemia, an intravenous infusion of 10–20 mg elemental calcium per kg or 1–2 ml/kg of a 10% calcium gluconate solution should be provided over 5–10 minutes with close electrocardiographic monitoring. As pointed out earlier, calcitriol also should be administered because the prior lack of renal hydroxylase stimulation due to inadequate PTH stimulation is likely to have led to reduced calcitriol circulating levels. Calcitriol may be administered intravenously at a daily dose of 0.25 μg initially and increased up to a maximum of 2 μg/day in 2–3 divided dosages depending on the response of the serum calcium concentration, which should be closely monitored. Divided dosages are preferable because of the short half-life of calcitriol and the need to obtain a prolonged response.

Maintenance Phase

Hypoparathyroidism due to Deficient PTH Production Logic would dictate that patients who suffer from hypoparathyroidism ideally should be treated by hormone replacement rather than the indirect therapeutic regimen outlined earlier. The present availability of synthetic PTH now makes this potentially possible; however, use of PTH has been approved only recently for adults and remains experimental in children. A recent study (148) has shown clear benefit of hormone replacement over the usual regimen, especially in terms of the risk of nephrocalcinosis and declining renal function. The mean urinary calcium excretion in PTH-treated patients was within the normal range throughout the duration of the study.

A careful analysis of the patient's usual dietary intake is essential to ensure adequate daily calcium and relatively low inorganic phosphate intakes. Vitamin D preparations are the main drugs in the treatment of hypo-calcemia, along with supplemental calcium (at least 1 g/day of elemental calcium). For treatment of symptomatic hypocalcemia, please follow the guidelines described earlier. Cholecalciferol and ergocalciferol are the least expensive preparations but have the longest durations of action and may result in prolonged toxicity during hypercalcemic episodes because of their storage in fat tissue. Calcitriol is the treatment of choice because it has the advantage of not requiring renal 1α-hydroxylation, which is decreased in hypoparathyroidism, and has the shorter half-life that minimizes the risk of prolonged toxicity. Starting dose of calcitriol is usually 20–100 ng/kg/day in 2–3 divided doses; or one can start calcitriol at 0.25 μg per day and raise the dose in increments of 0.25 μg until normocalcemia is achieved, over a minimum of 3 days. Dihydrotachysterol (DHT), which requires only 25-hydroxylation in the liver to be fully active, is prescribed at higher doses (10–40 μg/kg/day) because its relative activity is 1/1000 that of calcitriol; DHT's half life is 7 days with the full effect of a dose reached in 10–20 days. With the loss of the calcium-retaining effect of PTH, the increased intestinal calcium absorption following vitamin D supplementation results in increased filtered calcium and calcium excretion. Urinary calcium excretion may increase well before serum calcium normalizes. Hypercalciuria and nephrocalcinosis may develop if high-normal calcium levels are maintained for prolonged periods. If the serum calcium level is normalized and the serum phosphorus level remains greater than 6 mg/dL, a nonabsorbable antacid may be added. Dietary phosphorus intake should be decreased by avoiding dairy products that are high in phosphorus.

Prevention of hypercalciuria and the resulting nephrocalcinosis is most important for patients with hypercalciuric hypocalcemia caused by activating mutations of the CaSR gene. It is recommended that affected asymptomatic patients should not be treated routinely with vitamin D. Hydrochlorothiazide therapy at a dose of 0.5–2 mg/kg/day in affected symptomatic children can reduce the urinary calcium excretion, allow reduction of the vitamin D dose, and correct the hypocalcemia. Potassium supplementation may be required to treat the thiazide-induced hypokalemia.

Monitoring Close follow-up is required in the first month of treatment and then every 3–6 months after calcium and phosphate levels have stabilized. If hypercalcemia develops, vitamin D supplementation is stopped, and a dose 10% to 20% lower than the previous dose is started, with close follow-up of the serum calcium level for several weeks.

Pseudohypoparathyroidism There are no major differences in treatment between hypoparathyroidism and pseudohypoparathyroidism. Maintenance therapy includes calcitriol therapy at 0.01–0.04 µg/kg/day or DHT at 10–40 µg/kg/day, with or without calcium supplementation.. The goal of treatment is to maintain calcium concentration in the low to midnormal range (8.5–9.5 mg/dL) to avoid nephrocalcinosis associated with hypercalciuria. Patients with PHP require lower doses of vitamin D and have less risk of treatment-related hypercalciuria; it is assumed that in PHP, the endogenous PTH may stimulate renal calcium reabsorption in the presence of normalized calcitriol levels. Frequent evaluation of serum calcium and urinary calcium-to-creatinine excretion at 3-month intervals is necessary for dose adjustment and prevention of hypercalcemia and hypercalciuria. Treatment with vitamin D and/or calcium corrects hyperphosphatemia to a high-normal phosphate level. Patients with PHP require lower doses of vitamin D, and phosphate-binding gels are not necessary. Treatment of patients with hypothyroidism due to PHP-Ia or PHP-Ib is similar to that for patients with primary hypothyroidism. The same applies to patients with PHP-Ia and hypogonadism or growth failure due to gonadotropins or GH resistance.

HYPERCALCEMIA

Approximately half the total calcium in the extracellular fluid is bound to plasma proteins, mostly to albumin, whereas the remainder of calcium is free and represents the active form of calcium. Low albumin concentrations will decrease the total calcium with the concentration of the ionized calcium (iCa) remaining normal. A change in serum albumin of 1 g/dL results in a parallel change in the iCa concentration of 0.2 mmol/L. Normal serum calcium (8.5–10.5 mg/dL) and iCa (1.8–1.34 mmol/L) levels in infants and children are similar to those in adults. Hypercalcemia is present when serum calcium is more than 2.75 mmol/L (11 mg/dL) or when iCa is more than 1.4 mmol/L (5.6 mg/dL).

Hypercalcemia during infancy and in children is rare. Some of the causes of hypercalcemia (Table 39-4) include the following: 1) Williams syndrome, a syndrome with multisystem involvement including peculiar elfin-like facies, supravalvular aortic stenosis and peripheral-organ arterial stenoses, hypotonia, and cognitive delays. Williams syndrome is caused by the deletion of contiguous genes at 7q11.23. Hypercalcemia is present in 15% of affected patients during infancy and usually resolves between 2–4 years of age. However,

TABLE 39-4 Causes of Hypercalcemia

Neonatal hypercalcemia

Maternal excess vitamin D intake
Maternal hypocalcemia
   Hypoparathyroidism
   Pseudohypoparathyroidism
Williams syndrome
Excessive calcium intake
Vitamin D toxicity
Hypophosphatemia
Renal tubular acidosis
Neonatal Bartter syndrome

Infant/child hypercalcemia

Heterozygous inactivating mutation of CaSR (FHH)
Nutritional hypervitaminosis D
Inflammation-associated
Lymphoma
Hypophosphatemia
Thiazide diuretics
Idiopathic infantile hypercalcemia
Juvenile rheumatoid arthritis
Williams syndrome
Renal tubular acidosis
Infantile hypothyroidism
Bartter syndrome
Primary hyperparathyroidism
   Familial
      Multiple endocrine neoplasia syndrome
      Familial isolated primary
      PTHR gain-of function mutation (Jansen syndrome)
      Neonatal, severe (homozygous inactivating mutation of CaSR)
      Neonatal, self-limited with hypercalcuria
Secondary hyperparathyroidism
   Renal failure
   Chronic hyperphosphatemia

adults with hypercalciuria and ectopic calcium deposits have been described (149). 2) Familial hypocalciuric hypercalcemia (FHH). Heterozygous iactivating mutations of the gene controlling synthesis of the CaSR have been reported to cause a syndrome called *benign familial hypercalcemia* (FHH) in the heterozygous form and neonatal hyperparathyroidism in the homozygous state (122). In FHH, at normal serum calcium concentrations, the parathyroid gland senses a deficiency and is stimulated to secrete PTH; the remaining, responsive CaSRs are sufficient to reduce PTH secretion, thus minimizing the degree of hypercalcemia. The same process occurs in the renal tubule due to partial deficiency of CaSRs, which thus drives excess reabsorption of calcium in response to a perceived but nonexistent hypocalcemia.

Transient neonatal hypercalcemia may occur in infants born to hypocalcemic mothers whose underlying condition (i.e., hypoparathyroidism or PHP) is poorly controlled. The

decreased in utero supply of calcium from the hypocalcemic mother to the fetus leads to fetal hypocalcemia, fetal parathyroid hyperplasia, and fetal skeletal demineralization. Persistence of fetal parathyroid hyperplasia after birth may present with hypercalcemia or normocalcemia with elevated instead of decreased phosphate concentrations.

Hypercalcemia secondary to hypervitaminosis D is seen most often as a complication of vitamin D overtreatment of hypoparathyroidism, PHP, hypophosphatasia, and secondary hyperparathyroidism of renal osteodystrophy. In particular, children with renal osteodystrophy have a higher incidence of hypercalcemia when they are on treatment with calcitriol versus treatment with ergocalciferol or cholcalciferol. Children with PHP or hypoparathyroidism develop hypercalcemia during treatment at a lower rate than children with renal osteodystrophy independent of the vitamin D preparation. Infants born to mothers ingesting excessive vitamin D may develop hypercalcemia.

Subcutaneous fat necrosis in neonates with complicated delivery can be associated with violaceous discoloration and inflammation of the skin with mononuclear and giant cell infiltration at the pressure sites; hypercalcemia also may develop within days or weeks of delivery. The mechanism of hypercalcemia is thought to be elevated production of calcitriol by macrophages, and increased prostaglandin E activity at the lesion site has been seen in patients (150,151).

Hypercalcemia associated with malignancy includes affected patients with T-cell lymphoma/leukemia and can be due to elevated PTHrP, calcitriol, or PTH produced by the tumors or activated alveolar macrophages, as in sarcoidosis. Other conditions associated with hypercalcemia, suppressed PTH, and calcitriol levels include 1) Addison disease due to the antagonistic properties of glucocorticoids on calcium absorption and bone mobilization, as well the coexistence of dehydration in untreated adrenal insufficiency, 2) prolonged immobilization precipitated by loss of weight bearing and caused by an increase in osteoclastic bone resorption, 3) pheochromocytoma most commonly due to coexisting hyperparathyroidism in patients affected with multiple endocrine neoplasia type IIA (MEN IIA) (however, in cases of isolated pheochromocytoma, hypercalcemia may be caused by the effect of elevated catecholamines on bone turnover or due to secretion of PTHrP by the tumor), and 4) thyrotoxicosis due to the direct effect of thyroid hormones on bone turnover, increasing bone resorption rates. Medications associated with hypercalcemia include 1) excessive intake of vitamin A (hypervitaminosis A) most likely due to osteoclast-mediated bone resorption, 2) thiazide diuretics by increasing proximal tubular calcium reabsorption and decreasing plasma volume, and 3) lithium carbonate, which causes hypercalcemia associated with elevated PTH levels. Rare causes of hypercalcemia have been reported, including infantile hypothyroidism and oxalosis.

Pathophysiology and Manifestations Since the normal relationship of the extracellular $[Ca^{2+}]$ to the cytosolic concentration is 10^3–10^4 to 1, maintained by both energy (ATP)–dependent and electrogenic pumps, a significant increase in the extracellular calcium concentration threatens this normal relationship. In turn, the ability of the cell to maintain the normal compartmentalization of its calcium content depends on the transport of calcium out of the cell, as well as the ability to restore sarcolemmal stores and to bind excess calcium, chiefly to calmodulin. It is self-evident that sarcolemmal storage is finite, as is the binding capacity of preexisting calmodulin. Energy-dependent transport is, by definition, both concentration- and energy-limited; electrogenic transport is also concentration-dependent. Hence, exceeding the latter's capacities has significant ramifications for cellular function. In general, hypercalcemia has the effect of impairing cardiac and smooth muscle contractility; this adequately explains the hypertension, arrhytmias, shortened QT interval, and gut-associated clinical symptoms such as constipation and bowel hypomolity; however, the pancreatitis is probably more related to microcalcinosis. Chronic hypercalcemia in young infants and children may present with failure to thrive, irritability, gastrointestinal reflux, abdominal pain, and anorexia.

The genitourinary (GU)–related effects of hypercalcemia are the result of multiple factors. Calcium directly inhibits the action of antidiuretic hormone (ADH) on the collecting tubules, thus causing polyuria and dehydration. The vasoconstriction caused by elevated calcium reduces renal blood flow and glomerular filtration, the latter reduction being worsened by the dehydration. Increased calcium concentration and diminished urine flow contribute to the likelihood of nephrocalcinosis. Finally, the patient attempts to compensate for dehydration by increasing fluid intake (polydipsia).

The nervous system implications of hypercalcemia remain poorly understood; however, there are some data that provide insight. Formenti et al. (153) have reported on the effects of increased calcium concentration in cultures of rat thalamic neurons. In this preparation, as calcium was increased, there was a change in discharge pattern from single spike to burst,

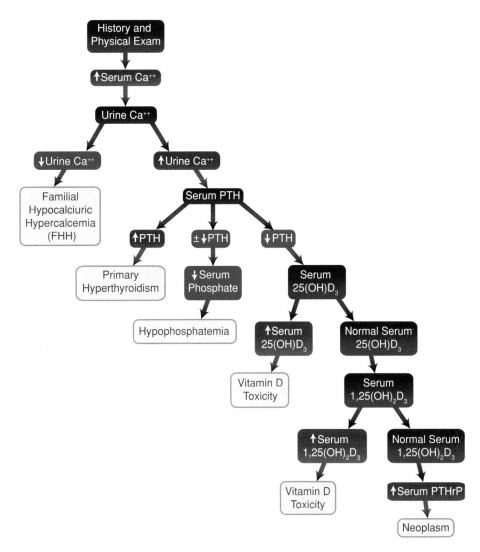

FIGURE 39-9. Algorithm for the diagnosis of hypercalcemia.

and the data were interpreted to show a correlation between hypercalcemia and the clinical findings of somnolence and lethargy. In a more recent report, Chen et al. (154) have reported on a patient with hypercalcemic-induced seizures who at the time of the seizures had magnetic resonance imaging (MRI) changes consistent with vasoconstrictive abnormalities, as shown by cerebral angiography. All changes were reversed following treatment of both the seizures and the hypercalcemia.

Diagnosis Laboratory evaluation of hypercalcemia includes measurement of total and ionized calcium, phosphorus, intact PTH, 25(OH)D$_3$, 1,25(OH)$_2$D$_3$, and spot urine for the calcium-to-creatinine ratio. Hypercalcemia and increased (or nonsuppresed) PTH suggest that the etiology of hypercalcemia is of parathyroid origin, including primary and tertiary hyperparathyroidism, as well as FHH. In general, hypercalcemia, elevated PTH, and no history of renal failure suggest primary hyperparathyroidism, except for the very rare cases where there is elevated

production of PTH by neoplasms; when renal failure is present, tertiary hyperparathyroidism is the cause of elevated PTH and hypercalcemia. FHH should be suspected in the absence of symptoms and a urinary calcium-to-creatinine ratio of less than 0.01.

Skeletal x-rays may show osteolytic lesions attributable to hyperparathyroidism or neoplasias. Abdominal ultrasound (US), including renal US, is recommended to evaluate for malignancies and nephrocalcinosis; nephrocalcinosis on renal US suggests primary hyperparathyroism. Figure 39-9 presents a diagnostic algorithm of other causes of hypercalcemia.

Treatment of Hypercalcemia Mild hypercalcemia, defined as a serum concentration of total calcium of 12 mg/dL or less, usually is asymptomatic and generally requires no immediate intervention. Patients are encouraged to increase their fluid intake, discontinue drugs such as thiazides that may contribute to hypercalcemia, and restrict calcium intake.

Moderate hypercalcemia, with serum levels below 13.5 mg/dL, usually is associated with symptoms and will require treatment. Rehydration with intravenous normal saline at twice maintenance will restore normal circulating volume, increase glomerular filtration rate (GFR), and improve calcium excretion. Saline infusion increases calcium excretion by increasing glomerular filtration of calcium and decreasing both proximal and distal tubular reabsorption of sodium and calcium. Addition of furosemide at a dose of 1 mg/kg intravenously every 6–8 hours will further enhance calcium excretion (induced diuresis should be followed by additional fluid input as well). Furosemide acts on the thick ascending loop of Henle to inhibit both sodium and calcium reabsorption. Furosemide treatment is discontinued when the calcium level is below 12 mg/dL. In severe hypercalcemia, where the serum calcium concentration exceeds 13.5 mg/dL, addition of bisphosphonate treatment (Pamidronate 1–2 mg/kg intravenously over 4 hours) will diminish bone reabsorption and assist in reducing the serum concentration of calcium. It is critical to prevent recurrent dehydration during treatment, so intake and output monitoring is an essential part of treatment. Also, in severe cases, electrocardiographic monitoring is called for, and rapid evaluation of parathyroid function, when abnormal, should result in an emergency parathyroidectomy. When there are CNS-associated symptoms, especially in view of the frequency of infiltrative disease as an etiology, other causes must be evaluated as a part of the clinical workup.

Glucocorticoid therapy can be effective in hypercalcemia due either to subcutaneous fat necrosis or to hematological malignancies and sarcoidosis. Glucocorticoids can be used in refractory cases of vitamin D intoxication in addition to measures that increase volume expansion and calciuresis. Hypercalcemia of thyrotoxicosis responds to β-blockers and resolves after correction of thyrotoxicosis. Hypercalcemia associated with adrenal insufficiency responds to volume replenishment and glucocorticoid treatment.

After correction of acute hypercalcemia, a high-sodium diet promotes renal calcium excretion, and oral furosemide therapy at 1–2 mg/kg/day divided in two or three divided doses may be of benefit.

PRIMARY HYPERPARATHYROIDISM

Hyperparathyroidism is characterized by excessive secretion of PTH leading to severe hypercalcemia, hypocalciuria, hypophosphatemia, and hyperphosphaturia.

Causes of Hyperparathyroidism

Primary hypeparararathyroidism (PHPT) is rare in children, but it can be seen with fair regularity in adults, the comparative incidence being approximately 1 in 100 (155). In both age groups, most cases are sporadic, and the most common cause in both groups is adenoma, accounting for approximately 50% to 60% of cases in children (155). The remainder of the causes of PHPT in children are accounted for by multiple endocrine neoplasia syndromes, MEN I and MEN II, with hyperparathyroidism being the most common feature of MEN I syndrome (see Chapter 46), hyperparathyroidism–jaw tumor (HPT-JT) syndrome, and familial isolated hyperparathyroidism (FIHP). HPT-JT is a rare syndrome with autosomal dominant inheritance associated with hyperparathyroidism, malignant parathyroid tumors, jaw ossifying tumors, renal cysts, hamartomas, Wilms tumors, and uterine tumors; the cause of HPT-JT is heterozygous inactivating germline mutations of the HPRT2 gene (hypoxanthine phosphoribosyltransferase 2) that encodes a tumor suppressor protein termed *parafibromin* and is mapped to 1q25-q31 (156). There is an additional entity known as *familial isolated hyperparathyroidism* (FIHP), in which there is a family history of isolated hyperparathyroidism and adenomatous changes in the parathyroid glands. FIHP is genetically heterogeneous, and in some cases, germline mutations of the HPRT2 gene have been identified along with menin and CaSR genes (157,158). For this reason, patients with FIHP and a nonestablished genetic basis should be considered at risk for parathyroid malignancy because it is possible that they carry a germline HRPT2 mutation.

Neonatal PHPT results from homozygous inactivating mutations of the CaSR gene and presents with severe hypercalcemia and skeletal disease. Certain inactivating mutations of the CaSR gene can present with neonatal hypercalcemia in the heterozygous state. Neonatal hypercalcemia may be seen in Jansen metaphyseal dysplasia, a rare autosomal dominant disorder characterized by short-limbed dwarfism and mottled calcifications in the distal end of the long bones. Jansen syndrome is caused by constitutively active mutations in the parathyroid hormone receptor (PTHR). Characteristic facial features include micrognathia, prominent eyes, high skull vault, hypertelorism, wide-open cranial sutures, and high arched palate. Other findings are choanal atresia, enlarged joints, flexion contractures of the knees and hip, normal IQ, hearing loss, and short stature.

Chronic renal disease in children may lead to hypersecretion of PTH; this "secondary" hy-perparathyroidism may persist beyond renal transplant. The term *secondary hyperparathyroidism* applies to states of increased PTH secretion deriving from some primary cause of hypocalcemia. Secondary hyperparathyroidism, when prolonged, may result in unregulated function of a parathyroid gland or a parathyroid adenoma; the resulting increase in circulating PTH is called *tertiary hyperparathyroidism*. The cellular mechanism that leads to this clinical situation is poorly understood. The critical difference between secondary and tertiary hyperparathyroidism is that the serum calcium is normal or low in secondary hyperparathyroidism, whereas calcium is elevated in tertiary hyperparathyroidism.

As glomerular filtration decreases below about 70 mL/min/1.73 m^2, 1α-hydroxylation begins to diminish, with a resulting fall in calcitriol synthesis. As a consequence, intestinal calcium absorption decreases with development of mild hypocalcemia and slightly increased PTH over time. As glomerular filtration falls further to 30–40 mL/min/1.73 m^2, PTH levels have risen with increasing degrees of hypocalcemia, and phosphate retention has increased. Treatment of hyperphosphatemia may involve the use of aluminum salts and would impair calcium absorption further, leading to enhanced or "secondary" PTH secretion. Continuation of this process leads to parathyroid chief cell hyperplasia due to combined stimulation by hypocalcemia, hyperphosphatemia, and diminished calcitriol production and consequent loss of normal regulatory mechanisms for PTH secretion, resulting in tertiary hyperparathyroidism. The critical difference between secondary and tertiary hyperparathyroidism is that the plasma calcium level is low or normal in secondary hyperparathyroidism, whereas it is elevated in tertiaty hyperparathyroidism due to the development of adenoma or hyperplasia of the parathyroid glands.

In X-linked hypophosphatemia (discussed later in this chapter), a disease in which renal tubular phosphate reabsorption is impaired, the direct inhibitory effect of phosphate on the parathyroid gland is exerted; thus, despite a low to low-normal serum calcium level in most patients, secondary hyperparathyroidism is uncommon, and serum PTH levels are in the normal range. However, tertiary hyperparathyroidism can develop in patients with hypophosphatemic rickets as a result of prolonged treatment with phosphate supplements, which induce transient hypocalcemia. The intermittent hypocalcemia in the presence of relative calcitriol deficiency can induce parathyroid gland hyperplasia.

Secondary hyperparathyroidism develops in vitamin D deficiency as a consequence of impaired calcium absorption and low serum calcium concentration, which creates a stimulus for PTH secretion. As long as the vitamin D deficiency persists, the parathyroid gland will respond to the combined stimulus of hypocalcemia and reduced circulating calcitriol. Secondary neonatal hyperparathyroidism is the cause of neonatal hypercalcemia, as discussed earlier, and develops in infants of mothers with hypocalcemia during pregnancy.

Whatever the genesis of the increase in circulating PTH hormone, the net effect is the same—PTH exerts both anabolic and catabolic effects on bone. If the increase in PTH is mild and intermittent, bone formation is enhanced because the consequent hypercalcemia seems to enhance osteoclast apoptosis (23), and the increased PTH stimulates formation of calcitriol. On the other hand, if the increase in PTH is persistent and long term, its hyperphosphaturic effect over time creates a significant negative phosphate balance that impairs the ability of the osteoblast to form new bone. The hyperphosphaturic effect of PTH on the renal tubule also can cause precipitation of calcium phosphate stones (nephrolithiasis) due to the combination of increased phosphate and calcium in the glomerular filtrate.

Clinical Presentation The most common presentation of PHPT is asymptomatic mild hypercalcemia. Hypercalcemia may be noted incidentally during evaluation for some other problem, as usually happens in patients with *familial hypocalciuric hypercalciuria* (FHH). In contrast to severe hypocalcemia, the symptoms of severe hypercalcemia are far more diverse, extending to virtually all systems. One commonly notes anorexia and nausea, abdominal pain, constipation, and rarely, acute pancreatitis among gastrointestinal (GI) system findings. Peptic disease may be present if PHPT is part of MEN I syndrome. Skeletal changes on x-rays include subperiosteal resorption of the tubular bones and destructive changes of the ends of the long bones (Figure 39-10). Nephrocalcinosis (diffuse deposition of calcium–phosphate compexes in the parenchyma and nephrolithiasis are renal complications, with nephrolithiasis still being the most common complication of PHPT (Figure 39-11). Polydipsia and polyuria are common symptoms referable to the GU system, whereas fatigue, weakness, somnolence, lethargy, stupor, and coma delineate the effects on the neurologic system.

Hypertension is common, and electrocardiography often exhibits a shortened QT interval without changes in the T wave. Bradycardia and first-degree atrioventricular block and other arrhythmias may occur. In general,

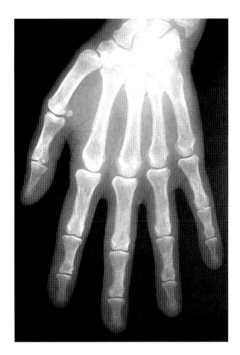

FIGURE 39-10. Hyperparathyroidism. The hand radiograph demonstrates the typical radial resorptive pattern involving the middle phalanges seen in hyperparathyroidism.

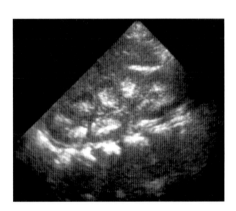

FIGURE 39-11. Nephrocalcinosis. Ultrasound of the kidney demonstrates multiple echogenic foci in the medulla of the kidney consistent with medullary nephrocalcinosis.

the development of symptoms correlates with the calcium levels and with how rapidly the calcium levels rise.

Neonatal PHPT may have a severe presentation at birth with the total calcium level between 20 and 30 mg/dL and skeletal changes.

Diagnosis Family and medical history is important to rule out inherited causes of hyperparathyroidism such as MEN I or MEN II syndrome or FHH. Dietary history of calcium and vitamin D intake should be documented in order to rule out low calcium intake and/or vitamin D deficiency as cause of secondary hyperparathyroidism and excess calcium intake and/or vitamin D toxicity as a cause of hypercalcemia. Laboratory evaluation

should include measurement of serum calcium (total and ionized forms), intact PTH, $25(OH)D_3$, $1,25(OH)_2D_3$, serum phosphate, urinary calcium and creatinine (spot urine), and alkaline phosphatase. PHPT is characterized by elevated total and ionized calcium levels, elevated PTH, hypophosphatemia, increased calcitriol concentration, low-normal $25(OH)D_3$ levels, increased alkaline phosphatase, and increased urinary calcium and creatinine in a 24-hour urine collection or in spot urine. Bone density studies are sensitive in detecting early skeletal changes. Renal US and abdominal x-rays can be used as baseline assessments of nephrolithiasis and nephrocalcinosis. If supported by conventional laboratory data, additional studies should include ultrasound and computed tomographic (CT) scaning of the neck and technetium-99m-sestamibi scintigraphy.

Biochemical abnormalities in Jansen metaphyseal dysplasia include elevated serum calcium, elevated alkaline phosphatase with low intact PTH levels, and elevated urinary cAMP due to the constitutional activation of the PTHR.

In vitamin D toxicity, intact PTH levels are low, phosphate levels are normal or elevated, and alkaline phosphatase activity is usually low. Serum and urinary calcium is high, circulating $25(OH)D_3$ is elevated, and $1,25(OH)_2D_3$ is normal. The low PTH levels in vitamin D toxicity explain the normal or elevated phosphorus levels (i.e., absence of the phosphaturic effect of PTH).

In FHH, a disorder caused by heterozygous inactivating mutations of the CaSR gene, the impaired calcium sensor drives increased PTH secretion and renal tubular calcium reabsorption. Calcitriol is low or normal, and serum phosphate may be reduced as a result of inappropriate PTH secretion. PTH levels are normal or high normal in the presence of hypercalcemia due to a higher than normal set point of parathyroid calciostat. Serum alkaline phosphatase is in the normal range. Magnesium levels tend to be elevated. Spot urine for the calcium-to-creatinine ratio shows a value 0.01 mg/mg creatinine or less, which further differentiates FHH from primary hyperparathyroidism, in which this ratio will be 0.03 or higher. Hypocalciuric hypercalcemia also may be found in one of the parents of patients with FHH because the majority of cases are inherited as an autosomal dominant trait. Genetic testing for CaSR abnormalities is still performed in research laboratories. Pedigree investigations and standard laboratory data, as outlined earlier, are likely to be sufficient to establish the diagnosis of FHH.

In patients with chronic renal failure, a central factor in development of secondary hyperparathyroidism is the lack of functional renal mass, leading to decreased ability to carry out the 1α-hydroxylation reaction. Hence these children evidence low circulating calcitriol levels and consequent hypocalcemia. Circulating $25(OH)D_3$ concentration is normal or just slightly low in these patients if dietary intake is sufficient. There is an accompanying hyperphosphatemia that derives in part from reduced glomerular filtration and thus abnormal regulation of phosphate handling in the renal tubule. The combination of persistent hypocalcemia, low calcitriol, and hyperphosphatemia stimulates the parathyroid chief cells and results in hyperparathyroidism and renal osteodystrophy. The latter condition will result in increased serum alkaline phosphatase as well, and of course, chronic renal failure will cause an elevated serum creatinine. In distinguishing renal disease from vitamin D deficiency, renal function testing (i.e., BUN and creatinine) are of obvious benefit because vitamin D–deficient children have normal renal function. Vitamin D deficiency, by definition, will manifest in low circulating $25(OH)D_3$ concentrations, coupled with low calcitriol as well. Serum alkaline phosphatase will be elevated, whereas serum phosphate will be low. The low serum calcium and calcitriol elicit a secretory response from the parathyroid chief cells, causing an elevated PTH and lower serum phosphate secondary to the renal tubular phosphaturia induced by PTH.

Surgery PHPT, which is usually caused by a parathyroid adenoma and is not subject to the usual physiological controls, surgical excision is the treatment of choice in patients with symptomatic disease, such as kidney stones and skeletal changes. It is important to establish the diagnosis of hyperparathyroidism due to MEN I or MEN II prior to surgery because these patients tend to have generalized involvement of the parathyroid glands. As techniques for identification and localization of these tumors have improved, the excision itself has become simpler, to the point of becoming a same-day surgical procedure performed through a minor incision. Insofar as possible, a subtotal parathyroidectomy should be performed to avoid permanent hypoparathyroidism.

Patients with asymptomatic PHPT in accordance with a National Institutes of Health (NIH) concensus statement in 2002 are recommended to have surgery if they have any of the following indications: 1) serum calcium level 1–1.6 mg/dL above normal, 2) kidney stones or hypercalciuria with 24-hour urinary calcium excretion above 400 mg/day, 3) reduced creatinine clearance by 30%, 4) reduced bone density (T-score less than 2.5 SDs

at any site), 5) age younger than 50 years, and 6) impossible or undesirable medical surveillance (e.g., coexisting illness) (159). Patients with FHH are not candidates for surgery because they do not develop nephrolithiasis or bone disease and therefore must be distinguished carefully from those with PHPT. However, neonatal hyperparathyroidism due to homozygous CaSR-inactivating mutations is a true surgical emergency.

Therapy after Parathyroidectomy There is a significant likelihood of postoperative hypocalcemia that may be quite severe and acute. In order to avoid the dangers of an acute hypocalcemic event postoperatively, patients should be given an intravenous maintenance dose of calcium gluconate (500 mg/kg/24 h) with close monitoring of blood calcium concentration and electrocardiographic pattern. If hypocalcemia persists after the second postoperative day, calcitriol may be started. In most cases, postoperative hypocalcemia is transient and does not require long-term therapy.

DISORDERS OF HYPOPHOSPHATEMIA

Mild to moderate hypophosphatemia is defined as a serum phosphate concentration of 1.5–3.5 mg/dL or 0.48–1.12 mmol/L and is usually asymptomatic (160). Severe hypophosphatemia is defined as a serum phosphate concentration of less than 1.5 mg/dL or 0.48 mmol/L and often is symptomatic, demanding prompt medical attention. In infants, normal serum phosphate concentrations can be as high as 7 mg/dL (160). Thus, in the first 6 months of life, hypophosphatemia is suggested at serum concentrations of 4–5 mg/dL.

Pathophysiology The causes of hypophosphatemia are complex (Table 39-5), arising from the following major mechanisms alone or in combination: 1) increased renal phosphate excretion, 2) decreased intestinal absorption, and 3) increased intestinal loss. Hypophosphatemia also may arise from phosphate shifting from extracellular compartment to cells and bones.

Severe hypophosphatemia occurs when decreased absorption is aggravated by an intracellular shift such as may occur in diabetic ketoacidosis, alcohol intoxication, severe burns, and refeeding syndromes (160). Phosphate-binding antacids used in treating peptic ulcers and total parenteral nutrition with insufficient phosphate contents are some other causes of severe hypophosphatemia (161).

Increased phosphate excretion is one of the hallmarks of hyperparathyroidism due to the phosphaturic effect of elevated PTH. In *chronic renal failure*, PTH becomes elevated

TABLE 39-5   Causes of Hypophosphatemia
Increased phosphate excretion
Hyperparathyroidism
Corticosteroid therapy
X-linked hypophosphatemia
Fanconi syndrome
Hypomagnesemia
Hyperaldosteronism
Volume expansion
Diuresis
Diuretics
Postobstructive diuresis
Decreased intestinal absorption
Dietary deficiency of phosphate
Vitamin D deficiency and vitamin D resistance
*Phosphate-binding antacids**
Increased intestinal loss
Vomiting
Various malabsorption states
Phosphate shift to cells and bones
Carbohydrate loading (glucose, fructose, etc.)
*Total parenteral nutrition**
Androgen therapy
Bone resynthesis
Recovery from hypothermia
Respiratory alkalosis
Gram-negative sepsis
Hyperventilation
Heat stroke
Thyrotoxicosis
Hepatic coma
Hypocalcemic periodic paralysis
Mixed mechanisms of decreased absorption and intracellular shift
*Diabetic ketoacidosis**
*Alcohol intoxication and withdrawal**
*Severe burns**
*Refeeding syndrome**
Miscellaneous
Oncogenic hypophosphatemia
Acute gout

*Severe causes of hypophosphatemia are denoted by asterisk and italics.

when the GFR falls below 50% of normal as a response to the hypocalcemia (162). However, phosphate wasting as a response to elevated circulating PTH fails to occur because the renal tubules in chronic kidney insufficiency are resistant to the effects of PTH; thus the subsequent phosphate retention results in hyperphosphatemia. Hypophosphatemia is encountered often after kidney transplantation because the increased PTH production from the hyperplastic parathyroid glands now exerts its effect on the normal, healthy kidney allograft, causing a marked increase in phosphate excretion.

Primary tubular defects such as X-linked hypophosphatemia (161) will be discussed in a separate section later in this chapter.

Fanconi syndrome, a secondary type of proximal renal tubular acidosis, is characterized by reduced renal proximal tubular reabsorption of phosphate and generalized aminoaciduria and potassium and bicarbonate wasting (162). *Volume expansion* following treatment of diabetic polyuria increases phosphate excretion for unexplained reasons. *Diuresis* following the use of diuretics or in postobstructive diuresis may promote phosphaturia, resulting in hypophosphatemia (160).

Decreased intestinal absorption of phosphate follows vitamin D deficiency and vitamin D resistance, excessive use of phosphate-binding antacids to treat peptic ulcers, and chronic vomiting and malabsorption states, such as steatorrhea, recurrent pancreatitis, and hepatic cirrhosis.

Phosphate shifting from the extracellular to the intracellular compartment and bones during carbohydrate loading such as glucose or fructose infusions may result in severe hypophosphatemia, especially in the setting of preexisting malnutrition and starvation (163–166). Intracellular shifting results from androgen therapy by an unknown mechanism, perhaps related to increased synthesis of phosphocreatine, bone resynthesis, and recovery from hypothermia. Respiratory alkalosis stimulates this intracellular phosphate shift also by poorly understood mechanism(s). Thus hypophosphatemia is encountered in the *respiratory alkalosis* induced by gram-negative sepsis, hyperventilation, heat stroke, thyrotoxicosis, hepatic coma, and hypocalcemic periodic paralysis.

Simultaneous decreased absorption and intracellular shift are seen often in diabetic ketoacidosis, alcohol intoxication, severe burns, and refeeding syndrome after starvation. Because of nausea and vomiting, patients with *diabetic ketoacidosis* already have dietary deficiency of phosphate (167). In addition, the metabolic acidosis promotes release of intracellular phosphate, which shifts into the extracellular spaces in the presence of insulin deficiency. Hyperphosphaturia follows and is aggravated by the coexisting osmotic diuresis of glycosuria and ketonuria. With insulin therapy, an intracellular shift of phosphate occurs to promote glycolysis and oxidative phosphorylation. Unintended acceleration of phosphaturia results from reexpansion of extracellular fluids often associated with the aggressive use of intravenous therapy. The severe hypophosphatemia often is accompanied by hypokalemia in treating diabetic ketoacidosis. Prompt replacement of both phosphate and potassium deficits is indicated.

Patients with *alcohol intoxication and withdrawal* often present with severe hypophosphatemia secondary to preexisting poor intake, vomiting, and coexisting hypomagnesemia. An intracellular phosphate shift is secondary to respiratory and metabolic alkalosis caused by delirium tremens, intercurrent sepsis, nasogastric suction, or diuretic-induced hypokalemia. It is worth noting that the hypophosphatemia may be mild on admission but often becomes severe after a few days of intravenous therapy not too far different from that described in diabetic ketoacidosis patients (discussed earlier).

Patients with *third-degree burns* tend to hyperventilate, resulting in respiratory alkalosis (168). The hypophosphatemia from respiratory alkalosis and the acceleration of glycolysis usually is encountered a few days after injury.

Refeeding hypophosphatemia after prolonged starvation was first seen in concentration camp victims at the end of the World War II, in whom, when refeeding was applied overzealously, edema, oliguria, and death were seen. No data on serum values were available from the chaotic conditions of the time. Recent studies on refeeding of patients with anorexia, however, have showed profound hypophosphatemia resulting from decreased intestinal uptake by the sparse epithelium and intracellular shift as the phosphate is used in new tissue formation.

Oncogenic hypophosphatemia results from phosphaturia secondary to increased production of fibroblast growth factor 23 (FGF-23). The latter is a potent phosphaturic substance produced by mesenchymal tumors that reduces the tubular reabsorption of phosphate (169).

The mechanism whereby *acute gout* is associated with hypophosphatemia is unclear at this point.

The *pathophysiological consequences of severe hypophosphatemia* are summarized in Table 39-6. There is significant impairment in carbohydrate metabolism and insulin

TABLE 39-6 Clinical and Laboratory Findings in Severe Hypophosphatemia	
Endocrine/metabolic findings Impaired carbohydrate metabolism, insulin insensitivity, increased 1, 25 dihydroxy-vitamin D **Skeletal muscle and cardiovascular findings** Clinical 　Weakness 　　Proximal myopathy 　　Rhabdomyolysis 　　Cardiomyopathy Laboratory 　Elevated creatine phosphokinase (CK) and aldolase 　Abnormal electromyelogram **Respiratory findings** Clinical 　Hypo- or hyperventilation 　Respiratory failure Laboratory 　Decreased vital capacity **Hematological findings** Red cells 　Impaired glycolysis 　Increased rigidity 　Hemolysis 　Reduced 2,3-DPG White cells 　Impaired phagocytosis Platelets 　Impaired function 　Thrombocytopenia	**Neurological findings** Clinical 　Encephalopathy 　Paresthesia Laboratory 　EEG anomalies 　Elevated cerebrospinal fluid protein **Gastrointestinal findings** Clinical 　Anorexia 　Nausea and vomiting 　Dysphagia 　Ileus Laboratory 　Increased absorption of calcium, phosphate, and magnesium due to elevated 1,25-dihydroxyvitamin D **Skeletal findings** Clinical 　Arthralgia 　Bone pain, joint stiffness, pseudofractures, osteomalacia/rickets Laboratory 　Osteomalacia 　Osteopenia 　Decreased bone calcium, phosphate, and magnesium **Renal findings** Clinical 　Stone (rare) Laboratory 　Hypophosphatemia, hypermagnesuria, glucosuria, bicarbonaturia, hypercalciuria **Liver findings** Abnormal liver function tests

insensitivity and increased production of $1,25(OH)_2D_3$ metabolites. It remains unclear as to whether the insulin insensitivity is a consequence of the phosphate deficit. The most important skeletal muscle and cardiovascular consequence of severe hypophosphatemia is rhabdomyolysis, which may lead to acute kidney failure. The cardiomyopathy of severe hypophosphatemia is potentially life-threatening. Encephalopathy and paresthesia are noted neurological complications of severe hypophosphatemia. Anorexia, nausea and vomiting, dysphagia, and ileus are encountered. Long-term hypophosphatemia causes arthralgia, bone pain, joint stiffness, pseudofractures, and osteomalacia/rickets.

Clinical Signs and Symptoms Since phosphate is intrinsic to so many cellular processes, depletion of cellular phosphate has wide-ranging effects (see Table 39-6) (160,161). Acute reduction results in muscle weakness, hyporeflexia, tremors, and occasionally, cranial nerve palsies, confusion, and coma. A slower, more chronic reduction in phosphate levels causes paresthesia, hypo- or areflexia, seizures, cardiorespiratory failure, hemolytic anemia, and rhabdomyolysis. Given the role of phosphate in oxidative metabolism, it is not surprising that such highly oxidative tissues as nerve and muscle are severely affected. In addition, the reciprocal relationship between phosphate and calcium (see below) disturbs to some extent calcium-dependent processes.

Diagnosis Laboratory evaluation of the patient with hypophosphatemia should include fractional excretion of phosphate, measurement of tubular maximum rate of phospharte reabsorption (T_mP) in relation to GFR (T_mP/GFR), spot urine for calcium-to-creatinine ratio, serum total and ionized calcium, PTH, and vitamin D metabolites. Considering that most referrals to the pediatric endocrinologist for workup of chronic hypophosphatemia are associated with renal wasting of phosphate, an estimation of the fractional excretion of phosphate is justified. A 24-hour urine collection gives a more accurate result; short of that, an early-morning urine sample may serve the purpose, but the urine needs to be obtained within 2 hours of the serum sample. The fractional excretion of phosphate is calculated by the formula

$$\text{(Urine phosphate)} \times \text{(plasma creatinine)} \times (100)/\text{(plasma phosphate)} \times \text{urinary creatinine)}$$

Normally, the fractional excretion of phosphate is less than 5% and ranges up to 20% depending on dietary phosphate intake. In the presence of hypophosphatemia, however, fractional excretion of phosphate should drop to single digits; if it exceeds 15% in the pres-

ence of hypophosphatemia, the diagnosis of renal phosphate wasting is established.

The T_mP in relation to GFR is the most reliable quantitative estimate of the overall tubular transport capacity; T_mP/GFR is 4–5.9 mg/dL in children aged 6–14 years of age and declines to 2.8–4.2 mg/dL by 20 years of age. T_mP/GFR is calculated by the formula

$$\text{Plasma phosphate} - \text{(urine phosphate} \times \text{serum creatinine)/urinary creatinine}$$

Hypophosphatemia with elevated serum and urinary calcium, elevated PTH levels, normal $25(OH)D_3$, and elevated $1,25(OH)2D_3$ suggests PHPT. On the other hand, persistently low serum and urinary calcium, hypophosphatemia, and elevated PTH suggest secondary hyperparathyroidism due to the following: 1) vitamin D deficiency if $25(OH)D_3$ levels are low, 2) vitamin D–resistant rickets type I if $25(OH)D_3$ levels are normal and $1,25(OH)_2D_3$ are low, 3) vitamin D–resistant rickets type II if both $25(OH)D_3$ and $1,25(OH)_2D_3$ are elevated, and 4) malabsorption if $25(OH)D_3$ is low and $1,25(OH)_2D_3$ is normal or elevated.

Hypophosphatemia with phosphaturia, normal serum and urinary calcium, normal PTH, and normal $25(OH)D_3$ and $1,25(OH)_2D_3$ levels suggests X-linked hypophosphatemic rickets, autosomal dominant hypophosphatemic rickets (ADHR), tumor-induced osteomalacia (TIO), and fibrous dysplasia, which all are disorders associated with phosphaturia and elevated serum levels of FGF-23. Hypophosphatemia with phosphaturia, normal serum and urinary calcium, normal or elevated PTH levels, normal $25(OH)D_3$, low or normal $1,25(OH)_2D_3$, normal serum anion gap, glucosuria, increased urinary bicarbonate excretion, and generalized aminoaciduria suggests renal Fanconi syndrome.

Imaging Studies With chronic hypophosphatemia, skeletal x-rays are needed to follow osteopenia, osteomalacia, and rickets. To rule out parathyroid adenoma, US of the neck has been used. Technetium-99m scan to rule out ectopic parathyroid gland also may be indicated.

Treatment Hypophosphatemia with plasma phosphate levels above 2 mg/dL does not require treatment. Appropriate treatment of hypophosphatemia is aimed at preventing mild, asymptomatic hypophosphatemia from progressing to severe, life-threatening hypophosphatemia. The underlying conditions risking severe hypophosphatemia must be identified. These include phosphate-binding antacids, total parenteral nutrition, diabetic ketoacidosis, alcohol intoxication, severe burns, and refeeding syndromes (161).

It is important to note that there is often a delay of a few days from admission of an alcoholic patient with mild hypophosphatemia before progression to profound hypophosphatemia. These patients have such long-standing nutritional deficiencies that when an intravenous glucose infusion is given for rehydration or refeeding, in order to prevent the development of severe hypophosphatemia, oral phosphate supplementation at a daily dose of 15–20 mg/kg of body weight should be given concurrently; oral phosphate can be given in a dose up to 3 g/day. In general, 1 g of oral phosphate would raise the serum phosphate level by 1.5 mg/dL in 1–2 hours. If oral phosphate supplements or skim milk is not tolerated, then intravenous phosphate supplementation at a dose of 10 mg/kg of body weight per day should be administered to prevent the development of severe hypophosphatemia. Whole milk is an excellent source of phosphate, potassium, calcium, and magnesium. The fat and lactose contents of whole milk, however, make it less well tolerated by severely malnourished individuals. Skim milk has the same phosphate content but less fat content and may be better tolerated. Another alternative for phosphate supplementation is the use of a buffered sodium phosphate enema (Fleet enema) in both children and adults.

Diabetic ketoacidosis of short duration (a few days) may not have sustained significant phosphate deficiency (167). In contrast, patients with prolonged diabetic ketoacidosis of several weeks would have mobilized and depleted their intracellular phosphate, resulting in more significant total-body phosphate deficiency. Such patients are at greater risk of severe hypophosphatemia, especially on initiating insulin and intravenous fluid therapy. Phosphate supplementation promotes normalization of intracellular 2,3-diphosphoglycerate and improvement of mental acuity. In such patients, a dose of intravenous phosphate of 15–20 mg/kg of body weight per day can be given for a few days until mental acuity improves and oral dosage can be given in place of the intravenous therapy (161).

Intravenous phosphate therapy is complicated by diuresis and diarrhea, which give rise to volume depletion and hypotension. Thus careful intake/output chartings are required; body weight and the blood pressure need to be monitored carefully. The diuresis may induce other electrolyte loss, giving rise to secondary complications such as hypokalemia, hyponatremia, hypocalcemia, and hypomagnesemia.

Intravenous phosphate therapy is contraindicated in patients with kidney failure because such therapy precipitates hyperphosphatemia. Parenteral phosphate therapy is contraindicated in hypocalcemia, hypercalcemia, or hyperkalemia. If oral phosphate therapy is used, careful monitoring of the serum phosphate concentration is required.

To recapitulate, the oral route of phosphate supplementation is preferred. The underlying disorders should be treated. Risk factors that increase the risk of progressing to severe hypophosphatemia should be identified and treated. Kidney failure is a contraindication to phosphate therapy. Treatment should be discontinued once the serum phosphate concentration rises above 2 mg/dL or when hypocalcemia (serum calcium <8 mg/dlL) is encountered.

DISORDERS OF HYPERPHOSPHATEMIA

Hyperphosphatemia is defined as a serum phosphate concentration above 5 mg/dL (1.6 mmol/L) in older children and adults and above 6 mg/dL in children younger than 2 years of age.

Pathophysiology The causes of hyperphosphatemia can be categorized (Table 39-7) according to the following mechanisms: 1) decreased GFR or increased renal reabsorption of phosphate, 2) increased phosphate loads, and 3) increased intestinal absorption.

Decreased GFR, as encountered in acute and chronic renal failure, impairs excretion of phosphate and gives rise to significant hyperphosphatemia (170). Under normal circumstances, the capacity of the uncompromised kidneys can adjust to most phosphate loads. In renal failure, hyperphosphatemia develops when the GFR is less than 25% of normal.

Defects in renal excretion of phosphate in the absence of renal failure can be seen in hypoparathyroidism and pseudohypoparathyroidism.

Increased renal tubular reabsorption of phosphate is seen in tumoral calcinosis (171), a rare autosomal recessive or autosomal dominant disorder in which progressive deposition of basic calcium phosphate crystals in periarticular spaces and soft tissues causes a disabling disease of soft tissue calcification, especially around the extensor surfaces of the joints. Ulceration of the tumor gives rise to sinus tracts and the risk of intercurrent infections. Despite the high serum calcium–phosphate product, systemic osteopenia is seen in patients with tumoral calcinosis.

Familial forms of tumoral calcinosis due to homozygous loss-of-function mutations in the FGF-23 or GALNT3 gene have been described (172–173). The disorder usually is seen in young black males and is characterized by normal response of the kidney to PTH and inappropriately normal or elevated $1,25(OH)_2D_3$ levels.

TABLE 39-7 Causes of Hyperphosphatemia

Decreased glomerular filtration rate

Acute and chronic kidney failure

Increased phosphate loads

Endogenous loads
    Cellular shift in diabetic ketoacidosis
    Lactic acidosis
    Tissue hypoxia
    Rhabdomyolysis
    Cytotoxic therapy of neoplasms
    Hemolysis
    Malignant hyperthermia
Exogenous loads
    Enemas and laxatives
    Vitamin D intoxication
    Parenteral phosphate
    Blood transfusions
    White phosphorus burns

Increased tubular reabsorption of phosphate

Parathyroid dysfunction
    Hypoparathyroidism
    Pseudohypoparathyroidism
    Transient parathyroid resistance of infancy
Endocrine dysfunction
    Tumoral calcinosis
    Hyperthyroidism
    Juvenile hypogonadism
    Postmenopausal state
    Acromegaly
    High ambient temperature
    Bisphosphonate etidronate

Miscellaneous

Hyperostosis

Massive tissue breakdown following rhabdomyolysis, cytotoxic therapy of neoplasms, or hemolysis are associated with increased endogenous phosphate loads, which may overwhelm the kidney's ability to cope; the common denominator in these diverse conditions is the release of intracellular phosphate and potassium into the extracellular compartment causing hyperphosphatemia, hyperkalemia, and often hypocalcemia.

Increased enteral phosphate absorption from vitamin D intoxication, excess parenteral phosphate administration, blood transfusion, and phosphorous burns can be the causes of increased exogenous phosphate loads. Hyperphosphatemia also may develop in laxative abusers because most enemas and laxatives are high in phosphate content (160).

Less common causes of hyperphosphatemia include *hyperthyroidism* (174), *juvenile hypogonadism*, *postmenopausal state*, and excessive circulating GH as seen in *acromegaly*. Reduced phosphate excretion is seen in conditions of *high ambient temperature*, as in desert climates, a response for which the mechanism is unclear. Mild hyperphosphatemia may follow the ad-

ministration of *bisphosphonate etidronate* in treating patients with osteopenia. The new generation of bisphosphonates (aminophosphonates) does not have this side effect.

Hyperphosphatemia is seen in patients with *hyperostosis*, a rare autosomal recessive and autosomal dominant disorder presenting in late childhood with mandible enlargement. Nerve compressions give rise to facial palsy and deafness.

Clinical Signs and Symptoms There is a reciprocal relationship between serum concentrations of calcium and phosphate: When one goes up, the other goes down. The pathophysiological consequences of severe hyperphosphatemia include 1) ectopic calcification, when the high calcium–phosphate ratio exceeds 70, and 2) hypocalcemic tetany, seizures, hypotension, and cardiac arrhythmia (168), when there is an acute drop in serum ionized calcium, such as may occur in the early phases of tumor lysis and severe rhabdomyolysis. Pulmonary dysfunctions follow the calcification of lung parenchyma and the alveolar lining. The effects of hyperphosphatemia on the intestinal system include nausea, vomiting, hematemesis, and ileus.

Hyperphosphatemia in chronic renal failure contributes indirectly to the development of secondary hyperparathyroidism and renal osteodystrophy by promoting hypocalcemia; hyperphosphatemia decreases $1,25(OH)_2D_3$ levels via inhibition of the activity of 1α-hydroxylase in the kidney, resulting in decreased intestinal calcium absorption and a state of skeletal resistance. It is the hypocalcemia that directly stimulates the parathyroid gland (175). In end-stage renal failure, the high serum calcium–phosphate product may lead to subcutaneous deposition of calcium, which may progress to intense pruritus.

One of the most significant consequences of severe hyperphosphatemia is the risk of acute renal failure. The massive tissue breakdown and release of phosphate secondary to rhabdomyolysis, myoglobinuria, crush injury, thermal burns, and chemotherapy in neoplastic diseases cause severe hyperphosphatemia. The hyperuricemia and hypovolemia associated with many of these conditions aggravate the risk of acute renal failure (176).

Generally, a surfeit of phosphate alone has minimal acute effects, apart from the signs and symptoms associated with the underlying cause.

Diagnosis The diagnostic workup of hyperphosphatemia includes determinations of serum calcium, magnesium, and other electrolytes. To exclude hypoparathyroidism and pseudohypoparathyroidism, serum PTH, $25(OH)D_3$, and $1,25(OH)_2D_3$ should be measured, as well as vitamin D metabolites.

It should be noted that spurious hyperphosphatemia may be encountered due to the following disorders interfering with phosphate measurements: hyperlipidemia, hyperbilirubinemia, and hyperglobulinemia. Measurement of serum lipids, bilirubin, and albumin would be justified if spurious hyperphosphatemia is suspected.

Electrocardiogram and Radiological Imaging

On electrocardiograms, QT intervals are prolonged. Radiological imaging of the hands, wrists, knees, and ankles to document the severity of renal osteodystrophy is recommended. If the calcium–phosphate product exceeds 70, radiological imaging to detect soft tissue calcifications may need to be considered. If acromegaly is a cause of the hyperphosphatemia, MRI of the pituitary with gadolinium enhancement would evaluate the pituitary for possible GH-secreting pituitary adenoma.

Treatment The *sine qua* non of therapy for hyperphosphatemia of any etiology is reduction of intake, which should be restricted to 800 mg/day with intravenous hydration to ensure adequate volume for diuresis (160). The omnipresence of phosphate in natural foods, however, can make such a restricted diet unpalatable and frequently unacceptable to children especially. Thus addition of a phosphate-binding material to the diet is advisable; neither aluminum- nor citrate-containing materials are recommended for use in children. Either calcium carbonate or calcium acetate is acceptable, the former being administered most frequently at a safe dose of 5 g/day with meals.

RICKETS AND OSTEOMALACIA

Pathophysiology Rickets is a generalized bone disorder associated with disruption in the endochondral ossification of the growth plate in children whose epiphyses have not yet fused. Rickets is also associated with osteomalacia, a delay in the mineralization of preformed osteoid at the trabecular, endosteal, and periosteal bone surfaces.

Osteoid noncalcification results from lack of the three essential substances: vitamin D, calcium, and phosphate. The latter two substances may become insufficient due to poor diet, starvation, or malabsorption. Vitamin D is activated in the skin by ultraviolet light as cholecalciferol, then at the liver into 25-hydroxyvitamin D, and finally, in the kidney into 1,25-dihydroxyvitamin D. Any interruption due to organ failure or genetic resistance at each of these pathways results in vitamin D insufficiency. Growing children can have rickets and osteomalacia, whereas adults, whose epiphyses have fused, only can have osteomalacia.

Most notably in the midst of the Industrial Revolution of the 19th century, an epidemic of rickets occurred in Europe from smoke pollution and lack of sunlight in the inner-city populations and factory workers. The use of irradiated plant steroids and fish liver oil supplements eliminated this epidemic by the turn of the 20th century. Unfortunately, the risk of rickets is returning in our century from a constellation of almost the same reasons in developing countries. In developed countries, the populations are also beginning to experience an increasing incidence of rickets partly from pollution but also from breast-fed infants of mothers with insufficient sunlight, the use of vegan diets without milk intake, and in some countries from lactose intolerance. Darker, pigmented skin, lack of sunlight, and no dietary supplementation of these essential substances increase the risks even further. Physicians caring for such patients need to be vigilant in recognizing the nonspecific and vague symptoms of the softening and weakening bones: lower extremity bowing, tender bone and dental deformities, muscular cramps, and hypocalcemic tetany.

Preterm and low-birth-weight infants are at high risk for metabolic bone disease from calcium and phosphate deficiency, especially if they are breast-fed or if they are on medications such as loop diuretics and corticosteroids. Mineral accretion in utero reaches a peak during the third trimester of pregnancy; typically, daily calcium skeletal accretion is 2.5–3.0 mmol/kg and that of phosphate is 2 mmol/kg (177). To match this calcium intake from breast milk would require an intake of 400 mL/kg, twice the maximum normal intake of a premature baby (178). In addition, breast milk has very little vitamin D (usually no more than 25 IU/L), which is inadequate to satisfy the infant's requirements (179). Neonatal osteopenia occurs in 30% of very low-birth-weight (<1250 g) premature infants of less than 28 weeks' gestation. The widespread use of breast-milk fortifiers and preterm formulas enriched with calcium, phosphate, and vitamin D has led to a decrease in bone disease, and frank rickets is uncommon in developed countries nowadays.

Clinical Presentation Rickets presents most often in infancy and at puberty, highlighting its association with periods of rapid growth (particularly the development of bone and teeth).

The pathological changes of rickets lead to the gradual softening of bone. The bone-related clinical manifestations include genu varum (bowed legs) or genu valgum (knocked knees) in ambulatory infants, swollen costochondral junctions of ribs (the classical beading sign of rachitic rosary), indentation of the lower anterior thoracic wall (Harrison's groove), involution of the ribs and protrusion of the sternum (pigeon chest), bowing of the arms, enlarged wrists, expansion of cranial bones relative to facial bones (frontal bossing), softening of the occipital area (craniotabes), delayed closing of fontanelles, and impaired development of teeth (delayed eruption, enamel hypoplasia, and greater subsceptibility to caries in the first dentition).

In general terms, the clinical features of rickets are associated most often with deformities of the skeletal system. However, other systems, such as the muscular and immune systems, also may be involved, particularly in rickets due to vitamin D deficiency. For example, the clinical manifestations of hypocalcemia (i.e., tetany, apneic episodes, stridor, and convulsions) may be the only presenting features in an infant. Delayed motor development with hypotonia may be present in the absence of hypocalcemia. Also, heterogeneous diseases from disorders of the liver and kidney, celiac disease, and other malabsorptive disorers to hereditary renal tubular diseases, as well as starvation, all may present with rickets in the child and osteomalacia in the adult.

Radiographical imaging of the long bones showing cupping, splaying, and fraying of the metaphysis leads to the diagnosis of rickets (Figure 39-12).

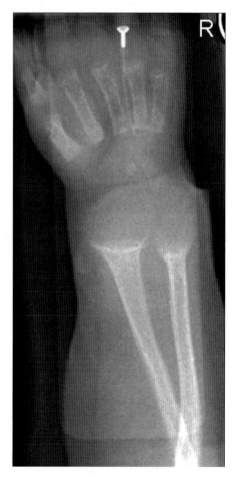

FIGURE 39-12. Rickets. A widened physis and cupping and fraying with irregularity of the distal metaphysis are present in this radiograph of the forearm.

We have organized the presentation of rickets into the following groups according to the calcium–phosphate product. Using milligrams per milliliter as the unit, a calcium concentration of 10 mg/mL multiplied by a phosphate concentration of 5 mg/mL gives the normal calcium–phosphate product of 50 mg/mL.

RICKETS WITH LOW SERUM CALCIUM–PHOSPHATE PRODUCT

Vitamin D deficiency, vitamin D–dependent rickets, nutritional calcium or phosphate deficiency, X-linked hypophosphatemia, hyposphosphatemia due to renal tubular acidosis, Fanconi syndrome, use of phosphate-binding antacids, and tumor-induced osteomalacia are forms of rickets and osteomalacia associated with a low serum calcium–phosphate product of less than 50 mg/dL.

Rickets due to Vitamin D Deficiency, Impaired Vitamin D Action, or Vitamin D Resistance

Vitamin D deficiency is the most common cause of rickets because it prevents the efficient absorption of dietary calcium and phosphorus, which gives rise to softening of the bones; rachitic changes typically are associated with 25(OH)D$_3$ levels of less than 20 ng/dL (range 15–20 ng/dL) (see Figure 39-13). However, a large number of infants, children, and adolescents can be vitamin D–insufficient without apparent skeletal abnormalities with 25(OH)D$_3$ levels between 21 and 29 ng/dL (179–181). Vitamin D is found in only small quantities in the diet (e.g., in oily fish or fish liver oil), and normal levels are maintained through formation from 7-dehydrocholesterol in the skin under the influence of the UVB in sunlight. The most common causes of vitamin D–deficient rickets in infants and young children are dark-pigmented skin, little exposure to sunlight, little or no vitamin D supplementation in mother or child, and exclusive breast-feeding (182). Vitamin D stores in infants are closely related to the the vitamin D status of the mother. A breast-fed infant whose mother is vitamin D–deficient most likely will develop rickets. Even breast-fed infants born to vitamin D–replete mothers develop vitamin D deficiency within 8 weeks of delivery in the absence of vitamin D supplementation (183,184). Rachitic changes may be seen in infants born to mothers who are severely malnourished or have malabsorption, particularly celiac disease.

Some other reasons for the increasing prevalence in older infants and toddlers may include 1) prolonged breast-feeding without vitamin D supplementation of dark-skinned children living in higher latitudes (182), 2) increased use of day-care facilities where

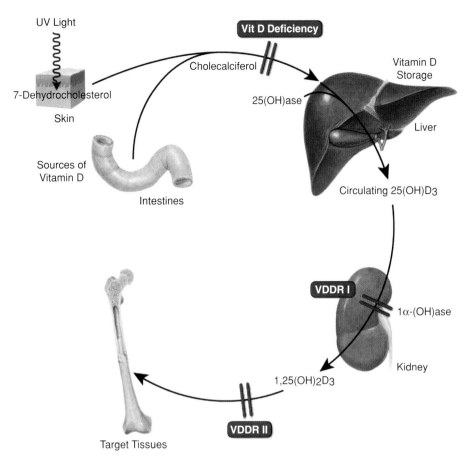

FIGURE 39-13. Rickets due to vitamin D deficiency and VDDRI and VDDRII. Vitamin D deficiency, leading to depleted 25(OH)D$_3$ stores, can be caused by inadequate intake, inadequate sunlight exposure, malabsorption, liver disease or seizure medications (impaired 25(OH)ase activity). In VDDR type I, 1,25(OH)$_2$D$_3$, is not formed due to impaired enzymatic activity of 1α(OH)ase. In VDDR type II, the active form of vitamin D is formed, but the target tissues are unresponsive due to defects in the Vitamin D receptor (VDR).

children spend the most of their time indoors, 3) macrobiotic diets and soy health food beverages that may be low in vitamin D or interfere with calcium uptake (185), and 4) increased pollution.

Pathophysiology In a vitamin D–deficiency state, only 10% to 15% of dietary calcium and 50% to 60% of dietary phosphorus are absorbed, resulting in decreased ionized calcium levels (186), which are sensed by the CaSRs in the parathyroid glands. This causes an increase in the expression, synthesis, and secretion of PTH. PTH, like 1,25(OH)$_2$D$_3$, enhances the expression of RANKL on osteoblasts to increase the production of mature osteoclasts to mobilize calcium from the skeleton and at the kidney increases reabsorption of calcium at both the proximal and distal convoluted tubules while decreasing phosphorus reabsorption. In addition, PTH stimulates the production of 1,25(OH)$_2$D$_3$ at the kidney. The serum calcium level usually is normal in the vitamin D–deficient infant or child, and it is only when the calcium stores in the skeleton are totally depleted that such an infant or child will become hypocalcemic. However, the phosphorus level is low, result-

ing in inadequate calcium–phospate product and impairing the mineralization of the osteoid laid down by osteoblasts.

Clinical Presentation Since vitamin D deficiency predominantly affects the areas of rapid bone growth, it is seen most often in patients under 18 months of age, with the majority presenting at between 4 and 12 months of age. Bone deformity and pseudofractures ensue due to loss of mechanical strength of bone structure. Patients complain of bone pains and muscle weakness. Weight loss is noted. The excess osteoid accumulation gives rise to loss of calcification and marked widening of epiphyseal osteoid seams. Besides bone changes, pneumonia may be present at diagnosis probably due to the rachitic changes in the chest and may also be a result of the role of vitamin D in the immune system.

Laboratory Evaluation Infants typically present with normal to low-normal serum calcium levels, low-normal or low fasting serum phosphorus levels, elevated alkaline phosphatase levels, and low 25(OH)D$_3$ levels. Because secondary hyperparathyroidism stimulates the kidneys to produce 1,25(OH)$_2$D$_3$, the levels of this compound are normal to elevated, which emphasizes why measurement of 1,25(OH)$_2$D$_3$ is of no value in diagnosing vitamin D deficiency.

Treatment A cumulative dose of 100,000–600,000 IU (2.5–15 mg) of vitamin D (ergocalciferol or cholecalciferol) with adequate calcium intake will effectively treat and cure rickets (187). New consensus guidelines for treatment of rickets (not yet published) suggests 1,000 IU/day for infants less than one month old, 1,000–5,000 IU/day for infants 1–12 months old, and higher than 5,000 IU for children older than 12 months old for 8 to 12 weeks; then the recommended maintenance dose is 400–1000 IU. If compliance is an issue 100,000 to 600,000 IU (0.25–15 mg), can be given as a single oral or intramuscular dose or as a weekly dose of 50.000 IU (1.25 mg) for eight weeks in older children and adults (186,187), or over 1–5 days in children older than one month of age, followed by maintenance dosing. High dose of vitamin D every 3 months can be repeated if poor compliance persists even with maintenance dosing. In small children a 50.000 IU capsule may be soaked in water to soften it and administer the intact capsule in blended food (187) or a 25,000 or 50,000 IU tablet may be crushed. Vitamin D can also be administered as 100,000 IU of Vitamin D every 2 hours over a 12 hour period (187). Parenteral form of Vitamin D is not currently available. Typically, calcium and phosphorus levels will normalize within 6–10 days and PTH within 1–2 months. Normalization of alkaline phosphatase and radiological abnormalities may take as long as 3–6 months depending on the severity of the deficiency but radiological changes may be observed in one week. Alkaline phosphatase levels may increase in the short term as bone formation increases. With 'stoss' therapy a biochemical response occurs in one week or two. Elemental calcium at a dose of 40–75 mg/kg/day in three divided doses is recommended in the initial phase to avoid hypocalcemia secondary to "hungry bone" syndrome, especially with 'stoss' therapy. It is advised to start at a higher dose and wean down to the lower end of the range over 2–4 weeks. In addition to calcium, calcitriol may be necessary at doses 20–100 ng/kg/day in 2–3 divided doses until normalization of calcium. Calcium is stopped when PTH and 25(OH)D levels have normalized and Vitamin D supplementation has been decreased to 400 IU a day during remineralization of the bone matrix. Following vitamin D treatment and healing of the osteomalacia, there is reappearance of the calcification front (188–190).

Of note, there is emerging literature suggesting that vitamin D$_2$ and vitamin D$_3$ should not be considered equivalent. Although vitamin D$_2$ at very high doses can prevent infantile rickets, the inefficiency of vitamin D$_2$ compared with vitamin D$_3$ on a per-mole basis at increasing 25(OH)D$_3$ concentration is well documented, and thus vitamin D$_2$ should not be used for supplementation or fortification of foods (191). Vitamin D$_2$ is available (1) as 200 µg/ml (8000 IU/ml) in propylene glycol solution, (2) as 1250 µg (50.000) gelcaps and (3) as 625 µg (25.000 IU) and 1250 µg (50.000 IU) tablets. Drisdol, Calciferol, Flintstones and Garfield vitamins and Prenatal and Women's multivitamins are vitamin D$_2$ preparations. Cholecalciferol or vitamin D$_3$ preparations are Poly-Vi-Sol and Delta D (1mg of vitamin D$_3$ equals 40.000 IU). Please see table for calcium preparations.

Monitoring of Treatment Careful monitoring includes measurement of serum calcium, phosphate, 25(OH)D$_3$, intact PTH, alkaline phosphatase, and spot urine calcium-to-creatinine ratio to detect hypercalciuria. In growing children, the preceding lab tests should be repeated every 6–8 weeks until a therapeutic response has been observed.

Prevention of Vitamin D Deficiency Regular and sensible sun exposure during the sunny months of the year can prevent vitamin D deficiency in infants and young children. Current recommended vitamin D intake to prevent rickets is 400 IU daily. However, breast-fed neonates (especially of dark skinned mothers) and children who are on vitamin D–deficient diets may respond well to oral doses of 800–1500 IU/day all year up to age 2 years and during the winter months up to age 5 years without any signs of vitamin D intoxication (192). All children on seizure medications should receive 400 IU of vitamin D and 1 g/day of elemental calcium supplementation; institutionalized children with decreased sunlight exposure may require vitamin D supplementation up to 2000 IU/day. Anticonvulsant drugs such as phenobarbital, phenytoin, primidone, and carbamazepine increase the activity of the P450 enzyme system, which increases vitamin D catabolism.

Vitamin D–Dependent Rickets (VDDR) Types I and II

These are rare autosomal recessive disorders caused by mutations in the 1α(OH)ase enzyme and vitamin D receptor (VDR) genes and present with similar clinical, radiological, and biochemical features of vitamin D deficiency (164). In VDDR type I, the active form of Vitamin D, 1α,25(OH)$_2$D$_3$, is not formed due to impaired enzymatic activity of 1α(OH)ase, whereas in the VDDR type II, the active form of vitamin D is formed, but the target tissues are unresponsive due to defects in the VDR (see Figure 39-13). The gene for the 1α(OH)ase enzyme has been cloned and mapped to the 12q13.3 chromosomal region, and several mutations have been described (193,194). The gene of the VDR also has been cloned and mapped to the 12q12-14 chromosomal region.

Clinical Presentation Affected patients with either VDDR type I or VDDR type II may present with rickets and/or hypocalcemic seizures during the first year of age. However, some patients with VDDR type II may have alopecia beginning in the first year of life; the severity of the alopecia may range from sparse hair to total alopecia without eyelashes. Clinical findings of rickets in both disorders are similar to those of nutritional rickets.

Laboratory Evaluation Patients with both forms develop biochemical findings of secondary hyperparathyroidism secondary to hypocalcemia due to impaired vitamin D activation (VDDR type I) or resistance (VDDR type II). Hypophosphatemia due to an increase in renal phosphate clearance, elevated alkaline phosphatase, and normal circulating levels of 25(OH)D$_3$ is common in both disorders; the normal 25(OH)D$_3$ level differentiates these patients from patients with rickets due to vitamin D deficiency. In patients affected with VDDR type I, the levels of 1,25(OH)$_2$D$_3$ are undetectable or markedly reduced, whereas patients affected with VDDR type II have markedly elevated 1,25(OH)$_2$D$_3$ levels. Generalized aminoaciduria may be observed in both forms probably due to secondary hyperparathyroidism.

Treatment Lifelong administration of 1,25(OH)$_2$D$_3$ (calcitriol), along with normal calcium intake, is the treatment of choice in VDDR type I. The initial dose of calcitriol is 0.5–1.5 µg/day.

The response to pharmacological doses of cholecalciferol, ergocalciferol, or calcitriol in patients with VDDR type II is variable, with some responding to calcitriol doses of 12.5–20 µg/day and elemental calcium supplementation of about 2 g/day. Patients with severe resistance may respond to administration of large amounts of calcium (195). Efficacy of treatment and compliance are monitored by measurement of intact PTH, serum calcium and phosphorus, and alkaline phosphatase.

Hypophosphatemic Rickets

X-linked hypophosphatemic rickets, autosomal dominant hypophosphatemic rickets (ADHR), autosomal recessive hypophosphatemic rickets (ARHR), tumor-induced osteomalacia (TIO), and fibrous dysplasia are all disorders associated with hypophosphatemia due to defects in the renal tubular reabsorption of filtered phosphate and elevated serum levels of FGF-23 (196). Inadequate levels of inorganic phosphate impair the function of mature osteoblasts (bone matrix ossification) resulting in rickets; formation of mature bone involves the precipitation of hydroxyapatite [3Ca$_3$(PO$_4$)$_2$:Ca(OH)$_2$] crystals.

X-linked hypophosphatemic rickets (XLH rickets) is the most common familial form of hypophosphatemic rickets, previously denoted as *vitamin D–resistant rickets*, with an estimated prevalence of 1:20,000 births (161). XLH rickets is caused by loss-of-function mutations of the PHEX gene, which stands for *phosphate-regulating with homology to endopeptidase on the X chromosome.* The PHEX gene has been mapped to the Xp22.1 chromosomal region and encodes a membrane-bound endopeptidase expressed primarily in the osteoblasts of bone and teeth (197). This loss-of-function mutation of the PHEX gene gives rise to the increased concentration of serum FGF-23 (198) because PHEX seems to be responsible for the degradation of the FGF-23, which is a phosphaturic peptide (phosphatonin); FGF-23 appears to be the leading phosphatonin that accounts for the biochemical phenotype of the XLH rickets patients (199).

Autosomal dominant hypophosphatemic rickets (ADHR) is a less frequent cause of hypophosphatemic rickets and is the result of activating mutations in the FGF-23 gene, causing an increase in the plasma levels of FGF-23 and phosphaturia. The FGF-23 gene has been cloned and mapped to the chromosomal region 12p13 (200). Somatic mosaicism and germline mosaicism for PHEX gene mutations may mimic autosomal dominant transmission of XLH rickets (201).

Tumor-induced osteomalacia (TIO) is an acquired form of hypophosphatemic rickets caused by unregulated and excessive secretion of FGF-23 from generally benign mesenchymal or mixed connective tissue tumors, mostly occurring in the head and neck (202,203).

Autosomal recessive hypophosphatemic rickets (ARHR) is a rare cause of hypophosphatemic rickets that results from mutations of the DMP1 gene, which encodes dentin matrix acidic phosphoprotein and is mapped to chromosomal region 4q21 (204,205).

Hereditary hypophosphatemic rickets with hypercalciuria (HHRH) is an autosomal recessive disorder most likely of renal phosphate reabsorption. Mutations of the closely related sodium–phosphate cotransporter genes SLC34A1 and SLC34A3, which are predominantly expressed in the kidney and appear to play a key role in renal phosphate handling, have been identified in affected families. Both genes are mapped to chromosomal region 9q34 (206,207). As with other phosphate-wasting disorders, HHRH is characterized by reduced tubular reabsorption of phosphate (TRP) and hypophosphatemia. However, in contrast to the characteristics of XLH rickets and ADHR, serum levels of 1,25(OH)$_2$D$_3$ in HHRH are appropriately elevated in response to hypophosphatemia despite suppressed parathyroid function. Increased 1,25(OH)$_2$D$_3$ levels enhance intestinal absorption of calcium and, subsequently, hypercalcemia and hypercalciuria.

X-linked recessive hypophosphatemic rickets (XRHR) is a form of X-linked hypercalciuric nephrolithiasis that consists of a group of disorders characterized by generalized aminoaciduria, glycosuria, low-molecular-weight proteinuria, hypercalciuria, nephrocalcinosis, and renal insufficiency. Mutations of the CLCN5 gene have been identified in affected family members of kindreds with Dent disease, X-linked recessive nephrolithiasis, and X-linked recessive hypophosphatemic rickets (208–210,211).

The CLCN5 gene encodes a new member of the CLC family of voltage-gated chloride channels and has been mapped to chromosomal region Xp11.22

Fibrous dysplasia (FD) also can be associated with hypophosphatemic hyperphosphaturic rickets due to excessive production of FGF-23 by osteoprogenitor cells and osteoblasts (208). The disease may involve one bone or multiple bones or even the entire skeleton. The base of the skull and the proximal metaphyses of the femora are the most commonly involved skeletal sites. All forms of FD are caused by activating missense mutations of the GNAS gene, encoding the α subunit of the stimulatory G protein (G$_s$α). FD can be associated with café-au-lait spots and hyperactivity of the endocrine system, presenting with precocious puberty, hyperthyroidism, GH excess, and Cushing syndrome. FD, when associated with one or more of the extraskeletal manifestations, is called *McCune–Albright syndrome.*

Some other causes of rickets include *Fanconi syndrome*, a disorder of renal proximal tubules in which there is decreased reabsorption of phosphorus, glucose, amino acids, and bicarbonate. Hypophosphatemia and the presence of metabolic acidosis contribute to the bone disease in patients with Fanconi syndrome, who can present with growth failure and rickets. As in XLH rickets, the plasma concentration of 1,25(OH)$_2$D$_3$ is decreased or normal in Fanconi syndrome, which is inappropriate in relation to the degree of hypophosphatemia. PTH can be normal or elevated, 25(OH)D$_3$ is normal, and alkaline phosphatase is elevated. Metabolic disorders affecting ATP production can lead to Fanconi syndrome because renal proximal tubule epithelial cells have a high metabolic requirement; hereditary fructose intolerance, cystinosis, mitochondrial disorders, glycogen storage diseases, and tyrosinemia are some of the underlying metabolic causes of Fanconi syndrome (212).

Clinical Presentation The main clinical manifestations of hypophosphatemic rickets are similar to those observed in nutritional rickets. Children with XLH rickets are asymptomatic until they start walking, when they develop bone pain, progressive deformities (particularly of the lower extremities), and stunted growth. Dentition may be delayed in very young children; older children may experience multiple dental abscesses affecting multiple noncarious primary or permanent teeth. The teeth in XLH rickets are characterized by enlarged pulp chambers, dentin dysplasia, and dentinal clefts. Abscesses are formed when the pulp is infected by bacteria invading through the enamel cracks and dentinal clefts of the teeth. The severity of XLH rickets is variable among affected individuals of the same family, and there is not a good correlation between phenotype and genotype (213).

Patients with ADHR may present either during infancy with renal phosphate wasting and rickets or after puberty with renal wasting, bone pain, fatigue, weakness, pseudofractures, and/or stress fractures. Affected females may develop hypophosphatemia shortly after they give birth. Unlike patients with rickets due to vitamin D deficiency, craniotabes and rachitic rosary are not seen in XLH rickets or ADHR. In ADHR, because of incomplete penetrance of the disease, there is great variability in the age of onset of the biochemical and clinical manifestations; occasionally, resolution of the phosphate-wasting defect has been noted (200).

In TIO, characteristic clinical manifestations include bone pain, muscle weakness, fractures, and osteomalacia or rickets and may be present for years before the causal tumor is identified.

Patients with ARHR present with similar clinical and biochemical findings to those of XLH rickets or ADHR, including elevated levels of FGF-23. Severe osteosclerosis combined with coarse and thickened calvaria and broad and undermodeled ribs and clavicles has been described in older patients.

Patients with HHRH have similar clinical presentation to the other forms of hypophosphatemic rickets; however, because of the increased calcium absorption, they eventually develop hypercalcemia, hypercalciuria, and nephrocalcinosis. Obligate carriers have been described to have borderline hypercalciuria but do not have hypophosphatemia or rickets.

Patients with XRHR have urinary loss of low-molecular-weight proteins as the most consistent abnormality, which is present in all affected males and in almost all female carriers of the disorder. Other signs of impaired proximal renal tubule reabsorption, such as generalized aminoaciduria and glucosuria, are variable and can be intermittent. Urinary acidification is normal in over 80 of patients, and when it is abnormal, it has been attributed to hypercalciuria or nephrocalcinosis.

Children affected with FD may present with facial asymmetry due to abnormal growth of the craniofacial bones and neurological symptoms due to bony encroachment on cranial nerves. They also may have symptoms characteristic of associated endocrinopathies and of rickets secondary to hypophosphatemia.

Laboratory Evaluation Characteristic biochemical findings in XLH rickets, ADHR, ARHR, and TIO include hypophosphatemia, hyperphosphaturia, and elevated alkaline phosphatase, which precedes hypophosphatemia. Serum creatinine, calcium, intact PTH, and $25(OH)D_3$ are all normal. In XHR rickets, ADHR, ARHR, TIO, and other hypophosphatemic rickets associated with increased activity of FGF-23, such as FD, plasma calcitriol is inappropriately normal or reduced despite the hypophosphatemia, which is a known stimulus of $25(OH)D_3$ 1α-hydroxylase activity; the reason for the inappropriately normal or low levels of $1,25(OH)_2D_3$ is not clearly understood. Of note, FGF-23 levels generally are elevated in TIO, but normal levels do not rule out TIO (203).

HHRH can be distinguished from XHR rickets, ADHR, ARHR, and TIO because it is associated with low intact PTH levels, elevated calcitriol levels, normal to low FGF-23 levels, elevated calcium levels, and hypercalciuria.

Patients with XRHR also have high levels of $1,25(OH)_2D_3$, increased intestinal calcium absorption, elevated calcium levels, and hypercalciuria. However, the increased urinary excretion of low-molecular-weight protein distinguishes patients with XRHR from patients with HHRH.

In the various forms of hypophosphatemic rickets, renal tubular reabsorption of phosphate (TRP) in a first urine specimen is low (60%).

If TIO is suspected, imaging should include cranial CT scan and MRI of the facial sinuses and mandible. A penetreotide or [111I]octreotide scan would help to localize the tumor (214). A technetium-99m scan is useful for evaluation of fibrous dysplasia.

Treatment Treatment consists of phosphate supplementation at 40–100 mg/kg/day, with a target phosphate level of at least 3.1 mg/dL. Phosphate should be administered very frequent intervals (four to six times a day) because of the very short life of each dose, and the total daily dose should not exceed 3 g/day. Neutra-Phos-K (250 mg elemental phosphorus per capsule) is the most commonly used

phosphate agent. Phosphate capsules or pills are preferred over liquid phosphate preparations because of the slower phosphorus absorption. The diarrhea on initiation of treatment subsides with time. Phosphate should not be administered with milk because the calcium contained in the milk interferes with the intestinal absorption of the phosphate. Patient compliance is confirmed easily because the total amount absorbed is excreted in a 24-hour period in the urine. Because phosphate administration alone will result in hypocalcemia, stimulating PTH secretion and phosphaturia, calcitriol at supraphysiological doses is added to the treatment; starting dose is 20 ng/kg/day up to 70 ng/kg/day divided in two doses, with the higher dose given at night because of the tendency toward nocturnal hyperparathyroidism (215). With adequate therapy, the elevated serum alkaline phosphatase levels decline and eventually normalize, particularly if treatment is started in the first months of life. However, levels may never completely normalize in a patient who starts treatment after 2 years of age.

The two most common complications of therapy include nephrocalcinosis and hyperparathyroidism. Hydrochlorothiazide diuretic and the potassium-sparing amiloride have been used as adjunctive therapy in the treatment of hypercalciuria and nephrocalcinosis. To avoid the risk of nephrocalcinosis, phosphate supplementation at no higher than 70 mg/kg/day has been advocated. Maintenance of good oral hygiene and regular dental care for topical fluoride application and pit and fissure sealants are important to prevent abscess formation. GH therapy, after rickets are controlled, at a dose of 0.35 mg/kg/week in patients with impaired growth or delayed diagnosis may be beneficial (216).

The accurate diagnosis of HHRH has important therapeutic implications. Unlike for XLH rickets and ADHR, phosphate supplementation alone can cause a complete remission of HHRH, whereas the addition of vitamin D can create complications, such as hypercalcemia, nephrocalcinosis, and renal damage. Long-term phosphate supplementation alone results in reversal of the clinical and biochemical abnormalities in HHRH, with the exception of the decreased renal phosphate reabsorption.

Monitoring of Treatment Evaluation should include serum calcium, phosphorus, alkaline phosphatase, intact PTH, and 24-hour urine for calcium-to-creatinine ratio every 3 months and renal US annually. Urinary calcium excretion in a 24-hour urine specimen should be less than 4 mg/kg/day. The calcium-to-creatinine ratio in a spot urine specimen should be less than 0.7 during the first year of age and less than 0.3 after the first year of life (217).

RICKETS WITH NORMAL OR HIGH SERUM CALCIUM–PHOSPHATE PRODUCT

Renal Osteodystrophy

Renal osteodystrophy and hypophosphatasia are associated with normal or elevated serum calcium phosphate product (>50 mg/dL), respectively. *Renal osteodystrophy* is a common bone disease in children with chronic kidney failure that is characterized by rickets or osteomalacia, with patients/parents reporting bone pain and growth retardation. The serum calcium level is normal until late in the course of chronic kidney failure. The serum phosphate level becomes elevated earlier in the course (175). Thus the serum calcium–phosphate product may be normal or high depending on the time the patient presents during the course of kidney failure.

The proximal renal tubule is the site where the 1α-hydroxylase gene at 12q13.3 is expressed, facilitating the conversion of $25(OH)D_3$ to $1,25(OH)_2D_3$. Expression of the 1α-hydroxylase gene is modulated by various factors, including calcium, phosphate, PTH, and insulin-like growth factors.

As renal function continues to deteriorate, the ability of the kidneys to produce $1,25(OH)_2D_3$ is impaired, resulting in poor absorption of calcium and phosphate. With the GFR reduced to 50% of normal in these children, serum PTH begins to rise in all patients (175).

When kidney function falls below 25% of normal, hyperphosphatemia and metabolic acidosis ensue because the failing kidneys can no longer adequately excrete the endogenous and exogenous loads of phosphate and hydrogen ions from endogenous metabolism. Serum alkaline phosphatase becomes elevated after the GFR declines to less than 25% of normal (175). The hyperparathyroidism, metabolic acidosis, and inadequate $1,25(OH)_2D_3$, as well as CaRS insensitivity associated with chronic kidney failure, contribute to the development of renal osteodystrophy.

The serum calcium level usually is maintained at normal concentrations until the GFR deteriorates to 5% of normal (175). This ability to maintain normal extracellular calcium homeostasis until so late in chronic kidney failure is due to rapid responses of intestinal, bone, and kidney to changes in PTH and $1,25(OH)_2D_3$.

Adynamic bone (low turnover rate) and osteomalacia are seen in 20% of end-stage kidney disease children and adolescents with secondary hyperparathyroidism receiving intermittent calcitriol treatment (218) (see Figure 39-14). The reduced osteoblastic activity

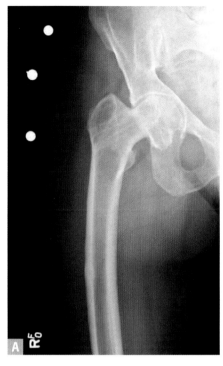

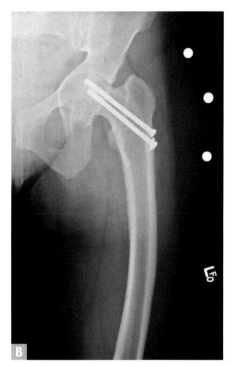

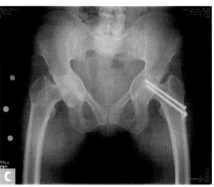

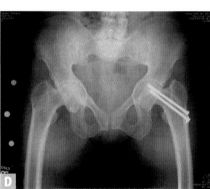

FIGURE 39-14. Osteomalacia. Bilateral bowing deformity in a patient on renal dialysis. The focal transverse lucencies are Looser zones; abnormally unmineralized osteoid is deposited, giving the characteristic appearance.

and lower bone turnover rate in adynamic renal osteodystrophy are reflected in the low or inappropriately normal serum concentrations of PTH and alkaline phosphatase.

It is crucial to optimal outcome that development of renal osteodystrophy be anticipated in the child with chronic renal failure. Renal osteodystrophy is often underrecognized because the earlier symptoms and signs are nonspecific. For example, the muscle weakness, bone pain, and growth retardation of renal osteodystrophy sometimes are mistaken for common aches and growing pains.

Soft tissue calcifications, commonly seen in adult end-stage kidney failures, are beginning to be recognized in greater frequency in children and adolescents. The extraskeletal soft tissue calcifications affect vascular, periarticular, and visceral sites. Cardiac calcifications, especially on the mitral and aortic valves, are seen in half of adult dialysis patients (219). Corresponding data in children are

being collected. Vascular calcifications are associated with higher mortality rates, especially from cardiac and cerebrovascular events.

Bone disease persists in children after successful kidney transplantation due to the need to use immunosuppressive agents (especially high-dose corticosteroid) to control acute and chronic rejection. A quarter of the patients have evidence of secondary hyperparathyroidism, and 10% show adynamic bone formation (220).

Treatment of renal osteodystrophy is aimed at maintaining the serum calcium and phosphate levels as close to normal as possible in order to prevent the development of secondary hyperparathyroidism and the extraskeletal depositions of calcium. Dietary phosphate restriction to less than 1200 mg phosphate per day aims to keep the serum calcium–phosphate product to 55 mg/dL or less. Poor palatability of diet as a result of these dietary restrictions prevents long-term patient com-

pliance. The addition of calcium-containing phosphate binders usually becomes necessary, with calcium carbonate being the most commonly prescribed agent, given together with meals in order to maximize its phosphate-binding efficiency and to minimize the absorption of calcium. The dosage, starting at 500–1000 mg elemental calcium per square meter per day, should be adjusted to maintain normal calcium and phosphate serum concentrations. Aluminum-containing binders are contraindicated in children because of the risk of aluminum toxicity. The combined calcium intake from dietary ingestion and phosphate binder should not exceed 2500 mg/day; the serum calcium and phosphate concentrations must be monitored every month for the first 3 months and then every 3 months thereafter.

When the GFR is 60 mL/min, PTH levels should be monitored very carefully. If PTH levels are elevated and $1,25(OH)_2D_3$ levels are decreased, calcitriol therapy is indicated, starting at 10–50 ng/kg/day (221). The dose can be increased progressively to maintain the PTH concentration within acceptable values. Paricalcitol, a new vitamin D analogue, is preferred for the therapy of renal osteodystrophy because it is believed to have lesser toxicity than calcitriol; paricalcitol suppresses parathyroid gland activity and has the least effect on intestinal calcium and phosphate absorption (222,223). Serum calcium concentrations are measured 1 month after starting calcitriol therapy and then quarterly. If hypercalcemia is encountered, calcitriol should be discontinued and resumed at the same dosage every other day or at a dose 0.25 μg lower than previous maintenance dose only when normocalcemia is reestablished.

Calcimimetic agents are coming into use, particularly in patients who are resistant to calcitriol or in whom hypercalcemic episodes prohibit its continued use (224). The mechanism of action of these medications is by signaling the parathyroid gland through stimulation of the CaSR (225) that serum calcium is normal, thus reducing further the tendency toward hyperparathyroidism. These agents have not yet been used extensively in children.

After renal transplantation, many patients continue to experience the ramifications of secondary hyperparathyroidism. A recent investigation suggests that the higher the pretransplant ionized calcium, the greater is this risk (226).

Parathyroidectomy is indicated when vitamin D therapy fails to control hyperparathyroidism. The "hungry bone" syndrome with high calcium uptake into the skeleton may follow parathyroidectomy. Calcitriol may be needed for a few days after surgery. If the serum calcium level falls below 8.5 mg/dL, calcium gluconate will be needed intravenously to provide 100 mg of elemental calcium per hour for the first 4–6 hours. Thereafter, it is adjusted to maintain calcium at normal levels. Hypophosphatemia may coexist, but phosphate supplementation should be avoided in order not to aggravate the hypocalcemia, unless the phosphate is less than 2 mg/dL. Then the aim is to maintain the serum phosphate level at 3.5–4.5 mg/dL.

Hypophosphatasia

Hypophosphatasia is a rare inherited disorder characterized by defective bone mineralization and a deficiency of tissue-nonspecific (TNSALP) alkaline phosphatase activity (227). Hypophosphatasia is caused by mutations in the TNSALP gene, which is localized to chromosomal region 1p36.1 (228).

Although TNSALP is normally present in all tissues, hypophosphatasia affects predominantly the skeleton and the teeth, and all forms have premature loss of dentition. The phenotypic spectrum of the disease is wide ranging, from an affected stillborn without any evident mineralization to pathological fractures developing only late in adulthood. Depending on the age of diagnosis, five clinical forms are recognized: perinatal, infantile, childhood, adult, and odontohypophosphatasia. The severe forms of the disease, perinatal and infantile, are transmitted through autosomal recessive inheritance, whereas the childhood type, odontohypophosphatasia, and the adult type are transmitted by both autosomal recessive and autosomal dominant inheritance. Odontohypophosphatasia is characterized by premature exfoliation of primary teeth with intact roots and/or severe dental carries not associated with abnormalities of the skeletal system.

Clinical Presentation Perinatal hypophosphatasia manifests during gestation with extreme skeletal hypomineralization and short, deformed limbs apparent at birth and rarely with bony spurs protruding from major long bones (Figure 39-15). Most affected newborns survive only briefly.

In the infantile form, the infant may appear normal at birth, but by 6 months of age, the poor feeding, failure to thrive, wide fontanels, and hypotonia usually bring the child to medical attention. At the same time, bone changes may be present, which appear as small areas of uncalcified metaphyses as in rickets, varying degrees of calcification of the skull, and a tendency to develop angular fractures of growing bone shafts. Hypercalcemia and hypercalciuria can cause recurrent vomiting and nephrocalcinosis. Despite open fontanels, functional craniosynostosis can occur

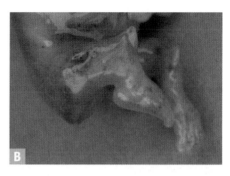

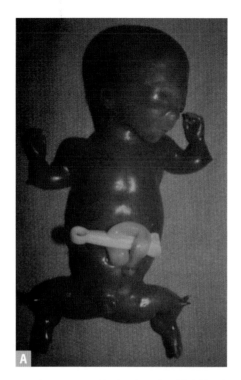

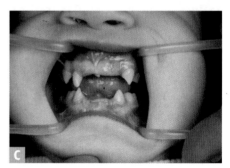

FIGURE 39-15. Hypophosphatasia. *Perinatal* (lethal form in **A, B**): Extreme skeletal hypomineralization and short, deformed limbs occur in utero. Though rare, it also can present with bony spurs protruding from major long bones. *Dental* (**C**): Premature loss of deciduous teeth.

(229). About 50% of patients die within the first year, and prognosis seems to improve if they survive beyond infancy. The bone deformity of the chest makes these patients prone to respiratory complications.

Patients affected with the childhood form may present with a history of delayed walking, waddling gait, bone pain, premature loss of dentition (with the incisors often being affected first), and frequent fractures.

The adult form shows pseudofractures and poor healing of stress fractures, especially at the metatarsus. In the odontohypophosphatemic form, premature loss of the teeth is the only finding.

Laboratory Evaluation Affected patients have a low serum alkaline phosphatase level and elevated phosphoethanolamine, inorganic pyrophosphate, and pyridoxal-5-phosphate in the serum and urine. The measurement of inorganic pyrophosphate in blood and urine is a research test. Radiological evaluation shows generalized undermineralization and rachitic changes, which are more marked in the perinatal form. Genetic testing is available.

Treatment Affected patients do not respond to standard treatment of rickets, which should be avoided because it exaggerates the hypercalcemia. Marrow cell transplantation has been used for treatment of the infantile form of hypophosphatasia (230). Therefore, treatment is supportive, and genetic counseling is indicated in all forms of hypophosphatasia.

OTHER METABOLIC BONE DISORDERS

Metabolic bone disorders with rickets and osteomalacia were discussed earlier. To round out consideration of metabolic bone disorders, we shall now focus here on neonatal osteopenia, hyperphosphatasia, osteoporosis, osteogenesis imperfecta, and osteopetrosis.

Hyperphosphatasia

Hyperphosphatasia, also known as *juvenile Paget disease*, is a rare high-bone-turnover congenital bone disease with extremely elevated alkaline phosphatase levels and normal calcium and phosphate levels; affected children are normal at birth but develop progressive long bone deformities, fractures, vertebral collapse, skull enlargement due to massively thickened calvarium, and deafness. The phenotypic variability ranges from presentation in infancy with severe progressive deformity to presentation in late childhood with minimal deformity. Most cases are caused by defects of the TNFRSF11B (tumor necrosis factor receptor superfamily, member 11B) gene that encodes osteoprotegerin (OPG), an important paracrine modulator of RANKL-mediated bone resorption (231,232).

Normally, RANKL (receptor activator of the nuclear factor κ-B ligand) binds to RANK-activating osteoclasts to reabsorb bone. In conjunction, osteoblasts secrete a soluble decoy receptor, osteoprotegerin (OPG), that inhibits the differentiation of osteoclast precursors by binding to RANKL. Defects in the TN-FRSF11B gene result in OPG deficiency and favor bone resorption because more RANKL is available for binding to RANK on osteoclasts. At present, treatment is far from optimal and consists of calcitonin to reduce bone turnover and bisphosphonate to inhibit bone resorption (233). Therapy with recombinant osteoprotegerin has shown promising results (234).

Osteoporosis

Osteoporosis arises from multiple causes (Table 39-8) and is characterized by susceptibility to long bone fractures, often secondary to nonconsequential, mild trauma. A detailed discussion of all the causes of osteoporosis is beyond the scope of this chapter.

TABLE 39-8   Classification of Osteoporosis
Immobolization
Primary
Osteogenesis imperfecta
Hyperphosphatasia
Old age
Secondary
Endocrine causes
Corticosteroid therapy
Adrenocortical tumor
Hyperthyroidism
Hypogonadism
Progeria
Acromegaly
Metabolic anomalies
Osteopetrosis
Ehlers-Danlos syndrome
Homocystinuria
Marfan syndrome
Menke syndrome
Rily–Day syndrome
Malabsorption
Celiac disease
Alcoholism
Cystic fibrosis
Anorexia nervosa
Vitamin C deficiency
Cirrhosis of liver
Hematological causes
Leukemia
Lymphoma
Multiple myeloma
Waldenstrom macroglobulinemia
Long-term heparin therapy
Genetic causes
Down syndrome
Turner syndrome
Rheumatoid disorders
Rheumatoid arthritis
Juvenile arthritis

Osteogenesis Imperfecta

Osteogenesis imperfecta (OI) is the most common genetic cause of osteoporosis and results from a defect in type I collagen fibers in bones and connective tissues. The majority of OI types are due to mutations in the (collagen, type I, α-1) gene on chromosome 17q21 and the (collagen, type II, α-2) gene on chromosome 7q22.1 (234). The incidence is 1 in 30,000 live births in type I, 1 in 60,000 live births in type II, and 1 in 70,000 live births in type III. Type IV is too rare for the incidence rate to be estimated. Most mutations causing OI occur de novo, and in most cases, recurrence of OI in a family with unaffected parents is due to parental gonadal mosaicism.

OI is frequently associated with blue sclerae, dental malformations (dentinogenesis imperfecta), and progressive hearing loss (236,237). Based on both clinical and radiological findidngs, OI is classified into four types (Sillence classification) (238); however, recently types V–VIII have been proposed. Although these types have continued the Sillence numeration, they are characterized based on bone histology, and their phenotype can be part of OI type IV or type II–III (239–241).

All four types are transmitted by autosomal dominant inheritance, except for type IIB (242–245) and type VIII (245). In type IIB OI, the defect involves the cartilage-associated protein (CRTAP), whereas in type VIII, the defect involves the prolyl 3-hydroxylase 1 (P3H1), the product of the LEPRE1 (leucine and proline enriched proteoglycan 1) gene, which hydroxylates a single proline, pro986, of the collagen type I α$_1$-chain (COL1A1) and forms a hydroxylation complex with CRTAP and cyclophilin B. Because the enzymatic activity in the 3-hydroxylation complex resides in P3H1, its absence results in severe bone dysplasia. The phenotype of patients with proposed OI type VIII overlaps with Sillence lethal type II/severe type III osteogenesis imperfecta, presenting with severe osteoporosis, shortened long bones, and a soft skull with wide-open fontanel. However, in contrast to the classical blue sclerae, triangular face, and narrow thorax of severe and lethal osteogenesis imperfecta, patients with type VIII OI have white sclerae, a round face, and a short, barrel-shaped chest.

OI type I is the mildest form of the disorder and subclassified into type IA (with dentinogenesis imperfecta [DI]) and type IB (without DI). Type IA is more severe than type IB, with a higher fracture rate, often occurring in childhood, and a greater chance of growth impairment. Overall characteristics show no long bone deformity, mild bone fragility, joint hyperextensibility, blue sclerae, kyphoscoliosis, easy bruisability, and in 50% of patients a mild hearing loss that may begin in the later teen years and progress to profound hearing loss.

OI type II is the most severe form of OI, commonly being lethal during the perinatal period. There are two forms: Type IIA is caused by mutations in the COL1A1 gene or the COL1A2 gene and is inherited in an autosomal dominant fashion. Type IIB is caused by mutation in the CRTAP gene and is inherited in an autosomal recessive manner. Overall, type II demonstrates extreme bone fragility resulting in intrauterine fractures, and few patients survive beyond the perinatal period. Affected patients are born prematurely, SGA, with extremely osteoporotic long bones and skull. Anterior and posterior fontanels are wide open. Death is usually secondary to respiratory failure and pneumonias.

Affected patients with *OI type III* have full life span expectancy and a progressively deforming disorder with severe bone fragility, with 50% of patients suffering from in utero fractures (see Figure 39-16). At birth, they present with limb shortening, triangular facies,

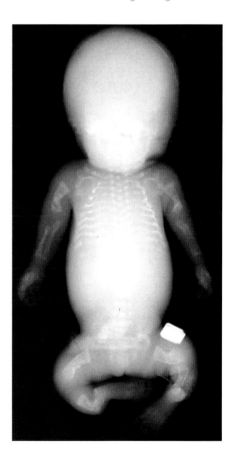

FIGURE 39-16. This newborn radiograph demonstrates the classic shortened, widened and thinned cortices of the long bones characteristic of osteogenesis imperfecta. Note the beaded appearance of the ribs and overall demineralization of the skeleton.

frontal bossing, and blue sclerae. Their long bones are so soft that they will deform from normal muscle tension. Final adult height is severely compromised.

OI type IV is the moderately severe form with osteoporotic long bones and compromised final adult height; many of these patients are responsive to GH therapy. Fractures are rare in utero. DI may be present. Both OI type III and OI type IV present with normal sclerae and normal hearing, and in both subtypes, fractures decrease after puberty.

The *diagnosis* of OI usually is made clinically based on the characteristic stigmata (236,237). Prenatally severe type II or III OI is difficult to distinguish from thanatropic dysplasia, camptomelic dysplasia, and achondrogenesis type I. During the neonatal period, OI type III and infantile hypophosphatasia may present similarly; however, infantile hypophosphatasia is characterized by a low alkaline phosphatase level and spurs extending from the sides of the knees and elbow joints. The skeletal features and joint laxity of OI types III and IV may overlap with Ehlers-Danlos syndrome.

The presence of metaphyseal corner fractures suggests battered child syndrome because these fractures are rare in OI types III and IV but common in child abuse cases. True skull, sternal, and scapular fractures, bucket handle fractures, and repeated healing and remineralization on serial x-rays are also rare in OI and seen more often in battered child syndrome.

Confirmation of the diagnosis is through mutation detection by direct sequencing. DNA testing can be used for prenatal diagnosis when mutations of the affected proband have been identified. By 15 weeks' gestation, US has been useful in revealing limb-length anomalies. Skin biopsy for fibroblast culture can evaluate collagen biochemistry through gel electrophoresis, especially in patients with OI type I, who synthesize a reduced amount of structurally normal type I collagen due to a null mutation of COL1A1; in these patients, genetic testing will show no gene abnormalities, but skin biopsy and electrophoresis will show an increase in the COL3:COL1 ratio.

Treatment of osteogenesis imperfecta is complex (245) and consists of: care for respiratory and other infections, surgical management of fractures and bone deformities, and physical therapy to improve joint mobility and increase muscle strength. Swimming should be encouraged, and vocational education programs should be designed for the parents.

GH therapy has shown to improve linear growth in OI type III. Administration of bisphosphonate has shown enhanced bone turnover and decreased bone loss (245–247).

Osteopetrosis

Pathophysiology *Osteopetrosis*, also known as *Albers–Schonberg* or *marble bone disease*, is a heterogeneous group of heritable disorders in which gene defects that mostly affect the functional capacity of mature osteoclasts result in defective bone resorption by osteoclasts and increased skeletal mass due to abnormally dense bone (249,250). Osteoclastic bone resorption is a tightly regulated process during which protons and proteases are secreted into the sealing zone of osteoclasts on bone (Howship lacunae) to dissolve bone minerals and digest the organic matrix. Subsequently, the degraded bone matrix components and dissolved bone minerals are transported within vesicles through the cytoplasm and leave the osteoclast cell via exocytosis at the basolateral membrane, which is at the opposite site of the ruffled border or resorptive membrane of the cell. Osteopetrosis is divided into three main forms based on the mode of inheritance, age of onset, severity, and associated clinical symptoms: 1) autosomal recessive infantile malignant osteopetrosis (ARO), 2) autosomal recessive intermediate mild osteopetrosis, and 3) autosomal dominant adult-onset benign osteopetrosis (ADO).

The incidence of ARO is 1 in 200,000 to 1 in 300,000 population and is 10 times higher in Costa Rica (251). More than three genes are involved in the etiology of this type of severe osteopetrosis. *T-cell immune regulator 1* (TCIRG1) gene defects account for 50% to 60% of cases with ARO (251,252). The TCIRG1 gene encodes the A3 subunit of the vacuolar ATPase proton pump (V-ATPase), which is located in the ruffled border of the osteoclast membrane and releases protons in the resorbing lacunae, resulting in acidification of the bony surface and initiating solubilization of the hydroxyapatite crystals and subsequent degradation of the bone matrix.

A less frequent genetic cause of ARO (10% to 15%) is homozygous or compound heterozygous null mutations in the CLCN7 gene encoding chloride channel 7 (CLCN7) (253,254). CLCN7 resides in the ruffled border membrane of the osteoclast and seems to preserve the electroneutrality of the ruffled border, allowing the V-ATPase to acidify the extracellular resorption lacunae.

A third gene involved in ARO is the gray lethal (GL) gene, which was found initially to be mutated in the gray lethal osteopetrotic mouse (255). This gene encodes an osteopetrosis-associated transmembrane protein 1 (OSTM1) or GAIP interacting protein N terminus (GIPN), which is suggested to have a role in cytoskeletal reorganization and development of the ruffled border.

Patients with ARO present at birth or within the first year of life with brittle bones, pancytopenia due to deficient hematopoiesis (the medullary cavity is filled with endochondral new bone, limiting the available space for hematopoietic cells), and neurological impairment. Bony encroachment of the optic, occulomotor, and facial nerves can result in progressive blindness and deafness, facial palsy, and difficulties with swallowing and feeding. Nasal congestion caused by malformation of the mastoid and paranasal sinuses can be an early symptom. Other clinical findings may include hepatosplenomegaly as a result of extramedullary hematopoiesis, nystagmus, dental abnormalities, failure to thrive, macrocephaly, intercurrent infections, and especially osteomyelitis and rickets due to the inability of osteoclasts to maintain a normal calcium–phosporus balance in the extracellular fluid.

The *autosomal recessive intermediate mild osteopetrosis* form has been described in kindreds with recessive mutations of the CLCN7 gene; whether the CLCN7 gene is the only gene involved in this form of osteopetrosis needs to be established (253–255).

Affected patients may present with recurrent fractures, thickening and sclerosis of the calvaria, unilateral facial palsy, dental abnormalities, osteomyelitis and short stature, mild to moderate anemia, extramedullary hematopoiesis, mandibular prognathism, and proptosis; deafness also can be present. The outcome is less severe, and life expectancy is higher than in ARO.

The *autosomal dominant forms*—ADO, ADO-I, ADO-II, and ADO-III—of osteopetrosis have a delayed presentation, and half the patients with this variant of osteopetrosis are asymptomatic. The diagnosis is often made incidentally, picked up by x-rays for evaluation of fractures or unrelated conditions. The frequency of ADO has been estimated to be 1 in 100,000 to 1 in 500,000 population. Two genes so far have been identified as having a role in ADO pathogenesis. Gain-of-function mutations of the low-density lipoprotein receptor 5 (LDLR5) gene, which belongs to a family of cell surface proteins that bind and internalize ligands in the process of receptor-mediated endocytosis, have been identified in ADO-I. This subform is characterized by diffuse osteosclerosis, more predominant in the cranial vault, and low fracture rate. Affected patients have a normal height, proportion, intelligence, and longevity. Flattened forehead and elongated mandible may be seen during the adolescent years (249).

Heterozygous mutations of the CLCN7 gene, which probably act in a dominant-negative way, have been identified in some cases of ADO-II (252,257,258). *ADO-II* is characterized by generalized osteosclerosis that is more pronounced in some skeletal sites such as the spine and pelvis. ADO-II is rare and is characterized by thickening of the spine and vertebral endplate, producing the classical sandwich vertebra appearance. The classical bone-within-bone appearance is present in most but not all skeletal sites. Fractures are common and heal slowly. Osteomyelitis, particularly of the mandible, can develop, as well as hearing loss, bilateral optic atrophy, facial palsy, anemia, and fractures. Although other forms of osteopetrosis are considerably more severe, the name *benign osteopetrosis* previously used for ADO-II probably is a misnomer (250).

The cause of the *ADO-III*, which is characterized by osteosclerosis of the distal appendicular skeleton and the skull, has not been identified (260). A minority of patients with osteopetrosis has a defect in the carbonic anhydrase II gene (CAII) and present with a less severe form of osteopetrosis, renal tubular acidosis, short stature, developmental delay, cerebral calcifications, cranial nerve compressions, increased frequency of fractures, dental abnormalities, and no hematological abnormalities. Mutations in the CAII gene impair the ability of the osteoclast to produce protons that are necessary for the acidification and resorption of the bone (261). A transient form of infantile osteopetrosis has been described, with spontaneous resolution of the radiographical findings by 28 months or age (262).

Diagnosis The characteristic radiological findings of osteopetrosis are generalized osteosclerosis (see Figure 39-17), clubbed and splayed metaphyses, lucent bands at the distal long bones, and development of endobone, which appears radiographically as a bone within bone. The severity and site of involvement depend on the type of osteopetrosis, as described earlier.

There is not an association of abnormal biochemical markers and osteopetrosis, except for elevated TRAP (tartrate-resistant acid phosphatase) in ADO-II and the associated biochemical findings of renal tubular acidosis in osteopetrosis due to CAII gene defects (263).

In ARO, because of 1) absence of genotype–phenotype correlations, 2) diversity of the disease-causing mutations, and 3) existence of at least one unidentified gene, negative mutational analysis of all three genes does not rule out the disease.

Treatment Bone marrow transplantation from allogeneic donors or HLA-identical siblings usually is considered for treatment of the infantile malignant osteopetrosis (264). In addition to bone marrow transplantation for congenital osteopetrosis, high-dose calcitriol therapy can ameliorate the symptoms

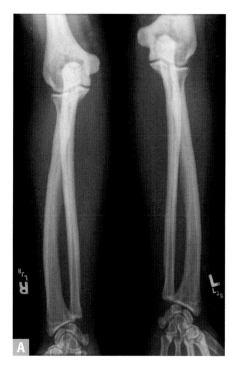

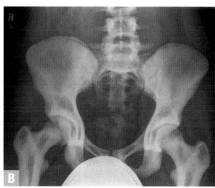

FIGURE 39-17. Osteopetrosis. The cortices demonstrate relative thickening consistent with osteopetrosis. In some extreme cases, the marrow space is never formed due to osteoclast arrest.

of osteopetrosis in 25% of patients. Calcitriol helps to stimulate dormant osteoclasts to increase bone resorption. The initial dose of calcitriol is 15 ng/kg/day, with maintenance dose of 5–40 ng/kg/day (265). Dietary calcium restriction has been used in conjunction with calcitriol with dramatic improvement in some cases; however, some patients became refractory to calcitriol treatment (265). Subcutaneous injections of interferon-γ have been used to reduce intercurrent infections (266). The oral antiviral agent lamivudine is undergoing clinical trials. Erythropoietin has been used to correct anemia in some patients. Despite the bone deformities and other limitations, with good medical and surgical care, many patients with the ADO forms of osteopetrosis lead productive careers, and some enjoy a normal life expectancy.

REFERENCES

1. Friedenstein AJ, Chaliakhjan RK, Latsinik NV, et al. Stromal cells responsible for transferring the microenvironment of the hemopoietic tissues: Cloning in vitro and retransplantation in vivo. *Transplantation* 1974;17:331–340.
2. Owen M. Lineage of osteogenic cells and their relationship to the stromal system. In: Peck WA, ed. *Bone Mineral Research*, Vol. 3. Amsterdam: Elsevier; 1985;1–25.
3. Triffit JT. The stem cell of the osteoblast. In: Bilezikian JP, Paisz LG, Rodan GA, eds. *Principles of Bone Biology*. San Diego: Academic Press; 1996:39–50.
4. Schor AM, Canfield AE, Sutton AB, et al. Pericyte differentiation. *Clin Orthop.* 1995;313:81–91.
5. Rosen V, Cox K, Hattersley G. Bone morphogenetic proteins. In: Bilezikian JP, Paisz LG, Rodan GA, eds. *Principles of Bone Biology.* San Diego: Academic Press; 1996:661–671.
6. Nijweide PJ, Burger EH, Klein-Nulend J, et al. The osteocyte. In: Bilezikian JP, Raisz LG, Rodan GA, eds. *Principles of Bone Biology.* San Diegi: Academic Press; 1996:115–126.
7. Mariotti G. The structure of bone tissues and the cellular control of their deposition. *Ital J Anat Embryol.* 1996;101:25–79.
8. Managolas SC, Jilka RL, Bellido T, et al. Interleukin-6-type cytokines and their receptors. In: Bilezikian JP, Raisz LG, Rodan GA, eds. *Principles of Bone Biology.* San Diego: Academic Press; 1996:701–713.
9. Roodman GD. Advances in bone biology: the osteoclast. *Endocr Rev.* 1996;17:308–332.
10. Nesbitt SA, Horton MA. Trafficking of matrix collagens through bone-resorbing osteoclasts. *Science.* 1997;276:270–273.
11. Salo J, Lehenkari P, Mulari M, et al. Removal of osteoclast bone resorption products by transcytosis. *Science.* 1997;276:270–273.
12. Parfitt AM. Osteonal and hemi-osteonal remodeling: The spatial and temporal framework for signal traffic in adult human bone. *J Cell Biochem.* 1994;55:273–286.
13. Hughes DE, Dai A, Tiffee JC, et al. Estrogen promotes apoptosis of murine osteoclasts mediated by TGF-β. *Nat Med.* 1996;2:1132–1136.
14. Jilka RL, Weinstein RS, Bellido T, et al. Osteoblast programmed cell death (apoptosis): Modulation by growth factors and cytokines. *J Bone Miner Res.* 1998;13:793–802.
15. Brown EM, Gamba G, Riccardi D, et al. Cloning and characterization of an extracellular Ca²⁺-sensing receptor from bovine parathyroid. *Nature.* 1993;366:575–580.
16. Kifor O, MacLeod RJ, Diaz R, et al. Regulation of MAP kinase by calcium-sensing receptor in bovine parathyroid and CaR-transfected HEK293 cells. *Am J Physiol Renal Physiol.* 2001;280:F291–302.
17. Pearce SHS, Brown EM. The genetic basis of endocrine disease: Disorders of calcium ion sensing. *J Clin Endocrinol Metab.* 1996;81:2030–2035.
18. DeLuca F, Baron J. The Ca²⁺-sensing receptor: Molecular biology and clinical importance. *Curr Opin Pediatr.* 1998;10:435–440.
19. Chang W, Tu C, Chen TH, et al. Expression and signal transduction of calcium-sensing

receptors in cartilage and bone. *Endocrinology.* 1999;140:5883–5893.

20. Yamaguchi T, Chattopadhyay N, Kifor O, et al. Expression of extracellular calcium-sensing receptor in human osteoblastic MG-63 cell line. *Am J Physiol Cell Physiol.* 2001;280:C382–393.

21. Chattppadhyay N, Yano S, Tfelt-Hansen J, et al. Mitogenic action of calcium-sensing receptor on rat calvarial osteoblasts. *Endocrinology.* 2004;145:3451–3462.

22. Kanatani M, Sugimoto T, Kanzawa M, et al. High extracellular calcium inhibits osteoclast-like cell formation by directly acting on the calcium-sensing receptor existing in osteoclast precursor cells. *Biochem Biophys Res Commun.* 1999;261:144–148.

23. Lorget F, Kamel S, Mentaverri R, et al. High extracellular calcium concentrations directly stimulate osteoclast apoptosis. *Biochem Biophys Res Commun.* 2000;268:899–903.

24. Greenfield EM, Bi Y, Miyauchi A. Regulation of osteoclast activity. *Life Sci.* 1999;65:1087–1102.

25. Suda T, Takahashi N, Udagawa N, et al. Modulation of osteoclast differentiation and function by the new members of the tumor necrosis factor receptor and ligand families. *Endocr Rev.* 1999;20:345–357.

26. Greenfield EM, Horowitz MC, Lavish SA. Stimulation by parathyroid hormone of interleukin-6 and leukemia inhibitory factor expression is an immediate-early gene response induced by cAMP signal transduction. *J Biol Chem.* 1996;271:10984–10989.

27. Grey A, Mitnick M, Shapses S, et al. Circulating levels of interleukin-6 and tumor necrosis factor-α are elevated in primary hyperparathyroidism and correlate with markers of bone resorption: A clinical research center study. *J Clin Endocrinol Metab.* 1996;81:3450–3454.

28. Greenfield EM, Shaw SM, Gornik SA, et al. Adenyl cyclase and interleukin-6 are downstream effectors of parathyroid hormone resulting in stimulation of bone resorption. *J Clin Invest.* 1995;96:1238–1244.

29. Gao Y, Morita I, Maruo N, et al. Expression of IL-6 receptor and GP-130 in mouse bone marrow cells during osteoclast differentiation. *Bone.* 1998;22:487–493.

30. Lowik C, van der Pluijm G, Bloys H, et al. Parathyroid hormone (PTH) and PTH-like protein stimulate interleukin-6 production by osteogenic cells: A possible role of interleukin-6 in osteoclastogenesis. *Biochem Biophys Res Commun.* 1989;162:1546–1552.

31. Roodman GD. Interleukin-6: an osteotropic factor? *J Bone Miner Res.* 1992;7:475–478.

32. Swarthout JT, D'Alonzo RC, Selvamurugan N, et al. Parathyroid hormone–dependent signaling pathways regulating genes in bone cells. *Gene.* 2002;282:1–17.

33. Cooke NE, Haddad JG. Vitamin D–binding protein (Gc-globulin). *Endocr Rev.* 1989; 10:294–307.

34. Dueland S, Holmberg I, Berg T, et al. Uptake and 25-hydroxylation of vitamin D_3 by isolated rat liver cells. *J Biol Chem.* 1981;256:10430–10434.

35. Cheng JB, Levine MA, Bell, NH, et al. Genetic evidence that the human CYP2R1 enzyme is a key vitamin D 25-hydroxylase. *Proc Natl Acad Sci USA.* 2004;101:7711–7715.

36. Bouillon R, Van Assche FA, Van Baelen H, et al. Influence of the vitamin D–binding protein on the serum concentration of 1,25-dihydroxyvitamin D_3: Significance of the free 1,25-dihydroxyvitamin D_3 concentration. *J Clin Invest.* 1981;67:589–596.

37. Nykjaer A, Dragun D, Walther D, et al. An endocytic pathway for renal uptake and activation of the steroid 25-(OH) vitamin D_3. *Cell.* 1999;96:507–515.

38. Adams JS, Chen H, Chun RF, et al. Novel regulators of vitamin D action and metabolism: Lessons learned at the Los Angeles Zoo. *J Cell Biochem.* 2003;88:308–314.

39. Liu W, Yu WR, Carkling T, et al. Regulation of gp330/megalin expression by vitamins A and D. *Eur J Clin Invest.* 1998;28:100–107.

40. Kumar R. Vitamin D metabolism and mechanisms of calcium transport. *J Am Soc Nephrol.* 1990;1:30–42.

41. Monkawa T, Yoshida T, Wakino S, et al. Molecular cloning of cDNA and genomic DNA for human 25-hydroxyvitamin D_3 1α-hydroxylase. *Biochem Biophys Res Commun.* 1997;239:527–533.

42. Miyamoto K, Kesterson RA, Yamamoto H, et al. Structural organization of the human vitamin D receptor chromosomal gene and its promoter. *Mol Endocr.* 1997;11:1165–1179.

43. Ecarot B, Desbarats M. 1,25-$(OH)_2D_3$ down-regulates expression of PHHEX, a marker of the mature osteoblast. *Endocrinology.* 1999;140:1192–1199.

44. Panda DK, Miao D, Bolivar I, et al. Inactivation of the 25-hydroxyvitamin D 1α-hydroxylase and vitamin D receptor demonstrates independent and interdependent effects of calcium and vitamin D on skeletal and mineral homeostasis. *J Biol Chem.* 2004;279:16754–16766.

45. Khosla S. Minireview: The OPG/RANKL/RANK system. *Endocrinology.* 2001;142:5050–5055.

46. Kondo T, Kitazawa R, Maeda S, et al. 1,25-Dihydroxyvitamin D_3 rapidly regulates the mouse osteoprotegrin gene through dual pathways. *J Bone Miner Res.* 2004;19:1411–1419.

47. Takeda S, Yoshizawa T, Nagai Y, et al. Stimulation of osteoclast formation by 1,25-dihydroxyvitamin D requires its binding receptor (VDR) in osteoblastic cells: Studies using VDR knockout mice. *Endocrinology.* 1999;140:1005–1008.

48. Carlberg C. Ligand-mediated conformational changes of the VDR are required for gene transactivation. *J Steroid Biochem Mol Biol.* 2004;89:227–232.

49. Jurutka PW, Whitfield GK, Hsieh JC, et al. Molecular nature of the vitamin D receptor and its role in regulation of gene expression. *Rev Endocrinol Metab Disord.* 2001;2:203–216.

50. Rachez C, Freedman LP. Mechanisms of gene regulation by vitamin D_3 receptor: A network of coactivator interactions. *Gene.* 2000;246:9–21.

51. Van Abel M, Hoenderop JG, van der Kemp AW, et al. Regulation of the epithelial Ca^{2+} channels in small intestine as studied by quantitative mRNA detection. *Am J Physiol Gastrointest Liver Physiol.* 2003;285:G78–85.

52. Bouillon R, van Cromphaut S, Carmeliet G. Intestinal calcium absorption: Molecular vitamin D–mediated mechanisms. *J Cell Biochem.* 2003;88:332–339.

53. Vennekens R, Hoenderop JG, Prenen J, et al. Permeation and gating properties of the novel epithelial Ca^{2+} channel. *J Biol Chem.* 2000;275:3963–3969.

54. Van Cromphant SJ, Dewerchin M, Hoenderop JG, et al. Duodenal calcium absorption in vitamin D receptor knockout mice: Functional and molecular aspects. *Proc Natl Acad Sci USA.* 2001;98:13324–13329.

55. Glendenning P, Ratajczak T, Dick IM, et al. Calcitriol upregulates expression and activity of the 1β isoform of the plasma membrane calcium pump in immortalized distal kidney tubular cells. *Arch Biochem Biophys.* 2000;380:126–132.

56. Garret JE, Tamir H, Kifor O, et al. Calcitonin-secreting cells of the thyroid express an extracellular calcium receptor gene. *Endocrinology.* 1995;136:5202–5211.

57. Martin TJ, Udagawa N. Hormonal regulation of osteoclast function. *TEM.* 1998;9:6–12.

58. Wada S, Udagawa N, Akatsu T, et al. Regulation by calcitonin and glucocorticoids of calcitonin receptor gene expression in mouse osteoclasts. *Endocrinology.* 1997;138:521–529.

59. Favus MJ. Intestinal absorption of calcium, magnesium and phosphorus. In: Coe FL, Favus MJ, eds. *Disorders of Bone and Mineral Metabolism.* New York: Raven Press; 1992:57–81.

60. Berndt TJ, Schiavi S, Kumar R. "Phosphatonins" and the regulation of phosphorus homeostasis. *Am J Physiol Renal Physiol.* 2005;289:F1170–1182.

61. Laires MJ, Monteiro CP, Bicho M. Role of cellular magnesium in health and human disease. *Frontiers Biosci.* 2004;9:262–276.

62. Dai L-J, Ritchie G, Kerstan D, et al. Magnesium transport in the renal distal convoluted tubule. *Physiol Rev.* 2001;81:51–84.

63. Naylor KE, Iqbal P, Fledelius C, et al. The effect of pregnancy on bone density and bone turnover. *J Bone Miner Res.* 2000;15:129–137.

64. Black AJ, Topping J, Durham B, et al. A detailed assessment of alterations in bone turnover, calcium homeostasis, and bone density in normal pregnancy. *J Bone Miner Res.* 2000;15:557–563.

65. Kovacs CS. Commentary: Calcium and bone metabolism in pregnancy and lactation. *J Clin Endocrinol Metab.* 2001;86:2344–2348.

66. Dahlman T, Sjoberg HE, Bucht E. Calcium homeostasis in normal pregnancy and puerperium: A longitudinal study. *Acta Obstet Gynaecol Scand.* 1994;73:393–398.

67. Seely EW, Brown EM, DeMaggio DM, et al. A prospective study of calciotropic hormones in pregnancy and postpartum: Reciprocal changes in serum intact parathyroid hormone and 1,25-dihydroxyvitamin D. *Am J Obstet Gynnecol.* 1997;176:214–217.

68. Gaboury CL, Woods, LL. Renal reserve in pregnancy. *Semin Nephrol.* 1995;15:449–453.

69. Kent GN, Price RI, Gutteridge DH, et al. Effect of pregnancy and lactation on

maternal bone mass and calcium metabolism. *Osteoporosis Int.* 1993;3:44S–47.

70. Gallecher SJ, Fraser WD, Owens OJ, et al. Changes in calciotrophic hormones and biochemical markers of bone turnover in normal human pregnancy. *Eur J Endocrinol.* 1994;131:369–374.

71. Ritchie LD, Fung EB, Halloran BP, et al. A longitudinal study of calcium homeostasis during human pregnancy and lactation and after resumption of menses. *Am J Clin Nutr.* 1998;67:693–701.

72. Schauberger CW, Pitkin RM. Maternal-perinatal calcium relationships. *Obstet Gynecol.* 1979;53:74–76.

73. Delivoria-Papadopoulos M, Battaglia FC, Bruns PD, et al. Total, protein-bound, and ultrafilterable calcium in maternal and fetal plasmas. *Am J Physiol.* 1967;213:363–366.

74. Robinson NR, Sibley CP, Mughal MZ, et al. Fetal control of calcium transport across the rat placenta. *Pediatr Res.* 1989;26:109–115.

75. Kovacs CS, Lanske B, Hunzelman JL, et al. Parathyroid hormone–related peptide (PTHrP) regulates fetal-placental calcium transport through a receptor distinct from the PTH/PTHrP receptor. *Proc Natl Acad Sci USA.* 1996;93:15233–15238.

76. Kovacs CS, Chafe LL, Fudge NJ, et al. PTH regulates fetal blood calcium and skeletal mineralization independently of PTHrP. *Endocrinology.* 2001;142:4983–4993.

77. Ron M, Menczel J, Schwartz L, et al. Vitamin D_3 metabolites in amniotic fluid in relation with maternal and fetal sera in term pregnancies. *J Perinat Med.* 1987;15:282–290.

78. Sagges G, Baroncelli GI, Bertelloni S, et al. Intact parathyroid hormone levels during pregnancy, in healthy term neonates, and in hypocalcemic preterm infants. *Acta Paediatr Scand.* 1991;80:36–41.

79. Kovacs CS, Kronenberg HM. Maternal-fetal calcium and bone metabolism during pregnancy, puerperium, and lactation. *Endocr Rev.* 1997;18:832–872.

80. Largo RH, Waelli R, Duc G, et al. Evaluation of perinatal growth. *Helv Paediatr Acta.* 1980;35:419–436.

81. Hoegler W, Schmid A, Raber G, et al. Perinatal bone turnover in term human neonates and the influence of maternal smoking. *Pediatr Res.* 2003;53:817–822.

82. Ducy P, Desbois C, Boyce B, et al. Increased bone formation in osteocalcin-deficient mice. *Nature.* 1996;382:448–452.

83. Linarelli LG. Newborn urinary cyclic AMP and developmental renal responsiveness to parathyroid hormone. *Pediatrics.* 1972;50: 14–23.

84. Mallet E, Basuyau JP, Brunelle P, et al. Neonatal parathyroid secretion and renal receptor maturation in premature infants. *Biol Neonate.* 1978;33:304–308.

85. Giles MM, Fenton MH, Shaw B, et al. Sequential calcium and phosphorus balance studies in preterm infants. *J Pediatr.* 1987;110:591–598.

86. Hollis BW, Lowery JW, Pittard WB, et al. Effect of age on the intestinal absorption of vitamin D_3–palmitate and nonesterified vitamin D_2 in the term human infant. *J Clin Endocrinol Metab.* 1996;81: 1385–1388.

87. Borowitz SM, Granrud GS. Ontogeny of intestinal phosphate absorption in rabbits. *Am J Physiol.* 1992;262:G847–853.

88. Bistarkis L, Voskaki I, Lambadaridis J, et al. Renal handling of phosphate in the first six months of life. *Arch Dis Child.* 1986;61: 677–681.

89. Karlen J, Rane S, Aperia A. Tubular response to hormones is blunted in weanling rats. *Acta Physiol Scand.* 1990;138:443–449.

90. Woda C, Mulroney SE, Halaihel N, et al. Renal tubular sites of increased phosphate transport and NaPi-2 expression in the juvenile rat. *Am J Physiol Regul Integr Comp Physiol.* 2001;280:1524–1533.

91. Hallak M, Cotton DB. Transfer of maternally administered magnesium sulfate into the fetal compartment of the rat: Assessment of amniotic fluid, blood and brain. *Am J Obstet Gynecol.* 1993;169:427–431.

92. Bezanilla F. The voltage sensor in voltage-dependent ion channels. *Physiol Rev.* 2000;80:555–592.

93. Niggli E. Localized intracellular calcium signaling in muscle: Calcium sparks and calcium quarks. *Annu Rev Physiol.* 1999;61:311–335.

94. Catterall WA. Structure and regulation of voltage-gated Ca^{2+} channels. *Annu Rev Cell Dev Biol.* 2000;16;521–555.

95. Meissner G. Ryanodine receptor/Ca^{2+} release channels and their regulation by endogenous effectors. *Annu Rev Physiol.* 1994;56:485–508.

96. Bers DM. Cardiac excitation-contraction coupling. *Nature.* 2002;415:198–205.

97. Ringer S. A further contribution regarding the influence of the blood on the contraction of the heart. *J Physiol.* 1983;4:29–42.

98. Armstrong CM, Bezanilla FM, Horowicz P. Twitches in the presence of ethylene glycol bis(β-aminoethyl ether)-N,N′-tetra-acetic acid. *Biochim Biophys Acta.* 1972;267:605–608.

99. Philipson KD, Nicoll DA. Sodium-calcium exchange: A molecular perspective. *Annu Rev Physiol.* 2000;62:111–133.

100. Langer GA. Calcium and the heart: Exchange at the tissue, cell and organelle levels. *FASEB J.* 1992;6:893–902.

101. Lee WK, Vargas A, Barnes J, et al. The Kenny-Caffey syndrome: Growth retardation and hypocalcemia in a young boy. *Am J Med Genet.* 1983;14:773–782.

102. Sanjad SA, Sakati NA, Abu-Osaba Y. Congenital hypoparathyroidism with dysmorphic features: A new syndrome (abstract). *Pediatr Res.* 1988;23:271A.

103. Bowl MR, Nesbit MA, Harding B, et al: An interstitial deletion-insertion involving chromosomes 2p25.3 and Xq27.1, near SOX3, causes X-linked recessive hypoparathyroidism. *J Clin Invest.* 2005;115: 2822–2831.

104. Ahonen P, Myllaerniemi S, Sipilae I, et al. Clinical variation of autoimmune polyendocrinopathy-candidiasis-ectodermal dystrophy (APECED) in a series of 68 patients. *N Engl J Med.* 1990;322:1829–1836.

105. Glazebrook GA. Efect of decicurie doses of radioactive iodine-131 on parathyroid function. *Am J Surg.* 1987;154:368–373.

106. Valsamis HA, Arora SK, Labban B, et al. Antiepileptic drugs and bone metabolism.

Nutr Metab. www.nutritionandmetabolism.com/contents/3/1/36,2006.

107. Champallou C, Basuyau JP, B, Veyret C, et al. Hypocalcemia following pamidronate administration for bone metases of solid tumor: Three case reports. *J Pain Sympt Manag.* 2003;25:185–190.

108. Monaco G, Pignata C, Rossi E, et al: George anomaly associated with 10p deletion. *Am J Med Genet.* 1991;39:215–216.

109. Lai MMR, Scriven PN, Ball C, et al: Simultaneous partial monosomy 10p and trisomy 5q in a case of hypoparathyroidism. *J Med Genet.* 1992;29:586–588.

110. Hasegawa T, Hasegawa Y, Aso T, et al: HDR syndrome (hypoparathyroidism, sensorineural deafness, renal dysplasia) associated with del(10)(p13). *Am J Med Genet.* 1997;73: 416–418.

111. Van Esch H, Groenen P, Nesbit MA, et al: GATA3 haplo-insufficiency causes human HDR syndrome. *Nature.* 2000;406:419–422.

112. Muroya K, Hasegawa T, Ito Y, et al: GATA3 abnormalities and the phenotypic spectrum of HDR syndrome. *J Med Genet.* 2001;38:374–380.

113. Franceschini P, Bogetti G, Girardo E, et al: Kenny-Caffey syndrome in two sibs born to consanguineous parents: Evidence for an autosomal recessive variant. *Am J Med Genet.* 1992;42:112–116.

114. Kelly TE, Blanton S, Saif R, et al. Confirmation of the assignment of the Sanjad-Sakati (congenital hypoparathyroidism) syndrome (OMIM 241419) locus to chromosome 1q42-43. *J Med Genet.* 2000;37:63–64.

115. Diaz GA, Kahn KTS, Gelb BD. The autosomal recessive Kenny-Caffey syndrome locus maps to chromosome 1q42-43. *Genomics.* 1998;54:13–18.

116. Sanjad SA, Sakati NA, Abu-Osba YK, et al. A new syndrome of congenital hypoparathyroidism, seizure, growth failure and dysmorphic features. *Arch Dis Child.* 1991;66: 193–196.

117. Sunthornthepvarakul T, Churesigaew S, Ngowngarmratana S. A novel mutation of the signal peptide of the preproparathyroid hormone gene associated with autosomal recessive familial isolated hypoparathyroidism. *J Clin Endocrinol Metab.* 1999,84: 3792–3796.

118. Parkinson DB, Thakker RV. A donor splice site mutation in the parathyroid hormone gene is associated with autosomal recessive hypoparathyroidism. *Nat Genet.* 1992;1:149–152.

119. Arnold A, Horst SA, Gardella TJ, et al: Mutation of the signal peptide-encoding region of the preproparathyroid hormone gene in familial isolated hypoparathyroidism. *J Clin Invest.* 1990;86:1084–1087.

120. Kanemura Y, Hiraga S, Arita N, et al. Isolation and expression analysis of a novel human homologue of the *Drosophila* glial cells missing (gcm) gene. *FEBS Lett.* 1999;442:151–156.

121. Ding C, Buckingham B, Levine MA. Familial isolated hypoparathyroidism caused by a mutation in the gene for the transcription factor GCMB. *J Clin Invest.* 2001;108:1215–1220.

122. Lienhardt A, Bai M, Lagarde JP, et al. Activating mutations of the calcium-sensing

receptor: Management of hypocalcemia. *J Clin Endocrinol Metab.* 2001;86:5313–5323.

123. Yang T, Hassan S, Huang YG, et al. Expression of PTHrP, PTH/PTHrP receptor and Ca^{2+} sensing receptor along the rat nephron. *Am J Renal Physiol.* 1997;272:F751–758.

124. Harvey JN, Barnett D. Endocrine dysfunction in Kearns-Sayre syndrome. *Clin Endocrinol (Oxf).* 1992;37:97–103.

125. Shanske S, Tang Y, Hirano M, et al. Identical mitochondrial DNA deletion in a woman with ocular myopathy and in her son with Pearson syndrome. *Am J Hum Genet.* 2002;71: 679–683.

126. Zlotogora J, Shapiro MS. Polyglandular autoimmune syndrome type I among Iranian Jews. *J Med Genet.* 1992;29:824–826.

127. Aaltonen J, Bjorses P, Sandkuijl L, et al. An autosomal locus causing autoimmune disease: Autoimmune polyglandular disease type I assigned to chromosome 21. *Nat Genet.* 1994;8:83–87.

128. Chase LR, Slatopolsky E. Secretion and metabolic effects of parathyroid hormone in patients with severe hypomagnesemia. *J Clin Endocrinol Metab.* 1974;38:363–371.

129. Agus ZS. Hypomagnesemia. *J Am Soc Nephrol.* 1999;10:1616–1622.

130. Albright F, Burnett CH, Smith PH, et al. Pseudo-hypoparathyroidism: An example of "Seabright-Bantam syndrome." Report of three cases. *Endocrinology.* 1942;30:922–932.

131. Mantovani G, Maghnie M, Weber G, et al. Growth hormone–releasing hormone resistance in pseudohypoparathyroidism type Ia: New evidence for imprinting of the Gsα gene. *J Clin Endocrinol Metab.* 2003;88:4070–4074.

132. Davies SJ, Hughes HE. Imprinting in Albright's hereditary osteodystrophy. *J Med Genet.* 1993;30:101–103.

133. Wilson LC, Oude Luttikhuis MEM, Clayton PT, et al. Parental origin of Gs-α gene mutations in Albright's hereditary osteodystrophy. *J Med Genet.* 1994;31:835–839.

134. Liu J, Erlichman B, Weinstein LS. The stimulatory G protein α-subunit Gs-α is imprinted in human thyroid glands:implication for thyroid function in pseudohypoparathyroidism types IA and IB. *J Clin Endocrinolo Metab.* 2003;88:4336–4341.

135. Yu S, Yu D, Lee E, et al. Variable and tissue-specific hormone resistance in heterotrimeric Gs protein α-subunit (Gs-α) knockout mice is due to tissue-specific imprinting of the Gs-α gene. *Proc Nat Acad Sci USA.* 1998;95:8715–8720.

136. Bastepe M, Frolich LF, Hendy GN, et al. Autosomal dominant pseudohypoparathyroidism type Ib is associated with a heterozygous microdeletion that likely disrupts a putative imprinting control element of GNAS. *J Clin Invest.* 2003;112:1255–1263.

137. Bastepe M, Frolich LF, Linglart A, et al. Deletion of the NESP55 diferentially methylated region causes loss of maternal GNAS imprints and pseudohypoparathyroidism type Ib. *Nat Genet.* 2005;37: 25–27.

138. Linglart A, Gensure RC, Olney RC, et al. A novel STX16 deletion in autosomal dominant pseudohypoparathyroidism type Ib redefines the boundaries of a cis-acting imprinting control element of GNAS. *Am J Hum Genet.* 2005;76:804–814.

139. Bastepe M, Lane AH, Juppner H. Parental uniparental isodisomy of chromosome 20q and the resulting changes in GNAS1 methylation as a plausible cause of pseudohypoparathyroidism. *Am J Hum Genet.* 2001;68:1283–1289.

140. Farel Z, Brothers VM, Brickman AS, et al. Pseudohypoparathyroidism: Inheritance of deficient receptor-cyclase coupling activity. *Proc Nal Acad Sci USA.* 1981;78:3098–3102.

141. Linglart A, Carel JC, Garabedian M, et al. GNAS lesions in pseudohypoparathyroidism 1a and 1c: Genotype phenotype relationship and evidence of the maternal transmission of the hormonal resistance. *J Cin Endocrinol Metab.* 2002;87:189–199.

142. De Sanctis L, Romagnolo D, Olivero M, et al. Molecular analysis of the GNAS1 gene for the correct diagnosis of Albright hereditary osteodystrophy and psudohypoparathyroidism. *Pediatr Res.* 2003;53:749–755.

143. De Sanctis L, Vai S, Andreo MR, et al. Brachydactyl in 154 genetically characterized pseudohypoparathyroidism type Ia patients. *J Clin Endocrinol Metab.* 2004;89: 1650–1655.

144. Stone MD, hosking DJ, Garcia-Himmelstine C, et al. The renal response to exogenous parathyroid hormone in treated pseudohypoparathyroidism. *Bone.* 1993;14:727–735.

145. Stirling HF, darling JA, Barr DG. Plasma cyclic cAMP response to intravenous parathyroid hormone in pseudohypoparathyroidism. *Acta Paediatr Scand.*1991;80:333–338.

146. Miura R, Yumita S, Yoshinaga K, et al. Response of plasma 1,25-dihydroxyvitamin D in the human PTH(1–34) infusion test: An improved index for the diagnosis of idiopathic hypoparathyroidism and pseudohypoparathyroidism. *Calcif Tissue Int.*1990;46:309–313.

147. Hedeland H, Berntorp K, Arheden K, et al. Pseudohypoparathyroidism type I and Albright's hereditary osteodystrophy with a proximal 15q chromosomal deletion in mother and daughter. *Clin Genet.* 1992;42:129–134.

148. Winer K, Ko CW, Reynolds JC, et al. Long-term treatment of hypoparathyroidism: A randomized, controlled study comparing parathyroid hormone(1–34) versus calcitriol and calcium. *J Clin Endocrinol Metab.* 2003;88:4214–4220.

149. Morris CA, Leonard CO, Dills C, et al: Adults with Williams syndrome. *Am Med Genet.* 1990;6:102–107.

150. Sharata H, Postellon DC, Hashimoto K. Subcutaneous fat necrosis, hypercalcemia and prostaglandin E. *Pediatr Dermatol.* 1995;12:43–47.

151. Kruse K, Irle U, Uhlig R. Elevated 1,25-dihydroxyvitamin D serum concentrations in infants with subcutaneous fat necrosis. *J Pediatr.*1993;122:460–463.

152. Jacobs TB, Bilezikian JP. Rare causes of hypercalcemia. *J Clin Endocrinol Metab.* 2005;90:6316–6322.

153. Formenti A, De Simoni A, Arrigoni E, et al. Changes in extracellular Ca^{2+} can affect the pattern of discharge in rat thalamic neurons. *J Physiol.* 2001;535:33–45.

154. Chen T-H, Huang C-C, Chang Y-Y, et al. Vasoconstriction as the etiology of hypercalcemia-induced seizures. *Epilepsia.* 2004;45:551–554.

155. Kollars J, Zarroug AE, van Heerden J, et al. Primary hyperparathyroidism in pediatric patients. *Pediatrics.* 2005;115:974–980.

156. Carpten JD, Robbins CM, Villablanca A, et al: HRPT2 encoding parafibromin is mutated in hyperparathyroidism–jaw tumor syndrome. *Nat Genet.* 2002;32:676–680.

157. Warner J, Epstein M, Sweet A, et al. Genetic testing in familial isolated hyperparathyroidism: Unexpected results and their implications. *J Med Genet.* 2004;41: 155–160.

158. Simonds WF, Robbins Cm, Agarwal SK, et al. Familial isolated hyperparathyroidism is rarely caused by germline mutation in HRPT2, the gene for the hyperparathyroidism-jaw tumor syndrome. *J Clin Endocrinol Metab.* 2004;89:96–102.

159. Bilezikian JP, Potts JT, Fuleihan GEH, et al. Summary statement from a workshop on asymptomatic primary hyperparathyroidism: A perspective for the 21st century. *J Clin Endoctinol Metab.* 2002;87:5353–5361.

160. Chan JCM, Bell NH. Disorder of phosphate metabolism. In: Chan JCM, Gill JR, eds. *Kidney Electrolyte Disorders.* New York: Churchill Livingstone; 1990:223–260.

161. Roth KS, Chan JCM. Hypophosphatemic rickets. eMedicine Specialties.Pediatrics. Endocrinology: An Online Medical Reference. eMedicine from WebMD; accessed April 5, 2006.

162. Hsu SY, Tsai IJ, Tsau YK. Comparison of growth in primary Fanconi syndrome and proximal renal tubular acidosis. *Pediatr Nephrol.* 2005;20:460–464.

163. Parsonage MJ, Wilkins EG, Snowden N, et al. The development of hypophosphataemic osteomalacia with myopathy in two patients with HIV infection receiving tenofovir therapy. *HIV Med.* 2005;6:341–346.

164. Day SL, Leake Date HA, Bannister A, et al. Serum hypophosphatemia in tenofovir disoproxil fumarate recipients is mulfactorial in origin, questioning the utility of its monitoring in clinical practice. *J AIDS.* 2005;38:301–304.

165. Lyman D. Undiagnosed vitamin D deficiency in the hospitalized patient. *Am Fam Phys.* 2005;71:299–304.

166. Ketzman DK. Medical complications in adolescents with anorexia nervosa: A review of the literature. *Int J Eating Disord.* 2005;37: S52–59.

167. Keller U, Berger W. Prevention of hypophosphatemia by phosphate infusion during treatment of diabetic ketoacidosis and hyperosmolar coma. *Diabetes.* 1980;29:87–92.

168. Popovitzer MM, Knochel JP, Kumar R. Disorders of calcium, phosphorus, vitamin D, and parathyroid hormone activity. In: Schrier RW, ed. *Renal Electrolyte Disorders,* 4th ed. Boston: Little, Brown; 1992:287–369.

169. Berndt TJ, Schiavi S, Kumar R. "Phosphatonins" and the regulation of phosphorus homeostasis *Am J Physiol Renal Physiol.* 2005;289:F1170–1182.

170. Ritz E, Gross ML, Dikow R. Role of calcium-phosphorous disorders in the

progression of renal failure. *Kidney Int.* 2005;99:S66–70.

171. Araya K, Fukumoto S, Backenroth R, et al. A novel mutation in fibroblast growth factor 23 gene as a cause of tumoral calcinosis. *J Clin Endocrinol Metab.* 2005;90:5523–5527.

172. Topaz O, Shurman DL, Bergman R, et al. Mutations in GALNT3, encoding a protein involved in O-linked glycosylation, cause familial tumoral calcinosis. *Nat Genet.* 2004;36:579–581.

173. Benet-Pages A, Orlik P, Strom TM, et al. An FGF23 missense mutation causes familial tumoral calcinosis with hyperphosphatemia. *Hum Mol Genet.* 2005;14:385–390.

174. Yamashita H, Yamazaki Y, Hasegawa H. Fibroblast growth factor-23 in patients with Graves' disease before and after antithyroid therapy: Its important role in serum phosphate regulation. *J Clin Endocrinol Metab.* 2005;90:4211–4215.

175. Chan JCM, Goplerud JM, Papadopoulou ZL, Novello AC. Kidney failure in childhood. *Int J Paediatr Nephrol.* 1981;2:201–222.

176. Williams DM, Sreedhar SS, Mickell JJ, et al. Acute renal failure: A pediatric experience over 20 years. *Arch Pediatr Adolesc Med.* 2002;156: 803–900.

177. Ziegler EE, O'Donnell Am, Nelson SE, et al. Body composition of the reference fetus. *Growth.* 1976;40:329–311.

178. Wharton B, Bishop N, et al. Rickets. *Lancet.* 2003;362:1389–1400.

179. Hollis, BW, Wagner CL. Assessment of dietary vitamin D requirements during pregnancy and lactation. *Am J Clin Nutr.* 2004;79:717–726.

180. Lee JM, Smith JR, Phillip BL, et al. Vitamin D deficiency in a healthy groups of mothers and newbon infants. *Clin Pediatr.* 2007;46:42–44.

181. Gordon CM, Depeter KC, Feldman HA, et al. Prevalence of vitamin D deficiency among healthy adolescents. *Arch Pediatr Adolesc Med.* 2004;158:531–537.

182. Kreiter SR, Schwaraz RP, Kirkman HN, et al. Nutritional rickets in African-Americanbreast-fed infants. *J Pediatr.* 2000;137:153–157.

183. Sale BL, Devlin EE, Lapillone A, et al. Perinatal metabolism of vitamin D. *Am J Clin Nutr.* 2000;71:1317S–1324.

184. Mughal MZ, Salama H, Greenway T, et al. Lesson of the week: Florid rickets associated with prolonged breast-feeding without vitamin D supplementation. *Br Med J.* 1999:318:39–40.

185. Carvalho NF, Kenney RD, Carrington PH, et al. Severe nutritional deficiencies in toddlers resulting from health food milk alternatives. *Pedaitrics.* 2001;107:E46.

186. Holick M. Resurrection of vitamin D deficiency and rickets: Science in medicine. *J Clin Invest.* 2006;116(8):2062–2072.

187. Shah BR, Finberg L. Single-dose therapy for nutritional vitamin D deficiencyrickets: A preferred method. *J Pediatr.* 1994;125:487–490.

188. Hanley DA, Davison KS. Vitamin D insufficiency in North America. *J Nutr.* 2005;135:332–337.

189. Hatun S, Ozkan B, Orbak Z, et al. Vitamin D deficiency in early infancy. *J Nutr.* 2005;135:279–282.

190. Pettifor JM. Rickets and vitamin D deficiency in children and adolescents. *Endocrinol Metab Clin North Am.* 2005;34:537–553.

191. Houghton LA, Vieth R, et al. The case against ergocalciferol (vitamin D₂) as a vitamin supplement. *Am J Clin Nutr.* 2006;84:694–697.

192. Garabedian M, Ben-Mekhbi H. Rickets and vitamin D deficiency. In: Hollick MF, ed. *Vitamin D Physiology, Molecular Biology, and Clinical Applications.* Princeton, NJ: Humana Press; 1999:273–286.

193. Wang JT, Lin CJ, Burridge SM, et al. Genetics of vitamin D 1α-hydroxylase deficiency in 17 families. *Am J Hum Genet.* 1998;63:1694–1702.

194. Malloy PJ, Hochberg Z, Tiosano D, et al. The molecular basis of hereditary 1,25-dihydroxyvitamin D₃–resistant rickets in seven related families. *J Clin Invest.* 1990;86:2071–2079.

195. Hochberg Z, Tiosano D, Even L. Calcium therapy for calcitriol resistant rickets. *J Pediatr.* 1992;121:803–808.

196. Ward LM. Renal phosphate-wasting disorders in childhood. *Pediatr Endocr Rev.* 2005;2:342–350.

197. Guo R, Quarles LD. Cloning and sequencing of human PEX from a bone cDNA library: Evidence for its developmental stage-specific regulation in osteoblasts. *J Bone Miner Res.* 1997;12:1009–1017.

198. Cho HY, Lee BH, Kang JH, et al. A clinical and molecular genetic study of hypophosphatemic rickets in children. *Pediatr Res.* 2005;58:329–333.

199. Jonsson KB, Zahradnik R, Larsson T, et al. Fibroblast growth factor 23 in oncogenic osteomalacia and X-linked hypophosphatemia. *N Engl J Med.* 2003;348:1656–1663.

200. Econs MJ, McEnery PT, Lennon F, et al. Autosomal dominant hypophosphatemic rickets is linked to chromosome 12p13. *J Clin Invest.* 1997;100:2653–2657.

201. Goji K, Ozaki K, Sadewa AH, et al. Somatic and germline mosaicism for a mutation of the PHEX gene can lead to genetic transmission of X-linked hypophosphatemic rickets that mimics an autosomal dominant trait. *J Clin Endocrinol Metal.* 2006;91:365–370.

202. Carpenter TO. Oncogenic osteomalacia, a complex dance of factors. *N Engl J Med.* 2003;348:1705–1708.

203. Imel EA, Peacock M, Pitukcheewanont P, et al. Sensitivity of fibroblast growth factor 23 measurements in tumor induced osteomalacia. *J Clin Endocrinol Metab.* 2006;91:20055–20061.

204. Lorenz-Depiereux B, Bastepe M, Benet-Pages A, et al. DMP1 mutations in autosomal recessive hypophosphatemia implicate a bone matrix protein in the regulation of phosphate homeostasis. *Nat Genet.* 2006;38:1248–1250.

205. Feng JQ, Ward LM, Liu S, et al. Loss of DMP1 causes rickets and osteomalacia and identifies a role for osteocytes in mineral metabolism. *Nat Genet.* 2006;38:1310–1315.

206. Lorenz-Depiereux B, Benet-Pages A, Eckstein G, et al. Hereditary hypophosphatemic rickets with hypercalciuria is caused by mutations in the sodium-phosphate cotransporter gene SLC34A3. *Am J Hum Genet.* 2006;78:193–201.

207. Bergwitz C, Roslin NM, Tieder M, et al. SLC34A3 mutations in patients with hereditary hypophosphatemic rickets with hypercalciuria predict a key role for the sodium-phosphate cotransporter NaP(i)-IIc in maintaining phosphate homeostasis. *Am J Hum Genet.* 2006;78:179–192.

208. Lloyd SE, Pearce SH, Fisher SE, et al. A common molecular basis for three inherited kidney stone diseases. *Nature.* 1996;379: 445–449.

209. Gambaro G, Vezzoli G, Casari G, et al. Genetics of hypercalciuria and calcium nephrolithiasis: From the rare monogenic to the common polygenic forms. *Am J Kidney Dis.* 2004;44:963–986.

210. Oudet C, Martin-Coignard D, Pannetier S, et al. A second family with XLRH displays the mutation S244L in the CLCN5 gene. *Hum Genet.* 1997;99:781–784.

211. Yamamoto T, Imanishi Y, Kinoshita E, et al. The role of fibroblast growth factor 23 for hypophosphatemia and abnormal regulation of vitamin D metabolism in patients with McCune-Albright syndrome. *J Bone Miner Metab.* 2005;23:231–237.

212. Tebben P, Thomas L, Kumar R. Fanconi syndrome and renal tubular acidosis. In: Favus M, ed. *Primer on the Metabolic Bone Diseases and Disorders of Mineral Metabolism.* 2006. Am Soc Bone Min Res, Wash, DC.

213. Holm IA, Nelson AE, Robinson BG, et al. Mutational analysis and genotype phenotype correlation of the PHEX gene in X-linked hypophosphatemic rickets. *J Clin Endocrinol Metab.* 2001;86:3889–3899.

214. Carpenter TO. Oncogenic osteomalacia, a complex dance of factors. *N Engl J Med.* 2003;348:1705–1708.

215. Carpenter TO, Mitnick MA, Ellison A, et al. Nocturnal hyperparathyroidism: A frequent cause of X-linked hypophosphaatemia. *J Clin Endocrinol Metab.* 1994;78:1378–1383.

216. Ariceta G, Langman CB. Growth in X-linked hypophosphatemic rickets. *Eur J Pediatr.* 2007;166:303–309.

217. Kruse K, Hinkel GK, Griefahn B. Calcium metabolism and growth during early treatment of children with X- linked hypophosphatemic rickets. *Eur J Paediatr.* 1998;157:894–900.

218. Hendy GN, Hruska KA, Mathew S, et al. New insights into mineral and skeletal regulation by active forms of vitamin D. *Kidney Int.* 2006;69:218–223.

219. Fox CS, Vasan RS, Parise H, et al. Mitral annular calcification predicts cardiovascular morbidity and mortality. The Framingham Heart Study. *Circulation.* 2003;107: 1492–1456.

220. Monier-Faugere M, Mawad H, Qi Q, et al. High prevalence of low bone turnover and occurrence of osteomalacia after kidney transplantation. *J Am Soc Nephrol.* 2000;11:1093–1099.

221. Chan JCM, McEnery PT, Chinchilli VM, et al. A prospective, double-blind study of growth failure in children with chronic renal insufficiency and the effectiveness of treatment with calcitriol versus dihydrotachysterol. *J Pediatr.* 1994;124:520–528.

222. Sprague SM, Llach F, Abdahl M, et al. Paricalcitol versus calcitriol in the treatment

of secondary hyperparathyroidism. *Kidney Int.* 2003;63:1483–1490.

223. Teng M, Wolf M, Lowrie E, et al. Survival of patients undergoing hemodialysis with paricalcitol or calcitriol therapy. *N Engl J Med.* 2003;349:446–456.

224. Goodman WG, Hladik GA, Turner SA, et al. The calcimimetic agent AMG 073 lowers plasma parathyroid hormone levels in hemodialysis patients with secondary hyperparathyroidism. *J Am Soc Nephrol.* 2002;13:1017–1024.

225. Tfelt-Hansen J, Brown EM. The calcium-sensing receptor in normal physiology and pathophysiology: A review. *Crit Rev Clin Lab Sci.* 2005;42:35–70.

226. Evenpoel P, Claes K, Kuypers D, et al. Natural history of parathyroid function and calcium metabolism after kidney transplantation: A single-center study. *Nephrol Dial Transplant.* 2004;19:181–187.

227. Taillandier A, Sallinen SL. Brun-Heath I, et al. Childhood hypophosphatasia due to a de novo missense mutation in the tissue-nonspecific alkaline phosphatase gene. *J Clin Endocrinol Metab.* 2005;90:2436–2439.

228. Greenberg CR, Evans JA, McKendry-Smith, S, et al. Infantile hypophosphatasia: Localization within chromosome region 1p36.1-34 and prenatal diagnosis using linked DNA markers. *Am J Hum Genet.* 1990;46:286–292.

229. Barcia JP, Strife CF, Langman CB. Infantile hypophosphatasia: Treatment options to control hypercalcemia, hypercalciuria and chronic bone demineralization. *J Pediatr.* 1997;130:825–828.

230. Whyte MP, Kurtzberg J, McAlister WH, et al. Marrow cell transplantation for infantile hypophosphatasia. *J Bone Miner Res.* 2003;18:624–636.

231. Chong B, Hegde M, Faukner M, et al. Idiopathic hypophosphatasia and TNFRSF11B mutation: Relationship between phenotype and genotype. *J Bone Miner Res.* 2005;12:2095–2104.

232. Cundy T, Hegde M, Naot D, et al. A mutation in the gene TNFRSF11B encoding osteoprotegerin causes an idiopathic hyperphosphatasia phenotype. *Hum Mol Genet.* 2002;11:2119–2127.

233. Tiegs RD. Paget's disease of bone: Indications for treatment and goals of therapy. *Clin Ther.* 1997;19:1309–1329.

234. Cundy T, Davidson J, Rutland MD, et al. Recombinant osteoprotegerin for juvenile Paget's disease. *N Engl J Med.* 2005;353:918–923.

235. Marini JC, Forlino A, Cabral WA, et al. Consortium for osteogenesis imperfecta mutations in the helical domain of type I collagen: Regions rich in lethal mutations align with collagen binding sites for integrins and proteoglycans. *Hum Mutat.* 2007;28:209–221.

236. Marini JC. Osteogenesis imperfecta. In: Favus M, ed. *Primer on the Metabolic Bone Diseases and Disorders of Mineral Metabolism.* 2006.

237. Rauch F, Glorieux FH. Osteogeneis imperfecta. *Lancet.* 2004;363:1377–1385.

238. Sillence DO, Senn A, Danks DM. Genetic heterogeneity in osteogenesis imperfecta. *J Med Genet.* 1979;16:101–116.

239. Glorieux FH, Rauch F, Plotkin H, et al. Type V osteogenesis imperfecta: A new form of brittle bone disease. *J Bone Miner Res.* 2000;15:1650–1658.

240. Glorieux FH, Ward Lm, Bauch F, et al. Osteogenesis impergecta type VI: A form of brittle bone disease with a mineralization defect. *J Bone Miner Res.* 2000;17:12–18.

241. Ward LM, Rauch F, Travers R, et al. Osteogenesis imperfecta type VII: An autosomal recessive form of brittle bone disease. *Bone.* 2002;31:12–18.

242. Cabral WA, Chang W, Barnes AM, et al. Prolyl 3-hydroxylase 1 deficiency causes a recessive metabolic bone disorder resembling lethal/severe osteogenesis imperfecta. *Nat Genet.* 2007;39:359–365.

243. Barnes AM, Chang W, Morello R, et al. Deficiency of cartilage-associated protein in recessive lethal osteogenesis imperfecta. *N Engl J Med.* 2006;355:2757–2764.

244. Morello R, Bertin TK, Chen Y, et al. CRTAP is required for prolyl 3-hydroxylation and mutations cause recessive osteogenesis imperfecta. *Cell.* 2006;127:291–304.

245. Rauch F, Glorieux FH. Treatment of children with osteogenesis imperfecta. *Curr Osteoporos Rep.* 2006;4:159–164.

246. Glorieux FH, Rauch F, Ward LM, et al. Alendronate in the treatment of pediatric osteogenesis imperfecta. *J Bone Miner Res.* 2004;19:1043.

247. Gatti D, Antoniazzi F, Prizzi R, et al. Intravenous neridronate in children with osteogenesis imperfecta: A randomized, controlled study. *J Bone Miner Res.* 2005;5:758–763.

248. Letocha AD, Cintas HL, Troendle JF, et al. Controlled trial of paminodrate in children with types III and IV osteogenesis imperfecta confirms vertebral gains but not short-term functional improvement. *J Bone Miner Res.* 2005;20:977–986.

249. Tolar J, Teitelbaum Sl, Orchard PJ, et al. Osteopetrosis. *N Engl J Med.* 2004;351:2839–2349.

250. Balemans W, Wesenbeeck LV, Hul Wv. A clinical and molecular overview of the human osteopetroses. *Calcif Tissue Int.* 2005;77:263–274.

251. Fasth A, Porras O. Human malignant osteopetrosis: Pathophysiology, management and the role of bone marrow transplantation. *Pediatr Transplant.* 1999;3:102–107.

252. Frattini A, Orchard PJ, Sobacchi C, et al. Defects in TCIRG1 subunit of the vacuolar proton responsible for a subset of human autosomal recessive osteopetrosis. *Nat Genet.* 2000;25:343–346.

253. Frattini A, Pangrazio A, Suzani L, et al. Chloride channel CLCN7 mutations are responsible for severe recessive, dominant,

and intermediate osteopetrosis. *J Bone Miner Res.* 2003;18:1740–1747.

254. Kornak U, Kasper D, Bosl MR, et al. Loss of the CLCN7 chloride channel leads to osteopetrosis in mice and man. *Cell.* 2001;104:205–215.

255. Campos-Xavier AB, Saraiva JM, Ribeiro LM, et al. Chloride channel 7 (CLCN7) gene mutations in intermediate autosomal recessive osteopetrosis. *Hum Genet.* 2003;112:186–189.

256. Chalhoub N, Benachenhou N, Rajapurohitam V, et al. Gray-lethal mutation induces severe malignant autosomal recessive osteopetrosis in mouse and human. *Nat Med.* 2003;9:399–406.

257. Van Wesenbeeck L, Cleiren E, Gram J, et al. Six novel missense mutations in the LDL receptor-related protein 5 (LRP5) gene in different conditions with an increased bone density. *Am J Hum Genet.* 2003;72:763–771.

258. Cleiren E, Benichou O, Van Jul E, et al. Albers-Schonberg disease (autosomal dominant osteopetrosis, type II) results from mutations in the CICN7 chloride channel gene. *Hum Mol Genet.* 2001;10:2861–2867.

259. Waguespack SG, Koller DL, White KE, et al. Chloride channel 7 (CLCN7) gene mutations and autosomal dominant osteoporosis, type II. *J Bone Miner Res.* 2003;18:1513–1518.

260. Kovacs CS, Lambert RG, Lavoie GJ, et al. Centrifugal osteopetrosis: Appendicular sclerosis with relative sparing of the vertebrae. *Skeletal Radiol.* 1995;24:27–29.

261. Sly WS, Whyte MP, Sundaram V, et al. Carbonic anhydrase II deficiency in 12 families with the autosomal recessive syndrome of osteopetrosis with renal tubular acidosis and cerebral calcification. *N Engl J Med.* 1985;313:139–145.

262. Monaghan BA, Kaplan FS, August CS, et al. Transient infantile osteopetrosis. *J Pediatr.* 1991;118: 252–256.

263. Waguespack SG, Hui SL, White K E, et al. Measurement of tartrate-resistant acid phosphatase and the brain isoenzyme of creatine kinase accurately diagnoses type II autosomal dominant osteopetrosis but does not identify gene carriers. *J Clin Endocrinol Metab.* 2002;87:2212–2217.

264. Gerritsen EJA, Vossen JM, Fasth A, et al. Bone marrow transplantation for autosomal recessive osteopetrosis: A report from the Working Party on Inborn Errors of the European Bone Marrow Transplantation Group. *J Pediatr.* 1994;125:896–902.

265. Key L, Carnes D, Cole S, et al. Treatment of congenital osteopetrosis with high-dose calcitriol. *N Engl J Med.* 1984;310:409–415.

266. Key LL Jr, Rodriguiz RM, Willi SM, et al. Long-term treatment of osteopetrosis with recombinant human interferon gamma. *N Engl J Med.* 1995;332:1594–1599.

CHAPTER 40

Disorders of Mineral Metabolism (Iron, Copper, Zinc, and Molybdenum)

David M. Koeller, MD

Copper, zinc, iron, and molybdenum are essential metals that must be acquired from the diet. Their roles vary from electron transfer and oxygen transport to the determination and maintenance of protein structure. There are hundreds of metalloproteins that function in many aspects of cellular metabolism. Thus it is not surprising that abnormalities of metal homeostasis can present with a broad range of clinical symptoms. Disorders of metal metabolism can be divided into three main categories characterized by either an excess, a deficiency, or a defect in intracellular metal metabolism. Disorders characterized by excess metal include hereditary hemochromatosis and Wilson disease, which result from toxic accumulation of iron and copper, respectively. Menkes disease and acrodermatitis enteropathica are examples of disorders that result from metal deficiency (i.e., copper and zinc, respectively). The third group of disorders is represented by molybdenum cofactor deficiency, which is caused by defective intracellular synthesis of a molydbenum-containing pterin. The varying pathophysiology of these disorders is also reflected in the variable response to therapy, which ranges from complete cure in acrodermatitis enteropathica to the virtual absence of effective treatment options in molybdenum cofactor deficiency.

DISORDERS OF COPPER METABOLISM

Overview of Copper Metabolism

Copper is a redox active metal (i.e., it is capable of functioning in electron-transfer reactions) that is required for the activity of many critical enzymes functioning in a wide variety of metabolic pathways. Consequently, copper deficiency has numerous effects on metabolism. Copper excess also has significant clinical consequences, which result from the ability of copper to transfer electrons to oxygen and generate toxic oxygen free radicals. The Recommended Daily Allowance (RDA) for copper ranges from 200 µg/day in infants to 900 µg/day in adults, and to avoid toxicity, copper intake should not exceed 10 mg/day (1). Copper is absorbed from the gut via hCTR1, a plasma membrane copper transporter (2). hCTR1 is also required for copper uptake from the circulation in nonintestinal cells. Within the cytoplasm, copper is bound by metallochaperones, which are proteins that deliver copper to the sites where it is used and also prevent toxicity (Figure 40-1). Three metallochaperones have been identified in humans (3). The copper chaperone for superoxide dismutase 1 (CCS) delivers copper to the enzyme Cu-Zn superoxide dismutatase, which breaks down superoxide in the cytosol and mitochondrial intermembrane space. COX17 (copper chaperone for cytochrome c oxidase) delivers copper to the mitochondrion for the assembly of cytochrome C oxidase. ATOX1 (antioxidant-1) delivers copper to intracellular copper transporters (ATP7A/MNK and ATP7B/WND), which transport copper into the trans-Golgi network (TGN). In enterocytes, transport of copper into the TGN by MNK (Menkes protein) is required for the export of dietary copper into the systemic circulation. In the liver, copper delivered to the TGN by WND (Wilson's disease protein) is used for the synthesis of secreted copper proteins such as ceruloplasmin. Excess copper is exported into the bile, which occurs via the fusion of vesicles derived from the TGN to the plasma membrane, resulting in the export of copper into the canilicular space. Over 90% of the copper in the blood is bound to ceruloplasmin. Though historically believed to function as a serum copper transport protein, the primary function of ceruloplasmin is in iron homeostasis (see below). The circulating pool of copper that is available for use by the tissues is bound to histidine and other amino acids. When dietary copper intake exceeds the systemic need, the excess accumulates in the liver and can be eliminated from the body via secretion into the bile. Thus total-body copper homeostasis is maintained via a balance between copper absorption from the gut and loss via biliary excretion. The specific mechanisms for sensing and regulating total-body copper levels are an active area of investigation and have not been elucidated completely. The two most common inherited disorders of copper metabolism affect either the absorptive (Menkes disease) or excretory (Wilson disease) phases of copper homeostasis.

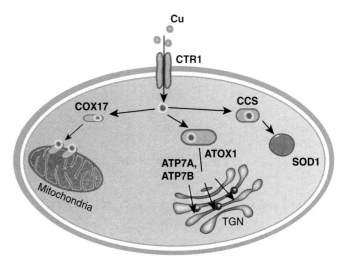

FIGURE 40-1. Intracellular copper trafficking. Copper enters the cell via the plasma membrane transporter CTR1 and is subsequently distributed within the cell via proteins known as copper chaperones. Copper is delivered to the mitochondrion by COX17, and to Cu-Zn superoxide dismutase (SOD1) via CCS. Copper destined for the trans golgi network (TGN) is delivered by ATOX1 to an ATP dependent transporter (ATP7A/MNK, ATP7B/WND) and subsequently transported across the membrane.

Hereditary Iron Overload Syndromes

AT-A-GLANCE

Hereditary iron overload syndromes share the common feature of excessive absorption of dietary iron. They are caused by mutations in genes that function in normal iron homeostasis, resulting in a disruption of the normal tight control the body maintains on iron levels. These disorders demonstrate significant variability in the nature of their symptoms, the organs involved, and age of symptom onset. Juvenile hemochromatosis is a rare disorder that presents in the 2nd to 3rd decade with hypogonadotropic hypogonadism and heart failure. Diagnosis in the 4th or 5th decades with fatigue, arthralgia, loss of libido, and impotence is the most common presentation of hereditary hemochromatosis.

DISORDER	INCIDENCE	GENE	PROTEIN	INH.	LOCUS	OMIM
HFE-related hereditary hemochromatosis	3–5:1000	HFE	HFE	AR	6p21.3	235200 (HFE type 1)
Juvenile hemochromatosis	Rare	HJV	Hemojuvelin	AR	1q21	602390 (HFE type 2A)
Juvenile hemochromatosis	Rare	HAMP	Hepcidin	AR	19q13.1	602390 (HFE type 2B)
TfR2-related hereditary hemochromatosis	Rare	TfR2	Transferrin receptor 2	AR	7q22	604250 (HFE type 3)
Ferroportin-related hereditary iron overload	Rare	SLC40A1	Ferroportin	AD	2q32	606069 (HFE type 4)

DISORDER	LABORATORY FINDINGS	CLINICAL PRESENTATION
HFE-related hereditary hemochromatosis (HFE type 1)	↑ serum ferritin ↑ transferrin saturation (>45%) Elevated liver iron	Onset in the 4th to 5th decade with fatigue, arthralgia, loss of libido, and impotence; associated findings include hepatomegaly, increased skin pigmentation, diabetes mellitus, abdominal pain, and cardiomyopathy
Juvenile hemochromatosis (HFE type 2A)	↑ serum ferritin ↑ transferrin saturation (>45%) Elevated liver iron	Hypogonadotropic hypogonadism; heart failure and diabetes presenting in the 2nd to 3rd decade
Juvenile hemochromatosis (HFE type 2B)	↑ serum ferritin ↑ transferrin saturation (>45%) Elevated liver iron	Hypogonadotropic hypogonadism; heart failure and diabetes presenting in the 2nd to 3rd decade
TfR2-related hereditary hemochromatosis (HFE type 3)	↑ serum ferritin ↑ transferrin saturation (>45%) Elevated liver iron	Onset in the 4th to 5th decade with fatigue, arthralgia, loss of libido, and impotence; associated findings include hepatomegaly, increased skin pigmentation, diabetes mellitus, abdominal pain, and cardiomyopathy
Ferroportin-related hereditary iron overload (HFE yype 4)	↑ serum ferritin ↑ transferrin saturation in later stages Accumulation of iron in Kupffer cells and macrophages	Onset in the 4th to 5th decade with fatigue, arthralgia, loss of libido, and impotence; associated findings include hepatomegaly, increased skin pigmentation, diabetes mellitus, abdominal pain, and cardiomyopathy; may have poor tolerance to therapeutic phlebotomy

AR = autosomal recessive; AD = autosomal dominant.

Disorders of Copper Metabolism

Copper is an essential trace element that is required for the activity of many essential enzymes, including cytochrome oxidase in the mitochondrial electron transport chain. The most common inherited disorder of copper metabolism is Wilson disease, which results in the accumulation of copper in the liver and hepatocellular damage. Copper also accumulates in the basal ganglia of the brain and can result in an extrapyramidal movement disorder and psychiatric symptoms. Menkes disease is a rare disorder of copper metabolism that results in severe systemic copper deficiency. Affected patients present as infants with an array of symptoms that are caused by the decreased activity of many copper-dependent enzymes.

DISORDER	OCCURENCE	GENE	LOCUS	OMIM
Wilson disease	Rare	WND, ATP7B	13q14.3-q21.1	606882
Menkes disease	Rare	MNK, ATP7A	Xq12-q13	309400
Occipital horn syndrome (X-linked cutis laxa)	Rare	MNK, ATP7A	Xq12-q13	304150
Aceruloplasminemia	Very rare	CP	3q23-q24	117700

DISORDER	BIOCHEMICAL ABNORMALITIES	CLINICAL PRESENTATION
Wilson disease	↑ 24-h copper excretion (urine) ↓ Copper (blood) ↓ Ceruloplasmin (blood)	Pediatric patients most commonly present with liver disease in the 1st or 2nd decade of life; hepatosplenomegaly, jaundice, and symptoms of hepatitis are the most common findings; some children may present with neurological symptoms, including dystonia, deterioration of school performance, and changes in behavior, with no evidence of liver disease; after adolescence, the disease presents more commonly with neurological symptoms and may mimic Parkinson disease; symptoms include progressive extrapyramidal signs, such as rigidity, dysarthria, dysphagia, drooling, and intellectual deterioration
Menkes disease	↑ HVA:VMA ratio (urine) ↑ DOPA:DHPG ratio (serum and CSF) ↓ Copper (blood) ↓ Ceruloplasmin (blood)	The most characteristic feature is the sparse and depigmented hair, with a texture similar to steel wool; in infants, lethargy, hypotonia, hypothermia, and feeding difficulties may be evident within a few days of birth; many affected infants appear relatively normal or have only subtle nonspecific symptoms during the first few months of life; wormian bones, osteoporosis, bladder diverticula, and tortuous blood vessels are frequent; severe developmental impairment and seizures are common
Occipital horn syndrome	NI–↑ HVA:VMA ratio (urine) NI–↑ DOPA:DHPG ratio (serum and CSF) NI–↓ Copper (blood) NI–↓ Ceruloplasmin (blood)	Primarily a disorder of connective tissues; symptoms include lax skin and joints, bladder diverticula, inguinal hernias, arterial tortuosity, and mild mental retardation; some patients also have symptoms of autonomic dysfunction, such as orthostatic hypotension, due to decreased dopamine β-hydroxylase activity
Acerulo plasminemia	↓ Copper (blood) ↓ Ceruloplasmin (blood) ↓ Iron (serum) Anemia	Ceruloplasmin plays an essential role in iron metabolism, and its absence results in the accumulation of iron in the pancreas, basal ganglia, and retina; the primary symptoms are diabetes mellitus, an extrapyramidal movement disorder, and retinal degeneration; a mild anemia with a decreased serum iron level and iron accumulation in the liver also may be seen

HVA:VMA = homovanillic-acid-to-vanillylmandelic-acid ratio; DOPA:DHPG = dihydroxyphenylalanine-to-dihydroxyphenylglycol ratio; CP = ceruloplasmin; CSF = cerebrospinal fluid.

Disorders of Zinc Metabolism

Zinc is a relatively abundant trace element that is required for the function of enzymes such as mitochondrial CuZn–superoxide dismutase, which is important for dealing with oxidative stress, and alkaline phosphatase, which is essential for healthy bones. Zinc is also an essential component of a large number of transcription factors that regulate genes controlling normal cellular growth and differentiation. Severe zinc deficiency results in dermatitis, diarrhea, alopecia, and failure to thrive. The skin lesions are erythematous and may be vesicular and crusted. Notably, these are indistinguishable from lesions seen in biotin deficiency. Secondary infection is common.

DISORDER	OCCURENCE	GENE	LOCUS	OMIM
Acrodermatitis enteropathica	Rare	ZIP4	8q24.3	607059
Reduced breast-milk zinc	Very rare	Unknown	Unknown	608118

DISORDER	BIOCHEMICAL ABNORMALITIES	CLINICAL PRESENTATION
Acrodermatitis enteropathica	↓ Zinc (blood)	Breast-fed infants typically present after weaning, whereas formula-fed babies may present in the first few months of life; the symptoms of zinc deficiency include alopecia, dermatitis, diarrhea, irritability, and failure to thrive
Reduced breast-milk zinc	↓ Zinc (blood) ↓ Zinc (mother's breast milk)	Symptoms are only seen in breast-fed infants, who may present any time while still breast-feeding; symptoms are the same as those seen in other forms of zinc deficiency and may resolve spontaneously after weaning

Disorders of Molybdenum Metabolism

Molybdenum is an essential trace element that is required for the activity of three enzymes, sulfite oxidase, xanthine dehydrogenase, and aldehyde oxidase. It is used for the synthesis of the molybdenum cofactor, which is a modified pterin required by these enzymes. Patients with inherited disorders that affect the synthesis of the molybdenum cofactor typically present in the newborn period with seizures and severe neurological symptoms. Similar symptoms are seen in patients with an isolated deficiency of sulfite oxidase.

DISORDER	OCCURENCE	GENE	LOCUS	OMIM
Molybdenum cofactor deficiency	Rare	MOCS1, MOCS2, GEPH	6p21.3, 5q11, 14q24	603930
Sulfite oxidase deficiency	Rare	SUOX	12q13.2	272300

DISORDER	BIOCHEMICAL ABNORMALITIES		CLINICAL PRESENTATION
Molybdenum cofactor deficiency	↑ Sulfite (urine); ↑ S-Sulfocysteine (blood, urine); ↑ Taurine (blood, urine); ↑ Thiosulfite (urine); ↑ Xanthine (urine) ↑ Hypoxanthine (urine)	↓ uric acid (blood, urine) ↓ sulfate (urine) ↓ cysteine (blood) ↓ homocysteine (blood)	Severe neonatal seizures, often refractory to treatment; feeding problems, abnormal muscle tone; dysmorphic facial features, including hypertelorism, a small nose, puffy cheeks and lips, a long philtrum, progressive microcephaly; lens dislocation is seen in approximately 50% of patients but may not be present in neonates; renal xanthine stones; milder cases may present in later infancy or childhood
Sulfite oxidase deficiency	↑ Sulfite (urine); ↑ S-Sulfocysteine (blood, urine); ↑ Taurine (blood, urine); ↑ Thiosulfite (urine)	↓ sulfate (urine) ↓ cysteine (blood) ↓ homocysteine (blood)	Severe neonatal seizures, often refractory to treatment; feeding problems, abnormal muscle tone; dysmorphic facial features, including hypertelorism, a small nose, puffy cheeks and lips, a long philtrum, progressive microcephaly; lens dislocation is seen in approximately 50% of patients but may not be present in neonates; milder cases may present in later infancy or childhood

MOCS1 = molybdenum cofactor synthesis-1; MOCS2 = molybdenum cofactor synthesis-2; GAPH = gephyrin; SUOX = sulfite oxidase.

MENKES DISEASE

Menkes disease is a very rare X-linked disorder of copper metabolism with an incidence of approximately 1 in 250,000 population (4) resulting from mutations in the ATP7A gene, which encodes an adenosine triphosphate (ATP)–dependent copper transporter (ATP7A or MNK). The MNK protein is found in almost all cells of the body, the liver being a notable exception (see section on Wilson disease). MNK plays an essential role in intestinal copper absorption, transporting copper taken up by the enterocytes from the gut into the blood. MNK is present in the placenta, where it is believed to function in fetal copper absorption (5). MNK is also believed to be important for the transport of copper into the central nervous system (CNS). MNK is expressed in mouse cerebrovascular endothelial cells, which form part of the blood–brain barrier (6). The loss of functional MNK in Menkes disease results in the accumulation of copper in the placenta and intestinal lining and severe systemic copper deficiency that begins even before birth. In addition to its role in systemic copper uptake, MNK also functions in intracellular copper homeostasis, transporting copper from the cytosol into the TGN. Copper is required in the TGN for the assembly of lysyl oxidase, which is secreted from the cell, as well as dopamine β-hydroxylase, peptidylglycine α-amidating monooxygenase, and tyrosinase, which are localized to intracellular vesicles formed within the Golgi network.

Clinical Features Menkes disease results in severe developmental delay and failure to thrive. Drowsiness, lethargy, hypotonia, hypothermia, and feeding difficulties may be evident within a few days of birth. However, many affected infants appear relatively normal or have only subtle nonspecific symptoms during the first few months of life. The most characteristic feature is the sparse and depigmented hair, with a texture similar to steel wool, leading to the term *Menkes kinky hair syndrome*. The individual hairs have a corkscrew-like microscopic appearance, termed *pili torti* (Figure 40-2). This can be easily missed in affected infants who have very little hair. The clinical features of Menkes disease are a direct result of the loss of function of copper-dependent enzymes. Tyrosinase deficiency results in hypopigmentation of the skin and hair. Peptidylglycine α-amidating monooxygenase (PAM) is required for activation of a large number of neuropeptides (e.g., gastrin, vasoactive intestinal peptide, melanocyte-stimulating hormone, thyrotropin-releasing hormone, cholecystokinin, vasopressin, corticotropin-releasing

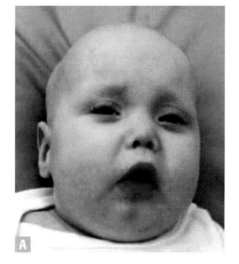
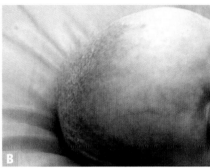
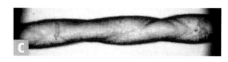
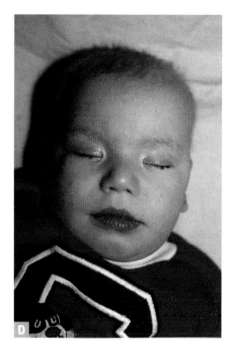

FIGURE 40-2. Clinical features of Menkes disease. **A.** Characteristic facies include pudgy cheeks, pale skin, sparse hair, and a bowed upper lip. **B.** Hair is hypopigmented and has a steel wool–like texture. **C.** Magnified image of an individual hair demonstrating the twisting morphology (pili torti). **D.** A milder form of Menkes disease is also seen.

hormone, and calcitonin). PAM catalyzes the C-terminal amidation of these peptide hormones, which is required for their full bioactivity. PAM deficiency leads to a broad spectrum of neuroendocrine derangements. Deficiency of lysyl oxidase affects collagen crosslinking, resulting in osteoporosis, flared metaphyses, and fractures. Wormian bones are also common. Arteries often are torturous, and the ureters and bladder wall are weakened and dilated, all as a consequence of abnormal collagen synthesis. The rupture of weakened intracranial blood vessels frequently results in subdural hematomas and death and may suggest nonaccidental trauma. Deficiency of dopamine β-hydroxylase results in a reduced ability to make norepinephrine and epinephrine, which results in hypothermia and orthostatic hypotension. CNS degeneration, characterized by abnormalities of myelin, and cerebral and cerebellar atrophy are likely due to decreased cytochrome oxidase activity. Seizures are common in affected males, and death usually occurs in the first decade.

A well-characterized variant of Menkes disease associated with milder mutations in the ATP7A gene is the *occipital horn syndrome*, also known as *X-linked cutis laxa* (7). The occipital horn syndrome is a disorder of connective tissues characterized by lax skin and joints, bladder diverticula, inguinal hernias, arterial tortuosity, and mild mental retardation. Ossification within the tendons that attach the trapezius and sternocleidomastoid muscles to the skull gives rise to the pathognomonic occipital horns, which can be felt by palpation and demonstrated radiographically. Patients have a deficiency of lysyl oxidase activity as a result of the defect in copper transport to the TGN. Some patients also have symptoms of autonomic dysfunction, such as orthostatic hypotension, due to decreased dopamine β-hydroxylase activity. The variability in the phenotype likely reflects differences in residual function of the MNK transporter.

Females heterozygous for a mutation in the ATP7A gene may show mild symptoms depending on X inactivation but usually are normal (8). Pili torti is present in approximately 50% of obligate carriers, but its absence, which can be caused by random X inactivation, does not exclude carrier status.

TABLE 40-1 Menkes Disease	
Laboratory Findings	
Decreased	**Increased**
Copper (B)	Urine HVA:VMA ratio
Ceruloplasmin (B)	Serum and CSF DOPA/
Norepinephrine	DHPG ratio

Diagnosis The primary biochemical abnormalities are decreased serum levels of copper and ceruloplasmin (see Table 40-1). Ceruloplasmin is a serum ferroxidase that functions in iron metabolism and requires copper for its enzymatic activity. It is made predominantly in the liver and is very unstable in the absence of bound copper. As a result of the severe copper deficiency in Menkes disease, most of the ceruloplasmin made by the liver is degraded rapidly, resulting in a low serum level. However, because the blood levels of copper and ceruloplasmin are low in normal infants and may overlap with those of affected patients, this is an unreliable approach to diagnosis in this age group. In contrast, abnormal levels of metabolites in the catecholamine biosynthetic pathway, which accumulate secondary to dopamine β-hydroxylase deficiency, can be detected in the blood, urine, and cerebrospinal fluid (CSF) of young infants and are the preferred approach to diagnosis (10). The demonstration of an increased accumulation of radioactive copper by cultured fibroblasts also can be used for diagnosis, but this test is not readily available. Causative mutations are split almost evenly between single-nucleotide substitutions (50%) and larger insertions, deletions, and rearrangements (9). In approximately a third of patients, the disease is due to a new mutation. Because of the large number of mutations that have been identified in the ATP7A gene, molecular diagnosis usually is not practical but is the preferred approach to prenatal diagnosis if a disease-causing mutation can be identified in a family.

Treatment As a result of the defect in absorption of copper from the gut, oral copper supplementation is not effective. In contrast, parenteral administration of copper histidine can normalize serum levels of copper and ceruloplasmin rapidly. However, most of the enzymes that require copper as a cofactor are intracellular, and it is difficult to evaluate the adequacy of treatment, particularly in the brain. When begun prior to the onset of severe neurological symptoms, copper histidine has been shown to improve neurological outcome and decrease seizure activity (11,12). The dosage of copper histidine used in published reports varies from 200–1000 μg (given subcutaneously) twice

per week, up to daily injections (7). Response to therapy is based on clinical symptoms and monitoring of serum copper and ceruloplasmin levels. Care must be taken to avoid liver toxicity due to excess copper accumulation, which can be monitored by 24-hour urine copper excretion with a goal of a level in the high-normal range (normal 20–50 μg/day), monitoring of serum transaminase levels, and liver biopsy. Long-term follow-up of one series of treated patients demonstrated improvement in neurological status but significant residual connective tissue problems, leading the authors to conclude that the therapy still should be considered experimental (11). A single unsuccessful attempt at in utero copper treatment also has been reported (13). Patients with residual activity of the MNK ATPase, as suggested by milder symptoms, are predicted to have a better response to therapy (12,13). There is no practical way to measure the activity of ATP7A in a clinical setting; the residual activity is inferred by the severity of symptoms.

WILSON DISEASE

Wilson disease is an autosomal recessive disorder caused by mutations in the ATP7B gene. The Wilson disease protein (ATP7B or WND) is a copper-transporting ATPase that is homologous to the Menkes disease protein. Like MNK, WND is localized to the TGN and transports copper delivered by the metallochaperone ATOX1. The differences in clinical symptoms between Menkes and Wilson diseases are largely a result of the different tissue distributions of the two proteins. WND is found primarily in the liver, whereas MNK is expressed in nonhepatic tissues. A lack of MNK results in severe copper deficiency due to an inability of copper absorbed from the gut to be transported out of the enterocyte and into the systemic circulation. In Wilson disease, the loss of functional WND blocks the ability of hepatocytes to transport copper into the TGN, disrupting both ceruloplasmin synthesis and biliary copper excretion and resulting in the accumulation of excess copper in hepatocytes and a reduction of serum ceruloplasmin. WND is also expressed in the brain, although its exact role in brain copper metabolism is still poorly defined (14).

Clinical Features Wilson disease was known originally as *hepatolenticular degeneration* due to its symptoms of liver cirrhosis and basal ganglia degeneration. However, pediatric patients present most commonly with liver disease, which usually becomes evident in the first or second decade. In childhood and early adolescence, hepatosplenomegaly, jaundice, and symptoms of hepatitis are the most common findings. Wilson disease should be con-

sidered in any pediatric patient presenting with acute liver failure, particularly when accompanied by a hemolytic anemia, which results from the rapid release of copper from dying hepatocytes. Dystonia, characteristic of damage to the basal ganglia, when seen in association with liver dysfunction, is highly suggestive of Wilson disease. Some children may present with only neurological manifestations and no evidence of liver disease. Deterioration of school performance and changes in mood and behavior are common initial symptoms. After adolescence, the disease presents more commonly with neurological symptoms. Progressive extrapyramidal signs, including rigidity, dysarthria, dysphagia, drooling, and intellectual deterioration, may mimic Parkinson disease. The pathophysiology of these symptoms of basal ganglia dysfunction is uncertain but may be related to the observation that ceruloplasmin and WND are both expressed in the brain. Psychiatric symptoms ranging from mania to depression, paranoia, and anxiety are also common. Occasionally, flapping tremor (asterixis), schizophrenic behavior, or the renal Fanconi syndrome may be the presenting feature. A brown or green ring around the corneal limbus in the eye, the *Kayser–Fleischer ring*, is a characteristic feature that is caused by copper deposition in Descemet's membrane.

Diagnosis The diversity of symptoms and broad age range of initial presentation require that the potential diagnosis of Wilson disease be considered in many clinical settings. Wilson disease should be considered in any child with unexplained liver disease, neurological/psychiatric dysfunction, or hemolytic anemia. The best diagnostic test is a determination of 24-hour urine copper excretion, which is elevated (>100 μg/24 h; normal 20–50 μg) in nearly all symptomatic patients (15). In normal persons, the majority of serum copper is bound to ceruloplasmin, which is not filtered in the glomerulus and thus does not enter the urine. In contrast, in patients with Wilson disease, ceruloplasmin levels are decreased, and non-protein-bound copper, which is excreted into the urine, is elevated (see Table 40-2). There is also expression of WND in the kidney tubules, but its role in renal copper clearance is unknown. Presymptomatic patients and carriers can have intermediate levels of copper excretion

TABLE 40-2 Wilson Disease	
Laboratory Findings	
Decreased	**Increased**
Copper (B)	24-hour urine copper
Ceruloplasmin (B)	

(50–100 µg/day) and may require a liver biopsy and direct measurement of copper content for definitive diagnosis (15). Plasma copper and ceruloplasmin levels usually are low, but this finding is not specific for Wilson disease, being seen in liver disease of other etiologies. Serum copper and ceruloplasmin levels may be normal in some patients, making such tests unreliable for diagnosis. A Kayser–Fleischer ring, which can be identified by slit-lamp examination, is nearly always present in patients with neurological and psychiatric symptoms. It is rarely present in pediatric patients, particularly in the absence of neurological symptoms. Although singly not 100% effective for diagnosis, the combined determination of 24-hour urine copper excretion, serum copper and ceruloplasmin level and a slit-lamp examination is unlikely to miss a true Wilson disease patient (16).

Many different mutations have been identified, and there is evidence for significant phenotypic variability within families (17). This is due in part to environmental factors, such as the diet, that can significantly influence the rate of accumulation of excess copper and timing of symptom onset. The large number of disease-causing mutations makes DNA diagnosis impractical at present.

Treatment Current treatments can prevent or reverse many symptoms, resulting in striking clinical improvement. Therefore, it is imperative to establish the diagnosis and begin treatment of Wilson disease as early as feasible. Treatment must be tailored to the individual patient based on symptomatology. In pediatric patients with minimal liver dysfunction, zinc acetate (Galzin), combined with a diet restricted in high-copper-containing foods (e.g., shellfish and chocolate), is highly effective. Oral zinc induces metallothionein expression in enterocytes, which bind to copper and block its absorption (18). This affects the absorption of dietary copper, as well as the reabsorption of copper contained in salivary and gastrointestinal secretions, resulting in a net loss of copper. Dosing is based on age and weight, and patients should be monitored twice a year by 24-hour urine copper excretion, with a goal of a level in the high-normal range (normal 20–50 µg/day). Pediatric patients in particular must be monitored carefully for signs of copper deficiency, which can be detected by the presence of a hypochromic, microcytic anemia (reviewed in 19). Patients presenting with significant liver disease should receive trientine (Syprine), a copper chelator, in addition to zinc (20). The recommended initial dose is 500–750 mg/day for pediatric patients and 750–1250 mg/day for adults given in divided doses two, three, or four times daily. This may be increased

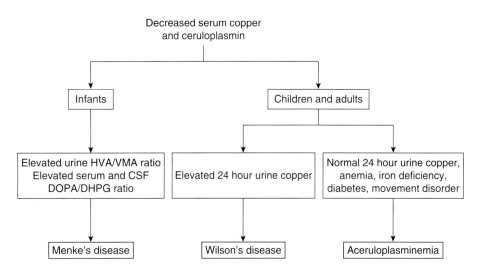

FIGURE 40-3. Flow diagram for patients presenting with decreased serum copper and ceruloplasmin. HVA = homovanillic acid; VMA = vanillylmandelic acid; DOPA = dihydroxyphenylalanine; DHPG = dihydroxyphenylglycol.

to a maximum of 2000 mg/day for adults or 1500 mg/day for pediatric patients age 12 or under. Trientine must be given on an empty stomach at least 1 hour before or 2 hours after a meal. For patients with neurological or psychiatric symptoms, a recently developed chelator, tetrathiomolybdate, is effective in halting and in many cases reversing symptoms (21). This agent is not yet approved by the Food and Drug Administration (FDA) but is available as an investigational new drug at selected centers. Chelation therapy with oral D-penicillamine historically has been the most frequent approach to therapy, but because of significant toxicity, its use is decreasing. D-Penicillamine should not be used initially in patients with neurological dysfunction because of the risk of worsening of neurological dysfunction with onset of therapy (22). Patients with significant liver and/or neurological disease should be referred to a center with extensive experience in the treatment of Wilson disease. Liver transplantation is indicated for patients with progressive hepatic insufficiency associated with cirrhosis and for those in fulminant hepatic failure. Successful liver transplant results in complete correction of copper homeostasis and reversal of most neurological dysfunction.

RARE DISORDERS OF COPPER METABOLISM

Aceruloplasminemia is a rare autosomal recessive disorder due to mutations in the ceruloplasmin gene (23). Ceruloplasmin is a copper-containing ferroxidase that is required for the mobilization of iron from reticuloendothelial cells into the systemic circulation. In addition to the liver, expression of ceruloplasmin also has been demonstrated in astrocytes, where it functions in CNS iron metabolism.

Accumulation of iron in the pancreas, basal ganglia, and retina is responsible for the

primary symptoms of aceruloplasminemia, which include diabetes mellitus, an extrapyramidal movement disorder, and retinal degeneration. Excess iron deposits also are seen in the liver. Plasma copper levels are low secondary to the ceruloplasmin deficiency (see Figure 40-3 for an algorithm distinguishing Menke's, Wilson's and aceruloplasminemia, all of which decreased levels of both serum copper and ceruloplasmin). The abnormalities of iron metabolism result in a mild anemia and decreased serum iron level. Fresh-frozen plasma contains ceruloplasmin and has been used as therapy at a dose of 450 mL weekly, as reported on a single patient (24).

Studies in mice have shown that mutations of the copper transporter CTR1 (the mouse homologue of hCTR1) and the metallochaperone ATOX1 result in severe systemic copper deficiency (25,26). Mutations in these genes have not yet been identified in human patients, but it is likely that in the future these and other genes required for normal copper homeostasis will be shown to be associated with inherited human disease.

DISORDERS OF ZINC METABOLISM

Overview of Zinc Metabolism

Zinc is required for the function of a large number of proteins, including enzymes of cellular metabolism (e.g., CuZn–superoxide dismutase and alkaline phosphatase) and a large number of transcription factors controlling normal cellular growth and differentiation. Zinc's importance for normal health is reflected in its relatively high RDA, which ranges from 2 mg/day in infants to near 10 mg/day in adults (27). Severe zinc deficiency results in dermatitis, diarrhea, alopecia, and failure to thrive. The skin lesions are erythematous and may be vesicular and crusted, resembling those seen in biotinidase deficiency. They have an acral distribution, particularly around the nose, mouth, eyes, and anus. Secondary infection is common and is exacerbated by the immune dysfunction associated with zinc deficiency (28). Milder degrees of zinc deficiency can result in growth failure, diarrhea, pulmonary and other infections, and neuropsychological impairment (29). Although rare in industrialized societies, zinc deficiency can be seen in patients with cystic fibrosis, Crohn disease, and other malabsorption states. Iatrogenic zinc deficiency is a potential risk in patients on chronic hyperalimentation and modified diets, such as those used to treat many inborn errors of metabolism. The diagnosis of zinc deficiency is indicated by a serum zinc level of less than 50 μg/dL (7.6 μmol/L).

ACRODERMATITIS ENTEROPATHICA

Pathophysiology Intestinal zinc absorption occurs via a two-step process, the first being transport from the intestinal lumen into the enterocyte across the apical membrane, and the second being the export of zinc across the basolateral membrane into the portal circulation. Acrodermatitis enteropathica is a rare autosomal recessive disorder of zinc absorption caused by a loss of function of the apical membrane zinc transporter hZIP4 (30). A mutation of the basolateral zinc transporter also would be predicted to result in a block to intestinal zinc absorption, but no patients with such a mutation have been described. There have been several reports of infants developing severe zinc deficiency due to a decreased zinc content in their mother's milk (31). This is believed to be due to a mutation in a mammary gland zinc transporter, but the affected gene has not been identified. A similar defect in mouse mammary gland zinc transport, which is called *lethal milk,* is due to a mutation in the ZnT4 zinc transporter (32).

Clinical Features Acrodermatitis enteropathica is an inherited disorder of zinc absorption that results in severe zinc deficiency. Breast-fed infants typically present around the time of weaning, whereas those receiving infant formula may be symptomatic within the first month of life. This difference is due to the greater bioavailability of zinc in human milk as compared with formula (33). Babies of mother's with depressed breast milk zinc levels may present prior to or after weaning depending on factors such as prematurity and size. This disorder can be diagnosed by measurement of the zinc content of the mother's milk. The symptoms of acrodermatitis entero-

pathica are similar to those seen in other forms of zinc deficiency and may include alopecia, dermatitis, diarrhea, irritability, and failure to thrive. The diagnosis is made on the basis of a low serum zinc level (<50 μg/dL) .

Treatment Treatment with 10 mg/kg/day of zinc sulfate or zinc gluconate results in rapid reversal of symptoms and clearing of the skin lesions within several weeks (34). Following normalization of serum zinc levels, lifelong maintenance therapy at 1–2 mg/kg/day is required (35).

DISORDERS OF IRON METABOLISM

Overview of Iron Metabolism

Iron is an essential nutrient, but due to its redox properties, it has significant potential for toxicity. There are no mechanisms for iron excretion; thus regulation of the body's iron content is controlled at the level of intestinal absorption. The RDA for iron is age- and gender-dependent, ranging from 12 mg/day at 12 months to 8 mg/day in adult males. In menstruating females, it increases to 18 mg/day and, during pregnancy, to 27 mg/day (1). The total-body iron content of an adult is about 3–4 g, of which 40% to 60% is in hemoglobin, 10% to 20% is in myoglobin and tissue enzymes, and 10% to 40% is bound to the iron storage protein ferritin. Newborn infants have total-body iron levels of about 250–400 mg. In the blood, iron is bound to transferrin, which is imported into cells via a specific transferrin receptor. Inside the cell, iron that is not needed immediately is bound and stored by ferritin, which serves to detoxify iron by decreasing its ability to participate in redox reactions and preventing the formation of toxic reactive oxygen species.

Intestinal iron absorption is mediated by two membrane-bound iron transporters. Divalent metal transporter 1 (DMT1), on the apical enterocyte membrane, imports iron from the gut lumen, and ferroportin transports it into the bloodstream at the basolateral membrane (36) (Figure 40-4). Dietary iron that enters the mucosal cells of the gut has two possible fates. It can be either released into the systemic circulation or retained and subsequently lost when the enterocyte

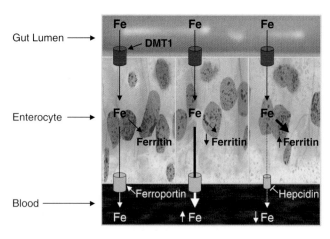

FIGURE 40-4. Schematic diagram of intestinal iron absorption. Iron (Fe) from the gut lumen enters the enterocyte via divalent metal transporter 1 (DMT1), which is located on the luminal membrane. Imported iron can be either exported to the blood by ferroportin, which is located on the basolateral enterocyte membrane, or bound by ferritin and retained (*left panel*). When systemic iron levels are low, most imported iron is released to the circulation, with little retained in ferritin (*middle panel*). When body iron stores are high, hepcidin is produced by the liver, which results in reduction of ferroportin levels and decreased iron release to the circulation (*right panel*).

is sloughed from the villous. Under normal circumstances, the amount of iron that enters the circulation is tightly regulated in response to systemic need. This regulation is mediated by the peptide hormone hepcidin, which is secreted by the liver and binds to ferroportin, targeting the protein for degradation and thus reducing enterocyte iron efflux (37). Inherited disorders that disrupt the normal homeostatic regulation of iron absorption can result in either iron deficiency or overload.

HEREDITARY HEMOCHROMATOSIS

Hemochromatosis is one of the most frequent genetic disorders of Caucasians, with an incidence of 3–5 per 1000 population. The most common form results from mutations in the HFE gene and is inherited as an autosomal recessive condition. Patients have total-body iron levels which are 5–10 times normal (15–40 g), which results from increased iron absorption from the gut. Onset of clinical features is typically at 30–50 years of age in males but is delayed in female patients as a result of menstrual blood loss, which slows the rate of excess iron accumulation. Rare forms can present during the 2nd or 3rd decade and may be identified in children serendipitously during routine laboratory testing of iron status.

Clinical Features Homozygosity for an HFE mutation is found in approximately 5 of every 1000 Caucasians (38). However, the penetrance of clinical symptoms is quite low, with estimates ranging from 50% to as low as 1% (38,39). Furthermore, in symptomatic patients, there is significant variability in the clinical phenotype, varying from an isolated elevation of the serum transferrin saturation to the complete symptom complex.

The most common presenting symptoms in adults are fatigue, arthralgia, loss of libido, and impotence. Associated findings include hepatomegaly, increased skin pigmentation, diabetes mellitus, abdominal pain, and cardiomyopathy (40). Iron accumulation in the liver results in cirrhosis and may lead to hepatocellular carcinoma. Diabetes results from pancreatic iron accumulation. The first symptoms in juvenile-onset forms are commonly hypogonadotropic hypogonadism and heart failure. The pathology in hemochromatosis is a direct result of tissue iron deposition and is believed to be due to the iron-catalyzed generation of toxic oxygen radicals.

Diagnosis Because of the low penetrance of an HFE mutation, biochemical measures of iron status must be used for diagnosis. A persistent elevation of the fasting transferrin saturation (>45% for 1 year) will identify 98% of affected patients (40). The transferrin saturation is elevated even when the level of ferritin and total-body iron stores are normal, allowing for diagnosis prior to the onset of clinical symptoms. Decisions regarding initiation of treatment should be based on measures of total-body iron load and symptoms. Most patients with an elevated transferrin saturation and normal ferritin level do not require therapy but should be reevaluated yearly. When the ferritin becomes elevated (≥200 µg/L in premenopausal women and ≥300 µg/L in men and postmenopausal women) or in the presence of liver disease, therapy should be begun. A liver biopsy may be required in patients with elevated liver enzymes to determine the level of iron accumulation and to evaluate for the presence of cirrhosis. Techniques for the quantitation of hepatic iron by magnetic resonance imaging (MRI) also have been developed and likely will have an increased role in the future (46,47).

Among those with clinical symptoms, approximately 90% are homozygous for the substitution of a tyrosine for cysteine at position 282 (C282Y) in HFE, 1% to 2% are homozygous for a histidine-to-aspartate mutation at position 63 (H63D), and 2% to 4% are compound heterozygotes for these two mutations (41). Carriers of HFE mutations can have biochemical abnormalities such as an elevated transferrin saturation and ferritin but rarely have symptoms (42). In addition to HFE, three other genes are associated with autosomal recessive iron overload. Mutations in the transferrin receptor 2 gene (TFR2) result in an adult-onset disorder very similar to that resulting from HFE mutations (43). TFR2 is expressed primarily in the liver, where

it is believed to function as a sensor of total-body iron status (44,45). Juvenile-onset iron overload is associated with mutations in the genes for hemojuvelin (HJV) and hepcidin (HAMP). In juvenile hemochromatosis, symptoms begin as early as the second decade and frequently result in death by age 30 due to heart failure (43) (see Figure 40-5 for a diagnostic algorithm of the different types of HFE).

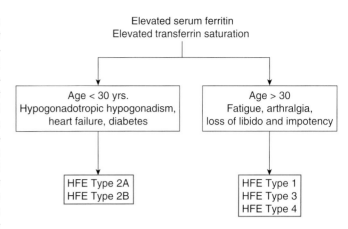

FIGURE 40-5. Flow diagram for patients presenting with elevated serum ferritin and transferrin saturation.

Treatment Fortunately, the iron that accumulates in hemochromatosis can be mobilized readily, allowing for treatment via repeated phlebotomy. Each pint of blood removes around 200–250 mg iron. Monitoring of therapy is done by following the serum ferritin level, which should be maintained in the low-normal range. The long-term prognosis for patients who begin treatment before significant tissue damage occurs (e.g., hepatic cirrhosis, and diabetes mellitus) is excellent, and in some reported series, outcome is no different from that in unaffected persons. However, much of the damage that occurs in hemochromatosis is irreversible, emphasizing the need for early diagnosis and treatment. Because of the high incidence and excellent response to early therapy, population screening for hereditary hemochromatosis has been considered.

RARE DISORDERS OF IRON METABOLISM

A rare autosomal dominant iron-overload disorder is caused by mutations in the gene for the plasma membrane iron transporter ferroportin (SLC40A1) (48). In these patients, iron accumulates in macrophages of the liver and spleen with relative sparing of hepatocytes. Patients have a low transferrin saturation and may develop iron-deficiency anemia. Diagnosis is made on the basis of an elevated serum ferritin level in the absence of other known liver disease or inflammatory process. Ferritin elevation may be seen as early as the first decade (43).

Neonatal hemochromatosis results from the accumulation of excess iron in utero and can result in fetal death or acute liver failure shortly after birth. The liver demonstrates cirrhosis, fatty infiltration, and bile duct proliferation with hemosiderin deposits. The pancreas, adrenals, thyroid, and myocardium also may be affected. The etiology of this disorder is

uncertain, but several studies support a role for maternal immunization against a fetal antigen (49,50), as seen by the high recurrence rate (up to 80%) and incidence in maternal half-siblings. A trial of high-dose intravenous immunoglobulin treatment of mothers with a previously affected child demonstrated improved survival and a reduced severity of liver dysfunction (49). However, this approach will require further study before it becomes standard therapy. The only other therapy that has been employed successfully is liver transplant.

Pantothenate kinase–associated neurodegeneration (PKAN) is a progressive movement disorder characterized by dystonia, chorea, athetosis, and developmental deterioration associated with iron deposition in the basal ganglia. The reason for the localization of the pathology is unknown; PANK2 is expressed in the basal ganglia as well as in other regions of the brain that do not show iron accumulation (51). The disorder is caused by mutations in the PANK2 gene, which encodes pantothenate kinase 2, an enzyme believed to function in coenzyme A biosynthesis (52). A defect in mitochondrial lipid metabolism has been proposed to have a role in the pathophysiology of PKAN, but the specific metabolic consequences of PANK2 deficiency and the molecular basis for the brain iron accumulation are still undefined (51). PKAN is inherited as an autosomal recessive disorder, and there is currently no effective therapy. Death in the second decade is typical.

Atransferrinemia is a very rare autosomal recessive disorder due to mutations in the transferrin gene. Patients have a hypochromic anemia that is resistant to iron therapy but can be treated by infusion of plasma that contains transferrin. Excess iron accumulation occurs in the myocardium and liver. A similar clinical phenotype also has been reported in a single patient believed to have a mutation in the DMT1 gene (53).

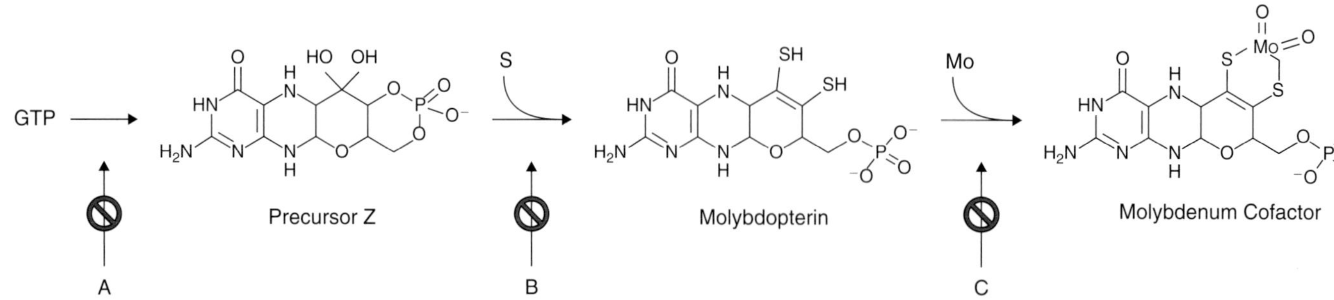

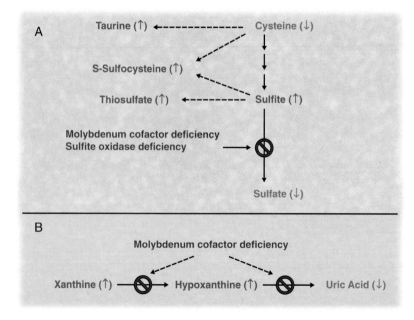

FIGURE 40-6. Biosynthesis of the molybdenum cofactor. Deficiencies in three steps of molybdenum cofactor biosynthesis have been identified via analysis of patient samples. Complementation group A patients are unable to synthesize precursor Z from GTP. Patients in group B cannot convert precursor Z to molybdopterin. Group C patients are unable to form the molybdenum cofactor from molybdopterin.

DISORDERS OF MOLYBDENUM METABOLISM

Overview of Molybdenum Metabolism

Molybdenum is an essential trace element with an RDA ranging from 3 μg/day in infants to 45 μg/day in adults (27). Molybdenum is well absorbed in the gut, and dietary deficiency is very rare. Molybdenum is required for the activity of three enzymes, sulfite oxidase, xanthine dehydrogenase, and aldehyde oxidase. The functionally active form of molybdenum is called the *molybdenum cofactor*, and it consists of a molybdenum atom bound to a modified pterin (molybdopterin). Biosynthesis of the molybdenum cofactor occurs in five steps. The first four steps generate the molybdopterin, and the final step is the addition of molybdenum to the pterin ring. Studies of patient fibroblasts have identified three complementation groups (Figure 40-6). Complementation group A patients are deficient in the conversion of GTP to precursor Z and carry mutations in the MOCSI gene (molybdenum cofactor synthesis-1). Group B patients cannot convert precursor Z to molybdopterin and carry mutations in the MOCS2 (molybdenum cofactor synthesis-2) gene that abrogates conversion of the precursor Z to molybdopterin. Group C patients are unable to form the molybdenum cofactor from molybdopterin due to mutations in the gephyrin gene (GEPH) that encodes the gephyrin protein, which catalyzes the insertion of molybdenum into molybdopterin (54). Mutations affecting the genes required for molybdenum cofactor biosynthesis all result in a similar clinical phenotype called *molybdenum cofactor deficiency.*

MOLYBDENUM COFACTOR DEFICIENCY

Clinical Features The most common presentation of molybdenum cofactor deficiency is with severe neonatal seizures (55). Infants may appear normal at birth but subsequently develop feeding problems, seizures, and abnormalities of muscle tone. The seizures typically are generalized and resistant to therapy. Many patients die in the neonatal period, but those who survive have severe developmental problems and rarely live beyond the third year of life. Brain imaging demonstrates abnormalities of the white matter, enlargement of the ventricles and CSF spaces, and subcortical cysts that may mimic postanoxic encephalopathy (56–58). A single patient has been studied by MR spectroscopy and was found to have decreased N-acetyl-aspartate and increased lactate levels (59). Pathological studies demonstrate severe neuronal loss and astrogliosis in the cortex and cystic changes in the white matter (60). The pathophysiology of these changes is uncertain, but they may be due to a direct excitotoxic effect of the sulfite- and sulfur-containing amino acids that accumulate as a result of the lack of sulfite oxidase activity (60). Dysmorphic facial features, including hypertelorism, a small nose, puffy cheeks and lips, a long philtrum, and progressive microcephaly, usually are present (61). Lens dislocation is seen in approximately 50% of patients but may not be present in neonates (62). The loss of xanthine dehydrogenase activity results in an elevated excretion of xanthine and can lead to renal stones. The majority of patients with molybdenum cofactor deficiency present as neonates, but milder forms with a later onset also have been reported (63).

An isolated deficiency of sulfite oxidase results in a clinical phenotype very similar to that in the severe form of molybdenum cofactor deficiency. This disorder results from a mutation in the gene for sulfite oxidase (SUOX) and does not affect molybdenum cofactor synthesis or the activity of xanthine dehydrogenase and aldehyde oxidase. Based on this observation, it is believed that most of the symptoms seen in molybdenum cofactor deficiency, especially the cerebral atrophy, are related to the lack of sulfite oxidase activity.

Biochemical Effects and Diagnosis Deficiency of sulfite oxidase, which functions in the cysteine degradation pathway, leads to the accumulation of taurine, sulfite, thiosulfite, and S-sulfocysteine (Figure 40-7; see also

FIGURE 40-7. Biochemical effects of molybdenum cofactor deficiency (**A,B**) and isolated sulfite oxidase deficiency (**A**). Metabolites are increased (↑) or decreased (↓) as indicated.

TABLE 40-3	Sulfite Oxidase Deficiency
Laboratory Findings	
Decreased	**Increased**
Sulfate (U)	Sulfite (U)
Cysteine (B)	*S*-Sulfocysteine (B, U)
Homocysteine (B)	Taurine (B, U)
	Thiosulfite (U)

TABLE 40-4	Molybdenum Cofactor Deficiency
Laboratory Findings	
Decreased	**Increased**
Uric acid (B, U)	Sulfite (U)
Sulfate (U)	*S*-Sulfocysteine (B, U)
Cysteine (B)	Taurine (B, U)
Homocysteine (B, U)	Thiosulfite (U)
	Xanthine (B)
	Hypoxanthine (U)

Table 40-3). Cysteine levels are decreased secondary to reaction with sulfite and formation of *S*-sulfocysteine. Total serum homocysteine is also very low in patients lacking sulfite oxidase activity (64,65). Urine sulfite can be detected by a sulfite dipstick, but fresh urine must be used to avoid loss via oxidation to sulfate and a false-negative result. A more stable marker is urine *S*-sulfocysteine, which is the preferred metabolite for diagnosis. Urine thiosulfite also can be measured but has a high rate of false-positive results due to cross-reaction of commonly used antibiotics (66).

Xanthine dehydrogenase functions in purine degradation, catalyzing the conversion of hypoxanthine to xanthine and xanthine to uric acid. Loss of enzymatic activity leads to markedly decreased levels of both serum and urine uric acid (see Table 40-4). Consequently, the determination of serum uric acid level is an excellent screening test in infants with neonatal seizures of unknown etiology. However, in some affected infants, particularly those with later onset or milder symptoms, the level of uric acid may be within the low-normal range and result in a false-negative test (67). There is also a significant elevation of xanthine and a more modest increase in hypoxanthine, which can be detected by measuring oxypurines in either urine or blood (68). Determination of oxypurines and uric acid allows differentiation between molybdenum cofactor deficiency and isolated sulfite oxidase deficiency (see Figure 40-8).

Based on the results of biochemical testing, definitive enzymatic studies then can be performed on cultured fibroblasts. This is im-

portant not only for diagnosis but also for genetic counseling. Both molybdenum cofactor deficiency and sulfite oxidase deficiency are inherited as autosomal recessive disorders and thus have a 25% recurrence risk. Prenatal diagnosis can be done by measurement of sulfite oxidase activity in cultured amniocytes or tissue obtained by CVS (69).

Treatment The seizures associated with molybdenum cofactor deficiency are difficult to control, and no specific therapies are yet available. Direct administration of molybdenum cofactor is not practical due to its instability. In contrast, the use of a stable precursor has been reported to be effective in a mouse model of molybdenum cofactor deficiency (70). Use of a diet with reduced levels of sulfur-containing amino acids (e.g., cysteine and methionine) has been successful in two patients with a mild form of sulfite oxidase deficiency, resulting in a decrease of urinary thiosulphate and *S*-sulphocysteine (71). Both patients grew normally with no signs of neurological deterioration. Based on the hypothesis that *S*-sulfocysteine may cause excitotoxicity via activation of NMDA receptors, one patient was treated with dextromethorphan (12.5 mg/kg/d), an NMDA receptor inhibitor, resulting in decreased seizures and improvement in the electroencephalogram (72). No further use of this approach has been reported. Overall, the therapeutic options in molybdenum cofactor deficiency are very limited, and as a result, the outcome is usually poor.

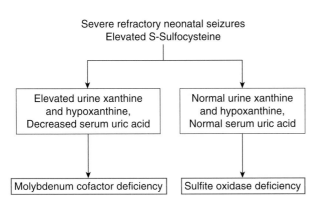

FIGURE 40-8. Flow diagram for patients presenting with refractory seizures and elevated *S*-sulfocysteine.

REFERENCES

1. Trumbo P, Yates AA, Schlicker S, et al. Dietary reference intakes: Vitamin A, vitamin K, arsenic, boron, chromium, copper, iodine, iron, manganese, molybdenum, nickel, silicon, vanadium, and zinc. *J Am Diet Assoc.* 2001;101:294–301.
2. Lee J, Pena MM, Nose Y, et al. Biochemical characterization of the human copper transporter CTR1. *J Biol Chem.* 2002;277: 4380–4397.
3. Prohaska JR, Gybina AA. Intracellular copper transport in mammals. *J Nutr.* 2004;134: 1003–1006.
4. Tonnesen T, Kleijer WJ, Horn N. Incidence of Menkes disease. *Hum Genet.* 1991;86:408–410.
5. Hardman B, Manuelpillai U, Wallace EM, et al. Expression and localization of Menkes and Wilson copper transporting ATPases in human placenta. *Placenta.* 2004;25:512–517.
6. Qian Y, Tiffany-Castiglioni E, Welsh J, et al. Copper efflux from murine microvascular cells requires expression of the menkes disease Cu-ATPase. *J Nutr.* 1998;128:1276–1282.
7. Kaler SG, Gallo LK, Proud VK, et al. Occipital horn syndrome and a mild Menkes phenotype associated with splice site mutations at the MNK locus. *Nat Genet.* 1994;8:195–202.
8. Kaler SG. Menkes disease. *Adv Pediatr.* 1994;41:263–304.
9. Stenson PD, Ball EV, Mort M, et al. Human Gene Mutation Database (HGMD): 2003 update. *Hum Mutat.* 2003;21:577–581.
10. Kaler SG, Gahl WA, Berry SA, et al. Predictive value of plasma catecholamine levels in neonatal detection of Menkes disease. *J Inherit Metab Dis.* 1993;16:907–908.
11. Christodoulou J, Danks DM, Sarkar B, et al. Early treatment of Menkes disease with parenteral copper-histidine: Long-term follow-up of four treated patients. *Am J Med Genet.* 1998;76:154–164.
12. Kaler SG, Das S, Levinson B, et al. Successful early copper therapy in menkes disease associated with a mutant transcript containing a small in-frame deletion. *Biochem Mol Med.* 1996;57:37–46.
13. Kaler SG, Buist NR, Holmes CS, et al. Early copper therapy in classic Menkes disease patients with a novel splicing mutation. *Ann Neurol.* 1995;38:921–928.
14. Barnes N, Tsivkovskii R, Tsivkovskaia N, et al. The copper-transporting ATPases, Menkes and Wilson disease proteins, have distinct roles in adult and developing cerebellum. *J Biol Chem.* 2005;280:9640–9645.
15. Brewer GJ. Recognition, diagnosis, and management of Wilson disease. *Proc Soc Exp Biol Med.* 2000;223:39–46.
16. Gow PJ, Smallwood RA, Angus PW, et al. Diagnosis of Wilson's disease: An experience over three decades. *Gut.* 2000;46:415–419.
17. Panagiotakaki E, Tzetis M, Manolaki N, et al. Genotype-phenotype correlations for a wide spectrum of mutations in the Wilson disease gene (ATP7B). *Am J Med Genet.* 2004;131A:168–173.
18. Brewer GJ, Dick RD, Johnson VD, et al. Treatment of Wilson's disease with zinc: XV. Long-term follow-up studies. *J Lab Clin Med.* 1998;132:264–278.
19. Brewer GJ, Dick RD, Johnson VD, et al. Treatment of Wilson's disease with zinc: XVI.

Treatment during the pediatric years. *J Lab Clin Med.* 2001;137:191–198.

20. Askari FK, Greenson J, Dick RD, et al. Treatment of Wilson's disease with zinc: XVIII. Initial treatment of the hepatic decompensation presentation with trientine and zinc. *J Lab Clin Med.* 2003;142:385–390.

21. Brewer GJ, Johnson V, Dick RD, et al. Treatment of Wilson disease with ammonium tetrathiomolybdate: II. Initial therapy in 33 neurologically affected patients and follow-up with zinc therapy. *Arch Neurol.* 1996;53:1017–1025.

22. Brewer GJ, Terry CA, Aisen AM, et al. Worsening of neurologic syndrome in patients with Wilson's disease with initial penicillamine therapy. *Arch Neurol.* 1987;44:490–493.

23. Gitlin JD. Aceruloplasminemia. *Pediatr Res.* 1998;44:271–276.

24. Yonekawa M, Okabe T, Asamoto Y, et al. A case of hereditary ceruloplasmin deficiency with iron deposition in the brain associated with chorea, dementia, diabetes mellitus and retinal pigmentation: Administration of fresh-frozen human plasma. *Eur Neurol.* 1999;42:157–162.

25. Hamza I, Faisst A, Prohaska J, et al. The metallochaperone Atox1 plays a critical role in perinatal copper homeostasis. *Proc Natl Acad Sci USA.* 2001;98:6848–6852.

26. Lee J, Prohaska JR, Thiele DJ. Essential role for mammalian copper transporter Ctr1 in copper homeostasis and embryonic development. *Proc Natl Acad Sci USA.* 2001;98: 6842–6847.

27. Panel on Micronutrients. *Dietary Reference Intakes.* Washington: Institute of Medicine; 2001.

28. Fraker PJ, King LE, Laakko T, et al. The dynamic link between the integrity of the immune system and zinc status. *J Nutr.* 2000;130:1399S–1406.

29. Hambidge M. Human zinc deficiency. *J Nutr.* 2000;130:1344S–1349.

30. Wang K, Zhou B, KuoYM, et al. A novel member of a zinc transporter family is defective in acrodermatitis enteropathica. *Am J Hum Genet.* 2002;71:66–73.

31. Michalczyk A, Varigos G, Catto-Smith A, et al. Analysis of zinc transporter, hZnT4 (Slc30A4), gene expression in a mammary gland disorder leading to reduced zinc secretion into milk. *Hum Genet.* 2003;113:202–210.

32. Huang L, Gitschier J. A novel gene involved in zinc transport is deficient in the lethal milk mouse. *Nat Genet.* 1997;17:292–297.

33. Krebs NF, Westcott J. Zinc and breast-fed infants: If and when is there a risk of deficiency? *Adv Exp Med Biol.* 2002;503:69–75.

34. Mancini AJ, Tunnessen WW Jr. Picture of the month: Acrodermatitis enteropathica-like rash in a breast-fed, full-term infant with zinc deficiency. *Arch Pediatr Adolesc Med.* 1998;152:1239–1240.

35. Perafan-Riveros C, Franca LF, Alves AC, et al. Acrodermatitis enteropathica: Case report and review of the literature. *Pediatr Dermatol.* 2002;19:426–431.

36. Andrews NC. A genetic view of iron homeostasis. *Semin Hematol.* 2002;39:227–234.

37. Nemeth E, Tuttle MS, Powelson J, et al. Hepcidin regulates iron efflux by binding to ferroportin and inducing its internalization. *Science.* 2004;306:2090–2093.

38. Beutler E, Felitti VJ, Koziol JA, et al. Penetrance of 845GnA (C282Y) HFE hereditary haemochromatosis mutation in the USA. *Lancet.* 2002;359:211–218.

39. Bulaj ZJ, Ajioka RS, Phillips JD, et al. Disease-related conditions in relatives of patients with hemochromatosis. *N Engl J Med.* 2000;343:1529–1535.

40. Powell LW, George DK, McDonnell SM, et al. Diagnosis of hemochromatosis. *Ann Intern Med.* 1998;129:925–931.

41. Beutler E, Bothwell TH, Charlton RW, et al. Hereditary hemochromatosis. In: Scriver CR, Beaudet AL, Sly WS, Valle D, eds. *The Metabolic and Molecular Bases of Inherited Disease,* 8th ed., Vol. II. New York: McGraw-Hill; 2001:3127–3161.

42. Bulaj ZJ, Griffen LM, Jorde LB, et al. Clinical and biochemical abnormalities in people heterozygous for hemochromatosis. *N Engl J Med.* 1996;335:1799–1805.

43. Pietrangelo A. Hereditary hemochromatosis: A new look at an old disease. *N Engl J Med.* 2004;350:2383–2397.

44. Johnson MB, Enns CA. Diferric transferrin regulates transferrin receptor 2 protein stability. *Blood.* 2004;104:4287–4293.

45. Robb A, Wessling-Resnick M. Regulation of transferrin receptor 2 protein levels by transferrin. *Blood.* 2004;104:4294–4299.

46. St Pierre TG, Clark PR, Chua-anusorn W, et al. Noninvasive measurement and imaging of liver iron concentrations using proton magnetic resonance. *Blood.* 2005;105:855–861.

47. Alustiza JM, Artetxe J, Castiella A, et al. MR quantification of hepatic iron concentration. *Radiology.* 2004;230:479–484.

48. Montosi G, Donovan A, Totaro A, et al. Autosomal-dominant hemochromatosis is associated with a mutation in the ferroportin (SLC11A3) gene. *J Clin Invest.* 2001;108:619–623.

49. Whitington PF, Hibbard JU. High-dose immunoglobulin during pregnancy for recurrent neonatal haemochromatosis. *Lancet.* 2004;364:1690–1698.

50. Schoenlebe J, Buyon JP, Zitelli BJ, et al. Neonatal hemochromatosis associated with maternal autoantibodies against Ro/SS-A and La/SS-B ribonucleoproteins. *Am J Dis Child.* 1993;147:1072–1075.

51. Kotzbauer PT, Truax AC, Trojanowski JQ, et al. Altered neuronal mitochondrial coenzyme A synthesis in neurodegeneration with brain iron accumulation caused by abnormal processing, stability, and catalytic activity of mutant pantothenate kinase 2. *J Neurosci.* 2005;25:689–698.

52. Zhou B, Westaway SK, Levinson B, et al. A novel pantothenate kinase gene (PANK2) is defective in Hallervorden-Spatz syndrome. *Nat Genet.* 2001;28:345–349.

53. Priwitzerova M, Pospisilova D, Prchal JT, et al. Severe hypochromic microcytic anemia caused by a congenital defect of the iron transport pathway in erythroid cells. *Blood.* 2004;103:3991–3992.

54. Reiss J. Genetics of molybdenum cofactor deficiency. *Hum Genet.* 2000;106:157–163.

55. Slot HM, Overweg-Plandsoen WC, Bakker HD, et al. Molybdenum-cofactor deficiency: an easily missed cause of neonatal convulsions. *Neuropediatrics.* 1993;24:139–142.

56. Schuierer G, Kurlemann G, Bick U, et al. Molybdenum-cofactor deficiency: CT and MR findings. *Neuropediatrics.* 1995;26:51–54.

57. Topcu M, Coskun T, Haliloglu G, et al. Molybdenum cofactor deficiency: Report of three cases presenting as hypoxic-ischemic encephalopathy. *J Child Neurol.* 2001; 16:264–270.

58. Bakker HD, Abeling NG, ten Houten R, et al. Molybdenum cofactor deficiency can mimic postanoxic encephalopathy. *J Inherit Metab Dis.* 1993;16:900–901.

59. Salvan AM, Chabrol B, Lamoureux S, et al. In vivo brain proton MR spectroscopy in a case of molybdenum cofactor deficiency. *Pediatr Radiol.* 1999;29:846–848.

60. Salman MS, Ackerley C, Senger C, et al. New insights into the neuropathogenesis of molybdenum cofactor deficiency. *Can J Neurol Sci.* 2002;29:91–96.

61. Johnson JL, Duran M. Molybdenum cofactor deficiency and isolated sulfite oxidase deficiency. In: Scriver CR, Beaudet AL, Sly WS, Valle D, eds. *The Metabolic and Molecular Bases of Inherited Disease,* 8th ed., Vol. II. New York: McGraw-Hill; 2001:3163–3177.

62. Lueder GT, Steiner RD. Ophthalmic abnormalities in molybdenum cofactor deficiency and isolated sulfite oxidase deficiency. *J Pediatr Ophthalmol Strabis.* 1995;32:334–337.

63. Hughes EF, Fairbanks L, Simmonds HA, et al. Molybdenum cofactor deficiency-phenotypic variability in a family with a late-onset variant. *Dev Med Child Neurol.* 1998;40:57–61.

64. Sass JO, Nakanishi T, Sato T, et al. New approaches towards laboratory diagnosis of isolated sulphite oxidase deficiency. *Ann Clin Biochem.* 2004;41:157–159.

65. Sass JO, Kishikawa M, Puttinger R, et al. Hypohomocysteinaemia and highly increased proportion of S-sulfonated plasma transthyretin in molybdenum cofactor deficiency. *J Inherit Metab Dis.* 2003;26:80–82.

66. Mann G., Kirk JM. Antibiotic interference in urinary thiosulphate measurements. *J Inherit Metab Dis.* 1994;17:120–121.

67. Simmonds HA, Hoffmann GF, Perignon JL, et al. Diagnosis of molybdenum cofactor deficiency. *Lancet.* 1999;353:675.

68. van Gennip AH, Abeling NG, Stroomer AE, et al. The detection of molybdenum cofactor deficiency: Clinical symptomatology and urinary metabolite profile. *J Inherit Metab Dis.* 1994;17:142–145.

69. Johnson JL. Prenatal diagnosis of molybdenum cofactor deficiency and isolated sulfite oxidase deficiency. *Prenat Diagn.* 2003;23:6–8.

70. Schwarz G, Santamaria-Araujo JA, Wolf S, et al. Rescue of lethal molybdenum cofactor deficiency by a biosynthetic precursor from *Escherichia coli. Hum Mol Genet.* 2004;13: 1249–1255.

71. Touati G, Rusthoven E, Depondt E, et al. Dietary therapy in two patients with a mild form of sulphite oxidase deficiency: Evidence for clinical and biological improvement. *J Inherit Metab Dis.* 2000;23:45–53.

72. Kurlemann G, Debus O, Schuierer G. Dextromethorphan in molybdenum cofactor deficiency. *Eur J Paediatr.* 1996;155:422–423.

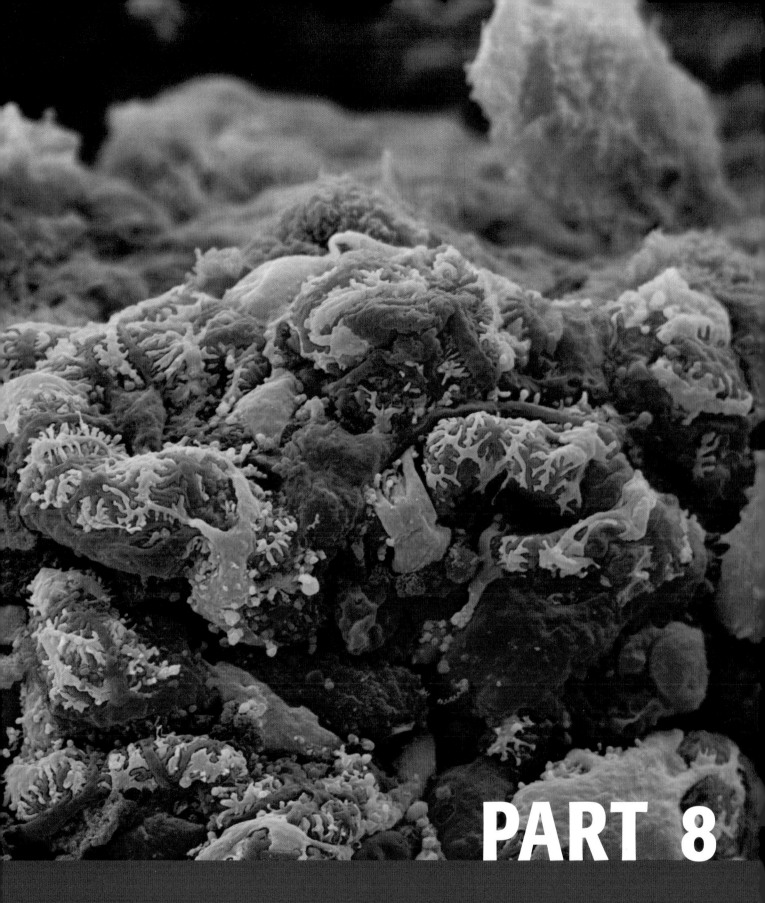

PART 8

Disorders of Water Metabolism and Transport Systems

IN THIS PART

Previous page: Image of the loops of a kidney-corpuscle from the cortex.

CHAPTER 41

Disorders of Water Metabolism

Tim Cheetham, MD
Stephen Ball, PhD, FRCP

Water is the largest constituent of the human body, representing about 60% of a person's body weight. Approximately 65% of total-body water is intracellular, with the remaining 35% extracellular water, which is further divided into smaller intravascular (plasma) and larger extravascular (interstitial) compartments. While the solute compositions of intracellular and extracellular fluids are markedly different, most cell membranes are permeable to water; therefore, the total solute concentration is very similar between the two compartments. Sodium is the major solute and determinant of the osmolality of plasma and other extracellular fluids because its concentration in these compartments is high, and it is restricted from entering into cells. The osmolality of intracellular fluid and cell volume, which are essential for its survival, depend on the osmolality of extracellular fluid, which itself is in a constant state of exchange with the environment. That most cells cannot withstand significant volume changes to function properly highlights the crucial importance of keeping extracellular fluid osmolality within a precise and narrow range.

The extracellular fluid osmolality, and in particular, plasma osmolality (Posm), in humans is maintained through the regulation of thirst and secretion of the antidiuretic hormone arginine vasopressin (AVP). Both thirst and AVP release are influenced by similar stimuli (i.e., changes in Posm and pressure–volume changes). An increase in extracellular osmolality stimulates thirst and vasopressin secretion, which lead to water intake and a decrease in urinary water loss.

The osmotic threshold for AVP secretion is slightly lower than that for thirst perception, permitting maximum use of the antidiuretic mechanism to preserve water balance and lower dependence on the thirst mechanism and constant water supply. Under normal circumstances, water balance and maintenance of plasma osmolality are achieved mainly by AVP-regulated free water excretion and less by thirst-regulated water intake.

NORMAL PHYSIOLOGY

The Neurohypophysis and Vasopressin

Vasopressin (AVP), a nonapeptide (Figure 41-1), is the major determinant of renal solute-free water excretion. It is produced by secretory neurons residing in the supraoptic nuclei (SON) and paraventricular nuclei (PVN) of the hypothalamus (highlighted in Figure 41-2). The neurons project along the supraoptic–hypophyseal tract and terminate in the posterior pituitary. The generation and release of AVP hormone from the axon terminal are the consequence of the processing and cleavage of a large precursor molecule (preproAVP) encoded by the arginine vasopressin–neurophysin II gene (AVP-NPII gene) (Figure 41-3). PreproAVP consists of a signal peptide, the AVP moiety, a tripeptide linker, a binding protein (neurophysin), a dipeptide linker, and a glycosylated peptide known as *copeptin*. Cleavage of the signal peptide occurs as

preproAVP translocates into the endoplasmic reticulum. Dimerization then takes place as the molecules pass into the neurosecretory granules from the Golgi apparatus. Further oligomerization and processing occur as the neurosecretory granules move along toward the axon terminal, with cleaved neurophysin II and copeptin bound noncovalently to AVP. Exocytosis and release of the mature AVP–neurophysin complex from the nerve endings in the posterior pituitary follow neurotransmitter-induced depolarization. The AVP–neurophysin complex then dissociates to release free hormone. Mature AVP has a circulating half-life of some 5–15 minutes. Some of the vasopressinergic PVN neurons terminate in the hypophyseal–portal bed of the hypothalamus and cosecrete corticotrophin-releasing factor (CRF) as well as AVP. AVP and CRF production by these neurons is subject to negative-feedback control by glucocorticoids (see the section on vasopressin release below).

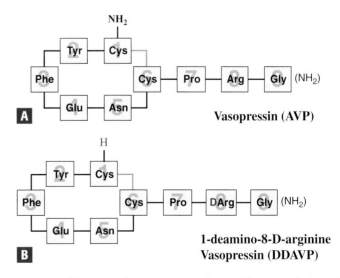

FIGURE 41-1. A to **B.** (A.) Arginine vasopressin (AVP) & (B.) Desamino-D-arginine vasopressin (DDAVP) Diagrammatic representation of the AVP nono-peptide highlighting cyclical structure and di-sulphide bridge between cysteine residues at positions 1 and 6. Replacement of L-arginine with D-arginine at position 8 and amino-terminal deamidation at position 1 (highlighted in red) result in the analogue DDAVP which has more potent and prolonged antidiuretic activity.

Disorders of Water Metabolism

AT-A-GLANCE

The disorders of water metabolism typically result from abnormalities of vasopressin (AVP) production or action or from excessive fluid intake (primary polydipsia). The term *diabetes insipidus* refers to the excessive passage of dilute urine, which may reflect abnormally low AVP production (central diabetes insipidus [CDI]), impaired AVP action (nephrogenic diabetes insipidus [NDI]), or excessive fluid intake (primary polydipsia [PP]). CDI and NDI can reflect specific genetic defects but also may be acquired. In CDI, the acquired causes are frequently destructive processes that damage the hypothalamus (e.g., trauma and tumors), whereas acquired NDI typically reflects metabolic derangement such as hyperglycemia, hypercalcemia, or hypokalemia or renal disease. Treatment of CDI usually includes the administration of the AVP analogue desmopressin (DDAVP). Managing the inherited forms of NDI can be difficult and usually involves reducing urine output by the combined use of a thiazide diuretic and a prostaglandin synthetase inhibitor. PP is not uncommon in the young child.

The disorders of water balance also will encompass the production of AVP and atrial natriuretic peptide (ANP) and/or brain natriuretic peptide (BNP) leading to hyponatremia. Both usually occur in association with intercurrent illness or surgery. Recently, it has been recognized that a genetic defect causing constitutive activation of the AVP receptor also can lead to persistent hyponatremia (nephrogenic syndrome of inappropriate antidiuresis [NSIAD]).

DISORDER	OCCURENCE	GENE	LOCUS	OMIM
Central diabetes insipidus (CDI)	3:100,000*			
Familial isolated CDI				
Autosomal dominant		AVP-NPII	20p13	125700
Autosomal recessive		AVP-NPII	20p13	125700
Developmental syndrome with midline defects				
Septo-optic dysplasia	Rare	HESX1	3p21.2-p21.1	182230
Holoprosencephaly	1:16,000			
Loci potentially associated with CDI include:				
HPE1		HPE1	21q22.3	236100
HPE2		SIX3	2p21	603714
HPE3		SHH	7q36	600725
HPE4		TGIF	18p11.3	602630
HPE5		ZIC2	13q32	603073
HPE6		HPE6	2q37.1-q37.3	605934
HPE7		PTCH	9q22.3	601309
HPE8		HPE8	14q13	609408
In association with ant. pituitary hormone def.	Rare	N/A		
DIDMOAD (WFS1)	Very rare	Wolframin	4p16.1	606201
Nephrogenic diabetes insipidus (NDI)	1:250,000*			
Familial NDI				
X-linked	~1:200,000	AVPR2	Xq28	304800
Autosomal recessive		AQP2	12q13	222000
Autosomal dominant		AQP2	12q13	125800
Primary polydipsia	Relatively common			
NSIAD	Unknown	AVPR2	Xq28	#300539
SIADH		N/A		
Cerebral salt wasting (ANP/BNP production)		N/A		

*Including genetic causes.

Acquired causes of CDI	Acquired causes of NDI
Trauma (neurosurgery, head injury, hypoxemic/ischemic brain damage)	Osmotic diuresis (diabetes mellitus)
Tumors (craniopharyngioma, germinoma, optic glioma, pinealoma)	Metabolic (hypercalcemia, hypokalemia)
Autoimmune	Chronic renal disease, after obstructive uropathy
Lymphocytic neurohypophysitis	Sickle cell disease
Granuloma (TB, sarcoid, Langerhans' cell histiocytosis)	Drugs (lithium, amphotericin, demeclocycline)
Infections (congenital CMV, toxoplasmosis, encephalitis, meningitis)	
Idiopathic	

DISEASE	FINDINGS		CLINICAL PRESENTATION FIRST YEAR OF LIFE	CHILDHOOD & ADOLESCENCE
Familial isolated CDI	↑ sNa	↓ uNa	Irritability, increased thirst, heavy diapers; dehydrated patients may generate relatively concentrated urine	Evolving polyuria and polydipsia
	↑ sOsm	↓ uOsm		
	↑ renin	↑ aldo		
	↓ AVP			
Familial isolated CDI + midline defects	↑ sNa	↓ uNa	Irritability, increased thirst, heavy diapers; look for other evidence of CNS dysfunction, including anterior pituitary hormone deficiencies	
	↑ sOsm	↓ uOsm		
	↑ renin	↑ aldo		
	↓ AVP			
Acquired CDI	↑ sNa	↓ uNa	Sudden or evolving polyuria and polydipsia; patients not usually fussy about type of fluid; look for evidence of associated anterior pituitary dysfunction	
	↑ sOsm	↓ uOsm		
	↑ renin	↑ aldo		
	↓ AVP			
Familial NDI (X-linked)	nl/ ↑ sNa	↓ uNa	Irritability, increased thirst, heavy diapers	
	nl/ ↑ sOsm	↓ uOsm		
	nl K	↑ AVP		
	nl Ca	nl glucose		
Familial NDI (AR)			Polyuria and polydipsia in early life but less profound than in the X-linked form	Usually presents before 5 years of age; nonclassical form may present in childhood or adolescence
Acquired causes of NDI	? ↑ Glucose	? ↑ Ca	Drug history important; assess renal function as well as glucose, calcium, and potassium	
	? ↑ Creat	? ↑ K		
	nl/ ↑ sNa	↓ uNa		
	nl/ ↑ sOsm	↓ uOsm		
	↑ AVP			
Primary polydipsia	↓ sNa	↓ uNa		Typically prefer flavored drinks to water. Risk of hyponatremia and seizures at the time of intercurrent illness
	nl/ ↓ sOsm	nl/ ↓ uOsm		
	nl K	↓ AVP		
NSIAD	↓ sNa	↑ uNa	Low serum sodium; increased by fluid restriction	Electrolytes may be normal in later life
	↓ sOsm	↑ uOsm		
	↓ renin	nl aldo		
	↓ BUN	↓ Hct		
SIADH	↓ sNa	↑ uNa	Patients have increased weight gain, moist mucous membranes, decreased urine output with increased urine specific gravity.	
	↓ sOsm	↑ uOsm		
	nl/ ↓ K	↓ uric acid		
	↓ renin	nl aldo		
	↓ BUN	Hct		
	↑ BNP	↑ ANP		
Cerebral salt wasting	↓ sNa	↑ uNa(>100meq/L)	Polyuric and volume depleted; frequently there is an associated CNS insult or pathology; CSWS usually appears in the first week after brain injury and spontaneously resolves in 2–4 weeks; PRA and aldosterone may be "paradoxically" low	
	↑ sOsm	↓ uOsm		
	nl/ ↓ K	nl uric acid		
	↓ renin	↓ aldo		
	↑ BUN	↑ Hct		
	↑ BNP	↑ ANP		

CDI = cranial diabetes insipidus; NDI = nephrogenic diabetes insipidus; NSIAD = nephrogenic syndrome of inappropriate antidiuresis, SIADH = syndrome of inappropriate ADH (AVP) production; Na = sodium; K = potassium; Ca = calcium; BUN = blood urea nitrogen; creat = creatinine; sOsm = serum osmolality; uOsm = urine osmolality; Aldo = aldosterone; nl = normal; uNa = urinary sodium; Hct = hematocrit; CSWS = cerebral salt wasting; AR = autosomal recessive; PRA = plasma renin activity; ANP = atrial natriuretic peptide; BNP = brain natriuretic peptide.

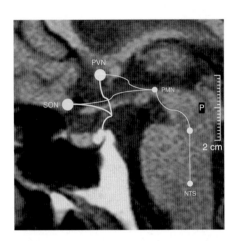

FIGURE 41-2. The neurohypophysis and its afferent connections. The neurohypophysis highlighting the position of the PVN and SON in relation to the posterior pituitary. Vasopressinergic neurones project from both nucleii to the posterior pituitary via the supraoptic hypophyseal tract. Volume and baro-sensitive afferents project to the hypothalamic nucleii via the Nucleus Tractus Solitarius (NTS) and Paramedian Nucleus (PMN).

Vasopressin Action

Water homeostasis is maintained by balancing fluid intake governed by the sensation of thirst and by reducing water excretion through the kidney via the countercurrent mechanism and antidiuretic effect of AVP. The anatomical arrangement of the renal tubules and vascular elements is such that both tubules and medullary vessels (vasa recta) run from the cortex to the papillary tip of the medulla and then loop back to the cortex. The reversal of the tubular fluid allows countercurrent multiplication and countercurrent exchange to take place, resulting in concentration of the urine.

AVP's antidiuretic function and formation of concentrated urine is achieved by increasing water permeability, and thus reabsorption of free water at the level of the collecting ducts, by allowing equilibration of the tubular urine with the hyperosmolar milieu of the renal medulla. The increase

in water permeability of the renal collecting tubules is mediated by binding of AVP to the G protein–coupled type 2 AVP receptor (V2-R) on the basal aspect of the renal collecting tubular cell, activation of adenyl cyclase, and generation of cyclic adenosine monophosphate (cAMP) with subsequent activation of protein kinase A and phosphorylation of the water-channel protein aquaporin 2 (AQP-2). Phosphorylated AQP-2 then forms homotetramers in subapical vesicles within the cytoplasm that fuse with the cell membrane of the luminal surface (Figure 41-4). These channels result in a large increase in water permeability and allow water to diffuse from the lumen of the nephron into the cells of the collecting duct along a concentration gradient. Other AVP-independent aquaporins, AQP-3 and AQP-4, are expressed on the basolateral surface of the collecting-duct epithelium and are responsible primarily for the subsequent passage of water from within the cell into the hypertonic medullary renal interstitium and circulation (1). The movement of water in excess of solute will result in the production of a more concentrated urine. AQP-1 is expressed in proximal tubular epithelium, the thin descending limb of the loop of Henle, and the vasa recta of the kidney. It is also required for maximum renal concentrating ability, but by an alternative, AVP-independent mechanism.

VASOPRESSIN RELEASE AND THE PHYSIOLOGY OF WATER HOMEOSTASIS

Normal serum *osmolality* is maintained primarily through the regulation of AVP release and thirst, whereas the maintenance of body fluid *volume* is governed principally by the mechanisms controlling sodium excretion, such as the renin–angiotensin system. The threshold for AVP production is approxi-

mately 280 mOsm/L, and a rise in plasma solute concentration (plasma osmolality) above this value will increase AVP release. A decrease in plasma osmolality below this set point will suppress AVP secretion (Figure 41-5). This osmoregulatory process is extremely sensitive, and even a 1% change in serum osmolality can alter AVP release. The major mediator of hemodynamic changes to the hypothalamic nuclei (SON and PVN) originates from baroreceptors of the carotid sinus, atria, and the aortic arch. Baroregulation of AVP release is not as sensitive as osmoregulation because a change in mean arterial blood pressure or circulating volume of 5% to 10% is necessary before AVP is released; release of AVP increases exponentially when the 5% to 10% threshold is exceeded (Figure 41-6). Chronic volume depletion can lead to baroregulatory inputs overriding osmoregulatory drive, resulting in increased water resorption at the expense of hemodilution in an attempt to bolster circulating volume. Other nonosmoregulatory factors influencing AVP production include nausea, vasovagal reactions, hypoglycemia, cortisol, and drugs such as carbamazepine.

Under normal conditions, water balance is maintained by controlling renal water excretion so that plasma osmolality is confined to around 280–295 mOsm/kg. Maximum antidiuresis is achieved with plasma AVP concentrations around 2–4 pmol/L (Figure 41-7). Increases in plasma osmolality above 300 mOsm/kg will increase plasma AVP levels further, but this rise will not result in further urine concentration because of a finite water channel expression and medullary concentration gradient. In this situation, water balance is conserved by ingestion of fluid driven by thirst. The sensation of thirst is under osmotic control similar to that of AVP, and there is a linear relationship between thirst perception and plasma osmolality, assuming an intact thirst mechanism.

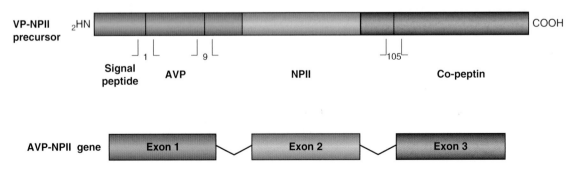

FIGURE 41-3. The vasopressin-neurophsin II (AVP-NPII) gene, the preprovasopressin precursor (preproAVP) and its relationship to vasopressin (AVP). Schematic representation of the AVP-NPII gene exons and their protein product precursor. Numbers reflect amino acid position in relation to first amino acid of VP. SP = signal peptide; VP = vasopressin; NP = neurophysin.

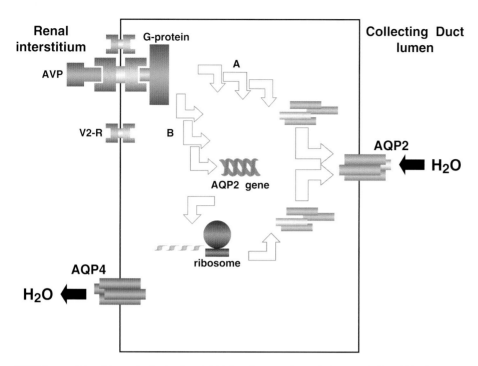

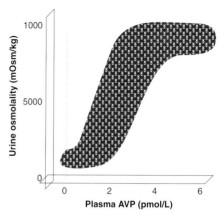

FIGURE 41-7. The relationship between plasma AVP (pAVP) and urine osmolality. Normogram describing the relationship of plasma AVP concentration to urine concentration in healthy adults. Maximum urine concentration is achieved at plasma AVP concentrations of 2–4 pmol/l. Further increases in plasma AVP above this level do not produce additional increases in urine concentration.

FIGURE 41-4. AVP and the renal collecting duct. AVP binds to the G-protein coupled V2-R on the interstitial cell surface, triggering a two-pronged intracellular signal transduction cascade. One arm of the cascade (A) increases the rate at which preformed AQP2 monomers are assembled into homo-tetramers and inserted into the luminal surface of the cell as functional water channels. The second arm stimulates the production of new AQP2 monomers by enhancing AQP2 gene transcription and formation of new AQP2 protein. AQP2 channels facilitate the movement of water from the lumen into the collecting duct cell along a concentration gradient. AQP4 is the predominant channel facilitating movement of water from the collecting duct cell into the renal interstitium. AQP4 activity does not require AVP, while the expression of AQP2 is dependent upon the action of AVP.

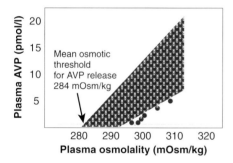

FIGURE 41-5. Relationship between plasma osmolality (pOsm) and plasma AVP (pAVP). Normogram describing the relationship of plasma osmolality to plasma AVP levels. There is a linear relationship between plasma osmolality and plasma AVP concentrations in the physiological range. The relationship has two additional important characteristics: a threshold osmolality above which AVP is released (the osmolar threshold) and the sensitivity of the osmoregulatory system —as depicted by the slope of the line. Though there is some inter-individual variation (as depicted by the shaded area), the relationship is remarkably constant within an individual over time.

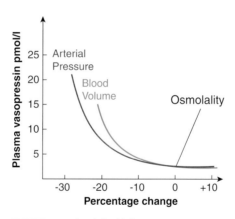

FIGURE 41-6. The relationship between percentage change in blood osmolality (black line), blood volume (green) and arterial blood pressure (red) and vasopressin release.

Fluid Balance in Childhood

During infancy and early childhood, there is a steady increase in intracellular water and a reduction in extracellular and total-body water. Renal concentrating ability is reduced in infancy, with a maximum urine osmolality around 300 mOsm/kg at term rising to around 650 mOsm/kg by 2 months of age. A relatively high surface area and associated increased insensible losses necessitate a high fluid intake in the young child. Infants with decreased oral intake or diarrhea or those given a high solute load are at risk of hypernatremic dehydration because of the relatively high insensible loss and reduced urine concentrating ability (2). The discrepancy between fluid intake and urine output (mL/kg) becomes less pronounced as the infant matures and insensible losses decrease. The relationship between plasma osmolality and AVP production in young children differs from that in the adult, with a shift in the relationship to the left reflecting more pronounced AVP production in response to a rising plasma osmolality (3). The relationship between plasma AVP and urine osmolality is similar in children and adults.

DIABETES INSIPIDUS

Diabetes insipidus is defined as the passage of large volumes of dilute urine (in excess of 2 L/m²/24 h, or approximately 150 mL/kg/24 h at birth, 110 mL/kg/24 h at 2 years of age, and 40 mL/kg/24 h in the older child and adult). The polyuric disorders of water balance can be caused by abnormalities of any of the three factors that determine water balance (i.e., vasopressin production, vasopressin action, and thirst). Some authors restrict the diagnosis of diabetes insipidus to patients with polydipsia and polyuria due to AVP deficiency or resistance, but in this chapter, the more literal meaning will be used (the siphon-like passage of insipid/weak urine), which also encompasses patients with an increased fluid intake that is not related primarily to either of these mechanisms. The causes of diabetes insipidus therefore are as follows:

- *Neurogenic, hypothalamic, or central diabetes insipidus* (CDI), where there is a partial or complete deficiency of osmoregulated AVP secretion
- *Nephrogenic diabetes insipidus* (NDI), where there is partial or total renal resistance to circulating AVP
- *Primary polydipsia* (PP), where there is excessive, inappropriate fluid intake

Central Diabetes Insipidus

Pathophysiology CDI is an abnormality of urine concentrating ability due to deficient secretion of AVP with main clinical features including polyuria and polydipsia. Central nervous system (CNS) defects causing CDI can be genetic or aquired and may involve one or more of the following factors of AVP regulation and synthesis: hypothalamic osmoreceptors, supraoptic (SON) or paraventricular (PVN) nuclei, and the supraoptic–hypophyseal tract. The majority of patients with CDI have lesions of the pituitary gland or of the PVN and SON nuclei; the osmoreceptor cells in the anterior hypothalamus usually are not impaired, and the thirst mechanism is intact.

Genetic defects may affect AVP production alone, or it can be a component of a more generalized abnormality of CNS development. Familial CDI is rare, accounting for about 5% of all patients. Mutations of the AVP gene encoding the large AVP precursor molecule have been identified. The AVP gene is mapped on chromosome 20 (20p13). The mode of inheritance is autosomal dominant with a high degree of penetrance: autosomal recessive inheritance has also been described (4). Degeneration of the AVP-synthesizing magnocellular neurons of the SON and PVN nuclei secondary to accumulation of the abnormal gene product in the endoplasmic reticulum appears to be the cause of familial CDI (5). Clinical manifestations may occur in infancy but usually develop at the ages of 5–10 years.

Wolfram or DIDMOAD syndrome consists of central diabetes insipidud (DI), diabetes mellitus (DM), optic atrophy (OA), and deafness (D). Wolfram syndrome may be inherited in an autosomal recessive pattern due to mutations in the gene encoding wolframin (WFS1; locus 4p16) or may be due to mitochondrial deletions. Other clinical manifestations of Wolfram syndrome include hydronephrosis, atonia of the bladder, ataxia, peripheral neuropathy, and mental retardation (6); however, only insulin-dependent diabetes mellitus and bilateral progressive optic atrophy are necessary to make the diagnosis of DIDMOAD syndrome. Patients with DIDMOAD syndrome usually present in early childhood with diabetes mellitus as the first manifestation.

Congenital abnormalities of midline brain development such as septo-optic dysplasia, holoprosencephaly, and familial pituitary hypoplasia with absent pituitary stalk may be associated with inherited forms of AVP deficiency (7) (see At-a-Glance page).

Acquired CDI is due to destructive lesions of the AVP-secreting neurons either directly or through retrograde degeneration from surgical interruption of AVP axons, which travel from the hypothalamus to the posterior pituitary, terminating at various sites within the stalk and the gland; the closer the lesions of the AVP axons are to the hypothalamus, the greater is the permanent loss of AVP secretion. Aquired causes (8,9) include trauma, neurosurgical interventions, neoplasms, and infiltrative autoimmune and infectious diseases. Between 30% and 50% of the acquired cases are called *idiopathic* because no etiology can be found (10). The most common form of CDI is the one following trauma or surgery to the hypothalamic–pituitary region. Usually local edema as a result of traction and/or manipulation of the pituitary stalk results in transient polyuria that begins 2–6 hours after surgery and resolves as edema diminishes in 6–7 days. In some postoperative patients, the polyuria may be followed by a phase of antidiuresis resulting in normal urinary output or the syndrome of inappropriate antidiuretic hormone secretion (SIADH) due to the release of AVP-peptide from the damaged stalk. During a third phase, the patient then may return to normal or develop persistent CDI after a period of days or weeks as damaged neurones recover or die (the triple-phase response). Frequently, permanent diabetes insipidus, either partial or complete, develops without the triple-phase response.

Germinomas and pinealomas are the most common CNS tumors presenting with CDI because they typically arise near the base of the hypothalamus. Germinomas can be very small and undetectable by magnetic resonance imaging (MRI) for several years following the onset of polyuria. Large-size craniopharyngiomas and gliomas may present with CDI before surgery. Infiltrative diseases such as Langerhans' cell histiocytosis (LCH) and lymphocytic hypophysitis also may present with CDI. About 10% of the patients with histiocytosis, particularly those with multisystem involvement, develop CDI with characteristic MRI changes (thickening of the pituitary stalk). Other acquired causes include hypoxic brain injury, autoimmunity (11), leukemia, and infection (congenital cytomegalovirus [CMV] infection and toxoplasmosis).

Clinical Presentation CDI tends to develop suddenly and usually is acquired. Family history, nevertheless, is important because of the inherited nature of some forms of diabetes insipidus. There is a wide range of severity, from mild degrees that may escape early detection to patients with profound polyuria of up to 400 mL/kg/24 h. By the time symptoms develop, much of the brain's ability to produce AVP has been lost. Infants may present with nonspecific symptoms such as poor feeding, failure to thrive, irritability (due to dehydration and hypernatremia), constipation, fever without apparent cause, and excessively wet diapers from urination. Infants who are breast-fed may present later than those who are bottle-fed. Affected breast-fed infants are less susceptible to hypernatremia because breast milk has less osmotic load than formula, requiring less obligate water loss via the kidney for excretion of the daily osmotic load.

Older children classically present with polyuria, polydipsia, nocturia, and sometimes nocturnal enuresis. The diagnosis may be delayed in children, who, by increasing their fluid intake, maintain normal water balance and sodium levels. However, the very young child without free access to fluids is at increased risk of dehydration and hypernatremia.

Children with severe CDI who have polyuria during the day and night prefer fluids with a low solute content (e.g., tap, toilet, or bath water), and they are not fussy about the fluid source. Growth retardation can occur in CDI but usually is not as pronounced as in NDI (12).

The physical examination can provide important clues about possible underlying diagnoses. An assessment of the child's nutritional status and an examination of the skeleton, skin, abdomen, and CNS, including funduscopy, are particularly important because of the possibility of cranial tumors and systemic diseases such as LCH.

Patients with midline defects of brain development and destructive lesions may also have anterior pituitary hormone deficiencies, including adrenocorticotropic hormone (ACTH) deficiency. Concomitant ACTH and cortisol deficiency may mask the symptoms of CDI because glucocorticoids increase the water permeability of the distal nephron and inhibit AVP production. Polyuria then may become apparent when corticosteroid replacement therapy is commenced.

Investigations and Diagnosis Baseline investigation of a child with polyuria and polydipsia should include serum electrolytes, blood urea nitrogen, glucose, calcium, random serum osmolality, hemoglobin A1c (HbA1c), liver function tests, and a complete blood count (CBC). Random urine should be obtained for urine osmolality, urine electrolytes, urinalysis for glucose and protein, urine specific gravity, and microscopy. TORCH titers should be drawn in patients suspected of congenital infections.

An elevated baseline serum sodium and elevated urinary sodium excretion with low urine osmolality suggests diabetes insipidus (CDI or NDI) (13). A urine specific gravity of 1.005 or less and a urine osmolality less than 200 mOsm/kg is the hallmark of diabetes insipidus. Random plasma osmolality generally is greater than 287 mOsm/kg; however, one should keep in mind that young infants generally exhibit a constitutional hyposthenuria. Hypernatremia due to extrarenal hypotonic losses (e.g., gastrointestinal [GI] losses or "third spacing") is distinguished from diabetes insipidus because it is associated with a low urine sodium and maximally concentrated urine (>700 mmol/kg). During interpretation of the laboratory evaluation of a patient suspected of having diabetes insipidus, one should keep in mind the following: 1) the measurement of plasma osmolality may not be as accurate as the measurement of serum sodium in many laboratories, so a single plasma osmolality without an associated serum sodium should be interpreted with caution; 2) patients with diabetes insipidus and normal fluid intake and thirst mechanism have normal basal plasma osmolality and serum sodium; 3) the osmolality of an early morning urine sample obtained at home can be helpful, but it is difficult to interpret without a concomitant serum osmolality; 4) children with CDI (and NDI) can concentrate their urine when in a volume-contracted state (Figure 41-8); and, 5) osmolality or urine specific gravity of a random urine sample can be normal in patients with partial CDI or NDI. Parents of patients suspected of having diabetes insipidus can be prepared to measure input and output at home in oder to confirm the presence of polydipsia and polyuria before an admission for a water-deprivation test is pursued; however, fluid intake should not be restricted until a diagnosis has been made. The 24-hour fluid intake and urinary volume can be determined relatively easily in the older child. Measurement of urinary osmolality

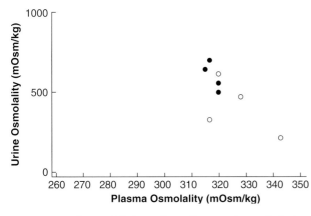

FIGURE 41-8. Urine Osmolality in 2 patients with untreated CDI and NDI. A comparison of Urine and Plasma Osmolalities in a patient with longstanding, untreated CDI (O) and a patient with longstanding, untreated NDI (O). This illustrates the capacity of the kidney to produce relatively concentrated urine when serum osmolality is high and circulating volume is reduced.

TABLE 41-1   Protocol of Water-Deprivation/Desmopressin Test

Preparation
- Fluid given over night before test
- Avoid caffeine
- Weigh patient
- Liase with laboratory before test begins

Dehydration phase
- Draw blood and collect urine for osmolality and electrolyte measurements and urine volume measurement at 8 A.M.
- Restrict fluids—a 4- to 8-hour fast usually will suffice.
- Weigh patient at 2 hourly intervals.
- Collect blood and urine for osmolality and volume measurements at regular intervals—ideally every 2 hours. Assess results as soon as they are available because it may be possible to terminate the test.
- Stop test if weight loss exceeds 5% of starting weight or if thirst becomes intolerable.

Renal desmopressin response
This test can be undertaken separately and does not have to follow the dehydration phase of a water-deprivation test.
- Administer 1-10 μg DDAVP solution intranasally or inject intramuscular, subcutaneous, or intravenous desmopressin (DDAVP) 0.4 μg (<2 years of age) to 1 μg (>2 years of age). Monitor fluid intake carefully because of the potential for hyponatremia in the patient with primary polydipsia. Oral desmopressin 50–200 μg also can be used.
- Collect urine for osmolality and volume with measurement of serum osmolality at regular 4- to 6-hour intervals.

and creatine in a 24-hour urine collection during unrestricted fluid intake would allow determination of total solute excretion (urine osmolality × urinary volume) and differentiate diabetes insipidus from diabetes mellitus or other forms with increased renal solute loss; patients with diabetes insipidus have normal solute excretion (normal solute is 35 mOsm/kg/day in infants and young children and decreases to 20 mOsm/kg/day in older children and adults).

In infants, parents usually are able to assess intake, but measuring urinary output can be challenging. Weighing of diapers can help to gauge fluid output.

Overall, a serum osmolality of greater than 300 mOsm/kg and a urine osmolality of less than 300 mOsm/kg are characteristic of diabetes insipidus; a serum osmolality of less than 270 mOsm/kg and/or a urine osmolality of greater than 600 mOsm/kg make the diagnosis of diabetes insipidus unlikely. When the diagnosis of diabetes insipidus is questionable, a period of observation with documentation of fluid balance and behavior in an inpatient unit can be very helpful.

Water-Deprivation Test The ability of the CNS to make and the kidney to respond to AVP can be investigated by a water-deprivation test (Table 41-1). Care is required in very young children, and it is important to allow free access to fluid before starting fluid restriction and to supervise the patient closely to avoid surreptitious drinking during the test. Vital signs should be monitored throughout the study. The deprivation test should start in the morning so that the child can be supervised adequately, and the laboratory should be aware of the need to provide rapid feedback of urine and plasma osmolalities. A standard 8- to 12-hour deprivation test protocol is detailed in Chapter 49. Test interpretation is outlined on Table 41-2. Plasma osmolality within the normal reference range (280–295 mOsm/kg), combined with a urine osmolality of greater than 750 mOsm/kg during the dehydration phase (or urine:serum osmolality ratio greater than approximately 2.6), excludes significant water imbalance. With prompt feedback, many tests can be terminated in the first few hours. The test also should be stopped prematurely if body weight loss exceeds 5% of the baseline value or if the patient is symptomatic (e.g., pallor, hypotension, and tachycardia).

Water-deprivation test interpretation is usually more straightforward in patients with severe CDI; patients with more subtle defects of AVP production may have equivocal results

TABLE 41-2 Interpretation of Fluid-Deprivation and Desmopressin Tests in Polyuric Patients

Urine Osmolality(mOsm/kg)

After Fluid Deprivation	After Desmopressin	Diagnosis
<300	>750	CDI
<300	<300	NDI
>750	>750	PP
300–750	<750	? Partial CDI, ? partial NDI, ? PP

Note: The majority of children with urine osmolalities of 600 or more at the time of a normal serum osmolality do not have CDI or NDI. PP = primary polydipsia.

at the end of a water-deprivation test (Figure 41-9 and Table 41-2).

Renal Response to Desmopressin Administration Administration of desmopressin (DDAVP) can be used to evaluate maximal renal concentrating capacity and distinguish NDI from CDI; patients with complete or partial CDI show an increase in the urine osmolality with the DDAVP test, whereas patients with NDI show no increase in urine osmolality. The test can be performed either in the morning after an overnight fast or at the end of the water-deprivation test. Sometimes, if investigations confirm diabetes insipidus, an assessment of renal responsiveness can be conducted at a later stage, providing the child with an opportunity to recover and avoiding the need for sample collection in the evening or overnight. DDAVP can be administered at a dose of 10 μg in infants and 20 μg in children intranasally or subcutaneously at a dose of 0.5 μg/m². After emptying the bladder, the patient receives the appropriate dose of DDAVP, and urine is collected hourly, if possible, for 4 hours, with osmolality measured in each urine specimen. In CDI, urine osmolality typically will rise in excess of 600–700 mOsm/kg. Unfortunately, the test does not always neatly distinguish between partial CDI and primary polydipsia.

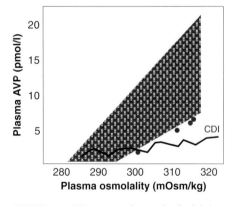

FIGURE 41-9. AVP response to hypertonic saline infusion. Changes in plasma AVP in response to an infusion of 5% saline. The shaded area depicts the range of response in normal individuals. The solid line represents the typical response in a patient with CDI.

Urinary AQP-2 concentrations (i.e., AVP-regulated water channels) are low in patients with CDI (14). While levels have been used as a guide to the renal response to AVP, the assay with appropriate reference ranges is not widely available, so this is primarily a research tool.

Other Investigative Tools

Hypertonic Saline Infusion If a diagnosis has not been reached following the water-deprivation test, then it may be appropriate to conduct a hypertonic saline infusion study to assess the ability of the hypothalamus–pituitary to produce AVP in response to a rising serum osmolality. Hypertonic 5% saline (850 mmol/L) is infused over a period of 2 hours at a rate of 0.05 mL/kg/minute or until a plasma osmolality of 300 mOsm/kg is achieved with AVP measured sequentially (15). Normograms describing the relationship between osmolality and AVP can be used to determine whether a child has CDI. The limited availability of a reliable AVP assay, the relatively large sample volume needed for AVP measurement, and the practical difficulties that may accompany the administration of irritant hypertonic saline solution to children need to be taken into consideration. It is best to avoid this test in the very young. Figure 41-10 demonstrates the normal response of healthy adults and the subnormal AVP diagnostic of CDI. Healthy children may have a more exaggerated AVP response than adults.

DDAVP Trial If it is still unclear whether a child has partial CDI, then some physicians will consider a trial of DDAVP administration. After a period of 2–4 days during which weight, plasma sodium, urine volume, and osmolality are monitored, the patient is given a small dose of oral, intranasal, subcutaneous, or intramuscular desmopressin (DDAVP) daily for about 7–10 days. An initial dose of 50–100 μg by mouth, 2.5–10 μg intranasally, or 0.3–0.5 μg subcutaneously in the young child or 100–200 μg orally, 10 μg intranasally, or 0.5–1 μg subcutaneously in the teenager is appropriate. Patients with CDI can be exquisitely sensitive to DDAVP

initially, so the effects of a first dose need to be established before a second dose is given. Measurements are continued during the desmopressin trial and for a few days after stopping the drug. Patients with CDI will experience an improvement in thirst and polyuria, whereas plasma sodium will remain in the normal range. There will be no clinical or biochemical response in those with NDI.

Further Investigation of the Patient with CDI The cause of CDI needs to be established, although many of the investigations described are likely to have been performed already. Tumor markers (e.g., alpha-fetoprotein and human chorionic gonadotropin) should be measured because they can be elevated in germinomas. An MRI of the pituitary, hypothalamus, and surrounding structures should be performed to look for pituitary and parapituitary masses, craniopharyngioma, germinoma, or pituitary stalk abnormalities. In many patients (70% or more) with CDI, there is loss of the normal hyperintense signal on T1-weighted MRI images of the posterior pituitary, although this may also be a feature of NDI and may be seen in a small minority of healthy subjects (~10%). In CDI, this is due to reduced AVP production and in NDI, to enhanced release. The signal usually will be normal in primary polydipsia. Children with acquired CDI who have a normal MRI at baseline should have serial imaging because of the possibility of evolving disease (16,17). A skeletal survey should be conducted if LCH is suspected. Genetic studies to identify mutations in the precursor AVP molecule (AVP-NPII, chromosome 20p13) or mutations in the gene encoding wolframin (WFS1) on chromosome 4p may be undertaken if familial CDI or Wolfram syndrome is suspected.

Treatment Intact thirst mechanism and significantly increased fluid intake will maintain normal plasma osmolality and prevent hyponatremia in diabetes insipidus patients. The following example shows the high amount of fluids that a patient with diabetes insipidus has to drink to maintain normal plasma osmolality and serum sodium: A patient with diabetes insipidus, maximum urine concentrating ability at 100 mOsm/kg, and a body surfase area of 1 m² would have to drink 5 L of water for his or her kidney to excrete a normal obligate solute load of 500 mOsm/m², as well as 500 mL/m²/day of water to compensate for insensible losses.

Desmopressin Two minor structural alterations to the AVP molecule (see Figure 41-1) result in a synthetic analogue, desmopressin (DDAVP), that has prolonged antidiuretic

Polyuria and Polydipsia

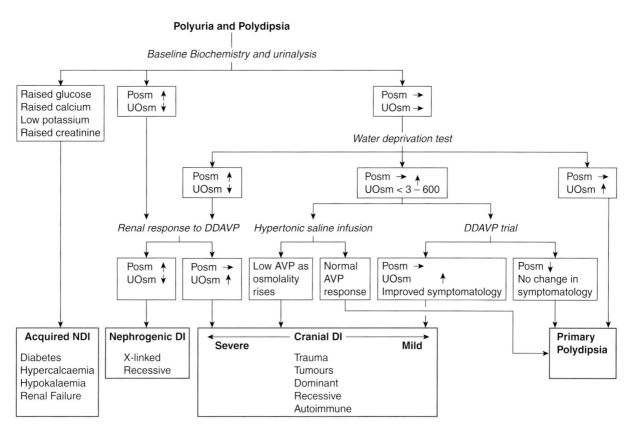

FIGURE 41-10. Flow diagram highlighting the major investigative pathways in patients presenting with polyuria and polydipsia in childhood and adolescence.

action and minimal pressor activity. Desmopressin can be administered orally, intranasally, or parenterally. There are wide individual variations in the doses required to reduce fluid intake to normal (18). When initiating DDAVP therapy, it is safer to start with one bedtime dose and titrate the size and frequency of dosage based on the patient's response to therapy. If the dose is effective but does not last long, the dose should be increased, or a second morning dose should be added.

Daily requirements for the oral preparation in older children vary from 100–1200 μg in two or three divided doses; for the intranasal route, around 2–40 μg, usually in two divided doses; and for the parenteral/subcutaneous route, 0.1–1 μg in one or two divided doses. The onset of action for DDAVP via the parenteral route is a few minutes; for the oral route, 1 hour; and for the intranasal route, 15–30 minutes. Forms for intranasal route administration include a nasal spray pump or a rhinal tube. The nasal spray administers 10 μg per spray. The fixed dose per spray does not allow small adjustments in infants and children who require doses of DDAVP of less than 10 μg. The administration of DDAVP with a rhinal tube requires the drawing of the DDAVP dose into the flexible rhinal tube, placing the tube in the nostril, and blowing the dose through the tube to the nose using

the other end of the rhinal tube. Nasal absorption of DDAVP can be affected by upper respiratory congestion. Patients who have been AVP-depleted typically are very sensitive to DDAVP, and it is wise to start with a low dose that can be increased as necessary. As little as 0.5 μg of the nasal solution administered once daily may suffice in neonates with CDI, and the hospital pharmacy can prepare a manageable volume by diluting standard DDAVP solution. This can then be administered by 1-mL syringe, which will allow a small quantity to be dropped accurately into the supine child's nostrils.

In infants, the risk of hyponatremia during treatment with DDAVP is increased due to their increased fluid intake because they receive all their caloric intake through formula. Oral DDAVP is becoming increasingly popular in infancy and in young children due to the relatively shorter half-life of oral DDAVP compared with the parental or nasal forms, which may reduce the likelihood of overtreatment and hyponatremia (19). DDAVP tablets can be dispersed in water, and a dose of 5–25 μg can be administered once daily and can be increased, as required, to a twice-daily regimen; this is a reasonable starting dose in this age group. The new sublingual "melt" DDAVP formulation may prove to be particularly useful in children with CDI (60- and 120-μg DDAVP melt preparations are ap-

proximately equivalent to 100- and 200-μg DDAVP tablets, respectively). A period of careful observation and monitoring is required as the dose is adjusted. The treatment of small children with diabetes insipidus can be very difficult, with rapid changes in osmolality. It is important for the family to be closely involved from the onset so that they are able to gauge what is an appropriate fluid intake and urine output. It is safer to under- rather than overdose an infant with CDI because regular access to fluid, including water, will allow them to compensate for a relatively high urine output. Dilutional hyponatremia with an associated risk of extrapontine myelinolysis is the only potential hazard with desmopressin administration. The likelihood of hyponatremia can be reduced by allowing a periodic "breakthrough" in the urine output. GI upset may reduce the activity of the orally administered drug. A child with a surface area of 1 m² still will require approximately 800 mL to 1 L of fluid daily despite maximally concentrated urine.

Other Therapies for CDI Children with partial CDI also can be treated with chlorpropramide or carbamazepine. These drugs appear to sensitize the renal tubule to the actions of the remaining endogenous AVP. Chlorpropramide is used in a dose of up to 200–350 mg daily. The impact of this medication on blood glucose levels needs to be taken into consideration. Carbamazepine has been used in a dose of 200 mg once or twice daily. It is important to be aware of the potentiating effect of carbamazepine on DDAVP action in children with CDI and CNS disease who are on this medication to control seizures. These drugs are used rarely now because of the efficacy of DDAVP.

The Child with CDI and Hypothalamic Adipsic Syndrome The child with CDI and adipsia or hypodipsia presents a difficult treatment challenge because the ability both to produce AVP and to osmoregulate by drinking is compromised. Adipsia in children with CDI is usually the effect of a tumor or surgical treatment in the area around the hypothalamus. Management of adipsic patients with CDI, initially in the hospital setting, consists of: 1) minimizing urinary water losses by treating with DDAVP: and, 2) ensuring that daily fluid intake does not exceed urinary and insensible losses. After discharge, frequent electrolyte measurement and daily weights would allow determination of appropriate basal fluid intake to maintain normal water homeostasis (20).

Perioperative Management of Patients with CDI Children with preexisting CDI or those who developed CDI postoperatively due to procedures close to hypothalamic–pituitary area should be managed with short-acting aqueous AVP (half life 5–10 minutes) and fluid restriction or intravenous fluid therapy without DDAVP until they are able to take fluids orally. Intravenous DDAVP should not be used in the acute management of CDI because of the risk of water intoxication due to its long half life (8–12 hours).

The protocol described below is based on the fact that antidiuresis with AVP is essentially an "all or none" phenomenon and uses continuous aqueous AVP infusion to produce a "functional SIADH" state along with fluid restriction and administration of a normal saline solution for initial treatment (21). The protocol is as follows: Aqueous AVP infusion (Pittressin) is started at 0.5 mU/kg/h and titrated upward in 0.5 mU/kg/h increments every 5 to 10 minutes until urinary output decreases to less than 2 mL/kg/h. Once a urinary output of less than 2 mL/kg/h is achieved, the AVP infusion may be adjusted downward. During surgery and perioperatively, normal saline at two-thirds maintenance (approximately 1000 mL/m²/d) is administered to prevent volume overload and hyponatremia, especially in the presence of full antidiuresis; additional normal saline may be given to replace blood loss and maintain hemodynamic stability. Hourly monitoring of urinary output and serum concentrations should be performed until urinary output is controlled, and it then can be changed to every 2 to 4 hours. Of note, chil-

dren, who are euvolemic and in a state of functional SIADH will continue to produce urine (~0.5 mL/kg/h). Anuria in the presence of tachycardia and decreased blood pressure signals hypovolemia and is an indication for additional fluids. Children with known diabetes insipidus, when they are able to take adequate oral fluid intake, should resume DDAVP therapy; children with adequate fluid intake but at risk for developing diabetes insipidus postoperatively should stop both intravenous fluids and AVP infusion and should not start DDAVP until they demonstrate evidence of recurrent polyuria. During the observation period, the fluid input is linked to urine output and calculated insensible loss; weight, serum sodium, and urine osmolality will help to confirm that input is not "driving" urine production. Single doses of DDAVP should be administered when polyuria develops.

In young children at risk for CDI following neurosurgery, fluid therapy without DDAVP may be preferred. This approach allows the postoperative assessment of thirst sensation, diabetes insipidus development, or emergence of the SIADH phase of the triple-phase response to neurosurgical injury. The fluid protocol is as follows: A background 5% dextrose–0.2 N saline infusion (40 mL/m²/h) is used to approximate insensible loss plus the urine production necessary to excrete the average daily solute load (if urine were maximally concentrated). Extra fluid then is administered as 5% dextrose (D₅) if hourly urine output exceeds this infusion rate, up to a maximum (including the baseline infusion) of 120 mL/m²/h. For example, if the urinary output is 50 mL/h, 10 mL (50–40) of the urinary output will be replaced with D₅. With this regimen, the patient with diabetes insipidus is kept in a mildly volume-contracted state (serum sodium in the 150 mEq/L range), allowing the physician to assess thirst, development of diabetes insipidus, or SIADH postoperatively.

Patients with diabetes insipidus who require high volumes of fluids during chemotherapy may be better managed with aqueous AVP as an intravenous drip (0.1 mU/kg/h) or 2.5–10 U intramuscularly or subcutaneously bid/qid prn (22). Whatever the circumstances and strategy employed, the importance of a strict assessment of input and output coupled with regular monitoring of electrolytes every 4 to 6 hours should be emphasized.

Nephrogenic Diabetes Insipidus

Pathophysiology Nephrogenic diabetes insipidus (NDI) is caused by the inability of the renal collecting ducts to absorb water in response to AVP. Urine osmolality is inappro-

priately low and does not increase in response to AVP. NDI can result from genetic defects that reduce the capacity of the kidney to reabsorb water, or it may be secondary to the impact of acquired diseases on renal function. NDI can be inherited through an X-linked recessive mode due to mutations of the gene that encodes the vasopressin V2 receptor (V2-R) in renal collecting duct cells (most frequent cause, accounting for 90% of such cases) or through autosomal inheritance due to mutations in the gene that encodes the water channel protein AQP-2 (approximately 10% of kindreds). As a consequence of one of these defects, the ducts do not respond appropriately to AVP. Normally, AVP is transported in the blood to receptor sites on the basolateral surface of the collecting-duct membrane. Through G protein–adenylate cyclase coupling, activation of the AVP receptor increases cAMP production and stimulates protein kinase A, leading to increased recycling of the protein aquaporin in the plasma membrane. In the presence of AVP stimulus, exocytic insertion of aquaporin into the apical or luminal surface of the tubule cell occurs. Aquaporin enhances water entry into the cell from the lumen. Absence of the AVP receptor does not allow this process to take place, causing inhibition of water uptake and polyuria. Alternatively, defective or absent aquaporin impairs the process in the presence of normal V2-Rs.

Acquired causes of AVP-resistant polyuria and polydipsia include type 1 diabetes mellitus, in which there is a reduction in the osmotic gradient necessary for the action of AVP across the renal tubule, as well as hypercalcemia and hypokalemia due to impaired tubular responses to AVP. Other causes of acquired NDI include chronic renal failure, sickle cell disease, drugs (e.g., lithium, demeclocycline, and amphotericin), and postobstructive uropathy.

Molecular studies of kindreds with X-linked NDI have identified mutations or deletions in the V2-R located on Xq28 (23,24). The V2-R is a classical seven-domain transmembrane protein, and the genetic defects in the V2-R gene map to the extracellular, transmembrane, and intracellular domains. Most are associated with a severe clinical phenotype. Both autosomal recessive and autosomal dominant patterns of inheritance are observed with AQP-2 gene mutations (mapped on chromosome 12q). Autosomal dominant mutations cause NDI because the abnormal gene product interferes with the actions of protein encoded by the normal gene in a dominant-negative manner (25,26). Patients with AQP-1 defects are unable to concentrate urine maximally but not to a point where they develop polyuria (27).

Clinical Features Most of the affected males with the X-linked form of NDI present within the first 2.5 years of life. Main symptoms at clinical presentation include polyuria, polydipsia, hypernatremic dehydration, vomiting and anorexia, failure to thrive, unexplained fever, and constipation. Failure to thrive reflects the very low maximum urine osmolality in most children with this disorder, in whom the desire to drink exceeds the desire for nutrition. Patients with NDI may have a dilated renal tract and be susceptible to urinary tract infection. Severe hydronephrosis with a small rupture of the urinary tract after a minor trauma and episodes of acute urine retention have been described. Height standard deviation (SD) scores for age remain below the 50th centile in the majority of patients, whereas weight for height SD scores show catch-up after several years of being underweight. Most patients are found to have normal intelligence; this is in contrast to the belief that mental retardation is the most frequent long-term sequela of NDI. Except for a possibly milder phenotype in patients with an AVPR2 G185C mutation, no clear relationship between clinical and genetic data has been found (28).

Interestingly, some heterozygous females also have polyuria and polydipsia, which may reflect differences in X-inactivation pattern within the nephron (29). Patients with the autosomal form of NDI present during infancy with similar symptomatology (30). Polyuria with episodes of hypernatremic dehydration and rapid changes in extra- and intracellular osmolality may affect neurodevelopment in patients with either form of NDI. Breast-fed infants affected with NDI may present later than those who are bottle-fed because of the reduced osmotic load of breast milk.

Investigations and Diagnosis If the patient is suspected to have NDI, a 24-hour urine volume and *ad libitum* fluid intake should be documented. Urinalysis for microorganisms, glucose, and protein is important to exclude infection, diabetes mellitus, and a tubuloglomerulopathy. Measurement of electrolytes, calcium, blood urea nitrogen (BUN), and creatinine and review of drug history will exclude aquired causes of NDI. A baseline serum sodium and osmolality may be normal or raised in untreated NDI. Urine osmolality needs to be compared with a concomitant serum sample because children with NDI can concentrate their urine when in a volume-contracted state (see Figure 41-8).

Further Investigation of Patients with Suspected NDI

Water-Deprivation Test Interpretation is usually relatively straightforward in patients with the genetic forms of NDI. Serum osmolality is high normal or elevated in the presence of dilute urine at a relatively early stage of the test. Measurement of plasma AVP may help (elevated values for a given urine/serum osmolality), although the diagnosis of NDI is usually established before the assay result is available.

Renal Response to Desmopressin Administration Patients with X-linked NDI will not respond to DDAVP administration, so urine remains dilute, typically with an osmolality less than 200 mOsm.

Other Investigative Tools

Hypertonic Saline Infusion This investigation is rarely required. Some patients with NDI will have AVP values in the normal reference range initially, although values may be inappropriately elevated for a given urine osmolality. As serum osmolality rises, AVP levels also are more likely to be abnormally high.

DDAVP 'Trial' There will be a minimal or typically no clinical or biochemical response in those with the genetic forms of NDI because DDAVP cannot bind to the V2-R.

Renal Tract Imaging Patients with NDI may have a dilated urinary tract, and a renal ultrasound examination should be conducted in all these patients (31).

Genetic Testing Genetic testing is available for both X-linked and autosomal forms of NDI.

Treatment Effective treatment of NDI is still challenging, except for those forms which are drug-induced or related to metabolic disorders. Withdrawal of the drug or correction of the metabolic disturbance often reverses the renal resistance to AVP, but correction may take a number of weeks.

The treatment consists of prevention of dehydration by ensuring *ad libitum* fluid intake and by decreasing polyuria through reduction of urinary solute load by salt restriction combined with administration of a thiazide diuretic (e.g., hydrochlorothiazide 3 mg/kg/d). Thiazide diuretics inhibit the NaCl cotransporter in the distal convoluted tubule. Enhanced sodium excretion leads to a reduced circulating volume and a reduction in glomerular filtration rate (GFR). The reduced GFR enhances proximal tubular sodium and water reabsorption. A reduced urine output is the consequence of the fall in sodium and water delivery to the collecting ducts. There is also recent evidence that thiazides may increase water resorption in the collecting ducts directly. Thiazides may need to be administered with a potassium-sparing agent such as amiloride (0.3 mg/kg/d) (32). This approach can reduce urine output by 40% in infants. A similar reduction in urine flow may be achieved with the prostaglandin synthetase inhibitor indomethacin given in doses of 1.5–3.0 mg/kg. The addition of high-dose desmopressin to the combination of a thiazide and indomethacin may be considered in some patients and may reduce urine output still further.

Primary Polydipsia

Pathophysiology Primary polydipsia is an uncommon clinical disorder characterized by compulsive water drinking in the absence of a physiological stimulus to drink. Psychiatric illness or hypothalamic defects leading to an increased thirst are uncommon causes in children. The excessive water drinking suppresses AVP secretion and induces polyuria. In primary polydipsia, the polydipsia precedes and is the cause of the polyuria, in contrast to CDI or NDI, where the polyuria precedes and is the cause of the polydipsia. The synthesis of, secretion of, and nephron sensitivity to ADH and the osmoreceptor response are all intact. Primary polydipsia is well tolerated unless hyponatremia supervenes.

Investigations and Diagnosis The hallmark of this disease is plasma hypoosmolarity ($\leq$270 mOsm/L) in the presence of polyuria and the ability to form a maximally concentrated urine when deprived of water or when ADH is administered. Patients usually remain normonatremic despite large fluid intakes but eventually may develop hyponatremia if water intake exceeds 10 L/m^2/d in children and 4 L/m^2/d in neonates due to following mechanisms: 1) obligatory "sodium loss" in the large volumes of urine voided; 2) decreased renal medulla hypertonicity due to washout of the renal medulla by the large volumes of water; and, 3) concomitant nonosmoregulated AVP release. A clue for primary polydipsia can be a dramatic reduction in fluid intake accompanying the switch from flavored 'juice' to water (patients with CDI or NDI will continue to consume large quantities of water).

Water-Deprivation Test A healthy, young child with pronounced daytime polydipsia and low or low-normal sodium at baseline who has minimal weight loss, decreased urinary output, and maintenance of a normal serum sodium and osmolality on deprivation testing most likely has primary polydipsia.

A normal or high-normal serum osmolality and a urine osmolality of less than 600 mOsm/kg are not uncommon following an 8-hour fast in a child who has primary polydipsia. This is probably so because after prolonged polyuria of any cause, the renal interstitial solute is "washed out," resulting in some degree of renal resistance to AVP action due to reduction of the osmotic gradient across the distal renal tubular cell.

DDAVP Trial Children with primary polydipsia may continue to drink, in contrast to those with CDI, and therefore are at risk of hyponatremia if their fluid intake is not curtailed. If primary polydipsia is a possible diagnosis, then it is wise to conduct this assessment in the hospital so that fluid balance and behavior can be monitored carefully and so that desmopressin can be stopped if hyponatremia develops.

Treatment The management of primary polydipsia consists of reducing water intake, searching for the underlying psychological or psychiatric causes, and beginning behavioral modification.

SYNDROME OF INAPPROPRIATE ADH SECRETION

Pathophysiology Hyponatremia usually reflects sodium loss or water overload. Inappropiate elevation of AVP (SIADH) is one of the least common causes of hyponatremia in children and is characterized by nonosmotically driven elevation of AVP in the absence of hemodynamic disturbance or any other nonosmotic stimulus for AVP release. An example of appropriate elevation of AVP in response to nonosmotic stimulus and in the presence of hyponatremia is the case of intravascular volume depletion secondary to gastroenteritis, where the baroregulated AVP production compensates for the hypovolemia by an increase in water retention.

The hyponatremia of SIADH is secondary to increased total-body water with decreased total-body sodium. Accumulation of excess water due to inappropriately elevated AVP results in suppression of plasma renin activity and aldosterone and stimulation of atrial natriuretic peptide (ANP) production in an effort to prevent further volume expansion; the preceding changes in aldosterone and ANP secretion explain the low and sometimes falling sodium in the circulation of the euvolemic patient with SIADH, in whom the urinary sodium excretion is increased (typically greater than 20–30 mEq/L).

Most pediatric patients have abnormal or inappropriate AVP production in association with an acute insult. Children at risk for SIADH therefore include those with CNS disorders (e.g., encephalitis, tuberculous meningitis, intracranial tumors and bleeds, and after hypothalamic–pituitary surgery) and children with pulmonary disease (e.g., asthma, cystic fibrosis, and empyema) and malignancies. SIADH also may be precipitated by drugs such

as vinblastin, vincristin, carbamezapine, chlorpropamide, and tricyclic antidepressants. Patients with SIADH but without an obvious cause may have an underlying intracranial neoplasm. Activating mutations of the AVP receptor with associated inappropriate AVP production and hyponatremia (i.e., nephrogenic syndrome of inappropriate antidiuresis) have been reported (33).

Clinical Features Abnormal AVP production as a part of SIADH should be considered in sick, hyponatremic patients who are not hypovolemic (i.e., have normal blood pressure and pulse without orthostatic changes), moist mucous membranes, normal skin turgor, no edema, and no polyuria. Symptoms of SIADH depend on the level of hyponatremia and the rate at which it develops. Symptoms are rare when the serum sodium is above 125 mEq/L. At a serum sodium concentration ranging between 125 and 130 mEq/L, predominant symptoms are gastrointestinal (e.g., nausea and vomiting). Acute onset of hyponatremia (in less than 48 hours) and a serum sodium concentration of less than 120 mEq/L may present with lethargy, disorientation, generalized seizures, reversible ataxia, papilledema, hypoactive reflexes, myoclonus, psychosis, and coma due to subsequent brain edema. In patients with SIADH and acute hyponatremia, the brain's adaptation to hypotonicity (a decrease in intracellular organic osmolytes) is not completed, making these patients prone to severe cerebral edema (34). Children who have gradual onset of hyponatremia due to SIADH or onset of hyponatremia longer than 48 hours (chronic hyponatremia) are usually asymptomatic due to the existing brain adaptation to low plasma osmolality.

Biochemical Findings Patients with hyponatremia due to SIADH have low plasma osmolality (<280 mOsm/kg) low anion gap, high urinary osmolality (>200mOsm/kg in the presence of hyponatremia; normal response of the kidney in presence of hyponatremia is a maximally diluted urine to values less than 100 mOsm/Kg), a relatively high urinary sodium (>20–30 mEq/L), increased fractional

sodium excretion in the urine (>1%), low renin and normal aldosterone levels, low to normal potassium levels normal thyroid function tests, and normal glucocorticoid function; BUN and serum uric acid levels tend to fall because of plasma dilution and increased excretion of nitrogenous products (Table 41-3).

Differential Diagnosis of Hyponatremia due to SIADH and Other Causes Patients with hyponatremia due to renal salt wasting are distinguished from patients with SIADH because they present with weight loss, elevated BUN increased anion gap, and elevated aldosterone and renin, in addition to high urinary sodium and increased fractional sodium excretion in the urine. Patients with isolated aldosterone deficiency or congenital adrenal hyperplasia due to enzymatic defects that affect aldosterone synthesis (e.g., 3β-hydroxy-steroid dehydrogenase deficiency [3β-HSD], 21-hydroxylase deficiency [21-OHD], and lipoid adrenal hyperplasia) differ from patients with SIADH or renal disease because they have hyperkalemia, elevated renin, and low aldosterone levels, as well as characteristic changes of adrenal steroid concentrations (see Chapter 27).

Hyponatremia associated with elevated renin and aldosterone, low urinary sodium (<10 mEq/L), and hypovolemia suggests extrarenal causes, in particular GI losses and "third spacing" of fluids. Hyponatremia with elevated renin and aldosterone, low urinary sodium (<10 mEq/L), and hypervolemia suggests disorders with decreased effective plasma volume, as seen in congestive heart failure, liver and kidney failure, and nephrotic syndrome. Patients with hypothyroidism or glucocorticoid deficiency due to secondary adrenal insufficiency have impaired free water clearance and present with hyponatremia and euvolemia.

Of note, elevated concentrations of triglycerides and hyperglycemia may cause factitious hyponatremia. During hyperglycemia, serum sodium concentration decreases 1.6 mEq/L for every 100 mg/dL increase in blood glucose

TABLE 41-3   Diagnostic Criteria of SIADH

- Hyponatremia (serum sodium <135 mEq/L)
- Decreased plasma osmolality (<280 mOsm/kg)
- Inappropriately elevated urinary osmolality (>100 mOsm/kg water) in presence of hyponatremia and decreased serum osmolality
- Elevated urine sodium concentration (>20–30 mEq/L) or increased fractional sodium excretion (>1%) during normal sodium and water intake
- Clinical euvolemia (absence of peripheral edema, congestive heart failure, cirrhosis, nephrotic syndrome, intravascular volume depletion)
- Normal renal, adrenal, and thyroid function

TABLE 41-4   Differentiation of SIADH versus SWS

SIADH		SWS
High	AVP	Low
Low	Serum uric acid	Normal
Low and concentrated	Urine output	Increased and dilute
Low	Aldosterone/renin	Low
20–30	Urinary Na concentration	40–100
Low	Hematocrit	High
Low	BUN/creatinine	High

concentration. Patients with severe hypothyroidism may develop hyponatremia because thyroid hormone is required for normal free water clearance.

Differentiating SIADH from Cerebral Salt Wasting Cerebral salt wasting syndrome (CSWS) is defined by the development of excessive natriuresis and subsequent hyponatremic dehydration in patients with intracranial disease. Differentiation of CSWS from SIADH, another common cause of hyponatremia in this setting, is critical to initiating appropriate therapy (Table 41-4).

The exact mechanism underlying renal salt wasting in this syndrome remains unclear. Excess of ANP or of the similar peptide brain natriuretic peptide (BNP) may be the primary underlying mechanism accounting for hyponatremia in patients with CNS lesions, hydrocephalus, or CNS surgery. Patients secreting excess ANP or BNP therefore will have excess renal sodium loss in the absence of primary renal pathology. The associated hyponatremia usually can be differentiated from SIADH by the presence of a marked natriuresis (urinary sodium typically > 100 mEq/L), polyuria, and hypovolemia. Patients with CSWS demonstrate orthostatic hypotension and have dry mucous membranes with weight loss and a negative fluid balance with increased anion gap and hypokalemia. Creatinine/BUN and hematocrit tend to be raised. AVP levels are low. Renin and aldosterone values usually are "paradoxically" low for a hypovolemic, sodium-depleted child. This presumably reflects an inhibitory effect of ANP/BNP. In contrast, patients with SIADH have euvolemia, elevated ANP levels but less natridiuresis, moist mucous membranes, weight gain, decreased hematocrit, BUN, and creatinine levels, and elevated AVP levels.

Management of the patient with SIADH involves fluid restriction, whereas the patient with cerebral salt wasting requires liberal quantities of isotonic saline. The potential for diagnostic confusion is self-evident, and the regular assessment of clinical signs and biochemistry will help to ensure that treatment is having the desired effect.

Treatment The cause of SIADH needs to be identified and managed. At the same time, a degree of fluid restriction is introduced to normalize serum sodium concentrations. Patients with chronic SIADH are treated by restriction of their oral fluid intake to 1000 mL/m^2; 500 mL/m^2 is needed for the excretion of a normal daily obligate renal solute loss of 500 mOsm/m^2 when urine is maximally concentrated (urine osmolality of 1000 mOsm/kg), plus another 500 mL/m^2 to account for insensible losses. In infants, in whom a fluid restriction may not provide adequate calories for growth, demeclocycline may be added (which causes nephrogenic diabetes insipidus by inhibiting transepithelial water transport). Salt administration is not effective in treating patients with SIADH because they have suppressed aldosterone and elevated ANP concentrations, resulting in natriuresis of the administered sodium.

Emergency Treatment In all symptomatic cases of hyponatremia in children, treatment should be implemented immediately, and water should be restricted (see Chapter 1). However, the aggressiveness of treatment depends on whether the episode of hyponatremia is acute or chronic. If hyponatremia is acute, rapid correction with 3% hypertonic saline (500 mmol/L) at 1–2 mL/kg/h for 2–3 hours should be initiated. Saline infusion should be stopped as soon as the patient becomes asymptomatic, regardless of the degree of hyponatremia. Electrolytes should be measured and the patient reassessed every 2 hours to ensure that the serum sodium concentration rises by no more than 10 mEq/L every 24 hours or 0.5 mEq/L/h. If the hyponatremia is chronic, hypertonic saline treatment should be implemented only until the serum sodium concentration is raised enough to correspond to an improvement in mental status. Particularly in patients with chronic hyponatremia, an overly rapid correction can result in demyelination syndrome or central pontine myelinosis (CPM) (35). CPM is characterized by spastic quadriparesis, pseudobulbar palsy, lethargy, behavioral changes, and al-

terations in cognition. In 10% of cases, myelinosis can be extrapontine, presenting with ataxia and movement disorders. CPM symptoms may occur 2–3 days after correction of hyponatremia, and the prognosis is variable (36). The risk of CPM is less in the reversal of acute hyponatremia than in the reversal of chronic hyponatremia.

Furosemide (1 mg/kg) may be used in conjunction with isotonic or hypertonic saline because it helps to maintain urine output and blocks secretion of ADH. However, in the presence of risk factors for CPM (e.g., hypokalemia, liver disease, malnutrition, and large burns), correction should be restricted to 10 mEq/L per 24 hours.

NEPHROGENIC SYNDROME OF INAPPROPIATE ANTIDIURESIS (NSIAD)

NSIAD is an X-linked disorder caused by gain-of-function mutations in the gene encoding the vasopressin V2 receptor with a clinical picture consistent with chronic SIADH but who have undetectable AVP levels. Affected patients have decreased serum osmolality, hyponatremia with inappropiately increased urine osmolality and urinary sodium, low or suppressed renin and normal aldosterone levels due to euvolemia. Female carriers seem not to be affected (37).

REFERENCES

1. King LS, Yasui M. Aquaporins and disease: lessons from mice to humans. *Trends Endocrinol Metab.* 2002;13:355–360.
2. Oddie S, Richmond S, Coulthard M. Hypernatremic dehydration and breast feeding: A population study. *Arch Dis Child.* 2001;85:318–320.
3. Robertson GL. Disorders of water balance. In: Brook CGD, Hindmarsh PC, eds. *Clinical Pediatric Endocrinology,* 3d ed. Malden, MA: Blackwell Science; 2001:193.
4. Willcutts MD, Felner E, White PC. Autosomal recessive familial neurohypophyseal diabetes insipidus with continued secretion of mutant weakly active vasopressin. *Hum Mol Genet.* 1999;8:1303–1307.
5. Wahlstrom JT, Fowler MJ, Nicholson WE, et al. A novel mutation in the preprovasopressin gene identified in a kindred with autosomal dominant neurohypophyseal diabetes insipidus. *J Clin Endocrinol Metab.* 2004;89:1963–1968.
6. Strom TM, Hortnagel K, Hofmann S, et al. Diabetes insipidus, diabetes mellitus, optic atrophy and deafness (DIDMOAD) caused by mutations in a novel gene (wolframin) coding for a predicted transmembrane protein. *Hum Mol Genet.* 1998;7:2021–2028.
7. Yagi H, Nagashima K, Miyake H, et al. Familial congenital hypopituitarism with central diabetes insipidus. *J Clin Endocrinol Metab.* 1994;78:884–889.

8. Wang LC, Cohen ME, Duffner PK. Etiologies of central diabetes insipidus in children. *Pediatr Neurol.* 1994;11:273–277.

9. Maghnie M, Cosi G, Genovse E, et al. Central diabetes insipidus in children and young adults. *N Engl J Med.* 2000;343:998–1007.

10. Maghnie M. Diabetes isipidus. *Horm Res.* 2003;59:42–54.

11. Pivonello R, De Bellis A, Faggiano A, et al. Central diabetes insipidus and autoimmunity: Relationship between the occurrence of antibodies to arginine vasopressin-secreting cells and clinical, immunological, and radiological features in a large cohort of patients with central diabetes insipidus of known and unknown etiology. *Journal of Clinical Endocrinol Metab.* 2003;88:1629–1636.

12. Nijenhuis M, van den Akker ELT, Zalm R, et al. Familial neurohypohysial diabetes insipidus in a large Dutch kindred: Effect of the onset of diabetes on growth in children and cell biological defects of the mutant vasopressin prohormone. *J Clin Endocrinol Metab.* 2001;86:3410–3420.

13. Richman RA, Post EM, Notman DN, et al. Simplifying the diagnosis of diabetes insipidus in children. *Am J Dis Child.* 1981;135:839–841.

14. Saito T, Ishikawa S, Ito T, et al. Urinary excretion of aquaporin-2 water channel differentiates psychogenic polydipsia from central diabetes insipidus. *J Clin Endocrinol Metab.* 1999;84:2235–2237.

15. Angelica M, Acerini CL, Cheetham TD, et al. Hypertonic saline test for the investigation of posterior pituitary function. *Arch Dis Child.* 1998;79:431–434.

16. Mootha SL, Barkovich AJ, Grumbach MM, et al. Idiopathic hypothalamic diabetes insipidus, pituitary stalk thickening, and the occult intracranial germinoma in children and adolescents. *J Clin Endocrinol Metab.* 1997;82:1362–1367.

17. Leger J, Velasquez A, Garel C, et al. Thickened pituitary stalk on magnetic resonance imaging in children with central diabetes insipidus. *J Clin Endocrinol Metab.* 1999;84:1954–1960.

18. Boulgourdjian EM, Martinez AS, Ropelato MG, et al. Oral desmopressin treatment of central diabetes insipidus in children. *Acta Paediatr.* 1997;86;1261–1262.

19. Rizzo V, Albanese A, Stanhope R. Morbidity and mortality associated with vasopressin replacement therapy in children. *J Pediatr Endocrinol.* 2001;14:861–867.

20. Ball SG, Vaidja B, Baylis PH. Hypothalamic adipsic syndrome: Diagnosis and management. *Clin Endocrinol (Oxf).* 1997;47: 405–409.

21. Wise-Faberowski L, Soriano-Sulpicio G, Ferrari L, et al. Perioperative management of diabetes insipidus in children. *J Neuroosurg Anesthesiol.* 2004;16:14.

22. Bryant WP, O'Marcaigh AS, Legder GA, et al. Aqueous vasopressin infusion during chemotherapy in patients with diabetes insipidus. *Cancer.* 1994;74:2589.

23. Bichet DG, Birnbaumer M, Lonergan M, et al. Nature and recurrence of AVPR2 mutations in X-linked nephrogenic diabetes insipidus. *Am J Hum Genet.* 1994;55:278–286.

24. Pasel K, Schulz A, Timmermann K, et al. Functional characterization of the molecular defects causing nephrogenic diabetes insipidus in eight families. *J Clin Endocrinol Metab.* 2000;85:1703–1710.

25. Hochberg Z, Lieburg AV, Even L, et al. Autosomal recessive nephrogenic diabetes insipidus caused by an aquaporin-2 mutation. *J Clin Endocrinol Metab.* 1997;82:686–689.

26. Mulders SM, Bichet DG, Rijss JPL, et al. An aquaporin-2 water channel mutant which causes autosomal dominant nephrogenic diabetes insipidus is retained in the Golgi complex. *J Clin Invest.* 1998; 102:57–66.

27. King LS, Choi M, Fernandez PC, et al. Defective urinary concentrating ability due to a complete deficiency of aquaporin-1. *N Engl J Med.* 2001;345:175–179.

28. van Lieburg AF, Knoers NV, Monnens LAH. Clinical presentation and follow-up of 30 patients with congenital nephrogenic diabetes insipidus. *J Am Soc Nephrol.* 1999;10: 1958–1964.

29. Van Lieburg AF, Verdijk MAJ, Schoute F, et al. Clinical phenotype of nephrogenic diabetes insipidus in females heterozygous for a vasopressin type 2 receptor mutation. *Hum Genet.* 1995;96:70–78.

30. van Lieburg AF, Verdijk MAJ, Knoers VVAM, et al. Patients with autosomal nephrogenic diabetes insipidus homozygous for mutations in the aquaporin 2 water-channel gene. *Am J Hum Genet.* 1994;55:648–652.

31. Shalev H, Romanovsky I, Knoers NV, et al. Bladder function impairment in aquaporin-2 defective nephrogenic diabetes insipidus. *Nephrol Dialysis Transplant.* 2004;19: 608–613.

32. Kirchlechner V, Loller DY, Seidl R, et al. Treatment of nephrogenic diabetes insipidus with hydrochlorothiazide and amiloride. *Arch Dis Child.* 1999;80:548–552.

33. Feldman BJ, Rosenthal SM, Vargas GA, et al. Nephrogenic syndrome of inappropriate antidiuresis. *N Engl J Med.* 2005; 352:1884–1890.

34. Sterns RH, Baer J, Ebersol S, et al. Organic osmolytes in acute hyponatremia. *Am J Physiol.* 1993;264:F833–836.

35. Karp BI, Laureno R. Pontine and extrapontine myelinolysis: A neurological disorder following rapid correction of hyponatremia. *Medicine (Baltimore)* 1993;72:359–373.

36. Verbalis JG, Martinez AJ. Neurological and neuropathological sequelae of correction of chronic hyponatremia. *Kidney Int.* 1991;39:1274–1282.

37. Feldman BJ, Rosenthal SM, Vargas GA, et al. Nephrogenic syndrome of inappropiate antiduresis. *New Eng. J. Med.* 2005; 35:1884–1890.

CHAPTER 42

Disorders of Membrane Transport

Karl S. Roth, MD

Disorders of membrane transport are perhaps the least well-recognized group of human genetic disorders, and study of the diseases comprising this category has contributed as much or more to our understanding of cell biology and metabolism as any other group of disorders discussed in this book. Indeed, one might make the cogent argument that it was one of these disorders that literally defined the term *inborn errors of metabolism* when Dr. Archibald Garrod introduced the phrase in 1908. In his Croonian Lecture to the members of the Royal Academy, Garrod proposed that there is a group of disorders, each one familial in nature, deriving from a specific abnormality of metabolism of a particular compound. As proof of his hypothesis, he offered examples of four distinct disorders, of which one was the membrane-transport disorder cystinuria.

It also should be recognized that the field of pharmacology is greatly beholden to our study of disorders of membrane transport, which has helped to shape the design of drugs such as calcium channel blockers, proton pump inhibitors, and receptor-blocking agents. Finally, it should be mentioned that the increased understanding of the biochemical composition and topology of cell membranes deriving from studies of these diseases has greatly informed investigations of acquired immune-deficiency syndrome (AIDS), as well as the development of antibiotic and antiviral agents. Our understanding of the pathophysiology of many diseases of the central nervous system has been furthered by knowledge of membrane biology that had its origins in investigations of transport disorders. Out of all these studies, two fundamental principles of membrane transport have emerged: membrane transport carriers have a substrate-binding specificity very much like enzymes, and in order to operate against a concentration gradient, there must be an energy source to drive the system.

Each of the disorders in this family is substrate-specific and usually is manifested by abnormally high levels of excretion in urine and/or stool of particular biological materials. This specificity gives the first clue to the underlying genetic nature of these disorders because biological specificity typically is based on the tertiary–quaternary structure of proteins, whose synthesis is genetically directed. The proteins involved in the group of transport disorders normally function to convey substrate either into or out of the cell or cellular organelles and thus must be located physically at or within the membrane. In fact, these proteins have different "domains," some of which are located at cell surfaces, either inner or outer, and others of which are literally embedded within the bilayer structure. As a group, membrane-transport disorders generally are monogenetic with a pattern of autosomal re-

cessive transmission. As with all general rules, there are a few exceptions to this statement. Some (e.g., cystic fibrosis) often have devastating consequences for the affected individual, whereas others, such as renal tubular glycosuria, are harmless variations of normal, generally discovered by accident.

DISORDERS OF RENAL HYDROGEN ION TRANSPORT

Disorders of renal hydrogen ion transport are generally thought of as renal tubular acidosis (RTA); the sine qua non of this term is a systemic acidosis (see Figure 42-1) that is

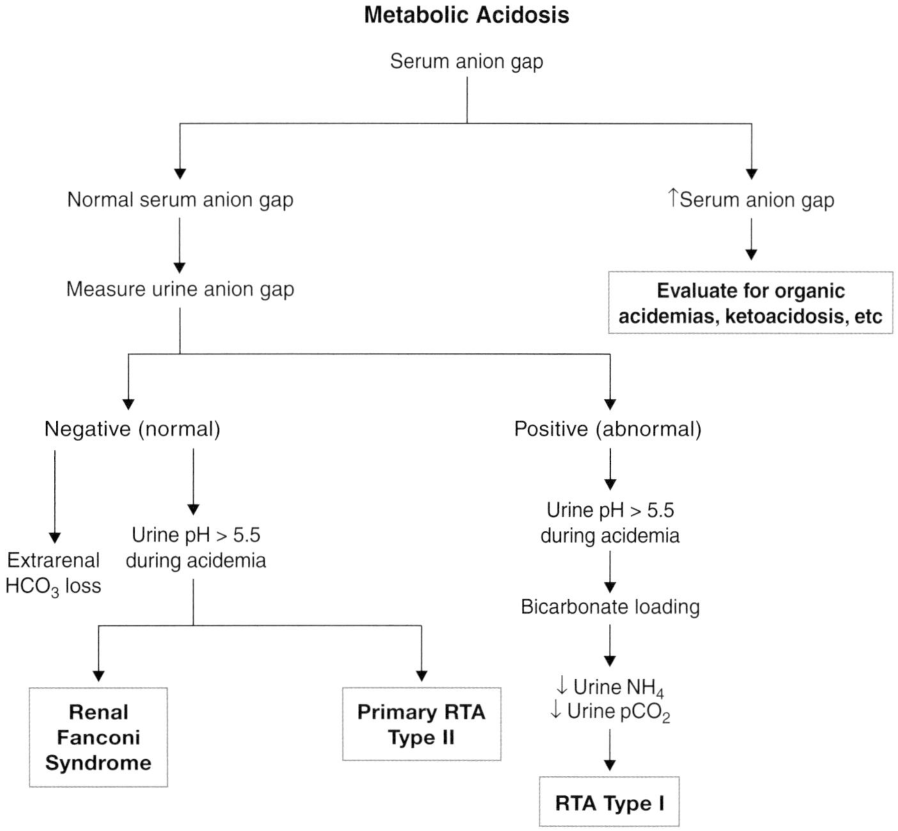

Metabolic Acidosis

Serum anion gap

Normal serum anion gap / ↑Serum anion gap

Normal serum anion gap → Measure urine anion gap

↑Serum anion gap → **Evaluate for organic acidemias, ketoacidosis, etc**

Negative (normal) / Positive (abnormal)

Negative (normal):
- Extrarenal HCO₃ loss
- Urine pH > 5.5 during acidemia

→ **Renal Fanconi Syndrome** / **Primary RTA Type II**

Positive (abnormal):
- Urine pH > 5.5 during acidemia
- Bicarbonate loading
- ↓ Urine NH₄, ↓ Urine pCO₂

→ **RTA Type I**

FIGURE 42-1. The presence of an anion gap, calculated as $AG = ([Na^+]) - ([Cl^-] + [HCO_3^-])$, permits an important diagnostic distinction in evaluating hypokalemic acidosis. If $AG \geq 16$, an immediate investigation should begin for organic acidemias or ketoacidosis from other sources, such as diabetes mellitus or toxic ingestion, etc. If the AG is normal, measurement of the urine anion gap will help in distinguishing between type I RTA and primary or secondary type II RTA.

Disorders Renal Hydrogen Ion Transport

AT-A-GLANCE

Disorders of renal hydrogen ion transport generally are grouped as renal tubular acidosis (RTA). As a group, they are defined clinically as conditions in which the urine pH is inappropriately high in relation to the blood pH, suggesting an inability of the kidney to acidify the urine adequately. Chief clinical manifestations are chronic, systemic acidosis accompanied by growth failure, rickets, muscle weakness, constipation, and nephrocalcinosis in type I. Type II generally is associated with a primary underlying disorder. Adequate alkali replacement is the chief form of therapy. The disorders, when primary, generally have a good prognosis; prognosis for an associated type II RTA depends on the nature of the underlying problem.

TYPES	OCCURRENCE	GENE	LOCUS	OMIM
Type I (distal)				
(AD)	N/A	SLC4A1	17q21-q22	179800
(AR)	N/A	ATPVOA4	7q33-q34	602722
(AR + deafness)	N/A	1ATP6V1B	2cen-q13	267300
Type II (proximal)	N/A	SLC4A4	4q21	603345

FORM	FINDINGS	CLINICAL PRESENTATION	
		BIRTH	CHILDHOOD & ADOLESCENCE
Type I (distal)	↑ pH (U) (6–7) ↓ K, bicarb (B) (10–15 mM) Cl (B), ↓ NH₄ (U) ↑ K, Ca (U) ↑ Urine calcium ↓ citrate (U)	Normal at birth; failure to thrive in first 2–3 months; may be tachypneic; may experience constipation; rickets frequently occurs along with nephrocalcinosis; systemic acidosis may be life-threatening	Vomiting and constipation are common; growth is poor; weakness may develop; long-term nephrocalcinosis may cause renal failure; in some patients sensorineural hearing loss may develop
Type II (proximal)	↑ pH (U) (7–7.5) ↓ K, bicarb (B) (15–20 mM) ↑ Cl (B), NI NH₄ (U) ↓ K (U), NI, Ca (U) ± NI citrate (U)	Persistent mild to moderate; hyperchloremic acidosis; vomiting, decreased caloric intake with growth impairment; constipation may occur together with polyuria	Delayed bone age; rickets or osteomalacia; hypokalemia with constipation and polyuria; nephrolithiasis, nephrocalcinosis rarely occur rickets or osteomalacia

Renal Fanconi Syndrome

The renal Fanconi syndrome is the clinical consequence of a generalized proximal renal tubular transport dysfunction. Hence a substantial proportion of those filtered molecules that normally are reabsorbed by the proximal tubule with great efficiency escape into the urine in increased amounts. These include bicarbonate, glucose, amino acids, phosphate, sodium, and calcium, among many. Hence the clinical consequences of the renal Fanconi syndrome are related to loss of these compounds; chief among these are type II RTA and rickets. Appearance of a primary renal Fanconi syndrome is quite rare, whereas most cases are secondary to an underlying genetic or acquired cause. These include entities such as infantile cystinosis, hereditary tyrosinemia, heavy-metal toxicity, etc.

TYPES	OCCURRENCE	GENE	LOCUS	OMIM
Primary	Very rare	N/A	15q15.3	134600
Secondary	Majority of cases	See Table 42-1	See Table 42-1	N/A

FORM	FINDINGS	BIRTH	CLINICAL PRESENTATION CHILDHOOD & ADOLESCENCE
Primary	$\uparrow$ pH (U); $\downarrow$ pH (B) $\downarrow$ Ca, K (B) $\downarrow$ Pi (B), $\uparrow$ glucose (U) $\uparrow$ amino acids (U)	Typically not clinically detectable	Gradual onset of RTA type II, glucosuria, aminoaciduria, phosphaturia, growth failure, proteinuria, hypokalemia, D-resistant rickets, renal function remains stable in childhood, occasionally declines in adults
Secondary	All as above, except may be reversible with treatment of under-lying disorder	Depends on primary disorder (genetic vs. acquired)	As in the primary form, a slow evolution occurs; no information available as to order of appearance In many cases (e.g., cystinosis) renal failure invariably occurs with time

Cystinosis

Cystinosis is defined separately here because it is among the most frequent underlying causes of secondary Fanconi syndrome but is not manifested as either failure to absorb cystine or an abnormal loss of cystine in urine. Rather, it is a membrane-transport defect manifested at the level of impaired egress of cystine from the lysosome. Thus, in tissues throughout the body (e.g., conjunctivae, thyroid, liver, kidney, and intestinal epithelium), there is on-going lysosomal cystine accumulation that eventually impairs parenchymal function. Earliest and most severe involvement occurs in the renal proximal tubule, causing metabolic acidosis (RTA type II), that is, glucosuria, aminoaciduria, phosphaturia, and polyuria.

With longer-term involvement, destruction of the renal parenchyma leads to an inability to add a 1 α-hydroxyl group to 25-hydroxycholecalciferol, causing vitamin D–resistant rickets. Early diagnosis improves the therapeutic result from use of oral cysteamine treatment, proven to delay and in some patients potentially prevent glomerular involvement.

TYPES	OCCURRENCE	GENE	LOCUS	OMIM
Infantile nephropathic	>90% of cases	CTNS	17p13	219800
Juvenile (onset)	<10% of cases	CTNS	17p13	219900
Adult onset (non-nephropathic)	<10% of cases	CTNS	17p13	219750

FORM	FINDINGS	BIRTH	CLINICAL PRESENTATION CHILDHOOD & ADOLESCENCE
Infantile nephropathic	Similar to renal Fanconi syndrome; also hypothryroidism, renal failure and vitamin D-resistant rickets	None	At $\pm$6 mos. infant will show some evidence of renal Fanconi syndrome; polyuria may cause dehydration with fever of unknown origin (FUO); decline in growth rate and failure to thrive; signs of photophobia; later there is delayed walking due to pain; vitamin-D resistant rickets cause pain and bowing; growth delay becomes striking; pt. becomes weak (hypokalemia) and develops renal failure, anemia, and clinical hypothyroidism
Juvenile onset	Same as infantile onset	None	Onset at above 10–12 years of age; course similar to above
Adult onset	Corneal crystals but without renal Fanconi, renal failure, or hypothyroidism	None	Asymptomatic, except for photophobia; no renal component

Disorders of Amino Acid and Sugar Transport

The disorders grouped in this category are those attributable to impaired membrane uptake of a specific substrate and which have clinical importance. There are many not included here that are innocuous and have no detectable adverse effects on the affected individual. An example of these is renal tubular glycosuria, included because of its potential for confusion with diabetes mellitus. Others can have catastrophic consequences, such as lysinuric protein intolerance, whereas some are quietly progressive, such as cystinuria, showing itself only as nephrolithiasis and/or renal failure.

TYPE	OCCURRENCE	GENE	LOCUS	OMIM
Cystinuria type I, II, III	1:7000(all types)	SLC3A1, SLC7A9	2p16.3, 19q13.1	220100, 600918
Lysinuric protein intolerance	1:60,000 in Finland	SLC7A7	14q11.2	222700
Hartnup disorder	1:14,000	SLC6A19	5p15	234500
GLUT1 deficiency	N/A	SLC2A1	1p35-p31.3	606777
Renal tubular glycosuria	N/A	SLC5A2	16p11.2	233100
Familial glucose-galactose malabsorption	N/A	SLC5A1	22q13.1	606824

FORM	FINDINGS	CLINICAL PRESENTATION	
		BIRTH	CHILDHOOD & ADOLESCENCE
Cystinuria, all types	Flat, hexagonal crystals in urine, + CNT urolithiasis, staghorn calculi; ↑ cystine, lysine, arginine, ornithine, citrulline	None	Often presents as renal colic in late adolescence, some cases may demonstrate a staghorn calculus
Lysinuric protein intolerance	↑ lysine (U), arginine, ornithine hyperammonemia, hepatic and/or renal insufficiency, alveolar proteinosis	Symptom-free if breast fed, when weaned develop anorexia, FTT, may lapse into coma if given protein PO or per NG tube	Pts. avoid dietary protein, show growth failure, hepatospleno-megaly, hypotonia, osteoporosis, poor hair growth and variable MR; may have periodic hyper-ammonemic crises, and develop renal or respiratory failure
Hartnup disease	↑ neutral amino acids (U) ↑ neutral amino acids (S)	Neutral aminoaciduria, may demonstrate eczema and chronic diarrhea	Pellagra-type rash, light-sensitive neutral aminoaciduria, cerebellar ataxia and emotional lability that may resemble psychosis
GLUT1 Deficiency	NI glucose (B) ↓ CSF glucose, lactate	Normal, begin seizing in early infancy, slowed cranial growth, developmental delay	Daily seizures, microcephaly, spasticity → hypotonia, ataxic gait, expressive language affected → comprehensive, speech slurred, mental retardation
Renal glucosuria	NI glucose (B) ↑ to ↑↑ glucose (U)	Normal	Normal
Familial glucose-galactose malab-sorption	± ↑ glucose (U) Abnormal BH_2T ↓ pH (B) + reducing substances in stool, ↓ pH (S)	Massive diarrhea, dehydration, severe acidosis	Asymptomatic on glucose-galactose free diet; otherwise, same as newborn

Disorders of Renal Ion Transport

This group of disorders includes abnormalities of membrane transport involving the ions of sodium, potassium, and chloride. The major diagnostic entities in this category are Bartter and Gitelman syndromes. Common to all are metabolic alkalosis and hyperreninism and hyperaldosteronism. hypertrophy of the juxtaglomerular apparatus with hyperreninism and hyperaldosteronism.

TYPE	OCCURRENCE	GENE	LOCUS	OMIM
Bartter type I	N/A	SLC12A1	15q15-21.1	601678
Bartter type II	N/A	ROMK	11q24	241200
Bartter type III	N/A	CLCNKB	1p36	607364
Gitelman syndrome	N/A	SLC12A3	16q13	263800

FORM	FINDINGS	CLINICAL PRESENTATION	
		BIRTH	CHILDHOOD & ADOLESCENCE
Bartter type I	$\uparrow$ UV; $\downarrow$ USG $\uparrow\uparrow\uparrow$ Ca, Na (U) $\uparrow$ K (U), $\uparrow\uparrow\uparrow$ Cl (U) $\uparrow$ pH (B), $\downarrow$ K (B) $\downarrow$ Cl (B), $\uparrow$ PRA (B) $\uparrow$ Aldo (B), $\uparrow$ Cl (AF) $\uparrow\uparrow\uparrow$ PGE (U)	Fetal polyhydramnios at 6 mos.; prematurity; polyuria, hyposthenuria; dehydration; FTT	Appropriately diagnosed and treated, type I evolves subsequently into type III, or classical Bartter
Bartter type II	Identical to type I	As in type I	As in type I
Bartter type III (classic Bartter's)	$\uparrow$ UV; $\downarrow$ USG $\pm$ Nl Ca (U), $\uparrow$ Na (U) $\uparrow$ Cl (U), $\uparrow$ pH (B) $\downarrow$ K, Cl (B) $\uparrow$ PRA, Aldo (B)	Not present	>1 yr. old onset of polyuria, polydipsia and salt craving, dehydration, vomiting and constipation, FTT, muscle weakness and cramping
Gitelman syndrome	Nl UV, USG $\downarrow$ Ca (U), $\uparrow$ Mg (U) $\pm$ Nl Na, Cl (U) $\pm\uparrow$ pH (B), $\downarrow$ K (B) $\pm\downarrow$ Cl (B), $\uparrow$ PRA $\uparrow$ Aldo (B)	Not present	Periodic muscle weakness, abdominal pain, vomiting, possible carpopedal spasms

UV = urine volume; USG = urine specific gravity; Ca = calcium; U = urine; Na = sodium; K = potassium; Cl = chloride; B = blood; PRA = renin; Aldo = aldosterone; AF = amniotic fluid; PGE = prostaglandin E; Mg = magnesium; FTT = failure to thrive; S = stool; CNT = cyanide nitroprusside test; BH_2T = breath hydrogen test; P_i = phosphate renal in origin, and it should be understood that there is more than one entity that may cause this finding. In broad concept, these disorders may be looked on as either failure to eliminate H^+ or impaired ability to handle HCO_3^- at the level of the renal tubule portion of the nephron, generally resulting in an inappropriately alkaline urine pH in relation to the blood pH (1). Depending on the anatomical location of the defect, the patient is said to have proximal RTA or distal RTA, types II and I, respectively. The physiological function of each of the two nephron segments fundamentally defines the nature of the defect (Figure 42-2). The proximal tubule is unable to achieve hydrogen ion excretion but is the primary site of *net* bicarbonate reabsorption; hence proximal RTA (pRTA) results from impairment of this process. Net hydrogen ion secretion occurs chiefly in the distal tubule; hence distal RTA (dRTA) is the

TABLE 42-1   Disorders Associated with Type II Renal Tubular Acidosis

		Renal Findings	
	Inherited	Treatable	Reversible
Cystinosis	Yes	Yes	No
Galactosemia	Yes	Yes	Yes
Fructose intolerance	Yes	Yes	Yes
Glycogenoses, types I & III	Yes	Yes	Yes
Lowe syndrome	Yes	No	No
Tyrosinemia type I	Yes	Yes	Yes
Wilson Disease	Yes	Yes	Yes
Mitochondropathies*	Yes	Partially	No
Outdated Tetracycline	No	Yes	Yes
Severe Burns	No	Yes	Yes
Heavy-metal toxicity	No	Yes	Yes

*Includes mtDNA deletions or depletion, cytochrome C oxidase, complex III or IV deficiencies.

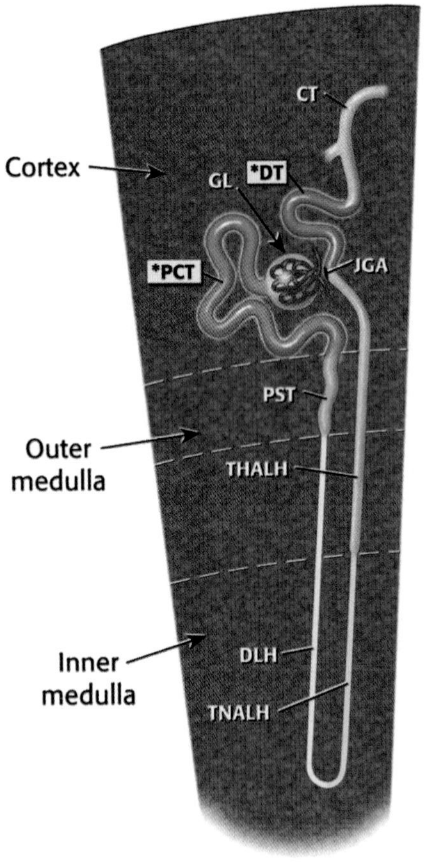

result of impaired H^+ secretion. While type I RTA generally is seen as a primary disorder, type II is often associated with other genetic or acquired disease (Table 42-1).

Proximal (Type II) Renal Tubular Acidosis

Primary Disorder The anatomical proximity of the glomerular complex to the proximal tubule presents the plasma ultrafiltrate directly to the brush-border surface of the transporting epithelial cells that line the tubular lumen. These cells are responsible for reclaiming a multitude of biologically important materials present in the ultrafiltrate in the short space of time required for the fluid to pass through. The process of diffusion is too slow and concentration-gradient-dependent to satisfy the need for adequate reclamation. Hence the cells of the proximal tubule have evolved tremendously active membrane transport systems, enabling rapid and specific uptake of materials that also can operate against a concentration gradient, the characteristics of active transport mentioned earlier. Among the materials contained in the ultrafiltrate that require uptake is bicarbonate, the primary body buffer.

Pathophysiology In a normal adult, approximately 85% of the more than 6000 mEq of daily filtered bicarbonate is returned to the blood by the proximal tubule. On the face of it, a significant reduction in the reabsorption process (bicarbonate wasting) should lead immediately to a systemic acidosis. However, the bicarbonate buffer system is an "open" one, with an immense capacity to compensate for losses via the lungs. Thus metabolic acidosis usually is blunted through pulmonary compensation, and for this reason,

a severe metabolic acidosis is seen infrequently in patients with primary type II RTA (2). Nevertheless, the body produces "fixed acid" as a consequence of metabolism that must be buffered in the blood until it can be eliminated through the action of the distal nephron, which is charged with net secretion of H^+. As a consequence, the more extreme signs of systemic acidosis, such as growth failure and osteomalacia, generally do not occur until late in the course of untreated disease. Nonetheless, loss of bicarbonate, by the laws of electrical neutrality, demands that a cation be lost on a mole-for-mole basis. This cation is usually potassium, but sodium is also lost to a smaller degree. In particular, it is the sodium loss that causes blood volume contraction and, as a result, a secondary release of aldosterone; thus potassium loss is exacerbated, and hypokalemia appears.

Most patients with type II RTA are affected by generalized tubular dysfunction caused by an additional underlying disorder that magnifies the clinical importance of the bicarbonate wasting (3). As shown in Figure 42-3, the process of HCO_3^- reabsorption is far more complex than simple transport of filtered bicarbonate across the brush-border surface, through the cell, and out the basolateral surface into the blood.

Primary proximal RTA is seen rarely after infancy; when found in isolation, it is likely the result of a mutation in the gene for the sodium bicarbonate cotransporter (NBC-1) molecule (see Figure 42-3) (2,3). Human gene cloning has demonstrated the presence of three isoforms (NBC-1, NBC-2, and NBC-3) in human kidney, but the functions of the latter two remain unclear (4–6). A defect in the cotransporter molecule would have no effect on the return of carbonic anhydrase–synthesized CO_2

FIGURE 42-2. The nephron unit. The complete nephron unit is shown, together with its orientation within the defined regions of the kidney. The portions of the nephron involved in the two major types of renal tubular acidosis are identified by an asterisk (*). GL = glomerulus; PCT = proximal convoluted tubule; PST = proximal straight tubule; DLH = descending limb of the loop of Henle; TNALH = thin ascending limb of the loop of Henle; THALH = thick ascending limb of the loop of Henle; JGA = juxtaglomerular apparatus; DT = distal tubule; CT = collecting tubule.

In figure: Cortex; Outer medulla; Inner medulla; CT; GL; *DT; *PCT; JGA; PST; THALH; DLH; TNALH

Proximal Tubule

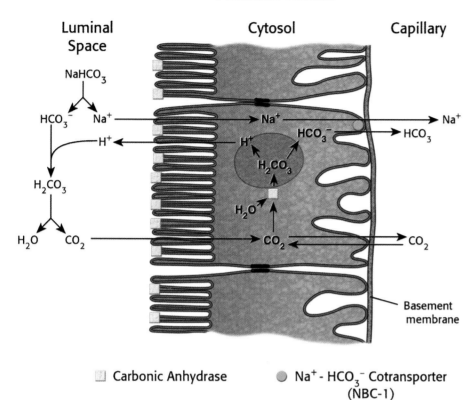

FIGURE 42-3. Proximal tubule cell. The complex process of bicarbonate reabsorption is shown. Proper function of the Na^+-HCO_3^- cotransporter (NBC-1) is critical to net delivery of bicarbonate from lumen to capillary. It also should be noted that carbonic anhydrase is present at two separate sites—the luminal surface and the cytosol—and is involved in the reabsorption process in both locations.

into blood achieved by diffusion, as shown, but it would impair net bicarbonate absorption. Consequently, the net bicarbonate wasting results from a backflow from the cytosol into the lumen rather than an inability to reclaim filtered bicarbonate. It is also noteworthy that the NBC protein is located at the basolateral membrane, illustrating the point that transport *out* of the cell can be as clinically important as uptake into it. Thus the classical concept of proximal RTA being caused by a reduction in the T_m for bicarbonate implying slower entry to the cell from the tubular lumen requires revision because there is no impairment of the brush-border uptake of bicarbonate.

Secondary proximal RTA is an altogether separate and distinct entity from the primary form of this disorder (2,3). Affected patients generally manifest signs of the underlying primary disorder such that RTA is a member of a group of associated findings. The primary disorder may be genetic or acquired (see Table 42-1); it is unclear whether the mechanism by which bicarbonate loss occurs is the same as that in the primary genetic disorder. The most common genetic cause of secondary type II RTA is the rare disease cystinosis, in which the complete renal Fanconi syndrome typically is seen. The calciuria and phosphaturia that are parts of the renal Fanconi syndrome serve to greatly amplify the impact of systemic acidosis on bone metabolism; hence

growth failure and rickets are seen frequently in secondary type II RTA.

Clinical Presentation The clinical presentation of type II RTA is characterized by a normal anion gap (Table 42-2), hyperchloremic metabolic acidosis, and associated failure to thrive secondary to retarded linear growth and anorexia. Calculation of the anion gap generally is determined as the difference between serum sodium (as the primary serum cation) and the sum of serum chloride plus serum bicarbonate (as the chief anions). A normal value is in the range of 10–16 depending on age, but in no case should it exceed 16. The hypokalemia due to potassium loss in the urine may provoke chronic constipation, whereas the water loss that follows the sodium and potassium excretion may cause polyuria. In essence, however, the findings are a "final common denominator" of chronic systemic acidosis of any etiology. Moreover, the extent of the acidosis may vary; classically, this was attributed to variability in the degree to which the T_m for bicarbonate was reduced. In fact, the ability of the distal tubule to achieve net hydrogen ion excretion, combined with pulmonary compensation, tends to blunt the effects on acid–base balance of a chronic bicarbonate loss. Indeed, the distal tubule's continued net secretion of hydrogen ion permits production of an acid urine even in the face of bicarbonate loss. For this reason alone, urine pH cannot be relied on as a diagnostic finding in type II RTA. In the more frequent circumstance, when the RTA is a secondary phenomenon, the clinical presentation of the underlying etiologic disorder (see Table 42-1) is often far more dramatic than that of the RTA itself.

TABLE 42-2   Conditions Presenting with Metabolic Acidosis and a Normal Anion GAP
Renal Bicarbonate Loss
Renal tubular acidosis type 1 (distal RTA)
Renal tubular acidosis type 2 (proximal RTA)
Carbonic anhydrase inhibitors
Early uremic acidosis
Hyperparathyroidism
Hypoaldosteronism (type IV RTA)
Gastrointestinal Bicarbonate Loss
Diarrhea
Small bowel fistula or surgical drainage
Ureterosigmoidostomy
Anion exchange resins
Calcium chloride
Other Causes
RTA type IV (acquired)—seen in obstructive uropathy and chronic renal failure
Hyperalimentation (excess lysine and arginine hydrochloride)

It is worthwhile to note that type II RTA is seen frequently in neonates, consistent with the fact that every infant at birth is less capable of bicarbonate reabsorption than an adult (2). Infants who are affected clinically by a transient metabolic acidosis on a renal basis may be manifesting a developmental variation in NBC-1 maturation as a basis for the finding. The acidosis usually will remit spontaneously within days. In a small number of babies, the acidosis may be persistent and severe enough to merit treatment to avoid anorexia and growth impairment, but this is not often the case.

Distal (Type I) Renal Tubular Acidosis

Primary Disorder (Recessive and Dominant): The distal tubule is responsible for elimination of "fixed acid," that is, those acidic anions that result from ordinary metabolic processes, such as sulfate, lactate, and phosphate (2). The average adult generates approximately 1 mEq/kg/day of such acids, which must be entirely eliminated to maintain pH homeostasis. In the bargain, the distal tubule accomplishes a net hydrogen ion excretion, sending the H^+ into the urine along with the anion while reclaiming sodium. Thus it follows logically that the distal tubule is key to urinary acidification, so impairment of this process will lead quickly to a very severe metabolic acidosis. It should be considered that lactate can be recycled for metabolism by conversion to pyruvate, but neither sulfate nor phosphate has an alternative metabolic route, thus creating an acidosis due to accumulation of inorganic anions with a normal anion gap. The primary disorder is inherited as either an autosomal recessive or an autosomal dominant trait; the gene loci for both are listed above (7,8).

Pathophysiology As mentioned earlier, the deficit in bicarbonate reabsorption seen in type II RTA does not generally result in severe acidosis because the distal tubule mitigates the disequilibration by net secretion of hydrogen ion. However, normal bicarbonate reabsorption in the proximal tubule will have virtually no effect on restoration of the acid–base disruption created by a failure of acid secretion at the distal tubule. Hence the degree of metabolic acidosis in type I RTA generally is quite severe and has much more serious systemic implications than does type II RTA. Key to the ability to achieve a very steep pH gradient between the cell and the lumen of the distal tubule is the capacity for direct secretion of hydrogen ion into the lumen independent of sodium flux (Figure 42-4). Powering this active process is an H^+-ATPase pump that directly expels a

Distal tubule

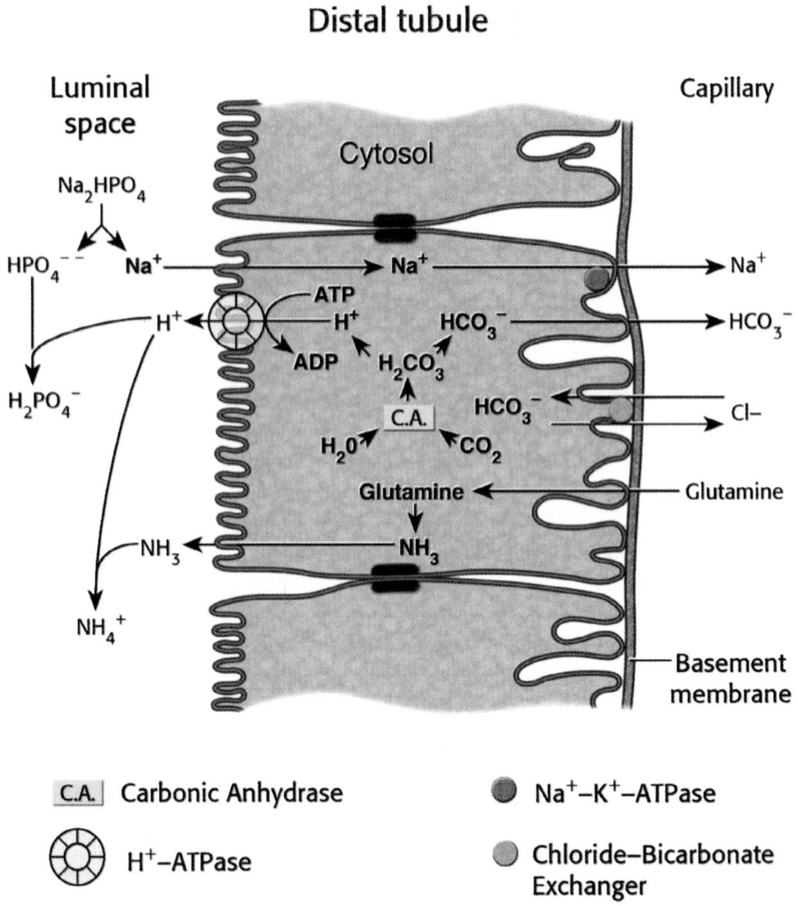

FIGURE 42-4. Distal tubule cell. The process of net acid secretion is shown here. Note that the more common, autosomal dominant form of RTA is a result of a functional deficit in the chloride–bicarbonate exchanger, whereas the autosomal recessive variant results from impaired function of the H^+-ATPase pump at the luminal surface.

hydrogen ion generated from the intracellular carbonic anhydrase–mediated synthesis of carbonic acid. Also contributing to this ability to create a steep pH gradient are the nonleaky tight junctions between the cells that prevent backflux from the lumen directly into the blood. Another unusual feature of the distal tubular cell is the ability to generate ammonia through the action of glutaminase on glutamine; ammonia diffuses freely through membranes and follows a concentration gradient into the lumen, where the expelled hydrogen ion is combined chemically with it to form the NH_4^+ radical. The latter then combines with the "fixed acids," phosphate, and sulfate so that the expelled hydrogen is also chemically retained within the lumen. This permits the distal tubule to increase the hydrogen ion concentration of the urine by up to 1000-fold (2).

At the molecular level, there appears to be a divergence in etiology between the dominant and recessive forms of type I RTA. The *dominant* pattern has been definitively demonstrated to be due to a defect in the antiluminal membrane molecule, the Cl^-–HCO_3^- exchanger; this transporter is responsible for

moving the bicarbonate generated intracellularly across the basement membrane into blood in exchange for a chloride ion to maintain electrical neutrality (7). When this function is impaired, the bicarbonate accumulates intracellularly; the effect of this is to reduce carbonic acid ionization and generation of H^+ for secretion, as well as to reduce the sodium reabsorption that normally follows the bicarbonate into the pericapillary space. In the majority of families thus far studied showing a *recessive* pattern, the molecular defect has been in the brush-border H^+-ATPase (3,8). In this case, inability of the proton pump to expel hydrogen ion into the tubular lumen reduces or eliminates the key ability of the distal tubule to establish and maintain a steep pH gradient.

Clinical Presentation The clinical presentation of dRTA mimics that of type II RTA to a large degree (1–3). There is a characteristic normal-anion-gap hyperchloremic metabolic acidosis associated with growth failure. Diminished sodium reabsorption (see above) leads to a secondary hyperaldosteronism, with the resulting sodium–potassium exchange causing hypokalemia. As in pRTA, the hypokalemia induces weakness and chronic constipation. In this regard, it should be pointed out that there is a disparate response to rehydration and pH correction between the two types of RTA (2). With dRTA, the volume correction relieves the hyperaldosteronism, which, in turn, reduces the sodium–potassium exchange and permits correction of the hypokalemia. However, with the massive sodium bicarbonate loss in pRTA, pH correction increases the potassium loss because of the consequent increased delivery of sodium bicarbonate to the distal tubule, which is the site of the sodium–potassium exchange.

A key difference between the two forms of RTA is the marked propensity for nephrocalcinosis in the distal type (2). This results from the rather severe degree of acidosis that is typical and is caused by the increased circulating ionized calcium displaced by the increased hydrogen ion concentration. The consequence is an increase in filtered calcium at the glomerular level. In addition, systemic acidosis inhibits citrate production by the mitochondria, which normally release this compound into urine; citrate acts as a solubilizer for calcium so that an increase in the filtered amount in the urine and decreased solubility combine to cause precipitation within the renal parenchyma and the collecting system. Hence nephrocalcinosis and renal failure are real factors in the natural history of untreated dRTA (2,3,8).

Diagnostic Approach Keeping in mind the fundamental definition of RTA—an inappropriate alkaline pH in relation to an acidotic serum pH—diagnostic evaluation follows some quite logical steps. The initial approach is to establish that the metabolic acidosis is a normal-anion-gap (see Table 42-2) hyperchloremic type and, in fact, that there is an inappropriate relationship by obtaining simultaneous serum and urine pH values. Once this has been established, the next sequential study is examination of the urinary citrate excretion, which is demonstrably lower than normal in dRTA and normal in pRTA. The difference between Pco_2 in urine and blood is directly proportional to the $[HCO_3^-]$ in the urine. This is so because the urinary bicarbonate is in equilibrium with dissolved CO_2 such that increases in urinary bicarbonate will be reflected in increases in solubilized carbon dioxide. Thus the distinction between the two types of RTA can be further confirmed by measurement of both urine and blood Pco_2 concentrations. In patients with pRTA, urine bicarbonate is increased, and the difference will be greater than 20 mm Hg, whereas patients with dRTA do not have increased urine bicarbonate concentration, and the difference

will be less than 15 mm Hg. Additional testing can be done by intravenous arginine hydrochloride administration, which should cause maximal hydrogen ion excretion, forcing the normal kidney to produce urine of pH less than 5.5; if a patient with RTA produces urine with a pH of less than 5.5 under these conditions, dRTA can be ruled out.

Another frequently overlooked means of distinction between RTA types I and II is use of the urinary anion gap. This value is equal to the sum (urine $[Na^+]$ + urine $[K^+]$) − urine $[Cl^-]$. In order to understand the utility of this calculation, it is necessary to remember that the distal tubule uses ammonium formation for the excretion of H^+ and that the ammonium ion generally is excreted as NH_4Cl. Thus, although ammonium is an "unmeasured" cation, increased chloride excretion in an acidotic patient probably represents a corresponding increase in ammonium excretion. From the formula, then, it is anticipated that a normal individual will decrease the urine anion gap in a state of acidosis because the distal tubule will increase hydrogen ion excretion as ammonium, and the urine chloride will rise correspondingly. So too in a patient with type II RTA will the normal distal tubular response take place and the urine anion gap decrease. *However, where the distal tubule is incapable of increased hydrogen ion excretion, as in type I RTA, there will be no change in the urine anion gap in the face of systemic acidosis.* It also should be noted that because chloride excretion is normally quite high, the urinary anion gap may be a negative value, so the term *decreased* actually refers to a larger number.

Other studies, which must not be overlooked, include blood urea nitrogen (BUN) and creatinine, as well as a renal ultrasound. The latter is particularly important in type I RTA with the marked propensity for nephrocalcinosis, which may lead to renal compromise.

Treatment The therapeutic focus in both forms of RTA is, of course, the metabolic acidosis from which all complications of the disorders arise. Consequently, alkali supplementation is the basis for treatment of both proximal and distal RTA. In type II RTA, daily losses of bicarbonate may be as great as 20 mmol/kg, requiring massive doses of replacement alkali. Tolerance to such large doses of sodium bicarbonate is restricted because of palatability; the alternative medication is the more palatable sodium citrate, although in the quantities needed even this may be poorly received, especially in younger patients. In treatment of type I RTA, use of citrate has an underlying rationale beyond the replenishment of depleted buffer base: the presence of citrate in urine acts as a calcium

solubilizer, thus reducing the risk of nephrocalcinosis and consequent renal damage. Following elimination of the systemic acidosis by alkali administration, growth rate should accelerate if renal impairment has not ensued. Close follow-up during the accelerated growth phase is essential to ensure continued adequate base replacement.

RENAL FANCONI SYNDROME

The initial case descriptions of renal Fanconi syndrome in the early 1930s focused on glycosuria and rickets, commenting as well on the significant growth failure seen in these patients. Inasmuch as the earliest published description in 1931 was authored by the Italian physician Fanconi, the renal syndrome continues to bear his name. Retrospectively, it is likely that one or more of the originally described patients may have been suffering from cystinosis (see below), of which the renal Fanconi syndrome is a prominent part. The clinical components of the renal Fanconi syndrome include glucosuria, bicarbonaturia (type II RTA), aminoaciduria, phosphaturia, natriuria, kaluria, and polyuria, all of which are the consequence of proximal tubular dysfunction. Although there have been reports of primary renal Fanconi syndrome, a secondary presentation is by far the most common. Diseases with which Fanconi syndrome is a secondary presentation has been reported are listed in Table 42-1; it should be noted that in some cases the tubular dysfunction is reversible. Moreover, the underlying causes of renal Fanconi syndrome can be either genetic or acquired disease (10).

Primary Disorder This form of the disorder, also known as *adult renal Fanconi syndrome*, usually is transmitted as an autosomal dominant trait in which glomerular disease can occur but is generally slowly progressive (11,12). Bone disease is often absent or mild, and due to the slow evolution of the tubular and glomerular dysfunctions, the diagnosis often is not made until adulthood. Also, it should be kept in mind that because of this slow evolution of findings, a diagnosis of "incomplete" Fanconi syndrome is sometimes made. Because of the multiple causes of a secondary Fanconi syndrome (see Table 42-1), age alone is insufficient as a determinant of primary versus secondary disease. Although relatively large family pedigrees have been reported in which individuals of every generation were affected, the true incidence in the population is not known.

Secondary Disorder The extraordinarily wide diversity of clinical situations in which one sees the secondary renal Fanconi syndrome compels the view that many or all primary conditions exert a common adverse effect on the proximal tubule (13). In addition, the gene loci of the various primary inherited disorders generally are quite remote from the gene locus of the primary renal Fanconi syndrome (see Table 42-1). For many conditions, this argument is further strengthened by the observation that where the primary disease is reversible by treatment, the renal manifestations also are reversed. However, at present, it is only possible to say that secondary Fanconi syndrome results from "renal tubular injury" resulting from the underlying disorder.

Pathophysiology The complete pathophysiologic sequence that underlies the generalized dysfunction of the renal Fanconi syndrome remains enigmatic. For instance, the generalized nature of the amino acid transport abnormalities would argue in favor of a common factor affecting carrier proteins with individual amino acid specificity. Since carrier proteins generally possess both intra- and extramembrane domains and bind sodium as well as specific substrate, one possible explanation for the observations is an alteration of membrane conformation leading to changes in binding of either sodium or substrate and failure to transport substrate into the cell. An alternative explanation could be that alterations in membrane permeability permit accumulated substrate to "leak" back into the tubular lumen. Other possibilities include an alteration in transport of accumulated substrate across the basolateral cell surface into blood forcing backleak across the brush-border (luminal) surface or basolateral permeability being so great that material "rushes" into the cell from the blood and forces backleak into the lumen. Finally, and most plausibly, there may be an adverse effect on the system by which active transport is energized such that any actively transported substrate would be affected by decreased energy supply and reduced cellular capacity for maintenance of a concentration gradient (10,13). This is supported by the observation that secondary renal Fanconi syndrome can be part of the multisystem presentation of mitochondropathies.

At a clinical level, the generalized transport dysfunction translates into some significant features: hyperchloremic metabolic acidosis and consequent poor physical growth, hypokalemia and muscle weakness, hypocalcemia and hypophosphatemia in association with rickets, and urinary electrolyte loss together with glucosuria leading to polyuria and sometimes severe dehydration. This is, of course, independent of any manifestations of underlying primary disorders, such as cystinosis or heavy-metal toxicity, for example. It should be mentioned that despite the striking urinary amino acid losses, these are minimal in rela-

tion to dietary intake, so there are no systemic consequences attributable to the aminoaciduria (10,13).

Clinical Presentation Glucosuria is thought to be the first manifestation of generalized proximal tubular dysfunction, although there has been no report of systematic study of the clinical evolution of the renal Fanconi syndrome. Moreover, it is unclear whether the evolution of the primary form of the disorder would be equivalent to that of the secondary form seen with a multiplicity of underlying disorders. It should be emphasized here that the glucosuria, like the aminoaciduria, is not reflected in low blood sugar concentration. Hence, if glucosuria is present as an isolated finding, prudence would dictate close follow-up to determine any further manifestation of the renal Fanconi syndrome. Likewise, if bicarbonaturia and hyperchloremic metabolic acidosis appear spontaneously, other tubular dysfunctions should be sought.

Perhaps the most striking clinical findings associated with the renal Fanconi syndrome are the growth failure and rickets that appear relatively late. Since both are as much a result of the metabolic acidosis as they are of urinary loss of calcium and phosphate, the early etiological evaluation of type II RTA, including a search for the renal Fanconi syndrome, can help to avoid such detrimental consequences (10,13,14).

Diagnostic Approach Given the numerous entities that may create a renal Fanconi syndrome as an associated clinical finding, it should be clear that the diagnosis of a primary Fanconi syndrome is one of exclusion. Among the primary inherited causes, cystinosis is the most common etiology of a renal Fanconi syndrome in childhood. Cystinosis can be diagnosed by documentation of corneal birefringent cystine crystals by slit-lamp examination. Other diagnostic tests include direct cystine assay of conjunctival or rectal biopsy specimens.

Among the acquired etiologies, probably the most common in childhood would be considered heavy-metal toxicity, specifically lead (15). Since determination of blood lead level is a routine part of good pediatric care, most children in the United States are screened for this. However, it should never be forgotten that a negative screen in infancy certainly can become positive in childhood, so repeat measurement in a patient with renal Fanconi syndrome is imperative.

The more obscure primary causes should be sought if the preceding workup is unrewarding. Obviously, family history will be helpful in Lowe syndrome, for example, which is transmitted as an X-linked trait, whereas hepatomegaly and recurrent hypo-

glycemia dominate the clinical presentation of glycogenoses, and severe liver disease and jaundice may lead to consideration of either tyrosinemia type I or Wilson disease. In children treated for malignancy with cisplatin, appearance of a renal Fanconi syndrome should not warrant an extensive etiological investigation.

Treatment Treatment of the primary Fanconi syndrome is purely symptomatic, unless there has been progression to glomerular injury, which then should prompt consideration of renal transplantation. Since the most troublesome manifestations of the renal condition are metabolic acidosis due to RTA and the threat of dehydration due to polyuria, alkali and electrolyte replacement should get the greatest attention. It has already been mentioned that neither the glucose nor the amino acid losses are important to nutritional balance, and the bone metabolic changes are primarily the result of persistent acidosis.

Treatments are available for many of the genetic and acquired primary etiologies that, when effective, may reverse the renal manifestations partially or completely. Hence to look on the renal Fanconi syndrome as the diagnostic gateway to treatment of a much more serious underlying condition would not be altogether wrong.

CYSTINOSIS

Since cystinosis is the most common cause of a secondary renal Fanconi syndrome in childhood, logic dictates a discussion of this rare inborn error following the preceding examination of the renal Fanconi syndrome itself. In keeping with conventional medical terminology, the name *cystinosis* denotes the extensive deposition of cystine crystals throughout the body. Of particular interest is the fact that this deposition has been clearly demonstrated to be present in utero with the identical tissue distribution as seen in the older child. Of course, the immediate implication of this is the feasibility of prenatal diagnosis, which has been available for many years.

Cystine is the oxidized dimer form of the sulfur amino acid cysteine (see Figure 42-5). Since the dimer is so readily and spontaneously formed in the presence of oxygen, it is easy to understand the resulting complexity of the cellular systems involved in regulating the balance between intracellular mono and dimer forms. It was this complexity that hampered efforts to understand the biochemical nature of the disorder for many years, until the elegant demonstration of the fundamental transport defect in the late 1980s. Thus, despite the clinical findings of generalized cystine storage, cystinosis is now firmly estab-

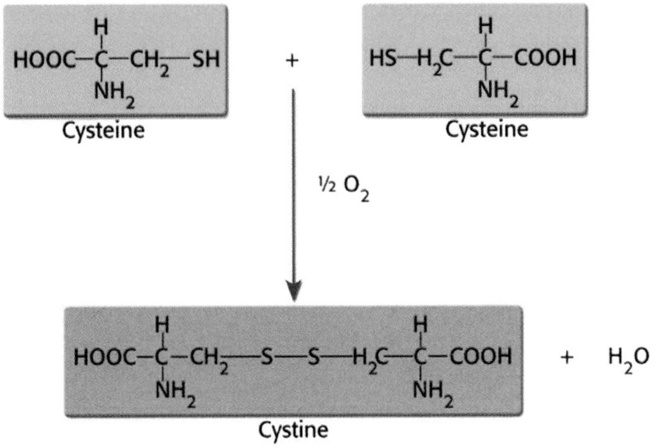

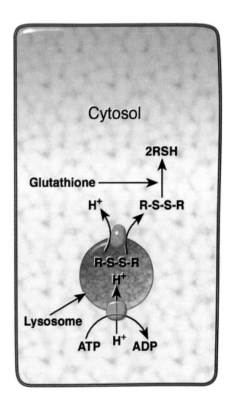

FIGURE 42-5. Dimerization of cysteine to cystine.

lished as a membrane-transport disorder involving the transport protein cystinosin (16–18).

"Classical" Nephropathic Cystinosis Otherwise known as *infantile nephropathic cystinosis*, this form of the disease accounts for the majority of cases, and the gene defect is transmitted as an autosomal recessive trait. Classical cystinosis inevitably results in development of renal failure by middle to late childhood, renal involvement generally being heralded by the appearance of the renal Fanconi syndrome (see above) (19). Electron microscopic studies many years ago defined the intracellular locus of the cystine deposition as intralysosomal, but investigators were misled by the original concept of the lysosome as the storage repository of all excess intracellular material. What was overlooked was the idea that entry into the lysosome might be carrier-mediated and bidirectional, so a defect in a carrier might account for the accumulation. Indeed, some very elegant studies finally defined the defect as one in which cystine enters but does not exit the lysosome properly.

"Variant" (Juvenile and Adult) Cystinosis These clinical forms, as is apparent from their names, are milder variants of the classical disease. The juvenile or adolescent form of the disease simply has a later onset than the infantile form, but eventually all the manifestations of the latter will appear, usually in the second decade of life or later (19). The adult form differs from the previous two in that while the photophobia created by the birefringent cystine crystal deposition in the eye is prominent, there is no renal involvement (20). It is now understood that these variants are the result of allelic mutations that all affect the same gene product but to a different degree of impairment in function (16–18).

Pathophysiology An understanding of the chemistry of the sulfur amino acids is essential to an explanation of the underlying pro-

cess by which cystine storage occurs. The monomer cysteine is quite soluble at physiological pH, even in the relatively acidic intracellular fluid. However, the –SH side chain is rather easily oxidized under physiological conditions, resulting in formation of the dimer form cystine. Cystine is one of the least soluble naturally occurring substances at physiological pH (and decreases further in solubility in the intracellular milieu), and the –S–S– bond is very stable. Thus it is apparent that there must be an intracellular mechanism by which the balance between the oxidized and reduced forms is maintained. The most potent cellular reducing agent is glutathione, which is generated on a constant basis to provide reducing equivalents for maintenance of this and other physiological systems. So efficient is this system that the predominant intracellular form of this sulfhydryl amino acid is the soluble monomer cysteine. Thus the presence of precipitated intracellular cystine crystals is extremely unusual and abnormal.

Our present understanding of the pathophysiology is based on a series of experimental studies that used isolated leukocytes or cultured fibroblasts and, subsequently, isolated lysosomes. Initially, it was demonstrated that by preloading normal and cystinotic leukocytes with labeled [^{35}S]cystine to equal, high concentrations, there was an infinitely slow loss of the radiolabel from cystinotic cells compared with normal cells, which lost half the label within about 45 minutes (21,22). Cultured skin fibroblasts showed the same results (23). Isolated lysosomes from normal and cystinotic cells reflected these findings, and by expressing the very early losses at various concentrations against time, it was shown that these "initial velocities" increased as a first-order equation until no further increase in rate could be demonstrated, confirming the saturable nature of the process and directly implicating carrier-mediated transport as the mediator (21,24,25). Conclusive evidence of this was presented by showing that radiolabeled cystine could be made to cross the normal lysosomal membrane more rapidly if there was a high concentration of unlabeled cystine on the opposite side of the membrane. Other experiments have demonstrated that reduction of the dimer cystine to the monomer cysteine made no difference

to the rate of egress, indicating that the carrier was specific for cystine. Still others have shown that egress of other amino acids from cystinotic lysosomes is normal, establishing the specificity of the carrier for the single amino acid. Thus, since cystine obviously can enter the cystinotic lysosome, the defect in cystinosis must reside in the inability of cystine to exit via the carrier (Figure 42-6) (21,24).

From the preceding, we may now view cystinosis as a lysosomal carrier defect in which cystine, once accumulated in the lysosome, is unable to exit, leading to further accumulation. It should be strongly emphasized that the entry phenomenon does not require an abnormally high intracellular cystine concentration, notwithstanding the experimental techniques used to demonstrate the defect. Thus there are no clinically detectable, abnormally elevated blood or urine cystine concentrations that might be interpreted as creating conditions for increased intracellular concentration.

Clinical Presentation Affected infants are indistinguishable from normal newborns, and early growth and development are entirely normal. It should be noted that renal function for the first several months of life is

FIGURE 42-6. Lysosomal cystine transport. The predominant form in cytosol is the monomer cysteine, maintained in the reduced form by the glutathione system, which provides reducing equivalents. Lysosomal cystine transport depends on the carrier molecule cystinosin and the entry of hydrogen ion by means of a H$^+$-ATPase pump as shown.

normal (19). Initial manifestations are variable but can include fevers of unknown origin secondary to polyuria and unrecognized dehydration, photophobia due to corneal cystine deposition, decreasing growth velocity as a consequence of bicarbonate wasting, and refusal to stand because of bone pain and rickets. It is worthy of note that all the preceding, except the photophobia, are directly attributable to the secondary renal Fanconi syndrome. As pointed out earlier, the renal Fanconi syndrome emerges with time, and it is unclear as to whether there is a predictable sequence in which the findings develop. Hence the same is true of cystinosis, the underlying etiology of the renal Fanconi syndrome in affected infants. On balance, cystinotic infants tend to be somewhat lighter in pigmentation than other family members; the reason for this remains unknown, but there is speculation that the melanosomes of melanocytes (structures analogous to lysosomes) may be impaired in their ability to form pigment.

Since in unrecognized cases renal failure usually does not supervene until the end of the first decade, other manifestations may appear due to the unabated deposition of cystine throughout the body. Growth failure persists and worsens, rickets and bowing of the lower extremities progress, photophobia worsens, and retinal lesions may develop, and there is increasing dysphagia and hypothyroidism. Of course, underlying these clinical findings are the associated manifestations of progressive renal failure, especially vitamin D resistance, proteinuria, hypoalbuminemia, malnutrition, muscle wasting and weakness, and additional growth failure. One can easily imagine the inanition, dwarfing, and chronically ill appearance of such a child.

The juvenile- or adolescent-onset variation of cystinosis only requires an adjustment based on age of onset to understand the presentation. Obviously, growth will be less affected in relation to the infantile type because onset is later. Although the polyuria of the associated renal Fanconi syndrome will be present, an older child is less prone to dehydration because of the ability to access fluids. Other complications secondary to cystine deposition will appear later, and renal failure usually is delayed until the second decade.

The adult-onset variant, on the other hand, resembles infantile nephropathic cystinosis only in that the corneal cystine deposition occurs with ensuing photophobia. Retinal lesions do not appear in this disorder, nor does the renal Fanconi syndrome or progressive renal failure (5). Consequently, although the gene map locus of the mutation is the same as the preceding two nephropathic forms of the disorder, the adult variant represents the mildest form of the disease (16–18).

Diagnostic Approach During routine office care, the manifestations most likely to draw the physician's attention are decreasing growth velocity in the latter half of the first year and unusual sensitivity to light, often first commented on by the parents. Any search for the etiology of slowed growth should include a urinalysis, which, in an affected infant, would be expected to show any or all of the following: glucose, protein, low specific gravity, and/or alkaline pH. Quantitative measurement of urinary amino acid excretion will show a large excess of virtually every one of the 21 naturally occurring compounds, thus providing definitive evidence of a renal Fanconi syndrome. The caveat here is that amino acid membrane-transport systems in the proximal tubule undergo development in the first year of life such that the very young infant may demonstrate a generalized amino aciduria as a developmentally normal phenomenon. Given that cystinosis is the most common cause of the renal Fanconi syndrome in childhood, the most rapid course to an etiological diagnosis is a slit-lamp examination of the eye with or without evidence of photophobia. The presence of corneal birefringent crystals is sufficient justification for determining the cystine content of leukocytes or establishing a fibroblast culture and quantitative measurement of the cystine content, which will be at least 10-fold greater than the normal range in affected cells. Obligate heterozygotes will evidence two- to fivefold the normal range of intracellular cystine content.

Given the pathophysiological implications of the renal Fanconi syndrome, prudence dictates an evaluation of the long bones for signs of rachitic changes, evaluation of the acid–base and calcium–phosphate status, and evaluation of renal function as well. It also should be kept in mind that as renal disease progresses, the vitamin D resistance will increase due to an inability to carry out the 1-hydroxylation of 25-OH-cholecalciferol to produce the active metabolite. In later stages of the disease, it is often necessary to use a synthetic dihydroxyvitamin D analogue to heal or prevent the recurrence of rickets.

Treatment Once the diagnosis is established, all patients should begin oral cysteamine treatment, which has been clearly demonstrated to have highly beneficial effects on preservation of glomerular function (19,26,27). Cysteamine is a compound with a free thiol group that is capable of reducing intracellular cystine and forming "mixed disulfide" compounds that exit the lysosome and the cell as well. After more than 30 years of treatment experience, it is now documented that compliant patients generally can deplete and maintain their white cell free cystine concentrations by greater than 80% of baseline. This depletion is also reflected in all body organs, with the exception of the eye, in which cystine accumulation continues unabated despite several years of oral cysteamine treatment. This situation has been addressed successfully by use of cysteamine eyedrops, which have been very effective in reducing crystalline deposits in the cornea and also may be used in the adult variant.

Naturally, since the kidney has long been recognized as the primary target organ in cystinosis, attention has been focused on the effectiveness of oral cysteamine in the preservation of renal function. Children started on oral cysteamine prior to age 2 years have shown normal developmental changes in creatinine clearance and continued normal renal function well past age 10, the age at which untreated subjects would be in chronic renal failure (19). Physical growth continues at a normal rate, and treated children progress through a normal puberty. Yet, with all this very encouraging evidence in hand, there remains the troubling and persistent renal Fanconi syndrome, suggesting some permanent renal tubular injury. We also lack firm proof that individuals with infantile nephropathic cystinosis treated successfully by age 2 will retain normal renal function over a normal life span. While this remains the treatment goal, renal allograft continues to be the only definitive solution to decreased renal function over many years.

Until the advent of successful renal transplantation techniques, all affected individuals experienced terminal renal failure for which dialysis was, at best, a palliative maneuver. The startling success of oral cysteamine therapy has greatly diminished the urgent need for either dialysis or allograft. The early experience with renal allograft in such patients was instructive because it became clear that the transplanted kidney did not reaccumulate cystine and therefore was to be considered a "cure" for the renal injury and ensuing failure in cystinosis. However, it rapidly became apparent that while obviating renal disease, the procedure did little to prevent continuing cystine accumulation and damage to the parenchyma of other organs. Thus the clinical focus in the care of a transplanted cystinotic child moved from the kidney to various other organs, such as thyroid, testis, and pancreas, and to gastrointestinal (GI) and pulmonary function, as well as neurological deterioration in some individuals. Posttransplantation continuation of oral cysteamine may be sufficient to forestall onset of dysfunction in these other areas, but experience is too scarce at this time to be definitive.

DISORDERS OF AMINO ACID AND SUGAR TRANSPORT

Cystinuria

As alluded to in the introductory section of this chapter, cystinuria was one of four human disorders to which Garrod gave the name *inborn errors* at the beginning of the 20th century. The initial understanding of the disease, originally described in 1810, represented urinary tract stone formation as a consequence of the increased presence of the amino acid dimer cystine in the urine. As distinct from the apparently complex disorder cystinosis, involving generalized storage of the same material throughout the body, cystinuria *per se* is the result of a membrane-transport defect confined to the kidney and intestine. Quantitative measurement of urinary amino acid excretion in affected individuals shows increased quantities of cystine and the dibasic amino acids lysine, arginine, and ornithine in proportions that vary depending on the nature of the gene defect. Unlike the larger family of autosomal recessive disorders to which cystinuria belongs, in this disorder carriers are often (but not always) at risk for clinical expression of the gene mutation. The search for the basis of a relationship between the genetic defect and clinical expression has been a long and difficult one that is not yet complete. Clinically, based on the specific combination of renal and intestinal transport defects in an affected individual, as well as the degree of urinary cystine and dibasic amino acid excretion, three distinct types (I, II, and III) are defined (Table 42-3). Type I is the *fully recessive type*, in which carriers do not express the defect clinically. Types II and III are referred to as *incompletely recessive forms*, in which there is carrier expression. Current belief is that the basis for this is allelic mutations of the SLC7A9 gene at 19q13.1 (28,29). As far as is known, morbidity is confined exclusively to urinary tract lithiasis. Given an approximate incidence of 1 in 7000 in the population at large, it can be seen that not only is it a remarkably common inherited disorder, but it also must account for a significant proportion of the adult stone-forming population.

Pathophysiology Cystine is a naturally occurring dimer of two cysteine residues linked through their sulfhydryl groups and formed under oxidizing conditions (see Figure 42-5). Cystine is a highly insoluble natural compound that has a solubility threshold of approximately 300 mg/L (1200 μM) at neutral pH. Cystinuric individuals may excrete more than 1 g of cystine per day, well above the solubility limit given the usual daily urine volume of 1–1.5 L. Cystine becomes diminishingly soluble under acid conditions, so it may precipitate either within the proximal tubule as water and bicarbonate are reclaimed or in the distal tubule

and collecting duct, where net hydrogen ion secretion may reduce the pH to as low as 5.0.

Moving beyond the original concept that cystinuria was a renal disease resulting in increased loss of cystine required the application of techniques for amino acid quantitation that did not exist before the mid-1900s. Prior to this, it had already been established by Brand and Cahill that oral cystine loading did not increase plasma cystine concentration, implying strongly the existence of an intestinal absorptive defect (30). It was then established that affected individuals also excreted immense quantities of the much more soluble dibasic amino acids in their urine. After demonstrating that the plasma concentrations of the structurally related amino acids cystine, lysine, arginine, and ornithine were normal in cystinuric individuals, Dent and Rose proposed that the increased urinary concentrations were the result of a renal membrane-transport defect (31). Extension of the earlier oral loading studies of Brand and Cahill demonstrated corresponding defects in the intestinal absorption of the dibasic amino acids. Thereafter, the focus of most investigations shifted to study of the more fruitful possibility that cystinuria was a membrane-transport disorder of genetic etiology. Subsequent direct demonstration of lack of uptake of radiolabeled cystine, lysine, and arginine by intestinal biopsy specimens from some, but not all, affected individuals provided irrefutable evidence of the intestinal absorptive defect, as well as helping to delineate various subtypes of the disorder (32).

Since circulating concentrations of cystine and the dibasics are normal, as with other blood amino acids, approximately 98% of that filtered appears in the glomerular filtrate. We now know of the existence of three membrane transport sites involved in renal tubular reclamation of filtered cystine and dibasic amino acids: 1) one shared by all four amino acids, 2) a specific high-affinity site for cystine, and 3) a high-affinity site shared only by the dibasic amino acids (Figure 42-7) (33).

TABLE 42-3 Clinical Distinction of Cystinuric Genotypes (I, II, and III)

Carriers	Amino Acid Excretion							
	Cystine		Lysine		Arginine		Ornithine	
	(U / S)		(U / S)		(U / S)		(U / S)	
I/N	N	N	N	N	N	N	N	N
II/N	++	++	+	++	+	++	+	+
III/N	+	+	+	+	+	+	+	+
Homozygotes								
I/I	+++	↑	+++	↑	+++	↑	+++	−
II/II	+++	N	+++	↑	+++	−	+++	−
III/III	+++	N	+++	N	+++	N	+++	−

U = urine; S = stool; N = normal; + ≈ 500 μmol/g creatinine.

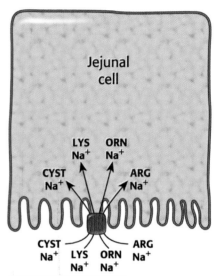

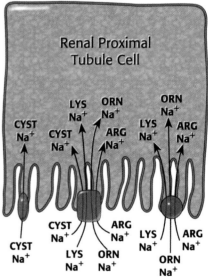

FIGURE 42-7. Cystine and dibasic amino acid transport in kidney and intestine. Three separate carriers exist in renal epithelium: a dedicated, high-affinity site exclusively for cystine, a system shared by cystine and the dibasic amino acids and a third system shared exclusively by the dibasic amino acids By contrast, jejunal cells possess only a single carrier for all four amino acids. Note that for all four species, there is Na+ cotransport.

It is the first transport site that is defective in cystinuria; since all four amino acids share the same site, each competes with the other. Consequently, the abnormal presence of large concentrations of lysine, arginine, and ornithine inhibits uptake of cystine from the tubular lumen. What permits some degree of cystine uptake is the immediate intracellular reduction in cysteine, so there is a small component of entry that is attributable to diffusion along the concentration gradient. The same transport system is defective in intestinal epithelium; however, it is thought that there is only the single system present in normal individuals, so impairment results in no measurable absorption of cystine or dibasic amino acids from the gut lumen in cystinuric individuals.

Of the four affected amino acids in cystinuria, cysteine (hence cystine) and ornithine are produced in the liver, and arginine is made by both the liver and the kidney; only lysine is essential for human nutrition. It is believed that cystinuric individuals avoid lysine deficiency by intestinal absorption of sufficient quantities of lysyl-dipeptides to supply their needs.

Clinical Presentation It has been known for many years that the amino acid membrane-transport systems of the proximal renal tubule undergo a maturational process; hence neonates may excrete high concentrations of cystine and dibasic amino acids, along with other amino acids, and thus confound attempts at accurate screening for cystinuria (34). However, while cystine urolithiasis has been reported in the cystinuric infant, presentation of the disorder in infancy is very rare. Typically, cystinuria is clinically silent until presentation in the 2nd and 3rd decades of life with the onset of renal colic. Not infrequently, irreparable damage to one or both kidneys already has taken place at this stage; large staghorn calculi may be present on initial evaluation. Usually, however, calculi are isolated, radiopaque, and recurrent. It is worthy of mention that calcium precipitation may form the nidus for a cystinuric stone, so chemical analysis of a stone showing a calcium component should not discount the importance of the presence of cystine. Thus the presentation of cystinuria cannot be distinguished clinically from that of any other cause of renal colic and/or recurrent urolithiasis. From a therapeutic point of view (see below), it is worth noting that cystine excretion in cystinurics varies directly with sodium excretion, which is not to say that there is a well-established cause-and-effect relationship.

Diagnostic Approach The first step in diagnosis is an awareness of the relative frequency of the disorder and thus a pursuit of its underlying presence in a patient with renal colic, recurrent urinary tract infection, or chronic renal failure of undetermined etiology with a history of urolithiasis. This should become a still higher priority in such cases as these where there is a similar family history. Initial morning urinalysis, even in the asymptomatic patient, will show the flat, hexagonal crystals of cystine; it is important to keep in mind that in this disorder even heterozygotes may be at risk for stone formation, so such a finding never must be ignored. An excellent chemical screening test for urinary cystine is the cyanide–nitroprusside reaction, which yields an unmistakable purple color in the presence of more than 75 mg/L. This chemical confirmation should be followed by a 24-hour urine collection for amino acid quantitation, which will be diagnostic. In addition, it is advisable to obtain an abdominal radiograph, even if the individual is asymptomatic, because cystine stones are radiopaque, and there is a tendency for the formation of large staghorn calculi that may remain clinically silent for years.

Treatment The two classical approaches to therapy rest squarely on physiological principles of solubility and pH. Since cystine has a maximum solubility of 300 mg/L, one obvious means of addressing the low solubility is to increase the urinary volume by increasing free water intake. Although theoretically quite effective, in practice, this approach is limited by the fact that some cystinuric patients excrete in excess of 1 g of cystine per day. It must be noted that this process continues over 24 hours based on renal circulation. Hence the patient must take in approximately 3.5 L of water per day, around the clock and every single day of life, which clearly detracts from the quality of life. Patient compliance with this regimen alone is not likely to be good, and years of therapeutic experience have provided confirmation of this. The second approach, using pH adjustment as a tool, takes advantage of the rapid increase in cystine solubility above pH 7. By adjusting the urinary pH through ingestion of alkali, the excreted cystine thus is made more soluble. There is some debate regarding the most advisable form of alkali to use, but it seems most advantageous to use citrate because the calcium-chelating action of citrate may be of help in reducing any tendency toward formation of a calcium nidus in alkaline urine. In addition to reduction of dietary sodium because of the direct relationship between excreted sodium and urine cystine, the use of potassium citrate is preferable to sodium bicarbonate for the production of alkaline urine.

Pharmacological treatment for cystinuria continues to rely on the simple principle of increasing solubility. The difference, however, is that the available compounds used for this purpose increase solubility by reducing the disulfide bond and then re-forming it with the drug to form more soluble molecules called *mixed disulfides*. As a consequence, the urine of a treated cystinuric patient will contain free cystine at a concentration below the solubility limit and a proportionately higher concentration of mixed disulfide compounds that are freely cleared in the kidney and do not precipitate. However, the drugs used, penicillamine, D-acetyl penicillamine, and mercaptopropionyl glycine, each have associated serious side effects seen in some, but not all, cystinuric patients. These include rashes, fever, arthralgia (separately or together, as in serum sickness), nephrotoxicity (e.g., nephrotic syndrome or rapidly progressive glomerulonephritis), pancytopenia, and various less serious complications. Most of these will resolve spontaneously on discontinuation of the drug, but many of them are serious enough that the risks should be faced only in patients who do not respond satisfactorily to classical treatment. Recent experience has been mixed in therapeutic trials of captopril, a sulfhydryl compound used in the treatment of hypertension that is generally well tolerated. In some studies it has been shown to be effective in reduction of free cystine excretion, whereas in others no effect could be demonstrated.

Monitoring of therapy should include the investigation of urinary pH (daily to weekly), hematuria, leukocyturia, and quantitative follow-up of urinary excretion of cystine, as well as ultrasonography of the kidneys in addition to clinical monitoring.

Lysinuric Protein Intolerance (Familial Protein Intolerance)

A discussion of lysinuric protein intolerance (LPI) follows logically from the earlier section on cystinuria because the urinary pattern of amino acid excretion is essentially the same but for the absence of cystine in LPI. Also as in cystinuria, the intestinal absorption of dibasic amino acids is impaired, illustrating once again the similarities of gene expression in kidney and intestinal epithelium. However, at this point, all similarity between the two entities ends. Initially described by Perheentupa and Visakorpi in 1965 as a disease of protein intolerance characterized by hyperammonemic coma and deficient transport of basic amino acids (35), the largest number of known patients with this disorder has been found in Finland. Due to the dramatic onset of coma, it was thought originally that LPI was likely a disorder of the urea cycle with an associated transport defect, but it is now clear that the transport defect is the primary abnormality. As study of cystinosis led to characterization of the first example of a lysosomal amino acid transport abnormality, investigation of LPI led to discovery of the first human disorder of an abnormality of epithelial basolateral surface amino acid transport. Transmitted as an autosomal recessive trait, the incidence in Finland is estimated at 1 in 60,000 population; the incidence in other countries is much lower and varies widely (36).

Pathophysiology Entry of amino acids from the intestine to the portal blood requires successful negotiation of the intestinal epithelium; this, in turn, poses at least two barriers, the luminal and basolateral membrane surfaces. The luminal surface of intestinal epithelial cells possesses a single transport system that is shared by cystine and the dibasic amino acids, unlike the kidney (Figure 42-7). Since cystine is derived from methionine metabolism, normal plasma cystine concentrations give no information about renal cystine handling in LPI. However, the ability of the kidney to reabsorb filtered cystine in LPI patients is clearly demonstrated by the conspicuous absence of significantly increased urinary cystine concentrations. By contrast, urinary excretion of lysine, arginine, and ornithine is massive, and plasma concentrations of all three are reduced substantially from normal in LPI patients (37). Failure of plasma concentrations to rise following an oral load implicates the intestinal absorptive process in accounting for the low plasma concentrations. However, an isolated deficiency of dibasic amino acid transport in the kidney and defective intestinal transport of these same compounds would require involvement of two distinct brush-border transport systems, each one on separate chromosomes. While such an explanation might be possible in a single, isolated individual, it is clearly inadequate to explain the dilemma of two autosomal recessive traits predictably appearing in multiple individuals in a pedigree.

The solution to the dilemma is contained in the fact that oral loading of patients with LPI with a lysyl-dipeptide, transported by a separate system, also did not enhance plasma lysine concentration (38). Dipeptides are known to be hydrolyzed within the intestinal cell after entry; hence failure of the free intracellular lysine to enter the plasma compartment strongly supported a postulate that the defect in LPI resided at the level of efflux across the basolateral membrane surface of the intestinal epithelium (Figure 42-8) (39). This defect also has been demonstrated to exist in the proximal renal tubule and cultured skin fibroblasts, and it is believed likely that it

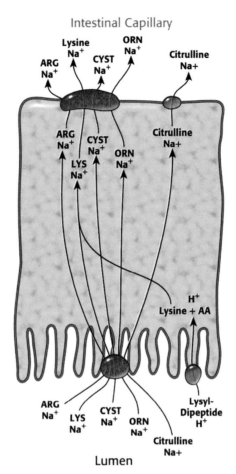

FIGURE 42-8. The basis for lysinuric protein intolerance. Uptake of cystine and dibasic amino acids in the intestine occurs by means of a single, shared carrier. Dipeptide uptake occurs by a separate carrier and intracellularly, the dipeptide is hydrolyzed to its separate components. Egress into the intestinal capillary of all these amino acids, with the exception of citrulline, which exits via a separate carrier requires a single basolateral carrier. For details of impaired function of the common carrier in LPI, see text.

also is present in hepatocytes (40). Thus lysine that enters the cell across the brush-border surface becomes "trapped" and backfluxes across the brush-border surface following a concentration gradient. Since arginine and ornithine share the same basolateral transport system, they accompany lysine into the urine. Cystine remains normal or near normal in the urine because transport of cystine at the basolateral surface in the renal tubule is independent of that of the others. Citrulline does not usually appear in elevated concentrations in the urine of LPI patients because this neutral amino acid does not share the basolateral system common to the other three. On the other hand, infusions of citrulline sufficient to produce citrullinuria in the LPI patient also will elevate urinary excretion of arginine and ornithine. The putative mechanism by which this occurs is renal conversion of citrulline to arginine and then ornithine, the latter two being unable to cross the basolat-

eral membrane and therefore appearing in the urine (41).

Although the mechanism underlying the significant hyperammonemia seen in these individuals remains somewhat obscure, normal urea cycle enzyme activities make it clear that it does not derive from any intrinsic abnormality in the urea cycle. Based on the preceding observations, it has been proposed that the extremely depressed circulating arginine and ornithine causes a hepatic mitochondrial ornithine "deficiency". This slows the urea cycle distal to carbamylphosphate synthase I and causes active production of orotic acid from carbamylphosphate II, excreted in urine after a protein load. This hypothesis is supported by the observation that intravenous infusion of arginine or ornithine or oral citrulline supplement will abort the hyperammonemia in a protein-loaded patient. There is no direct evidence for a hepatocytic "ornithine deficiency" in LPI, but the proposed mechanism is sufficient to a pathophysiological discussion. A further pathophysiological link is to arginine as the starting point of creatine synthesis.

Clinical Presentation As in so many other inborn errors with catastrophic outcomes, neonates with LPI typically are asymptomatic, especially if breast-fed, because of the relatively low protein content of human breast milk. Moreover, these infants are typically the outcomes of normal pregnancies, are of normal birth weight, and have normal newborn examinations; in the absence of neonatal metabolic screening, they are indistinguishable from all other infants. With advances in the feeding regimen and consequent increases in protein intake, the affected infant will begin to experience anorexia and vomiting and will show decreased growth and hepatosplenomegaly combined with muscular hypotonia. The relationship between increased protein density of the diet, greater frequency of vomiting, and slowed growth eventually presents as a full-blown failure to thrive; when combined with the marked hypotonia and organomegaly, a complete metabolic investigation is mandatory. Anemia and leukopenia are additional frequent findings, and serum ferritin is highly elevated.

The essential role of lysine in human nutrition is very widespread, inasmuch as lysine is present in most body proteins. Lysine is key to collagen formation, and a deficiency of lysine as occurs in LPI has an adverse impact on collagen and hence bone formation. As a result, pathological fractures are common in children with LPI, and the radiographical picture is one of manifest osteoporosis. The fractures usually are of long bones or vertebral compression and occur with the greatest frequency before age 5 years. Skeletal maturation is delayed, growth is impaired, the normal pubertal spurt generally is absent, yet adult height generally is less than 2 standard deviations (SD) below the mean because of the prolongation of bone growth.

Enlargement of the liver is common and is likely a result of the same essential amino acid deficiency that impairs bone growth. As in protein-deficient malnutrition (kwashiorkor), there is fatty degeneration, and inflammation is present; in some affected children who have died, autopsy findings suggest a degree of hepatic cirrhosis. Enlargement of the spleen has been found in some autopsies to be due to accumulation of amyloid material.

Perhaps the most worrisome finding in older patients and even some children has been the appearance of radiological changes consistent with pulmonary fibrosis, even in the absence of symptoms. Some individuals have had frank respiratory insufficiency, and lung biopsy/autopsy findings have shown changes of alveolar proteinosis or, in some, cholesterol granuloma formations. A second, later manifestation of LPI is renal glomerular involvement leading to diffuse, membranous or mesangial proliferative glomerulonephritis. The pathophysiology of these aspects of LPI remains completely obscure; although abnormal metabolism of an essential amino acid such as lysine could be the cause, these findings do not appear in patients suffering from prolonged protein malnutrition. Thus one is forced to conclude that while a lysine transport defect may be at fault, other factors clearly are involved. The susceptibility to severe hyperammonemic episodes decreases with age, and most affected adults have normal intelligence. Episodic psychiatric symptoms have been observed.

Diagnostic Approach It is important to recognize that LPI in an infant shares many of the symptoms of the urea cycle disorders; anorexia, vomiting, aversion to protein ingestion, irritability, somnolence, failure to thrive, orotic aciduria, and especially hyperammonemic coma are common to both. Thus a high index of suspicion for the urea cycle disorders also should account for LPI; hyperammonemia and orotic aciduria with a very low plasma ornithine, arginine, and lysine profile should elevate suspicion. The physical finding of hepatosplenomegaly may help in differentiation because organomegaly is not seen regularly in patients with urea cycle disorders. A urine amino acid profile showing massive amounts of lysine, arginine, and ornithine without cystine, together with the preceding, is diagnostic. Although many identified patients are Finnish, the disease has been found in many countries, so the

diagnostic possibility of LPI ought not to be discounted because of national origin.

In an undiagnosed older infant or young child undergoing evaluation for poor growth, a history of the preceding symptoms is vitally important to obtain and should suggest episodic hyperammonemia. In the course of such an evaluation, if long bone radiographs are obtained, the presence of osteoporosis should direct attention to the possibility of LPI. Once again, urine orotic acid and the plasma and urine amino acid profiles are diagnostic. Despite the rarity of LPI in relation to the family of urea cycle disorders, it is imperative that *all* potential metabolic causes of hyperammonemia be excluded before consideration of a force-feeding regimen to remedy apparent protein malnutrition, which would have devastating consequences.

Treatment Infants and young children with LPI are at risk of acute decompensation with hyperammonemia. This can be precipitated by any metabolic stress, such as fasting, a protein load, infection, anesthesia, or surgery. Early and consequent implementation of emergency treatment of intercurrent illnesses reduce the risk for hyperammonemic crises. All patients should have clear, detailed instructions of what to do (see Chapter 7).

Patients with LPI develop an early aversion to protein ingestion, a factor that may contribute further to the protein malnutrition deriving from a lysine deficiency directly related to the disease process. The reduced capacity of the urea cycle necessitates a protein-restricted diet that will be palatable and can reliably supply minimal needs for growth and development (see Chapter 7). This modality is basic to treatment of this disorder.

Given that defective intestinal malabsorption of lysine is the basis for this disorder, it is obvious that oral supplements of this amino acid are not likely to be helpful in therapy. The same holds true for arginine and ornithine; however, oral citrulline supplementation is well tolerated and quite effective in preventing many of the complications of LPI. The rationale for this regimen rests with the fact that citrulline, as a normal precursor to arginine and then ornithine in the urea cycle, when present in excess, will be converted to each in turn, thus alleviating the shortage of ornithine postulated to be the etiological factor in the hyperammonemia of this disease. Doses employed are 3–8 g/day, given with meals. Meeting minimal protein requirements with a low-protein diet while increasing the tolerance for protein by enhancing urea cycle activity with citrulline establishes the best possible protection for the affected individual against brain damage from hyperammonemia and enhances growth. However, there is no evidence for a protective

effect against the osteoporosis or the pulmonary or renal complications of the disease. It should be noted that the renal disease does not respond to high-dose steroids.

Hartnup Disorder

This autosomal recessive disorder of neutral amino acid transport is named for the family in whom the index cases were discovered (42,43,44). The defect is localized to renal and intestinal epithelium and came to medical attention originally in a patient who shared pellagra-like symptoms with his older sister. Virtually all neutral amino acids are lost to a variable degree in urine and/or feces as a consequence of the membrane-transport abnormality, the one of greatest significance being tryptophan. Originally thought of as an extremely rare condition, there are now reports from many countries, including Japan, Netherlands, Switzerland, and the United States, and the estimated overall incidence may be as high as 1 in 20,000 population. Interestingly, a large number of individuals identified through newborn screening and their affected family members are asymptomatic; the reasons for the apparent heterogeneity of clinical manifestations remain unclear, although several distinct mutations have been identified. It remains to be determined whether these are sufficient to explain the wide disparity in clinical picture among affected individuals.

Pathophysiology With the caveat that many genetically affected individuals apparently remain clinically normal without treatment, the chief manifestations of the disorder can be attributed to the massive loss of tryptophan in urine and feces (45). The category of neutral amino acids includes the important essential branched-chain amino acids (i.e., leucine, isoleucine, and valine), as well as threonine, and these compounds are transported by alternative systems that act to prevent deficiency. Tryptophan, categorized as an essential amino acid for humans, is therefore the only one of the amino acids lost that cannot be compensated through normal nutrition. One of the roles that tryptophan plays in metabolism is a limited conversion to niacin, thus making niacin the only "vitamin" that can be synthesized by the human body. Both nicotinamide dinucleotide (NAD) and nicotinamide dinucleotide phosphate (NADP) can be synthesized from tryptophan; NAD is used chiefly as a cofactor in oxidative pathways, such as the Krebs cycle, whereas NADP is important in lipogenesis and the pentose phosphate pathway, which is key to ribonucleotide synthesis. Perhaps the very central roles played in metabolism by the niacin-dependent pathways are what led to evolution of the ability to replace dietary deficiency with endogenous cofactor synthesis, to however limited an extent.

The defect is present at the brush-border surface of the renal tubular and intestinal epithelial cells. The basis for this defect is a mutation in the gene SLC6A19 resulting in an abnormal carrier, termed B^0AT1, that is responsible for sodium-dependent neutral amino acid transport across the brush-border surface (46,47). Expression of this gene is restricted to kidney, intestine, and skin; interestingly, affinity of the B^0AT1 protein carrier for tryptophan is rather low in relation to the other amino acids in the neutral group. If fed free amino acids, Hartnup patients show little to no plasma amino acid response, whereas if fed dipeptides consisting of the same amino acids, there is an increase in plasma concentrations (48,49). This points to defective free amino acid entry at the brush-border surface but normal transit across the basolateral surface once the dipeptide enters the cell and is hydrolyzed. Free filtration of neutral amino acids in the glomerulus leads to large amounts of these compounds presented to the tubular brush-border surface; defective uptake of tryptophan results in large urinary losses. Consequently, the combined losses of tryptophan hamper the ability of affected individuals to compensate marginal niacin intake by endogenous synthesis, leading to the clinical manifestations of niacin deficiency.

Clinical Presentation At the outset, it is important to reiterate the fact that many, if not most, genetically affected individuals show no overt manifestations of the disorder (50). Obligate heterozygotes also do not announce themselves by virtue of an aminoaciduria. To make matters even more confusing, there have been reports of individuals who have shown only urinary or only fecal losses (51). Thus the discussion of presentation here is directed at the classical picture of Hartnup disorder, as originally described.

The essential clinical features of Hartnup disorder, aside from the pathognomonic urinary amino acid excretion pattern, include a striking skin rash and cerebral ataxia. The rash is one that is identical to that seen in pellagra, the syndrome associated with dietary niacin deficiency, and appears on exposed surfaces (i.e., hands, face, and neck). It is erythematous, scaly, and crusted, and occasionally, there may be associated vesicle formation or desquamation. There may be a history of increasing dizziness, culminating in intermittent ataxia with a gait disturbance; frequent emotional instability and sometimes psychotic behavior also can be a part of the clinical presentation.

Diagnostic Approach Since the pathognomonic aminoaciduria is asymptomatic in and of itself, there would be no reason to engage in a diagnostic evaluation in an asymptomatic individual who was not related to a proband. However, in any individual who presents with pellagra-like skin lesions, Hartnup disorder should be considered in the differential diagnosis, especially because of its relative frequency in relation to dietary niacin deficiency, at least in the United States. The presence of emotional lability or bizarre psychiatric symptoms and/or gait disturbance should further heighten suspicion.

An exhaustive dietary history is imperative because there are foods that may interfere with normal metabolism of either dietary tryptophan or niacin; both sorghum and corn are examples of such foods, the former a common cause of pellagra in Java. Following this, a urinary amino acid profile should be obtained. If present, the pattern is clearly pathognomonic for Hartnup disorder; the urine will contain large quantities of alanine, asparagine, glutamine, histidine, isoleucine, leucine, phenylalanine, serine, threonine, tryptophan, tyrosine, and valine. The pattern differs from the "generalized aminoaciduria" seen in renal Fanconi syndrome by virtue of the conspicuous absence of all basic and acidic amino acids. By contrast, because of the normal capacity for absorption of dipeptides, the massive free amino acid losses are not reflected in depressed plasma concentrations.

Treatment Since the manifestations of the disorder are directly related to systemic niacin deficiency, as in pellagra, the therapeutic approach is directed at correction of this abnormality. Thus oral administration of supplemental nicotinamide reverses all clinical manifestations but will not affect the aminoaciduria. Consequently, supplementation will be required on a chronic basis to prevent recurrence of clinical symptoms. In an attempt to avoid the vasodilatory effects of large amounts of nicotinamide, therapy with the lipid-soluble tryptophan ethyl ester has been used successfully as an alternative means of increasing plasma tryptophan and alleviating symptoms.

GLUT1 Deficiency (DeVivo Syndrome)

This disorder, described initially by DeVivo and colleagues in 1991 (52), is the first of what will almost certainly become an entire family of conditions involving nutrient transport into the central nervous system (CNS). As a critically important metabolic fuel, the supply of glucose to cells cannot be left to simple diffusion alone; to date, five distinct glucose transporter proteins have been described (53).

Each one functions by facilitative diffusion that does not require energy and does not act against a concentration gradient yet acts to translocate glucose molecules across the lipid membrane barrier at a rate faster than simple diffusion would permit. One of these proteins, GLUT1, is present in erythrocytes and brain capillaries at a density approximately tenfold greater than any other tissues. It has been estimated that the GLUT1-containing brain capillaries transfer 10 times their weight in glucose per minute to the brain (52,54,55). This is critical to the highly active oxidative metabolism of the brain, which consumes glucose as its primary fuel. Of course, looked at from the opposite perspective, a deficiency of GLUT1-dependent glucose transfer by brain capillaries might be expected to have devastating consequences. These very consequences at the clinical level define the disease now recognized as autosomal dominant GLUT1 transporter deficiency. Although the true incidence is not known, a decade after the initial description, 54 patients had been identified, representing 28 distinct gene mutations (56,57).

Pathophysiology Until 1967, it was believed that brain metabolism was exclusively glucose-dependent; following the 1967 report of Owen et al., it has become common wisdom that during the slow transition from the postprandial state to one of fasting, the brain gradually transitions to a preference for ketone bodies, which do not require the GLUT1 transporter for entry (58). What is still unknown is whether there are regions within the brain that remain glucose-dependent even as the organ shifts overall to ketone body use (59,60). Such a possibility becomes particularly germane in respect to the therapeutic responses in this disorder, as discussed below. In any event, it is also well established that even in a ketone-consuming state, the brain retains a minimal glucose requirement, which represents that quantity necessary for generation of oxaloacetate to fuel the citric acid cycle.

The two critically important steps in initial glucose disposition are the cellular entry and conversion to glucose-6-phosphate. In the CNS, glucose transport as facilitated diffusion normally follows a concentration gradient from blood to cells and therefore is not rate-limiting for metabolism. Thus the normal rate-limiting step is phosphorylation, which creates a reservoir of unmetabolized glucose in the surrounding milieu. However, with decrease in the rate of facilitated diffusion due to restricted numbers of GLUT1 transporters, the reservoir is greatly diminished, and the rate of diffusion approaches more closely the rate of phosphorylation. Keeping in mind the fact that the brain's conversion from glucose to ketones for fuel is a slow, adaptive process, this now diminished reservoir places the brain at risk for glucose deprivation. It is this situation that leads to the clinical picture.

Clinical Presentation Onset of symptoms typically is at about 2 months of age; this would be consistent with the rapid postnatal growth of the brain that is seen normally and might be expected to place greater demand on glucose supply than the impaired transport system is able to supply (59,60). The usual first manifestation is a seizure, often myoclonic in appearance, and seizures become increasingly frequent as the infant grows older.

The key features of GLUT1 transporter deficiency are infantile-onset seizures and developmental delay, at least the first of which can be attributed with certainty to an episodic glucose deprivation in the brain. Together with the developmental delay, the growth of the cranium decelerates, and microcephaly is the rule in most reported patients. There may be varying degrees of spasticity and an ataxic gait, as well as toe-walking. Expressive language development is affected to a greater degree than is receptive development.

As the experience with affected children has grown, a spectrum of severity has emerged ranging from individuals who are developmentally normal between occasional seizures to severely disabled children who are unable to walk or talk. It has been hypothesized that there may be a correlation between genotype and phenotype that could account for this wide spectrum of variation. This theory requires for proof far greater experience with this disease than we have to date but remains a tantalizing explanation for the observations nonetheless.

Diagnostic Approach The sine qua non of diagnosis of GLUT1 transporter deficiency is the finding of a normal blood sugar concentration and an abnormally low cerebrospinal fluid (CSF) glucose concentration determined simultaneously. A ratio of blood to CSF sugar of less than 0.35 is considered suspicious (normal 0.65 ± 0.1). Although such a picture can be seen in bacterial meningitis or mitochondropathies, a distinguishing feature in relation to both these conditions is that in GLUT1 transporter deficiency the CSF lactate generally is below normal. Thus euglycemia in the face of low CSF glucose and lactate concentrations is virtually diagnostic of the disease. There are a number of ways to confirm the diagnosis, including evaluation of the uptake of a glucose analogue by erythrocytes, analysis of the gene product, and molecular probing of the gene itself.

Treatment The deficiency of GLUT1 transporters in the CNS effectively causes the brain to starve for glucose, leaving it entirely competent to adapt to ketone bodies for its metabolic fuel. Consequently, a ketogenic diet is the only effective treatment available. Supplementation of carbohydrate-free vitamins and minerals is essential. The diet needs to be introduced in a clinical setting and requires a pediatrician and dietician experienced with the diet in order to be successful. Outpatient follow-up needs to be close with an interdisciplinary team. Compliance is followed by measuring ketones in blood and urine. If ketones are inappropriately low, dietary instructions must be evaluated and possibly intensified. A possible pitfall is the high carbohydrate content of many medications.

This approach was attempted with the first patient described by DeVivo and associates at 71/2 months of age with rapid and complete success in cessation of seizures (52). However, the child remained microcephalic and developmentally delayed by 27 months with limited expressive language development. Whether or not this treatment rendered early in infancy will support normal development is a question requiring further clarification based on more experience.

An additional consideration is the fact that a chronic demand for ketone bodies generated by the diet also places considerable stress on the fatty acid catabolic pathway. A major factor in fatty acid catabolism is carnitine, which is important for entry of the fatty acid into the mitochondrion, where it is subjected to β-oxidation. Although carnitine is synthesized endogenously, such an unusual and chronic demand can outstrip the supply, so carnitine supplementation is recommended as well.

Finally, it should go without saying that GLUT1 inhibitors should be completely eliminated or avoided (61). Paradoxically, the first-line treatments for seizures in infancy are diazepam and phenobarbital, known to be inhibitors of GLUT1 transporter protein. Methyl xanthines, such as caffeine, chloral hydrate, and ethanol, are also known inhibitors. Valproate interferes with fatty acid oxidation and therefore is contraindicated. Topiramate, sultiam, and acetazolamid all inhibit the enzyme carbonicanydrase, which can result in an increase of metabolic acidosis.

Renal Tubular Glycosuria

Renal tubular glycosuria is most simply defined as the appearance of detectable glucose in urine with simultaneously normal blood sugar concentrations. No other hexose is found in excess in the urine of a patient with renal glycosuria, suggesting that the defect is specific for glucose. The most logical conclusion to reach from this is that the condition is due to a renal membrane transport defect for glucose. Originally thought to be transmitted as an autosomal dominant trait, the defect is now recognized to be an "incompletely" autosomal recessive trait, in which heterozygotes also may excrete glucose in urine (60). The true incidence is unknown because of a lack of active population screening studies. Although present as a genetic trait from birth, due to the benign nature of the disorder, it is frequently unrecognized until later in childhood when routine urinalysis indicates the presence of glucose.

Pathophysiology As a small organic molecule, glucose is freely filtered by the glomerulus and is almost completely cleared from the urine by the normal nephron; less than 0.05% of the daily filtered glucose load appears in the urine. About 90% of this load is removed from the filtrate by the proximal convoluted tubule and the remainder throughout the rest of the length of the nephron. Under usual circumstances, in a normal adult male, approximately 175 g of glucose is filtered through the glomerulus each day, so approximately 87.5 mg escapes reabsorption. Any impairment in the process that caused as little as a 1% daily loss would increase this to 1.75 g of glucose, thus illustrating the major impact of a small decrease in reabsorptive capacity.

Glucose transport across the luminal surface of the proximal convoluted tubule occurs by means of an energy-dependent, carrier-mediated, and Na^+-dependent mechanism (Figure 42-9) (61,62). Thus transport of glucose at this site is concentrative and proceeds against a concentration gradient. The driving force for this brush-border phenomenon is the Na^+,K^+-ATPase located at the inner basolateral membrane that pumps sodium out of and potassium into the cell. On the other hand, glucose exit from the tubule cell occurs by a separate process of sodium-independent facilitated diffusion along the concentration gradient (by definition) and expedited by separate carriers (GLUT2 and GLUT1). There is heterogeneity of brush-border transport along the length of the nephron as a consequence of the presence of two distinct carriers at the brush-border surface (63). In the early proximal tubule, there is a low-affinity, high-capacity sodium-dependent carrier (designated SGLT2) acting in tandem with the basolateral high-capacity GLUT2 carrier. This system gradually gives way in the late proximal tubule to a high-affinity, low-capacity sodium-dependent carrier (designated SGLT1) acting together with the high-affinity GLUT1 at the basolateral surface (64). From a physiological perspective, this is ideal because glucose is freely filtered and present in the early proximal tubule in concentrations equivalent to those of plasma. As the bulk

Proximal Tubule

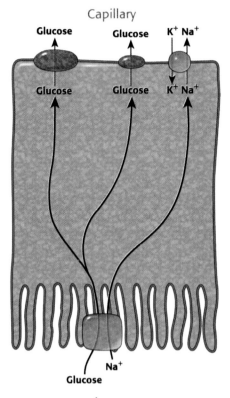

FIGURE 42-9. Glucose uptake in the proximal renal tubule. Entry of glucose at the luminal surface occurs by a sodium-dependent, energy-requiring carrier. The driving energy source is the antiluminal Na^+,K^+-ATPase. Glucose egress into the capillary is expedited by facilitated diffusion mediated by GLUT2 and GLUT1.

of this load is reabsorbed and the luminal concentration substantially reduced, higher-affinity binding is required for the transport of smaller amounts more distally.

Using intravenous glucose titration, two distinct types of renal glycosuria can be distinguished, designated types A and B. In type A, there is reduction of both the blood glucose concentration at which glucosuria occurs and the maximum rate of glucose reabsorption. It is likely (but not yet proven) that these observations reflect a defect of the SGLT2 transporter representing decreased low-affinity, high-capacity uptake in the early proximal tubule (65,66). By contrast, in type B, there is a normal maximal capacity, but glucose appears in the urine at a lower blood concentration than in the normal individual, suggesting a defect in the SGLT1 low-capacity, high-affinity transporter. While these explanations fit the observations, confirmation remains problematic because of the difficulties in justifying renal biopsy in essentially normal individuals affected by a curiosity of nature.

Clinical Presentation Affected individuals are completely symptom-free, although the eu-

glycemic renal loss of glucose can make the affected person slightly more prone to dehydration and earlier development of starvation ketosis.

Diagnostic Approach Since the disorder is benign, the diagnostic imperative is to distinguish it from other, more significant clinical problems. Initial recognition is usually as a result of the detection of isolated glucosuria in a random urinalysis from an otherwise well individual. The obvious major differential entities are diabetes mellitus and renal Fanconi syndrome; in each case, the benign clinical status of the patient dictates an early state of evolution. The obvious next step is to evaluate the state of the blood glucose concentration, which predictably will be normal. However, in early diabetes and at all stages of renal Fanconi syndrome, the blood sugar should be in the normal range, so some further investigation is merited. In a youngster at risk for type 1 diabetes, a 2-hour postprandial blood sugar test should be sufficient to distinguish abnormalities. If there is an equivocal result and a question remains, a glucose tolerance test may be obtained. Obviously, in renal glycosuria, all values will be completely within normal limits. It should be stated unequivocally that other than the need to establish a diagnosis, there is absolutely no connection between renal glycosuria and diabetes mellitus, nor does the one "morph" into the other, so the presence of a diagnosed renal glycosuria may not be used to qualify life or health insurance. Exclusion of the renal Fanconi syndrome will require a more extensive workup in order to exclude underlying causes (see above).

Treatment Due to the completely benign nature of this genetic disorder, no treatment is required.

Familial Glucose–Galactose Malabsorption

In contrast to other membrane-transport defects, familial glucose–galactose malabsorption (FGGM) is a very rare but life-threatening condition in neonates as a result of a catastrophic onset of diarrhea. The infant is unable to tolerate any diet containing glucose, galactose, or lactose (which is hydrolyzed to the former monosaccharides) but will thrive on a fructose-based formula. The disease is transmitted as an autosomal recessive trait; heterozygotes are not consistently affected (see below).

Pathophysiology The basis for the clinical picture is an inability to normally absorb the two hexoses glucose and galactose (69). Because the disaccharide lactose is hydrolyzed by the intestinal epithelium at the luminal surface

with the release of both glucose and galactose monomers and the disaccharide sucrose to yield glucose and fructose, lactose and sucrose are also offending substances. It should be noted here that this disease is distinct from lactase deficiency. Congenital lactase deficiency is likewise a rare condition. Since a significant proportion (35% to 45%) of a neonate's caloric intake consists normally of lactose, combined with a higher per kilogram of body weight water requirement, an inability to absorb the sugars will result in massive osmotic diarrhea with rapid deterioration. Of particular note in this regard is the fact that a direct link between sugar and water reabsorption has been established recently, a process that normally accounts for several liters of water reabsorption per day (70). The fact that removal of lactose from the diet without withdrawal of glucose and galactose will have no therapeutic impact clearly distinguishes this entity from lactase deficiency and implicates a specific membrane-transport defect.

Normal glucose and galactose entry from the intestinal lumen into the epithelial cell is mediated by the Na^+-dependent carrier SGLT1; exit into the blood at the basolateral surface occurs by facilitated diffusion along a concentration gradient mediated by the carrier GLUT2 (71,72). Using autoradiographic technique, Stirling and colleagues studied the entry of [^{14}C]galactose into intestinal biopsy specimens, incontrovertibly demonstrating a defect in entry and confirming the pathophysiological hypothesis that the massive diarrhea associated with the disease was specifically related to failure of enterocytes to take up the monosaccharides glucose and galactose (73,74). Deficiency of SGLT1 finally was confirmed by demonstrating pathogenic mutations.

Clinical Presentation Since glucose–galactose malabsorption is a genetic disorder, intolerance to dietary carbohydrate is manifested immediately after birth, on first feeding. Thus there is an abrupt onset of profuse, watery diarrhea following a lactose-, glucose-, or galactose-containing feeding. This diarrhea will lead to rapid dehydration, vascular collapse, shock, and death if not reversed rapidly by discontinuation of intestinal carbohydrate loading. Keeping in mind the frequent commonality of genetic expression in intestinal and renal cells and the fact that SGLT1 normally is expressed in renal tubular epithelium (75,76), there may be an associated renal glycosuria. Intestinal absorption of fructose and all amino acids is entirely normal, so proper choice of a formula containing fructose will result in abrupt remission and rapid return to a healthy state.

Diagnostic Approach The initial approach to evaluation should be a stool pH, expected in this case to be strongly acidic as a result of sugar-metabolizing bacterial action on the unabsorbed sugars. A breath hydrogen test will confirm the intestine's inability to absorb glucose and galactose quickly and noninvasively. With this evidence, there is no justification for intestinal biopsy because any histopathological changes observed will be secondary to the fundamental genetic defect.

Treatment The straightforward approach to treatment of this disorder is the elimination of dietary glucose, galactose, and lactose by provision of a fructose-based formula. Obviously, as the infant grows older, the diet will need to be tightly controlled because these sugars are widely distributed both in nature and in prepared foods. Thus, as solids are introduced, the assistance of an expert nutritionist is mandatory. With increased patient age, the tolerance of glucose, lactose, and sucrose increases.

ABNORMALITIES OF RENAL ION TRANSPORT

Bartter Syndrome

Bartter and associates published the first description of hyperplasia of the juxtaglomerular complex with hyperaldosteronism and hypokalemic alkalosis in 1962 (77). This publication initiated an intense interest in the molecular mechanisms of ion transport in the nephron that continues its momentum unabated to the present day. On clinical grounds, three distinct phenotypes have emerged since the original report: antenatal Bartter syndrome, classical Bartter syndrome (as first described), and Gitelman syndrome, which will be discussed separately. All can be defined as sharing the following characteristics: renal salt wasting, hypokalemic metabolic alkalosis (see Figure 42-10), normotensive hyperreninemia, hyperaldosteronism, and juxtaglomerular hyperplasia. In addition, all are transmitted as autosomal recessive traits. A great deal has been learned regarding the underlying molecular abnormalities in these disorders and thus the normal mechanisms of ion transport.

Antenatal Bartter Syndrome (Type I Bartter, Hyperprostaglandin E Syndrome)

This is the most severe form of Bartter syndrome, announcing itself by marked fetal polyuria causing polyhydramnios from the 6th month of gestation. Premature labor and delivery are the rule rather than the exception in this disorder. At 20 weeks of gestation, normal fetal urine output approximates 0.1 mL/minute and increases to 1.0 mL/minute at 40 weeks, only to fall back to 0.1 mL/minute

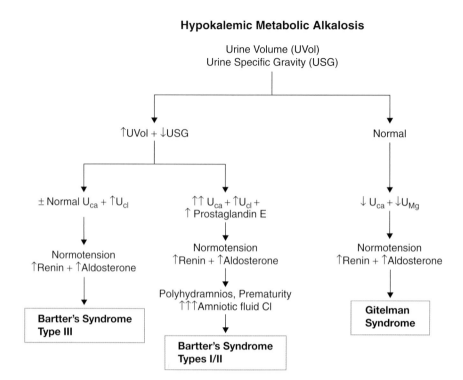

Hypokalemic Metabolic Alkalosis

Urine Volume (UVol)
Urine Specific Gravity (USG)

↑UVol + ↓USG → Normal

↑UVol + ↓USG branch:
- ± Normal U_{ca} + ↑U_{cl} → Normotension ↑Renin + ↑Aldosterone → **Bartter's Syndrome Type III**
- ↑↑ U_{ca} + ↑U_{cl} + ↑ Prostaglandin E → Normotension ↑Renin + ↑Aldosterone → Polyhydramnios, Prematurity ↑↑↑Amniotic fluid Cl → **Bartter's Syndrome Types I/II**

Normal branch:
- ↓ U_{ca} + ↓U_{Mg} → Normotension ↑Renin + ↑Aldosterone → **Gitelman Syndrome**

FIGURE 42-10. Hypokalemic metabolic alkalosis should immediately suggest the presence of either Bartter or Gitelman syndrome. The simplest means of distinction is measurement of urinary volume and specific gravity based on the pathophysiology (see text). Hypoexcretion of calcium and magnesium is characteristic of Gitelman syndrome and should be used as the next step in differentiation between the two, as shown.

in the neonatal state. In a newborn affected by type I Bartter syndrome, this urinary output may be as high as 2.5 mL/minute, emphasizing the degree of polyuria seen both intra- and extrauterinely in this disease. The amniotic fluid contains a markedly elevated concentration of chloride, indicating the early fetal abnormalities of electrolyte reabsorption by the nephron. Genetic transmission of this disorder follows an autosomal recessive pattern.

Pathophysiology Ion transport by the nephron is an exceedingly complex process involving many different carriers located in various sites along the length of the structure and situated in a number of discrete loci within the epithelial cells that line it. In Bartter syndrome type I, the defective gene is designated SLC12A1 and codes for a transport protein called Na^+-K^+-$2Cl^-$ cotransporter (NKCC2) (78–82). This carrier normally is situated at the luminal membrane of the thick ascending limb of the loop of Henle (Figure 42-11); luminal chloride uptake by NKCC2 is driven by low intracellular Na^+ and chloride concentrations created by the basolateral Na^+,K^+-ATPase and chloride channels (ClC-Kb) that extrude sodium and chloride across the basolateral surface (Figure 42-12). A fourth factor in this process is the ATP-requiring inwardly rectifying potassium (ROMK) channel located in the luminal membrane and recycling K^+ from the cell back to the tubular lumen. An additional

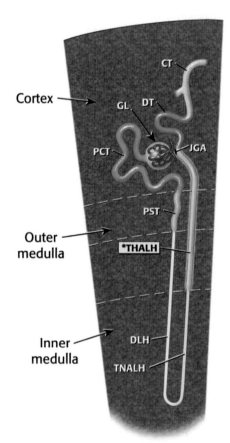

FIGURE 42-11. Nephron unit. The affected site of the nephron in antenatal Bartter's syndrome is the thick ascending limb of the loop of Henle (THALH), shown by an asterisk (*).

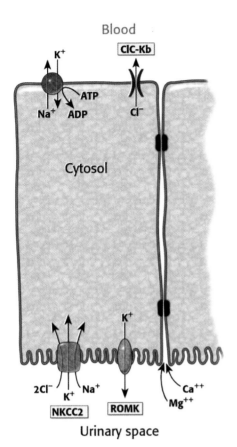

FIGURE 42-12. The transport defect in Bartter syndrome (types I, II, and III). Movement of chloride from the lumen to the cytosol takes place in the thick ascending limb of the loop of Henle via an Na$^+$-K$^+$-2Cl$^-$ cotransporter termed NKCC2. The driving force for this cotransport phenomenon derives from the antiluminal events of sodium–potassium exchange via a Na$^+$,K$^+$-ATPase and exit of Cl$^-$ through a chloride channel termed ClC-Kb. The function of the luminal potassium channel ROMK in returning potassium to the lumen enables the function of NKCC2. The luminal electropositivity generated by the simultaneous uptake of chloride and expulsion of potassium creates a driving force for paracellular movement of calcium and magnesium from lumen to blood. The molecular defect in type I Bartter syndrome is in the NKCC2 transporter; the defect in type II Bartter syndrome is in the ROMK potassium channel. Classical Bartter syndrome results from a defect in the antiluminal chloride channel, ClC-Kb.

feature of the ROMK channel function is that it generates the lumen-positive electrical gradient that energizes both calcium and magnesium reabsorption via paracellular pathways (83). The complexity of this overall process is such that a phenotypic abnormality due to a defect in one factor is not easily distinguished clinically from the phenotype associated with another impaired factor.

The most direct way to explain the pathophysiology of antenatal Bartter type I is that the dysfunctional NKCC2 leads to enhanced loss of urinary sodium, potassium, and chloride (84–86). In turn, there is a volume contraction that stimulates the renin–angiotensin axis and juxtaglomerular hypertrophy. The

potassium loss directly induces prostaglandin E$_2$ synthesis, which further adds to renin release and additional hypertrophy of the juxtaglomerular region (84). At least two major issues remain to be explained, however—why the amniotic fluid contains elevated chloride concentrations, whereas those of the other electrolytes are normal, and why the reabsorption of calcium and magnesium is so much more adversely affected in this form of Bartter syndrome than in others.

Clinical Presentation The presentation of antenatal Bartter syndrome is quite distinct from that of other forms of the syndrome (84,85). In the transition from the late second to the early third trimester of gestation, marked polyhydramnios appears as a consequence of fetal polyuria, often followed by premature birth. In the neonatal period, the infant manifests polyuria and iso/hyposthenuria, leading to severe, life-threatening dehydration. Failure to thrive is commonly associated with this form of Bartter syndrome. If the disorder is diagnosed and treated appropriately, the affected infant subsequently will evolve into a patient with all the features of classical Bartter syndrome (see below) (84).

Diagnostic Approach The rapid evolution of early third trimester polyhydramnios may alert the clinician to perform an amniocentesis, in which case measurement of chloride always should be a part of the chemical analysis of the fluid. In lieu of amniocentesis, in such cases, the chloride concentration of the fluid should be measured on delivery of the infant. On clinical laboratory examination of the newborn, the hallmark of the disease is hypokalemic metabolic alkalosis; hypochloremia is also present frequently, and there is marked hypercalciuria that often results in nephrocalcinosis. There is also severe urinary loss of sodium, potassium, and chloride accompanied by hyperaldosteronism and hyperreninism. However, the sine qua non of diagnosis given the preceding findings is demonstration of elevated systemic prostaglandin E, a feature that has led to the alternate naming of this disorder as *hyperprostaglandin E syndrome*.

Treatment Therapy is directed at the fundamental defect, which is urinary potassium loss as a consequence of impaired function of the NCCK2 transport carrier. Supplemental potassium is always required but alone cannot achieve adequate therapeutic effect because of the rapidity of urinary loss. Currently, the best available means for reducing potassium loss is to interrupt the production of excessive prostaglandin E by administration of the prostaglandin synthase inhibitor indomethacin. This drug should be used at dosages of 1.0–2.5 mg/kg/day (87). Even the lowest doses

have been reported in neonates to cause acute renal failure, which is quickly reversible with discontinuation (88); it is recommended that use of the drug in premature infants be delayed for 4–6 weeks after birth.. Higher doses, in the range of 3–5 mg/kg/day (not to exceed 150–200 mg/day), can be used in older children. Use of prenatal indomethacin has been reported from weeks 26–31 of gestation (88); results reportedly were good, although the rapid development of polyhydramnios on discontinuation at 31 weeks could be consistent with the natural history of the disease. The use of indomethacin prenatally is not without hazard because of the danger of premature constriction or closure of the ductus arteriosus. Shortly after the initiation of postnatal indomethacin treatment, serum potassium concentration rises in the face of reduced urinary losses, and serum aldosterone and renin concentrations fall toward normal. Adjustments to the indomethacin dosage should be made based on renal function, serum indomethacin levels, and urinary prostaglandin excretion. Assessment of urinary calcium excretion is also an important aspect of follow-up, and in patients in whom it remains elevated, periodic ultrasound of the kidneys is crucial to document nephrocalcinosis.

The use of rofecoxib, a cyclooxygenase-2 inhibitor, has been reported in an indomethacin-refractory case of antenatal Bartter syndrome (89), although this cannot be recommended without further study. Attempts to achieve a therapeutic effect by maternal indomethacin treatment and to avoid the extreme polyhydramnios and devastating fluid and salt losses will require further study before such therapy can be recommended.

Antenatal Bartter Syndrome Type II

This variant of Bartter syndrome is indistinguishable clinically from the antenatal form type I. The difference lies in the gene mutation and the resulting mutant protein; the former occurs on a distinctly different chromosome, whereas the latter affects the inward-rectifying apical potassium (ROMK) channel. Simon and colleagues were the first to report this distinct mutation in a number of different individuals from four kindreds, demonstrating the genetic heterogeneity of type I Bartter syndrome (90).

Pathophysiology The tight functional link between NCCK2 (see above) and ROMK in the medullary thick ascending loop of Henle easily explains the homogeneity of clinical phenotype shared between the two genotypes (86). While the Na$^+$-K$^+$-2Cl$^-$ cotransporter (NCCK2) is responsible for the cotransport of the three ions across the luminal surface into the epithelial cell, the enabling, favorable electrochemical gradient for K^+ is maintained by ROMK. Hence dysfunction in one branch of this functional "loop" impairs function of the other in direct proportion (see Figure 42-12). The result is urinary salt loss and all the attendant consequences, as addressed earlier.

Clinical Presentation Polyhydramnios, fetal and neonatal polyuria, hypokalemic metabolic alkalosis, and severe dehydration are identical to those seen in type I Bartter syndrome.

Diagnostic Approach Clinical laboratory parameters are indistinguishable from those of type I Bartter syndrome, including elevated prostaglandin E concentration. The sole distinction is the genotype.

Treatment Potassium supplementation and indomethacin treatment are instituted, as outlined earlier.

Classical Bartter Syndrome Type III

The so-called classical Bartter syndrome, as originally recognized and described, occurs beyond infancy and usually has its onset from ages 2–5 years. There is no pathognomonic history associated with prenatal events or serious illness; affected individuals are, by definition, normotensive. The gene mutation results in abnormal function of the chloride channel responsible for moving chloride ion from the cell into the blood (91,92). Since the gene defect is transmitted as an autosomal recessive trait, parents are unaffected clinically. An interesting feature of the classical variety has emerged over the years since its initial description—there is a wide heterogeneity of clinical expression not seen in the antenatal forms of the disease (92). The reasons underlying this difference remain unelucidated.

Pathophysiology Impairment of the basolateral surface chloride channel (ClC-Kb) function results in intracellular accumulation of chloride ion (84,86,93). This, in turn, adversely affects the normal electrogenic balance that encourages function of NKCC2 and entry of sodium, potassium, and chloride from the tubular lumen (see Figure 42-12). The consequence is, as in all forms of Bartter syndrome, increased urinary loss of salt with the attendant compensatory changes that result in hypochloremic metabolic alkalosis and normal blood pressure despite hyperreninism and hyperaldosteronism. It should be noted that in classical Bartter syndrome, as in the antenatal forms, there is elevation of prostaglandin E, which Bartter himself described. However, the increased prostaglandin E does not reach the levels seen in the

antenatal Bartter syndrome. It is thought that compensatory adjustments are made in the nephron for basolateral chloride transport because the salt losses are not as great as seen in the antenatal forms. Another important distinction lies in the absence of hypercalciuria and nephrocalcinosis in the classical form of the disorder; moreover, compensatory reabsorption in the proximal and distal tubule prevents marked hypocalcemia and, notably, hypomagnesmia, absence of which is an important differential diagnostic sign.

Clinical Presentation Onset of symptoms generally is after 1 year of age and includes polyuria, polydipsia, and salt hunger. In addition, vomiting and constipation may become manifest as development of hypokalemia progresses; there is also a tendency to dehydration secondary to the polyuria and salt loss. Untreated, failure to thrive becomes evident with time; some patients have been found to have associated growth hormone deficiency. Complaints of fatigue, muscle weakness, and cramping are common.

Diagnostic Approach Maintaining a high index of awareness is helpful because some patients are diagnosed from the starting point of a low serum potassium and an elevated total bicarbonate on an initial laboratory evaluation. Such studies certainly are warranted in a poorly growing child with polyuria and polydipsia, and the presence of a normal blood sugar concentration ought not to distract from these other possible abnormalities. Examination of urinary electrolyte excretion with demonstrable salt losses then may point the way to diagnosis by means of measuring serum aldosterone and renin levels.

Treatment As in other forms of Bartter syndrome, supplemental potassium is fundamental. Beyond this, indomethacin treatment (2–5 mg/kg/day) is less dramatically effective in the classical form than in the antenatal forms but necessary nonetheless. Long-term efficacy of indomethacin therapy is well established and relatively safe. Since urinary calcium excretion generally is not a problem in this form of Bartter syndrome, close follow-up of urine calcium concentration is not required, nor is periodic ultrasonic evaluation of the kidneys. However, it is important to monitor closely the serum potassium levels and to maintain great caution during any anesthetic procedures in an affected individual. Sudden death may result from severe potassium depletion due to urinary losses.

Gitelman Syndrome

As is immediately apparent from the gene locus, which is distinct from all others causing Bartter syndrome, Gitelman syndrome is

a separate entity that bears clinical similarity to the former. Initially described by Gitelman and associates in 1966 (94), this similarity has caused Gitelman syndrome to be viewed as a variant of Bartter syndrome in most authors' classifications. However, there are many reasons to doubt this, including the fact that prostaglandins are not elevated and the physical defect is located in the distal tubule compared with all Bartter variants, in which the defect is present in the thick ascending limb of the loop of Henle (95,96). The affected gene normally codes for a sodium–chloride transporter protein termed NCCT located at the luminal surface of the distal convoluted tubule (Figure 42-13). The carrier is also known as TSC, standing for *thiazide-sensitive cotransporter*, because chronic thiazide administration inhibits its function and produces many of the findings of the syndrome (97,98). Transmitted as an autosomal recessive trait, Gitelman syndrome is seen infrequently in pediatric-age patients.

Pathophysiology Functional impairment of the NCCT protein inhibits reabsorption of sodium and chloride in the distal convoluted tubule, which normally accounts for

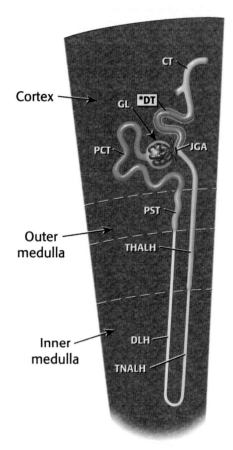

FIGURE 42-13. Region of nephron involvement in Gitelman syndrome. The nephron is shown with the distal tubule, the site of involvement in Gitelman syndrome, designated by an asterisk (*).

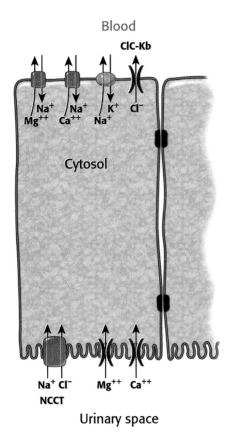

Blood

ClC-Kb

Na⁺ Na⁺ K⁺ Cl⁻
Mg⁺⁺ Ca⁺⁺ Na⁺

Cytosol

Na⁺ Cl⁻   Mg⁺⁺ Ca⁺⁺
NCCT

Urinary space

FIGURE 42-14. The transport defect in Gitelman syndrome. In the distal tubule cell, chloride transport into the cell is by means of a luminal NaCl cotransporter termed NCCT. Egress from the cell of each ion occurs by different means: Na⁺ exits by an antiluminal sodium–potassium ATPase; chloride exits via the chloride channel, ClC-Kb. The entry of Ca²⁺ and Mg²⁺ via voltage-regulated channels and exit via exchange with Na⁺ are speculative at this time. Gitelman syndrome is the result of a defect of either the NCCT transporter or the ClC-Kb chloride channel.

reabsorption of about 6% to 8% of the filtered sodium load (see Figure 42-14). The consequent increased delivery of sodium to the collecting tubule will reduce free water reabsorption and cause mild polyuria, the ensuing volume contraction thus promoting an aldosterone secretory response. As a result, there is enhanced distal tubular secretion of potassium and hydrogen ions, producing a hypokalemic metabolic alkalosis that mimics that of Bartter syndrome but usually is milder in degree. It is thought that the moderate nature of the homeostatic disruptions precludes the prostaglandin response seen in the latter disorder, so measured prostaglandin E levels are within normal limits (95). Key to understanding the reduction of urinary calcium seen in Gitelman syndrome is the presence of the basolateral membrane chloride channels, which permit continued exit of chloride from the cell in the face of reduced sodium–chloride entry, in effect hyperpolarizing the cell. Consequently, there is enhanced calcium entry across the luminal calcium

channels, whereas the reduced intracellular sodium concentration promotes basolateral exchange of sodium from blood for intracellular calcium. The typical increased magnesium excretion seen in Gitelman (and not in Bartter) syndrome remains unexplained because thiazide diuretics exert little effect on urinary magnesium content, suggesting that genetically impaired transporter function is also unlikely to be the cause (95,99). However, the increase in magnesium excretion is sufficient to cause frequent hypomagnesemia and therefore is a significant feature of the disease.

Clinical Presentation Although, as with any genetic disorder, Gitelman syndrome is present in infancy and childhood, clinical presentation before an affected individual reaches adulthood is infrequent. The mildness of the hypokalemic metabolic alkalosis may, absent other more remarkable findings, escape notice throughout childhood. In contrast to Bartter syndrome, in Gitelman syndrome, polyuria and growth impairment are not clinical manifestations. Indeed, the only likely findings are periodic muscle weakness, abdominal pain, and vomiting; on rare occasions, there may be carpopedal spasms. Historically, there is a notable absence of polyhydramnios and premature birth.

Diagnostic Approach On an initial laboratory investigation, one may note the presence of a mild hypokalemic metabolic alkalosis. In marked contrast to the hypocalcemia of Bartter syndrome, a patient with Gitelman syndrome will have normal serum calcium but be hypomagnesemic. Although both serum renin and aldosterone concentrations may be mildly increased, prostaglandin E will be normal. Assessment of urinary electrolytes will show excess potassium and magnesium; urinary excretion of calcium will be subnormal. Again, in contrast to Bartter syndrome, administration of furosemide in Gitelman syndrome will not cause increased calcium excretion, whereas the response in Bartter patients is to enhance urinary calcium excretion.

Treatment The basic therapeutic approach is to replace magnesium losses, which leads to correction of the calcium hypoexcretion and helps to normalize the serum potassium as well. Oral magnesium can be given in quantities up to 8 g/day; it is, however, a strong cathartic, so dosage is on an individual basis and should be monitored by measurement of serum magnesium concentrations and stool frequency and consistency. There is at least one report of magnesium intolerance, even at very low dosage, in three individuals in the same family, all suffering from Gitelman

syndrome (100). In these patients, the hypotension and polyuria were treated successfully with indomethacin and potassium supplements; what was not included in this report was the serum magnesium response to treatment. It is unlikely that there was any improvement because magnesium loss into the urine would have remained unaffected by this treatment. Some individuals may require potassium supplementation in addition to the magnesium in order to fully correct the deficit.

REFERENCES

1. Hanna JD, Scheinman JI, Chan JCM. The kidney in acid–base balance. *Pediatr Clin North Am.* 1995;42:1365–1395.
2. Roth KS, Chan JCM. Renal tubular acidosis: A new look at an old problem. *Clin Pediatr.* 2001;40:533–543.
3. Herrin JT. Renal tubular acidosis. In: Barrat TM, Avner ED, Harmon WE, ed. *Pediatric Nephrology,* 4th ed. Baltimore: Lippincott Williams & Wilkins; 1999.
4. Soleimani M, Burnham CE. Physiologic and molecular aspects of the Na⁺: HCO₃⁻ cotransporter in health and disease processes. *Kidney Int.* 2000;57:371–384.
5. Romero MF, Boron WF. Electrogenic Na⁺/ HCO₃⁻ cotransporters: Cloning and physiology. *Annu Rev Physiol.* 1999;61:699–723.
6. Boron WF, Fong P, Hediger MA, et al. The electrogenic Na/HCO₃ cotransporter. *Wien Klin Wochenschr.* 1997;109:445–456.
7. Karet FE, Gainza FJ, Gyory AZ, et al. Mutations in the chloride–bicarbonate exchanger gene AE1 cause autosomal dominant but not autosomal recessive distal renal tubular acidosis. *Proc Natl Acad Sci USA.* 1998;95:6337–6342.
8. Rodriguez-Soriano J. New insights into the pathogenesis of renal tubular acidosis: From functional to molecular studies. *Pediatr Nephrol.* 2000;14:1121–1136.
9. Caldas A, Broyer M, Deschaux M, et al. Primary distal tubular acidosis in childhood: Clinical study and long-term followup of 28 patients. *J Pediatr.* 1992;121:233–241.
10. Bergeron M, Gougoux A, Vinay P. The renal Fanconi syndrome. In: Scriver C, Beaudet A, Sly W, et al., eds. *The Metabolic and Molecular Bases of Inherited Disease,* 9th ed. New York: McGraw-Hill; 2001:Chapter 196.
11. Lichter-Konecki U, Broman KW, Blau EB, et al. Genetic and physical mapping of the locus for autosomal dominant renal Fanconi syndrome on chromosome 15q15.3. *Am J Hum Genet.* 2001;68:264–268.
12. Friedman AL, Trygstad CW, Chesney RW. Autosomal dominant Fanconi syndrome with early renal failure. *Am J Med Genet.* 1978;2:225–232.
13. Foreman JW, Roth KS. The human renal Fanconi syndrome: Then and now. *Nephrology.* 1989;51:301–306.
14. Bonnardeaux A, Bichet DG. Inherited disorders of the renal tubule. In: Brenner BM, ed. *The Kidney,* Vol. 2. Philadelphia: Saunders; 2000:1656–1698.

15. Diamond GL, Zalups RK. Understanding renal toxicity of heavy metals. *Toxicol Pathol.* 1998;26:92–103.

16. McDowell GA, Gahl WA, Stephenson LA, et al. Linkage of the gene for cystinosis to markers on the short arm of chromosome 17. *Nat Genet.* 1995;10:246–248.

17. Town M, Jean G, Cherqui S, et al. A novel gene encoding an integral membrane protein is mutated in nephropathic cystinosis. *Nat Genet.* 1998;18:319–324.

18. Touchman JW, Anikster Y, Dietrich NL, et al. The genomic region encompassing the nephropathic cystinosis gene (CTNS): Complete sequencing of a 200-kb segment and discovery of a novel gene within the common cystinosis-causing deletion. *Genome Res.* 2000;10:165–173.

19. Gahl WA, Thoene JG, Schneider JA. Cystinosis. *N Engl J Med.* 2002;347:111–121.

20. Anikster Y, Lucero C, Guo J, et al. Ocular nonnephropathic cystinosis: Clinical, biochemical, and molecular correlations. *Pediatr Res.* 2000;47:17–23.

21. Gahl WA, Tietze F, Bashan N, et al. Defective cystine exodus from isolated lysosome-rich fractions of cystinotic leucocytes. *J Biol Chem.* 1982;257:9570–9575.

22. Steinherz R, Tietze F, Gahl WA, et al. Cystine accumulation and clearance by normal and cystinotic leukocytes exposed to cystine dimethyl ester. *Proc Natl Acad Sci USA.* 1982;79:44–46.

23. Jonas AJ, Greene AA, Smith ML, et al. Cystine accumulation and loss in normal, heterozygous, and cystinotic fibroblasts. *Proc Natl Acad Sci USA.* 1982;79:44–42.

24. Jonas AJ, Smith ML, Schneider JA. ATP-dependent lysosomal cystine efflux is defective in cystinosis. *J Biol Chem.* 1982;257:13185–13188.

25. Pisoni RL, Thoene JG, Christensen HN. Detection and characterization of carrier-mediated cationic amino acid transport in lysosomes of normal and cystinotic human fibroblasts. *J Biol Chem.* 1985;260:4791–4798.

26. Gahl WA, Reed GG, Thoene JG, et al. Cysteamine therapy for children with nephropathic cystinosis. *N Engl J Med.* 1987;316:971–977.

27. Yudkoff M, Foreman JW, Segal S. Effects of cysteamine therapy in nephropathic cystinosis. *N Engl J Med.* 1981;304:141–145.

28. Calonge MJ, Nadal M, Calvano S, et al. Assignment of the gene responsible for cystinuria (rBAT) and of markers D2S119 and D2S177 to 2p16 by fluorescence in situ hybridization. *Hum Genet.* 1995;95:633–636.

29. Bisceglia L, Calonge MJ, Totaro A, et al. Localization, by linkage analysis, of the cystinuria type III gene to chromosome 19q13.1. *Am J Hum Genet.* 1997;60:617–616.

30. Brand E, Cahill GF. Further studies on metabolism of sulfur compounds in cystinuria. *Proc Soc Exp Biol Med.* 1934;33:1247.

31. Dent CE, Rose GA. Amino acid metabolism in cystinuria. *Q J Med.* 1951;20:205–219.

32. Thier SO, Fox M, Segal S, et al. Cystinuria. In vitro demonstration of an intestinal transport defect. *Science.* 1964;143:482–484.

33. Deves R, Boyd CAR. Transporters for cationic amino acids in animal cells: Dis-

covery, structure, and function. *Physiol Rev.* 1998;78:487–545.

34. Palacin M, Goodyer P, Nunes V, et al. Cystinuria. In: Scriver CR, Beaudet AL, Sly WS, et al., eds. *The Metabolic and Molecular Bases of Inherited Disease*, 9th ed. New York: McGraw-Hill; 2001:Chapter 191.

35. Perheentupa J, Visakorpi JK. Protein intolerance with deficient transport of basic amino acids. *Lancet.* 1965;2:813–816.

36. Norio R, Perheentupa J, Kekomaki M, et al. Lysinuric protein intolerance, an autosomal recessive disease: A genetic study of 10 Finnish families. *Clin Genet.* 1971;2:214–222.

37. Simell O, Perheentupa J. Renal handling of diamino acids in lysinuric protein intolerance. *J Clin Invest.* 1974;54:9–17.

38. Rajantie J, Simell O, Perheentupa J. Intestinal absorption in lysinuric protein intolerance: Impaired for diamino acids, normal; for citrulline. *Gut.* 1980;21:519–524.

39. Rajantie J, Simell O, Perheentupa J. Basolateral membrane transport defect for lysine in lysinuric protein intolerance. *Lancet.* 1980;1:1219–1221.

40. Rajantie J, Simell O. Lysinuric protein intolerance: Basolateral membrane transport defect in renal tubuli. *J Clin Invest.* 1981;67:1078–1082.

41. Palacin M, Bertran J, Chillaron J, et al. Lysinuric protein intolerance: mechanisms of pathophysiology. *Mol Genet Metab.* 2004;81: S27–37.

42. Kleta R, Romeo E, Ristic Z, et al. Mutations in SLC6A19, encoding B^0AT1, cause Hartnup disorder. *Nat Genet.* 2004;36:999–1002.

43. Seow HF, Broeor S, Broeor A, et al. Hartnup disorder is caused by mutations in the gene encoding the neutral amino acid transporter SLC6A19. *Nat Genet.* 2004;36:1003–1007.

44. Baron DN, Dent CE, Harris H, et al. Hereditary pellagra-like skin rash with temporary cerebellar ataxia, constant renal aminoaciduria and other bizarre biochemical features. *Lancet.* 1956;1:421–428.

45. Milne MD, Crawford MA, Girao CB, et al. The metabolic disorder in Hartnup disease. *Q J Med.* 1960;29:407–421.

46. Broer S, Cavanaugh JA, Rasko JEJ. Neutral amino acid transport in epithelial cells and its malfunction in Hartnup disorder. *Biochem Soc Trans.* 2005;33:233–236.

47. Verrey F, Ristic Z, Romeo E, et al. Novel renal amino acid transporters. *Annu Rev Physiol.* 2005;67:557–572.

48. Asatoor AM, Cheng B, Edwards KDG, et al. Intestinal absorption of two dipeptiddes in Hartnup disease. *Gut.* 1970;11: 380–387.

49. Shih VE, Bixby EM, Alper DH, et al. Studies of intestinal transport defect in Hartnup disease. *Gastroenterology.* 1971;61:445–453.

50. Mori E, Yamadori A, Tsutsumi A, et al. Adult-onset Hartnup disease presenting with neuropsychiatric symptoms but without skin lesions. *Rinsho Shinkeigaku.* 1989;29:687–692.

51. Scriver CR. Hartnup disease: A genetic modification of intestinal and renal transport of certain neutral alpha-amino acids. *N Engl J Med.* 1965;273:530–532.

52. DeVivo DC, Trifiletti RR, Jacobson RI, et al. Defective glucose transport across

the blood–brain barrier as a cause of persistent hypoglycorrhacia, seizures, and developmental delay. *N Engl J Med.* 1991;325:703–709.

53. Brown GK. Glucose transporters: Structure, function and consequences of deficiency. *J Inherit Metab Dis.* 2000;23:237–246.

54. Dick APK, Harik SI, Klip A, et al. Identification and characterization of the glucose transporter of the blood–brain barrier by cytochalasin B binding and immunological reactivity. *Proc Natl Acad Sci USA.* 1984;81:7233–7237.

55. Flier JS, Mueckler M, McCall AL, et al. Distribution of glucose transporter messenger RNA transcripts in tissues of rat and man. *J Clin Invest.* 1987;79:657–661.

56. DeVivo DC, Leary L, Wang D. Glucose transporter 1 deficiency syndrome and other glycolytic defects. *J Child Neurol.* 2002;17:3S15–3S25.

57. Wang D, Kranz-Eble P, DeVivo DC. Mutational analysis of GLUT1 (SLC2A1) in GLUT1 deficiency syndrome. *Hum Mutat.* 2000;16:224–231.

58. Owen OE, Morgan AP, Kemp HG, et al. Brain metabolism during fasting. *J Clin Invest* 1967;46:1589–1595.

59. Asano T, Shibasaki Y, Kasuga M, et al. Cloning of a rabbit brain glucose transporter cDNA and alteration of glucose transporter mRNA during tissue development. *Biochem Biophys Res Commun.* 1988;154:1204–1211.

60. Vannuci SJ, Clark RR, Koehler-Stec E, et al. Glucose transporter expression in the brain: Relationship to cerebral glucose utilization. *Dev Neurosci.* 1998;20:369–379.

61. Klepper J, Wang D, Fischbarg J, et al. Defective glucose transport across brain tissue barriers: A newly recognized neurological syndrome. *Neurochem Res.* 1999;24:587–594.

62. Elsas LJ, Busse D, Rosenberg LE. Autosomal recessive inheritance of renal glycosuria. *Metabolism* 1971;20:968–975.

63. Saktor B. Sodium coupled hexose transport. *Kidney Int.* 1989;36:342–350.

64. Thorens B. Facilitated glucose transporters in epithelial cells. *Annu Rev Physiol* 1993;55:591–608.

65. Kanai Y, Lee W-S, You G, et al. The human kidney low affinity Na(+)/glucose cotransporter SGLT2: Delineation of the major renal reabsorptive mechanism for D-glucose. *J Clin Invest.* 1994;93:397–404.

66. Turner RJ, Moran A. Hetreogeneity of sodium-dependent D-glucose transport sites along the proximal tubule: Evidence from vesicle studies. *Am J Physiol.* 1982;242: F406–414.

67. Pajor AM, Hirayama BA, Wright EM. Molecular evidence for two renal Na^+/glucose cotransporters. *Biochim Biophys Acta.* 1992;1106:216–220.

68. Van den Heuvel LP, Assink K, Willemsen M, et al. Autosomal recessive renal glucosuria attributable to a mutation in the sodium glucose cotransporter (SGLT2). *Hum Genet.* 2002;111:544–547.

69. Elsas LJ, Hillman RE, Patterson JH, et al. Renal and intestinal hexose transport in familial glucose–galactose malabsorption. *J Clin Invest.* 1970;49:576–585.

70. Loo DDF, Zeuthen T, Chandy G, et al. Cotransport of water by the Na$^+$/glucose cotransporter. *Proc Natl Acad Sci USA.* 1996;93:13367–13370.

71. Meinild A-K, Klaerke D, Loo DDF, et al. The human Na$^+$/glucose cotransporter is a molecular water pump. *J Physiol.* 1998;508:15–21.

72. Martin GM, Turk E, Lostao MP, et al. Defects in Na$^+$/glucose cotransporter (SGLT1) trafficking and function cause glucose–galactose malabsorption. *Nat Genet.* 1996;12:216–220.

73. Schneider AJ, Kinter WB, Stirling CE. Glucose–galactose malabsorption: Report of a case with autoradiographic studies of a mucosal biopsy. *N Engl J Med.* 1996;274:305.

74. Stirling CE, Schneider AJ, Wong M-D, et al. Quantitative radioautography of sugar transport in intestinal biopsies from normal humans and a patient with glucose–galactose malabsorption. *J Clin Invest.* 1972;51:438–451.

75. Turk E, Zabel B, Mundlos S, et al. Glucose/galactose malabsorption caused by a defect in the Na$^+$/glucose cotransporter. *Nature.* 1991;350:354–356.

76. Wright EM, Hirayama BA, Hazama A, et al. The sodium/glucose cotransporter (SGLT1). In: *Molecular Biology and Function of Carrier Proteins.* New York: Rockefeller University Press; 1993:230–241.

77. Bartter FC, Pronove P, Gill JR Jr, et al. Hyperplasia of juxtaglomerular complex with hyperaldosteronism and hypokalemic alkalosis. *Am J Med.* 1962;33:811–828.

78. Zelikovic I. Molecular pathophysiology of tubular transport disorders. *Pediatr Nephrol.* 2001;16:919–935.

79. International Collaborative Study Group for Bartter-like Syndromes. Mutations in the gene encoding the inwardly rectifying renal potassium channel, ROMK, cause the antenatal variant of Bartter syndrome: Evidence for genetic heterogeneity. *Hum Mol Genet.* 1997;6:17–26.

80. Vargas-Poussou R, Feldmann D, Vollmer M, et al. Novel molecular variants of the Na-K-2Cl cotransporter gene are responsible for antenatal Bartter syndrome. *Am J Hum Genet.* 1998;62:1332–1340.

81. Starremans PGJF, Kersten FFJ, Knoers NVAM, et al. Mutations in the human Na-K-2Cl cotransporeter (NKCC2) identified in Bartter syndrome type I consistently result in nonfunctional transporters. *J Am Soc Nephrol.* 2003;14:1419–1426.

82. Simon DB, Karet FE, Hamdam JM, et al. Bartter's syndrome, hypokalemic alkalosis with hypercalciuria, is caused by mutations in the Na-K-2Cl cotransporter NKCC2. *Nat Genet.* 1996;13:183–188.

83. Friedman PA. Codependence of renal calcium and sodium transport. *Annu Rev Physiol.* 1998;60:179–197.

84. Scheinman SJ, Guay-Woodford LM, Thakker RV, et al. Genetic disorders of renal electrolyte transport. *N Engl J Med.* 1999;340:1177–1187.

85. Peters M, Jeck N, Reinalter S, et al. Clinical presentation of genetically defined patients with hypokalemic salt-losing tubulopathies. *Am J Med.* 2002;112:183–190.

86. Guay-Woodford LM. Bartter syndrome: Unraveling the pathphysiologic enigma. *Am J Med.* 1998;105:151–161.

87. Amirlak I, Dawson KP. Bartter syndrome: An overview. *Q J Med.* 2000;93:207–215.

88. Martin K, Andreas L, Peter H, et al. Prenatal and postnatal management of hyperprostaglandin E syndrome after genetic diagnosis from amniocytes. *Pediatrics.* 1999;103:678–683.

89. Haas NA, Nossal R, Schneider CH, et al. Successful management of an extreme example of neonatal hyperprostaglandin-E syndrome (Bartter's syndrome) with the new cyclooxygenase-2 inhibitor rofecoxib. *Pediatr Crit Care Med.* 2003;4:249–251.

90. Simon DB, Karet FE, Rodriguez-Soriano J, et al. Genetic heterogeneity of Bartter's syndrome revealed by mutations in the K$^+$ channel, ROMK. *Nat Genet.* 1996;14:152–156.

91. Simon DB, Bindra RS, Mansfield TA, et al. Mutations in the chloride channel gene, CLCNKB, cause Bartter's syndrome type III. *Nat Genet.* 1997;17:171–178.

92. Konrad M, Vollmer M, Lemmink HH, et al. Mutations in the chloride channel gene CLCNKB as a cause of classic Bartter syndrome. *J Am Soc Nephrol.* 2000; 11:1449–1459.

93. Zelikovic I. Hypokalemic salt-losing tubulopathies: An evolving story. *Nephrol Dial Transplant.* 2003;18:1696–1700.

94. Gitelman HJ, Graham JB, Welt LG. A new familial disorder characterized by hypokalemia and hypomagnesemia. *Trans Assoc Am Phys.* 1966;79:221–235.

95. Scheinman SJ, Guay-Woodford LM, Thakker RV, et al. Genetic disorders of renal electrolyte transport. *N Engl J Med.* 1999;340:1177–1187.

96. Simon DB, Lifton RP. The molecular basis of inherited hypokalemic alkalosis: Bartter's and Gitelman's syndromes. *Am J Physiol.* 1996;40:F961–966.

97. Lemmink HH, KNoers MVAM, Karolyi L, et al. Novel mutations in the thiazide-sensitive NaCl cotransporter gene in patients with Gitelman syndrome with predominant localization to the C-terminal domain. *Kidney Int.* 1998;54:720–730.

98. Pollak MR, Delancy VB, Graham RM, et al. Gitelman's syndrome (Bartter's variant) maps to the thiazide-sensitive cotransporter gene locus on chromosome 16q13 in a large kindred. *J Am Soc Nephrol.* 1996;7:2244–2248.

99. Quamme GA. Renal magnesium handling: New insights in understanding old problems. *Kidney Int.* 1997;52:1180–1195.

100. Liaw LCT, Banerjee K, Coulthard MG. Dose related growth response to indometacin in Gitelman syndrome. *Arch Dis Child.* 1999;81:508–510.

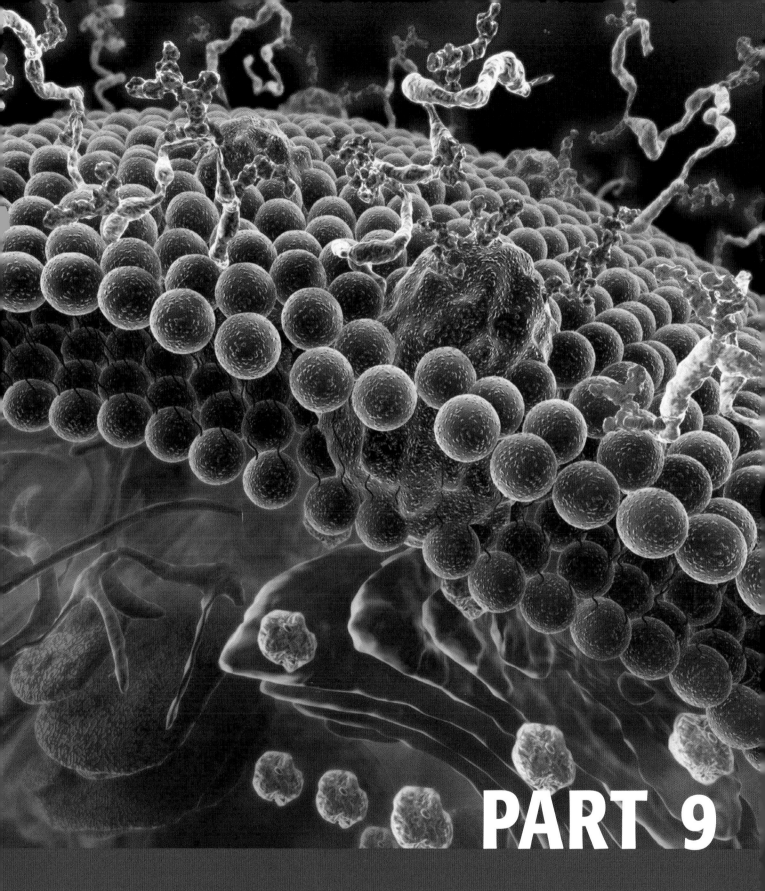

PART 9

Select Disorders of Complex Molecule Biosynthesis

Previous page: Computer generated image of the plasma membrane of a cell showing sugars (red) protruding from the outer surface. The sugars are linked to membrane proteins and lipids forming glycoprotein and glycolipid groups. These surface sugars act as receptors and are responsible for recognizing and binding molecules like hormones or toxins. The plasma membrane itself is formed of a lipid bilayer (green) with integral transmembrane proteins (purple). Inside the cell is a stack of Golgi apparatus (lower right) producing lysosomes (blue spheres).

CHAPTER 43

Lysosomal Disorders

Gregory M. Enns, MB, ChB

Robert D. Steiner, MD

Tina M. Cowan, PhD, FACMG

INTRODUCTION

Lysosomes are spherical organelles, contained by a single-layer membrane, that are present in all nucleated cells (1). Lysosomes originate in the Golgi apparatus, with the digestive enzymes manufactured in the the rough endoplasmic reticulum. An integral part of the intracellular recycling process, lysosomes contain hydrolytic enzymes that digest obsolete cell components and degrade complex cellular substrates such as glycoproteins, mucopolysaccharides (glycosaminoglycans), oligosaccharides, and lipids into simpler components in a stepwise manner. A block in the degradation of these substrates leads to abnormal accumulation of complex macromolecules within lysosomes.

Lysosomal disorders (LDs) are inherited conditions that are caused by defects in enzymes, enzyme activator proteins, membrane proteins, transporters, or enzyme targeting to the lysosome with resulting abnormal storage of complex macromolecules. When a lysosomal pathway is blocked, there is progressive accumulation of a variety of partially degraded intermediate metabolic products such as triglycerides, sterols, sphingolipids, sulfatides, sphingomyelin, gangliosides, and lipofuscins (2). The increasing storage of substrates within lysosomes results in impaired function of the affected organs. The pathological features of the various LDs depend on the nature of the stored substrate and the organs where storage occurs. Substrate accumulation occurs primarily in the organs where they are synthesized (e.g., liver, spleen, bone, and nervous system). This explains in part the varied organ involvement and symptomatology of these disorders. Defective targeting of lysosomal enzymes to lysosomes (e.g., I-cell disease), abnormal lysosomal membrane proteins (e.g., Danon disease), and defective egress of substrate (e.g., infantile sialic acid storage disease/Salla disease) also may cause

abnormal storage. As the lysosomes enlarge, cellular and organ function are increasingly impaired. The exact causes of such impairment, however, are still the subject of investigation. Because a wide range of clinical features are encountered in LDs, disease pathogenesis presumably involves the activation of various deleterious biochemical pathways or cellular processes. The release of acid hydrolases into the cytoplasm undoubtedly could cause cellular damage, but such an occurrence has not been clearly established. In theory, defective transport of substrates into and out of lysosomes secondary to abnormal storage may play a role in disease pathogenesis, especially in disorders that involve membrane lipids (e.g., sphingolipidoses). Dysregulation of apoptosis may cause disease manifestations in some LDs. Indeed, increased apoptosis has been noted in a number of the sphingolipidoses and in the neuronal ceroid lipofuscinoses. Gene profiling using microarrays has provided evidence for pathological microglial activation and subsequent reactive gliosis following neuronal cell death in GM_1 and GM_2 gangliosidoses and mucopolysaccharidoses types I and IIIB (6). These possible mechanisms of pathogenesis, of course, are not mutually exclusive, and various combinations may exist in a given LD.

All these disorders are inherited as autosomal recessive traits, with the notable exceptions of Hunter syndrome (MPS-II), Fabry disease, and Danon disease, which are X-linked conditions. There are more than 40 LDs, and each is rare. In aggregate, the incidence of LDs is about 1 in 7000 to 1 in 10,000 births (6). Each LD is caused by mutations in a specific gene. However, in most cases, numerous mutations have been described in different patients affected by the same condition. The prognosis usually cannot be determined on the basis of genotyping, although exceptions exist. Certain ethnic groups may show an increased prevalence of a given condition. Examples include an

increased occurrence of Tay-Sachs disease, Gaucher disease type 1, Niemann-Pick disease type A, and mucolipidosis IV in the Ashkenazi Jewish population and an increased frequency of infantile neuronal ceroid lipofuscinosis, Salla disease, and aspartylglucosaminuria in patients of Finnish descent. In such instances of increased prevalence in an ethnic group, typically only a few mutations are responsible for causing disease (7).

Classification of LDs is based on the major type(s) of stored substances present in a given condition. However, because lysosomal enzymes may degrade a variety of different substrates, resulting in a complex pattern of storage, in some cases classification is not straightforward. Major categories of LD include the mucopolysaccharidoses, sphingolipidoses, oligosaccharidoses (glycoproteinoses), and neuronal ceroid lipofuscinoses. Select disorders from each of these categories are described below. A comprehensive list of LDs is shown in the corresponding tables.

MUCOPOLYSACCHARIDOSES

Etiology/Pathophysiology The mucopolysaccharides are a heterogeneous group of macromolecules involved predominantly in the structural integrity of the extracellular matrix. They consist of unbranched polysaccharide chains containing both acidic and amino sugars and are also referred to as *glycosaminoglycans* or, when linked to proteins, *proteoglycans*. There is varied tissue distribution for the different mucopolysaccharides: keratan sulfate is found predominantly in cartilage, cornea, and intervertebral disks; dermatan sulfate is found in heart, blood vessels, and skin; and heparan sulfate is a component of lung, arteries, and cell surfaces in general.

Mucopolysaccharidoses (MPSs) are disorders resulting from defects in the stepwise

Lysosomal Disorders

AT-A-GLANCE

Lysosomal disorders (LDs) are a heterogeneous group of over 40 inherited disorders that individually are rare but as a group have an incidence of 1 in 7000 to 1 in 10,000 live births. LDs are caused by enzyme, enzyme activator, membrane transporter, or membrane protein defects that result in abnormal accumulation of complex macromolecules normally degraded in lysosomes. Multisystemic involvement and progressive disease are typical, although some disorders affect primarily a single organ system (e.g., skeletal or central nervous system). The extent and severity of the manifestations depend on the type and amount of substrate that accumulates. For most of these conditions, treatment is supportive. Enzyme-replacement therapy (ERT) and bone-marrow transplantation (BMT) have been successful in some LDs. Novel therapies include substrate-reduction therapy (SRT) by small molecules that can cross the blood–brain barrier (3, 4).

Mucopolysaccharidoses

The mucopolysaccharidoses are lysosomal storage disorders characterized by deficient degradation of mucopolysaccharides (glycosaminoglycans). Storage material consists of dermatan sulfate, heparan sulfate, keratan sulfate, chondroitin sulfate, or hyaluronan either in isolation or in various combinations depending on the underlying enzymatic defect. These conditions typically are multisystemic, with progressive involvement of the brain, visceral organs, and bone. Mental retardation is common, although not invariable. ERT has become avaliable for Hurler syndrome (MPS-IH), although efficacy has been limited because of the inability of the recombinant enzyme to cross the blood–brain barrier. BMT has been successful in altering the course of some of these disorders but is not curative. The pattern of pathological glycosaminoglycans in the various mucopolysaccharidoses are summarized below.

TYPES OF MUCOPOLYSACCHARIDOSES	OCCURRENCE	GENE	LOCUS	OMIM
Hurler syndrome (MPS-IH)	~1:100,000	IDUA	4p16.3	607014
Scheie syndrome (MPS-IS)	~1:1,000,000	IDUA	4p16.3	607016
Hurler-Scheie syndrome (MPS-III/S)	~1:300,000	IDUA	4p16.3	607015
Hunter syndrome (MPS-II)	~1:100,000	IDS	Xq28	309900
Sanfilippo syndrome type A (MPS-IIIA)	~1:130,000	SGSH	17q25.3	252900
Sanfilippo syndrome type B (MPS-IIIB)	~1:230,000	NAGLU	17q21	252920
Sanfilippo syndrome type C (MPS IIIC)	~1:1,400,000	Unknown		252930
Sanfilippo syndrome type D (MPS-IIID)	~1:1,000,000	GNS	12q14	252940
Morquio syndrome type A (MPS-IVA)	~1:200,000	GALNS	16q24.3	253000
Morquio syndrome type B (MPS-IVB)	~1:250,000	GLB1	3p21.33	230500
Maroteaux-Lamy syndrome (MPS-VI)	~1:200,000	ASB	5q11-q13	253200
Sly syndrome (MPS-VII)	~1:1,500,000	GUSB	7q21.11	253220
Hyaluronidase deficiency (MPS-IX)	–	HYAL1	3p21	607071

FORM	FINDINGS	CLINICAL PRESENTATION	
		Birth	Childhood & Adolescence
Hurler syndrome (MPS-IH)	↑ urine dermatan and heparan sulfate; ↓ α-L-iduronidase activity	Most appear normal, but hydrops fetalis may occur	Coarsening of features, hepatosplenomegaly, corneal clouding develops in infancy and progress; skeletal abnormalities (dysostosis multiplex), joint limitation, and short stature develop in childhood; progressive mental retardation occurs
Scheie syndrome (MPS-IS)	Same as MPS IH	Appear normal	Only mild systemic features occur; intelligence, lifespan, and stature are normal
Hurler–Scheie syndrome (MPS-IH/S)	Same as MPS IH	Appear normal	Features intermediate between MPS-IH and MPS-IS
Hunter syndrome (MPS-II)	↑ urine dermatan and heparan sulfate; ↓ iduronate sulfatase activity	Appear normal	Features are similar to MPS I, except that there is no corneal clouding and skin can appear "pebbly"

FORM	FINDINGS	CLINICAL PRESENTATION Birth	Childhood & Adolescence
Sanfilippo syndrome (MPS-IIIA)	↑ urine heparan sulfate; ↓ heparan N-sulfatase activity	Appear normal	Coarse features and relatively mild organomegaly occur in early childhood; progressive mental retardation and behavior problems occur in childhood
Sanfilippo syndrome (MPS-IIIB)	↑ urine heparan sulfate; ↓ α-N-acetylglucos-aminidase activity		
Sanfilippo syndrome (MPS-IIIC)	↑ urine heparan sulfate ↓ acetyl Co-A: α-glucos-aminidine acetyltransferase activity		
Sanfilippo syndrome (MPS-IIID)	↑ urine heparan sulfate; ↓ N-acetylglucosamine-6-sulfatase activity		
Morquio syndrome type A (MPS-IVA)	↑ urine keratan and chondroitin 6-sulfate; ↓ N-acetylgalactosamine-6-sulfatase activity	Most appear normal, but hydrops fetalis may occur	Intelligence is normal; mild to severe skeletal manifestations are present; corneal clounding and hearing impairment are common
Morquio syndrome type B (MPS-IVB)	↑ urine keratan and chondroitin 6-sulfate; ↓ β-galactosidase activity		
Maroteaux-Lamy syndrome (MPS-VI)	↑ urine dermatan sulfate; ↓ N-acetylgalactosamine-4-sulfatase activity (arylsulfatase B)	Appear normal	Intelligence is normal; skeletal manifestations are prominent and noticed at 6–24 months; corneal clouding, valvular heart disease, and spinal cord compression occur
Sly syndrome (MPS-VII)	↑ urine dermatan, heparan, and chondroitin 6-sulfate; ↓ β-glucuronidase activity	Most appear normal, but hydrops fetalis may occur	Coarse features, organomegaly and dysostosis multiplex are typical although and severity are variable
Hyaluronidase deficiency (MPS-IX)	↓ hyaluronidase activity	Only one patient described; intelligence is normal; short stature and nodular periarticular masses are present	

Disorders of Lysosomal Enzyme Localization

I-cell disease (mucolipidosis II) and pseudo-Hurler polydystrophy (mucolipidosis III) are both caused by defective targeting of lysosomal enzymes to ly-sosomes. Newly synthesized lysosomal enzymes are therefore secreted into the extracellular matrix instead of localizing to lysosomes. The clinical features of I-cell disease resemble those of Hurler syndrome, although onset is earlier. Pseudo-Hurler polydystrophy has a milder course.

TYPES OF LOCALIZATION DEFECTS	OCCURRENCE	GENE	LOCUS	OMIM
I-cell disease (mucolipidosis II)	~1:325,000	GNPTA	4q21-q23	607840
Pseudo-Hurler polydystrophy (mucolipidosis III)	–	GNPTA	4q21-q23	252600

FORM	FINDINGS	CLINICAL PRESENTATION Birth	Childhood & Adolescence
I-cell disease (mucolipidosis II)	Normal urine mucopolysaccarides, vacuolated lymphocytes, ↓ N-acetylglucosamine-1-transferase activity	Features may present at birth; hydrops fetalis may occur	Similar to MPS-IH, except coarse facies may be present at birth and this condition is more rapidly progressive
Pseudo-Hurler polydystrophy (mucolipidosis III)		Appear normal	More mild than I-cell disease; finger contractures, scoliosis, and short stature is present in childhood; a progressive skeletal dysplasia is typical; 50% have learning disabilities or mental retardation

Sphingolipidoses

The sphingolipidoses are characterized by abnormal storage of complex phospholipids that contain a sphingosine moiety. Sphingolipids are essential components of the cell membrane and are constantly being recycled. Although central nervous system involvement, with developmental regression, is present in many of these conditions, some feature only systemic involvement. ERT for Gaucher disease type 1 and Fabry disease has revolutionized the care of these individuals. Unfortunately, for most of the sphingolipidoses, therapy is supportive.

TYPES OF SPHINGOLIPIDOSES	OCCURRENCE	GENE	LOCUS	OMIM
G_{M2}-gangliosidoses				
Type A (Tay–Sachs disease)*	~1:200,000	HEXA	15q23-q24	272800
Type O (Sandhoff disease)	~1:400,000	HEXB	5q13	268800
Type AB (G_{M2}-activator deficiency)	–	GM2A	5q31-q33	272750
Niemann–Pick disease type A*	~1:250,000	SMPD1	11p15	275200
Neimann–Pick disease type B*	–	SMPD1	11p15	607608
Niemann–Pick disease type C	~1:200,000	NPC1	18q11-q12	257220
		NPC2	14q24.3	607625
Gaucher disease type 1*	~1:60,000	GBA	1q21	230800
Gaucher disease type 2	–	GBA	1q21	230900
Gaucher disease type 3	–	GBA	1q21	231000
Fabry disease	~1:120,000	GLA	Xq22	301500
Metachromatic leukodystrophy	~1:100,000	ARSA	22q13	250100
Saposin B deficiency	–	PSAP	10q22	249900
Multiple sulfatase deficiency	~1:1,400,000	SUMF1	3p26	272200
Globoid cell leukodystrophy (Krabbe disease)	~1:150,000	GALC	14q31	245200
GM1-gangliosidosis type I***	–	GLB1	3p21.33	230500
GM1-gangliosidosis type II	–	GLB1	3p21.33	230600
GM1-gangliosidosis type III	–	GLB1	3p21.33	230560
Farber lipogranulomatosis	–	ASAH	8p22-p21	228000

*Higher incidence in Ashkenazi Jewish population; ***Combined estimated incidence of approx. 1/100,000–1/300,000.

FORM	FINDINGS	CLINICAL PRESENTATION	
		Birth	Childhood & Adolescence
Tay–Sachs disease	↓ β-hexosaminidase A activity	Appear normal	Rapidly progressive neuro-degeneration, an exaggerated startle reflex, and a "cherry red" spot are typical; late- and adult-onset forms occur
Sandhoff disease	↑ urine oligosaccharides; ↓ β-hexosaminidase A & B activity	Appear normal	Similar to Tay–Sachs disease
GM₂-activator deficiency (AB variant)	↓ GM_2 activator	Appear normal	Similar to Tay–Sachs disease
Niemann–Pick disease type A	↓ sphingomyelinase activity	Most appear normal, but hydrops fetalis may occur	Hepatosplenomegaly develops in infancy; rapid neurodegeneration occurs; 50% have a "cherry red" spot
Niemann–Pick disease type B	↓ sphingomyelinase activity	Appear normal	Splenomegaly often noted; hepatomegaly and pulmonary involvement are typical; normal intelligence; hyperlipidemia is common
Niemann-Pick Disease Type C	↓ cholesterol esterification	Neonatal hepatitis may occur	Clinical features include hepatosplenomegaly, (which can be a mild and late finding), upward gaze palsy, developmental regression, seizures (rare), and ataxia

FORM	FINDINGS	Birth	CLINICAL PRESENTATION Childhood & Adolescence
Gaucher disease type 1	↓ β-glucosidase activity	Appear normal	Splenomegaly may appear, but some remain asymptomatic; avascular necrosis of the hip and growth retardation may occur
Gaucher disease type 2	↓ β-glucosidase activity	Hydrops fetalis and ichthyosis may occur	Neurodegeneration and hepatosplenomegaly occur in infancy or early childhood
Gaucher disease type 3	↓ β-glucosidase activity	Appear normal	Intermediate between types 1 and 2
Fabry disease	↓ α-galactosidase activity	Appear normal	Extremity pain and paresthesias common in childhood; asymptomatic corneal opacities and heart disease occur; renal failure in adulthood
Metachromatic leukodystrophy	↑ urine sulfatides ↓ arylsulfatase A activity	Appear normal	Progressive neurodegeneration, without organomegaly, occurs; late-infantile, juvenile, and adult forms exist
Saposin B deficiency	↑ urine sulfatides ↓ sulfatide activator protein	Appear normal	Similar to metachromatic leukodystrophy
Multiple sulfatase deficiency	↑ urine mucopolysaccharides and oligosaccharides; ↓ arylsulfatase A, B, & C activities; ↓ sulfamidase activity; ↓ iduronate-2-sulfatase activity	Hydrops fetalis may occur	Clinical features resemble various combinations characteristic of single sulfatase deficiencies, ranging from MPS-IH-like to metachromatic leukodystrophy-like
Krabbe disease	↓ β-galactocerebroside activity	Appear normal	Progressive neurodegeneration without organomegaly occurs
G$_{M1}$ gangliosidosis	↑ urine oligosaccharides Nl or slightly ↑ urine mucopolysaccharides ↓ β-Galactosidase	Most appear normal, but hydrops fetalis may occur	Neurodegeneration, coarse features. Type I: infantile hypotonia, hepatosplenomegaly, dysostosis multiplex, and "cherry red" spots (50%); infants to adults present with ataxia, dystonia, normal intelligence, or mental retardation
Farber lipogranulomatosis	↓ acid ceramidase acitivity	Appear normal	Typically presents in infancy with painful, deformed joints, subcutaneous nodules, and progressive hoarseness; visceral and neurologic involvement is variable

Sialic Acid Disorders

Sialic acid disorders are a heterogeneous group of conditions characterized by abnormal accumulation of N-acetyl-neuraminic acid (sialic acid) in lysosomes or the cytoplasm (sialuria). The biochemical defects and clinical phenotypes differ in each condition. Sialidosis is caused by neuraminidase deficiency. Galactosialidosis is associated with combined deficiency of β-galactosidase and neuraminidase secondary to a defect in lysosomal protective protein/cathepsin A. Infantile free sialic acid storage disease and Salla disease are caused by defective lysosomal membrane transport of sialic acid and other acidic monosaccharides. Sialuria has been described in only a handful of patients and is caused by impaired feedback inhibition of uridine diphosphate-N-acetylglucosamine 2-epimerase. Sialuria is inherited in an autosomal dominant fashion (the other conditions listed here are autosomal recessive). These condtions have a variable clinical phenotype, ranging from being similar to MPS-IH to isolated central nervous system involvement.

TYPES OF SIALIC ACID DISORDERS	OCCURRENCE	GENE	LOCUS	OMIM
Sialidosis (Mucolipidosis I)	~1:4,000,000	NEU1	6p21.3	256550
Galactosialidosis	–	PPGB	20q13	256540
Infantile sialic acid storage disease	~1:500,000	SLC17A5	6q14-q15	269920
Salla disease*	–	SLC17A5	6q14-q15	604369
Sialuria	–	GNE	9q12-p11	269921

*Higher incidence in Finnish population.

FORM	FINDINGS	CLINICAL PRESENTATION	
		Birth	Childhood & Adolescence
Sialidosis (Mucolipidosis I)	↓ neuraminidase activity	Most appear normal, but hydrops fetalis may occur	Variable features occur, ranging from MPS-IH-like to development of a "cherry red" spot and myoclonus in adolescence
Galactosialidosis	↑ urine sialic acid-containing oligosaccharides; ↓ neuraminidase activity; ↓ β-galactosidase activity	Most appear normal, but hydrops fetalis may occur	Coarse facial features, dysostosis multiplex and cherry red spots
Infantile sialic acid storage disease	↑ urine sialic acid	Hydrops fetalis may occur	Coarse features, profound mental retardation, and hepatosplenomegaly occur in infancy
Salla disease	↑ urine sialic acid	Most appear normal, but hydrops fetalis may occur	Ataxia and mental retardation occur in childhood; high incidence in Finland
Sialuria	↑ urine sialic acid	Appear normal	Coarse features, hepatosplenomegaly, and relatively mild intellectual involvement occur (sialic acid accumulates in the cytoplasm in this condition)

Oligosaccharidoses (glycoproteinoses)

Oligosaccharidoses are characterized by abnormal lysosomal storage of complex glycoproteins. Some of these disorders resemble classical mucopolysaccharidoses (e.g., α-mannosidosis, fucosidosis), whereas others primarily affect the central nervous system, similar to many sphingolipidoses (e.g., Schindler disease, aspartylglucosaminuria).

TYPES OF OLIGOSACCHARIDOSES	OCCURRENCE	GENE	LOCUS	OMIM
GM1-gangliosidosis type I***	–	GLB1	3p21.33	230500
GM1-gangliosidosis type II	–	GLB1	3p21.33	230600
GM1-gangliosidosis type III	–	GLB1	3p21.33	230560
G_{M2}-gangliosidoses				
Type A (Tay–Sachs disease)*	~1:200,000	HEXA	15q23-q24	272800
Type O (Sandhoff disease)	~1:400,000	HEXB	5q13	268800
Type AB (G_{M2}-activator deficiency)	–	GM2A	5q31-q33	272750
α-Mannosidosis	~1:1,000,000	MAN2B1	19cen-q12	248500
β-Mannosidosis	–	MANBA	4q22-q25	248510
Fucosidosis	–	FUCA1	1p34	230000
Sialidosis (mucolipidosis I)	~1:4,000,000	NEU1	6p21.3	256550
Galactosialidosis	–	PPGB	20q13 2	56540
Schindler disease	–	NAGA	22q11	104170
Aspartylglucosaminuria*	~1:2,000,000	AGA	4q32-q33	208400

*Higher incidence in Finnish population; ***Combined estimated incidence of approx. 1/100,000–1/300,000.

FORM	FINDINGS	CLINICAL PRESENTATION	
		Birth	Childhood & Adolescence
G_{M1}-gangliosidosis	↑ urine oligosaccharides, Nl ↑ urine mucopolysaccharides, ↓ β-galactosidase	Most appear normal, but hydrops fetalis may occur	Neurodegeneration, coarse features. Type I: infantile hypotonia, hepatosplenomegaly, dysostosis multiplex, and "cherry red" spots (50%); infants to adults present with ataxia, dystonia, normal intelligence, or mental retardation
Tay–Sachs disease	↓ β-hexosaminidase A activity	Appear normal	Rapidly progressive neurodegeneration, an exaggerated startle reflex, and a "cherry red" spot are typical

FORM	FINDINGS	Birth	CLINICAL PRESENTATION Childhood & Adolescence
Sandhoff disease	↑ urine oligosaccharides; ↓ β-hexosaminidase A & B activity	Appear normal	Similar to Tay–Sachs disease
G_{M2}-activator deficiency (AB variant)	↓ GM$_2$ activator	Appear normal	Similar to Tay–Sachs disease
α-Mannosidosis	↑ urine oligosaccharides ↓ α-mannosidase activity	Appear normal	Infantile MPS-IH-like, and milder juvenile/adult forms exist
β-Mannosidosis	↑ urine oligosaccharides; ↓ β-mannosidase activity	Appear normal	Variable features, ranging from infantile neurodegeneration to juvenile mental retardation; hearing loss, and angiokeratoma, may occur
Fucosidosis	↑ sweat sodium chloride; ↑ urine oligosaccharides; ↓ α-L-fucosidase	Appear normal	Infantile MPS-IH-like, and milder juvenile and adult forms exist; angiokeratomas are relatively common
Sialidosis (mucolipidosis I)	↓ neuraminidase activity	Most appear normal, but hydrops fetalis may occur	Variable features occur, ranging from MPS-IH-like to development of a "cherry red" spot; myoclonus in adolescence
Galactosialidosis	↑ urine sialic acid-containing oligosaccharides; ↓ neuraminidase activity; ↓ β-galactosidase activity	Most appear normal, but hydrops fetalis may occur	Coarse facial features, dysostosis multiplex and cherry red spots.
Schindler disease	↑ urine oligosaccharides ↓ α-N-acetylgalactos-aminidase activity	Appear normal	Variable features ranging from infantile neuraxonal dystrophy to mild impairment; angiokeratomas and mild intellectual impairment occur in an adult form
Aspartylglucosaminuria	↑ urine glycoasparigines; ↓ aspartylglucos-aminidase activity	Appear normal	Progressive neurodegeneration occurs from age 2–4 years; connective tissue changes lead to coarse features, thick calvarium, and osteoporosis

Neuronal Ceroid Lipofuscinoses

Neuronal ceroid lipofuscinoses (NCL) are severe, progressive neurodegenerative conditions that feature the accumulation of an autofluorescent waxy pigment (lipofuscin) in the lysosomes. These conditions may have onset anytime from infancy through adulthood. Typical features include developmental arrest and regression, microcephaly, blindness, and seizures.

TYPES OF NCL	OCCURRENCE	GENE	LOCUS	OMIM
Infantile NCL (Santavuori-Haltia disease)*	1:13,000	PPT1	1p32	256730
Late infantile NCL (Jansky-Bielschowshy disease)	~1/100,000	CLN2	11p15.5	204500
Juvenile NCL (Batten disease)	~1:170,000	CLN3	16p12.1	204200
Adult NCL (Kufs disease)	–	PPT1 CLN3, CLN4	1p32 16p12.1	204300

*Higher incidence in Finnish population.

FORM	FINDINGS	Birth	CLINICAL PRESENTATION Childhood & Adolescence
Infantile NCL (Santavuori-Haltia disease)	Normal blood and urine studies; ↓ palmitoyl-protein thioesterase activity	Appear normal	Progressive neurodegeneration and macular degeneration occur; death in childhood is typical
Late infantile NCL (Jansky-Bielschowshy disease)	Normal blood and urine studies; ↓ pepsinase activity	Appear normal	Slower progression than infantile NCL; death occurs between 10–15 years
Juvenile NCL (Batten disease)	Normal routine blood and urine studies	Appear normal	Neurologic and opthalmologic features in late childhood; death between 20 and 40 years is typical

Other Lysosomal Storage Disorders

There are a number of other lysosomal disorders that are more difficult to classify into a specific category on the basis of the type of material stored. These are listed below.

OTHER LYSOSOMAL STORAGE DISORDERS	OCCURRENCE	GENE	LOCUS	OMIM
Wolman disease	~1:530,000	LIPA	10q24-q25	278000
Cholesteryl ester storage disease	–	LIPA	10q24-q25	278000
Cystinosis (see Chapter 42)	~1:200,000	CTNS	17p13	219800
Pycnodysostosis	–	CTSK	1q21	265800
Pompe disease (glycogen storage disease type II)	~1:150,000	GAA	17q25	232300
Danon disease		LAMP2	Xq24	300257
Mucolipidosis IV	–	MCOLN1	19p13	252650

FORM	FINDINGS	Birth	CLINICAL PRESENTATION Childhood & Adolescence
Wolman disease	Nl plasma cholesterol and triglycerides; ↓ acid lipase activity	Hydrops fetalis; is typical onset hepatosplenomegaly is typical	Neonates have increased vomiting and diarrhea; anemia; abnormal development; calcification of adrenal glands; death usually by age 6 months
Cholesteryl ester storage disease	↑ plasma cholesterol + triglycerides; ↓ acid lipase activity	Hepatomegaly may be present	Onset varies from birth to second decade; progressive hepatomegaly; neurologic involvement and adrenal calcification are rare
Cystinosis (see Chapter 42)	Aminoaciduria, proteinuria, glycosuria; ↓K^+, ↓PO_4^{2-}, ↓ uric acid	Appear normal	Infants present with vomiting, failure to thrive, and polyuria; crystal keratopathy and hypothyroidism occur; milder variants present later
Pycnodysostosis	↓ cathepsin K activity	May have dysmorphic features	Short stature, dysmorphic features, osteosclerosis, and fractures
Pompe disease	↓ acid maltase activity	Appear normal	Cardiomegaly, hepatomegaly, hypotonia and weakness in early infancy; late-onset forms with skeletal muscle involvement and respiratory distress
Danon disease	↓ lysosomal associated membrane protein 2 (LAMP-2)	Appear normal	May appear in infancy with cardiomyopathy and myopathy; but typically presents in second decade
Mucolipidosis IV	Nl urine mucopolysaccharides mucopolysaccharides	Appear normal	Mental retardation, retinal degeneration, and corneal clouding

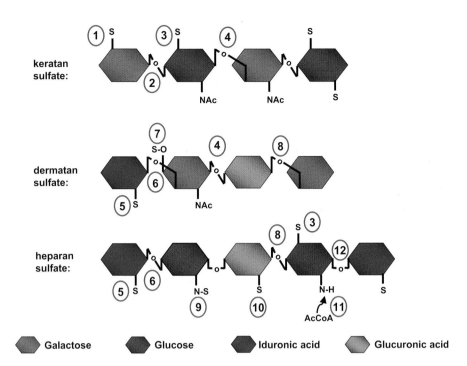

FIGURE 43-1. Representative structures of keratan sulfate, dermatan sulfate, and heparan sulfate. Numbers indicating specific enzymes and their corresponding disease states are 1) galactose-6-sulfatase (Morquio syndrome type A), 2) β-galactosidase (Morquio syndrome type B), 3) N-acetylglucosamine-6-sulfatase (Sanfilippo syndrome type D), 4) β-hexosaminidase A and B (Sandhoff disease), 5) iduronate sulfatase (Hunter syndrome), 6) α-iduronidase (Hurler, Scheie syndromes), 7) N-acetylgalactosamine-4-sulfatase (Maroteaux–Lamy syndrome), 8) β-glucuronidase (Sly syndrome), 9) heparan-N-sulfatase (Sanfilippo syndrome type A), 10) glucuronate sulfatase (disease unknown), 11) α-acetyl-CoA.α-glucosaminide acetyltransferase (Sanfilippo syndrome type C), 12) α-N-acetylglucosaminidase (Sanfilippo syndrome type B).

degradation of mucopolysaccharides due to enzymatic blocks at various points in the catabolic pathways of keratan, heparan, and dermatan sulfate and hyaluronan. There are 11 different known enzyme deficiencies leading to abnormal mucopolysaccharide storage, including four genetically distinct deficiencies leading to Sanfilippo syndrome and two leading to Morquio syndrome. All the MPSs are inherited in an autosomal recessive manner except Hunter syndrome (MPS-II), which is X-linked. In the current MPS classification scheme, MPS-V (formerly Scheie syndrome) and MPS-VIII are no longer recognized. Representative structures of the three major abnormally stored mucopolysaccharides—keratan sulfate, dermatan sulfate, and heparan sulfate—are shown in Figure 43-1.

Abnormal mucopolysaccharide storage leads to a variety of pathophysiological changes throughout the body. Somatic storage results in variable organomegaly (e.g., hepatomegaly and splenomegaly), coarsening of facial features, cardiac abnormalities (e.g., cardiomyopathy, valvular regurgitation, and narrowing of the coronary arteries), joint stiffness, progressive airway obstruction, hearing loss, corneal clouding leading to blindness, and short stature. Typical skeletal abnormalities, known as *dysostosis multiplex*, include vertebral

beaking, proximal pointing of the metacarpals, and the so-called J-shaped sella apparent on lateral skull x-ray.

Histological changes associated with the MPSs include large, empty-appearing vacuoles (Figure 43-2), inclusions resembling zebra bodies, and metachromatic granules (seen on staining with a cationic dye such as Alcian blue) representing lysosomes distended by stored material. Storage is seen in many cell types, including mononuclear

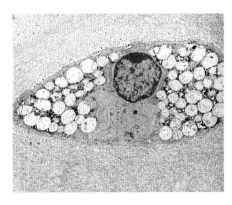

FIGURE 43-2. Abnormal lysosomal storage in a macrophage of a patient with Hurler syndrome. (Courtesy of Richard Sibley, M.D., Stanford University Pathology Department.)

phagocytic cells, endothelial cells, intimal smooth muscle cells, and fibroblasts. Depending on the specific disorder and the presence or absence of residual enzyme activity, storage also may be seen in other specialized cells, including hepatocytes and neurons. The definitive diagnosis is based on enzyme assays for the specific lysosomal enzymes and demonstration of deficient or significantly reduced (<10% of normal) enzyme activity. Assays can be performed using either leukocytes or cultured skin fibroblasts. More recently, the activities of several lysosomal enzymes, including α-iduronidase and α-glucosidase, have been reliably measured using dried blood spots (8), raising the possibility of presymptomatic screening for these disorders in the near future.

Clinical Presentation Although clinically heterogeneous, the MPSs generally are characterized by a period of normal growth and development, followed by progressive organomegaly (including hepatomegaly and splenomegaly), developmental delay in many of the disorders, skeletal abnormalities (dysostosis multiplex), and coarsening of facial features (9). Depending on the type and severity of the disorder, the age of presentation ranges from late infancy to adulthood. Other characteristic features include umbilical hernia, gibbus deformity, and short stature. Distinguishing features of each of the MPSs are summarized below.

MPS-I (Hurler, Hurler/Scheie, Scheie Syndromes; MPS-IH, MPS-IH/S, MPS-IS)

Type I MPSs encompass a wide phenotypic spectrum ranging from severe (Hurler syndrome) to mild (Scheie syndrome). Despite this clinical variability, all cases of MPS-I are caused by deficient activity of α-iduronidase (IDUA), which normally cleaves iduronate residues from dermatan sulfate and heparan sulfate. Deficient IDUA activity leads to abnormal storage of dermatan and heparan sulfate in multiple organs and tissues, including liver, spleen, connective tissue, and brain, as well as to abnormal urinary excretion of these compounds. More than 70 different IDUA mutations have been described to date (10). Those associated with the more severe Hurler phenotype are predominately nonsense mutations leading to a complete absence of enzyme activity, whereas those underlying milder phenotypes are often single-base substitutions. The distinction between Hurler, Scheie, and the intermediate phenotypes cannot be made by biochemical studies because all such patients excrete abnormal levels of dermatan and heparan sulfate, and all have similarly deficient IDUA activity when measured by typical laboratory assays employing an artificial enzyme substrate.

Patients with Hurler syndrome present early and with classical features of an MPS, including hepatosplenomegaly, coarse facial features, dysostosis multiplex, and developmental delay (9) (Figure 43-3). Patients often appear normal at birth but may have inguinal hernias. Hurler syndrome is often first suspected by the child's facial appearance, including coarsening of features and an enlarged tongue, with developmental delay apparent during the first year. Development may reach the functional level of a 2- to 4-year-old, followed by rapid decline and loss of milestones. Other features include recurrent ear and nose infections, short stature, cardiomyopathy, and communicating hydrocephalus with increased intracranial pressure, with death typically occurring in the first decade. At the other end of the spectrum, patients with Scheie syndrome typically are

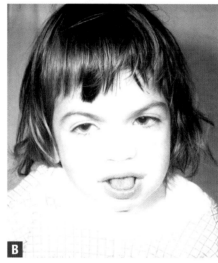

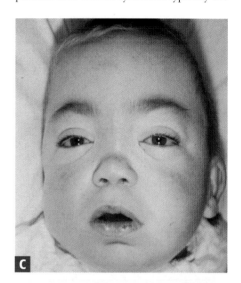

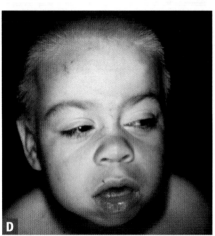

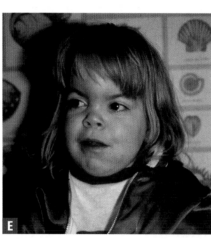

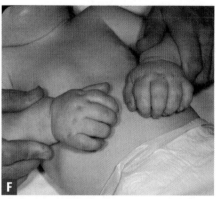

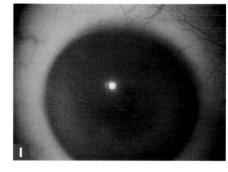

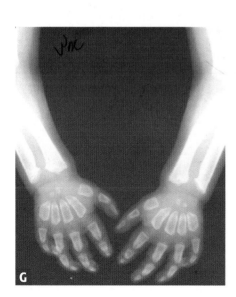

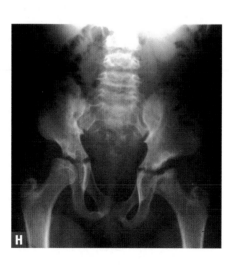

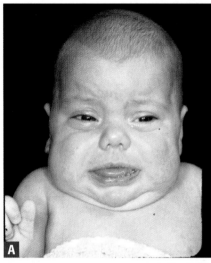

FIGURE 43-3. Hurler syndrome (MPS-IH). **A** to **E.** Examples of characteristic facies in Hurler syndrome (macrocephalic head with frontal bossing and scaphocephaly, flat face with coarse features, wide-set prominent eyes, full lips, protruding tongue, open mouth, flared nostrils, low nasal bridge, bushy eyebrows, thickened-coarse hair, and low set hairline). **F** to **G.** Clawhand deformity. **H.** Pelvic characteristics of Hurler syndrome (basilar portion of ilia, flared iliac crest, long femoral neck, and cox valga) in an 8-year-old patient. **I.** Close-up photo of the cloudy ornea feature found in Hurler syndrome. (Courtesy of Robert Gorlin, D.D.S., M.S., D.Sc., University of Minnesota Medial School.)

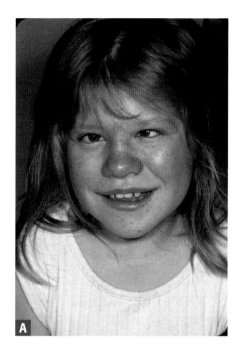
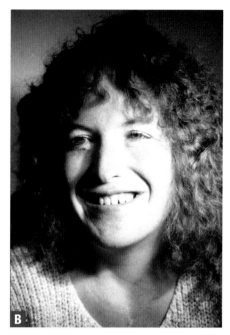
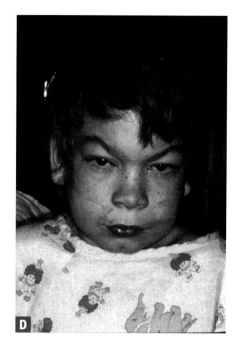
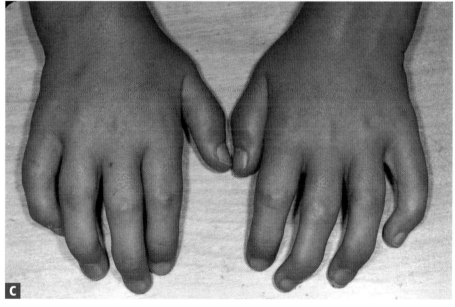
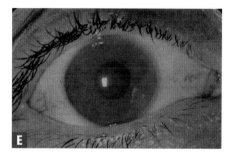

FIGURE 43-4. Hurler-Scheie phenotype (MPS-IH/S) is intermittent between Hurler and Scheie with the following characteristics: macrocephaly, low nasal bridge, prominent lips, micrognathia, mild to moderate claw-hand deformity, joint limitation without gibbus **(A** to **D),** and corneal clouding **(E).**

diagnosed in the second decade of life, with symptoms appearing after the age of 5 years. Symptoms include joint stiffness, mild claw-hand deformity, visual impairment due to corneal clouding, and a broadened or mildly coarse facial appearance (Figure 43-5). Other complications can include carpal tunnel syndrome, aortic valve disease, and deafness. Intelligence and lifespan are both characteristically normal in Scheie syndrome. Finally, Hurler/Scheie syndrome (MPS-IH/S) is used to describe an intermediate phenotype between the two extremes, including later age of onset and slower rate of progression than Hurler syndrome (Figure 43-4). Intelligence is normal or only mildly impaired, and survival is into adulthood.

Hunter Syndrome (MPS-II)

Hunter syndrome is the only MPS that is X-linked and results from deficient activity of iduronate-2-sulfatase (IDS), the enzyme that normally cleaves sulfate residues from the number 2 position of iduronate in the degradation of dermatan sulfate and heparan sulfate (see Figure 43-1). As with MPS-I, deficient IDS activity leads to abnormal storage of dermatan and heparan sulfate in multiple organs and tissues, including liver, spleen, connective tissue, and brain, as well as to abnormal urinary excretion of these compounds. The incidence of Hunter syndrome has been estimated at between 1 in 34,000 and 1 in 165,000 male births in various popu-

lations. Over 270 IDS mutations have been identified, many of which represent complex gene rearrangements (11). This vast spectrum of mutations underlies the wide clinical variability described in patients with Hunter syndrome.

As an X-linked recessive disorder, Hunter syndrome typically occurs only in males. However, rare females have been reported with Hunter syndrome resulting from nonrandom lyonization and preferential inactivation of the nonmutant X chromosome (12).

Hunter syndrome historically is divided into two discrete clinical entities, severe and mild, although the clinical phenotype is best represented as a continuum between

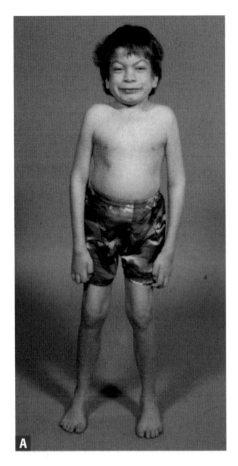
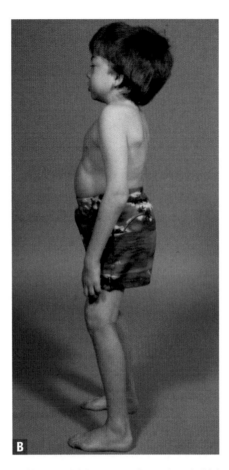
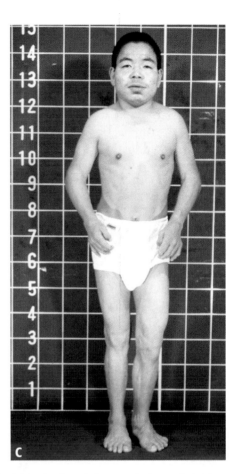

FIGURE 43-5. Characteristics of Scheie syndrome: broadened but milder coarse facial appearance (figures a,b) and mild claw hand deformity (figure c). (Courtesy of Robert Gorlin, D.D.S, M.S., D.Sc., University of Minnesota Medical School).

these extremes. Patients appear normal at birth, with the most severely affected males presenting between 2 and 4 years of age with coarsening of facial features, hepatosplenomegaly, short stature, joint stiffness, and progressive mental retardation. Persistent, asymptomatic skin lesions consisting of firm, hypopigmented papules on the back, chest, arms, and legs are also seen (13) (Figure 43-6). Corneas are characteristically clear, a feature that distinguishes Hunter syndrome from Hurler syndrome. In addition, disease progression tends to be slower than in Hurler syndrome. Patients with milder forms of Hunter syndrome may have normal intelligence and survival into adulthood, with somatic involvement similar to, but milder than, patients with more severe forms of the disorder.

MPS-IIIA, -B, -C, and -D (Sanfilippo Syndrome Types A, B, C, and D)

Sanfilippo syndrome results from a deficiency in one of the four different heparan sulfate–degrading enzymes, heparan-N-sulfatase (type A), α-N-acetylglucosaminidase (type B), acetyl coenzyme-A:α-glucosaminidine acetyl-transferase (type C), and N-acetylglucos-amine-6-sulfatase (type D). The combined incidence of Sanfilippo syndrome has been estimated at 1 in 58,000 live births (14), with types A and B being the most common and type D being extremely rare (15). All types of Sanfilippo syndrome are associated with abnormal storage of heparan sulfate, predominantly affecting the central nervous system (CNS). Patients typically present around 3–6 years of age with severe behavioral abnormalities, including hyperactivity and aggression, developmental delay, and mental retardation. In contrast to Hurler and Hunter syndromes, somatic findings are relatively mild and include little or no hepatosplenomegaly or claw-hand deformity, only mild skeletal abnormalities, and clear corneas. Hirsutism is often present, including coarse, thick hair and synophrys (Figure 43-7). In particular, type B is associated with a more severe course, including earlier onset and more pronounced neurological abnormalities than the other forms of the disorder (15). In addition to Sanfilippo syndrome, deviant, aggressive behavior is also prominent in patients with MPS-II (Hunter syndrome) and α-fucosidosis.

Morquio Syndrome (MPS-IVA and -B)

Morquio syndrome results from a deficiency in one of the two keratan sulfate–degrading enzymes, N-acetylgalactosamine-6-sulfatase (GALNS, MPS-IVA) and β-galactosidase (MPS-IVB) It is interesting to note that β-galactosidase is also the enzyme deficient in the sphingolipidosis G_{M1}-gangliosidosis due to the effects of different mutations on two sites with distinct substrate specificities (keratan sulfate and G_{M1}-ganglioside) of the same enzyme (16).

A deficiency of either GALNS or β-galactosidase leads to abnormal storage of keratan sulfate and its abnormal excretion in the urine. Because keratan sulfate is a component of cartilage, the disease predominately affects the skeletal system, leaving other tissues and the CNS relatively spared. Typical features include dwarfism with short trunk, scoliosis, and vertebral deformities, becoming apparent between 1 and 4 years of age and worsening over time (Figure 43-8). Odontoid hypoplasia is a universal finding and can lead to life-threatening atlantoaxial instability. Both mild and severe forms of both MPS-IVA and MPS-IVB have been described (17).

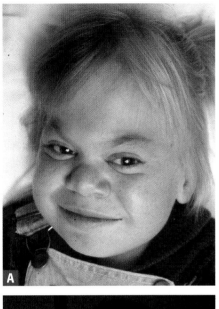

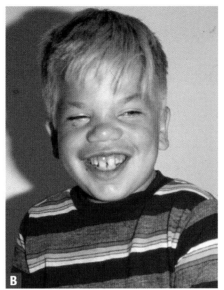

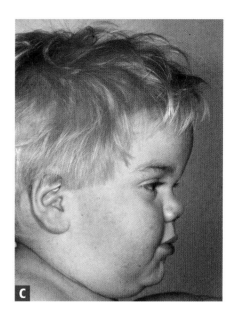

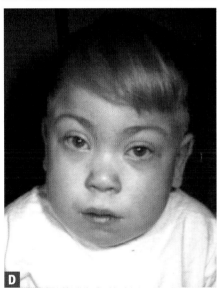

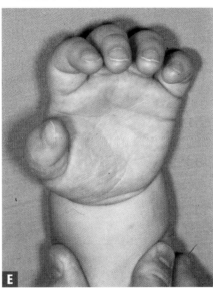

FIGURE 43-6. Characteristics of Hunter syndrome (MPS-II). While similarly enlarged head and coarse facies to MPS-IH, Hunter patients (MPS-II) bear more resemblance to family members than Hurler patients. Features include flat nose, depressed nasal bridge, enlarged tongue, and low hairline (**A** to **D**). Hunter patients do not have corneal clouding or gibbus. **E.** Claw-hand deformity with broad and stubby fingers. (Courtesy of Susan Berry, M.D., University of Minnesota Medical School.)

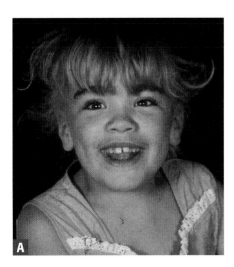

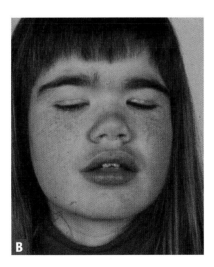

FIGURE 43-7. Characteristics of Sanfilippo syndrome (MPS-III). Mildly coarse facies with a slightly depressed nasal bridge and thickened lips, bushy eyebrows. Normal corneas. (Courtesy of Susan Berry, M.D., and Robert Gorlin, D.D.S., M.S., D.Sc., University of Minnesota Medical School.)

Maroteaux–Lamy Syndrome (MPS-VI)

Maroteaux–Lamy syndrome is caused by a deficiency of N-acetylgalactosamine-4-sulfatase, also known as *arylsulfatase B* (ARSB). This enzyme is involved in the degradation of dermatan sulfate, which has a wide tissue distribution but is not a component of the CNS. Accordingly, patients with Maroteaux–Lamy syndrome have a Hurler-like appearance but are distinguished by normal intelligence and lack of excretion of heparan sulfate. As with the other MPSs, a number of different molecular mutations in the ARSB gene underlie a broad range of clinical phenotypes ranging from severe to near normal (18–20). The population frequency of Maroteaux–Lamy syndrome has been estimated at 1 in 248,000 live births in Australia (21).

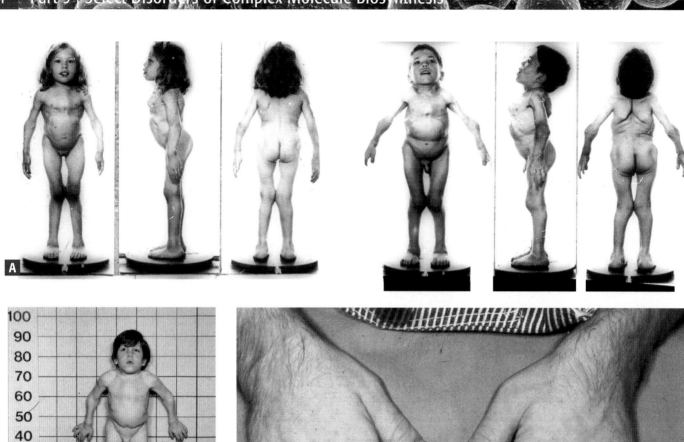

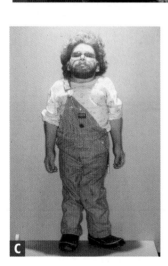

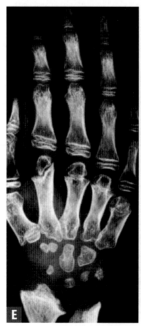

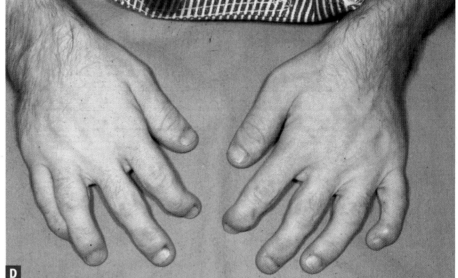

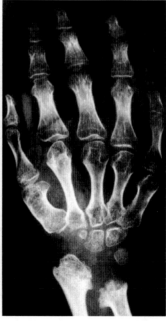

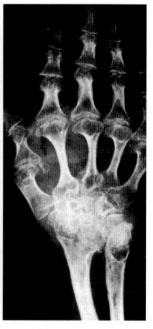

FIGURE 43-8. Characteristics of Morquio syndrome (MPS-IV). The most characteristic features of Morquio syndrome are the skeletal features. **A** to **D.** Reduced height due to shortened neck and trunk; pectus carinatum; joint laxity with enlarged wrists, marked kyphoscoliosis; thoracolumbar gibbus. **E.** The humerus, radius, ulna, and metacarpals are short, coarse, curved, and irregularly tabulated. (Courtesy of Susan Berry, M.D., and Robert Gorlin, D.D.S, M.S., D.Sc., University of Minnesota Medical School.)

Severely affected patients present in the first few years of life with growth delay, progressive joint restriction, coarse facial features, hepatosplenomegaly, and corneal clouding (Figure 43-9). Skeletal abnormalities, including short stature and a constellation of deformities known as *dysostosis multiplex*, are also characteristic. Cardiac abnormalities include aortic and mitral valvular dysfunction, resulting from abnormal accumulations of glycosaminoglycans, as well as cardiomyopathy. In severely affected patients, cardiac failure leads to death in the second or third decade. Recently, an adult patient was described with an attenuated phenotype of Maroteaux–Lamy syndrome involving abnormal inclusion bodies in leukocytes and mild hearing loss but normal height, joint mobility, and facial appearance, as well as normal findings on opthalomogical, cardiac, and skeletal examination (20).

Sly Syndrome (MPS-VII)

Sly syndrome is an extremely rare MPS caused by deficient activity of β-glucuronidase (GUSB), which normally cleaves glucuronide residues from dermatan sulfate, heparan sulfate, and chondroitin sulfate. Over 45 different mutations in the GUSB gene have been reported, the majority of which are point mutations (22).

Although first described in a 2-year-old boy with Hurler-like features (23), Sly syndrome is now recognized as having a wide phenotypic spectrum. In its most severe form, it is distinguished from the other MPSs by having a neonatal, or even fetal, age of onset. This form is characterized by dysostosis multiplex, hepatosplenomegaly, and coarse facial features sometimes apparent even at birth. Fetal

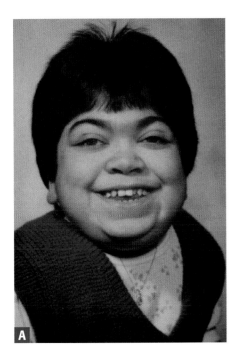

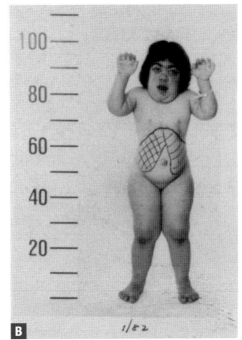

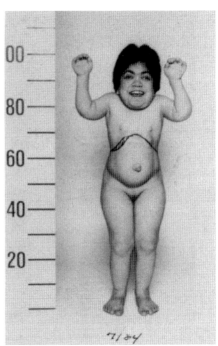

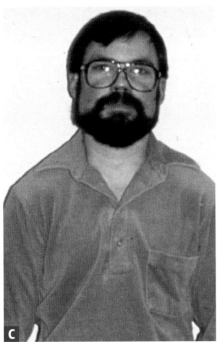

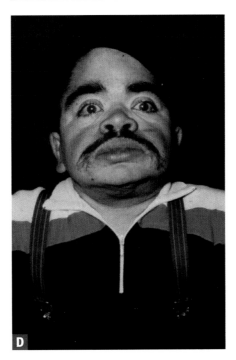

FIGURE 43-9. Characteristics of Maroteaux–Lamy syndrome (MPS-VI). Similar but milder coarse facies than patients with Hurler syndrome (low nasal bridge, hypertelorism, full cheek and lips, bushy eyebrows), patients with Maroteaux–Lamy may present with short stature, protruding abdomen, and hepatosplenomegaly. (Courtesy of Susan Berry, M.D., and Robert Gorlin, D.D.S., M.S., D.Sc., University of Minnesota Medical School.)

death from nonimmune hydrops fetalis has been reported in a number of patients (24). Milder patients have been described, including a child diagnosed at age 7 years with mild facial dysmorphism, short stature, corneal opacity, and mild mental retardation. This patient died suddenly at age 37 years from presumed cardiac arrest and represents the longest known survivor of Sly syndrome (25).

Hyaluronidase Deficiency (MPS-IX)

Hyaluronidase deficiency leads to the abnormal storage of hyaluronan (HA), a glycosaminoglycan of repeating disaccharide units of glucuronic acid and N-acetylglucosamine. It is abundant in extracellular matrix of connective tissue, particularly in synovial fluid and vitreous humor. The gene encoding hyaluronidase, HYAL1, is a member of a tandemly distributed family of genes encoding different hyaluronidase enzymes with distinct tissue distributions and substrate specificities (26).

Hyaluronidase deficiency has been described in only a single patient, a 14-year-old girl with nodular soft tissue periarticular masses affecting the joints of her ankles, knees, and fingers. Other features included cutaneous swelling, mild dysmorphic features, and short stature, with normal joint mobility and intelligence. Histological examination demonstrated abnormal HA storage in lysosomes in macrophages and fibroblasts and an abnormally elevated serum HA concentration (27).

Diagnosis
- Urine total mucopolysaccharide excretion is elevated.
- Excretion of specific mucopolysaccharides, fractionated by thin-layer chromatography, electrophoresis, or isoelectric focusing, is abnormal (Table 43-1).
- Deficient activity of specific lysosomal enzyme confirms the diagnosis.
- DNA testing is available by either gene sequencing or targeted mutation analysis for most of the disorders.

- MPS patients typically appear normal at birth.
- All disorders are characterized by a progressive (developmentally regressive) course.
- Mental retardation and severe visceral involvement are seen in Hunter and Hurler syndromes.
- Mental retardation and minimal visceral involvement are seen in Sanfilippo syndrome.
- Visceral involvement and normal intelligence are seen in Maroteaux–Lamy syndrome.
- Severe skeletal abnormalities and normal intelligence are seen in Morquio syndrome.

- Prenatal diagnosis is possible for the MPSs by enzyme assay on chorionic villus tissue or cultured amniocytes and by molecular studies in families where the underlying defect is known. Carrier testing, either by enzyme assay or molecular studies, is also feasible.
- Molecular testing is preferred for detecting carriers of the X-linked Hunter syndrome because of the influence of X-inactivation on iduronate sulfatase activity, which can lead to both false-positive and false-negative results.
- Encouraging new studies demonstrate the feasibility of identifying patients with these disorders presymptomatically by testing newborn screening blood spots using a tandem mass spectrometry–based approach (28). This is particularly important because treatment by enzyme replacement therapy (ERT) is most effective when initiated as early as possible, ideally before the onset of symptoms (see below).

Treatment Supportive management for the MPSs includes ventriculoperitoneal shunting for communicating hydrocephalus, spinal fusion for cord compression, adenoidectomy and tonsillectomy, hernia repair, corneal transplants, and median nerve release for carpal tunnel syndrome. Bone-marrow transplanta-

- Urine screening for abnormal mucopolysaccharides is a useful first-line test through the determination of total glycosaminoglycan concentration and the specific distribution of individual mucopolysaccharides.
- Urine screening by measurement of total mucopolysaccharides, without identification of specific mucopolysaccharide species, may miss some patients who have normal levels but an abnormal distribution of mucopolysaccharides.
- Diagnosis is established by specific enzyme assays in leukocytes or cultured fibroblasts.
- Carrier testing and prenatal diagnosis are available.

tion (BMT) is a therapy aimed at replacing the missing enzyme through introduction of an allogenic graft and has been performed with varying degrees of success on patients with MPS-I, -II, -III, -VI, and -VII. Improvement has been noted for many of the somatic abnormalities associated with the MPSs, including organomegaly, facial appearance, joint stiffness, and breathing difficulties (29). Skeletal and neurological outcomes are more variable, and in some cases, no effect of BMT on these systems is appreciated, especially for MPS-II and -III. For MPS-I, it appears likely that children under the age of 2 without significant developmental delay may benefit, whereas children with significant developmental delay may not achieve continuing mental development. Furthermore, the risks associated with poor engraftment and graft-versus-host disease have resulted in significant morbidity and mortality associated with this procedure. Complications of BMT specific to MPSs, such as myocardial infarction and pneumonitis, have been noted.

Enzyme-replacement therapy (ERT) is playing an increasingly important role in the treatment of the MPSs, although efficacy is limited because recombinant enzymes do not

TABLE 43-1	Glycosaminoglycans in Different MPSs							
	Mucopolysaccharidosis							Typical Clinical Findings, Affected Organ Systems
	I	II	III	IV	VI	VII	IX	
Dermatan sulfate	++	++			++	+		Skeleton + internal organs
Heparan sulfate	+	+	+			n – +		Mental retardation
Keratan sulfate				+				Skeleton
Chondroitin sulfate	+			(+)		+	++	

Adapted with permission from Zschocke J, Hoffmann GF. Pathological glycosaminoglycans in different MPSs. In: Vademecum Metabolicum: Manual of Metabolic Paediatrics, 2nd ed. Stuttgart: Schattauer; 2004.

cross the blood–brain barrier (30). Laronidase (Aldurazyme), or recombinantly produced α-iduronidase, has been approved by the Food and Drug Administration (FDA) as an ERT strategy for MPS-I, following an initial evaluation in a randomized, placebo-controlled study of 45 MPS-I patients. Promising early results show improved pulmonary function and endurance in this small cohort of patients, although with no clear evidence of CNS improvement (31). Specifically, ERT has been shown efficacious only in those more mildly affected MPS-I patients without CNS involvement (i.e., MPS-IH/S and MPS-IS). More detailed long-term studies of outcomes following laronidase treatment are currently underway.

Recently, ERT has also been approved for the treatment of MPS-II and -VI, with new approaches being evaluated for targeting directly to the CNS in MPS-I and -II and potentially for MPS-III. The development of an ERT strategy is also underway for MPS-IV (32,33).

DISORDERS OF LYSOSOMAL ENYZME LOCALIZATION

I-Cell Disease and Pseudo-Hurler Polydystrophy

Etiology/Pathophysiology I-cell disease (mucolipidosis type II, or ML-II) and pseudo-Hurler polydystrophy (mucolipidosis type III, or ML-III) are autosomal recessive disorders characterized by deficient activity of multiple lysosomal enzymes, including those involved in the catabolism of mucopolysaccharides, oligosaccharides, and sphingolipids (34). The term *mucolipidosis* reflects the constellation of clinical features shared by the mucopolysaccharidoses and sphingolipidoses, including organomegaly, coarse facies, restricted joint movement, and psychomotor retardation.

The primary defect for both ML-II and ML-III lies in the enzyme N-acetylglucosaminyl-1-phosphotransferase, which is required for proper posttranslational processing of lysosomal acid hydrolases and their subsequent import into lysosomes. During normal lysosomal biogenesis, phosphotransferase participates in the formation of a mannose-6-phosphate recognition marker on enzymes destined for the lysosomes. Absence of this marker leads to the inappropriate secretion of numerous lysosomal enzymes outside cells and to their deficiency inside lysosomes, where they would normally function at an acidic pH (see Figure 43-10). This, in turn, leads to abnormal storage of lysosomal substrates, including mucopolysaccharides, oligosaccharides, and sphingolipids and ultimately to cell toxicity and death (6).

Phosphotransferase itself is a multisubunited enzyme, with all reported cases of ML-II and some cases of ML-III due to mutations in the α-subunit gene. Other cases of ML-III have been shown to be genetically distinct and due to mutations in the γ-subunit gene. Patients with ML-II are more severely affected, whereas ML-III appears to have a later onset and milder course. There is good evidence for genotype/phenotype correlation, with ML-III patients retaining some residual phosphotransferase activity.

I-cell disease is so named because of characteristic inclusion bodies seen in the cytoplasm of fibroblasts and other cells of mesenchymal origin. These inclusions represent membrane-bound vacuoles containing electron-lucent or fibrillogranular material and include mucopolysaccharides, oligosaccharides, and lipids. Multiple organs and tissues are affected, including the skeletal, central nervous, muscular, and cardiac systems. In particular, the vacuolization of cells of the heart valves leads to valvular thickening and subsequent cardiac insufficiency. Patients with ML-III demonstrate intracellular inclusions similar to but not as prominent as those in ML-II.

Clinical Presentation Patients with I-cell disease present with many features of Hurler syndrome (MPS-I) but are distinguished from Hurler patients by earlier onset, more rapidly progressive course, prominent gingival hyperplasia, lack of excessive mucopolysacchariduria, and coarse facies at birth. Other presenting symptoms

- Most I-cell patients do not have abnormal mucopolysaccharide excretion.

- Diagnosis of either ML-II or ML-III is by demonstration of abnormally increased lysosomal enzyme activities in serum and decreased activities in cells.

- The distinction between ML-II and ML-III is made on clinical grounds, with ML-III patients presenting later and showing a milder disease progression.

include decreased birth weight and length, hypotonia, and joint immobility. The skeletal system of ML-II patients is severely affected, with abnormalities including anterior beaking and wedging of vertebral bodies, kyphoscoliosis, gibbus deformity, and widening of the ribs. ML-II patients may develop valvular disease associated with the presence of vacuolated fibroblasts in heart valves (35). Tracheal narrowing also can occur as a result of glycosaminoglycan deposition (36). Other abnormalities include psychomotor retardation and organomegaly (including liver, spleen, and heart). Death typically occurs between 5 and 8 years of age from pneumonia or congestive heart failure.

Patients with ML-III have a later onset of symptoms than those with ML-II, as well as a milder and more slowly progressive course. Onset is typically between 2 and 4 years of

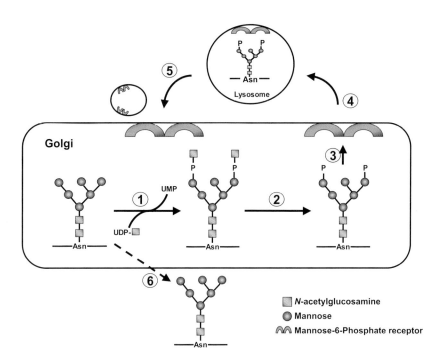

FIGURE 43-10. Targeting of lysosomal enzymes via the mannose-6-phosphate receptor: 1) transfer of *N*-acetylglucosamine-1-phosphate to mannose via phosphotransferase (defective in ML-II and ML-III), 2) removal of *N*-acetylglucosamine exposing the mannose-6-phosphate marker, 3) recognition and binding of lysosomal enzymes to the mannose-6-phosphate receptor, 4) transport of lysosomal enzymes to lysosomes, 5) recycling of mannose-6-phosphate receptors back to the Golgi membrane, 6) abnormal secretion of lysosomal enzymes that fail to acquire the mannose-6-phosphate marker, as in ML-II and ML-III.

TABLE 43-2   Laboratory Findings: ML-II and ML-III

Decreased	Increased
N-Acetylglucosamine-1-phosphotransferase activity	Mucopolysacchariduria (normal to mildly elevated)
	Serum β-hexosaminidase (10–20×)
	Serum arylsulfatase A (10–20×)

age, with survival possible into adulthood. Features include growth retardation, stiff joints, claw-hand deformity, mild coarsening of facial features, and mild psychomotor delay. In contrast to patients with ML-II, the skeletal dysplasia is slowly progressive over many years. Neurological involvement is also characteristically milder than in ML-II, with mental retardation reported in approximately 50% of ML-III patients.

Diagnosis

- Determination of lysosomal enzyme activity in serum (not in fibroblasts or cells) is useful in the diagnosis of I-cell disease because these enzymes are secreted out of the cells.

- Normal to mildly increased mucopolysacchariduria may be present (Table 43-2).

- Inclusion bodies (membrane-bound vacuoles) are found in fibroblasts.

- Assays for phosphotransferase activity are reliable but not widely available on a clinical basis.

- Prenatal diagnosis is accomplished by demonstration of increased lysosomal enzyme activities (e.g., β-hexosaminidase and arylsulfatase A) in cell-free amniotic fluid and decreased intracellular activities in cultured amniocytes.

Treatment There is no definitive treatment for either disorder. Supportive therapies include antibiotic treatment of recurrent respiratory infections, physical therapy for joint limitations, and hip-replacement surgery. BMT has been performed on a limited number of patients with I-cell disease, with apparent prevention of cardiopulmonary complications and continued neurocognitive development (37,38). Treatment of two ML-III patients with the bisphosphonate pamidronate resulted in significant improvement in mobility and reduction in bone pain (39).

SPHINGOLIPIDOSES

Tay-Sachs Disease and Sandhoff Disease: The G_{M2}-Gangliosidoses

Etiology/Pathophysiology The G_{M2}-gangliosidoses are autosomal recessive conditions that feature abnormal accumulation of ganglioside G_{M2} and other related glycolipids in neuronal lysosomes secondary to deficiency of β-hexosa-minidase. There are two forms of β-hexosa-minidase, Hex A (consisting of an α and a β subunit) and Hex B (consisting of two β subunits). Tay-Sachs disease is caused by mutations in the gene coding for the α subunit of β-hexosaminidase (Hex A deficiency). Sandhoff disease is caused by mutations in the gene encoding the β subunit of β-hexosaminidase (Hex A and Hex B deficiency) (see Figure 43-11). Both conditions are panethnic, although Tay-Sachs disease has a higher prevalence in the Ashkenazi Jewish population. In addition, G_{M2}-activator deficiency (also sometimes referred to as *variant AB*) results in a Tay-Sachs-like phenotype. G_{M2} activator forms a complex with gangliosides that is presented to β-hexosaminidase in order for hydrolysis to occur (40). The nervous system is the site of pathology in Tay Sachs disease. Membranous cytoplasmic bodies composed of G_{M2}-ganglioside, cholesterol, and phospholipids are found throughout the central and peripheral nervous systems. In Sandhoff disease, the nervous system pathology is similar to that seen in Tay-Sachs disease. However, additional storage material in Sandhoff disease is found in liver, spleen, lung, lymph nodes, and kidney. Nevertheless, such visceral storage usually does not lead to significant organomegaly. The pathogenesis of the G_{M2}-gangliosidoses is not clearly understood. Altered neuronal cell membrane ganglioside structure leading to abnormal neuronal connections and the formation of toxic compounds (e.g., lysoganglioside G_{M2}) may contribute to disease progression. Lysosphingolipids have been shown to inhibit protein kinase C and, in theory, may cause aberrant neuronal signal transduction. Recent experiments in mouse models have implicated CNS inflammation in disease pathogenesis in both G_{M2}- and G_{M1}-gangliosidoses (41).

Clinical Presentation The acute infantile forms of Tay-Sachs disease, Sandhoff disease, and G_{M2}-activator deficiency present similarly with weakness, usually appearing at between 3 and 5 months. Progressive loss of neurological function occurs insidiously at first. Hypotonia, poor head control, an exaggerated startle reflex, seizures, and blindness supervene. A cherry-red spot is typical on ophthalmological evaluation. Macrocephaly secondary to cerebral gliosis is noted from about age 18 months. Decerebrate posturing and eventual complete unresponsiveness occur in the second year. Death usually is caused by pneumonia and occurs at between 2 and 5 years of age.

Later-onset forms of Tay-Sachs disease and Sandhoff disease exist. Late-onset juvenile forms of G_{M2}-gangliosidoses typically present between the ages of 2 and 10 years with ataxia, dystonia, progressive spasticity, dementia, and increasing seizures. Affected individuals usually die in the second decade. Adult-onset forms of disease are even more insidious in progression. Patients may have normal intelligence, although other neurological problems, including dystonia, ataxia, and spinocerebellar degeneration, may occur. Psychiatric problems, including psychosis, are relatively common in late-onset forms Tay-Sachs disease and Sandhoff disease.

Diagnosis

- Urine oligosaccharide analysis may show an increase in N-acetylglucosaminyl oligosaccharides in Sandhoff disease (Table 43-3) but is normal in Tay-Sachs disease because such compounds are not stored in the latter.

- Decreased β-hexosaminidase A is present in plasma, leukocytes, fibroblasts, and tissues in Tay-Sachs disease. A combined deficiency of β-hexosaminidase A and β-hexosaminidase B is present in Sandhoff disease. Specific assays to detect G_{M2}-activator

β-Hexosaminidase isoenzymes

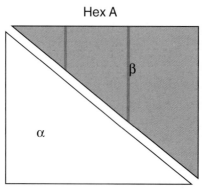

Hex A

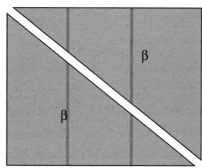

Hex B

FIGURE 43-11. Molecular mechanisms of Tay–Sachs and Sandhoff diseases.

TABLE 43-3 Laboratory Findings: Tay–Sachs/Sandhoff Diseases	
Decreased	**Increased**
β-Hexosaminidase activity	Tissue ganglioside G_{M2} content
	Urine *N*-acetylglucosaminyl oligosaccharides (Sandhoff)

activity or the amount of G_{M2}-activator protein are needed for a biochemical diagnosis of variant AB.

- Mutation analysis is widely available for the common Ashkenazi Jewish mutations. In this population, two mutations account for most cases of infantile onset Tay-Sachs disease.

- Healthy individuals have been identified who have an apparent deficiency of Hex A activity when measured by standard techniques. These pseudodeficient individuals have been detected most often as part of screening programs.

- Prenatal diagnosis is possible by measuring β-hexosaminidase activity in amniocytes or chorionic villi. If the mutations are known, DNA analysis is also possible. It is especially important to perform mutation analysis for alleles known to cause pseudodeficiency if parental mutations are not known so that a clinically unaffected fetus will not be mistaken for classic disease.

Treatment Therapy is supportive. ERT by intravenous infusion has been attempted in a few patients, but because enzyme does not cross the blood–brain barrier, this approach is ineffective (42). Bone marrow transplantation has been attempted, but with no clear success. Substrate-reduction therapy using N-butyldeoxynorjirimycin (Miglustat) has shown success in a mouse model of Tay-Sachs disease, and clinical trials are under way in late-onset forms of Tay-Sachs disease (43).

Niemann–Pick Disease Types A and B

Etiology/Pathophysiology Niemann–Pick disease (NPD) types A and B are autosomal recessive conditions caused by acid sphingomyelinase (ASM) deficiency, which leads to abnormal accumulation of sphingomyelin in lysosomes and secondary increases in cholesterol and other lipids. The more severe type A form is characterized by undetectable to less than 5% of normal ASM activity when measured in leukocytes or fibroblasts, whereas ASM activity in type B is usually higher, although some overlap exists. Sphingomyelin is a major component of the plasma membrane and membranes of subcellular organelles in most cell types. NPD types A and B are panethnic, but NPD type A has a relatively high prevalence in the Ashkenazi Jewish popula-

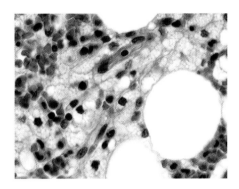

FIGURE 43-12. Bone marrow with focal aggregates of multivacuolated histiocytes typical of Neimann–Pick disease. This histiocyte morphology, however, is not specific for this disease. (Courtesy of Daniel Arber, M.D., Stanford University Pathology Department.)

tion. The monocyte–macrophage system is the site of the greatest storage of sphingomyelin. The stored material has a mulberry-like or honeycomb-like appearance in histiocytes. Such cells are often referred to as *foam cells* or *Niemann–Pick cells* (see Figure 43-12). Similar-appearing cells may be found in G_{M1}-gangliosidosis, Wolman disease, and cholesterol ester storage disease. In NPD type A, the spleen and lymph nodes may be completely filled with foam cells, but all organ systems have some degree of infiltration. Sphingomyelin and its downstream metabolic intermediates have important functions in cellular signal transduction. For example, sphingosine is a potent inhibitor of protein kinase C activity (the protein kinase C family of serine–threonine kinases is involved in multiple cell-signaling pathways). Ceramide is a lipid second messenger in diverse pathways involving apoptosis, cell division and differentiation, and sterol homeostasis. Lysosphingolipids also accumulate in NPD and may contribute to cell dysfunction and affect apoptosis. Therefore, NPD patients may have abnormalities in a variety of cell-signaling pathways that contribute to disease pathophysiology, although the precise defects remain to be elucidated. Massive accumulation of bis(monoacylglycero)phosphate also occurs, but the role this plays in disease pathogenesis is unclear.

Clinical Presentation NPD type A presents in infancy, usually within the first few months, with abdominal distension and hepatosplenomegaly. Nonimmune hydrops fetalis has been described (44). Feeding difficul-

ties, intermittent vomiting, and constipation are common. Developmental delay usually is present by 6 months, and regression occurs. Neurological features include hypotonia and weakness. In later stages, spasticity supervenes. Although about 50% of children will have a "cherry red" spot noted on ophthalmological examination, visual loss is rare. Lipid deposits may cause corneal and retinal opacification. Pulmonary involvement consisting of alveolar infiltration also may occur but is usually not a significant problem, although episodes of bronchitis and aspiration pneumonia may be severe. Growth is impaired, and osteoporosis is common; such features are likely secondary to poor nutrition and bone infiltration. These children usually succumb by age 3 years. Asphyxia or pneumonia may represent the terminal event.

In contrast, NPD type B is a milder condition with a more variable clinical presentation and course. For example, some may have significant organomegaly in infancy, whereas others only develop signs in later adulthood. However, most are diagnosed during infancy or childhood when hepatosplenomegaly is noted on a routine examination. Still milder forms are not detected until adulthood. Pulmonary involvement often develops, secondary to alveolar infiltration, and may be severe. In some cases, liver disease is severe and progresses to cirrhosis. Hyperlipidemia is common. Intelligence is normal. Interestingly, some patients with NPD type B have been noted to have "cherry red" maculae. Survival is usually into adulthood, although death may occur in childhood or adolescence. Significant liver involvement with cirrhosis, respiratory disease (e.g., pneumonia), and cor pulmonale may be life-threatening (45).

Diagnosis

- Decreased acid sphingomyelinase activity is present in peripheral blood leukocytes or fibroblasts (Table 43-4).

- Sometimes the diagnosis is made when Niemann–Pick cells are detected after a bone marrow biopsy is performed for suspected malignancy or a liver biopsy is undertaken to investigate hepatomegaly.

- X-rays may show osteoporosis and pulmonary alveolar infiltration.

- Decreased plasma high-density lipoprotein (HDL) cholesterol and increased triglycerides and low-density lipoprotein (LDL) cholesterol may occur (46) .

- Because three common alleles are responsible for over 90% of cases of NPD type A in the Ashkenazi Jewish population, molecular diagnosis may be relatively straightforward in this group. In contrast, diverse, "private" mutations typically are present in

TABLE 43-4 Laboratory Findings: Niemann–Pick Disease Types A and B

Decreased	Increased
Acid sphingomyelinase activity (<5% type A; <10% type B)	Tissue sphingolipid and cholesterol content
Hemoglobin/hematocrit	Plasma LDL cholesterol
Platelets	Plasma triglycerides

other ethnic groups, and only will be detected by DNA sequencing.

- ΔR608 is a "neuroprotective" (i.e., type B) mutation in the Ashkenazi Jewish population.
- Prenatal diagnosis is possible by measuring ASM activity in amniocytes or chorionic villi. If the mutations are known, DNA analysis is also possible.

Treatment In general, treatment is supportive for all types of NPD. Liver transplantation has had some success in severe nonneuropathic cases. Bone marrow transplantation has been performed in both types A and B. No change in the neurological course was noted in type A disease. ERT may be of benefit in the later-onset form of NPD. Improvement of organomegaly following bone marrow transplantation has been observed in NPD type B (47). A clinical trial using ERT is scheduled to start soon for NPD type B. Other treatments, including gene therapy, are currently under investigation.

Niemann–Pick Disease Type C

Etiology/Pathophysiology NPD type C is an autosomal recessive, panethnic condition caused by a defect in cellular cholesterol trafficking leading to late-endosomal/lysosomal storage of unesterified cholesterol. The majority (~90%) of affected individuals carry mutations in NPC1, a gene that encodes a protein that localizes in late endosomes and interacts with lysosomes in the trans-Golgi network. The exact function of NPC1 protein is unknown (48). A minority of patients carry mutations in HE1, which codes for a protein present in lysosomes and late endosomes that may play a role in the egress of cholesterol and glycolipids from lysosomes (49). Variant forms also exist. NPD type C is characterized by the presence of foam cells or sea-blue histiocytes in visceral organs and the CNS (50). Neurofibrillary tangles are seen in the CNS of patients who have a prolonged neurological course.

Clinical Presentation NPD type C is a progressive neurodegenerative disease that has wide clinical variability. Vertical supranuclear ophthalmoplegia (upward-gaze palsy), ataxia, dystonia, behavioral problems and dementia

- The molecular defects in NPD type C are different from the defect present in NPD types A and B.

are characteristic of the classical disease phenotype. Hepatosplenomegaly is variable but can be severe and represent the initial sign of underlying disease. Although most cases present in childhood, onset may vary from the neonatal period to adulthood. Severe, lethal neonatal liver disease (neonatal hepatitis) and hydrops fetalis may occur. Psychiatric illness, including dementia, is a common feature in adult variants. Most affected individuals die after one to three decades of steady deterioration.

Diagnosis

- An abnormal pattern of fibroblast cholesterol is seen by Filipin fluorescence staining.
- Abnormal cholesterol esterification is seen in cultured fibroblasts (Table 43-5).
- Foam cells or sea-blue histiocytes are present in many tissues.
- Polymorphous cytoplasmic bodies may be seen on electron microscopy of skin or conjunctiva.
- ASM activity may be normal, low, or even elevated.
- Variant forms exist in which biochemical studies are near normal. These forms can be detected using a fluorescent sphingolipid analogue (BODIPY-lactosylceramide) when analyzing fibroblasts.
- Mutation analysis is available.
- Prenatal diagnosis is possible by measuring ASM activity in amniocytes or chorionic villi. If the mutations are known, DNA analysis is also possible.

Treatment Definitive therapy is not available, so care and management are supportive. Substrate-reduction therapy with Miglustat, an inhibitor of glycosphingolipid

synthesis, has shown early encouraging results in a NPD type C patient and is under investigation (51).

Gaucher Disease

Etiology/Pathophysiology Gaucher disease is the most prevalent lysosomal disorder. A deficiency of β-glucocerebrosidase (β-glucosidase) results in storage of the lipid glucosylceramide, an intermediate in the catabolism of globoside and gangliosides. Gaucher disease can be somewhat artificially divided into three forms that can be differentiated by the relative degree of neurological involvement. In reality, there is probably a continuous spectrum of disease phenotypes, but the old classification is nevertheless useful. Although Gaucher disease type 1 is panethnic, it occurs most frequently in the Ashkenazi Jewish population (~1:1000). All forms of Gaucher disease are inherited in an autosomal recessive fashion. Lipid-laden cells (Gaucher cells) derived from the monocyte–macrophage system containing cytoplasm with a "wrinkled tissue paper" or "crumpled silk" appearance are characteristic. Liver, spleen, and brain (in neuronopathic forms) of affected individuals have shown markedly increased glucosylceramide content. In Gaucher disease type 1, Gaucher cells and glucosylceramide accumulate in the vascular periadventitial areas of the Virchow–Robinow spaces. Gaucher cells are especially prominent in spleen, liver sinusoids, hepatic Kupffer cells, and lymph nodes. Storage in the liver and spleen can lead to massive hepatosplenomegaly. Fibrosis in systemic organs and brain gliosis occur. Progressive accumulation of Gaucher cells in bone marrow, vascular compromise, and infarction lead to skeletal complications, including osteopenia, osteosclerosis, osteonecrosis (e.g., avascular necrosis of the femoral head), painful bone crises, and remodeling abnormalities. Gaucher cells can coalesce to form a pseudotumorous lesion (gaucheroma) that may resemble a chondrosarcoma. In neuropathic forms of Gaucher disease, significant amounts of glucosylceramide and glucosylsphingosine are present in the CNS.

Clinical Presentation Type 1 has a variable phenotype, ranging from asymptomatic individuals to children who have massive hepatosplenomegaly, pancytopenia, and severe skeletal abnormalities (52). Common presenting signs and symptoms include splenomegaly with associated hypersplenism, epistaxis, easy

TABLE 43-5 Laboratory Findings: Niemann–Pick Disease Type C

Decreased	Increased
Ability to synthesize cholesterol esters	Intracellular unesterified cholesterol

bruising, and hepatomegaly. Hypersplenism and bone marrow infiltration lead to pancytopenia. Although massive hepatomegaly may occur, hepatic failure or cirrhosis is rare. Growth retardation is often present in children, but bone lesions usually occur later than visceral involvement. Painful bone crises may occur, especially during childhood or adolescence. In children, acute hip involvement sometimes may be mistaken for Legg–Calvé–Perthe disease. Gaucher disease type 1 also has been misdiagnosed as lymphoma, leukemia, bleeding disorders, and osteomyelitis. Lung infiltration by Gaucher cells may happen in children, but this is a rare finding. Pulmonary hypertension, portal hypertension, and renal involvement are encountered rarely. Cancer, especially hematological malignancies, appears to be slightly more common in individuals who have Gaucher disease than in the general population.

Gaucher disease type 2 is a severe, progressive disorder that presents in infancy or early childhood with massive hepatosplenomegaly, failure to thrive, and progressive neurological dysfunction with spasticity, cortical thumbs, and opisthotonus. Strabismus and oculomotor apraxia may be the first sign of disease. Fetal hydrops and a congenital ichthyosis like rash also have been described (44).

Gaucher disease type 3 is intermediate in severity between types 1 and 2. Severe, early-onset massive organomegaly and slowly progressive neurological dysfunction are typical. Some affected individuals do not have massive organomegaly. This form is relatively common in the Norrbottnian region of Sweden.

Diagnosis

- Decreased β-glucosidase activity is present in peripheral blood leukocytes or fibroblasts (Table 43-6).

- Sometimes the diagnosis becomes evident when Gaucher cells are detected after a bone marrow biopsy is performed for suspected malignancy or a liver biopsy is undertaken to investigate hepatomegaly.

- Skeletal x-rays may reveal the characteristic "Erlenmeyer flask" deformity of the distal femur in Gaucher disease type 1.

- Because well-established genotype–phenotype correlations exist, mutation analysis is

often performed. For example, the 1226G (N370S) mutation is considered to be neuroprotective because it has never been detected in patients with neuronopathic disease. On the other hand, homozygosity for the 1448C (L444P) mutation is associated with neuronopathic disease, although there may be exceptions.

- Prenatal diagnosis is possible by measuring β-glucosidase activity in amniocytes or chorionic villi. If the mutations are known, DNA analysis is also possible.

Treatment ERT is the mainstay of treatment for type 1 disease (53). Therapy consists of bimonthly intravenous infusion of human β-glucosidase manufactured using recombinant DNA techniques. ERT improves anemia, thrombocytopenia, hepatosplenomegaly, and bone crises. Prolonged treatment over 2 or 3 years may be required for any noticeable improvement in skeletal disease. Severe skeletal manifestations can be prevented if ERT is begun before irreversible bone damage has occurred. Because presentation in childhood is indicative of moderate or severe disease, all children should be considered for ERT therapy, even those with isolated splenomegaly.

ERT also should be considered in those who have type 3 disease because of the relatively slow progression of neurological disease in these individuals. There is still debate whether the enzyme may reach the brain. Although a few type 2 patients have received ERT, such treatment has no effect on the devastating neurodegenerative course in this subtype and generally is not recommended.

N-Butyldeoxynorjirimycin (Miglustat) decreases the rate of synthesis of glucocerebroside, a sphingolipid that is involved in the synthesis of complex lipid formation in the pathway common to Gaucher, Fabry, Tay-Sachs, and Sandhoff diseases. Decreased synthesis of the stored compound (substrate-reduction therapy [SRT]) is an alternative treatment that has been approved recently for Gaucher disease type 1. Oral SRT with Miglustat improves hepatosplenomegaly and hematological parameters. Its effect on bone complications and the brain are unclear. Although SRT is not likely to replace ERT, it may prove to be a useful adjunctive therapy. Currently in the United States, Miglustat is

approved by the FDA for use only when ERT is not a therapeutic option.

Bisphosphonates (e.g., palmidronate) inhibit bone resorption and may prove useful in the management of advanced bone disease, especially when used in conjunction with ERT. Symptomatic treatment of complications, including analgesics for pain crises, repair of fractures, and joint replacement, is, of course, still important. However, with the advent of ERT, the current therapeutic goal is the *a priori* prevention of such complications. Although BMT has been performed in Gaucher disease type 1 patients in the past, such therapy is no longer recommended because of the availability of ERT. BMT also has been performed in type 2 and type 3 patients but has not changed the course of neurological deterioration. Gene therapy has shown promise *in vitro* and in animal models of Gaucher disease but is not yet ready for clinical application.

Fabry Disease

Etiology/Pathophysiology Fabry disease is an X-linked disorder of glycosphingolipid metabolism caused by defects in the lysosomal enzyme α-galactosidase A. This enzyme cleaves α-galactosyl moieties from a variety of substrates, predominately globotriaosylceramide [galactosyl($\alpha 1 \rightarrow 4$)galactosyl($\beta 1 \rightarrow 4$)glucosyl($\beta 1 \rightarrow 1'$)ceramide]. Other substrates include galabiosylceramide and blood group B substances. The enzyme is deficient in all tissues of affected males and variably deficient in heterozygous females, with most showing intermediate levels of α-galactosidase A activity. Fabry disease has been reported in numerous ethnic groups and occurs at an estimated frequency of 1 in 40,000 males. The incidence in females is unknown (54). Over 150 different mutations in the α-galactosidase A gene have been identified, including deletions, point mutations, gene rearrangements, and splice-site defects. Hemizygous males with partial residual enzyme activity have been described with later onset and milder course. Disease progression in females is variable and depends not only on the specific mutation but also on the pattern of X inactivation.

Abnormal storage of globotriaosylceramide occurs in lysosomes of the vascular endothelium, as well as in perithelial and smooth muscle cells of the heart and kidney. Less pronounced storage also occurs in connective tissue, cornea, and ganglion and perineural cells of the autonomic nervous system. This is seen as tissue deposits of crystalline glycosphingolipids that show birefringence, or the characteristic "Maltese cross" appearance, under polarization microscopy.

TABLE 43-6	Laboratory Findings: Gaucher Disease		
Decreased	**Increased**
β-Glucosidase activity	Angiotensin-converting enzyme
Hemoglobin/hematocrit	Total (nonprostatic) acid phosphatase
Platelets	Chitotriosidase
	Tissue glucocerbroside content

The primary tissues affected in Fabry disease are skin, kidney, nervous system, eye, and heart. Skin abnormalities are manifest as progressive teleangeictasia and angiokeratoma resulting from vascular damage in capillaries of the dermal papillae. Similarly, vascular abnormalities of the kidney, resulting from glycosphingolipid storage in the glomerulus and distal tubules, lead to progressive renal dysfunction and, without treatment, end-stage renal disease. Nervous system storage appears to be confined to the peripheral and central autonomic nerve cells, leading to paresthesias, extreme pain, hypohidrosis, and gastrointestinal symptoms. The CNS also can be involved in that strokes and brain white matter changes can occur. Glycosphingolipid deposits in the eye lead to a whorl-like dystrophic corneal pattern characteristic of Fabry disease. Damage resulting from deposition in myocardial cells and valvular fibrocytes leads to cardiomegaly, ventricular hypertrophy, valvular disease, and eventually, congestive heart failure.

Clinical Presentation Hemizygous males with no detectable α-galactosidase A activity typically present in childhood or adolescence with pain and paresthesis of the extremities, angiokeratoma, hypohidrosis, and corneal whorls. The episodic, painful crises associated with Fabry disease can be debilitating and often are triggered by fever, exercise, fatigue, or other external stress. Unfortunately, these symptoms in children typically do not lead to a diagnosis of Fabry disease but sometimes are ignored, misunderstood, or misdiagnosed as erythromyalgia or other conditions (55). Over time, increasing damage to the kidneys and heart leads to proteinuria, hypertension, lymphedema, and uremia, as well as angina, electrocardiographic (ECG) abnormalities, ventricular hypertrophy, valvular disease, and congestive heart failure. Increasing storage of glycosphingolipids in the brain can lead to transient ischemic attacks and strokes. Gastrointestinal manifestations include abdominal pain, constipation or diarrhea, difficulty gaining weight, and vomiting. Prior to the availability of treatment by dialysis or kidney transplantation, death typically occurred in the third to fifth decades of life from renal or cardiac complications. Even with dialysis and transplant, death by the fifth decade was not uncommon prior to the development of ERT (see below).

Variant forms of Fabry disease have been described with partial residual enzyme activity. These patients lack many of the characteristic features of the disease, with clinical findings often limited to mild proteinuria and cardiac abnormalities. Although specific

TABLE 43-7 Laboratory Findings: Fabry Disease

Decreased	Increased
α-Galactosidase A activity	Urinary protein
	Lipid-laden macrophages in bone marrow

α-galactosidase A gene mutations appear to be associated with the milder phenotype, these same mutations also have been seen in classically affected Fabry patients, suggesting that other factors modulating the expression of phenotype exist.

Heterozygous females can remain asymptomatic through early adulthood. The most common finding in these women is the characteristic whorl-like corneal dystrophy, seen in approximately 70% of heterozygotes. Some heterozygous females also experience angiokeratoma, hypohidrosis, and involvement of the cardiac, renal, and central nervous systems, and females have been described with clinical manifestations as severe as those seen in classically affected males. Almost all women heterozygous for Fabry disease eventually will show some signs or symptoms of the condition.

Diagnosis

- The diagnosis of Fabry disease is confirmed by the demonstration of absent or significantly reduced α-galactosidase A activity in plasma, leukocytes, or fibroblasts (Table 43-7).

- Other laboratory abnormalities associated with Fabry disease include proteinuria and other signs of renal dysfunction, birefringent lipid globules in urine (with characteristic "Maltese crosses"). and lipid-laden macrophages in bone marrow.

- Due to random X-inactivation, enzymatic diagnosis of heterozygous females is more problematic, and normal α-galactosidase A activity does not rule out heterozygous status (56).

- Molecular studies, including targeted mutation analysis, gene rearrangement studies, and gene sequencing, can be performed to confirm heterozygous status in females.

- Fabry disease is an X-linked disorder.

- Major clinical findings in males include painful crises, renal disease, cardiac abnormalities, and angiokeratoma.

- Many heterozygous females have characteristic whorl-like corneal dystrophy, and some women develop clinical manifestations as severe as those seen in males.

- Prenatal diagnosis is available by molecular analysis in families in which a Fabry mutation has been identified.

- Enzymatic testing in females is unreliable.

Treatment Conventional treatment of Fabry disease patients includes medical management of pain using various analgesics and dialysis and/or renal transplantation for progressive renal insufficiency. In addition, ERT is now widely available (57,58). This promising approach involves intravenous infusions with α-galactosidase A produced by recombinant DNA technology. The treatment, currently marketed as Fabrazyme (agalsidase beta), has recently received FDA approval as an orphan drug; while initial studies appear promising, the full range of clinical benefits and side effects with long-term use are still being evaluated (59,60). Pain is reduced significantly in patients, as well as reversal of hearing deficits, although long-term treatment may be needed for the latter. Further positive effects have been described for the cardiac, renal, and gastrointestinal systems. Replagal (agalsidase alpha) is an alternative ERT that is approved in many countries outside the United States. There are no differences in the administration mode (intravenously) or infusion rhythm (biweekly), but the pattern of glycosylation and the recommended doses differ.

Metachromatic Leukodystrophy

Etiology/Pathophysiology Metachromatic leukodystrophy (MLD) is an autosomal recessive condition caused by arylsulfatase A deficiency. Arylsulfatase A catalyzes the first step in the degradation of complex sulfated glycolipids that are present in myelin sheaths of central and peripheral neurons and in viscera to a lesser extent. Sulfatide accumulates in lysosomes and the plasma membrane of myelin. This increased plasma membrane sulfatide content alters the carefully regulated stoichiometry of membrane lipids and likely plays a crucial role in the demyelination process (61).

Clinical Presentation Late infantile, juvenile, and adult forms of MLD have been identified. The late infantile form is most common. Hypotonia, unsteady gait, and diminished reflexes are common presenting signs. Psychomotor regression with gradual

TABLE 43-8   Laboratory Findings: Metachromatic Leukodystrophy

Decreased	Increased
Arylsulfatase A activity	Tissue sulfatide content
	Urine sulfatide
	CSF sulfatide
	CSF protein (later in disease course)

worsening of cortical, cerebellar, and peripheral nerve function is typical. Children have increasing speech difficulties, optic atrophy, and feeding difficulties. Seizures occur in about 25%. Late disease is characterized by a decerebrate state. Survival beyond 8 years is rare.

Most juvenile MLD patients present before 6 years of age, but onset in teenage years may occur. Subtle behavioral disturbances, worsening school performance, and clumsiness are noted. Spasticity, ataxia, and extrapyramidal signs are common, as are seizures and optic atrophy. Although the course of disease is variable, most patients die by age 20 years.

Gradual deterioration in school or job performance, clumsiness, and incontinence occur in the rare adult-onset form of MLD. Psychiatric symptoms, such as personality changes, paranoia, auditory hallucinations, dementia, and schizophrenia, are relatively common.

Diagnosis

- Brain computed tomographic (CT) scanning and magnetic resonance imaging (MRI) show symmetrical low-density signal throughout the cerebral white matter. Mild cerebral atrophy may be present.

- Most patients have decreased motor nerve conduction velocity and diminished sensory nerve action potentials.

- Decreased arylsulfatase A activity is present in leukocytes and fibroblasts (Table 43-8).

- Mutation analysis is available, and over 80 pathogenic mutations have been identified.

- In the European population, 1% to 2% of individuals have arylsulfatase A "pseudodeficiency" (relatively low activity but normal phenotype). This can complicate enzymatic diagnosis, but specialized tests (e.g., sulfatide loading test) can overcome this difficulty.

- Prenatal diagnosis is possible by measuring arylsulfatase A activity in amniocytes or chorionic villi. If the mutations are known, DNA analysis is also possible.

Treatment   Treatment is supportive. BMT has been attempted in MLD without clear success (29). Other experimental therapies, including gene therapy, are currently under investigation.

Multiple Sulfatase Deficiency

Etiology/Pathophysiology   Multiple sulfatase deficiency (MSD) is an extremely rare autosomal recessive disorder characterized by the combined deficiency of all 12 known sulfatase enzymes (62). Six of the sulfatases have been localized to lysosomes, including iduronate-2-sulfatase (deficient in Hunter syndrome), sulfamidase (Sanfilippo syndrome type A), glucosamine-6-sulfatase (Sanfilippo syndrome type D), N-acetylgalactosamine-6-sulfatase (Morquio syndrome type A), arylsulfatase B (Maroteaux–Lamy syndrome), and arylsulfatase A (metachromatic leukodystrophy). Two additional sulfatases have been localized tentatively to lysosomes, but with unclear function or natural substrate. Finally, four sulfatases have been localized to the microsomes or to the Golgi network, including arylsulfatase C or steroid sulfatase (X-linked ichthyosis), arylsulfatase F (chondrodysplasia punctata), and two sulfatases of unknown function.

The primary defect in MSD lies in faulty posttranslational modification of a specific cysteine residue located at the catalytic site of all sulfatases to C_α-formylglycine (FGly). This modification is required for the expression of normal sulfatase activity and occurs in the endoplasmic reticulum during sulfatase synthesis and maturation. It is mediated by the enzyme FGE (FGly-generating enzyme), also known as *sulfatase modifying factor 1* (SUMF-1), which is encoded by a single gene on chromosome 3. Disease-causing mutations in SUMF-1 have been demonstrated in at least seven patients with MSD (63). Deficient activity of multiple sulfatases leads to abnormal lysosomal storage of their natural substrates, including mucopolysaccharides and sulfatides, in turn leading to pathological abnormalities characteristic of many of the single lysosomal enzyme defects. There is reduced activity of sulfatase enzymes, but typically some residual activity is present. A complex spectrum of clinical phenotypes has been described, with disease severity generally related to the degree of residual sulfatase activity.

Clinical Presentation   Patients with MSD present with findings resembling a combination of the single-sulfatase deficiencies, including metachromatic leukodystrophy, mucopolysaccharidoses, X-linked ichthyosis, and chondrodysplasia punctata. Specific features include neurological deterioration and developmental delay, as well as coarse facies, dysostosis multiplex, organomegaly, ichthyosis, and chondrodysplasia punctata. There is often a period of normal early development followed by rapid decline and early death. Several patients have been described who presented around 1 year of age with clinical features suggestive of Hunter syndrome and later were shown to have MSD (64). One patient presented at birth with dysmorphic features, hydrocephalus, chondrocalcificans congenita, and heart abnormalities and had excessive mucopolysacchariduria and profound deficiency of all sulfatases (65). The degree of clinical severity may be related to the amount of residual sulfatase activity present in cells.

Diagnosis

- The diagnosis of MSD is established by demonstrating reduced activities of multiple sulfatases, including arylsulfatases A, B, and C, as well as sulfamidase and iduronate-2-sulfatase, in leukocytes or cultured fibroblasts (Table 43-9).

- Significant residual activity of sulfatases may be present depending on the patient, varying from less than 10% to 90% of normal (14,66)

- It is not necessary to measure all the sulfatases for diagnostic confirmation. Practically, demonstration of deficiency of two or more sulfatases, under proper cell culture conditions and in the appropriate clinical setting, is considered diagnostic.

- Mutation analysis is available on a research basis. Numerous pathogenic mutations have been identified.

- Additional features of MSD include metachromatic degeneration of peripheral nerve myelin and abnormal leukocyte granulation.

TABLE 43-9   Laboratory Findings: Multiple Sulfatase Deficiency

Decreased	Increased
Activities of multiple sulfatases	Urinary excretion of mucopolysaccharides, oligosaccharides, and sulfatides
	CSF protein

- Prenatal diagnosis is possible through assays of sulfatases in chorionic villi or amniocytes.
- Direct analyses of FGE activity or SUMF-1 mutations are currently not available on a clinical basis.

- Urine screening for abnormal mucopolysaccharides is a useful first-line test.
- Diagnosis is established by enzyme assays of individual sulfatases.

Treatment No effective treatment for MSD currently exists. However, clinical trials are either planned or underway for enzyme replacement of many of the individual sulfatases, including those deficient in Hunter syndrome and Maroteaux–Lamy syndrome. This raises the possibility of a future ERT strategy for the treatment of at least some of the symptoms associated with MSD.

Krabbe Disease (Globoid Cell Leukodystrophy)

Etiology/Pathophysiology Krabbe disease is an autosomal recessive condition caused by deficiency of lysosomal galactosylceramidase. Galactosylceramide storage occurs in multinucleated macrophages (globoid cells) in the nervous system. Peripheral nerves are also affected. Near-complete loss of oligodendrocytes and myelin is present in terminal stages of disease. Galactosylsphingosine (psychosine) is a toxic metabolite that accumulates and plays a central role in disease pathogenesis, possibly by causing increased oligodentrocyte apoptosis. Brain psychosine levels appear to correlate with disease severity (67).

Clinical Presentation Affected infants typically present at between 3 and 6 months of age with nonspecific features, including irritability and increased sensitivity to stimuli. Rapid neurological degeneration follows. Patients are hypersensitive to sound, light, or touch, resulting in screaming and rigidity. Hypertonia and hyperreflexia are present early in the course, but patients progress to hypotonia and unresponsiveness. Blindness (secondary to optic atrophy), deafness, and a peripheral neuropathy are common. Microcephaly is common, but macrocephaly can also occur. Visceromegaly is not a feature. Seizures become more frequent with disease progression, and most patients die before age 2 years.

Later-onset (i.e., late infantile, juvenile, and adult) forms occur less frequently. Vision loss, ataxia, hemiparesis, and more insidious psychomotor regression are encountered in later-onset forms.

TABLE 43-10 Laboratory Findings: Krabbe Disease

Decreased	Increased
Galactosylceramidase activity	Brain psychosine content
	CSF protein

Diagnosis

- Brain CT scanning and MRI show symmetrical cerebral atrophy. White matter abnormalities, plaque-like high-intensity T2 signal on MRI, especially in the parieto-occipital region, may be present (Table 43-10).
- Electromyography and nerve conduction studies may show evidence of a peripheral neuropathy.
- Abnormalities in auditory brain stem response, sensory evoked potentials, and visual evoked potentials may occur.
- Decreased galactosylceramidase activity is present in leukocytes and fibroblasts.
- Mutation analysis is available for Krabbe disease, and over 60 pathogenic mutations have been identified.
- Prenatal diagnosis is possible by measuring galactosylceramidase activity in amniocytes or chorionic villi. If the mutations are known, DNA analysis is also possible.

Treatment Treatment is primarily supportive. BMT has shown some success in Krabbe disease if performed before extensive neurological damage has occurred, mainly in later-onset forms. Experimental therapies, including gene therapy, are under investigation.

G$_{M1}$-Gangliosidosis

Etiology/Pathophysiology G$_{M1}$-gangliosidosis is a rare autosomal recessive condition that is caused by lysosomal β-galactosidase deficiency and subsequent storage of ganglioside G$_{M1}$ and asialo derivatives in brain and viscera. Gangliosides are abundant in the CNS, and progressive storage leads to neurodegeneration. Distended histiocytes that may appear like Gaucher cells may be seen in viscera. Membranous cytoplasmic bodies are present in neurons, and various types of inclusions are found in glial cells. Cholinergic abnormalities and abnormal activities of phospholipase C and adenyl cyclase may be present. In mouse models, inflammatory cell infiltration has been noted, suggesting that inflammation also may play a role in disease pathogenesis (41).

Clinical Presentation Infantile (type 1), late infantile/juvenile (type 2), and adult (type 3) forms of G$_{M1}$-gangliosidosis exist. The infantile form is characterized by early developmental delay or arrest, dysmorphic features (i.e., coarse, thick skin, frontal bossing, gingival hypertrophy, and macroglossia), hepatosplenomegaly, and failure to thrive. As in the G$_{M2}$-gangliosidoses, an exaggerated startle reflex may be present. In addition, approximately 50% have a macular "cherry red" spot, and corneal clouding is common. Skeletal abnormalities, such as short, broad digits, kyphoscoliosis, and contractures, are common. Nonimmune hydrops fetalis and neonatal cardiomyopathy may occur (44). Initially, affected infants appear hypotonic, but spasticity supervenes as the disease progresses, and seizures are typical by 1 year. Death, often secondary to respiratory failure, occurs by 2 years of age.

Late-infantile/juvenile G$_{M1}$-gangliosidosis has a more insidious course. Cherry red spots, visceromegaly, and skeletal abnormalities usually are absent. Developmental delay typically is noted at approximately 1 year of age. Progressive decline in function, seizures, and abnormal movements may occur, leading to death at between 3 and 10 years of age.

Adult G$_{M1}$-gangliosidosis has an onset in the second or third decade. This appears to be the least common variant but may have an increased frequency in Japan (68). Early development is normal. Ataxia or speech abnormalities are common presenting signs and are followed by dystonia, spinocerebellar degeneration, and decreasing cognitive abilities. Dysmorphic features, seizures, cherry red spots, visceromegaly, and prominent skeletal abnormalities do not occur.

Diagnosis

- Urine oligosaccharide analysis may show an increase in galactose-containing oligosaccharides (Table 43-11).
- Decreased β-galactosidase activity is present in leukocytes, fibroblasts, and tissues. In infantile and late-infantile/juvenile variants, enzyme activity is less than 5% of

TABLE 43-11 Laboratory Findings: G$_{M1}$ Gangliosidosis

Decreased	Increased
β-Galactosidase activity	Tissue ganglioside G$_{M1}$ content
	Urine galactose-containing oligosaccharides

normal, and in the adult form, activity is 5% to 10%.

- Foam cells are present in tissue biopsy specimens but to a lesser extent than in Gaucher disease or NPD.
- Mutation analysis is available for G_{M1} gangliosidosis. Five common mutations in different ethnic groups have been identified.
- Different mutations in same gene (β-galactosidase) cause Morquio syndrome type B.
- Prenatal diagnosis is possible by measuring β-galactosidase activity in amniocytes or chorionic villi. If the mutations are known, DNA analysis is also possible.

- G_{M1}-gangliosidosis may present in childhood through the third decade.
- A cherry red spot is present in about half the cases.

Treatment Treatment is supportive. Gene therapy, SRT (the reduction of storage material by inhibiting synthetic enzymes using small molecules), and enhancement of mutant enzyme activity using chemical chaperones have shown preliminary success in animal models (69).

Farber Disease

Etiology/Pathophysiology Farber disease is a rare autosomal recessive disorder of lipid metabolism caused by deficient activity of lysosomal acid ceramidase. This enzyme participates in the normal degradation and turnover of ceramide, an important precursor of gangliosides, myelin, and membrane components. Ceramidase deficiency results in the abnormal accumulation of ceramide in lysosomes of multiple organs and tissues and to the progressive development of multiple ceramide-containing subcutaneous nodules (lipogranulomata). Granulomatous infiltrations can be seen in subcutaneous tissues and joints, as well as in other sites, including the larynx, liver, spleen, lung, and heart. Abnormal ceramide accumulation also is described in the nervous system in the majority of patients. Electron microscopy studies reveal Farber bodies, or characteristic curvilinear structures, in biopsied tissue (70). Thirteen mutations in the acid ceramidase (AC) gene have been described to date, with no clear genotype–phenotype correlation (71).

- Farber disease is characterized by the triad of painful, swollen joints, subcutaneous nodules, and progressive hoarseness.

TABLE 43-12 Laboratory Findings: Farber Disease

Decreased	Increased
Ceramidase activity	Lysosomal ceramide content
	Urinary ceramide
	Presence of Farber bodies on electron microscopy

Clinical Presentation Clinical manifestations of Farber disease have been divided into seven phenotypic subtypes. Types 1–5 reflect a spectrum of disease severities ranging from neonatal onset and early death to onset in later infancy and survival into the second decade. Characteristic symptoms involve a triad of painful, swollen joints, subcutaneous nodules (lipogranulomata), and progressive hoarseness (72). Nervous system involvement is seen in the majority of patients, including psychomotor delay, diminished reflexes, hypotonia, and seizures. Patients with type 4 disease present with severe neonatal hepatosplenomegaly and die before the development of the characteristic features of classical Farber disease. Types 6 and 7 have each been described only in single case reports, with type 6 representing a combination of Farber and Sandhoff diseases in a single patient and type 7 involving a combined deficiency of multiple lysosomal enzymes (including ceramidase) resulting from a complete deficiency of prosaposin (73,74).

Diagnosis

- Reduced or absent lysosomal ceramidase activity is seen in white blood cells, cultured skin fibroblasts, and amniocytes (Table 43-12).
- Abnormal ceramide accumulation is seen in cultured cells.
- Abnormal ceramide excretion occurs in urine.
- The presence of Farber bodies is seen in biopsy samples.

Treatment Treatment is supportive, and no effective therapy currently exists. BMT has been performed in two patients, resulting in resolution of somatic symptoms but without apparent effect on neurological features (75).

SIALIC ACID DISORDERS

Galactosialidosis

Etiology/Pathophysiology Galactosialidosis is a rare autosomal recessive disorder involving a combined deficiency of the lysosomal enzymes β-galactosidase and neuraminidase (also known as *sialidase*). The primary defect lies in a genetically distinct protective protein shared by the two enzymes, protective protein/cathepsin A (PPCA). PPCA is a multi-

catalytic enzyme with a variety of functions, including carboxypeptidase, deamidase, and esterase activities. Proper association of PPCA with β-galactosidase and neuraminidase during early lysosomal biogenesis is required for correct sorting and proteolytic processing of enzyme precursors. PPCA also plays a protective role against premature degradation of β-galactosidase and neuraminidase and is required for expression of neuraminidase catalytic activity (76–79).

Defective PPCA leads to functional deficiency of β-galactosidase and neuraminidase, which, in turn, leads to abnormal storage of sialyloligosaccharides in lysosomes and their excretion in urine. Ultrastructural analysis reveals membrane-bound vacuoles and membranous cytoplasmic bodies in multiple tissues, including nervous system (central, peripheral, and autonomic), retina, liver, kidney, skin, and lymphocytes. Foam cells can be seen in bone marrow. Three clinical subtypes of galactosialidosis are recognized—early infantile, late juvenile, and juvenile/adult—with growing evidence for the correlation of disease severity with PPCA genotype.

Clinical Presentation Patients with galactosialidosis have clinical features typical of many of the lysosomal storage disorders, including coarse facial features, hepatosplenomegaly, corneal clouding, and cherry red spots. Dysostosis multiplex, a complex constellation of skeletal abnormalities, is seen often and includes vertebral beaking, proximal pointing of the metacarpals, and the so-called J-shaped sella apparent on lateral skull x-ray. Patients with the early-infantile form present from birth to 3 months of age with fetal hydrops, edema, proteinuria, and telangiectasias. Organomegaly (including heart, liver, and spleen), vertebral abnormalities, and psychomotor delay also have been described in the majority of patients. The course is rapidly progressive, with death typically occurring in the first year of life from heart and renal complications. Late-infantile patients also present in the first months of life with many features seen in the early-infantile form but without severe neurological abnormalities (e.g., myoclonus and ataxia) and survival into adulthood. Mild mental retardation and transient seizures have been observed in some patients.

TABLE 43-13   Laboratory Findings: Galactosialidosis

Decreased	Increased
β-Galactosidase activity	Urine sialyloligosaccharides
Neuraminidase activity	

More than half of all galactosialidosis patients are characterized by the juvenile/adult form, with the majority of these being of Japanese origin. This category encompasses a broad spectrum of phenotypes, with a mean age of onset of 16 years. Features include coarse facies, heart involvement, myoclonus, ataxia, progressive neurological deterioration, cherry red spots or corneal clouding leading to loss of visual acuity, vertebral changes, and angiokeratomas. Hepatosplenomegaly occurs much less frequently than in patients with the earlier-onset forms. Survival is well into adulthood.

Diagnosis

- The diagnosis of galactosialidosis is established by demonstrating significantly reduced activities of both β-galactosidase and neuraminidase (typically 5% to 15% of normal) in leukocytes or cultured skin fibroblasts (Table 43-13).

- Assays of cathepsin A activity and direct detection of PPCA mutations are possible but not routinely available on a clinical basis.

- Mutation analysis is available only on a research basis. Five common mutations in different ethnic groups have been identified.

- Other laboratory findings seen in galactosialidosis include:
  - Increased urinary excretion of sialyloligosaccharides but not free sialic acid
  - Decreased carboxypeptidase-L/protective protein activity.
  - Foam cells in lymphocytes and bone marrow.
  - Membrane-bound fibrillogranular inclusions in fibroblasts.
  - Peripheral lymphocytes seen by electron microscopy.

- Prenatal diagnosis is possible by measurement of combined β-galactosidase/neuraminidase activity in cultured amniocytes. Carrier testing is not offered routinely but is theoretically possible by direct studies of PPCA function or DNA sequence.

Treatment There is currently no effective treatment for galactosialidosis, and management is mainly supportive. Gene therapy studies using cathepsin A knockout mice suggest the possibility of this treatment approach in the future (76).

Infantile Sialic Acid Storage Disease/Salla Disease

Etiology/Pathophysiology Infantile sialic acid storage disease (ISSD) and Salla disease are autosomal recessive conditions characterized by accumulation of free sialic (N-acetylneuraminic) acid in lysosomes. Salla disease is more common in the Finnish population. ISSD and Salla disease are allelic disorders caused by mutations in the SLC17A5 gene, which codes for sialin, an integral lysosomal membrane protein that transports free sialic acid. Sialin has high expression in heart, kidney, skeletal muscle, liver, brain, and placenta.

Clinical Presentation ISSD patients have a severe phenotype characterized by mental retardation, seizures, coarse facial features, cardiomegaly, hepatosplenomegaly, dysostosis multiplex, and early death (<2 years). Hydrops fetalis also has been described in ISSD. Salla disease, on the other hand, is milder, with patients often presenting between 3 and 9 months with hypotonia, truncal and limb ataxia, mild dysmorphic features, and developmental delay. Head MRI may show abnormal myelination. Organomegaly and skeletal anomalies, with the exception of calvarial thickening, do not occur in Salla disease (80). Adults commonly have coarse facial features, spasticity, seizures, ataxia, athetosis, and mental retardation.

Diagnosis

- Increased urine excretion of free sialic acid is seen (10-fold in Salla disease, 100-fold in ISSD) (Table 43-14).

- Increased free sialic acid is seen in leukocytes and cultured fibroblasts.

- If elevated urine free sialic acid is found, skin fibroblast analysis for determination of subcellular sialic acid content should be performed to distinguish between lysosomal (ISSD and Salla disease) and cytoplasmic (sialuria) accumulation.

- Mutation analysis is available only on a research basis.

- Prenatal diagnosis is possible by measuring free sialic acid in amniocytes or chorionic villus samples or by DNA-based testing.

Treatment Only symptomatic therapy is available for ISSD and Salla disease.

Sialuria

Etiology/Pathophysiology Sialuria is often mentioned alongside other disorders of sialic acid storage but is not a lysosomal disorder *per se*; free sialic acid is stored in the cytoplasm in this condition. Sialuria is a very rare autosomal dominant disorder in which normal feedback inhibition of UDP-N-acetylglucosamine (UDP-GlcNAc) 2-epimerase by CMP-sialic acid is lost, leading to massively increased synthesis of cytoplasmic free sialic acid. CMP-sialic acid, the end product of the sialic acid synthetic pathway, normally inhibits the function of UDP-GlcNAc 2-epimerase, leading to decreased sialic acid synthesis. In sialuria, the allosteric binding site for CMP-sialic acid in UDP-GlcNAc 2-epimerase is defective, leading to increased activity of this enzyme and abnormal accumulation of sialic acid in the cytoplasm. Periodic acid–Schiff positive–staining granules are present throughout the cytoplasm (81).

Clinical Presentation Presentation is in infancy with coarse and mildly dysmorphic facial features and hepatosplenomegaly. Seizures may occur. Developmental delay may be present but typically is mild. Mild dysostosis multiplex may be noted, but growth is normal (81).

Diagnosis

- There is increased leukocyte and cultured fibroblast free sialic acid content.

- Mutation analysis of a specific region (between codons 263 and 266) that codes for the allosteric binding site for CMP-sialic acid in the UDP-GlcNAc 2-epimerase gene is available only as a research test.

- Massive free sialic acid excretion in urine is seen (Table 43-15).

- In sialuria, free sialic acid accumulates in the cytoplasm.

Treatment Although only symptomatic treatment is available for sialuria, reported patients in general have done relatively well.

TABLE 43-14   Laboratory Findings: ISSD/Salla Disease

Decreased	Increased
	Urine free sialic acid

TABLE 43-15   Laboratory Findings: Sialuria

Decreased	Increased
	Urine free sialic acid
	UDP-GlcNAc 2-epimerase activity (activity may by normal)

OLIGOSACCHARIDOSES (GLYCOPROTEINOSES)

Disorders of Glycoprotein Degradation (Oligosaccharidoses)

Etiology/Pathophysiology Oligosaccharides are a structurally heterogeneous group of macromolecules that make up the carbohydrate portion of glycoproteins and consist of 10–20 sugar residues with a characteristic branched structure. Typical structures for complex and high-mannose oligosaccharides are shown in Figure 43-13. These molecules play an integral role in determining the specificity of protein structure, function, and antigenicity and are found throughout the body. The oligosaccharidoses are a group of disorders arising from enzymatic defects in the stepwise degradation of N-linked oligosaccharides, or oligosaccharides linked to protein through an asparagine residue. This degradation normally occurs by the action of 1) a series of exoglycosidases acting in sequential fashion at the nonreducing termini and 2) aspartylglycosaminidase, which cleaves the bond between asparagine and the adjacent sugar, N-acetylglucosamine (see Figure 43-14).

The diseases arising from enzymatic deficiencies in the degradative pathway of oligosaccharides are 1) α-mannosidosis, 2) β-mannosidosis, 3) fucosidosis, 4) sialidosis, and 5) aspartylglucosaminuria (82). These deficiencies lead to the abnormal accumulation of oligosaccharide structures terminating in a mannose (in either an α- or β-linkage), fucose, sialic acid, or N-acetylglucosamine residue, respectively. Because oligosaccharides also are found linked to sphingolipids and glycosaminoglycans, their abnormal degradation can lead to accumulations of these macromolecules as well. Vacuolated lymphocytes and foam cells have been described in all disorders except the mild form of sialidosis.

All the oligosaccharidoses follow an autosomal recessive pattern of inheritance, and all are very rare (except in Finland). Although most of them are panethnic, aspartylglucosaminuria occurs predominately in the Finnish population, where a single founder mutation in the AGA gene, C163S, accounts for 98% of disease alleles.

Abnormal urinary oligosaccharide excretion is seen in patients with oligosaccharidoses, as well as in some patients with mucolipidosis, sphingolipidoses, and glycogen storage disease. The specific pattern of oligosaccharide excretion, together with clinical symptoms, can be used to guide further diagnostic evaluations of specific enzyme deficiencies.

Clinical Presentation The abnormal storage of incompletely degraded oligosaccharides leads to clinical pathology similar to the mucopolysaccharidoses, including progressive mental retardation, hepatosplenomegaly, dysostosis multiplex, and coarse facial features (Figure 43-15). These disorders overlap sig-

nificantly with the mucopolysaccharidoses (MPSs), and the two groups often are considered together in the evaluation of patients. Characteristic features of each of the oligosaccharide storage disorders are summarized below.

α-Mannosidosis

Deficiency of α-mannosidase activity leads to incomplete degradation of high-mannose and complex oligosaccharides and to abnormal storage and urinary excretion of the partially degraded products (83). Both missense and nonsense mutations have been described in MANB, the gene that encodes α-mannosidase (84). This disorder historically is divided into type I (severe) and type II (mild) forms, representing endpoints of a broad spectrum of clinical phenotypes (85). Patients with the severe form of α-mannosidosis present in early infancy with rapidly progressive psychomotor delay, hepatosplenomegaly, facial coarsening, dysostosis multiplex, and hearing loss, with death typically occurring in the first decade (Figure 43-15). In contrast, patients with type II, or the juvenile-adult form of the disorder, experience onset of mental retardation during later childhood, after a period of normal early development. Hearing loss is particularly prominent, with milder skeletal abnormalities than in type I patients and survival possible into adulthood.

β-Mannosidosis

β-Mannosidase deficiency is an extremely rare autosomal recessive condition first recognized in goats and later identified in humans (86). It is associated with the abnormal storage and urinary excretion of specific mannose-containing compounds, particularly a disaccharide containing mannose and N-acetylglucosamine (87). Only a small number of patients with β-mannosidosis have been reported, and this disorder is probably underdiagnosed because it lacks many of the features characteristic of the other oligosaccharidoses. The majority of patients described to date have presented in the first year of life with respiratory infections, mental retardation, hearing loss, and angiokeratoma but without facial coarsening, hepatosplenomegaly, dystosis multiplex, or vacuolated lymphocytes. Because the disease is so rare, the phenotypic spectrum has not yet been fully characterized.

Fucosidosis

Fucosidosis is characterized by the abnormal accumulation of an incompletely degraded product consisting of fucose linked

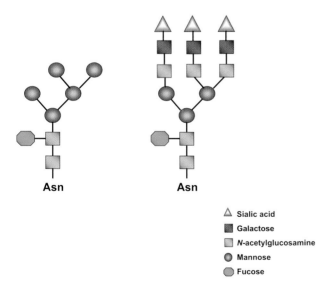

Sialic acid — △
Galactose — ■ (dark square)
N-acetylglucosamine — ■ (light square)
Mannose — ● (dark circle)
Fucose — ● (light circle)

FIGURE 43-13. Representative structure of oligosaccharides of the high-mannose (*left*) and complex (*right*) types.

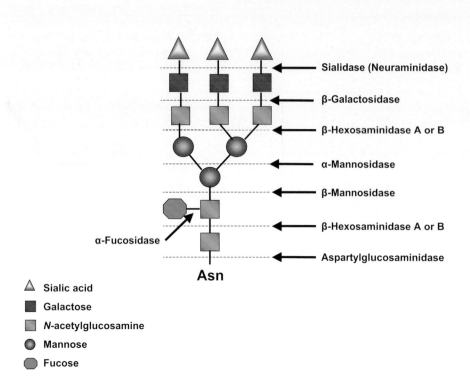

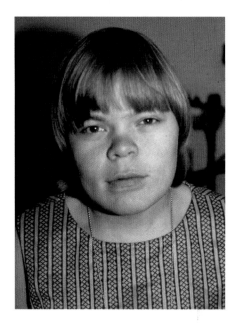

FIGURE 43-14. Stepwise degradation of asparagine-linked oligosaccharides.

FIGURE 43-15. Mannosidosis (oligosaccharidoses). Coarse facies with prominent supraorbital ridges, hypertelorism, broad-based nose, and prominent jaw.

to the N-acetylglucosamine residue attached to asparagine (88). As with α-mannosidosis, severe and mild subgroups of fucosidosis, designated types I and II, have been described. More than 22 different mutations in FUCA, the gene encoding fucosidase, have been described to date, with little or no genotype–phenotype correlation (89).

Patients with type I fucosidosis present in the first year of life with psychomotor retardation, coarse facial appearance, hepatosplenomegaly, and growth retardation. This form is also characterized by markedly increased sweat chloride concentration as well as variable seizures. Angiokeratomas, indistinguishable from those seen in Fabry disease, are also variably seen and increase in frequency in older patients. More mildly affected patients have onset of psychomotor retardation in the second or third year of life, with other features similar to, but milder than, those seen in type I. The natural history of fucosidosis has been reviewed for 77 patients, with 9% of patients dying before the age of 5 years and the majority surviving beyond the second decade (90). These authors suggest that fucosidosis is more appropriately characterized as a continuum of phenotypes rather than a dichotomous group of disorders.

Sialidosis (Mucolipidosis Type I)

Sialidosis is caused by deficient activity of sialidase (neuraminidase), leading to the abnormal storage of sialylated glycopeptides and oligosaccharides. The range of clinical phenotypes associated with sialidosis has been categorized as type I (adult onset), type II (childhood onset), and the congenital form. At least 34 unique mutations have

been described in NEUI, the gene encoding neuraminidase, and are associated with varying degrees of enzyme impairment (91).

Patients with sialidosis type I (also known as the *cherry red spot–myoclonus syndrome*) typically present after the second decade of life with gait abnormalities and visual disturbances, including color blindness and night blindness, but lack other somatic findings including hepatosplenomegaly and skeletal abnormalities. The visual abnormalities are associated with the presence of macular cherry red spots, similar to those seen in Tay-Sachs disease and other sphingolipid storage disorders. Myoclonus has been reported in the vast majority of patients and may be poorly controlled by medication. Patients with more severe forms of sialidosis have onset either apparent at birth (congenital form) or in infancy or early childhood (sialidosis type II). These forms are more often associated with hepatosplenomegaly, coarse facial features, dysostosis multiplex, and developmental delay but with variable ocular abnormalities and myoclonus. Congenital sialidosis is also associated with ascites or hydrops in the majority of patients.

Aspartylglucosaminuria

Aspartylglucosaminuria results from the inability to cleave the bond between asparagine and N-acetylglucosamine in the final step of oligosaccharide degradation due to a deficiency of aspartylglucosaminidase. Although panethnic, this disorder has an increased incidence in the Finnish population, where the majority of cases are due to a single, common mutation in the AGU gene.

Patients with aspartylglucosaminuria typically present in the first few years of life with frequent respiratory infections, hypotonia, and developmental (particularly speech) delay. Facial coarsening and hepatosplenomegaly are relatively mild, and the predominant symptoms are neurological. Patients may reach the developmental equivalent of 5–6 years, followed by rapid decline and severe mental retardation. Variable findings include seizures, osteoporosis, and mildly short stature. Survival is into adulthood, typically the fourth or fifth decade (92).

TABLE 43-16	Laboratory Findings: Oligosaccharidoses
Decreased	**Increased**
Activity of specific oligosaccharide-degrading enzyme	Urine oligosaccharides

Diagnosis

- The diagnosis of an oligosaccharidosis is suspected when results of urine screening tests show oligosaccchariduria, and is confirmed by specific enzyme assays (Table 43-16).

- Mutation analysis is available only on a research basis.

- Other laboratory findings include:
  - Vacuolated lymphocytes;
  - Abnormal oligosacchariduria;
  - Deficient activity of specific lysosomal enzyme.

- DNA testing is not widely available for any of the oligosaccharidoses except aspartylglucosaminuria, for which targeted analysis for the C163S mutation can be performed on patients of Finnish descent.

- Prenatal diagnosis is possible for all the oligosaccharidoses by enzyme analysis following either chorionic villus biopsy or amniocentesis, or by DNA testing in families where the disease-causing mutations are known.

- Presymptomatic diagnosis of α-mannosidosis had been demonstrated in newborn blood spots using a tandem mass spectrometry–based assay, and future studies are expected to expand the number of lysosomal disorders detectable by this technology. As with the mucopolysaccharidoses, early detection will be essential for optimal outcome as treatments become available.

Treatment Allogenic BMTs have been performed for several patients with α-mannosidosis, fucosidosis, and aspartylglucosaminuria (29,93). Correction of skeletal abnormalities and improvement of intelligence have been reported for α-mannosidosis, as well as some improvement in neurological function for fucosidosis. Results on BMTs for aspartylglucosaminuria have been encouraging but limited (93). No ERT trials are currently underway for treatment of the oligosaccharidoses.

- Urine screening for oligosaccharides is a useful first-line test.

- Diagnosis is established by specific enzyme assays in leukocytes or cultured fibroblasts.

- Carrier testing and prenatal diagnosis are possible.

NEURONAL CEROID LIPOFUSCINOSES

Etiology/Pathophysiology The neuronal ceroid lipofuscinoses (NCLs) constitute a group of at least eight inherited neurodegenerative disorders that are caused by various defects in enzymes or transmembrane proteins involved in lysosomal protein catabolism. As a group they are characterized by accumulation of heterogeneous autofluorescent material in brain and other tissues. They are relatively common conditions, with an overall incidence of 1 in 12,500 births. Defects in genes coding for palmitoyl:protein thioesterase 1 (PPT, CLN1), tripeptidylpeptidase 1 (TPP, CLN2), cathepsin D (CLN8), and transmembrane proteins of undetermined function (CLN3 and CLN5) have been identified (94). Mutations in CLN1 cause infantile neuronal ceroid lipofuscinosis (INCL), a panethnic disorder that occurs more frequently in the Finnish population. CLN2 mutations cause the classical late-infantile variant (LINCL), and CLN3 mutations cause juvenile-onset disease (JNCL, also known as *Batten disease*). The pattern of autofluorescent material storage, when viewed by electron microscopy, is characteristic for the various forms of NCL: granular osmiophilic deposits (GRODs) are found in INCL; curvilinear profiles, in classical LINCL; and fingerprint profiles, in JNCL. The storage material consists of protein (i.e., saposins and fragments of glial fibrillary acidic protein) and lipids in INCL. In LINCL and JNCL, the major protein component of the storage material is subunit c of the mitochondrial ATP synthase complex (complex V). Marked brain atrophy is present in the early-onset forms of disease. Although detailed mechanisms of pathogenesis are largely unknown, there is good evidence that the early neuronal cell death present in INCL and JNCL is caused, at least in part, by increased apoptosis secondary to abnormalities in signaling pathways necessary for cell survival. Activation of glial cell populations and glutamate excitotoxicity also may contribute to disease pathogenesis.

Clinical Presentation All forms of NCL are characterized by progressive neurological impairment, but age of onset and rate of deterioration differ depending on the type (95). Dysmorphic features and visceromegaly are absent. Children affected by INCL appear to develop normally until 6 to 12 months. Slowed head growth occurs at the mean age of 9 months. Cerebral atrophy is present on head imaging even before the onset of symptoms. Developmental arrest, mood changes, hypotonia, and ataxia are noted between 12 and 18 months of age. Vision problems often are noted by age 1 year, and blindness occurs by age 2 years. Microcephaly, macular degeneration, retinal pigment accumulation, myoclonic jerks, generalized convulsions, and unusual hand movements reminiscent of those seen in Rett syndrome are typical. The mean age of death is 6.5 years.

Myoclonic or generalized tonic–clonic seizures beginning between 2 and 4 years of age often are the first clear indication of disease in LINCL. Delayed speech is also common but usually does not cause much initial alarm. Developmental arrest, ataxia, retinitis pigmentosa, blindness, and dementia occur as disease progresses. Death occurs at between 10 to 15 years of age.

Visual impairment between 4 and 7 years of age usually is the first indication of disease in JNCL (Batten disease). Retinitis pigmentosa is present, and blindness occurs by 6 to 14 years of age. Impaired school performance progresses to mental retardation and dementia. Seizures often are present by age 10 years but are not invariable. Death typically occurs at between 10 and 30 years of age. Variant forms of NCL and an adult-onset form (Kufs disease) also exist.

Diagnosis

- Brain MRI shows early cerebral and cerebellar atrophy in INCL and classical LINCL, but may appear normal until about 10 years of age in JNCL. Features range from being similar to MPS-IH to primary CNS involvement (96).

- Electroretinography (ERG) and visual and somatosensory evoked potentials (SEPs) show abnormalities between about 1.5 and 2.5 years of age in INCL. Abnormalities occur later in other forms of NCL. For example, classical LINCL presents at between 2 and 4 years of age. ERG shows enlarged early components (giant waves) and an enlarged SEP is present in some patients. An extinguished ERG is present in almost all children with JNCL at the time of presentation (5–6 years of age), and SEPs may be decreased (95,97).

- Electron microscopic identification of the characteristic stored autofluorescent material patterns in circulating lymphocytes, skin, or conjunctival biopsies often leads to diagnosis.

TABLE 43-17 Laboratory Findings: Neuronal Ceroid Lipofuscinosis (Infantile and Late-Infantile)

Decreased	Increased
Palmitoyl:protein thioesterase 1 (INCL) or tripeptidylpeptidase 1 (LINCL) activities	Autofluorescent material storage on electron microscopy

- Decreased palmitoyl:protein thioesterase 1 (INCL) or tripeptidylpeptidase 1 (LINCL) activity is present in leukocytes and fibroblasts (Table 43-17).
- Mutation analysis is available on a clinical basis for INCL, classical and Finnish-variant LINCL, and JNCL. A single pathogenic mutation causes INCL in the Finnish population. Various mutations have been identified in other populations.
- Prenatal diagnosis is possible in INCL and classical LINCL by measuring PPT or TPP activity in amniocytes or chorionic villi. If the mutations are known, prenatal diagnosis via DNA analysis is also possible for any form of NCL.

Treatment Treatment for all forms of NCL is supportive. BMT has been attempted in INCL, LINCL, and JNCL but without proven efficacy. Gene therapy experiments have shown some success in animal models. A LINCL clinical trial has started using direct brain injection of an adeno-associated viral vector. Another trial using brain injection of neural stem cells for INCL and LINCL has also recently begun.

OTHER LYSOSOMAL STORAGE DISORDERS

Wolman Disease and Cholesteryl Ester Storage Disease

Etiology/Pathophysiology Wolman disease (WD) and cholesterol ester storage disease (CESD) are autosomal recessive conditions caused by mutations in different parts of the lysosomal acid lipase (LIPA) gene. Lysosomal acid lipase hydrolyzes cholesteryl esters and triglycerides that are delivered to lysosomes via the LDL receptor pathway, and therefore is of central importance in the control of plasma lipoprotein levels and the regulation of tissue lipid levels (98). In WD, massive storage of cholesteryl esters and triglycerides occurs in the liver, adrenal gland, and intestine. Milder lipid accumulation throughout the body occurs in CESD. Because acid lipase activity is higher in CESD compared with WD, it is possible that the difference in disease phenotypes is secondary to differential regulation of the LDL receptor. In CESD, enzyme activity is high enough to release at least some free cholesterol from lysosomes, which leads to down regulation of the LDL receptor gene. Subsequently, lysosomes are not overloaded with LDL-derived cholesteryl esters and triglycerides. In contrast, the LDL receptor is up regulated in Wolman disease, leading to excessive delivery of lipids to lysosomes and massive storage.

Clinical Presentation WD presents in the first two weeks of life with worsening vomiting and diarrhea, abdominal distension, hepatosplenomegaly, and cachexia. WD may present as nonimmune hydrops fetalis (44). Neurological development is not normal (weakness and abnormal reflexes occur), but the extent of the abnormalities is difficult to assess because of the early demise of these patients (99). Anemia also occurs by 1.5 months and may be severe. Marked calcification of the adrenal glands is a striking feature. Death typically occurs between 3 and 6 months of age.

CESD has variable features, with presentation ranging from the neonatal period to adulthood. Hepatomegaly, with or without splenomegaly, is a common feature. Other reported findings include recurrent abdominal pain, malabsorption, epistaxis, gastrointestinal bleeding, and clotting abnormalities. Severe premature atherosclerosis may be present. Neurological abnormalities are encountered rarely.

Diagnosis
- Calcification of the adrenal glands is present on abdominal x-rays in WD.
- Vacuolization of lymphocytes in blood and bone marrow may be present in WD.
- Lipid-laden foam cells are present in tissues.
- Decreased lysosomal acid lipase activity is present in leukocytes and fibroblasts (100) (Table 43-18).
- Mutation analysis is available on a research basis.

- Prenatal diagnosis is possible in WD by measuring acid lipase activity in amniocytes or chorionic villi. If the mutations are known, prenatal diagnosis via DNA analysis is also possible.

Treatment There is no effective therapy for either WD or CESD. HMG–CoA reductase inhibitors and bile acid–binding resins have been used to treat the hypercholesterolemia in CESD. Lovastatin (20 mg twice daily) was shown to reduce plasma cholesterol, triglycerides, and LDL cholesterol significantly in a patient with CESD (101). Liver transplantation for chronic liver failure has been performed in CESD. A patient with WD underwent BMT and was reported to be gaining developmental milestones at age 4 years (102). Other experimental therapies, including ERT and gene therapy, are being explored in animal models (103).

Pompe Disease (Glycogen Storage Disease Type II)

Etiology/Pathophysiology Pompe disease, also known as *glycogen storage disease type II* or *acid maltase deficiency*, is an autosomal recessive disorder of glycogen metabolism caused by defects in the lysosomal enzyme α-glucosidase (GAA). This enzyme cleaves α-1,4- and α-1,6-glucosidic linkages during the normal degradation of glycogen and, unlike other glycogen-metabolizing enzymes, functions optimally at an acidic pH. Pompe disease is therefore the only lysosomal storage disease that is also classified as a glycogen storage disorder. Unlike other glycogen storage diseases, since GAA is a lysosomal enzyme, hypoglycemia is not a feature in Pompe disease. Since Pompe disease is also a neuromuscular disorder, the categorization and nomenclature for this condition in textbooks and elsewhere can be confusing. For the purposes of this text, Pompe disease is classified as a lysosomal storage disorder. We feel that this is the most logical classification, especially with the possibility of ERT. For information on other glycogen storage disorders, please refer to Chapter 6. The combined incidence of Pompe disease for all ethnic groups has been estimated at 1 in 40,000 population, although it may occur more frequently among

TABLE 43-18 Laboratory Findings: Wolman Disease and Cholesteryl Ester Storage Disease

Decreased	Increased
Acid lipase activity ↓ 200-fold in WE ↓ 50- to 100-fold in CESD	Plasma cholesterol ± triglycerides (CESD)
	Plasma LDL (CESD)
	Apolipoprotein B (CESD)
	Tissue storage of cholesteryl esters and triglycerides

African Americans and in regions of Taiwan and the Netherlands.

Deficiency of GAA leads to abnormal storage of structurally normal glycogen in all tissues, with skeletal, cardiac, and smooth muscle affected predominately. A spectrum of clinical phenotypes exists, ranging from early onset (<1 year) to later onset extending into adulthood. Clinical severity is associated with the extent of glycogen storage, with the most severe forms showing massive accumulations of glycogen in heart, skeletal muscle, and liver, as well as more generalized involvement of other tissues, including the kidney and brain. The milder forms show more modest accumulations of glycogen that may be confined to skeletal muscle. Microscopic evaluation of muscle biopsies shows the presence of periodic acid–Schiff (PAS)–positive (i.e., glycogen-containing) vacuoles. These vacuoles also stain positively for the lysosomal enzyme acid phosphatase and in severe cases may contain acid mucins or glycolipids. In milder cases, usually those with later onset, there may be heterogeneous involvement of muscle tissue such that muscle biopsy may yield normal results. Multiple mutations in the GAA gene have been shown to underlie Pompe disease, with some evidence for limited genotype–phenotype correlations.

Clinical Presentation In the most severe cases, patients present in the first few months of life with marked hypotonia and progressive muscle weakness, cardiomegaly, macroglossia, and hepatomegaly. Feeding and respiratory abnormalities are common. Progressive accumulation of glycogen in cardiac muscle leads to increasing cardiac hypertrophy, with thickening especially of the left ventricular wall. A characteristic ECG finding of shortened PR interval and large QRS complexes is seen. Mental retardation usually is not a feature (104). Respiratory insufficiency occurs due to muscle weakness. Death is usually before 1 year of age, most often from cardiorespiratory complications (105,106). Atypical patients presenting in the first year of life with severe muscle involvement with or without cardiomyopathy and with longer survival also have been reported.

Later-onset forms of Pompe disease can present from early childhood through adulthood with varying degrees of muscle involvement, rates of progression, and extents of other organ involvement. Most patients presenting after the age of 2 years do not have obvious cardiomegaly or cardiomyopathy, and intelligence is normal. Features include delayed motor development, progressive proximal muscle weakness, and lordosis, kyphosis, and/or scoliosis. Adult-onset patients typically present with proximal muscle weak-

ness, with the lower limbs more affected than the upper, or may present only with respiratory involvement. Development of cardiomyopathy, even late in the disease process, is distinctly unusual. Sleep-disordered breathing is very common. Patients with these later-onset forms may be misdiagnosed with muscular dystrophy, polymyositis, or scapuloperoneal syndrome, especially limb-girdle muscular dystrophy. Death is usually from respiratory complications.

Diagnosis

- Pompe disease is diagnosed by the demonstration of absent or significantly reduced (typically <10% of normal) GAA activity in cultured fibroblasts or muscle (Table 43-19).

- Although standard GAA assays typically are not reliable in blood due to interference from other GAA isozymes, recent studies demonstrate the efficacy of using dried blood spots in an assay with a specific inhibitor of other α-glucosidases to diagnose patients with Pompe disease (107).

- GAA activity also can be measured accurately in blood lymphocytes if similar precautions are taken.

- Other findings associated with Pompe disease include:

  - Elevated serum creatine kinase (up to 10-fold normal in early-onset patients; can be normal in milder variants).
  - Elevated serum transaminases.
  - Abnormal excretion of a particular glucose-containing tetrasaccharide [α-D-Glc-(1→6)-, α-D-Glc-(1→4)-, α-D-Glc-(1→4)-D-Glc] detectable by oligosaccharide thin-layer chromatography screening.
  - Abnormal electromyographic studies, with normal nerve conduction velocity.
  - PAS-positive and acid phosphatase–positive vacuoles on muscle biopsy characteristic EKG pattern of prominent.
  - P waves, massive QRS wave and a shortened PR interval.

- DNA analysis is available for Pompe disease.

- Prenatal diagnosis is possible through measurements of GAA activity in amniocytes and chorionic villus biopsies and by DNA

TABLE 43-19   Laboratory Findings: Pompe Disease

Decreased	Increased
α-Glucosidase activity	Serum creatine kinasae (not universal)
	Serum transaminases
	Urine oligosaccharides

analysis in families where the GAA mutation(s) are known.

- Although newborns are not currently screened presymptomatically for Pompe disease, recent studies demonstrate the feasibility of including Pompe disease in newborn screening programs in the future (108).

Treatment ERT for Pompe disease using recombinant human GAA is available. Studies demonstrate significant improvement of cardiac and skeletal muscle function and prolonged survival in some, but clearly not all, classically presenting infants (105,111,112). Other management strategies are supportive and involve management of the respiratory, cardiac, and physical complications, although some studies suggest that dietary changes, including high-protein diet and L-alanine supplementation, may be useful in late-onset patients (109,110).

Pycnodysostosis

Etiology/Pathophysiology Pycnodysostosis is a rare autosomal recessive skeletal dysplasia resulting from deficient activity of cathepsin K. This lysosomal protease is normally present in high levels in osteoclasts and functions in the degradation of type I collagen and other bone matrix proteins (113). Cathepsin K deficiency results in a profound deterioration of bone quality, leading to skeletal osteosclerosis, short stature, and bone fragility (114). Demineralization of bone occurs normally, but with an impaired degradation of bone matrix proteins (115). Histological abnormalities include excessive thickening of cortical and trabecular bones on light microscopy, as well as abnormal lysosomal storage of partially degraded collagen fibrils within osteoclasts by electron microscopy. The gene encoding cathepsin K has been localized to chromosome 1q21, and several mutations underlying pycnodysostosis have been identified (114,116).

Clinical Presentation Clinical findings associated with pycnodysostosis include short stature, short limbs with bowing of the legs, characteristic facial appearance, and short, broad hands and feet. Other complications may include upper airway obstruction, growth hormone deficiency, hematological abnor-

TABLE 43-20 Laboratory Findings: Pycnodysostosis

Decreased	Increased
Degradation of bone matrix proteins	Bone density
Lysosomal cathepsin K activity	Lysosomal storage of partially degraded collagen fibrils within osteoclasts

TABLE 43-21 Laboratory Findings: Danon Disease

Decreased	Increased
LAMP-2 staining on immunohistochemistry	Creatine kinase
	Transaminases

malities (e.g., microcytic anemia and thrombocytopenia), and mandibular osteomyelitis. Increased bone density on x-ray examination is a characteristic finding. Craniofacial findings include large head, delayed closure of anterior and posterior fontanels, obtuse angle of the mandible, exophthalmos, and prominent, beaked nose. There is an increased tendency for fractures of the long bones, lumbar spondylolysis, and stress fractures at other sites, including clavicles, scapulae, and metatarsals. Numerous dental abnormalities have been described in patients with pycnodysostosis, including hypodontia, retention of deciduous teeth, and delayed eruption of permanent teeth. Lifespan typically is normal, although early death may result from orthopedic complications.

Diagnosis The diagnosis of pycnodysostosis is established from distinct clinical and radiological findings and must be distinguished from other skeletal dysplasias, including osteopetrosis, osteogenesis imperfecta, and others. Although enzyme assays for cathepsin K activity are not widely available, the diagnosis can be confirmed by either gene sequencing or targeted mutation analysis of the cathepsin K gene, CTSK (Table 43-20).

• The diagnosis of pycnodysostosis is made on clinical grounds, with molecular confirmation possible by identification of CTSK mutations.

Treatment No therapy currently exists to increase cathepsin K activity in pycnodysostosis patients. Management strategies include orthopedic and/or surgical interventions aimed at treating or minimizing orthopedic complications and prophylactic dental care. Growth hormone replacement therapy has resulted in increased linear growth in a small number of pycnodysostosis patients with growth hormone deficiency (117,118), although long-term follow-up has not been reported.

Danon Disease

Etiology/Pathophysiology Danon disease is a panethnic X-linked dominant disorder caused by a primary deficiency in lysosome-associated membrane protein 2 (LAMP-2). LAMP-2 is located in the inner side of the lysosomal membrane. The precise function of LAMP-2 is still under investigation, although it appears to play a role in protein importation into lysosomes and may protect the lysosomal membrane from proteolytic enzymes. Small autophagic basophilic vacuoles are present on muscle histology. Cardiomyocytes show severe vacuolation and degeneration (119).

Clinical Presentation Affected individuals are characterized by a clinical triad of cardiomyopathy, myopathy, and variable mental retardation. Cardiac symptoms, especially hypertrophic or dilated cardiomyopathy, dominate the presentation. Wolff–Parkinson–White syndrome is present in about a third of patients (119). Hepatomegaly may be present, especially in males. Transaminases and creatine kinase levels may be elevated. The clinical features are similar to those encountered in Pompe disease.

Diagnosis

• Basophilic vacuoles are seen in muscle fibers.

• Severe vacuolation and degeneration are seen in cardiomyocytes.

• LAMP-2 is absent on immunohistochemistry (Table 43-21).

• Acid α-1,4-glucosidase activity is normal in most male patients but may be increased.

• Mutation analysis is available only on a research basis.

• Most mothers of affected children have cardiac symptoms, although about 30% are asymptomatic.

Treatment Definitive therapy is not available, so care and management are supportive. Cardiac pacemaker insertion and cardiac transplantation have been performed (119).

Mucolipidosis IV

Etiology/Pathophysiology Mucolipidosis IV (ML-IV) is a rare autosomal recessive lysosomal storage disorder caused by mutations in the MCOLN1 gene. The condition is described as a mucolipidosis because there is storage of both lipids and water-soluble substances. There is no mucopolysacchariduria, although gangliosides and mucopolysaccharides accumulate in fibroblasts, and inclusions can be seen in many tissues, including conjunctivae. The defective protein, mucolipin 1, is a 580-amino-acid protein member of the transient receptor potential (TRP) family related to Ca^{2+} channels. Mucolipin-1 functions as a nonselective cation channel in expression systems (120–123). Lysosomal storage in ML-IV is attributed to a transport defect in the late steps of endocytosis.

Clinical Presentation ML-IV typically presents in infancy, with severe psychomotor retardation that becomes evident by 2–3 years of age. There is no facial dysmorphism or organomegaly, and skeletal changes are absent. ML-IV should be considered in infants and children with early onset of developmental delay whether static (ML-IV can be misdiagnosed as cerebral palsy) or with regression of previously acquired cognitive and motor skills (124). Affected individuals develop corneal clouding, retinal degeneration, and strabismus, with resulting visual impairment that is slowly progressive during the first decade. Severe visual impairment is present by adolescence. Episodic pain consistent with corneal erosions is common, but this symptom appears to decrease in frequency and severity with age (125). Brain MRI typically shows hypoplasia of the corpus callosum with absent rostrum and dysplastic or absent splenium, white matter signal abnormalities on T1-weighted images, and ferritin deposition in the thalamus and basal ganglia. Cerebellar atrophy is observed in older individuals (126). There is wide variability in severity of ML-IV. Patients can live well into the third decade, but the developmental ceiling reached is often 12–15 months. Rarely, atypical ML-IV manifests with less severe psychomotor retardation and/or ophthalmological involvement.

Diagnosis This condition is one of the Jewish genetic diseases, and approximately 75% of the patients described have been Ashkenazi Jewish. Mutations in MCOLN1 cause ML-IV, and two mutations account for 95% of disease alleles in Ashkenazi Jews

TABLE 43-22   Laboratory Findings: Mucolipidosis Type IV

Decreased	Increased
Iron	Gangliosides and mucopolysaccharides in fibroblasts
	Plasma gastrin concentration

(127,128). Mutation analysis for the two common mutations is available in clinical laboratories. Mutation analysis is the only definitive test for ML-IV. Sequencing of MCOLN1 with methods currently in use can detect mutations in most Ashkenazi Jews who do not have the common mutations, as well as most individuals of non–Ashkenazi Jewish heritage. Such testing is currently available on a research basis only.

- Elevated plasma gastrin concentration is seen in virtually all individuals with ML-IV (124,129) (Table 43-22).

- Biopsy of skin or conjunctiva shows accumulation of abnormal lamellar membrane structures and amorphous cytoplasmic inclusions in diverse cell types by ultrastructural analysis (130,131).

- Typical vacuoles can be demonstrated by PAS staining of conjunctival cells obtained with a swab (132).

- Iron deficiency is common, and iron deficiency anemia can be seen.

- Prenatal diagnosis is possible by mutation analysis in amniocytes or chorionic villi if the mutations in the family are known.

Treatment In general, treatment is supportive for ML-IV.

REFERENCES

1. Wilcox WR. Lysosomal storage disorders: The need for better pediatric recognition and comprehensive care. *J Pediatr.* 2004;144:S3–14.
2. Malatack JJ, Consolini DM, Bayever E, et al. The status of hematopoietic stem cell transplantation in lysosomal storage disease. *Pediatr Neurol.* 2003;29:391–403.
3. Desnick RJ. Enzyme replacement and beyond. *J Inherit Metab Dis.* 2001;24:251–265.
4. Platt FM, et al. Inhibition of substrate synthesis as a strategy for glycolipid lysosomal storage disease therapy. *J Inherit Metab Dis.* 2001;24:275–290.
5. Wraith JE. Lysosomal disorders. *Semin Neonatol.* 2002;7:75–83.
6. Futerman AH, van Meer G. The cell biology of lysosomal storage disorders. *Natl Rev Mol Cell Biol.* 2004;5:554–565.
7. Zinberg RE, Kornreich R, Edelmann L, et al. Prenatal genetic screening in the Ashkenazi Jewish population. *Clin Perinatol.* 2001;28:367–682.
8. Millington DS. Newborn screening for lysosomal storage disorders. *Clin Chem.* 2005;51:808–809.
9. Muenzer J. The mucopolysaccharidoses: A heterogeneous group of disorders with variable pediatric presentations. *J Pediatr.* 2004;144:S27–34.
10. Yogalingam G, Guo XH, Muller VJ, et al. Identification and molecular characterization of α-L-iduronidase mutations present in mucopolysaccharidosis type I patients undergoing enzyme replacement therapy. *Hum Mutat.* 2004;24:199–207.
11. Parkinson EJ, Muller V, Hopwood JJ, et al. Iduronate-2-sulphatase protein detection in plasma from mucopolysaccharidosis type II patients. *Mol Genet Metab.* 2004;81:58–64.
12. Tuschl K, Gal A, Paschke E, et al. Mucopolysaccharidosis type II in females: Case report and review of literature. *Pediatr Neurol.* 2005.32:270–272.
13. Lonergan CL, Payne AR, Wilson WG, et al. What syndrome is this? Hunter syndrome. *Pediatr Dermatol,* 2004;21:679–681.
14. Nelson J, Crowhurst J, Carey B, et al. Incidence of the mucopolysaccharidoses in western Australia. *Am J Med Genet A.* 2003;123:310–313.
15. van de Kamp JJ, Niermeijer MF, von Figura K, et al. Genetic heterogeneity and clinical variability in the Sanfilippo syndrome (types A, B, and C). *Clin Genet.* 1981;20:152–160.
16. Okumiya T, Sakuraba H, Kase R, et al. Imbalanced substrate specificity of mutant beta-galactosidase in patients with Morquio B disease. *Mol Genet Metab.* 2003;78:51–58.
17. Northover H, Cowie RA, Wraith JE. Mucopolysaccharidosis type IVA (Morquio syndrome): A clinical review. *J Inherit Metab Dis.* 1996;19:357–365.
18. Litjens T, Hopwood JJ. Mucopolysaccharidosis type VI: Structural and clinical implications of mutations in N-acetylgalactosamine-4-sulfatase. *Hum Mutat.* 2001;18:282–295.
19. Karageorgos L, Harmatz P, Simon J, et al. Mutational analysis of mucopolysaccharidosis type VI patients undergoing a trial of enzyme replacement therapy. *Hum Mutat.* 2004;23:229–233.
20. Brooks DA, Gibson GJ, Karageorgos L, et al. An index case for the attenuated end of the mucopolysaccharidosis type VI clinical spectrum. *Mol Genet Metab.* 2005;85:236–238.
21. Meikle PJ, Hopwood JJ, Clague AE, et al. Prevalence of lysosomal storage disorders. *JAMA.* 1999;281:249–254.
22. Tomatsu S, Orii KO, Vogler C, et al. Missense models [Gus$^{tm(E536A)Sly}$, Gus$^{tm(E536Q)Sly}$, and Gus$^{tm(L175F)Sly}$] of murine mucopolysaccharidosis type VII produced by targeted mutagenesis. *Proc Natl Acad Sci USA.* 2002;99:14982–14987.
23. Sly WS, Quinton BA, McAlister WH, et al. Beta-glucuronidase deficiency: Report of clinical, radiologic, and biochemical features of a new mucopolysaccharidosis. *J Pediatr.* 1973;82:249–257.
24. Cheng Y, Verp MS, Knutel T, et al. Mucopolysaccharidosis type VII as a cause of recurrent non-immune hydrops fetalis. *J Perinat Med.* 2003;31:535–537.
25. Storch S, Wittenstein B, Islam R, et al. Mutational analysis in longest known survivor of mucopolysaccharidosis type VII. *Hum Genet.* 2003;112:190–194.
26. Triggs-Raine B, Salo TJ, Zhang H, et al. Mutations in HYAL1, a member of a tandemly distributed multigene family encoding disparate hyaluronidase activities, cause a newly described lysosomal disorder, mucopolysaccharidosis IX. *Proc Natl Acad Sci USA.* 1999;96:6296–6300.
27. Natowicz MR, Short MP, Wang Y, et al. Clinical and biochemical manifestations of hyaluronidase deficiency. *N Engl J Med.* 1996;335:1029–1033.
28. Meikle PJ, Ranieri E, Simonsen H, et al. Newborn screening for lysosomal storage disorders: Clinical evaluation of a two-tier strategy. *Pediatrics.* 2004;114:909–916.
29. Krivit W, Peters C, Shapiro EG. Bone marrow transplantation as effective treatment of central nervous system disease in globoid cell leukodystrophy, metachromatic leukodystrophy, adrenoleukodystrophy, mannosidosis, fucosidosis, aspartylglucosaminuria, Hurler, Maroteaux–Lamy, and Sly syndromes, and Gaucher disease type III. *Curr Opin Neurol.* 1999;12:167–176.
30. Kakkis ED. Enzyme replacement therapy for the mucopolysaccharide storage disorders. *Exp Opin Invest Drugs.* 2002;11:675–685.
31. Wraith JE, Clarke LA, Beck M, et al. Enzyme replacement therapy for mucopolysaccharidosis I: A randomized, double-blinded, placebo-controlled, multinational study of recombinant human α-L-iduronidase (laronidase). *J Pediatr.* 2004;144:581–588.
32. Harmatz P, Whitley CB, Waber L, et al. Enzyme replacement therapy in mucopolysaccharidosis VI (Maroteaux–Lamy syndrome). *J Pediatr.* 2004;144:574–580.
33. O'Connor LH, Erway LC, Vogler CA, et al. Enzyme replacement therapy for murine mucopolysaccharidosis type VII leads to improvements in behavior and auditory function. *J Clin Invest.* 1998;101:1394–1400.
34. Neufeld EF. Lysosomal storage diseases. *Annu Rev Biochem.* 1991;60:257–280.
35. Martin JJ, Leroy JG, van Eygen M, et al. I-cell disease: A further report on its pathology. *Acta Neuropathol (Berl).* 1984;64:234–242.
36. Peters ME, Arya S, Langer LO, et al. Narrow trachea in mucopolysaccharidoses. *Pediatr Radiol.* 1985;15:225–228.
37. Grewal S, Shapiro E, Braunlin E, et al. Continued neurocognitive development and prevention of cardiopulmonary complications after successful BMT for I-cell disease: A long-term follow-up report. *Bone Marrow Transplant.* 2003;32:957–960.
38. Krivit W. Allogeneic stem cell transplantation for the treatment of lysosomal and peroxisomal metabolic diseases. *Springer Semin Immunopathol.* 2004;26:119–132.
39. Robinson C, Baker N, Noble J, et al. The osteodystrophy of mucolipidosis type III

and the effects of intravenous pamidronate treatment. *J Inherit Metab Dis.* 2002;25:681–693.

40. Mahuran DJ. Biochemical consequences of mutations causing the G$_{M2}$-gangliosidoses. *Biochim Biophys Acta.* 1999;1455:105–138.

41. Jeyakumar M, Thomas R, Elliot-Smith E, et al. Central nervous system inflammation is a hallmark of pathogenesis in mouse models of G$_{M1}$ and G$_{M2}$ gangliosidosis. *Brain.* 2003;126:974–987.

42. von Specht BU, Geiger B, Arnon R, et al. Enzyme replacement in Tay–Sachs disease. *Neurology.* 1979;29:848–854.

43. Platt FM, Neises GR, Reinkensmeier G, et al. Prevention of lysosomal storage in Tay–Sachs mice treated with N-butyldeoxynojirimycin. *Science.* 1997; 276:428–431.

44. Steiner RD. Hydrops fetalis: Role of the geneticist. *Semin Perinatol.* 1995;19:516–524.

45. Elleder M, Jirasek A. Niemann–Pick disease: Report on a symposium held in Hlava's Institute of Pathology, Charles University, Prague 2nd–3rd September, 1982. *Acta Univ Carol (Med) (Praha).*1983;29:259–267.

46. McGovern MM, Pohl-Worgall T, Deckelbaum RJ, et al. Lipid abnormalities in children with types A and B Niemann–Pick disease. *J Pediatr.* 2004;145:77–81.

47. Vellodi A, Hobbs JR, O'Donnell NM, et al. Treatment of Niemann–Pick disease type B by allogeneic bone marrow transplantation. *Br Med J (Clin Res Ed).* 1987;295:1375–1376.

48. Davies JP, Ioannou YA. Topological analysis of Niemann–Pick C1 protein reveals that the membrane orientation of the putative sterol-sensing domain is identical to those of 3-hydroxy-3-methylglutaryl-CoA reductase and sterol regulatory element binding protein cleavage-activating protein. *J Biol Chem.* 2000;275:24367–24374.

49. Millat G, Chikh K, Naureckiene S, et al. Niemann–Pick disease type C: Spectrum of HE1 mutations and genotype/phenotype correlations in the NPC2 group. *Am J Hum Genet.* 2001;69:1013–1021.

50. Fink JK, Filling-Katz MR, Sokol J, et al. Clinical spectrum of Niemann–Pick disease type C. *Neurology.* 1989;39:1040–1049.

51. Lachmann RH, te Vruchte D, Lloyd-Evans E, et al. Treatment with miglustat reverses the lipid-trafficking defect in Niemann–Pick disease type C. *Neurobiol Dis.* 2004; 16:654–658.

52. Mankin HJ, Rosenthal DI, Xavier R. Gaucher disease: New approaches to an ancient disease. *J Bone Joint Surg.* 2001;83A:748–762.

53. Barton NW, Brady RO, Dambrosia JM, et al. Replacement therapy for inherited enzyme deficiency: Macrophage-targeted glucocerebrosidase for Gaucher's disease. *N Engl J Med.* 1991;324:1464–1470.

54. Masson C, Cisse I, Simon V, et al. Fabry disease: A review. *Joint Bone Spine.* 2004;71:381–383.

55. Ries M, et al. Pediatric Fabry disease. *Pediatrics.* 2005.

56. Bennett RL, Hart KA, O'Rourke E, et al. Fabry disease in genetic counseling practice: recommendations of the National Society of Genetic Counselors. *J Genet Couns.* 2002;11:121–146.

57. Mignani R, Cagnoli L. Enzyme replacement therapy in Fabry's disease: Recent advances and clinical applications. *J Nephrol.* 2004;17:354–363.

58. Schiffmann R, Kopp JB, Austin HA, et al. Enzyme replacement therapy in Fabry disease: A randomized, controlled trial. *JAMA.* 2001;285:2743–2749.

59. Guffon N, Fouilhoux A. Clinical benefit in Fabry patients given enzyme replacement therapy: a case series. *J Inherit Metab Dis.* 2004;27:221–227.

60. Wilcox WR, Banikazemi M, Guffon N, et al. Long-term safety and efficacy of enzyme replacement therapy for Fabry disease. *Am J Hum Genet.* 2004;75:65–74.

61. Gieselmann V. Metachromatic leukodystrophy: Recent research developments. *J Child Neurol.* 2003;18:591–594.

62. Parenti G, Meroni G, Ballabio A. The sulfatase gene family. *Curr Opin Genet Dev.* 1997;7:386–391.

63. Dierks T, Dickmanns A, Preusser-Kunze A, et al. Multiple sulfatase deficiency is caused by mutations in the gene encoding the human C(α)-formylglycine generating enzyme. *Cell.* 2003;113:435–444.

64. Burk RD, Valle D, Thomas GH, et al. Early manifestations of multiple sulfatase deficiency. *J Pediatr.* 1984;104:574–578.

65. Burch M, Fensom AH, Jackson M, et al. Multiple sulphatase deficiency presenting at birth. *Clin Genet.* 1986;30:409–415.

66. Steckel F, Hasilik A, von Figura K. Synthesis and stability of arylsulfatase A and B in fibroblasts from multiple sulfatase deficiency. *Eur J Biochem.* 1985;151:141–145.

67. Suzuki K. Globoid cell leukodystrophy (Krabbe's disease): Update. *J Child Neurol.* 2003;18:595–603.

68. Nishimoto J, Nanba E, Inui K, et al. G$_{M1}$-gangliosidosis (genetic β-galactosidase deficiency): Identification of four mutations in different clinical phenotypes among Japanese patients. *Am J Hum Genet.* 1991;49:566–574.

69. Kasperzyk JL, El-Abbadi MM, Hauser EC, et al. N-Butyldeoxygalactonojirimycin reduces neonatal brain ganglioside content in a mouse model of G$_{M1}$ gangliosidosis. *J Neurochem.* 2004;89:645–653.

70. Schmoeckel C, Hohlfed M. A specific ultra-structural marker for disseminated lipogranulomatosis (Faber). *Arch Dermatol Res.* 1979;266:187–196.

71. Muramatsu T, Sakai N, Yanagihara I, et al. Mutation analysis of the acid ceramidase gene in Japanese patients with Farber disease. *J Inherit Metab Dis.* 2002;25:585–592.

72. Salo MK, Karikoski R, Hällström M, et al. Farber disease diagnosed after liver transplantation. *J Pediatr Gastroenterol Nutr.* 2003;36:274–277.

73. Fusch C, et al. A case of combined Farber and Sandhoff disease. *Eur J Pediatr.* 1989;148:558–562.

74. Paton BC, Schmid B, Kustermann-Kuhn B, et al. Additional biochemical findings in a patient and fetal sibling with a genetic defect in the sphingolipid activator protein (SAP) precursor, prosaposin: Evidence for a deficiency in SAP-1 and for a normal lysosomal neuraminidase. *Biochem J.* 1992;285:481–488.

75. Yeager AM, Uhas KA, Coles CD, et al. Bone marrow transplantation for infantile ceramidase deficiency (Farber disease). *Bone Marrow Transplant.* 2000;26:357–363.

76. Hiraiwa M. Cathepsin A/protective protein: An unusual lysosomal multifunctional protein. *Cell Mol Life Sci.* 1999;56:894–907.

77. Ostrowska H, Krukowska K, Kalinowska J, et al. Lysosomal high molecular weight multienzyme complex. *Cell Mol Biol Lett.* 2003;8:19–24.

78. Strehle EM. Sialic acid storage disease and related disorders. *Genet Test.* 2003;7:113–121.

79. Pshezhetsky AV, Ashmarina M. Lysosomal multienzyme complex: Biochemistry, genetics, and molecular pathophysiology. *Prog Nucl Acid Res Mol Biol.* 2001;69:81–114.

80. Suwannarat P. Disorders of free sialic acid. *Mol Genet Metab.* 2005;85:85–87.

81. Enns GM, Seppala R, Musci TJ, et al. Clinical course and biochemistry of sialuria. *J Inherit Metab Dis.* 2001;24:328–336.

82. Cantz M, Ulrich-Bott B. Disorders of glycoprotein degradation. *J Inherit Metab Dis.* 1990;13:523–537.

83. Bennet JK, Dembure PP, Elsas LJ. Clinical and biochemical analysis of two families with type I and type II mannosidosis. *Am J Med Genet.* 1995;55:21–26.

84. Gotoda Y, Wakamatsu N, Kawai H, et al. Missense and nonsense mutations in the lysosomal α-mannosidase gene (MANB) in severe and mild forms of α-mannosidosis. *Am J Hum Genet.* 1998;63:1015–1024.

85. Michalski JC, Klein A. Clycoprotein lysosomal storage disorders: α- and β-Mannosidosis, fucosidosis and α-N-acetylgalactosaminidase deficiency. *Biochim Biophys Acta.* 1999;1455:69–84.

86. Wenger DA, Sujansky E, Fennessey PV, et al. Human β-mannosidase deficiency. *N Engl J Med.* 1986;315:1201–1205.

87. Tjoa S, Wenger DA, Fennessey PV. Quantitative analysis of disaccharides in the urine of β-mannosidosis patients. *J Inherit Metab Dis.* 1990;13:187–194.

88. Michalski JC, et al. Characterization and 400-MHz ^{1}H-NMR analysis of urinary fucosyl glycoasparagines in fucosidosis. *Eur J Biochem.* 1991;201:439–458.

89. Willems PJ, Seo HC, Coucke P, et al. Spectrum of mutations in fucosidosis. *Eur J Hum Genet.* 1999;7:60–67.

90. Willems PJ, Gatti R, Darby JK, et al. Fucosidosis revisited: A review of 77 patients. *Am J Med Genet.* 1991;38:111–131.

91. Seyrantepe V, Poupetova H, Froissart R, et al. Molecular pathology of NEU1 gene in sialidosis. *Hum Mutat.* 2003;22:343–352.

92. Arvio P, Arvio M. Progressive nature of aspartylglucosaminuria. *Acta Paediatr.* 2002;91:255–257.

93. Malm G, Mansson JE, Winiarski J, et al. Five-year follow-up of two siblings with aspartylglucosaminuria undergoing allogeneic stem-cell transplantation from unrelated donors. *Transplantation.* 2004;78:415–419.

94. Cooper JD. Progress towards understanding the neurobiology of Batten disease or neuronal ceroid lipofuscinosis. *Curr Opin Neurol.* 2003;16:121–128.

95. Santavuori P, Vanhanen SL, Autti T. Clinical and neuroradiological diagnostic aspects of

neuronal ceroid lipofuscinoses disorders. *Eur J Paediatr Neurol.* 2001;5:157–161.

96. Vanhanen SL, Puranen J, Autti T, et al. Neuroradiological findings (MRS, MRI, SPECT) in infantile neuronal ceroid-lipofuscinosis (infantile CLN1) at different stages of the disease. *Neuropediatrics.* 2004;35:27–35.

97. Pampiglione G, Harden A. So-called neuronal ceroid lipofuscinosis: Neurophysiological studies in 60 children. *J Neurol Neurosurg Psychiatry.* 1977;40:323–330.

98. Anderson RA, Bryson GM, Parks JS. Lysosomal acid lipase mutations that determine phenotype in Wolman and cholesterol ester storage disease. *Mol Genet Metab.* 1999;68:333–345.

99. Crocker AC, Vawter GF, Neuhause EB, et al. Wolman's disease: Three new patients with a recently described lipidosis. *Pediatrics.* 1965;35:627–640.

100. Burton BK, Reed SP. Acid lipase cross-reacting material in Wolman disease and cholesterol ester storage disease. *Am J Hum Genet.* 1981;33:203–208.

101. Ginsberg HN, Le NA, Short MP, et al. Suppression of apolipoprotein B production during treatment of cholesteryl ester storage disease with lovastatin: Implications for regulation of apolipoprotein B synthesis. *J Clin Invest.* 1987;80:1692–1697.

102. Krivit W, Dusenbery K, Ben-Yoseph Y, et al. Wolman disease successfully treated by bone marrow transplantation. *Bone Marrow Transplant.* 2000;26:567–570.

103. Du H, Schiavi S, Levine M, et al. Enzyme therapy for lysosomal acid lipase deficiency in the mouse. *Hum Mol Genet.* 2001;10:1639–1648.

104. van den Hout HM, Hop W, van Diggelen OP, et al. The natural course of infantile Pompe's disease: 20 original cases compared with 133 cases from the literature. *Pediatrics.* 2003;112:332–340.

105. Van den Hout JM, Reuser AJ, de Klerk JB, et al. Enzyme therapy for Pompe disease with recombinant human α-glucosidase from rabbit milk. *J Inherit Metab Dis.* 2001;24:266–274.

106. Marsden D. Infantile onset Pompe disease: A report of physician narratives from an epidemiologic study. *Genet Med.* 2005;7:147–150.

107. Chamoles NA, Niizawa G, Blanco M, et al. Glycogen storage disease type II: Enzymatic screening in dried blood spots on filter paper. *Clin Chim Acta.* 2004;347:97–102.

108. Li Y, Scott CR, Chamoles NA, et al. Direct multiplex assay of lysosomal enzymes in dried blood spots for newborn screening. *Clin Chem.* 2004;50:1785–1796.

109. Slonim AE, Coleman RA, McElligot MA, et al. Improvement of muscle function in acid maltase deficiency by high-protein therapy. *Neurology.* 1983;33:34–38.

110. Bodamer OA, Haas D, Hermans MM, et al. L-Alanine supplementation in late infantile glycogen storage disease type II. *Pediatr Neurol.* 2002;27:145–146.

111. Amalfitano A, Bengur AR, Morse RP, et al. Recombinant human acid α-glucosidase enzyme therapy for infantile glycogen storage disease type II: Results of a phase I/II clinical trial. *Genet Med.* 2001;3:132–138.

112. Winkel LP, et al. Enzyme replacement therapy in late-onset Pompe's disease: A three-year follow-up. *Ann Neurol.* 2004;55:495–502.

113. Gelb BD, Shi GP, Chapman HA, et al. Pycnodysostosis, a lysosomal disease caused by cathepsin K deficiency. *Science.* 1996;273:1236–1238.

114. Fratzl-Zelman N, Valenta A, Roschger P, et al. Decreased bone turnover and deterioration of bone structure in two cases of pycnodysostosis. *J Clin Endocrinol Metab.* 2004;89:1538–1547.

115. Motyckova G, Fisher DE. Pycnodysostosis: Role and regulation of cathepsin K in osteoclast function and human disease. *Curr Mol Med.* 2002;2:407–421.

116. Hou WS, Brömme D, Zhao Y, et al. Characterization of novel cathepsin K mutations in the pro and mature polypeptide regions causing pycnodysostosis. *J Clin Invest.* 1999;103:731–738.

117. Darcan S, Akisü M, Taneli B, et al. A case of pycnodysostosis with growth hormone deficiency. *Clin Genet.* 1996;50:422–425.

118. Soliman AT, Ramadan MA, Sherif A, et al. Pycnodysostosis: Clinical, radiologic, and endocrine evaluation and linear growth after growth hormone therapy. *Metabolism.* 2001;50:905–911.

119. Sugie K, Yamamoto A, Murayama K, et al. Clinicopathological features of genetically confirmed Danon disease. *Neurology.* 2002;58:1773–1778.

120. Fares H, Greenwald I. Regulation of endocytosis by CUP-5, the *Caenorhabditis elegans* mucolipin-1 homolog. *Nat Genet.* 2001;28:64–68.

121. LaPlante JM, Falardeau J, Sun M, et al. Identification and characterization of the single channel function of human mucolipin-1 implicated in mucolipidosis type IV, a disorder affecting the lysosomal pathway. *FEBS Lett.* 2002;532:183–187.

122. Slaugenhaupt SA. The molecular basis of mucolipidosis type IV. *Curr Mol Med.* 2002;2:445–450.

123. Treusch S, Knuth S, Slaugenhaupt SA, et al. *Caenorhabditis elegans* functional orthologue of human protein h-mucolipin-1 is required for lysosome biogenesis. *Proc Natl Acad Sci USA.* 2004;101:4483–4488.

124. Altarescu G, Sun M, Moore DF, et al. The neurogenetics of mucolipidosis type IV. *Neurology.* 2002;59:306–313.

125. Newman NJ, Starck T, Kenyon KR, et al. Corneal surface irregularities and episodic pain in a patient with mucolipidosis IV. *Arch Ophthalmol.* 1990;108:251–254.

126. Frei KP, Patronas NJ, Crutchfield KE, et al. Mucolipidosis type IV: Characteristic MRI findings. *Neurology.* 1998;51:565–569.

127. Wang ZH, Zeng B, Pastores GM, et al. Rapid detection of the two common mutations in Ashkenazi Jewish patients with mucolipidosis type IV. *Genet Test.* 2001;5:87–92.

128. Goldin E, Stahl S, Cooney AM, et al. Transfer of a mitochondrial DNA fragment to MCOLN1 causes an inherited case of mucolipidosis IV. *Hum Mutat.* 2004;24:460–465.

129. Schiffmann R, Dwyer NK, Lubensky IA, et al. Constitutive achlorhydria in mucolipidosis type IV. *Proc Natl Acad Sci USA.* 1998;95:1207–1212.

130. Prasad A, Kaye EM, Alroy J. Electron microscopic examination of skin biopsy as a cost-effective tool in the diagnosis of lysosomal storage diseases. *J Child Neurol.* 1996;11:301–308.

131. Bargal R, Goebel HH, Latta E, et al. Mucolipidosis IV: Novel mutation and diverse ultrastructural spectrum in the skin. *Neuropediatrics.* 2002;33:199–202.

132. Smith JA, Chan CC, Goldin E, et al. Noninvasive diagnosis and ophthalmic features of mucolipidosis type IV. *Ophthalmology.* 2002;109:588–594.

Purine and Pyrimidine Metabolism

William L. Nyhan MD, PhD

METABOLIC INTERRELATION: SYNTHESIS AND DEGRADATION OF PURINES AND PYRIMIDINES

Purine and pyrimidine nucleotides are synthesized by both *de novo* and salvage pathways (Figures 44-1 and 44-2). The *de novo* pathways create these complex phosphorylated molecules from simple precursors, such as CO_2, glycine, and glutamine, in stepwise fashion, whereas the salvage pathways serve the reuse of purine and pyrimidine bases of metabolic and dietary sources. In purine metabolism, inosinic acid (inosine monophosphate (IMP)) is the central product of both pathways and is central to the interconversion to adenine and purine nucleotides (see Figure 44-1). Phosphoribosylpyrophosphate (PRPP) synthetase catalyzes the first step in the pathway of *de novo* purine synthesis; the next step, the amidotransferase reaction, is the first committed step. Purine salvage is catalyzed by the enzymes adenine phosphoribosyltransferase (APRT), adenosine kinase, and hypoxanthine–guanine phosphoribosyl transferase (HPRT). Other important interrelations include the conversion of adenosine monophosphate (AMP) to IMP, catalyzed by adenosine myoadenylate deaminase (AMPDA) and the adenylosuccinate lyase (ASL) reactions in which IMP is converted to AMP via adenylosuccinate (AMPS). The latter enzyme also catalyses the conversion of 5-phosphoribosyl-5-amino-4-imidazole-succinylcarboxamide (SAICAMP) to 5-phosphoribosyl-5-amino-4-imidazole-carboxamide(AICAMP). Adenosine is converted to inosine in the reaction catalyzed by adenosine deaminase (ADA). Purine nucleoside phosphorylase (PNP) catalyzes the conversion inosine to hypoxanthine; it also catalyzes the conversion of guanosine and the deoxy analogues to their bases. The conversion of hypoxoxanthine to xanthine and their conversion to uric acid is catalyzed by xanthine oxidase (XO). Uric acid is the endpoint of purine metabolism in humans.

De novo synthesis of pyrimidines begins with a carbamylphosphate synthetase 2 reaction. It is catalyzed by a different synthetase than the one involved in the urea cycle, but when carbamylphosphate accumulates as in ornithine transcarbamyl synthetase deficiency and other disorders of the urea cycle, pyrimidine synthesis accelerates, and orotic acid and uracil accumulate. The last two steps of the pyrimidine *de novo* pathway are catalyzed by uridine 5'-monophosphate (UMP) synthase (UMPS), which contains two catalytic activities, orotic acid phosphoribosyltransferase (OPRT) and orotidine monophosphate decarboxylase (OPC). Thus OPRT potentially can serve in pyrimidine salvage as well as in *de novo* synthesis. The functional enzyme in pyrimidine salvage is uracil phosphoribosyl transferase (UPRT), which serves the syntheses of UMP from uracil and also from cytosine, which first must be deaminated to uracil and ammonia. The pyrimidine-5'-nucleotidases (ses Figure 44-2) and uridine monophosphate hydrolase (UMH) include enzymes specific for pyrimidine nucleotides and the cytosolic high K_m enzyme, activated by ATP, for which both purine and pyrimidine monophosphates are substrates.

Pyrimidine base catabolism is initiated by the dihydropyrimidine dehydrogenase (DPD) reaction in which thymine and uracil are converted to their dihydro forms in a reversible reaction. Dihydrothymine and dihydrouracil are converted to ureidobutyric and ureidopropionic acid in the dihydropyrimidine amidohydrolase reaction mediated by dihydropyrimidinase (DHP)). These compounds then are converted to β-aminoisobutyric acid and β-alanine by ureidopropionase.

Rates of purine and pyrimidine synthesis and catabolism are controlled by the availability of substrates. Thus, in the presence of accumulated PRPP, as in HPRT deficiency and PRPP synthetase overactivity, purine synthesis and uric acid production are accelerated. Some reactions, such as APRT and HPRT, are inhibited by their products. The

amido transferase reaction in purine *de novo* synthesis is inhibited by both AMP and guanosine monophosphate (GMP).

Among disorders of purine and pyrimidine metabolism (1), heterogeneity in mutation leads to enzymes with varying degrees of abnormal activity from zero to hyperactivity. These different activities lead to quite different syndromes, even in defects of the same enzyme. Correlation of enzyme activity with clinical phenotype sometimes can be made by assay of the enzyme or the pathway in intact cultured cells. On the other hand, mutant enzymes usually are unstable and denature in cell lysates, in which assays often reveal zero activity despite evidence of partial residual activity *de novo*.

LESCH–NYHAN DISEASE

Etiology/Pathophysiology Lesch–Nyhan disease (2–7) was first described as a syndrome of hyperuricemia and cerebral dysfunction in 1964 in two brothers aged 4 and 8 years. The younger brother presented with hematuria and had had previous diagnoses of mental retardation and cerebral palsy, as did his brother. Both brothers exhibited what we called *choreoathetosis* and self-injurious behavior manifest predominantly by biting that was destructive of tissue.

The defect is a lack of activity of the enzyme HPRT (8) (see Figure 44-3). HPRT catalyzes the reaction in which the purine bases hypoxanthine and guanine are reused to form their respective nucleotides, IMP and GMP. The gene for HPRT is located on the X chromosome, and the disorder occurs almost exclusively in males, but a small number of females has been reported, most reflecting nonrandom inactivation of the normal X chromosome (9). Phenotypic heterogeneity in clinical expression is seen and correlates with varying degrees of residual HPRT activity (10). Patients with partial deficiency of HPRT usually are referred to as *partial variants*. The incidence for this group

Disorders of Purine and Pyrimidine Metabolism

AT-A-GLANCE

Inherited defects of purine and pyrimidine metabolism are all monogenic diseases and have been recognized in 14 different disorders, many of which are associated with neurological abnormalities. Lesch–Nyhan disease is the most common and best studied disorder in this group.

Purines and pyrimidines are the building blocks of the nucleic acids DNA and RNA. They are, as demonstrated by two inborn errors of metabolism, important for the development of the immune system. They form the cores of a number of cofactors involved in intermediary metabolism. The trinucleotides adenosine triphosphate (ATP) and guanosine triphosphate (GTP) are central to energy and signal transduction, whereas cyclic adenosine monophosphate (cAMP) mediates the action of hormones. The nucleosides adenosine and guanosine are involved in neurotransmission. It comes, therefore, as no surprise that the clinical manifestations of disorders of purine and pyrimidine metabolism are many and varied.

TYPES OF DISEASE	OCCURRENCE	GENE	LOCUS	OMIM
Hypoxanthine–guanine phosphoribosyl transferase deficiency	1:100,000 males	HPRT	Xq26-27	308000
PRPP synthetase overactivity	Rare	PRPS1 PRPS2	Xq22-24 Xp 22.2-22.3	311850 311860
AICA ribosiduria	Very rare	ATIC	?	–
Adenylosuccinate lyase deficiency	Rare	ASL	22q 1.3.1-1.3.2	103050
Adenine phosphoribosyltransferase deficiency	Rare	APRT	16q24.3	102600
Adenosine deaminase deficiency	Rare	ADA	20q 13.11	102700
Purine nucleoside phosphorylase deficiency	Rare	PNP	14q11-21	164050
Myoadenylate deaminase deficiency	1:5–8	AMPD1	1p 13-21	102770
Xanthine oxidase deficiency	Rare	XO	2p22	278300
Molybdenum cofactor deficiency	Very rare	MOCSIA MOCS1B MOCS2 GEPH	6p 21-3 ? 5q11 ?	252150 252160 – –
Orotic aciduria	Very rare	UMPS	3q13	258900
Pyrimidine nucleotide depletion syndrome	Very rare	?	?	–
Dihydropyrimidine dehydrogenase deficiency	Rare	DPD	1p22	274270
Dihydropyrimidinase deficiency	Rare	DP	8q22	222748
Ureidopropionase deficiency	Very rare	UP	22q11.2	210100

DISORDER	FINDINGS	CLINICAL PRESENTATION
Lesch–Nyhan disease	Hyperuricemia, uricosuria, deficiency of HPRT activity	Motor developmental disability, spasticity, dystonia, choreoathetosis, self-injurious behavior, gout, renal stone disease, urate nephropathy
HPRT partial variants	Hyperuricemia, uricosuria, deficiency of HPRT activity	Gout, renal stone disease, urate nephropathy
HPRT neurological variants	Hyperuricemia, uricosuria deficiency of HPRT activity	Lesch–Nyhan phenotype without SIB, normal intelligence

DISORDER	FINDINGS	CLINICAL PRESENTATION
PRPP synthetase overactivity	Hyperuricemia, uricosuria, abnormal (hyper) activity of PRPP synthetase	Gout, renal stone disease, urate nephropathy, sensorineural deafness
AICA ribosiduria	Positive Bratton–Marshall; ZTP accumulation; deficient activity of AICAR transformylase	Mental retardation, blindness, seizures
Adenylosuccinate lyase deficiency	Positive Bratton–Marshall; deficient activity of the lyase; accumulation of adenylosuccinate and SAICA riboside	Mental retardation, seizures
Adenine phosphoribosyl transferase deficiency	Dihydroxyadeninuria; deficiency of APRT activity	Renal stone disease
Adenosine deaminase deficiency	Deficient activity of ADA	Immunodeficiency (SCID)
Purine nucleoside phosphorylase deficiency	Hypouricemia, deficient activity of PNP	SCID
Myoadenylate deaminase deficiency	Increased CK, absence of NH_3 increase with ischemic exercise, deficient activity of AMPD in muscle	Pain or cramps after exercise
Xanthine oxidase deficiency	Hypouricemia, xanthinuria, deficiency of xanthine oxidase in liver or intestine	Urinary tract calculi
Molybdenum cofactor deficiency	Sulfituria, accumulation of sulfocysteine, deficient activity of xanthine oxidase and sulfite oxidase	Global developmental delay, seizures, urinary tract stone disease
Orotic aciduria	Orotic aciduria, UMP synthase deficiency	Megaloblastic anemia, neutropenia, susceptibility to infection, crystalluria
Pyrimidine nucleotide depletion	Uricosuria, hyperactivity of 5′-nucleotidase	Developmental delay, seizures, aggressive behavior
Pyrimidine 5′-nucleotidase deficiency	Defective activity of leukocyte 5′-nucleotidase	Hemolytic anemia
Dihydropyrimidine dehydrogenase deficiency	Uraciluria, thyminuria, deficient activity of DPD	Developmental delay, seizures, toxicity to 5-fluorouracil
Dihydropyrimidinase deficiency	Increased excretion of dihydrouracil, dihydrothymine, uracil, and thymine; deficient activity of dihydropyrimidinase	Mental retardation, seizures, toxicity to 5-fluorouracil
Ureidopropionase deficiency	Excretion of ureidopropionate and ureidobutyrate	Mental retardation, seizures

HPRT=hypoxanthine–guanine phosphoribosyl transferase; PRPP=phosphoribosylpyrophosphate; AICA=aminoimidazole carboxamide; AICAR=AICA riboside; ZTP=AICA ribotide; APRT=adenine phosphoribosyltransferase; ADA=adenosine deaminase; PNP=purine nucleoside phosphorylase; SCID=severe combined immunodeficiency; CK=creatine kinase; AMPD-adenylate deaminase; UMP=uridine monophosphate; DPD=dihydropyrimidine dehydrogenase.

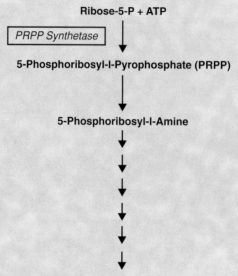
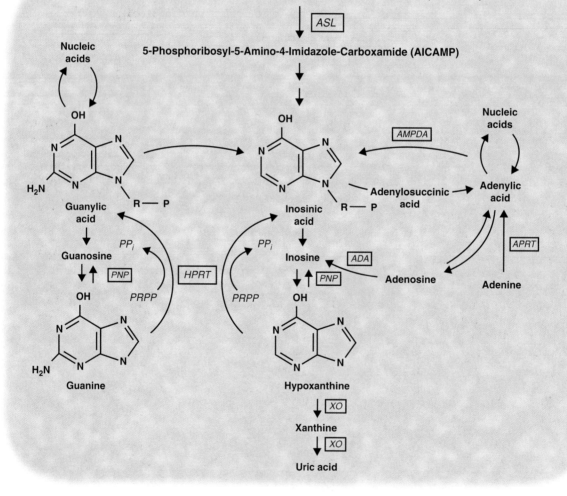

Normal Metabolism of Purines

FIGURE 44-1. Purine metabolism. Pathways of synthesis, salvage, interrelations, and degradation of purine nucleotides. The enzymatic steps in the boxes indicate the sites of the commonly encountered disorders of purine metabolism. Abbreviations include the hypoxanthine: guanine phosphoribosyl transferase (HPRT) reaction. This enzyme is the molecular defect in Lesch–Nyhan disease. ASL = adenylosuccinate lyase, APRT = adenine phosphoribosyltransferase; GMP = guanylic acid; IMP = inosinic acid; HPRT = hypoxanthine–guanine phosphoribosyl transferase; PRPP = phosphoribosylpyrophosphate; AICA = aminoimidazole carboxamide; AICAMP = AICAR = AICA ribotide = ZMP; SAICAMP = SAICAR = succinyl-AICAR; APRT = adenine phosphoribosyltransferase; ADA = adenosine deaminase; PNP = purine nucleoside phosphorylase; AMPDA = adenylate deaminase; XO = xanthine oxidase.

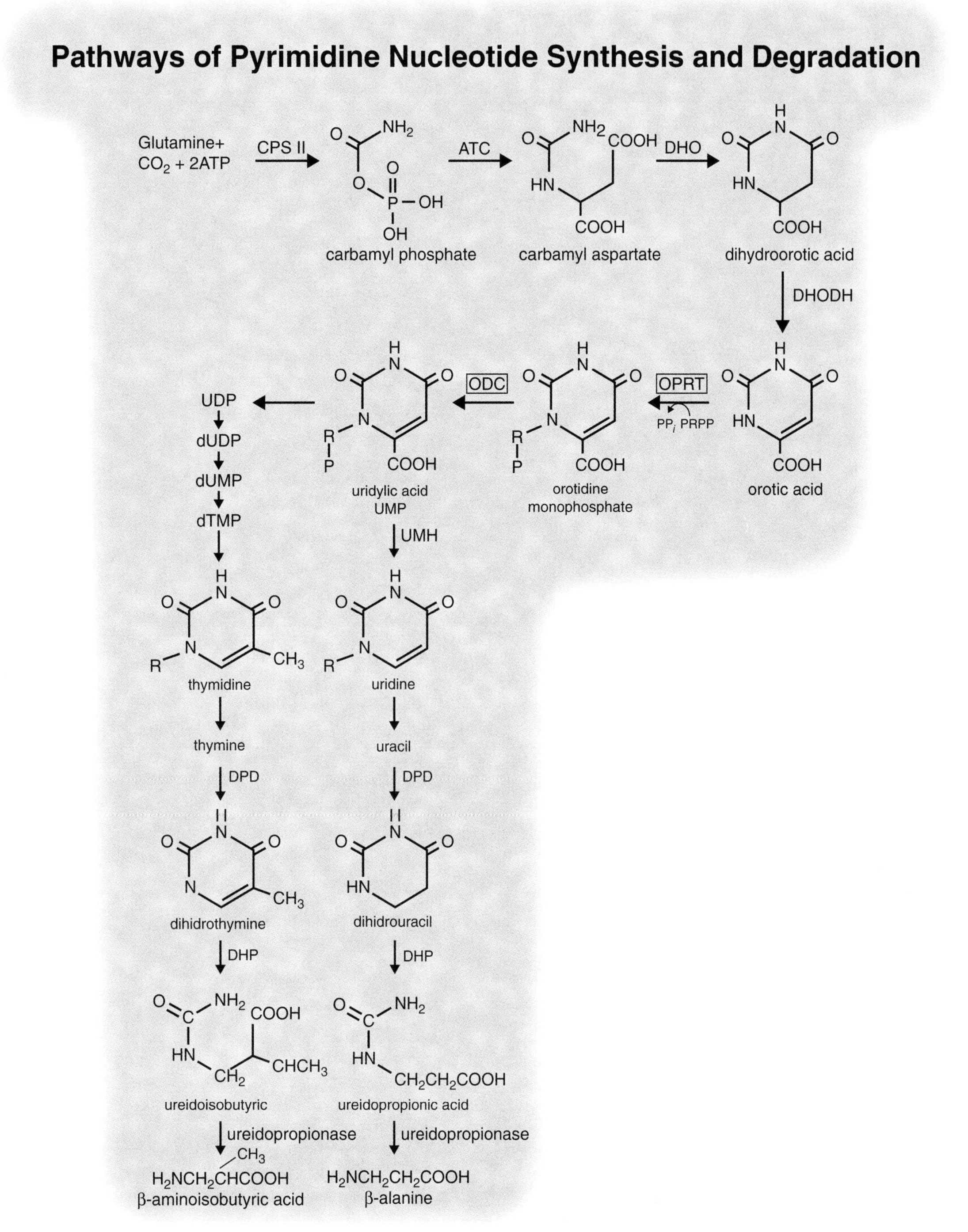

Pathways of Pyrimidine Nucleotide Synthesis and Degradation

FIGURE 44-2. Pathways of pyrimidine nucleotide synthesis and degradation. CPSII = carbamylphosphate synthetase II; ATC = aspartate transcarbamylase; DHO = dihydroorotase; DHODH = dihydroorotate dehydrogenase; OPRT = orotic acid phosphoribosyltransferase; ODC = orotidine 5-phosphate decarboxylase; UMH = UMP hydrolase; DHP = dihydropyrimidinase. UMP = uridine monophosphate; DPD = dihydropyrimidine dehydrogenase.

is not known, but it is much lower than for the classical Lesch–Nyhan disease. The life expectancy of most patients with partial HPRT deficiency is normal. The Lesch–Nyhan patient rarely survives the third decade, but the immediate cause of death is often unclear.

Because the gene for HPRT is on the X chromosome, heterozygous females are mosaics and have two populations of cells, one of which is deficient in HPRT activity. These carrier females usually are clinically asymptomatic. Several studies have shown, however, that some females heterozygous for partial defects have elevated serum levels of uric acid, and symptoms of hyperuricemia or gout in females have been attributed to heterozygosity for HPRT deficiency (11). Normal enzyme activity in hematopoietic tissues, uniformly found in Lesch–Nyhan heterozygotes,

probably is related to selection against HPRT-negative cells (12).

Clinical Manifestations Affected infants appear normal at birth and may develop normally for the first 4–8 months. The first sign of the disease is what is described as "orange sand" in the diapers, but the disease very seldom has been recognized on the basis of this crystalluria. Delayed development is

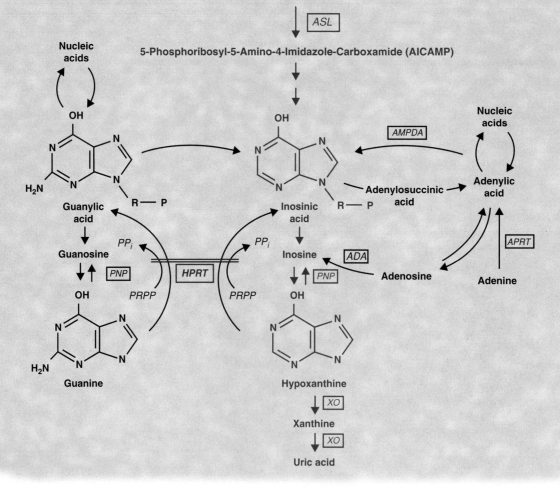
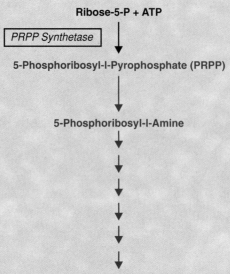

Deficiency of HPRT (Lesch-Nyhan Syndrome)

FIGURE 44-3. HPRT deficiency. The site of the molecular defect in the Lesch–Nyhan disease. ASL = adenylosuccinate lyase; APRT = adenine phosphoribosyltransferase; GMP = guanylic acid; IMP = inosinic acid; HPRT = hypoxanthine:guanine phosphoribosyl transferase; PRPP = phosphoribosylpyrophosphate; AICA = aminoimidazole carboxamide; AICAMP = AICAR = AICA ribotide = ZMP; SAICAMP = SAICAR = succinyl-AICAR; APRT = adenine phosphoribosyltransferase; ADA = adenosine deaminase; PNP = purine nucleoside phosphorylase; AMPDA = adenylate deaminase; XO = xanthine oxidase.

apparent within the first year, and the affected child does not learn to sit alone or loses this ability if it has been achieved. Patients with this disease do not learn to walk or even to stand unassisted. If securely fastened around the chest, the child is able to sit in a chair, and these children usually are encountered seated in a narrow wheelchair. Extrapyramidal signs develop during the first year. Involuntary movements are dystonic as well as choreic and athetoid. Opisthotonic arching of the back is a regular feature. Signs of pyramidal tract involvement develop during the first years, and the accompanying spasticity is severe and may lead to dislocation of the hips. Patients have hyperreflexia, ankle clonus, and positive Babinski responses, but abnormal or voluntary movements make reflexes difficult to elicit. Scissoring of the legs is common. Dysarthria and dysphagia are other features of the disease, and the dysarthria can combine with the motor defect to make proper assessment of cognitive development difficult. Many eat poorly, and most of them vomit. The vomiting becomes incorporated into the behavior. Height and weight are nearly always lower than normal (3). Mental development may be retarded; the IQ, as measured, may be 40–70. However, testing is made difficult by the behavior and the motor defect. Some patients have had normal cognitive function, and a few have been successful mainstream students. In a series of 15 patients with classical enzymatic phenotypes, mean IQ was 59 ± 15, and 10 of the 13 fell below 70 (13). The mean of 15 controls was 108 ± 9. There was scatter in performance on different tests with mild impairment of temporal orientation and recognition memory and with severe impairment of auditory divided attention and reasoning.

The aggressive, self-injurious behavior is one of the distinctive features of the classical Lesch–Nyhan phenotype, and in our experience, it has always been present (3). However, at least two exceptions to the rule have been reported from Spain (6). Patients bite their lips and fingers with resulting loss of tissue; there have been partial amputations of phalanges of the fingers or the tongue. Patients are not insensitive to pain but scream in pain when they bite and are usually relaxed only when securely restrained, preventing injury. Physical restraints and extraction of teeth are the only effective methods of prevention of the behavior. Aggressive behavior is also directed toward others. Patients bite, hit, or kick aggressively, but the motor defect limits the effectiveness of this behavior. Speech joins the behavior, and four-letter words are also common. The abnormal behavior appears to be compulsive and beyond the control of the patient, who often shows signs of remorse.

Hyperuricemia is characteristic; serum uric acid levels are usually between 5 and 10 mg/dL. The excretion of uric acid is 3–5 mg of uric acid per milligram of creatinine (controls have age-dependent excretions from a mean of 1.55 ± 0.7 mg of uric acid per milligram of creatinine in the first week of life to 0.37 ± 0.04 mg at 5–16 years of age).

Older children and adults excrete less than 1 mg uric acid per milligram of creatinine. The consistent finding of this elevated uric acid:creatinine ratio and its relative ease of measurement usually make it a useful initial screening test for this and other metabolic hyperuricemias (14,15), but urinary data for uric acid can be spuriously low as a result of bacterial contamination, and 24-hour collections at room temperature are especially suspect.

The clinical consequences of hyperuricemia are manifestations shared with gout: arthritis, tophi, hematuria, nephrolithiasis, urinary tract infection, and in untreated patients, renal failure. Patients also have manifested megaloblastic anemia, in some severe enough to require regular blood transfusions. Macrocytosis or megaloblastic changes in the marrow also have been found in the absence of clinical anemia.

The most significant pathological feature is the abnormality of the central nervous system (CNS). The patient with Lesch–Nyhan disease is normal in gross anatomy and in microscopic and electron microscopic histology. The accumulation of uric acid in soft tissue tophi yields an amorphous, powdery histological picture, whereas in joints, an inflammatory response surrounds crystallized needles of sodium urate that are then engulfed by leukocytes. The deposition of sodium urate in the renal parenchyma leads to an inflammatory response that ultimately leads to fibrosis and renal failure. In acute anuria, observed at times of dehydration, obstruction may be engendered by the precipitation of crystals of uric acid in the renal tubules or in the ureters.

Diagnosis A preliminary diagnosis of classical Lesch–Nyhan disease can be made on the basis of the phenotype. Choreoathetosis and spasticity in combination with the typical self-injurious behavior are almost diagnostic. In the case of partial HPRT deficiency, the clinical phenotype is less distinct. In virtually all instances of HPRT deficiency, hyperuricemia and increased excretion of uric acid are present. A serum concentration in a child of more than 4–5 mg/dL uric acid and a urine uric acid:creatinine ratio of 3–4 are supportive, but a definitive diagnosis requires analysis of HPRT enzyme activity, which is assayed in erythrocyte lysates. With this method, the

classical Lesch–Nyhan patient usually has an enzyme activity close to 0%, whereas patients with partial HPRT deficiency have values between 0% and 60%. Significantly, in this assay, the enzyme activity obtained for the partially HPRT-deficient patient shows little correlation with the clinical phenotype.

The intact-cell assay was developed as a more physiological approach that turned out to discriminate among the various clinical phenotypes of HPRT deficiency (10). In the intact-cell assay, HPRT enzyme activity is analyzed by incubation with labeled hypoxanthine or guanine with cultured fibroblasts, and subsequently, the labeled nucleotides are separated by high-pressure liquid chromatography. Because this assay provides a good correlation between enzyme activity and severity of the disease, it can be of great value in predicting the outcome of the disease in a newly diagnosed infant with no family history of HPRT deficiency. HPRT enzyme activity also can be measured in hair roots. This is employed most often in carrier detection. Molecular techniques also are used for diagnosis of HPRT deficiency, and they are valuable in the ascertainment of carriers and in prenatal diagnosis (16).

Biochemical and Molecular Features HPRT is a cytoplasmic enzyme expressed in every cell of the body; the highest levels are in the basal ganglia and testis. The defect is detectable in erythrocytes hemolysates and in cultured fibroblasts. It is measured most readily in erythrocyte lysates, in which quantitative assays yield virtually zero activity (8).

In HPRT deficiency, the underuse of hypoxanthine and guanine leads to increased excretion of the degradation product uric acid, and the accompanying underuse of PRPP gives rise to increased activity in the *de novo* pathway, increasing uric acid production. Plasma levels of hypoxanthine and xanthine are only slightly elevated because of the efficiency of hepatic xanthine oxidase, but this enzyme is not active in brain, and high levels of hypoxanthine are found in the cerebrospinal fluid (CSF). The other consequence of increased *de novo* pathway activity is the elevation in levels of 5-aminoimidazole-4-carboxamide (AICA) and its corresponding nucleoside (AICAR).

Treatment The excessive uric acid production in HPRT-deficient patients is treated effectively with daily administration of allopurinol. The amounts required are high. We start with 20 mg/kg in an infant or child newly diagnosed and seek to keep the serum uric acid concentration under 3 mg/dL. Once this level is achieved, we attempt to make the urinary oxypurines maximal in hypoxanthine and minimal in xanthine and uric acid. No medication is effective in treating the neurological or behavioral manifestations of the disease in classical Lesch–Nyhan patients. The only successful approaches to the self-injurious behavior have been physical restraint and removal of the teeth.

OTHER VARIANTS OF HPRT

Following recognition that the defect in Lesch–Nyhan disease was in HPRT, enzyme deficiency was found in patients with gout and with urinary tract calculi (17,18). It was thought initially that this population of patients with HPRT deficiency might be quite large, but this is not the case. Most patients with HPRT deficiency have Lesch–Nyhan disease, and most patients with gout do not have HPRT deficiency. Nevertheless, any patient with gout should be studied for the possibility of increased excretion of uric acid because the treatment of such a patient with a uricosuric agent such as probenecid can induce fatal renal shutdown. Assay for HPRT deficiency should be undertaken in any patient with overproduction hyperuricemia. The enzyme also should be assayed in any patient with uric acid calculi. In an infant or child with renal stones, it may be easier to obtain an assay of HPRT than of the nature of the calculus, especially since so many calculi are lost. Some variant enzymes display some residual activity in the erythrocyte assay, often more than 5% of control, making them readily distinguishable from the classical Lesch–Nyhan pattern, a distinction that is particularly important in assessing prognosis in a newly diagnosed young infant. These patients have been referred to as *partial variants*. The phenotype of patients with these partial variants of enzyme consists of manifestations that can be related directly to the accumulation of uric acid in body fluids, acute attacks of gouty arthritis, tophi, and renal urinary tract complications. The CNS and the behavior are normal. However, many patients with variant clinical phenotypes have zero activity in the erythrocyte assay, and such patients also display no activity in fibroblast lysates.

Distinction among variants became possible with the development methodology for the assessment of enzyme activity in intact cultured fibroblasts (10,19). The method permits assessment of the kinetic properties of HPRT. The K_m for hypoxanthine found in normal fibroblasts was identical to that of the purified human enzyme, and a number of kinetic variants have been reported (20). Patients with Lesch–Nyhan disease have displayed activity below 1.5% of normal, and the classical partial variants all had greater than 8% of control activity.

After testing of these two populations of HPRT-deficient patients, it became evident that there was a third group, and these patients had intermediate levels of enzyme activity in the whole-cell assay. We have called these intermediate patients *neurological variants*. Among the variants studied, one patient with a classical Lesch–Nyhan phenotype and 1.4% of control activity could be distinguished from other Lesch–Nyhan variants by the more normal behavior of his cells in selective media (21). This small but important group of patients usually is characterized by a neurological phenotype that is identical to that of the classical Lesch–Nyhan patient with spasticity, dystonia, and chorea. They are confined to wheelchairs and unable to walk. However, behavior is normal, and intelligence is normal or nearly normal.

Another phenotype with 7.5% of residual activity in the intact-cell assay and a different neurological picture was observed in a family whose HPRT variant we have called HPRT$_{Salamanca}$ (22). Four males in three generations had an identical phenotype, the most prominent feature of which was spastic diplegia. They all could walk, but gait was classically spastic. Hypertonicity and brisk deep tendon reflexes were more prominent in the lower extremity. Babinski responses were positive bilaterally. There was bilateral pes cavus and exaggerated lumbar lordosis. Mental retardation was mild. Tophaceous gout appeared by 32 years in a previously untreated patient.

In variant patients, missense mutations have been the rule, and the changes have been conservative. In the original patient of Catel and Schmidt (23,24), the mutation changed a valine to a glycine (25), which would not be expected to make a major difference in protein structure. Others had changes such as an isoleucine to a threonine. In these patients and in the partial or hyperuricemic variants, no deletions, stop codons, or major rearrangements were observed. In HPRT$_{Salamanca}$, there were two mutations: a T-to-G change at position 128 and a G-to-A change at position 130. These changes resulted in the substitution of two adjacent amino acids at positions 43 and 44, methionine to arginine and aspartic acid to asparagine. These mutations would not appear to be particularly conservative, but the phenotype probably was the mildest of the neurological variants observed. They may have reflected another observation that the milder mutations have tended to cluster at the amino-terminal end of the enzyme. Point mutations in Lesch–Nyhan patients have been more likely to be sited in areas important to substrate binding and catalytic activity.

Treatment   Allopurinol is the treatment of choice.

PHOSPHORIBOSYLPYRO-PHOSPHATE SYNTHETASE OVERACTIVITY

Etiology/Pathophysiology   Inherited variation in the PRPP synthetase protein molecule in which activity is greater than normal leads to hyperuricemia and uricosuria (26) (see Figure 44-4). Complications include nephropathy and hematuria, crystalluria, urinary tract calculi, and gouty arthritis. In some kindreds, affected members also had deafness (27,28).

Clinical Manifestations   In this disease, hyperuricemia and uricosuria are invariant. All the clinical features that are results of the accumulation of uric acid in body fluids are potential consequences of PRPP synthetase overactivity. Gouty arthritis has been reported with onset as early as 21 years of age (26). Renal colic has been observed, as well as the passage of calculi (29). One boy developed hematuria at the age of 2 months and was found to have crystalluria, hyperuricemia, and uricosuria (30). In families in which clinical onset is early, females may develop symptoms prior to menopause (31).

Deafness in some families has been associated with an abnormally active PRPP synthetase. In one family, there were three involved males, each of whom also had severe neurodevelopmental retardation (28). One of our patients was thought to be mentally retarded, and his behavior was thought to be autistic, but with time, it was apparent that he was deaf, and his behavior was quite appropriate.

Diagnosis   Increased amounts of uric acid in the blood and urine are the rule, and concentrations in serum may range from 8–12 mg/dL (26,27). In the initial proband (26), uric acid excretion was 2400 mg/24 h. Urinary excretion may range from 1.8–3.3 mg/mg of creatinine. Overproduction of purine *de novo* was documented by measuring the *in vivo* conversion of [^{14}C]glycine to urinary uric acid (27). In 7 days, 0.7% of the isotope of glycine administered was converted to uric acid—seven times the control level of 0.1%.

Biochemical and Molecular Features   Intact cultured fibroblasts in this disease incorporate purines, adenine, guanine, and hypoxanthine more rapidly into nucleotides than do controls (32), and incorporation of ^{14}C-labeled formate is also accelerated. These findings indicate the presence of increased intracellular concentrations of PRPP, and this may be the most reliable method of screening for the disease.

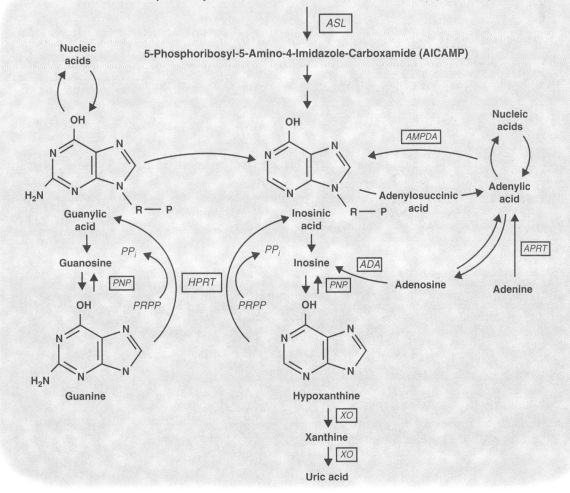
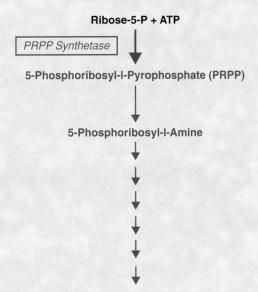

PRPP Synthetase Overactivity

FIGURE 44-4. PRPP synthetase hyperactivity. ASL = adenylosuccinate lyase; APRT = adenine phosphoribosyltransferase; GMP = guanylic acid; IMP = inosinic acid; AICA = aminoimidazole carboxamide; AICAMP = AICAR = AICA ribotide = ZMP; SAICAMP = SAICAR = succinyl-AICAR; HPRT = hypoxanthine:guanine phosphoribosyl transferase; PRPP = phosphoribosylpyrophosphate; APRT = adenine phosphoribosyltransferase; ADA = adenosine deaminase; PNP = purine nucleoside phosphorylase; AMPDA = Adenylate deaminase; XO = xanthine oxidase.

The enzyme defect is an altered PRPP synthetase structure that leads to superactive enzyme activity. Activity may be three times that of normal enzyme (29). In one of the families studied, increased enzyme activity was demonstrable only at low concentrations of phosphate, and there was diminished responsiveness to feedback inhibition by purine nucleotides (33). In another family, an elevated level of enzyme-specific activity was demonstrable over a wide range of phosphate concentrations, and feedback inhibition was normal (29). The amounts of immunoreactive enzyme protein may be normal. These observations indicate the presence in normal amounts of a protein in which structural alteration leads to increased specific activity. The data are consistent with the presence of two important sites on the enzyme, a catalytic site that may be altered by mutation and a regulatory site that may be altered by another. In one patient, the altered structure affected both catalytic and regulatory activities (32).

The altered PRPP synthetase, though hyperactive, also may be unstable; so diminished levels in old erythrocytes may be low or normal. Therefore, enzyme assay of erythrocyte lysates in this disease may be misleading (32).

PRPP synthetase (Figure 44-4) catalyzes the initial step in the de novo synthesis of purines in which ribose-5-P reacts with ATP to form PRPP. PRPP is the substrate for the first rate-limiting step in the 10-step reaction. Increased quantities of intracellular PRPP lead to overproduction of purine de novo and of IMP, which ultimately yields uric acid.

PRPP synthetase is coded for by two genes on the X chromosome at Xq 22-24 and Xp 22.2-22.3. The genes have been cloned and sequenced (34) and are referred to as PRPS1 and S2. A small number of point mutations has been defined in PRPS1 in patients with overactivity and altered allosteric properties of the enzyme. In 6 patients with overactivity of PRPP synthase, no mutation in the DNA of PRPS1 or S2 was found. Instead, there were increased quantities of the S1 isoform, whose physical and catalytic properties were normal (35). The PRPP synthetase gene is on the X chromosome (33). It may be fully expressed in females, or it may be fully recessive. This could reflect different degrees of lyonization; on the other hand, it is easier for an overactive than a deficient enzyme to function as an X-linked dominant.

The cDNA of human S_1 PRPP synthetase encodes transcripts of 2.3 kb and a protein of 317 amino acids. PRPS1 and S2 cDNAs have 80% nucleotide sequence identity. In six male patients with overactivity of PRPP synthetase and resistance to purine nucleotide feedback,

there was single-base transition that led to single-amino-acid changes (35,36).

An entirely different variation in PRPP synthetase has been described (37) in an infant with markedly decreased activity of PRPP synthetase in erythrocytes. The patient was severely retarded mentally and had a megaloblastic anemia. PRPP synthetase deficiency led to low levels of uric acid in blood and urine and large amounts of orotic acid in the urine, which would be consistent with a shortage of PRPP substrate for the orotic acid phosphoribosyltransferase (OPRT) reaction.

Treatment Allopurinol is the treatment of choice in any overproduction hyperuricemia, including the PRPP synthetase defects. Treatment of abnormalities in PRPP synthetase is simpler than that of HPRT deficiency. This is because in the presence of normal HPRT activity, there is extensive reuse of hypoxanthine accumulating behind the block in xanthine oxidase, leading to a substantial decrease in total purine excretion.

5-AMINO-4-IMIDAZOLECARBOXAMIDE (AICA) RIBOSIDURIA

Etiology/Pathophysiology This newly described disorder of purine biosynthesis (38) was discovered in a 4-year-old with congenital blindness, developmental delay, and dysmorphic features. Its discovery was the result of a screening test of the urine with the Bratton–Marshall reaction. This riboside is the dephosphorylated counterpart of aminoimidazolecarboxamide ribotide (AICAR), an intermediate in a later step of purine biosynthesis de novo (see Figure 44-5). The defect is in the activity of AICAR transformylase.

Clinical Manifestations The screening test was done to evaluate the patient as an instance of unexplained mental retardation. She had been blind from birth, and the electroretinogram was markedLy abnormal. Retardation was profound. In addition, she had epileptic seizures. Dysmorphic features included a prominent forehead, bushy eyebrows, low-set ears, anteverted nostrils, and a wide mouth. Concentrations in blood of cholesterol and fatty acids were low.

Biochemical/Enzyme Characteristics The patient was thought initially to have adenylosuccinate lyase deficiency, but high-pressure liquid chromatography (HPLC) of the urine revealed no evidence of the key metabolites adenylosuccinate and succinyl-AICAR (SAICAR). AICAR is also known as ZMP, and this compound and its di- and-triphosphates were found to accumulate in erythrocytes.

The very large peak of ZMP was in contrast with control erythrocytes, in which the compound was not detected. Incubation of patient fibroblasts with AICA riboside led to a huge accumulation of AICAR, again unlike controls. These data indicated the presence of a defect in the conversion of AICAR to formyl-AICAR (FAICAR). This conversion is catalyzed by a bifunctional enzyme, AICAR tranformylase/IMP cyclohydrolase (ATIC). In patient fibroblasts, the transformylase was profoundLy deficient, whereas the cyclohydrolase activity was 40% of control.

Genetic/Molecular Features The ATIC gene contains seven exons coding for IMP cyclohydrolase and nine coding for ACAR tranformylase. Sequencing of the ATIC gene revealed a maternally derived frame shift in exon 2 and a paternally derived missense mutation K426R in nucleotide 1277 in the transformylase region. Expression of recombinant enzyme carrying K426R yielded evidence of zero transformylase activity.

The discovery of this disorder emphasizes the importance of a search for inborn enzymes of purine and pyrimidine metabolism in patients with unexplained mental retardation or neurological abnormalities.

Treatment Treatment is supportive. Specific treatment has not been devised.

ADENYLOSUCCINATE LYASE DEFICIENCY

Etiology/Pathophysiology Adenylosuccinate lyase deficiency, first described by Jacken and Van Den Berghe (39) in 1984, was immediately interesting because patients displayed autistic behavior. However, many searches among autistic populations have failed to confirm this association. Mental retardation and seizures are major manifestations.

The deficient enzyme adenylosuccinate lyase (adenylosuccinase [ASL]) catalyzes the eighth step in the de novo synthesis of purines, in which SAICAR (SAICAMP) is converted to AICAR (AICAMP, or ZMP) (40,41) (see Figure 44-6). The enzyme also catalyzes the conversion of adenylosuccinate to AMP in purine nucleotide interconversion, forming AMP (42). The gene has been mapped to human chromosome 22q1.3.1-1.3.2 (43). The human cDNA has been cloned, and a point mutation was discovered in the index family (44). A number of different missense mutations has been found, most of them in compound heterozygotes, the most common being R426H (45).

Clinical Manifestations Psychomotor retardation is the only constant manifestation of the phenotype (39,42,46,47). Seizures have

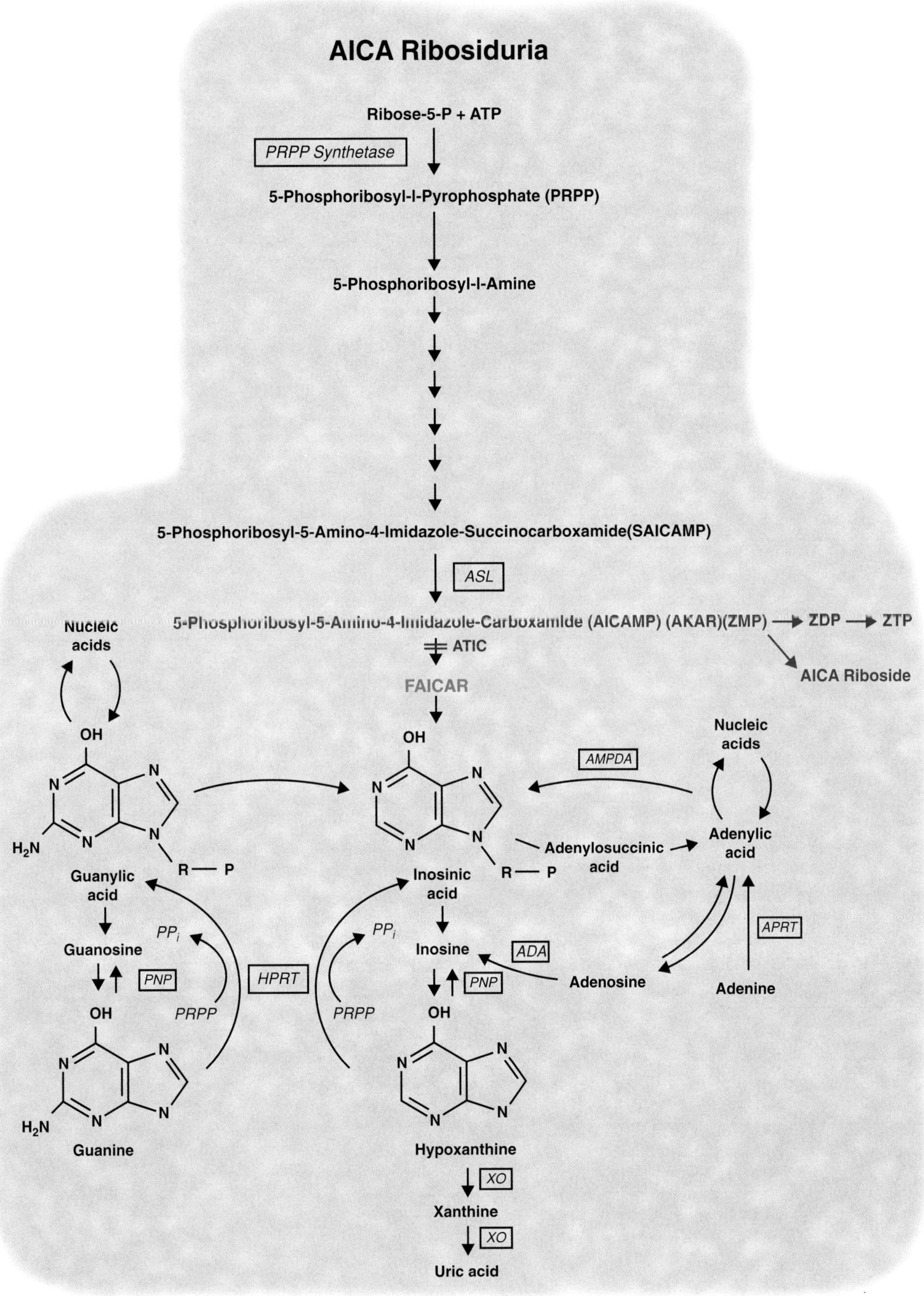

FIGURE 44-5. AICA ribosiduria. ASL = adenylosuccinate lyase; ATIC = AICAR tranformylase/IMP cyclohydrolase; APRT = adenine phosphoribosyltransferase; GMP = guanylic acid; IMP = inosinic acid; HPRT = hypoxanthine:guanine phosphoribosyl transferase; PRPP = phosphoribosylpyrophosphate; AICA = aminoimidazole carboxamide; AICAMP = AICAR = AICA ribotide = ZMP; FAICAR = formyl-AICAR; SAICAMP = SAICAR = succinyl-AICAR; APRT = adenine phosphoribosyltransferase; ADA = adenosine deaminase; PNP = purine nucleoside phosphorylase; AMPDA = adenylate deaminase; XO = xanthine oxidase.

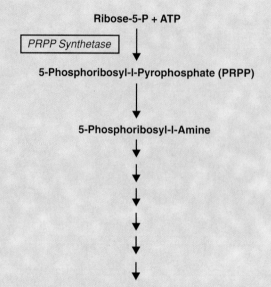
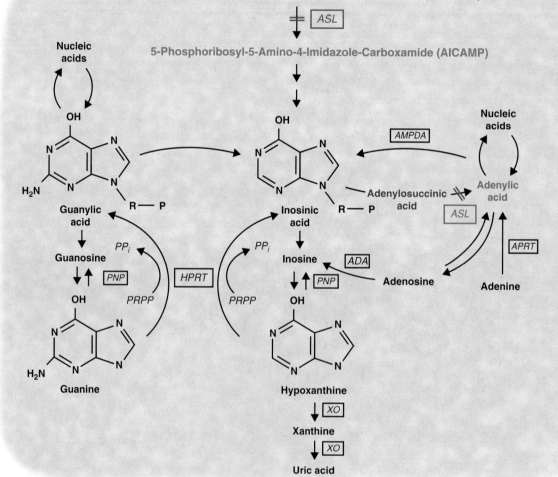

FIGURE 44-6. Adenylosuccinate lyase deficiency. ASL = adenylosuccinate lyase; APRT = adenine phosphoribosyltransferase; GMP = guanylic acid; IMP = inosinic acid; HPRT = hypoxanthine:guanine phosphoribosyl transferase; PRPP = phosphoribosylpyrophosphate; AICA = aminoimidazole carboxamide; AICAMP = AICAR = AICA ribotide; SAICAMP = SAICAR = succinyl-AICAR; APRT = Adenine phosphoribosyltransferase; ADA = Adenosine deaminase; PNP = Purine nucleoside phosphorylase; AMPDA = Adenylate deaminase; XO = xanthine oxidase.

occurred in many; early-onset seizures have been associated with death in infancy (48). Autistic features in some have included absence of eye contact, repetitive behavior, temper tantrums, and self-injurious behavior, none of them rare in retarded individuals. Retardation of growth and muscle wasting also have been observed (40). In most patients, mental retardation has been severe (49), but there have been a few exceptions with milder delay (40,46).

Biochemical/Enzymatic Characteristics A distinctive feature of ASL deficiency that simplifies the detection of this disorder is the accumulation of adenylosuccinate and SAICA riboside, the dephosphorylated products of the substrates for the defective enzyme. These compounds give a positive Bratton–Marshall reaction (50). Confirmation of this positive screening test is done by identification of adenylosuccinate and SAICA riboside in urine or blood, usually by HPLC (39). Both compounds are also elevated in the CSF, where concentrations are 20- to 100-fold those of plasma and are as high as 500 μmol/L (39,51). Urinary excretions range from 25–700 mmol/mol of creatinine (39,40,51).

The enzyme generally has been assayed by following the conversion of adenylosuccinate to AMP spectrophotometrically. Deficiency of activity has been documented in liver, fibroblasts, and lymphocytes (52).

Genetics/Molecular Features The disorder is autosomal recessive. Molecular analysis in the first reported Moroccan family with four affected children (39,40) indicated homozygosity for a point mutation resulting in a serine-to-proline change (S438P). Heterozygosity was documented in the parents. Another mutation in a gypsy patient (53), G1279A, converted a well-conserved arginine at 401 to histidine. Other missense mutations, a 39-bp deletion and a splice-site mutation and a nonsense mutation, have been described, indicating a high degree of molecular heterogeneity.

Treatment Specific therapy is not available. Seizures are treated with anticonvulsant agents.

ADENINE PHOSPHORIBOSYLTRANSFERASE (APRT) DEFICIENCY

Etiology/Pathophysiology Deficiency of APRT, first reported in 1976 (54,55), is one of the causes of urinary tract stones in children (56). Calculi are composed of 2,8-dihydroxyadenine and may be mistaken for those of uric acid when colorimetric tests for uric acid are employed. These assays have been replaced largely by uricase or HPLC, but it pays to check because clinical chemistry laboratories do not list their methodology on the order form.

The disease may be first recognized in adults, particularly in Japan, where the disease is more common (57).

Clinical Manifestations Deficiency of APRT owes its clinical expression entirely to the insolubility of 2,8-dihydroxyadenine, which leads to nephrolithiasis and nephropathy (58,59). The severity of the disease is quite variable, ranging from asymptomatic to life-threatening renal disease. Onset of symptoms has ranged from birth to 74 years (57). Patients may have hematuria, dysuria, crystalluria, or urinary tract infection, as well as calculi. Patients may have renal colic or urinary retention. Acute renal failure may be caused by dehydration in the presence of crystalluria. This may be reversible, but the long-term outcome may be chronic renal failure leading to dialysis or renal transplantation (59).

Plain roentgenograms of the abdomen usually are negative because 2,8-dihydroxyadenine stones, like those of uric acid, are radiolucent. Abdominal ultrasound or intravenous urography should identify radiolucent stones.

Biochemical/Enzymatic Features APRT catalyzes the conversion of adenine to its mononucleotide (AMP), so it is a purine salvage enzyme (see Figure 44-7). Deficiency of APRT is readily documented by assay of erythrocyte lysates. There may be no activity, or in some patients there is residual activity up to 10% to 25% of control activity.

Deficiency of APRT leads to accumulation of adenine, which is oxidized in the presence of xanthine oxidase to 2,8-dihydroxyadenine, which is very insoluble. The excretion of adenine and 2,8-dihydroxyadenine occurs in a ratio of 1:1.5. 8-Hydroxyadenine is excreted in lesser amounts

Genetic/Molecular Features APRT deficiency is transmitted in an autosomal recessive fashion. The gene is localized to chromosome 16q24.3 (60). It has been cloned and sequenced, and a number of mutations has been identified (61), including three mutations that account for 96% of the mutant alleles found in Japan (62).

Many patients are compounds of two mutant alleles. A T insertion in intron 4 at the splice donor site has been found in five families from Europe and the United States; it leads to abnormal splicing and loss of exon 4 in the mRNA (63) and creates an MseI restriction site that is useful in diagnosis.

Among Japanese patients with the milder phenotype, the most common mutation is a T-to-C mutation that changes methionine 136 to threonine (M136T) (62). Three mutations account for 95% of the mutant alleles in Japanese patients (62).

Treatment Therapy is aimed at reducing the formation of 2,8-dihydroxyadenine by the use of a low-purine diet and allopurinol (56,58). A dose of allopurinol of 10 mg/kg/day up to 300 mg in an adult has virtually eliminated 2,8-dihydroxyadenine from the urine (58,64). A high fluid intake is prudent. Alkali therapy is not beneficial; the solubility of 2,8-dihydroxyadenine is not altered by changes of urinary pH in the range obtainable physiologically. Stones may be treated with lithotripsy.

ADENOSINE DEAMINASE DEFICIENCY

Etiology/Pathophysiology The association of adenosine deaminase (Figure 44-8) (ADA) deficiency and severe combined immunodeficiency disease (SCID)(65) provides clear evidence of the importance of purine nucleotides in immunodeficiency. The discovery came during review of polymorphic markers in candidates for bone marrow transplantation for SCID (65). One and then a second unrelated patient were found to be deficient in ADA. Within a year, there were many immunodeficient patients with ADA deficiency (66). Gilbert and her colleagues used the same approach to discover purine nucleoside phosphorylase deficiency (see below).

ADA is an enzyme of purine interrelations that converts adenosine to inosine (see Figure 44-8). This is an important reaction because adenosine is not a substrate for nucleoside phosphorylase, which converts inosine and guanosine to hypoxanthine and guanine. ADA is distributed widely in animal tissues. ADA and purine nucleoside phosphorylase (PNP) deficiencies represent enzymatic defects that affect primarily cells of the immune system. The mechanism appears to be the accumulation of purine nucleotides and deoxynucleotides that are toxic to T and B cells (67).

Clinical Manifestations Patients with classical ADA deficiency have a distinct syndrome of SCID. They have both defective immmunoglobulins or bone marrow–derived B-cell function and defective cell-mediated immunity or thymus-derived T-cell function. Patients with B-cell immunodeficiency have infections caused by organisms such as the *Pneumococcus* with capsules as well as some viruses. Patients with T-cell or cell-mediated immunodeficiency have infections caused by opportunistic organisms, such as *Monilia*. In the first months of life, patients with SCID present with failure to thrive and diarrhea (65,67,68). Severe bacterial and viral infections occur very early.

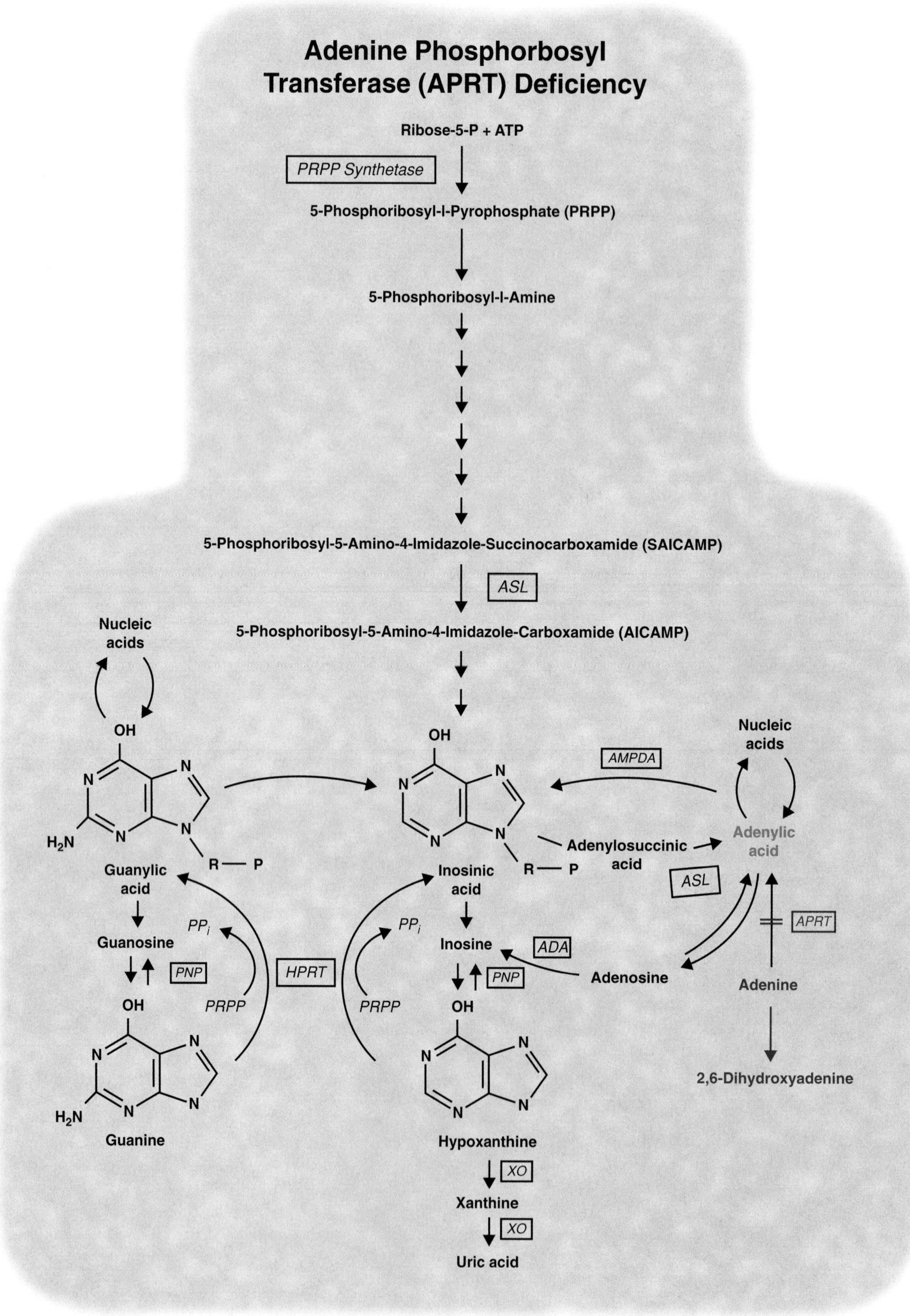

FIGURE 44-7. Adenine phosphoribosyltransferase deficiency. ASL = adenylosuccinate lyase; APRT = adenine phosphoribosyltransferase; GMP = guanylic acid; IMP = inosinic acid; HPRT = Hypoxanthine-guanine phosphoribosyl transferase; PRPP = phosphoribosylpyrophosphate; AICA = aminoimidazole carboxamide; AICAMP = AICAR = AICA ribotide = ZMP; SAICAMP = SAICAR = succinyl-AICAR; APRT = Adenine phosphoribosyltransferase; ADA = Adenosine deaminase; PNP = Purine nucleoside phosphorylase; AMPDA = Adenylate deaminase; XO = xanthine oxidase.

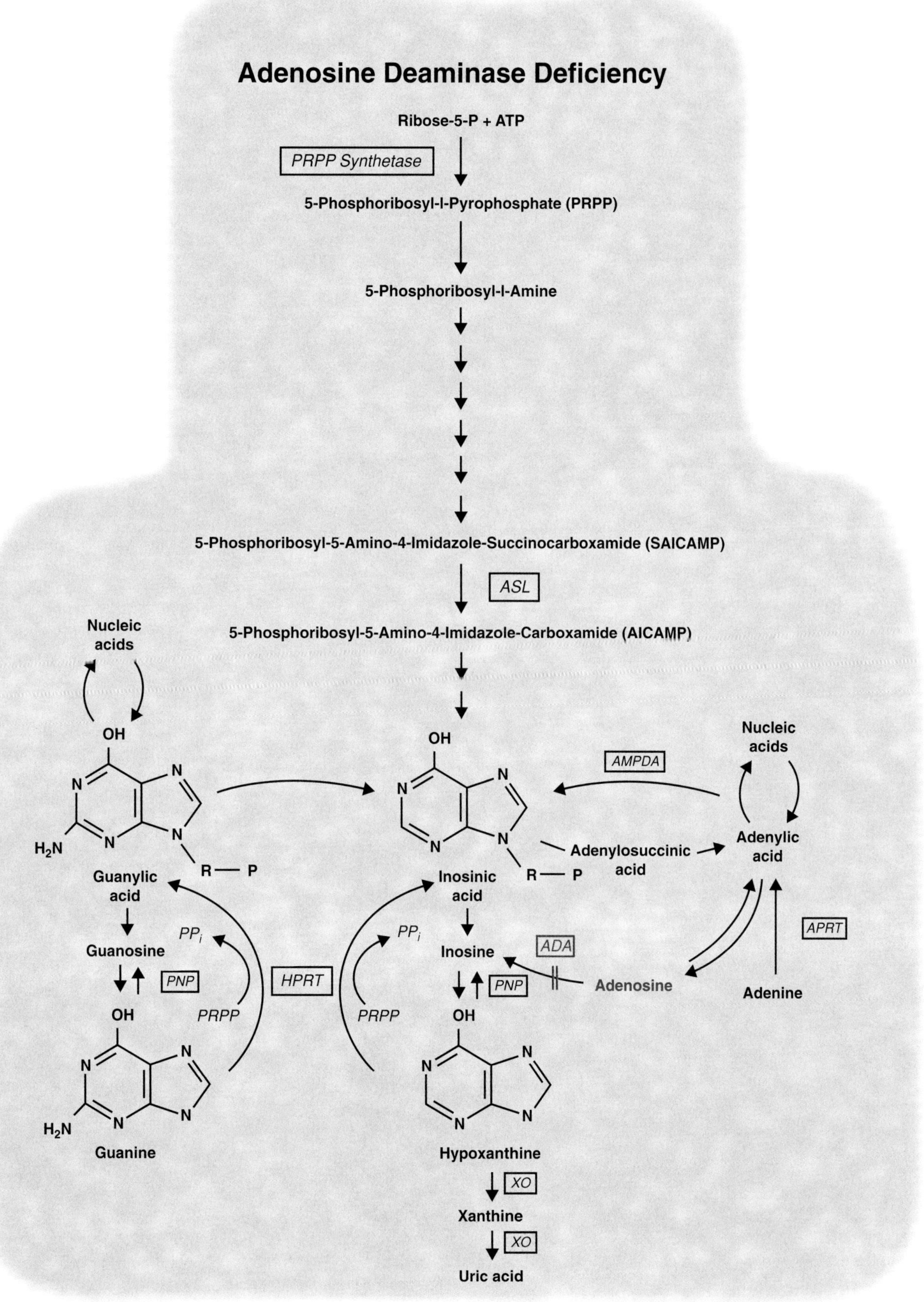

FIGURE 44-8. Adenosine deaminase deficiency. ASL = adenylosuccinate lyase; APRT = adenine phosphoribosyltransferase; GMP = guanylic acid; IMP = inosinic acid; HPRT = Hypoxanthine-guanine phosphoribosyl transferase; PRPP = phosphoribosylpyrophosphate; AICA = aminoimidazole carboxamide; AICAMP = AICAR = AICA ribotide = ZMP; SAICAMP = SAICAR = succinyl-AICAR; APRT = Adenine phosphoribosyltransferase; ADA = Adenosine deaminase; PNP = Purine nucleoside phosphorylase; SCID = Severe combined immunodeficiency; AMPDA = Adenylate deaminase; XO = xanthine oxidase.

Extensive candidiasis is the rule. A SCID triad is thrush, diarrhea, and pneumonia. Many have bacterial infections of the skin, and recurrent otitis media is common, as is pneumonia. Many patients have died, often of infections with opportunistic organisms.

Patients are at risk for the development of graft-versus-host disease from blood transfusion or for disseminated disease following immunization with live-attenuated vaccines, such as poliomyelitis. Known patients are better immunized with Salk inactivated vaccine. Patients surviving infancy may have pulmonary insufficiency, a consequence of repeated infection.

Autoimmune disease is also a feature of ADA deficiency, including autoimmune thyroid insufficiency, autoimmune thrombocytopenia, and fatal autoimmune hemolytic anemia.

Neurological abnormalities may occur in ADA deficiency. They may be the consequence of the type of life-threatening disease seen in these patients, but in some, neurological abnormality has appeared to be an intrinsic feature. Patients have had spasticity, nystagmus, tremors, dystonic posturing, athetosis, hypotonia, and head lag (69,70). In at least one patient, improvement was documented after successful treatment with enzyme replacement (70). Developmental delay has been reported to be more prevalent in ADA-deficient patients with SCID than in ADA-normal patients with SCID (69).

Hepatic dysfunction observed in this disease may be a consequence of infection. Many patients have elevated transaminase levels. Recurrent hepatitis has led to chronic hepatobiliary disease. B-cell lymphomas have been related to infection with Epstein-Barr virus.

There is also a bony dysphasia in this disease (71). The sacroiliac notch may be large, and the acetabular angle may be reduced. The ribs are flared, enlarged anteriorly, and cupped at the costochondral ends. There is platyspondyly. Growth arrest lines may be unusually thick. Roentgenograms of the bones also may reveal profound osteoporosis and vertebral compression fractures. Most patients have chronic pulmonary disease, such as in infections with *Pneumocystis carinii*.

Examination of the blood reveals profound lymphopenia. Total lymphocyte count may be less than 500/μL.

Skin tests for delayed hypersensitivity are deficient, and skin tests for *Candida* are negative in patients with florid candidiasis. The response of lymphocytes in vitro to phytohemagglutinin and other lectins is reduced or absent, and the formation of T-cell rosettes is poor. All the immunoglobulins in these patients are decreased, and the antibody response to an immunizing antigen is faulty.

Pathological examination of the thymus at autopsy has revealed a very small organ with little differentiation into lobules. No Hassall corpuscles are seen.

Biochemical/Enzyme Characteristics ADA catalyzes the irreversible deamination of adenosine (see Figure 44-8) to form inosine and of deoxyadenosine to form deoxyinosine. ADA may be assayed in the erythrocyte, and there is no detectable activity in most patients (67). A screening test permits the diagnosis on spots of dried blood in neonatal screening.

In ADA deficiency, adenosine and 2'-deoxyadenosine accumulate in plasma, and large amounts of deoxyadenosine are excreted in the urine. Prenatal diagnosis has been accomplished by assay of the enzyme in cultured amniocytes and chorionic villus samples (72). In heterozygous carriers for ADA deficiency, levels of enzyme activity are about half the normal level (72), but detection of carriers by enzyme assay in erythrocytes or fibroblasts is not reliable.

Genetic/Molecular Features ADA deficiency is autosomal recessive. The gene is on chromosome 20q13.11 (73). It has been cloned and sequenced, and a considerable number of mutations has been identified (74,75), most of them single-amino-acid changes. In a family in which the mutation is known, this is a reliable approach to carrier detection and prenatal diagnosis.

Heterogeneous pattern of mutations causes deficient enzyme activity, and most patients are compounds of two different mutant genes. A 329V mutation, a relatively common mutation, has been found in a number of unrelated patients (74); so has R211H. Splice-site mutations, such as a G-to-A change in IVS10 that inserts 100 amino acids, have been observed in patients with more indolent disease, suggesting that alternate splicing may provide useful amounts of the wild-type enzyme (76,77).

Treatment Bone marrow transplantation is the definitive treatment of ADA deficiency (78). Enzyme-replacement therapy has been developed using bovine ADA conjugated to polyethylene glycol (PEG-ADA) (79). Intramuscular PEG-ADA treatment restores immune competence. PEG-ADA also has been employed to prepare very ill patients for transplantation. ADA deficiency also has been treated by gene therapy, in which hematopoietic cells of the patient are recipients for gene transfer of human ADA genes and then are infused. To date, all patients so treated also have received PEG-ADA, making the issue of expression of ADA difficult to assess.

PURINE NUCLEOSIDE PHOSPHORYLASE DEFICIENCY

Etiology/Pathophysiology Purine nucleoside phosphorylase (PNP, see Figure 44-9) deficiency causes a clinical syndrome of SCID indistinguishable from that of ADA deficiency. This disorder also was discovered by Enid Gilbert and her colleagues (80,81). PNP catalyzes the reversible phosphorolytic cleavage of inosine and guanosine to their respective bases hypoxanthine and guanine. Deoxyinosine and deoxyguanosine are also substrates. The disease is a rare autosomal recessive disorder.

Clinical Manifestations PNP deficiency is unique among immunodeficiency diseases because it presents with impressive hypouricemia. Concentrations of uric acid in blood may be under 1 mg/dL, and urinary excretion of uric acid is also reduced (80,82). Patients may have SCID, but some have had cellular immunodeficiency with normal humoral immunity. They may present early in infancy with viral infections, such as disseminated varicella. They also may have recurrent of otitis media, diarrhea, sinusitis, or pneumonia (83). One patient died of generalized vaccinia following vaccination (84).

Patients are lymphopenic, and lymphocyte response to phytohemagglutinin is deficient. The thymic shadow is absent on roentgenograms. Immunoglobulins may be normal or low. Neurological abnormalities have been observed in about half the patients (85,86) Varying degrees of developmental delay have been associated with spastic tetraparesis, hypotonia or hypertonia, ataxia, and tremor. Autoimmune disorders have been observed, particularly hemolytic anemia (87), but also thrombocytopenia, neutropenia, systemic lupus, and CNS vasculitis. B-cell lymphomas have been reported (86).

Biochemical/Molecular Features The enzyme deficiency can be demonstrated in erythrocyte lysates or cultured fibroblasts (88,89). The activity in intact erythrocytes correlates more closely with phenotypic severity than that of lysates (89). Prenatal diagnosis may be made by assay of cultured amniocytes or chorionic villus cells (90–92). Heterozygotes may have intermediate levels of activity.

In the presence of PNP deficiency, levels of inosine and guanosine and their deoxy counterparts are elevated in blood and urine.

Treatment The definitive treatment is bone marrow transplantation from a histocompatible donor (93), which also can improve neurological symptoms.

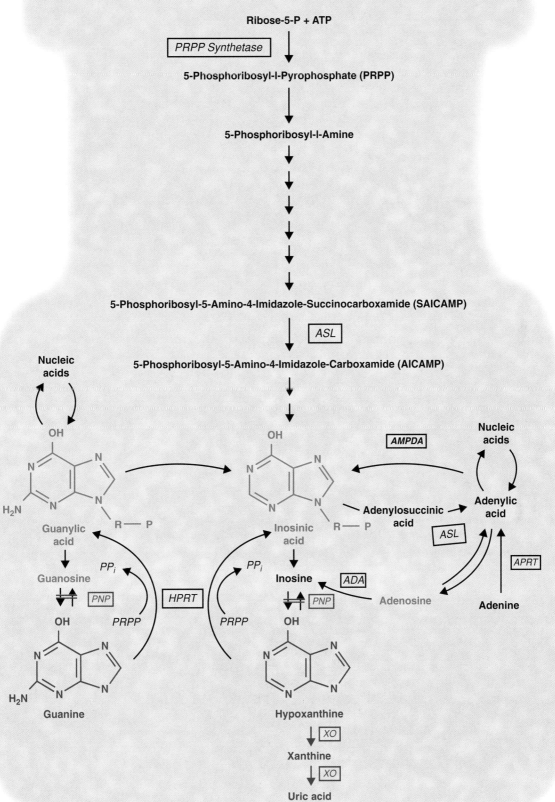

FIGURE 44-9. Purine nucleoside phosphorylase deficiency. ASL = adenylosuccinate lyase; APRT = adenine phosphoribosyltransferase; GMP = guanylic acid; IMP = inosinic acid; HPRT = Hypoxanthine-guanine phosphoribosyl transferase; PRPP = phosphoribosylpyrophosphate; AICA = aminoimidazole carboxamide; AICAMP = AICAR = AICA ribotide = ZMP; SAICAMP = SAICAR = succinyl-AICAR; APRT = Adenine phosphoribosyltransferase; ADA = Adenosine deaminase; PNP = Purine nucleoside phosphorylase; AMPDA = Adenylate deaminase; XO = xanthine oxidase.

MYOADENYLATE DEAMINASE DEFICIENCY

Etiology/Pathophysiology Inherited deficiency of myoadenylate deaminase is associated with pain or cramps in muscle following exercise (94). Many affected individuals are asymptomatic. Deficiency of the enzyme has been found in 2% of a large number of muscle biopsies submitted for pathological analysis (95). Affected individuals all have been homozygous for a C-to-T transition at nucleotide 34 that changes glutamine to a stop codon (Q12X) (96).

Variable expression can be explained by the fact that there is alternative splicing of the AMPDA1 gene that removes exon 2 containing the mutation and leads to a catalytically active enzyme (97,98). There are other AMPDA isozymes, one of which, AMPDA3, also expresses in muscle (99). There also may be hybrid AMPDA1/AMPDA3 enzymes (99).

Clinical Manifestations Patients with AMPDA1 deficiency characteristically develop myalgia, cramps, or fatigue following vigorous or even moderate exercise. They do not develop muscle wasting, and the histological appearance of muscle is unremarkable. A majority of patients have been male. An increase in creatine kinase in the blood is seen in about half the patients, but in some this increase occurs only following exercise. Myoglobinuria has been observed rarely (100,101). The electromyogram may be normal.

The onset of symptoms maybe in infancy, but more often it is in adolescence or adulthood. A much more severe disease was reported in 11 families in Finland (102). The phenotype included hypotonia, visual failure, and mental retardation.

The nosology of the disease has been confused by the description of what has been called *acquired myoadenylate deaminase deficiency* (103), in which heterozygotes for the common transition at nucleotide C34T have another disease, myopathy, collagen disease, or chronic licorice ingestion that further reduces enzyme activity. The E isozyme coded for by AMPDA3 is found in erythrocytes. Complete deficiency of erythrocyte AMPDA activity has been described in asymptomatic individuals in Japan (104).

The forearm ischemic exercise test, which assesses for an absence of the normal rise in venous ammonia, is a useful screening test (105,106).

Biochemical/Enzyme Characteristics The enzyme aminohydrolase (AMP) deaminase catalyzes the conversion of AMP to IMP and

NH₃. This enzyme with adenylosuccinate synthetase and adenylosuccinate lyase constitutes the purine nucleotide cycle (see Figure 44-10). The activities of the three enzymes are much greater in skeletal muscle than in other tissues, and that of aminohydrolase deaminase (AMPDA) is 100 times that of the other two (107,108). Flux through the cycle in muscle increases with exercise, providing energy through the citric acid cycle and rapid repletion of adenosine triphosphate (ATP).

Genetic/Molecular Features The gene AMPDA1 is located on the short arm of chromosome at 1p13-21 and contains 16 exons over 23 kb (109). Diagnosis classically has been made by assay of enzyme activity in biopsied muscle. Immunoreactive AMPDA1 protein is undetectable. The C34T mutation abolishes a Mae II restriction site, providing a simple diagnostic test (96,106,109). It also can be used for heterozygote detection.

Treatment Prudent restriction of exercise usually is effective in avoiding symptomatology. Efforts to increase replenishment of ATP pools have been recommended (107), and there are conflicting reports that the administration of ribose in doses up to 200 mL/kg/h to increase PRPP synthesis decreases symptoms (110,111). Measures, as yet undiscovered, to increase the rate of alternate splicing to remove exon 2 or to increase expression of the AMPD3 gene might be expected to be therapeutic.

XANTHINE OXIDASE DEFICIENCY–HEREDITARY XANTHINURIA

Etiology/Pathophysiology Hereditary xanthinuria is an inborn error of purine metabolism that results from deficiency of xanthine (see Figure 44-11) oxidase. The deficiency leads to very low levels of uric acid in body fluids, and many patients are recognized because of hypouricemia. In patients with what has been referred to as type I disease, there is isolated deficiency of xanthine oxidase, and patients can oxidize allopurinol to oxypurinol because this conversion is catalyzed by aldehyde oxidases. Type II patients are both deficient in the activity of oxidase and cannot metabolize allopurinol (112). A third group of patients has deficient activity of sulfite oxidase as well, and they have molybdenum cofactor deficiency (see below).

Clinical Features More than half the recognized patients are asymptomatic. They usually are ascertained because of hypouricemia or because of an affected relative. Those

with symptoms usually have xanthine calculi. These may lead to hematuria, renal colic, urinary tract infection, and hydronephrosis (113). This constellation ultimately can lead to uremia and renal failure, but most patients have a more benign course. Stones also may lead to acute renal failure, even in childhood (114–116). Pains or cramps in muscles, particularly after stressful exercise, which increases purine nucleotide turnover in muscle, have been observed in some patients (117–119). In this situation, crystals of xanthine have been found in muscle. Crystals of xanthine are not found in joints, and there are no deposits in the renal parenchyma.

Xanthine calculi are not radiopaque except when calcium is codeposited. They may be found by ultrasound or by pyelography. They may be identified chemically by HPLC, infrared or mass spectrometry, or x-ray crystallography.

Biochemical/Molecular Characteristics The diagnosis usually is made by assays of the xanthine and the other oxypurines in the urine. In the presence of a low-purine diet, normal oxypurine excretion is 2–3 mmol (500 mg)/24 h, and more than 90% is uric acid; the ratio of hypoxanthine to xanthine is 1.4:1. In xanthinuria, the total is 1–2 mmol/24 h, uric acid is very low, and the ratio of hypoxanthine to xanthine 1:4 (120). Plasma concentrations of xanthine may be 10–40 times the normal level of 1 μmol/L (120).

The deficient activity of xanthine oxidase has been demonstrated in biopsied liver and intestine. An *in vivo* method of demonstrating xanthine oxidase deficiency is by measuring urinary pterin and isoxanthopterin after oral tetrahydrobiopterin administration (121). The distinction between type I and type II xanthinuria usually is made by measuring plasma oxypurinol 90 minutes after administration of 300 mg oral allopurinol; oxypurinol formation indicates type I (122).

Mutations in the gene for xanthine oxidase have been demonstrated in type I xanthinuria in three Japanese patients (123). A C682G mutation changed arginine 228 to a stop codon. A fourth patient also had a stop codon.

Treatment In the presence of normal HPRT, most of the xanthine found in the urine is thought to come from the action of guanase on guanine (112,122,124,125). It is thought that treatment with allopurinol to inhibit residual activity of xanthine oxidase would be ineffective in reducing urinary xanthine, but this has not been studied systematically. A diet low in purines and a high fluid intake appear prudent. Stones may be treated with lithotripsy.

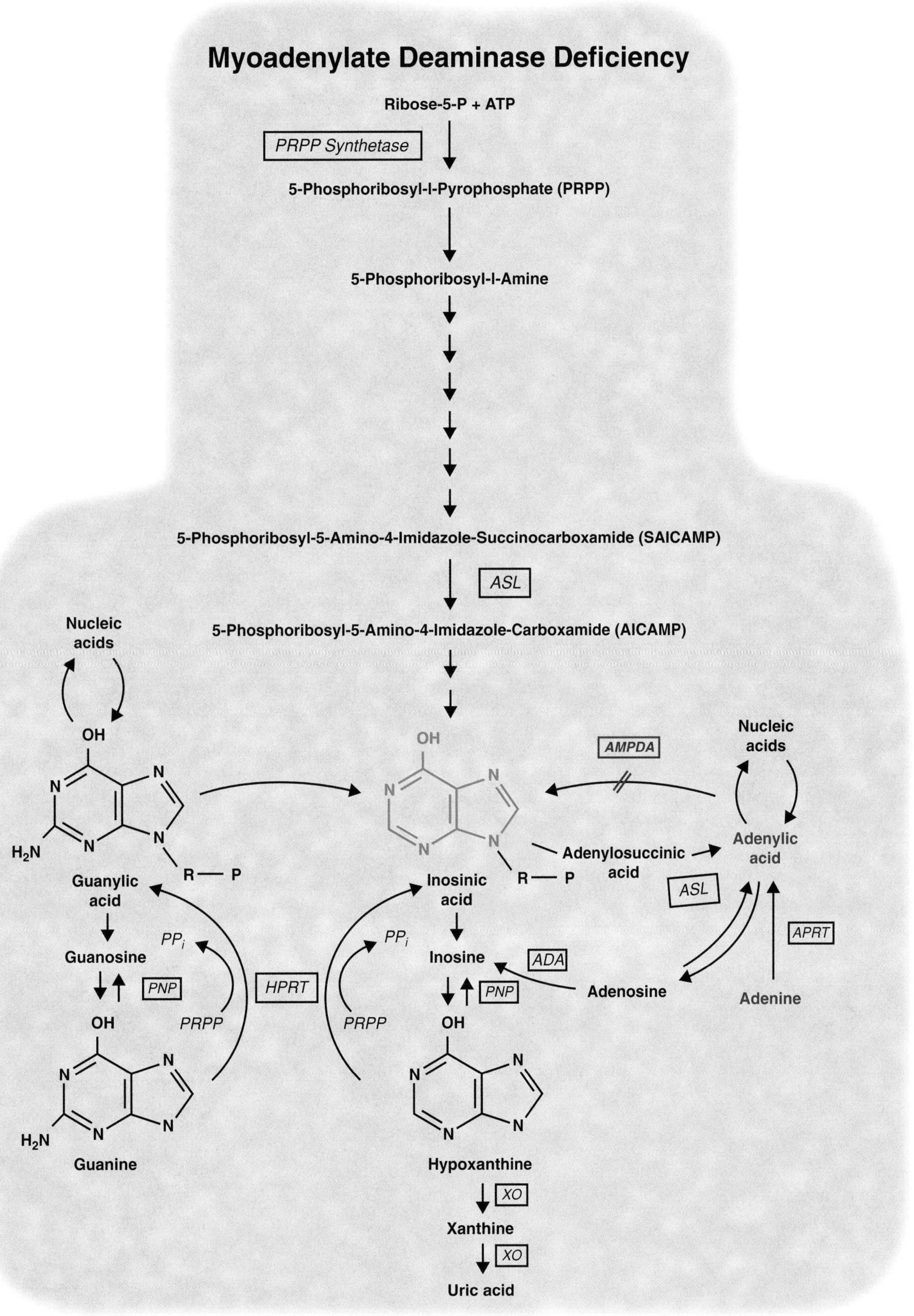

FIGURE 44-10. Myoadenylate deaminase deficiency. ASL = adenylosuccinate lyase; APRT = adenine phosphoribosyltransferase; GMP = guanylic acid; IMP = inosinic acid; HPRT = Hypoxanthine-guanine phosphoribosyl transferase; PRPP = phosphoribosylpyrophosphate; AICA = aminoimidazole carboxamide; AICAMP = AICAR = AICA ribotide = ZMP; SAICAMP = SAICAR = succinyl-AICAR; APRT = Adenine phosphoribosyltransferase; ADA = Adenosine deaminase; PNP = Purine nucleoside phosphorylase; AMPDA = Adenylate deaminase; XO = xanthine oxidase.

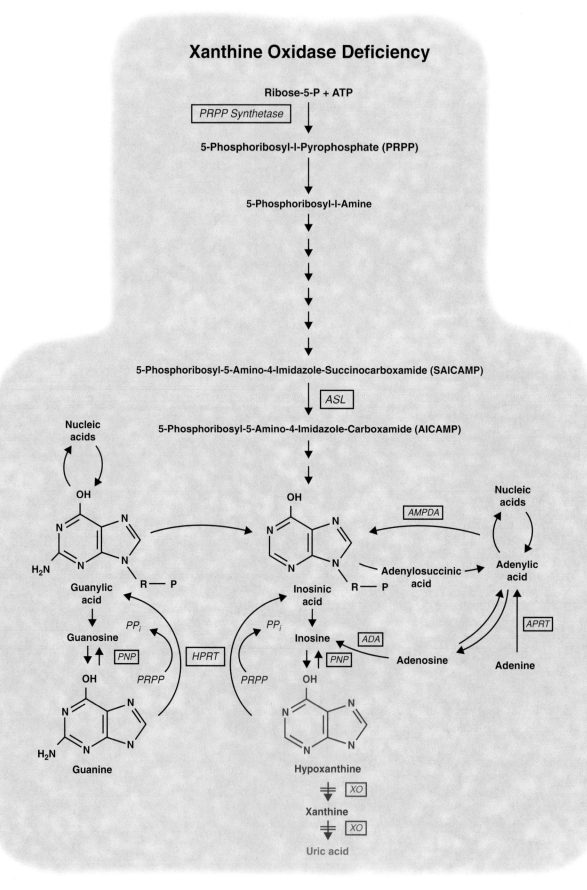

FIGURE 44-11. Xanthine oxidase deficiency. ASL = adenylosuccinate lyase; APRT = adenine phosphoribosyltransferase; GMP = guanylic acid; IMP = inosinic acid; HPRT = Hypoxanthine-guanine phosphoribosyl transferase; PRPP = phosphoribosylpyrophosphate; AICA = aminoimidazole carboxamide; AICAMP = AICAR = AICA ribotide = ZMP; SAICAMP = SAICAR = succinyl-AICAR; APRT = Adenine phosphoribosyltransferase; ADA = Adenosine deaminase; PNP = Purine nucleoside phosphorylase; AMPDA = Adenylate deaminase; XO = xanthine oxidase.

MOLYBDENUM COFACTOR AND ISOLATED SULFITE OXIDASE DEFICIENCY

Etiology/Pathophysiology Deficiency of the molybdenum cofactor results in a combined deficiency of xanthine oxidase and sulfite oxidase. A molybdenum-containing cofactor serves as cofactor for three enzymes: xanthine oxidase, aldehyde oxidase, and sulfite oxidase. Patients affected with molybdenum cofactor or isolated sulfite oxidase deficiency usually have a devastating disease of the CNS that is attributable to deficiency of the latter enzyme.

Clinical Manifestations Deficiency of xanthine oxidase and sulfite oxidase was first described in 1978 (126). The classical presentation is with severe neonatal seizures, often status epilepticus (127–130). This is also the presentation of severe isolated deficiency of sulfite oxidase. Many have died early in infancy. Seizures are difficult to control with anticonvulsant medications. There may be feeding difficulties early, but patients surviving the neonatal period may feed well and grow normally. Axial hypotonia and extremity hypertonicity are characteristic. Deep tendon reflexes are brisk, and there may be ankle clonus. The Babinski response is positive. Seizures are tonic–clonic, but later patients may develop myoclonus. Mental retardation is global.

Patients surviving the neonatal period develop subluxed ocular lenses (131,132). They also may have nystagmus, cortical blindness, enophthalmos, spherophakia, or coloboma of the iris. The facial appearance of these patients is similar (133). Dysmorphic features include a long face, puffy cheeks, widely spaced eyes, elongated palpebral fissures, and a long philtrum. Microcephaly maybe progressive, but the head may appear small even in patients in whom the circumference is within normal limits. Some have developed hydrocephalus.

The electroencephalogram (EEG) may reveal focal or generalized dysrhythmia. We have observed a burst-suppression pattern in the neonatal period.

Neuroimaging studies may reveal decreased density of the white matter. Soon the overwhelming appearance is that of atrophy. Thalamic calcifications have been observed (134). Pathology of the brain is that of atrophy and microgyria (135) with underlying severe loss of neurons and white matter.

Biochemical/Enzyme Characteristics Hypouricemia due to deficiency of xanthine oxidase is a readily detected feature by which these patients may be recognized. A caution is that in the neonatal period, when these patients

usually present with intractable seizures, uric acid levels are higher, so this may be misleading. Analysis of the urine for oxypurines yields information on the impressive xanthinuria. Hypoxanthine is also elevated. In isolated sulfite oxidase deficiency, purine metabolites are normal.

Sulfituria is another characteristic. Sulfite oxidase is the terminal enzyme in the oxidative degradation pathway of sulfur-containing amino acids. This disease provides an argument for the continued use of sulfite dipsticks in programs of screening for metabolic disease. Fresh urine is important because of oxidation of sulfite to sulfate (136). A refrigerated sample still may be positive for up to 4 days and a frozen one for up to 7 days.

The key component is S-sulfocysteine, which is markedly elevated in the urine. It is best assayed by tandem mass spectrometry. The compound is formed by direct reaction of sulfite with cysteine. Urinary thiosulfate is also increased. Urinary sulfate should be decreased, but adequate normative data for children are not available. Lactic acidemia has been observed in a rare later-onset patient with what appeared to be static encephalopathy (137).

Enzyme assay is done most conveniently for sulfite oxidase because it is expressed in cultured fibroblasts (130). Deficiency of both enzymes has been documented in liver. Prenatal diagnosis has been accomplished by assay of sulfite oxidase activity in chorionic villus cells (138). It also may be done by assay for S-sulfocysteine in amniotic fluid.

The molybdenum cofactor is a small molecule in which molybdenum is complexed with a unique pterin, molybdopterin. It is a cofactor for aldehyde oxidase, as well as the other two enzymes. It is synthesized in a series of steps from a guanosine phosphate. The gene MOCS1 (6p21.3) which results through alternative splicing in two products MOCS1A and MOCS1B is required for the conversion to precursor Z, which is converted to molybdopterin. This is catalyzed by a two-subunit molybdopterin synthase. Two more genes are required for the addition of molybdenum, among them the gene for geophyrin. The activities of cofactor in three patients' livers have been studied using rat liver demolybdosulfate oxidase, and all were completely deficient (139,140).

Genetic/Molecular Features The diseases is autosomal recessive. Patients with molybdenum cofactor deficiency have been found to fall into two complementation groups. Those in group A are defective in early steps in the pathway and have mutations in MOCS1 (138). Those in group B are deficient in the molybdopterin synthase step, coded for by MOCS2 (5q11), and a number of mutations

has been described. In another patient a frame-shift deletion has been found in geophyrin. The majority of mutations identified have been at the MOCS1 locus on chromosome 6 (141). Prenatal diagnosis has been carried out by analysis of a splice-site mutation in MOCS1 (142). In addition, in isolated sulfite oxidase deficiency, mutations were identified in the human sulfite oxidase gene in cell lines from patients.

Treatment No effective therapy has been devised. Diets low in methionine (XMet, SHS) have been effective in milder isolated sulfite oxidase–deficient patients. Vigabatrin or other anticonvulsants may be used in the chronic control of seizures.

OROTIC ACIDURIA

Etiology/Pathophysiology Orotic aciduria is an inherited disorder of *de novo* pyrimidine biosynthesis (see Figure 44-2). It was studied initially in detail in a single patient who died of overwhelming varicella at 2 1/2 years (143). Extensive studies carried out on the family established its genetic transmission as autosomal recessive and localized the metabolic defect (144). The defective enzyme uridine 5'-monophosphate (UMP) (see Figure 44-12) synthase contains in one polypeptide coded for by a single gene (145,146) the activities of two enzymes, orotic acid phosphoribosyltransferase (OPRT) and orotidine-5'-monophosphate (ODC) decarboxylase, that catalyze the last two steps of UMP synthesis.

Clinical Manifestations Orotic aciduria is a rare disease characterized by megaloblastic anemia that is resistant to therapy with vitamin B_{12}, folic acid, or ascorbic acid (147–149). Leukopenia or neutropenia has been present in most patients. Platelet counts have been normal. A devastating response to what is usually mild infection is seen often in megaloblastic anemias of early life, and immunodeficiency has been documented in some patients (150), along with diarrhea and stomatitis.

The feature that led to the original recognition of the condition was crystalluria (143). Crystals precipitated on standing at room temperature and were particularly prominent at times of acute illness when the patient reduced fluid intake. Urethral and ureteral obstructions have been observed on the basis of precipitated crystals (148,151). Hematuria, azotemia, and renal colic have been seen (148,150,151).

Retardation of physical and intellectual development has been observed (148,152) but not invariably because treatment has become available (151). On the other hand, one patient had delayed development and oculomotor dyspraxia without hematological abnormalities (153).

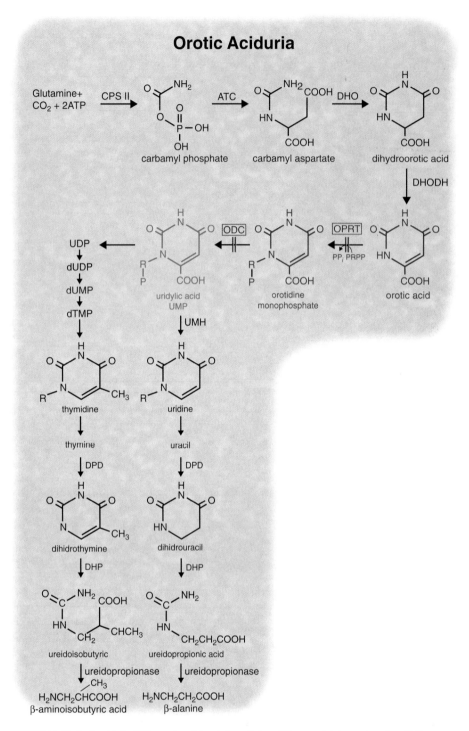

Orotic Aciduria

FIGURE 44-12. Orotic aciduria. CPSII = carbamylphosphate synthetase; ATC = aspartate transcarbamylase; DHO = dihydroorotase; DHODH = dihydroorotate dehydrogenase; OMP = orotidine monophosphate; OPRT = orotic acid phosphoribosyltransferase; ODC = orotidine 5-phosphate decarboxylase; UMH = UMP hydrolase; DPD = dihydropyrimidine dehydrogenase; DHP = dihydropyrimidinase; UMP = uridine monophosphate.

The hair may be sparse and fail to grow, and the fingernails have been noted not to grow. Untreated patients may be pale, fail to thrive, and develop recurrent serious infections.

Biochemical/Enzyme Features In orotic aciduria, only orotic acid is found in excess in the urine. Levels of orotic acid in the urine have ranged from 1–10 mmol/mol of creatinine, whereas normal individuals excrete less than 10 μmol/mol of creatinine (147,154). Increased excretion of orotic acid has been observed in heterozygotes.

The activities of both enzymes, OPRT and ODC, are deficient in erythrocytes, leukocytes, and cultured patient's fibroblasts. Heterozygotes have intermediate levels of activity, but they cannot always be distinguished reliably from normal (155). The distinction bewteen type 2 orotic aciduria, because of a patient with demonstrable deficiency of the decarboxylase, and normal OPRT activity seems artificial now that it is clear that there is only one gene and one protein.

Genetics/Molecular Features The UMP synthase gene has been localized to chromosome 3q13. The gene contains six exons spanning approximately 15 kb. Two patients had a C378T missense mutation (P92S); in one, a T961A mutation also was missense (I286N). In another family, two alleles contained R96G and V109G (156). The patient with no megaloblastic anemia had a T928G mutation (I310V) (153).

Treatment Orotic aciduria represents metabolic pyrimidine "starvation" in humans. The therapeutic effect of uridine is supportive of this hypothesis. Excellent remission has been obtained regularly with doses of 50–300 mg/kg/day; some patients relapsed with less than 100 mg/kg, and only one required more than 200 mg/kg (150,157,158). Hematological response is accompanied by weight gain and improvement in activity and well-being. Orotic aciduria has not yet been treated with triacetyluridine, but it doubtless would be effective because its oral bioavailability is higher.

PYRIMIDINE NUCLEOTIDE DEPLETION AND OVERACTIVE CYTOSOLIC 5'-NUCLEOTIDASE

Etiology/Pathophysiology A syndrome has been observed in six patients in whom increased degradation of purine and pyrimidine nucleotides is associated with a phenotype that has been attributed to pyrimidine nucleotide depletion (159). The activity of 5'-nucleotidase was found to be increased in cultured fibroblasts.

Clinical Manifestations Patients have had developmental delay, seizures, and alopecia. There was evidence of mild immunodeficiency; infections, particularly sinusitis, have been recurrent. Some patients have had ataxia, an awkward gait, and mildly impaired fine motor control. Speech problems, including slurring and tremulous intonation, have been consistent features. Each has had a striking pattern of hyperactive and aggressive behavior, along with distractibility and an inability to focus. Two have had scaling dermatosis. Macrocytic anemia was found in two patients.

Biochemical/Enzyme Features Each patient has had decreased quantities of uric acid in the urine. Reported amounts ranged from 0.41–0.76 mg/mg of creatinine (160), all lower than controls of that age (161).

Cultured fibroblasts were found to incorporate orotic acid or uridine poorly into nucleotides. Enzymatic analysis revealed six- to eightfold increased activity of 5'-nucleotidase tested with purine or pyrimidine monophosphate. The enzyme was the cytosolic high K_m enzyme usually activated by ATP, and this activation was found to be defective in the patients.

Genetic/Molecular Features The disease has to date been found in different families and in patients of both sexes. It is likely to be autosomal recessive. Analysis of the gene for 5'-nucleotidase has failed to reveal any molecular abnormalities, suggesting that the overactivity is secondary to a molecular defect not yet identified.

Treatment Treatment with uridine was found to ameliorate most of the manifestations of the disease. More recently, patients have been treated with triacetyl uridine, which has much better oral bioavailability than uridine and releases uridine into the blood and tissues. In this disorder, as in hereditary orotic aciduria, the therapeutic principle appears to be the supply of needed pyrimidine nucleotide via salvage of the nucleoside.

PYRIMIDINE-5'-NUCLEOTIDASE DEFICIENCY

Etiology/Pathophysiology Pyrimidine-5'-nucleotidase deficiency was reported as a cause of hemolytic anemia by Valentine and colleagues in 1974 (162). The enzyme is specific for pyrimidine nucleotides; hydrolysis of purine nucleotides is normal in this disease (163). There may be two cytosolic pyrimidine-5'-nucleotidases, only one of which is important for hydrolysis of nucleotides in erythrocytes (164).

Clinical Manifestations Patients present in infancy or early childhood with jaundice and anemia (162,165–168). The spleen may be enlarged, and sometimes the liver, and there may be basophilic stippling of erythrocytes. Anemia may be chronically mild or moderate, with hemoglobin concentrations approximately 10 mg/dL, but exacerbations of severe hemolysis occur with infections or pregnancy, leading to hemoglobin levels of 5 mg/dL. Reticulocyte concentrations may be as high as 45%. The plasma bilirubin is unconjugated. Haptoglobin may be decreased and erythrocyte glutathione increased. Hemoglobinuria occurs (167), and kidneys may be enlarged and accumulate iron. Two patients had an acute aplastic crisis following an infection with parvovirus (168). Reported hypotonia and mental retardation (166) could be unrelated.

Biochemical/Enzyme Features Erythrocyte concentrations of pyrimidine nucleotides may be three to six times normal (166), particularly those of cytidine (160). The high concentration of nucleotides in erythrocytes makes it possible to diagnose this disorder by nuclear magnetic resonance (NMR) spectroscopy (170). It also makes for a screening procedure useful in diagnosis by measuring the ultraviolet absorption maximum of deproteinated erythrocytes. There is a shift from the normal wavelength of 256–257 nm to 266–270 nm (165,171).

The activity of the enzyme is reduced to 0% to 30% of normal levels (167); some relatively high levels may be a function of the fact that the enzyme is much more active in young cells, and these patients have a high proportion of reticulocytes.

Genetic/Molecular Features The disease is autosomal recessive. Heterozygotes as a group have intermediate levels of erythrocyte enzyme, but overlap makes a normal level insecure. Altered kinetic properties of the enzyme in some families make the occurrence of different mutations probable.

Treatment No specific therapy has been developed. Management should be that of any hemolytic anemia. Splenectomy does not seem to help.

DIHYDROPYRIMIDINE DEHYDROGENASE DEFICIENCY

Etiology/Pathophysiology Dihydropyrimidine dehydrogenase (DPD see Figure 44-13) catalyzes the first step in the degradation of the pyrimidine bases uracil and thymine. NADPH is a cofactor, and the dehydro-products are dihydrouracil and dihydrothymine. 5-Fluorouracil (5-FU) and other 5'-substituted analogues, such as bromo- and nitrouracils, are also substrates, and therefore, patients with cancer treated with 5-FU may develop severe toxicity to the usual chemotherapeutic doses if they have deficiency of DPD (172). Although severe DPD deficiency is rare, as many as 5% of patients may have deficiency that could lead to life-threatening toxicity; therefore, testing has been recommended prior to the use of 5-FU.

Clinical Manifestations Most patients with severe deficiency of DPD have presented with developmental delay or seizures or both (173–178). Most appeared normal at birth. A few have been thought to have normal intelligence. Autistic behavior has been observed in a few. Some have had mild learning disabilities, but some have been severely retarded (177). Microcephaly, increased deep tendon reflexes, and monoplegia have been observed. One patient had multiple subdural hematomas (179). Ocular abnormalities have been found in one patient who also had the Kearns–Sayre mtDNA deletion and in others.

Another group of patients has been discovered, even as late as 40 years of age, because of toxic reactions to 5-FU (179–181). Reactions include severe neurological dysfunction and loss of speech and ability to move extremities. Magnetic resonance imaging (MRI) was consistent with demyelination. Death has been observed. Two patients discovered in this way had been in excellent heath prior to the development of a tumor.

Biochemical/Enzyme Features In nonchemotherapy patients, the diagnosis is first suspected in study of the urine, which reveals large amounts of uracil and thymine. Levels 1000 times normal have been found (174). Uracil excretion has ranged from 56–683 mmol/mol of creatinine, and thymine, 7–439 mmol/mol of creatinine. In some, 5-hydroxymethyluracil has been found in amounts as high as 54 mmol/mol of creatinine. Isotope dilution gas chromatography mass spectrometry (GCMS) analysis of amniotic fluid for uracil and thymine has been employed successfully in prenatal diagnosis (182). Plasma levels of 20–25 μM are 100 times normal.

Deficiency of the enzyme may be documented in liver, erythrocytes, leukocytes, or cultured fibroblasts (174,183). Levels may be 0% to 5% of normal. Heterozygotes have had levels of 30% to 80% of normal (173). Studies of enzyme activity are important for diagnosis because uraciluria and thyminuria may occur in other conditions, such as dihydropyrimidinase deficiency (see below) and hyperammonemia, as in urea cycle defects and the breakdown of pseudouridine, often excreted in cancer patients. In patients uncovered because of 5-FU toxicity, levels of enzyme activity have ranged from undetectable to 30% of control (180,184).

Genetic/Molecular Features Deficiency of DPD is autosomal recessive. Despite intermediate values in heterozygotes, carriers cannot be distinguished reliably from normal individuals by enzyme assay. If the mutation in a family is known, molecular detection of heterozygosity and prenatal diagnosis are reliable. Patients with clinical symptoms of DPD deficiency are homozygous. Those uncovered because of 5-FU toxicity may be homozygous or heterozygous.

The gene has 23 exons and has been mapped to chromosome 1p22 (185). A splice-site mutation IVS14+1GnA that leads to skipping of exon 14 is relatively common in European populations (186,187). This causes loss of a restriction site and provides a rapid test for the mutation; it has been

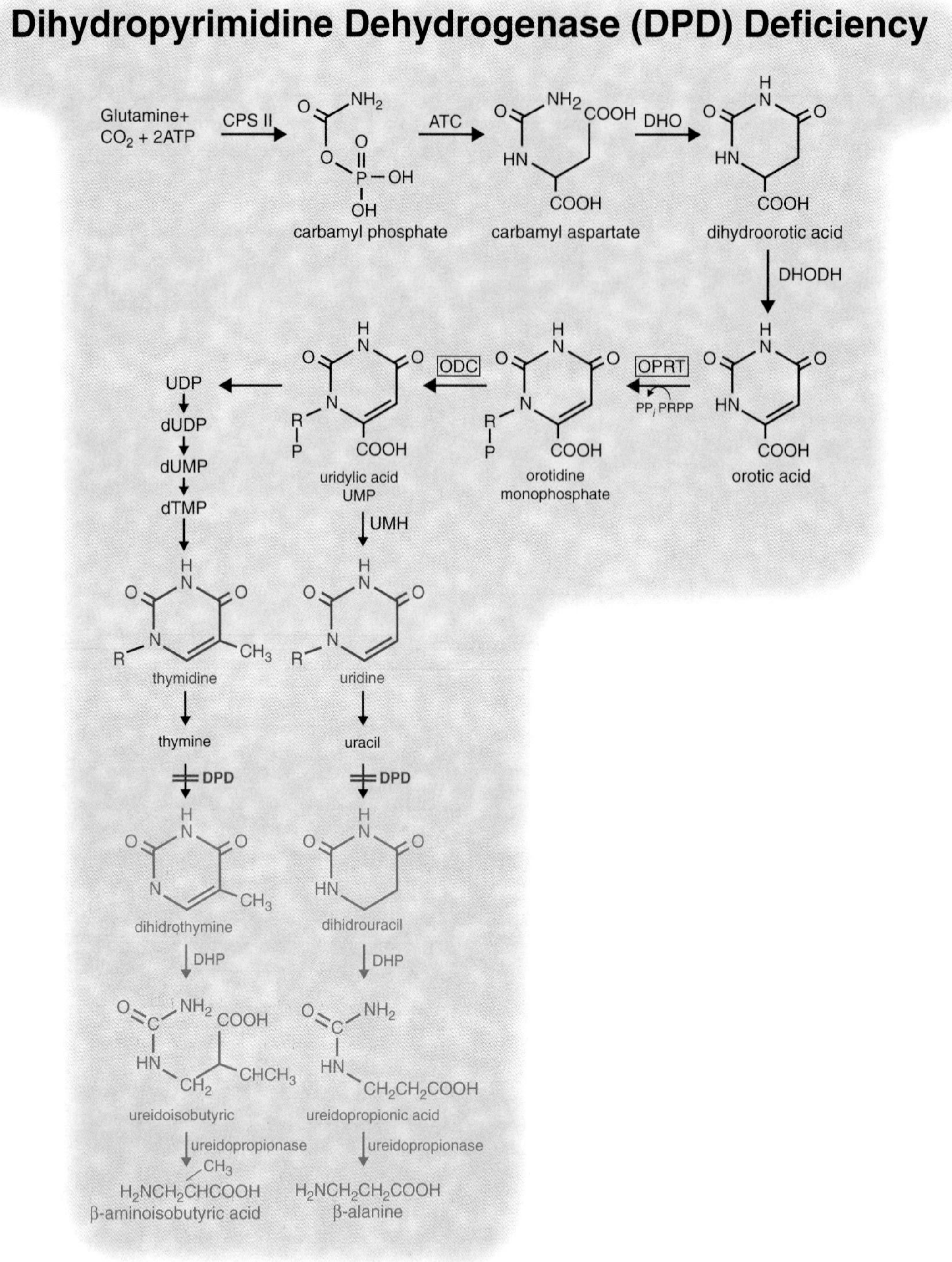

Dihydropyrimidine Dehydrogenase (DPD) Deficiency

FIGURE 44-13. Dihydropyrimidine dehydrogenase deficiency. CPSII = carbamylphosphate synthetase; ATC = aspartate transcarbamylase; DHO = dihydroorotase; DHODH = dihydroorotate dehydrogenase; OMP = orotidine monophosphate; OPRT = orotic acid phosphoribosyltransferase; ODC = orotidine 5-phosphate decarboxylase; UMH = UMP hydrolase; DPD =dihydropyrimidine dehydrogenase; DHP = dihydropyrimidinase; UMP = uridine monophosphate.

proposed as a screening method for the avoidance of 5-FU toxicity in these populations (DPD1). A small number of other mutations has been discovered.

Treatment Specific treatment has not been defined. Convulsions are readily treated with anticonvulsants. The avoidance of toxicity from chemotherapy may be lifesaving.

DIHYDROPYRIMIDINASE DEFICIENCY (DIHYDROPYRIMIDINURIA)

Etiology/Pathophysiology Dihydropyrimidinase (DHP) deficiency leads to accumulations of dihydrouracil and dihydrothymine, as well as uracil and thymine. The disease has been encountered much less frequently than DDP

deficiency (188). The phenotype is not yet clear, but patients have had seizures and mental retardation (189).

Clinical Manifestations Patients with dihydropyrimidinuria have been ascertained by analysis of pyrimidines in the urine of patients with epilepsy and mental retardation. Microcephaly has been observed (188).

Another had intractable diarrhea and microvillous atrophy. The lack of other manifestations makes it likely that this was coincidence (190). One patient (189) had only one attack of seizures; otherwise, he developed normally. Two patients detected by a screening program in Japan were well (191,192).

As in the case of DPD deficiency, these patients can be suspected to be susceptible to 5-FU toxicity, but this has not been observed.

Biochemical/Enzyme Features   Dihydropyrimidinase catalyzes the conversion of dihydrouracil and dihydrothymine to ureidopropionic and ureidobutyric acids (see Figure 44-14). It is expressed in liver and kidney as a tetramer with four subunits of 54 kDa. The diagnosis is made by study of the pyrimidines of the urine. There are large amounts of uracil and thymine and larger amounts of their dihydro derivatives.

The defective activity of the enzyme is documented by assay of biopsied liver (188). This is important because in the presence of bacteria, as in urinary tract infection, dihydropyrimidines may be converted to their carbamoylamine products (193).

Genetic/Molecular Features   The disease is autosomal recessive. Consequently, it has been observed in Turkish and Pakistanian families reported from Europe. The gene has been mapped to chromosome 8q22 (194). It contains 10 exons. Mutation analysis indicated a frame-shift mutation in exon 5; 812–814 insA causes a shift at codon 272 and termination at codon 287 (194). Expression yielded very low activity of the enzyme. This also was true of five missense mutations. W360R alters the region needed for assembly of the tetramer, and expressions yielded profound deficiency of immunoprecipitable enzyme (194,195).

Treatment   Supplementation with β-alanine has been tried, but results are not available.

UREIDOPROPIONASE DEFICIENCY

Etiology/Pathophysiology   β-Ureidopropionase catalyzes the third step in the catabolism of uracil and thymine, the conversions of ureidopropionic and ureidobutyric acids to β-alanine and β-aminoisobutyric acid (see Figure 44-15). A 17-month-old girl, product of consanguineous parents, was reported (196) who had large amounts of the two ureido (N-carbamyl) amino acids in her urine.

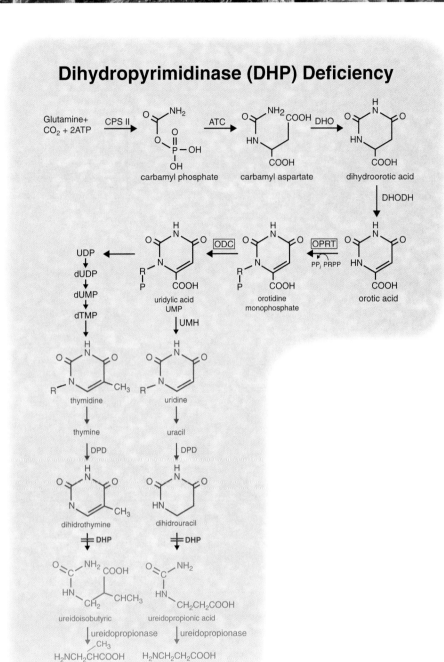

FIGURE 44-14. Dihydropyrimidinase deficiency. CPSII = carbamylphosphate synthetase; ATC = aspartate transcarbamylase; DHO = dihydroorotase; DHODH = dihydroorotate dehydrogenase; OMP = orotidine monophosphate; OPRT = orotic acid phosphoribosyltransferase; ODC = orotidine 5-phosphate decarboxylase; UMH = UMP hydrolase; DPD = dihydropyrimidine dehydrogenase; DHP = dihydropyrimidinase; UMP = uridine monophosphate.

Clinical Manifestations   The index patient (196) had severe developmental delay, hypotonia, and dystonia. She had optic atrophy and microcephaly. MRI showed aphasia of the cerebellar vermis, hypoplasia of the brain stem, and a thin corpus callosum. Three additional patients (197) presented with severe seizure disorders and developmental delay. Metabolic acidosis was present, as well as an elevated level of lactic acid in blood and CSF. Computed tomographic (CT) scan and ultra-

sound of the brain were unremarkable. It is conceivable that patients with a complete β-ureidopropionase deficiency are also at risk of developing severe 5-FU toxicity.

Biochemical/Enzyme Features   Analysis of the urine reveals moderately elevated levels of dihydrouracil and dihydrothymine, as well as of carbamylalanine and carbamyl-aminoisobutyric acid (196,197). The enzyme is expressed only in liver. It is a hexamer of 43-kDa

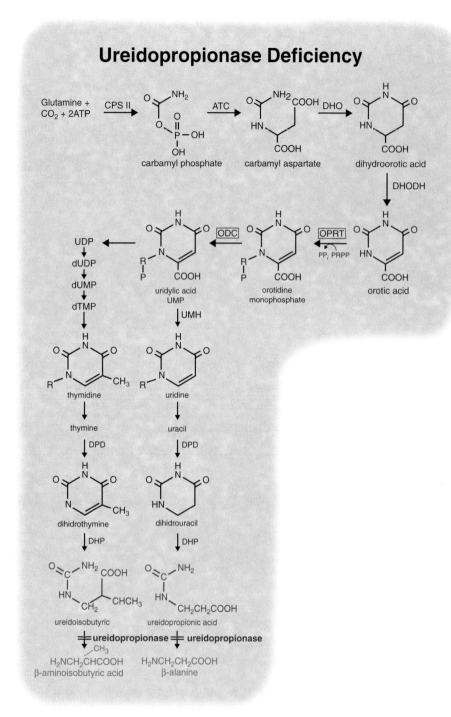

FIGURE 44-15. Ureidopropionase deficiency. CPSII = carbamylphosphate synthetase; ATC = aspartate transcarbamylase; DHO = dihidroorotase; DHODH = dihydroorotate dehydrogenase; OMP = orotidine monophosphate; OPRT = orotic acid phosphoribosyltransferase; ODC = orotidine 5-phosphate decarboxylase; UMH = UMP hydrolase; DPD = dihydropyrimidine dehydrogenase; DHP = dihydropyrimidinase; UMP = uridine monophosphate.

subunits. Deficiency of activity in biopsied liver has been documented in two patients (196,197). In another patient, biopsied liver revealed no enzyme activity or protein.

Elevated excretion of ureidopropionate also has been found in propionic acidemia (198). It appears that ureidopropionase is inhibited by propionic acid. It also may be found in DPH deficiency in the presence of a urinary tract infection (193).

Genetic/Molecular Features The disease is autosomal recessive. Three mutations have been defined, two splice-site mutations (IVS1-2AnG and IVS8-1GnA) and one missense mutation (A85E).

Treatment Treatment has not been defined. Supplementation of β-alanine did not result in clinical improvement.

REFERENCES

1. Hoffmann GF, Nyhan WL, Zschocke J, et al. *Core Handbooks in Pediatrics: Inherited Metabolic Diseases.* Philadelphia: Lippincott Williams & Wilkins; 2002
2. Lesch M., Nyhan WL. A familial disorder of uric acid metabolism and central nervous system function. *Am J Med.* 1964; 36:561–570.
3. Nyhan WL, Ozand P. *Atlas of Metabolic Disease,* 2nd ed. London: Arnold; 2005.
4. Christie R, Bay C, Kaufman IA, et al. Lesch–Nyhan disease: Clinical experience with nineteen patients. *Dev Med Child Neurol.* 1982;24:293.
5. WL Nyhan, HA Jinnah, JC Harris, et al. (updated November 2007) Lesch-Nyhan Syndrome in GeneReviews at Gene Tests: Medical Genetics Information Resource [database online]. Copyright, University of Washington, Seattle. 1997–2007. Available at http://www.genetest.org.
6. Puig GJ, Torres RJ, Mateos FA, et al. The spectrum of hypoxanthine–guanine phosphoribosyltransferase (HPRT) deficiency: Clinical experience based on 22 patients from 18 Spanish families. *Medicine.* 2001;80:102.
7. Seegmiller JE, Rosenbloom FM, Kelley WN. Enzyme defect associated with a sex-linked human neurological disorder and excessive purine synthesis. *Science.* 1967; 155:1682–1684.
8. Crawhall JC, Henderson JF, Kelley WN. Diagnosis and treatment of the Lesch–Nyhan syndrome. *Pediatr Res.* 1972;6:504.
9. De Gregorio L, Nyhan WL, Serafin E, et al. An unexpected affected female patient in a classical Lesch–Nyhan family. *Mol Genet Metab.* 2000;69:263–268.
10. Page T, Bakay B, Nissinen E, et al. Hypoxanthine guanine phosphoribosyl transferase variants: Correlation of clinical phenotype with enzyme activity. *J Inherited Metab Dis.* 1981;4:203–206.
11. Puig JG, Mateos FA, Torres RJ, et al. Purine metabolism in female heterozygotes for hypoxanthineguanine phosphoribosyltransferase deficiency. *Eur J Clin Invest.* 1998;28:950–957.
12. Nyhan WL, Bakay B, Connor JD, et al. Hemizygous expression of glucose-6-phosphate dehydrogenase in erythrocytes of heterozygotes for the Lesch–Nyhan syndrome. *Proc Natl Acad Sci USA.* 1970;65:2114.
13. Schretlen DJ, Harris JC, Park KS, et al. Neurocognitive functioning in Lesch–Nyhan disease and partial hypoxanthine–guanine phosphoribosyltransferase deficiency: *J Int Neurol Soc.* 2001;7:805–812.
14. Kaufman JM, Greene ML, Seegmiler JE. Urine uric acid to creatinine ratio: Screening test for disorders of purine metabolism. *Pediatrics.* 1968;73:583–592.
15. Ohdoi C, Nyhan WL, Kuhara T. Chemical diagnosis of Lesch–Nyhan syndrome using gas chromatography–mass spectrometry detection. *J Chromatogr.* 2003;792:123–130.
16. Jinnah HA, De Gregorio L, Harris JC, et al. The spectrum of inherited mutations causing HPRT deficiency: 75 new cases and a review of 196 previously reported cases. *Mutat Res.* 2000;463:309–326.

17. Kelley WL, Greene ML, Rosenbloom FM, et al. Hypoxanthine–guanine phosphoribosyltransferase deficiency in gout: A review. *Ann Intern Med.* 1969;70:155–206.

18. Kogut MD, Donnell GN, Nyhan WL, et al. Disorder of purine metabolism due to partial deficiency of hypoxanthine–guanine phosphoribosyltransferase. *Am J Med.* 1970;48:148–161.

19. Bakay B, Nissinen E, Sweetman L. Analysis of the radioactive and non-radioactive purine bases, nucleosides and nucleotide, by high-speed chromatography on a single column. *Anal Biochem.* 1978;86:65–77.

20. Page T, Bakay B, Nyhan WL. Kinetic studies of normal and variant hypoxanthine phosphoribosyltransferases in intact fibroblasts. *Anal Biochem.* 1982;122:144–147.

21. Page T, Broock RL, Nyhan WL, et al. Use of selective media for distinguishing variant forms of hypoxanthine phosphoribosyl transferase. *Clin Chim Acta.* 1986;154:195–202.

22. Page T, Nyhan WL, Morena de Vega V. Syndrome of mild mental retardation, spastic gait, and skeletal malformations in a family with partial deficiency of hypoxanthineguanine phosphoribosyltransferase. *Pediatrics.* 1987;79:713–717.

23. Catel VW, Schmidt J. Uber familiar gichtische Diathese in Verbindung mit zerebralen und renalen Symptomen bei einem Kleinkind. *Dtsch Med Wochenschr.* 1959;84:2145–2147.

24. Bakay B, Nissinen E, Sweetman L, et al. Utilization of purines by an HPRT variant in an intelligent, nonmutilative patient with features of the Lesch–Nyhan syndrome. *Pediatr Res.* 1979;13:1365–1370.

25. Sege-Peterson K, Chambers J, Page T, et al. Characterization of mutations in phenotypic variants of hypoxanthine–guanine phosphoribosyltransferase deficiency: *Hum Mol Genet.* 1992;1:427–432.

26. Sperling O, Eilma G, Persky-Brosh S, et al. Accelerated erythrocyte 5-phosphoribosyl-1-pyrophosphate synthesis: A familial abnormality associated with excessive uric acid production and gout. *Biochem Med.* 1972;6:310.

27. Nyhan WL, James JA, Teberg AJ, et al. A new disorder of purine metabolism with behavioral manifestations. *J Pediatr.* 1969;74:20–27.

28. Simmonds HA, Webster DR, Wilson J, et al. Evidence of a new syndrome involving hereditary uric acid overproduction, neurological complications and deafness. In: DeBruyn CHMM, Simmonds HA, Muller MM, eds. *Purine Metabolism in Man,* Vol. IV. New York: Plenum Press; 1984:97–102.

29. Becker MA, Meyer LJ, Seegmiller JE. Gout with purine overproduction due to increased phosphoribosylpyrophosphate synthetase activity. *Am J Med.* 1973;55:232.

30. DeVries A, Sperling O. Familial gouty malignant uric acid lithiasis due to mutant phosphoribosyltransferase synthetase. *Urologe A.* 1973;12:153.

31. Becker MA, Puig JG, Mateos FA, et al. Inherited superactivity of phosphoribosylpyrophosphate synthetase: Association of uric acid overproduction and sensorineural deafness. *Am J Med.* 1986;85:383.

32. Becker MA, Raivio KO, Bakay B, et al. Variant human phosphoribosylpyrophosphate synthetase altered in regulatory and catalytic functions. *J Clin Invest.* 1980;65:109–120.

33. Sperling O, Boer P, Persky-Brosh S, et al. Altered kinetic property of erythrocyte phosphoribosylpyrophosphate synthetase in excessive purine production. *Eur J Clin Biol Res.* 1972;17:73.

34. Becker MA, Smith PR, Taylor W, et al. The genetic and functional basis of purine nucleotide feedback-resistant phosphoribosylpyrophosphate synthetase superactivity: *J Clin Invest.* 1995;96:2133.

35. Taira M, Ishijima S, Kita K, et al. Nucleotide and deduced amino acid sequences of two distinct cDNAs for rat phosphoribosylpyrophosphate synthetase. *J Biol Chem.* 1987;262:14867.

36. Roessler BJ, NMosal JM, Smith PR, et al. Human X-linked phosphoribosylpyrophosphate synthetase superactivity is associated with distinct point mutations in the PRPS1 gene. *J Biol Chem.* 1993;268:26476.

37. Wada Y, Nishimura Y, Tanabu M, et al. Hypouricemic, mentally retarded infant with a defect of 5-phosphoribosyl-1-pyrophosphate synthetase of erythrocytes. *Tohuku J Exp Med.* 1974;113:149.

38. Marie S, Heron B, Bitoun P, et al. AICA-ribosiduria: A novel inborn error of purine biosynthesis caused by mutation of ATIC. *J Inherited Metab Dis.* 2001,27.

39. Jaeken J, Van den Berghe G. An infantile autistic syndrome characterized by the presence of succinylpurines in body fluids. *Lancet.* 1984;2:1058.

40. Jaeken J, Wadman SK, Duran M, et al. Adenylosuccinase deficiency: An inborn error of purine nucleotide synthesis. *Eur J Pediatr.* 1988;148:126.

41. Lowy BA, Ben-Zion, D. Adenylosuccinase activity in human and rabbit erythrocyte lysates. *J Biol Chem.* 1970;245:3043.

42. Van den Berghe G, Bontemps F, Vincent MF, et al. The purine nucleotide cycle and its molecular defects. *Prog Neurobiol.* 1992;39:547.

43. Fon EA, Demczuk S, Delattre O, et al. Mapping of the human adenylosuccinate lyase (ADSL) gene to chromosome 22q1.2.2-q1.3.2. *Cytogenet Cell Genet.* 1993;64:201.

44. Stone RL, Aimi J, Barshop BA, et al. A mutation in adenylosuccinate lyase associated with mental retardation and autistic features. *Nat Genet.* 1992;1:59.

45. Marie S, Race V, Nassogne M-C, et al. Mutation of a nuclear respiratory factor 2 binding site in the 5' untranslated region of the ADSL gene in three patients with adenylosuccinate lyase deficiency. *Am J Hum Genet.* 2002;71:14.

46. Jaeken JF, Van der Bergh F, Vincent MF, et al. Adenylosuccinase deficiency: A newly recognized variant. *J Inherited Metab Dis.* 1992;15:416.

47. Van den Bergh F, Vincent MF, Jaeken J, et al. Residual adenylosuccinase activities in fibroblasts of adenylosuccinase-deficient children: Parallel deficiency with adenylosuccinate and succinyl-AICAR in profoundly retarded patients and on parallel deficiency in a mildly retarded girl. *J Inherited Metab Dis.* 1993;16:415.

48. Köhler M, Assmann B, Bräutigam C, et al. Adenylosuccinase deficiency: Possibly underdiagnosed encephalopathy with variable clinical features. *Eur J Paediatr Neurol.* 1999;3:3.

49. Van den Berghe G, Vincent MF, Jaeken J. Inborn errors of the purine nucleotide cycle: Adenylosuccinase deficiency. *J Inherited Metab Dis.* 1997;20:193.

50. Laikind PK, Seegmiller JE, Gruber HE. Detection of 5'-phosphoribosyl-4-(N-succinylcarboxamide)-5-aminoimidazole in urine by use of the Bratton–Marshall reaction: Identification of patients deficient in adenylosuccinate lyase activity. *Anal Biochem.* 1986;156:81.

51. De Bree PK, Wadman SK, Duran M, et al. Diagnosis of inherited adenylosuccinase deficiency by thin-layer chromatography of urinary imidazoles and by automated cation exchange column chromatography of purines. *Clin Chim Acta.* 1986;156:279.

52. Van den Bergh F, Vincent MF, Jaeken J, et al. Radiochemical assay of adenylosuccinase: Demonstration of parallel loss of activity toward both adenylosuccinate and succinylaminoimidazole carboxamide ribotide in liver of patients with the enzyme defect. *Anal Biochem.* 1991;193:287.

53. Kmoch S, Hartmannova H, Krijt J, et al. Adenylosuccinase deficiency: Identification of a new disease-causing mutation. *J Inherited Metab Dis.* 1996;19:13.

54. Simmonds HA, Van Acker KJ, Cameron JS, et al. The identification of 2,8-dihydroxyadenine, a new compound of urinary stones. *Biochem J.* 1976;157:485.

55. Debray H, Cartier P, Temstet A, et al. Child's urinary lithiasis revealing a complete deficit in adenine phosphoribosyltransferase. *Pediatr Res.* 1976;10:762.

56. Barratt TM, Simmonds HA, Cameron JS, et al. Complete deficiency of adenine phosphoribosyltransferase: A third case presenting as renal stones in a young child. *Arch Dis Child.* 1979;54:25.

57. Kamatani N, Terai C, Kuroshima S, et al. Genetic and clinical studies on 19 families with adenine phosphoribosyltransferase deficiencies. *Hum Genet.* 1987;75:163.

58. Greenwood MC, Dillon MJ, Simmonds HA, et al. Renal failure due to 2,8-dihydroxyadenine urolithiasis. *Eur J Paediatr.* 1982;138:346.

59. Fye KH, Sahota A, Hancock DC, et al. Adenine phosphoribosyltransferase deficiency with renal deposition of 2,8-dihydroxyadenine leading to nephrolithiasis and chronic renal failure. *Arch Intern Med.* 1993;153:767.

60. Kahan B, Held KR, DeMars R. The locus for human adenine phosphoribosyltransferase on chromosome no. 16. *Genetics.* 1974;78:1143.

61. Sahota A, Chen J, Stambrook PJ, et al. Mutational basis of adenine phosphoribosyltransferase deficiency. *Adv Exp Med Biol.* 1991;309B:73.

62. Kamatani N, Hakoda M, Otsuka S, et al. Only three mutations account for almost all of defective alleles causing adenine phosphoribosyltransferase deficiency in Japanese patients. *J Clin Invest.* 1992;90:130.

63. Chan J, Sahota A, Martin GF, et al. Analysis of germline and in vivo somatic mutations in the human adenine phosphoribosyltransferase genes: Mutational hotspots at the intron 4 splice donor site and at codon 87. *Mutat Res.* 1993;287:217.

64. Simmonds HA, Cameron JS, Barratt TM, et al. Purine enzyme defects as a cause of acute renal failure in childhood. *Eur J Urol.* 1989;14:493.

65. Giblett ER, Anderson JE, Cohen F, et al. Adenosinedeaminase deficiency in two patients with severely impaired cellular immunity. *Lancet.* 1972;2:1067.

66. Pollara B, Pickering RJ, Meuwissen HJ. Combined immunodeficiency disease associated with adenosine deaminase deficiency, an inborn error of metabolism. *Pediatr Res.* 1973;7:362.

67. Hirschhorn R. Overview of biochemical abnormalities and molecular genetics of adenosine deaminase deficiency. *Pediatr Res.* 1993;33:S35.

68. Parkman R, Gelfand EW, Rosen FS, et al. Severe combined immunodeficiency and adenosine deaminase deficiency. *N Engl J Med.* 1975;292:714.

69. Stephan JL,Vlekova V, Le Deist F, et al. A retrospective single center study of clinical presentation and outcome in 117 patients. *J Pediatr.* 1993;123:564.

70. Hirschhorn R, Papageorgiou PS, Kesariwala HH, et al. Amelioration of neurologic abnormalities after "enzyme replacement" in adenosine deaminase deficiency. *N Engl J Med.* 1980;303:377.

71. Wolfson JJ, Cross VF. The radiographic findings in 49 patients with combined immunodeficiency. In: Meuwissen HJ, Pickering RJ, Pollara B, Porter IH, eds. *Combined Immunodeficiency Disease and Adenosine Deaminase Deficiency: A Molecular Defect.* New York: Academic Press; 1975:225.

72. Hirschhorn R, Beratis N, Rosen FS, et al. Adenosine deaminase deficiency in a child diagnosed prenatally. *Lancet.* 1975;1:73.

73. Petersen MB, Tranebjaerg L, Tommerup N, et al. New assignment of the adenosine deaminase gene locus to chromosome 20q13.11 by study of a patient with interstitial deletion 20q. *J Med Genet.* 1987;24:93.

74. Hirschhorn R, Ellenbogen A, Tzall S. Five missense mutations at the adenosine deaminase locus (ADA) detected by altered restriction fragments and their frequency in ADA: Patients with severe combined immunodeficiency (ADA-SCID). *Am J Med Genet.* 1992;42:201.

75. Markert ML. Molecular basis of adenosine deaminase deficiency. *Immunodeficiency.* 1994;5:141.

76. Santisteban I, Arredondo-Vega FX, Kelly S, et al. Novel splicing, missense, and deletion mutations in 7 adenosine deaminase deficient patients with late/delayed onset of combined immunodeficiency disease: Contribution of genotype to phenotype. *J Clin Invest.* 1993;92:820.

77. Arredondo-Vega FX, Santisteban I, Kelly S, et al. Correct splicing despite a GnA mutation at the invariant first nucleotide of a 5' splice site: A possible basis for disparate clinical phenotypes in siblings with adenosine deaminase (ADA deficiency. *Am J Hum Genet.* 1994;54:820.

78. Buckley RH. Breakthroughs in the understanding and therapy of primary immunodeficiency. *Pediatr Clin North Am.* 1994;41:665.

79. Hershfield MS, Chaffee S, Sorensen RU. Enzyme replacement therapy with polyethylene glycol–adenosine deaminase in adenosine deaminase deficiency: Overview and case reports of three patients, including two new receiving gene therapy. *Pediatr Res.* 1993;33:S42.

80. Giblett ER. ADA and PNP deficiencies: How it all began. *Ann NY Acad Sci.* 1985;451:1.

81. Giblett ER, Ammann AJ, Wara DW, et al. Nucleoside–phosphorylase deficiency in a child with severe defective T-cell immunity and normal B-cell immunity. *Lancet.* 1975;1:1010.

82. Simmonds HA, Sahota A, Potter CF, et al. Purine metabolism and immunodeficiency: Urinary purine excretion as a diagnostic screening test in adenosine deaminase and purine nucleoside phosphorylase deficiency. *Clin Sci Mol Med.* 1978;54:579.

83. Ammann AJ. Immunologic aberrations in purine nucleoside phosphorylase deficiencies. In: Elliot K, Whelan J, eds. *Enzyme Defects and Immune Dysfunction.* Ciba Foundation Symposium 68. New York: Excerpta Medica: 1979:55.

84. Virelizier JL, Hamet M, Ballet JJ, et al. Impaired defense against vaccinia in a child with T-lymphocyte deficiency associated with inosine phosphorylase defect. *J Pediatr.* 1978;92:358.

85. Simmonds HA, Fairbanks LD, Morris GS, et al. Central nervous system dysfunction and erythrocyte guanosine triphosphate depletion in purine nucleoside phosphorylase deficiency. *Arch Dis Child.* 1987;62:385.

86. Watson AR, Evans DK, Marsden HB, et al. Purine mucleoside phosphorylase deficiency associated with a fatal lymphoproliferative disorder. *Arch Dis Child.* 1981;56:563.

87. Rich KC, Arnold WJ, Palella T, et al. Cellular immune deficiency with autoimmune hemolytic anemia in purine nucleoside phosphorylase deficiency. *Am J Med.* 1979;67:172.

88. Chu SY, Cashion P, Jiang M. Purine nucleoside phosphorylase in erythrocytes: Determination of optimum reaction conditions. *Clin Biochem.* 1989;22:3.

89. Fairbanks JD, Simmonds HA, Webster DR. Usefullness of intact erythrocyte studies in the diagnosis of inherited purine and pyrimidine defects. In: Nyhan WL, Thompson LF, Watts RWF, eds. *Purine and Pyrimidine Metabolism in Man,* Vol. V, Part A: *Clinical Aspects Including Molecular Genetics.* New York: Plenum Press; 1986:101–107.

90. Dooley T, Fairbanks LD, Simmonds HA, et al. First trimester diagnosis of adenosine deaminase deficiency. *Prenat Diagn.* 1987;7:561.

91. Carapella De Luca E, Stegagno M, Dionisi Vici C, et al. Prenatal exclusion of purine nucleoside phosphorylase deficiency. *Eur J Pediatr.* 1986;145:51.

92. Durandy A, Peter MO, Freycon F, et al. Early prenatal diagnosis of inherited severe immunodeficiencies linked to enzyme deficiencies. *J Pediatr.* 1987;111:595.

93. Classen CF, Schulz AS, Sigl-Kraetzig M, et al. Successful HLA-identical bone marrow transplantation in a patient with PNP deficiency using busulfan and fludarabine for conditioning. *Bone Marrow Transplant.* 2001;28:93–96.

94. Fishbein WN, Armbrustmacher VW, Griffin JL. Myoadenylate deaminase deficiency: A new disease of muscle. *Science.* 1978;200:545.

95. Mercelis R, Martin J-J, de Barsy T,et al. Myoadenylate deaminase deficiency: Absence of correlation with exercise intolerance in 452 muscle biopsies. *J Neurol.* 1987;234.

96. Morisaki T, Gross M, Morisaki H, et al. Molecular basis of AMP deaminase deficiency in skeletal muscle. *Proc Natl Acad Sci USA.* 1992;89:6457.

97. Mineo I, Clarke PRH, Sabina RL, et al. A novel pathway for alternative splicing: Identification of an RNA intermediate that generates an alternative 5' splice donor site not present in the primary transcript of AMPD1. *Mol Cell Biol.* 1990;10:5271.

98. Morisaki H, Morisaki T, Newby LK, et al. Alternative splicing: A mechanism for phenotypic rescue of a common inherited defect. *J Clin Invest.* 1993;91:2275.

99. van Kuppevelt THv, Veerkamp JH, Fishbein WN, et al. Immunolocalization of AMP-deaminase isozymes in human skeletal muscle and cultured muscle cells: Concentration of isoform M at the neuromuscular junction. *J Histochem Cytochem.* 1994;42:861.

100. Tonin P, Lewis P, Servidei S, et al. Metabolic causes of myoglobinuria. *Ann Neurol.* 1990;27:181.

101. Zimmer C, Altenkirch H, Dorfumller-Kuchlin S, et al. Type 2a fiber rhabdomyolysis in myoadenylate deaminase deficiency. *J Neurol.* 1991;238:31.

102. Raivio KO, Santavuori P, Somer H. Metabolsim of AMP in muscle extracts from patients with deficient activity of myoadenylate deaminase. In: DeBruyn CHMM, Simmonds HA., Mullter M., eds. *Purine Metabolsim in Man,* Vol. IV. New York: Plenum Press; 1984:431.

103. Fishbein WN. Myoadenylate deaminase deficiency: Inherited and acquired forms. *Biochem Med.* 1985;33:158.

104. Ogasawara N, Goto H, Yamada Y, et al. Deficiency of erythrocyte type isozyme of AMP deaminase in human. In: Nyhan WL, Thompson LF, Watts RWF, eds. *Purine and Pyrimidine Metabolism in Man,* Vol. V, Part A: *Clinical Aspects Including Molecular Genetics.* New York: Plenum Press; 1986:123.

105. Valen PA, Nakayama DA, Veum JA, et al. Myadenylate deaminase deficiency: Diagnosis by forearm ischemic exercise testing. In: Nyhan WL, Thompson LF, Watts RWF, eds. *Purine and Pyrimidine Metabolism in Man,* Vol. V, Part B: *Basic Science Aspects.* New York: Plenum Press; 1986:525.

106. Baumeister FAM, Gross M, Wagner DR, et al. Mayoadenylate deaminase deficiency with severe rhabdomyolysis. *Eur J Pediatr.* 1993;152:513.

107. Sabina RL, Swain JL, Patten BM, et al. Disruption of the purine nucleotide cycle: A potential explanation for muscle dysfunction

in myoadenylate deaminase deficiency. *J Clin Invest.* 1980;66:1419.

108. Lowenstein JM. Ammonia production in muscle and other tissues: The purine nucleotide cycle. *Physiol Rev.* 1972;52:382.

109. Norman B, Mahnke-Zizelman DK, Vallis A, et al. Genetic and other determinants of AMP deaminase activity in healthy adult skeletal muscle. *J Appl Physiol.* 1998;85:1273.

110. Zollner N, Reiter S, Gross M, et al. Myoadenylate deaminase deficiency: Successful symptomatic therapy by high-dose oral administration of ribose. *Klin Wochenschr.* 1986;64:1281.

111. Lecky BRF. Failure of D-ribose in myoadenylate deaminase deficiency. *Lancet.* 1983;1:193.

112. Reiter S, Simmonds HA, Zollner N, et al. Demonstration of a combined deficiency of xanthine oxidase and aldehyde oxidase in xanthinuric patients not forming oxypurinol. *Clin Chim Acta.* 1990;187:221.

113. Carpenter TO, Lebowitz RL, Nelson D, et al. Hereditary xanthinuria presenting in infancy with nephrolithiasis. *J Pediatr.* 1986;109:307.

114. Bradbury MG, Henderson M, Brocklebank JT, et al. Acute renal failure due to xanthine stones. *Pediatr Nephrol.* 1995;9:476.

115. Bradbury MG, Henderson M, Brocklebank JT, et al. Acute renal failure due to xanthine stones. *Pediatr Nephrol.* 1995;9:476.

116. Simmonds HA, Cameron JS, Barratt TM, et al. Purine enzyme defects as a cause of acute renal failure in childhood. *Pediatr Nephrol.* 1989;3:433.

117. Chalmers RA, Watts RW, Bitensky L, et al. Microscopic studies on crystals in skeletal muscle from two cases of xanthinuria. *J Pathol.* 1969;99:45.

118. Landaas S, Borch K, Aagaard E. A new case with hereditary xanthinuria: Response to exercise. *Clin Chim Acta.* 1989;181:119.

119. Parker R, Snedden W, Watts RW. The quantitative determination of hypoxanthine and xanthine ("oxypurines") in skeletal muscle from two patients with congenital xanthine oxidase deficiency (xanthinuria). *Biochem J.* 1970;116:317.

120. Kojiima T, Nishina T, Kitamura M, et al. Biochemical studies on the purine metabolism of four cases with hereditary xanthinuria. *Clin Chim Acta.* 1984;137:189.

121. Blau N, de Klerk KJ, Thony B, et al. Tetrahydrobiopterin loading test in xanthine dehydrogenase and molybdenum cofactor deficiencies. *Biochem Mol Med.* 1996;58:199.

122. Yamamoto T, Higashino K, Kono N, et al. Metabolism of pyrazinamide and allopurinol in hereditary xanthine oxidase deficiency. *Clin Chim Acta.* 1989;180:169.

123. Ichida K, Amaya Y, Kamatani N, et al. Identification of two mutations in human xanthine dehydrogenase gene responsible for classical type I xanthinuria. *J Clin Invest.* 1997;99:2391.

124. Simmonds HA, Levin B, Cameron JS. Variations in allopurinol metabolism by xanthinuric subjects. *Clin Sci Mol Med.* 1974;47:839.

125. Salti IS, Kattuah N, Alam S, et al. The effect of allopurinol on oxypurine excretion in xanthinuria. *J Rheumatol.* 1976;3:201.

126. Duran M, Beemer FA, van der Heiden C, et al. Combined deficiency of xanthine oxidase and sulphite oxidase: A defect of molybdenum metabolism or transport? *J Inherited Metab Dis.* 1978;1:175.

127. Wadman SK, Duran M, Beemer FA, et al. Absence of hepatic molybdenum cofactor: An inborn error of metabolism leading to a combined deficiency of sulphite oxidase and xanthine dehydrogenase. *J Inherited Metab Dis.* 1983;6:78.

128. Ogier H, Saudubray JM, Charpentier C, et al. Double deficit en sulfite et xanthine oxidase, cause d'encephalopathie due a une anomalie hereditaire du metabolism edu molybden. *Ann Med Interne (Paris).* 1982;133:594.

129. Munnich A, Saudubray JM, Charpentier C, et al. Multiple molybdoenzyme deficiencies due to an inborn error of molybdenum cofacotor metabolism: Two additional cases in a new family. *J Inherited Metab Dis.* 1983;6:95.

130. Endres W, Shin YS, Gunther R, et al. Report on a new patient with combined deficiencies of sulphite oxidase and xanthine dehydrogenase due to molybdenum cofactor deficiency. *Eur J Paediatr.* 1988;148:246–249.

131. Lueder GT, Steiner RD. Ophthalmic abnormalities in molybdenum cofactor deficiency and isolated sulfite oxidase deficiency. *J Pediatr Ophthalmol Strabismus.* 1995;32:334.

132. Parini R, Briscioli V, Caruso U, et al. Spherophakia associated with molybdenum cofactor deficiency. *Am J Med Genet.* 1997;73:272.

133. de Klerk JBC, Bakker HD, Beemer FA, et al. Facial dysmorphism in molybdenum cofactor deficiency/sulfite oxidase deficiency. *Enzyme Protein.* 1996;49:185.

134. Slot HMJ, Overweg-Plandsoen WCG, Bakker HD, et al. Molybdenum-cofactor deficiency: An easily missed cause of neonatal convulsions. *Neuropediatrics.* 1993;24:139.

135. Roth A, Nogues C, Monnet JP, et al. Anatomopathological findings in a case of combined deficiency of sulphite oxidase and xanthine oxidase with a defect of molybdenum cofactor. *Virchows Arch (Pathol. Anat).* 1985;405:379.

136. Ker K, Potter M. Urine sulfite assay: How important is the "freshness" of urine samples? *Mol Gene Metab.* 2004;81:173.

137. Kleppe S, Shinawi M, Hunter J, et al. Atypical clinical and biochemical presentation in a patient with molybdenum cofactor deficiency. *Mol Gene Metab.* 2004;81:174.

138. Johnson J. Prenatal diagnosis of molybdenum cofactor deficiency and isolated sulfite oxidase deficiency. *Prenat Diagn.* 2003;23:6–8.

139. Johnson JL, Jones HP, Rajagopalan KV. Molecular basis of the biological function of molybdenum: Molybdenum-free sulfite oxidase from livers of tungsten-treated rats. *J Biol Chem.* 1974;249:5046.

140. Johnson JL, Jones HP, Rajagopalan KV. In vitro reconstitution of demolybdosulfite oxidase by a molybdenum cofactor from rat liver and other sources. *J Biol Chem.* 1977;252:4994.

141. Shalata A, Mandel H, Reiss J, et al. Localization of a gene for molybdenum cofactor deficiency, on the short arm of chromosome 6, by homozygosity mapping. *Am J Hum Genet.* 1998;63:148–154.

142. Reiss J. Prenatal diagnosis of molybdenum cofactor deficiency and isolated sulfite oxidase deficiency. *Prenat Diagn.* 1999;19:386.

143. Huguley C, Bain J, Rivers S, et al. Refractory megaloblastic anaemia associated with excretion of orotic acid. *Blood.* 1959;14:615.

144. Fallon H, Smith LJ, Graham J, et al. A genetic study of hereditary orotic aciduria. *N Engl J Med.* 1964;270:878.

145. Smith LJ, Sullivan M, Huguley C. Pyrimidine metabolism in man: IV. The enzymatic defect of orotic aciduria. *J Clin Invest.* 1961;40:656.

146. Suttle D, Bugg B, Winkler J, et al. Molecular cloning and nucleotide sequence for the complete coding region of UMP synthase. *Proc Natl Acad Sci. USA.* 1988;84:1754.

147. Becroft D, Phillips L. Hereditary orotic aciduria and megaloblastic anaemia: A second case with response to uridine. *B Med J.* 1965;1:547.

148. Haggard ME, Lockhart LH. Megaloblastic anemia and orotic aciduria: A hereditary disorder of pyrimidine metabolism responsive to uridine. *Am J Dis Child.* 1967;113:733.

149. Rogers L, Warford L, Patterson B, et al. Hereditary orotic aciduria: I. A new case with family studies. *Pediatrics.* 1968;42:415.

150. Girot R, Hamet M, Perignon J-L, et al. Cellular immune deficiency in two siblings with hereditary orotic aciduria. *N Engl J Med.* 1983;308:700.

151. Tubergen D, Krooth R, Heyn R. Hereditary orotic aciduria with normal growth and development. *Am J Dis Child.* 1984;118:1333.

152. Soutter J, Yu J, Lovric A, et al. Hereditary orotic aciduria. *Aust Paediatr J.* 1970;6:47.

153. Fairbanks LD, Marinaki AM, Besley GTN, et al. A point mutation resulting in hereditary orotic aciduria with neurological deficits but no megaloblastic anaemia. Bruges, Belgium. Eighth Symposium, European Society: Purine & Pyrimidine Metabolism in Man. 2001:59.

154. Alvarado C, Livingston L, Jones M, et al. Uridine-responsive hypogammaglobulinemia and congenital heart disease in a patient with hereditary orotic aciduria. *J Pediatr.* 1988;113:867.

155. Fox R, Wood M, Royse-Smith D, et al. Hereditary orotic aciduria: Types I and II. *Am J Med.* 1973;55:791.

156. Suchi M, Mizuno H, Kawai Y, et al. Molecular cloning of the human UMP synthase gene and characterization of point mutations in two hereditary orotic aciduria families. *Am J Hum Genet.* 1997;60:525.

157. Mcclar R, Black M, Jones M, et al. Neonatal diagnosis of orotic aciduria: An experience with one family. *J Pediatr.* 1983;102:85.

158. Sumi S, Suchi M, Kidouchi K, et al. Pyrimidine metabolism in hereditary orotic aciduria. *J Inherited Metab Dis.* 1997;20:104.

159. Page T, Yu A, Fontanesi J, et al. Developmental disorder associated with increased cellular nucleotidases activity. *Proc Natl Acad Sci USA.* 1997;94:11601.

160. Page T, Yu A, Fontenessi J, et al. A syndrome of seizures and pervasive developmental disorder associated with excessive cellular nucleotidases activity. New York: Plenum Press; 1998.

161. Kaufman JM, Greene ML, Seegmiller JE. Urine uric acid to creatinine ratio: A screening test for inherited disorders of purine metabolism. *J Pediatr.* 1968;73:583.

162. Valentine WN, Fink K, Paglia DE, et al. Hereditary hemolytic anemia with human erythrocyte pyrimidine 5'-nucleotidase deficiency. *J Clin Invest.* 1974;54:866.

163. Paglia DE, Valentine WN. Characteristics of a pyrimidine specific 5'-nucleotidase in human erythrocytes. *J Biol Chem.* 1975;250:7973.

164. Hirono A, Fujii H, Miyajima H, et al. Three families with hereditary hemolytic anemia and pyrimidine 5'-nucleotidase deficiency: electrophoretic and kinetic studies. *Clin Chim Acta.* 1983;130:189.

165. Torrance JD, Karabus CD, Shinier M, et al. Haemolytic anaemia due to erythrocyte pyrimidine 5'-nucleotidase deficiency. *S Afr Med J.* 1977;52:671.

166. Harley EH, Berman P. Diagnostic and therapeutic approaches in pyrimidine 5'-nucleotidase deficiency. In: DeBruyn CHMM, Simmonds, HA., Mullet MM, eds. *Purine Metabolism in Man*, Vol. IV. New York: Plenum Press; 1984:103.

167. Tomoda A, Noble NA, Lachant NA, et al. Hemolytic anemia in hereditary 5'-nucleotidase deficiency: Nucleotide inhibition of glucose-6-phosphate dehydrogenase and the pentose phosphate shunt. *Blood.* 1982;60:1212.

168. Paglia D, Fink K, Valentine W. Additional data from two kindreds with genetically-induced deficiencies of erythrocyte pyrimidine nucleotidases. *Acta Haematol (Basel).* 1980;63:262.

169. Rechavi G, Vonsover A, Manor Y, et al. Aplastic crisis due to human B-19 parvovirus infection in red cell pyrimidine-5'-nucleotidase deficiency. *Acta Haematol (Basel).* 1989;82:46.

170. Kagimoto T, Shirono K, Higaki T, et al. Detection of pyrimidine 5'-nucleotidase deficiency using HP' or P" nuclear magnetic resonance. *Experientia.* 1986;42:69.

171. International Committee for Standardization in Hematology. Recommended screening test for pyrimidine-5'-nucleotidase deficiency. *Clin Lab Haematol.* 1989;11:55.

172. Salgueiro N, Veiga I, Fragoso M, et al. Mutations in exon 14 of dihydropyrimidine dehydrogenase and 5'-fluorouracil toxicity in Portuguese colorectal cancer patients. *Genet Med.* 2004;6:102.

173. Berger R, Stoker-de-Vries, Wadman SK, et al.: Dihydropyrimidine dehydrogenase deficiency leading to thymine-uraciluria: An inborn error of pyrimidine metabolism. *Clin Chim Acta.* 1984;141:227.

174. Bakkeren JAJM, De Abreau RA, Sengers RCA, et al. Elevated urine, bood and cerebrospinal fluid levels of uracil and thymine in a child with dihydrothymine dehydrogenase deficiency. *Clin Chim Acta.* 1984;140:247.

175. DeAbreau RA, Bakkeren JAJM, Braakhekke J, et al. Dihydrothymine dehydrogenase deficiency in a family, leading to elevated levels of uracil and thymine. In: Nyhan WL, Thompson LF., Watts RWE, eds. *Purine and Pyrimidine Metabolism in Man*, Vol. V, Part A: *Clinical Aspects Including Molecular Genetics*. New York: Plenum Press; 1986:77.

176. Van Kuilenburg A, Vreken P, Abeling N, et al. Genotype and phenotype in patients with dihydropyrimidine dehydrogenase deficiency. *Hum Genet.* 1999;104:1.

177. Van Gennip A, Abeling N, Stoomer A, et al. Clinical and biochemical findings in six patients with pyrimidine degradation defects. *J Inherited Metab Dis.* 1994;17:130.

178. Henderson M, Ward K, Simmonds H, et al. Dihydropyrimidines deficiency presenting in infancy with severe developmental delay. *J Inherited Metab Dis.* 1993;16:574.

179. Diasio RB, Reaves TI, Carpenter JT. Familial deficiency of dihydropyrimidine dehydrogenase: Biochemical basis for familial pyrimidinemia and severe 5'-fluorouracil-induced toxicity. *J Clin Invest.* 1988;81:47.

180. Diasio R, Beavers T, Carpenter J. Familial deficiency of dihydropyrimidine dehydrogenase. *J Clin Invest.* 1988;81:47.

181. Shehata N, Pater A, Tang S-H. Prolonged severe 5'-fluorouracil associated neurotoxicity in a patient with dihydropyrimidine dehydrogenase deficiency. *Cancer Invest.* 1999;17:201.

182. Van Gennip A. Screening for inborn errors of purine and pyrimidine metabolism by bidimensional TLC and HPLC. In: Zwieg G, Sherma J, Krstulovic A, eds. *Handbook of Chromatography*, Vol. 1, Part A. Boca Raton, FL: CRC Press; 1987.

183. Van Kuilenburg A, Van Lenthe H, Van Gennip A. Identification and tissue-specific expression of a NADH-dependent activity of dihydropyrimidine dehydrogenase deficiency in man. *Anticancer Res.* 1996;16:389.

184. Harris B, Carpenter J, Diasio R. Severe 5'-fluorouracil toxicity secondary to dihydropyrimidine dehydrogenase deficiency: A potentially more common pharmacogenetic syndrome. *Cancer.* 1991;68:499.

185. Takai S, Fernandez-Salguero P, Kimura S, et al. Assignment of the human dihydropyrimidine dehydrogenase gene (DPYD) to chromosome region 1p22 by fluorescence in situ hybridization. *Genomics.* 1994;24:613.

186. Meinsma R, Fernandez-Salguero P, Van Kuilenburg A, et al. Human polymorphism in drug metabolism: Mutation in the dihydropyrimidine dehydrogenase gene results in exon skipping and thymine uraciluria. *DNA Cell Biol.* 1995;14:1.

187. Vreken P, Van Kuilenburg A, Meinsma R, et al. A point mutation in an invariant splice donor site leads to exon skipping in two unrelated Dutch patients with dihydropyrimidine dehydrogenase deficiency. *J Inherited Metab Dis.* 1996;19:645.

188. Van Gennip A, Abeling N, Vreken P, et al. Inborn errors of pyrimidine degradation: Clinical, biochemical and molecular aspects. *J Inherited Metab Dis.* 1997;20:203.

189. Wang L, Strittmatter S. Brain CRMP forms heterotetramers similar to liver dihydropyrimidinase. *J Neurochem.* 1997;69:2261.

190. Assmann B, Hoffmann GF, Wagner L, et al. Dihydropyrimidinase deficiency and congenital microvillous atrophy: Coincidence or genetic relation? *J Inherited Metab Dis.* 1997;20:681.

191. Ohba S, Kidouchi K, Sumi S, et al. Dihydropyrimidinuria: The first case in Japan. *Adv Exp Med Biol.* 1994;370:383.

192. Sumi S, Kidouchi K, Hayashi K, et al. Dihydropyrimidinuria without symptoms. *J Inherited Metab Dis.* 1996;19:701.

193. Van Gennip A, Busch S, Wizinga L, et al. Application of simple chromatographic methods for the diagnosis of pyrimidine degradation. *Clin Chem.* 1993;39:380.

194. Hamajima N, Kouwaki M, Vreken P, et al. Dihydropyrimidinase deficiency: Structural organization, chromosomal localization, and mutation analysis of the human dihydropyrimidinase gene. *Am J Hum Genet.* 1998;63:717.

195. Hamajima N, Matsuda K, Sakata S, et al. A novel gene family defined by human dihydropyrimidines and three related proteins with differential tissue distribution. *Gene.* 1996;180:157.

196. Assmann B, Gohlich-Ratmann G, Bräutigam C, et al. Presumptive ureidopropionase deficiency as a new defect in pyrimidine catabolism found with in vitro H-NMR spectroscopy. *J Inherited Metab Dis.* 1998;21:1.

197. Van Kuilenburg ABP, Meinsma R, Beke E, et al. b-Ureidopropionase deficiency: An inborn error of pyrimidine degradation associated with neurological abnormalities. *Hum Mol Genet.* 2004;13:2793.

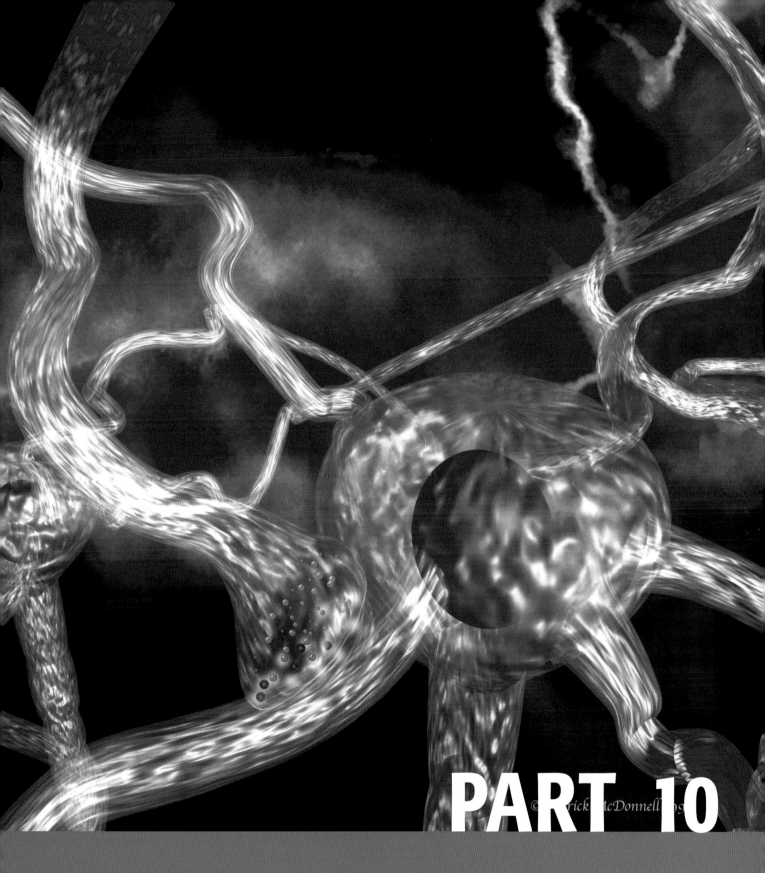

© rick McDonnell '9

PART 10

Neurotransmitter Deficiencies

IN THIS PART

Previous page: Nerve synapses.

CHAPTER 45

Neurotransmitter Disorders

Keith Hyland, PhD
K. Michael Gibson, PhD, FACMG
Radhakant Sharma, PhD
Johan L.K. van Hove, PhD, MBA
Georg F. Hoffmann, MD, Univ.-Prof. Dr. med., Prof. h.c. (RCH)

Brain function depends on the capacity for neurons within interconnecting neuronal circuitry to excite or inhibit one another. Excitation and inhibition are achieved through synaptic transmission, which, in turn, is mediated by chemical messengers called *neurotransmitters*. Neurotransmission may be thought of as translation of an electrical signal to a chemical signal (mediated by the neurotransmitter) and back to an electrical signal. In the mammalian brain, the primary excitatory neurotransmitters meeting these criteria are acetylcholine and glutamic acid, whereas gamma-aminobutyric acid (GABA), together with glycine, act as the major inhibitory neurotransmitters. The biogenic amines are also critically important chemical neurotransmitters. These include the catecholamines (i.e., dopamine, norepinephrine, and epinephrine) and the indoleamines (i.e., serotonin and melatonin).

Neurotransmitters are involved in many brain functions, including the regulation of body temperature and pain threshold and control of behavior and motor function, neuronal excitation and inhibition, memory, and a host of other processes. Alterations in glycine, GABA, glutamate, serotonin, norepinephrine, and dopamine levels have been implicated in diverse neurological disorders, including depression, dementia, schizophrenia, Parkinson's disease, epilepsy, Huntington's disease, and autism. Treatment by modulation of receptor function and neurotransmitter chemistry is well established in neurology and psychiatry. Experimental treatment modalities include human neuronal stem cell therapy as well as gene therapy.

Our ability to diagnose disorders of neurotransmitter metabolism is hampered because of our limited understanding of the interplay of neurotransmitters with their multitude of receptors and because the primary diagnostic matrix available is cerebrospinal fluid (CSF) which is only a distant mirror of the metabolic processes in the brain.

CSF analysis only mirrors the overall disturbance of neurotransmitter biosynthesis or degradation and does not necessarily reflect metabolic processes specific to localized brain structures and/or function. Differentiated functions of the brain are determined primarily by a magnitude of different receptors in contrast to the limited number of neurotransmitters. Genetic defects of neurotransmitter receptor subtypes are only now rapidly emerging as a new group of disorders that cause a wide range of neurological and psychiatric symptoms. The first such defect recognized was in the α_1-subunit of the glycine receptor causing hyperekplexia (1). Since then, defects in the GABAA1-, GABAB1-, and GABAG2-receptors and in the α_4-subunit and β_2-subunit of the nicotinic acetylcholine receptor have been shown to cause familial seizure disorders. The same holds true for genetic defects of the glutamate transporter causing severe neonatal epileptic encephalopathy. Diagnosis of some of these disorders may be aided by specific abnormalities of neurotransmitter metabolites in CSF, e.g., reduced levels of GABA in children suffering from hyperekplexia, but primarily, diagnosis rests on molecular analyses.

Monogenic defects of neurotransmission have become recognized as a cause of severe, progressive encephalopathies, mostly of early onset. The diagnosis is based almost exclusively on the quantitative determination of the neurotransmitters or their metabolites in CSF, that is, the amino acids glutamate, glycine, and GABA, the acidic metabolites of the biogenic monoamines, and individual pterin species (2).

For the purpose of this text, the monoamine disorders encompass the inherited diseases that affect serotonin and/or catecholamine (dopamine and norepinephrine) metabolism. These include the deficiencies of tyrosine hydroxylase (TH), aromatic L-amino acid decarboxylase (AADC), monoamine oxidase (MAO), and dopamine β-hydroxylase (DβH), together with dominantly inherited GTP cyclohydrolase 1 (GTPCH) deficiency and sepiapterin reductase (SR) deficiency, the latter being the defects of tetrahydrobiopterin (BH₄) metabolism that do not lead to hyperphenylalaninemia. A folinic acid–responsive seizure disorder is discussed in the light of other monoamine disorders because a marker for the disease appears on the analytical system used to measure monoamine metabolites (3). The underlying etiology of this disorder remains to be elucidated.

The metabolism of pyridoxine is linked closely to the monoamines because it is the cofactor required for AADC activity. Deficiencies of pyridox(am)ine 5′-phosphate oxidase (pyridoxal phosphate–dependent epilepsy), hypophosphatasia, L-Δ^1-pyrroline-5-carboxylate dehydrogenase (hyperprolinemia type II), and piperideine-6-carboxylate dehydrogenase (pyridoxine-dependent epilepsy) are the four proven monogenic disorders.

Disorders of GABA metabolism include deficiencies of 4-aminobutyrate aminotransferase (GABA-transaminase [GABA-T]) and succinate semialdehyde dehydrogenase (SSADH). Both have been documented using enzymatic and molecular techniques (4). Disorders of GABA synthesis may exist but have not been proven convincingly, such as homocarnosinosis (associated with serum carnosinase deficiency and documented in only a single Flemish family using CSF analysis).

Glycine is a major neurotransmitter and neuromodulator in the brain with both inhibitory and excitatory effects. Nonketotic hyperglycinemia (NKH, glycine encephalopathy) is a disorder caused by deficient activity of the glycine cleavage enzyme system—the most important catabolic enzyme of glycine metabolism. As a consequence, brain glycine levels increase. The glycine cleavage enzyme system consists of four subunits. Mutations have been reported in the genes coding for the P-, T-, and H-protein subunits. The disorder is characterized by elevated

Neurotransmitter Disorders

AT-A-GLANCE

Monogenic defects of neurotransmission have become recognized as a cause of severe, progressive encephalopathies mostly of early onset. The diagnosis is based almost exclusively on the quantitative determination of the neurotransmitters and their metabolites in cerebrospinal fluid (CSF).

The monoamine disorders include the deficiencies of tyrosine hydroxylase (TH), aromatic L-amino acid decarboxylase (AADC), monoamine oxidase (MAO), and dopamine β-hydroxylase (DβH), together with dominantly inherited GTP cyclohydrolase 1 (GTPCH) deficiency and sepiapterin reductase (SR) deficiency. The metabolism of pyridoxine is closely linked to the monoamines. Deficiencies of pyridox(am)ine-5'-phosphate oxidase (pyridoxal-phosphate-dependent epilepsy), hypophosphatasia, L-Δ^1-pyrroline-5-carboxylate dehydrogenase (hyperprolinemia type II), and piperideine-6-carboxylate dehydrogenase (pyridoxine-dependent epilepsy) are the four proven monogenic disorders. Disorders of GABA metabolism include deficiencies of 4-aminobutyrate aminotransferase (GABA-transaminase [GABA-T]) and succinate semialdehyde dehydrogenase (SSADH).

Nonketotic hyperglycinemia (NKH, glycine encephalopathy) is a disorder caused by deficient activity of the glycine cleavage enzyme system. The disorder is characterized by elevated glycine in plasma, urine, and CSF. The increase in CSF is disproportionally high, resulting in an elevated CSF:plasma glycine ratio, which is diagnostic. The most important biosynthetic pathway for glycine synthesis is via serine hydroxymethyltransferase. Serine itself is synthesized from the glycolytic intermediate 3-phoshoglycerate. The first step in the serine synthesis is catalyzed by 3-phosphoglycerate dehydogenase. Deficiency of this enzyme leads to a serine-deficiency disorder. Biochemically, serine and glycine are reduced in CSF, and there is hypomyelination and seizures.

The clinical presentation of neurotransmitter disorders can be quite distinctive, and specific investigations should not be performed routinely in every child with an unexplained encephalopathy presenting after 1 year of age. Patients with GABA-T deficiency usually present with early-onset severe encephalopathy, dominated by seizures refractory to treatment. NKH patients can have a similar neonatal episode of coma, apnea, and seizures. Defects of glutamate transport lead to a similar clinical picture. Folinic acid–responsive seizures or defects in pyridoxine metabolism also present similarly; however, rational therapies have been developed with satisfactory or even excellent success.

Defects in the biosynthesis of dopamine generally result in progressive extrapyramidal movement disorders, especially parkinsonism–dystonia and chorea. The spectrum of individual symptoms and course of disease, however; is wide, ranging from intermittent focal dystonia to severe, lethal infantile encephalopathies.

The hallmark of SSADH deficiency is an increase of 4-hydroxybutyric acid in urine and CSF. The clinical symptoms are variable, and the main findings of mental retardation, delayed speech, and hypotonia are rather unspecific. Seizures, ataxia, and behavioral abnormalities (especially hyperkinesia and/or aggressive behavior) occur in 30% to 70% of patients.

NKH is the second most common amino acid disorder after phenylketonuria. Most patients have neonatal neurological depression with coma, apnea, seizures, and a burst–suppression pattern on EEG. They tend to recover spontaneously within 2 weeks. Thereafter, patients develop moderate to profound mental retardation and a seizure disorder. Based on age at presentation, patients are categorized as neonatal onset or late onset. Patients with serine deficiency due to 3-phosphoglycerate dehydrogenase deficiency have congenital microcephaly. They develop severe psychomotor retardation with spastic tetraparesis and severe microcephaly. Seizures usually start in infancy as West syndrome with hypsarrythmia, later developing in multiple seizure pattern with multifocal epileptiform discharges.

Recently an international support group, the Pediatric Neurotransmitter Disease (PND) Association, has been established as a nonprofit organization that has been instrumental in helping to provide information and to link families and professionals involved in the diagnosis, care, and research related to neurotransmitter disorders. The association's board of directors and medical and scientific advisory board reviews all contents, resources, and medical information posted on the website, located at www.pndassoc.org The NKH International Family Network Information website (www.nkh-network.org/) provides an international resource for NKH patients with active chapters in North America and Germany.

TYPES OF DISORDER	OCCURENCE	GENE	LOCUS	OMIM
Monoamines				
GTP cyclohydrolase 1 def. Segawa disease, dopa-responsive dystonia (GTPCH)	80%	GCH1	14q22.1-q22.2	128230
Sepiapterin reductase def. (SPR)	~2%	SPR	2p14-p12	182125
Tyrosine hydroxylase def. (TH)	5%	TH1* TH2* TH3* TH4*	11p15.5	191290
Aromatic L-amino acid decarboxylase def. (AADC)	5%	DDC	7p12.1-p12.3	608643
Monoamine oxidase def. (MAO)	Very rare	MAO-A	Xp11.4-p11.3	309850
Dopamine β-hydroxylase def. (DβH)	~1%	DBH	9q34.3	223360
Folinic acid–responsive seizures	Very rare	Unknown		

*Alternately spliced products.

TYPES OF DISORDER	OCCURENCE	GENE	LOCUS	OMIM
B_6				
Pyridoxine-dependent epilepsy	~1:350.000	Antiquitin	5q31.2-3	266100
Hyperprolinemia type II	Very rare	ALDH4A1	1p.36	239510
Pyridoxal-phosphate-dependent epilepsy	Very rare	PNPO	17q21.2	603287
GABA				
GABA-T deficiency	Very rare	GABA-T	16p13.3	137150
SSADH deficiency	<1:200.000	SSADH (AlDH5a1)	6p22	271980
Glycine (nonketotic hyperglycinemia)	1:60,000			
P-protein deficiency	70%	GLDC	9p22	238300
T-protein deficiency	25%	AMT	3p21.1-2	238310
H-protein deficiency	<1%	GCSH	16q24	238330
Other	5%	Unknown	–	605899
Transient	Very rare	Unknown	–	605899
Serine				
3-Phosphoglycerate dehydrogenase deficiency	Rare	PHGDH	1q12	601815

Monoamine Disorders

DISORDER	FINDINGS (BLOOD/URINE)	FINDINGS (SPINAL FLUID)	BIRTH	CLINICAL PRESENTATION INFANCY, CHILDHOOD & ADOLESCENCE
GTPCH (dominant)	↑ Phe/Tyr ratio and ↑ biopterin to oral Phe loading (B)	↓ HVA, ↓ BH_4 ±↓ 5-HIAA, ↓ Neop	None	Progressive parkinsonism–dystonia, hypotonia, tremor, dyskinesias, rigidity, bradykinesia, ataxia, spasticity, torticollis, writer's cramp, akinesia
SR	↑ Prolactin (B) ↑ Phe/Tyr ratio and ↑ biopterin to oral Phe loading (B)	↓ HVA, ↑ BH_2 ↓ 5-HIAA, ↑ SEP ↓ BH_4	None	Progressive parkinsonism–dystonia, hypotonia, dyskinesia, ataxia, psychomotor retardation, myoclonus, choreoathetosis, seizures, hypertonia, microcephaly, tremor
TH	↑ Prolactin (B)	↓ HVA ↓ MHPG	Possibility of prematurity, hypoglycemia, fetal distress	Progressive parkinsonism–dystonia, chorea, truncal hypotonia, oculogyric crises, ptosis of the eyelids, temperature instability, excessive sweating, feeding difficulties, hypersalivation, GER, irritability, mental retardation, truncal hypotonia, limb hypertonia, seizures, rigidity
AADC	↑ 3-OMD (B, U) ↑ L-Dopa (B,U) ↑ 5HTP (B,U) ↑ Vanillactic acid (U) ↑ Prolactin (B) ↑ DA (U) ↓ Serotonin (B) ↓ NE (B), AADC activity (B)	↓ HVA ↓ 5-HIAA ↑ 3-OMD ↑ L-Dopa ↑ 5-HTP	Possibility of prematurity, hypoglycemia, irritability, feeding difficulties, temperature instability; hypotonia, ptosis of the eyelids, miosis	Progressive dystonia, chorea, oculogyric crises, truncal hypotonia, limb hypertonia, ptosis of the eyelids, temperature instability, excessive sweating, feeding difficulties, hypersalivation, GER, torticollis, irritability, mental retardation

HVA = homovanillic acid; 5-HIAA = 5-hydroxyindoleacetic acid; SEP = sepiapterin; 3-OMD = 3-O-methyldopa; 5-HTP = 5-hydroxytryptophan; Neop = neopterin; BH_4 = tetrahydrobiopterin; BH_2 = 7,8-dihydrobiopterin; NE = norepinephrine; E =epinephrine; MHPG = 3-methoxy-4-hydroxyphenylglycol; NM = normetanephrine; 3-MT = 3-methoxytyramine; VMA = vanillylmandelic acid; Phe = phenylalanine; Tyr = tyrosine; DA = dopamine; GER = gastrointestinal reflux. *Appears on the monoamine metabolite chromatographic system. **Dexamethasone stimulated fibroblasts.

Monoamine Disorders

DISORDER	FINDINGS (BLOOD/URINE)	FINDINGS (SPINAL FLUID)	BIRTH	CLINICAL PRESENTATION INFANCY, CHILDHOOD & ADOLESCENCE
MAO-A	↑ NM (U) ↑ 3-MT (U), ↑ Tyramine (U) ↑ Serotonin (B) ↓ VMA (U) ↓ HVA (U) ↓ 5-HIAA (U) ↓ MHPG (U), ↓ MAO activity**	↓ HVA, ↓ 5-HIAA ↓ MHPG	None	Mild mental retardation and behavioral abnormalities; stereotypic hand movements, flushing (carcinoid syndrome)
DβH	↓ NE (B) ↓ E (B) ↓ MHPG (B) ↑ DA (B) ↑ L-Dopa (B)	↓ MHPG ↑ HVA	Ptosis of the eyelids, hypothermia, hypoglycemia	Orthostatic hypotension
Folinic acid–responsive seizures	None	↑ Tyrosine ↑ Tryptophan ↑ Methionine ↑ Valine ↑ Isoleucine ↑ Glutamine ↑ Histidine ↑ Leucine ↑ Unknown compound*	Neonatal fatal epileptic encephalopathy	

HVA = homovanillic acid; 5-HIAA = 5-hydroxyindoleacetic acid; SEP = sepiapterin; 3-OMD = 3-O-methyldopa; 5-HTP = 5-hydroxytryptophan; Neop = neopterin; BH_4 = tetrahydrobiopterin; BH_2 = 7,8-dihydrobiopterin; NE = norepinephrine; E = epinephrine; MHPG = 3-methoxy-4-hydroxyphenylglycol; NM = normetanephrine; 3-MT = 3-methoxytyramine; VMA = vanillylmandelic acid; Phe = phenylalanine; Tyr = tyrosine; DA = dopamine; GER = gastrointestinal reflux. *Appears on the monoamine metabolite chromatographic system. **Dexamethasone stimulated fibroblasts.

B_6 Disorders

DISORDER	FINDINGS (BLOOD/URINE)	FINDINGS (SPINAL FLUID)	BIRTH	CLINICAL PRESENTATION INFANCY, CHILDHOOD & ADOLESCENCE
Pyridoxine-dependent epilepsy	↑ Pipecolic acid (B,U)	↑ Glutamate ↑ Pipecolic acid ↑ L-Δ^1-piperideine-6-carboxylate ↓ Free GABA	Neonatal fatal epileptic encephalopathy	Variants: 1) Late onset, i.e., later than 28 days 2) Neonatal onset, initial response to conventional anticonvulsant therapy 3) Neonatal onset, response to pyridoxine initially negative, later positive
Hyperprolinemia type II	↑ Proline (B,U) ↑ Glycine (U) ↑ L-Δ^1-pyrroline-5-carboxylate (B,U)	↑ Proline ↑ L-Δ^1-pyrroline-5-carboxylate ↑ L-Δ^1-pyrroline-3-hydroxy-5-carboxylate	None	Febrile convulsions, epilepsy, (mild) mental retardation
Pyridoxal-phosphate-dependent-epilepsy (pyridox(am)ine-5′-phosphate oxidase deficiency)	↑ 3-OMD (B, U) ↑ Vanillactic acid (U) ↑ Prolactin (B) ↑ Threonine (B,U) ↑ Glycine (B,U)	↓ HVA ↓ 5-HIAA ↑ 3-OMD ↑ L-Dopa ↑ 5-HTP ↑ Lactate ↑ Threonine ↑ Glycine ↑ Taurine ↑ Histidine ↓ Arginine	Neonatal fatal epileptic encephalopathy prematurity, hypoglycemia, (lactic) acidosis	No developmental progress, severe epileptic encephalopathy

HVA = homovanillic acid; 5-HIAA = 5-hydroxyindoleacetic acid; 3-OMD = 3-O-methyldopa; 5-HTP = 5-hydroxytryptophan; GABA = γ-aminobutyrate.

GABA Disorders

DISORDER	FINDINGS (BLOOD/URINE)	FINDINGS (SPINAL FLUID)	CLINICAL PRESENTATION	
			BIRTH	INFANCY, CHILDHOOD & ADOLESCENCE
GABA-T deficiency	↑ β-Alanine ↑ Free GABA ↓ GABA-T activity***	↑ Total GABA ↑ HC ↑ β-Alanine ↑ Free GABA	Neonatal epileptic encephalopathy	Severe psychomotor retardation, leukodystrophy, accelerated growth, hypotonia, hyperreflexia, high-pitched cry
SSADH deficiency	↑ GHB (B, U) ↑ DHHA (U)	↑ Total GABA ↑ GHB ↑ DHHA	None	Mild to moderate psychomotor retardation, impaired language development, absent speech, ataxia, hypotonia, behavioral disturbances, hyporeflexia, seizures

GABA = γ-aminobutyrate; GHB = γ-hydroxybutyrate; DHHA = 4,5-dihydroxyhexanoic acid; HC = homocarnosine; ***Leucocytes, liver.

NKH

DISORDER	FINDINGS (BLOOD/URINE)	FINDINGS (SPINAL FLUID)	CLINICAL PRESENTATION	
			NEONATAL PERIOD	CHILDHOOD & ADOLESCENCE
Neonatal NKH, severe	↑ Plasma glycine ↑ CSF:plasma glycine ↑ CSF glycine ratio (>0.08)	None	Neonatal period: obtundation developing into coma, hypotonia, neonatal seizures, and burst suppression on EEG, apnea (often transient lasting up to 2 weeks)	No developmental progress Development of severe seizures over the first 2 years, requiring multiple anticonvulsants. Brain malformations possible
Neonatal NKH, moderate	↑ Plasma glycine ↑ glycin ↑ CSF:plasma glycine ratio (>0.08)	None		Some developmental progress, but moderate to severe mental retardation. Seizures: mild, responding to a single anticonvulsant
Late-onset NKH, severe	↑ Plasma glycine ↑ glycine ↑ CSF:plasma glycine ratio (>0.06)	None	Often starting in infancy with increasingly severe seizures; occasionally, degenerative course in late infancy or early childhood	No developmental progress. Development of severe seizures over the first 2 years, requiring multiple anticonvulsants
Late-onset NKH, mild	↑ Plasma glycine ↑ glycine ↑ CSF:plasma glycine ratio	CSF glycine and CSF/plasma glycine ratio tend to be lower (ratio can be ≤0.06)	Starting in infancy or childhood	Moderate to mild mental retardation Mild seizure disorder in some
Transient NKH	↑ Plasma glycine ↑ glycine ↑ CSF:plasma glycine ratio (>0.08)	Normalization after months	Neonatal coma and seizures, or infantile seizures	Normal outcome or mental retardation
Mild NKH	↑ Plasma glycine ↑ glycine ↑ CSF:plasma glycine ratio (>0.08)	Biochemistry persists	Neonatal coma and seizures	Normal outcome

Molecular Variants of NKH

DISORDER	FINDINGS	ENZYMOLOGY GLYCINE CLEAVAGE ENZYME ASSAY	GLYCINE EXCHANGE ASSAY
P-protein deficiency	↑ Plasma glycine ↑ glycine ↑ CSF:plasma glycine ratio	Deficient	Deficient
T-protein deficiency	↑ Plasma glycine ↑ glycine (tends to be lower) ↑ CSF:plasma glycine ratio glycine (tends to be lower)	Deficient, small residual activity	Normal
H-protein deficiency	↑ Plasma glycine ↑ glycine ↑ CSF:plasma glycine ratio	Deficient	?
Other	↑ Plasma glycine ↑ glycine ↑ CSF:plasma glycine ratio	Deficient	?

Serine Synthesis Defect

DISORDER	FINDINGS (BLOOD)	FINDINGS (SPINAL FLUID)	BIRTH	CLINICAL PRESENTATION INFANCY, CHILDHOOD & ADOLESCENCE
3-Phospho-glycerate dehydrogenase deficiency	↓ Serine when fasting Low-normal glycine	↓ Serine ↓ Glycine ↓ 5-Methyltetrahydrofolate	Microcephaly, congenital	Seizures from infancy (cataracts, hypogoniadism, absent myelination, megaloblastic anemia) Severe psychomotor retardation, spastic tetraparesis (nystagmus)

glycine in plasma, urine, and CSF. The increase in CSF is disproportionally high, resulting in an elevated CSF:plasma glycine ratio, which is diagnostic.

The most important biosynthetic pathway for glycine synthesis is the serine hydroxymethyltransferase. L-Serine is a primary precursor for the synthesis of phospholipids (through phosphatidylserine) and for ceramides and sphingomyelins. These are very important constituents of myelin in the brain. In certain brain regions, L-serine is in equilibrium with D-serine, which functions as a neurotransmitter. Serine itself is synthesized from the glycolytic intermediate 3-phoshoglycerate. The first step in serine synthesis is catalyzed by 3-phosphoglycerate dehydrogenase. Deficiency of this enzyme leads to a serine-deficiency disorder. Biochemically, serine and glycine are reduced in CSF, and there is hypomyelination and seizures.

The clinical presentation of neurotransmitter disorders can be quite distinctive, and specific investigations should not be performed routinely in every child with an unexplained encephalopathy presenting after 1 year of age. Patients with GABA-T deficiency usually present with early-onset severe encephalopathy, dominated by seizures refractory to treatment. NKH patients can have a similar neonatal episode of coma, apnea, and seizures. Defects of glutatmate transport lead to a similar clinical picture. Folinic acid–responsive seizures or defects in pyridoxine metabolism also present similarly; however, rational therapies have been developed with satisfactory or even excellent success.

The defects in monoamine neurotransmitter metabolism result in a wide variety of signs and symptoms depending on the site of the metabolic block. Defects in the biosynthesis of dopamine generally result in progressive extrapyramidal movement disorders, especially parkinsonism–dystonia and chorea. The spectrum of individual symptoms and course of disease, however, are wide, ranging from intermittent focal dystonia to severe, lethal infantile encephalopathies. Defects of dopamine β-hydroxylase lead to orthostatic hypotension, becoming most obvious in adolescence, and monoamine oxidase deficiency does not affect movement but rather leads to psychiatric symptoms and aggressive behavior.

The hallmark of succinic semialdehyde dehydrogenase deficiency is an increase of 4-hydroxybutyric acid in urine and CSF. The clinical symptoms are variable, and the main findings of mental retardation, delayed speech, and hypotonia are rather unspecific. Seizures, ataxia, and behavioral abnormalities (especially hyperkinesia and/

or aggressive behavior) occur in 30% to 70% of patients.

NKH is the second most common amino acid disorder after phenylketonuria. Patients can have neonatal neurological depression with coma, apnea, seizures, and a burst-suppression pattern on electroencephalogram (EEG). They tend to recover spontaneously within 2 weeks. Thereafter, patients develop moderate to profound mental retardation and a seizure disorder. Based on age at presentation, patients are categorized as neonatal onset or late onset. Based on outcome, patients are categorized as severe NKH, making no developmental progress, or moderate NKH, making some developmental progress. Patients with the late-onset disorder can have stable severe or moderate NKH, or they can have a neurodegenerative course. A few patients are known with a seemingly transient form of the NKH in which the biochemical abnormalities disappear in infancy. In additon, there are rare patients with mild NKH who have presented with typical biochemical abnormalities and a neonatal presentation but with normal outcome.

Patients with serine deficiency due to 3-phosphoglycerate dehydrogenase deficiency have congenital microcephaly. They develop severe psychomotor retardation with spastic tetraparesis and severe microcephaly. Seizures usually start in infancy as West syndrome with hypsarrythmia, later developing in multiple-seizure pattern with multifocal epileptiform discharges. Magnetic resonance imaging (MRI) is characterized by striking delayed or absent myelination and reduction in white matter volume with subsequent cortical and subcortical atrophy. Variable symptoms include cataracts, hypogonadism, megaloblastic anemia, and nystagmus.

DIAGNOSTIC APPROACH

The regulation of neurotransmitter metabolism is finely tuned and is governed by the rates of neurotransmitter synthesis and degradation and by receptor status. The overall functioning of monoamine neurotransmission can be examined by determining the levels of neurotransmitter metabolites in CSF. Even borderline changes can be diagnostic. It is important that CSF be collected using strictly standardized protocols and that metabolite values be compared with adequate age-related reference ranges because there are craniocaudal gradients of metabolite concentrations, as well as diurnal, catamenal sex- and age-dependent variations (5,6). For several reasons, there are very few laboratories that provide neurotransmitter metabolite analysis. First, the very low

concentrations of metabolites in CSF require the use of extremely sensitive analytical methods. Second, very specific sample collection and handling procedures are necessary to preserve the metabolites and to aid interpretation of values. Laboratories have their own reference values that differ from each other because of variations in the technique of CSF sampling and the precise aliquot used for analysis (5). Last, a lumbar puncture is needed to obtain the sample. As a consequence, only a small number of patients have been diagnosed, and few pediatricians and neurologists have become familiar with the broad clinical spectrum and the diagnostic approach to neurotransmitter disorders.

In summary, we suspect a substantial underdiagnosis of neurotransmitter disorders (2,7). However, we do not imply that neurotransmitter disorders are a major cause of encephalopathies of unknown origin. They will remain relatively rare conditions requiring a complex diagnostic approach and experienced guidance of therapy. The situation will be improved by a better understanding of the pathophysiology of these disorders, a clearer recognition of the limitations of the biochemical and molecular diagnostic approaches, and especially a strengthened liaison between clinicians and laboratories.

In the diagnostic workup of a suspected neurometabolic disorder, a lumbar puncture should complement the results of intensive metabolic analyses in blood and urine and careful evaluation of neuroimaging studies (2,7).

The clinical symptomatology of neurotransmitter disorders as listed in Table 45-1 is not meant to be taken as a checklist in the workup of a patient suffering from an encephalopathy of unknown origin. It can only guide the decision in the context of a combination of symptoms. The "broadest" single indication for CSF investigations of neurotransmitter disorders including biogenic monoamines, glycine, and GABA is severe neonatal/infantile epileptic encephalopathy.

CSF investigations for the diagnosis of neurotransmitter disorders cannot and should not be separated from the broader scope of CSF investigations for neurometabolic disorders (Table 45-2). The CSF sample should be free from contamination with blood or serum also from breakdown of the blood–brain barrier. Therefore, red blood cell count and protein in CSF always should be measured and found normal for proper

• Blood and urine first! No multisystem disease!

TABLE 45-1　Main Symptomatology of Neurotransmitter Disorders

- Early-onset seizures–refractory to conventional treatment

　　Nonketotic hyperglycinemia → glycine in CSF and plasma

　　GABA-T deficiency → GABA in CSF

　　Vitamin B_6–dependent epilepsy → therapeutic trial of vitamin B_6

　　Pyridox(am)ine-5′-phosphate oxidase deficiency → therapeutic trial of pyridoxal phosphate

　　Folinic acid–responsive seizures → therapeutic trial of folinic acid

- Hypokinesia, hypomimia, truncal hypotonia*
- Dystonia–parkinsonism*
- Distal chorea *
- Rigidity*
- Hyperreflexia
- Diurnal variation*
- Ataxia*[†]
- Tremor*
- Oculogyric crises*
- Ptosis, miosis*
- Hypersalivation*
- Temperature instability, sweating, restlessness*
- Hypoglycemia (neonates)*
- Signs of autonomic dysfunction*
- Abnormal behavior, including aggression and hyperactivity (MAO-A deficiency)*[†]
- Severe progressive encephalopathy *[†]
- Neonatal apnea[§]
- Agenesis of the corpus callosum, hydrocephalus[§]
- Progressive seizure disorder in infancy[‡]
- Microcephaly with absent to very delayed myelination[¶]
- Profound hypotonia[§]

*Suggestive of defects that affect monoamine metabolism (serotonin and/or catecholamines [dopamine and norepinephrine]) including defects of tetrahydrobiopterin metabolism. Diagnosis is through determination of biogenic amines and pterins in CSF.

[†]Suggestive of succinate semialdehyde dehydrogenase (SSADH) deficiency (4-hydroxybutyric aciduria). Diagnosis is through determination of organic acids in urine.

[‡]Suggestive of nonketotic hyperglycinemia and defects of pyridoxal metabolism or of serine deficiency.

[§]Suggestive of nonketotic hyperglycinemia.

[¶]Suggestive of serine-deficiency syndrome.

TABLE 45-2　CSF Investigations for Neurotransmitter Disorders

Cells, protein, immunoglobulin classes, and glucose (plus plasma glucose and evaluation of blood–brain barrier)

Lactate, pyruvate

Amino acids (plus plasma obtained simultaneously)

Biogenic monoamines metabolites

Individual pterin species

5-Methyltetrahydrofolate

- Each newborn with severe neonatal/infantile epileptic encephalopathy should have a lumbar puncture and receive consecutive therapeutic trials of vitamin B_6 (100 mg intravenously in a single dose, to be followed by 30 mg/kg/day for 3 days), folinic acid (3–5 mg/kg of body weight per day for 3 days), and pyridoxal 5′-phosphate (30 mg/kg of body weight per day in three doses for 3 days) (see Table 45-1).

analysis of amino acids in CSF requires especially sensitive methods and expert interpretation. Normal levels of plasma glycine and serine should not be taken as an indicator that the patient does not have a disorder of glycine or serine, and the analysis must be completed by CSF analysis.

It already has been elucidated that reliable results of specialized CSF investigations can be obtained only if the appropriate protocol is adhered to strictly. This should be discussed beforehand with the neurometabolic laboratory.

BH_4 cofactor deficiency may be restricted to the CNS, and pterin (BH_4 and neopterin) analysis in the CSF should be included whenever biogenic monoamines are investigated. Free GABA can be determined only in samples that have been shock frozen at the bedside in dry ice or liquid nitrogen. Samples must be taken at a certain time of the day and have to be collected in a specific order with fixed amounts of CSF collected per fraction. This is so because of diurnal variations and a caudocranial concentration gradient for many metabolites. It is therefore essential to label the CSF samples (fractions) that are sent to the laboratory exactly. Exact documentation is of utmost importance and must include all special features such as deviation from the protocol, sample color, all medications, and present-day clinical conditions such as fever, etc. Good clinical and sample information can make the difference between making or missing a diagnosis.

The use of certain medications, such as valproate, the sedative 4-hydroxybutyrate, dopamine or serotonin receptor agonists, serotonin reuptake inhibitors, or carbidopa/levodopa (Sinemet), is very important in the interpretation of the results of the CSF analyses, and this information must be shared with the laboratory.

- CSF samples must be stored at −70°C or, as an intermediate measure, on dry ice or liquid nitrogen. The analyses of some substances (e.g., pterins, serotonin, and catecholamines) require the addition of certain chemicals to the respective sample tubes.

interpretation. Amino acids and glucose always should be analyzed in parallel in plasma because ratios are relevant for the diagnosis of some disorders, for example, glucose transport protein deficiency and nonketotic hyperglycinemia. Levels of amino acids and glucose in plasma can change rapidly, and ratios should be calculated only on samples obtained at the same time as the lumbar puncture. You can easily double the serum glycine with a bit of food in an hour, let alone in a few days later. The

DISORDERS OF MONOAMINE METABOLISM

Etiology/Pathophysiology Disorders affecting biogenic monoamine neurotransmitter metabolism arise from inherited defects affecting the biosynthesis or catabolism of serotonin and/or the catecholamines. Defective enzyme activity may occur due to mutations in the genes coding for the individual proteins or to defective production of the obligatory cofactors, tetrahydrobiopterin (BH_4) or pyridoxal 5'-phosphate. The phenotypic spectrum in this group of disorders is large and depends on the site of the defect within the pathways (see below).

The catecholamines (i.e., norepinephrine, dopamine, and epinephrine) and serotonin are formed from the amino acids tyrosine and tryptophan, respectively. The pathway for the synthesis and catabolism of the monoamines and the sites of known defects are shown in Figure 45-1. The first step in their synthesis requires the hydroxylation of the amino acids using the enzymes tyrosine hydroxylase (TH) and tryptophan hydroxylase to yield L-dopa and 5-hydroxytryptophan. These are decarboxylated by pyridoxal 5'-phosphate, requiring aromatic L-amino acid decarboxylase (AADC) to form dopamine and serotonin. In noradrenergic neurons, dopamine can be further hydroxylated by the enzyme dopamine

β-hydroxylase (DβH) to yield norepinephrine, and in the pineal gland, serotonin can form melatonin. Following release of the active monoamines, they act on their appropriate receptors and then are either taken back into the presynaptic terminals and restored in vesicles or are catabolized via the action of monoamine oxidase (MAO) and catechol-O-methyltransferase. Dopamine forms homovanillic acid (HVA), serotonin 5-hydroxyindoleacetic acid (5-HIAA), and norepinephrine 3-methoxy-4-hydroxyphenylglycol (MHPG). These are released into CSF, and their measurement in this compartment reflects the overall turnover of the individual neurotransmitters (8).

The initial hydroxylation steps catalyzed by tryptophan hydroxylase and TH require BH_4 as a cofactor. This pterin compound is formed in a three-step pathway from guanosine triphosphate (GTP). The first and rate-limiting reaction is catalyzed by GTP cyclohydrolase (GTPCH) and leads to the production of dihydroneopterin triphosphate. This compound can be dephosphorylated intracellularly to form dihydroneopterin, which is exported and may undergo oxidation to form neopterin. The dihydroneopterin triphosphate then is converted to 6-pyruvoyltetrahydropterin (6-PTP) by 6-pyruvoyltetrahydropterin synthase (6-PTPS).

Finally, sepiapterin reductase (SR) catalyzes the reaction to form BH_4. During the hydroxylation of tyrosine and tryptophan, BH_4 is oxidized to quinonoid dihydrobiopterin, which is reduced back to the active cofactor via the action of dihydropteridine reductase. Since BH_4 is also required for hydroxylation of phenylalanine to tyrosine in the liver, most defects of BH_4 metabolism cause hyperphenylalaninemia, which is diagnosed on neonatal screening. Dominantly inherited GTPCH defi-

ciency and the autosomal recessive SR deficiency both lead to reduced levels of BH_4 within the CNS without significantly affecting phenylalanine metabolism in the liver. However, turnover of serotonin and the catecholamines in the brain are both severely reduced in SR deficiency, whereas in the dominantly inherited GTPCH deficiency, a decreased dopamine turnover is more prominent.

The pathophysiology of the disorders of monoamine metabolism is associated with their diverse range of function and is in some cases specific to the individual disorder. Within the CNS, they provide control of psychomotor function, being involved, for example, in the regulation of motor coordination, processing of sensory input, reward-driven learning, arousal, emotional stability, memory, appetite, mood, sleep, vomiting, and secretion of anterior pituitary and other hormones. Peripherally, their involvement includes regulation of vascular tone and blood flow, control of ion and water transport in the kidneys, control of motility in the gastrointestinal tract, control of thermoregulation, and modulation of pain mechanisms. A broad allocation of clinical symptomatology to a deficiency of individual monoamines is attempted in Table 45-3.

Differential Diagnosis Deficiencies of GTPCH, SR, TH, and AADC result in similar clinical phenotypes caused by dopamine deficiency. The pattern of monoamine metabolites, BH_4, and neopterin in CSF allows distinction between these disorders (9) (Table 45-4). The BH_4 deficiencies and AADC deficiency lead to low levels of HVA, MHPG, and 5-HIAA in CSF. BH_4 metabolism is normal in AADC deficiency, but in dominantly inherited GTPCH deficiency and SR deficiency, there are characteristic changes in the pterins. GTPCH leads to low levels of both BH_4 and neopterin in CSF (10). In SR deficiency, there is accumulation of 7,8-dihydrobiopterin and sepiapterin (11), and BH_4 levels are reduced. Further evidence for GTPCH and SR deficiencies can be obtained by finding abnormal phenylalanine:tyrosine ratios in plasma after oral phenylalanine loading (12).

TABLE 45-3 Clinical Features Associated with Biogenic Monoamines Deficiency

- *General:* Progressive/severe encephalopathy
- *Dopamine deficiency:* Parkinsonism-dystonia, dyskinesia and hypokinesia, dystonia and chorea, tremor, truncal hypotonia/limb hypertonia, deterioration during the day, hypersensitivity to L-dopa, oculogyric crises, miosis, ptosis, hypomimia, hypersalivation, growth retardation
- *Norepinephrine deficiency:* Axial hypotonia, cerebellar symptoms, ptosis, impaired orthostasis (blood pressure), hypoglycemia
- *Serotonin deficiency:* Insomnia, depression, disturbance of temperature regulation (fever, profuse sweating), disturbed intestinal motility

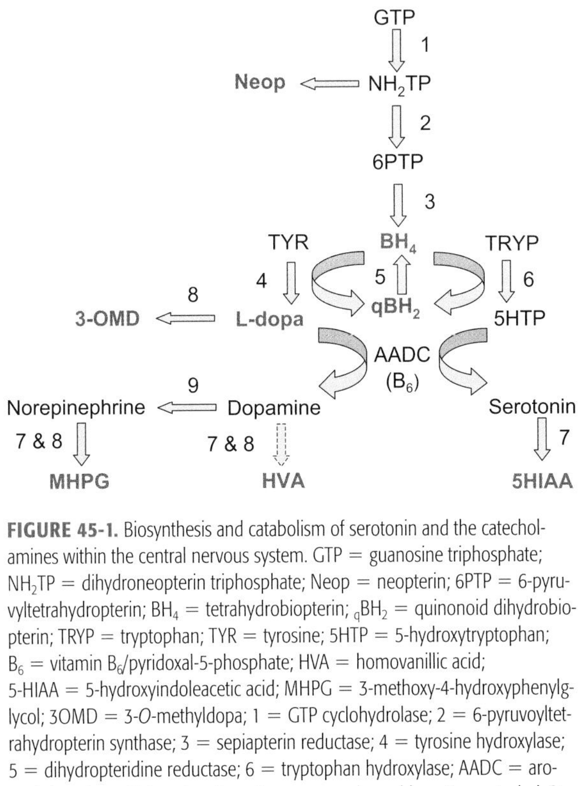

FIGURE 45-1. Biosynthesis and catabolism of serotonin and the catecholamines within the central nervous system. GTP = guanosine triphosphate; NH_2TP = dihydroneopterin triphosphate; Neop = neopterin; 6PTP = 6-pyruvyltetrahydropterin; BH_4 = tetrahydrobiopterin; $_qBH_2$ = quinonoid dihydrobiopterin; TRYP = tryptophan; TYR = tyrosine; 5HTP = 5-hydroxytryptophan; B_6 = vitamin B_6/pyridoxal-5-phosphate; HVA = homovanillic acid; 5-HIAA = 5-hydroxyindoleacetic acid; MHPG = 3-methoxy-4-hydroxyphenylglycol; 3OMD = 3-O-methyldopa; 1 = GTP cyclohydrolase; 2 = 6-pyruvoyltetrahydropterin synthase; 3 = sepiapterin reductase; 4 = tyrosine hydroxylase; 5 = dihydropteridine reductase; 6 = tryptophan hydroxylase; AADC = aromatic L-aminoacid decarboxylase; 7 = monoamine oxidase; 8 = catechol-O-methyltransferase; 9 = dopamine-hydroxylase. The dashed lines indicate more than one step. Compounds in purple are the metabolites measured in CSF to assess the integrity of the serotonin and catecholamine pathways.

TABLE 45-4 Pattern of CSF metabolites in Disorders of Monoamine Metabolism

Defect	BH₄	BH₂	Neop	HVA	5-HIAA	3OMD	MHPG	SEP
GTPCH (D)	↓	N	↓	±↓	±↓	N	↓	N
GTPCH (R)	↓	N	↓	↓	↓	N	↓	N
SR	±↓	↑	±↑	↓	↓	N	↓	↑
TH	N	N	N	↓	N	N	↓	N
AADC	N	N	N	↓	↓	↑	↓	N
MAO-A	N	N	N	↓	↓	N	↓	N
D-β-H	N	N	N	↑	N	N	↓	N

Confirmation of deficiencies of GTPCH and SR can be obtained by enzyme analysis in cytokine-stimulated and unstimulated fibroblasts, respectively (11,13).

TH deficiency leads to low levels of the catecholamine metabolites HVA and MHPG in CSF (14) with normal BH₄ and neopterin profiles. Low CSF HVA concentrations also can be found secondary to some as yet undefined events (15). There are no easily accessible tissues where TH activity can be measured, so confirmation of TH deficiency relies on detection of mutations within the TH gene.

In AADC deficiency, there is accumulation of the AADC substrates L-dopa and 5-hydroxytryptophan together with 3-O-methyldopa. In addition, vanillactate accumulates in urine. This pattern, together with very low levels of 5-HIAA and HVA in CSF, is only seen when there is defective activity of AADC (16). However, low activity can occur either due to mutations in the AADC gene (17) or due to defective synthesis of its cofactor pyridoxal-5'-phosphate (18). The two forms can be distinguished because glycine and threonine are elevated in CSF and plasma in the cofactor deficiency and plasma AADC activity is decreased in the primary defect. Clinically, the two forms also can be distinguished because pyridox(am)ine-5'-phosphate oxidase deficiency presents with intractable neonatal seizures (18,19), which are not a feature when there is a defect in the AADC protein.

Patients with folinic acid–responsive seizures do not have abnormalities in neurotransmitter metabolites in CSF, but these patients are recognized because two additional compounds appear on the neurotransmitter metabolite chromatographic trace. In addition, there are elevations of certain amino acids in CSF, these being tyrosine, tryptophan, methionine, valine, isoleucine, glutamine, histidine, and leucine (20).

Isolated monoamine oxidase A deficiency was first described in one Dutch family (21). Diagnosis was inferred from a finding of elevated urinary levels of the monoamine oxidase A substrates normetanephrine, 3-methoxytyramine, and tyramine in combination with reduced amounts of the monoamine oxidase products vanillylmandelic acid, HVA, MHPG, and 5-HIAA (21–23). Confirmation of monoamine oxidase A deficiency was obtained by measurement of the activity of this enzyme in dexamethasone-stimulated fibroblasts (21).

Patients with DβH deficiency present with orthostatic hypotension in adolescence (24,25). There is no evidence of other neurological defects, either central or peripheral. Diagnosis is made by measurement of plasma catecholamine profiles in conjunction with physiological tests of autonomic function. There are absent or low levels of norepinephrine and epinephrine and their metabolites in plasma, CSF, and urine. Plasma dopamine concentrations are elevated, and there is a two- to threefold increase in L-dopa. Confirmation of diagnosis relies on mutation analysis.

Dominantly Inherited GTP Cyclohydrolase Deficiency

Etiology/Pathophysiology Dominantly inherited GTP cyclohydrolase deficiency, otherwise known as *Segawa disease, hereditary progressive dystonia with diurnal fluctuation,* or *dopa-responsive dystonia,* is caused by mutations scattered throughout the GCH1 gene (9,26). The mutations affect the activity of the enzyme within dopaminergic neurons in the brain and lead to decreased levels of BH₄ and subsequently dopamine (see Figure 45-2) and a decrease in the steady-state concentration of tyrosine hydroxylase protein within the striatum (27).

Molecular Variants GTPCH is encoded by a single-copy gene,

GCH1, located on chromosome 14q22.1-q22.2 and composed of six exons spanning about 30 kb. There is great allelic heterogeneity and evidence to suggest a relatively high spontaneous mutation rate of the GTPCH gene (28). To date, 78 cases are listed in the BIOMDB database (29). Changes at the DNA level have involved missense mutations, deletions, base transition at the splice acceptor site of intron 1, base transition at the conserved consensus sequence GT at the 5' end of intron 2 that led to skipping of the entire exon 2 in the mature mRNA, and nonsense mutations. In numerous cases, mutations have not been found in either the coding exons or the exon/intron boundaries, and it is assumed that mutation may exist in the untranslated or regulatory portion of the gene or result in large deletions in the GCH1 gene (30).

Clinical Presentation Dominantly inherited GTP cyclohydrolase deficiency is an eminently treatable condition. Early recognition therefore is of crucial importance. Presentation in children usually occurs within the first decade of life, with a mean age of onset of symptoms being about 7 years (range 16 months to 13 years) (31). The first symptom is usually postural dystonia of one leg, with progression to all limbs, followed by action dystonia and hand tremor within the next 10–15 years, during which time

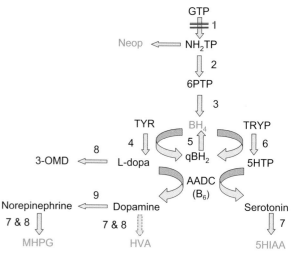

FIGURE 45-2. GTP cyclohydrolase deficiency and its laboratory consequences. All reduced metabolite levels are depicted in green. GTP = guanosine triphosphate; NH₂TP = dihydroneopterin triphosphate; Neop = neopterin; 6PTP = 6-pyruvyltetrahydropterin; BH₄ = tetrahydrobiopterin; qBH₂ = quinonoid dihydrobiopterin; TRYP = tryptophan; TYR = tyrosine; 5HTP = 5-hydroxytryptophan; B₆ = vitamin B₆/pyridoxal-5-phosphate; HVA = homovanillic acid; 5-HIAA = 5-hydroxyindoleacetic acid; MHPG = 3-methoxy-4-hydroxyphenylglycol; 3OMD = 3-O-methyldopa; 1 = GTP cyclohydrolase; 2 = 6-pyruvoyltetrahydropterin synthase; 3 = sepiapterin reductase; 4 = tyrosine hydroxylase; 5 = dihydropteridine reductase; 6 = tryptophan hydroxylase; AADC = aromatic L-aminoacid decarboxylase; 7 = monoamine oxidase; 8 = catechol-O-methyltransferase; 9 = dopamine-hydroxylase. The dashed lines indicate more than one step.

cognition remains intact. Occasionally, in older children, the first signs may start in the arms or be torticollis or writer's cramp (focal dystonia). The dystonia frequently is asymmetrical and accompanied by parkinsonian features, such as reduced facial expression or slowing of fine finger movements. Diurnal fluctuation normally is present, with symptoms improving after nighttime sleep or bed rest. The variation in presenting symptoms is, however, large and may include minor muscle cramps, an early nonprogressive course, delayed attainment of motor milestones, or spastic diplegia (32). In others, presentation was with an apparent primary torsion dystonia that was responsive to anticholinergic agents (33) or with a myoclonus–dystonia syndrome (34). Of the patients who present at the average age with the typical dystonic gait disorder, 20% also have hyperreflexia and apparent extensor plantar responses, as well as other clinical features suggesting spasticity.

Prominent upper motor neuron findings, including spastic diplegia, have led in many cases to an initial diagnosis of cerebral palsy (35). Presentation is not limited to childhood because the first signs can be the occurrence of tremor or parkinsonian-like features in later life (32), and a patient has been described in whom the first symptom was an adult-onset oromandibular dystonia (36). Penetrance is reduced, and many carriers of a mutant gene are asymptomatic. The frequency of symptoms is three- to fourfold higher in females than in males (32). A psychiatric component of this disorder is not well documented, but the presence of depressive disorder and obsessive–compulsive disorder is noted with high frequency in patients older than 20 years of age. Abnormal sleep also is seen (37).

Compound heterozygotes exist (see Chapter 14). The clinical course is more severe. However, hyperphenylalaninemia also may be absent in compound heterozygotes.

Diagnosis In classical cases with prominent dystonia of the lower limbs, marked diurnal variation, and worsening of the symptoms after exercise, the clinical diagnosis of GTPCH deficiency is easily made, and diagnosis can be considered certain in the presence of dramatic and sustained response to L-dopa. However, the diagnosis can be a real challenge in unusual cases. A positive clinical

- Developmental assessments are notoriously difficult in children with motor disability. A diagnosis of GTPCH deficiency should not be ruled out because of an applied label of "cognitively impairment."

- Most mutations are random and spontaneous.
- Mutant allele carriers can be totally asymptomatic
- Prenatal diagnosis is unnecessary because this is a treatable condition.
- Newborn screening is unavailable currently.

response to low-dose L-dopa is the cornerstone of diagnosis but does not by itself prove GTPCH deficiency because TH deficiency and other dystonia syndromes, including juvenile parkinsonism (caused by mutations in the *parkin* gene) and some secondary dystonias, may respond in a similar manner. Another mistake is to expect a dramatic, immediate response in *every* patient with GTPCH deficiency, although this is usually the case. The therapeutic trial of cocareldopa (Sinemet, L-dopa plus a peripheral decarboxylase inhibitor) must be adequate, that is, at the maximally tolerated dose up to 10 mg/kg/day of L-dopa divided into at least four doses for at least 3 months.

Diagnosis of GTPCH deficiency can be ascertained by determining BH_4, neopterin, and HVA in CSF. All levels usually are decreased, although occasionally individual low-normal values may be obtained. Unfortunately, the biochemical analysis of BH_4 and its precursor neopterin, which is the most diagnostic metabolite, is undertaken in only few laboratories worldwide, which limits its usefulness in routine clinical practice. Additional support for the diagnosis can be obtained by performing an oral phenylalanine loading test (12). Elevated plasma phenylalanine:tyrosine ratios after oral loading are very suggestive of a problem in BH_4 metabolism. False-positive results may be found in a phenylketonuria (PKU) heterozygote, however. This can be excluded if biopterin is also analyzed in the plasma samples. In PKU heterozygotes, biopterin inceases above 18 nmol/L (cutoff), whereas its increase is less in GTPCH deficiency (9).

Confirmation of the diagnosis can be achieved by enzyme analysis in cultured skin fibroblasts (38) or by mutation analysis. Unfortunately, the potential usefulness of the elegant enzyme analysis, which could be considered the "gold standard" for diagnosis, is currently restricted to two European specialist laboratories. The wide distribution of the mutations, as well as the fact that some patients carry two mutations, makes it necessary to sequence the entire coding region of the GCH-1 gene. This has hampered the introduction of direct sequencing of the GCH-1 gene into clinical practice as a means of diagnostic genetic testing. Puzzlingly, only half of all patients with classical GTPCH deficiency have detectable mutations of GCH-1 in the coding region or the splice sites. Sequence analysis of both the upstream promoter region and the sequence around the poly-A signal at the downstream end of GCH-1 has been performed in some mutation-negative cases. Mutations in the promoter region were found in only two of the cases analysed and remain of uncertain significance because the mRNA of these patient was not available for mRNA expression analysis. Recent evidence suggests that at least some patients with classical dominantly inherited GTPCH deficiency, in whom mutations could not be detected by conventional sequencing, arise as a result of large deletions in the GCH-I gene (30).

Treatment/Prognosis Treatment following diagnosis relies on L-dopa in combination with 10% to 25% carbidopa. Amounts administered have varied from 3–10 mg/kg/day divided into three to four doses, with the effectiveness of treatment being monitored by clinical outcome. Infants usually require smaller doses of 1–3 mg/kg/day divided into three to four doses. Therapy should be introduced slowly and increased in steps of not more than 1 mg/kg over days to weeks. The psychiatric and sleep components of GTPCH deficiency probably relate to subtle serotonin and/or melatonin deficiencies. Treatment with 5-HTP/carbidopa, monoamine oxidase inhibitors, or serotonin reuptake inhibitors may be beneficial (e.g., fluoroxitin). In contrast to other forms of parkinsonism, L-dopa does not need to be increased over years, and drug-related movement disorders do not occur. In general, the overall prognosis is excellent.

Sepiapterin Reductase Deficiency

Etiology/Pathophysiology Severe SR deficiency is caused by autosomal recessively inherited mutations in the SR gene (11). A milder form presenting as dopa-responsive dystonia also has been described that was caused by a heterozygous base change in the 5′ untranslated region of SPR (39). The reduced SR activity leads to BH_4 deficiency within the brain and consequently decreased levels of serotonin and the catecholamine neurotransmitters (see Figure 45-3). Peripheral hyperphenylalaninemia is not present because other enzymes replace SR activity in the liver and other peripheral tissues (40). The monoamine neurotransmitter deficiency in SR deficiency can be explained by two mechanisms. The first relates to the lack of sufficient production of BH_4. The second involves inhibition of tyrosine and tryptophan hydroxylases by 7,8-dihydrobiopterin

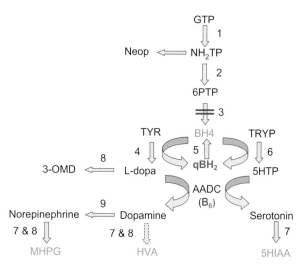

FIGURE 45-3. Sepiapterin reductase deficiency and its laboratory consequences. Elevated metabolite levels are depicted in blue, reduced levels in green. GTP = guanosine triphosphate; NH_2TP = dihydroneopterin triphosphate; Neop = neopterin; 6PTP = 6-pyruvyltetrahydropterin; BH_4 = tetrahydrobiopterin; $_qBH_2$ = quinonoid dihydrobiopterin; TRYP = tryptophan; TYR = tyrosine; 5HTP = 5-hydroxytryptophan; B_6 = vitamin B_6/pyridoxal-5-phosphate; HVA = homovanillic acid; 5-HIAA = 5-hydroxyindoleacetic acid; MHPG = 3-methoxy-4-hydroxyphenylglycol; 3OMD = 3-O-methyldopa; 1 = GTP cyclohydrolase; 2 = 6-pyruvoyltetrahydropterin synthase; 3 = sepiapterin reductase; 4 = tyrosine hydroxylase; 5 = dihydropteridine reductase; 6 = tryptophan hydroxylase; AADC = aromatic L-aminoacid decarboxylase; 7 = monoamine oxidase; 8 = catechol-O-methyltransferase; 9 = dopamine-hydroxylase. The dashed lines indicate more than one step.

that accumulates in SR deficiency (11). BH_4 is also required for the activity of all forms of nitric oxide synthase (NOS) (41). In the presence of low levels of BH_4, the NOS reaction becomes uncoupled and leads to the formation of peroxynitrite. Peroxynitrite is a potent oxidizing radical that may be involved in central pathophysiology of SR deficiency.

Molecular Variants The SPR gene spans a region of 4–5 kb located on chromosome 2p14-12 (42); the coding region is comprised of three exons (43). Mutations have been identified in all 12 patients with SR deficiency reported recently. Two were missense mutations (R150G and P163L), one was a premature termination codon (Q119X), one was a 5-bp deletion leading to frameshift and premature termination codon at amino acid 152, and one was a splicing mutation (IVS2-2AnG). All mutations in the coding region are located in exon 2, whereas the intronic mutation is located in the splicing acceptor AG dinucleotide preceding exon 3. Steinberger and colleagues (36,39) reported a patient with a mild form of dopa-responsive dystonia who was shown to be heterozygote for a mutation in the 5′ untranslated region of the SPR gene (a G-to-A transition 13 nucleotides before the ATG), whereas the coding region was normal.

Clinical Presentation Since the original decription in 2001, close to 20 cases of SR deficiency have been described. Symptoms in all but one case have started in the first few months of life with hypotonia. Symptoms have included progressive dystonia, chorea, oculogyric crises, tremor, spasticity, microcephaly, growth retardation, depressive and aggressive behavior, and psychomotor retardation. (Figure 45-4) Diurnal variation is mostly present (45). Signs of autonomic dysfunction have included hypersalivation, temperature instability, lethargy, hypersomnolence, and episodes of sweating and pallor. Less frequently reported were bulbar signs (e.g., drooling, dysarthria, and abnormal tongue movements) (44), "ataxia" (probably not cerebellar ataxia nor sensory ataxia but dystonic gait), occasional seizures, growth retardation, and Gower sign. In one, presentation was initially with toe walking. This disappeared before puberty, but at age 15 years, abnormal finger movements developed, followed by gait abnormalities, dystonia, and tremor (39). All the patients were diagnosed after 2 years of age due to a lack of hyperphenylalaninemia and consequently a negative newborn screen. At this time, dystonia was the main clinical feature, with parkinsonian signs (i.e., tremor, bradykinesia, rigidity, and cogwheel motions) appearing in the older patients.

Diagnosis Diagnosis relies on the measurement of tetrahydrobiopterin, 7,8-dihydrobiopterin, HVA, and 5-HIAA in CSF. Concentrations of HVA, 5-HIAA, and tetrahydrobiopterin are decreased. Levels of 7,8-dihydrobiopterin are elevated. Sepiapterin is not detected by the regularly used methods used in the investigation of biogenic monoamine metabolites in CSF but can be determined reliably in a few specialized laboratories. Its presence is diagnostic of the disorder. All patients tested so far also have had abnormal phenylalanine loading test results. Confirmation of the diagnosis is achieved by

- Prenatal diagnosis is possible where mutations have been established. It will be considered unnecessary in most circumstances because this is a treatable condition.

- Newborn screening is unavailable.

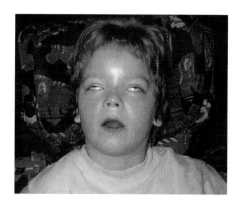

FIGURE 45-4. Oculogyric crisis. Oculogyric crises reflect dystonic eye movements and can occur due to deficiencies of GTPCH, SR, TH, and AADC. They are often mistaken as seizures. The child depicted at age 8 years suffered from TH deficiency. (Reproduced with permission from Hoffmann et al., 2003, ref. 44.)

measurement of SR activity in cultured skin fibroblasts or by mutation analysis (38).

Treatment/Prognosis Treatment following diagnosis relies on L-dopa in combination with carbidopa and 5-hydroxytryptophan. Amounts administered have varied from 1–10 mg/kg/day in three or four doses. 5-Hydroxytryptophan is given in similar but usually somewhat less amounts (1–9 mg/kg/day in three or four doses). L-Dopa/carbidopa/5-hydroxytryptophan therapy should be introduced slowly and increased in steps of not more than 1 mg/kg over days to weeks. Some patients do not tolerate 5-hydroxytryptophan due to gastrointestinal side effects. In these patients, monotherapy with L-dopa/carbidopa may be sufficient. Additional supplementation of BH_4 may be considered.

The effectiveness of treatment is monitored clinically by repeated careful evaluation by a (pediatric) neurologist, including video documentation and follow-up of metabolite concentrations by consecutive lumbar punctures in the morning before the medication (at least yearly). L-Dopa/carbidopa/5-hydroxytryptophan therapy may reduce CSF folates (CH_3-group trapping by L-dopa to 3-O-methyl-dopa), requiring folinic acid (5-formyltetrahydrofolate) substitution (15 mg/day). In some patients with high prolactin before L-dopa supplementation, prolactin levels can aid monitoring of therapy.

- Effectiveness of treatment is monitored by clinical outcome and measurement of prolactin in serum and HVA and 5-HIAA levels in CSF. Prolactin levels can change in response to stress. To obtain reliable values, three determinations should be done hourly. If these are in agreement, the value is to be trusted.

Therapy leads to marked improvement of movement control, muscle tone, eye movements, gait, and speech. Improvement continues over years with excellent final results in some patients. Sleep disturbance was described in most patients and was ameliorated to some degree by 5-hydroxytryptophan.

Experience is limited to a few patient-years, with no adult patient known. There appears no need to increased L-dopa over years, and no drug-related movement disorders have been observed. The overall prognosis appears good, although intellectual function may remain below average (45).

Tyrosine Hydroxylase Deficiency

Etiology/Pathophysiology TH deficiency is an autosomal recessive disorder leading to reduced production of L-dopa and consequently a deficiency of dopamine, norepinephrine, and epinephrine. TH catalyzes the hydroxylation of L-tyrosine to L-dihydroxyphenylalanine (L-dopa), the rate-limiting step in the biosynthesis of the catecholamines dopamine, norepinephrine, and epinephrine (see Figure 45-5). The iron-containing mixed-function oxidase requires molecular oxygen and BH_4 for activity. The enzyme is expressed in the central and peripheral nervous systems, in particular in the brain and adrenal medulla. A critical role for TH in prenatal development and for postnatal survival is shown by

the nonviability of TH-deficient knockout mice (46). The pathophysiology in the brain in TH deficiency is related to the roles of dopamine in the control of movement, cognition, emotion/affect, and neuroendocrine, pituitary gland hormone (prolactin and growth hormone), and parathyroid hormone secretion. Dopamine concentrations are also high in the kidney, where dopamine is involved in control of ion and water transport. In the gastrointestinal tract it controls motility. Absence of norepinephrine can lead to hypoglycemia, ptosis, cerebellar symptoms, and decreased blood pressure.

Molecular Variants The human gene for TH (47) is localized to chromosome 11p15.5 (48). The coding region is comprised of 14 exons. Differential splicing using two splice donor sites in the first exon and inclusion or exclusion of the second exon (49) leads to the formation of four different forms of TH mRNA and protein (50).

The first indication of primary genetic TH deficiency in humans was provided in 1994 by Clayton and coworkers and was confirmed by demonstrating a point mutation in exon 5 (L205P) of the TH gene (51). Thereafter, TH deficiency caused by a different mutation in exon 11 (Q381K) with a relatively high residual enzyme activity of 15% (52) was identified in two siblings described as suffering from recessive L-dopa-responsive dystonia. A different point mutation in exon 6 (R233H) could be identified in five patients with autosomal recessive L-dopa-responsive infantile parkinsonism (53), as well as seven different novel mutations in children with the initial diagnoses of spastic paraplegia (54), recessive L-dopa-responsive dystonia (55), and L-dopa-responsive progressive encephalopathy (56).

Clinical Presentation Patients with TH deficiency have variable clinical phenotypes. Most present with progressive infantile encephalopathy with motor retardation and fluctuating extrapyramidal and ocular and vegetative symptoms (44). TH deficiency also can cause L-dopa-responsive dystonia and has become incorporated into classifications of dystonias as the cause of recessive L-dopa-responsive dystonia. However, clear differences are obvious between GTPCH deficiency or Segawa-like patients, who typically present in childhood with

walking problems due to dystonia of the lower limbs or much later with a Parkinson-like disease, and the majority of patients with TH deficiency, in whom several cerebral and possibly cerebellar systems are affected. Diurnal fluctuation, which is a hallmark of Segawa syndrome, generally is not prominent in TH deficiency (Table 45-5).

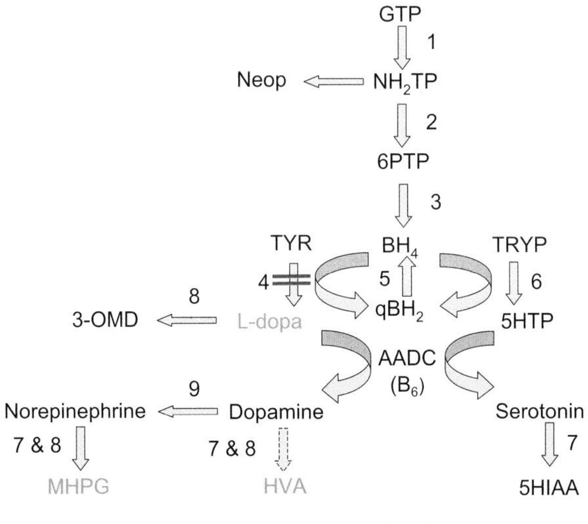

At the severe end of the spectrum of TH deficiency, virtually no movements are observed, including no dystonic movements. The first clinical impression of these infants, who generally hold a frog-like position, is that of a neuromuscular disorder. However, increased deep tendon reflexes and pyramidal tract signs point to cerebral dysfunction. Oculogyric crises (see Figure 45-4) develop. Miosis may be present but may go undiagnosed because of prominent ptosis. It is important to stress that such patients also show symptoms of significant catecholamine deficiency, such as hypoglycemia and inadequate stress responses. There is an obvious tendency to preterm birth with troublesome cardiorespiratory perinatal adaptation. It is reasonable to assume that a number of patients die undiagnosed perinatally or even prenatally. After the neonatal period, difficult-to-control and potentially life-threatening paroxysmal periods of general malaise with lethargy and vegetative symptoms of irritability, sweating, and drooling can occur. Growth can be compromized and bone age severely delayed, suggestive of an impaired secretion pattern and/or stimulation of growth hormone (GH).

Surprisingly, some infants with TH deficiency can develop normally until an arrest of motor development with a characteristic combination of neurological symptoms before or around 1 year of age. Hypokinesia, marked truncal hypotonia, a mask face, oculogyric crises, myoclonic jerks, and an extrapyramidal tremor develop progressively. The latter three can be mistaken as epileptic phenomena. After infancy, muscle tone increases progressively. Contractures, failure to thrive, and immobilization may develop; (dystonic) cerebral palsy is a likely descriptive (mis)diagnosis.

Some patients who did not develop extrapyramidal symptoms in the first year of life were able to walk independently and followed a clinical course best summarized as spastic paraplegia. Their symptoms resolved completely following L-dopa supplementation, and they are by now healthy and

FIGURE 45-5. Tyrosine hydroxylase deficiency and its laboratory consequences. Reduced metabolite levels are depicted in green. GTP = guanosine triphosphate; NH_2TP = dihydroneopterin triphosphate; Neop = neopterin; 6PTP = 6-pyruvyltetrahydropterin; BH_4 = tetrahydrobiopterin; qBH_2 = quinonoid dihydrobiopterin; TRYP = tryptophan; TYR = tyrosine; 5HTP = 5-hydroxytryptophan; B_6 = vitamin B_6/pyridoxal-5-phosphate; HVA = homovanillic acid; 5-HIAA = 5-hydroxyindoleacetic acid; MHPG = 3-methoxy-4-hydroxyphenylglycol; 3OMD = 3-O-methyldopa; 1 = GTP cyclohydrolase; 2 = 6-pyruvoyltetrahydropterin synthase; 3 = sepiapterin reductase; 4 = tyrosine hydroxylase; 5 = dihydropteridine reductase; 6 = tryptophan hydroxylase; AADC = aromatic L-aminoacid decarboxylase; 7 = monoamine oxidase; 8 = catechol-O-methyltransferase; 9 = dopamine-hydroxylase. The dashed lines indicate more than one step.

- Prenatal diagnosis is possible where mutations have been established.

- Newborn screening is unavailable.

TABLE 45-5 Symptomatology of TH Deficiency versus Dominantly Inherited GTPCH Deficiency

	TH Deficiency	GTPCH Deficiency
Mean age of onset of symptoms	4 months	7 years
Fetal distress	+	−
Progression	+ +	+
Diurnal fluctuation	− (+)	+ +
Focal limb dystonia	− (+)	+ +
Generalized dystonia	+	− (+)
Rest or postural tremor	+	+ +
Bradykinesia	−	+ +
Hypokinesia	+ +	− (+)
Truncal hypotonia	+ +	−
Rigidity	− (+)	+ +
Pyramidal tract signs	+	− (+)
Hypomimia	+	−
Bilaterale ptosis	+	−
Oculogyric crises	+	−
Paroxysmal sweating	+	−
Hypersalivation	+	−
Scoliosis	− (+)	+ +
Retarded growth	+ +	− (+)
Mental retardation	+	−

+ = pathologic; − = not present, i.e. normal.

independently living adults. Others may have no pyramidal tract or ocular signs but progressive extrapyramidal symptoms including dystonia and rigidity (55). In several patients, TH deficiency has led to infantile-onset parkinsonism (53,55,57).

Diagnosis Diagnosis relies on a characteristic metabolite constellation: low concentrations of metabolites of dopaminergic neurotransmission, HVA, and MHPG in the presence of normal concentrations of the serotonin metabolite 5-HIAA (14). A finding of elevated plasma prolactin also points to a central dopamine deficiency because the release of prolactin normally is inhibited by central dopamine concentrations. Confirmation of the diagnosis by mutation analysis is always required because secondary decreases of the dopaminergic system are found in several unrelated conditions, such as mitochondrial encephalopathies, generalized hypoxia, and severe epileptic encephalopathies (15). Enzyme analysis is not possible in TH deficiency because tissues expressing enzyme activity, brain and adrenal medulla, are difficult to obtain.

Treatment/Prognosis The principal treatment of TH deficiency relies on bypassing the metabolic block using L-dopa (1–10 mg/kg/day in two to six divided doses). Some patients respond readily to low-dose L-dopa treatment, some require higher doses, and some do not respond at all or suffer from intolerable adverse effects such as irritability, dyskinesias, mainly hyperkinesia and ballism, and/or nausea (44,58).

For a successful therapeutic trial with L-dopa, some points have to be taken into account:

- L-Dopa has to be administered in combination with an L-dopa-decarboxylase inhibitor (25% of L-dopa daily dosage, if the total daily dose is below 400 mg/day, 10% of L-dopa daily dosage above 400 mg/day).

- L-Dopa treatment has to be started carefully and slowly. Individual steps of increments should not be more than 1 mg/kg/day to avoid dyskinesias and irritability due to dopamine receptor hypersensitivity. Slow-release preparations may be better tolerated by ensuring constant L-dopa levels. In early diagnosed, severe cases, initial doses should be as low as 0.25 mg/kg/day in two to six divided doses. In such patients, L-dopa can be increased only very very slowly, sometimes over several years.

- Effectiveness of treatment is monitored by clinical outcome and measurement of prolactin in serum and HVA levels in CSF.

- An L-dopa trial should last at least 6 months with sufficient doses (10 mg/kg/day) before its effect is judged.

- L-Dopa/carbidopa therapy may reduce CSF folates (CH$_3$-group trapping by L-dopa to 3-O-methyl-dopa), requiring folinic acid (5-formyltetrahydrofolate) substitution (15 mg/day).

Combination of L-dopa substitution with anticholinergic treatment (Trihexiphenidyl) or adjunctive treatment of L-dopa substitution with inhibitors of monoamine oxidase B such as Selegelin, COMT inhibitors such as Entacapone, and dopamine agonists such as bromocriptine are helpful therapeutic combinations in some patients. Monitoring of therapy requires repeated careful clinical evaluation by a (pediatric) neurologist, including video documentation and follow-up of CSF HVA, 5-HIAA, and 5-MTHF concentrations by consecutive lumbar punctures in the morning before the medication (at least yearly). In some patients with high prolactin before L-dopa supplementation, prolactin levels can aid monitoring of therapy. Treatment in early infancy may require monitoring and correction of hypoglycemia.

Response to treatment appears variable and depends on the severity of the disease (58). The early-onset encephalopathic forms may respond poorly, whereas later onset forms that present with dystonia may have complete resolution of the symptoms (59). Despite all therapeutic interventions, the disease course still can be lethal (44).

Aromatic l-Amino Acid Decarboxylase Deficiency

Etiology/Pathophysiology Aromatic L-amino acid decarboxylase (AADC) deficiency is caused by autosomal recessively inherited mutations in the DDC gene (17,60). The enzyme is required for the synthesis of both serotonin and the catecholamines; therefore, a deficiency leads to low levels of all these neurotransmitters and accumulation of 3-O-methyldopa, 5-hydroxytryptophan, and L-dopa in CSF, plasma, and urine (Figure 45-6). The methylation of L-dopa leads to the formation of 3-O-methyldopa. The increased requirement for methyl groups reduces the levels of S-adenosylmethionine within the CNS and sometimes reduces the levels of 5-methyltetrahydrofolate (61). No anatomical abnormalities are present, and computed tomographic (CT) scanning and magnetic resonance imaging (MRI) show a normal brain or slight cerebral atrophy. The neurological symptoms are attributed to the severe deficiency of biogenic amine neurotransmitters.

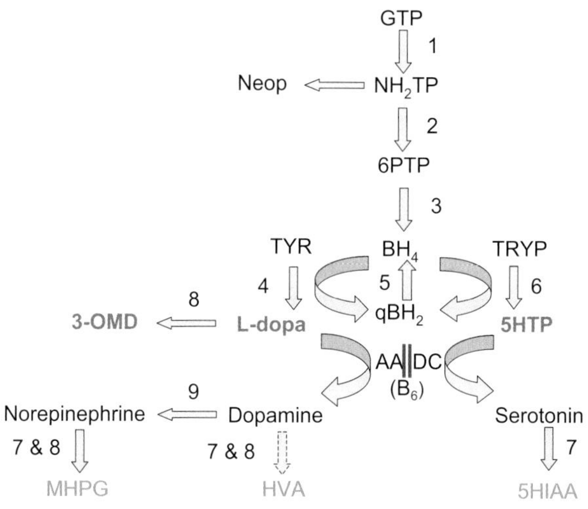

FIGURE 45-6. Aromatic L-amino acid decarboxylase deficiency and its laboratory consequences. Elevated metabolite levels are depicted in blue, reduced levels in green. GTP = guanosine triphosphate; NH_2TP = dihydroneopterin triphosphate; Neop = neopterin; 6PTP = 6-pyruvyltetrahydropterin; BH_4 = tetrahydrobiopterin; $_qBH_2$ = quinonoid dihydrobiopterin; TRYP = tryptophan; TYR = tyrosine; 5HTP = 5-hydroxytryptophan; B_6 = vitamin B_6/pyridoxal-5-phosphate; HVA = homovanillic acid; 5-HIAA = 5-hydroxyindoleacetic acid; MHPG = 3-methoxy-4-hydroxyphenylglycol; 3OMD = 3-O-methyldopa; 1 = GTP cyclohydrolase; 2 = 6-pyruvoyltetrahydropterin synthase; 3 = sepiapterin reductase; 4 = tyrosine hydroxylase; 5 = dihydropteridine reductase; 6 = tryptophan hydroxylase; AADC = aromatic L-aminoacid decarboxylase; 7 = monoamine oxidase; 8 = catechol-O-methyltransferase; 9 = dopamine hydroxylase. The dashed lines indicate more than one step.

Clinical Presentation Over 20 cases of AADC deficiency have been found since the initial description of the index family (16). Two reviews have been published (62,63). Approximately half the patients had feeding difficulties, autonomic dysfunction, and hypotonia in the neonatal period (62). Patients then typically present in the first few months of life with dystonia or intermittent limb spasticity, axial and truncal hypotonia, extreme irritability, oculogyric crises, and psychomotor retardation. Autonomic symptoms have included ptosis, miosis, temperature instability, paroxysmal sweating, nasal congestion, hypotension, and gastroesophageal reflux (64). In a milder case, psychomotor retardation was first noted at 9 months of age. Hypotonia, short periods of hypertonicity, and oculogyric crises were present, but even without treatment, the child could sit and communicate nonverbally by the age of 2 years (65). Another untreated child had autism as the major symptom (66).

Molecular Variants The human DDC gene is encoded by a single-gene copy that is over 85 kbp in length. It is located on chromosome 7p12.1-p12.3 and contains 15 exons (67). The enzyme requires pyridoxal phosphate as cofactor and is a homodimer composed of identical subunits with a molecular mass of 53.9 kDa (68). Differential splicing leads to two forms of AADC mRNA that code for a single amino acid sequence. These mRNA's differ in their 5' untranslated regions and are encoded by two distinct exons, exon N1 being designated the neuronal type and exon L1 the nonneuronal type. The two forms of mRNA are produced by alternative use of these two first exons. Alternative splicing also exists in the coding region of the human AADC mRNA. Differential splicing in this area leads to the formation of a short-version transcript that lacks exon 3 and appears not to have any enzyme activity (69). Genomic sequencing of the DDC gene has revealed 23 mutations. Sixteen were missense mutations causing single-amino-acid substitutions. A S250F missense mutation was present on 10 alleles, suggesting that this might be a fairly common mutation. Two lead to formation of premature stop codons. In one family, three patients investigated showed an L-dopa-responsive movement disorder. Sequencing revealed a homozygous G-to-A substitution converting glycine to serine at position 102 (G102S) in exon 3. Kinetic studies and analysis of the protein structure revealed that the mutation increased the K_m apparent for L-dopa, altering the protein configuration near to the substrate-binding site (60).

Diagnosis Diagnosis relies on the measurement of HVA, 3-OMD, and 5-HIAA in CSF. Concentrations of HVA and 5-HIAA are decreased, whereas 3-OMD levels are elevated. Additionally, L-dopa, and 5-hydroxytryptophan are also elevated in plasma and CSF, and in urine, there is a small elevation of vanillactic acid. Confirmation of the diagnosis is by enzyme assay in plasma (70). A severe deficiency of pyridoxal-5'-phosphate can lead to similar metabolite changes in CSF, but in these cases, enzyme activity in plasma is either normal or elevated (18,19).

Treatment/Prognosis The main goal is to increase monoaminergic transmission. This has been attempted using dopamine agonists (e.g., pergolide, pramipexole, bromocriptine, and ropinirole), anticholinergic treatment (Trihexiphenidyl) and/or nonselective MAO inhibitors (e.g., tranylcypromine, selegiline and phenelzine). Response to treatment is variable, but outcome appears to be better in males than in females (62). All patients have received vitamin B_6, but no sustained effects have been reported. L-Dopa substrate–responsive AADC deficiency has been described (60,71). A trial with L-dopa therefore might be considered in all patients with AADC deficiency.

The overall prognosis is guarded. About half the patients stabilize on individual treatment regiments and aquire different degrees of motor and psychosocial skills. Others do not show any sustained improvements (62). Despite all therapeutic interventions, the disease course still can be lethal.

Monoamine Oxidase A Deficiency

Etiology/Pathophysiology Monoamine oxidase (MAO) catalyzes the oxidative deamination of a wide variety of monamines, including serotonin, the catecholamines, and many minor amines (72). Two forms of the enzyme are expressed in most tissues, and these are classified as MAO-A and MAO-B depending on their sensitivity to inhibitors and preferential affinity for substrates. The genes for both are mapped to the X chromosome. A point mutation in MAO-A has been described; loss of enzyme activity leads to accumulation of the monoamine neurotransmitters and decreased levels of their metabolites in body fluids and compartments (see Figure 45-7) (21). The accumulation of monoamines probably is involved in the aggressive phenotype found in the one family described with MAO-A deficiency. Aggressive behavior is also a feature of the MAO-A knockout mouse (73).

Clinical Presentation MAO-A deficiency was described originally in a large Dutch family (74). Early presentation details were not given. Males within the family had mild mental retardation and a tendency toward stereotyped hand movements (e.g., hand wringing, plucking, or fiddling) and behavioral problems with repeated occurrences of aggression that included attempted rape, repeated fighting, stabbing, arson, exhibitionism, voyeurism, and sexual advances to female family members (74).

- Effectiveness of treatment is monitored by clinical outcome.

- Prenatal diagnosis is possible where mutations have been established.

- Newborn screening is unavailable.

- Prenatal diagnosis is possible where mutations have been established.

- Newborn screening is unavailable.

- There are no effective treatment for MAO-A deficiency.

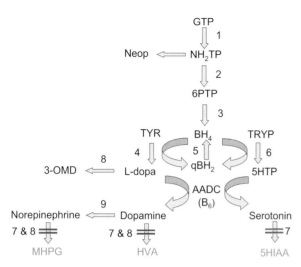

FIGURE 45-7. Monoamine oxidase deficiency and its laboratory consequences. Reduced metabolite levels are depicted in green. GTP = guanosine triphosphate; NH_2TP = dihydroneopterin triphosphate; Neop = neopterin; 6PTP = 6-pyruvyltetrahydropterin; BH_4 = tetrahydrobiopterin; $_qBH_2$ = quinonoid dihydrobiopterin; TRYP = tryptophan; TYR = tyrosine; 5HTP = 5-hydroxytryptophan; B_6 = vitamin B_6/pyridoxal-5-phosphate; HVA = homovanillic acid; 5-HIAA = 5-hydroxyindoleacetic acid; MHPG = 3-methoxy-4-hydroxyphenylglycol; 3OMD = 3-O-methyldopa; 1 = GTP cyclohydrolase; 2 = 6-pyruvoyltetrahydropterin synthase; 3 = sepiapterin reductase; 4 = tyrosine hydroxylase; 5 = dihydropteridine reductase; 6 = tryptophan hydroxylase; AADC = aromatic L-aminoacid decarboxylase; 7 = monoamine oxidase; 8 = catechol-O-methyltransferase; 9 = dopamine-hydroxylase.

Molecular Variants MAO-A has been mapped to the X chromosome in the p11.23–11.4 region (75). The human gene extends over 80 kb and is composed of 15 exons (76). The cDNA that encodes human MAO-A has been cloned. The deduced amino acid sequence shows MAO-A to have a subunit weight of 59.7 kDa (77). There are two species of MAO-A mRNA, 2.1 and 4.3 kb. The longer message has an extension of 2.2 kb in the 3' noncoding region that is contained entirely within exon 15. The two messages probably arise from alternative use of two polyadenylation sites present in the same exon (76).

A single mutation has been found in the index family with MAO-A deficiency. This was a single-base substitution (CnT) at nucleotide 936 leading to the formation of a premature stop codon (Q296X) (21).

Diagnosis MAO-A deficiency should be considered in males who show prominent behavioral disturbance, especially if there is a family history and linkage to proximal Xp. A second diagnostic angle is symptomatic hyperserotoninemia in the absence of carcinoid. Diagnosis of MAO-A deficiency is achieved by analysis of urinary monoamines and their metabolites. Either 24-hour or spot urines can be used for testing (22). Concentrations of MAO-A substrates (i.e., normetanephrine, 3-methoxytyramine, and tyramine) are elevated, and concentrations of the MAO-A products (i.e., vanillylmandelic acid, homovanillic acid, and 5-hydroxyindolacetic acid) are decreased (21). It is important that subjects not eat amine-rich foods such as bananas or dates in the period prior to testing. Confirmation of the diagnosis can be obtained by measurement of MAO-A activity in dexamethasone-stimulated fibroblasts (74).

Treatment/Prognosis Treatment for MAO-A deficiency is experimental. Cyproheptadine hydrochloride and sertraline hydrochloride have been used. Sertraline hydrochloride should be introduced slowly because of the risk of causing the serotonin syndrome. Dietary intervention by avoiding foods rich in amines may be beneficial. MAO-A deficiency does not carry a risk of substantial or even life-threatening complications. It is possible that hypertensive crises may result through an increased sensitivity to dietary or pharmacological amines (21,74).

Dopamine β-Hydroxylase Deficiency

Etiology/Pathophysiology DβH catalyzes the hydroxylation of dopamine to norepinephrine within noradrenergic neurons. Recessively inherited mutations in the DβH gene lead to decreased enzyme activity and lowered levels of norepinephrine within central and autonomic noradrenergic neurons (Figure 45-8). The disorder is characterized by sympathetic noradrenergic denervation and adrenomedullary failure. The central consequences appear minimal, but the norepinephrine deficiency in the autonomic neurons leads to the appearance of severe orthostatic hypotension, noradrenergic failure, and ptosis of the eyelids in adolescence (24,78).

Clinical Presentation To date, 12 patients with DβH deficiency have been reported. Patients presented in adolescence with severe orthostatic hypotension, noradrenergic failure, and ptosis of the eyelids. During childhood, fatigue, episodes of fainting, syncope, and exercise intolerance generally were present. Physical and cognitive function was normal. Sexual function is normal in females, but in males, ejaculation is retrograde (24,78). Several other clinical features, such as blepharoptosis, hyperflexible joints, high palate, sluggish deep tendon reflexes, and a mild normocytic anemia, have been described (79).

Molecular Variants The human DβH gene has been mapped to chromosome 9q34 (80). It is approximately 23 kbp in length and is composed of 12 exons. Alternative use of two polyadenylation sites in exon 12 generates two different mRNA types designated type A (2.7 kb) and type B (2.4 kb) that differ only in the 3' untranslated region. Type A contains a 3' extension of 300 bp at the end of type B. Both mRNAs encode the same amino acid sequence of 603 amino acid residues with a molecular mass of 64.9 kDa (81). The final protein is a homotetramer with two atoms of copper per subunit.

A polymorphism (-1021CnT) has been located in the 5' flanking region of the DβH gene, and homozygosity has been associated with very low plasma enzyme activities (82); however, it is not yet clear whether this is associated with a pathological phenotype. In

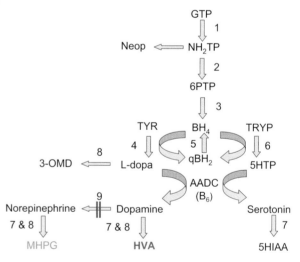

FIGURE 45-8. Dopamine β-hydroxylase deficiency and its laboratory consequences. Elevated metabolite levels are depicted in blue, reduced levels in green. GTP = guanosine triphosphate; NH_2TP = dihydroneopterin triphosphate; Neop = neopterin; 6PTP = 6-pyruvyltetrahydropterin; BH_4 = tetrahydrobiopterin; $_qBH_2$ = quinonoid dihydrobiopterin; TRYP = tryptophan; TYR = tyrosine; 5HTP = 5-hydroxytryptophan; B_6 = vitamin B_6/pyridoxal-5-phosphate; HVA = homovanillic acid; 5-HIAA = 5-hydroxyindoleacetic acid; MHPG = 3-methoxy-4-hydroxyphenylglycol; 3OMD = 3-O-methyldopa; 1 = GTP cyclohydrolase; 2 = 6-pyruvoyltetrahydropterin synthase; 3 = sepiapterin reductase; 4 = tyrosine hydroxylase; 5 = dihydropteridine reductase; 6 = tryptophan hydroxylase; AADC = aromatic L-aminoacid decarboxylase; 7 = monoamine oxidase; 8 = catechol-O-methyltransferase; 9 = dopamine-hydroxylase.

- Newborn screening is unavailable.

two families, a T-to-C transversion in the splice donor site of the DβH intron 1 that leads to a premature stop codon on one allele is associated with a missense mutation in exon 2 on the other allele in one affected patient and missense mutations on the other allele in exons 1 and 6 in the second patient (83,84).

Diagnosis DβH deficiency should be considered in any adult with chronic orthostatic hypotension, with a devastating orthostatic hypotension being characteristic in adults. There are a multitude of conditions that can lead to acute or chronic orthostatic hypotension. DβH deficiency is classified as a primary autonomic neuropathy. Conditions that lead to chronic failure of the autonomic nervous system therefore are included in the primary differential diagnosis. These include the Bradbury–Eggleston syndrome, a peripheral autonomic failure, the Shy–Drager syndrome, multiple-system atrophy causing central autonomic failure, and the Riley–Day syndrome, a familial dysautonomia. Autonomic neuropathy also may occur secondary to other easily recognizable systemic diseases such as diabetes, porphyria, or amyloidosis. Biochemically, DβH deficiency is different from all other recognized conditions with orthostatic hypotension or autonomic dysfunction. Failure to produce norepinephrine and the consequent lack of end product inhibition of TH leads to a norepinephrine:dopamine ratio of less than 0.1, and such a finding is pathognomonic for the disease (24,25). An increase in blood pressure and correction of the orthostatic hypotension in response to dihydroxyphenylserine are also diagnostic. This compound is decarboxylated by AADC to yield norepinephrine (NE), and its administration leads to an increase in plasma NE concentrations (85). Between 3% and 4% of the normal adult population has near-zero levels of plasma DβH (86); therefore, plasma enzyme measurement in isolation cannot be used to make a positive diagnosis.

Treatment/Prognosis DβH deficiency is treated with dihydroxyphenylserine (DOPS). This compound is decarboxylated by aromatic L-amino acid decarboxylase to form NE, which is taken up and stored in the noradrenergic neurons. Administration of 250–500 mg of DOPS twice daily produces an increase in blood pressure and sustained relief of the orthostatic symptoms. Without appropriate treatment, postural hypotension can lead to significant injuries or even death. Treatment with DOPS greatly reduces this danger.

Folinic Acid–Responsive Seizures

Etiology/Pathophysiology Folinic acid–responsive seizures were identified during the course of a study to investigate biogenic amine metabolism in neonates and infants with epileptic encephalopathies. Fewer than 10 patients have been identified, in whom analysis of CSF constantly revealed a large peak on the HPLC system used routinely for determination of biogenic amine metabolites (20). The unknown was not present in more than a thousand CSF samples investigated from neonates and infants with a wide variety of neurological conditions. Retrospectively, a metabolite related to medications could be excluded. However, the metabolic basis for this disorder remains unclear. A primary defect in folate metabolism is unlikely, leaving the hypothesis of a primary disturbance in an intermediate pathway that requires folate as a cofactor.

Clinical Presentation All patients presented with severe epileptic encephalopathy. Onset of myoclonic and clonic seizures is early, from the 2nd hour to a few days of life. Seizures may be ameliorated by high-dose multiple-anticonvulsant therapy but still are likely to progress to status epilepticus and coma. Without specific treatment with folinic acid, seizures will be controlled only partially by multiple-anticonvulsant therapy. Psychomotor development will be severely impaired. In two children, a transient dilatative cardiomyopathy was diagnosed in the first week of life that disappeared during the following months (20). In three families, previous sibships have suffered and died from a similar seizure disorder, which points to an inherited basis of the condition.

Diagnosis The diagnosis of folinic acid–responsive seizures is primarily a clinical diagnosis, similar to the diagnosis of pyridoxine-dependent or pyridoxal-phosphate-dependent epilepsies. It is based on a positive response to a therapeutic trial of folinic acid. There is no established protocol for a trial of folinic acid. Doses of 3–5 mg/kg of body weight per day in three doses have been successful. Since folinic acid–responsive seizure disorder is a treatable condition, a high index of suspicion is warranted. Each newborn with severe neonatal/infantile epileptic encephalopathy should have a lumbar puncture and immediately receive consecutive therapeutic trials of vitamin B_6, pyridoxal-5'-phos-

phate, and folinic acid. Folinic acid usually is given in conjunction with antiepileptic drugs. In this situation, cessation of seizure activity in response to folinic acid would be suggestive, but not conclusive, of folinic acid–responsive seizures. To confirm the diagnosis, folinic acid therapy would have to be withdrawn, followed by seizures that again respond to folinic acid. Alternatively, treatment could be continued until breakthrough seizures occur that respond promptly to an increase in folinic acid corresponding to the increase in body weight during growth. In one infant with folinic acid–responsive seizures, the response was only partial despite an increase of folinic acid up to 50 mg four times a day. In all other known patients, the response was marked to dramatic. Breakthrough seizures responded to increased doses of folinic acid. The differential diagnosis is wide, including all major causes of neonatal seizures. Inborn errors of metabolism that can present identically are nonketotic hyperglycinemia and the deficiencies of sulfite oxidase, adenylosuccinate lyase, and GABA transaminase and certain types of congenital disorders of glycosylation. There are biochemical markers available. However, the increases in concentration of amino acids in CSF are only moderate and can be missed or misinterpreted easily. Increases of the unknown compound on the monoamine metabolite chromatographic system could be considered the "gold standard" for diagnosis, but currently, this approach is restricted to one specialist laboratory.

Treatment/Prognosis Successful treatment was achieved with 3–5 mg of folinic acid per kilogram of body weight per day in three doses. Doses need to be increased and adjusted to body weight during growth. Patients probably require lifelong supplementation. Obvious criteria to increase the doses are breakthrough seizures. In all patients reported, folinic acid therapy was initiated many weeks after the onset of seizures. It can be assumed that folinic acid will not reverse preexisting brain damage caused by late diagnosis and treatment. All patients known show some degree of developmental delay despite good seizure control after introducing folinic acid. Serial cognitive assessment is recommended. In one child, only a partial reduction of seizures could be achieved, and the child died at the age of 2.5 months.

- Prenatal diagnosis is unavailable.
- Newborn screening is unavailable.

- Effectiveness of treatment is monitored by clinical outcome.

DISORDERS OF VITAMIN B₆ METABOLISM

Etiology/Pathophysiology Pyridoxal-5'-phosphate is an essential cofactor of transamination and decarboxylation reactions in various pathways, including serotonin and dopamine biosynthesis. It is synthesised from dietary pyridoxal, pyridoxamine, and pyridoxine. The conversion of pyridoxine and pyridoxamine to the active cofactor, pyridoxal-5'-phosphate, requires the activity of a kinase and then of pyridox(am)ine 5'-phosphate oxidase; synthesis of the active cofactor from dietary pyridoxal or pyridoxal phosphate requires the kinase only (Figure 45-9). The three biologically active 2-methylpyridine derivatives collectively carry the generic name *vitamin B₆*.

In the mouse, neurotransmitter metabolism can be regulated by modulation of the synthesis of pyridoxal 5'-phosphate, and failure to maintain pyridoxal phosphate levels results in epilepsy (87). In humans, pyridoxine deficiency causes peripheral neuritis, dermatitis, anemia, and relevant to neurotransmitter disorders, irritability, restlessness, hyperacusis, and convulsions in the CNS. One monogenic disorder in humans is located directly within the synthesis of pyridoxal-5'-phosphate: pyridoxal-phosphate-dependent epilepsy due to pyridox(am)ine-5'-phosphate oxidase deficiency (88). In hypophosphatasia, the transport of pyridoxal-5'-phosphate across the cellular membrane is severely impaired, effectively resulting in intracellular pyridoxal-5'-phosphate deficiency and, again, seizures. In two other neurometabolic diseases, pyridoxine-dependent epilepsy (piperideine-6-carboxylate dehydrogenase deficiency) and hyperprolinemia type II, intermediates accumulating because of the primary defect scavenge pyridoxal-phos-phate and lead to pyridoxal-5'-phosphate deficiency (88) (see Figure 45-9).

Pyridoxine-Dependent Epilepsy

Etiology/Pathophysiology In 1954, Hunt and colleagues described the first patient with a seizure disorder that "occurred spontaneously and was corrected solely by the administration of pyridoxine." He already coined the term *pyridoxine dependency* to distinguish this entity from pyridoxine deficiency. Among the numerous enzymatic reactions in which pyridoxal-5'-phosphate is involved is glutamic acid decarboxylase, which converts glutamate to GABA, the principal inhibitory neurotransmitter in the mammalian CNS. It was tempting to speculate that pyridoxine-dependent epilepsy is caused by a primary molecular defect in this enzyme (89,90). In contrast to pyridox(am)ine-5'-phosphate oxidase (PNPO) deficiency (see below), there are no indications of disturbances of other enzymatic reactions requiring pyridoxal-5'-phosphate, and intrinsic vitamin B₆ levels are normal. However, recently, the enzymatic defect could be pinpointed to a piperideine-6-carboxylate dehydrogenase located in the degradation pathway of lysine, the accumulating intermediate L-Δ^1-piperideine-6-carboxylate scavenging pyridoxal phosphate (91). It also was recognized that pipecolic acid and L-Δ^1-piperideine-6-carboxylate accumulate before the primary block and can be found elevated in body fluids. A similar pathomechanism is responsible for pyridoxal deficiency in hyperprolinemia type II, where L-Δ^1-pyrroline-3-hydroxy-5-carboxylate is accumulating in addition to proline and as a side effect resulting from treatment with the tuberculostatic drug isoniacid. It has yet to be proven that all forms of pyridoxine dependency are genetically homogeneous.

Clinical Presentation In the classical presentation, pyridoxine-dependent epilepsy usually begins within the first week of life, the latest within 28 days (89). In some patients, intrauterine convulsions are reported. The familiy history may reveal previous siblings who have suffered and died from a similar disorder. Seizures can be of different types, including those commonly associated with structural brain pathology (e.g., focal seizures and infantile spasms). Unfortunately, there is no consistent electrographic pattern unique to this patient population. Continuous and discontinuous backgrounds, suppression burst-like patterns, and hypsarrhythmia all have been observed. Pyridoxine-dependent seizures may be ameliorated but are never controlled even by high-dose multiple-anticonvulsant therapy. Only specific treatment with pyridoxine leads to rapid ceasation of the seizures.

Pyridoxine-dependent seizures can be heterogeneous in their presentation, and sometimes idiopathic epilepsies respond to treatment with pyridoxine. In addition to the classical presentation within the first days of life, there are at least three atypical presentations:

- Late onset, that is, later than 28 days
- Neonatal onset but with an initial response to conventional anticonvulsant therapy
- Neonatal onset with initially negative but a later sustained positive response to pyridoxine

In fact, atypical presentations may be more common than the classical neonatal form.

Diagnosis Pyridoxine-dependent epilepsy is a clinical diagnosis based on a positive response to a therapeutic trial of pyridoxine (89). Since it is a treatable condition, a high index of suspicion is warranted. Each newborn with severe neonatal/infantile epileptic encephalopathy should have a lumbar puncture and immediately receive consecutive therapeutic trials of vitamin B₆, pyridoxal-5'-phosphate, and folinic acid.

There is no universal protocol for a pyridoxine trial. The dose required is variable, and higher doses may be necessary to control seizures, at least initially. In classical cases, we suggest a starting dose of 100 mg intravenously. If there is no response within 24 hours, the dose should be repeated (and possibly increased up to 500 mg in total) before being sure about pyridoxine nonresponsiveness. If there is uncertainty about at least a partial response, pyridoxine should be continued at 30 mg/kg/day for 7 days before final conclusions are drawn.

Initially, pyridoxine is given often in conjunction with antiepileptic drugs. In this situation, cessation of seizure activity in response to pyridoxine can be suggestive but may not be conclusive, especially in atypical presentations. To confirm the diagnosis, pyridoxine therapy would have to be withdrawn, fol-

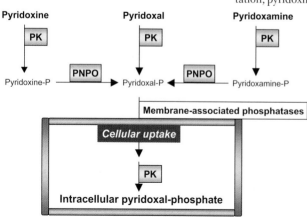

FIGURE 45-9. B₆ metabolism. Pyridoxal phosphate (P) is synthesised from dietary pyridoxal, pyridoxamine, and pyridoxine by pyridoxal kinase (PK) and pyridox(am)ine-5'-phosphate oxidase (PNPO).

- All patients with difficult-to treat seizures starting before 2 years of age should have a trial of pyridoxine (usually given orally in this circumstance).

- Prenatal diagnosis is possible where mutations have been established.

- Newborn screening is unavailable.

- Each newborn with severe neonatal/infantile epileptic encephalopathy should have a lumbar puncture and then immediately receive consecutive therapeutic trials with vitamin B$_6$, pyridoxal-5'-phosphate, and folinic acid.

- Pyridoxine may cause apnea and prolonged cerebral depression after the initial dose. Resuscitation equipment and intensive-care facilities should be available.

- Effectiveness of treatment is monitored by clinical outcome.

lowed by seizures that again respond to pyridoxine. Alternatively, treatment could be continued until breakthrough seizures occur that respond promptly to an increase in pyridoxine corresponding to the increase of body weight during growth.

The differential diagnosis of pyridoxine-dependent epilepsy is wide, including all major causes of neonatal seizures. Inborn errors of metabolism that can present identically are nonketotic hyperglycinemia, sulfite oxidase, adenylsuccinate lyase, GABA transaminase deficiencies, and certain types of congenital disorders of glycosylation. In cases where seizures respond to pyridoxine beyond the neonatal period, pyridoxine deficiency should be kept in mind. Pyridoxine deficiency can be caused by dietary insufficiency (e.g., gastrointestinal malabsorptive states), liver diseases, increased metabolic demands (e.g., hyperthyroidism), or leukemia or can be iatrogenic (e.g., isoniazid therapy). In addition to CNS dysfunction, pyridoxine deficiency also results in peripheral neuritis, dermatitis, and anemia.

Pipecolic acid measurement in plasma and CSF now provides a sensitive diagnostic marker for pyridoxine-responsive seizures (91,92). Pipecolic acid is situated in the primarily affected pathway of lysine degradation. Finally, enzyme assay and mutation analysis can prove the diagnosis.

Treatment/Prognosis Successful treatment requires 5–30 mg of pyridoxine per kilogram of body weight per day in one dose. Doses need to be increased and adjusted to body weight during growth. Patients require lifelong supplementation. Obvious criteria to increase the doses are breakthrough seizures. In many patients, specific therapy is not instituted within a few days or even weeks of symptoms. Pyridoxine will not reverse preexisting brain damage caused by late diagnosis or treatment, and many patients show some degree of mental impairment. Neurological disability (including seizures) will require treatment in its own right. There is evidence that lower doses of pyridoxine, while controlling seizures, still may not prevent the development of cognitive impairment. Serial cog-

nitive assessment is recommended. High doses of pyridoxine carry the risk of producing skin photosensitivity and a peripheral sensory neuropathy, which must be weighted against the anticipated neurodevelopmental benefit. Doses of up to 1 g/day can be regarded as safe in older children. If there is a positive family history of pyridoxine-dependent seizures, maternal treatment in utero is indicated.

Hyperprolinemia Type II (L-Δ^1-Pyrroline-5-Carboxylate Dehydrogenase Deficiency)

Etiology/Pathophysiology Hyperprolinemia type II had long been delineated as being caused by a recessively inherited defect in the second step of proline and hydroxyproline degradation. Proline is first oxidized by proline oxidase, a deficiency of which causes the clinically benign phenotype hyperprolinemia type I. The product of this reaction is L-Δ^1-pyrroline-5-carboxylate, which converts spontaneously and is in equilibrium with glutamic acid γ-semialdehyde. The next enzyme, L-Δ^1-pyrroline-5-carboxylate dehydrogenase, is defective in hyperprolinemia type II (93,94). The accumulating L-Δ^1- pyrroline-3-hydroxy-5-carboxylate and L-Δ^1-pyrroline-3-hydroxy-5-carboxylate combine with pyridoxal-5'-phosphate in a reaction known as *Knoevenagel condensation* (91). The scavenged pyridoxal-5'-phosphate is no longer metabolically available, and with time, the body may get depleted of pyridoxal-5'-phosphate.

Clinical Presentation Only a few patients with hyperprolinemia type II have been identified, and it has long been debated if there is any clinical phenotype. Initially, hyperprolinemia type I, which has no phenotype, and hyperprolinemia type II were not separated, and in addition, individuals with hyperprolinemia type II often have no clinical manifestations. On investigation of larger cohorts of affected individuals, it became obvious that hyperprolinemia type II could lead to a phenotype. Epilepsy in childhood was found in greater than 50%, with the seizures being mostly of grand mal in type (93). The epilepsy disappears in adulthood, and most adults with hyperprolinemia type II have no symptoms from

their disease. Furthermore, there is no evidence that maternal hyperprolinemia type II compromises fetal development.

Diagnosis Hyperprolinemia type II is suspected on grounds of highly elevated levels of proline in body fluids. The plasma concentrations always exceed 1500 μmol/L. Proline levels in plasma, CSF, and urine usually are higher in hyperprolinemia type II than in hyperprolinemia type I. Whereas proline is the only amino acid elevated in plasma and CSF, glycine and hydroxyproline also are found elevated in urine. These three amino acids share a common renal tubular transport system; when one is present in high amounts, the tubular reabsorption of the other two is impaired, and therefore, their urinary excretion is enhanced. Hyperprolinemia type II can be distinguished unequivocally from hyperprolinemia type I by demonstration of elevated levels of L-Δ^1-pyrroline-5-carboxylate. The diagnosis also can be reached by enzyme assay and/or molecular analysis.

Treatment/Prognosis No specific treatment is usually required. However, on demonstration of hyperprolinemia type II in a child with a seizure disorder, treatment with 5–30 mg of pyridoxine per kilogram of body weight per day in one dose should be started.

Pyridoxal-Phosphate-Dependent Epilepsy (Pyridox(am)ine-5'-Phosphate Oxidase Deficiency)

Etiology/Pathophysiology Pyridoxal-phosphate-dependent epilepsy due to pyridox(am)ine-5'-phosphate oxidase (PNPO) deficiency has been delineated recently in three families with five (by family history nine) children suffering from genetically proven neonatal epileptic encephalopathy (88). CSF and urine analyses indicated reduced activities of several pyridoxal-phosphate-dependent enzymes. Specifically, biochemical findings indicated combined deficiencies of aromatic L-amino acid decarboxylase, threonine dehydratase, ornithine δ-aminotransferase, and the glycine cleavage enzyme. In addition, the patients displayed variable lactic acidemia as well as a tendency to hypoglycemia. The encephalopathy that dominated the clinical picture was resistant to treatment with pyridoxine but ceased with administration of pyridoxal-5'-phosphate. Without PNPO, pyridoxine and pyridoxamine cannot be converted into pyridoxal-5'-phosphate, leaving pyridoxal phosphate as the only source of the active cofactor (see Figure 45-9). In addition to the impairment of aromatic L-amino acid decarboxylase, threonine dehydratase, ornithine (-aminotransferase, and the glycine cleavage enzyme, mitochondrial energy metabolism can be assumed to be compromised in PNPO deficiency because the mitochondrial aspartate shuttle that transports reducing equivalents to the mitochondria requires a pyridoxal-phosphate-dependent aspartate aminotransferase in the cytosol as well as in the mitochondria. This may explain the elevated blood lactate levels noted in affected patients. Furthermore, glycogenolysis likely is reduced because glycogen phosphorylase uses pyridoxal-5′-phosphate as a cofactor. Additionally, conversion of lactate to glucose during fasting may be impaired because in the fasting state the citric acid cycle in the liver is supplied by the carbon skeletons of glucogenic amino acids, and these are produced by pyridoxal-5′-phosphate-dependent reactions. Both mechanisms can be seen to disturb glucose homeostasis and explain the clinically observed hypoglycemia. It remains to be seen whether GABA metabolism is also disturbed because glutamic acid decarboxylase (GAD) is also a vitamin B_6–requiring enzyme.

Clinical Presentation All PNPO-deficient patients have had a very severe and acute early neonatal presentation with convulsions, myoclonus, rotatory eye movements, sudden clonic contractions, hypoglycemia, and (lactic) acidosis (88). Seizures were resistant to conventional anticonvulsant therapy. EEG showed a burst-suppression pattern. In all three families identified, previous sibships suffered and died from a similar neurometabolic disorder. Pyridoxal-5′-phosphate given by nasogastric tube is dramatically effective in stopping the seizures and improving the appearance of the EEG. It is important to note that patients all were born prematurely between 22 and 35 weeks' gestation. Fetal distress was common, as were "signs of asphyxia," and all but one had a low Apgar score and/or required intubation. Early (lactic) acidosis and hypoglycemia were observed. Thus PNPO deficiency must enter the differential diagnosis of hypoxic–ischemic encephalopathy (HIE) in a prematurely born infant.

Still unpublished are observations of neonates and infants with epileptic encephalopathy unresponsive to treatment with conventional antiepileptic drugs who were not born prematurely and did not not show suspicious metabolic findings but responded dramatically to pyridoxal-5′-phosphate and were shown to have mutations in the pyridox(am)ine-5′-phosphate

- Prenatal diagnosis is possible where mutations have been established.

- Newborn screening is unavailable.

oxidase gene (Hoffmann, unpublished observation). In view of success to treatment with pyridoxal phosphate as the only reliable diagnostic test and in analogy with pyridoxine-dependent epilepsy, we suggest calling this disorder primarily *pyridoxal-phosphate-dependent epilepsy*.

Diagnosis Pyridoxal-phosphate-dependent epilepsy, respectively, PNPO deficiency, is a very severe acute (neuro-) metabolic disorder. The clinical history of previously diagnosed patients reveals numerous misdiagnoses in all three known families. The differential diagnosis is wide, including all major causes of neonatal seizures, especially hypoxic–ischemic encephalopathy (HIE), in a prematurely born infant. Pyridoxal-phosphate-dependent epilepsy also should be a candidate in the differential diagnosis of Ohtahara syndrome. Additional inborn errors of metabolism that can present identically are nonketotic hyperglycinemia, the deficiencies of sulfite oxidase and adenylsuccinate lyase, GABA transaminase deficiencies, and certain types of congenital disorders of glycosylation. PNPO deficiency may have a complex biochemical phenotype, but characteristic biochemical findings may be missing (88). Unfortunately, the most characteristic changes are found by CSF analysis with a biochemical pattern indicative of AADC deficiency. Concentrations of HVA, 5-HIAA, and MHPG are all decreased in association with increased concentrations of L-dopa, 5-hydroxytryptophan, and 3-OMD. In urine, vanillactic acid can be found elevated by organic acid analysis. Activity of AADC in plasma was found to be normal or even increased. Additional biochemical abnormalities included raised CSF levels of glycine (in all five patients published), threonine (four of five), taurine (four of five), histidine (five of five), and low arginine (three of five). Since most patients to date were born prematurely at between 22 and 35 weeks' gestation, a biochemical test not requiring a lumbar puncture would be desirable. Unfortunately, changes of amino acids in plasma or urine in premature infants are variable. Possibly the elevation of vanillactic acid in urine detectable by organic acid analysis can help in pinpointing the disorder. However, the elevations generally are slight, and laboratories will not automatically search for this compound unless specifically instructed. The only reliable diagnosis of pyridoxal-phosphate-dependent epilepsy is the positive response to the drug. Following this positive response, mutation anaylyis can verify the diagnosis.

Treatment/Prognosis Successful treatment of pyridoxal-phosphate-dependent epilepsy is achieved with doses of 30–60 mg pyridoxal-

Pyridoxal-5′-phosphate may cause apnea and prolonged cerebral depression after the initial dose. Resuscitation equipment and intensive-care facilities must be available. Effectiveness of treatment is monitored by clinical outcome and measurement of prolactin in serum and serotonin and dopamine metabolites in CSF.

5′-phosphate per kilogram of body weight per day in four doses. Doses need to be increased and adjusted to body weight during growth. Patients probably require lifelong supplementation. Obvious criteria to increase the doses are breakthrough seizures. So far, specific therapy has been instituted successfully in only one patient 2 weeks after onset of symptoms. All other patients had died without specific therapy within the first months of life. The treated patient had significant developmental delay at 21 months of age but was in a stable condition (88). With regard to treatment and prognosis, many questions are open. Pyridoxal-5′-phosphate, while controlling seizures, still may not prevent the development of cognitive impairment. In one patient, an autopsy revealed brain damage that probably was prenatal in onset (88). Serial cognitive assessments are recommended. If there is a positive family history of pyridoxal-phosphate-dependent epilepsy, maternal treatment during pregnancy may be tried on an experimental basis.

DISORDERS OF GABA METABOLISM

Etiology/Pathophysiology The pathway of GABA synthesis and degradation in the CNS (Figure 45-10) links neurotransmitter degradation with energy production via the Krebs cycle and electron-transport chain. Once released into the synaptic cleft, the major chemical transmitters (glutamate = excitatory; GABA = inhibitory) mediate synaptic transmission via postsynaptic receptor binding. On release, transmitters undergo reuptake by the presynaptic neuron for further metabolism. Three enzymes are involved directly in GABA homeostasis (see Figure 45-10). Glutamic acid decarboxylase (GAD), a pyridoxine-dependent enzyme, catalyzes the irreversible decarboxylation of glutamate to GABA. Two forms of GAD exist, GAD_{65} and GAD_{67}, transcribed from different genes with discrete regional localizations (95,96). GABA is metabolized in a two-step sequence, catalyzed by pyridoxine-dependent GABA transaminase (GABA-T, a reversible reaction that generates succinate semialdehyde), and NAD^+-dependent succinate semialdehyde

A. GABA Synthesis and Degradation in the CNS

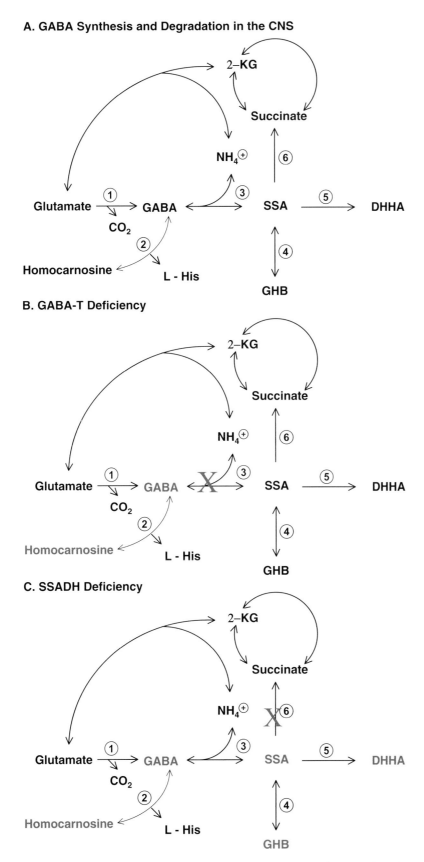

B. GABA-T Deficiency

C. SSADH Deficiency

FIGURE 45-10. Biosynthesis and catabolism of the major excitatory/inhibitory transmitters glutamate and GABA in the central nervous system. Numbered enzymes include 1) glutamic acid decarboxylase (GAD), 2) carnosinase (possibly identical to serum carnosinase), 3) GABA-transaminase, 4) succinate semialdehyde reductase, 5) an uncharacterized reaction converting succinate semialdehyde to 4,5-dihydroxyhexanoic acid (DHHA), 6) succinate semialdehyde dehydrogenase (SSADH, AlDH5a1). GABA = 4-aminobutyric acid; His = histidine; SSA = succinate semialdehyde; GHB = γ-hydroxybutyrate; NH_4^+ = ammonium ion; and 2-KG = 2-ketoglutarate.

dehydrogenase (SSADH; AlDH5a1, an irreversible reaction that produces succinic acid). There is 1:1 stoichiometry between glutamate and GABA turnover because each GABA molecule entering the Krebs cycle as succinate produces one molecule of glutamate (2-ketoglutarate is the nitrogen acceptor for the GABA-T reaction; see Figure 45-10). This replenishing, or anaplerotic, cycle is frequently referred to as the *GABA shunt* pathway in brain (97,98).

Neurological disease, mild to severe, might be expected in disorders with altered GABA degradation. In the developing brain, GABA may be excitatory and depolarizing (99). Prior to the onset of synaptic inhibition, early GABAergic synaptic events activate calcium channels and regulate gene expression via second-messenger pathways (100). Other GABAergic signals appear to mediate chemotactic/chemokinetic actions of trophically released GABA (101). Alterations in GABA release would be predicted to have significant physiological sequelae in terms of neuron migration because developing neurons are exquisitely sensitive to GABA concentrations (99,101,102). In addition to GABA, SSADH-deficient patients accumulate γ hydroxybutyrate (GHB), a short-chain fatty acid with an extensive pharmacological fingerprint (103). In normal CNS, GHB levels are approximately 1–4 μM in discrete regions; conversely, the CSF derived from patients reveals concentrations of 1 mM or higher, sufficient to saturate high- and low-affinity GHB receptors and induction of receptor desensitization with chronic exposure (96,104). GHB is also a weak $GABA_B$ receptor agonist at millimolar concentrations (105). Individuals who ingest GHB illicitly display the neurological features seen in SSADH-deficient patients, including ataxia, hypotonia, seizures, and behavioral disturbances (106).

Differential Diagnosis

With only two documented families, the phenotype of GABA-T deficiency remains to be established. Nonetheless, severe neonatal epileptic encephalopathy appears the leading presentation, and imaging of affected individuals might lead to a tentative diagnosis of idiopathic leukodystrophy. SSADH-deficient patients have carried provisional diagnoses of cerebral palsy, autism-spectrum disorder, and/or idiopathic mental retardation (107,108). The presence of a seizure disorder may add an additional confound. For GABA-T deficiency, CSF amino acid analysis with particular focus on GABA (free and total) appears necessary, perhaps explaining the low number of identified patients. SSADH deficiency is readily documented by detection of increased GHB in the urine organic acid profile. Both disorders may be confirmed by enzyme assay in leukocytes isolated from whole blood, with molecular genetic confirmation.

GABA-Transaminase Deficiency

Etiology/Pathophysiology GABA-T deficiency is an autosomal recessive disorder resulting in excessive accumulation of GABA in the CNS. The enzyme is expressed in CNS and the periphery (i.e., liver, kidney, platelets, and leukocytes), enabling analysis in peripheral tissues in suspected patients.

Molecular Variants Medina-Kauwe and coworkers (1999) used a full-length rat GABA-T cDNA (GenBank U29701) to isolate the corresponding human cDNA from a pancreatic islet cDNA library (GenBank U80226). Interspecies deduced amino acid sequence revealed 88% homology. The human cDNA was employed to isolate a genomic clone encoding human GABA-T from a pWE15 cosmid library (109). Restriction mapping indicated that the human GABA-T gene was contained within approximately 16.5 kb of nucleotide sequence. A single causative mutation was identified in the index family, substituting a highly conserved arginine with lysine at amino acid 220. This arginine resides within a highly conserved amino acid triad, His–Gly–Arg, that has been shown to stabilize pyridoxal-5'-phosphate binding. No molecular variants are currently known.

Clinical Presentation Clinical manifestations observed in two families with three affected children included neonatal epilepsy, hypotonia, lethargy, hyperreflexia, poor feeding, severe retardation of psychomotor development, and high-pitched cry ("cat cry"). Linear growth in two siblings was accelerated (110). The patients continued with generalized epileptiform paroxysms, developed severe developmental delay, and died at between 5 months and 2 years of age. CT scan demonstrated significant ventricular enlargement. In two siblings, a tentative diagnosis of idiopathic leukodystrophy was made, whereas the third patient had agenesis of the corpus callosum and cerebellar hypoplasia.

Diagnosis CSF amino acid analysis demonstrates significantly elevated levels of GABA (both free and total), as well as β-alanine and homocarnosine. Quantitation of free GABA is not trivial and is offered using accurate stable-isotope dilution methodology in only a small number of highly specialist laboratories (111). Plasma levels of these amino acids are also increased, but not as significantly as elevations detected in CSF. A similar pattern of metabolites was described in a single patient with hyper-β-alaninemia (112). In this pa-

- Prenatal diagnosis is possible by enzyme assay in amniocytes and chorionic villi and where mutations have been established.

- Newborn screening is unavailable.

tient, a deficiency of β-alanine transaminase was suggested but never demonstrated. It appears possible that hyper-β-alaninemia is a variant form of GABA-T deficiency. High levels of GABA, as well as of β-alanine and homocarnosine, are also seen in patients treated with the antiepileptic medication γ-vinyl-GABA (Vigabatrin), an inhibitor of GABA-T. Elevations of GABA in other metabolic diseases are rare and far smaller than in GABA-T deficiency, for example, in SSADH deficiency or glutaric aciduria type I. They can be recognized only by quantitation of free GABA by stable-isotope dilution methodology and cannot cause confusion in diagnosis.

Treatment/Prognosis There are no effective and no specific treatments available. Therapeutic trials with pyridoxine had no clinical effect. Despite all therapeutic interventions, all patients succumbed within the first months of life.

Succinic Semialdehyde Dehydrogenase Deficiency

Etiology/Pathophysiology Succinic semialdehyde dehydrogenase deficiency, synonymous with 4-hydroxybutyric aciduria, is an autosomal recessive disorder in the second step of the conversion of GABA to succinic acid. First identified in 1981, it is a rare neurometabolic disorder with approximately 350 diagnosed patients worldwide. In addition to accumulation of GABA in CSF, patients also demonstrate elevated concentrations of GHB, the biochemical hallmark of this disease. Presumably, GHB accumulates from enzymatic transformation of accumulated succinic semialdehyde in response to the metabolic block (see Figure 45-10). Accumulation of GABA and GHB makes SSADH deficiency one of the few heritable disorders in which two neuropharmacologically active compounds accumulate (113). The enzyme is expressed in CNS and in peripheral tissues (i.e., liver and leukocytes).

Clinical Presentation The clinical phenotype of SSADH deficiency is heterogeneous, even within sibships. The cardinal clinical features include language delay, ataxia, hypotonia, and mental retardation. Seizures have been documented in about 50% of patients, but the extent of subclinical seizures remains unknown. Generalized seizures appear to be the

most prevalent, and in particular tonic–clonic seizures, although absence and myoclonic seizures has been reported. Additional manifestations may include hyporeflexia, behavioral problems (i.e., aggression and anxiety), strabismus, oculomotor dyspraxia, nonspecific gastrointestinal problems, and poor feeding in the neonatal period. EEG may show spike-wave discharges and generalized slowing, and imaging indicates a preferential increase in T2-weighted signaling in the globus pallidus bilaterally (107,108).

Molecular Variants The human SSADH gene, composed of 11 exons spanning approximately 38 kb of genomic sequence, resides on chromosome 6p22. Two major SSADH mRNA isoforms (1827 and 5225 nucleotides, respectively) derive from a single transcription start site and arise from the use of alternative polyadenylation sites. Polymorphic variations identified in the human coding sequence include 1) a C-to-T transition in exon 3 (c.538C>T), leading to a His–Tyr substitution at amino acid position 180 (H180Y), 2) a C-to-T transition at position 545 (c.545C>T), leading to a Pro–Leu substitution at amino acid position 182 (P182L), 3) an A-to-G transition in exon 7 (c.1115A>G), leading to an Asn Ser substitution at amino acid position 372 (N372S), and 4) a complex dinucleotide microsatellite in the noncoding region at the 5' end of IVS 6 (114,115). A number of mutations have been identified in 10 exons, including missense, nonsense, frameshift, insertion, and deletion alleles. Exon 4B (39 nucleotides) was not identified in our earlier work (116) and is predicted to encode a 13-amino-acid sequence; no mutations have been identified in this exon.

Diagnosis A definitive clinical diagnosis of SSADH deficiency is impossible because the most common manifestations, delayed development of motor, mental, and fine motor skills, are not unique to SSADH deficiency but occur in a variety of cerebellar syndromes or encephalopathies in childhood. Diagnosis usually is achieved by demonstration of increased concentrations of GHB in urine by urinary organic acid analysis. GHB is also increased in other physiological fluids, including plasma and CSF (117). Isotope dilution analysis maybe required for reliable diagnosis, especially in older patients, because of the age-dependent decline of urinary excretion. In addition, the finding of increased 4,5-dihydroxyhexanoic acid in the urine organic acid profile supports the diagnosis. Dicarboxylic aciduria has been noted and may indicate a secondary inhibition of mitochondrial fatty acid β-oxidation or propionyl–coenzyme A metabolism by succinic semialdehyde or its related metabolites. Several patients manifested elevated urinary glycolic acid and glycinuria, and in one, a transient CSF glycine elevation was documented.

Confirmatory enzyme assays are obtained by analysis of SSADH activity in extracts of leukocytes isolated from whole blood (118). Iatrogenic administration of GHB (Somsanit) for sedation purposes results in marked accumulation in all body fluids. Somsanit is well recognized in pediatric practice as a safe and efficient sedative. Its use for sedation for cerebral MRI and lumbar puncture in the diagnostic workup of an unknown childhood encephalopathy has resulted in diagnostic confusion when use of this drug was not reported to the metabolic laboratory (119). The substance disappears completely from plasma within 2–4 hours and from urine within 8 hours of intake.

Treatment/Prognosis Vigabatrin (Sabril; γ-vinyl-GABA) has been used extensively to treat patients. Seizures and behavioral disturbances are the main therapeutic targets. Intuitively, the use of this medication (not approved by the Food and Drug Administration [FDA] in the United States) is logical, in that suicide inhibition of GABA-T should lead to decreased production of GHB and elevated levels of CNS GABA (see Figure 45-10). Repetitive analysis of CSF from patients receiving vigabatrin has verified these expected alterations (120). However, studies in a murine knockout model of SSADH deficiency suggest that elevation of GABA in a disorder in which GABA is already increased beyond the physiological range may not be prudent (121,122). Further, ocular abnormalities have been associated with the use of vigabatrin (123). As noted earlier, the use of vigabatrin is empirical. It has had inconsistent efficacy and actually detrimental results in some patients (124). Methylphenidate, thioridizine, risperidal, fluoxetine, and benzodiazepines have been useful in problems of anxiety and behavior. Symptomatic treatment for seizures using carbamazepine and lamotrigene has demonstrated some clinical efficacy (107,108). The prognosis of SSADH deficiency is garded. Encephalopathy is slowly progressive, becoming static in most patients. Life expectancy does not appear to be substantial reduced.

Prenatal Diagnosis Prenatal diagnosis is available through analysis of GHB concentration in amniotic fluid, in addition to assay of SSADH activity in amniocytes and chorionic villi (fresh biopsy or cultured cells) (125). Molecular prenatal diagnosis also has been performed in those families for which causative mutations have been identified (126,127).

NONKETOTIC HYPERGLYCINEMIA

Etiology/Pathophysiology Nonketotic hyperglycinemia (NKH), an autosomal recessive condition, is caused by defects of the glycine cleavage enzyme, the main catabolic route of glycine (128). The glycine cleavage enzyme activity is high in liver, brain, and placenta. In the brain, it keeps glycine levels very low, resulting in a typically low CSF:plasma glycine ratio. Glycine is connected to multiple biochemical pathways (Figure 45-11). Via the formation of methylene tetrahydrofolate, the glycine cleavage enzyme, in conjunction with the glycine serine hydroxymethyltransferase, is one of the main donors of one-carbon-group metabolites.

Both the enzyme and its metabolite glycine have to be transported into the mitochondrion for the reaction to take place. The glycine cleavage system consists of four protein subunits: the P-protein, the H-protein, the T-protein, and the L-protein (Figure 45-12) (128,129). The P-protein must contain the active form of pyridoxal phosphate. The H-protein must be lipoylated to be active (130). In the first step of glycine metabolism, the P-protein catalyzes a pyridoxal-phosphate-dependent decarboxylation with release of CO_2 and transfers the aminomethyl group onto the lipoic acid of the H-protein. The T-protein transfers the α-carbon as a methyl group from the H-protein onto tetrahydrofolate to methylene tetrahydrofolate with release of ammonia. Finally, the H-protein is reoxidized to the disulfide form by the L-

protein. In contrast to plants, in humans, the L-protein is a distinct protein from the E3 component of the ketoacid decarboxylases. The biochemical sequence of reactions is shown in the accompanying Figure 45-12.

In the brain, all three protein components (P, T, and H) are present together in astrocytes in the forebrain and cerebellum and to a lesser extent in spinal cord (131). Neurons do not have the P-protein.

Clinically, NKH is characterized by elevated glycine levels in plasma and CSF, with elevation typically greater in CSF than in plasma. All symptoms are exclusively neurological, including mental retardation, hypotonia, seizures, and brain malformations.

Pathological examination of the brain in patients with NKH shows pronounced spongiosis with gliosis and markedly large astrocytes in myelinated areas (132–134). Electron microscopy shows the spongiotic microvacuolation to consist of splitting of the myelin lamellae. The spongiosis is limited to the already myelinated areas, but mega-astrocytic gliosis is also present in unmyelinated regions of the white matter. Myelination is delayed but progressive without evidence of myelin breakdown. Peripheral nerves are unaffected. Migrational abnormalities have been observed in the cerebellum and the olivary nucleus, and in some cases there was loss of Purkinje and granular neurons. No abnormalities were reported in cortical neurons.

On MRI of the brain, patients with severe NKH can have agenesis or hypoplasia of the corpus callosum (135,136). They can have

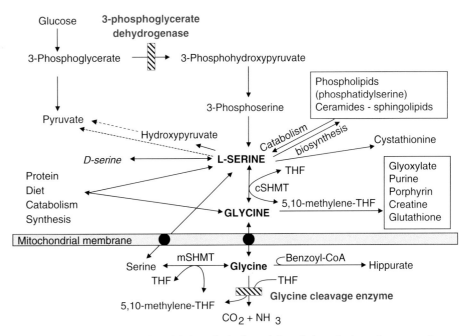

FIGURE 45-11. Biochemical connections of glycine and serine in metabolism. Glycine and serine are interconnected with multiple reactions in metabolism. THF = tetrahydrofolate; cSHMT = cytosolic serine hydroxymethyltransferase; mSHMT = mitochondrial serine hydroxymethyltransferase; 5,10-methyleneTHF = 5,10-methylenetetrahydrofolate; benzoyl–CoA = benzoyl–coenzyme A.

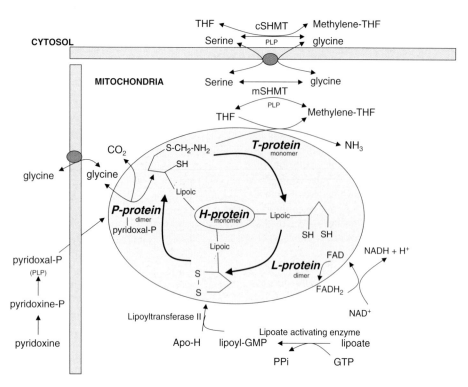

FIGURE 45-12. The glycine cleavage enzyme system. The glycine cleavage system is a complex intramitochondrial multiprotein system. Some components require several steps for activation. THF = tetrahydrofolate; methylene-THF = 5,10-methylene-tetrahydrofolate; cSHMT = cytosolic serine hydroxymethyltransferase; mSHMT = mitochondrial serine hydroxymethyltransferase; NAD = nicotine adenine dinucleotide; FAD = flavine adenine dinucleotide; lipoyl-GMP = lipoyl-guanosine-monophosphate; GTP = guanosine triphosphate; HC = homocarnosine.

malformations of the posterior fossa presenting as hydrocephalus and a retrocerebellar cyst (137). Cortical and cerebellar atrophy is seen primarily in older patients (136). Delayed myelination and particularly restricted diffusion on diffusion-weighted MRI images is seen in regions typically affected by spongiosis, such as the dorsal brain stem, cerebral peduncles, and posterior limb of the corpus callosum (138). A peak corresponding to glycine + myoinositol can be seen in the 3.5 ppm region on long-echo-time water-suppressed magnetic resonance spectroscopic sequences corresponding to concentrations between 3 and 8 mM (139).

The pathophysiology of this disorder is not yet known. Glycine is a neurotransmitter; it is also pivotal in a number of biochemical reactions in the brain. In glycinergic synapses, glycine acts as an inhibitory neurotransmitter (128). Neurotransmision at these receptors is inhibited by strychnine. In the spinal cord, these glycinergic synapses inhibit the muscle reflex, contributing to the hypotonia in NKH patients. Glycinergic inhibitory receptors are present in the respiratory center in the brain stem, where they slow the respiratory cycle (140), contributing to the apnea in the neonatal period in NKH patients. These inhibitory glycine receptors are glycine-gated chloride channels, which are composed of α and

β subunits ($\alpha_3\beta_2$) and a cytoplasmic anchoring subunit. The neonatal form of the glycine receptor subunit α_2, with lower affinity for strychnine, is replaced by the adult-type α_1 subunit within 2–3 weeks of birth (141). Glycine is an allosteric activator of the NMDA type of the excitatory glutamate receptor (142). Glycine increases the sensitivity of this receptor for activation by its neurotransmitter glutamate. Increased activity at the NMDA receptor has been suggested as a possible mechanism for seizures in NKH and can contribute to the mental retardation (143). Blockers of the NMDA receptor, such as dextromethorphan (144) and felbamate, have proven antiepileptic properties in patients with NKH. Finally, glycine acts as a neurotransmitter on some less characterized neurotransmitter receptors. The NMDA receptor subunit NR1 coexpressed with the NR3A and NR3B subunits forms an excitatory glycinergic receptor that is unaffected by glutamate and inhibited by D-serine (145). NR3B subunits are restricted to motorneurons, but NR3A receptors are expressed more widely. They function as excitatory glycine receptors. Certain strychnine-inhibitable glycinergic receptors, including subunits of the glycinergic inhibitory receptor, also are present in cortical neurons, in the hippocampus, and in Cajal–Retzius cells (141,146). They seem

important for neuronal migration. However, very little is presently known about the functionality of either one of these newly described glycine-sensitive receptors.

The contribution of the biochemical alterations due to the enzyme deficiency in NKH has received very little attention. Homocysteine tends to be mildly elevated in CSF, and serine levels tend to be lower, although these findings are not correlated with outcome (147). Glycine metabolism is compartmentalized between the mitochondrion and the cytosol. The glycine cleavage system, together with serine hydroxymethyltransferase, is the main one-carbon donor in the mitochondria, but the functional consequences of this deficiency have not been investigated.

Clinical Presentation The incidence of non-ketotic hyperglycinemia is estimated at 1 in 60,000 births, making it the second most frequent disorder of amino acid metabolism (148). It is present worldwide. An increased frequency is known in northern Finland (149) and in certain Arabs in Israel (150,151). The clinical presentation of NKH can be divided based on both the age at presentation and the severity of the affectation on follow-up.

Neonatal-Onset NKH (128,152) The pregnancy and delivery generally are uneventful. In retrospect, some mothers report having felt hiccupping in utero. Patients with neonatal-onset NKH present in the first days of life with increasing lethargy, ineffective sucking, and poor feeding, developing into a deep coma between the first and the eighth day of life. Patients are markedly hypotonic. Most patients have neonatal seizures with hiccupping and myoclonic spasms and a burst–suppression pattern on EEG. Apnea, or a very slow breathing rate, develops around the third day of life in two-thirds of patients, usually necessitating artificial ventilation. Spontaneous breathing resumes typically in the second week of life. During the second half of the first month of life, patients tend to regain some alertness and have better feeding.

Severe Neonatal NKH Patients with the severe form of NKH rapidly loose whatever gains they make in the next months. They develop signs of spasticity with early pyramidal tract signs. They develop seizures of increasing severity, initially consisting of hypsarrhythmias and myoclonic spasms, later developing into multifocal seizures. By the end of the first year, most patients require multiple anticonvulsant medications for seizure control. Development is extremely poor, with no grasping, sitting, or contact with the environment. Feeding through a G-tube is often required. Most patients with congenital malformations belong to this category of severe neonatal NKH.

Mild Form of Neonatal NKH In two different surveys, up to 15% of NKH patients with neonatal presentation have a different clinical course (152,153). They have a better recovery in the first 2 months of life after the neonatal period with increased wakefulness and delayed signs of corticospinal tract involvement. They have a milder seizure disorder, usually controlled by benzoate therapy or by a single anticonvulsant medication. Most of these patients make developmental progress. They learn to grasp and to sit. Several of them learned to walk and communicate usually with sign language. They are still mentally retarded, with developmental quotients varying between 10 and 60. They can have similar symptoms as described in late-onset mild NKH. There is evidence for a lower glycine index in these less affected patients (154). Two families had less severe mutations with residual activity.

The distinction between these two groups in outcome is somewhat artificial (154). Occasional patients are known to have an intermediary outcome between these two groups. Also, in a few patients, a striking neurodegenerative course has been seen at a later age (varying from late infancy to toddler years), transforming an apparently better developing child into one with a severe form of NKH.

The age at death of patients who survive the neonatal period has ranged from 2 months to more than 15 years (152). One study suggests that female patients have a worse prognosis for development and survival than males (152). This must be confirmed in future studies.

Late Presentation Patients with a late-onset presentation do not have a phase of neurological depression in the neonatal period. They can present in infancy or in childhood. According to final neurodevelopmental outcome and severity of seizure disorder, they can be classified into severe and mild late-onset cases.

Late-Onset Severe NKH Several patients had a severe neurodegenerative course of NKH with the development of severe mental retardation, severe seizures, and spasticity (155). This neurodegerative course occurred after 2–6 months of normal neurological development. The disease in these patients is similar to that in patients with the severe form of neonatal NKH but without the neonatal presentation.

Mild Late-Onset NKH These patients present with mild mental retardation and a mild seizure disorder that is usually controlled by benzoate or a single anticonvulsant medication. They often have marked hyperactivity, chorea, and intermittent mild ataxia (156,157). Expressive speech is more impaired than receptive language. They can have episodes of delirium, decreased consciousness up to coma, and vertical gaze palsy. Symptoms can be worsened by infections or by the use of valproate (158). Some patients remain stable throughout life; others gradually develop a spinocerebellar syndrome with optic atrophy (159). Several, but not all, patients had a lower CSF:plasma glycine ratio, varying between 0.02 and 0.08, that is, even a normal CSF glycine concentration in a single patient (160,161). In some patients, residual glycine cleavage enzyme activity has been documented.

Transient NKH A few patients have been described with the neonatal clinical presentation of NKH and with the biochemical abnormalities of increased glycine in plasma and CSF (162,163). After 2–4 months, the biochemical signs of elevated glycine disappear, constituting the essential definition of the transient form. Some patients have had normal developmental outcome; some patients had severe mental retardation.

Only a dozen patients with the transient form are known, compared with many patients with typical NKH, making the frequency of the transient form less than 1% of cases. Of the 12 reported patients, several did not have follow-up CSF glycine levels measured, making it possible that they represent mild cases in which the plasma glycine levels at times can be normal. Others responded well to treatment with pyridoxine, making a disorder of pyridoxine metabolism a possibility.

Asymptomatic or Transiently Symptomatic NKH A few patients have been described with initial clinical and biochemical features of NKH who later had normal developmental outcome and absence of seizures (150,151). In contrast to the transient form, they have persistent biochemical signs of elevated glycine. Residual activity (32%) and a mild mutation (A802V in GLDC) were documented in one family. This phenotype likely represents the milder extreme of the mild form of neonatal NKH.

Pulmonary Hypertension Several patients with NKH, varying in neurological presentation from severe neonatal presentation to neurologically asymptomatic, have developed severe and often fatal pulmonary hypertension (164). In many patients, the diagnosis was confirmed by deficient glycine cleavage enzyme activity. Mutation analysis has not been reported.

Maternal Nonketotic Hyperglycinemia An adult woman with NKH had two uncomplicated pregnancies, and the children were normal (165).

Prognosis Within families, the severity of NKH seems to be concordant, suggesting a genetic basis for the clinical severity (152). Preliminary results indicate the existence of a genotype—phenotye correlation. This aspect will require more systematic study.

Diagnosis

- Glycine is elevated in plasma and urine. Elevation of glycine in plasma can vary throughout the day and can be normal at times.

- Glycine is elevated in CSF, almost always greater than 30 µM, except in some mild late-onset patients. Glycine levels decline rapidly in the CSF during the first 2 months of life in both normal controls and affected patients.

- The CSF:plasma glycine ratio is elevated. The normal ratio of CSF to plasma glycine is less than 0.04. Most patients with NKH have a CSF:plasma glycine ratio 0.08 or more; some patients with mild NKH can have a CSF:plasma glycine ratio lesss than 0.08 (161).

- Urinary organic acids are normal. Small increases in acylglycines are sometimes seen.

- The diagnosis of nonketotic hyperglycinemia must be confirmed by enzyme assay or molecular analysis.

- The rapid development of spasticity in infancy, a severe seizure disorder, and a need for high doses of benzoate to correct the plasma glycine level characterize patients with poor neurodevelopmental outcome.

- Patients with the neonatal presentation who continue to breath after the second week of life are unlikely to die from apnea. Decisions regarding withdrawal of support should be made in the first week of life.

- The following considerations are important when counseling patients with neonatal NKH: Transient NKH and transiently symptomatic NKH are very rare and rarely affect decision making. Most patients with NKH have a dismal prognosis, but up to 15% of patients with this phenotype make varying degrees of developmental progress.

- The presence of malformations is usually associated with poor outcome. A CSF:plasma glycine ratio of 0.07 or less is often associated with a better outcome.

- Hyperglycinemia can present in the following disorders and conditions and should be differentiated from NKH (166).
- Organic acidurias, such as propionic and methylmalonic aciduria, have elevated glycine levels. They are often, but not always, associated with ketoacidosis and hyperammonemia, unlike in NKH. The mechanism of hyperglycinemia in these patients is through inhibition of glycine cleavage enzyme at the liver. Patients with these disorders (ketotic hyperglycinemia) have a normal CSF:plasma glycine ratio. In addition, glyceric aciduria can present clinically and biochemically similarly to NKH.
- Patients on valproate treatment. Valproate treatment can raise the CSF glycine levels substantially (up to more than 60 μM) and the CSF:plasma glycine ratio, leading to a false diagnosis of NKH. Levels should be repeated after discontinuation of valproate.
- Threonine levels are not elevated, excluding pyridoxal-phosphate-responsive encephalopathy, where CSF glycine may be elevated.
- Blood or serum contamination from a traumatic spinal tap and breakdown of the blood–brain barrier. Due to the large gradient of glycine from blood to CSF, even a very small contamination of CSF with blood can result in a substantial elevation of CSF glycine and in an erroneous raise of CSF-to-plasma glycine ratio. Similarly, breakdown of the blood–brain barrier can be associated with an elevated CSF:plasma glycine ratio. Therefore, a normal CSF rbc count and protein concentration are required for correct interpretation of the glycine level.
- Abnormal liver function. Profound liver dysfunction (very prolonged PT) can cause elevated plasma glycine levels.

Enzyme Assay The enzyme deficiency can be measured reliably only in liver biopsy or in a biopsy of the placenta or chorionic villus. Since the enzyme is unstable, tissue samples must be frozen immediately and shipped frozen. Enzyme assays in Epstein–Barr virus (EBV)–transformed lymphoblasts are unreliable, having missed severely affected patients. There are two assays that measure different aspects (167–169).

In the *glycine cleavage enzyme assay*, tissue homogenate is incubated with radioactive [1-^{14}C]glycine, and the release of radioactive [^{14}C]CO_2 is measured. This assay measures the overall activity of the glycine cleavage enzyme. The enzyme assay shows severely reduced to absent enzyme activity in NKH.

Generally, patients with very mild outcome and patients with defects in the T-protein can have mild residual activity (169).

The *glycine exchange reaction* involves incubation of tissue homogenate with radioactive carbon dioxide and following the incorporation into radioactive glycine. This reaction measures the reverse reaction of the P-protein, including the H-protein but without the T-protein. It therefore can be used to discriminate between a deficiency in the T-protein and a deficiency in P- or H-protein activity. The glycine exchange reaction typically is deficient in patients with P-protein defects but normal in patients with T-protein defects This assay requires a substantial amount of liver tissue usually obtained by open liver biopsy.

Enzymatic studies have estimated that a deficiency of P-protein is present in approximately 80% of patients, T-protein in 15% of patients, and H-protein in 5% of patients (143,168).

Prenatal diagnosis is made commonly through enzyme assay in direct uncultured chorionic villi. This test carries a 1% risk of a false diagnosis of an unaffected individual (168,170). Sufficient chorionic villus material must be obtained to avoid a low-activity result leading to a false diagnosis of an affected patient. When the mutation is known, prenatal diagnosis is also possible by molecular means.

Molecular Variants

- NKH due to P-protein deficiency
- NKH due to T-protein deficiency
- NKH due to H-protein deficiency

The P-protein, T-protein, and H-protein are encoded by the GLDC, the AMT, and the GCSH genes, respectively (128). The GLDC gene, encoding the P-protein, on chromosome 9p22 has 25 exons. There is an interfering processed pseudogene, and sequencing analysis must be done genomically. The AMT gene, encoding the T-protein, on chromosome 3p21 has 9 exons, and the GCSH gene, encoding the H-protein, has 5 exons. The gene for the L-protein is unknown at present. Of patients with NKH in which a mutation could be identified, approximately 26% of patients have defects in the AMT gene, and the remaining patients have defects in the GLDC gene (168). Very rare patients have been reported with a defect in the GCSH gene. In approximately 5% of patients, a defect was not found in these three genes using current methods.

Most patients have private mutations, with few recurring mutations (168). In the GLDC gene, the R515S in exon 12 and deletions around exon 1 have been reported in 5% and 10% of the alleles, respectively. In the Finnish population, S564I and G761R represent 70%

- Confirmation of diagnosis by enzyme assay and/or molecular analysis is highly advisable to facilitate future prenatal diagnosis.
- Blood or serum contamination of CSF is the most common reason for erroneous diagnosis of NKH.
- Prenatal diagnosis is possible by enzyme assay in uncultured CVS or by mutation analysis if a mutation has been identified in the index case.
- There are few recurring mutations, making molecular diagnosis tedious. A mutation could not be identified in some patients, in which case enzyme assay remains the only way for prenatal diagnosis. This should be taken into account when making decisions about the method of diagnostic verification in the proband.

and 8% of the alleles, respectively (168,149). Genomic deletions of one or more exons of the GLDC gene constitute more than 20% of the alleles. In the AMT gene, R320H is a frequently recurring mutation, often found in association with E211K polymorphism on the same allele (171). The mutations I106T, H42R, and IVS7-1GnA have recurred in patients. In three Japanese patients, D276H in combination with 183delC was found. Patients with mutations in the AMT gene may have slightly higher residual enzyme activity on the glycine cleavage enzyme assay (171). There is no difference in severity or clinical presentation between patients with a defect in the AMT or the GLDC gene.

Treatment Treatment of patients with NKH has focused on lowering of the plasma glycine levels with sodium benzoate with or without a glycine-restricted diet, interference with the overactivity of glycinergic neurotransmitter receptors, and symptomatic treatment including anticonvulsant therapy (128). None of the current treatment strategies changes the neurodevelopmental course or prevents or ameliorates the mental retardation. Withdrawal of artificial ventilation and intensive-care support should be discussed with the parents of neonates in the apneic phase. However, once breathing resumes, most patients survive for many years. In surviving patients, treatment can improve the quality of life substantially.

Benzoate, after activation to benzoylcoenzyme A, conjugates with glycine in liver and kidney to form hippurate, which is excreted readily in the urine. Benzoate treatment at high doses removes large amounts of glycine and lowers plasma glycine levels (172–174). The dose required ranges from 500–750 mg/kg/day for severely affected patients and from

200–500 mg/kg/day for more mildly affected patients (172). The dose may vary depending on the glycine index of the individual patient. Benzoate therapy should be initiated at the low end of the dose range and increased every few days until effective glycine levels have been obtained. At high benzoate doses or low glycine levels, measuring serum benzoate levels can help to avoid toxicity. A benzoate dose above 750 mg/kg/day has been associated with toxicity and should be avoided (174). Overdosing of benzoate causing severe toxicity usually is seen when serum benzoate levels exceed 3 mM. Administration should be divided into at least three but preferably four to six doses per day. It should be given as capsules or dissolved in water but not as free powder to avoid mucosal irritation. Monitoring efficacy of benzoate treatment is done by measuring plasma glycine levels, typically obtained at least 2 hours after the first dose of the day (154). Typically, symptomatic improvement is seen when plasma glycine levels are between 120 to 280 µM.

In patients with mild NKH, either of neonatal or late onset, lowering plasma glycine results in a reduction or complete cessation of seizures, improves alertness, and prevents episodes of stupor, agitation, and hallucinations (152,154,157,173,174). The dose used in these mildly affected patients typically ranges from 200–450 mg/kg/day. In patients with severe NKH, benzoate therapy improves alertness and can reduce the severity of the seizure disorder, but patients still need multiple anticonvulsant medications in addition to control seizures. In these patients, restriction of glycine in the diet can help to control the glycine levels when used in association with high-dose benzoate therapy (>600 mg/kg/day) (154). At these high doses, gastric irritation due to benzoate is very frequent, and gastric protection with H_2-antihistamine or proton pump inhibitors is recommended (144).

Seizures in the infantile period respond well to benzodiazepines (175). In severely affected patients, additional anticonvulsant medications usually are required in late infancy. Blocking the NMDA receptor with dextromethorphan results in improved seizure control (144,176). The pharmacokinetics of dextromethorphan vary widely between individual patients, but 5 mg/kg/day divided in three doses provides a starting point. It is particularly effective in patients with mild NKH, whose seizures are not controlled with benzoate. A number of anticonvulsant medications have been used in patients with severe NKH. In rare patients with severe therapy-resistant seizures, felbamate, which is a blocker of the glycinergic site of the NMDA receptor (177), has been effective. Cautious

- Benzoate treatment is most effective in controlling symptoms in mild NKH patients but can improve seizure control in severely affected patients.

- The dose of benzoate should be increased gradually and titrated to the individual needs of the patient. Monitoring CSF glycine is not needed in the follow-up of treatment.

- No current therapy changes the course of the mental retardation.

- Valproate should be avoided in patients with mild NKH.

monitoring of the hepatic and hematological side effects is necessary. Valproate, which inhibits the glycine cleavage enzyme, should be avoided in patients with mild NKH; if used, it can elicit severe symptoms (158).

Most patients with severe NKH need G-tube feeding (152). Gastroesophageal reflux develops frequently in these patients, and many patients benefit from an early added Nissen fundoplication. Recurrent bronchitis is a major problem, and bronchopneumonia is frequently the cause of death. Hydrocephalus occurs in some patients in infancy and requires ventriculoperitoneal shunting (137). For patients with mild NKH, management of the hyperactivity can be a major challenge. Treatment with benzoate and imipramine has been suggested in the literature, but they are not always effective (157,178).

Psychosocial Support NKH is a devastating neurometabolic disorder that requires considerable effort in caring for parents. The NKH International Family Network (www.nkh-network.org/) is a patient association that provides support for families throughout the world.

SERINE-DEFICIENCY DISORDERS

3-Phosphoglycerate Dehydrogenase Deficiency

Etiology/Pathophysiology Serine is synthesized from the glycolytic intermediate 3-phosphoglycerate by 3-phosphoglycerate dehydogenase (179) (see Figure 45-12). Deficiency of this enzyme leads to a serine-deficiency disorder. In the brain, serine is synthesized primarily endogenously, and deficiency of the enzyme results in reduced levels of serine in the CSF (180). In the brain, the enzymes of the serine biosynthetic pathway are restricted to glial cells and most notably to the astrocytes (181). In vitro studies have shown that L-serine is also an important neurotrophic factor involved in dendritogenesis and neuronal survival (181). L-Serine is a well-known precursor

for nucleotide synthesis. In the CNS, serine has additional important functions (179), such as being the precursor of the neurotransmitters D-serine and glycine and one of the components of ceramides and phosphatidylserine, both important components of myelin. Phosphatidylserine is made by base-exchange reaction of serine with phosphatidylethanolamine. The first step in the biosynthesis of sphingolipids is the condensation of palmitoyl-CoA with L-serine to form 3-ketodihydrosphingosine. From this structure, the ceramides and gangliosides are formed. The highest concentration of sphingolipids occurs in the white matter of the CNS, and deficiencies in synthesis result in severe neurological disease. The role of serine as a one-methyl donor through the serine hydroxymethyltransferase enzymes is evident from the low levels of 5-methylfolate in the patients with 3-phosphoglycerate dehydrogenase deficiency (182).

Clinical Presentation Patients with 3-phosphoglycerate dehydrogenase deficiency present with congenital microcephaly (180, 182–185). Longitudinal monitoring of an affected fetus showed reduction in brain growth after the 20th week of gestation (186) and very little head growth after birth, leading to severe microcephaly. Patients develop severe psychomotor retardation, spastic tetraparesis with adducted thumbs, and hyperexcitability. Seizures usually start in infancy (ages 2–14 months) and may include West syndrome (187) or later development of tonic, atonic, myoclonic, or atypical laughing seizures. The EEG shows hypsarrhytmia or severe multifocal seizures on a poor background. Variable symptoms observed in some patients includes cataracts, hypogonadism, megaloblastic anemia, and nystagmus.

MRI of the brain shows a striking reduction in white matter volume and very delayed to absent mylination. The cerebral white matter on T2-weighted images has a higher signal intenstity than the cortex, indicative of a lack of myelin (188). There is cortical and subcortical atrophy. MRS showed a decreased level of N-acetylaspartate/creatine and an increased level of choline/creatine in the white matter and to a lesser extent in the cortex.

- Serine deficiency should be suspected in patients with congenital microcephaly, infantile seizures.

- Serine should be examined in the CSF. The CSF amino acid analysis should not be limited to glycine only.

- Plasma amino acids should not be relied on to exclude this treatable disorder.

Diagnosis Biochemically, the condition is characterized by serine deficiency, particularly in the brain (180,182–185). CSF serine is severely reduced to less than 14 μM (normal CSF serine 42–86 μM if younger than 1 year of age).

- Plasma serine is reduced in a fasting sample (28–64 μM, normal controls 70–187 μM). However, nonfasting levels can be normal, and the diagnosis can be missed easily when only plasma amino acids are examined.
- Glycine in CSF is often decreased 1–4 μM (normal 4–15 μM if younger than 1 year of age).
- 5-Methylfolate in CSF can be reduced to half normal levels (e.g., 33–46 nM for normal, 64–182 nM if younger than 1 year of age) (182).
- The condition should be confirmed by enzyme assay or by mutation analysis.
- The enzyme activity can be assayed spectrophotometrically in fibroblasts (185).

Molecular Variants The PHGD gene is located on chromosome 1q12. Most patients have shown homozygosity for a common mutation, V490M, that has occurred independently on different genetic backgrounds or a rarer mutation, V425M. Both mutations have substantial residual activity (up to 50%) (189,190).

Treatment Treatment with substitution of serine has shown remarkable effects (180, 182–186). Serine levels and glycine levels in the CSF may normalize. Patients have been treated with 400–500 mg/kg/day divided into four to six doses. Doses above 550 mg/kg/day have led to adverse symptoms (183). This has been related to a block of neutral amino acid blood–brain barrier transport and reverses on lowering the serine dose. Some patients with persistent symptoms such as seizures have been treated with glycine 200–300 mg/kg/day in addition to serine supplementation (182). Treatment with folinic acid has been suggested due to the low CSF 5-methylfolate levels.

After 1 to 2 weeks of treatment, the seizures stop. The EEG improves after a few months, and evoked potentials improve (187). On MRI, the white matter shows myelination and increase in volume (188). In some patients, there is an associated catch-up growth of the head circumference. There can be some progression in development, particularly when treated early in infancy.

Prenatal treatment from the 29th week of pregnancy by giving the mother 190 mg/kg/day resulted in restoration of head growth and normal birth (186). Subsequent treatment of the child with 400 mg/kg/day of l-serine resulted in normal neurological development

and developmental outcome. This report strongly illustrates the importance of serine in prenatal development.

Other Serine Deficiency Disorders

A single patient has been described with 3-phosphoserine phosphatase deficiency (191). Plasma and CSF studies showed decreased serine levels. This patient also had Williams syndrome. It is unclear what symptoms, if any, can be attributed to this deficiency. Treatment with L-serine was followed by catch-up growth of the head circumference. Deficiency of phosphoserine aminotransferase, the second step in the biogenesis of serine, has been described in two siblings with the same phenotype of microcephaly and seizures (192). There was a similar response to early treatment with serine and glycine supplementation.

A single patient with progressive axonal polyneuropathy, seizures, ichtyosis, and growth retardation had low serine levels in plasma and, to a lesser extent, in CSF (180). Treatment with L-serine resulted in improvement in the ichtyosis and strength. The gene or the enzyme defect is unknown.

REFERENCES

1. Becker C. Glycine receptors: Molecular heterogeneity and implications for disease. *Neuroscientist.* 1995;1:130–141.
2. Hoffmann GF, Surtees RA, Wevers RA. Cerebrospinal fluid investigations for neurometabolic disorders. *Neuropediatrics.* 1998;29:59–71.
3. Torres OA, Miller VS, Buist NM, et al. Folinic acid–responsive neonatal seizures. *J Child Neurol.* 1999;14:529–532.
4. Gibson KM, Jacobs C. Disorders of beta- and gamma-amino acids in free and peptide linked forms. In: Scriver CR, Beaudet AL, Sly WS, et al., eds. *The Metabolic and Molecular Bases of Inherited Disease,* 8th ed. New York: McGraw-Hill; 2001:2079–2105.
5. Bräutigam C, Weykamp C, Hoffmann GF, et al. Neurotransmitter metabolites in CSF: An external quality control scheme. *J Inherited Metab Dis.* 2002;25:287–298.
6. Hyland K, Surtees RA, Heales SJ, et al. Cerebrospinal fluid concentrations of pterins and metabolites of serotonin and dopamine in a pediatric reference population. *Pediatr Res.* 1993;34:10–14.
7. Assmann B, Surtees R, Hoffmann GF. Approach to the diagnosis of neurotransmitter diseases exemplified by the differential diagnosis of childhood-onset dystonia. *Ann Neurol.* 2003;54:S18–24.
8. Wester P, Bergstrom U, Eriksson A, et al. Ventricular cerebrospinal fluid monoamine transmitter and metabolite concentrations reflect human brain neurochemistry in autopsy cases. *J Neurochem.* 1990;54:1148–1156.
9. Blau N, Thony B, Cotton RG, et al. Disorders of tetrahydrobiopterin and related biogenic amines. In: Scriver CR, Beaudet AL, Sly WS, et al., eds. *The Metabolic and Molecular Bases of Inherited Disease,* 8th ed. New York: McGraw-Hill; 2001:1725–1776.
10. Niederwieser A, Blau N, Wang M, et al. GTP cyclohydrolase I deficiency, a new enzyme defect causing hyperphenylalaninemia with neopterin, biopterin, dopamine, and serotonin deficiencies and muscular hypotonia. *Eur J Paediatr.* 1984;141:208–214.
11. Bonafe L, Thony B, Penzien JM, et al. Mutations in the sepiapterin reductase gene cause a novel tetrahydrobiopterin-dependent monoamine-neurotransmitter deficiency without hyperphenylalaninemia. *Am J Hum Genet.* 2001;69:269–277.
12. Hyland K, Fryburg JS, Wilson WG, et al. Oral phenylalanine loading in dopa-responsive dystonia: A possible diagnostic test. *Neurology.* 1997;48:1290–1297.
13. Blau N, Bonafe L, Thony B. Tetrahydrobiopterin deficiencies without hyperphenylalaninemia: Diagnosis and genetics of dopa-responsive dystonia and sepiapterin reductase deficiency. *Mol Genet Metab.* 2001;74:172–185.
14. Bräutigam C, Wevers RA, Jansen RJ, et al. Biochemical hallmarks of tyrosine hydroxylase deficiency. *Clin Chem.* 1998;44:1897–1904.
15. Van Der Heyden JC, Rotteveel JJ, Wevers RA. Decreased homovanillic acid concentrations in cerebrospinal fluid in children without a known defect in dopamine metabolism. *Eur J Paediatr Neurol.* 2003;7:31–37.
16. Hyland K, Surtees RA, Rodeck C, et al. Aromatic L-amino acid decarboxylase deficiency: Clinical features, diagnosis, and treatment of a new inborn error of neurotransmitter amine synthesis. *Neurology.* 1992;42:1980–1988.
17. Chang YT, Mues G, McPherson JD, et al. Mutations in the human aromatic L-amino acid decarboxylase gene. *J Inherited Metab Dis.* 1998;21:4.
18. Clayton PT, Surtees RA, DeVile C, et al. Neonatal epileptic encephalopathy. *Lancet.* 2003;361:1614.
19. Bräutigam C, Hyland K, Wevers R, et al. Clinical and laboratory findings in twins with neonatal epileptic encephalopathy mimicking aromatic L-amino acid decarboxylase deficiency. *Neuropediatrics.* 2002;33:113–117.
20. Hyland K, Buist NR, Powell BR, et al. Folinic acid responsive seizures: A new syndrome? *J Inherited Metab Dis.* 1995;18:177–181.
21. Brunner HG, Nelen M, Breakefield XO, et al. Abnormal behavior associated with a point mutation in the structural gene for monoamine oxidase A. *Science.* 1993;262:578–580.
22. Abeling NG, van Gennip AH, van Cruchten AG, et al. Monoamine oxidase A deficiency: Biogenic amine metabolites in random urine samples. *J Neural Transm Suppl.* 1998;52:9–15.
23. Lenders JW, Eisenhofer G, Abeling NG, et al. Specific genetic deficiencies of the A and B isoenzymes of monoamine oxidase are characterized by distinct neurochemical and clinical phenotypes. *J Clin Invest.* 1996;97:1010–1019.
24. Man in 't Veld AJ, Boomsma F, Moleman P, et al. Congenital dopamine–β-hydroxylase

deficiency: A novel orthostatic syndrome. *Lancet.* 1987;1:183–188.

25. Robertson D, Haile V, Perry SE, et al. Dopamine β-hydroxylase deficiency: A genetic disorder of cardiovascular regulation. *Hypertension* 1991;18:1–8.

26. Ichinose H, Ohye T, Takahashi E, et al. Hereditary progressive dystonia with marked diurnal fluctuation caused by mutations in the GTP cyclohydrolase I gene (see comments). *Nat Genet.* 1994;8:236–242.

27. Furukawa Y, Nygaard TG, Gutlich M, et al. Striatal biopterin and tyrosine hydroxylase protein reduction in dopa-responsive dystonia. *Neurology.* 1999;53:1032–1041.

28. Furukawa Y, Lang AE, Trugman JM, et al. Gender-related penetrance and de novo GTP-cyclohydrolase I gene mutations in dopa-responsive dystonia. *Neurology.* 1998;50:1015–1020.

29. Blau N, Thony B. BIOMDB: International database of mutations causing tetrahydrobiopterin deficiencies, www.bh4.org/biomdb1.html, 2005.

30. Furukawa Y, Guttman M, Sparagana SP, et al. Dopa-responsive dystonia due to a large deletion in the GTP cyclohydrolase I gene. *Ann Neurol.* 2000;47:517–520.

31. Segawa M, Nomura Y, Nishiyama N. Autosomal dominant guanosine triphosphate cyclohydrolase I deficiency (Segawa disease). *Ann Neurol.* 2003;54:S32–45.

32. Nygaard TG. Dopa-responsive dystonia: Delineation of the clinical syndrome and clues to pathogenesis. *Adv Neurol.* 1993;60:577–585.

33. Jarman PR, Bandmann O, Marsden CD, et al. GTP cyclohydrolase I mutations in patients with dystonia responsive to anticholinergic drugs. *J Neurol Neurosurg Psychiatry.* 1997;63:304–308.

34. Leuzzi V, Carducci C, Carducci C, et al. Autosomal dominant GTP-CH deficiency presenting as a dopa-responsive myoclonus–dystonia syndrome. *Neurology.* 2002;59:1241–1243.

35. Nygaard TG, Waran SP, Levine RA, et al. Dopa-responsive dystonia simulating cerebral palsy. *Pediatr Neurol.* 1994;11:236–240.

36. Steinberger D, Topka H, Fischer D, et al. GCH1 mutation in a patient with adult-onset oromandibular dystonia. *Neurology.* 1999;52:877–879.

37. Van Hove JL, Stock GJ, Matthijs G, et al. Expanded motor and psychiatric phenotype in autosomal dominant Segawa syndrome due to GTP cyclohydrolase deficiency. *J Neurol Neurosurg Psychiatry.* 2006;77:18–23.

38. Bonafe L, Thony B, Leimbacher W, et al. Diagnosis of dopa-responsive dystonia and other tetrahydrobiopterin disorders by the study of biopterin metabolism in fibroblasts. *Clin Chem.* 2001;47:477–485.

39. Steinberger D, Blau N, Goriuonov D, et al. Heterozygous mutation in 5′-untranslated region of sepiapterin reductase gene (SPR) in a patient with dopa-responsive dystonia. *Neurogenetics.* 2004;5:187–190.

40. Iino T, Tabata M, Takikawa S, et al. Tetrahydrobiopterin is synthesized from 6-pyruvoyl-tetrahydropterin by the human aldo-keto reductase AKR1 family members. *Arch Biochem Biophys.* 2003;416:180–187.

41. Tayeh MA, Marletta MA. Macrophage oxidation of L-arginine to nitric oxide, nitrite, and nitrate: Tetrahydrobiopterin is required as a cofactor. *J Biol Chem.* 1989;264:19654–19658.

42. Ichinose H, Katoh S, Sueoka T, et al. Cloning and sequencing of cDNA encoding human sepiapterin reductase: An enzyme involved in tetrahydrobiopterin biosynthesis. *Biochem Biophys Res Commun.* 1991;179:183–189.

43. Ohye T, Hori TA, Katoh S, et al. Genomic organization and chromosomal localization of the human sepiapterin reductase gene. *Biochem Biophys Res Commun.* 1998;251:597–602.

44. Hoffmann GF, Assmann B, Bräutigam C, et al. Tyrosine hydroxylase deficiency causes progressive encephalopathy and dopa-nonresponsive dystonia. *Ann Neurol.* 2003;54:S56–65.

45. Neville BG, Parascandalo R, Farrugia R, et al. Sepiapterin reductase deficiency: A congenital dopa-responsive motor and cognitive disorder. *Brain.* 2005;128:2291–2296.

46. Zhou QY, Quaife CJ, Palmiter RD. Targeted disruption of the tyrosine hydroxylase gene reveals that catecholamines are required for mouse fetal development. *Nature.* 1995;374:640–643.

47. Grima B, Lamouroux A, Boni C, et al. A single human gene encoding multiple tyrosine hydroxylases with different predicted functional characteristics. *Nature.* 1987;326:707–711.

48. Craig SP, Buckle VJ, Lamouroux A, et al. Localization of the human tyrosine hydroxylase gene to 11p15: Gene duplication and evolution of metabolic pathways. *Cytogenet Cell Genet.* 1986;42:29–32.

49. Kobayashi K, Kaneda N, Ichinose H, et al. Structure of the human tyrosine hydroxylase gene: Alternative splicing from a single gene accounts for generation of four mRNA types. *J Biochem (Tokyo).* 1988;103:907–912.

50. Lewis DA, Melchitzky DS, Haycock JW. Four isoforms of tyrosine hydroxylase are expressed in human brain. *Neuroscience.* 1993;54:477–492.

51. Ludecke B, Knappskog PM, Clayton PT, et al. Recessively inherited L-dopa-responsive parkinsonism in infancy caused by a point mutation (L205P) in the tyrosine hydroxylase gene. *Hum Mol Genet.* 1996;5:1023–1028.

52. Knappskog PM, Flatmark T, Mallet J, et al. Recessively inherited L-dopa-responsive dystonia caused by a point mutation (Q381K) in the tyrosine hydroxylase gene. *Hum Mol Genet.* 1995;4:1209–1212.

53. van den Heuvel LP, Luiten B, Smeitink JA, et al. A common point mutation in the tyrosine hydroxylase gene in autosomal recessive L-dopa-responsive dystonia in the Dutch population. *Hum Genet.* 1998;102:644–646.

54. Furukawa Y, Graf WD, Wong H, et al. Dopa-responsive dystonia simulating spastic paraplegia due to tyrosine hydroxylase (TH) gene mutations. *Neurology.* 2001;56:260–263.

55. Swaans RJ, Rondot P, Renier WO, et al. Four novel mutations in the tyrosine hydroxylase gene in patients with infantile parkinsonism. *Ann Hum Genet.* 2000;64:25–31.

56. Bräutigam C, Steenbergen-Spanjers GC, Hoffmann GF, et al. Biochemical and molecular genetic characteristics of the severe form of tyrosine hydroxylase deficiency. *Clin Chem.* 1999;45:2073–2078.

57. Wevers RA, de Rijk-van Andel JF, Brautigam C, et al. A review of biochemical and molecular genetic aspects of tyrosine hydroxylase deficiency including a novel mutation (291delC). *J Inherited Metab Dis.* 1999;22:364–373.

58. de Lonlay P, Nassogne MC, van Gennip AH, et al. Tyrosine hydroxylase deficiency unresponsive to L-dopa treatment with unusual clinical and biochemical presentation. *J Inherited Metab Dis.* 2000;23:819–825.

59. Furukawa Y, Kish SJ, Fahn S. Dopa-responsive dystonia due to mild tyrosine hydroxylase deficiency. *Ann Neurol.* 2004;55:147–148.

60. Chang YT, Sharma R, Marsh JL, et al. Levodopa-responsive aromatic L-amino acid decarboxylase deficiency. *Ann Neurol.* 2004;55:435–438.

61. Bräutigam C, Wevers RA, Hyland K, et al. The influence of L-dopa on methylation capacity in aromatic L-amino acid decarboxylase deficiency: Biochemical findings in two patients. *J Inherited Metab Dis.* 2000;23:321–324.

62. Pons R, Ford B, Chiriboga CA, et al. Aromatic L-amino acid decarboxylase deficiency: Clinical features, treatment, and prognosis. *Neurology.* 2004;62:1058–1065.

63. Swoboda KJ, Saul JP, McKenna CE, et al. Aromatic L-amino acid decarboxylase deficiency: Overview of clinical features and outcomes. *Ann Neurol.* 2003;54:S49–55.

64. Swoboda K, Hyland K, Goldstein D, et al. Clinical and therapeutic observations in aromatic L-amino acid decarboxylase deficiency. *Neurology.* 1999;53:1205–1211.

65. Abeling NG, van Gennip AH, Barth PG, et al. Aromatic L-amino acid decarboxylase deficiency: A new case with a mild clinical presentation and unexpected laboratory findings. *J Inherited Metab Dis.* 1998;21:240–242.

66. Burlina AB, Burlina AP, Hyland K, et al. Autistic syndrome and aromatic L-amino acid decarboxylase (AADC) deficiency. *J Inherited Metab Dis.* 2001;24:34.

67. Albert VR, Allen JM, Joh TH. A single gene codes for aromatic L-amino acid decarboxylase in both neuronal and non-neuronal tissues. *J Biol Chem.* 1987;262:9404–9411.

68. Nagatsu T. Genes for human catecholamine-synthesizing enzymes. *Neurosci Res.* 1991;12:315–345.

69. Chang YT, Mues G, Hyland K. Alternative splicing in the coding region of human aromatic L-amino acid decarboxylase mRNA. *Neurosci Lett.* 1996;202:157–160.

70. Hyland K, Clayton PT. Aromatic L-amino acid decarboxylase deficiency: Diagnostic methodology. *Clin Chem.* 1992;38:2405–2410.

71. Fiumara A, Brautigam C, Hyland K, et al. Aromatic L-amino acid decarboxylase deficiency with hyperdopaminuria: Clinical and laboratory findings in response to different therapies. *Neuropediatrics.* 2002;33:203–208.

72. Weyler W, Hsu YP, Breakefield XO. Biochemistry and genetics of monoamine oxidase. *Pharmacol Ther.* 1990;47:391–417.

73. Cases O, Seif I, Grimsby J, et al. Aggressive behavior and altered amounts of brain

serotonin and norepinephrine in mice lacking MAOA. *Science.* 1995;268:1763–1766.

74. Brunner HG, Nelen MR, van ZP, et al. X-linked borderline mental retardation with prominent behavioral disturbance: Phenotype, genetic localization, and evidence for disturbed monoamine metabolism. *Am J Hum Genet.* 1993;52:1032–1039.

75. Lan NC, Heinzmann C, Gal A, et al. Human monoamine oxidase A and B genes map to Xp 11.23 and are deleted in a patient with Norrie disease. *Genomics.* 1989;4:552–559.

76. Chen ZY, Hotamisligil GS, Huang JK, et al. Structure of the human gene for monoamine oxidase type A. *Nucl Acids Res.* 1991;19:4537–4541.

77. Bach AW, Lan NC, Johnson DL, et al. cDNA cloning of human liver monoamine oxidase A and B: Molecular basis of differences in enzymatic properties. *Proc Natl Acad Sci USA.* 1988;85:4934–4938.

78. Robertson D, Goldberg MR, Onrot J, et al. Isolated failure of autonomic noradrenergic neurotransmission: Evidence for impaired beta-hydroxylation of dopamine. *N Engl J Med.* 1986;314:1494–1497.

79. Timmers HJ, Deinum J, Wevers RA, et al. Congenital dopamine–β-hydroxylase deficiency in humans. *Ann NY Acad Sci.* 2004;1018:520–523.

80. Craig SP, Buckle VJ, Lamouroux A, et al. Localization of the human dopamine β-hydroxylase (DBH) gene to chromosome 9q34. *Cytogenet Cell Genet.* 1988;48:48–50.

81. Kobayashi K, Kurosawa Y, Fujita K, et al. Human dopamine β-hydroxylase gene: Two mRNA types having different 3′-terminal regions are produced through alternative polyadenylation. *Nucl Acids Res.* 1989;17:1089–1102.

82. Zabetian CP, Anderson GM, Buxbaum SG, et al. A quantitative-trait analysis of human plasma-dopamine β-hydroxylase activity: Evidence for a major functional polymorphism at the DBH locus. *Am J Hum Genet.* 2001;68:515–522.

83. Garland EM, Hahn MK, Ketch TP, et al. Genetic basis of clinical catecholamine disorders. *Ann NY Acad Sci.* 2002;971:506–514.

84. Kim CH, Zabetian CP, Cubells JF, et al. Mutations in the dopamine–β-hydroxylase gene are associated with human norepinephrine deficiency. *Am J Med Genet.* 2002;108:140–147.

85. Biaggioni I, Robertson D. Endogenous restoration of noradrenaline by precursor therapy in dopamine–β-hydroxylase deficiency. *Lancet* 1987;2:1170–1172.

86. Dunnette J, Weinshilboum R. Inheritance of low immunoreactive human plasma dopamine–β-hydroxylase: Radioimmunoassay studies. *J Clin Invest.* 1977;60:1080–1087.

87. Gachon F, Fonjallaz P, Damiola F, et al. The loss of circadian PAR bZip transcription factors results in epilepsy. *Genes Dev.* 2004;18:1397–1412.

88. Mills PB, Surtees RA, Champion MP, et al. Neonatal epileptic encephalopathy caused by mutations in the PNPO gene encoding pyridox(am)ine-5′-phosphate oxidase. *Hum Mol Genet.* 2005;14:1077–1086.

89. Baxter P. Pyridoxine-dependent and pyridoxine-responsive seizures. *Dev Med Child Neurol.* 2001;43:416–420.

90. Baxter P. Pyridoxine-dependent and pyridoxine-responsive seizures. In: Baxter P, ed. *Vitamin Responsive Conditions in Paediatric Neurology.* London: MacKeith Press,2005:166–175.

91. Mills PB, Struys E, Jakobs C, et al. Mutations in antiquitin in individuals with pyridoxine-dependent seizures. *Nat Med.* 2006;12:307–309.

92. Plecko B, Hikel C, Korenke GC, et al. Pipecolic acid as a diagnostic marker of pyridoxine-dependent epilepsy. *Neuropediatrics* 2005;36:200–205.

93. Flynn MP, Martin MC, Moore PT, et al. Type II hyperprolinaemia in a pedigree of Irish travelers (nomads). *Arch Dis Child.* 1989;64:1699–1707.

94. Geraghty MT, Vaughn D, Nicholson AJ, et al. Mutations in the Δ^1-pyrroline-5-carboxylate dehydrogenase gene cause type II hyperprolinemia. *Hum Mol Genet.* 1998;7:1411–1415.

95. Bu DF, Erlander MG, Hitz BC, et al. Two human glutamate decarboxylases, 65-kDa GAD and 67-kDa GAD, are each encoded by a single gene. *Proc Natl Acad Sci USA.* 1992;89:2115–2119.

96. Maitre M. The γ-hydroxybutyrate signaling system in brain: Organization and functional implications. *Prog Neurobiol.* 1997;51:337–361.

97. Hassel B, Johannessen CU, Sonnewald U, et al. Quantification of the GABA shunt and the importance of the GABA shunt versus the 2-oxoglutarate dehydrogenase pathway in GABAergic neurons. *J Neurochem.* 1998;71:1511–1518.

98. Kornberg HL. The role and control of the glyoxylate cycle in *Escherichia coli. Biochem J.* 1966;99:1–11.

99. van den Pol AN, Gao XB, Patrylo PR, et al. Glutamate inhibits GABA excitatory activity in developing neurons. *J Neurosci.* 1998;18:10749–10761.

100. Owens DF, Boyce LH, Davis MB, et al. Excitatory GABA responses in embryonic and neonatal cortical slices demonstrated by gramicidin perforated-patch recordings and calcium imaging. *J Neurosci.* 1996;16:6414–6423.

101. Behar TN, Li YX, Tran HT, et al. GABA stimulates chemotaxis and chemokinesis of embryonic cortical neurons via calcium-dependent mechanisms. *J Neurosci.* 1996;16:1808–1818.

102. Miranda-Contreras L, Itez-Diaz P, Pena-Contreras Z, et al. Levels of amino acid neurotransmitters during neurogenesis and in histotypic cultures of mouse spinal cord. *Dev Neurosci.* 2002;24:59–70.

103. Wong CG, Gibson KM, Snead OC III. From the street to the brain: Neurobiology of the recreational drug γ-hydroxybutyric acid. *Trends Pharmacol Sci* 2004;25:29–34.

104. Snead OC III. Evidence for a G protein–coupled γ-hydroxybutyric acid receptor. *J Neurochem.* 2000;75:1986–1996.

105. Lingenhoehl K, Brom R, Heid J, et al. γ-Hydroxybutyrate is a weak agonist at recombinant GABA(B) receptors. *Neuropharmacology.* 1999;38:1667–1673.

106. Wong CG, Chan KF, Gibson KM et al. Gamma-hydroxybutyric acid: Neurobiology and toxicology of a recreational drug. *Toxicol. Rev.* 2004;23:3–20.

107. Pearl PL, Gibson KM. Clinical aspects of the disorders of GABA metabolism in children. *Curr Opin Neurol.* 2004;17:107–113.

108. Pearl PL, Wallis DD, Gibson KM. Pediatric neurotransmitter diseases. *Curr Neurol Neurosci Rep.* 2004;4:147–152.

109. Medina-Kauwe LK, Tobin AJ, De Meirleir L, et al. 4-Aminobutyrate aminotransferase (GABA-transaminase) deficiency. *J Inherited Metab Dis.* 1999;22:414–427.

110. Jaeken J, Casaer P, de Cock P, et al. Gamma-aminobutyric acid transaminase deficiency: A newly recognized inborn error of neurotransmitter metabolism. *Neuropediatrics.* 1984;15:165–169.

111. Kok RM, Howells DW, van den Heuvel CC, et al. Stable isotope dilution analysis of GABA in CSF using simple solvent extraction and electron-capture negative-ion mass fragmentography. *J Inherited Metab Dis.* 1993;16:508–512.

112. Scriver CR, Pugsley TA, Davis MD. Hyper-β-alaninemia associated with β-aminoaciduria and γ-aminobutyric aciduria, somnolence and seizures. *N Engl J Med.* 1966;274:635–643.

113. Wong CG, Bottiglieri T, Snead OC III: GABA, γ-hydroxybutyric acid, and neurological disease. *Ann Neurol.* 2003;54:S3–12.

114. Akaboshi S, Hogema BM, Novelletto A, et al. Mutational spectrum of the succinate semialdehyde dehydrogenase (ALDH5A1) gene and functional analysis of 27 novel disease-causing mutations in patients with SSADH deficiency. *Hum Mutat.* 2003;22:442–450.

115. Blasi P, Boyl PP, Ledda M, et al. Structure of human succinic semialdehyde dehydrogenase gene: Identification of promoter region and alternatively processed isoforms. *Mol Genet Metab.* 2002;76:348–362.

116. Chambliss KL, Hinson DD, Trettel F, et al. Two exon-skipping mutations as the molecular basis of succinic semialdehyde dehydrogenase deficiency (4-hydroxybutyric aciduria). *Am J Hum Genet.* 1998;63:399–408.

117. Gibson KM, Aramaki S, Sweetman L, et al. Stable isotope dilution analysis of 4-hydroxybutyric acid: An accurate method for quantification in physiological fluids and the prenatal diagnosis of 4-hydroxybutyric aciduria. *Biomed Environ Mass Spectrom.* 1990;19:89–93.

118. Gibson KM, Lee CF, Chambliss KL, et al. 4-Hydroxybutyric aciduria: Application of a fluorometric assay to the determination of succinic semialdehyde dehydrogenase activity in extracts of cultured human lymphoblasts. *Clin Chim Acta* 1991;196:219–221.

119. Wolf NI, Haas D, Hoffmann GF, et al. Sedation with 4-hydroxybutyric acid: A potential pitfall in the diagnosis of SSADH deficiency. *J Inherited Metab Dis.* 2004;27:291–293.

120. Gibson KM, Jakobs C, Ogier H, et al. Vigabatrin therapy in six patients with succinic semialdehyde dehydrogenase deficiency. *J Inherited Metab Dis.* 1995;18:143–146.

121. Gibson KM, Schor DS, Gupta M, et al. Focal neurometabolic alterations in mice deficient for succinate semialdehyde dehydrogenase. *J Neurochem.* 2002;81:71–79.

122. Hogema BM, Gupta M, Senephansiri H, et al. Pharmacologic rescue of lethal seizures in mice

deficient in succinate semialdehyde dehydrogenase. *Nat Genet.* 2001;29:212–216.

123. Gross-Tsur V, Banin E, Shahar E, et al. Visual impairment in children with epilepsy treated with vigabatrin. *Ann Neurol.* 2000;48:60–64.

124. Matern D, Lehnert W, Gibson KM, et al. Seizures in a boy with succinic semialdehyde dehydrogenase deficiency treated with vigabatrin (gamma-vinyl-GABA). *J Inherited Metab Dis.* 1996;19:313–318.

125. Gibson KM, Baumann C, Ogier H, et al. Pre- and postnatal diagnosis of succinic semialdehyde dehydrogenase deficiency using enzyme and metabolite assays. *J Inherited Metab Dis.* 1994;17:732–737.

126. Aligianis IA, Farndon PA, Gray RG, et al. Prenatal diagnosis of succinate semialdehyde dehydrogenase deficiency in non-identical twins. *J Inherited Metab Dis.* 2002;25:517–518.

127. Hogema BM, Akaboshi S, Taylor M, et al. Prenatal diagnosis of succinic semialdehyde dehydrogenase deficiency: Increased accuracy employing DNA, enzyme, and metabolite analyses. *Mol Genet Metab.* 2001;72:218–222.

128. Hamosh A, Johnson MV. Nonketotic hyperglycinemia. In: Scriver CR, Beaudet AL, Sly WS, et al., eds. *The Metabolic and Molecular Bases of Inherited Disease,* 8th ed. New York: McGraw-Hill; 2001:2065–2078.

129. Kikuchi G. The glycine cleavage system: Composition, reaction mechanism, and physiological significance. *Mol Cell Biochem.* 1973;1:169–187.

130. Fujiwara K, Suzuki M, Okumachi Y, et al. Molecular cloning, structural characterization and chromosomal localization of human lipoyltransferase gene. *Eur J Biochem.* 1999;260:761–767.

131. Sato K, Yoshida S, Fujiwara K, et al. Glycine cleavage system in astrocytes. *Brain Res.* 1991;567:64–70.

132. Agamanolis DP, Potter JL, Herrick MK, et al. The neuropathology of glycine encephalopathy: A report of five cases with immunohistochemical and ultrastructural observations. *Neurology.* 1982;32:975–985.

133. Brun A, Borjeson M, Hultberg B, et al. Neonatal nonketotic hyperglycinemia: A clinical, biochemical and neuropathological study including electronmicroscopic findings. *Neuropadiatrie.* 1979;10:195–205.

134. Dalla BB, Aicardi J, Goutieres F, et al. Glycine encephalopathy. *Neuropadiatrie.* 1979;10:209–225.

135. Dobyns WB. Agenesis of the corpus callosum and gyral malformations are frequent manifestations of nonketotic hyperglycinemia. *Neurology.* 1989;39:817–820.

136. Press GA, Barshop BA, Haas RH, et al. Abnormalities of the brain in nonketotic hyperglycinemia: MR manifestations. *Am J Neuroradiol.* 1989;10:315–321.

137. Van Hove JL, Kishnani PS, Demaerel P, et al. Acute hydrocephalus in nonketotic hyperglycemia. *Neurology.* 2000;54:754–756.

138. Khong PL, Lam BC, Chung BH, et al. Diffusion-weighted MR imaging in neonatal nonketotic hyperglycinemia. *Am J Neuroradiol.* 2003;24:1181–1183.

139. Huisman TA, Thiel T, Steinmann B, et al. Proton magnetic resonance spectroscopy of the brain of a neonate with nonketotic hyperglycinemia: In vivo–in vitro (ex vivo) correlation. *Eur Radiol.* 2002;12:858–861.

140. Schmid K, Bohmer G, Gebauer K. Glycine receptor–mediated fast synaptic inhibition in the brain stem respiratory system. *Respir Physiol.* 1991;84:351–361.

141. Betz H. Glycine receptors: Heterogeneous and widespread in the mammalian brain. *Trends Neurosci.* 1991;14:458–461.

142. Johnson JW, Ascher P. Glycine potentiates the NMDA response in cultured mouse brain neurons. *Nature.* 1987;325:529–531.

143. Tada K, Kure S. Nonketotic hyperglycinaemia: Molecular lesion, diagnosis and pathophysiology. *J Inherited Metab Dis.* 1993;16:691–703.

144. Hamosh A, Maher JF, Bellus GA, et al. Long-term use of high-dose benzoate and dextromethorphan for the treatment of nonketotic hyperglycinemia. *J Pediatr.* 1998;132:709–713.

145. Chatterton JE, Awobuluyi M, Premkumar LS, et al. Excitatory glycine receptors containing the NR3 family of NMDA receptor subunits. *Nature.* 2002;415:793–798.

146. Okabe A, Kilb W, Shimizu-Okabe C, et al. Homogenous glycine receptor expression in cortical plate neurons and Cajal-Retzius cells of neonatal rat cerebral cortex. *Neuroscience.* 2004;123:715–724.

147. Van Hove JL, Lazeyras F, Zeisel SH, et al. One-methyl group metabolism in nonketotic hyperglycinaemia. Mildly elevated cerebrospinal fluid homocysteine levels. *J Inherited Metab Dis.* 1998;21:799–811.

148. Applegarth DA, Toone JR, Lowry RB. Incidence of inborn errors of metabolism in British Columbia, 1969–1996. *Pediatrics.* 2000;105:e10.

149. Kure S, Takayanagi M, Narisawa K, et al. Identification of a common mutation in Finnish patients with nonketotic hyperglycinemia. *J Clin Invest.* 1992;90:160–164.

150. Boneh A, Degani Y, Harari M. Prognostic clues and outcome of early treatment of nonketotic hyperglycinemia. *Pediatr Neurol.* 1996;15:137–141.

151. Korman SH, Boneh A, Ichinohe A, et al. Persistent NKH with transient or absent symptoms and a homozygous GLDC mutation. *Ann Neurol.* 2004;56:139–143.

152. Hoover-Fong JE, Shah S, Van Hove JL, et al. Natural history of nonketotic hyperglycinemia in 65 patients. *Neurology.* 2004;63:1847–1853.

153. Hennermann JP, Baruf JM, Monch E. Clinical variation in nonketotic hyperglycinemia. *J Inherited Metab Dis.* 2001;24:35.

154. Van Hove JL, Vande Kerckhove K, Hennermann JP, et al. Benzoate treatment and the glycine index in nonketotic hyperglycinemia. *J Inherited MetabDis.* 2005; 28:651–663.

155. Trauner DA, Page T, Greco C, et al. Progressive neurodegenerative disorder in a patient with nonketotic hyperglycinemia. *J Pediatr.* 1981;98:272–275.

156. Steiner RD, Sweetser DA, Rohrbaugh JR, et al. Nonketotic hyperglycinemia: atypical clinical and biochemical manifestations. *J Pediatr.* 1996;128:243–246.

157. Wiltshire EJ, Poplawski NK, Harrison JR, et al. Treatment of late-onset nonketotic hyperglycinemia: Effectiveness of imipramine and benzoate. *J Inherited Metab Dis.* 2000;23:15–21.

158. Hall DA, Ringel SP. Adult nonketotic hyperglycinemia (NKH) crisis presenting as severe chorea and encephalopathy. *Mov Disord.* 2004;19:485–486.

159. Steiman GS, Yudkoff M, Berman PH, et al. Late-onset nonketotic hyperglycinemia and spinocerebellar degeneration. *J Pediatr.* 1979;94:907–911.

160. Jackson AH, Applegarth DA, Toone JR, et al. Atypical nonketotic hyperglycinemia with normal cerebrospinal fluid to plasma glycine ratio. *J Child Neurol.* 1999;14:464–467.

161. Jaeken J, de Koning TJ, Van Hove JL. Disorders of GABA, glycine, serine and proline. In: Blau N, Blaskovics M, Gibson KM, eds. *Physician's Guide to the Laboratory Diagnosis of Metabolic Diseases,* 2d ed. Berlin: Springer; 2003:123–140.

162. Aliefendioglu D, Tana AA, Coskun T, et al. Transient nonketotic hyperglycinemia: Two case reports and literature review. *Pediatr Neurol.* 2003;28:151–155.

163. Luder AS, Davidson A, Goodman SI, et al. Transient nonketotic hyperglycinemia in neonates. *J Pediatr.* 1989;114:1013–1015.

164. Catalatepe S, van Marter LJ, Kozakewich H, et al. Pulmonary hypertension associated with nonketotic hyperglycinemia. *J Inherited Metab Dis.* 2000;25:137–144.

165. Ellaway CJ, Mundy H, Lee PJ. Successful pregnancy outcome in atypical hyperglycinaemia. *J Inherited Metab Dis.* 2001;24:599–600.

166. Korman SH, Gutman A. Pitfalls in the diagnosis of glycine encephalopathy (nonketotic hyperglycinemia). *Dev Med Child Neurol.* 2002;44:712–720.

167. Applegarth DA, Toone JR. Nonketotic hyperglycinemia (glycine encephalopathy): Laboratory diagnosis. *Mol Genet Metab.* 2001;74:139–146.

168. Applegarth DA, Toone JR. Glycine encephalopathy (nonketotic hyperglycinaemia): Review and update. *J Inherited Metab Dis.* 2004;27:417–422.

169. Toone JR, Applegarth DA, Coulter-Mackie MB, et al. Biochemical and molecular investigations of patients with nonketotic hyperglycinemia. *Mol Genet Metab.* 2000;70:116–121.

170. Applegarth DA, Toone JR, Rolland MO, et al. Non-concordance of CVS and liver glycine cleavage enzyme in three families with non-ketotic hyperglycinaemia (NKH) leading to false-negative prenatal diagnoses. *Prenat Diagn.* 2000;20:367–370.

171. Toone JR, Applegarth DA, Levy HL, et al. Molecular genetic and potential biochemical characteristics of patients with T-protein deficiency as a cause of glycine encephalopathy (NKH). *Mol Genet Metab.* 2003;79:272–280.

172. Van Hove JL, Kerckhove KV, Hennermann JB, et al. Benzoate treatment and the glycine index in nonketotic hyperglycinaemia. *J Inherited Metab Dis.* 2005;28:651–663.

173. Van Hove JL, Kishnani P, Muenzer J, et al. Benzoate therapy and carnitine deficiency in nonketotic hyperglycinemia. *Am J Med Genet.* 1995;59:444–453.

174. Wolff JA, Kulovich S, Yu AL, et al. The effectiveness of benzoate in the management of seizures in nonketotic hyperglycinemia. *Am J Dis Child.* 1986;140:596–602.

175. Matalon R, Michals K, Naidu S, et al. Treatment of nonketotic hyperglycinemia with diazepam, choline and folinic acid. *J Inherited Metab Dis.* 1982;5:3–5.

176. Deutsch SI, Rosse RB, Mastropaolo J. Current status of NMDA antagonist interventions in the treatment of nonketotic hyperglycinemia. *Clin Neuropharmacol.* 1998;21:71–79.

177. Kleckner NW, Glazewski JC, Chen CC, et al. Subtype-selective antagonism of N-methyl-D-aspartate receptors by felbamate: Insights into the mechanism of action. *J Pharmacol Exp Ther.* 1999;289:886–894.

178. Neuberger JM, Schweitzer S, Rolland MO, et al. Effect of sodium benzoate in the treatment of atypical nonketotic hyperglycinaemia. *J Inherited Metab Dis.* 2000;23:22–26.

179. de Koning TJ, Snell K, Duran M, et al. L-Serine in disease and development. *Biochem J.* 2003;371:653–661.

180. de Koning TJ, Poll-The BT, Jaeken J. Continuing education in neurometabolic disorders: Serine deficiency disorders. *Neuropediatrics.* 1999;30:1–4.

181. Furuya S, Tabata T, Mitoma J, et al. L-Serine and glycine serve as major astroglia-derived trophic factors for cerebellar Purkinje neurons. *Proc Natl Acad Sci USA.* 2000;97:11528–11533.

182. de Koning TJ, Duran M, Dorland L, et al. Beneficial effects of L-serine and glycine in the management of seizures in 3-phosphoglycerate dehydrogenase deficiency. *Ann Neurol.* 1998;44:261–265.

183. Häusler MG, Jaeken J, Monch E, et al. Phenotypic heterogeneity and adverse effects of serine treatment in 3-phosphoglycerate dehydrogenase deficiency: Report on two siblings. *Neuropediatrics.* 2001;32:191–195.

184. Jaeken J, Detheux M, Van Maldergem L, et al. 3-Phosphoglycerate dehydrogenase deficiency and 3-phosphoserine phosphatase deficiency: Inborn errors of serine biosynthesis. *J Inherited Metab Dis.* 1996;19:223–226.

185. Jaeken J, Detheux M, Van ML, et al. 3-Phosphoglycerate dehydrogenase deficiency: An inborn error of serine biosynthesis. *Arch Dis Child.* 1996;74:542–545.

186. de Koning TJ, Klomp LW, van Oppen AC, et al. Prenatal and early postnatal treatment in 3-phosphoglycerate-dehydrogenase deficiency. *Lancet.* 2004;364:2221–2222.

187. Pineda M, Vilaseca MA, Artuch R, et al. 3-Phosphoglycerate dehydrogenase deficiency in a patient with West syndrome. *Dev Med Child Neurol.* 2000;42:629–633.

188. de Koning TJ, Jaeken J, Pineda M, et al. Hypomyelination and reversible white matter attenuation in 3-phosphoglycerate dehydrogenase deficiency. *Neuropediatrics.* 2000;31:287–292.

189. Klomp LW, de Koning TJ, Malingre HE, et al. Molecular characterization of 3-phosphoglycerate dehydrogenase deficiency: A neurometabolic disorder associated with reduced L-serine biosynthesis. *Am J Hum Genet.* 2000;67:1389–1399.

190. Pind S, Slominski E, Mauthe J, et al. V490M, a common mutation in 3-phosphoglycerate dehydrogenase deficiency, causes enzyme deficiency by decreasing the yield of mature enzyme. *J Biol Chem.* 2002;277:7136–7143.

191. Jaeken J, Detheux M, Fryns JP, et al. Phosphoserine phosphatase deficiency in a patient with Williams syndrome. *J Med Genet.* 1997;34:594–596.

192. Hart CE, Race V, Achouri Y, et al. Phosphoserine aminotransferase deficiency: a novel disorder of the serine biosynthesis pathway. *Am J Hum Genet.* 2007;80:931–937.

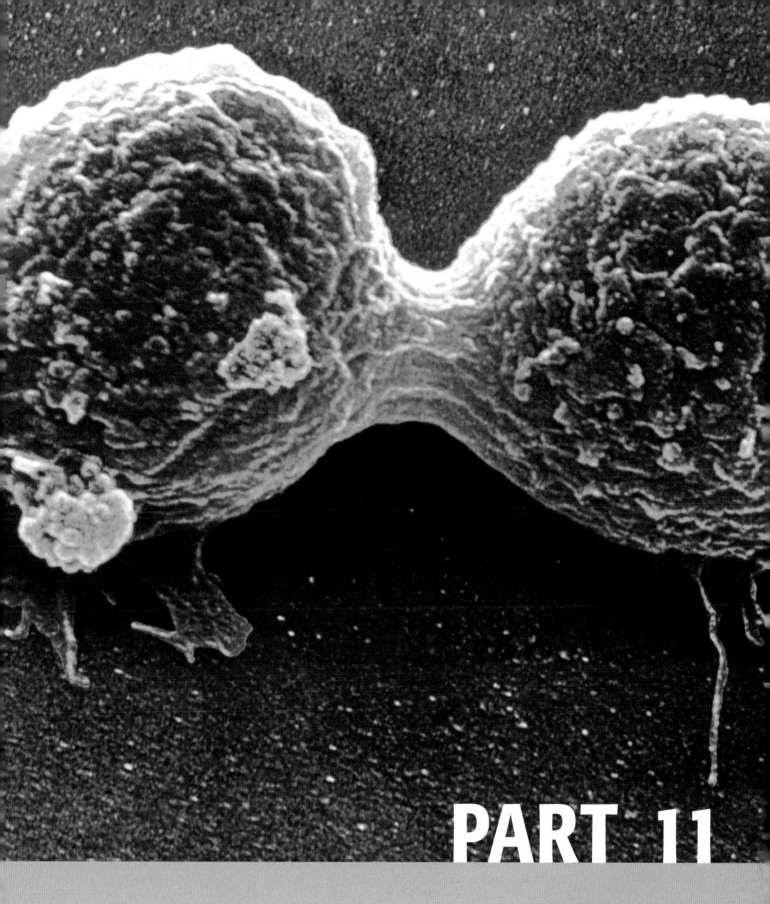

PART 11

Endocrine-Related Neoplasias

IN THIS PART

Previous page: Colored scanning electron micrograph (SEM) of two cancer cells in the final stage of cell division.

CHAPTER 46

Endocrine-Related Cancer*

Constantine A. Stratakis, MD, D(Med)Sci
Karel Pacak, MD, PhD, DSc
Jordan Pinsker, MD*
Andrew J. Bauer, MD*

THYROID TUMORS AND CANCER

Thyroid carcinoma is the most common endocrine tumor in children (and in adults); approximately 10% of thyroid cancers are diagnosed before 21 years of age. In children, the female:male ratios are age-specific, with a 1:6 female:male ratio from ages 5–9 years, a 1:1 female:male ratio for ages 10–14, and a 5:2 female:male ratio for ages 15–19, the later being the peak incidence of the disease (1). Similar to adults, the most common presentation is an asymptomatic nodule noted on physical examination; however, thyroid nodules are reported much less frequently in children, and the risk of malignant disease appears to be much higher, with 20% to 50% of pediatric nodules found to have carcinoma compared with 10% to 14% of adults (2). In addition, at diagnosis, up to 90% of children have regional lymph node metastasis, and up to 20% have lung metastasis (3–19).

There is some suggestion that two subpopulations in the pediatric age warrant greater concern secondary to increased incidence and aggressiveness of disease: children diagnosed with thyroid cancer prior to 10 years of age and children with a history of previous radiation exposure, either from environmental accidents or from therapeutic treatment of oncologic disease (20–22). In both groups, there is an increased risk to develop both thyroid nodules or malignancy, with relative risks for the later being reported as high as 27 to 53 times greater than in children without a history of radiation exposure (20,21). With aggressive surgical intervention and radioiodine ablation, most children with thyroid carcinoma typically experience excellent long-term prognosis; however, close monitoring and transition in care at adulthood are essential because 25% of cancers may recur, at times after many years of apparently negative studies (6,8–12,22).

Histology, Etiology, and Natural History

Differentiated thyroid carcinoma (DTC) is the most common form of thyroid cancer in children; 70% to 80% of these tumors are papillary thyroid carcinomas (PTCs), whereas the rest are follicular thyroid carcinomas (FTCs) (3–5). In children with a history of radiation exposure, both PTCs and FTCs are found, but similar to spontaneous tumors, the majority of radiation-induced thyroid cancers have PTC-like histological characteristics (23). It has become clear that the thyroid gland in children exhibits increased sensitivity to small doses of radiation; in addition, the latency with which a child develops thyroid nodules or cancer decreases the younger the child is at the time of radiation exposure (24,25).

FTC is more common in the adolescent age group compared with children younger than 10 years of age; adolescents diagnosed with FTC, have less frequent regional lymph node and distant metastasis. Interestingly, however, even with these apparent differences, both PTC and FTC share similarly excellent rates of disease-free survival (3,4,8,15,19,26). With the release of an updated classification system that now classifies the "follicular variant of papillary" cancer as another form of PTC, it is predicted that there may be a slight increase in the overall reported incidence of PTC (27). It is unclear right now whether these changes in histopathpological classification are of any clinical significance.

Despite the similar histology of DTC in children when compared with adults, the molecular signature of childhood DTC differs considerably when compared with adults. In adults, *BRAF* and *ras* mutations are found commonly, and when present, *ret/PTC1* mutations often portend more aggressive disease. In children, ret/PTC mutations are more common, and does not appear to be a corre-lation between the presence of *ret/PTC* rearrangements and radiation exposure or clinical behavior (28,29).

Inherited forms of pediatric thyroid cancer also occur and comprise approximately 5% of reported PTC cases (30). These include various forms of familial nonmedullary thyroid carcinoma (29,30), Cowden disease (AD inheritance; multiple hamartomas, breast cancer, and colon cancer, caused by mutations of the *PTEN* gene) (32–35), Gardner syndrome (AD inheritance; familial adenomatoid polyposis, desmoid tumors, lipomas; *APC* gene) (36,37), and Carney complex (AD inheritance; lentiginoses, pituitary adenomas, primary pigmented nodular adrenocortical disease, testicular tumors; *PRKAR1A* and *CNC2* genes, as discussed later in this chapter) (38).

Anaplastic or undifferentiated thyroid cancer (UTC) is extraordinarily rare in children, making up a less than 1% of the total in all reported series; however, as in adults, UTC has a poor prognosis.

Clinical Presentation Children ultimately diagnosed with thyroid cancer typically present with an asymptomatic thyroid mass that is most commonly discovered during routine physical examination for school or participation in a sports program, on follow-up examination for a history of autoimmune thyroiditis, or following a request from a family member that felt the mass. At diagnosis, metastasis to local lymph nodes occurs in up to 90% of children, and more than half the patients with PTC present with cervical neck mass, often without history of a palpable thyroid lesion (10–14). Thus, while thyroid cancer in children is uncommon, it is extremely important to consider DTC as part of the differential diagnosis of persistent cervical adenopathy. Other symptoms including dysphagia, hoarseness, or neck pain that typically are reported in adults are found less commonly

---

*The opinions and assertions contained herein are the private views of the authors and are not to be construed as official or as reflecting the opinions of Walter Reed Army Medical Center, the Uniformed Services University of the Health Sciences, the Department of the Army, or the Department of Defense.

Endocrine-Related Cancer

AT-A-GLANCE

Endocrine-related cancer is extraordinarily rare in children. Most endocrine tumors in children are benign; pituitary, thyroid, and adrenal adenomas are by far the most common endocrine masses in childhood. Sporadic (nonfamilial) carcinomas in children are mostly thyroid and adrenal. Most other endocrine malignant tumors in children occur in the context of genetic conditions predisposing to multiple neoplasias: multiple endocrine neoplasia types 1 and 2 (MEN-1 and MEN-2), McCune–Albright syndrome (MAS), Carney complex, von Hippel–Lindau (VHL) disease, Peutz–Jeghers syndrome (PJS), Cowden disease (CD), hereditary hyperparathyroidism and jaw-tumor syndrome HPT-JT. Occasional sporadic parathyroid cancer, malignant testicular and ovarian tumors, and pheochromocytomas or other paragangliomas also have been reported, each in a handful of cases in the pediatric age group.

DISORDER	OCCURRENCE	GENE	LOCUS	OMIM
Pituitary adenomas	~0.1:1 million/year	Various	Several	
Thyroid follicular adenomas	0.1% of all tumors	Various	Several	
Adrenal adenomas	Rare	Various	Several	
Bilateral adrenal hyperplasias	Rare	PRKAR1A, other	17q23-q24	188830
Thyroid cancer	Rare	RET-PTC, other	Several	
Adrenal cancer	Rare	TP53, other	17p, other	
MEN-1	Rare	MEN1	11q13	131100
MEN-2	Rare	RET	10q11.2	162300, 171400
McCune–Albright syndrome (MAS)	Rare	GNAS	20q13.2	174800
Carney complex (CNC)	Rare	PRKAR1A, other	17q23-q24, 2p16, 17p13.1	160980, 605244
Peutz–Jeghers syndrome	Rare	STK11/LKB1	19p13.3	175200
von Hippel–Lindau disease	Rare	VHL	3p26-p25	193300
Cowden disease	Rare	PTEN	10q23.31, 10q22.3	158350
Hyperparathyroidism/jaw tumors	Very rare	HRPT2	1q25-q31	145001
Pheochromocytoma	1/100, 000	VHL, RET, SDH-D, SDH-B, GDNF	3p26-p25, 10q11.2, 11q23, 1p36.1-p35, 5p13.1-p12	171300, 606537, 164761, 602690, 185470, 600837
Hereditary paragangliomas	Very rare	SDH-B, -C and -D	1p36, 1q21, 11q23	16800, 605373, 602690, 605373, 185470
Carney–Stratakis syndrome	Very rare	SDH-B, -C and -D	1p, 1q, 11q	#606864

DISEASE	FINDINGS LABORATORY	CLINICAL PRESENTATION
Pituitary tumors	↑ ACTH, ↑ F, ↑ GH, ↑ PRL	Prolactinomas account for 40% of all pituitary tumors; more common in females and during adolescence; females present with delayed puberty, amenorrhea, irregular menses, galactorrhea; males typically present with headaches, visual loss, growth or pubertal arrest and other signs of hypopituitarism. GH tumors can be part of MEN-1, MAS or CNC; account for 3% of intracranial tumors; tend to be hormonally active in children presenting with accelerated growth (gigantism). Children with ACTH secreting tumors present with obesity, decreased growth rate due to Cushing disease.
Thyroid tumors and cancer	Normal TSH, free T_4	Most common endocrine tumor in children; typically present with asymptomtic nodule in routine follow-up; high risk of malignancy; if malignant, 90% chance of regional lymph node metastasis

DISEASE	FINDINGS LABORATORY	CLINICAL PRESENTATION
Adrenal hyperplasias adenomas or, cancer	↑ serum and urine free cortisol, ↑ serum DHEA-S, ↑ 24 hour urinary 17-OHCS and 17-KS	Can present at all ages with peaks before age 5 years and in the 4th to 5th decade of life; female predominance; children can present with growth acceleration, precocious puberty, and virilization; Cushing syndrome; low-renin hypertension; hypoglycemia; and non-glucocorticoid related insulin resistance are rare, but may also be present
MEN-1	↑ PTH, high calcium PRL, or fasting gastrin	Unheard of in infancy. Autosomal dominant disorder characterized by tumors of the parathyroid, pituitary, pancreas and other gastrointestinal tumors; usually presents after 10 years of age and hyperparathyroidism is usually the first manifestation; pituitary tumors have been reported as early as 5 years of age; gastrinoma does not usually develop before 12 years and insulinoma has developed as early as 5 years
MEN-2	↑ PTH, ↑ calcium ↑ plasma or urinary metanephrines, ↑ calcitonin	Pheochromocytoma has been reported in infancy but usually occurs in adulthood; medullary thyroid carcinoma in situ may be detected as early as the end of the first year of life, although asymptomatic; usually presents after 5 years of age with local and/or metastatic medullary thyroid carcinoma; pheochromocytoma(s) may lead to hypertension and/or abdominal discomfort; hyperparathyroidism is rarely symptomatic
McCune–Albright syndrome	↑ free T$_4$, ↑ GH and/or PRL, ↑ F and other steroid hormones	During infancy can present with cafe-au-lait skin lesions, bone tumors and signs of early puberty; Cushing syndrome present almost exclusively in infancy; symptoms of hyperthyroidism, hyperparathyroidism, gigantism, or acromegaly at any age; during childhood the first manifestation usually is precocious puberty; thyroid cancer is rare; sarcomas and/or other tumors may develop later
Carney complex	↑ GH, ↑ PRL, ↑ serum and urinary F, Nl thyroid and gonadal function	During infancy lentigines and other skin lesions, Cushing syndrome, heart myxoma presenting with brain hemorrhage/stroke and other tumors may be present; mean age of presentation 10–20 years; during childhood, Cushing syndrome, heart and other myxomas, nevi and other pigmented skin lesions, thyroid cancer, gigantism or acromegaly, bone tumors, schwannomas and other lesions may develop
Peutz–Jeghers syndrome	The only hormonal abnormality may be hyperestrogenemia in boys due to testicular Sertoli cell tumors; normal thyroid function tests	Pigmented lesions and hanartomatous polyps may be present in infancy, but usually presents after 5 years of age with polyps, diverticula, and skin pigmented lesions; unusual presentations include young boys with gynecomastia and precocious puberty due to testicular Sertoli cell tumors; the latter may be become malignant in later life; adolescents may develop thyroid and other cancers (breast, ovarian)
Von Hippel–Lindau disease	↑ plasma and urinary normetanephrine	In infancy hemangioblastomas may be picked up coincidentally, and a pheochromocytoma may be symptomatic; usually presents in late childhood with hypertension (due to pheochromocytoma) or one of the tumors associated with the disease; malignant pheochromocytoma is unusual but occurs; renal cancer is one of the main tumors of the disease
Pheochromo-cytoma	↑ plasma and urinary metanephrines	Extremely rare during infancy and almost always with genetic predisposition; in childhood usually familial pheochromocytoma is found; some can be more aggressive and have predisposition to develop malignant disease (especially those associated with SDHB gene mutation); present with hypertension, tachycardia, and other symptoms related to catecholamine overproduction
Hereditory paraganglioma Carney–Stratakis syndrome	↑ plasma and urinary metanephrines	Extremely rare during infancy and always with genetic predisposition; children may also present with gastrointestinal tumors in the Carney-Stratakis syndrome; older children may present with masses, secreting paragangliomas or pheochromocytomas and hypertension, or in Carney–Stratakis syndrom, with gastrointestinal tumors and/or sarcomas

ACTH = adrenocorticotropin; PRL = prolactin; GH = growth hormone; PTH = parathyroid hormone; Nl = normal; 17-OHCS = 17-hydroxycorticosteroids; 17-KS = 17-ketosteroids; DHEA-S = dihydroepiandrosterone-sulfate in children at the time of presentation with any type of thyroid cancer.

Diagnosis The reported prevalence of thyroid nodules in children is less than 2%; however, this number may reflect an underrepresentation of the true prevalence because not all children have careful routine thyroid examinations (39). However the detection of a nodule in the thyroid of a child is worrisome because, unlike in adults, these nodules have an up to 50% chance of being cancerous.

Evaluation of a child with a thyroid nodule or persistent cervical adenopathy includes thyroid ultrasound to assess the size, number, centricity (i.e., bilateral, multicentric, or focal), and other characteristics (e.g., cystic, solid, or mixed) of the nodule, followed by fine-needle biopsy (FNA). In the majority of cases, the use of cervical computed tomographic (CT) scans or magnetic resonance imaging (MRI) to assess local or regional disease is not indicated, and if used, it is extremely important to avoid iodine-containing contrast solutions because they can alter uptake and effectiveness of radioactive iodine and may delay future treatments. Baseline chest x-ray and chest CT scans are relatively insensitive for the detection of pulmonary metastasis; these studies are often normal in children despite the presence of pulmonary disease in 6% to 20% of cases. The postablation ^{131}I scan appears to be the most sensitive test for the detection of pulmonary disease (11,18,40). The previously routine use of scintigraphic procedures to characterize a nodule as "hot," "warm," or "cold" is now in decline. Reports of malignant lesions found in warm or hot nodules blur these classical distinctions, and as such, they cannot be relied on to ultimately define the risk of malignancy (41–44).

Overall, FNA is now the primary tool for diagnosis of thyroid cancer in children. The use of local anesthesia should be considered; in younger patients, systemic sedation is warranted and increases the likelihood of obtaining adequate material for diagnosis. The ability to detect malignant cells prior to being in the operating room allows for greater planning and counseling for the family, clinician, and surgeon. If the FNA results are equivocal, a repeat FNA procedure or even surgery should be considered due to the relatively increased risk of malignancy in chidren (2,45–47): up to 50% compared with 10% to 14% reported in adults. Thus only the most benign and definitive FNA results should be trusted for further management. Accordingly, diagnostic results from preoperative FNA in a child with a thyroid nodule may obviate the need for frozen-section examination of the tissue during surgical removal of the mass (lobectomy).

There are several exceptions to this general approach. We have had several adolescent girls referred for suppressed thyrotropin levels with minimal signs or symptoms of hyperthyroidism that on thyroid scan were found to have an autonomous nodule. In this situation, thyroid scanning may be helpful in tailoring the treatment plan, alleviating the need for total thyroidectomy. A second group, on the other side of the risk spectrum, consists of children with thyroid nodules with a history of exposure to radiation. These children should have a careful annual thyroid examination, and based on the clinical findings, initial diagnosis, age at the time, dose and field of radiation, and serial thyroid ultrasound examinations should be considered. If nodules develop in these children, they are often multiple, and because of the increased risk of malignancy, it is not unreasonable to recommend surgery without any additional preoperative evaluation.

Treatment

Surgery Treatment of thyroid cancer in children is similar to that in adults, with surgical resection followed by radioiodine therapy being the most effective initial approach. Controversy exists concerning the extent of surgery (19,48–52), but DTC in children is often multifocal and bilateral, and in the hands of a surgeon experienced with pediatric thyroidectomy, near-total or total thyroidectomy with removal of local lymph nodes is associated with low risk of complications and reduced risk of persistent or recurrent disease (4,6–8,15,17).

The most frequent complications of aggressive thyroid surgery are permanent hypoparathyroidism and recurrent laryngeal nerve damage. Removal of the entire thyroid and suspicious lymph nodes provides distinct advantages for follow-up, most importantly allowing for the most efficient use of radioiodine therapy and improving the sensitivity of detecting residual or persistent disease on posttreatment scans (4–6,8,17). The excellent prognosis that most children with DTC experience is expected only when total thyroidectomy and ^{131}I are used to treat residual and recurrent disease.

[131]I Ablation The incorporation of ^{131}I ablation as a postoperative therapeutic modality has become commonplace, with the goal of treatment being to eliminate any thyroid remnants from the cervical region. When successful, the ablative dose reduces remaining malignant cells and allows for the more effective use of surveillance methods, including ^{131}I scanning and serum thyroglobulin measurements.

The ablative dose of [131]I (radioactive iodine [RAI]) usually is administered 4–6 weeks after surgery, allowing time for the patient to recover and for wound healing to take place. Thyroid hormone replacement therapy should be started after surgery, using triiodothyronine (T3, 25–75 μg/day). Two weeks before the scheduled ^{131}I dose, the T3 should be stopped and a low iodine diet initiated, allowing for optimal absorption of the [131]I. A serum thyrotropin (TSH) determination should be performed before the administration of ^{131}I, and if most (if not all) thyroid tissue was removed at surgery, TSH should be at least 30 μU/mL. Because of the associated decreased quality of life and the concern that an elevated TSH level may serve as a proliferative factor for any remaining malignant thyroid cells, some centers have started using recombinant human TSH (rhTSH) to prepare adult patients for ablation. More recently, this has been studied in children using similar dosing (0.9 mg given 24 hours apart) with similar results (53). Prospective studies are needed to more adequately determine the safety and efficacy of this practice.

There are two schools of thought in deciding on the ablative ^{131}I dose. A relatively small dose of just less than 30 mCi allows the patient to remain as an outpatient and may result in ablation of up to 93% of any residual thyroid tissue (54). Unfortunately, in patients with greater amounts of residual thyroid tissue and/or with metastatic disease, this low dose is less effective, and an increased risk of later recurrences has been observed. Alternatively, one can give a larger dose of ^{131}I, typically 80–150 mCi. The advantages of the higher dose include a greater efficacy on eliminating residual thyroid cells, serving as an initial treatment for metastatic disease, as well as allowing for identification and localization of metastatic disease in a postablation whole-body scan done 7–10 days postablation.

Six months after RAI ablation, children should be reevaluated for residual disease. Currently, levothyroxine hormone withdrawal is instituted 3–6 weeks prior to this evaluation, with a goal of having the TSH concentration greater than 40 mIU/L; at the same time that levothyroxine is stopped, T3 therapy at 25–75 μg per day is started and continued until two weeks before a whole-body scan (WBS) is to be performed in an effort to avoid a prolonged hypothyroid state; T3 has a shorter serum half-life (1 day compared with 5–7 days for T4); in children, two weeks of levothyroxine withdrawl without T3 supplementation may also be adequate to raise TSH levels at this range (55). At the same time that T3 is discontinued, patients are also placed on a low-iodine diet in an effort to optimize update of the [131]I. This somewhat complicated approach with its associated side effects may be avoided if the 2-week withdrawal regimen (55) or rhTSH become more commonplace, but until prospective studies are performed and the sensitivity and specificity of these techniques to detect residual or recurrent disease are known, use of the traditional approach is advised.

Two days prior to the potential ^{131}I dose, determinations of serum TSH, thyroglobulin (Tg), and human chorionic gonadotropin (β-hCG, for any adolescent female to rule-out pregnancy) are done, and if the TSH is adequately elevated, a WBS is performed. Depending on availability, ^{123}I should be used in place of ^{131}I for the WBS because it causes less thyroid cell injury, improving the efficacy of the RAI treatment dose (56). Therapy is indicated based on clinical suspicion of disease and radiological evidence of disease. If available, dosimetry should be performed to provide the safest, most effective RAI dose. In the absence of dosimetry, 100–125 mCi of ^{131}I for disease confined to the cervical region and 125–150 mCi for pulmonary metastasis are reasonable doses to consider.

Annual physical examinations, thyroid hormone withdrawal scans, and stimulated serum Tg levels should be performed. Patients are considered free of disease when their Tg level is undetectable and scans are negative for 2 consecutive years. Cumulative doses of less than 600 mCi have been associated with a twofold decrease in relapse and improved disease-free survival; however, despite aggressive surgical and radioiodine therapy, the overall recurrence rate of thyroid cancer in children is high at 15% to 25% (3–9,17,19).

Side effects from ^{131}I are relatively rare in children. Acutely ill patients may experience nausea and vomiting, thyroiditis, and inflammation of salivary glands (sialoadenitis); the latter is decreased by the use of careful attention to hydration and measures to increase salivary flow during the exposure. With larger doses, bone marrow suppression also may occur that typically normalizes by 2 months. There have been rare reports of leukemia developing after repeated high-dose ^{131}I given over a short period of time (57). Other malignancies reported after high-dose ^{131}I therapy include breast (58), bladder, and colorectal cancer (59).

Lastly, gonadal toxicity is another potential long-term toxic effects of ^{131}I and should be discussed with the family prior to therapy. In the first year after therapy, adolescent girls and young women may experience menstrual irregularities; boys and young men may have transient elevation of follicle-stimulating hormone (FSH) (60–64). Decreased fertility has not been observed; it is generally recommended that male patients of repro-ductive age should wait at least 4 months after treatment before attempting fatherhood, and females should wait at least 1 year before attempting to become pregnant. In addition, postpubertal male patients receiving doses greater than 400 mCi should be counseled on consideration of sperm banking.

Thyroid Hormone Replacement All children with thyroid cancer need to be placed on suppressive doses of thyroid hormone, with a goal of having the TSH concentration at 0.01–0.02 μU/mL (65). This typically can be accomplished with a dose of thyroxine of 2.1–4.5 μg/kg/day. Release from suppressive therapy is individualized based on determination of when the patient appears to be in remission. Patients must be counseled and followed closely for the associated potential negative impact that this therapy can have on bone density, particularly important during this period of peak bone mass acquisition (66).

Treatment Summary In summary, prognosis for children diagnosed with differentiated cancer (PTC or FTC) is good, with low disease-specific mortality compared with other pediatric cancers (10–16,67,68). However, even with aggressive initial therapy, up to a third of patients may experience recurrence of disease sometimes at 10 or more years after diagnosis, with pregnancy appearing to be a time of increased risk (3,4,8,17,19). Total thyroidectomy with ablation appears to be the most prudent approach to initial treatment, with a 10-fold increase in disease-free survival when compared with nontotal thyroidectomy and a 5-fold reduction in risk of recurrence with the use of ^{131}I ablation (17). Children should be followed with annual examinations, stimulated or rhTSH-induced Tg levels, and thyroid scans. Unfortunately, there continues to be a paucity of information on children followed for 20 years or more after treatment.

ADRENOCORTICAL CANCER

Malignant neoplasms of the adrenal cortex account for 0.05% to 0.2% of all cancers, with an approximate prevalence of 2 new cases per 1 million population per year (69–71). Adrenocortical cancer (ACC) occurs at all ages, from early infancy to the eighth decade of life (69,72–75). A bimodal age distribution has been reported, with the first peak occurring before the age of 5 years and the second in the fourth to fifth decade. In all published series, females predominate, accounting for 65% to 90% of the reported cases. Several studies have shown a left-sided prevalence in adrenal cancer; however, others have reported a right-sided preponderance. In approximately 2% to 10% of the patients, adrenal cancer is found bilaterally (76). Overall, there appears to be a higher prevalence of ACC among patients with incidentally discovered adrenal masses than in the general population (77). Among the radiologically detectable masses, independently of size, 1 in 1500 lesions may be an adrenal carcinoma, but in children, this number is probably much higher (76). Using the 5-cm-diameter cutoff as the most commonly accepted criterion for clinical investigation of an adrenal tumor in adults, carcinoma may be found in as many as 7% of patients with adrenal lesions larger than 5 cm; tumors over 12 cm in size have a 25% or higher chance of being malignant (76,78,79). Although the incidence of adrenal incidentalomas appears to be higher in some familial neoplasia syndromes such as multiple endocrine neoplasia type 1 (MEN-1) (80) and familial adenomatous polyposis (FAP) (81), it is unclear whether this finding is accompanied by a higher predisposition to adrenal cancer. In some areas of the world, such as in southern Brazil, a higher incidence of adrenal cancer, especially in children, has been documented, propably due to environmental mutagens (82).

In a recent series of 11 patients (3 boys and 8 girls) with a median age of 7 years, three histologically proven carcinomas were less than 5 cm in maximal width. Overall, the cutoff criterion of 5 cm does not apply in children, and any adrenal tumor should be considered suspicious for ACC (83,84).

Unlike adults, most pediatric patients with ACC present with a hormonal syndrome that may make their detection easier and lead to their early surgical resection and medical treatment. Other features, including a different genetic background and a better prognosis, differentiate ACC in chidlren from that in adults (83,85,86) (see below).

Clinical Presentation Adrenocortical tumors can be hormonally silent or hormone-secreting. The clinical presentation of ACC can be variable, and patients can present with symptoms of a specific hormonal syndrome or with nonspecific symptoms in up to 30% of the cases, such as nonspecific abdominal or dorsal pain due to mass effect (87,88). In children older than 5 years of age, more than 60% of ACCs are hormonally active (83,84,86,89). This number may be higher if subtle, asymptomatic biochemical abnormalities are sought in patients with adrenal carcinoma. Inactive steroid precursors, such as pregnenolone, 17α-hydroxypregnenolone (17OHPreg), and 11-deoxycortisol (S), or their metabolites can be found in the circulation and the urine, respectively (85). Occasionally, patients may have ACCs that secrete deoxycorticosterone

(DOC) or corticosterone (B) and present with low-renin, low-aldosterone hypertension and hypokalemic alkalosis in the absence of hypercortisolism (90).

Virilization and/or precocious puberty that is due to hypersecretion of adrenal androgens is the most common endocrine manifestation of a hormone-secreting ACC in children, particularly in patients younger than 5 years of age, where it is the presenting symptom in 95% of cases (85). Cushing syndrome is present in 30% to 40% of patients with adrenal cancer. Multiple hormones can be produced by a single tumor, leading to a mixed clinical picture (e.g., Cushing syndrome plus virilization) (76,85,91,92). Feminization, hyperaldosteronism, hypoglycemia, non-glucocorticoid-related insulin resistance, and polycythemia are other rare endocrine or paraneoplastic phenomena observed in patients with ACC (76,85).

A palpable mass is present in approximately half the patients with ACC at the time of diagnosis (85). Local invasion, which may be present in more than 20% of the patients at the time of diagnosis, commonly involves the kidneys and inferior vena cava (17,77). Additional metastatic disease may be found in the retroperitoneal lymph nodes, lungs, liver, or bone (87,88).

Laboratory Evaluation

Depending on the presentation, the laboratory investigation should aim at diagnosing the specific hormonal syndrome. Cushing syndrome should be diagnosed by baseline 24 hour urinary free cortisol (UFC) excretion, androgen-producing tumors by urinary 17-ketosteroids (17-KS), and feminizing tumors by measuring serum estradiol (E_2) or estrone (E_1). Cortisol- or androgen-producing tumors fail to suppress hormonal production on dexamethasone testing, but this is usually not necessary when baseline levels are consistently elevated in a patient with a large intra-abdominal tumor and an easily recognizable clinical syndrome. Often patients will present with precocious puberty that will be isosexual or heterosexual depending on the type of hormone produced and the sex of the patient. Tumors that produce mineralocorticoids are rare; suppressed plasma renin activity and high serum aldosterone concentrations, along with refractory hypokalemia, are diagnostic of these cancers. Hypokalemia and alkalosis also may be present in patients with severe Cushing syndrome independently of whether the tumor is a mixed glucocorticoid and mineralocortisoid hormone producer or an isolated glucocorticoid producer, because at high levels cortisol can occupy and stimulate the mineralocorticoid hormone receptor.

CT scan of the abdomen is the preferred imaging method to detect adrenocortical tumors. MRI and positron-emission tomographic (PET) scanning both have been used to detect the primary tumor or metastatic lesions.

Molecular Investigations Adenomas and carcinomas are mostly monoclonal lesions, and genetic changes at specific loci in the genome have been shown to be necessary for adrenal tumorigenesis (93,94). These include the genes coding for p53, KIP2/p57, insulin-like growth factor type II (IGF-2), angiotensin II, endothelin 1, diminuto/Dwarf-1, adrenomedullin, urotensin II, novH, and cAMP early repressor (95).

Comparative genomic hybridization (CGH) analysis has shown genetic aberrations in adrenocortical tumors (ACTs), with the most common being gains of chromosomes 4 and 5 and losses of chromosomes 11 and 17, whereas 9q34 amplification was seen in eight of nine tumors from Brazilian children (96,97).

Fluorescent in situ hybridization (FISH) investigation has shown frequent alterations and polyploidy in ACTs but also in benign adrenal tumors, particularly those associated with hyperaldosteronism (97–99).

Treatment

Surgery Although ACC is a rare tumor, it tends to be quite aggressive and carries a very poor prognosis, which appears to depend little on the initial presentation (70,85). In cases where adrenal cancer is expected, an open approach provides a better opportunity for margin-free resection and resection of isolated metastases and thus is the preferred surgical approach (76,85,100).

Chemotherapy Medical therapy of ACC consists mainly of o,p'-DDD (1,1-dichloro-diphenyl-dichloroethane, Mitotane), which has therapeutic effects in approximately 30% of patients (101). o,p'-DDD, appears to decrease hormone secretion in steroid-producing tumors; however, data to support that it significantly improves survival are lacking. Efforts to use other chemotherapeutic agents, either alone or in combination, generally have not been more effective than o,p'-DDD alone, although some recent studies have suggested that combination chemotherapy plus o,p'-DDD induced at least partial response in up to 50% of patients (102).

Therapy with o,p'-DDD may be initiated as an adjuvant to surgical treatment or for patients with inoperable cancer (85,91,103–105). o,p'-DDD is given at maximally tolerated oral doses (up 10 g/m^2/day). It ameliorates the endocrine syndrome in approximately two-thirds of the patients,

whereas tumor regression or arrest of growth has been observed in as many as one-third of patients. Although mean survival time does not appear to be altered, there are patients with unresectable carcinomas who achieved long-term survival on o,p'-DDD. The side effects include nausea, vomiting, diarrhea, skin reactions, and neurological manifestations, primarily lethargy, somnolence, dizziness, and muscle weakness. Other chemotherapeutic agents such as cisplatin, 5-fluorouracil, suramin, doxorubicin, and etoposide may be useful (76,85,106–110). Occasionally, for the correction of hypercortisolism, steroid synthesis inhibitors (e.g., aminoglutethimide, metyrapone, trilostane, and ketoconazole) or glucocorticoid antagonists (RU 486) are required (70,85). Patients taking o,p'-DDD may develop hypoaldosteronism or hypocortisolism, and thus fludrocortisone or hydrocortisone should be added as needed. Radiation therapy can be helpful for palliation of metastases.

Prognosis ACC tends to be quite aggressive and carries a very poor prognosis (mean survival of approximately 18 months), which appears to depend little on the initial presentation (70,85). However, children with ACC generally have a better prognosis than adult patients (83,85,86). Highly aggressive tumors can progress rapidly within a few months. With aggressive surgical therapy, the mean survival increases to 48 months, and survival as long as 10 years has been described for some patients receiving vigilant monitoring and aggressive surgery for local recurrences or distant metastases (100,103–105,109,111–114). Cures have been achieved for patients operated on at the early stages of adrenal cancer while the tumor was still encapsulated (70,83,85,86,109).

MULTIPLE ENDOCRINE NEOPLASIA TYPE 1

Pathophysiology and Presentation

Familial MEN-1 is an autosomal dominant disorder with variable penetrance characterized by tumors of the parathyroids, anterior pituitary, pancreas, and other locations of the gastrointestinal tract, and other tissues. The MEN-1 gene, menin, which is located on chromosome 11q13, was identified in 1997 (115). Individuals affected by MEN-1 inherit a menin inactivated allele (first hit); tumorigenesis in specific tissues follows inactivation of the remaining normal allele (second hit). MEN-1 is regarded as an endocrinopathy presenting in young adulthood (116). As with many hereditary tumors, MEN-1 typically presents earlier than sporadic tumors of the same tissue type. The age disparity at presentation is striking for MEN-1-related hyperparathyroidism (third versus sixth decade in sporadic cases) but less pronounced for gastrinoma and insulinoma (fourth versus fifth decade in each) (117). By contrast, there has been no apparent age difference for the onset of MEN-1-associated and sporadic prolactinoma (fourth decade) (118–120). The age of clinical onset of treatable MEN-1-related tumors is an important factor in formulating biochemical and DNA screening recommendations.

Hyperparathyroidism is usually the earliest and most common endocrine manifestation of MEN-1, with hypercalcemia being an almost universal finding at the time of MEN-1 diagnosis (119,121,122). Clinically evident hyperparathyroidism in MEN-1 has been reported at ages 5 and 7 years (123) and several times at age 8 years (119,124). However, no morbidity has been reported from early hyperparathyroidism in MEN-1. MEN-1-associated prolactinomas have been reported previously in children aged 10–13 years (125–127). Growth hormone (GH)–producing adenomas in MEN-1 have been described in early adolescence (127), whereas a somatomammotroph adenoma was reported recently in a 5-year-old boy (128). Gastrinoma, the other defining feature of MEN-1 (123,124,126), has not been seen earlier than age 12. MEN-1-related insulinoma has been described as early as age 6 (129).

Laboratory Evaluation

Patients with known MEN-1 should be screened annually, starting in childhood (after the age of 5 years), for the main manifestations of the disorder. Careful monitoring of the growth rate and annual screening of plasma ionized calcium and serum intact parathyroid hormone (i-PTH) in children of families with MEN-1, who are known mutation carriers is recommended. If the growth rate is increased as in acromegaly, or decreased as in prolactinomas, Cushing disease, or Cushing syndrome, appropriate tests are ordered. The latter tumors can also be associated with an increase in weight gain. Routine screening for pituitary tumors in the absence of symptoms is not necessary until late childhood or early adolescence (ages 10–15 years) because they occur only rarely before these ages. Similarly, fasting gastrin, C-peptide, and plasma insulin determinations and serial prolactin measurements (obtained every 20 minutes for 1 hour through an indwelling catheter that has been inserted an hour before the sampling to avoid stress-related, falsely elevated levels) and pituitary or abdominal imaging are not necessary until adolescence. Although such biochemical testing may be done annually thereafter, imaging may be done only as needed and when the presence of a tumor is suggested by clinical symptoms or laboratory testing; clinical symptoms such as hypoglycemia, delayed puberty, irregular menses, gynecomastia, galactorrhea, weight gain, moon facies, hirsutism, abnormal visual fields, decrease in school performance, suggest a pituitary tumor and should be followed by an MRI of the pituitary with gadolinium. Depending on the size of the pituitary tumor, symptoms of secondary adrenal insufficiency may also be present. If hypoglycemia or peptic ulcer disease are the presenting symptoms, abdominal imaging is necessary to screen for insulinoma and gastrinoma, respectively; however insulinomas and gastrinomas are extraordinarily rare in children with MEN-1. In young adults with MEN-1, in addition to the annual biochemical testing prescribed earlier, annual imaging of the abdomen (and the pancreas in particular) may be obtained; pituitary imaging may be obtained in the absence of symptoms or suggestive biochemical testing no more frequently than every 5 years to avoid false-positive studies and unnecessary follow-up testing.

Molecular Genetics and Recommendations for Screening
Identification of the MEN-1 gene was first achieved by positional cloning (115), and mutation testing is now available at several centers (116,117). The main candidates for MEN-1 mutational analysis include the index cases with MEN-1, their unaffected relatives, and some cases with features atypical for MEN-1. There have been more than 150 mutations in menin; they are spread almost equally along the length of the gene without any apparent genotype–phenotype correlation (115–117,128). Some mutations occur more frequently than others, but there are no obvious "hot spots" in the nine coding exons of the gene. The mutations that are more frequent involve exons 83, 84, 209–211, and 514–516, which contain unstable DNA sequences (e.g., dinucleotide repeats or poly(C) tracts). A small number of MEN-1 kindreds do not have mutations in the MEN-1 gene, but since there is no obvious genetic heterogeneity in the syndrome, it is likely that mutations in these families and sporadic cases are in the noncoding regions of the gene (130). The recent recognition of significant morbidity from MEN-1 at young ages (128), the need for carrier testing in large families with known mutations, and advances in molecular testing will probably lead to more frequent genetic testing in the future.

Treatment
The treatment of tumors associated with MEN-1 in children is mainly surgical, with the exception of prolactinomas and the medical management of Zollinger–Ellison syndrome (ZES). Gigantism may be treated by somatostatin analogues and dopamine agonists (128), as in adult patients with similar tumors, but the primary approach would be by transsphenoidal surgery (TSS). Orally administered dopamine agonists are the main treatment for prolactinomas, and only occasionally may a macroprolactinoma that is not responsive to medical treatment and causes symptoms or continues to grow need to be excised by TSS.

Medical gastrectomy by omeprazole or ranitidine and other proton-pump inhibitors or H_2-blockers, respectively, is all that is required for the treatment of hypergastrinemia. Surgery should be avoided as the primary treatment of ZES.

Hyperparathyroidism is treated surgically if a serum calcium level consistently above 12 mg/dL or when nephrolithiasis or bone loss is evident. Since hyperparathyroidism is the most common and earlier-appearing manifestation of MEN-1, near-total parathyroidectomy is not unusual in late adolescence in menin mutation carriers with severe hyperparathyroidism. The alternative surgical method of total parathyroidectomy and reimplantation of parathyroid tissue in the nondominant forearm does not offer significant advantages: The rate of recurrent hypercalcemia after both procedures approaches 50% in MEN-1 patients in cohorts with long follow-up.

Other tumors associated with MEN-1 that are symptomatic or have the potential of being malignant, such as insulinoma or the rare case of a malignant gastrinoma, are also approached surgically.

MULTIPLE ENDOCRINE NEOPLASIA TYPE 2

Pathophysiology and Presentation

The three MEN-2 syndromes are the phenotypic expressions of variants of activating mutations in the RET proto-oncogene, a tyrosine kinase receptor (131). Thus all clinical manifestations of the MEN-2 syndromes reflect the inappropriate transduction of this growth- and survival-promoting signal in the neural crest–derived tissues that naturally express RET (132). The primary and most common lesion of the MEN-2 syndromes is medullary thyroid cancer (MTC); it is present in up to 95% of patients with MEN-2 and is preceded by hyperplasia of the calcitonin-secreting thyroid parafollicular C cells (132,133). Histological evidence of MTC in more than 95% of obligate gene carriers is present by age 35 years. Calcitonin provocative testing is not as specific for MTC as was believed initially because a small fraction of persons with normal calcitonin provocative testing were shown to be obligate noncarriers of their kindred's characteristic RET mutation. Conversely, those classified as being affected on the basis of C cell hyperplasia alone should be reevaluated with *RET* testing to allow accurate counseling about their children's risk for MEN-2 (132,133).

Pheochromocytoma typically affects 50% to 60% of MEN-2A kindreds with a high rate of bilaterality but a low rate of extra-adrenal sites or malignancy. The tumor is commonly present in MEN-2B and absent by definition in familial medullary thyroid cancer (FMTC). A yearly program for pheochromocytoma that uses urinary catecholamines and metabolites to screen can effectively identify tumors at an early stage (<2 cm), before the development of hypertension or other adverse sequelae. Laparoscopic adrenalectomy is now the method of choice for the surgical removal of a pheochromocytoma.

Parathyroid disease is detected clinically in 10% to 15% of patients with MEN-2A. Recently, two variants of MEN-2A with distinctive nonendocrine manifestations have been recognized. MEN-2A with cutaneous lichen amyloidosis, which is characterized by pruritic lesions composed of subepidermal keratin deposits over the scapular region (134), and MEN-2A with partial or extensive Hirschsprung syndrome, which represents another distinct clinical syndrome (135). Patients with this disease exhibit evidence of both *RET* hyperfunction and hypofunction in a tissue-specific fashion (136). Expanding the clinical spectrum of the MEN-2 syndromes are the distinctive skeletal findings found in virtually all MEN-2B patients: elongated facies with a long, relatively thin nose, proliferation of corneal nerves, mucosal neuromas of the lips and tongue, and gastrointestinal ganglioneuromas (136) see Figure 46-1 A to E. In addition, these patients frequently have aggressive tumors, both MTC and pheochromocytoma. These manifestations all appear to stem from abnormal proliferation of neural crest elements during fetal and postnatal life and may be orchestrated by a hyperfunctioning *RET* tyrosine kinase receptor (137).

Laboratory Evaluation

In known carriers of a *RET* mutation, other than prophylactic thyroidectomy (see below), annual screening for pheochromocytoma should be performed after age 5, along with a serum ionized calcium measurement; usually hyperparathyroidism in these patients does not develop until later childhood or adolescence, so, if necessary, one can limit the screening to that for pheochromocytoma *only* between the ages 5 and 10 years. Plasma catecholamines are the best screening test for pheochromocytoma (see below). An ionized calcium level that is elevated should be followed by measurements of parathyroid hormone.

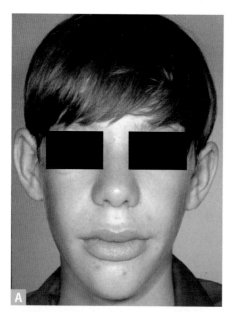
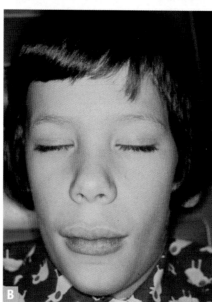
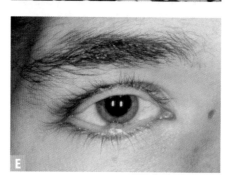
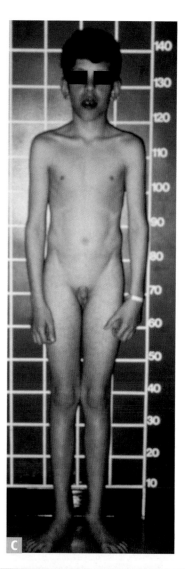
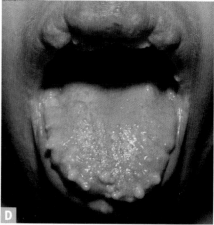

FIGURE 46-1 **A** to **E.** Spectrum of phenotypic features in patients with MEN-2B (thickened lips and eyelids; eversion of upper eyelids; palpebral conjuctiva neuroma; ganglioneuromas of the tongue; marfanoid habitus)

Molecular Genetics and Recommendations for Screening Analyzing the *RET* gene in the MEN-2A and FMTC syndromes revealed that most of the patients had mutated one of five cysteine codons in exons 10 and 11; however, isolated FMTC also was caused by mutations in the first tyrosine kinase domain of the receptor (137). The cysteine-to-arginine change in codon 634 of the *RET* protein appears to be the most common mutation in the MEN-2 syndromes and is also found in the few kindreds with MEN-2A that have pheochromocytoma and hyperparathyroidism but no other clinical manifestations. In MEN-2A/Hirschsprung disease, most kindreds have mutations in codons 609, 618, and 620. In MEN-2B, the mutations are in the tyrosine kinase domain.

Over the past 35 years, there has been a substantial improvement in survival in MEN-2 families, an improvement largely attributable to the success of family screening programs, first provocative biochemical tests, and more recently, detection of *RET* gene mutations (131–133). *RET* gene analysis has superseded older methods because of its high sensitivity and specificity, utility in younger children, and much higher degree of patient acceptance (137). A typical screening program for known MEN-2A and FMTC kindreds is to initiate testing for *RET* mutations at 2 years of age. In the case of MEN-2B, it is generally possible to recognize the characteristic mucosal neuroma phenotype within the first 2 years of life. Prophylactic thyroidectomy is now recommended for all patients who test positive for most disease-causing mutations of the *RET* gene. In addition to established MEN-2 kindreds, 6% to 8% of MTC patients with no apparent family history of the disorder harbor germline *RET* mutations and thus may have offspring at risk. On the basis of this figure, it appears prudent to offer germline *RET* analysis to everyone with apparent sporadic MTC.

Finally, mutations of *RET* and some of its ligands, including glial-derived nerve growth factor (GDNF), have been found in approximately half the 10% of familial cases of Hirschsprung disease and its variants (138,139). However, screening for *RET* gene mutations (and mutations of its ligands) for familial Hirschsprung disease does not seem to affect clinical care for this disease, which usually presents in infancy or early childhood.

Treatment Other than prophylactic thyroidectomy, most other tumors associated with MEN-2 are also treated surgically. As in MEN-1, hyperparathyroidism is treated surgically when necessary (see above) by near-total parathyroidectomy (or by total parathyroidectomy and reimplantation of parathyroid tissue in the nondominant forearm). The rate of recurrent hypercalcemia is less in MEN-2 that in MEN-1 after these procedures but does not differ substantially between them. Pheochromocytomas are removed preferably laparoscopically today; more on the treatment of pheochromocytomas is provided later in this chapter.

CARNEY COMPLEX

Pathophysiology and Presentation

Carney complex (CNC) was first reported in 1985; the syndrome described the association of heart myxomas and lentigines with pituitary-independent Cushing syndrome caused by an unusual adrenal pathology (140–146). The latter was characterized by multiple, small, pigmented, adrenocortical nodules and internodular cortical atrophy; the disease was shown to be primary and bilateral and is now commonly referred to as *primary pigmented nodular adrenocortical disease* (PPNAD). In the late 1980's, several patients were described with PPNAD and various combinations of myxomas affecting multiple organs (e.g., heart, skin, and breast), spotty skin pigmentation (e.g., lentigines and blue nevi), and tumors of three endocrine organs (i.e., adrenal, pituitary, and testis) (142–144). Subsequently, the syndrome was shown to be transmitted in a manner consistent with dominant inheritance (145,146).

Cushing syndrome in CNC is the most common endocrine manifestation and is always caused by PPNAD. Patients with CNC often present with a variant Cushing syndrome called *atypical* (ACS) (147) that is characterized by an asthenic rather than obese body habitus caused by severe osteoporosis, short stature, and muscle and skin wasting. ACS was recognized as early as 1956 and since has been described in several patients with Cushing syndrome (148–150). Patients with ACS tend to have normal or near-normal 24-hour free cortisol production (UFC), but this is characterized by the absence of the normal circadian rhythmicity of this hormone (147–153). Occasionally, patients present with *periodic Cushing syndrome* (PCS), a variant of Cushing syndrome that is found frequently in children with CNC (151,153). All patients with PPNAD and classical Cushing syndrome and most patients with ACS or PCS respond to dexamethasone with a paradoxical rise of cortisol production (151,153). In a recent study of the largest series reported to date (153), all patients with PPNAD responded to the graded administration of dexamethasone during the classical Liddle's test with a rise in both urinary free cortisol and 17-hydroxycorticosteroid (17-OHCS) production. The test may be used diagnostically for the identification of PPNAD, even in patients who have normal baseline cortisol levels and do not have clinical stigmata of Cushing syndrome.

About 10% of patients with CNC have a GH-secreting pituitary adenoma that results in acromegaly. Although most of the known patients with this condition had macroadenomas, a number of recently investigated cases show that abnormal 24-hour GH and prolactin secretion can precede the development of a pituitary tumor in CNC (154,155). The disorder, therefore, provides the unusual opportunity for prospective screening of affected patients without clinical acromegaly.

Hyperplasia appears to be present in the pituitary gland of all patients with CNC, acromegaly, and a GH-producing microadenoma operated on to date (156).

Endocrine involvement in CNC also includes three types of testicular tumors: large cell, calcifying Sertoli cell tumor (LCCSCT), adrenocortical rests, and Leydig cell tumor (157). More than three-quarters of affected male patients have one or more of these masses. LCCSCT may secrete estrogens and cause precocious puberty, gynecomastia, or both (157). Since 1985, three new components of the syndrome have been identified: psammomatous melanotic schwannoma, epithelioid blue nevus, and ductal adenoma of the breast (158–160). Thyroid follicular neoplasms, both benign and malignant, also have been found in a number of patients (161).

Laboratory Evaluation

The recommended clinical surveillance of patients with CNC differs based on age group. For postpubertal pediatric and adult patients, we recommend annual echocardiogram (this study may be needed biannually for adolescent patients with a history of excised myxoma), testicular and thyroid ultrasound, and UFC and serum IGF-1 levels. For prepubertal pediatric patients, we recommend annual echocardiogram (biannually for patients with a history of excised myxoma) and testicular ultrasound for boys. If close monitoring of growth rate and pubertal staging indicates other abnormalities, such as possible Cushing syndrome, appropriate testing should be done as needed. For PPNAD leading to Cushing syndrome, in addition to UFC, we recommend diurnal cortisol determinations (11:30 p.m., 12:00 midnight, and 7:30 and 8:00 a.m. sampling) and/or a dexamethasone stimulation test (modified Liddle's test, as per Stratakis et al. [10]), and an adrenal CT scan. For gigantism/acromegaly, in addition to serum IGF-1 determinations, pituitary MRI and a 3-hour oral glucose tolerance test (oGTT) may be obtained. For psammomatous melanotic schwannoma, MRI of the brain, spine, chest, abdomen, retroperitoneum, and/or pelvis may be necessary.

Molecular Genetics and Recommendations for Screening Genetic heterogeneity has been confirmed in this syndrome with at least two loci. The locus on 17q22-24 harbors the *PRKARIA* gene coding for the type IA regulatory subunit (RIα) of protein kinase A (PKA) as the gene responsible for CNC in most families that mapped to chromosome 17 and some sporadic cases of the disease (162–164). Almost all CNC-responsible mutations lead to truncation of the protein. A defective cyclic nucleotide–dependent pathway had long been considered a candidate mechanism for the various manifestations of CNC (141,165), including tumors similar to those of McCune–Albright syndrome (155,157) and paradoxical responses to hormonal stimuli (153). An overresponsive PKA enzyme is now considered the most likely mechanism underlying tumorigenesis in CNC.

Identification of the gene causing CNC on chromosome 17 left a group of families that appear to map collectively to chromosome 2 (although none of them with a LOD score over 3) for which the syndrome has not been elucidated molecularly (166,167). There are also families that seem to map neither to chromosome 2 nor to chromosome 17, allowing for a third possible locus harboring gene(s) responsible for the complex. In tumors from patients with CNC, genetic changes of the chromosome 2p16 locus, including both copy-number gain and loss, have been identified (168). Interestingly, these changes are shared by both chromosome 2– and chromosome 17–mapping families, indicating, perhaps, a common molecular mechanism (168).

Clinical and biochemical screening for CNC remains the "gold standard" for the diagnosis of CNC. Molecular testing for *PRKAR1A* mutations is not recommended at present for all patients with CNC but may be advised for detection of affected patients in families with known mutations of that gene to avoid unnecessary medical surveillance of noncarriers.

PEUTZ-JEGHERS SYNDROME (PJS)

Pathophysiology and Presentation

The hallmark of this syndrome is the presence of pigmented spots on the lips, which are first present in early childhood (169,170). These lesions are associated with gastrointestinal hamartomatous polyps (171). Gastrointestinal cancers are frequent in PJS; they may arise from genetic changes known to occur in colorectal carcinoma and other tumors because the PJS-responsible gene(s) function as tumor suppressor(s) (171,172). PJS patients are also at an increased risk for breast, ovarian, testicular, uterine, and cervical cancers, as well as nonmalignant lesions in these tissues (171–176). A 49-year follow-up of the Harrisburg family, the kindred originally described by Jeghers et al., revealed that PJS is a premalignant condition associated with significant morbidity and increased mortality (177). Among the 12 affected family members, 10 underwent 75 polypectomies, and 2 developed gastric cancer and duodenal carcinoma, respectively. Other investigators found that cancer developed in 15 of 31 patients from 13 unrelated families; the overall incidence of carcinoma in patients with PJS

varies from 20% to 50%, and it appears at a relatively early age (173–179).

Among the nongastrointestinal neoplasms associated with PJS, endocrine tumors are the most frequent (173–182). These include thyroid nodules and cancer (180) and genital tract neoplasms (181,182). The latter include, in female patients with PJS, ovarian neoplasms from both the epithelium and stromal cells and adenoma malignum of the cervix and adenocarcinoma of the endometrium. Male patients with PJS often have Leydig cell tumors or a Sertoli cell tumor that is uniquely found in PJS and CNC (157): large cell calcifying Sertoli cell tumor (LCCSCT) (183). LCCSCT in PJS, as in CNC, may be associated with increased aromatization of adrenal or testicular androgens, which produces estradiol and other estrogens (estrone, in particular) that may lead to precocious puberty and prepubertal or peripubertal gynecomastia (183).

Molecular Genetics Most PJS families have been linked to 19p13.3; the PJS gene at 19p13.3 is *STK11* (for serine threonine kinase 11) also known as *LKB1* (184,185). More than half the families with PJS have mutations in this gene, although the percentage varies greatly from one study to the next (186–191). *STK11/LKB1* is a novel serine–threonine kinase containing nine exons; The kinase domain of the *STK11/LKB1* gene is highly conserved between mouse and human (192,193). Although it has been suggested that mouse Lkb1 is a nuclear protein, wild-type *STK11/LKB1* shows both nuclear and cytoplasmic localization. A number of recent studies have elucidated the effects of inherited *STK11/LKB1* mutations in PJS kindreds based on the functional domains of the protein; in most cases, elimination of the kinase activity underlies the molecular cause of the phenotype (194). Genetic heterogeneity in PJS appears not to be accompanied by clinical heterogeneity because there are no known differences between the families that map to 19p13.3 and have *STK11/LKB1* mutations and those that map elsewhere or do not have mutations in that gene (194,195).

COWDEN DISEASE (CD)

CD is associated with hamartomas and tumors of ecto-, meso- and endodermal origin affecting multiple organs (196–198). Thyroid and breast masses, hamartomatous polyps, and mucocutaneous lesions (e.g., oral papillomatosis, acral keratosis, and multiple fibromas) occur consistently in this syndrome, which is also associated with anomalies of the skeletal and nervous systems (198). CD was first mapped to chromosome 10 (197); mutations in the tumor-suppressor gene *PTEN* on

10q were found shortly after that (199–201). CD is allelic to Ruvalcaba–Myhre–Smith, Bannayan–Zonana, or Bannayan–Riley–Ruvalcaba syndrome, which is also associated with hamartomatous intestinal polyposis, lentiginosis of the genitalia and developmental defects (e.g., macrocephaly and eye and skeletal anomalies), and myopathy (200,201). Both syndromes are due to mutations of the *PTEN* gene on chromosome 10 (199–201), although genetic heterogeneity may exist.

VON HIPPEL–LINDAU DISEASE (VHLD)

VHLD is a multiple-tumor syndrome that affects the pancreas (pancreatic cysts) and the adrenal medulla (pheochromocytoma) (202). However, the main components of the syndrome are nonendocrine and include renal carcinoma and cysts and tumors of the cerebellum, spinal cord, eyes, and epididymis (202). The *VHL* gene has tumor-suppressor functions and is located on chromosome 3p (202–204). Sporadic pheochromocytomas may harbor *VHL* mutations (205).

PHEOCHROMOCYTOMA

Pathophysiology and Presentation

Pheochromocytomas are chromaffin cell tumors that produce, store, metabolize, and secrete catecholamines. The metabolism of catecholamines is a more consistent process than that of catecholamine secretion (206,207). Nearly 80% to 85% of pheochromocytomas arise from the adrenal medulla, whereas about 15% to 20% arise from extra-adrenal chromaffin tissue called *paragangliomas*. Paragangliomas are divided into two groups: those that arise from parasympathetic-associated tissues, most commonly along cranical and vagus nerves (e.g., glomus tumors, chemodectomas, and carotid body tumors), and those that arise from sympathetic-associated chromaffin tissue (often designated *extra-adrenal pheochromocytomas*) (208).

Pheochromocytoma has been labeled the "great mimic" because there are numerous reports in the literature of unusual presentations of benign or metastatic pheochromocytomas that require emergency intervention. Emergency situations are either the result of organ-specific actions of catecholamines produced in high quantity by the tumor or the consequence of complications related to tumor localization (209).

Paroxysmal hypertension represents a frequent clinical dilemma, particularly when these bouts are of abrupt onset and severe (blood pressure >200/110 mm Hg). Although severe paroxysmal hypertension always should raise suspicions of pheochromocytoma (especially when other symptoms such as palpitations, sweating, and pallor are present), it also can reflect a clinical entity called *pseudopheochromocytoma*.

Pseudopheochromocytoma refers to the large majority of individuals (most often women) with severe paroxysmal hypertension, whether normotensive or hypertensive between episodes, in whom pheochromocytoma has been ruled out (208–211). Pseudopheochromocytoma is a heterogeneous clinical condition subdivided into primary and secondary forms. In contrast to the primary form, the secondary form is associated with various pathologies (e.g., hypoglycemia, epilepsy, and baroreceptor failure), medications, and drug abuse. The most common clinical characteristics of this syndrome in many cases might be attributable to a short-term activation of the sympathetic nervous system. In contrast to pheochromocytoma, patients with pseudopheochromocytoma more often present with panic attacks or anxiety, flushing, nausea, and polyuria. Another important feature distinctive from pheochromocytoma are the circumstances under which episodes occur. In pheochromocytoma, symptoms usually are unprovoked, whereas in pseudopheochromocytoma, they usually follow some identifiable events. It is important, therefore, in questioning these patients, to search for specific provocative factors that may have precipitated these episodes. Similar to pheochromocytoma, episodes may last from a few minutes to several hours and may occur daily or once every few months. Between episodes, blood pressure is normal or may be mildly elevated. Pseudopheochromocytoma is sometimes successfully treatable by antihypertensive drugs, antidepressants, or antianxiety drugs or psychotherapy.

Incidence of Familial Pheochromocytoma
Pheochromocytomas may occur sporadically or as part of hereditary syndrome. According to the latest studies, among patients with apparently sporadic pheochromocytoma, up to 24% of tumors may be inherited (212–214). Hereditary syndromic pheochromocytoma is associated with MEN-2A or MEN-2B, neurofibromatosis type 1 (NF-1), and VHL syndrome. Familial nonsyndromic pheochromocytoma and paraganglioma (derived from both sympathetic and parasympathetic tissue) is associated with germline mutations of genes encoding succinate dehydrogenase subunits B, C, and D. In general, the traits are inherited in an autosomal dominant pattern (212).

Genetics of Pheochromocytoma
Patients with MEN-2-related pheochromocytoma often lack hypertension or symptoms (occurs only in about 50%) (215). MEN-2-related pheochromocytomas are characterized by production of epinephrine only or epinephrines together with norepinephrine and therefore are best detected by elevations of plasma or urinary metanephrine, usually but not always in association with elevations of normetanephrine and parent catecholamines. MEN-2-related pheochromocytomas almost always are intra-adrenal, often bilateral, and they are rarely malignant (<5%) (216,217). In addition, as with most epinephrine-secreting pheochromocytomas, hypertension, when present, is more likely to be paroxysmal than sustained. For these reasons, the diagnosis is easy to miss.

Overall, fewer than 30% of patients with VHL germline mutation develop a pheochromocytoma (218,219). Pheochromocytomas as part of the VHL syndrome have an exclusively noradrenergic phenotype, reflecting lack of production of epinephrine. Biochemical diagnosis therefore is best achieved from elevations of plasma or urinary normetanephrine. These tumors are mainly located intra-adrenally and are in about 50% of patients bilateral with a less than 5% incidence of metastasis.

Since pheochromocytomas in VHL patients do not express glucagon receptors, the glucagon test is not useful for diagnosis. These tumors are found commonly based on periodic annual screening or during searches for other tumors that are part of this syndrome. Therefore, when detected, these tumors are commonly small and often fail to be detected by nuclear imaging methods. Furthermore, about 80% of pheochromocytomas found in VHL patients during screening are asymptomatic and not associated with hypertension.

Recently, pheochromocytoma susceptibility has been associated with germline mutations of the succinate dehydrogenase gene family (SDH) (213,214,220). The SDH genes (SDHA, SDHB, SDHC, and SDHD) encode the four subunits of complex II of the mitochondrial electron transport chain (221,222). Most pheochromocytomas, usually in extra-adrenal location, are associated with mutations of SDHD and SDHB genes. Nonfunctional paragangliomas that do not produce, metabolize, or secrete catecholamines and that appear to arise from parasympathetic tissue also may occur secondary to mutations of SDHB, SDHD, or rarely of SDHC genes. Mutations of the SDHA gene do not appear to cause pheochromocytomas or paragangliomas. In recent studies, it has been found that about 4% to 12% of apparently sporadic pheochromocytomas and in up to 50% of familial pheochromocytomas have either SDHD or SDHB mutation (223). Currently, there is a strong association of SDHD and SDHB mutations with the presence of extra-adrenal multifocal pheochromocytoma (212,224,225).

Recently, it has been suggested that all patients younger than 50 years of age with either solitary extra-adrenal or multifocal pheochromocytoma (not found initially in the adrenal gland) should undergo genetic testing to search for mutations of SDH genes (212,213). It also has been suggested that these patients have periodic follow-up including yearly measurement of plasma or urinary metanephrines (212). In addition to the hereditary paraganglioma syndromes, paragangliomas can be associated with gastrointestinal stromal tumors or sarcomas in the context of Carney Triad and the newly described Carney–Stratakis syndrome.

Metastatic Pheochromocytoma The incidence reported for malignant pheochromocytoma ranges depending on the genetic background and tumor localization from 3% to 36% of pheochromocytoma patients (226–230). Patients with SDHB mutations have a particularly high incidence of metastatic pheochromocytoma. Malignant disease has an overall 5-year survival rate of 50% (226,227). Patients with malignant pheochromocytoma, particularly those with metastases occurring secondary to extra-adrenal pheochromocytoma, may present with more dopamine-producing tumors than patients with intra-adrenal pheochromocytoma (231). In some of these patients, specific imaging studies (e.g., 6-[^{18}F]fluorodopamine PET scanning or [$^{123/131}$I]metaiodobenzylguanidine) are negative, but [^{18}F]fluorodeoxyglucose PET scanning can be important.

Biochemical Diagnosis of Pheochromocytoma The diagnosis of a pheochromocytoma depends on biochemical evidence of excessive catecholamine (i.e., norepinephrine and epinephrine) production by the tumor. Such evidence is best obtained during initial testing by measurements of urinary fractionated metanephrines or plasma free metanephrines (207,228). Plasma free metanephrines have a higher specificity but the same sensitivity compared to urinary fractionated metanephrines and may offer the preferred test, but this also depends on the proficiency of the testing laboratory in providing accurate results, free of analytical interference; high sensitivity indicates a low rate of false-negative results and high specificity indicates a low rate of false-positive results. Since missing the diagnosis of pheochromocytoma (due to low diagnostic sensitivity e.g., if catecholamines are measured) can have catastrophic consequences, we recommend measurements of plasma free metanephrines as the initial biochemical test to confirm or rule out pheochromocytoma, with measurements of urinary fractionated metanephrines providing the next test. Measurements of

TABLE 46-1   Drugs That May Cause False-Positive Elevations of Plasma and Urinary Catecholamines or Metanephrines

	Catecholamines		Metanephrines	
	NE	E	NMN	MN
Tricyclic antidepressants				
Amitriptyline (Elavil), imipramine (Topfranil), nortriptyline (Aventyl)	+++	−	+++	−
α-Blockers (nonselective)				
Phenoxybenzamine (Dibenzyline)	+++	−	+++	−
α-Blockers (α₁-selective)				
Doxazosin (Cardura), terazosin (Hytrin), prazosin (Minipress)	+	−	−	−
β-Blockers				
Atenolol (Tenormin), metoprolol (Lopressor), propranolol (Inderal), labetolol (Normadyne)*	+	+	+	+
Calcium channel antagonists				
Nifedipine (Procardia), amlodipine (Norvasc), diltiazem (Cardizem), verapamil (Calan)	+	+	−	−
Vasodilators				
Hydralazine (Apresoline), isosorbide (Isordil, Dilatrate), minoxidil (Loniten)	+	−	Unknown	
Monoamine oxidase inhibitors				
Phenelzine (Nardil), tranylcypromine (Parnate), selegiline (Eldepryl)	−	−	+++	+++
Sympathomimetics				
Ephedrine, pseudoephedrine (Sudafed), amphetamines, albuterol (Proventil)	++	++	++	++
Stimulants				
Caffeine (coffee,* tea), nicotine (tobacco), theophylline	++	++	Unknown	
Miscellaneous				
Levodopa, carbidopa (Sinemet)*	++	−	Unknown	
Cocaine	++	++	Unknown	

NE = norepinephrine; E = epinephrine; NMN = normetanephrine; MN = metanephrine; +++ = substantial increase; ++ = moderate increase; + = mild increase if any; − = little or no increase.

*A drug that also can cause direct analytical interference with some methods.

plasma free metanephrines also can help to predict tumor size and location (229). This additional information may be useful for guiding diagnostic decision making before and after tumor-localization procedures.

The conditions under which blood or urine samples are collected can be crucial to the reliability and interpretation of test results. Blood for measurement of plasma free metanephrines or catecholamines should be collected with patients supine for at least 15–20 minutes before sampling. To avoid any stress associated with the needle stick, samples ideally should be collected through a previously inserted intravenous line. Patients should have refrained from nicotine and alcohol use for at least 12 hours, and to minimize analytical interference, they should have fasted overnight before blood sampling. This is not required when the mass-spectrometry method is used. Depending on the laboratory method used for measurement of plasma free metanephrines, patients may have to avoid acetaminophen for at least 5 days before sampling. Tricyclic antidepressants and phenoxybenzamine increase plasma and urinary norepinephrine and normetanephrine and represent the most common causes of medication-associated false-positive results in patients tested for pheochromocytoma (Table 46-1).

In patients with renal failure, pheochromocytoma can be excluded reliably based on normal values for plasma free metanephrines; this is in contrast to conjugated metanephrines, which are cleared by the kidneys and show large increases associated with renal failure (230).

Although measurements of plasma free normetanephrine and metanephrine provide a sensitive test for the diagnosis of pheochromocytoma, these measurements may fail to detect tumors that produce predominantly dopamine (patients with these tumors usually do not present with any cardiovascular symptoms that are normally seen in tumors secreting epinephrine or norepinephrine) (231). Measurement of plasma free methoxytyramine (metabolite of dopamine) or dopamine can be used to detect these rare tumors, which usually are found extra-adrenally; in contrast, measurement of urinary dopamine is much less reliable due to derivation of the urinary amine mainly from circulating dihydroxyphenylalanine, not dopamine (231).

Imaging of Pheochromocytoma The imaging test of choice is the CT scan, which usually localizes about 95% of all pheochromocytomas. MRI is also a very reliable imaging method, identifying over 95% of pheochromocytomas, and it is sometimes preferred for the localization of extra-adrenal pheochromocytomas, especially those in unusual locations. MRI also should be the initial imaging method of choice in children, pregnant women, patients with a documented allergy to contrast dye, and in patients in whom no additional radiation exposure is desired (232).

There is some debate about whether functional imaging should be used as a 2nd step after CT scan or MRI to confirm that the tumor is indeed a pheochromocytoma. Several important considerations affect the choice of additional functional imaging studies. First, although this tumor is localized most often in the adrenal gland, the adrenal gland is also the site of many benign adrenal tumors (adenomas); in the general population, between 5% and 10% may be expected to have such masses. Second, about 50% of adrenal pheochromocytomas produce near exclusively norepinephrine, this representing the same pattern as in extra-adrenal pheochromocytomas. Thus, whereas production of epinephrine (best detected by an increases in metanephrine) indicates an adrenal location, exclusive production of norepinephrine (best indicated by increases in normetanephrine with normal metanephrine) may reflect either an adrenal or extra-adrenal location. Third, about 10% of patients have metastatic pheochromocytoma at initial diagnosis; those with primary tumors larger than 5 cm are at particular risk. Fourth, in patients with previous surgeries (especially in the abdomen), the presence of postoperative tissue changes (e.g., tissue fibrosis and adhesions) and surgical clips often precludes correct localization of recurrent or metastatic pheochromocytomas using CT scan or MRI. Fifth, about 20% to 30% of pheochromocytomas are familial, and these tumors often are multiple. Based on the preceding, we advise additional use of functional imaging studies for localization of most cases of biochemically proven pheochromocytoma. Exceptions may include small (<5 cm) adrenal masses associated with elevations of plasma or urine metanephrine (practically all epinephrine-producing pheochromocytomas are found in the adrenal gland or are recurrences of previously resected adrenal tumors).

Currently, metaiodobenzylguanidine scintigraphy (MIBG scan) is used to locate and confirm pheochromocytoma and rule out metastatic disease. The specificity of MIBG is about 95% to 100%, but this technique offers suboptimal sensitivity (78% to 83%) with the ^{131}I-labeled agent. ^{123}I-MIBG scintigraphy provides superior image quality and seems to be especially useful for detecting recurrent or metastatic pheochromocytoma (208).

Other imaging modalities that can be used to locate pheochromocytoma include a new method, PET scanning using 6-[^{18}F]fluorodopamine or 6-[^{18}F]fluorodopa,

that has been introduced recently (233). This method offers an excellent visualization of primary and metastatic pheochromocytoma, and 6-[^{18}F]fluorodopamine PET scanning was found to be superior to [^{123}I]-MIBG and Octreoscan, especially for localization of metastatic lesions or tumors that are very difficult to localize (e.g., previous surgical procedure) (234). In patients with rapidly progressing metastatic pheochromocytoma, MIBG and 6-[^{18}F]fluorodopamine functional imaging studies sometimes can be be negative, and in these situations, [^{18}F]fluorodeoxyglucose or Octreoscan may be useful. Otherwise, these two methods should not be used for initial functional imaging.

Management

Laparoscopic surgery is now the technique of first choice for resection of adrenal and extra-adrenal pheochromocytomas. Observational studies have shown clearly that the laparoscopic procedure decreases postoperative morbidity, hospital stay, and expense compared with the conventional transabdominal technique for tumor removal. Due to the high incidence of bilateral adrenal disease in hereditary pheochromocytoma, partial adrenalectomies are advocated in these patients, thereby avoiding the morbidity associated with medical adrenal replacement.

Preparation of the patient for surgery requires adequate preoperative medical treatment to minimize operative and postoperative complications. Exposure to high levels of circulating catecholamines during surgery may cause hypertensive crises and arrhythmias, which can occur even when patients are normotensive and asymptomatic preoperatively. All patients with pheochromocytoma therefore should receive appropriate preoperative medical management to block the effects of released catecholamines.

Phenoxybenzamine (Dibenzyline), an α-adrenoceptor blocker, is used most commonly for preoperative control of blood pressure. The drug is administered orally at a dose of 10–20 mg twice daily for 10–14 days before surgery (higher doses may be necessary to control symptoms of catecholamine overproduction). At some centers, a supplemental dose (0.5–1.0 mg/kg) is administered at midnight before surgery, in which case appropriate safeguards are required to avoid orthostatic hypotension. Intravenous fluids usually are administered to adequately replaced blood volume. Alternatives to phenoxybenzamine for preoperative blockade of catecholamine-induced vasoconstriction include calcium channel blockers and selective α_1-adrenoceptor blocking agents, such as terazosin (Hytrin) and doxazosin (Cardura).

A β-adrenoceptor blocker (usually atenolol, starting does is about 12.5–25 mg/day) may be used for preoperative control of arrhythmias, tachycardia, or angina. However, loss of β-adrenoceptor-mediated vasodilatation in a patient with unopposed catecholamine-induced vasoconstriction can result in dangerous increases in blood pressure. Therefore, β-adrenoceptor blockers never should be employed without first blocking α-adrenoceptor-mediated vasoconstriction (see Table 46-1).

PROLACTINOMA IN CHILDREN

Pathophysiology and Presentation

In adults, prolactin-secreting tumors account for approximately 40% of all pituitary tumors, and over 90% of these are microprolactinomas (235). In children and adolescents, prolactinomas account for only 1% of pediatric intracranial masses, but they account for approximately 50% of pediatric pituitary adenomas (236). Overall, 6% of all pituitary adenomas occur in patients younger than 20 years of age (236). It is believed that pituitary adenomas arise from a monoclonal origin, but attempts at discovering a mutational etiology have not been successful, with only modifications in expression of various oncogenes or suppressors, including PTTG, HMGA2, and FGF-R type 4, being found in atypical, aggressive tumors (237).

Prolactin-producing tumors in children are more common in females, the majority occurring during the adolescent years (238). At diagnosis, females typically present with delayed puberty, amenorrhea, irregular menses, galactorrhea, and other signs of hypogonadism. Males have a higher incidence of macroprolactinomas (238,239) and more often present with neuropthalmological abnormalities, including cranial nerve dysfunction, headaches, and visual loss (240). Growth or pubertal arrest and other signs of hypopituitarism also may be present (240). Gynecomastia is not a common sign.

The differential diagnosis of elevated prolactin in children is quite large because many factors can lead to a loss of dopaminergic suppression of the pituitary lactotropes with resulting secondary hyperprolactinemia. Secondary causes include neurogenic causes (e.g., emotional stress, nipple stimulation, and chest wall lesions), medications (e.g., phenothiazines, metoclopramide, and centrally acting antihypertensives), or mechanical processes (e.g., craniopharyngioma, Rathke cleft cyst, nonfunctioning adenoma, and infiltrative processes). Large, nonfunctioning adenomas that compress the pituitary stalk almost always lead to prolactin levels in the range of 25–100 µg/L, sometimes as high as 200 µg/L.

Inherited conditions leading to prolactinomas in children include MEN-1, CNC, and familial isolated pituitary adenomas (239). It is important to note that in MEN-1 (see above), 60% of pituitary tumors are prolactinomas. Although less common, anterior pituitary adenoma can be the first clinical manifestation of MEN-1, with the youngest reported case being in a 5-year-old with a pituitary lactotroph–somatotroph macroadenoma, as already mentioned.

Evaluation

Evaluation of hyperprolactinemia is often difficult because many secondary causes of elevated serum prolactin levels exist. Several endocrine disorders, including hypothyroidism, that are thought to be caused by increased thyrotropin-releasing hormone (TRH)– or GH-secreting adenomas and Cushing disease all may have associated hyperprolactinemia. Polycystic ovarian syndrome (PCOS) may have associated mild hyperprolactinemia, and hyperprolactinemia may cause a PCOS-type picture (241). Serum prolactin levels also may be elevated in renal failure secondary to decreased clearance.

Microprolactinomas generally raise prolactin levels to greater than 100 µg/L, but there is overlap between prolactin levels seen with microprolactinomas and those of secondary hyperprolactinemia, with a range of 50–200 µg/L. Macroprolactinomas typically are associated with levels of greater than 200 µg/L and can exceed 1000 µg/L.

Given the varied causes and presentations of hyperprolactinemia, including stress, an elevated random prolactin determination should be repeated, fasting, after placement of an indwelling catheter. In patients with a discrepancy between clinical findings and elevated prolactin level, it is useful to measure macroprolactin. Macroprolactin is a bioinactive, large antigen–antibody complex form of prolactin that typically comprises less than 1% of measured prolactin but does crossreact with most prolactin assays. The macroprolactin level my be elevated in some individuals with no pathology and may lead to unnecessary worry and evaluation. However, while controversy exist as to the significance, up to 15% of patients may be found to have pituitary adenomas (242).

Treatment Treatment of childhood microprolactinomas is similar to that of adults. Bromocriptine (2.5–7.5 mg/day PO divided bid; occasionally doses up to 10–15 mg/day are required), cabergoline (0.25–1 mg/day PO twice weekly), pergolide (0.25–1 mg/day PO twice weekly), or quinagolide (0.05–0.1 mg/day PO for microprolactinoma; up to 0.5 mg/day for macroprolactinoma), dopamine agonists, may normalize secretion of prolactin and reduce tumor size. Common side effects of bromocriptine include gastrointestinal upset and postural hypotension. These side effects occur less commonly with cabergoline, which can be dosed twice weekly and may be more effective than bromocriptine. Data from adults show that 25% of patients will have no recurrence when stopping bromocriptine 24 months after normalizing prolactin levels (243). In one study, 60% of patients had normal prolactin levels after withdrawing cabergoline, although some patients redeveloped gonadal dysfunction later on (244). TSS is another option, with a 60% to 90% success rate, but it is more effective for smaller tumors with lower prolactin levels. However, there appears to be a higher incidence of recurrence with long-term follow-up (245). Given the effectiveness and limited side effects of dopamine agonists, medical treatment usually is the preferred option.

The treatment of macroprolactinomas is similar, but patients often require higher doses of bromocriptine or cabergoline. Reduction in tumor size, decrease in prolactin levels, and restoration of anterior pituitary function usually begin in a few weeks but can take months to years to complete. After tumor size has decreased by 50% and prolactin levels have been stable for 2 years, a gradual taper of dopamine agonists can be started. The recurrence rate is high if medications are stopped. For nonresponders to treatment, TSS can be attempted but is rarely curative. Radiation therapy also has been used but can result in hypopituitarism, damage to the optic nerve, and neurological dysfunction.

GH-SECRETING TUMORS IN CHILDREN

Pathophysiology and Presentation

Gigantism is the pediatric expression of acromegaly caused by the effects of excess GH on a skeleton with open epiphyseal growth plates. In children, it is an exceedingly rare condition and, when diagnosed, should trigger the clinician to consider associated disorders, including MEN-1 (128,246), McCune–Albright syndrome (MAS) (246,247), and CNC (248). GH-secreting pituitary adenomas also may occur sporadically (249–251), and GH excess may occur secondarily to dysregulation of GH-releasing hormone (GHRH) signaling caused by a neighboring mass, such as an optic glioma found in NF-1 (252). Isolated familial somatotropinoma (IFS) describes families with at least two members having gigantism or acromegaly where MEN-1, CNC, and MAS has been excluded (253). Recently, mutations of the AIP gene were found in patients with IFS.

Overall, pituitary adenomas account for approximately 3% of intracranial tumors diagnosed in children. Pituitary tumors in children are more likely to be macroadenomas and biochemically active than in adults. Most, approximately 50% to 60%, secrete prolactin (PRL); close to 1% to 10% secrete GH (249, 254), whereas the remaining adenomas are mixed adrenocorticotropin hormone (ACTH)–producing and nonsecreting tumors. Mammosomatotropic tumors are common (consisting of GH- and PRL-secreting cells). Similar to other pituitary tumors, it is believed that these tumors arise from monoclonal origin (251).

Children with gigantism present with accelerated growth. For many children, the relative tall stature may not be viewed negatively, and because of this, they may not come to early medical attention unless they have associated constitutional findings, such as headache, visual disturbances, pubertal delay, or menstrual irregularities (secondary to combined GH and PRL secretion). On physical examination, acromegalic features may be present, including coarse facial features with broadened nose, large hands and feet with thick fingers and toes, obesity, and organomegaly. Several monogenic hereditary causes of tall stature also exist, including Sotos syndrome, Weaver syndrome, Marfan syndrome, homocystinuria, and others, but these syndromes are characteristically associated with nonaccelerating tall stature, developmental delay, unique dysmorphic features, and absent biochemical abnormalities.

Evaluation

In the child with accelerating linear growth, endocrine disorders are more common than hereditary causes of tall stature. In the absence of signs and symptoms of precocious puberty or hyperthyroidism, GH, IGF-1, and PRL should be determined because these tumors are often of mammosomatotrophic origin. Prolactin levels typically are more than 200 µg/L but may be in the macroprolactinoma range of more than 1000 µg/L (1 µg/L = 2.6 mU/L). IGF-1 levels typically are elevated for age but may be normal. In these cases, serial overnight GH sampling may show loss of pulsatility, and in all cases, GH levels will not suppress (<0.04 µg/L) on oral glucose tolerance testing (128,255). Radiographic evaluation should include a bone age (to rule out precocious puberty) and cranial MRI.

Genetic evaluation should be considered if the family history is consistent with an autosomal dominantly inherited MEN syndrome, including MEN-1 (tumors of the parathyroids, enteropancreas, and anterior pituitary; MEN-1 allele), CNC (spotty skin pigmentation, cardiac tumors, primary pigmented nodular adrenocortical disease, and other endocrine tumors; PRKAR1A), or NF-1 (café-au-lait spots, more than two neurofibromas of any type or one plexiform neurofibroma, freckling in the axillary or inguinal region, and optic glioma; NF-1). If the family history is consistent with IFS, analysis of the chromosome 11q13 region should be performed (253). Lastly, while somatic mutations in the gsp oncogene, the GNAS gene (α-subunit of the stimulatory G protein Gs), may be found in up to a third of sporadic GH-secreting tumors in adults (256,257), they appear to have a lower prevalence in sporadic somatotroph adenomas found in children and adolescents (246). In children presenting with a GH-secreting tumor and found to have an activating mutation in gsp, if not already being followed for MAS (i.e., café-au-lait spots, polyostotic fibrous dysplasia, and precococious puberty), further evaluation and follow-up for this sporadically inherited syndrome should be undertaken.

Treatment   The goal of treatment of GH- and GH/PRL-secreting pituitary adenomas in children is similar to that in adults: reduction in biochemical abnormalities with the least possible damage to the hypothalamic–pituitary axis. Unfortunately, in children, these tumors are often larger in size and more locally invasive (258). Transsphenoidal surgery is often the initial treatment of choice because it may be curative for small, circumscribed tumors and may be of clinical benefit to decompress tumors off the optic chiasm (258,259). However, due to the inherent size and invasiveness of these tumors, persistent or recurrent disease is common, and multimodal therapy with pharmacologic agents is indicated, often both before and after surgery. Permanent partial or complete hypopituitarism is reported to occur in approximately 6% to 19% of children who undergo primary transsphenoidal surgery (259).

Medical therapy also has been shown to be effective at reducing tumor size as well biochemical abnormalities. There is increasing experience with the somatostatin analogues octreotide (initial: 50–500 μg subcutaneously tid; doses of 300–600 μg/day or higher rarely result in additional benefit) and its longer-acting form, octerotide-LAR (10–30 mg intramuscularly q28d), both of which have been associated with reduced GH, IGF-1, and PRL levels, as well as reduction in size of the tumor (250,260,261). Side effects of these medications include nausea, diarrhea, flatulence, and an increased incidence of gall-

stones. More recently, in two case reports, the GH-receptor agonist pegvisomant (loading dose: 40 mg subcutaneously; maintenance dose: 10 mg/day subcutaneously, which may be increased or decreased every 4–6 weeks by 5-mg increments, as determined by IGF-I levels; maximal dose: 30 mg/day), which has been used more extensively in adult patients, was reported to lower IGF-1 levels in patients who were unresponsive to traditional therapies (262,263). Bromocriptine and cabergoline, dopamine agonists (see the prolactinoma section for dose), have a long safety record and are used widely as adjunctive therapy for patients with mammosomatotrophic tumors (247). For patients who have failed surgical and multimodal medical therapy, radiation therapy can be considered but should be used only in extreme, persistent cases secondary to the associated latent efficacy and risks of cerebral microaneurysms, cerebral radionecrosis, and secondary tumor induction (259).

REFERENCES

1. Ries LAG, Smith MA, Gurney JG, et al., eds. *Cancer Incidence and Survival Among Children and Adolescents: United States SEER Program 1975–1995*. NIH Pub. No. 99-4649. Bethesda, MD: National Cancer Institute SEER Program; 1999:Chap. XI.
2. Corrias A, Einaudi S, Chiorboli E, et al. Accuracy of fine needle aspiration biopsy of thyroid nodules in detecting malignancy in childhood: Comparison with conventional clinical, laboratory, and imaging approaches. *J Clin Endocrinol Metab.* 2001;86:4644–4648.
3. Kumar A, Bal CS. Differentiated thyroid cancer. *Ind J Pediatr.* 2003;70:707–713.
4. Giuffrida D, Scollo C, Pellegriti G, et al. Differentiated thyroid cancer in children and adolescents. *J Endocrinol Invest.* 2002;25:18–24.
5. Lee YM, Lo CY, Lam KY, et al. Well-differentiated thyroid carcinoma in Hong Kong Chinese patients under 21 years of age: A 35 year experience. *J Am Coll Surg.* 2002;194:711–716.
6. Brink JS, van Heerden JA, McIver B, et al. Papillary thyroid cancer with pulmonary metastases in children: Long-term prognosis. *Surgery.* 2000;128:881–887.
7. Landau D, Vini L, A'Hern R, et al. Thyroid cancer in children: The Royal Marsden Hospital experience. *Eur J Cancer.* 2000;36:214–220.
8. Chow SM, Law S, Mendenhall WM, et al. Differentiated thyroid carcinoma in childhood and adolescence: Clinical course and role of radioiodine. *Pediatr Blood Cancer.* 2004;42:176–183.
9. Powers PA, Dinauer CA, Tuttle RM, et al. Tumor size and extent of disease at diagnosis predict the response to initial therapy for papillary thyroid carcinoma in children and adolescents. *J Pediatr Endocrinol Metab.* 2003;16:693–702.
10. Samuel AM, Sharma SM. Differentiated thyroid carcinomas in children and adolescents. *Cancer.* 1991;67:2186–2190.
11. Ceccarelli C, Pacini F, Lippi F, et al. Thyroid cancer in children and adolescents. *Surgery.* 1988;104:1143–1148.
12. Viswanathan K, Gierlowski TC, Schneider AB. et al Childhood thyroid cancer: Characteristics and long-term outcome in children irradiated for benign conditions of the head and neck. *Arch Pediatr Adolesc Med.* 1994;148:260–263.
13. Harness JK, Thompson NW, McLeod MK, et al. Differentiated thyroid carcinoma in children and adolescents. *World J Surg.* 1992;16:47–54.
14. Schlumberger M, De Vathaire F, Travagli JP, et al. Differentiated thyroid carcinoma in childhood: Long-term follow-up of 72 patients. *J Clin Endocrinol Metab.* 1987;65:1088–1094.
15. Welch-Dinauer CA, Tuttle RM, Robie DK, et al. Clinical features associated with metastasis and recurrence of differentiated thyroid cancer in children, adolescents and young adults. *Clin Endocrinol.* 1998;49:619–628.
16. Lamberg BA, Karkinen-Jaaskelainen M, Franssila KO. Differentiated follicle-derived thyroid carcinoma in children. *Acta Paediatr Scand.* 1989;78:419–425.
17. Jarzab B, Junak D, Wloch J, et al. Multivariate analysis of prognostic factors for differentiated thyroid carcinoma in children. *Eur J Nucl Med.* 2000;27:833–841.
18. Bal CS, Kumar A, Chandra P, et al. Is chest x-ray or high-resolution computed tomography scan of the chest sufficient investigation to detect pulmonary metastasis in pediatric differentiated thyroid cancer? *Thyroid.* 2004;14:217–25.
19. Haveman JW, Van Tol KM, Rouwe CW, et al. Surgical experience in children with differentiated thyroid carcinoma. *Ann Surg Oncol.* 2003;10:15–20.
20. Hung W, Sarlis NJ. Current controversies in the management of pediatric patients with well-differentiated nonmedulllary thyroid cancer: A review. *Thyroid.* 2002;12:683–702.
21. Sklar C, Whitton J, Mertens A, et al. Abnormalities of the thyroid in survivors of Hodgkin disease: Data from the Childhood Cancer Survivor Study. *J Clin Endocrinol Metab.* 2000;85:3227–3232.
22. Tucker MA, Morris Jones PH, Boice JD, et al. Therapeutic radiation at a young age is linked to secondary thyroid cancer. *Cancer Res.* 1991;51:2885–1888.
23. Mahoney MC, Lawvere S, Falkner KL, et al. Thyroid cancer incidence trends in Belarus: Examining the impact of Chernobyl. *Int J Epidemiol.* 2004;33:1025–1033.
24. Bhatia S, Yasui Y, Robison LL, et al. High risk of subsequent neoplasms continues with extended follow-up of the late effects study group. *J Clin Oncol.* 2003;21:4386–4394.
25. Farahati J, Demidchik EP, Biko J, et al. Inverse association between age at the time of radiation exposure and extent of disease in cases of radiation-induced thyroid carcinoma in Belarus. *Cancer.* 2000;88:1470–1476.
26. Farahati J, Bucsky P, Parlowsky T, et al. Characteristics of differentiated thyroid

carcinoma in children and adolescents with respect to age, gender, and histology. *Cancer.* 1997;80:2156–2162.

27. LiVolsi VA, Albores-Saavedra J, Asa SL, et al. Papillary carcinoma. In: DeLellis RA, Lloyd RV, Heitz PU, Eng C, eds. *Pathology and Genetics of Tumors of Endocrine Organs (World Health Organization Classification of Tumors).* Lyon: IARC Press; 2004:57–66.

28. Fenton CL, Lukes Y, Nicholson D, et al. The ret/PTC mutations are common in sporadic papillary thyroid carcinoma of children and young adults. *J Clin Endocrinol Metab.* 2000;85:1170–1175.

29. Elisei R, Romei C, Vorontsova T, et al. RET/PTC rearrangements in thyroid nodules: Studies in irradiated and not irradiated, malignant and benign thyroid lesions in children and adults. *J Clin Endocrinol Metab.* 2001;86:3211–3216.

30. Ozaki O, Ito K, Kobayashi K, et al. Familial occurrence of differentiated, nonmedullary thyroid carcinoma. *World J Surg.* 1988;12:565–571.

31. Sturgeon C, Clark OH. Familial nonmedullary thyroid cancer. *Thyroid.* 2005;15: 588–593.

32. Hemminki K, Eng C, Chen B. Familial risks for nonmedullary thyroid cancer. *J Clin Endocrinol Metab.* 2005;90:5747–5753; e-pub July 2005.

33. Eng C. Role of PTEN, a lipid phosphatase upstream effector of protein kinase B, in epithelial thyroid carcinogenesis. *Ann NY Acad Sci.* 2002;968:213–221.

34. Marsh DJ, Coulon V, Lunetta KL, et al. Mutation spectrum and genotype-phenotype analyses in Cowden disease and Bannayan–Zonana syndrome, two hamartoma syndromes with germline PTEN mutation. *Hum Mol Genet.* 1998;7:507–515.

35. Liaw D, Marsh DJ, Li J, et al. Germline mutations of the PTEN gene in Cowden disease, an inherited breast and thyroid cancer syndrome. *Nat Genet.* 1997;16:64–67.

36. Perrier ND, van Heerden JA, Goellner JR, et al. Thyroid cancer in patients with familial adenomatous polyposis. *World J Surg.* 1998;22:738–742; discussion 743.

37. Bell B, Mazzaferri EL. Familial adenomatous polyposis (Gardner's syndrome) and thyroid carcinoma: A case report and review of the literature. *Dig Dis Sci.* 1993;38:185–190.

38. Stratakis CA, Kirschner LS, Carney JA. Clinical and molecular features of the Carney complex: Diagnostic criteria and recommendations for patient evaluation. *J Clin Endocrinol Metab.* 2001;86:4041–4046.

39. Bentley AA, Gillespie C, Malis D. Evaluation and management of a solitary thyroid nodule in a child. *Otolaryngol Clin North Am.* 2003;36:117–128.

40. Fassina AS, Rupolo M, Pelizzo MR, Casara D. Thyroid cancer in children and adolescents. *Tumori.* 1994;80:257–262.

41. Hopwood NJ, Kelch RP. Thyroid masses: approach to diagnosis and management in childhood and adolescence. *Pediatr Rev.* 1993;14:481–487.

42. Hung W, Anderson KD, Chandra RS, et al. Solitary thyroid nodules in 71 children and adolescents. *J Pediatr Surg.* 1992;27: 1407–1409.

43. Lugo-Vicente H, Ortiz VN. Pediatric thyroid nodules: Insights in management. *Bol Assoc Med PR.* 1998;90:74–78.

44. Belfiore A, Giuffrida D, La Rosa GL, et al. High frequency of cancer in cold thyroid nodules occurring at young age. *Acta Endocrinol (Copenh).* 1989;121:197–202.

45. Degnan BM, McClellan DR, Francis GL. An analysis of fine-needle aspiration biopsy of the thyroid in children and adolescents. *J Pediatr Surg.* 1996;31:903–907.

46. Raab SS, Silverman JF, Elsheikh TM, et al. Pediatric thyroid nodules: Disease demigraphics and clinical management as determined by fine needle aspiration biopsy. *Pediatrics.* 1995;95:46–49.

47. Amrikachi M, Ponder TB, Wheeler TM, et al. Thyroid fine-needle aspiration biopsy in children and adolescents: Experience with 218 aspirates. *Diagn Cytopathol.* 2005;32:189–192.

48. Kowalski LP, Filho JG, Pinto CA, et al. Long-term survival rates in young patients with thyroid carcinoma. *Arch Otolaryngol Head Neck Surg.* 2003;129:746–749.

49. Robie DK, Welch-Dinauer C, Tuttle RM, et al. The impact of initial surgical management on outcome in young patients with differentiated thyroid cancer. *J Pediatr Surg.* 1999;33:1134–1140.

50. Welch-Dinauer CA, Tuttle MR, Robie DK, et al. Extensive surgery improves recurrence-free survival for children and young patients with class I papillary thyroid carcinoma. *J Pediatr Surg.* 1999;34:1799–1804.

51. Borson-Chazot F, Causeret S, Lifante JC, et al. Predictive factors for recurrence from a series of 74 children and adolescents with differentiated thyroid cancer. *World J Surg.* 2004;28:1088–1092.

52. Thompson GB, Hay ID. Current strategies for surgical management and adjuvant treatment of childhood papillary thyroid carcinoma. *World J Surg.* 2004;28:1187–1198.

53. Iorcansky S, Herzovich V, Qualey RR, et al. Serum thyrotropin (TSH) levels after recombinant human TSH injections in children and teenagers with papillary thyroid cancer. *J Clin Endocrinol Metab.* 2005;90:6553–6555.

54. Van Wyngaarden M, McDougall IR. What is the role of 1100 MBq (<30 mCi) radioiodine ^{131}I in the treatment of patients with differentiated thyroid cancer? *Nucl Med Commun.* 1996;17:199–207.

55. Kuijt WJ, Huang SA. Children with differentiated thyroid cancer achieve adequate hyperthyrotropinemia within 14 days of levothyroxine withdrawal. *J Clin Endocrinol Metab.* 2005;90:6123–6125.

56. Yaakob W, Gordon L, Spicer KM, et al. The usefulness of iodine-123 whole-body scans in evaluating thyroid carcinoma and metastases. *J Nucl Med Technol.* 1999;27:279–281.

57. Maxon HR III, Smith HS. Radioiodine-131 in the diagnosis and treatment of metastatic well differentiated thyroid cancer. *Endocrinol Metab Clin North Am.* 1990;19:685–715.

58. Green DM, Edge SB, Penetrante RB, et al. In situ breast carcinoma treatment during adolescence for thyroid cancer with radioiodine. *Med Pediatr Oncol.* 1995;24:82–86.

59. Rubino C, de Vathaire F, Dottorini ME, et al. Second primary malignancies in thyroid cancer patients. *Br J Cancer.* 2003;89:1638–1644.

60. Edmonds CJ, Smith T. The long-term hazards of the treatment of thyroid cancer with radioiodine. *Br J Radiol.* 1986;59:45–51.

61. Hyer S, Vini L, O'Connell M, et al. Testicular dose and fertility in men following ^{131}I therapy for thyroid cancer. *Clin Endocrinol (Oxf).* 2002;56:755–758.

62. Pacini F, Gasperi M, Fugazzola L, et al. Testicular function in patients with differentiated thyroid carcinoma treated with radioiodine. *J Nucl Med.* 1994;35:1418–1422.

63. Vini L, Hyer S, Al-Saadi A, et al. Prognosis for fertility and ovarian function after treatment with radioiodine for thyroid cancer. *Postgrad Med J.* 2002;78:92–93.

64. Casara D, Rubello D, Piotto A, et al. Pregnancy after high therapeutic doses of iodone-131 in differentiated thyroid cancer: Potential risks and recommendations. *Eur J Nucl Med.* 1993;20:192–194.

65. Hung W, Sarlis NJ. Current controversies in the management of pediatric patients with well-differentiated nonmedulllary thyroid cancer: A review. *Thyroid.* 2002;12:683–702.

66. Radetti G, Castellan C, Tato L, et al. Bone mineral density in children and adolescent females treated with high doses of L-thyroxine. *Horm Res.* 1993;39:127–131.

67. Zimmerman D, Jay ID, Gough IR, et al. Papillary thyroid carcinoma in children and adults: Long-term follow-up of 1039 patients conservatively treated at one institution during three decades. *Surgery.* 1988;104: 1157–1166.

68. Samaan NA, Schultz PN, Hickey RC, et al. The results of various modalities of treatment of well differentiated thyroid carcinoma: A retrospective review of 1599 patients. *J Clin Endocrinol Metab.* 1992;75:714–720.

69. Kloos RT, Gross MD, Francis IR, et al. Incidentally discovered adrenal masses. *Endocr Rev.* 1995;16:460–484.

70. Latronico AC, Chrousos GP. Extensive personal experience: Adrenocortical tumors. *J Clin Endocrinol Metab.* 1997;82:1317.

71. Ross NS, Aron DC. Hormonal evaluation of the patient with an incidentally discovered adrenal mass. *N Engl J Med.* 1990;323:1401.

72. Cagel PT, Hough AJ, Pysher TJ. Comparison of adrenal cortical tumors in children and adults. *Cancer.* 1986;57:2235.

73. Didolkar MS, Bescher RA, Elias EG, et al. Natural history of adrenal cortical carcinoma: A clinicopathologic study of 42 patients. *Cancer.* 1981;47:2153.

74. King DR, Lack EE. Adrenal cortical carcinoma: A clinical and pathologic study of 49 cases. *Cancer.* 1979;44:239.

75. Kloos RT, Gross MD, Francis IR, et al. Incidentally discovered adrenal masses. *Endocr Rev.* 1995;16:460.

76. Beuschlein F, Schulze E, Mora P, et al: Steroid 21-hydroxylase mutations and 21-hydroxylase messenger ribonucleic acid expression in human adrenocortical tumors. *J Clin Endocrinol Metab.* 1998;83:2585.

77. Demeure MJ, Somberg LB. Functioning and nonfunctioning adrenocortical carcinoma: Clinical presentation and therapeutic strategies. *Surg Oncol Clin North Am.* 1998;7:791.

78. Terzolo M, Osella G, Ali A, et al. Adrenal incidentaloma, a five year experience. *Minerva Endocrinol.* 1995;20.69–78.

79. Gruppo Piemontese Incidentalomi Surrenalici. *Arch Surg.* 1997;132:914.

80. Kasperlik-Zaluska AA, Migdalska BM, Makowska AM. Incidentally found adrenocortical carcinoma: A study of 21 patients. *Eur J Cancer.* 1998;34:1721.

81. Skogseid B, Rastad J, Gobl A, et al. Adrenal lesion in multiple endocrine neoplasia type 1 *Surgery* 1995;118·1077

82. Marchesa P, Fazio VW, Church JM, et al. Adrenal masses in patients with familial adenomatous polyposis. *Dis Colon Rectum.* 1997;40:1023.

83. Sandrini R, Ribeiro RC, DeLacerda L. Childhood adrenocortical tumors. *J Clin Endocrinol Metab.* 1997;82:2027.

84. Stratakis CA, Chrousos GP: Cushing syndrome and disease. In: Finberg L, ed. *Saunder's Manual of Pediatric Practice.* Philadelphia: Saunders; 1998:807.

85. Stratakis CA, Chrousos GP: Endocrine tumors. In: Pizzo PA, Poplack DG, eds. *Principles and Practice of Pediatric Oncology.* Philadelphia: Lippincott–Raven; 1997:947.

86. Teinturier C, Pauchard MS, Brugieres L, et al. Clinical and prognostic aspects of adrenocortical neoplasms in childhood. *Med Pediatr Oncol.* 1999;32:106.

87. Barzilay JI, Pazianos AG. Adrenocortical carcinoma. *Urol Clin North Am.*1989;16:457.

88. Pommier RF, Brennan MF. An eleven-year experience with adrenocortical carcinoma. *Surgery.* 1992;112:963.

89. Chundler RM, Kay R. Adrenocortical carcinoma in children. *Urol Clin North Am.* 1989;16:469.

90. Fraser R, James VHT, Landon J, et al. Clinical and biochemical studies of a patient with a corticosterone-secreting adrenocortical tumor. *Lancet.* 1968;2:116.

91. Flack MR, Chrousos GP. Neoplasms of the adrenal cortex. In: Holland JF, ed. *Cancer Medicine,* 4th ed. New York: Lea & Febiger; 1996:1563.

92. Luton JP, Cerdas S, Billaud L, et al. Clinical features of adrenocortical carcinoma, prognostic factors, and the effect of Mitotane therapy. *N Engl J Med.* 1990;322:1195.

93. Beuschlein F, Reincke M, Karl M, et al. Clonal composition of human adrenocortical neoplasms. *Cancer Res.* 1994;54:4927.

94. Bornstein S, Stratakis CA, Chrousos GP. Recent advances in adrenocortical tumors. *Ann Intern Med.* 1999;130:759.

95. Stratakis CA. Genetics of adrenocortical tumors: Gatekeepers, landscapers and conductors in symphony. *Trends Endocrinol Metab.* 2003;14:404–410.

96. Kjellman M, Kallioniemi OP, Karhu R, et al. Genetic aberrations in adrenocortical tumors detected using comparative genomic hybridization correlate with tumor size and malignancy. *Cancer Res.* 1996;56:4219.

97. Figueiredo BC, Stratakis CA, Sandrini R, et al. Comparative genomic hybridization analysis of adrenocortical tumors of childhood. *J Clin Endocrinol Metab.* 1999;84:1116.

98. Sidhu S, et al. Comparative genomic hybridization analysis of adrenocortical tumors.

J Clin Endocrinol Metab. 2002;87:3467–3474.

99. Shono T, et al. Analysis of numerical chromosomal aberrations in adrenal cortical neoplasms by fluorescence in situ hybridization. *J Urol.* 2002;168:1370–1373.

100. Steingart DE. Treating adrenal cancer. *Endocrinologist.* 1992;2:149.

101. Hahner S, Fassnacht M. Mitotane for adrenocortical carcinoma treatment. *Curr Opin Invest Drugs.* 2005;6:386–394.

102. Berruti A, Terzolo M, Sperone P, et al. Etoposide, doxorubicin and cisplatin plus Mitotane in the treatment of advanced adrenocortical carcinoma: A large prospective phase II trial. *Endocr Relat Cancer.* 2005;12:657–666.

103. Barzon L, Fallo F, Sonino N, et al. Adrenocortical carcinoma: Experience in 45 patients. *Oncology.* 1997;54:490.

104. Becker D, Schumacher OP. o,p'-DDD therapy in invasive adrenocortical carcinoma. *Ann Intern Med.* 1975;82:677.

105. Hoffman DL, Mattox VR. Treatment of adrenocortical carcinoma with o,p'-DDD. *Med Clin North Am.* 1972;56:999.

106. Berruti A, Terzolo M, Pia A, et al. Mitotane associated with etoposide, doxorubicin, and cisplatin in the treatment of advanced adrenocortical carcinoma: Italian Group for the Study of Adrenal Cancer. *Cancer.* 1998;83:2194.

107. Fallo F, Pilon C, Barzon L, et al. Effects of taxol on the human NCI-H295 adrenocortical carcinoma cell line. *Endocr Res.* 1996;22:709.

108. Fallo F, Pilon C, Barzon L, et al. Paclitaxel is an effective antiproliferative agent on the human NCI-H295 adrenocortical carcinoma cell line. *Chemotherapy.* 1998;44:129.

109. Freeman DA. Adrenal carcinoma. *Curr Ther Endocrinol Metab.* 1997;6:173.

110. La Rocca RV, Stein CA, Danesi R, et al. Suramin in adrenal cancer: Modulation of steroid hormone production, cytotoxicity in vitro, and clinical antitumor effect. *J Clin Endocrinol Metab.* 1990;71:497.

111. Bellantone R, Ferrante A, Boscherini M, et al. Role of reoperation in recurrence of adrenal cortical carcinoma: Results from 188 cases collected in the Italian National Registry for Adrenal Cortical Carcinoma. *Surgery.* 1997;122:1212.

112. Khorram-Manesh A, Ahlman H, Jansson S, et al. Adrenocortical carcinoma: Surgery and mitotane for treatment and steroid profiles for follow-up. *World J Surg.* 1998;22:605.

113. Lack E: *Atlas of Tumor Pathology: Tumors of the Adrenal Gland and Extra-Adrenal Paraganglia.* Washington, DC: Armed Forces Institute of Pathology, 1997.

114. Weiss LM. Comparative histologic study of 43 metastasizing and nonmetastasizing adrenocortical tumors. *Am J Surg Pathol.* 1984;8:163.

115. Chandrasekharappa SC, Guru SC, Manickam P, et al. Positional cloning of the gene for multiple endocrine neoplasia type 1. *Science.* 1997;276:404–407.

116. Marx SJ, Agarwal SK, Kester MB, et al. Multiple endocrine neoplasia type 1: Clinical and genetic features of the hereditary

endocrine neoplasias. *Rec Prog Horm Res.* 1999;54:397–438.

117. Marx SJ. Multiple endocrine neoplasia type 1. In: Bilezikian JP, Levine MA, Marcus R, eds. *The Parathyroids.* New York: Raven Press; 2000.

118. Trump D, Farren B, Wooding C, et al. Clinical studies of multiple endocrine neoplasia type 1 (MEN1). *Q J Med.* 1996;89:653–669.

119. Vasen HF, Lamers CB, Lips CJ. Screening for the multiple endocrine neoplasia syndrome type I: A study of 11 kindreds in The Netherlands. *Arch Intern Med.* 1989;149:2717–2722.

120. Skarulis MC, Marx S, Spiegel AM, et al. Multiple endocrine neoplasia type 1: Clinical and genetic topics. *Ann Intern Med.* 1998;129:484–494.

121. Lamers CB, Froeling PG. Clinical significance of hyperparathyroidism in familial multiple endocrine adenomatosis type I (MEN I). *Am J Med.* 1979;66:422–424.

122. Marx SJ, Vinik AI, Santen RJ, et al. Multiple endocrine neoplasia type I: Assessment of laboratory tests to screen for the gene in a large kindred. *Medicine.* 1986;65:226–241.

123. Ballard HS, Frame B, Hartsock RJ. Familial multiple endocrine adenoma-peptic ulcer complex. *Medicine.* 1964;43:481–516.

124. Betts JB, O'Malley BP, Rosenthal FD. Hyperparathyroidism: A prerequisite for Zollinger Ellison syndrome in multiple endocrine adenomatosis type 1. Report of a further family and a review of the literature. *Q J Med.* 1980;49:69–76.

125. Scheithauer BW, Laws ER Jr, Kovacs K, et al. Pituitary adenomas of the multiple endocrine neoplasia type I syndrome. *Semin Diagn Pathol.* 1987;4:205–211.

126. Shepherd JJ. The natural history of multiple endocrine neoplasia type 1: Highly uncommon or highly unrecognized? *Arch Surg.* 1991;126:935–952.

127. O'Brien T, O'Riordan DS, Gharib H, et al. Results of treatment of pituitary disease in multiple endocrine neoplasia, type I. *Neurosurgery.* 1996;39:273–278; discussion 278–279.

128. Stratakis CA, Schussheim DH, Freedman SM, et al. Pituitary macroadenoma in a 5-year-old: An early expression of multiple endocrine neoplasia type 1. *J Clin Endocrinol Metab.* 2000;85:4776–4780.

129. Giraud S, Zhang CX, Serova-Sinilnikova O, et al. Germline mutation analysis in patients with multiple endocrine neoplasia type 1 and related disorders. *Am J Hum Genet.* 1997;63:455–467.

130. Thakker RV. Multiple endocrine neoplasia: Syndromes of the twentieth century. *J Clin Endocrinol Metab.* 1998;83:2617–2620.

131. Gagel RF. RET protooncogene mutations and endocrine neoplasia: A story intertwined with neural crest differentiation. *Endocrinology.* 1996;137:1509–1511.

132. Eng C, Clayton D, Schuffenecker I, et al. The relationship between specific RET proto-oncogene mutations and disease phenotype in multiple endocrine neoplasia type 2. International RET mutation consortium analysis. *JAMA.* 1996;276:1575–1579.

133. Edery P, Eng C, Munnich A, et al. RET in human development and oncogenesis. *Bioessays*. 1997;19:389–395.

134. Gagel RF, Levy ML, Donovan DT, et al. Multiple endocrine neoplasia type 2A associated with cutaneous lichen amyloidosis. *Ann Intern Med*. 1989;111:802–806.

135. Borrego S, Eng C, Sanchez B, et al. Molecular analysis of the ret and GDNF genes in a family with multiple endocrine neoplasia type 2A and Hirschsprung disease. *J Clin Endocrinol Metab*. 1998;83:3361–3364.

136. Eng C, Mulligan LM. Mutations of the RET proto-oncogene in the multiple endocrine neoplasia type 2 syndromes, related sporadic tumours, and Hirschsprung disease. *Hum Mutat*. 1997;9:97–109.

137. Hoff AO, Cote J, Gagel RF. Multiple endocrine neoplasias. *Annu Rev Physiol*. 2000;62:377–411.

138. Angrist M, Bolk S, Hallushka M, et al. Germline mutations in glial-derived neurotrophic factor (GDNF) and RET in a Hirschsprung disease patient. *Nat Genet*. 1996;14:341–344.

139. Decker RA, Peacock ML, Watson P. Hirschsprung disease in MEN 2A: Increased spectrum of RET exon 10 genotypes and strong genotype–phenotype correlation. *Hum Mol Genet*. 1998;7:129–134.

140. Carney JA, Gordon H, Carpenter PC, et al. The complex of myxomas, spotty pigmentation, and endocrine overactivity. *Medicine*. 1985;64:270–283.

141. Stratakis CA. Genetics of Carney complex and related familial lentiginoses, and other multiple tumor syndromes. *Frontiers Biosci*. 2000;5:353–366.

142. Salomon F, Froesh ER, Hedinger CE. Familial Cushing syndrome (Carney complex) (letter). *N Engl J Med*. 1990;322:1470.

143. Shenoy BV, Carpenter PC, Carney JA. Bilateral primary pigmented nodular adrenocortical disease: Rare cause of the Cushing syndrome. *Am J Surg Pathol*. 1984;8:335–344.

144. Schweizer-Cagianut M, Froesch ER, Hedinger CE. Familial Cushing's syndrome with primary adrenocortical microadenomatosis (primary adrenocortical nodular dysplasia). *Acta Endocrinol (Copenh)*. 1980;94:529–535.

145. Carney JA, Hruska LS, Beauchamp GD, et al. Dominant inheritance of the complex of myxomas, spotty pigmentation and endocrine overactivity. *Mayo Clin Proc*. 1986;61:165–172.

146. Carney JA, Young WF. Primary pigmented nodular adrenocortical disease and its associated conditions. *Endocrinologist*. 1992;2:6–21.

147. Mellinger RC, Smith RW. Studies of the adrenal hyperfunction in 2 patients with atypical Cushing's syndrome. *J Clin Endocrinol Metab*. 1955;16:350–366.

148. Kracht J, Tamm J. Bilaterale kleiknotige Adenomatose der Nebennierenrinde bei Cushing-Syndrom. *Virchows Arch Pathol Anat*. 1960;333:1–9.

149. Levin ME. The development of bilateral adenomatous adrenal hyperplasia in a case of Cushing's syndrome of eighteen years' duration. *Am J Med*. 1966;40:318–324.

150. De Moor P, Roels H, Delaere K, et al. Unusual case of adrenocortical hyperfunction. *J Clin Endocrinol Metab*. 1965;25:612–620.

151. Sarlis NJ, Chrousos GP, Doppman JL, et al. Primary pigmented nodular adrenocortical disease (PPNAD): Reevaluation of a patient with Carney complex 27 years after unilateral adrenalectomy. *J Clin Endocrinol Metab*. 1997;82:2037–2043.

152. Gomez-Muguruza MT, Chrousos GP. Periodic Cushing's syndrome in a short boy: Usefulness of the ovine corticotropin releasing hormone test. *J Pediatr*. 1989;115:270–273.

153. Stratakis CA, Sarlis NJ, Kirschner LS, et al. Paradoxical response to dexamethasone assists with the diagnosis of primary pigmented nodular adrenocortical disease (PPNAD). *Ann Intern Med*. 1999;131:585–591.

154. Watson JC, Stratakis CA, Bryant-Greenwood PK, et al. Neurosurgical implications of Carney complex. *J Neurosurg*. 2000;92:413–418.

155. Raff SB, Carney JA, Krugman D, et al. Prolactin secretion abnormalities in patients with the "syndrome of spotty skin pigmentation, myxomas, endocrine overactivity and schwannomas" (Carney complex). *J Pediatr Endocrinol Metab*. 2000;13:373–379.

156. Pack S, Kirshner LS, Pak E, et al. Pituitary tumors in patients with the "complex of spotty skin pigmentation, myxomas, endocrine overactivity and schwannomas" (Carney complex): Evidence for progression from somatomammotroph hyperplasia to adenoma. *J Clin Encocrinol Metab*. 2000;85:3860–3865.

157. Premkumar A, Stratakis CA, Shawker TH, et al. Testicular ultrasound in Carney complex. *J Clin Ultrasound*. 1997;25:211–214.

158. Carney JA. Psammomatous melanotic schwannoma: A distinctive, heritable tumor with special associations, including cardiac myxoma and the Cushing syndrome. *Am J Surg Pathol*. 1990;14:206–222.

159. Carney JA, Toorkey BC. Ductal adenoma of the breast with tubular futures: A probable component of the complex of myxomas, spotty pigmentation, endocrine overactivity, and schwannomas. *Am J Surg Pathol*. 1991;15:722–731.

160. Carney JA, Stratakis CA. Ductal adenoma of the breast (letter). *Am J Surg Pathol*. 1996;20:1154–1155.

161. Stratakis CA, Courcoutsakis N, Abati A, et al. Thyroid gland abnormalities in patients with the "syndrome of spotty skin pigmentation, myxomas, and endocrine overactivity" (Carney complex). *J Clin Endocrinol Metab*. 1997;82:2037–2043.

162. Casey M, Mah C, Merliss AD, et al. Identification of a novel genetic locus for familial cardiac myxomas and Carney complex. *Circulation*. 1998;98:2560–2566.

163. Kirschner LS, Carney JA, Pack S, et al. Mutations in the gene encoding the type Ia regulatory subunit of the protein kinase A (PRKARIA) in patients with Carney complex. *Nat Genet*. 2000;26:89–92.

164. Scott JD. Cyclic nucleotide–dependent protein kinases. *Pharmacol Ther*. 1991;50:123–145.

165. DeMarco L, Stratakis CA, Boson WL, et al. Sporadic cardiac myxomas and tumors from patients with Carney complex are not associated with activating mutations of the Gsα gene. *Hum Genet*. 1996;98:185–188.

166. Stratakis CA, Carney JA, Lin JP, et al. Carney complex, a familial multiple neoplasia and lentiginosis syndrome: Analysis of 11 kindreds and linkage to the short arm of chromosome 2. *J Clin Invest*. 1996;97:699–705.

167. Kirschner LS, Sandrini F, Monbo J, et al. Genetic heterogeneity and spectrum of mutations of the PRKAR1A gene in patients with the Carney complex. *Hum Mol Genet*. 2000;12:3037–3046.

168. Taymans SE, Kirschner LS, Pack S, et al. YAC–BAC contig of the Carney complex (CNC) critical region on 2p16 and copy number gain of 2p16 in CNC tumors: Evidence for a novel oncogene? *Am J Hum Genet*. 1999;65:A326.

169. Peutz JL. Very remarkable case of familial polyposis of mucous membrane of intestinal tract and nasopharynx accompanied by peculiar pigmentation of skin and mucous membrane (Dutch). *Nederl Maandschr Geneesk*. 1921;10:134–146.

170. Jeghers H, McKusick VA, Katz KH. Generalised intestinal polyposis and melanin spots of the oral mucosa, lips and digits. *N Engl J Med*. 1949;241:993–1005 and 1031–1036.

171. Hemminki A. The molecular basis and clinical aspects of Peutz–Jeghers syndrome. *Cell Mol Life Sci*. 1999;55:735–750.

172. Hemminki A, Tomlinson I, Markie D, et al. Localisation of a susceptibility locus for Peutz–Jeghers syndrome to 19p using comparative genomic hybridisation and targeted linkage analysis. *Nat Genet*. 1997;15:87–90.

173. Boardman LA, Thibodeau SN, Schaid DJ, et al. Increased risk for cancer in patients with the Peutz–Jeghers syndrome. *Ann Intern Med*. 1998;128:896–899.

174. Westerman AM, Wilson JHP. Peutz–Jeghers syndrome: Risks of a hereditary condition. A clinical review. *Scand J Gastroenterol*. 1999;230:64–70.

175. Giardello FM, Welsh SB, Hamilton SR, et al. Increased risk of cancer in the Peutz–Jeghers syndrome. *N Engl J Med*. 1987;316:1511–1514.

176. Hizawa K, Iida M, Matsumoto T, et al. Cancer in Peutz–Jeghers syndrome. *Cancer*. 1993;72:2777–2781.

177. Foley TR, McGarrity TJ, Abt AB. Peutz–Jeghers syndrome: A clinicopathologic survey of the "Harrisburg family" with a 49-year follow up. *Gastroenterology*. 1988;95:1535–1540.

178. Rustgi AK. Hereditary gastrointestinal polyposis and nonpolyposis syndromes. *N Engl J Med*. 1994;331:1694–702.

179. Spigelman AD, Murday V, Phillips RKS. Cancer and Peutz–Jeghers syndrome. *Gut*. 1989;30:1588–1590.

180. Pathomvanich A, Koch C, Stratakis CA. Thyroid abnormalities in Peutz–Jeghers syndrome: Report of new observation and review of the literature. *J Endocrinol Genet*. 1999;1:47–49.

181. Young RH, Scully RE. Mucinous ovarian tumors associated with mucinous adenocarcinomas of the cervix: Clinicopathologic analysis of 16 cases. *Int J Gynecol Pathol*. 1988;7:99–111.

182. Young RH, Welch WR, Dickersin GE, et al. Ovarian sex stromal tumor with annular tubules: Review of 74 cases including 27 with Peutz–Jeghers syndrome and 4 with adenoma malignum of the cervix. *Cancer.* 1982;50:1384–1402.

183. Young S, Gooneratne S, Straus FH, et al. Feminizing Sertoli cell tumors in boys with Peutz–Jeghers syndrome. *Am J Surg Pathol.* 1995;19:50–58.

184. Hemminki A, Markie D, Tomlinson I, et al. A serine/threonine kinase gene defective in Peutz–Jeghers syndrome. *Nature.* 1998;391:184–187.

185. Jenne DE, Remann H, Nezu J, et al. Peutz–Jeghers syndrome is caused by mutations in a novel serine threonine kinase. *Nat Genet.* 1998;18:38–43.

186. Westerman AM, Entius MM, Boor PPC, et al. Novel mutations in the *LKB1/STK11* gene in Dutch Peutz–Jeghers families. *Hum Mutat.* 1999;13:476–481.

187. Wang ZJ, Churchman M, Avizienyte E, et al. Germline mutations of the LKB1 (STK11) gene in Peutz–Jeghers patients. *J Med Genet.* 1999;36:365–368.

188. Resta N, Simone C, Mareni C, et al. STK11 mutations in Peutz–Jeghers syndrome and sporadic colon cancer. *Cancer Res.* 1998;58:4799–4801.

189. Jiang CY, Esufali S, Berk T, et al. STK11/LKB1 germline mutations are not identified in most Peutz–Jeghers syndrome patients. *Clin Genet.* 1999;56:136–141.

190. Ylikorkala A, Avizienyte E, Tomlinson IPM, et al. Mutations and impaired function of LKB1 in familial and non-familial Peutz–Jeghers syndrome and a sporadic testicular cancer. *Hum Mol Genet.* 1999;8:45–51.

191. Boardman LA, Couch FJ, Burgart LJ, et al. Genetic heterogeneity in Peutz–Jeghers syndrome. *Hum Mutat.* 2000;16:23–30.

192. Su JY, Erikson E, Maller JL. Cloning and characterization of a novel serine/threonine protein kinase expressed in early *Xenopus* embryos. *J Biol Chem.* 1996;271:14430–14437.

193. Smith DP, Spicer J, Smith A, et al. The mouse Peutz–Jeghers syndrome gene Lkb1 encodes a nuclear protein kinase. *Hum Mol Genet.* 1999;8:1479–1485.

194. Mehenni H, Gehrig C, Nezu J, et al. Loss of LKB1 kinase activity in Peutz–Jeghers syndrome, and evidence for allelic and locus heterogeneity. *Am J Hum Genet.* 1998;63:1641–1650.

195. Mehenni H, Blouin JL, Radhakrishna U, et al. Peutz–Jeghers syndrome: Confirmation of linkage to chromosome 19p13.3 and identification of a potential second locus, on 19q13.4. *Am J Hum Genet.* 1997;61:1327–1334.

196. Liaw D, Marsh DJ, Li J, et al. Germline mutations of the PTEN gene in Cowden disease, an inherited breast and thyroid cancer syndrome. *Nat Genet.* 1997;16:64–67.

197. Nelen MR, Padberg GW, Peeters EAJ, et al. Localization of the gene for Cowden disease to chromosome 10q22-23. *Nat Genet.* 1996;13:114–116.

198. Eng C. Genetics of Cowden syndrome: Through the looking glass of oncology. *Int J Oncology.* 1998;12:701–710.

199. Nelen MR, van Staveren WCG, Peeters EAJ, et al. Germline mutations in the PTEN/MMAC1 gene in patients with Cowden disease. *Hum Mol Genet.* 1997;6:1383–1387.

200. Marsh DJ, Kum JB, Lunetta KL, et al. PTEN mutation spectrum and genotype–phenotype correlations in Bannayan–Riley–Ruvalcaba syndrome suggest a single entity with Cowden syndrome. *Hum Mol Genet.* 1999;8:1461–1472.

201. Longy M, Coulon V, Duboue B, et al. Mutations of PTEN in patients with Bannayan–Riley–Ruvalacaba phenotype. *J Med Genet.* 1998;35:886–889.

202. Linehan WM, Lerman MI, Zbar B. Identification of the von Hippel–Lindau (VHL) gene. *JAMA.* 1995;273:564–570.

203. Latif F, Tory K, Gnarra J, et al. Identification of the von Hippel–Lindau disease tumor suppressor gene. *Science.* 1993;260:1317–1320.

204. Richards FM, Webster AR, McMahon R, et al. Molecular genetic analysis of von Hippel–Lindau disease. *J Intern Med.* 1998;243:527–533.

205. Bar M, Friedman E, Jakobovitz O, et al. Sporadic phaeochromocytomas are rarely associated with germline mutations in the von Hippel–Lindau and RET genes. *Clin Endocrinol (Oxf).* 1997;47:707–712.

206. Eisenhofer G, Lenders JW, Pacak K. Biochemical diagnosis of pheochromocytoma. *Front Horm Res.* 2004;31:76–106.

207. Lenders JW, Pacak K, Walther MM, et al. Biochemical diagnosis of pehochromocytoma: Which test is best? *JAMA.* 2002;287:1427–34.

208. Lenders JW, Eisenhofer G, Mannelli M, et al. Pheochromoctyoma. *Lancet.* 2005;366:665–75.

209. Brouwers FM, Lenders JW, Eisenhofer G, et al. Pheochromocytoma as an endocrine emergency. *Rev Endocrinol Metab Disord.* 2003;4:121–128.

210. Kuchel O. Pseudopheochromocytoma. *Hypertension.* 1985;7:151–158.

211. Kuchel O. New insights into pseudopheochromocytoma and emotionally provoked hypertension. In: Mansoor GA, ed. *Secondary Hypertension.* Totowa, NJ: Humana Press, 2004.

212. Bryant J, Farmer J, Kessler LJ, et al. Pheochromocytoma: The expanding genetic differential diagnosis. *J Natl Cancer Inst.* 2003;95:1196–1204.

213. Neumann HP, Bausch B, McWhinney SR, et al. Germline mutations in nonsyndromic pheochromocytoma. *N Engl J Med.* 2002;346:1459–1466.

214. Gimenez-Roquelo AP, Favier J, Rustin P, et al. Mutations in the SDHB gene are associated with extra-adrenal and/or malignant phaeochromocytomas. *Cancer Res.* 2003;63:5615–5621.

215. Eisenhofer G, Walther MM, Huynh TT, et al. Pheochromocytomas in von Hippel–Lindau syndrome and multiple endocrine neoplasia type 2 display distinct biochemical and clinical phenotypes. *J Clin Endocrinol Metab.* 2001;86:1999–2008.

216. Pacak K, Ilias I, Adams KT, et al. Biochemical diagnosis, localization and management of pheochromocytoma: Focus on multiple endocrine neoplasia type 2 in relation to other hereditary syndromes and sporadic forms of the tumour. *J Intern Med.* 2005;257:60–68.

217. Gertner ME, Kebebew E. Multiple endocrine neoplasia type 2. *Curr Treat Options Oncol.* 2004;5:315–325.

218. Maher ER. Von Hippel–Lindau disease. *Curr Mol Med.* 2004;4:833–842.

219. Hes FJ, Hoppener JW, Lips CJ. Clinical review 155: Pheochromocytoma in Von Hippel–Lindau disease. *J Clin Endocrinol Metab.* 2003;88:969–974.

220. Gimenez-Roqueplo AP, Favier J, Rustin P, et al. Functional consequences of a SDHB gene mutation in an apparently sporadic pheochromocytoma. *J Clin Endocrinol Metab.* 2002;87:4771–4774.

221. Astrom K, Cohen JE, Willett-Brozick JE, et al. Altitude is a phenotypic modifier in hereditary paraganglioma type 1: Evidence for an oxygen-sensing defect. *Hum Genet.* 2003;113:228–237.

222. Baysal BE. Genomic imprinting and environment in hereditary paraganglioma. *Am J Med Genet C Semin Med Genet.* 2004;129:85–90.

223. Astuti D, Latif F, Dallol A, et al. Gene mutations in the succinate dehydrogenase subunit SDHB cause susceptibility to familial pheochromocytoma and to familial paraganglioma. *Am J Hum Genet.* 2001;69:49–54.

224. Gimm O, Armanios M, Dziema H, et al. Somatic and occult germ-line mutations in SDHD, a mitochondrial complex II gene, in nonfamilial pheochromocytoma. *Cancer Res.* 2000;60:6822–6825.

225. Benn DE, Croxson MS, Tucker K, et al. Novel succinate dehydrogenase subunit B (SDHB) mutations in familial phaeochromocytomas and paragangliomas, but an absence of somatic SDHB mutations in sporadic phaeochromocytomas. *Oncogene.* 2003;22:1358–1364.

226. O'Riordain DS, Young WF Jr, Grant CS, et al. Clinical spectrum and outcome of functional extraadrenal paraganglioma. *World J Surg.* 1996;20:916–921.

227. John H, Ziegler WH, Hauri D, et al. Pheochromocytomas: Can malignant potential be predicted? *Urology.* 1999;53:679–683.

228. Sawka AM, Jaeschke R, Singh RJ, et al. A comparison of biochemical tests for pheochromocytoma: Measurement of fractionated plasma metanephrines compared with the combination of 24-hour urinary metanephrines and catecholamines. *J Clin Endocrinol Metab.* 2003;88:553–558.

229. Eisenhofer G, Lenders JW, Goldstein DS, et al. Pheochromocytoma catecholamine phenotypes and prediction of tumor size and location by use of plasma free metanephrines. *Clin Chem.* 2005;51:735–744.

230. Eisenhofer G, Huysmans F, Pacak K, et al. Plasma metanephrines in renal failure. *Kidney Int.* 2005;67:668–677.

231. Eisenhofer G, Goldstein DS, Sullivan P, et al. Biochemical and clinical manifestations of dopamine-producing paragangliomas: Utility of plasma methoxytyramine. *J Clin Endocrinol Metab.* 2005;90:2086–2075.

232. Ilias I, Pacak K. Current approaches and recommended algorithm for the diagnostic

localization of pheohcromocytoma. *J Clin Endocrinol Metab.* 2004;89:479–491.

233. Pacak K, Eisenhofer G, Carrasquillo JA, et al. 6-[^{18}F]Fluorodopamine positron emission tomographic (PET) scanning for diagnostic localization of pheochromocytoma. *Hypertension.* 2001;38:6–8.

234. Ilias I, Yu J, Carrasquillo JA, et al. Superiority of 6-[^{18}F]fluorodopamine positron emission tomography versus [^{131}I]metaiodobenzylguanidine scintigraphy in the localization of metastatic pheochromocytoma. *J Clin Endocrinol Metab.* 2003;88:4083–4087.

235. Schlechte JA. Clinical practice: Prolactinoma. *N Engl J Med.* 2003;349:2035–2041.

236. Haddad SF, VanGilder JC, Menezes AH. Pediatric pituitary tumors. *Neurosurgery.* 1991;29:509–514.

237. Spada A, Mantovani G, Lania A. Pathogenesis of prolactinomas. *Pituitary.* 2005;8: 7–15.

238. Lafferty AR, Chrousos GP. Pituitary tumors in children and adolescents. *J Clin Endocrinol Metab.* 1999;84:4317–4323.

239. Ciccarelli A, Daly AF, Beckers A. The epidemiology of prolactinomas. *Pituitary.* 2005;8:3–6.

240. Fideleff HL, Boquete HR, Sequera A, et al. Peripubertal prolactinomas: Clinical presentation and long-term outcome with different therapeutic approaches. *J Pediatr Endocrinol Metab.* 2000;13:261–267.

241. Lane DE. Polycystic ovary syndrome and its differential diagnosis. *Obstet Gynecol Surv.* 2006;61:125–35.

242. Strachan MW, Teoh WL, Don-Wauchope AC, et al. Clinical and radiological features of patients with macroprolactinaemia. *Clin Endocrinol (Oxf).* 2003;59:339–346.

243. Passos VQ, Souza JJ, Musolino NR, et al. Long-term follow-up of prolactinomas: Normoprolactinemia after bromocriptine withdrawal. *J Clin Endocrinol Metab.* 2002;87:3578–3582.

244. Colao A, Di Sarno A, Cappabianca P, et al. Withdrawal of long-term cabergoline therapy for tumoral and nontumoral hyperprolactinemia. *N Engl J Med.* 2003;349: 2023–2033.

245. Losa M, Mortini P, Barzaghi R, et al. Surgical treatment of prolactin-secreting pituitary adenomas: Early results and long-term outcome. *J Clin Endocrinol Metab.* 2002;87:3180–3186.

246. Metzler M, Luedecke DK, Saeger W, et al. Low prevalence of Gsα mutations in somatotroph adenomas of children and adolescents. *Cancer Genet Cytogenet.* 2006;166: 146–151.

247. Akintoye SO, Chebli C, Booher S, et al. Characterization of gsp-mediated growth hormone excess in the context of McCune–Albright syndrome. *J Clin Endocrinol Metab.* 2002;87:5104–5112.

248. Bossis I, Voutetakis A, Matyakhina L, et al. A pleiomorphic GH pituitary adenoma from a Carney complex patient displays universal allelic loss at the protein kinase A regulatory subunit 1A (PRKARIA) locus. *J Med Genet.* 2004;41:596–600.

249. Pandey P, Ojha BK, Mahapatra AK. Pediatric pituitary adenoma: A series of 42 patients. *J Clin Neurosci.* 2005;12:124–127.

250. Ayuk J, Sheppard MC. Growth hormone and its disorders. *Postgrad Med J.* 2006;82:24–30.

251. Eugster EA, Pescovitz OH. Gigantism. *J Clin Endocrinol Metab.* 1999;84:4379–4384.

252. Drimmie FM, MacLennan AC, Nicoll JA, et al. Gigantism due to growth hormone excess in a boy with optic glioma. *Clin Endocrinol (Oxf).* 2000;53:535–538.

253. Soares BS, Eguchi K, Frohman LA. Tumor deletion mapping on chromosome 11q13 in eight families with isolated familial somatotropinoma and in 15 sporadic somatotropinomas. *J Clin Endocrinol Metab.* 2005;90:6580–6587.

254. Cannavo S, Venturino M, Curto L, et al. Clinical presentation and outcome of pituitary adenomas in teenagers. *Clin Endocrinol (Oxf).* 2003;58:519–527.

255. Melmed S, Casanueva F, Cavagnini F, et al. Consensus statement: Medical management of acromegaly. *Eur J Endocrinol.* 2005;153:737–740.

256. Landis CA, Masters SB, Spada A, et al. GTPase inhibiting mutations activate the alpha chain of Gs and stimulate adenylyl cyclase in human pituitary tumours. *Nature.* 1989;340:692–696.

257. Vallar L, Spada A, Giannattasio G. Altered Gs and adenylate cyclase activity in human GH-secreting pituitary adenomas. *Nature.* 1987;330:566–568.

258. Abe T, Tara LA, Ludecke DK. Growth hormone–secreting pituitary adenomas in childhood and adolescence: Features and results of transnasal surgery. *Neurosurgery.* 1999;45:1–10.

259. Flitsch J, Ludecke DK, Stahnke N, et al. Transsphenoidal surgery for pituitary gigantism and galactorrhea in a 3.5 year old child. *Pituitary.* 2000;2:261–267.

260. Otsuka F, Mizobuchi S, Ogura T, et al. Long-term effects of octreotide on pituitary gigantism: Its analgesic action on cluster headache. *Endocr J.* 2004;51:449–452.

261. Schoof E, Dorr HG, Kiess W, et al. Five-year follow-up of a 13-year-old boy with a pituitary adenoma causing gigantism: Effect of octreotide therapy. *Horm Res.* 2004;61:184–189.

262. Rix M, Laurberg P, Hoejberg AS, et al. Pegvisomant therapy in pituitary gigantism: Successful treatment in a 12-year-old girl. *Eur J Endocrinol.* 2005;153:195–201.

263. Main KM, Sehested A, Feldt-Rasmussen U. Pegvisomant treatment in a 4-year-old girl with neurofibromatosis type 1. *Horm Res.* 2006;65:1–5.

CHAPTER 47

Endocrine Problems in Pediatric Cancer Survivors

Thomas Moshang, Jr., MD
Sogol Mostoufi-Moab, MD

Radiation, chemotherapy, surgery, and bone-marrow transplantation (BMT) all negatively affect endocrine function. Radiation destroys both cancer cells and normal tissue. Tumors themselves can also impact endocrine function prior to radiation. Direct radiation to the brain, gonads, thyroid, or bone can cause primary injury. Multiple hormones may be affected from the central nervous system (CNS) radiation doses used commonly to treat childhood brain tumors. Persistant ovarian failure occurs in approximately 6% of female survivors of childhood cancer; also, infants born of women who received uterine irradiation as children are more likely to be preterm or have a low birth weight. In 32 children and adults who received an average of 54 Gray units (Gy) of radiation (1 gray = 100 rad) to the hypothalamus and pituitary as part of their brain tumor treatment, 28% had one hormone deficiency, 25% lacked two hormones, 25% lacked three hormones, and 12% lacked four hormones. Fewer than 10% of the subjects had all hormone systems intact (1). The hypothalamus is more sensitive to the effects of radiation than the pituitary gland. Of the pituitary hormones, growth hormone (GH) is the most likely to be affected, followed by gonadotropins, adrenocorticotropic hormone (ACTH), and then thyrotropin (TSH). Prolactin and vasopressin functions are not altered by radiation but by tumor effects or surgery (2). GH deficiency is the most common manifestation of neuroendocrine injury following cranial irradiation.

The toxic effects of chemotherapy during the acute phase of cancer treatment are well known. Children often experience malaise, cachexia, lethargy, electrolyte disturbances, hyperglycemia, and growth arrest. Most often these acute effects resolve with the cessation of treatment, but growth failure may persist. The mechanisms are not completely clear. Chemotherapy, particularly with the aklylating chemotherapeutic agents, is known to cause primary gonadal damage (3–6). However, chemotherapy is not known to cause either precocious puberty or gonadotropin deficiency.

While BMT has provided increased survival for a number of children with malignant disease, many survivors of BMT have significant growth failure, primary and/or secondary hypothyroidism, and gonadal failure.

GROWTH FAILURE AND GROWTH HORMONE DEFICIENCY

Pathophysiology and Prevalence GH deficiency is a relatively common endocrine problem in childhood cancer survivors (7). Radiation is the most significant risk factor, particularly if the patient is less than 4 years of age. A number of studies demonstrate growth deceleration or short stature in 40% to 70% of children treated with radiation for brain tumors (8–12), as well as subnormal physiologic GH secretion (13) or decreased GH concentrations following provocative stimuli (8–11,14). Children with non–brain tumor cancers treated with cranial irradiation, such as patients with leukemia or facial tumors, often develop GH deficiency (15,16). Total-body irradiation in preparation for BMT also can result in diminished GH secretion, with isolated GH deficiency observed with radiation doses as low as 10 Gy (17). The frequency of radiation-induced GH deficiency in fact may be underestimated because the reported numbers could be influenced by the test used to assess GH secretion, that is, physiological versus pharmacological tests (18), as well as not testing children because of marginally normal growth velocities. In addition, early onset of puberty is common after cranial radiation, further reducing final adult height. The younger the child is at the time of radiation, the greater likelihood there is for earlier onset of puberty.

The effects of irradiation on GH function are dose-dependent. In children with leukemia, the pubertal increase in spontaneous GH secretion is diminished with a radiation dose greater than 18 Gy, whereas above 24 Gy, all spontaneous GH secretion is decreased. Above 27 Gy, the GH response to provocative stimuli may be blunted (14). However, even high-dose cranial irradiation can be associated with incongruently normal GH responses to provocative stimuli in the presence of deficient spontaneous secretion of GH (8).

GH deficiency following cranial irradiation not only depends on the cumulative dosage but also on the fraction sizes of radiation over time interval, the age of the patient, and the time interval between treatment and evaluation of GH production. A larger fraction size of radiation administered over a shorter time interval is more likely to cause GH deficiency than smaller fraction sizes administered over longer periods of time (14,19). In younger children, the same doses of radiation are more likely to cause GH deficiency (20,21) than comparable doses given to older children. Note that while GH deficiency may not develop immediately after radiation, it has been shown to develop progressively over time (22,23). Several studies suggest that 80% to 85% of children treated with significant doses of irradiation will fail provocative GH testing by 2 years after radiation treatment (14) or during adolescence (24), indicating a need for continued surveillance. It is important to recognize, however, that children still may grow normally despite failing GH provocative stimulation tests (25). In particular, children with hypothalamic–chiasmatic glioma, for reasons not yet determined, often grow normally following significant radiation exposure (2).

Chemotherapy also may influence growth, by inhibiting insulin growth factor 1 (lgF-1) production by the liver. (26). Protocols using melphalan appeared to impair growth significantly (27), whereas protocols using busulfan and cyclophosphamide without total-body irradiation for acute myeloproliferative disease resulted in significantly better growth in children (28–30). Most studies indicate

Endocrine Problems of Childhood Cancer Survivors

AT-A-GLANCE

By 2010, it is estimated that approximately 1 in 700 adults will be childhood cancer survivors. These individuals are at increased risk for a variety of health problems, and endocrine dysfunction (7) affects approximately 40% of all long-term survivors. In some cases, the cause is the cancer itself, as in hormone-producing tumors (Sertoli–Leydig cell tumors or adrenal carcinoma) or tumors that disrupt hormone secretion (craniopharyngioma). In the majority of cases, it is the curative treatment that is damaging because radiation and chemotherapy have a negative effect on multiple endocrine systems. Whether or not "late effects" or therapy-related sequelae occur depends on several factors, including the type of cancer, the type of treatment received, and the patient's age at treatment.

ENDOCRINE PROBLEM	OCCURRENCE	CAUSE
Growth hormone deficiency	40–80%	• Pituitary–hypothalamic tumors • Cranial irradiation (doses > 24 Gy or lesser doses in younger patients)
Central precocious puberty	20%	• Hypothalamic brain tumors • Cranial irradiation (12–18 Gy, but higher doses of 23–39 Gy also may be causative)
Central (secondary) gonadal failure	30–40%	• Cranial irradiation (>40 Gy)
Primary gonadal failure	100%	• Direct gonadal irradiation (>0.4 Gy or 400 cGy in adult males)
A. Males–infertility	Unknown	• Alkylating chemotherapy
Hormonal dysfunction	Infrequent	• Direct gonadal irradiation with 10 Gy
B. Females–fertility	Unknown	• Abdominal irradiation (>10 Gy) • Alkylating chemotherapy
Hormonal dysfunction	Infrequent	• Alkylating chemotherapy
Primary hypothyroidism	30–80%	• Direct neck irradiation (10–20 Gy) • Spinal irradiation >30 Gy
Secondary (central) hypothyroidism	15–65%	• Cranial irradiation
Diabetes insipidus	100%	• Pituitary stalk surgery
Central salt wasting	10–20%	• Acute complication of brain tumor, surgery, increased CNS pressure, radiation treatment
ACTH insufficiency	10–20%	• Pituitary or hypothalamic tumor • Surgery • High-dose radiation (>50 Gy)
Decreased bone growth/osteoporosis	Unknown	• Radiation, chemotherapy • Bone-marrow transplant • Growth hormone deficiency
Metabolic syndrome	Unknown	• Irradiation, perhaps chemotherapy • Growth hormone deficiency

that chemotherapy alone does not cause GH deficiency, alter hypothalamic–pituitary–target gland axes, or exacerbate skeletal disproportion. However, chemotherapy in combination with radiation may have a deleterious effect on growth (31,32). Children with medulloblastoma treated with chemotherapy and craniospinal irradiation grow worse than similar patients treated with identical doses of craniospinal irradiation alone (31). The time interval before diagnosis of GH deficiency following treatment for medulloblastoma in 22 children treated with craniospinal radiation and adjuvant chemotherapy was 3.5 years compared with 5.1 years in 7 children treated with radiation alone (Moshang, unpublished observations). This synergism is also observed in other areas of neurodevelopment, where radiation damage to hearing and intelligence is increased by the addition of chemotherapy (33). Glucocorticoids are known to inhibit growth through a number of mechanisms, including altered bone metabolism, loss of bone calcium, decreased gut absorption of calcium and phosphorus, and competitive antagonism to GH action.

Spinal radiation is part of the treatment of brain tumors to prevent spinal relapse and is associated with disproportionate growth (decreased upper to lower segment ratios) and an adverse effect on final adult height due to direct effect on spine and growth plates (8,34). The younger age at the time of radiation, the greater is the loss in growth potential due to impaired spinal growth (34).

Growth outcome following total-body irradiation for BMT preconditioning is variable, ranging from significant growth failure to achievement of normal adult height, albeit generally shorter than expected based on pretreatment heights and midparental heights. These variations in adult height outcomes probably are related to a number of factors, including the type of malignancy, the cancer and preconditioning chemotherapy and radiation regimens (i.e., dose and fractionation), and the age of the patient. There is a significant relationship between the age of the child at BMT and subsequent growth velocity, with a significantly worse growth outcome in the younger transplanted child (27,35).

In a study of patients with neuroblastoma and BMT treatment, more than 50% responded poorly to standard doses (0.3 mg/kg/week) of GH, suggesting GH resistance (36). Similarly, other investigators have found normal or high levels of insulin-like growth factor 1 (IGF-1) in poorly growing children following BMT, suggesting IGF-1 resistance (37). Whether higher than usual doses of GH might overcome the GH insensitivity is not known.

Diagnosis and Surveillance Children should be seen by a pediatric endocrinologist early following cancer therapy and followed regularly to establish a pattern of growth surveillance. Acute growth failure is common during the initial and early phases of cancer therapy, and poor growth often persists for a year or longer after completion of cancer treatments. This initial phase of poor growth probably is due to the acute toxic effects of irradiation or chemotherapy, including glucocorticoid therapy. There may or may not be a subsequent period of catch-up growth, followed by a decline in growth velocity in patients with GH deficiency. Interval growth velocity should be calculated at each visit because growth deceleration is frequently an earlier sign of GH deficiency than short stature. Comparison of actual growth velocity with standard growth velocity charts and attention to the timing and magnitude of the expected pubertal growth spurt are important factors in the clinical assessment of growth in cancer survivors, especially adolescents.

Accurate determinations of standing height, using a stadiometer with at least three determinations at each visit, should be done every 6 months. Sitting height and arm-span measurements should be determined, and upper segment (sitting height) to lower segment (standing height minus sitting height) ratios should be calculated to uncover disproportionate growth (34). Growth data from the primary pediatrician should be obtained to determine growth patterns prior to the diagnosis of malignancy. Parental heights should be determined to establish a target height based on midparental heights.

Children who demonstrate growth deceleration or, in the case of pubertal children, who fail to grow at normal pubertal growth velocities despite clinical findings of developing secondary sexual characteristics need evaluation for GH deficiency. Initial screening studies should aim to exclude other medical causes of growth failure and include routine serum chemistry and hematological profiles, erythrocyte sedimentation rate, thyroid function tests, (free T_4 and TSH) and a hand–wrist radiograph for determination of skeletal age. Routine skeletal age progression is useful for monitoring progression of physiological maturation. However, normal bone age progression in a cancer survivor who is failing to grow is not unusual and should not deter one's clinical judgment that evaluation of growth failure is indicated. Serum concentrations of testosterone, estradiol sensitive, and gonadotropin levels, as determined by ultrasensitive assays (38), should be monitored in boys and girls who are of pubertal age or showing signs of pubertal development.

Measurement of serum IGF-1 and IGFBP-3 has become standard in the evaluation of growth in children. Serum concentrations of IGF-1 and IGFBP-3 exhibit little diurnal variation, accurately reflect spontaneous GH secretion, and have been reported to be up to 95% sensitive and specific for diagnosing GH deficiency in children (39–41). However, serum IGF-1 levels often are reduced in children with malnutrition and other catabolic diseases, and considerable overlap in IGF-1 levels exists between short normal children and children with true GH deficiency. Furthermore, a number of studies have demonstrated that IGF-1 and IGFBP-3 concentrations may be less accurate in diagnosing GH deficiency in children with brain tumors (42) and in children treated with cranial irradiation (43,44). In a series of 72 children with GH deficiency and brain tumors, normal IGF-1 levels were found in 27% of patients, and normal IGFBP-3 levels were found in 50%. IGF-1 and IGFBP-3 levels were particularly ineffective in predicting GH deficiency in pubertal children and in children with hypothalamic–chiasmatic glioma, of whom 33% had precocious puberty (42). Puberty, whether normal or precocious, may mask true GH deficiency. The increase in gonadal steroids both improves growth velocity, hiding the clinical finding of poor growth, and increases serum concentrations of IGF-1 and IGFBP-3 (45–47), masking the biochemical markers of GH deficiency.

Clinical judgment in conjunction with laboratory testing should be used to make the diagnosis of GH deficiency. The clinical diagnosis takes into account the location of the tumor, extent of pituitary resection or cranial irradiation, growth velocity of the patient, pubertal stage, bone age, IGF-1 and IGFBP-3 levels, and the results of provocative GH testing. Some GH-deficient children with signs of growth failure may demonstrate neurosecretory GH dysfunction and growth deceleration despite normal levels of growth factors and normal GH responses to provocative secretagogues (14).

Treatment Although GH therapy has been successful in improving growth in GH-deficient children following tumor treatment (48,49), adult height still is likely to fall short of midparental target height even with GH therapy (32,50). This is true especially for children who have received chemotherapy in addition to cranial irradiation (32,50) or who have received radiation to the spine (32,50,51) and for children following BMT (52). The decreased effectiveness of GH in such patients is multifactorial, including delay in receiving GH (pending assurance of cancer remission), direct skeletal injury from irradiation, resistance to GH therapy, and early puberty.

The dose of GH may influence adult height. GH therapy in cancer survivors is initiated at a dose of 0.3 mg/kg/week as it has been shown that they grow better on this GH dose compared to patients treated with a GH dose of 0.15 mg/kg/week (53). Similarly, children with medulloblastoma treated with a GH dose of 0.3 mg/kg/week (50) achieved a height significantly taller than brain tumor survivors treated with 0.15 mg/kg/week (32).

Although untested, the use of pubertal dosing might overcome poor GH response. Doses as high as 0.7 mg/kg/week during puberty result in greater growth in GH-deficient children than that achieved with standard GH doses (54), perhaps by mimicking the normal increase in GH that occurs during puberty (55,56). Furthermore, in children who received spinal irradiation, the loss in spinal growth is greatest during puberty (51). Final height in children in early puberty can be improved with the addition of a gonadotropin-releasing hormone (GnRH) agonist to the GH therapy to restrain normal puberty and delay epiphyseal closure (57). Aromatase inhibitors (AI) such as Anastrozole and Letrozole may have a promising role in prepubertal GH deficient children with advanced bone age. AI may increase final adult height by prolonging the period of growth as they delay bone maturation and epiphyseal closure.

GH therapy in patients who received total-body irradiation or spinal irradiation has not been shown to increase the incidence of scoliosis or kyphosis but rather increase the severity of these conditions caused by irradiation, as noted by a greater need for orthopedic intervention (58). There is more need for bracing and surgical intervention in patients on GH compared with the general adolescent population. It is not known whether a higher dose of GH during puberty further aggravates spinal deformities.

Risk of Recurrence or Second Cancer

A waiting period of 1 year after completion of tumor therapy and with no evidence of further tumor growth is recommended by the Lawson Wilkins Pediatric Endocrinology Society before initiating GH therapy (59). Some would wait 2 years before initiation of GH therapy (60). Craniopharyngioma is a benign tumor, and patients can be treated when it is clear that the tumor is stable (often 1 year after surgery). However, despite the fact that the tumor is benign, the recurrence rate is significant. The potential mitogenic stimulation of GH causing tumor recurrence is a serious concern and should be discussed with the family. However, most outcome studies (57–65) suggest that GH therapy does not increase the

incidence of recurrence in patients with CNS tumors such as craniopharyngioma, medulloblastoma, and hypothalamic glioma, the three most common pediatric brain tumors or other tumors such as rhabdomyosarcoma, neuroblastroma and leukemia. Treatment with GH may increase risk of secondary solid tumors but the overall risk remains small and appears to diminish over time (66). Meningiomas are the most common secondary neoplasia in GH-treated cancer survivors, all of whom receive cranial irradiation. Although meningiomas may develop after cranial irradiation (67), a true effect of GH can not be ruled out as meningiomas express GH/IGF-1 receptors. There is a shorter latency period between radiation and meningioma in GH-treated patients.

Cancer surveillance should be monitored closely, including appropriate imaging studies after initiation of GH therapy (such as a repeat MRI with contrast material in brain tumor patient within 6 months). Further, IGF-1 levels should be monitored and GH dose adjusted so that the IGF-1 level does not exceed 2 SDs of that appropriate for Tanner stage and gender.

GH for the Young Adult

For young-adult cancer survivors with known GH deficiency, it is generally recommended that GH treatment be continued for life to reduce risks for cardiovascular mortality and other features of the metabolic syndrome, as well as to improve bone mineral density. Patients with childhood-onset GHD should be retested 3 months after stopping GH therapy to determine whether GH therapy should continue through adulthood. However, patients with severe organic GHD and multiple pituitary hormone deficiencies can be excluded from retesting in accordance to a consensus statement by the GH Research Society (69). Although there is not much data regarding the transition to adult GH therapy in cancer survivors, GH therapy may improve cardiac systolic function, body composition and may decrease the prevalence of metabolic syndrome (68–69).

The "gold standard" for testing for GH deficiency in the adult patient is the insulin tolerance test (ITT), with a peak GH < 3µg/l being diagnostic of GH deficiency (70). Because many cancer survivors, especially brain tumor patients, are at risk for hypoglycemic seizures during ITT due to underlying seizure disorders the combination of GHRH and arginine has been suggested to provide concordant results with ITT (71); a recent study comparing the two tests in young-adult medulloblastoma survivors showed that GHRH–arginine testing often will misdiagnose GH sufficiency compared with the results by ITT (72). Therefore, the optimal way

to diagnose GH deficiency in young adults after cranial irradiation remains ITT until other provocative GH stimulation tests are shown to be concordant with ITT.

CENTRAL AND PERIPHERAL DISTURBANCES IN PUBERTY FOLLOWING CANCER THERAPY

Pathophysiology and Prevalence Precocious puberty can occur following either low- or high-dose cranial radiation, or it can be related directly to the tumor type or the tumor location. Patients with chiasmatic or hypothalamic glioma, pinealoma, hypothalamic hamartoma, and ependymoma may present with precocious puberty. Hypothalamic hamartoma causes precocious puberty due to production of GnRH, but the other tumors probably disrupt hypothalamic–pituitary mechanisms that control the onset of puberty. Except for hypothalamic harmatoma, it is unusual for brain tumors to present with isolated precocious puberty without other CNS signs or symptoms.

In patients with leukemia, doses of 18 Gy to the brain result in a significant number of survivors with early puberty (72,73). In patients with medulloblastoma, who generally are treated with 30 Gy to the hypothalamus, early puberty is also common (as much as 90% in one study) (74), indicating that either high- or low-dose cranial radiation can disrupt neuroendocrine control of puberty.

Gonadotropin deficiency with lack of onset or progression of puberty is more common than precocious puberty following high-dose cranial irradiation. In children with hypothalamic–chiasmatic glioma, following high-dose cranial radiation, 25% to 33% of patients demonstrate hypogonadotropic hypogonadism, including some children who presented initially with precocious puberty (2). Precocious puberty is likely to be due to injury that alters regulation of the onset of puberty, but ionizing radiation eventually is destructive, thereby causing gonadotropin deficiency.

Direct gonadal irradiation, most often because of leukemic infiltration, typically results in permanent primary gonadal failure. In an ethically questionable study on normal adult male incarcerated volunteers, spermatogonia were damaged at radiation doses as low as 0.2 Gy (200 cGy) (75). Even with doses of less than 10 Gy, damage can occur to testicular germ cells and ovarian follicular cells (76,77). Prepubertal gonads appear to be somewhat less radiosensitive, although there are no studies indicating the degree of sensitivity or insensitivity of gonads to radiation. Following direct radiation to the gonads during childhood, follicle-stimulating hormone (FSH) serum concentrations may be elevated in the presence of normal luteinizing hormone (LH) levels and normal development of secondary sexual characteristics, indicating follicular or spermatogonia damage with preservation of sex steroid producing cells. This clinical observation suggests that spermatogonia and ova are more likely to be injured with radiation and chemotherapy than sex steroids producing cells. Alkylator chemotherapy may result in irregular menses or irreversible amenorrhea.

Women surviving childhood cancer, excluding brain tumors, have evidence for poor ovarian development, even when they have not received abdominal radiation or alkylating chemotherapy (6). The combination of radiotherapy and chemotherapy, even with the exclusion of alkylating agents, may be particularly detrimental to gonadal function. A study by Larsen and colleagues evaluated adult women treated for pediatric cancers and found diminished ovarian volume as well as decreased numbers of follicles, even in women with spontaneous menstrual cycles and those treated only with nonalkylating agents and radiation above the diaphragm (7). These findings suggest that women followed into adulthood after having survived pediatric cancer therapy are at risk for premature ovarian failure. Data from the Childhood Cancer Survivor Study (CCSS) showed acute ovarian failure (AOF) within 5 years of tumor diagnosis in 6.3 % of 3390 women aged over 18 years (3). Identified risk factors for AOF were older age at tumor diagnosis, Hodgkin's lymphoma, ovarian radiation less or equal of 10Gy or alkylating agents at ages 13–20 years, when compares with survivors without AOF.

Diagnosis and Surveillance Accurate assessment of the pubertal stage and growth rate should be done in all children at each visit to identify those with aberrant developmental patterns. Yearly radiographs of the hand and wrist should be performed for the determination of the skeletal age as an assessment of physiological maturation in children surviving cancer. With clinical findings of either sexual precocity or delay, laboratory assessment includes the measurement of serum levels of prolactin, testosterone, and/or estradiol, LH and FSH, and a bone age. Primary hypogonadism will be reflected by elevated gonadotropins, especially FSH. The usefulness of inhibin B and anti-Müllerian hormone has not yet been established in the evaluation of gonadal function in adolescent cancer survivors.

Treatment in Early Puberty Precocious puberty is treated with long-acting GnRH agonists, which, if initiated early, contribute to improvements in final height outcome (78). Adequacy of suppression is demonstrated by serial clinical assessment, bone age radiographs, and in boys, documentation of prepubertal serum testosterone levels. In girls, suppression of the hypothalamic-pituitary-gonadal axis is indicated by LH and FSH levels less than 0.3–0.5 mIU/ml. Gonadotropins levels should be measured three months after the initiation of GnRH agonist therapy and then at frequent intervals (3–4 months). Parents are instructed to bring the dose of GNRH to the clinic so that gonadotropin levels and sex steroids are measured before the dose is given (see Chapter 33) (79). If there appears to be lack of suppression of LH/FSH levels, the dose may need to be either given more frequently, such as every 3 weeks, or increased further. Parents and patients with precocious puberty due to brain tumor or to cranial irradiation should be informed of subsequent development of hypogonadotropic hypogonadism.

In children who also have GH deficiency, the onset of puberty, even at an appropriate age, may interfere with the response to GH therapy by limiting the time available for catch-up growth, and thus puberty may need to be suppressed. The combined use of a long-acting GnRH agonist with GH has been demonstrated to improve adult height in cranial radiation patients with GH deficiency (57,80). Aromatase inhibitors also may delay bone maturation and epiphyseal closure and their role needs to be explored.

Treatment in Delayed Puberty or Sexual Arrest Male hormone replacement during pubertal years is accomplished through monthly doses of intramuscular testosterone enanthate or cypionate, starting at 50 mg and increasing gradually over 2–3 years to 200 mg every 2–4 weeks (see Chapter 37). Transdermal testosterone patches and gels appropriate for adult males are available and may produce more consistent serum levels of testosterone in older adolescents who have completed growth and sexual maturation. There are ongoing studies using transdermal gels to determine appropriate dosing during puberty as to prevent premature epiphyseal fusion. Female hormone replacement usually is initiated with low doses of conjugated estrogens. Premarin 0.3 mg or ethinyl estradiol 2 µg is used and increased over the next 1–2 years, after which a progestin such as medroxyprogesterone acetate or Provera is added for 5–7 days each month to induce bleeding (see Chapter 36). Estrogen patches with estradiol concentrations low enough for use in prepubertal girls can be used instead of conjugated estrogen pills, such as starting with a once-a-week 0.014-mg patch. The dose can be increased subsequently to 0.025 mg every

6 months until menstrual bleeding occurs. Once cycling has been induced, it is generally more convenient in adolescents to use one of the estrogen–progestin combination oral contraceptive pills. Monitoring of gonadal steroid replacement usually is accomplished clinically, although trough testosterone levels may provide useful information for dose titration in males. Assessment of skeletal maturation every 6 to 12 months will assure normal bone maturation and final adult height. It is important to note that children treated with cranial irradiation have significant risk for seizures, radiation angiitis, cerebrovascular bleeding, and thrombosis. Therefore, the risks of thrombosis and vascular problems associated with estrogen therapy in girls may be increased.

In patients with secondary hypogonadism, fertility may be possible and a referral should be facilitated during the reproductive years. Children treated with direct gonadal irradiation or alkylating chemotherapeutic agents most likely will develop infertility. There are experimental trials attempting to preserve fertility for sexually immature patients by using GnRH agonists or cryopreservation of gonadal tissue. In two recent articles traditional and recent developments for fertility options and preservation are described as well as the recommendations of American Society of Clinical Oncology on fertility preservation in cancer patients (81,82). Parents and hypogonadal patients should be explained that gonadal steroid–replacement therapy most likely will be necessary for the greater part of adult life to maintain bone mineral density, vaginal and prostate secretion, libido, energy, and quality of life.

HYPOTHYROIDISM

Pathophysiology and Prevalence Hypothyroidism in cancer survivors can be primary, secondary, or mixed. Direct radiotoxic effects to thyroid tissue result in primary hypothyroidism. Irradiation to the head and neck for treatment of brain tumors produces permanent primary hypothyroidism in about 16% to 30% of patients (8,82,83). Primary hypothyroidism is seen in 60% to 80% of patients receiving direct neck irradiation for lymphoma (84–88). This effect appears to be dose-related, with a threshold effect of approximately 10 Gy (87) resulting in elevation of TSH known as *subclinical hypothyroidism* and clinically significant thyroid dysfunction at about 20 Gy (82, 87). The peak incidence of primary hypothyroidism following irradiation is noted after 2–4 years, but thyroid dysfunction may develop after as many as 25 years following radiotherapy (88,89). Primary hypothyroidism is rarely isolated in cancer survivors; only 18% of patients with mild primary hypothyroidism had mild TSH elevation alone; the remainder also had hypothalamic–pituitary hormone deficiencies as well (84).

Central hypothyroidism is recognized to occur in as many as 65% of patients with brain and nasopharygeal tumors and 15% of patients following cranial irradiation for leukemia. *Mixed hypothyroidism* refers to children following cranial or craniospinal (>30 Gy) or a BMT preparatory regimen in whom there is elevation of TSH with a combined absence of the nocturnal TSH surge, suggesting both a peripheral and central pathology (90); however mixed hypothyroidism is not always associated with raised basal TSH. A low normal free T_4 values (in the lowest third of the normal range) is highly suspicious of central or mixed hypothyroidism. If raised daytime TSH values used as the sole criterion for hypothyroidism, most cases of central hypothyroidism and mixed hypothyroidism will be missed and the diagnosis will be delayed until the slow down of growth velocity.

Chemotherapy generally has not been implicated in thyroid dysfunction, although one study showed an increase in TSH levels in 44% of patients with Hodgkin lymphoma treated only with chemotherapy (91). This finding has not been substantiated by other studies. However, a number of chemicals, such as various halogens, minerals (lithium), and anticonvulsant drugs, can interfere with thyroid function. Many of these drugs are part of the medical armamentarium used in treating various late effects of cancer survivors.

Diagnosis and Surveillance Many of the symptoms and signs of hypothyroidism are nonspecific and overlap with the side effects of cancer therapy, with the most frequent complaints being fatigue, lack of energy, and lethargy. Hypotension and/or bradycardia may be noted on examination. The more classical signs and symptoms of hypothyroidism, including constipation, myxedema, and cold intolerance, usually are not found in children following cancer treatment. Mild primary hypothyroidism should be suspected in children with mildly elevated TSH and T_4 levels within normal limits, when there is a slow down of the growth velocity in children or poor response to GH therapy. Thyroid replacement therapy even in mild hypothyroidism would improve growth velocity (90). Therefore, laboratory monitoring of thyroid function should be done routinely. Using baseline FT_4 and TSH alone, 92% of those with central hypothyroidism and 27% of those with mixed hypothyroidism can be missed by standard laboratory screening (90). Monitoring for decline in free thyroxine (FT_4) and rise in serum TSH, and early recognition of either

primary or mixed hypothyroidism is clinically valuable. TSH surge and TRH tests, will differentiate between primary and mixed hypothyroidism. Normally, TSH secretion occurs in a circadian pattern with lower concentrations in the afternoon, a nocturnal surge beginning after 1900 h, and higher concentrations between 2200 h and 0400 h. Both children and adults normally experience a nocturnal surge in TSH of 50–300% as a normal circadian event.

The most sensitive indicator of central and mixed hypothyroidism is a blunted or absent nocturnal surge of TSH, with a TSH response to thyrotropin-releasing hormone (TRH) that is often normal or prolonged (90). Both tests are necessary for the identification of all cases of central or mixed hypothyroidism. However, nocturnal studies often are difficult, and at present, synthetic TRH for diagnostic evaluation of thyroid axis in hypothalamic–pituitary disorders is no longer available. Thus, determination of thyroid function generally will be based only on TSH and free thyroxine (T_4). In patients treated with cranial irradiation, in whom hypothyroidism is more likely to be secondary or tertiary, the clinician can only rely on free T_4 values and clinical judgment if nocturnal surge of TSH can not be evaluated. Since the patient's baseline free T_4 level prior to cancer diagnosis and treatment generally is not known, low-normal values of free T_4 may indicate a need for thyroid hormone replacement.

Treatment Treatment of children with hypothyroidism typically is initiated at doses of 2–3 μg of L-thyroxine per kilogram per day. Despite norlmalization of thyroid function tests, many of these patients may continue to complain of lethargy and lack of energy. The addition of a small amount triiodothyronine (T_3) might be a useful adjunct to therapy, yet at this time it still remains an open question. Repeat thyroid studies should be obtained 6–8 weeks after the initiation of therapy or dose change and, in stable patients, once or twice yearly. Free T_4 levels should be maintained in the upper half of the normal range. TSH in patients with secondary or tertiary hypothyroidism is low and they do not need to be measured. In children with primary or mixed hypothyroidism, maintenance of TSH levels in the lower half of the normal range (<3.0 μU/mL) is an appropriate assessment for adequacy of thyroid treatment.

ADRENAL INSUFFICIENCY

Pathophysiology and Prevalence Primary adrenal insufficiency is not a consequence of cancer treatment except when the malignancy involves the adrenal gland or when the

use of ketoconazole is required to treat opportunistic fungal infections. Prolonged use of glucocorticoids as part of chemotherapy or to treat graft-versus-host disease following BMT results in suppresion of the hypothalamic-pituitary-adrenal (HPA) axis. Permanent ACTH deficiency can develop following central irradiation or when brain tumors or brain surgery cause panhypopituitarism. Clinical ACTH deficiency is uncommon in patients receiving less than 50 Gy to the hypothalamus and pituitary, but more subtle defects in the hypothalamic–pituitary–adrenal axis may be seen with doses between 35 and 50 Gy, such as decreased ACTH levels in response to either metyrapone or corticotropin-releasing hormone (CRH) stimulation testing. ACTH deficiency is reported to occur in 18% to 35% of patients (22,92).

Diagnosis and Surveillance The signs and symptoms of adrenal insufficiency following cancer therapy tend to be nonspecific. In general, following cranial irradiation, ACTH deficiency is not manifested by electrolyte or cardiovascular disturbances but often by lethargy, failure to thrive, and anorexia.

Routine determination of early-morning cortisol levels to monitor for adrenal insufficiency can miss up to 25% of patients who otherwise would be detected by dynamic tests of the hypothalamic–pituitary–adrenal (HPA) axis. Insulin tolerance testing, for evaluation of the HPA axis may be associated with an increased risk of hypoglycemic seizure in brain tumor survivors, who already may have an underlying seizure disorder. CRH testing soon after irradiation may be normal in children with early dysfunction of the HPA axis. Thus the low-dose (1 μg) ACTH stimulation test is preferred (93). A normal cortisol response to this test which is a peak cortisol level >18 μg/dl or 500 nmol/l, reassuring for that moment in time, that clinical concerns prompted adrenal evaluation. However, because the effects of radiation on the brain can manifest years later, repeated dynamic testing of the HPA axis may be necessary (94).

Treatment In children with demonstrated adrenal insufficiency, which is almost always secondary or tertiary, the lowest dose of glucocorticoids to alleviate symptoms of lethargy, anorexia, nausea, or vomiting is recommended. Persistence of symptoms with doses higher than physiological replacement (10–15 mg/m²/day) or even with "stress dosing" (30–50 mg/m²/day) probably is not due to adrenal insufficiency. In fact, many children with biochemical evidence of adrenal insufficiency based on CRH or low-dose ACTH testing are asymptomatic and do very well without daily glucocorticoid replacement. However, this latter group of patients must be counseled to use stress doses of glucocorticoids with an illness.

There is no clear consensus regarding the duration of adrenal suppression following high-dose glucocorticoid therapy and the optimal protocol for weaning of hydrocortisone (95). In general, maintenance oral hydrocortisone treatment of 8–12 mg/m^2/day should be initiated in children who have received prolonged high-dose glucocorticoids for cancer therapy. Maintenance hydrocortisone then is weaned slowly, with a gradual tapering of 10% to 20% of the total daily dose over a number of weeks. During this time, families should be instructed to give stress doses of hydrocortisone during stress or illness; stress doses of hydrocortisone, typically are three to five times the maintenance dose.

EFFECTS OF CANCER THERAPY ON BONE

Pathophysiology and Prevalence Decreased bone density, skeletal deformities, avascular necrosis are some of effects of cancer therapy on bone. Direct radiation to bone, cranial radiation (decreased bone formation secondary to GH deficiency), gonadal failure (increased bone resorption due to decreased sex steroids), methotrexate and corticosteroids, all can cause bone damage. Some primary or metastatic cancers damage bone directly. More commonly, bone injury is due to radiotherapy. Certain cancers, such as medulloblastoma, require spinal irradiation to prevent or treat metastases to the spinal cord. Children about to undergo BMT often will be prepared with total-body irradiation. The mechanisms of radiation-induced injury to bone are many but mostly involve altered chondroblastic activity. Epiphyseal injury arrests chondrogenesis, whereas metaphyseal injury decreases the absorptive processes and leads to decreased trabeculation. In contrast, diaphyseal injury results in faulty bone modeling through altered periosteal activity (96). Blood vessels supplying the bones also can be damaged, compounding the primary bone injury by poor blood support for healing. Spinal irradiation can cause scoliosis by attenuating spinal growth with fibrosis of adjacent muscle tissue. Adult height thus is compromised by the loss of vertebral height, scoliosis, and muscle atrophy.

Relatively long limbs compared with a short trunk often characterize adult stature in cancer survivors treated with craniospinal irradiation. There may be a decreased upper to lower segment ratio (8) or a sitting height lower than the mean for age-matched normal children (11). This disproportionate reduction in spinal growth becomes most evident during puberty (51). Although most of the observed radiation-induced skeletal effects occur in the spine, these effects may extend to other bones. Because the skeletal tissue is injured, growth failure may be resistant to GH therapy (36). One study in patients treated with craniospinal irradiation demonstrated improved adult height using high doses of GH, but the sitting height was still impaired, suggesting that the limbs responded better to GH than the trunk (50).

Injury to bone is further manifested by decreased bone mineral content in adults surviving cancer treatment as children. In young adults treated for childhood leukemia, osteopenia has been documented in patients with no evidence of GH deficiency (97). Radiation clearly is a cause of osteopenia (98). GH deficiency per se also has an adverse effect on bone mineral density, and thus, for many young-adult survivors of childhood cancer, the combination of GH deficiency and radiotherapy translates into a significant risk for osteopenia and osteoporosis.

Diagnosis and Surveillance Adult patients surviving childhood cancer should have periodic dual-energy x-ray absorption (DXA) scans. There are questions about the best approach in children, and at present, there are very few studies in the pediatric age range that evaluate bone density in cancer survivors. Part of the difficulty arises from the techniques used for studying bone density. The most acceptable technique, DXA, has serious limitations, including a paucity of normative data for children, especially data correcting for height or pubertal development (99). Therefore, the degree of decreased bone mineral density due to GH deficiency, compared with the degree directly related to the toxic effects of cancer treatment is still not clear. Developing techniques such as peripheral quantitative computed tomography with appropriate age, gender, and pubertal standards may provide better assessment of bone health in children.

Treatment Good nutrition, sufficient calcium and vitamin D intake, and physical activity are essential. GH therapy and sex hormone replacement in GH-deficient patients with gonadal failure may improve bone density. There are sufficient data to suggest that significant injury to bone formation is due to cancer therapy per se and not just GH deficiency or other hormonal deficiencies. Therefore, it follows that hormonal therapy may not completely restore bone mineral health and that it may be necessary to use other means, including biphosphonates, to permit children to develop normal peak bone density as young adults (98).

DIABETES INSIPIDUS AND SIADH

Pathophysiology and Prevalence Diabetes insipidus (DI) is a common occurrence following neurosurgery in the area of the pituitary stalk or due to tumors of the pituitary or hypothalamus such as hypothalamic germinoma. Following surgery involving the pituitary stalk, DI is almost a certainty. In tumors involving the pituitary stalk, such as craniopharyngioma or germinoma, the onset of DI is more variable. Symptoms of DI include excessive thirst and urination, free water loss with dilute urine, and dehydration. Biochemical findings include hypernatremia, increased serum osmolality, decreased urinary osmolality and decreased urinary sodium loss (see Chapter 41).

Acutely following surgery, there also can be temporary inappropriate vasopressin secretion (SIADH). It is typically transient and occurs in the immediate postoperative period in the setting of increased intracranial pressure or injury to the infundibular stalk. Late SIADH, occurring many years after cranial radiation, may be due to cerebrovascular hemorrhage and/or stroke from radiation angiitis due to changes in intracranial pressure or CNS infection. SIADH is characterized by oliguria, hyponatremia, increased urinary sodium loss (>20–30 meq/l), decreased serum osmolality and inappropriately increased urine osmolality (>200 mOsm/kg).

Diagnosis and Surveillance Fluid balance, including urine output, always should be monitored closely in the postoperative period following neurosurgery. Chronically, for brain tumor patients or those who have received central irradiation, a careful history for evidence of problems with fluid balance should be obtained at every visit, and the patient and/or family should be informed of symptoms that require medical attention. Profuse dilute urine output and elevated serum sodium levels suggest the diagnosis of DI. Formal water deprivation testing, in which controlled dehydration is employed to stimulate the secretion of antidiuretic hormone, is seldom necessary.

Treatment Treatment of DI involves hormone replacement with a long-acting synthetic form of antidiuretic hormone, such as desmopressin (DDAVP), via an intranasal solution or spray or an oral tablet (see Chapter 41). Adequacy of vasopressin replacement is assessed by monitoring serum electrolytes, fluid intake, weight and urine output. In patients with an intact thirst-sensing mechanism, the goal of treatment is to reduce urinary volume and frequency. This is usually accomplished with once-nightly or

TABLE 47-1   Findings in Inadequately Treated DI, Fluid Overload or Vasopressin Excess, SIADH, and Salt Wasting

	DI–Inadequate Treatment	Excess Water or Vasopressin	SIADH	Salt Wasting
Serum sodium	High	Low	Low	Low
Urine sodium	Low	Low	High	High
Urine output	Excessive	Normal or low	Oliguric	Excessive
Hydration	Dehydrated	Mild edema	Mild edema	Dehydrated
Treatment	Increase vasopressin	Restrict fluid and vasopressin	Fluid restriction	Replace with sodium and water as necessary; withhold vasopressin

twice-daily dosing of intranasal or oral DDAVP. Families are instructed to withhold subsequent dosing of DDAVP until the previous dose has worn off, readily noted by an increase in urination. In infants and children with impaired thirst due to hypothalamic damage to the thirst center, as is often seen in large hypothalamic gliomas or other brain injury the management is more complex. Caregivers typically are asked to keep a log of fluid input and urinary output. Base water replacement, using the child's age and body surface area, is calculated, and supplemental water is given for excessive urine output.

If a child receiving vasopressin for DI suddenly develops hyponatremia without polyuria and dehydration, water intoxication due to overtreatment with vasopressin is more likely, but SIADH should also be considered. The treatment is water restriction in either case. Vasopressin excess caused by inappropriate medication dosing is likely to resolve quickly, whereas SIADH may be more persistent and likely will be accompanied by other evidence of central pathology.

Vigilant monitoring of fluid input and output and serum sodium is necessary because the resolution of SIADH often is followed by the onset of persistent DI.

CENTRAL SALT WASTING

Pathophysiology and Prevalence A major concern in the posttreatment surveillance of patients with DI is the patient who develops sudden polyuria despite previously good control on synthetic vasopressin replacement (DDAVP). In many cases, polyuria is due to vasopressin insufficiency either because of noncompliance or because of inadequate medication dose. However, patients with DI and polyuria, who are compliant and on appropriate DDAVP dose, need to be assessed for the possibility of salt and water wasting.

There are chemotherapeutic agents that cause renal tubular salt wasting, but more commonly, salt wasting is central in etiology due to CNS injury or increased intracranial

pressure. Brain natriuretic peptide (BNP) and atrial natriuretic peptide (ANP) are released inappropriately in this condition, resulting in excessive urinary losses of sodium (>100 meq/L) water, hyponatremia, and dehydration (100,101). Coincident DI and cerebral salt wasting in childhood survivors of brain tumors does occur, complicating even further the diagnosis (102). Salt wasting in children with DI is dangerous when the condition is not recognized. Continued excessive urination is interpreted as insufficient vasopressin replacement, and repeated doses of DDAVP are given inappropriately, worsening the hyponatremia and increasing the risk of hyponatremic seizures.

Diagnosis and Surveillance Increased free water loss due to inadequate vasopressin therapy should be suspected in patients with increased urinary output, increased serum osmolality, hypernatremia and decreased urinary sodium. Salt wasting should be suspected when excessive urination persists despite vasopressin administration. Patients with both DI and salt wasting may have low to low normal serum sodium, decreased serum osmolality, increased urinary sodium loss, weight loss and dehydration with elevated BNP and ANP levels. Measurement of atrial natriuretic peptide or brain natriuretic peptide generally is not available in the acute setting to aid in the diagnosis and treatment. Table 47-1 summarizes the differences in SIADH, salt wasting, DI, and fluid overload.

Treatment For treatment of central salt wasting, vasopressin should be withheld while sufficient salt and water are provided to restore volume and sodium depletion due to continuing polyuria. Because these children often have concomitant vasopressin insufficiency, the urinary output can be very large, and replacement fluids will be equally voluminous, which often creates a strong desire by the clinician to use vasopressin to decrease urination. However, medical caretakers must restrain from using vasopressin in patients with salt wasting because it will only worsen the hyponatremia by causing retention of free

water. Constant clinical and laboratory evaluation is an absolute necessity, to correct the urinary losses of fluids and electrolytes.

OBESITY AND METABOLIC SYNDROME

Pathogenesis and Prevalence Survivors of childhood cancer are at risk for obesity due to hypothalamic damage from tumor, surgery and irradiation, hormonal deficiencies (GH and gonadal hormones), corticosteroid therapy, altered behavior, energy utilization and sleep patterns. Hypothalamic damage due to craniopharyngioma itself and its treatments (surgery and/or irradiation) is invariably associated with refractory hypothalamic obesity.

Decreased activity with increased sleepiness due to either reduced melatonin secretion or orexin deficiency can exacerbate hypothalamic deficiency. Melatonin therapy has been shown to decrease daytime sleepiness (103,104). A retrospective cohort of 1,765 adult survivors of childhood ALL showed a significant association between treatment with cranial irradiation of 20 Gy or more and obesity, especially in girls treated at age 9 years or younger (105); another study involving 618 ALL children found that those diagnosed at age 13 years or younger had an increase in their body mass index (BMI) regardless of whether they had received cranial irradiation (106); similarly another retrospective study showed that age (<6 years) and BMI at diagnosis, rather than type of CNS treatment received, predicted adult weight in long term cancer survivors of childhood hematologic malignancies. Of note, in this study high risk patients who received 24 Gy of cranial irradiation were more likely to be males, older at diagnosis and with higher BMI in comparison to the patients that received 18 Gy or high dose intrathecal methotrexate (107).

Total body irradiation in preparation for hematopoietic cell transplant (HCT) is associated with increased risk for diabetes but no increase in obesity when HCT survivors were compared to their siblings (108). These reports show that cancer survivors face metabolic disturbances that resemble the metabolic syndrome or syndrome X. The *metabolic syndrome* or *syndrome X*, which is characterized by central obesity, hypertension, insulin resistance, glucose intolerance, and dyslipidemia, is associated with a substantially increased risk for type 2 diabetes mellitus and atherosclerotic cardiovascular disease (109–110). While little is known about the pathogenesis of metabolic syndrome in childhood cancer survivors, there are similarities in features of metabolic syndrome and the symptoms of GH deficiency in adults, including central obesity, insulin resistance, and increased cardiovascular mortality (111). Antineoplastic agents and irradiation also may play a role in the development of metabolic syndrome (112).

Diagnosis and Surveillance Biannual assessment of weight and body-mass index (BMI) with clinical assessment of central fat distribution should be performed, along with measurement of blood pressure, fasting lipid profile, and fasting glucose and insulin levels. Oral glucose tolerance testing also should be considered in patients at high risk for insulin resistance and the metabolic syndrome.

Treatment Patients should receive ongoing counseling about healthy diet and exercise patterns. Hypertension, hyperlipidemia, and diabetes, if present, should be treated according to standard protocols. It has not yet been demonstrated that lifelong GH treatment will alter the increased risk of the metabolic syndrome or cardiovascular disease in GH-deficient subjects.

REFERENCES

1. Constine LS, Wolf PD, Cann D, et al. Hypothalamic–pituitary dysfunction after radiation for brain tumors. N Engl J Med. 1993;328:87–94.
2. Collett-Solberg PF, Sernyak H, Satin-Smith M, et al. Endocrine outcome in long term survivors of low grade hypothalamic chiasmatic glioma. Clin Endocrinol. 1997;47:79–85.
3. Chematily W, Mertens AC, Mitby P, et al. Acute ovarian failure in the childhood cancer survivor study. J Clin Endocrinol Metab 2006;91:1723–1728.
4. Chapman RM. Effect of cytotoxic therapy on sexuality and gonadal function. Semin Oncol. 1982;9:84–94.
5. Byrne J, Fears TR, Gail MH, et al. Early menopause in long term survivors of cancer during adolescence. Am J Obstet Gynecol. 1992;166:788–793.
6. Larsen C, Muller J, Schmiegelow K, et al. Reduced ovarian function in long-term survivors of radiation- and chemotherapy-treated childhood cancer. J Clin Endocrinol Metab. 2003;88:5307–5314.
7. Rutter MM, Rose SR. Long-term sequelae of childhood cancer. Curr Opin Pediatr 2007;19:480–487.
8. Oberfield SE, Allen JC, Pollack J, et al. Long-term endocrine sequelae after treatment of medulloblastoma: Prospective study of growth and thyroid function. J Pediatr. 1986;108:219–223.
9. Ahmed SR, Shalet SM, Beardwell CG. The effects of cranial irradiation on growth hormone secretion. Acta Pediatr Scand. 1985;75:255–260.
10. Nivot S, Benelli C, Clot JP, et al. Nonparallel changes of growth hormone (GH) and insulin-like growth factor-1, insulin-like growth factor binding protein-3, and growth hormone binding protein, after craniospinal irradiation and chemotherapy. J Clin Endocrin Metab. 1994;78:597–601.
11. Pasqualini T, Diez B, Domene H, et al: Long-term endocrine sequelae after surgery, radiotherapy, and chemotherapy in children with medulloblastoma. Cancer. 1987;59:801–806.
12. Bongers ME, Francken AB, Rouwe C, et al. Reduction of adult height in childhood acute lymphoblastic leukemia survivors after prophylactic cranial irradiation. Pediatr Blood Cancer. 2005;45:139–143.
13. Blatt J, Bercu BB, Gillin JC, et al. Reduced pulsatile growth hormone secretion in children after therapy for acute lymphoblastic leukemia. J Pediatr. 1984;104:182–186.
14. Shalet SM. Radiation and pituitary dysfunction. N Engl J Med. 1993;328:131–133.
15. Clayton PE, Shalet SM, Morris-Jones PH, et al. Growth in children treated for acute lymphoblastic leukemia. Lancet. 1988;1:460–462.
16. Lam KSL, Tse VKC, Wang C, et al. Effects of irradiation on hypothalamic–pituitary function: A 5 year longitudinal study in patients with nasopharyngeal carcinoma. Q J Med. 1991;78:165.
17. Ogilvy-Stuart AL, Clark DJ, Wallace WH, et al: Endocrine deficit after fractionated total body irradiation. Arch Dis Child. 1992;67:1107–1110.
18. Darzy KH, Shalet SM. Radiation-induced growth hormone deficiency. Horm Res. 2003;59:S1–11.
19. Withers HR. Biologic basis for altered fractionation schemes. Cancer. 1985;55:2086–2091.
20. Kirk JA, Stevens MM, Menser MA, et al. Growth failure and growth hormone deficiency after treatment for acute lymphoblastic leukemia. Lancet. 1987;1:190–193.
21. Sklar CA. Growth and pubertal development in survivors of childhood cancer. Pediatrics. 1991;18:53–60.
22. Duffner PK, Cohen ME, Voorhess ML, et al. Long term effects of cranial irradiation on endocrine function in children with brain tumors: A prospective study. Cancer. 1985;56:2189–2193.
23. Meacham LR, Mason PW, Sullivan KM. Auxologic and biochemical characterization of the three phases of growth failure in pediatric patients with brain tumors. J Pediatr Endocrinol Metab. 2004;17:711–717.
24. Kim RJ, Janss A, Shanis D, et al. Adult heights attained by children with hypothalamic/chiasmatic glioma treated with growth hormone. J Clin Endocrinol Metab. 2004;89:4999–5002.
25. Shalet SM, Price DA, Beardwell CG, et al. Normal growth despite abnormalities in growth hormone secretion in children treated for acute leukemia. J Pediatr. 1979;94:719–722.
26. Price DA, Morris MJ, Rosell KV, et al: The effects of antileukaemic drugs on somatomedic production and cartilage responsiveness to somatomedin in vitro. Pediatr Res. 1981;15:1553.
27. Willi SM, Cooke K, Goldwein J, et al. Growth in children after bone marrow transplantation for advanced neuroblastoma compared with growth after transplantation for leukemia or aplastic anemia. J Pediatr. 1992;120:726–732.
28. Afify Z, Shaw PJ, Clavano-Harding A, et al. Growth and endocrine function in children with acute myeloid leukaemia after bone marrow transplantation using busulfan/cyclophosphamide. Bone Marrow Transplant. 2000;25:1087–1092.
29. Shankar SM, Bunin NJ, Moshang T Jr. Growth in children undergoing bone marrow transplantation after busulfan and cyclophosphamide conditioning. J Pediat Hematol Oncol. 1996;18:362–366.
30. Bozzola M, Giorgiani G, Locatelli F, et al. Growth in children after bone marrow transplantation. Horm Res. 1993;39:122–126.
31. Olshan JS, Gubernick J, Packer RJ, et al. The effects of adjuvant chemotherapy on growth in children with medulloblastoma. Cancer. 1992;70:2013–2017.
32. Ogilvy-Stuart AL, Shalet S. Growth and puberty after growth hormone treatment after irradiation for brain tumours. Arch Dis Child. 1995;73:141–146.
33. Schell MJ, McHaney VA, Green AA, et al. Hearing loss in children and young adults receiving cisplatin with or without prior cranial irradiation. J Clin Oncol. 1989;76:754–760.
34. Shalet SM, Gibson B, Swindell R, et al. Effect of spinal irradiation on growth. Arch Dis Child. 1987;62:461–464.
35. Sanders JE, Pritchard S, Mahoney P, et al. Growth and development following marrow transplantation for leukemia. Blood. 1986;68:1129–1135.
36. Olshan J, Willi S, August C, et al. Growth hormone function and treatment following bone marrow transplant for neuroblastoma. Bone Marrow Transplant. 1993;12:381–385.
37. Brauner R, Adan L, Souberbielle JC, et al. Contribution of growth hormone deficiency to the growth failure that follows bone marrow transplantation. J Pediatr. 1997;130:785–792.
38. Neely EK, Hintz RL, Wilson DM, et al. Normal ranges for immunochemiluminometric gonadotropin assays. J Pediatr. 1995;127:40–46.
39. Blum WF, Ranke MR, Kietzman K, et al. A specific radioimmunoassay for the growth hormone (GH)–dependent somatomedin-binding protein: its use for diagnosis of GH deficiency. J Clin Endocrinol Metab. 1990;70:1292–1298.
40. Blum WF, Albertsson-Wikland K, Rosberg S, et al. Serum levels of insulin-like growth

factor I (IGF-I) and IGF binding protein 3 reflect spontaneous growth hormone secretion. *J Clin Endocrinol Metab.* 1990;76:1610–1616.

41. Rosenfeld RG, Wilson DM, Lee PDK, et al. Insulin-like growth factors I and II in evaluation of growth retardation. *J Pediatr.* 1986;109:428–433.

42. Weinzimer SA, Homan SA, Ferry RJ, et al. Serum IGF-I and IGFBP-3 concentrations do not accurately predict growth hormone deficiency in children with brain tumors. *Clin Endocrinol.* 1991;51:339–345.

43. Sklar C, Sarafoglou K, Whittam E. Efficacy of insulin-like growth factor binding protein-3 in predicting the growth hormone response to provocative testing in children treated with cranial irradiation. *Acta Endocrinol.* 1993;129:511–515.

44. Tillmann V, Buckler JMH, Kibirige MS, et al. Biochemical tests in the diagnosis of childhood growth hormone deficiency. *J Clin Endocrinol Metab.* 1997;82:531–535.

45. Rosenfield RL, Furlanetto R, Bock D. Relationship of somatomedin-C concentrations to pubertal changes. *J Pediatr.* 1983;10:723–728.

46. Pescovitz OH, Rosenfeld RG, Hintz RL, et al. Somatomedin-C in accelerated growth of children with precocious puberty. *J Pediatr.* 1985;107:20–25.

47. Rosenfield RL, Furlanetto R. Physiologic testosterone or estradiol induction of puberty increases somatomedin-C. *J Pediatr.* 1985;107:415–417.

48. Vassilopoulou-Sellin R, Klein MJ, Moore BD III, et al. Efficacy of growth hormone replacement therapy in children with organic growth hormone deficiency after cranial irradiation. *Horm Res.* 1995;43:188–193.

49. Clayton PE, Shalet SM, Price DA. Response to growth hormone treatment in children with central nervous system malignancy. In: Ranke MB, Gunnarson R, eds. *Progress in Growth Hormone Therapy: 5 Years of KIGS.* Mannheim: Verlag; 1994:173–189.

50. Xu W., Janss AJ, Moshang T Jr. Adult height and sitting height in children surviving medulloblastoma. *J Clin Endocrinol Metab.* 2003;88:4677–4681.

51. Clayton PE, Shalet SM. The evolution of spine growth after irradiation. *Clin Oncol.* 1991;3:220–222.

52. Cohen A, Rovelli A, Van-Lint MT, et al. Final height of patients who underwent bone marrow transplantation during childhood. *Arch Dis Child.* 1996;74:437–440.

53. Brownstein CM, Mertens AC, Mitby PA, et al. Factors that affect final height and change in height standard deviation scores in survivors of childhood cancer treated with growth hormone: A report from the childhood cancer survivor study. *J Clin Endocrinol Metab.* 2004;89:4422.

54. Mauras N, Attie KM, Reiter EO, et al. High dose recombinant human growth hormone (GH) treatment of GH-deficient patients in puberty increases near-final height: A randomized, multicenter trial. *J Clin Endocrinol Metab.* 2000;85:3653–3660.

55. Juul A, Bang P, Hertel NT, et al. Serum insulin-like growth factor-I in 1030 healthy children, adolescents, and adults: Relation to age, sex, stage of puberty, testicular size, and body mass index. *J Clin Endocrinol Metab.* 1990;78:744–752.

56. Martha PM Jr, Gorman KM, Blizzard RM, et al. Endogenous growth hormone secretion and clearance rates in normal boys, as determined by deconvolution analysis: Relationship to age, pubertal status and body mass. *J Clin Endocrinol Metab.* 1992;74:336–344.

57. Adan L, Souberbielle JC, Zucker JM, et al. Adult height in 24 patients treated for growth hormone deficiency and early puberty. *J Clin Endocrinol Metab.* 1997;82:229–233.

58. Wang ED, Drummond DS, Dormans JP, et al. Scoliosis in patients treated with growth hormone. *J Pediatr Orthop.* 1997;17:708–711.

59. Wilson TA, Rose SR, Cohen P, et al. Update of guidelines for the use of growth hormone in children; the Lawson Wilkins Pediatric Endocrinology Society Drug and Therapeutics Commitee. *J Pediatr* 2003;143:415–421.

60. Savage LI, Murray RD. Late effects of cancer therapy on growth and GH. *Int Growth Monitor* 2006;16:2–7.

61. Moshang T Jr, Chen Rundle A, Graves DA, et al. Brain tumor recurrence in children treated with growth hormone: The National Cooperative Growth Study experience. *J Pediatr.* 1996;128:S4–7.

62. Darendeliler F, Karagiannis G, Wilton P, et al. Recurrence of brain tumors in patients treated with growth hormone: analysis of KIGS (Pfizer International Growth Database). *Acta Paediatr* 2006; 95:1284–1290.

63. Packer RJ, Boyett JM, Janss AJ, et al. Growth hormone replacement therapy in children with medulloblastoma: Use and effect on tumor control. *J Clin Oncol.* 2001;15;19:480–487.

64. Sklar CA, Mertens AC, Mitby P, et al. Risk of disease recurrence and second neoplasms in survivors of childhood cancer treated with growth hormone: A report from the Childhood Cancer Survivor Study. *J Clin Endocrinol Metab.* 2002;87:3136–3141.

65. Ergun-Longmire B, Mertens AC, Mitby P, et al. growth hormone treatment and risk of second neoplasm in the childhood cancer survivor. *J Clin Endocrinol Metab* 2006;91:3494–3498.

66. Neglia JP, Robison LL, Stoval M, et al. New primary neoplasms of the central nervous system in survivors of childhood cancer: a report from the Childhood Cancer Survivor Study. *J Natl Cancer Inst* 2006;98:1528–1537.

67. Murray RD, Darzy KH, Gleeson HK, et al. GH-deficient survivors of childhood cancer: GH replacement during adult life. *J Clin Endocrinol Metab.* 2002;87:129–135.

68. Folin C, Thilen U, Ahren b, et al. Improvement in cardiac systolic function and reduced prevalence of metabolic syndrome after 2 years of growth hormone(GH) treatment in GH- deficient adult survivors of childhood-onset of acute lymphoblastic leukemia. *J Clin Endocrinol Metab* 2006; 91:1872–1875.

69. Growth Hormone Research Society. Consensus guidelines for the diagnosis and treatment of growth hormone deficiency in childhood and adolescence: Summary statement of the Growth Hormone Research Society. *J Clin Endocrin Metab.* 2000;85:3990–3993.

70. Darzy KH, Aimaretti G, Wieringa G, et al. The usefulness of the combined growth hormone (GH)–releasing hormone and arginine stimulation test in the diagnosis of radiation-induced GH deficiency is dependent on the post-irradiation time interval. *J Clin Endocrin Metab.* 2003;88:95–102.

71. Ham JN, Ginsberg J, Hendell C, et al. Growth hormone–releasing hormone plus arginine stimulation testing in young adults treated in childhood with cranio-spinal radiation therapy. *Clin Endocrinol.* 2005;62:628–632.

72. Gleeson HK, Shalet SM. The impact of cancer therapy on the endocrine system in survivors of childhood brain tumors. *Endocr Relat Cancer.* 2004;11:589–602.

73. Leiper AD, Stanhope R, Kitching P, et al. Precocious and premature puberty associated with treatment of acute lymphoblastic leukemia. *Arch Dis Child.* 1987;62:1107–1112.

74. Xu W, Janss AJ, Packer RJ, et al. Endocrine outcome in children with medulloblastoma (PNET) treated with 18 Gy craniospinal radiation therapy (CSRT). *Neurooncology.* 2004;6:113–118.

75. Rowley MJ, Leach DR, Warner GA, et al. Effect of graded doses of ionizing radiation on the human testis. *Radiat Res.* 1974;59:665–678.

76. Shalet SM, Beardwell CG, Jacobs HS, et al. Testicular function following irradiation of the human prepubertal testis. *Clin Endocrinol.* 1978;9:483–490.

77. Stillman RJ, Schinfield JS, Schiff I, et al. Ovarian failure in long-term survivors of childhood malignancy. *Am J Obstet Gynecol.* 1981;139:62–66.

78. Paul D, Conte FA, Grumbach MM, et al. Long term effect of gonadotropin-releasing hormone agonist therapy on final and near-final height in 26 children with true precocious puberty treated at a median age of less than 5 years. *J Clin Endocrinol Metab.* 1995;80:546–551.

79. Leiper AD, Stanhope R, Preece MA, et al. Precocious or early puberty and growth failure in girls treated for acute lymphoblastic leukaemia. *Horm Res.* 1988;30:72–76.

80. Thomas BC, Stanhope R, Leiper AD. Gonadotropin releasing hormone analogue and growth hormone therapy in precocious and premature puberty following cranial irradiation for acute lymphoblastic leukaemia. *Horm Res.*1993;39:25–29.

81. Nieman CL, Kazer R, Brannigan RE, et al. Cancer survivors and infertility: a review of a new problem and novel answers. *J Support Oncol* 2006;4:171–178.

82. Lee SJ, Schover LR, Partridge AH, et al. American Society of Clinical Oncology recommendations on fertility preservation in cancer patients. *J Clin Oncol* 2006; 24:2917–2931.

83. Oberfield SE, Sklar C, Allen J, et al. Thyroid and gonadal function and growth of long-term survivors of medulloblastoma/PNET. In: Green DM, D'Angio GJ, eds. Late Effects of Treatment for Childhood Cancer. New York: *Wiley–Liss;* 1992:55.

84. Rose SR, Lustig RH, Pitukcheewanont P, et al. Diagnosis of Hidden Central Hypothyroidism in Survivors of Childhood Cancer. *J Clin Endocrinol Metab.* 999;84:4472–4479.

85. Shalet SM, Rosenstock JD, Beardwell CG, et al. Thyroid dysfunction following external irradiation to the neck for Hodgkin's disease in childhood. *Radiology.* 1997;28:511–515.

86. Kaplan MM, Garnick MB, Gelber R, et al. Risk factors for thyroid abnormalities after neck irradiation for childhood cancer. *Am J Med.* 1983;74:272–280.

87. Devney RB, Sklar CA, Nesbit ME, et al. Serial thyroid function measurements in children with Hodgkin's disease. *J Pediatr.* 1984;105:223–227.

88. Hancock SL, Cox RS, McDougall JR. Thyroid diseases after treatment of Hodgkin's disease. *N Engl J Med.* 1991;325:599–605.

89. Schmiegelow M, Feldt-Rasmussen U, Rasmussen HK, et al. A population-based study of thyroid function after radiotherapy and chemotherapy for childhood brain tumor. *J Clin Endocrinol Metab.* 2003;88:136–140.

90. Rose SR. Cranial irradiation and central hypothyroidism. *Trends Endocrinol Metab.* 2001;12:97–104.

91. Sutcliffe SB, Chapman R, Wrigley PFM. Cyclical combination chemotherapy and thyroid function in patients with advanced Hodgkin's disease. *Med Pediatr Oncol.* 1981;9:439–448.

92. Oberfield SE, Nirenberg A, Allen JC, et al. Hypothalamic–pituitary–adrenal function following cranial irradiation. *Horm Res.* 1997;47:9–16.

93. Rose SR, Lustig RH, Burstein S, et al. Diagnosis of ACTH deficiency. Comparison of Overnight Metyrapone Test to Either Low-Dose or High-Dose ACTH Test. *Horm Res* 1999;52:73–79.

94. Rose SR, Danish RK, Kearney NS, et al. ACTH deficiency in childhood cancer isurvivors. *Pediatr Blood Cancer.* 45:808–813;2005.

95. Fass B. Glucocorticoid therapy for non-endocrine disorders: Withdrawal and "coverage." *Pediatr Clin North Am.* 1979;26:251–256.

96. Goldwein JW. Effects of radiation therapy on skeletal growth in childhood. *Clin Orthop.* 1991;262:101–107.

97. Vassilopoulou-Sellin R, Brosnan P, Delpassand A, et al. Osteopenia in young adult survivors of childhood cancer. *Med Pediatr Oncol.* 1999;32:272–278.

98. Odame I, Duckwork J, Talsma D, et al. Osteopenia, physical activity and health-related quality of life in survivors of brain tumors treated in childhood. *Pediat Blood Cancer.* 2006;46:357–362.

99. Leonard MB, Zemel BS. Current concepts in pediatric bone disease. *Pediatr Clin North Am.* 2002;49:143–173.

100. Ganong CA, Kappy MS. Cerebral salt wasting in children: The need for recognition and treatment. *Am J Dis Child.* 1993;147:167–169.

101. Kappy MS, Ganong CA. Cerebral salt wasting in children: The role of atrial natriuretic hormone. *Adv Pediatr.* 1996;43:271–308.

102. Ferry RJ Jr, Kesavulu V, Kelly A, et al. Hyponatremia and polyuria in children with central diabetes insipidus: Challenges in diagnosis and management. *J Pediatr.* 2001;138:744–747.

103. Nishino S, Ripley B, Overeem S, et al. Hypocretin (orexin) deficiency in human narcolepsy. *Lancet* 2000;355:39–40.

104. Muller HL, Handwerker G, Gebhardt U, et al. Melatonin treatment in obese patients with childhood craniopharyngioma and increased daytime sleepiness. cancer Causes Control 2006;17:583–589.

105. Dalton VK, Rue M, Silverman LB, et al. Height and weight in children treated for acute lymphoblastic leukemia. Relationship to CNS trreatment. *J Clin Oncol* 2003;21:2953–2960.

106. Oeffinger KC, Mertens AC, Sklar CA, et al. Obesity in adult survivors of childhood acute lymphoblastic leukemia: A report from the Childhood Cancer Survivor Study. *J Clin Oncol.* 2003;17:1359–1365.

107. Razzouk BI, Rose SR, Hongeng S, et al. Obesity in Survivors of Childhood Acute lymphoblastic Leukemia and lymphoma. *J Clin Oncol* 2007; 25:1183–1189.

108. Baker KS, Ness KK, Steinberger J, et al. Diabetes, hypertension, and cardiovascular events in survivors of hematopoietic cell transplantation: a report from the bone marrow transplantation survivor study. *Blood* 2007;109:1765–1772.

109. Oeffinger KC, Mertens AC, Sklar CA, et al. Chronic Health Conditions in Adult Survivors of Childhood Cancer. *N Engl J Med* 2006;355:1572–1582.

110. Nuver J, Smit AJ, Postma A, et al. The metabolic syndrome in long-term cancer survivors: An important target for secondary preventive measures. *Cancer Treat Rev.* 2002;28:195–214.

111. Johannsson G, Bengtsson BA. Growth hormone and the metabolic syndrome. *J Endocrinol Invest.* 1999;22:41–46.

112. Huddart RA, Norman A, Shahidi M, et al. Cardiovascular disease as a long-term complication of treatment for testicular cancer. *J Clin Oncol.* 2003;21:1513–1523.

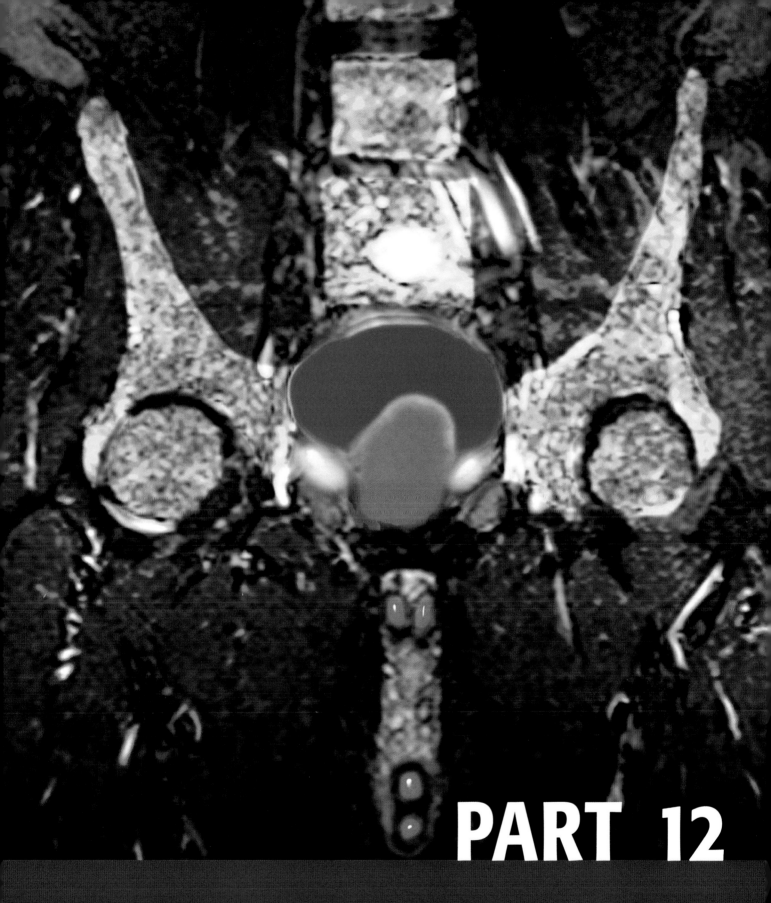

PART 12

Endocrine and Metabolic Laboratory and Radiology Tests

IN THIS PART

Previous page: Color enhanced coronal view of the male pelvis obtained by Magnetic Resonance Imaging.

CHAPTER 48

Laboratory Investigations of Inborn Errors of Metabolism

Tina M. Cowan, PhD, FACMG
Chunli Yu, MD, FACMG

This chapter presents practical guidelines for the laboratory testing of the inborn errors of metabolism. Although some tests are readily available in major hospital laboratories or commercial reference laboratories, others are offered by only a small number of laboratories worldwide (and sometimes only in a single laboratory). A number of useful resources exist for identifying laboratories performing such esoteric testing, including GeneClinics (www.geneclinics.org), the University of California San Diego Biochemical Genetics Test List (http://biochemgen.ucsd.edu/UCSDW3BG/), and the Metabolic Center at the University of Heidelberg (www.stoffwechsel.uni-hd.de). A general overview of testing strategies for the evaluation of specific metabolic disorders is shown in Table 48-1. Providers are urged to contact the testing laboratory prior to specimen collection for specific instructions and information about newly available tests.

METABOLIC SCREENING TESTS

Test Description Simple metabolic screening begins with general inspection of the urine, including color, odor, and pH. A number of urine spot tests are available to provide a rapid, although relatively crude, indication of abnormal metabolite excretion. These tests often are offered as part of a "metabolic screening panel," with the composition of specific panels varying widely among laboratories. Although they are inexpensive and easy to perform, they are also significantly limited in both sensitivity and specificity. The most commonly used spot tests for various metabolic disorders are listed in Table 48-2 and include the ferric chloride test for phenylketonuria (PKU) and tyrosinemia, the nitroprusside–cyanide test for cystinuria and homocystinuria, and the silver–nitroprusside test for homocystinuria. Other screening procedures such as thin-layer chromatography (TLC) and paper chromatography can be used to detect gross elevations in amino acid concentrations

but are inadequate for detecting more subtle abnormalities. Abnormal decreases in amino acid levels also will not be detected by this approach.

Indications The usefulness of the metabolic screening tests is limited, and these tests are not appropriate for the workup of an acutely ill patient. Most laboratories have replaced these tests with newer technologies, such as quantitative amino acid analysis. However, in certain settings, particularly the evaluation of an older patient with nonspecific findings such as developmental delay or mental retardation, abnormal spot-test results can give useful clues that a more extensive metabolic workup may be warranted. Specifically, the sulfite dipstick can be useful in diagnosing sulfite oxidase or molybdenum cofactor deficiencies, although this test is reliable only in fresh urine and should be performed at the bedside.

Sample Requirements Specific sample requirements vary by laboratory. Testing typically requires 10–20 mL of urine (either first-morning or random) collected in a clean container without preservatives and stored frozen prior to analysis. The sample need not be collected in a sterile fashion.

Interpretation Positive spot tests are revealed by specific changes in color and/or clarity on addition of the test reagent. These tests can yield false-negative results from dilute urine and/or modest elevations of metabolites, as well as false-positive results from interference from certain medications (e.g., antibiotics, intravenous glucose, and contrast dye).

For qualitative fractionation procedures such as TLC, amino acids are detected with ninhydrin staining, and the resulting pattern is visually compared with that of normal controls and, when possible, abnormal samples from previously diagnosed patients. This detects gross changes in amino acid concentrations, but false-negative results can arise in cases of more subtle disturbances. Drug interference also can yield false-positive results.

Abnormal screening results always should be followed by more specific metabolic studies. The choice of follow-up testing is guided by the clinical picture and results of other laboratory investigations and typically includes quantitative amino acid analysis, urine organic acid analysis by gas chromatography/mass spectrometry (GC/MS), acylcarnitine profile, and others. Even with normal screening results, more detailed metabolic studies often are warranted depending on the clinical situation.

AMINO ACID TESTS

Free amino acids can be evaluated in plasma, urine, or cerebrospinal fluid (CSF) depending on the clinical concern. Plasma amino acids are evaluated to identify primary disorders of amino acid metabolism (e.g., PKU, citrullinemia) and to monitor treatment efficacy in previously diagnosed patients. Plasma amino acids are also evaluated as part of a comprehensive workup in patients suspected of having a broad range of metabolic disorders, particularly the urea cycle disorders and organic acidemias, and often reveal secondary disturbances that help to guide further diagnostic testing. Urine amino acids are evaluated to identify generalized or specific disorders of renal amino acid transport (e.g., renal Fanconi syndrome, cystinuria), and CSF amino acids are evaluated to identify disorders of amino acid metabolism that affect the central nervous system (e.g., glycine encephalopathy).

Quantitative Amino Acid Analysis

Test Description The "gold standard" for quantitative amino acid analysis is a dedicated amino acid analyzer using ion-exchange high-pressure liquid chromatography (HPLC) with ninhydrin detection. These systems measure the concentrations of 30–40 amino acids in a single analysis. Because of the increased sensitivity and specificity, most laboratories with automated systems offer this

TABLE 48-1   Testing Strategies for the Evaluation of Metabolic Disorders

Disease	Screening and diagnostic tests	Additional confirmatory studies
Amino acids disorders		
Phenylketonuria	AA (P), pterins (U), DHPR activity (RBC)	DNA sequencing (*PAH*)
Tyrosinemia (Types I, II and III)	AA (P, U), OA (U), succinylacetone (U), AFP (S)	Targeted mutation analysis or sequencing (*FAH*) (tyrosinemia type I)
Maple Syrup Urine Disease	AA (P), OA (U)	BCKAD enzyme assay (cultured cells), DNA sequencing (*BCKDHA, BCKDHB, DBT*), targeted mutation analysis (*BCKDHA, BCKDHB*) for Menonites and Jewish
Glycine Encephalopathy	AA (P, CSF), CSF/Plasma glycine ratio	GCS enzyme assay (liver), GCS subunit gene sequencing (*GLDC, AMT* and *GCSH*)
Urea Cycle Defects	AA (P, U), OA (U), orotic acid (U)	Enzyme assays (liver, F or RBC), mutation analysis
Homocystinuria due to CBS Deficiency	AA (P), total homocysteine (P)	CBS enzyme assay (F) and/or mutation analysis
Organic acids disorders		
Methylmalonic Acidemia	OA (U), AA (P), ACP (P), Carn (P), MMA (S), total homocysteine (P)	Complementation studies (F) DNA sequencing (*MUT, MMAA, MMAB* and *MMACHC*)
Propionic Acidemia	OA (U), AA (P), ACP (P), Carn (P)	PCC enzyme assay (B or F) and/or DNA sequencing (*PCCA, PCCB*)
Isovaleric Acidemia	OA (U), AA (P), ACP (P), Carn (P)	Targeted mutation analysis or DNA sequencing
Multiple Carboxylase Deficiency	OA (U), AA (P), ACP (P), Carn (P), biotinidase activity (S)	HCS enzyme assay, individual carboxylase enzyme assays (B or F) and/or DNA sequencing (*HLCS* and *BTD* genes)
3-Methylcrotonyl-CoA Carboxylase Deficiency	OA (U), AA (P), ACP (P), Carn (P)	3MCC enzyme assay (B or cultured cells) and/or DNA sequencing (*MCC1* and *MCC2* genes)
Glutaric Acidemia Type I	OA (U), AA (P), ACP (P,U), Carn (P), glutaric and 3-hydroxyglutaric acids (P, U)	Glutaryl-CoA dehydrogenase enzyme assay (F) and/or DNA sequencing
Fatty acid oxidation disorders		
Short-Chain Acyl-CoA Dehydrogenase Deficiency	ACP (P), OA (U), AG (U), Carn (P)	Targeted mutation analysis and/or DNA sequencing, fatty acid oxidation flux (F)
Medium-Chain Acyl-CoA Dehydrogenase Deficiency	ACP (P), OA (U), AG (U), Carn (P)	Targeted mutation analysis and/or DNA sequencing
Very Long-Chain Acyl-CoA Dehydrogenase Deficiency	ACP (P), OA (U), Carn (P)	DNA sequencing, fatty acid oxidation flux (F), enzyme assay (B)
Long-Chain Hydroxyacyl-CoA Dehydrogenase/ Trifunctional Protein Deficiency	ACP (P), OA(U), Carn (P)	Targeted mutation analysis and/or DNA sequencing (*HADHA, HADHB*), TFP enzyme assay (F)
Carnitine Uptake Defect	Carn (P,U)	Carnitine transporter activity (F), DNA sequencing
Carnitine Palmitoyltransferase I Deficiency	ACP (P), Carn (P), CPT I enzyme assay (F)	DNA sequencing or targeted mutation analysis (for Innuits)
Carnitine Palmitoyltransferase II/Carnitine Acylcarnitine Translocase Deficiency	ACP (P), Carn (P)	CPT II and CACT enzyme assays (F) and/or DNA sequencing
Mitochonrial Disorders		
Disorders of Pyruvate Metabolism	Lactate, pyruvate (B), ketones (B), ACP (P), Carn (P), AA (P), OA (U)	Enzyme assays for PC and PDH, DNA sequencing (*PDHA1*)
Tricarboxylic Acid Cycle Disorders	Lactate, pyruvate (B), ketones (B), ACP (P), Carn (P), AA (P), OA (U)	Assays for TCA cycle enzyme activities
Disorders of the Mitochondrial Respiratory Chain	Lactate, pyruvate (B), ketones (B), ACP (P), Carn (P), AA (P), OA (U), mt DNA panels	nDNA analysis and mtDNA sequencing
Peroxisomal Disorders		
Peroxisomal Biogenesis Disorders (Zellweger Spectrum Disorders)	VLCFA (P), plasmalogens (RBC), pipecolic acid (P, U), bile acids (P,U)	Fibroblasts studies including VLCFA oxidation, catalase distribution, plasmalogen synthesis, complementation, specific enzyme activities; mutation analysis
Rhizomelic Chondrodysplasia (Type I, II and III)	VLCFA (P), plasmalogens (RBC), phytanic acid (P)	Phytanic acid oxidation, plasmalogen synthesis (F), GHAPAT, AGPS enzyme assays (F), mutation analysis (*PEX7, GNPAT, AGPS*)
X-Llinked Adrenoleukodystrophy	VLCFA (P), adrenal function (P)	VLCFA (F), mutation analysis (ABCD1)

TABLE 48-1   Testing Strategies for the Evaluation of Metabolic Disorders *(continued)*

Disease	Screening and diagnostic tests	Additional confirmatory studies
Lysosomal Disorders		
Sphingolipidoses	Specific enzyme assays (L, F)	Mutation analysis
Mucopolysaccharidoses	MPS screening (U), specific enzyme assays (L, F)	Mutation analysis
Oligosaccharidoses	OS screening (U), specific enzyme assays (L, F)	Mutation analysis
Neurotransmitter disorders		
Disorders of Serotonin, Catecholamine and BH$_4$ Metabolism	Neurotransmitters metabolites profile (CSF)	Enzyme assays, mutation analysis. Phenylalanine loading test (GTPCH or SR deficiencies)
Carbohydrate Disorders		
Glycogen Storage Disorders	Glycogen content, specific enzyme assays	Mutation analysis
Galactosemia (GALT, GALE and GALK deficiency)	Reducing sugars (U), Gal-1-P(RBC), Galactitol (U) GALT, GALE and GALK enzyme assays (RBC)	GALT targeted mutation plus sequencing analysis
Hereditary Fructose Intolerance	Reducing sugars (U), OA(U), lactate (P)	Enzyme assay and/or mutation analysis
Congenital Disorders of Glycosylation	Transferrin isoforms (S)	Mutation analysis and/or enzyme assays
Purine/Pyrimidine Disorders		
	Purine, pyrimidine metabolites (U), Pyrimidine nucleotides (RBC)	Enzyme assays and/or mutation analysis

AA = amino acids; ACP = acylcarnitine profile; AFP = α-fetoprotein; AG = acylglycines; AGPS = alkyldihydroxyacetonephosphate synthase; B = blood; BCKAD = branched-chain α-ketoacid dehydrogenase complex; CACT = carnitine acylcarnitine translocase; Carn = carnitine, free and total; CBS = cystathionine-α-synthase; CPT I = carnitine palmitoyltransferase I; CPT II = carnitine palmitoyltransferase II; CSF = cerebrospinal fluid; DBT = dihydrolipoamide branched-chain transacylase; DHAPAT = Dihydroxyacetone phosphate acyltransferase; DHPR = dihydropteridine reductase; F = fibroblasts; Gal-1-P = galactose-1-phosphate; GALE = UDP-galactose 4-epimerase; GALK = galactokinase; GALT = galactose-1-phosphate uridyltransferase; GCS = glycine cleavage system; GTPCH = GTP cyclohydrolase; HCS = holocarboxylase synthetase; L = leukocytes; 3 MCC = 3-methylcrotonyl-CoA carboxylase; MMA = methylmalonic acid; MPS = mucopolysaccharides; mtDNA = mitochondrial DNA; nDNA = nuclear DNA; OA = organic acids; OS = oligosaccharides; P = plasma; PC = pyruvate carboxylase; PCC = propionyl-CoA carboxylase; PDH = pyruvate dehydrogenase complex; RBC = red blood cells; S = serum; SR = sepiaterin reductase; TCA = tricarboxylic acid cycle; TFP = trifunctional protein; U = urine; VLCFA = very long chain fatty acids.

test routinely in lieu of metabolic spot tests or other qualitative studies.

Less comprehensive amino acid profiling can be done using other HPLC methods, GC/MS, and most recently, tandem mass spectrometry (MS/MS). These benefit from more rapid turnaround times but are limited in their ability to separate and accurately quantitate specific compounds. Targeted analysis of specific amino acids in dried blood spots is used widely to monitor the treatment of patients with metabolic disorders such as PKU and maple syrup urine disease (MSUD). Amino acid quantitation by MS/MS is part of many newborn screening programs; in this case, abnormal results must be followed by comprehensive analysis on a dedicated amino acid analyzer.

Indications   Indications for testing are diverse, reflecting a variety of different causes. Typical presentations include: 1) overwhelming neonatal illness (particularly if accompanied by ketosis, hyperammonemia, metabolic acidosis, or hypoglycemia); 2) history of recurrent metabolic decompensation; 3) neurological abnormalities (including seizures, hypotonia, lethargy, coma, developmental delay, or unexplained mental retardation); 4) failure to thrive; 5) history of a previously affected

TABLE 48-2   Urinary Spot Tests

Test Name or Reagent	Condition Identified by Positive Result (Compound Identified)
Ferric Chloride	• PKU (phenylpyruvic acid) • Tyrosinemia (*p*-hydroxyphenylpyruvic acid) • Liver disease (*p*-hydroxyphenylpyruvic acid) • MSUD (branch chain α-ketoacids) • Alkaptonuria (homogentisic acid) • Histidinemia (imidazolepyruvic acid) • Ketosis (acetoacetate)
Dinitrophenylhydrazine (DNPH)	• MSUD (branched chain α-ketoacids) • PKU (phenylpyruvic acid) • Tyrosinemia (*p*-hydroxyphenylpyruvic acid) • Liver disease (*p*-hydroxyphenylpyruvic acid) • Lactic acidosis (pyruvate, α-ketoglutarate) • Ketosis (acetoacetate)
Cyanide-Nitroprusside	• Cystinuria (cystine) • Homocystinuria (homocystine) • γ-glutamyl cycle disorders (glutathione)
Nitrosonapthol	• Tyrosinemia (*p*-hydroxyphenylpyruvic acid) • Liver disease (*p*-hydroxyphenylpyruvic acid) • Parental infusion (*N*-acetyltyrosine)
Reducing Substances (Clinitest)	• Galactosemia (galactose, galactose-1-phosphate) • Diabetes (glucose) • Hereditary Fructose Intolerance (fructose) • Renal Fanconi Syndrome (glucose)
Sulfite Test	• Sulfite oxidase and molybdenum cofactor deficiencies (reliable in fresh urine only)

sibling; and 6) follow-up of an abnormal new-born screening result.

Sample Requirements The preferred specimen in most cases is plasma, particularly for newborns and young infants in whom the evaluation of urine is often unreliable. Urine is useful for detecting specific disorders of renal transport, such as cystinuria and lysinuric protein intolerance, as well as more generalized renal tubular dysfunction. Analysis of CSF is important in evaluations for glycine encephalopathy (formerly known as *nonketotic hyperglycinemia*) and the serine-deficiency disorders. Specific specimen requirements vary by laboratory, including collection tubes and sample volumes.

- *Plasma or Serum.* Morning fasting blood or preprandial samples are preferred. For young infants, blood should be collected just before the next scheduled feeding. Most laboratories require plasma to be collected in either sodium or lithium heparan. Separate plasma or serum from cells by centrifugation as soon as possible, and store the sample frozen prior to analysis.

- *Urine.* Quantitative assessment of amino acid excretion is most reliable using a 24-hour collection. However, due to the impractical nature of collecting a 24-hour sample, particularly for infants, a random urine specimen is also valid for reflecting renal tubular reabsorption because normalizing amino acid levels to creatinine concentration. Testing typically requires collection of 10–20 mL of urine (either first-morning or random) in a clean container without preservatives, although smaller volumes also may be acceptable. Samples should be stored frozen prior to analysis.

- *CSF.* Collect CSF in a sterile container without additives, and store frozen prior to analysis. Samples submitted for the evaluation of glycine encephalopathy or serine-deficiency disorders must be accompanied by a simultaneously obtained plasma sample for calculation of CSF:plasma ratios.

Interpretation Amino acid patterns for the more commonly encountered conditions are presented in Table 48-3. Typical reports include quantitative data for each of the compounds measured (typically 30–40) and an age-matched reference range. Nonstandard amino acids such as carnosine (in carnosinemia), alloisoleucine (in MSUD), argininosuccinic acid (in argininosuccinate lyase deficiency), and homocitrulline (in hyperammonemia–hyperornithinemia–homocitrullinuria [HHH] syndrome) may be reported when present. The interpretation includes an explanation of results, possible diagnoses, and recommendations for further testing, including other metabolic studies, enzyme assays, and/or molecular analyses when appropriate.

Amino acid patterns can be influenced by a number of factors, such as diet, nutritional status, medications, and inappropriate sample processing. For example, total parental nutrition and certain infant formulas can lead to nonspecific elevations of numerous amino acids. Elevations of branched-chain amino acids can be induced by decreased protein intake or increased catabolism, such as by prolonged fasting or vomiting. Elevation of plasma glycine, a feature of glycine encephalopathy, can be seen secondary to administration of valproate, carbamazepine, and certain antidepressants. Amino acid abnormalities also can arise as a consequence of a secondary disturbance, such as hyperalaninemia secondary to lactic acidosis or elevations of methionine, tyrosine, and phenylalanine in cases of liver dysfunction. Therefore, it is critical that all relevant clinical, medication, and diet history be communicated to the laboratory for optimal interpretation of results.

TABLE 48-3   Disease Patterns of Amino Acids

Amino Acid Pattern	Condition
Alloisoleucine (P) ↑, Valine, Isoleucine and Leucine (P) ↑	Maple Syrup Urine Disease
Arginine (P) ↑	Arginase deficiency
Citrulline (P) ↑↑	Argininosuccinic acid synthetase deficiency (Citrullinemia type I)
Citrulline (P) ↑, Methionine, Tyrosine, Arginine (P) ↑	Citrin deficiency (Citrullinemia type II)
Citrulline (P) ↑, Argininosuccinic acid (P, U) ↑	Argininosuccinic acid lyase deficiency
Cysteine (U) ↑↑, Arginine, Lysine, Ornithine (U) ↑	Cystinuria
Glyine (P) ↑	Glycine encephalopathy (with ↑↑ CSF glycine) Organic acidemias (e.g., propionic academia, methylmalonic academia) Certain medications (e.g., valproate)
Gutamine (P) ↑, Citrulline (P) ↓ or normal, Arginine (P) ↓ or normal	Ornithine transcarbamoylase deficiency (with ↑↑ orotic acid) Carbamoyl phosphate synthetase I deficiency N-acetylglutamate synthetase deficiency
Lysine (U) ↑↑, Arginine, Ornithine (U) ↑	Lysinuric protein intolerance
Methionine (P) ↑, Homocysteine (P) ↑	Cystathionine-β-synthase deficiency
Methionine (P) ↑	S-adenosylmethionine transferase deficiency (MAT I/III, MAT II) S-adenosylhomocysteine hydrolase deficiency Transient hypermethioninemia Liver dysfunction and/or certain formulas (secondary finding)
Ornithine (P) ↑↑	Ornithine aminotransferase deficiency (gyrate atrophy of choroid and retina)
Ornithine (P) ↑, Homocitrulline (P, U) ↑	Hyperornithinemia-hyperammonemia-homocitrullinuria (HHH) syndrome
Phenylalanine (P) ↑, Tyrosine (P) ↓ or normal	Phenylketonuria Hyperphenylalaninemia BH$_4$ deficiency
Phosphoethanolamine (U) ↑	Hypophosphatasia
Proline (P) ↑	Hyperprolinemia types I & II
Tyrosine (P) ↑	Tyrosinemia (types I, II and III) Transient neonatal tyrosinemia Liver dysfunction (secondary finding)

P = plasma; U = urine; CSF = cerebrospinal fluid; BH$_4$ = tetrahydrobiopterin

ORGANIC ACID ANALYSIS

Urine organic acid determinations are ordered as part of a comprehensive evaluation in patients suspected of having a broad range of metabolic disorders. This workup also should include routine chemistry studies and plasma amino acid analysis and often investigations of acylcarnitines and free and total carnitine. Urine organic acid analysis identifies primary disorders of organic acid metabolism, including many inborn errors of intermediates of amino acids, purines, pyrimidines, and fatty acids.

Test Description Testing is by GC/MS following extraction of compounds from urine by organic solvents or silicic acid. The sample volume is adjusted based on creatinine concentration prior to extraction. Organic acids are analyzed as their trimethylsilane (TMS) derivatives and identified by chromatographic retention time and mass spectra. For optimal detection of keto acids, including succinylacetone, pyruvate, and certain intermediates of branched-chain amino acid metabolism, an oximation step via the addition of hydroxylamine or a similar agent during sample preparation is required. Testing can be performed by either qualitative or quantitative methods, and both are equally appropriate for the detection of patients with organic acidemias. Quantitative testing, in which peak areas are related to standard curves generated for each of the reported compounds, may be more useful in the follow-up of previously diagnosed patients, although there is wide interlaboratory variability in quantitative results.

Specific organic acids (e.g., methylmalonic acid, glutaric acid, and succinylacetone) can be monitored in known patients using other techniques such as MS/MS and stable-isotope-dilution analysis. Such targeted analyses are appropriate for the follow-up of previously diagnosed patients but should not be ordered in lieu of a more comprehensive organic acid screen during an initial workup.

Indications Together with other metabolic studies, particularly plasma amino acid and acylcarnitine profile analyses, urine organic acid analysis should be undertaken in patients suspected of having a wide range of disorders of amino acid (including urea cycle intermediates), organic acid, fatty acid, and carbohydrate metabolism. Typical indications include: **1)** overwhelming neonatal illness, including altered mental status, tachypnea, vomiting, metabolic acidosis (including lactic acidosis and ketosis), hypoglycemia, and hyperammonemia; **2)** history of recurrent or episodic metabolic decom-

pensation; **3)** neurological abnormalities, including seizures, hypotonia, lethargy, coma, developmental delay, or unexplained mental retardation; **4)** specific clinical findings associated with particular disorders, such as macrocephaly in Canavan disease and glutaric acidemia type I and neonatal liver dysfunction in tyrosinemia type I; **5)** failure to thrive; **6)** history of a previously affected sibling; and **7)** follow-up of an abnormal newborn screening result.

Sample Requirements Organic acids are analyzed in urine, from either a random void or, ideally, a first-morning specimen, collected in a clean container without preservatives. Ideally, specimens should be collected during the time of acute illness because abnormal metabolite levels often decrease, sometimes to near-normal concentrations, when the patient is well. Samples should be frozen as soon as possible after collection and stored frozen prior to analysis.

In specific situations, such as the monitoring of patients with methylmalonic acidemia, targeted analytes are analyzed in plasma collected from heparanized whole blood. Separate plasma by centrifugation, and store frozen prior to analysis.

Interpretation Organic acid patterns associated with various metabolic diseases are summarized in Table 48-4. An optimal interpretation depends not only on recognition of disease patterns but also an awareness of secondary influences from clinical status, diet, and certain medications. Clinical influences include liver dysfunction or prematurity (both associated with abnormal elevation of tyrosine metabolites), ketosis, cardiac abnormalities, and gastrointestinal abnormalities such as short-gut syndrome. Diets supplemented with medium-chain triglycerides, common for some infant formulas, leads to abnormal elevations of certain fatty acid intermediates. Artifacts also can arise from total parental nutrition (leading to a marked elevation of N-acetyltyrosine), chocolate, and gelatin desserts such as Jello (which contains adipic acid and an additive), as well as from plastic specimen containers, soaps, lotions, and metabolites from gut bacteria. Many medications, including acetaminophen, valproate, and chloral hydrate, also can lead to abnormal findings.

Abnormal results indicative of a particular metabolic disorder should be followed by specific enzyme assays when possible. Molecular studies to delineate specific mutations are becoming increasingly available on either a clinical or research basis and should be pursued when feasible.

ANALYSIS OF CARNITINE AND ACYLCARNITINES

Carnitine testing includes the evaluation of free carnitine, total carnitine, and the ratio of esterified to free carnitine (acyl:free ratio). This test identifies patients with primary disorders of carnitine transport (i.e., carnitine uptake deficiency) and the carnitine cycle (e.g., carnitine palmitoyl transferase 1), as well as secondary disturbances in carnitine levels arising from disorders of organic acid or fatty acid metabolism, or disorders of renal function because carnitine is reabsorbed by the kidney. Carnitine (β-hydroxy, γ-trimethylaminobutyric acid) is required for fatty acid β-oxidation of long-chain fats and is conjugated to abnormal acids in the mitochondrion, which leads to the accumulation of abnormal acylcarnitine species in certain inborn errors of metabolism.

Acylcarnitine profile analysis reveals abnormalities in levels of specific acylcarnitine species from chain length C_2 (acetylcarnitine) to C_{18} (stearylcarnitine) and identifies disorders of fatty acid β-oxidation and some disorders of organic acid metabolism (1,2). Examples of disorders identified include medium-chain acyl-CoA dehydrogenase (MCAD), (elevated C_6, C_8, and $C_{10:1}$ acylcarnitines) and long-chain 3-hydroxyacyl-CoA dehydrogenase (LCHAD) deficiencies (elevated $C_{16:OH}$ and $C_{18:OH}$), carnitine palmitoyltransferase II and carnitine/acylcarnitine translocase deficiencies, and propionic acidemia (C_3), isovaleric acidemia (C_5), and others. Acylcarnitine profile analysis is often performed in conjunction with plasma amino acid and urine organic acid analysis and free and total carnitine determination. It is also being used with increasing frequency in neonatal screening programs, allowing early recognition of a variety of fatty acid oxidation and organic acid disorders (3).

Carnitine (Free and Total)

Test Description Carnitine analysis involves the direct measurement of free carnitine and the measurement of total carnitine following alkaline hydrolysis of the acylcarnitines by potassium hydroxide. The fraction of total carnitine representing the acylcarnitines (also called the *esterified fraction*) is determined by subtraction. Urine carnitine is normalized to creatinine concentration. Results also include a calculation of the ratio of acyl to free carnitine. Several approaches can be used to determine carnitine levels, including spectrophotometric and radioenzymatic methods (4,5), as well as analyses using HPLC, stable-isotope-dilution MS/MS (6), and specific chemistry analyzers (7). Carnitine determination should be performed in cases of known

TABLE 48-4   Disease Patterns of Organic Acids

Organic Acids Patterns	Conditions
Intermediates of aromatic amino acid metabolism	
Homogentisic acid	Alkaptonuria
4-Hydroxycyclohexyacetate	Hawkinsinuria
4-Hydroxyphenylpyruvic, 4-hydroxyphenyllactic, 4-hydroxyphenylacetic acids, succinyl acetone	Tyrosinemia type I
4-Hydroxyphenylpyruvic, 4-hydroxyphenyllactic, 4-hydroxyphenylacetic acids	Tyrosinemia types II and III (with N-acetyltyrosine) Liver disease
Phenylpyruvic acid, phenyllactic acid, phenylacetic acid, 2-hydroxyphenylacetic acids	Phenylketonuria
Intermediates of branched chain amino acid metabolism	
3-Hydroxyisovaleric acid, isovalerylglycine	Isovaleric acidemia
3-Hydroxyisovaleric acid, 3-methylcrotonylglycine	3-Methylcrotonyl-CoA carboxylase deficiency
3-Hydroxyisovaleric acid, 3-methylcrotonylglycine, 3-hydroxypropionic acid, lactic acid, methylcitric acid	Holocarboxylase synthetase deficiency or biotinidase deficiency
3-Hydroxy-3-methylglutaric acid, 3-methylglutaconic acid, 3-methylglutaric acid, 3-hydroxyisovaleric acid	3-Hydroxy-3-methylglutaryl-CoA lyase deficiency
3-Hydroxypropionic acid, methylcitric acid, propionylglycine, and tiglylglycine	Propionyl-CoA carboxylase deficiency
Isobutyrylglycine	Isobutyryl-CoA dehydrogenase deficiency
2-Ketoisocaproic acid, 2-keto-3-methylvaleric acid, 2-ketoisovaleric acid, 2-hydroxyisovaleric acid	Maple Syrup Urine Disease
2-Methylbutyrylglycine	2-Methylbutyryl-CoA dehydrogenase deficiency
3-Methylglutaconic acid, 3-methylglutaric acid, 3-hydroxyisovaleric acid	3-Methylglutaconic aciduria (3-MethylglutaconylCoA hydratase deficiency)
2-Methyl-3-hydroxybutyric acid, 2-methylacetoacetic acid, tiglylglycine	3-Oxothiolase deficiency (T_2 deficiency)
Methylmalonic acid, 3-hydroxypropionic acid, methylcitric acid, tiglylglycine	Methylmalonyl-CoA mutase deficiency
Methylmalonic acid, methylcitric acid, ± tiglylglycine, ± 3-hydroxypropionic acid	Methylmalonic acidemia variants (Cbl A, Cbl B) Combined methylmalonic acidemia and homocystinuria (Cbl C, Cbl D, Cbl F, Transcobalamin-II or vitamin B_{12} deficiencies)
Intermediates of fatty acid oxidation	
Dicarboxylic acids (octenedioic, decenedioic, adipic, suberic, and sebacic acids)	Most of the fatty acids oxidation disorders while symptomatic, except for disorders of the carnitine cycle
Ethylmalonic acid, methylsuccinic acid	Short-chain acyl-CoA dehydrogenase deficiency
Glutaric acid, 2-hydroxyglutaric acid, ethylmalonic acid, isovalerylglycine, hexanoylglycine, suberylglycine	Multiple acyl-CoA dehydrogenase deficiency
Hexanoylglycine, suberylglycine, phenylpropionylglycine	Medium-chain acyl-CoA dehydrogenase deficiency
3-Hydroxydicarboxylic acids, dicarboxylic acids	Long-chain hydroxyacyl-CoA dehydrogenase/Trifunctional protein deficiency
Miscellaneous Disorders	
N-acetylaspartic acid	Canavan disease
Fumaric acid	Fumarase deficiency
Glutaric acid, 3-hydroxyglutaric acid	Glutaric acidemia type I
D-Glyceric acid	D-Glyceric aciduria
4-Hydroxybutyric acid	Succinic semialdehyde dehydrogenase deficiency
Mevalonic acid, mevalonolactone	Mevalonic aciduria
5-Oxoproline (pyroglutamic acid)	Glutathione synthetase deficiency
Oxalic acid, glycolic acid, glyoxylic acid	Hyperoxaluria type I
Oxalic acid, L-glyceric acid	Hyperoxaluria type II

or suspected primary (i.e., carnitine uptake defect) or secondary (e.g., organic acidemias, fatty acid oxidation disorders, and renal losses) carnitine deficiency. An abnormal acyl:free ratio is an indication for an acylcarnitine profile if this has not been performed already in order to identify the abnormal acyl species.

Indications Indications for testing include lethargy or hypotonia, myopathy (either cardiac or skeletal), hypoglycemia, hypoketosis, metabolic acidosis, hyperammonemia, elevated liver transaminases, hepatomegaly, recurrent episodes of hepatic dysfunction, a clinical suspicion of a fatty acid oxidation defect (see "Acylcarnitine Profile"), clinical suspicion of an organic acidemia (see "Organic Acid Analysis"), renal dysfunction, a positive family history, or positive newborn screening result with decreased free carnitine and/or abnormal acylcarnitine profile. This test is often ordered in conjunction with acylcarnitine profile and organic acid analysis.

Sample Requirements The most common sample type is serum or plasma. Specific requirements vary by laboratory; general guidelines are given below:

- *Plasma or serum.* Most laboratories require plasma to be obtained from green-top (sodium or lithium heparan) tubes. Separate plasma or serum from cells by centrifugation as soon as possible, and store frozen prior to analysis.
- *Urine.* Collect a random urine sample in a clean container without preservatives. Store frozen prior to analysis. Urine as well as plasma carnitine concentrations are evaluated in patients suspected of having a primary disorder of carnitine transport.

Interpretation Results include quantitation of free and total carnitine and a calculation of the ratio of acyl to free carnitine. This ratio, when abnormally elevated, can indicate an underlying metabolic disorder and should be followed up with organic acid and acylcarnitine profile analysis when warranted clinically. Significantly decreased levels of plasma free and total carnitine, together with abnormal elevations in urine, are indicative of primary carnitine deficiency (however, the urine carnitine concentration may be in the normal range because the plasma carnitine concentration is so low).

Acylcarnitine Profile

Test Description Acylcarnitines typically are determined by MS/MS following stable-isotope dilution with internal standards and less frequently by HPLC and GC/MS methods. Compounds are analyzed most often as their butyl or methyl derivatives but are sometimes analyzed underivatized. Quanti-

tative results of 20–30 different acylcarnitines are provided along with comparison with age-matched controls.

Indications Indications include: 1) neurological abnormalities (including hypotonia, lethargy, coma, and seizures) presenting at any age, particularly if accompanied by hypoglycemia, hypoketosis, metabolic acidosis, hyperammonemia, elevated liver transaminases, and hepatomegaly; 2) recurrent episodes of hepatic dysfunction; 3) cardiomyopathy presenting at any age; 4) myopathy, exercise intolerance, or rhabdomyolysis; 5) infant of a mother with acute fatty liver of pregnancy (AFLP) or hypertension, elevated liver enzymes, and low platelet (HELLP) syndrome; 6) positive newborn screening result of abnormal acylcarnitine profile; and 7) positive family history, including history of sudden unexplained death, apparent life-threatening event (ALTE), or Reye syndrome.

Sample Requirements This test is performed routinely in serum or plasma, as well as on dried blood spots collected on filter-paper cards. It is performed less frequently in urine, although this may be a more sensitive approach

for detecting certain metabolic disorders, such as glutaric acidemia type I (8). Specific requirements vary by laboratory; general guidelines are given below:

- *Plasma or serum.* Most laboratories require plasma to be collected in either sodium or lithium heparan. Separate plasma or serum from cells by centrifugation as soon as possible, and store frozen prior to analysis.
- *Dried blood spot.* Completely fill two to three circles with blood on a newborn screening filter card. Allow to air-dry.
- *Urine.* Testing requires a random urine sample obtained in a clean container and without preservatives. Store frozen prior to analysis.

Interpretation Disorders indicated by specific acylcarnitine abnormalities are summarized in Table 48-5. It is important to note that results may be compromised when free carnitine levels are low; in these cases, retesting is often recommended following initiation of carnitine supplementation. Certain medications (e.g., valproate, cefotaxime, and pivalic acid–based antibiotics) can lead to artifactual findings.

TABLE 48-5	Abnormal Acylcarnitine Levels and Associated Disorders	
Designation	**Acylcarnitine Name**	**Disorder**
$C_0 \downarrow$	Free Carnitine	Carnitine Uptake Defect
		Secondary carnitine deficiencies in organic acidemia and fatty acid oxidation disorders
$C_3 \uparrow$	Propionyl	Propionic acidemia
		Methylmalonic acidemia
		Multiple carboxylase deficiency (with $C_{5\text{-OH}}$)
$C_4 \uparrow$	Butyryl	Short-chain acyl-CoA dehydrogenase deficiency
		Multiple acyl-CoA dehydrogenase deficiency (with C_5, C_6 and others)
	Isobutyryl	Isobutyryl-CoA dehydrogenase deficiency
$C_5 \uparrow$	Isovaleryl	Isovaleric acidemia
	Methylbutyryl	2-Methylbutyryl-CoA dehydrogenase deficiency
$C_{5\text{-OH}} \uparrow$	3-Hydroxyisovaleryl	β-Methylcrotonyl-CoA carboxylase deficiency
		3-Hydroxy-3-methylglutaryl-CoA lyase deficiency
		Holocarboxylase synthetase/Biotinidase deficiency
	3-Hydroxy-2-methylbutyryl	3-Oxothiolase deficiency
$C_5DC \uparrow$	Glutaryl	Glutaric acidemia type I
$C_8 \uparrow$	Octanoyl	Medium-chain acyl-CoA dehydrogenase deficiency (with C_6, C_{10}, $C_{10:1}$)
$C_{14:1} \uparrow$	Tetradecenoyl	Very long-chain acyl-CoA dehydrogenase deficiency (with C_{14}, $C_{14:2}$, C_{16})
$C_{16} \uparrow$	Palmitoyl	Carnitine palmitoyltransferase II deficiency (with $C_{18:1}$, C_{18})
		Carnitine acylcarnitine translocase deficiency (with $C_{18:1}$, C_{18})
$C_{16\text{-OH}} \uparrow$	3-Hydroxypalmitoyl	Long-chain hydroxyacyl-CoA dehydrogenase (with $C_{18:1\text{-OH}}$)
		Mitochondrial trifunctional protein deficiency (with $C_{18:1\text{-OH}}$)

LABORATORY EVALUATION OF MITOCHONDRIAL DISORDERS

The mitochondrial myopathies encompass a heterogeneous group of disorders arising from primary defects of pyruvate metabolism (i.e., pyruvate dehydrogenase complex, pyruvate carboxylase), enzymatic defects of the tricarboxylic acid (TCA) cycle, disorders of the mitochondrial respiratory chain, and defects in proteins involved in the assembly and maintenance of normal mitochondrial structure and function.

Many tests can be applied to the workup of a mitochondrial patient, and no single approach has emerged as optimal in all cases. An overview of tests used in the evaluation of mitochondrial disorders is shown in Table 48-6. Noninvasive tests frequently are initiated before pursuing those requiring invasive procedures for sample collection, with the precise course of action often dictated by clinical findings, available specimens, and locally available tests (9).

Clinical findings leading to the suspicion of a mitochondrial disorder are broad and nonspecific. Although these disorders are associated most often with myopathy (either skeletal or cardiac), they can affect any organ system, including brain, kidney, eyes, ears, and endocrine function, as well as overall growth and development. Presentation can range from severe neonatal illness and death to mild symptoms in adults. In general, mitochondrial disorders should be considered in patients with persistent lactic acidosis, hypotonia, muscle weakness or pain, exercise intolerance, cardiomyopathy or cardiac conduction defects, developmental delay, failure to thrive, seizures, hearing or visual loss, pancreatic abnormalities, or diabetes. A family history of maternal inheritance indicates the possibility of a mitochondrial disorder arising from defects in mitochondrial DNA.

METABOLIC STUDIES

Blood Lactate, Pyruvate, and the Lactate:Pyruvate Ratio

The identification of lactic acidosis is often the first clue leading to a more comprehensive mitochondrial workup. Lactate and pyruvate typically are measured enzymatically on dedicated chemistry analyzer instruments.

Sample Requirements Specific requirements vary by laboratory. Testing generally is performed on plasma obtained from a gray-top (sodium fluoride/potassium oxalate) tube from blood collected without the use of a tourniquet. Samples for pyruvate determination require immediate treatment with perchloric acid prior to centrifugation. Separate plasma, and freeze as soon as possible.

Interpretation Elevated lactate can be seen in primary disorders of pyruvate metabolism, abnormalities of the TCA cycle, and other mitochondrial disorders, including primary deficiencies of the respiratory chain complexes. Lactic acidosis also can be seen in disorders of gluconeogenesis or secondary to hypoxia, cardiac defects, sepsis, and other inborn errors of metabolism (e.g., organic acidemias). A lactate:pyruvate ratio more than 20 is suggestive of a mitochondrial respiratory chain disorder, whereas a ratio of less than 20 indicates that a block may be upstream of the respiratory chain. It is important to note that normal lactate and lactate:pyruvate ratio do not exclude the possibility of a mitochondrial disorder. In some patients with neurological symptoms, lactate elevations may be found only in CSF and/or by NMR spectroscopy of the brain.

Urine Organic Acids

Urine organic acids are analyzed by GC/MS (see "Organic Acid Analysis" for test description and specimen requirements) in patients suspected of having a mitochondrial disorder.

Interpretation The pattern of organic acid excretion in mitochondrial patients may be normal but often shows variably elevated lactate, pyruvate (when analyzed following oximation), ketone bodies, medium-chain dicarboxylic acids (e.g., adipic, suberic, and sebacic acids), ethylmalonic, 3-methylglutaconic acid, α-ketoglutaric and aconitic acids, and in particular, fumaric and malic acids (10).

Abnormal patterns should be followed up by additional studies, including specific enzyme assays and/or DNA studies as appropriate. Because normal results do not exclude the possibility of a mitochondrial disorder, additional testing also should be sought in any patient with clinically suspected mitochondrial disease regardless of organic acid findings.

Plasma Amino Acids

Amino acids are analyzed on an amino acid analyzer using ion-exchange chromatography (see "Quantitative Amino Acid Analysis" for test description and specimen requirements) in patients suspected of having a mitochondrial disorder.

Interpretation Abnormally elevated alanine can be seen secondary to lactic acidosis and should be followed up by blood lactate and pyruvate determinations. Elevations of citrulline and lysine are seen in pyruvate carboxylase deficiency. Abnormal patterns should be followed up by additional studies, including specific enzyme assays and/or DNA studies as appropriate. In patients with neurological symptoms, elevation of alanine and threonine in CSF can be diagnostic.

Plasma Carnitine and Acylcarnitine Profile

See "Analysis of Carnitine and Acylcarnitines." Patients with mitochondrial disorders often show decreased levels of free and total carnitine with an elevated ratio of acyl:free carnitine. The acylcarnitine profile may be normal, but some mitochondrial respiratory patients have profiles similar to patients with disorders of mitochondrial fatty acid oxidation (11,12).

Plasma Ketones (β-Hydroxybutyrate and Acetoacetate)

Plasma ketones are evaluated as a routine chemistry test and may be paradoxically elevated postprandially in patients with mitochondrial disorders. More specific studies of plasma β-hydroxybutyrate, acetoacetate, and their ratio are useful in estimating mitochondrial NAD/NADH and may be abnormally elevated in defects of the respiratory chain and reduced in pyruvate carboxylase deficiency.

MICROSCOPY STUDIES

Test Description Examination of mitochondria by light or electron microscopy is used to identify abnormalities in mitochondrial structure and function. Histological studies on cryostat sections of biopsied muscle involve the use of essential stains, including modified Gomori trichrome (to detect subsarcolemmal collections of mitochondria, seen

---

TABLE 48-6   Tests for Mitochondrial Disorders

- **Metabolic studies**

  Blood and CSF lactate, pyruvate

  Urine organic acids

  Plasma amino acids

  Plasma carnitine and acylcarnitine profile

  Plasma ketones (β-hydroxybutyrate and acetoacetate)

- **Microscopy**

- **Analysis of enzymes upstream of the mitochondrial respiratory chain**

  Pyruvate dehydrogenase complex, pyruvate carboxylase

  Other TCA enzymes

- **Studies of the mitochondrial respiratory chain**

  Respiratory chain enzyme analysis

  Respiratory chain structural analysis

- **DNA studies**

  Mitochondrial DNA studies

  Nuclear DNA studies

as "ragged red fibers"), cytochrome oxidase (COX, to detect respiratory chain complex IV activity), succinate dehydrogenase (SDH, complex II), and NADH dehydrogenase (a general indicator of oxidative phosphorylation). Transmission electron microscopy (TEM) can be used to evaluate mitochondrial ultrastructure, inclusion bodies, and cristae morphology (13), but its usefulness in the diagnostic evaluation of mitochondrial patients has been questioned because of increased expense and lack of specificity (14).

Sample Requirements Obtain samples by open muscle biopsy and process within 30 minutes of collection. Histology studies require approximately a $1 \times 0.5 \times 0.5$ cm piece of muscle, from which a very small portion $(0.2 \times 0.1 \times 0.1$ cm) can be placed in glutaraldehyde and the remainder snap-frozen for cryosections. Additional muscle should be obtained for enzymology and DNA studies (see below).

Interpretation The modified Gomori trichrome stain reveals increases in subsarcolemmal red staining representing ragged-red fibers (RRFs), a classical finding in mitochondrial disease. RRFs are seen more commonly in disorders affecting mitochondrial protein synthesis, such as the myoclonic epilepsy and ragged red fiber (MERRF) disease, and are seen rarely in other disorders, such as Leigh syndrome with an underlying complex I deficiency. They are also rarely, if ever, encountered in patients younger than 3 years of age (14). On the other hand, RRFs can be a nonspecific finding in a variety of unrelated conditions, including aging and other myopathies, and their presence alone cannot be taken as diagnostic of a mitochondrial disorder. A strong increase in SDH activity can indicate mitochondrial proliferation in disorders such as mitochondrial encephalopathy, lactic acidosis and stroke-like episodes (MELAS). RRFs with strong SDH activity but COX negativity indicate a disorder of mitochondrial protein synthesis, whereas those that are COX-positive are characteristic of MELAS or other defects of mitochondrial structural genes (excluding COX) (14). It is important to note that some patients with mitochondrial myopathy have completely normal muscle histology.

ANALYSIS OF ENZYMES UPSTREAM OF THE MITOCHONDRIAL RESPIRATORY CHAIN

Pyruvate Dehydrogenase Complex, Pyruvate Carboxylase, and TCA-Cycle Enzyme Assays

Test Description Enzymatic methods employing specific radioactive substrates are used to measure activities of pyruvate dehydrogenase complex (PDHC) and pyruvate carboxylase (PC). Less frequently, the TCA-cycle enzymes fumarase and α-ketoglutarate dehydrogenase are assayed in patients with characteristic organic acid findings of abnormally elevated fumarate or α-ketoglutarate, respectively.

Indications In addition to lactic acidosis and a clinical picture suggestive of mitochondrial dysfunction, patients with PC deficiency have characteristically elevated citrulline and lysine by plasma amino acid analysis. Fumarase and α-ketoglutarate dehydrogenase are assayed in patients with organic acid abnormalities (see above).

Sample Requirements PC and PDHC enzyme assays typically are performed on cultured fibroblasts obtained from a skin biopsy. Some laboratories also offer testing on liver or other tissues or in leukocytes or transformed lymphoblasts from blood collected in an ACD (yellow-top) tube. Laboratories should be contacted for specific requirements prior to sample collection.

Interpretation Enzyme activities are evaluated together with appropriate positive and negative controls to exclude the possibility of artifactual results. Significantly reduced or absent enzyme activity is indicative of a specific disorder, but partial deficiencies still may have pathological significance and must be interpreted in the clinical context of the patient.

STUDIES OF THE MITOCHONDRIAL RESPIRATORY CHAIN

Mitochondrial Respiratory Chain Enzyme Assays

Test Description Functional studies of the respiratory chain complexes are performed using spectrophotometric or polarographic determinations of respiratory chain activity in the presence or absence of various oxidative substrates or inhibitors. This allows for differentiation between the activities of all the complexes except complex V, as well as coenzyme Q. Citrate synthase, a mitochondrial matrix enzyme, typically is measured to control for specimen integrity.

Sample Requirements The preferred sample is fresh muscle. Obtain a minimum of 150–200 mg of muscle (skeletal or cardiac). When samples must be shipped to an outside laboratory, freeze immediately in liquid nitrogen and ship on dry ice. Testing also can be performed in cultured skin fibroblasts obtained from a skin biopsy (15).

Interpretation Significant residual enzyme activity is often present in patients with mitochondrial enzymopathies, and it can be difficult to interpret the clinical significance of modest decreases. False-negative results may arise in frozen muscle (16). Results must be considered carefully in the context of the patient's clinical history because false-negative or false-positive conclusions could result otherwise. A significant number of patients with mitochondrial disorders will have normal respiratory chain activities in fibroblasts, and these patients should be followed up with studies in muscle whenever warranted clinically. Normal enzymology in either fibroblasts or muscle does not rule out a mitochondrial disorder, and for some patients, the diagnosis will continue to be strongly suspected on clinical grounds alone.

Respiratory Chain Structural Analysis

Monoclonal antibodies against specific respiratory chain subunits have become available for use recently in either Western blot analysis or immunocytochemistry studies in cultured cells or immunohistochemistry studies in frozen tissue sections (17). Their clinical utility has been reported recently in the identification of patients with a significant reduction or absence of entire respiratory chain complexes (15). This approach does not detect abnormalities in which the complexes are intact but nonfunctional, such as with mutations that alter catalytic activity without diminishing protein abundance. However, when results are considered together with other histological, enzymatic, and clinical findings, these monoclonal antibodies represent a new and valuable tool in the identification of mitochondrial patients.

DNA STUDIES

Test Description *Mitochondrial DNA* (mtDNA) can be evaluated for known point mutations, deletions or large DNA sequence rearrangements, or generalized mtDNA depletion (18). Point mutations include those described in patients with MELAS, LHON, MERRF, NARP, and other syndromes. Testing is by allele-specific methods such as restriction fragment-length polymorphism (RFLP) analysis and allele-specific oligonucleotide hybridization (ASO). When mtDNA mutations are not detected by these methods, other mutation-scanning techniques can be employed, such as single-strand conformation polymorphism (SSCP) analysis, temporal temperature-gradient gel electrophoresis (TTGE), and denaturing high-performance liquid chromatography (DHPLC). Abnormalities detected by these methods are followed up by direct mtDNA sequencing. Large rearrangements, including large deletions associated with Kearns–Sayre syndrome, chronic progressive external opthalmoplegia (CPEO), and others, typically are detected by Southern blot analysis, but polymerase chain reaction (PCR)–based techniques also can be used. Generalized mitochondrial depletion (as well as mitochondrial proliferation) is evaluated by a quantitative assessment of mtDNA copy number, either by Southern analysis or by real-time quantitative PCR analysis.

Nuclear DNA (nDNA) mutations leading to mitochondrial myopathies have been described in genes encoding subunits of the mitochondrial respiratory chain complexes themselves (for complexes I and II), genes involved in the synthesis of specific respiratory chain elements (e.g., SURF1, SCO1, SCO2, and COX10), and genes involved in intergenomic communication (e.g., POLG and TK2) (19). These mutations are identified by direct sequencing of genomic DNA following PCR amplification of relevant regions.

Sample Requirements DNA testing (either mtDNA or nDNA) is performed from whole-blood samples collected with EDTA anticoagulant. mtDNA testing further may require the collection of muscle because certain mutations are not evident in blood and may be detected only in DNA isolated from muscle. A minimum of 50 mg of muscle is required for mutation analysis.

Interpretation The identification of a known pathogenic mutation in a patient with consistent clinical findings serves to establish the diagnosis. It is often less straightforward to attribute clinical significance to novel DNA changes identified through gene scanning or sequencing approaches, and conclusions must be reached after considering the predicted biochemical consequences of the mutation, as well as the clinical history of the patient. Because some mtDNA mutations are tissue-specific, the lack of identification of a mutation in one tissue does not rule out its presence in another. Heteroplasmy also can complicate results interpretation, particularly because mtDNA mutations at low copy number may go undetected by direct sequencing. If a novel mtDNA mutation is obtained in a patient, the mother's mitochondrial DNA should be analyzed to help determine the likelihood that the detected change is pathogenic.

TESTS FOR PEROXISOMAL DISORDERS

The following laboratory tests are appropriate for the screening and diagnosis of patients with peroxisomal disorders, including 1) the Zellweger spectrum disorders (i.e., Zellweger syndrome [ZS], neonatal adrenoleukodystrophy [NALD], and infantile Refsum disease [IRD]), 2) disorders of peroxisomal β-oxidation (i.e., X-linked adrenoleukodystrophy [XALD] and

deficiencies of acyl-CoA oxidase 1 [ACOX1], D-bifunctional protein [DBP], and 2-methyl-acyl-CoA-racemase [AMACR]), 3) disorders of peroxisomal α-oxidation (i.e., adult Refsum disease), 4) disorders of peroxisomal ether-phospholipid biosynthesis (i.e., rhizomelic chondrodysplasia punctata [RCDP types 1, 2, and 3]), and 4) disorders of glyoxylate detoxification (i.e., hyperoxaluria type I [PHI]).

Indications for peroxisomal testing are broad, reflecting the heterogeneous nature of these disorders. Clinical hallmarks include neurological dysfunction and deterioration, often accompanied by dysmorphic features, hypotonia, hepatomegaly, liver and kidney dysfunction, growth failure, and cataracts. The RCDP group of disorders is clinically distinct and characterized by abnormal shortening of the proximal limbs.

The diagnostic strategy is dictated by the clinical presentation of the patient and often begins with biochemical evaluations in plasma (for very-long-chain fatty acids [VLCFA], phytanic acid, and others) and/or plasmalogen content in erythrocytes (specifically for RCDP), followed by more detailed studies in fibroblasts and finally molecular studies to identify causative mutations (20). Carrier and prenatal testing are available in many cases. An overview of tests available for the peroxisomal disorders is shown in Table 48-7.

BIOCHEMICAL TESTS

Very Long-Chain Fatty Acids (VLCFA), Phytanic Acid and Pristanic Acid

Test Description VLCFA, or fatty acids of carbon length C_{22}–C_{26}, are evaluated in plasma by GC/MS. VLCFA testing often includes the evaluation of phytanic acid, a saturated 20-carbon branched-chain fatty acid of dietary origin, and pristanic acid, a 19-carbon product of phytanic acid metabolism.

Indications VLCFA determination is often the first-line test in the evaluation of a suspected peroxisomal disorder, including patients with the Zellweger spectrum disorders and disorders of β-oxidation. For these patients, testing also may include bile acid intermediates (i.e., DHCA and THCA) and erythrocyte plasmalogen content. Phytanic and pristanic acid evaluations are specifically indicated in patients with a clinical suspicion of RCDP (including proximal limb shortening) and Refsum disease (i.e., visual loss, anosmia, deafness, and ataxia).

Specimen Requirements Most laboratories require the collection of 1–3 mL of whole blood in a lavender-top (EDTA) tube. Fasting or preprandial samples are preferred. Ship whole

TABLE 48-7   Tests for Peroxisomal Disorders
• **Biochemical tests**
Very long chain fatty acids (VLCFA) (plasma or fibroblasts)
Phytanic acid (plasma)
Pristanic acid (plasma)
Plasmalogen content (erythrocytes)
Pipecolic acid (plasma or urine)
Bile acid intermediates (plasma)
Dihydroxycholestenoic acid (DHCA)
Trihydroxycholestenoic acid (THCA)
• **Fibroblast studies**
Functional tests
β-Oxidation of $C_{26:0}$ and pristanic acid
α-Oxidation of phytanic acid
Plasmalogen synthesis
Complementation studies
Catalase distribution
Enzyme assays
Dihydroxyacetonephosphate acyltransferase (RCDP type 2)
Alkyldihydroxyacetonephosphate synthase (RCDP type 3)
Acyl-CoA oxidase
D-Bifunctional protein
Phytanic acid oxidase
Pristanic acid oxidase
• **DNA studies**

blood via overnight courier at room temperature, or separate plasma and ship on dry ice.

Interpretation Elevations of plasma $C_{26:0}$ (hexacosanoic acid) and the ratio of $C_{26:0}$ to $C_{22:0}$ (docosanoic acid) are indicative of Zellweger syndrome or a related disorder. Patients with Zellweger syndrome also have characteristically elevated plasma phytanic acid, pipecolic acid, and bile acid intermediates and reduced plasmalogen content. VLCFA elevations are also seen in X-ALD, ACOX1 deficiency, and DBP deficiency, and additional diagnostic tests, guided by the clinical history, will serve to establish the diagnosis.

Abnormal VLCFA results should be followed by more specific studies in fibroblasts for a disorder of either peroxisomal biogenesis or β-oxidation. Next-line testing includes evaluations of fibroblast plasmalogen synthesis, VLCFA oxidation, oxidation of phytanic and pristanic acids, and catalase distribution. Abnormalities in multiple peroxisomal functions indicate one of the Zellweger spectrum disorders, which can be further delineated by complementation studies in fibroblasts. Confirmation by molecular analysis is possible in some cases once the complementation group has been established. When fibroblast studies indicate an isolated defect in peroxisomal β-oxidation, the identification of mutations in the ABCD1 gene confirms a diagnosis of X-ALD. Enzymatic assays for fibroblast ACOX1 and DBP activities will reveal single-enzyme deficiencies in the β-oxidation pathway, which can be confirmed by molecular analysis of the ACOX1 and DBP genes, respectively.

Elevations of phytanic acid (with normal or decreased levels of pristanic acid) are seen in RCDP type 1 and Refsum disease, although this is a variable finding and depends on dietary intake. For patients suspected of having adult Refsum disease, follow-up studies include evaluation of α-oxidation of phytanic acid in cultured fibroblasts and molecular analysis of the PAHX/PHYH gene.

Pristanic acid (together with DHCA and THCA) is elevated in patients with AMACR deficiency, which can be confirmed by molecular analysis of the AMACR gene. Pristanic acid is also elevated (together with VLCFAs) in patients with DBP deficiency but is normal in ACOX1 deficiency.

Plasmalogen Content

Test Description and Indications Erythrocyte plasmalogen content is evaluated by GC as a comprehensive screening test for RCDP in patients with characteristic clinical findings, including proximal limb shortening, and, together with VLCFA and other biochemical markers, in patients being evaluated for Zellweger syndrome.

Specimen Requirements Testing requires the collection of 3–5 mL of whole blood in a purple-top (EDTA) tube. Ship whole blood via overnight courier at room temperature, or separate erythrocytes and ship on dry ice. Contact laboratory for specific instructions prior to collection.

Interpretation Erythrocyte plasmalogen content is decreased significantly in Zellweger syndrome and in all types of RCDP. A finding of decreased plasmalogens together with abnormally elevated phytanic acid is consistent with RCDP type 1, whereas normal phytanic acid levels suggest RCDP types 2 or 3. Patients should be further evaluated for RCDP by more detailed studies of plasmalogen biosynthesis and enzymatic activities in cultured fibroblasts, followed by molecular testing for specific mutations in the PEX 7, DHAPAT (dihydroxyacetonephosphate acyltransferase), and AGPS (alkyldihydroxyacetonephosphate synthase) genes. Plasmalogen levels are normal in the other peroxisomal disorders, including NALD, X-ALD, deficiencies of ACOX1, DBP and AMACR, and Refsum disease.

Pipecolic Acid

Test Description and Indication Abnormal elevations of pipecolic acid, a minor intermediate of lysine metabolism, are detected by GC/MS in plasma or urine. Testing is indicated for patients with clinical suspicion of one of the Zellweger spectrum disorders.

Specimen Requirements Testing requires 1 mL of plasma or 10 mL of urine. For plasma, collect whole blood in a purple-top (EDTA) tube, and ship at room temperature via overnight courier. Collect urine in clean container, and ship on wet or dry ice.

Interpretation Pipecolic acid levels are elevated levels in the Zellweger spectrum disorders (i.e., ZS, NALD, and IRD) together with elevated VLCFAs, bile acid intermediates, and phytanic and pristanic acids and decreased plasmalogen content. Pipecolic acid is also elevated in vitamin B_6–dependent epilepsy.

Bile Acid Intermediates (DHCA and THCA)

Testing for bile acid intermediates is offered by only a few laboratories worldwide and is performed in plasma or urine by GC/MS and stable-isotope dilution. DHCA and THCA levels are elevated in the Zellweger spectrum disorders, DBP deficiency, and AMACR deficiency but are normal in all types of RCDP, X-ALD, ACOX deficiency, and adult Refsum disease. Analysis of bile acids and bile alcohols is the only definitive method for identifying inborn errors of bile acid synthesis.

FIBROBLAST STUDIES

Studies in fibroblasts are available for the evaluation of VLCFA β-oxidation, catalase distribution, peroxisomal plasmalogen synthesis, and enzymatic activities of dihydroxyacetonephosphate acyltransferase, alkyldihydroxyacetonephosphate synthase, acyl-CoA oxidase, D-bifunctional protein, phytanic acid oxidase, and pristanic acid oxidase. Complementation studies also can be performed to delineate the specific abnormality in patients with peroxisomal biogenesis defects. Practically speaking, these tests are performed in only a few laboratories worldwide; contact the laboratory for specific specimen requirements prior to sample collection. Deficiencies in enzyme activity and/or peroxisomal function should be followed up with molecular studies whenever possible.

DNA STUDIES

Mutation analysis and/or direct gene sequencing are available to confirm mutations in the following genes:

- PEX1, PXMP3 (PEX2), PXR1 (PEX5), PEX6, PEX10, PEX12, PEX13, PEX14, PEX15, PEX16, PEX19 and PEX26 (peroxisomal biogenesis disorders)
- PEX7 (RCDP type 1)
- DHAPAT (RCDP type 2)
- AGPS (RCDP type 3)
- ABCD1 (X-linked adrenoleukodystrophy)

Testing for mutations in other genes may be available on a research basis in a select number of laboratories.

TESTS FOR LYSOSOMAL STORAGE DISORDERS

Testing for lysosomal storage disorders identifies patients with specific lysosomal enzyme deficiencies included in the broad categories of sphingolipidoses, mucopolysaccharidoses, and oligosaccharidoses (Chapter 43). For patients suspected of having a mucopolysaccharidosis or oligosaccharidosis, the laboratory evaluation can be streamlined by performing urine screening tests in order to narrow the differential diagnosis prior to evaluating specific enzymes. Most sphingolipid disorders cannot be approached in this way, and the selection of specific enzyme assays is based on clinical presentation of the patient. Evaluation of a skin biopsy by electron microscopy detects abnormal storage material in almost all disorders.

Urine Screening Tests (Mucopolysaccharides and Oligosaccharides)

Test Description

Mucopolysaccharides (MPSs) Total urinary MPSs (also known as glycosaminoglycans [GAGs]) can be evaluated by simple spot tests using reagents such as dimethylmethylene blue (DMB), Alcian blue, and Toluidine blue. For quantitative tests such as the DMB-binding method, values must be compared with age-dependent reference ranges. When abnormal elevations are detected, fractionation by TLC or electrophoresis is performed to identify abnormal excretion of dermatan sulfate, heparan sulfate, keratan sulfate, or chondroitin-6-sulfate. Results are compared with banding patterns from known patients with Hunter or Hurler, Sanfilippo, Morquio, Maroteaux–Lamy and Sly syndromes.

Oligosaccharides Urinary oligosaccharides are separated by TLC, and the resulting bands are visualized by orcinol, a nonspecific reagent that detects all sugars, and resorcinol, which detects sialic acid–containing carbohydrate residues. Banding patterns are compared with those of known patients with α- or β-mannosidosis, fucosidosis, sialidosis, G_{M1}-gangliosidosis, and others.

Indication Urine screening should be undertaken in patients with clinical suspicion of a mucopolysaccharidosis or oligosaccharidosis, including organomegaly, developmental regression, coarse facial features, or dysostosis multiplex.

Specimen Requirements Collect 2–5 mL of random urine in a clean container without preservatives for the MPS spot test and oligosaccharide TLC. MPS TLC requires collection of 10–15 mL of urine. Store frozen, and ship to the laboratory on dry ice.

Interpretation Urine spot tests for total MPSs can yield both false-positive and false-negative results, particularly in very young infants. Significant abnormalities should be followed up with MPS fractionation, which identifies patients with Hunter, Hurler, or Scheie syndrome (i.e., elevated excretion of heparan and dermatan sulfate), Sanfilippo syndrome types A, B, C, and D (heparan sulfate), Morquio syndrome types A and B (keratan sulfate), Maroteaux–Lamy syndrome (i.e., dermatan sulfate), Sly syndrome (variable excretion of heparan, dermatan, and chondroitin sulfate), or multiple sulfatase deficiency (elevated excretion of heparan, dermatan, and chondroitin sulfate). Distinct oligosaccharide TLC banding patterns are seen in patients with α- or β-mannosidosis, α-fucosidosis, G_{M1}- gangliosidosis, galactosialidosis, Sandhoff disease, Schindler disease, aspartylglucosaminuria, sialidosis, and the free sialic acid transport disorders, although the pattern may be only weakly positive and is best interpreted in the context of clinical history. Any abnormality should be confirmed by enzyme testing to establish the diagnosis. False-negative results can occur with both MPS and oligosaccharide TLC, and enzyme studies always should be pursued in patients with a strong clinical suspicion regardless of urine screening results.

Lysosomal Enzyme Assays

Test Description Lysosomal enzyme deficiencies are diagnosed using assays with commercially available artificial substrates based on flurometric, spectrophotometric, or radioactive methods. Some laboratories allow the selection of individual enzyme tests, whereas others evaluate a panel of enzymes based on the clinical history of the patient (21). The one disorder not diagnosed by traditional enzyme assays is Niemann–Pick disease type C, for which testing is based on filipin staining and light microscopy in cultured fibroblasts, or on demonstration of abnormal cholesterol esterification in cultured fibroblasts.

Many of the lysosomal enzymes can be assayed for the purposes of carrier detection in families with an affected proband. In these cases, testing should include appropriate family members (i.e., the proband and obligate heterozygotes, if available) as positive controls and healthy, unrelated individuals as negative controls. Enzymatic carrier testing is less reliable for the X-linked disorders Hunter syndrome and Fabry disease.

Indications Lysosomal testing is indicated in patients with progressive mental retardation and developmental delay, loss of milestones, organomegaly (particularly hepatosplenomegaly, other neurological abnormalities including seizures and ataxia), eye findings (cherry-red spot, visual loss), coarse facial features, or skeletal abnormalities (dysostosis multiplex). Among the sphingolipidosis, enzyme deficiencies most often associated with neurological findings are β-galactosidase (G_{M1}- gangliosidosis), β-hexosaminidase (Tay–Sachs and Sandhoff diseases), arylsulfatase A (metachromatic leukodystrophy), and β-galactocerebrosidase (Krabbe disease), and these four enzymes are often considered together in a diagnostic evaluation. Those associated with more visceral involvement, particularly hepatosplenomegaly, are β-glucocerebrosidase (Gaucher disease) and sphingomyelinase (Niemann–Pick disease types A and B).

Sample Requirements Many laboratories require the shipment of one or more control samples collected at the same time as the patient sample. Most tests are performed in mixed leukocytes isolated from whole blood; specific collection volumes and tube types vary by laboratory. Refrigerate blood after collection, and keep cool during shipment; blood should be received by the testing laboratory within 24 hours of collection. Some laboratories require that a leukocyte pellet be prepared by dextran sedimentation and shipped on dry ice.

Plasma or serum assays require the collection of 3–5 mL of blood in a green- or red-top tube. Centrifuge as soon as possible, separate and freeze plasma or serum, and ship to the laboratory on dry ice.

For fibroblasts assays, culture cells obtained from a skin biopsy to confluence (size and number of flasks vary by laboratory) and ship via overnight express at room temperature. Many laboratories require certification that cells are free of *Mycoplasma* contamination. Contact individual laboratories before shipping any prenatal samples.

Interpretation Absent or significantly reduced (<10% of normal) enzyme activity establishes the diagnosis in most cases. Exceptions occur in cases of enzyme pseudodeficiency, in which deficient *in vitro* enzyme activity is seen in clinically unaffected individuals. Pseudodeficiency has been reported for a number of diseases, including metachromatic leukodystrophy, Tay–Sachs disease, Fabry disease, Sly syndrome, and others. Questions of pseudodeficiency should be followed up with clinical correlations and molecular studies as appropriate. For many enzymes, intermediate (approximately 50% normal) activities can be suggestive of carrier status, but this should be interpreted only by a laboratory with significant experience in carrier detection for the disorder in question. In rare cases, normal *in vitro* enzyme activity can be seen in patients with clinically significant *in vivo* enzyme deficiency, such as for activator protein deficiencies associated with G_{M2}-gangliosidosis, metachromatic leukodystrophy, and Gaucher disease.

DNA Studies

Confirmation of molecular mutations is becoming increasingly widespread for many lysosomal storage disorders. DNA studies should be pursued only after a specific enzyme deficiency has been established and are rarely appropriate for primary diagnostic evaluations. Testing is by both allele-specific methods and gene sequencing and requires blood from a purple-top (EDTA) tube.

NEUROTRANSMITTER STUDIES

Biochemical studies are performed to evaluate for disorders of catecholamine (e.g., dopamine, epinephrine, and norepinephrine) and serotonin metabolism, including deficiencies of tyrosine hydroxylase, aromatic L-amino acid decarboxylase (AADC, or dopa decarboxylase), dopamine-β-hydroxylase, and the pterin defects without hyperphenylalaninemia (see Chapter 45). The metabolic end products homovanillic acid (HVA), 5-hydroxyindoleacetic acid (5-HIAA), and 3-methoxy-4-hydroxyphenylglycol (MHPGP) are released into CSF, and their measurement in this compartment reflects the overall turnover of the individual neurotransmitters (22). Neurotransmitter disorders arising from defects in tetrahydrobiopterin (BH_4) cofactor metabolism (e.g., GTP cyclohydroase, 6-pyruvoyltetrahydropterin synthase [PTPS], and sepiapterin reductase and dihydropteridine reductase deficiencies) are also evaluated. For most of the disorders, including the BH_4-related disorders that do not involve hyperphenylalaninemia, abnormalities are revealed only through testing of CSF. A comprehensive evaluation of neurotransmitter disorders should include the determination of all end products, including HVA, 5-HIAA, MHPGP, 3-O-methyldopa (3-OMD), 5-hydroxytryptophan (5-HTP), and the pterin species.

Test Description Intermediates of neurotransmitter metabolism (HVA, 5HIAA,

5HTP and 3-O-methyldopa [3OMD]) and biopterin metabolism (BH$_4$, dihydrobiopterin [BH$_2$] and total neopterin) are evaluated in CSF by HPLC and a combination of electrochemical and fluorescence detection. Depending on the pattern of results, follow-up testing should include enzyme analysis and DNA studies (either targeted mutation analysis or gene sequencing) to confirm the diagnosis. Phenylalanine loading studies are used to evaluate for dopa-responsive dystonia due to GTP–cyclohydroase deficiency or sepiapterin reductase deficiency; this test consists of an oral phenylalanine challenge followed by measurements of the plasma phenylalanine:tyrosine ratio by amino acid analysis. Ideally, pterins are also determined (23). Practically speaking, testing for neurotransmitter disorders is performed in only a few laboratories worldwide and in a single laboratory in the United States (see www.geneclinics.org or www.stoffwechsel.uni-hd.de).

Indications The full phenotypic spectrum of the neurotransmitter disorders is unknown but includes neonatal seizures, progressive dystonia, limb rigidity, ataxia, hypotonia, orthostatic hypotension, oculogyric crises, ptosis, and temperature instability.

Sample Requirements *CSF (for 5-HIAA, 3-OMD, l-Dopa, HVA, 5-HTP, MHPG, BH4, BH2, and Neopterin)* Contact the laboratory for specific CSF collection protocol and tube requirements. In general, CSF for BH$_4$ must be collected into a tube containing antioxidants. Blood-contaminated samples are unstable unless the tube is immediately centrifuged and the clear supernatant separated from red blood cells. Freeze at –70°C, and ship on dry ice.

Interpretation Decreased CSF levels of HVA and MHPG with normal 5-HIAA are suggestive of tyrosine hydroxylase deficiency. Decreased levels of BH$_4$ and neopterin, with variably decreased HVA and 5-HIAA, indicate GTP–cyclohydrolase deficiency, either dominant or recessive, whereas decreased BH$_4$, HVA, and 5-HIAA with elevated BH$_2$ indicate a deficiency of dihydropyrimidine reductase or sepiapterin reductase. Sepiapterin is not detected in routine investigations of biogenic monoamine metabolites in CSF but can be determined reliably in a few specialized laboratories. Its presence is diagnostic of sepiapterin reductase deficiency. Decreased levels of HVA and 5-HIAA with abnormally elevated 3-OMD suggest a deficiency of AADC. Dopamine-β-hydroxylase deficiency is suggested by abnormally low levels of norepinephrine, epinephrine, and MHPG with markedly elevated dopamine and L-dopa. Presumed enzyme deficiencies should be followed up by enzyme assay and

DNA mutation analysis of the relevant coding regions whenever possible.

TESTS FOR DISORDERS OF CARBOHYDRATE METABOLISM
Glycogen Storage Disorders

The glycogen storage disorders (GSDs) encompass a broad clinical spectrum of hepatic and/or myopathic presentations (see Chapter 6). Diagnostic evaluations for a particular GSD are guided by the clinical presentation, together with results of routine laboratory studies, including glucose, lactate, ketones, triglycerides, cholesterol, liver enzymes (AST/ALT), creatine kinase, uric acid, bilirubin, and prothrombin time. Specific enzyme assays are available for all the GSD, and molecular confirmation is available for most.

Indications for testing for the GSDs with predominantly hepatic involvement (GSD types I, III, VI, and IX) include fasting ketotic hypoglycemia, hyperuricemia, lactic acidosis, and growth retardation, whereas those primarily involving the muscle (GSD types II, V, and VII) are characterized by cardiomyopathy (in the early-onset form of GSD-II) or later-onset weakness and exercise intolerance. Patients with GSD-IV can have both hepatic and cardiac involvement, including hepatic failure, cirrhosis, and cardiomegaly.

Glycogen Content and Specific Enzyme Assays

Test Description Table 48-8 summarizes the enzyme assays and tissue requirements for diagnostic testing of the GSDs. Assays for

glycogen content and structure and specific enzymatic activities are performed in homogenates of biopsied liver or muscle tissue and less frequently in cultured fibroblasts. Enzyme activities and glycogen content are determined directly in tissue homogenates and compared with both positive and negative controls.

Specimen Requirements Contact the laboratory for specific requirements prior to specimen collection; general guidelines are as follows:

- *Liver.* Obtain at least 15 mg total weight via percutaneous or open liver biopsy. Freeze immediately in liquid nitrogen, and ship on dry ice.
- *Muscle.* Obtain 150–200 mg of muscle (skeletal or cardiac, depending on indication); freeze immediately, and ship on dry ice.
- *Fibroblasts.* Obtain skin biopsy in sterile culture medium; ship directly at room temperature or culture to confluence prior to shipping.

Interpretation Glucose infusion around the time of a biopsy can artificially elevate the liver glycogen content. Absent or significantly reduced activity of a particular enzyme serves to establish the diagnosis. Assays in chorionic villi or amniocytes may be suitable for prenatal diagnosis in some cases, but contact the laboratory prior to the collection of any prenatal samples. Enzyme assays generally are not appropriate for carrier testing.

DNA Studies

Targeted mutation analysis and/or direct DNA sequencing are performed for GSD

TABLE 48-8	Diagnostic testing for the glycogen storage disorders (GSD)		
Disorder	**Enzyme tested**	**Tissue**	**DNA testing**
GSD 0	Glycogen syntthase	Liver	Targeted mutation analysis or direct sequencing
GSD Ia	Glucose-6-phosphatse	Liver	Targeted mutation analysis or direct sequencing
GSD Ib/c	Glucose-6-translocase	Liver	Targeted mutation analysis or direct sequencing
GSD II	α-glucosidase	Fibroblasts Muscle Blood spot	Targeted mutation analysis
GSD III	Amylo-1,6-glucosidase (debrancher)	Liver	Targeted mutation analysis or linkage analysis
GSD IV	Branching enzyme	Liver Muscle Fibroblasts	Not available
GSD V	Myophosphorylase	Muscle	Targeted mutation analysis
GSD VI	Liver phosphorylase	Liver	Targeted mutation analysis or direct sequencing
GSD VII	Muscle phosphofructokinase	Muscle	Targeted mutation analysis
GSD IX	Liver phosphorylase kinase	Liver	Targeted mutation analysis or direct sequencing

types 0, 1a, 1b, II, III, V, VI, VII, and IX but not for GSD type IV in the US.

Specimen Requirements Testing requires collection of 10 mL of whole blood in a lavender-top (EDTA) tube. Ship at room temperature via overnight courier. DNA studies also may be performed on prenatal samples (chorionic villi or amniocytes) in families in whom pathogenic mutations have been identified.

Interpretation Identification of pathogenic mutations serves to confirm the diagnosis, but absence of detectable mutations in a targeted analysis does not rule one out. For these cases, complete sequencing of either the entire coding region or selected exons may be warranted to identify new mutations.

DISORDERS OF GALACTOSE METABOLISM

Testing for disorders of galactose metabolism (Table 48-9) identifies patients with deficiencies of galactokinase (GALK), galactose-1-phosphate uridyltransferase (GALT), and UDP-4-epimerase (GALE), the three major enzymes of the Leloir pathway (see Chapter 9). This workup is often initiated following an abnormal newborn screening result for classical galactosemia (GALT deficiency) through identification of reduced GALT activity and/or abnormally elevated galactose metabolites (galactose and galactose-1-phosphate [gal-1-P]) in dried blood spots. For states that include galactose metabolites in newborn screening, abnormalities also can indicate either GALK or GALE deficiency. Clinical findings suggestive of classical galactosemia in the neonate include poor feeding, jaundice, vomiting, liver dysfunction, increased bleeding tendency, and septicemia (particularly due to *Escherichia coli*). Galactokinase deficiency is associated with ocular cataracts but not with other systemic findings. The vast majority of GALE-deficient patients are clinically well and are identified only by newborn screening, whereas a very small number have

TABLE 48-9 Galactose-Related Tests

- **Detection of galactose metabolites**
  Urine reducing sugars (Clinitest)
  RBC galactose-1-phosphate
- **Enzyme assays**
  Galactokinase
  Galactose-1-phosphate uridyltransferase (GALT)
  UDP-galactose-4′-epimerase
- **GALT isozyme studies** (electrophoresis or isoelectric focusing)
- **GALT DNA analysis**

clinical symptoms ranging from mild to severe and similar to those of classical galactosemia.

Urine Reducing Sugars (Clinitest)

Test Description Reducing sugars are detected via the conversion of cupric sulfate to cupric oxide, leading to a color change that varies according to the amount of reducing sugars present.

Indications This screening test is used as a rapid indicator of the possibility of galactosemia but should not replace quantitative red cell assays for GALT activity and gal-1-P, particularly in patients with clinical suspicion of classical galactosemia.

Sample Requirements Collect 1–2 mL of random urine in a clean container and without preservatives.

Interpretation The color change associated with a positive result is compared with a color chart provided by the manufacturer. Reducing sugars giving a positive result include glucose, galactose, fructose, lactose, and pentose. False-positive results can occur with certain medications and treatments, including some antibiotics and intravenous glucose administration, whereas false-negative results can result from a dilute urine sample. Negative results also are seen in galactosemia patients who are not consuming galactose.

RBC Galactose-1-Phosphate (Gal-1-P)

Test Description The quantitative evaluation of gal-1-P in red blood cells traditionally is performed using spectrophotometric methods. Newer methods using GC/MS or MS/MS are becoming increasingly widespread.

Indications Quantitative gal-1-P determination is ordered as part of the initial workup in patients suspected of having GALT or GALE deficiency either by newborn screening or by clinical presentation. It is also used to monitor the treatment efficacy of known patients on a galactose-restricted diet.

Sample Requirements Testing typically requires the collection of 3–5 mL of whole blood in a heparanized (green-top) tube, and the same specimen generally can be used for enzyme assays. Some laboratories require that the red cells be washed in normal saline and shipped on dry ice; contact individual laboratories for specific requirements. Because the assay is performed on red blood cells, testing will not be reliable in patients who have been recently transfused.

Interpretation Results include gal-1-P concentration as well as a reference range. Classical galactosemia patients on a galactose-

mia-free diet still may have modest elevations of gal-1-P. There is no universally accepted gal-1-P target range for treated galactosemics or galactosemia variants.

ENZYME ASSAYS

Galactokinase

Test Description Erythrocyte galactokinase activity is determined radioactively using hemolysates from washed red blood cells.

Indications Testing is indicated for patients with elevated galactose metabolites and normal GALT activity detected by newborn screening and in patients with cataracts, particularly if also accompanied by positive urine reducing sugars.

Sample Requirements Testing is performed on red blood cell hemolysates prepared from 3–5 mL of whole blood collected in a heparanized (green-top) tube. Contact individual laboratories for specific requirements.

Interpretation Patients with galactokinase deficiency have significantly reduced or absent enzyme activity, whereas intermediate activity levels suggest the possibility of galactokinase heterozygote.

Galactose-1-Phosphate Uridyltransferase (GALT)

Test Description GALT activity can be determined in red cell hemolysates using spectrophotometric, fluorometric, or radioactive approaches. All methods are appropriate for the diagnosis of classical galactosemia, but the radioactive method has the greatest sensitivity at lower activities and is the most reliable for identifying GALT variants with partial residual activity.

Indications Testing is indicated for patients with abnormal newborn screening results for galactosemia, in patients suspected clinically of having classical galactosemia, and in relatives of an affected individual to determine carrier status. Galactosemia carrier testing also can be done using molecular methods once the specific mutation(s) in a family have been identified.

Sample Requirements Testing is performed on red blood cell hemolysates prepared from 3 to 5 mL whole blood collected in a heparanized (green-top) tube. Contact individual laboratories for specific requirements.

Interpretation Patients with classical galactosemia have zero or near-zero levels of red cell GALT activity. A reduction of activity to approximately 50% of normal indicates that the patient is either a heterozygote for classical galactosemia (G/N) or a homozygote for the

Duarte galactosemia variant; 25% normal activity is indicative of compound heterozygote for classical galactosemia and the Duarte variant (D/G). Because GALT activities associated with the different genotypes can overlap, results suggesting the presence of one or more variant alleles should be followed up with GALT isozyme studies and/or DNA analysis to identify particular galactosemia variants.

UDP-Galactose-4′-Epimerase

Test Description GALE activity can be determined in red cell hemolysates spectrophotometrically or radioactively.

Indications Testing is indicated for patients with elevated galactose metabolites detected by newborn screening, in patients with an identified elevation of red blood cell (RBC) gal-1-P and normal GALT activity, and in patients with clinical symptoms suggestive of classical galactosemia but normal GALT activity.

Sample Requirements Testing is performed on RBC hemolysates prepared from 3–5 mL of whole blood collected in a heparanized (green-top) tube. Contact individual laboratories for specific requirements.

Interpretation Significantly reduced or absent RBC GALE activity is indicative of GALE deficiency, but the pathological significance of this may be difficult to interpret in light of reported patients with isolated RBC GALE deficiency and apparently normal phenotype (24). In cases where generalized, clinically significant GALE deficiency is suspected, enzyme determinations in other tissues such as cultured fibroblasts or transformed lymphoblasts may be warranted.

GALT Isozyme Studies (Electrophoresis or Isoelectric Focusing)

Test Description This test detects the presence of abnormal GALT isozymes associated with Duarte, the most common variant of the enzyme. RBC lysates are subjected to electrophoresis or isoelectric focusing, and GALT bands are visualized following staining with a GALT-specific activity stain.

Indications GALT isozyme analysis is indicated for patients with reduced RBC GALT activity, ranging from 25% of normal (suggestive of D/G compound heterozygote) to 75% of normal (suggestive of D/N heterozygote). Similar information can be obtained from DNA mutation analysis and the detection of N314D, the mutation associated with the abnormal electrophoretic banding phenotype of Duarte (25).

Sample Requirements Isozyme analysis can be performed on the same blood sample submitted for GALT activity assays (see above).

Interpretation The Duarte variant gives rise to abnormally migrating GALT bands on isoelectric focusing (four bands compared with the normal six) or electrophoresis (three bands compared with the normal one). Because staining is activity-dependent, patients with GALT deficiency will not show any isozyme bands, and the bands resulting from D/G will be relatively faint but still interpretable.

GALT DNA Analysis

Test Description GALT mutations are identified in galactosemic patients using allele-specific techniques to screen for known mutations or DNA sequencing to identify novel mutations. For patients clinically suspected of having classical galactosemia, DNA analysis should be undertaken only after GALT deficiency has been established enzymatically.

Sample Requirements DNA typically is isolated from blood collected in either a lavender-top (EDTA) or yellow-top (ACD solution A) tube. Some laboratories also perform testing on DNA isolated from a dried blood spot. Contact individual laboratories for specific specimen information.

Interpretation The detection of previously described GALT mutations confirms the diagnosis in a patient and also enables molecular testing of other family members for carrier detection and prenatal diagnosis. Most laboratories offer targeted testing for 6–10 specific GALT mutations, corresponding to a detection rate of 70%–80% of galactosemia alleles in Caucasian patients and fewer in other ethnic groups. For patients with deficient GALT activity for which no pathogenic mutations are detected by targeted analysis, DNA sequencing is used to identify novel mutations. It is important to remember that DNA changes identified in this way may represent benign polymorphisms with no impact on protein structure and function; the predicted consequences of each identified mutation must be considered carefully before clinical significance can be concluded.

DISORDERS OF FRUCTOSE METABOLISM

Screening and diagnostic tests for disorders of fructose metabolism (Table 48-10) identify patients with hereditary fructose intolerance (HFI, or aldolase B deficiency), a relatively common disorder of fructose metabolism, and fructose-1,6-biphsophatase (FBP) deficiency, a rare disorder of gluconeogenesis (see Chapter 10).

Indications for testing include: 1) onset of hypoglycemia, metabolic acidosis, vomiting, and failure to thrive after ingestion of fructose-containing foods; 2) avoidance of fruits and sugar

TABLE 48-10 Tests for Fructose Disorders

• **Urine reducing sugars**
  Clinitest
  Monosaccharide thin-layer chromatography

• **Fructose tolerance test**
• **Specific enzyme assays** (HFI and FBP deficiency)
• **DNA studies** (HFI)

(sucrose); and 3) hepatomegaly associated with episodes of hypoglycemia, ketosis, and lactic acidosis. Patients with FBP deficiency also show a characteristic pattern of organic acid excretion of lactic aciduria and ketonuria with abnormal elevations of glycerol when ill.

Urine Reducing Sugars

Clinitest See "Urine Reducing Sugars, Clinitest" (Disorders of Galactose Metabolism).

Monosaccharide TLC This test fractionates sugars from urine of patients with positive results by Clinitest in order to identify which reducing sugar (i.e., glucose, lactose, fructose, galactose, or pentose) is elevated. This test is often bypassed in patients with a strong clinical suspicion of a fructose disorder in favor of more specific diagnostic tests (see below).

Fructose Tolerance Test

This is an invasive test in which patients are infused with a 20% fructose solution at a dose of 200 mg/kg, and blood is collected pretreatment and at regular intervals over the next 2 hours (26). In many countries, intravenous fructose is no longer available. It can not be substituted by oral fructose. Samples are evaluated for glucose, phosphate, magnesium, and uric acid. In patients with HFI or FBP deficiency, fructose infusion results in characteristic hypoglycemia and hypophosphatemia, along with hyperuricemia and hypermagnesemia. This test should be administered in a controlled hospital setting by experienced personnel and only while the patient is well.

Specific Enzyme Assays

Enzyme assays for aldolase B and fructose-1,6-bisphosphatase are used to confirm the diagnosis of HFI and fructose-1,6-bisphosphatase deficiency, respectively. Testing requires a liver biopsy with collection of at least 15 mg of tissue, frozen immediately in liquid nitrogen. Contact the laboratory for specific instructions prior to specimen collection.

DNA Studies (HFI)

Mutation analysis for aldolase B deficiency tests for the three most common aldolase B mutations, accounting for at least 75% of known HFI alleles in Caucasians. This is often used as the first line of testing before other invasive procedures are performed. Detection of disease-causing mutations establishes the diagnosis of HFI, but negative results do not rule out the disorder.

CONGENITAL DISORDERS OF GLYCOSYLATION

The congenital disorders of glycosylation (CDG) are associated with abnormal serum transferrin glycoforms resulting from defective synthesis of N-linked oligosaccharide structures. CDG subtypes are distinguished by enzyme assay and the identification of mutations in specific genes of the N-linked oligosaccharide synthetic pathway when such testing is available. Enzyme assays are available for phosphomannomutase (PMM) and phosphomannose isomerase (PMI), as well as the steadily increasing number of additional subtypes.

Clinical features associated with the CDGs are broad. Testing generally is indicated in patients with one or more of the following: mental and psychomotor retardation, generalized dysmyelinization, unusual fat deposits on the buttocks before 1 year of age, inverted nipples, protein-losing enteropathy, hypoglycemia, cerebellar abnormalities, stroke-like episodes, or optic atrophy.

Serum Transferrin Isoforms

Test Description Serum transferrin isoforms typically are evaluated using isoelectric focusing, although other techniques, including capillary electrophoresis and MS/MS, are also used. It is important to note that other commercially available assays for carbohydrate-deficient transferrin, widely used in clinical chemistry laboratories for the evaluation of excessive alcohol consumption, are not appropriate for the identification of CDG patients.

Specimen Requirements Typical collection requires 1 mL of blood in a red-top tube. Centrifuge and freeze serum, and ship on dry ice. EDTA plasma can give false false-negative results due to iron chelation.

Interpretation Normal transferrin contains biantennary glycans linked to asparagines with four sialic acid residues (tetrasialotransferrin). Abnormal patterns associated with CDGs reflect a decrease of tetrasialotransferrin and abnormal increases of asialo-, mono-sialo-, disialo-, and trisialotransferrin fractions. Testing may be unreliable in patients younger than 3 weeks of age and will not detect patients with CDG-IIb or CDG-IIc. Abnormal patterns can be associated with other conditions, including chronic alcoholism, classical galactosemia, and hereditary fructose intolerance. Genetic variants of transferrin itself also can cause a shift in isoelectric focusing. This can be differentiated from CDGs by repeat-

ing the electrophoresis after neuraminidase treatment, which removes the glycan from the transferrin protein, and also by studying the parents. Rare false-negative results have been reported for patients with CDG1a.

DNA Studies

Test Description Targeted mutation analysis and mutation-scanning studies are available for the detection of patients with CDG types Ia, Ib, Ic, Id, Ie, If, Ig, Ih, and Ii. Other genes associated with CDGs may be evaluated on a research basis.

Specimen Requirements Collect 3–5 mL of whole blood in a lavender-top (EDTA) tube. Transport via overnight courier at room temperature.

Interpretation Molecular analysis detects approximately 100% of PMM2 mutations associated with CDG-Ia and MPI mutations associated with CDG-Ib. The detection rate for mutations associated with the other types of CDG is unknown.

TESTS FOR DISORDERS OF PURINE AND PYRIMIDINE METABOLISM

Screening and diagnostic tests (Table 48-11) are available for the evaluation of patients with disorders of purine and pyrimidine metabolism, including PP-ribose-P synthetase (PRPS) superactivity, deficiencies of purine nucleoside phosphorylase (PNP), adenine phosphoribosyltransferase (APRT), adenosine deaminase (ADA), hypoxanthine–guanine phosphyribosyltransferase (HGPRT), adenosine monophosphate deaminase (AMPDA), adenylosuccinate lyase (ADSL), and xanthine oxidase (XO), as well as hereditary orotic aciduria (UMP–synthase deficiency), and deficiencies of dihydropyrimidine dehydrogenase (DHPD), dihydropyrimidinase (DHPA), and uridine monophosphate hydrolase (5'-nucleotidase deficiency).

Uric Acid

Test Description Uric acid, the end point of purine catabolism, is measured spectrophotometrically in urine, plasma, or serum or as part of a more comprehensive screen via HPLC with detection by ultraviolet (UV) light or MS/MS (see below). Measurements in urine typically are expressed as a ratio with creatinine.

Sample Requirements Specific collection instructions and containers vary by laboratory. Urine can be tested using either a random sample or 24-hour collection. For plasma or serum, collect and centrifuge whole blood, and separate from cells; freeze and send to the laboratory on dry ice.

TABLE 48-11	Tests for Purine and Pyrimidine Disorders

- **Uric acid** (urine, serum or plasma)
- **Succinylpurines** (urine or CSF)
- **Orotic acid** (urine)
- **General screening** for purine and pyrimidine metabolites (urine)
- **Specific enzyme assays**
- **DNA studies**

Interpretation Uric acid is elevated in HGPRT deficiency and PPRPS superactivity and is decreased in XO, molybdenum cofactor, and PNP deficiencies. Uric acid levels also are decreased in the urine of patients with pyrimidine nucleotide depletion syndrome due to increased 5'-nucleotidase activity (27). Patients with HGPRT deficiency presenting in acute renal failure may have normal uric acid excretion when expressed on a creatinine basis but elevated uric acid levels in blood. Patients with glycogen storage disease type I (von Gierke disease) have secondary elevations of uric acid. Other conditions associated with hyperuricemia include leukemia and other malignancies, endocrine disorders, infections, poisoning, acute illness, and alcohol ingestion.

Succinylpurines

Succinylpurines are evaluated in patients suspected of having adenylosuccinate lyase (ADSL) deficiency, a disorder associated with elevations of the succinylpurines succinylaminoimidazole carboxamide ribose (SAIC-R) and succinyladenosine (S-Ado) in body fluids. Testing also detects patients with aminoimidazolecarboxamide ribotide (AICAR) transformylase deficiency, a recently described disorder of purine biosynthesis associated with abnormal elevations of AICAR (28).

Test Description The Bratten–Marshall test is a relatively crude spot test in which sulfonamides react with the Bratten–Marshall reagent [N-(1-naphthyl)-ethylene diamine dihydrochloride] to yield a colored product that is detected spectrophotometrically. Separation of succinylpurines by HPLC with UV detection gives a more sensitive and specific indication of abnormalities.

Indications Succinylpurine screening is indicated for patients with unexplained psychomotor retardation or mental retardation, seizures, and autistic characteristics, typically in the absence of dysmorphic features.

Sample Requirements Random urine or CSF, stored and shipped frozen.

Interpretation Sulfa drugs can yield false-positive results on the Bratten–Marshall test.

Abnormal elevations of SAIC-R and S-Ado by HPLC are diagnostic for ADSL deficiency.

Orotic Acid

Abnormal elevations of orotic acid are seen in patients with hereditary orotic aciduria (UMPS deficiency). Orotic acid is also elevated in patients with certain urea cycle defects, particularly ornithine transcarbamylase deficiency.

Test Description Orotic acid can be measured by a variety of techniques, including spectrophotometry, gas chromatography, and MS/MS.

Indications This test is indicated for patients with megaloblastic anemia unresponsive to vitamin B_{12} or folate therapy, crystalluria, and urinary obstructions and in patients with hyperammonemia and a suspected urea cycle defect.

Sample Requirements Urine; collection volumes vary by laboratory. Freeze in clean container without preservatives.

Interpretation The finding of marked orotic aciduria in patients with vitamin B_{12}- and folate-unresponsive megaloblastic anemia is consistent with a diagnosis of hereditary orotic aciduria (UMPS deficiency). Males with ornithine transcarbamoylase deficiency also have marked orotic aciduria, whereas heterozygous females may have less pronounced elevations. Orotic acid is also elevated in argininosuccinic acid synthase deficiency (citrullinemia type 1) and argininosuccinic acid lyase deficiency but not in carbamoyl phosphate synthase 1 deficiency or N-acetylglutamate synthase deficiency. It is also elevated in lysinuric protein intolerance, a disorder of dibasic amino acid transport. Finally, levels are affected by other factors, including hematological status, reticu-

locytosis, iron, and agents such as allopurinol and 5-azauridine.

General Screening for Purine and Pyrimidine Metabolites

Test Description Metabolites are detected in urine via HPLC with UV spectrophotometry or MS/MS or by TLC. Screening panels vary by laboratory and may include the detection of adenine, xanthine, hypoxanthine, adenosine, deoxyadenosine, guanosine, inosine, succinyladenosine and uric acid (purine metabolites), and orotic acid, uracil, and thymine (pyrimidine metabolites). Two additional pyrimidine metabolites, dihydrouracil and dihydrothymine, are detected by GC/MS (see "Organic Acid Analysis") or MS/MS (29).

HPLC methods are used to detect abnormal elevations of pyrimidine nucleotides (UDP-glucose, UDP-N-acetylglucosamine, and CDP-choline, UTP, and CTP) in erythrocytes of patients with uridine monophosphate hydrolase (UMPH) deficiency (or 5'-nucleotidase deficiency).

Indications Testing for purine and pyrimidine disorders should be included in a broad investigation for inborn errors of metabolism, particularly in patients with renal stones or renal failure, mental retardation, developmental delay, seizures, unexplained immunodeficiency, hemolytic anemia, or gouty arthritis.

Sample Requirements A minimum of 3 mL of urine, stored frozen without preservatives, is needed. The detection of pyrimidine nucleotides requires plasma or serum, stored frozen.

Interpretation Purine disorders and their associated metabolite disturbances are listed in Table 48-12. Uric acid levels are increased in PPRPS superactivity and in HGPRT deficiency

and decreased in deficiencies of PNP, xanthine dehydrogenase, and MCD. Elevations of adenosine and deoxyadenosine are indicative of ADA deficiency, guanosine and inosine of PNP deficiency, and xanthine and hypoxanthine of xanthine dehydrogenase deficiency. AMPDA deficiency may be associated with normal levels of purine metabolites but is distinguished by an elevated ratio of lactate to ammonia during ischemic exercise (30).

Abnormalities associated with disorders of pyrimidine metabolism are listed in Table 48-13. Marked elevations of orotic acid in patients with hypochromic megaloblastic anemia are characteristic of UMP-synthase deficiency or hereditary orotic aciduria. Elevations of uracil and thymine, with normal findings on routine laboratory investigations, indicate DHPD deficiency. Detection of the unusual metabolites dihydrouracil and dihydrothymine, with moderate elevations of uracil and thymine, is indicative of DHPA deficiency. Deficiency of the last enzyme in the pathway, ureidopropionase, leads to elevations of ureidopropionate, β-alanine, and ureidoisobutyrate in addition to the previous four metabolites. Elevation of the pyrimidine nucleotides, and particularly UDP-glucose, are consistent with uridine monophosphate hydrolase deficiency (5'-nucleotidase deficiency).

Specific Enzyme Assays

For the purine-related disorders, diagnostic enzyme assays are available to confirm suspected cases of ADA, PNP, HGPRT, and APRT deficiency. These tests are based on radiochemical methods using either whole blood (3–5 mL, collected in a heparinized tube) or cultured fibroblasts. HGPRT also can be assayed using dried blood spots on

TABLE 48-12	**Metabolite profiles in disorders of purine metabolism.**									
	Uric Acid	Adenine	Xanthine	Hypoxan-thine	Adenosine	Deoxy-adenosine	Guanosine	Inosine	Succinyl-adenosine	Other
ADA	N				↑	↑				
AMPDA										↑ Lactate/NH_3 during ischemic exercise
PNP	↓						↑	↑		
XD	↓		↑	↑						
MCD	↓		↑	↑						
HGPRT	↑			↑						
APRT	N	↑								↑ 2,8-Dihydroxy-adenine
ADSL	N								↑	↑ SAICA-R
PPRPS	↑			↑						

N = normal; ADA = adenosine deaminase deficiency; AMPDA = adenosine monophosphate deaminase; PNP = purine nucleosidase phosphorylase deficiency; XD = xanthine dehydrogenase deficiency; MCD = molybdenum cofactor deficiency; HGPRT = hypoxanthine-guanine phosphoribosyltranseferase deficiency; APRT = adenine phosphoribosyltransferase deficiency; ADSL = adenylosuccinate lyase deficiency; PPRPS = phosphoribosylpyrophosphate synthetase superactivity; SAICA-R = succinylaminoimidazole carboxamide ribose.

TABLE 48-13   Metabolite Profiles in Disorders of Pyrimidine Metabolism

	Orotic Acid	Uracil	Thymine	5-Hydroxy-methyluracil	Dihydrouracil	Dihydrothymine	Other
UMPS	↑						Hypochromic megaloblastic anemia
DHPD		↑	↑	↑			Other routine chemistry tests normal
DHPA		±↑	±↑		↑	↑	
UMPH							↑ Pyrimidine nucleotides

UMPS = uridine monophosphate synthase deficiency; DHPD = dihydropyrimidine dehydrogenase deficiency; DHPA = dihydropyrimidinase deficiency; UMPH = uridine monophosphate hydrolase deficiency (5'-nucleotidase deficiency).

filter paper. For patients with hyperuricemia but normal HGPRT and APRT activities, PPRPS superactivity is suspected. Confirmation of muscle-specific AMPDA activity requires enzymatic assay in muscle samples.

Confirmation of UMP-synthase deficiency involves demonstrating significantly reduced or absent activities of orotic acid phosphoribosyltransferase (OPRT) and orotidine-5'-monophosphate decarboxylase (ODC), the two catalytic activities associated with enzyme UMP-synthase, in lysed erythrocytes and fibroblasts. Activity of DHPD and the other enzymes of pyrimidine degradation are measured in leukocytes or cultured fibroblasts.

DNA Studies

Identification of specific DNA mutations is available on a clinical basis for molybdenum cofactor deficiency and HGPRT deficiency using gene-sequencing and/or mutation-scanning techniques. Mutations in other genes may be identified on a research basis in a small number of laboratories worldwide.

REFERENCES

1. Millington DS, Kodo N, Norwood DL, et al. Tandem mass spectrometry: A new method for acylcarnitine profiling with potential for neonatal screening for inborn errors of metabolism. *J Inherited Metab Dis.* 1990;13:321–324.
2. Rashed MS. Clinical applications of tandem mass spectrometry: Ten years of diagnosis and screening for inherited metabolic diseases. *J Chromatogr B Biomed Sci Appl.* 2001;758: 27–48.
3. Schulze A, Lindner M, Kohlmuller D, et al. Expanded newborn screening for inborn errors of metabolism by electrospray ionization-tandem mass spectrometry: Results, outcome, and implications. *Pediatrics.* 2003; 111:1399–1406.
4. McGarry J, Foster D. An improved and simplified radio-isotopic assay for the determination of free and esterified carnitine. *J Lipid Res.* 1976;17:277–281.
5. Schmidt-Sommerfeld E, Werner D, Penn D. Carnitine plasma concentrations in 353 metabolically healthy children. *Eur J Pediatr.* 1988;147:356–360.
6. Stevens RD, Hillman SL, Worthy S, et al. Assay for free and total carnitine in human plasma using tandem mass spectrometry. *Clin Chem.* 2000;46:727–729.
7. Ghoshal AK, Soldin SJ. Determination of total and free plasma carnitine concentrations on the Dade Behring dimension RxL: Integrated chemistry system. *Clin Chim Acta.* 2005;361:80–85.
8. Tortorelli S, Hahn SH, Cowan TM, et al. The urinary excretion of glutarylcarnitine is an informative tool in the biochemical diagnosis of glutaric acidemia type I. *Mol Genet Metab.* 2005;84:137–143.
9. Wolf NI, Smeitink JA. Mitochondrial disorders: A proposal for consensus diagnostic criteria in infants and children. *Neurology.* 2002;59:1402–1405.
10. Barshop BA. Metabolomic approaches to mitochondrial disease: Correlation of urine organic acids. *Mitochondrion.* 2004;4:521–527.
11. Sim KG, Hammond J, Wilcken B. Strategies for the diagnosis of mitochondrial fatty acid beta-oxidation disorders. *Clin Chim Acta.* 2002;323:37–58.
12. Sim KG, Carpenter K, Hammond J, et al. Acylcarnitine profiles in fibroblasts from patients with respiratory chain defects can resemble those from patients with mitochondrial fatty acid beta-oxidation disorders. *Metabolism.* 2002;51:366–371.
13. Bourgeois JM, Tarnopolsky MA. Pathology of skeletal muscle in mitochondrial disorders. *Mitochondrion.* 2004;4:441–452.
14. Vogel H. Mitochondrial myopathies and the role of the pathologist in the molecular era. *J Neuropathol Exp Neurol.* 2001;60:217–227.
15. Kramer KA, Oglesbee D, Hartman SJ, et al. Automated spectrophotometric analysis of mitochondrial respiratory chain complex enzyme activities in cultured skin fibroblasts. *Clin Chem.* 2005;51:2110–2116.
16. Janssen AJ, Smeitink JA, van den Heuvel LP. Some practical aspects of providing a diagnostic service for respiratory chain defects. *Ann Clin Biochem.* 2003;40:3–8.
17. Capaldi RA, Murray J, Byrne L, et al. Immunological approaches to the characterization and diagnosis of mitochondrial disease. *Mitochondrion.* 2004;4:417–426.
18. Shanske S, Wong LJ. Molecular analysis for mitochondrial DNA disorders. *Mitochondrion.* 2004;4:403–415.
19. DiMauro S, Gurgel-Giannetti J. The expanding phenotype of mitochondrial myopathy. *Curr Opin Neurol.* 2005;18:538–542.
20. Wanders RJ. Metabolic and molecular basis of peroxisomal disorders: A review. *Am J Med Genet A.* 2004;126:355–375.
21. Wenger DA, Coppola S, Liu SL. Lysosomal storage disorders: Diagnostic dilemmas and prospects for therapy. *Genet Med.* 2002;4: 412–419.
22. Hyland K. The lumbar puncture for diagnosis of pediatric neurotransmitter diseases. *Ann Neurol.* 2003;54:S13–17.
23. Hyland K, Nygaard TG, Trugman JM, et al. Oral phenylalanine loading profiles in symptomatic and asymptomatic gene carriers with dopa-responsive dystonia due to dominantly inherited GTP cyclohydrolase deficiency. *J Inherited Metab Dis.* 1999;22:213–215.
24. Wasilenko J, Lucas ME, Thoden JB, et al. Functional characterization of the K257R and G319E-hGALE alleles found in patients with ostensibly peripheral epimerase deficiency galactosemia. *Mol Genet Metab.* 2005;84:32–38.
25. Elsas LJ, Dembure PP, Langley S, et al. A common mutation associated with the Duarte galactosemia allele. *Am J Hum Genet.* 1994;54:1030–1036.
26. Steinmann B, Gitzelmann R. The diagnosis of hereditary fructose intolerance. *Helv Paediatr Acta.* 1981;36:297–316.
27. Nyhan WL. Disorders of purine and pyrimidine metabolism. *Mol Genet Metab.* 2005;86:25–33.
28. Marie S, Heron B, Bitoun P, et al. AICA-ribosiduria: a novel, neurologically devastating inborn error of purine biosynthesis caused by mutation of ATIC. *Am J Hum Genet.* 2004;74:1276–1281.
29. Duran M, Dorland L, Meuleman EE, et al. Inherited defects of purine and pyrimidine metabolism: Laboratory methods for diagnosis. *J Inherited Metab Dis.* 1997;20:227–236.
30. Tarnopolsky M, Stevens L, MacDonald JR, et al. Diagnostic utility of a modified forearm ischemic exercise test and technical issues relevant to exercise testing. *Muscle Nerve.* 2003;27:359–366.

CHAPTER 49

Endocrine Testing

Bradley S. Miller, MD, PhD, FAAP
Irene Hong McAtee, MD, FAAP, MSCR

TESTING METHODOLOGY

Some of the most common tests used to diagnose endocrinological disorders are antibody-based immunological assays. Selection of an assay for measurement of a particular biochemical substance should be determined by the biological variability of the analyte, the ability of the assay to distinguish the analyte from similar compounds (i.e., similar steroid hormone, partial peptides, etc.), the ability of the assay to avoid interfering substances (i.e., blocking antibodies), and the variability of the assay measurement (intra-assay and inter-assay test variability). Age- and Tanner stage–specific normative data are important for certain biochemical assays. Normative data should be specific to the assay in question. For example, measurement of the analyte in the normative population by two different methods (i.e., immunoradiometric assay [IRMA] and liquid chromatography/tandem mass spectrometry [LC/MS/MS]) is likely to yield significantly different ranges. Clinicians should be aware of the biological variability of the analytes being measured, as well as the limitations of the specific assays used in their local and reference laboratories. At times, clinicians may expect more from an assay than it is capable of producing.

A two-way dialogue between the provider and the laboratory director(s) can be helpful in obtaining the most useful laboratory results and understanding the limitations of the available assays. Because of excellent specific-

ity and improving sensitivity, LC/MS/MS is being used increasingly for commercial laboratory analyses (Table 49-1).

COMPETITIVE IMMUNOASSAYS

Radioimmunoassays (RIAs), Fluorescence Immunoassays (FIAs), and Chemiluminescence Immunoassays (CIAs)

Purpose RIAs have been one the main tools for quantifying peptide hormones for more than 30 years and previously were considered the "gold standard" (1–4). These techniques represent a major advancement from earlier methods of hormone detection, such as bioassays, that studied the ways *in vivo* or *in vitro* systems reacted to a hormone's action (5).

Protocol In this assay, the hormone in the patient's blood competes with a *radiolabeled antigen* (called a *tracer*) for binding sites on a fixed amount of antibody that is specific for that hormone. The antibody solution usually is diluted to a concentration that would bind approximately half the tracer if none of the patient's hormone were present (6). The reaction is calibrated at each lab using standards with known concentrations of antigens (3,6). Other immunoassays do not use radioactivity but instead employ fluorometric or chemiluminescent signals to quantify the reaction (7,8).

Interpretation The more unlabeled hormone that is present, the less radiolabeled tracer will be bound to the antibody (3). This process produces a dose–response curve that is converted with specialized statistical programs into clinically interpretable concentrations of hormones (6).

Comments The precision of these assays depends on many factors, including the method used to separate bound from unbound hormone after the binding reaction, type of antibody used, and type of signal or label used to

quantify the reaction (3,6). Precision for these RIAs is worse at very low and very high hormone concentrations (6), and the RIA will not be able to differentiate alternate forms of a hormone if they have the same antibody-binding site (e.g., it may not be able to differentiate active from inactive fragments of parathyroid hormone [PTH]).

Enzyme-Linked Immunosorbent Assays (ELISAs)

Purpose ELISAs are similar to RIAs, but instead of radioactivity, enzyme activity is used to detect hormone levels (3,5). ELISAs are used widely because they are more rapid and eliminate the need for the complicated storage and surveillance of radioisotopes (3–5).

Protocol In the competitive form of this assay, the hormone in the patient's blood competes with an *antigen labeled with an enzyme* for binding sites on a fixed amount of antibody that is specific for that hormone. Then unbound reactants are washed away, and the antibody–hormone complex is incubated with a substance that produces a light-absorbent product (3). A spectrophotometer is used to measure the amount of hormone that is linked to the enzyme and bound to the antibody (5).

Interpretation The process is similar to RIAs, except that the dose–response curve involves enzyme activity rather than radioactivity (3). Interpretation depends on the standards used and the type of enzyme used, commonly horseradish peroxidase (3,5).

Comments There are many forms of ELISAs (1,3). For instance, instead of being incubated with light-absorbent substrates, the antibody–hormone complex may be incubated with chemiluminescence-producing substrates, and the enzyme activity then is measured with a luminometer (3,8). Enzyme-enhanced chemiluminescence produces more constant light emission and therefore is measured more reliably (8).

TABLE 49-1   Testing Methodologies

Competitive immunoassays
  Radioimmunoassays (RIAs)
  Chemiluminescence immunoassays (CIAs)
  Fluorescence immunoassays (FIAs)
  Enzyme-linked immunosorbent assay (ELISA)

Sandwich immunoassays (IRMAs)
  Immunoradiometric assays (IRMAs)
  Immunochemiluminescence assays (ICMAs)

Dialysis

Liquid chromatography/tandem mass spectrometry (LC/MS/MS)

SANDWICH IMMUNOASSAYS

Immunoradiometric Assays (IRMAs) and Immunochemiluminescent Assays (ICMAs)

Purpose Unlike the RIAs, in which a limited amount of antibody is presented relative to the amount of hormone, immunometric assays present a large amount of antibody in order to bind as much hormone as possible (3,6). Sandwich immunoassays (IRMA and ICMA) are more specific than RIAs because they bind two different sites and thus can distinguish more precisely between hormones with similar subunits, for example, the α subunits of luteinizing hormone (LH) and follicle-stimulating hormone (FSH) (4,6).

Protocol Sandwich immunoassays require a hormone that is large enough to bind two kinds of antibodies: 1) a *capture antibody* directed against the hormone that is also attached to a solid phase so that the whole complex is "extracted" out of the sample and 2) a *radioactively labeled signal antibody* that is also directed against the hormone and binds to the capture antibody–hormone complex (6).

Interpretation As in RIAs, the hormone level is calculated by generating a dose–response curve (e.g., signal versus concentration) and by comparing the amount of antibody-bound tracer to reference standards (3,6). ICMAs use enzymatic signal amplification detected via luminometer.

Comments If the concentration of hormone is so high that it approaches the effective binding capacity of the capture antibody, then the signal no longer increases or actually may decrease if the hormone exceeds the binding capacity. This is called the *high-dose hook effect* and can be confirmed by diluting the specimen (6). The accuracy of sandwich immunoassays also can be decreased by the presence of endogenous heterophile antibodies that mimic the hormone, which would yield falsely high results, or that react with the assay's antibodies to block the hormone from binding, which would give falsely low results (6).

DIALYSIS

Purpose To measure hormone concentrations in situations where both free and protein-bound hormone would be measured by antibody methods or where interfering antibodies are suspected.

Protocol The dialysis chamber has two cells containing assay buffer separated by a semipermeable membrane. The size of the pores in the membrane will determine the molecular weight of compounds able to cross the membrane. Assay buffer is added to both cells. The patient's serum is placed in the sample cell. Free hormone escapes the sample cell by crossing the membrane down the concentration gradient into the assay cell until equilibrium is established. Protein- or antibody-bound hormone is too large to cross the membrane through the pores. Free hormone is determined by analyzing the assay chamber. Centrifugal ultrafiltration across a semipermeable membrane also may be used to separate free from protein-bound hormone.

Interpretation Values are compared with those of matched controls.

Comments This method is not performed routinely because it is so labor-intensive, but it can be used in special situations. For example, when the free thyroxine (T$_4$) measured by standard methodology does not correlate with clinical findings and interfering antibodies are suspected, one can order a free T$_4$ level by dialysis. In addition, free or bioavailable testosterone may be measured by dialysis to remove the contribution of sex hormone–binding globulin to total testosterone.

LIQUID CHROMATOGRAPHY/ TANDEM MASS SPECTROMETRY (LC/MS/MS)

Purpose LC/MS/MS uses two separation techniques and an identification technique to determine the presence of an analyte.

Protocol Samples typically are autoinjected into the liquid chromatograph, which separates the analytes based on their ability to interact with the solid phase of the column. As the separated analytes are eluted from the chromatography column, they enter the tandem mass spectrometer. The first mass spectrometer is used to select compounds of the appropriate molecular weight to enter the collision cell between the mass spectrometers. Inside the collision cell, the analyte is split into specific fragments based on the chemical characteristics of the analyte. The molecular weights of the fragments are determined by the second mass spectrometer. The pattern of fragmentation is used to identify the analyte (9,10).

Interpretation Internal standards, typically containing stable, nonradioactive isotopes such as deuterium, are mixed with the sample prior to injection and used to quantify the analytes. Quantitated values are compared with normative data.

Comments The sensitivity of this method for certain compounds is comparable with that of IRMA/ICMA. However, normative pediatric data need to be obtained. As the availability of appropriate, cost-effective standards increases, LC/MS/MS is likely to see increased use. This method typically is limited to compounds with small molecular weights (<2000 kDa). However, improvements in mass spectrometry or use of different forms of ionization may allow analysis of larger molecules (11).

TESTS OF ADRENAL FUNCTION

Tests of adrenal function include those designed to determine whether glucocorticoid excess is present (e.g., Cushing syndrome), to localize the cause of glucocorticoid excess (ACTH-dependent versus ACTH-independent), to diagnose adrenocortical insufficiency (e.g., Addison disease), and tests diagnose congenital adrenal hyperplasia (CAH) (Table 49-2).

TABLE 49-2 Tests of Adrenal Function
Tests to determine whether glucocorticoid excess (Cushing syndrome) is present
24-hour urinary free cortisol (UFC)
Midnight salivary or plasma cortisol
Overnight low-dose dexamethasone suppression test
Tests to localize the cause of excessive glucocorticoid production
ACTH measurement
Low-dose/high-dose dexamethasone suppression test
CRH stimulation test with or without dexamethasone
Metyrapone test
Tests to evaluate adrenocortical insufficiency (Addison disease)
8 a.m. plasma cortisol and ACTH concentration
Low-dose ACTH stimulation test
High-dose ACTH stimulation test
Metyrapone test
Tests to diagnose congenital adrenal hyperplasia (CAH)
High-dose ACTH stimulation test
17-Hydroxyprogesterone (17OHP)
cyp21 analysis

TESTS TO DETERMINE WHETHER GLUCOCORTICOID EXCESS (CUSHING SYNDROME) IS PRESENT

Establishing the presence of excessive gluco-corticoid production is not necessarily straightforward. Of the many hormone tests available, none has 100% sensitivity or specificity, and multiple tests usually are necessary to determine a diagnosis. Often the morning cortisol and adrenocorticotropic hormone (ACTH) concentrations are within the normal range, but subtle elevations in the evening concentrations or loss of normal diurnal variation are found. Several common conditions such as obesity, stress, and depression can alter the function of the hypothalamic–pituitary–adrenal axis and produce a laboratory picture suggestive of cortisol excess (pseudo-Cushing syndrome).

Generally, the combination of normal 24-hour urinary free cortisol excretion plus an appropriately low late-evening plasma/serum concentration or salivary cortisol level rules out Cushing syndrome. In addition, subjects with pseudo-Cushing syndrome usually will have normal suppression of morning cortisol concentrations following low-dose dexamethasone administration the night before.

If these tests are *normal*, it is highly unlikely that the subject has true glucocorticoid excess, although episodic cortisol secretion can be missed, and further testing may be required if clinical suspicion is high. If these tests are *abnormal*, further testing is required to localize the source of the problem: central ACTH production, ectopic ACTH production, or a primary (ACTH-independent) adrenal problem.

24-Hour Urinary Free Cortisol (UFC)

Purpose UFC reflects the integrated 24-hour plasma free cortisol concentration. This is less susceptible to false-negative results than measuring random or timed plasma cortisol concentrations because cortisol concentrations vary throughout the day and because hypercortisolism may be intermittent. It is also not affected by corticosteroid binding globulin concentrations (12).

Protocol Three 24-hour urine collections are performed. UFC is measured along with urinary creatinine to verify the adequacy of the collection. UFC may be measured by immunoassay, high-performance liquid chromatography (HPLC), or less commonly and more expensively, MS combined with gas chromatography or HPLC. For children, the urinary cortisol excretion is corrected for body surface area (13).

Interpretation UFC greater than four times the normal upper limit is considered clearly diagnostic for Cushing syndrome. A less striking elevation may be found in pregnancy or pseudo-Cushing states (12). Usually the upper limit of normal is 100 μg/day (275.86 nmol/day) in adults and 80 μg/m²/day in children (15–20 μg/g or 4.68–6.24 nmol/mmol creatinine in normal children; up to 40 μg/g or 12.48 nmol/mmol creatinine in obese children).

Comments This cannot be used as a single screening test for Cushing syndrome because UFC may not be elevated in mild hypercortisolism and may miss these early diagnoses (13), or it may be elevated in pseudo-Cushing states.

Late-Night Cortisol Concentration (Plasma or Salivary)

Purpose This test demonstrates the presence of the normal late-evening nadir in cortisol level.

Protocol Plasma cortisol can be measured between 11 p.m. and midnight if drawn through a previously inserted line in a sleeping patient. It is important to prevent stress during the procedure so that cortisol concentrations are not elevated iatrogenically.

Saliva is collected between 11 p.m. and midnight by the patient or parent, either as a one-time screen or with repeated measurements over time to diagnose cyclic Cushing syndrome. Salivary cortisol is a noninvasive method of assessing cortisol levels (14). Saliva is collected by wetting a cotton roll (salivette) in the mouth for 1–2 minutes (15). Patients should avoid consumption of products containing citric acid and dairy products for 60 minutes prior to collection. The sample may be kept at room temperature up to 1 week. On arrival in the laboratory, salivettes are centrifuged to recover saliva. Saliva then is frozen until analysis by immunoassay (16).

Interpretation For plasma cortisol, some investigators use an evening cortisol concentration of 1.8 mg/dL (50 nmol/L) as the upper limit of normal (17). However, to eliminate pseudo-Cushing syndrome, some investigators use a level of 7.5 mg/dL (207 nmol/L) (18). Reference ranges specific for age and time of day have been developed and are lab-dependent (www.esoterix.com, http://labguide.fairview.org/).

Salivary cortisol concentrations are much lower than those measured in serum (Table 49-3). Measurement of an 11 p.m. salivary cortisol has been shown to be 100% sensitive and 95% specific for the diagnosis of Cushing syndrome in children using a cutoff

TABLE 49-3 Normative data for Salivary Cortisol[†]		
Prepubertal children		
8 a.m.:	0.17–1.2 mg/dL	[4.7–33 nmol/L]
4 p.m.:	0.10–0.33 mcg/dL	[2.8–9.1 nmol/L]
11 p.m.:	0.03–0.19 mg/dL	[0.8-5.2 nmol/L]
Adults		
8 a.m.:	0.18–0.95 mg/dL	[5.0–26.2 nmol/L]
4 p.m.:	0.10–0.28 mg/dL	[2.8–7.7 nmol/L]
11 p.m.:	0.05–0.17 mg/dL	[1.4-4.7 nmol/L]

†www.esoterix.com

of 0.19 mg/dL (5.5 nmol/L) established in normal obese children (19).

Comments These tests are not useful in children younger than 3 years of age, who may not have established a pattern of diurnal variation. The concentration of cortisol in the saliva is highly correlated with plasma cortisol, and salivary cortisol is stable at room temperature for 1 week. Because of the ease of collection and the fact that it can be done at home, this test may be the wave of the future in cortisol testing once more commercial assays become available. It should be performed in conjunction with other tests until larger studies validate its use.

Overnight Low-Dose Dexamethasone Suppression Test

Purpose This study is used in addition to the other screening tests to diagnose Cushing syndrome. In contrast to UFC measurement and the late-night cortisol level, this is a functional assay demonstrating normal negative feedback on the hypothalamic–pituitary–adrenal axis.

Protocol

1. Between 11 p.m. and midnight, 20 μg/kg (maximum 1 mg) dexamethasone is given orally (19).
2. At 8 a.m. the following morning, a fasting plasma cortisol level is measured.

Interpretation Dexamethasone, by negative feedback, should suppress the normal nocturnal surge in ACTH and the resulting morning rise in cortisol. Normal suppression is defined as a cortisol level of less than 1.8 μg/dL (50 nmol/L).

Comments The low-dose dexamethasone test should not be used as the sole criterion to exclude the diagnosis of endogenous hypercortisolism because this test can appropriately suppress concentrations of plasma cortisol and urinary steroids in those with mild or early Cushing syndrome (20). Alternatively, this test can be falsely positive (fail to suppress) in people with pseudo-Cushing states, increased corticosteroidbinding globulin (estrogen treatment), illness, and medications enhancing hepatic dexamethasone metabolism, including phenytoin (13).

TESTS TO LOCALIZE THE CAUSE OF EXCESSIVE GLUCOCORTICOID PRODUCTION

ACTH Plasma Measurement

Purpose To differentiate central (Cushing disease) ACTH hypersecretion, secretion of ACTH by an ectopic tumor, or a primary adrenal source of glucocorticoid excess.

Protocol Because proteases rapidly digest ACTH in plasma, blood should be collected in a prechilled heparin or EDTA tube and transported rapidly to the laboratory on ice. The tube preferably should be plastic because ACTH adheres to glass (21). Two-site immunoradiometric assays are the most reliable and sensitive, detecting ACTH levels below 10 pg/mL (2 pmol/L).

Interpretation ACTH concentrations of less than 5–10 pg/mL (1–2 pmol/L) suggest an ACTH-independent cause (adrenal Cushing) for cortisol excess, with central suppression of ACTH. However, ACTH levels may not be fully suppressed in some patients with adrenal Cushing and intermittent or relatively low secretion of cortisol. Concentrations generally are normal or in the high-normal range in Cushing disease, whereas they are often substantially elevated (>200 pg/ml, 44 pmol/L) in the case of ACTH-producing ectopic tumors.

Comments There is often considerable overlap in ACTH concentrations between Cushing disease and ectopic ACTH-secreting tumors.

Low-Dose/High-Dose Dexamethasone Suppression Test

Purpose To determine whether normal feedback inhibition of ACTH and cortisol production occurs when dexamethasone is given to help localize the cause of Cushing's syndrome.

Protocol

1. There are several variations of this test. The classical test takes 6 days—2 days each for baseline assessment, low-dose dexamethasone, and high-dose dexamethasone. During each 2-day period, two 24-hour urine collections are obtained for urinary free cortisol, and 8 a.m. ACTH and cortisol concentrations are measured. During the two low-dose days, dexamethasone 5–7.5 µg/kg/dose every 6 hours is given orally (up to 0.5 mg per dose). During the high-dose

days, dexamethasone 20–30 µg/kg/dose is given orally every 6 hours (up to 2 mg per dose).

2. Alternatively, a 2-day low-dose test may be used instead of the overnight dexamethasone in the initial evaluation of cortisol excess.

3. Some investigators do an overnight high-dose dexamethasone suppression test instead of the 2-day test. This involves giving a single dexamethasone dose of 80 µg/kg (up to 8 mg) at midnight and measuring the 8 a.m. ACTH and cortisol concentrations.

Interpretation Normal suppression generally is defined as a plasma cortisol concentration of less than 1.8 µg/dL (50 nmol/L) and a UFC of less than 10 µg (27 nmol/L).

Comments Normal individuals and those with pseudo-Cushing syndrome usually suppress after low-dose dexamethasone. Pituitary adenomas usually retain some degree of normal responsiveness to feedback inhibition, and 80% to 90% of pituitary adenomas are at least partially suppressed by high doses of dexamethasone (13). Ectopic tumors usually function completely independently of central control and are resistant to glucocorticoid suppression, although there are exceptions (e.g., certain neuroendocrine tumors such as carcinoid tumors of the pancreas). Primary adrenal lesions usually do not respond to dexamethasone suppression, although there are exceptions (e.g., some cases of multinodular adrenal hyperplasia).

CRH Stimulation Test With or Without Dexamethasone

Purpose Different investigators have suggested this test for different purposes, such as distinguishing normal individuals from those with pseudo-Cushing or mild Cushing disease, differentiating ACTH-independent from ACTH-dependent disease, distinguishing pituitary from hypothalamic disease, or during inferior petrosal sinus sampling, to determine the side of a pituitary microadenoma.

Protocol

1. Infuse synthetic ovine or human corticotropin-releasing hormone (CRH) 1 µg/kg intravenously, up to 100 µg.

2. Measure ACTH and plasma cortisol concentrations before and 15–45 minutes after CRH infusion.

3. If done in conjunction with dexamethasone, give dexamethasone 5–7.5 µg/kg/dose (0.5 mg maximum) by mouth every 6 hours beginning at noon on day 1 and continuing until 6 a.m. on day 3 and give the CRH at 8 a.m., 2 hours after the last dexamethasone dose.

Interpretation Normally, both ACTH and cortisol rise after CRH administration. Because most pituitary adenomas retain normal CRH responsiveness, no response suggests but does not prove an ectopic or adrenal source. After dexamethasone, normal individuals and those with pseudo-Cushing syndrome suppress plasma cortisol concentrations to less than 1.8 µg/dL (50 nmol/L), whereas those with Cushing disease may not completely suppress.

Interpretation of these tests depends on the type of CRH used, the time points measured, and the points chosen as normal cutoffs, varying between a 35% and a 50% rise above baseline for ACTH and between 14% and 20% rise above baseline for cortisol (17,22,23).

Comments This method has been validated with ovine-sequence CRH rather than human-sequence CRH. Because of the low cutoff, highly sensitive cortisol assays must be used. There is a high degree of individual variation in response that limits the utility of this test. It is also quite expensive. CRH has been suggested for use in diagnosing adrenal insufficiency as well but has not been well validated for this purpose (22).

Metyrapone Test

Purpose Metyrapone, which blocks the enzyme responsible for converting 11-deoxycortisol to cortisol (11β-hydroxylase), is another test used to distinguish Cushing disease (where appropriate response to cortisol feedback inhibition is often maintained) from adrenal disease or ectopic ACTH secretion. It also can be used to document lack of appropriate ACTH secretion in secondary adrenal insufficiency.

Protocol

1. Give metyrapone 30 mg/kg with food (to minimize gastrointestinal upset) at midnight.

2. The next morning at 8–9 a.m., measure 11-deoxycortisol, cortisol, and ACTH concentrations (22).

Interpretation When 11β-hydroxylase is inhibited, there is a buildup of the precursor 11-deoxycortisol, decreased cortisol concentrations, and a compensatory increase in ACTH concentrations due to a lack of negative feedback. In Cushing disease, the pituitary generally still responds to lack of negative feedback by increasing ACTH secretion. Generally, ACTH concentrations do not rise in the case of a primary adrenal problem or ectopic ACTH secretion.

Comments This test is used more widely in Europe to diagnose secondary adrenal insufficiency because metyrapone is difficult to obtain in the United States. The test could precipitate an adrenal crisis.

TESTS TO EVALUATE ADRENAL INSUFFICIENCY (ADDISON DISEASE)

Early Morning Plasma Cortisol and ACTH Concentrations

Purpose Early morning plasma cortisol and ACTH concentrations are the first-line screening tests to rule out adrenal insufficiency.

Protocol Several different specific and sensitive techniques are used to measure cortisol, including RIA, IRMA, and HPLC, with HPLC being the most specific (21). See the section on ACTH measurement above.

Interpretation Adrenal insufficiency is likely if the morning cortisol concentration is less than 3 μg/dL (83 nmol/L). Adrenal insufficiency is very unlikely if morning cortisol concentration is greater than18 μg/dL (500 nmol/L) (24,25). In adrenal insufficiency due to primary adrenal failure, the ACTH is significantly elevated.

Comments Because cortisol is secreted in a pulsatile manner, and many patients will have levels between 3 and 18 μg/dL (83 and 500 nmol/L), additional functional testing likely will be needed, as described below. Different laboratories may use different techniques and so have different cutoffs.

In some cases, measurement of cortisol and ACTH concentrations, together with the clinical picture, gives a clear diagnosis, but often dynamic testing, as described below, is necessary.

High-Dose ACTH (ACTH 1–24) Stimulation Test

Purpose In this test, a supraphysiological dose of ACTH (Cosyntropin) is given to directly test the adrenal glands' response. This test is used to diagnose primary adrenal insufficiency with 95% specificity and 97% sensitivity. However, this test only has 57% sensitivity and 95% specificity for secondary adrenal insufficiency (24).

Protocol

1. Give ACTH, 250 μg, intravenous push at any time of day. For children younger than 2 year of age, give ACTH 15 μg/kg up to a maximum of 250 μg. The subject does not need to be fasting.

2. Measure serum or plasma cortisol concentration before and 30 (optional) and 60 minutes after ACTH.

Interpretation If the stimulated cortisol concentration is less than 18 μg/dL (500 nmol/L),

then primary or secondary adrenal insufficiency is suspected (24). An increase from baseline concentration of less than 9 μg/dL (248 nmol/L) has been used to predict poor outcome in critically ill people but has been questioned recently in the critical-care literature (26).

Comments In a recent meta-analysis, healthy controls had stimulated cortisol concentrations ranging from 15–80 μg/dL (415–2200 nmol/L), so overlap exists between normal and adrenal insufficient levels in response to high-dose ACTH (24,25). Also, the cortisol concentration can be affected by several factors, including concentration of corticosteroid-binding globulin, time of day, and stress level.

Low-Dose ACTH (ACTH 1–24) Stimulation Test

Purpose This test is used most often to demonstrate recovery from glucocorticoid suppression. These subjects may respond to the supraphysiological stimulation of the high-dose ACTH stimulation test, which thus could give a false impression of hypothalamic–pituitary–adrenal competency.

Protocol

1. Give ACTH, 1 μg, intravenously in the morning (when the normal response would be expected to be the highest).

2. Measure serum or plasma cortisol concentration before and 30 (optional) and 60 minutes after ACTH.

Interpretation There is no consensus on the cutoff used to diagnose adrenal insufficiency, although classically a cortisol concentration of less than 18 μg/dL (500 nmol/L) is used (24,25). A recent literature review concluded that a *normal* result on the *low*-dose ACTH test is more likely to exclude adrenal insufficiency, whereas an *abnormal* result on the *high*-dose ACTH test is more likely to diagnose adrenal insufficiency correctly (25).

Comments Because there are no commercial formulations for 1 μg ACTH (only ampules of 250-μg doses exist), mistakes can be made in dilution and administration, especially since some of the dose may adhere to plastic intravenous tubing (25).

Insulin Tolerance Test

Purpose Some consider this the "gold standard" for dynamic testing of adrenal hypofunction because profound symptomatic hypoglycemia activates the hypothalamic–pituitary axis to increase ACTH secretion. However, this test is fraught with the risks of hypoglycemia and hypokalemia. Therefore, it is not used widely in children.

Protocol

1. Infuse regular insulin 0.1–0.15 U/kg intravenously to achieve hypoglycemia as low as 40 mg/dL (2.2 mmol/L) (25).

2. Measure glucose and cortisol concentrations at baseline and 30 and 60 minutes later.

3. Monitor carefully for the symptoms of hypoglycemia (especially seizures), and have a physician standing by to treat.

Interpretation Adrenal insufficiency is suspected when the cortisol concentration is less than 18 μg/dL (497–520 nmol/L).

Comments Some people without adrenal insufficiency can have concentrations below 18 μg/dL (497 nmol/L), and some people with adrenal insufficiency can have concentrations above this cutoff (27,28). Therefore, interpretation of this test is not absolutely clear-cut, and the side effects can be prohibitive. This test should not be used in people who are at risk for seizure or myocardial insufficiency.

Metyrapone Test

This test was described earlier under "Tests to Localize the Cause of Excessive Glucocorticoid Production." In the case of secondary adrenal insufficiency, 11-deoxycortisol concentrations rise and cortisol concentrations fall, but ACTH concentrations fail to rise. It can be used to evaluate the integrity of the hypothalamic–pituitary axis after trauma or prolonged steroid use.

TESTS TO DIAGNOSE CONGENITAL ADRENAL HYPERPLASIA

High-Dose Cosyntropin Stimulation Test

Purpose This test is done to diagnose the various forms of congenital adrenal hyperplasia.

Protocol The protocol was defined earlier under "Tests to Evaluate Adrenocortical Insufficiency (Addison disease)."

Interpretation Each screening laboratory establishes its own cutoffs, which should be adjusted for prematurity and low birth weight to improve predictive value (29).

Comments The general principle is that steroid precursors proximal to an enzyme defect will accumulate, and their circulating concentrations will be elevated, whereas steroids distal to the defect will be diminished. With partial defects, baseline steroid concentrations may be equivocal, but ACTH stimulation increases steroidogenesis and amplifies defects. Absolute steroid concentrations can be evaluated, as well as ratios of pre- and postenzyme steroid concentrations.

17-Hydroxyprogesterone (17-OHP)

Purpose This sensitive and specific test is used to screen newborns for the most common form of congenital adrenal hyperplasia, 21-hydroxylase deficiency (30). It is also used to monitor treatment of congenital adrenal hyperplasia.

Protocol

1. For screening, capillary blood should be collected from the newborn at 48–72 hours of age (usually by heel stick) on a filter-paper blood-spot card and sent to the screening laboratory in a timely manner.

2. For monitoring treatment, venipuncture is usually used to collect blood.

3. Ether extraction commonly precedes immunoassay (RIA or FIA) in order to avoid interference by metabolites that falsely increase reported concentrations of 17-OHP (31). However, Swedish investigators reported that extraction did not increase specificity or sensitivity of screening and added cost and report time (32).

Interpretation Each screening laboratory establishes its own cutoffs, which should be adjusted for prematurity and low birth weight to improve predictive value (29).

Comments To decrease false-positive results and increase specificity in mass newborn screening, some states are beginning second-tier steroid profiling using MS/MS on blood spots (9), which measures in addition to 17-OHP, cortisol and androstenedione levels.

CYP21 Analysis

Purpose The genetic basis for 21-hydroxylase deficiency has been studied in detail, ranging from deletion to sequence aberrations in *cyp21* alleles (32).

Protocol

1. Blood should be collected not only from the child but also from the parents for DNA interpretation.

2. Common techniques include allele-specific PCR and direct DNA sequencing.

Interpretation Disease severity and final adult height can be correlated with the type of *CYP21* mutation (32,33).

Comments Gene analysis is not necessary for the diagnosis of 21-hydroxylase deficiency but should be used in genetic counseling, and confirmation of the diagnosis and form of CAH, salt wasting vs. simple virilizing vs. non

TABLE 49-4 Test of Calcium and Bone Homeostasis
Tests for measuring calcium homeostasis
Total calcium
Ionized calcium
Parathyroid hormone assays
PTH-related protein (PTHrP) assays
Urine calcium:creatinine ratio
Tests of vitamin D status
25-OHD radioimmunoassay
25-OHD chemiluminescent assay
25-OHD mass spectrometry
1-25(OH)$_2$D radioimmunassay
Markers of bone turnover
Osteocalcin
Bone-specific alkaline phosphatase (BAP)
N-telopeptides (NTx)

classical as there is a good correlation between genotype and phenotype (33).

TESTS OF CALCIUM AND BONE HOMEOSTASIS

Tests of calcium and bone homeostasis include those designed to measure calcium homeostasis, vitamin D status, and bone turnover (Table 49-4).

TESTS FOR MEASURING CALCIUM HOMEOSTASIS

Total Calcium

Purpose Calcium is the most abundant cation in the body and the fifth most abundant element in the body (34,35). These tests measure total serum calcium, both protein-bound and ionized (free).

Protocol In many clinical laboratories, calcium is measured by photometric analysis, which measures the colored products formed on binding with calcium, and by ion-selective electrodes (ISE), which are described below in the measurement of ionized calcium (34).

Interpretation Normal concentrations of calcium vary widely between institutions depending on methodology.

Comments Because EDTA has high affinity for binding calcium, serum should not be drawn in tubes with EDTA (34). The patient's protein status also affects measurement of total calcium. For instance, if total calcium is elevated, simultaneous albumin concentrations or ionized calcium should be measured to exclude pseudohypercalcemia (36). If the patient has abnormal levels of albumin (either high or low), then a corrected total calcium may be calculated from the following equa-

tion, although measurement of the ionized calcium is likely more informative (34):

- Corrected total calcium(mg/dL) = measured total calcium (mg/dL) + {0.8 × [4 − albumin (g/dL)]}

Ionized Calcium

Purpose These tests measure only the ionized, or free, fraction of calcium, which is not bound to proteins, comprises about half of total serum calcium, and is finely controlled by parathyroid hormone (PTH) and 1,25-(OH)$_2$ vitamin D (34,36).

Protocol Clinical laboratories use free calcium analyzers (which use potentiometers) and calcium ion-selective electrodes (ISEs) to measure ionized calcium. Calcium ISEs use a complex system of liquid membranes containing an ion-selective calcium sensor and an external reference electrode, which creates an electrochemical cell across which a potential difference is measured and translated into free calcium concentration (34).

Interpretation Reference ranges for ionized calcium vary widely depending on the calcium analyzer.

Comments Calibration of the reference solutions and temperature affect measurement of ionized calcium. Also, as with total calcium, heparin is the only recommended anticoagulant for collection of blood for ionized calcium, because EDTA, citrate, and oxalate can decrease free calcium levels (34). Acid–base disorders also affect the fraction of ionized calcium in the serum (35).

Parathyroid Hormone Assay: Fragment Assays, IRMA, and ICMA

Purpose PTH circulates as an intact 84-amino-acid hormone that includes the active N-terminal and inactive fragments that contain only the C terminus or the middle two-thirds of the molecule known as the midregion (36,37). Two-site immunoassays with antibody binding to both the N- and C-terminal ends can distinguish between the intact molecule and fragments (36).

Protocol Traditionally, RIAs were the "gold standard" for measurement of PTH levels and are classified by the fragments they recognize, for example, C-terminal, N-terminal, or midregion (34,38,39). These assays can be difficult to interpret because inactive fragments have longer half-lives, especially in renal patients, so they represent a larger part of the immunoreactivity in the serum than the intact form of PTH. The competitive RIAs do not distinguish between PTH and nonparathyroid peptides with PTH activity (34,38).

In contrast, double-antibody two-site immunoradiometric (IRMA) and two-site immunochemiluminometric (ICMA) assays have been shown to be both highly sensitive and specific for distinguishing PTH from PTH-related protein (37). Newer automated methods using direct immunochemiluminescent sandwich assays are highly correlated with RIA but have improved specificity (39).

Interpretation Clinical decision limits are assay-specific (39). PTH should be measured simultaneously with the calcium level for proper interpretation (39,40). Rapid (15-minute turnaround time) intraoperative PTH measurement by IRMA has been developed to increase success rates of parathyroidectomy; classically, if all hypersecreting parathyroid tissue has been removed, then the PTH concentration 5–10 minutes after removal will be less than 50% of baseline values (41).

Comments Care should be taken when ordering and interpreting PTH levels because the less reliable competitive radioimmunoassays are still used in some clinical laboratories (34,37,38,40). Furthermore, recent studies have shown that some of the newer "intact PTH" immunometric assays may crossreact to detect N-truncated forms of PTH (amino acid sequence 7–84), so some advocate the use of only "bioactive whole PTH assays" or "cyclase-activating PTH assays," which measure only PTH that contains all 84 amino acids (42).

PTH-Related Protein (PTHrP) Radioimmunoassays and Two-Site Assays

Purpose These tests measure PTH-related protein (PTHrP), which is the most common cause of hypercalcemia in malignancy (36,43).

Protocol RIAs can measure PTHrP for the N-terminal, midregion, or C-terminal domain (43,44). However, two-site assays that use radioimmunometric, immunofluorometric, and chemiluminescent methods are more specific and more sensitive (43,44).

Interpretation Plasma PTHrP concentrations are high in patients with hypercalcemia due to malignancy (43,44).

Comments Multiple tumors, particularly solid tumors such as squamous carcinoma, renal carcinoma, and breast cancer, may produce PTHrP. Tumor production of normal PTH is rare but does occur (36,43).

Urine Calcium:Creatinine Ratio

Purpose Ionized calcium is excreted, whereas protein-bound calcium is not. Urine calcium excretion is useful in evaluating hypercalcemia, defining hypercalciuria, and assessing PTH activity.

Protocol It is measured in a random, fasting morning, or 24 hour sample.

Interpretation The calcium:creatinine ratio is age-dependent, approaching 2 or more in preterm infants, 1 in full-term infants, about 0.5 by 2 years of age, and 0.2–0.3 in children age 8 years and older.

Comments Conditions in which renal calcium excretion is increased include high dietary intake of calcium, hypercalcemia, saline diuresis, loop diuretic use, and acidosis. Calcium excretion is decreased by PTH, PTHrP, hypocalcemia, thiazide diuretics, and renal insufficiency. The calcium:creatinine ratio is lower in familial hypocalciuric hypocalcemia than in hyperparathyroidism.

TESTS OF VITAMIN D STATUS

25-OH Vitamin D: Radioimmunoassay

Purpose The precursor 7-dehydrocholesterol is converted to cholecalciferol (vitamin D_3) in the skin by ultraviolet (UV) light, which is then hydroxylated in the liver to produce 25-OHD, which is the major storage form of vitamin D in the body (36,45). Several tests measure 25-OHD, including RIA, CIA, and MS.

Protocol Traditionally, RIAs are the "gold standard" for measurement of 25-OHD levels. Since 1993, RIAs have used a ^{125}I-labeled tracer to detect 25-OHD (46). The ^{125}I-based RIA kit by DiaSorin appears to be more accurate than other kits because it quantitates not only cholecalciferol (vitamin D_3) from endogenous synthesis in the epidermis but also ergocalciferol (vitamin D_2) from exogenous dietary supplementation (47); vitamin D_2's bioequivalence to vitamin D_3 has not been established (48). Newer automated methods using direct competitive immunochemiluminescent assays highly correlate with RIAs (39).

Interpretation/Comments Reference values for 25-OHD vary not only by assay but also by season, latitude, age, and race (39). In the United States National Health and Nutrition Examination Survey (NHANES III, 1988–1994), mean 25-OHD concentrations in 18,875 adolescents and adults using the DiaSorin RIA were highest in non-Hispanic whites and lowest in non-Hispanic blacks (49). The same study found that deficiency is

relatively uncommon (25-OHD < 17.5 nmol/L), but insufficiency (25-OHD < 17.5–62.5 nmol/L) is common, especially in winter in the northern latitudes (49).

25-OH Vitamin D: Mass Spectrometry

Purpose Liquid chromatography–tandem mass spectrometry (LC/MS/MS) has been proposed as a reference method to validate routine immunoassays because it avoids problems caused by the binding of 25-OHD$_3$ to vitamin D–binding globulin (48).

Protocol In contrast to HPLC with UV detection and GC/MS, LC/MS/MS requires simpler sample preparation and shorter analytical run times (48).

Interpretation/Comments LC/MS/MS is being studied in multiple centers in order to create an international reference standard for 25-OHD$_3$ measurement (48).

25-OH Vitamin D: Chemiluminescent Protein-Binding Assay (CLPBA)

Purpose This test can be used to determine 25-OHD levels using automated methods, as opposed to labor-intensive HPLC (50,51).

Protocol This test measures 25-OHD with chemiluminescence instead of radioactivity, with less turnaround time (1 hour), and with less manual handling because of primary tube sampling (51).

Interpretation/Comments One-third of samples in patients with hip fractures showed discordant values between CLPBA and RIA, and both underestimate levels of 25-OHD compared with HPLC (51).

1,25-(OH)$_2$ Vitamin D Radioimmunoassay

Purpose After the liver hydroxylates vitamin D$_3$ to 25-OHD, it is hydroxylated again in the kidney to 1,25-(OH)$_2$D, which is the most biologically active form of vitamin D (34,45).

Protocol The 1,25-(OH)$_2$ vitamin D ^{125}I radioimmunoassay has been validated to be sensitive and specific in identifying normal individuals from those who have low levels of 1,25-(OH)$_2$D (45).

Interpretation Low levels of 1,25-(OH)$_2$ vitamin D are associated with hypocalcemia and rickets (34,45).

Comments This assay has minimal (<0.01%) cross-reactivity with 25-OHD, and results are not affected by freezing and thawing samples (45).

MARKERS OF BONE TURNOVER

Markers of bone formation are measured in the serum, whereas markers of bone breakdown are measured in the urine. The most common markers are listed below. These are generally used for research purposes in population studies and not for clinical decision making in individual patients.

Osteocalcin

Purpose Osteocalcin is a 49-amino-acid protein that is synthesized and secreted by the osteoblast. It constitutes about 20% of the noncollagenous protein of bone matrix, and serum levels represent an accurate index of bone formation (52).

Protocol Many commercial assays are available to measure serum osteocalcin, including ELISA, IRMA, and RIA (53).

Interpretation Normal standards are laboratory- and age-specific (54,55).

Comments Falsely reduced values can be produced by hemolysis (which releases proteases that degrade osteocalcin), lipemia (because lipids bind ostecalcin instead of allowing it to react to immunoassays), and increased freeze–thaw cycles (53). Increased concentrations are found in conditions with decreased glomerular filtration rates and correlate with increased serum creatinine (53,56).

Bone-Specific Alkaline Phosphatase

Purpose Total alkaline phosphatase (ALP) is one of the most common indices of bone formation and can be used in monitoring the therapy of rickets and renal osteodystrophy (53). Eighty percent of the total-body ALP derives from bone, whereas the rest derives primarily from the liver (52). The osteoblast synthesizes and sheds into the serum a bone-specific form of ALP (BAP).

Protocol Methods have been developed to differentiate between bone and liver sources of ALP, such as heat denaturation, gel electrophoresis, immunoassays, and IRMAs (53).

Interpretation Normal standards are both age- and laboratory-specific (57).

Comments Because many tests have some crossreactivity with liver ALP, liver involvement should be excluded when high BAP is found (53).

N-Telopeptides (NTx)

Purpose The collagen type I cross-linked N-telopeptides (NTx) are derived from degradation of bone collagen and are not further metabolized. Thus they are direct markers of bone resorption (52).

TABLE 49-5   Tests of Glucose Metabolism

Tests to evaluate diabetes risk or diagnose diabetes
  Type 1 diabetes autoantibodies
  HLA type
  Oral glucose tolerance test (OGTT)
Tests to evaluate β-cell function
  Measurement of first-phase insulin secretion
    Intravenous glucose tolerance test (IVGTT)
    Glucagon stimulation
    Arginine stimulation
  Hyperglycemic clamp
  Models derived from glucose and insulin levels
    HOMA β-cell index
    Insulinogenic index
  Mixed-meal tolerance test
Tests to measure insulin sensitivity
  Hyperinsulinemic, euglycemic clamp
  Minimal-model frequently sampled IVGTT
  Surrogate models of insulin sensitivity
    HOMA-IR
    QUICKI
    Insulin sensitivity index
Tests to evaluate hypoglycemia
  The "critical blood sample" after prolonged supervised fast
  Glucagon stimulation test
  Hypoglycemic clamp

Protocol NTx is measured in the urine with an ELISA, either in the second morning void or in a 24-hour urine collection (53).

Interpretation Normal standards are both age- and laboratory-specific (52,58–60).

Comments Urinary NTx are elevated in conditions of increased bone turnover such as metastatic malignancies, hyperthyroidism, and acromegaly (53).

TESTS OF GLUCOSE METABOLISM

Tests of glucose metabolism include those designed to evaluate diabetes risk or diagnose diabetes, those that evaluate β-cell function, those that measure insulin sensitivity, and those that evaluate hypoglycemia (Table 49-5). Many of these tests are used primarily in clinical research settings.

TESTS TO EVALUATE DIABETES RISK OR DIAGNOSE DIABETES

Type 1 Diabetes Autoantibodies and HLA Type

Purpose These studies can be done to identify individuals at high risk for development of type 1 diabetes or to help make a diagnosis when it is not clear whether a subject has autoimmune or another type of diabetes. Specific autoantibodies have been shown to be highly

---

predictive of development of type 1 diabetes. Certain HLA types confer higher risk of diabetes, whereas others are considered protective (see Chapter 20 for further discussion).

Protocol While many antibodies have been studied and are available in research laboratories, those currently available that are used most commonly clinically include antibodies to GAD65 (glutamic acid decarboxylase), ICA-512 (also called IA-2, neurosecretory granules found in β and other cells), IAA (insulin autoantibodies), and ICA (cytoplasmic islet cell antibodies). These are measured in serum. HLA type is measured in whole blood, and the specimen requires special handling.

Interpretation The pathogenic significance of the autoantibodies is unclear—they may be participants in the autoimmune process or, more likely, they are simply markers of β-cell damage. In a patient with known diabetes, the presence of at least one marker usually is considered sufficient to characterize the diabetes as type 1. However, about 4% of patients in North American and Europe described as having type 2 diabetes are GAD antibody–positive (61). Compared with other subjects with type 2 diabetes, these individuals are less insulin-resistant, have more favorable lipid levels, and have a lower prevalence of the metabolic syndrome. This type of diabetes also has been called *latent autoimmune diabetes in adults* (LADA) or *type 1.5 diabetes*, and it is not clear whether it should be considered type 2 diabetes, type 1 diabetes, or a completely separate diabetes category.

Nondiabetic subjects with autoantibodies are at high risk for development of diabetes, but disease progression is not inevitable. The more autoantibodies that are present, the greater is the risk.

Comments This is a rapidly changing field. Over the next several years, large multinational studies such as the National Institutes of Health–sponsored TrialNet will help to better define the role of these tests in predicting and diagnosing diabetes.

Oral Glucose Tolerance Test

Purpose The oral glucose tolerance test (OGTT) can be used to determine the presence of type 2 diabetes in individuals in whom fasting or random levels are not diagnostic and to diagnose impaired glucose tolerance. It is sometimes used to evaluate the degree of glucose intolerance and hyperinsulinemia in subjects with the metabolic syndrome.

Protocol

1. The test is performed in the morning between 7 and 10 a.m. Patients must have been fasting for at least 8 hours and must

have consumed a reasonable amount of carbohydrate (minimum of 200 g/day) for 3 days preceding the test. An intravenous line is inserted for blood drawing.

2. Time 0: Draw a fasting glucose and insulin (and/or C-peptide) level. Then give glucose (standard beverage provided through the pharmacy), 1.75 g/kg up to a maximum of 75 g, consumed within 5 minutes.

3. Determine glucose and insulin (and/or C-peptide) levels every 30 minutes for 2 hours (times 30, 60, 90, and 120 minutes) after the start of the glucose ingestion.

Interpretation Fasting plasma glucose

- <100 mg/dL (5.6 mmol/L)—normal
- 100–125 mg/dL (5.6–6.9 mmol/L)— impaired fasting glucose
- ≥126 mg/dL (7.0 mmol/L)—diabetes

Two-hour glucose

- <140 mg/dL (7.8 mmol/L)—normal
- 140–199 mg/dL (7.8-11.1 mmol/L)— impaired glucose tolerance
- ≥200 mg/dL (11.1 mmol/L)—diabetes

Comments The test has high sensitivity and specificity, and the criteria are universally accepted and understood worldwide. However, it is subject to intraindividual variability (62). In 1997, the American Diabetes Association Expert Committee on the Diagnosis and Classification of Diabetes Mellitus acknowledged that the OGTT was a valid way to diagnosis diabetes but discouraged its use for diagnostic purposes in clinical practice because of inconvenience, less reproducibility, and greater cost than a simple fasting glucose determination (63). Since that report, others have challenges the stance because the OGTT is the only reliable method of diagnosing impaired glucose tolerance or diabetes without fasting hyperglycemia, and thus, youth and adults at risk for diabetes and the metabolic syndrome might be missed by a simple fasting glucose determination (64,65). This issue may be particularly relevant in the pediatric population, where those with fasting hyperglycemia may represent only a small fraction of patients with abnormal glucose tolerance.

TESTS TO EVALUATE β-CELL FUNCTION

Measurement of First-Phase Insulin and/or C-peptide Secretion

Purpose The intravenous glucose tolerance test (IVGTT) and glucagon and arginine stimulation tests are done to measure acute insulin and/or C-peptide secretion as an indicator of β-cell function. The hyperglycemic clamp assesses β-cell function by measuring the response to sustained hyperglycemia.

Protocol

- Intravenous glucose tolerance test:

1. Fasting insulin (and/or C-peptide) and glucose levels are measured. The fasting glucose must be less than 115 mg/dL (5.7 mmol/L) for the test to be accurate (66).

2. Dextrose (0.3 g/kg) is given by intravenous push in less than 30 seconds.

3. Insulin (and/or C-peptide) levels are measured at 1, 3, 4, 5, 7, and 10 minutes.

- Glucagon stimulation test

1. Fasting insulin (and/or C-peptide) and glucose levels are measured.

2. Glucagon (1 mg) is given by intravenous push in less than 30 seconds.

3. Insulin (and/or C-peptide) levels are measured at 1, 2, 4, 6, 8, and 10 minutes.

4. Subjects may become nauseated.

- Arginine stimulation test

1. Fasting insulin (and/or C-peptide) and glucose levels are measured.

2. Arginine (5 g) is given by intravenous push in less than 30 seconds.

3. Insulin (and/or C-peptide) levels are measured each minute for 10 minutes.

4. Subjects may experience a brief metallic taste.

5. The higher the baseline glucose level, the greater is the insulin secretion in response to arginine. Potentiation tests measure the slope of sequential responses to arginine at increasing glucose concentrations. The values after arginine stimulation at glucose levels greater than 450 mg/dL (24.4 mmol/L) can be used to determine the maximal acute insulin response (AIR_{max}).

- Hyperglycemic clamp

1. Glucose ($D_{20}W$ or $D_{50}W$) is infused to elevate the blood glucose concentration to the desired supraphysiological level. The infusion rate is determined by measuring blood glucose levels at the bedside at 5-minute intervals and adjusting the infusion as needed to maintain the desired degree of hyperglycemia.

2. Once steady state is achieved, insulin levels are measured to determine the β-cell response. Insulin secretion between subjects can be compared at a similar level of hyperglycemia.

3. This test is often started with an IVGTT, which allows measurement of first-phase insulin secretion and also rapidly pushes blood glucose levels into the desired hyperglycemic range.

Interpretation The insulin response within the first 10 minutes after stimulation is called the *first-phase insulin response* (FPIR) or the *acute insulin response* (AIR). It can be measured as the area under the curve or as peak level minus baseline. It represents release of insulin from an immediately accessible β-cell pool. As damage to the cell occurs, this pool is lost. Impairment or absence of the FPIR occurs before the onset of hyperglycemia and thus is an early indicator of β-cell damage.

For all of these tests, insulin levels generally are measured in subjects who have never received exogenous insulin therapy. Those who have received insulin therapy often develop insulin antibodies, which may interfere with the insulin assay. For these subjects, measurement of C-peptide levels is preferable. Because C-peptide has a longer half-life than insulin, somewhat different results are achieved.

Comments These tests generally are done by experienced investigators as part of research protocols.

Models of β-Cell Function Derived from Glucose and Insulin Levels

Purpose Various models have been developed to estimate β-cell function from fasting or OGTT-derived glucose and/or insulin levels. Two of the most commonly used models are the HOMA β-cell index and the insulinogenic index.

Protocol

1. The homeostasis model assessment (HOMA β-cell index) is calculated as (67)

$$\frac{[\text{Fasting insulin } (\mu U/mL) \times 20]}{[\text{fasting glucose } (mmol/L) - 3.5]}$$

2. The insulinogenic index (I/G30) uses the increment above basal in insulin and glucose concentrations during the first 30 minutes of the OGTT and is calculated as (68)

$$\frac{[\text{Insulin } (30 \text{ min}) - \text{insulin } (0 \text{ min})]}{[\text{glucose } (30 \text{ min}) - \text{glucose } (0 \text{ min})]}$$

Interpretation These models are used to compare differences in β-cell function (insulin secretion) between populations. They are attractive for epidemiological studies because they are convenient and inexpensive. They should be interpreted with caution, however, in populations with abnormal glucose metabolism.

Comments In individuals with normal glucose tolerance, these surrogate measures correlate reasonably well with more accurate measures of β-cell function, such as first-phase insulin secretion or the hyperglycemic clamp (69). In subjects with abnormal glucose tolerance, however, they may not be accurate because they may be more dependent on fasting glucose levels than on insulin secretion, and because the relationship between fasting glucose and insulin is not linear and does not change in parallel with worsening of glucose tolerance (70).

The Mixed-Meal Tolerance Test

Purpose This test is a more physiological indicator of β-cell function than the OGTT because carbohydrates, amino acids, and fats all stimulate insulin secretion directly and indirectly via the incretin gut hormones.

Protocol

1. The test is performed in the morning between 7 and 10 a.m. Patients must have been fasting for at least 8 hours.

2. Time 0: Draw a fasting glucose and insulin (and/or C-peptide) level. Then give a standardized liquid mixed meal. One protocol uses Boost® HP 6 mL/kg (maximum 360 mL), to be ingested within 5 minutes. Other protocols have used Sustacal®.

3. Determine glucose and insulin (and or C-peptide) levels at times 15, 30, 60, 90, and 120 minutes after the start of ingestion of the mixed meal.

Interpretation The peak C-peptide level, the peak C-peptide minus basal C-peptide level, or the area under the C-peptide curve can be used as a measure of β-cell function.

Comments This test usually is performed to evaluate residual C-peptide secretion in subjects with diabetes. The response to the mixed meal may be normal in some patients with abnormal glucose tolerance because the impaired β cell responds differently to glucose than to fat and protein.

TESTS TO EVALUATE INSULIN SENSITIVITY

The Hyperinsulinemic Euglycemic Clamp

Purpose This test is considered the "gold standard" for measurement of insulin sensitivity (71).

Protocol

1. Briefly, exogenous insulin is infused continuously at a predetermined constant rate (based on weight or body surface area) to achieve a desired plasma level. The assumption usually is made that it takes about 150 minutes to achieve steady state

(equilibration between vascular and interstitial insulin levels).

2. Glucose levels are measured at the bedside at 5- to 10-minute intervals, and a dextrose infusion is adjusted as needed to "clamp" the plasma glucose at a predetermined physiological level. Once the steady-state insulin concentration is achieved, the amount of exogenous glucose infused reflects the amount of glucose being used by the body (R_d = rate of glucose disappearance) and reflects the individual's sensitivity to insulin.

3. Insulin sensitivity M is calculated as the average milligram per kilogram per minute of glucose infused over 30–40 minutes after steady state is achieved.

4. Potassium phosphate is often also infused in order to prevent an acute drop in plasma potassium levels associated with insulin-induced intracellular shifts.

5. Stable isotopes or radioisotopes may be infused to measure suppression by insulin of hepatic glucose production (hepatic insulin sensitivity) (72).

Interpretation M, the milligrams per kilogram per minute of glucose required to maintain euglycemia during steady-state insulin infusion, is a measure of total body insulin sensitivity (a combination of peripheral glucose uptake and suppression of hepatic glucose production). A higher M value, meaning that more glucose is required, is a measure of greater insulin sensitivity. M often is normalized to lean body mass because muscle is the primary tissue involved in insulin-induced glucose uptake. When isotopes are used during the clamp, it is possible to calculate hepatic glucose production separately.

Comments This test requires a clinical research center or similar facility and specially trained nurses and physicians. It is relatively inexpensive, in that there are few laboratory assays performed, but it is extremely labor-intensive and is generally performed by a physician.

The Minimal-Model FSIVGTT

Purpose Bergman's minimal-model assessment of insulin sensitivity uses computer-based mathematical modeling of glucose and insulin levels during a frequently sampled intravenous glucose tolerance test to derive measurement of insulin sensitivity (S_I = a measure of total-body glucose disposal), glucose effectiveness (S_G = insulin-independent glucose uptake), the acute insulin response (AIR), and the disposition index (DI, i.e., AIR × S_I, a description of the relation between insulin secretion and resistance) (73). Measures of insulin sensitivity obtained with the model are closely correlated

with measures obtained with the euglycemic clamp (74).

Protocol

1. At time 0, glucose (0.3 g/kg) is injected over 30 seconds with time 0 set at the end of the injection. Glucose and insulin are measured at −10, −5, 0, 2, 3, 4, 5, 6, 8, 10, 12, 14, 16, 19, 22, 24, 26, 28, 30, 40, 50, 60, 70, 90, 100, 120, 140, 160, and 180 minutes.

2. The original model was modified because it more accurately measures the effect of insulin when greater levels of insulin are present. Either a bolus of intravenous tolbutamide (300 mg, 5 mg/kg) at time 20 minutes or exogenous insulin (4 mU/kg/minute) infused during time 20–25 minutes is added to increase the insulin level (75).

3. Accuracy in timing is critical.

4. A 90-minute version of the test (−30, −15, 0, 1, 2, 3, 4, 5, 6, 8, 10, 12, 14, 16, 19, 22, 23, 24, 25, 27, 30, 35, 40, 50, 60, 70, and 90 minutes) has been validated in children (76).

Interpretation Glucose and insulin levels are entered into a computer program that can be purchased. Normal values are published for adults and children and by race (76–78). Extreme insulin resistance is not well measured with this model because the calculations require a measurable effect of insulin on glucose levels.

Comments This test requires a clinical research center or similar facility. It is expensive because of the multiple insulin assays, but it can be performed by a trained nurse and thus requires less physician time than the clamp.

Fasting Insulin Levels

Purpose Fasting insulin levels are sometimes used as a surrogate measure of insulin resistance.

Protocol A fasting sample is measured in a non-stressed individual.

Interpretation Levels of 15 μU/mL (107.6 pmol/L) or greater generally are considered indicative of insulin resistance.

Comments The fasting insulin level correlates strongly with insulin resistance measured by the euglycemic clamp (M) because both are highly dependent on the level of body fatness (79). Fasting insulin does not have the same discriminatory power as M, however, because it does not show the same differences between males and females or between Tanner stages (80) and because M and fasting insulin differ in their relation to cardiovascular risk factors (79). The lack of comparability between M and fasting insulin may be explained by the fact that determination of insulin resistance with the euglycemic clamp is an experimentally controlled model that isolates insulin resistance, whereas fasting insulin represents an active, integrated biological system of which insulin sensitivity is only one variable.

Surrogate Models of Insulin Sensitivity

Purpose Surrogate models of insulin sensitivity are simple tests that often are used in large epidemiological studies because the euglycemic clamp and the FSIVGTT are laborious or expensive and require special clinical research facilities.

Protocol Multiple models to estimate insulin resistance exist using the fasting insulin and glucose levels with or without other levels obtained during the OGTT. Three of the most common methods are HOMA-IR, QUICKI and Insulin sensitivity index (see Models of Estimating Insulin Resistance).

Models of Estimating Insulin Resistance

1. HOMA-IR (homeostasis model assessment—insulin resistance) (67):

$$\frac{\text{glu 0 min (mmol/L)} \times \text{ins 0 min (μU/mL)}}{22.5}$$

2. QUICKI (quantitative insulin sensitivity check index) (81):

$$\frac{1}{\log(\text{ins 0 min}) + \log(\text{glu 0 min})}$$

3. Insulin sensitivity index (82):

$$\frac{10,000}{\sqrt{(\text{ins 0 min} \times \text{glu 0 min}) \times (\text{mean glu} \times \text{mean in})}}$$

Interpretation These models are heavily dependent on the fasting insulin level, which correlates strongly with insulin resistance but is not the same thing (see earlier comments under fasting insulin). In subjects with normal glucose tolerance, a linear relationship is observed between fasting glucose and insulin levels, and the surrogate models may provide a reasonable estimate of insulin sensitivity (69). The linear relationship is not seen in subjects with abnormalities in fasting glucose or abnormal glucose tolerance (70) or in overweight youth at risk for the development of type 2 diabetes (83).

Comments The convenience of these models makes them attractive for epidemiological studies. Models depending on fasting glucose or insulin levels may be of limited usefulness, however, in the setting of abnormal glucose tolerance or prediabetes. They should be confined to population studies and not be used for clinical assessment of insulin sensitivity in an individual.

TESTS FOR EVALUATION OF HYPOGLYCEMIA

The "Critical Blood Sample" after Prolonged Supervised Fast

Purpose This is a collection of blood samples that should be drawn acutely when the child is hypoglycemic in order to investigate the etiology of the hypoglycemia. Defects in fatty acid oxidation, glycogen metabolism, gluconeogenesis, and ketone body metabolism; deficiencies of counter-regulatory hormones, such as growth hormone and cortisol; and hyperinsulinism present with hypoglycemia during fasting or stress (84,85).

Protocol Ideally, the critical blood sample should be drawn when the child first presents with hypoglycemia before treatment is instituted. However, in cases where intravenous or oral glucose is given before the critical sample is drawn, urine still can be analyzed for ketones and urinary organic acids. Therefore, it is often necessary to admit the child to a hospital setting to perform a prolonged controlled fast to induce hypoglycemia under physician supervision.

During admission to the hospital, monitor the child's blood sugar frequently by fingerstick. Frequency of fingerstick blood sugar test depends on the age and the rate of decrease in blood sugar, but often testing every hour is necessary, or sooner if the child becomes symptomatic. When the child becomes hypoglycemic, immediately draw the serum critical sample, including confirmatory blood glucose, insulin, serum β-hydroxybutyrate (preferably on an instantaneous blood ketone meter), lactate, cortisol, growth hormone, ammonia (on ice), and free fatty acids (84,85) (Table 49-6). The level of hypoglycemia at which this critical sample should be drawn is debated to be less than 40 or 60 mg/dL (2.2 and 3.3 mmol/L) (84,85). After collecting this critical sample, a glucagon stimulation test (see below) may be both diagnostic and therapeutic.

Interpretation Differential diagnoses of hypoglycemia usually are divided into ketotic versus nonketotic hypoglycemia. Detectable insulin levels in the face of hypoglycemia or suppressed fatty acid and ketone levels (even if insulin levels are low) indicate hyperinsulinism. The level of insulin that is considered too high is debated (84–86).

Comments Care should be taken when allowing a child to fast in order to provoke hypoglycemia. Fasting should be avoided if fatty oxidation defect is suspected. Preparation is key, including placing intravenous access on admission to the hospital, having immediate access to intramuscular glucagon in case of loss of intravenous access, and assembling the appropriate types of blood collection tubes at the bedside (Table 49-6).

Glucagon Stimulation Test

Purpose This test is performed at the time of hypoglycemia not only to help elucidate the etiology of the hypoglycemia but also to treat it (85). In particular, it distinguishes between glycogen storage defects and hyperinsulinism (85,86).

Protocol At the time of hypoglycemia, administer glucagon intramuscularly or subcutaneously. Check blood glucose immediately prior to glucagon administration and 30 minutes after. There is little consensus on the dosage of glucagon to be used, ranging from 30–100 μg/kg to a single dose of 0.5–1 mg (85,86).

Interpretation A positive response consists of a rise in the serum glucose of more than 30 mg/dL (1.7 mmol/L) 30 minutes after glucagon administration, which indicates that the patient is able not only to store glycogen but also to mobilize the stores from the liver. A positive response suggests insulin excess as the etiology of hypoglycemia. Lack of a response to glucagon suggests that the patient may have a glycogen storage disease or that the patient is malnourished with depleted glycogen stoores.

Comments Be careful to monitor the child for rebound hypoglycemia after glucagon administration because glycogen stores will be depleted (85). In addition, glucagon administration can cause nausea, vomiting, and abdominal pain.

TABLE 49-6   Critical Sample Details for Evaluation of Hypoglycemia

Test	Tube Type	Min.Vol.	Method	Significance
Glucose*	Green (Li heparin)	0.2 mL	Colorimetric reflectance spectrophotometry; glucose oxidase	Glucose levels are monitored by meter at the bedside to provide immediate feedback, but these are not absolutely accurate in hypoglycemia, so laboratory confirmation is necessary.
Insulin*	Red/black or gold (gel)	1.2 mL	Chemiluminescent immunoassay	Insulin levels should be suppressed in hypoglycemia, although the level that defines hyperinsulinism is debated. An exception is the child with chronically hyperstimulated insulin secretion, such as the infant in the neonatal intensive-care unit receiving a high glucose infusion rate (GIR) in total parenteral nutrition or the undernourished child receiving continuous gastrostomy tube feedings. These children may have iatrogenic hypersecretion of insulin if the GIR is not weaned slowly.
β-Hydroxybutyrate by blood ketone meter*	Can be performed at bedside, or transport whole blood to lab in heparinized syringe; green (Li heparin) tube also acceptable, but *cannot* be centrifuged.	0.1 mL	β-Hydroxybutyrate dehydrogenase reaction (Medisense Precision Xtra)	In hypoglycemia, fatty acids are metabolized to provide energy, which produces ketones, mainly β-hydroxybutyrate. Insulin suppresses ketone formation, so hypoglycemia without ketonemia indicates hyperinsulinism. Alternatively, lack of ketones could indicate defects in fatty oxidation including primary carnitine deficiency or defects in ketogenesis (86); malnurished infants, may have decreased ketones because of lack of substrate.
Growth hormone*	Red/black or gold (gel)	0.8 mL	Chemiluminescent immunoassay	Growth hormone (GH) is an important counterregulatory hormone for maintaining fasting blood glucose levels in infants, so levels should rise in hypoglycemia. Low levels of GH should provoke investigation of hypopituitarism, including serum levels of other pituitary hormones and a pituitary MRI. GH deficiency should be confirmed with GH stimulation testing.
Cortisol*	Red/black or gold (gel)	0.5 mL	Chemiluminescent immunoassay	Cortisol is an important counterregulatory hormone in hypoglycemia, so low levels should provoke an investigation of hypopituitarism as described above. A low-dose (1 μg) cosyntropin stimulation test should be performed if cortisol deficiency is suspected.
Free fatty acids*	Red/black or gold (gel)	0.6 mL	Spectrophotometric	In hypoglycemia, adipose tissue is broken down to fatty acids to provide energy and ketones through fatty oxidation. Insulin suppresses free fatty acid formation, so hypoglycemia with low levels of free fatty acids (and ketones) indicates hyperinsulinism. Alternatively, high free fatty acid levels and inappropriate low ketones for the degree of hypoglycemia indicate a defect in fatty acid oxidation.
Lactate*	Green (Li heparin) on ice; collect without the use of a tourniquet or within 3 minutes of applying the tourniquet, but before releasing the tourniquet. Deliver to laboratory immediately.	0.2 mL	Colorimetric reflectance spectrophotometry (lactate oxidase); lactate electrode	Elevated lactate levels can indicate defects in gluconeogenesis, glycogen storage disease (type I), ketone synthesis defects, mitochondrial disease, organic acidemias, and fatty oxidation defects (86).
Ammonia†	Green (Li heparin) on ice; deliver sample to laboratory within 5 minutes of collection	0.2 mL	Colorimetric reflectance spectrophotometry (bromophenol blue)	Elevated ammonia levels along with evidence of hyperinsulinism suggest an activating mutation in glutamate dehydrogenase (GDH), which was formerly known as leucine-sensitive hypoglycemia. The two- to fivefold increase in ammonia is usually asymptomatic but should be confirmed with multiple measurements because falsely elevated levels of ammonia are common, especially if the sample is not placed on ice immediately. Organic acidemias and fatty oxidation defects may have elevated ammonia levels.

(Continued)

TABLE 49-6 Critical Sample Details for Evaluation of Hypoglycemia *(Continued)*

Test	Tube Type	Min.Vol.	Method	Significance
IGFBP-1†	Red	0.5 mL	ICMA by Esoterix	While hypoglycemia increases insulin-like growth factor–binding protein 1, insulin decreases IGFBP-1 (87). Therefore, low levels of IGFBP-1 in the face of hypoglycemia suggest hyperinsulinism.
C-peptide†	Red/black or gold (gel)	0.6 mL	Chemiluminescent immunoassay	A suppressed C-peptide level in the presence of an elevated insulin level suggests exogenous insulin administration.
Quantitative plasma amino acids†	Green (Li heparin).	0.7 mL	High-performance ion-exchange liquid chromatography	Quantitative plasma amino acids are measured to assess substrate availability and check for defects in gluconeogenesis. For instance, in fasting hypoglycemia, low alanine with high ketones and low lactate can indicate glycogen synthase deficiency (86).
Urine organic acids†	Urine can be collected by any appropriate method and placed in any nonreactive container (typically a plastic urine cup)	Not to exceed 4 mL	GC/MS	Urine organic acids are measured to rule out organic acidemias, dicarboxylic aciduria (fatty oxidation defects), characteristic metabolites in ketolytic defects, or defects of ketone synthesis and the Krebs cycle. The first urine after hypoglycemia, even if it follows glucose administration, can be sent for organic acid analysis.
Free and total serum carnitine	Red/black or gold (gel)	1.4 mL	Spectrophotometry	Carnitine carries long- and very-long-chain fatty acids into the mitochondria for oxidation. During each cycle of fatty β- oxidation, acetyl CoA is released and is either directed to the Krebs cycle or to the liver for ketone synthesis. Low ketones and high free fatty acids indicate enzymatic defects in fatty oxidation, including carnitine cycle defects and primary carnitine deficiency. Patients with fatty oxidation disorders or organic acidemias develop secondary carnitine deficiency because carnitine binds the accumulated metabolites to be excreted in the urine. Free and total carnitine levels can be measured even after glucose administration. Abnormal ratio of free carnitine to esterified carnitne may indicate carnitine cycle defects (CPT-I, CPT-II, carnitine translocase defects).

Note: Tube types, minimal volumes, and methods are reported for the Fairview Diagnostic Laboratories at the University of Minnesota as of March 2005 and should be confirmed for specific institutions.
*Send immediately while the child is hypoglycemic.
†If volume must be minimized, then can be drawn at the discretion of the physician.

The Hypoglycemic Clamp

Purpose This test usually is used in the clinical research setting to study counterregulatory or neurocognitive responses to hypoglycemia.

Protocol Insulin and glucose are infused continuously at predetermined rates to achieve a constant state of hypoglycemia. Frequent monitoring of blood glucose, potassium, and insulin is done. If this study is performed to evaluate the integrity of the counterregulatory response, then glucagon, epinephrine, norepinephrine, growth hormone, and cortisol levels are measured. The hypoglycemic clamp also can be used to evaluate cognitive function during hypoglycemia. Protocols differ by investigational question.

Interpretation Interpretation differs based on investigational question.

Comments Because of the frequent monitoring, adjustment of insulin infusion rates, the need for multiple intravenous access sites, and safety concerns while inducing hypoglycemia, this type of study requires highly trained personnel in a clinical research center and usually is performed by a physician.

TESTS OF GROWTH HORMONE SUFFICIENCY AND EXCESS

The tests specific to the evaluation of the growth hormone (GH)–insulin-like growth factor (IGF) cascade include assays of individual components of this system and GH provocation testing. The individual components of the GH–IGF cascade that have been investigated for their relationship to growth include GH, IGF-1, IGF-2, six different IGF- binding proteins (IGFBPs), GH-binding protein (GHBP), and the acid labile subunit (ALS) of the IGF ternary complex. Serum levels of IGF-1, IGFBP-3, and ALS are directly GH-dependent. Analyses of these various components are difficult due to assay methodology and biological variability (Table 49-7).

TABLE 49-7 Tests of Growth Hormones Sufficiency and Excess

Tests for determining growth hormone sufficiency
Growth hormone assays
Growth hormone provocative testing
Insulin-like growth factor 1 (IGF-1)
IGF-binding protein 3 (IGFBP-3)
IGF generation test
IGF-binding protein 2 (IGFBP-2)
Growth hormone–binding protein
Acid-labile subunit
12- or 24-hour growth hormone sampling

Tests for determining growth hormone excess
Insulin-like growth factor 1 (IGF-1)
Oral glucose tolerance test
TRH stimulation test

TESTS FOR DETERMINING GROWTH HORMONE SUFFICIENCY

Growth Hormone Assays

Purpose These tests are used to detect and quantify GH in serum.

Protocol Currently, the most sensitive assays use a two-site IRMA with recombinant GH or pituitary-derived GH as the standard.

Interpretation Due to the pulsatility of GH secretion, random GH values are not helpful. This assay is used in the setting of frequent sampling to measure spontaneous or stimulated GH release.

Growth Hormone Provocative Testing

Purpose Due to the pulsatility of pituitary GH secretion, it is rarely useful to analyze random levels of GH (88). Therefore, GH secretory reserve, as a surrogate marker for GH deficiency, typically is assessed by peak response to provocative stimuli. At least 34 provocative tests in 189 different combinations have been used to assess pituitary secretion of GH (89). A brief description of commonly used protocols is provided below.

Protocols Due to the suppressive impact of food intake on GH secretion, each of these provocative tests is best performed in the fasting state. They may be performed sequentially or on separate days. Intravenous access is necessary for medication administration and/or to facilitate frequent blood sampling in these tests.

- *Arginine.* Arginine is infused over 30 minutes (0.5 g/kg up to 30 g). Serum GH levels are measured at 20-minute intervals for 2 hours (90).

  Proposed mechanism: By reduction of the tonic levels of somatostatin, a GH-release inhibitor, arginine potentiates the GH-releasing action of GH-releasing hormone (GHRH) (89). Arginine also may facilitate GH release by causing the release of insulin and glucagon from the pancreas.

  Adverse reactions: Nausea, anaphylaxis, metallic taste.

  Comments: Arginine is available from Pfizer, Inc. through its R-Gene 10 Complimentary Program (1-866-485-1359). This test may follow a clonidine stimulation test. Ornithine has been substituted for arginine in France.

- *Clonidine.* An oral dose of clonidine (5 μg/kg up to 200 μg) is followed by measurements of serum GH at 30-minute intervals for 2 hours (91).

Proposed mechanism: Clonidine, an α-adrenergic agonist; stimulates hypothalamic GHRH secretion.

Adverse reactions: Hypotension, somnolence.

- **GHRH.** Give GHRH (1 μg/kg) intravenously. Collect samples for GH determination at 0, 15, 30, 60, 90, and 120 minutes (92).

  Proposed mechanism: GHRH directly stimulates pituitary release of GH.

  Adverse reactions: Flushing, injection-site pain, tightness in chest, pallor, headache.

  Comment: GHRH alone has low sensitivity. The sensitivity and reproducibility of GHRH testing is improved by combining it with arginine or pyridostigmine. In a patient who fails a GHRH test, a normal response to GHRH testing after priming with daily injections of GHRH is suggestive of a hypothalamic lesion. Absence of improvement suggests a primary pituitary defect (89).

- *GHRH–Arginine.* Give GHRH (1 μg/kg) intravenously, followed by an infusion of arginine (0.5 g/kg up to 30 g) over 30 minutes. Collect samples for GH determination at 0, 15, 30, 60, 90, and 120 minutes (92).

  Proposed mechanism: GHRH directly stimulates pituitary release of GH. Arginine-induced release of insulin and glucagon from the pancreas potentiates GHRH-stimulated GH secretion and is felt to improve reproducibility.

  Adverse reactions: Flushing, injection-site pain, nausea, anaphylaxis, tightness in chest, pallor, headache, metallic taste.

- *Glucagon.* Give glucagon (15 μg/kg up to 1 mg) by rapid infusion intravenously (93,94). Collect samples for GH determination at 0, 2, 5, 10, 20, 30, 40, 50, and 60 minutes.

  Proposedm Mechanism: Glucagon has been proposed to directly stimulate GH secretion. In addition, glucagon is felt to stimulate GH secretion by rebound hypoglycemia following glucagon-induced hyperglycemia.

  Adverse reactions: Nausea, vomiting, abdominal pain (less in infants).

  Comment: GH response is enhanced when glucagon is coupled with a β-blocker such as propranolol (89,95,96). Peak response typically is seen before 20 minutes (93).

- *Insulin-induced hypoglycemia.* Plasma or blood glucose and GH concentrations are measured at baseline and at 15-minute intervals for 2 hours following rapid infusion of insulin. The dose of regular insulin to achieve hypoglycemia (<45 mg/dL, or 2.48 mmol/L) is 0.075–0.1 U/kg given by rapid intravenous infusion. If baseline blood glucose is less than 70 mg/dL (3.85 mmol/L) or

there is a high suspicion of panhypopituitarism, 0.050 U/kg of regular insulin should be used (97).

Proposed mechanism: Insulin-induced hypoglycemia reduces the tonic levels of somatostatin, a GH-release inhibitor, and may stimulate α-adrenergic receptors to promote hypothalamic GHRH secretion (89).

Adverse reactions: Hypoglycemia can result in seizures. There has been significant morbidity as well as several deaths associated with use of this test in children.

Comments: This test should be used with due caution and appropriate observation. Intravenous dextrose should be readily available for emergency administration.

- *L-Dopa.* L-Dopa may be administered orally either alone or in combination with a decarboxylase inhibitor. L-Dopa may be given alone at a dose of 10 mg/kg (minimum 200 mg and maximum 500 mg) (98,99). Blood is collected at 30-minute intervals for 2 hours. There is a commercially available combination of L-Dopa (250 mg) and the decarboxylase inhibitor, carbidopa (25 mg). The decarboxylase inhibitor reduces metabolism of L-dopa to dopamine and improves its efficacy at each dosage level (125, 250 or 500 mg L-dopa) (100).

  Proposed mechanism: L-Dopa increases GH secretion through dopaminergic and α-adrenergic pathways.

  Adverse reactions: Nausea, vomiting, vertigo.

  Comments: There is a high rate of false-negative results with L-dopa. L-Dopa may be combined with arginine. L-Dopa is difficult to obtain for testing.

Interpretation GH deficiency has been defined as a peak response of GH to provocative stimuli below an arbitrary cutoff value. The current cutoff value accepted by most pediatric endocrinologists and third-party payers is less than 10 ng/mL (10 μg/L). Using the potent stimulus GHRH–arginine, GH deficiency has been described as a peak response of less than 20 ng/mL (101). Adolescents may have higher GHRH–arginine–induced peaks of GH stimulation than adults. A cutoff of 24 ng/mL (24 μg/L) was shown to have 86% sensitivity in adolescents with GH deficiency (102).

Comments Provocative GH testing was developed as a diagnostic tool to justify patient selection during an era of short supply of GH obtained from cadaveric pituitary extracts. The GH Research Society (GRS) has supported GH stimulation testing as the "gold standard" for the diagnosis of GH deficiency (103). This has been referenced in other consensus guidelines from the American Association of Clinical Endocrinologists (AACE) and Lawson Wilkins Pediatric

Endocrinology Society (LWPES) (104,105). However, in an era of sufficient GH supply, GH stimulation testing has been a controversial topic due to safety, lack of reproducibility, and a lack of correlation with the growth response to GH therapy. A lack of specificity has been shown by studies that report that a number of children with normal growth patterns had abnormally low responses to provocative stimuli (false-negative rate 10% to 20%) (89). Repeat stimulation testing of children with the same stimulus and separate stimuli on subsequent occasions has been shown to produce disparate results (106,107). The appropriate cutoff to determine GH deficiency in an individual patient also has been a controversial topic. This value has increased with the availability of GH from 5 to 7 to 10 ng/mL (μg/L) in most centers. However, these cutoff values have not been adjusted for improvements in the assay methods or for changes in the accepted standards (108). GH stimulation testing is expensive and can be dangerous. Despite these negative aspects of GH stimulation testing, it remains the "gold standard" supported by the GRS and is expected by many insurance agencies prior to approval of GH therapy for the diagnosis of GH deficiency. In addition, there still may be a role for use of GH stimulation testing in predicting the development of metabolic complications of GH deficiency in children and adults. GHRH–arginine and insulin-induced hypoglycemia have been reported to be the best methods of GH stimulation testing (101). The combination of anthropometric measurements, radiographic bone age, and assays of serum concentrations of IGF-1 and IGFBP-3 have been proposed as an alternate diagnostic strategy for diagnosis of GH insensitivity (109).

Insulin-Like Growth Factor 1 (IGF-1)

Purpose IGF-1 is produced in a GH-dependent fashion. The majority of IGF-1 is produced in the liver and circulates in the blood as a protein-bound complex. IGF-1 in the circulation is more stable than GH and reflects GH activity.

Protocol Serum or plasma is separated from cells and frozen. Multiple commercial assays are available that use two-site IRMA, ELISA, and ICMA methodology. The use of an extraction method prior to analysis is important due to the presence of high-affinity IGF-binding proteins in the serum.

Interpretation IGF-1 concentrations have been shown to be age- and sex-dependent and rise in a fashion that mimics the growth chart until skeletal maturation (110). The availability of an age- and Tanner stage–appropriate reference population for normative data for each assay is crucial to interpretation of this test. Reporting values as standard deviation scores (SDS) for a particular reference population is particularly helpful. Normative data with standard deviations are published for one commercial assay by age (111) and Tanner stage (Diagnostic Systems Laboratories, Austin, TX) (112). SDS calculators for several commercial laboratories are available or in development. Despite concerns about the biological variability of IGF-1 measurements, this test has gained acceptance for use in the diagnosis of GH deficiency. When the IGF-1 concentration is above –1 SDS, a diagnosis of GH deficiency is very unlikely (113). When the IGF-1 concentration is below –2 SDS, GH deficiency is much more likely. The combination of low IGF-1 concentration and low IGFBP-3 concentration has been shown to be very specific for GH insensitivity, especially in children younger than 10 years of age (114). The IGF-1 concentration also has been used to guide GH therapy. Studies have shown that GH-treated children with IGF-1 concentrations in the upper normal range have a greater growth response than children with IGF-1 concentrations at the mean or below.

Comments The measurement of "true free" IGF-1 has been a difficult process (115). IGF-1 concentrations can be low in the setting of poor nutrition and chronic illness (89).

IGF Binding Protein-3 (IGFBP-3)

Purpose The majority of IGFBP-3 is produced in the liver in a GH-dependent fashion and circulates in the blood as a protein-bound complex. IGFBP-3 in the circulation is more stable than GH and reflects GH activity. In combination with IGF-1, this test provides a useful assessment of the activity of the GH axis.

Protocol Serum or plasma is separated from cells and frozen. Multiple commercial assays are available that use two-site IRMA, ELISA, and ICMA methodology.

Interpretation Like IGF-1, IGFBP-3 concentrations also increase with age, although less strikingly (116). Interpretation of the reported assay values is most accurate if age-, sex-, and Tanner stage–appropriate reference ranges are available. Reporting values with SDS is particularly helpful. IGFBP-3 measurement can be affected by proteolysis. Proteolytic fragments of IGFBP-3 may be detected differentially by independent assays due to the specificity of the antibodies employed (117). Detection of the IGFBP-3 fragments may be relevant depending on the ability of the fragment to bind IGF-1. IGFBP-3 concentrations below –2 SDS are consistent with a diagnosis of GH insensitivity (114). IGFBP-3 concentrations are monitored frequently during GH therapy. The molar ratio of IGF-1 to IGFBP-3 may provide some clinically useful estimate of "free," or bioactive, IGF-1.

IGF Generation Test

Purpose The IGF generation test is a classical endocrine provocative test that has been used for several decades to evaluate GH sensitivity (118). The validity of IGF generation tests for differentiating between different etiologies of short stature and predicting response to GH therapy has been debated. In addition, the reproducibility of this test has been questioned. Recent publications have provided normative data for the IGF generation test with comparisons with subjects with GH deficiency, idiopathic short stature (ISS), and GH insensitivity (splice mutation E180) (119–122). Generation of IGF-1 and IGFBP-3 showed excellent positive and negative predictive value for determining a diagnosis of GH insensitivity (120,121). In addition, the responses of subjects with ISS to GH were found to differ qualitatively from the other populations studied (122). This difference in generation of IGF-1 and IGFBP-3 in individuals with ISS following GH treatment is supportive of partial GH insensitivity as a cause of ISS.

Protocol Multiple protocols for generation of IGF-1 and IGFBP-3 have been described (120,123–125). In the protocol described by Buckway and colleagues (120), the subject receives daily injections of GH (low dose 0.025 mg/kg/day; high dose 0.050 mg/kg/day) in the evening for 4 or 7 days. IGF-1 and IGFBP-3 concentrations are obtained in the fasting state on the morning of days 1 (prior to the first dose), 5 (short protocol), and 8 (long protocol).

Interpretation Blum and colleagues established the response criteria for the IGF generation test (125). A normal response to GH treatment was indicated by an increment of at least 15 μg/L (1.96 nmol/L) IGF-1 or 0.4 mg/L (140 nmol/L) IGFBP-3 over baseline values. Using these criteria, Buckway and colleagues (120) showed that the IGF-1 response to the high-dose long protocol (0.05 mg/kg/day for 7 days) has the best sensitivity (91%) and specificity (97%) for identifying individuals with GH insensitivity. The shorter protocol also has good specificity but poorer sensitivity. The utility of the test improves when using a combination of the responses of IGF-1 and IGFBP-3 than when analyzing either factor separately with a combined sensitivity of 91% and specificity of 100%. Using an IGF-1 response at either 5 or 8 days of less than –2.5 SDS, the IGF generation test has been shown to differentiate between primary IGF deficiency (GH insensitivity) due to the GH receptor mutation E180 and secondary IGF deficiency (GH deficiency) with excellent sensitivity (95.7%) and specificity (95.7%) (119).

Comments The IGF generation test is an important tool for the evaluation of children with extreme short stature for GH insensitivity. In this population, the high-dose long protocol performs best. Although there is good evidence that the IGF generation test can differentiate between GH insensitivity due to the E180 splice mutation of the GH receptor and other etiologies of short stature, it is not clear if this can be extended to other forms of GH insensitivity. Differentiating the quantitative IGF generation response of normal children from children with GH deficiency or ISS has been problematic because it is difficult to apply a constant cutoff value to variable responses seen in partial GH deficiency. The ability of the IGF generation test to predict response to GH therapy has not been established and requires further study.

IGF Binding Protein-2 (IGFBP-2)

Purpose IGFBP-2 is a high-affinity IGF-binding protein present in circulation. The regulation of IGFBP-2 is unclear.

Protocol Serum or plasma is separated from cells and frozen. A two-site ELISA is available commercially.

Interpretation This assay has been used primarily in the research setting because of its utility in predicting the growth response to GH therapy. Although the levels of IGFBP-2 are not regulated directly by GH, they are inversely related to GH secretory response at baseline. However, baseline IGFBP-2 levels have a positive correlation with the first-year response to GH therapy (126).

Growth Hormone Binding Protein (GHBP)

Purpose GHBP represents the cleaved extracellular domain of the GH receptor (GHR). Evaluation of GHBP levels can provide information about the number of cell-surface GHRs. This information can be used as one component in the estimation of GH sensitivity. GHR mutations may affect the production of the GHR and GHBP. The most common GHR mutations result in undetectable levels of GHR and GHBP. However, forms of partial GH insensitivity have been shown to involve mutations of the GHR that lead normal or elevated levels of cell surface GHRs and serum GHBP due to impaired function of the GHR and truncations, leaving only the extracellular domain of the GHR (127–130).

Protocol Serum or plasma is separated from cells and frozen. A two-site ELISA is available commercially.

Interpretation Age-related normative data are available (Esoterix, Calabassas Hills, CA, www.esoterix.com). Very low or very high concentrations of GHBP are suggestive of a GHR mutation (129). GHBP concentrations also have been reported to be low in the setting of poor nutrition (131).

Acid-Labile Subunit (ALS)

Purpose ALS is produced in the liver in a GH-dependent fashion and circulates in the blood as a protein-bound complex. ALS forms a ternary complex with IGF-1 and IGFBP-3 to prolong their biological half-life in the serum (132,133).

Protocol Serum or plasma is separated from cells and frozen. A two-site ELISA is available commercially.

Interpretation Age-related normative data are available (134,135) (Esoterix, Calabassas Hills, CA, www.esoterix.com). Assays of ALS have not been found to be useful in the routine evaluation of abnormal growth. However, two patients with relative short stature have been described with ALS deficiency (136) (Ron Rosenfeld, personal communication).

12- or 24-Hour Growth Hormone Sampling

Purpose Due to the pulsatile nature of the pituitary release of GH, quantification of spontaneous GH secretion has been attempted by frequent sampling (88). Normative data for GH secretory profiles have been described for periods ranging from 3–24 hours.

Protocol These studies require hospitalization. The most common protocol has been a 12-hour overnight collection. Blood collection should begin at least 2–3 hours after the evening meal because of a suppressive effect of food on GH secretion. GH concentrations are obtained every 20–30 minutes. The resulting data are used to generate an estimate of 12- or 24-hour secretion.

Interpretation Algorithms have been designed to characterize these data (137,138). Day-to-day reproducibility of this test is poor but may be better than GH stimulation testing. When compared with GH stimulation testing, spontaneous GH secretion profiles have been described as having poorer sensitivity (139). However, the specificity is also questionable because as many as one in four normal children will have low GH values on overnight secretion testing (140). A 12-hour GH secretion test has been felt to be the most reliable assessment of neurosecretory dysfunction of GH secretion. Therefore, this test should be considered in patients who have had brain

tumors, especially of the suprasellar/hypothalamic region and/or cranial irradiation.

TESTS FOR DETERMINING GROWTH HORMONE EXCESS

Insulin-Like Growth Factor 1 (IGF-1)

Purpose The majority of IGF-1 is produced in the liver in a GH-dependent fashion and circulates in the blood as a protein-bound complex. IGF-1 in the circulation is more stable than GH and reflects GH activity. IGF-1 levels are elevated in acromegaly. Normalization of IGF-1 levels is a target of acromegaly therapy.

Protocol Serum or plasma is separated from cells and frozen. Multiple commercial assays are available that use two-site IRMA, ELISA, and ICMA methodology. The use of an extraction method prior to analysis is important due to the presence of high-affinity IGF-binding proteins in the serum.

Interpretation IGF-1 levels have been shown to be age- and sex-dependent and to risc in a fashion that mimics the growth chart until skeletal maturation (110). The availability of an age- and Tanner stage–appropriate reference population for normative data for each assay is crucial to interpretation of this test. Reporting values as SDS for a particular reference population is particularly helpful. IGF-1 serum concentrations greater than +2 SDS in the setting of unexpected rapid growth and prominent facial and extremity features are highly suggestive of excess GH production. The target of treatment of acromegaly is to return the IGF-1 level to the mean (141).

Oral Glucose Tolerance Test

Purpose To evaluate the ability of a glucose load to suppress GH secretion.

Protocol After overnight fast, patients receive an oral glucose challenge (1.75 grams/kg, up to 75 grams). GH is measured at 30-minute intervals for 2 hours.

Interpretation Normal subjects experience suppression of GH concentration (nadir) below 0.30 μg/L with current highly sensitive GH assays. Determination of 3-hour spontaneous GH secretion may yield similar findings (142).

TRH Stimulation Test

Purpose In normal individuals, thyrotropin-releasing hormone (TRH) has no effect on GH release. However, in acromegaly, TRH administration has the paradoxical effect of increasing GH secretion. This effect is likely

TABLE 49-8	Tests of Pubertal Disorders and Sexual Differentiation

Tests to evaluate gonadal function
Testosterone, total and free
Estradiol
Sex hormone–binding globulin (SHBG)
hCG stimulation test
Progesterone withdrawal
Tests to assess gonadotropin secretion
Luteinizing hormone (LH, lutropin)
Follicle-stimulating hormone (FSH)
GnRH stimulation test

due to inhibition of the elevated somatostatin tone in acromegalics (143).

Protocol TRH (200 µg) is infused intravenously over 5 minutes, and blood samples for GH assay are collected at time −15, 0 (baseline) and 20, 30, and 60 minutes after the infusion began (144).

Interpretation A positive test for GH excess would be determined if there is an increase in GH at least 50% above baseline or peak concentrations more than 6 µg/L above baseline.

Comments TRH is no longer available in the United States.

TESTS OF PUBERTAL DISORDERS AND SEXUAL DIFFERENTIATION

Tests of pubertal disorders and sexual differentiation include those designed to evaluate gonadal function and those that assess central gonadotropin secretion (Table 49-8).

TESTS TO EVALUATE GONADAL FUNCTION

Testosterone, Total

Purpose Useful in determining testicular function in males at baseline and in response to human chorionic gonadotropin (hCG), and gonadotropin-releasing hormone (GnRH) analogue stimulation and in assessing hyperandrogenic states in females. Testosterone concentrations are helpful in monitoring testosterone-replacement therapy for hypogonadism and gonadotropin agonist therapy for precocious puberty.

Protocol Organic extraction is performed on serum or plasma to denature protein to facilitate release of testosterone from sex hormone–binding globulin (SHBG). Chromatographic separation is undertaken to separate similar crossreactive species such as conjugated metabolites of testosterone. The separated samples are analyzed by TR/FIA, RIA, or MS/MS (145).

Interpretation In males, basal levels greater than 10 pg/mL (34.67 pmol/L) are consistent with puberty. A GnRH-stimulated testosterone level diagnostic of central precocious puberty has not been established. Age-, gender-, and Tanner stage–specific normative data are available.

Comments More sensitive assays are necessary when assessing testosterone production in peripubertal males and in females.

Testosterone, Free

Purpose Useful in assessing hyperandrogenic states in females (146).

Protocol Multiple methods of determining bioavailable or free testosterone have been developed. Bioavailable testosterone includes free testosterone and testosterone that is weakly bound to albumin. The primary means of separating free and protein-bound testosterone are dialysis and ammonium sulfate precipitation. Free testosterone is also estimated by several methods.

Dialysis: After collection of serum, the unbound testosterone is separated from protein-bound testosterone using a dialysis cell overnight at 37°C. Following dialysis, the samples may be subjected to immunoassay. Sensitivity may be enhanced by using larger volumes of serum, lower volumes of antibody, and longer incubation times (146). Alternatively, chromatography may be performed to improve immunoassay sensitivity following dialysis (147). HPLC/MS/MS is also a sensitive and specific method of detecting testosterone following dialysis.

Ammonium sulfate precipitation: After collection of serum, testosterone is removed by addition of charcoal. Tracer-labeled testosterone is added. SHBG-bound testosterone is precipitated by the addition of cold ammonium sulfate. The remaining bioavailable (unbound or weakly bound) tracer-labeled testosterone is quantified (148).

Estimation: The free androgen index (FAI) (149) is calculated as follows: FAI = total testosterone/SHBG × 100. Other estimations of free testosterone are also available.

Interpretation Values during puberty are unavailable. However, normative data for prepubertal children and adults are available for various assays. Low levels of free testosterone are suggestive of hypogonadism. Elevated levels of free testosterone are seen in polycystic ovary syndrome and other hyperandrogenic syndromes.

Comments The equilibrium dialysis method is considered the "gold standard." However,

values obtained with ammonium sulfate precipitation correlate well with those obtained by equilibrium dialysis (148).

Estradiol, Ultrasensitive

Purpose In prepubertal and peripubertal females, this sensitive assay is useful in determining the level of ovarian activity at baseline and in response to GnRH analogue stimulation. In males, this assay may be useful in assessing aromatase activity. Estrogen concentrations also may be monitored during gonadotropin agonist therapy for precocious puberty.

Protocol Serum is subjected to HPLC using a Sephadex LH-20 chromatography matrix to separate similar compounds. An immunoassay using antibodies specific for 17β-estradiol is used to quantify estradiol following chromatographic separation (150).

Interpretation In females, basal levels greater than 10 pg/mL (3.67 pmol/L) are consistent with puberty, and GnRH-stimulated levels greater than 40 pg/mL (14.68 pmol/L) are consistent with central puberty. In males, pubertal concentrations do not exceed those for adult males (<80 pg/mL, or 29.37 pmol/L).

Comments Pharmaceutical derivatives of estrogen may not be identified by this technique. Typical estradiol assays are not sufficiently sensitive to detect early pubertal levels accurately but may be useful for assessing menstrual irregularities. At this time, ultrasensitive cell bioassays developed to measure minute estrogen levels have been used for research purposes but have not been developed for commercial use (151).

Sex Hormone–Binding Globulin (SHBG)

Purpose SHBG is the major sex steroid–binding protein present in the serum. It binds testosterone, dihydrotestosterone, and 17β-estradiol with high affinity. SHBG levels affect the bioavailability of sex hormones in serum (152). It is measured when total sex hormone levels do not correlate with clinical characteristics.

Protocol Diluted serum or plasma are assayed using two-site IRMA or ICMA. Dilution is necessary to avoid aggregation. An international SHBG standard is available as a reference. Time-resolved FIAs are also available (153).

Interpretation Age- and sex-specific normative data are available for each assay. SHBG levels are elevated in hyperthyroidism, pregnancy, and in patients receiving synthetic estrogen therapy. Low SHBG levels have been associated with androgen excess, insulin, glucocorticoids, GH, obesity, the metabolic syndrome, and increased cardiovascular risk (154).

Comments In the presence of low SHBG, total sex hormone concentrations may be normal despite elevation of free (active) levels.

Human Chorionic Gonadotropin (hCG) Stimulation Test

Purpose To evaluate gonadal androgen synthesis in males with suspected Leydig cell agenesis, anorchia, undescended testes, errors of testosterone synthesis, or 5 α-reductase deficiency. hCG stimulates the gonads, but not the adrenal glands, to produce androgens (155). This can be used in the evaluation of micropenis, vanishing testis syndrome, ambiguous genitalia, and testicular dysfunction to confirm the presence of functional male gonads.

Protocol Multiple protocols exist ranging from a one-time dose of 5000 IU/m^2, to 200–1500 IU on three consecutive days, to 1500 IU every other day for 15 days (156,157).

1. Patients do not need to be fasting before or during test.

2. The night prior to the test, some protocols require the patient to take dexamethasone 1 mg orally in order to suppress androstenedione production from the adrenal glands to better elucidate androstenedione synthesis from the testes.

3. Prior to the first hCG injection, measure testosterone, dihydrotestosterone, androstenedione, LH, FSH, estradiol, and dihydroepiandrosterone (DHEA).

4. Begin hCG injection regimen:

   a. 5000 IU/m^2 hCG intramuscularly (155); repeat hormonal analysis 72 hours later.

   b. 1500 IU hCG intramuscularly on days 1, 3 and 5; repeat hormonal analysis on day 6 (Esoterix Manual).

   c. 1500 IU hCG intramuscularly every 2 days for 15 days; repeat hormonal analysis on day 16.

   The total dose should not exceed 15,000 IU, with about 10,000 IU divided over several days probably being optimal, in order to achieve sufficient stimulation without excess virilization or bone age advancement (158).

Interpretation There is an age-dependent increase of testosterone and dihydrotestosterone to hCG in males with normal testicular function. A two- to threefold rise in testosterone following hCG stimulation is considered to be normal (157). In infants up to 6 months of age, the basal levels of testosterone are elevated, leading to a smaller in-

crease in hCG-stimulated testosterone. Abnormally low responses can be seen in conditions of testicular agenesis or dysfunction. In normal individuals, final testosterone concentrations should reach adult concentrations of greater than 300 ng/dL (10,402 pmol/L) after prolonged hCG exposure (159). The testosterone:dihydrotestosterone ratio (T:DHT) is helpful in the diagnosis of 5 α-reductase deficiency. Because of the reduced ability to convert testosterone to dihydrotestosterone in these individuals, the post-hCG T:DHT should be elevated. The normal T:DHT in infants is 1.5–17 (160). However, a cutoff of 10 has been used in infants to reduce the number of false-negative results (157). The T:DHT ratio becomes more pronounced with age. Normative data for regimen b is available at www.esoterix.com (Table 49-9).

Comments hCG has few side effects with one-time or short-term use. Long-term hCG may cause increased bone age, but this is usually not an issue in doses of 15,000 IU or less. Cryptorchid testes may descend with this dose, and testes previously not palpated or well visualized by ultrasound may become more apparent by virtue of the increased size.

Progesterone Withdrawal

Purpose Administration of progesterone in the presence of endogenous estrogen allows accumulation and stabilization of the endometrium. The response to progesterone withdrawal is a measure of estrogen status and the competence of the outflow tract (161).

Protocol The most common regimen is medroxyprogesterone acetate (MPA) administered orally (10 mg/day for 5–10 days). Other progesterone preparations and single-dose intramuscular progestins are also effective (162,163).

Interpretation Any uterine bleeding occurring 2 to 7 days after administration of progesterone is considered a positive test (161).

Comments The short course of MPA induces uterine bleeding in 93% of amenorrheic women (164).

TESTS TO ASSESS CENTRAL GONADOTROPIN SECRETION

Luteinizing Hormone and Follicle-Stimulating Hormone ICMA

Purpose Useful to assess pubertal status, gonadal function, menstrual irregularity, and pituitary function.

Protocol LH and FSH concentrations are measured in serum by a third-generation immunoassay (ICMA or TR/FIA) (165,166). LH generally is measured by a highly sensitive assay. An ultrasensitive assay is also available for FSH but is used less commonly due to wider variability of FSH values during the peripubertal period.

Interpretation Normative data are available for different phases of the menstrual cycle. LH and FSH levels may be monitored during gonadotropin agonist therapy for precocious puberty to confirm pituitary suppression prior to the next dose. Elevated basal gonadotropin levels are consistent with gonadal failure, and an increased LH:FSH ratio may be seen in some patients with polycystic ovary syndrome.

Comments The highly sensitive LH assay may detect early stages of puberty, although most investigators feel that GnRH stimulation testing is necessary to truly detect onset of central puberty (167).

GnRH Stimulation Test

Purpose This study is done to determine if central puberty has begun and may be used to monitor efficacy of gonadotropin releasing hormone agonist therapy.

Protocol Previously, a 1-hour stimulation test with the GnRH agonist Factrel was used, but since it is no longer available, other agonists such as leuprolide are being used.

1. Measure serum estradiol (in girls) and serum testosterone (in boys) concentrations at baseline.

2. Administer leuprolide acetate 10–20 μg/kg subcutaneously.

3. Measure serum LH and FSH at 0, 1, 2, and 3 hours after leuprolide administration. Some investigators recommend additional

TABLE 49-9 Normative Values for β-hCG Stimulation Test of Infants (1 week to 6 months)[†]

	Baseline			Post-hCG		
	Testosterone (ng/dL)	DHT (ng/dL)	T/DHT	Testosterone (ng/dL)	DHT (ng/dL)	T/DHT
Mean	190	43	4.4	395	76	7.2
Range	4–530	<2–60	2–8	180–735	13–183	1.5–15.5

[†]www.esoterix.com

TABLE 49-10	Tests of Thyroid Status

Tests to measure thyroid hormone concentrations and TSH
  Thyroid-stimulating hormone (TSH)
  Total triiodothyronine (T₃)
  Free thyroxine (FT₄)
Tests for autoimmune thyroid disease
  Thyroid-stimulating immunoglobulin (TSI)
  Thyroid receptor antibody (TRAb)
  Antithyroglobulin (ATG)
  Thyroid peroxidase antibodies (TPO)
Tests to measure central TSH secretion
  TSH diurnal testing
  TRH stimulation test

6-, 12-, and 18- to 24-hour LH and FSH timepoints (168).

4. Measure serum estradiol (in girls) and serum testosterone (in boys) concentrations 24 hours after administration of leuprolide.

Interpretation Normal ranges depend on laboratory methodology. In response to leuprolide, peak LH levels are seen at 1–3 hours, peak FSH levels occur at 3–6 hours, and peak E₂ or testosterone levels occur at 24 hours. Prior to the onset of puberty, there is no increase in FSH or LH in response to a single dose of GnRH. Once puberty is well established an LH:FSH ratio greater than 1 is expected, but early in puberty (whether normal or precocious), FSH may predominate (168).

Comments The leuprolide stimulation test has been used more widely to diagnose precocious puberty in girls than in boys. Cutoffs for normal versus pubertal ranges may vary by institution and practice. Overall an LH level of more than 8 IU/L and stimulated estradiol level of 50 pg/mL or greater signals puberty. Due to the amount of free leuprolide in depot preparations, suppressed LH and FSH levels measured at intervals after therapeutic injection may indicate adequate dosing.

TESTS OF THYROID STATUS

Tests of the hypothalamic–pituitary–thyroid axis include those designed to evaluate hypo- and hyperthyroidism, including measurement of thyroid hormones, thyroid-stimulating hormone (TSH), and thyroid autoantibodies (Table 49-10).

TESTS FOR MEASURING THYROID HORMONE LEVELS

Thyroid-Stimulating Hormone (TSH), Total Triiodothyronine (TT₃), Free Thyroxine (FT₄)

Purpose These studies establish hyperfunction and hypofunction of the thyroid gland.

Protocol All are measured in the serum. FT₄ represents the fraction of thyroid hormone that is not bound to protein and so is available to cause metabolic changes. The "gold standards" are equilibrium dialysis and ultrafiltration techniques, but these are complex to perform clinically (169). Laboratories most often use immunoassays in which a labeled analogue of T₄ competes with the patient's free hormone for binding with an antibody. TT₃ is measured in a similar fashion.

TSH is measured by a sandwich-type process in which an antibody that is typically directed against the α-subunit is used to anchor the TSH molecule, whereas other antibodies (typically antibodies against the β-subunit) are conjugated with an enzyme (in immunoenzymometric assay) or are radioiodinated (in immunoradiometric assay) (169).

Interpretation Age-specific laboratory normal values are available. This is particularly important in the newborn period, where physiologic elevation of TSH may be detected as an abnormality in the newborn screen if screening is performed too early.

Comments TSH can be affected by diurnal variation, with levels highest at night.

TESTS FOR AUTOIMMUNE THYROID DISEASE

Thyroid-Stimulating Immunoglobulin (TSI), Thyroid Receptor Antibody (TRAb), Antithyroglobulin Antibody (ATG), Thyroid Peroxidase Antibody (TPO)

Purpose Antibody measurement is performed to help diagnose autoimmune thyroiditis or Grave disease.

Protocol Antibodies are measured in the serum. Many techniques are available for measurement of the TPO and ATG autoantibodies, although agglutination using synthetic beads may be the most sensitive (169). Antibodies that bind the TSH receptor may stimulate receptor activation (TSI, also called *thyroid-stimulating antibodies* [TSAbs]) and block the binding of TSH to the receptor (thyroid stimulation–blocking antibodies [TBAs]). TRAbs can be measured by the radioreceptor thyrotropin-binding inhibition immunoglobulin (TBII) assay, in which the patient's immunoglobulin and labeled TSH compete for a common receptor binding site on the thyroid cell membrane (169). Although not as simple as the TBII assay, detection of TRAbs with TSH receptor stimulator activity (TSI or TSAb) can be accomplished through a bioassay that measures TSH receptor activation by quantifying the production of cAMP in cultured rat thyroid cells exposed to the patient's immunoglobulin G (IgG) in vitro (169).

Interpretation These antibodies should be negative in the serum of normal individuals. TRAbs, as measured by TSII assay, are positive in 95% of patients with Graves disease and decline with treatment (169). The TSII assay also can be positive in hypothyroid patients who have TSH receptor–blocking antibodies (TBA). While the bioassay is more specific for stimulation of the TSH receptor, this is seldom needed because the clinical circumstances generally direct interpretation of the laboratory results. Determination of the quality of TRAbs (TSI versus TBA) may hold promise in predicting remission following antithyroid drug treatment for Graves disease (170).

TPO antibodies are less specific; they are found in approximately 95% of patients with Hashimoto thyroiditis and approximately 75% of those with Graves disease (169). Thyroglobulin antibodies are the least specific of the three because they rarely appear without TPO, except in papillary thyroid carcinoma (169).

Comments Maternally transmitted TBAs can cause transient neonatal hypothyroidism. Levels of the antibody can be followed to determine when it is safe to discontinue thyroxine therapy. Placental transfer of maternal TSI or TBA can occur even in the absence of clinically apparent maternal thyroid disease. *Long-acting thyroid stimulator* (LATS) is the historical synonym for TSI and TSAbs.

TESTS OF CENTRAL TSH SECRETION

Previously, TRH stimulation testing was done to differentiate hypothalamic from pituitary hypothyroidism or to assess partial TSH deficiency. TRH is no longer available in the United States, so TSH diurnal testing has been devised as a screen for those who should have overnight sampling.

TSH Diurnal Testing

Purpose To detect partial TSH deficiency. Overnight sampling and diurnal variation have been used to test for this condition in patients with risk factors for TSH deficiency (such as brain tumor or radiation history) with free thyroxine levels in the lowest tertile of the normal range (171,172).

Protocol The TSH secretory profile requires hospitalization. TSH values are drawn hourly from 2–6 p.m. 1800 and 10 p.m. to 4 a.m. A more clinically practical test may be done by comparing a single TSH drawn between

3 and 5 p.m. (nadir) with a second TSH drawn between 9 p.m. and midnight (peak) (173) or 6 and 8 a.m. (peak) (S. Rose, personal communication).

Interpretation TSH deficiency is diagnosed by an absence of the evening rise in TSH. If the TSH peak (late evening or early morning) is not more than 50% higher than the TSH nadir (midafternoon), a diagnosis of TSH deficiency is supported (TSH peak < 1.5 mU/L × TSH nadir = partial TSH deficiency).

Comments This test is not as easy to interpret as the TRH test, but in one study, the result of TSH diurnal testing correlated well with previously available TRH stimulation test data (174). Due to the need for lifelong L-thyroxine supplementation in those with documented central TSH deficiency, obtaining a TSH secretory profile in the hospital should be considered in patients who have failed the diurnal screen.

TRH Stimulation Test

Purpose Dynamic hormone response test historically used to identify central hypothyroidism (171,175).

Protocol TRH (7 µg/kg up to a maximum dose of 200 µg) is infused intravenously over 5 minutes. Blood samples for TSH assay are drawn at time 0 (baseline) and 10, 15, 30, 45, 60, 90, 120, and 180 minutes after the infusion began (175).

Interpretation The interpretation of this test is based on the magnitude of the peak TSH response and its timing. In the setting of primary hypothyroidism, the TSH peak will be elevated compared with the normal range (8–25 mU/L) with normal peak timing (30 minutes). Individuals with central hypothyroidism have a delayed peak TSH response (usually >45 minutes) and a delayed return to baseline. In central hypothyroidism, the magnitude of the TSH response to TRH stimulation is often normal (171).

Comments This test has been found to have a high false-negative rate, with 30% to 90% of individuals with central hypothyroidism having normal TSH peak magnitude and timing (171). TRH is no longer available in the United States.

TESTS FOR DETERMINING WATER HOMEOSTASIS

Tests of water homeostasis are designed to differentiate between central diabetes insipidus, nephrogenic diabetes insipidus, and primary polydipsia (176–178). These tests analyze the ability of the posterior pituitary to produce

TABLE 49-11   Tests for Determining Water Homeostasis

Serum and urine osmolality

Urine specific gravity

Water-deprivation test

Vasopressin challenge

Serum vasopressin levels

vasopressin and the kidney to respond to vasopressin (Table 49-11).

TESTS FOR MEASURING WATER HOMEOSTASIS

Serum and Urine Osmolality

Purpose This test is used to determine the solute concentration of a fluid. The clinical application typically is to determine the concentrating ability of the kidney or the presence of an excessive serum solute load.

Protocol The refrigerated sample is subjected to micro-osmometry by determining the freezing-point depression. Freezing-point osmometers take advantage of the physiochemical properties of solutions. An increase in solute concentration reduces the freezing point of a solution.

Interpretation The normal range for serum osmolality is 275–295 mOsm/kg. This is usually tightly controlled, although the lower limit of serum osmolality may be lower in infants. Normal urine osmolality ranges from 100–1200 mOsm/kg depending on the state of hydration.

Comments Micro-osmometry is a technique that requires expensive instrumentation. However, due to the imprecision of specific gravity, this method should be used to evaluate water homeostasis.

Urine Specific Gravity

Purpose This test is used to estimate the solute concentration of a fluid. The clinical application typically is to determine the concentrating ability of the kidney.

Protocol Specific gravity is estimated by several methods: weight, refractometry, and test strips. The most common method is the use of test strips. For the weight method, urine samples of measured volume are compared with distilled water on a precision balance. Refractometry uses the prism of a clinical refractometer calibrated with distilled water. Test strips use a colorimetric determination of specific gravity.

Interpretation The specific gravity of distilled water is 1.000. Specific gravity values increase

as the urine becomes more concentrated. The normal range of urine specific gravity is 1.001–1.035.

Comments Urine specific gravity is too imprecise to be a useful diagnostic test for diabetes insipidus. Of the methods described, urine specific gravity measured by refractometry correlates best with osmometry.

Water-Deprivation Test

Purpose After obtaining a thorough clinical history and baseline evaluation of urine (i.e., osmolality and glucose) and serum (i.e., osmolality, glucose, sodium, potassium, and calcium), the water-deprivation test is a key component in the diagnostic evaluation of a child with polyuria and polydipsia (177,178).

Protocol A water-deprivation test should be performed under close medical supervision with careful attention to detail. Children should be allowed free access to water prior to the test. Beginning in the morning, the child is restricted from access to water. Vital signs are monitored carefully throughout the study. Eight hours of water deprivation typically is sufficient to obtain diagnostic results. At baseline, obtain an accurate weight, urine (i.e., osmolality and volume), and serum (i.e., antidiuretic hormone [ADH], osmolality, and electrolytes). Repeat weight, urine (i.e., osmolality and volume), and serum (i.e., osmolality and electrolytes) determinations should be obtained every 1–2 hours. Serum ADH also should be determined at baseline and at hours 4 and 8 or at termination of the test. The test should be terminated if weight loss exceeds 5% of starting weight, thirst becomes intolerable, vital signs are unstable, or urine osmolality exceeds 1000 mOsm/kg. The test may be prolonged until the urine osmolality becomes stable (<10% change between consecutive voids), as long as the child has not lost more than 5% of body weight, has normal vital signs, and appears well hydrated. Termination of the water-deprivation test often is followed immediately by the vasopressin challenge.

Interpretation If a child is able to concentrate the urine to an osmolality of more than 1000 mOsm/kg or stable concentration more than 600 mOsm/kg, there is no evidence of diabetes insipidus. Serum osmolality exceeding 300 mOsm/kg with urine osmolality less than 600 mOsm/kg is diagnostic of diabetes insipidus. The vasopressin challenge is necessary to determine if the diabetes insipidus is central or nephrogenic.

Comments Some centers recommend evaluation of urine sodium during the water-deprivation test.

Vasopressin Challenge

Purpose This test is used to determine the responsiveness of the kidney to vasopressin.

Protocol The vasopressin challenge frequently is performed immediately following a water-deprivation test. Desmopressin acetate (DDAVP, 0.025 µg/kg up to 1 µg subcutaneously or 0.25 µg/kg up to 10 µg intranasally) is administered. Urine volume and osmolality are monitored with each void. The duration of monitoring may be determined by the test results. The patient is allowed to consume a volume of liquid equal to the urine volume lost during the water-deprivation test.

Interpretation If a child is able to concentrate the urine to an osmolality of more than 750 mOsm/kg following DDAVP, central diabetes insipidus is diagnosed. If the urine osmolality in response to DDAVP is less than 300 mOsm/kg, nephrogenic diabetes insipidus is present. If the urine osmolality is between 300 and 750 mOsm/kg following DDAVP administration, the possibility of a partial form of central or nephrogenic diabetes insipidus or primary polydipsia (with disruption of the renal concentrating gradient) remains. The serum ADH levels may be helpful in differentiating between these conditions.

Comments In indeterminate cases, some centers recommend the measurement of vasopressin during infusion of hypertonic saline to assess central vasopressin production (179). Patient, parents, and medical staff should be aware of the acute effects of subcutaneous vasopressin. On administration, patients can have transient symptoms of pallor, headache, vertigo, sweating, nausea, and vomiting. These effects are seen less frequently with intranasal administration.

Serum Vasopressin Levels

Purpose To determine production of arginine vasopressin by the posterior pituitary.

Protocol EDTA–plasma is separated from cells as soon as possible following collection and frozen for shipping. Multiple commercial RIAs are available.

Interpretation Following water deprivation, ADH levels should be elevated in children who are normal or have nephrogenic diabetes insipidus or primary polydipsia. The actual ADH values vary depending on the assay used. For adults with normal osmolarity, the normal range is 0.7–3.8 pg/mL, or 0.64–3.51 pmol/L (www.esoterix.com).

Comments Sample volume may be a limiting factor. These assays require at least 1 mL per time point. In the past, availability of a reliable assay was limited. Current RIAs are reliable, but not approved by the Food and Drug Administration (FDA).

REFERENCES

1. Ekins RP. Ligand assays: From electrophoresis to miniaturized microarrays. *Clin Chem.* 1998;44:2015.
2. Report of the Expert Committee on the Diagnosis and Classification of Diabetes Mellitus. *Diabetes care.* 1997;20:1183.
3. Gill S, Hayes F, Sluss P. Issues in endocrine immunoassay. In: Hall J, Nieman LK, eds. *Contemporary Endocrinology: Handbook of Diagnostic Endocrinology.* Totowa, NJ: Humana Press; 2003:1–22.
4. Lowry PJ, Linton EA, Hodgkinson SC. Analysis of peptide hormones of the hypothalamic pituitary adrenal axis using "two-site" immunoradiometric assays. *Horm Res.* 1989;32:25.
5. Albertson BD. Hormonal assay methodology: Present and future prospects. *Clin Obstet Gynecol.* 1990;33:591.
6. Klee G. Laboratory techniques for recognition of endocrine disorders. In: Larsen P, ed. *Williams Textbook of Endocrinology.* Philadelphia: Saunders; 2003:65–80.
7. Barnard G. The development of fluorescence immunoassays. *Prog Clin Biol Res.* 1988;285:15.
8. Pazzagli M, et al. Immunoassays monitored by chemiluminescence. *Prog Clin Biol Res.* 1988;285:61.
9. Lacey JM, et al. Improved specificity of newborn screening for congenital adrenal hyperplasia by second-tier steroid profiling using tandem mass spectrometry. *Clin Chem.* 2004;50:621.
10. Minutti CZ, et al. Steroid profiling by tandem mass spectrometry improves the positive predictive value of newborn screening for congenital adrenal hyperplasia. *J Clin Endocrinol Metab.* 2004;89:3687.
11. Lacey JM, et al. Rapid determination of transferrin isoforms by immunoaffinity liquid chromatography and electrospray mass spectrometry. *Clin Chem.* 2001;47:513.
12. Boscaro M, Barzon L, Sonino N. The diagnosis of Cushing's syndrome: Atypical presentations and laboratory shortcomings. *Arch Intern Med.* 2000;160:3045.
13. Arnaldi G, et al. Diagnosis and complications of Cushing's syndrome: A consensus statement. *J Clin Endocrinol Metab.* 2003;88:5593.
14. Gunnar MR, Vazquez DM. Low cortisol and a flattening of expected daytime rhythm: Potential indices of risk in human development. *Dev Psychopathol.* 2001;13:515–538.
15. Hessl D, et al. Cortisol and behavior in fragile X syndrome. *Psychoneuroendocrinology.* 2002;27:855–872.
16. Kirschbaum C, et al. Cortisol and behavior: 1. Adaptation of a radioimmunoassay kit for reliable and inexpensive salivary cortisol determination. *Pharmacol Biochem Behav.* 1989;34:747–751.
17. Newell-Price J, et al. Optimal response criteria for the human CRH test in the differential diagnosis of ACTH-dependent Cushing's syndrome. *J Clin Endocrinol Metab.* 2002;87:1640.
18. Papanicolaou DA, et al. A single midnight serum cortisol measurement distinguishes Cushing's syndrome from pseudo-Cushing states. *J Clin Endocrinol Metab.* 1998;83:1163.
19. Martinelli CE Jr, et al. Salivary cortisol for screening of Cushing's syndrome in children. *Clin Endocrinol.* 1999;51:67.
20. Findling JW, Raff H, Aron DC. The low dose dexamethasone suppression test: A reevaluation in patients with Cushing's syndrome. *J Clin Endocrinol Metab.* 2004;89:1222.
21. Miller W. The adrenal cortex. In: Sperling M, ed. *Pediatric Endocrinology,* 2nd ed. Philadelphia: Saunders; 2002:385–438.
22. Nieman LK, et al. A simplified morning ovine corticotropin-releasing hormone stimulation test for the differential diagnosis of adrenocorticotropin-dependent Cushing's syndrome. *J Clin Endocrinol Metab.* 1993;77:1308–1312.
23. Invitti C, et al. Diagnosis and management of Cushing's syndrome: Results of an Italian multicentre study. Study Group of the Italian Society of Endocrinology on the Pathophysiology of the Hypothalamic-Pituitary-Adrenal Axis. *J Clin Endocrinol Metab.* 1999;84:440.
24. Dorin RI, Qualls CR, Crapo LM. Diagnosis of adrenal insufficiency. *Ann Intern Med.* 2003;139:194.
25. Nieman LK. Dynamic evaluation of adrenal hypofunction. *J Endocrinol Invest.* 2003;26:74.
26. Marik PE. Unraveling the mystery of adrenal failure in the critically ill. *Crit Care Med.* 2004;32:596.
27. Lindholm J, Kehlet H. Re-evaluation of the clinical value of the 30 min ACTH test in assessing the hypothalamic-pituitary-adrenocortical function. *Clin Endocrinol (Oxf).* 1987;26:53.
28. Tsatsoulis A, et al. Adrenocorticotropin (ACTH) deficiency undetected by standard dynamic tests of the hypothalamic-pituitary-adrenal axis. *Clin Endocrinol (Oxf).* 1988;28:225.
29. Olgemoller B, et al. Screening for congenital adrenal hyperplasia: Adjustment of 17OPH cutoff values to both age and birth weight markedly improves the predictive value. *J Clin Endocrinol Metab.* 2003;88:5790.
30. Clayton PE, et al. Consensus statement on 21-hydroxylase deficiency from the European Society for Paediatric Endocrinology and the Lawson Wilkins Pediatric Endocrine Society. *Horm Res.* 2002;58:188–195.
31. Wong T, et al. Identification of the steroids in neonatal plasma that interfere with 17α-hydroxyprogesterone (17-OPH) radioimmunoassays. *Clin Chem.* 1992;38:1830.
32. Nordenstrom A, et al. Neonatal screening for congenital adrenal hyperplasia: 17OPH levels and CYP21 genotypes in preterm infants. *Pediatrics.* 2001;108:E68.
33. Balsamo A, et al. CYP21 genotype, adult height, and pubertal development in 55 patients treated for 21-hydroxylase deficiency. *J Clin Endocrinol Metab.* 2003;88:5680.

34. Endres D, Rude R. Mineral and bone metabolism. In: Burtis C, Ashwood E, eds. *Tietz Textbook of Clinical Chemistry*, 3rd ed. Philadelphia: Saunders; 1999:1395–1457.

35. Robertson WG, Marshall RW. Calcium measurements in serum and plasma: Total and ionized. *CRC Crit Rev Clin Lab Sci*. 1979;11:271.

36. Leder B, Finkelstein J. Hyper- and hypocalcemia. In: Hall J, Nieman L, eds. *Handbook of Diagnostic Endocrinology*. Totowa, NJ: Humana Press; 2003:239–256.

37. Endres DB, et al. Immunochemiluminometric and immunoradiometric determinations of intact and total immunoreactive parathyrin: Performance in the differential diagnosis of hypercalcemia and hypoparathyroidism. *Clin Chem*. 1991;37:162.

38. Endres DB, et al. Measurement of parathyroid hormone. *Endocrinol Metab Clin North Am*. 1989;18:611.

39. Souberbielle JC, et al. Assay-specific decision limits for two new automated parathyroid hormone and 25-hydroxyvitamin D assays. *Clin Chem*. 2005;51:395.

40. Marx SJ. Hyperparathyroid and hypoparathyroid disorders. *N Engl J Med*. 2000;343:1863.

41. Sokoll LJ. Measurement of parathyroid hormone and application of parathyroid hormone in intraoperative monitoring. *Clin Lab Med*. 2004;24:199.

42. Blumsohn A, Al Hadari A. Parathyroid hormone: What are we measuring and does it matter? *Ann Clin Biochem*. 2002;39:169.

43. Strewler GJ. The parathyroid hormone-related protein. *Endocrinol Metab Clin North Am*. 2000;29:629.

44. Burtis WJ, et al. Immunochemical characterization of circulating parathyroid hormone-related protein in patients with humoral hypercalcemia of cancer. *N Engl J Med*. 1990;322:1106.

45. Clive DR, et al. Analytical and clinical validation of a radioimmunoassay for the measurement of 1,25-dihydroxy vitamin D. *Clin Biochem*. 2002;35:517.

46. Hollis BW, et al. Determination of vitamin D status by radioimmunoassay with an ^{125}I-labeled tracer. *Clin Chem*. 1993;39:529.

47. Hollis BW. Comparison of commercially available ^{125}I-based RIA methods for the determination of circulating 25-hydroxyvitamin D. *Clin Chem*. 2000;46:1657.

48. Vogeser M, et al. Candidate reference method for the quantification of circulating 25-hydroxyvitamin D$_3$ by liquid chromatography-tandem mass spectrometry. *Clin Chem*. 2004;50:1415.

49. Looker AC, et al. Serum 25-hydroxyvitamin D status of adolescents and adults in two seasonal subpopulations from NHANES III. *Bone*. 2002;30:771.

50. MacFarlane GD, et al. Evaluation of 25-OH vitamin D in chronic renal failure and end stage renal disease subjects. *J Steroid Biochem Mol Biol*. 2004;89–90:619.

51. Glendenning P, et al. Issues of methodology, standardization and metabolite recognition for 25-hydroxyvitamin D when comparing the DiaSorin radioimmunoassay and the Nichols Advantage automated chemiluminescence protein-binding assay in hip fracture cases. *Ann Clin Biochem*. 2003; 40:546.

52. de Ridder CM, Delemarre-van de Waal HA. Clinical utility of markers of bone turnover in children and adolescents. *Curr Opin Pediatr*. 1998;10:441.

53. Calvo MS, Eyre DR, Gundberg CM. Molecular basis and clinical application of biological markers of bone turnover. *Endocr Rev*. 1996;17:333.

54. Cioffi M, et al. Serum osteocalcin in 1634 healthy children. *Clin Chem*. 1997;43:543.

55. Slemenda CW, et al. Reduced rates of skeletal remodeling are associated with increased bone mineral density during the development of peak skeletal mass. *J Bone Miner Res*. 1997;12:676–682.

56. Friedman AL, et al. Serum osteocalcin concentrations in children with chronic renal insufficiency who are not undergoing dialysis. Growth Failure in Children with Renal Diseases Study. *J Pediatr*. 1990; 116:S55.

57. Tobiume H, et al. Serum bone alkaline phosphatase isoenzyme levels in normal children and children with growth hormone (GH) deficiency: A potential marker for bone formation and response to GH therapy. *J Clin Endocrinol Metab*. 1997;82:2056.

58. Bollen AM, Eyre DR. Bone resorption rates in children monitored by the urinary assay of collagen type I cross-linked peptides. *Bone*. 1994;15:31.

59. Hanson DA, et al. A specific immunoassay for monitoring human bone resorption: Quantitation of type I collagen cross-linked N-telopeptides in urine. *J Bone Miner Res*. 1992;7:1251.

60. Mora S, et al. Bone turnover in neonates: Changes of urinary excretion rate of collagen type I cross-linked peptides during the first days of life and influence of gestational age. *Bone*. 1997;20:563.

61. Zinman B, et al. Phenotypic characteristics of GAD antibody-positive recently diagnosed pateints with type 2 diabetes in North American and Europe. *Diabetes*. 2004;53:3193–3200.

62. Mooy JM, et al. Intra-individual variation of glucose, specific insulin and proinsulin concentrations measured by two oral glucose tolerance tests in a general Caucasian population: The Hoorn study. *Diabetologia*. 1996;39:298–305.

63. Expert Committee on the Diagnosis and Classification of Diabetes Mellitus. Report of the Expert Committee on the Diagnosis and Classification of Diabetes Mellitus. *Diabetes Care*. 1997;20:1183–1197.

64. Gomez-Diaz R, et al. Lack of agreement between the revised criteria of impaired fasting glucose and imparied glucose tolerance in children with excess body weight. *Diabetes Care*. 2004;27:2229–2233.

65. Blake DR, et al. Impaired glucose toleracne, but not impaired fasting glucose, is associated with increased levels of coronary heart disease risk factors. *Diabetes*. 2004;53: 2095–2100.

66. Vague P, Moulin J-P. The defective glucose sensitivity of the B cell in non-insulin-dependent diabetes: Improvement after twenty hours of normoglycaemia. *Metabolism*. 1982;31:139–142.

67. Matthews DR, et al. Homeostasis model assessment: insulin resistance and B-cell function from fasting plasma glucose and insulin concentrations in man. *Diabetologia*. 1985;28:412–419.

68. Phillips DI, et al. Understanding oral glucose tolerance: comparisons of glucose or insulin measurement during the oral glucose tolerance test with specific measurements of insulin resistance and insulin secretion. *Diabetes Med*. 1994;11:286–292.

69. Gungor N, et al. Validation of surrogate estimates of insulin sensitivity and insulin secretion in children and adolescents. *J Pediatr*. 2004;144.

70. Tripathy D, et al. Contribution of insulin-stimulated glucose uptake and basal hepatic insulin sensitivity to surrogate measures of insulin sensitivity. *Diabetes Care*. 2004;27:2204–2210.

71. DeFronzo RA, Tobin JD, Andres R. Glucose clamp technique: A method for quantifying insulin secretion and resistance. *Am J Physiol*. 1979;237:E214–223.

72. Finegood DT, Bergman RN, Vranic M. Estimation of endogenous glucose production during hyperinsulinemic-euglycemic glucose clamps. *Diabetes*. 1987;36:914–924.

73. Bergman RN, Phillips LS, Cobelli C. Physiologic evaluation of factors controlling glucose disposition in man: Measurement of insulin sensitivity and beta-cell sensitivity from the response to intravenous glucose. *J Clin Invest*. 1981;68:1456–1467.

74. Bergman RN, et al. Equivalence of the insulin sensitivity index in man derived by the minimal model and the euglycemic glucose clamp. *J Clin Invest*. 1987;79:790–800.

75. Finegood DT, Hramiak IM, Dupre J. A modified protocol for estimation of insulin sensitivity with the minimal-model of glucose kinetics in patients with insulin-dependent diabetes. *J Clin Endocrinol Metab*. 1990;70:1538–1549.

76. Cutfield WS, et al. The modified minimal model: Application to measurement of insulin sensitivity in children. *J Clin Endocrinol Metab*. 1990;70:1644–1650.

77. Gower BA, et al. Contribution of insulin secretion and clearance to glucose induced insulin concentration in African-American and Caucasian children. *J Clin Endocrinol Metab*. 2002;87:2218–2224.

78. Sunehag AI, et al. Glucose production, gluconeogenesis and insulin sensitivity in children and adolescents: An evaluation of their reproducibility. *Pediatr Res*. 2001;50:115–123.

79. Sinaiko AR, et al. Insulin resistance syndrome in childhood: Associations of the euglycemic insulin clamp and fasting insulin with fatness and other risk factors. *J Pediatr*. 2001;139:700–707.

80. Moran A, et al. Insulin resistance during puberty: Results from clamp studies in 357 children. *Diabetes*. 1999;48:2039–2044.

81. Katz A, et al. Quantitative insulin sensitivity check index: A simple, accurate method for assessing insulin sensitivity in humans. *J Clin Endocrinol Metab*. 2000;85:2402–2410.

82. Matsuda M, DeFronzo RA. Insulin sensitivity indices obtained from oral glucose tolerance testing. *Diabetes Care*. 1999;22: 1462–1470.

83. Weigensberg MJ, Cruz ML, Goran MI. Association between insulin sensitivity and post-glucose challenge plasma insulin values in overweight Latino youth. *Diabetes Care.* 2003;26:2094–2099.

84. Dekelbab BH, Sperling MA. Hyperinsulinemic hypoglycemia of infancy: The challenge continues. *Diabetes Metab Res Rev.* 2004;20:189.

85. Aynsley-Green A, et al. Practical management of hyperinsulinism in infancy. *Arch Dis Child.* 2000;82:F98.

86. Saudubray JM, et al. Genetic hypoglycaemia in infancy and childhood: Pathophysiology and diagnosis. *J Inherited Metab Dis.* 2000;23:197.

87. Levitt Katz LE, et al. Insulin-like growth factor binding protein-1 levels in the diagnosis of hypoglycemia caused by hyperinsulinism. *J Pediatr.* 1997;131:193–199.

88. Albertsson-Wikland K, Rosberg S. Analyses of 24-hour growth hormone profiles in children: Relation to growth. *J Clin Endocrinol Metab.* 1988;67:493.

89. Sizonenko PC, et al. Diagnosis and management of growth hormone deficiency in childhood and adolescence: 1. Diagnosis of growth hormone deficiency. *Growth Horm IGF Res.* 2001;11:137.

90. Parker ML, Hammond JM, Daughaday WH. The arginine provocative test: an aid in the diagnosis of hyposomatotropism. *J Clin Endocrinol Metab.* 1967;27:1129.

91. Gil-Ad I, Topper E, Laron Z. Oral clonidine as a growth hormone stimulation test. *Lancet.* 1979;2:278.

92. Gelato MC, et al. Growth hormone (GH) responses to GH-releasing hormone during pubertal development in normal boys and girls: Comparison to idiopathic short stature and GH deficiency. *J Clin Endocrinol Metab.* 1986;63:174.

93. Weber B, Helge H, Quabbe HJ. Glucagon-induced growth hormone release in children. *Acta Endocrinol (Copenh).* 1970;65:323–341.

94. Stimmler L, Snodgrass G. The plasma growth hormone response to i.v. Glucagon administration. *Clin Sci.* 1971;40:28P–29P.

95. Parks JS, et al. Growth hormone responses to propranolol-glucagon stimulation: A comparison with other tests of growth hormone reserve. *J Clin Endocrinol Metab.* 1973;37:85–92.

96. AvRuskin TW, Tang SC, Juan CS. The glucagon infusion test and growth hormone secretion. *J Pediatr.* 1975;86:102–106.

97. Kaplan SL, et al. Growth and growth hormone: I. Changes in serum level of growth hormone following hypoglycemia in 134 children with growth retardation. *Pediatr Res.* 1968;2:43.

98. Hayek A, Crawford JD. L-Dopa and pituitary hormone secretion. *J Clin Endocrinol Metab.* 1972;34:764–766.

99. Laron Z, Josefsberg Z, Doron M. Effect of L-dopa on the secretion of plasma growth hormone in children and adolescents. *Clin Endocrinol (Oxf).* 1973;2:1–7.

100. Fevang FO, et al. The effect of L-dopa with and without decarboxylase inhibitor on growth hormone secretion in children with short stature. *Acta Paediatr Scand.* 1977;66:81–84.

101. Ghigo E, et al. Reliability of provocative tests to assess growth hormone secretory status: Study in 472 normally growing children. *J Clin Endocrinol Metab.* 1996;81:3323.

102. Maghnie M, et al. GHRH plus arginine in the diagnosis of acquired GH deficiency of childhood onset. *J Clin Endocrinol Metab.* 2002;87:2740–2744.

103. Growth Hormone Research Society. Consensus guidelines for the diagnosis and treatment of growth hormone (GH) deficiency in childhood and adolescence: Summary statement of the GH Research Society. GH Research Society. *J Clin Endocrinol Metab.* 2000;85:3990.

104. Gharib H, et al. American Association of Clinical Endocrinologists medical guidelines for clinical practice for growth hormone use in adults and children—2003 update. *Endocr Pract.* 2003;9:64–76.

105. Wilson TA, et al. Update of guidelines for the use of growth hormone in children: The Lawson Wilkins Pediatric Endocrinology Society Drug and Therapeutics Committee. *J Pediatr.* 2003;143:415–421.

106. Eddy RL, et al. Human growth hormone release: Comparison of provocative test procedures. *Am J Med.* 1974;56:179.

107. Siegel SF, et al. Comparison of physiologic and pharmacologic assessment of growth hormone secretion. *Am J Dis Child.* 1984;138:540.

108. Reiter EO, et al. Variable estimates of serum growth hormone concentrations by different radioassay systems. *J Clin Endocrinol Metab.* 1988;66:68.

109. Gandrud LM, Wilson DM. Is growth hormone stimulation testing in children still appropriate? *Growth Horm IGF Res.* 2004;14:185.

110. Juul A, et al. Serum insulin-like growth factor I in 1030 healthy children, adolescents, and adults: Relation to age, sex, stage of puberty, testicular size, and body mass index. *J Clin Endocrinol Metab.* 1994;78:744.

111. Brabant G, et al. Serum insulin-like growth factor I reference values for an automated chemiluminescence immunoassay system: Results from a multicenter study. *Horm Res.* 2003;60:53.

112. Moran A, et al. Association between the insulin resistance of puberty and the insulin-like growth factor-I/growth hormone axis. *J Clin Endocrinol Metab.* 2002;87:4817.

113. Ranke MB, et al. Significance of basal IGF-I, IGFBP-3, and IGFBP-2 measurements in the diagnostics of short stature in children. *Horm Res.* 2000;54:60.

114. Juul A, Skakkebaek NE. Prediction of the outcome of growth hormone provocative testing in short children by measurement of serum levels of insulin-like growth factor I and insulin-like growth factor binding protein 3. *J Pediatr.* 1997;130:197.

115. Juul A, et al. Free insulin-like growth factor I serum levels in 1430 healthy children and adults, and its diagnostic value in patients suspected of growth hormone deficiency. *J Clin Endocrinol Metab.* 1997;82:2497.

116. Juul A, et al. Serum levels of insulin-like growth factor (IGF)-binding protein-3 (IGFBP-3) in healthy infants, children, and adolescents: The relation to IGF-I, IGF-II, IGFBP-1, IGFBP-2, age, sex, body mass index, and pubertal maturation. *J Clin Endocrinol Metab.* 1995;80:2534.

117. Diamandi A, et al. Immunoassay of insulin-like growth factor-binding protein-3 (IGFBP-3): New means to quantifying IGFBP-3 proteolysis. *J Clin Endocrinol Metab* 2000;85:2327.

118. Rosenfeld RG, et al. Insulin-like growth factor (IGF) parameters and tools for efficacy: The IGF-I generation test in children. *Horm Res.* 2004;62:37.

119. Rosenfeld R, et al. The IGF-1 SDS generation test: A diagnostic test to identify rhGH-responsive patients. ICE Meeting, April 2004 Lisbon, Portugal.

120. Buckway CK, et al. The IGF-I generation test revisited: A marker of GH sensitivity. *J Clin Endocrinol Metab.* 2001;86:5176.

121. Buckway CK, et al. Insulin-like growth factor binding protein-3 generation as a measure of GH sensitivity. *J Clin Endocrinol Metab.* 2002;87:4754.

122. Selva KA, et al. Reproducibility in patterns of IGF generation with special reference to idiopathic short stature. *Horm Res.* 2003;60:237.

123. Rosenfeld RG, Rosenbloom AL, Guevara-Aguirre J. Growth hormone (GH) insensitivity due to primary GH receptor deficiency. *Endocr Rev.* 1994;15:369.

124. Rudman D, et al. Children with normal-variant short stature: treatment with human growth hormone for six months. *N Engl J Med.* 1981;305:123.

125. Blum WF, et al. Improvement of diagnostic criteria in growth hormone insensitivity syndrome: Solutions and pitfalls. Pharmacia Study Group on Insulin-like Growth Factor I Treatment in Growth Hormone Insensitivity Syndromes. *Acta Paediatr.* 1994;399:117.

126. Ranke MB, et al. Relevance of IGF-I, IGFBP-3, and IGFBP-2 measurements during GH treatment of GH-deficient and non-GH-deficient children and adolescents. *Horm Res.* 2001;55:115.

127. Iida K, et al. Functional characterization of truncated growth hormone (GH) receptor (1–277) causing partial GH insensitivity syndrome with high GH-binding protein. *J Clin Endocrinol Metab.* 1999;84:1011–1016.

128. Milward A, et al. Growth hormone (GH) insensitivity syndrome due to a GH receptor truncated after Box1, resulting in isolated failure of STAT 5 signal transduction. *J Clin Endocrinol Metab.* 2004;89:1259.

129. Woods KA, et al. A homozygous splice site mutation affecting the intracellular domain of the growth hormone (GH) receptor resulting in Laron syndrome with elevated GH-binding protein. *J Clin Endocrinol Metab.* 1996;81:1686–1690.

130. Rosenfeld RG, Buckway CK. Growth hormone insensitivity syndromes: Lessons learned and opportunities missed. *Horm Res.* 2001;55:36.

131. Postel-Vinay MC, Saab C, Gourmelen M. Nutritional status and growth hormone-binding protein. *Horm Res.* 1995;44:177.

132. Guler HP, et al. Insulin-like growth factors I and II in healthy man: Estimations of half-lives and production rates. *Acta Endocrinol.* 1989;121:753.

133. Baxter RC. Circulating levels and molecular distribution of the acid-labile subunit of the high molecular weight insulin-like growth factor-binding protein complex. *J Clin Endocrinol Metab.* 1990;70:1347.

134. Juul A, et al. The acid-labile subunit of human ternary insulin-like growth factor binding protein complex in serum: Hepatosplanchnic release, diurnal variation, circulating concentrations in healthy subjects, and diagnostic use in patients with growth hormone deficiency. *J Clin Endocrinol Metab.* 1998;83:4408.

135. Nimura A, et al. Acid-labile subunit (ALS) measurements in children. *Endocr J.* 2000;47:S111.

136. Domene HM, et al. Deficiency of the circulating insulin-like growth factor system associated with inactivation of the acid-labile subunit gene. *N Engl J Med.* 2004;350:570.

137. Merriam GR, Wachter KW. Algorithms for the study of episodic hormone secretion. *Am J Physiol.* 1982;243:E310.

138. Martha PM Jr, et al. Endogenous growth hormone secretion and clearance rates in normal boys, as determined by deconvolution analysis: Relationship to age, pubertal status, and body mass. *J Clin Endocrinol Metab.* 1992;74:336.

139. Rose SR, et al. The advantage of measuring stimulated as compared with spontaneous growth hormone levels in the diagnosis of growth hormone deficiency. *N Engl J Med.* 1988;319:201.

140. Lanes R. Diagnostic limitations of spontaneous growth hormone measurements in normally growing prepubertal children. *Am J Dis Child.* 1989;143:1284.

141. Biermasz NR, et al. Determinants of survival in treated acromegaly in a single center: Predictive value of serial insulin-like growth factor I measurements. *J Clin Endocrinol Metab.* 2004;89:2789.

142. Grottoli S, et al. Three-hour spontaneous GH secretion profile is as reliable as oral glucose tolerance test for the diagnosis of acromegaly. *J Endocrinol Invest.* 2003;26:123.

143. De Marinis L, et al. Preoperative growth hormone response to thyrotropin-releasing hormone and oral glucose tolerance test in acromegaly: A retrospective evaluation of 50 patients. *Metabolism.* 2002; 51:616–621.

144. Ronchi CL, et al. Long-term evaluation of postoperative acromegalic patients in remission with previous and newly proposed criteria. *J Clin Endocrinol Metab.* 2005;90: 1377–1382.

145. Fiet J, et al. Development of a highly sensitive and specific new testosterone time-resolved fluoroimmunoassay in human serum. *Steroids.* 2004;69:461.

146. Sinha-Hikim I, et al. The use of a sensitive equilibrium dialysis method for the measurement of free testosterone levels in healthy, cycling women and in human immunodeficiency virus-infected women. *J Clin Endocrinol Metab.* 1998;83:1312.

147. Torma A, et al. A method for measurement of free testosterone in premenopausal women involving equilibrium dialysis, chromatography, and radioimmunoassay. *Steroids.* 1995;60:285.

148. Morris PD, et al. A mathematical comparison of techniques to predict biologically available testosterone in a cohort of 1072 men. *Eur J Endocrinol.* 2004;151:241.

149. Wilke TJ, Utley DJ. Total testosterone, free-androgen index, calculated free testosterone, and free testosterone by analog RIA compared in hirsute women and in otherwise-normal women with altered binding of sex-hormone-binding globulin. *Clin Chem.* 1987;33:1372.

150. Gupta D, Attanasio A, Raaf S. Plasma estrogen and androgen concentrations in children during adolescence. *J Clin Endocrinol Metab.* 1975;40:636.

151. Klein KO, et al. Use of an ultrasensitive recombinant cell bioassay to determine estrogen levels in girls with precocious puberty treated with a luteinizing hormone-releasing hormone agonist. *J Clin Endocrinol Metab.* 1998;83:2387.

152. Hammond GL. Molecular properties of corticosteroid binding globulin and the sex-steroid binding proteins. *Endocr Rev.* 1990;11:65.

153. Kim MR, et al. Serum prostate specific antigen, sex hormone binding globulin and free androgen index as markers of pubertal development in boys. *Clin Endocrinol.* 1999;50:203.

154. Thaler M, et al. Immunoassay for sex hormone-binding globulin in undiluted serum is influenced by high-molecular-mass aggregates. *Clin Chem.* 2005;51:401.

155. Zachmann M. Evaluation of gonadal function in childhood and adolescence. *Helv Paediatr Acta.* 1974;34:53.

156. Forest MG. Pattern of the response of testosterone and its precursors to human chorionic gonadotropin stimulation in relation to age in infants and children. *J Clin Endocrinol Metab.* 1979;49:132.

157. Ng KL, Ahmed SF, Hughes IA. Pituitary-gonadal axis in male undermasculinisation. *Arch Dis Child.* 2000;82:54.

158. Saez JM, Bertrand J. Studies on testicular function in children: plasma concentrations of testosterone, dehydroepiandrosterone and its sulfate before and after stimulation with human chorionic gonadotrophin. *Steroids.* 1968;12:749.

159. Chasalow FI, et al. An improved method for evaluating testosterone biosynthetic defects. *Pediatr Res.* 1984;18:759.

160. Pang S, et al. Dihydrotestosterone and its relationship to testosterone in infancy and childhood. *J Clin Endocrinol Metab.* 1979;48:821.

161. Kiningham RB, Apgar BS, Schwenk TL. Evaluation of amenorrhea. *Am Fam Phys.* 1996;53:1185.

162. McIver B, Romanski SA, Nippoldt TB. Evaluation and management of amenorrhea. *Mayo Clin Proc.* 1997;72:1161.

163. Apgar BS, Greenberg G. Using progestins in clinical practice. *Am Fam Phys.* 2000;62:1839.

164. Battino S, et al. Factors associated with withdrawal bleeding after administration of oral dydrogesterone or medroxyprogesterone acetate in women with secondary amenorrhea. *Gynecol Obstet Invest.* 1996;42:113.

165. Goji K. Twenty-four-hour concentration profiles of gonadotropin and estradiol (E_2) in prepubertal and early pubertal girls: The diurnal rise of E_2 is opposite the nocturnal rise of gonadotropin. *J Clin Endocrinol Metab.* 1993;77:1629.

166. Goji K, Tanikaze S. Spontaneous gonadotropin and testosterone concentration profiles in prepubertal and pubertal boys: Temporal relationship between luteinizing hormone and testosterone. *Pediatr Res.* 1993;34:229.

167. Neely EK, et al. Normal ranges for immuno-chemiluminometric gonadotropin assays. *J Pediatr.* 1995;127:40.

168. Garibaldi LR, et al. The relationship between luteinizing hormone and estradiol secretion in female precocious puberty: Evaluation by sensitive gonadotropin assays and the leuprolide stimulation test. *J Clin Endocrinol Metab.* 1993;76:851.

169. Volpe R. Rational use of thyroid function tests. *Crit Rev Clin Lab Sci.* 1997;34:405.

170. Wallaschofski H, et al. Prediction of remission or relapse for Graves' hyperthyroidism by the combined determination of stimulating, blocking and binding TSH-receptor antibodies after the withdrawal of antithyroid drug treatment. *Horm Metab Res.* 2002;34:383–388.

171. Rose SR. Cranial irradiation and central hypothyroidism. *Trends Endocrinol Metab.* 2001;12:97.

172. Rose SR. Endocrinopathies in childhood cancer survivors. *Endocrinologist.* 2003;13:488.

173. Rose SR. Disorders of thyrotropin synthesis, secretion, and function. *Curr Opin Pediatr.* 2000;12:375.

174. Rose SR, et al. Hypothyroidism and deficiency of the nocturnal thyrotropin surge in children with hypothalamic-pituitary disorders. *J Clin Endocrinol Metab.* 1990;70:1750.

175. Rose SR, et al. Diagnosis of hidden central hypothyroidism in survivors of childhood cancer. *J Clin Endocrinol Metab.* 1999;84:4472.

176. Baylis PH, Cheetham T. Diabetes insipidus. *Arch Dis Child.* 1998;79:84.

177. Cheetham T, Baylis PH. Diabetes insipidus in children: Pathophysiology, diagnosis and management. *Paediatr Drugs.* 2002;4:785.

178. Dashe AM, et al. A water deprivation test for the differential diagnosis of polyuria. *JAMA.* 1963;185:699.

179. Mohn A, et al. Hypertonic saline test for the investigation of posterior pituitary function. *Arch Dis Child.* 1998;79:431–434.

CHAPTER 50

Radiographic Imaging

Kumud Sane, MD
Shashikant M. Sane, MD

DIAGNOSTIC IMAGING IN PEDIATRIC ENDOCRINOLOGY

Diagnostic imaging is a critical part of contemporary medicine. Since the discoveries of x-rays in 1895, plain radiography has evolved into several imaging modalities, such as ultrasonography (US), scintigraphy (NM), computed tomographic (CT) scanning, magnetic resonance imaging (MRI), and positron-emission tomographic (PET) scanning. The limited role of imaging in the evaluation of patients with endocrine disorders of only two to three decades ago has given way to a richness of opportunity to improve patient care through imaging.

Each modality has its strengths and weaknesses. Plain radiography is best in evaluating the metabolic abnormalities of the skeleton including skeletal maturation. US provides anatomical information without ionizing radiation. NM is used primarily for functional imaging of the thyroid and parathyroid gland. It is also useful in adrenal and pancreatic tumors. CT scanning and MRI provide high-resolution cross-sectional imaging, improving the detection and localization of the source of endocrine hyperfunction or endocrine pathology responsible for failure of hormone production. Recent advances of multislice spiral CT scanning and MRI give multiplanar images that frequently are diagnostic. In addition, these images can be useful for subsequent three-dimensional (3D) reconstruction in select patients. CT scanning involves radiation but can be accomplished rapidly, obviating the need for sedation. CT scanning is excellent in detecting calcification. MRI has superior tissue contrast which improves lesion detection without ionizing radiation to the patient. The downside of MRI is the frequent need for sedation, the high cost and the increased acquisition time leading to breathing/motion artifact.

These diagnostic modalities usually are complementary to one another for the demonstration of normal anatomy or physiology in health or disease. Although functional abnormalities can be assessed, the main usefulness of diagnostic imaging is in the evaluation of masses. It is critical that the primary physician/endocrinologist and the radiologist communicate before setting the course for imaging workup.

Finally, let this be a word of caution: Present-day multislice, multiplanar CT and MRI images are so breathtaking that through a seductive display of anatomical detail, incidental abnormalities frequently are recognized. One needs to deal with these "incidentalomas" by a thoughtfully balancing of potential benefits and risks.

HYPOTHALAMIC-PITUITARY IMAGING

Anatomy and Physiology The pituitary gland occupies the sella turcica, a cup-shaped depression in the basisphenoid bone. The roof of the sella is formed by the diaphragma sella, a fold of dura that is perforated to allow passage of the pituitary stalk. This stalk, also known as *infundibulum*, connects the hypothalamus to the pituitary, joining the gland at the junction of the anterior and posterior lobes of the pituitary. These lobes are embryologically, physiologically, and anatomically distinct. The anterior lobe or adenohypophysis is the largest part, comprising nearly 75% of total pituitary volume. It arises from an invagination of Rathke's pouch from the primitive oral cavity. It is composed of glandular cells that produce growth hormone (GH), thyroid-stimulating hormone (TSH), adrenocorticotropic hormone (ACTH), prolactin (PRL), follicle-stimulating hormone (FSH), luteinizing hormone (LH), and melanin-stimulating hormone. The release of these hormones is mediated by the hypothalamus. On T2- and unenhanced T1-weighted MRI images, the adenohypophysis is isointense relative to gray matter.

The posterior lobe of the pituitary, infundibular stalk, and paraventricular hypothalamic nuclei form the neurohypophysis. These structures are derived from diencephalic neuroectoderm. The axon terminals of the hypothalamic neurons release antidiuretic hormone (ADH). Oxytocin and vasopressin are synthesized in the hypothalamus, coupled with carrier proteins known as *neuro-physins* and enveloped by phospholipid membranes to form vesicles that are then transported to the posterior pituitary through the infundibular stalk. The posterior pituitary is normally hyperintense on T1-weighted MRI images. This is called the *bright spot* or *high signal* which is a distinctive feature because aside from fat, few things are hyperintense on T1-weighted un-enhanced images. The bright spot in neurohypophysis may be due to vasopressin storage within the neurosecretory vesicles. (Figure 50-1). Absent high

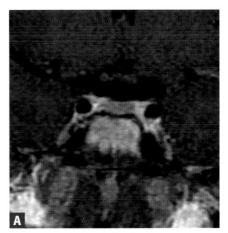

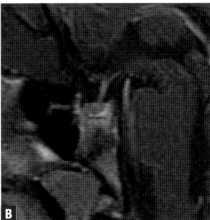

FIGURE 50-1. A to **B.** Normal pituitary shown on (A) coronal and (B) sagittal T1 weighed MRIs post gadolinium contrast. (B) T pituitary stalk with the posterior pituitary appearing brighter wrapping around underneath the anterior pituitary can be seen in the sagittal image.

Radiographic Imaging

AT-A-GLANCE

Diagnostic imaging is a critical part of contemporary medicine. Since the discovery of x-rays in 1895, plain radiography has evolved into several imaging modalities, such as ultrasonography (US), scintigraphy (NM), computed tomography (CT), magnetic resonance imaging (MRI), and positron-emission tomography (PET).

Each modality has its strengths and weaknesses. Plain radiography is best in evaluating the metabolic abnormalities of the skeleton, including skeletal maturation. US provides anatomical information without ionizing radiation. NM is used primarily for functional imaging of the thyroid and parathyroid gland. It is also useful in adrenal and pancreatic tumors. CT scanning and MRI provide high-resolution cross-sectional imaging, improving the detection and localization of the source of endocrine hyperfunction or endocrine pathology responsible for failure of hormone production. Recent advances of multislice spiral CT scanning and MRI give multiplanar images that are frequently diagnostic. In addition, these images can be useful for subsequent 3D reconstruction in select cases. CT scanning involves radiation but can be accomplished rapidly, obviating the need for sedation. CT scanning is excellent at detecting calcification. MRI involves no ionizing radiation and is not hampered by bone artifacts, as is CT scanning, but MRI frequently needs sedation.

These diagnostic modalities usually are complementary to one another for the demonstration of normal anatomy or physiology in health or disease. Although functional abnormalities can be assessed, the main usefulness of diagnostic imaging is in the evaluation of masses. It is critical that the primary physician/endocrinologist and the radiologist communicate before setting the course on imaging workup.

PITUITARY–HYPOTHALAMUS	TEST(S) (IN ORDER OF PRIORITY)	FINDINGS/COMMENTS
Hypopituitarism	MRI of brain and hypothalamic pituitary area	Lesions of pituitary gland are seen in three planes; size, position of gland, and posterior pituitary signal are helpful in making the diagnosis; midline defects and optic nerves are visualized well; need for sedation and immobilization make it difficult for young children
	CT scan of brain and hypothalamic pituitary area	Useful in detecting calcification; need for sedation is less obligatory.
	US of head and brain	Useful in newborns and infants with open anterior fontanel; no exposure to radiation; sedation is not required; ventricular size and hemorrhage can be assessed with ease.
Brain and pituitary tumors Craniopharingioma	CT scan of brain and hypothalamic area	Useful in detecting calcification in sellar and suprasellar tumors; cystic component can be seen as rim in the lesion. Helpful in preoperative planning (anatomical structures, approach to tumor.)
Pituitary adenoma/germinoma	MRI of pituitary and hypothalamus	Suprasellar and sellar tumors are detected on MRI; Contrast IV gadolinium helps in detecting small pituitary adenomas. Germinomas are seen in pineal area.
Langerhans' cell histiocytosis	MRI of brain and pituitary	Pituitary lesions include thickening of the pituitary stalk and absence of hyperintense posterior pituitary signal.

THYROID	TEST(S) (IN ORDER OF PRIORITY)	FINDINGS/COMMENTS
Congenital hypothyroidism	Scintigraphy (^{123}I or ^{99m}Tc pertechnetate)	Scintigraphy more likely to find ectopic or very small gland, although US can be accurate in the hands of a very experienced practitioner.
Acquired hypothyroidism		Generally, there is mild enlargement of gland, decreased uptake, irregular and mottled pattern in 50% but early on may be homogeneous; nodules may be present and should be regarded with suspicion of malignancy;
Hyperthyroidism		Iodine-123 uptake is increased at 4 hours and may be at 24 hours; scintigraphy may not be necessary unless toxic adenoma or large multinodular goitre is present.
Nodule	Ultrasound	*Cystic nodule:* Usually benign; if cyst does not move easily or layers in different positions, biopsy should be performed. *Solid nodule:* Usually but not always benign adenoma; hypoechoic halo around the nodule indicates benign. *Mixed echoic nodule:* Usually but not always benign adenoma or nodular goiter. Hypoechoic: May be benign, but this is the most common finding in malignancy. *Isoechoic nodule:* 25% are malignant; pattern often found in follicular adenoma and carcinoma.
	Scintigraphy (^{123}I)	Depending on the degree of radionuclide accumulation, nodules can be classified as cold (20% to 30% malignant), warm, or hot (which are usually benign); iodine-123 uptake is useful for followup S/P thyroid surgery for malignancy.
Large thyroid mass (thyroid cancer; metastasis)	CT and/or MRI	The lack of idodinated contrast medium is an advantage of MRI, but the specificity of MRI is not different from that of multiplanar CT; CT more sensitive for identifying calcification

PARATHYROID	TEST(S) (IN ORDER OF PRIORITY)	FINDINGS/COMMENTS
Parathyroid adenoma/ hyperparathyroidism	Scintigraphy (99tm sestamibi and thallium-201)	Early and delayed images after 4 hours will detect parathyroid glands; double agents as Tc sestamibi and pertechnate can be beneficial to detect parathyroid lesions; ectopic glands can be presrent in neck and chest; absolute immobilization during study is required.
	Parathyroid CT	Large hyperplastic gland or adenoma can be detected.

ADRENAL	TEST(S) (IN ORDER OF PRIORITY)	FINDINGS/COMMENTS
Adrenal insufficiency	Ultrasound	Diffuse adrenal enlargement in newborn with CAH and ambiguous genitalia; bilateral adrenal hemorrhage in neonates can be diagnosed; lipoid glands in rare form of CAH; calcified glands in Wolman disease.
Adrenal tumors	Iodine 123 meta-iodobenzylguanidine (MIBG) scintigraphy	Useful to detect neuroblastoma and pheochromocytoma. Primary as well as metastatic lesions can be seen.
	CT scan with or without contrast	Contrast agents should be used with caution in adrenal medullary lesions. Adrenal adenoma in Cushing syndrome can be detected on CT scan; adenoma as small as 2-5 mm in diameter can be detected on CT; calcification in adrenal lesions best detected on CT.

PANCREATIC	TEST(S) (IN ORDER OF PRIORITY)	FINDINGS/COMMENTS
Pancreatic tumors—Islet cell tumor	CT scan of pancreas with and without contrast	Islet cell tumors are more common; tumor shows less attenuation than pancreatic tissue; Intravenous contrast material will enhance the tumor image.
Gastrinoma/glucagonoma/ VI Pomas/somastatinoma	CT of pancreas	Usually malignant with metastasis; larger tumors measure 4–7 cm in diameter; cystic changes and calcifications are common; they are hormonally active; hormonally inactive tumors are large (> 8 cm) and cause local pain and metastasis. VI Pomas are vasoactive intestinal peptide–secreting tumors.

GONADAL	TEST(S) (IN ORDER OF PRIORITY)	FINDINGS/COMMENTS
Ambiguous genitalia	Ultrasound of the pelvis and labial/scrotal area	Examination is performed through distended bladder; ovaries in newborn female show hypoechoic follicles; testes have a solid, homogeneous echoic structure; presence or absence of uterus with thin endometrial stripe is noted.
	Fluoroscopic genitography	Fluid-filled structure behind the bladder can be vagina in females or prostatic utricle in males; urethra, urinary bladder, vagina, and uterine cervical impression on the cephalic part of vagina can be seen.
	MRI of pelvis	Useful in demonstrating presence, absence, or any abnormality of genital structures; intrapelvic testes are better visualized.
Turner syndrome	Pelvic and abdominal ultrasound	Uterus may be prepubertal or smaller than normal size; ovaries nonvisualized or streak ovaries on one or both sides; renal abnormalities—single kidney or horseshoe kidney.
Primary amenorrhea	Pelvic ultrasound	Presence or absence of uterus; size, shape and maturation, as well as ovarian development, provides guidance to the etiology.
Ovarian neoplasm	Ultrasound of pelvis and abdomen	Localized mass in adnexal region; characters—cystic, solid, or combination; lymphadenopathy, obstructive uropathy, ascites, solid-organ metastasis can be detected.
	CT of pelvic organs	CT scan is of greater value in large ovarian tumors; it detects local invasion of the adjacent structures; presence of calcification, ossification, and tooth as seen in teratoma can be recognized with all modalities.

GONADAL	TEST(S) (IN ORDER OF PRIORITY)	FINDINGS/COMMENTS
Testes cryptorchidism	Ultrasound of testes	Most of undescended testes are in inguinal canal and can be located by US.
	MRI of testes	MRI will help to localize testes above the inguinal ring.
Testicular tumors	Ultrasound of testes	Testicular mass distinct from normal tissue or diffuse enlargement can be detected; variable echogenicity representing calcification, necrosis, and /or hemorrhage in tumors; cystic lesions are more common in large tumors.

SKELETAL	TEST(S) (IN ORDER OF PRIORITY)	FINDINGS/COMMENTS
Short stature	Plain radiograph of left hand and wrist; skeletal survey	Bone maturation can be assessed with single radiograph in child above age of 2 years and older; radiograph of hemiskeleton is needed for younger than two years; helpful for skeletal disorders of genetic and metabolic nature; type of bones affected—proximal, middle, or distal from torso are affected in different disorders; most useful in type of injury to cause breaks in bones.
Osteoporosis/osteomalacia /rickets	Plain radiography	Rickets can be diagnosed with plain radiograph of rapidly growing bones of the upper and lower extremities in children; delay in calcification of growth plates causes widening, fraying,cupping, and deformation of metaphyseal region.
	DEXA scan of total body and spine and long bones	Useful in assessing bone density; the comparisons for age, gender, and pubertal status are most important to interpret the results; serial examination can be helpful in interpreting the success or failure of treatment.

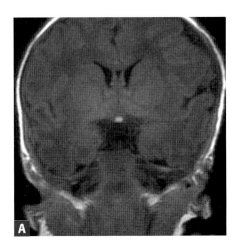

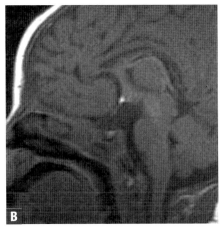

FIGURE 50-2. A to **B.** Ectopic neurohypophysis is shown as a "bright" spot on coronal and sagittal T1 weighed MRI images.

signal is often associated with central diabetes insipidus or compressive pituitary gland lesions. In 10% of cases, absent high signal may be a normal variant. An ectopic position of the posterior pituitary may be a normal variant but also can be associated with congenital pituitary GH deficiency or panhypopituitarism when there may be a small fossa and reduced amount of pituitary tissue (Figure 50-2).

The shape and size of the pituitary vary with age and sex. In neonates, the pituitary is rounder, brighter, and relatively larger during the first 2 months of life than in later infancy or childhood. This finding is thought to reflect the marked metabolic and hormonal activity that is characteristic of the neonatal period. In adults, the average height is 3.5–8 mm, and it is slightly larger in women than in men. In pubescent girls and pregnant or postpartum women, the gland enlarges and often appears spherical or upwardly convex and can reach 10–11 mm in height (1). The anterior pituitary also may appear hyperintense in pregnant or postpartum women. During pregnancy, there is a progressive linear increase in gland height of the mother, at an

approximate rate of 0.1 mm per week; the pituitary stalk may also increase in size throughout pregnancy but should never exceed 4 mm in diameter. Gland size should rapidly return to normal after the first postpartum week. Breast feeding has no apparent influence on the return of the gland to normal size. Pubertal males may have a slightly rounded, upwardly convex pituitary that measures 6–7 mm in height. The pituitary gland decreases in size with age. In addition to the normal physiological changes in the pituitary, the pituitary may enlarge during administration of exogenous estrogens, in central precocious puberty, with hypothalamic tumors, or with ectopic tumors secreting hypothalamic-releasing factors. It also can increase in size even to the extent of appearance of a mass secondary to end-organ failure (e.g., hypothyroidism) (2) (Figure 50-3).

Imaging Techniques

MRI and CT scanning are the main imaging modalities for evaluating the sella and parasellar region, with MRI being the preferred choice. MRI has significantly better soft tissue resolution than CT scanning and also avoids bony artifacts and ionizing radiation. The multiplanar capability of MRI allows direct imaging in all three planes. The current imaging protocols typically use sagittal and coronal T1-weighted spin-echo sequences. To achieve high spatial resolution, thin slices (2.5–3 mm) and a small field of view (16–20 cm) are used. The same sequences can be repeated after intravenous administration of gadolinium (Gd). Acquiring an additional dynamic T1-weighted spin-echo sequence within 1–2 minutes of injection of intravenous contrast material slightly improves the sensitivity of MRI for the detection of small pituitary adenomas.

There is still a role for CT scanning in imaging the hypothalamic–pituitary axis. There are a number of patients who cannot undergo MRI due to metallic objects in the area or the requirement for sedation during the procedure. CT scanning is also useful in detection of calcification, the presence of which occasionally can influence the differential diagnosis. CT scanning occasionally may contribute to preoperative planning, particularly with regard to the anatomy and pneumatization of the sphenoid bone. The helical CT scan data can be acquired in the axial plane with 0.5- or 1-mm resolution and images reformatted in coronal, axial, and sagittal planes for review. After the initial CT scan, the examination can be repeated after administration of intravenous iodinated contrast material (2 mL/kg, maximum to 100 mL).

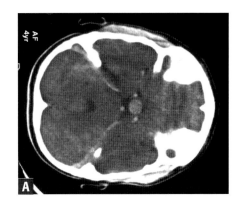

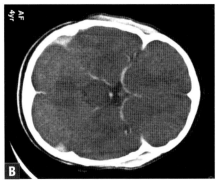

FIGURE 50-3. A to **B.** CT scans showing a pituitary mass in 4 year old child with hypothyroidism (A). After thyroxine replacement therapy mass resolves (B).

Pituitary Dwarfism

This is a heterogeneous group of conditions caused by complete or partial GH deficiency. It is postulated to result from an insult in utero or perinatal vascular injury to the infundibulum or lack of normal embryological development of both lobes of the pituitary gland. In nearly half the cases, there is a history of birth trauma, asphyxia, or breech delivery. Males are affected twice as frequently as females.

MRI is the preferred modality for diagnosis over CT scanning. Typical features include a small sella turcica ($< 200 \text{ mm}^3$), hypoplastic or, more often, an absent pituitary stalk, and an ectopic posterior pituitary lobe at the level of median eminence. A normal sella volume in the pediatric group is 240–500 mm³ and 240–1100 mm³ in adults.

Neoplasms

Tumors of the pituitary region also are commonly associated with pituitary dysfunction. Other symptoms may vary depending on the size, nature, and location of the tumor.

Craniopharyngioma

This is the most common pituitary tumor in childhood, accounting for 50% of all sellar and juxtasellar region tumors in children. They arise from remnants of the

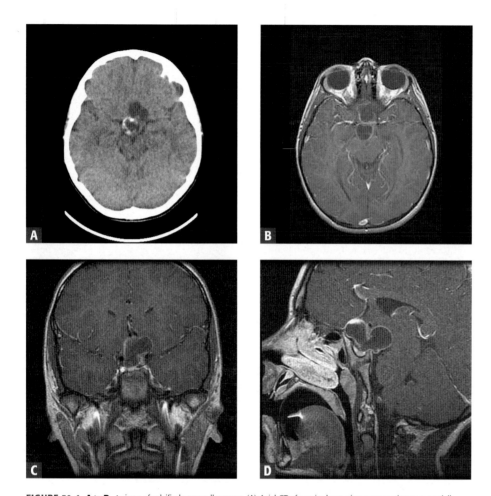

FIGURE 50-4. A to **D.** 4 views of calcified suprasellar mass. (A) Axial CT of craniopharyngioma presenting as a partially calcified cystic suprasellar mass. (B–D) T1 weighted axial, coronal and sagittal MRI images post gadolinium showing a predominantly suprasellar lobular mass. The lesion shows displacement of the optic chiasm and optic nerves, deviation of the floor of the third ventricle and splaying of the circle of Willis.

craniopharyngeal duct, anywhere along the pituitary stalk to the pituitary gland. They are hormonally inactive, but symptoms of vision loss, hormone dysfunction, and hydrocephalus can result from compression of pituitary gland, optic chiasm, and hypothalamus. Hypothalamic growth failure and diabetes insipidus are the most common endocrine manifestations.

Craniopharyngiomas have a characteristic appearance of at least a partially cystic, enhancing, and calcified mass in the sella or the suprasellar region (Figure 50-4), 70% are intra- and suprasellar, 20% are suprasellar only, and 10% are intrasellar only. Calcification is detected on CT scan in 90% of cases (3). On MRI, cysts can be identified in 95% of patients. The cyst contents may have a variable appearance, with both bright and dark signals on T1-weighted images, reflecting the differences in cholesterol and keratin contents of the cysts. More than 90% of craniopharyngiomas will show some degree of enhancement on CT scan, either of the solid portion of the lesion or of the rim of the cys-

tic component. Similar enhancement is also observed on MRI.

Rathke's Cleft Cysts

Rathke cleft cyst is a benign epithelium-lined cyst, that arises primarily within the sella turcica and is thought to originate from remnants of the Rathke's pouch. Rathke's pouch is the primordium of the pituitary gland and normally closes during fetal development, but a remnant often persists as a cleft that lies between the anterior and posterior lobes of the pituitary gland. Although similar in origin, these are seen less frequently than craniopharyngiomas. They are simple cysts with minimal, if any, enhancement of the cyst wall. They show no calcification or nodularity. Occasionally, debris may be present in the dependent portion of the mucoid fluid within the cysts. Although tiny Rathke's cleft cysts are seen frequently at autopsy, only the large ones present with the symptoms of pituitary dysfunction. (i.e., if they are large enough to compress the optic chiasm can vision loss occur).

Germinomas

Nearly 35% of intracranial germ cell tumors arise in the suprasellar area. Unlike pineal lesions, which have a strong male predominance, suprasellar tumors affect both sexes equally. Germinoma is the most common germ cell tumor and accounts for approximately 70% of all germ cell tumors and more than 50% of the pineal region. These suprasellar germinomas are of utmost importance because the early diagnosis can be lifesaving and can reduce the craniospinal radiation required to achieve cure. The most common presenting symptoms that result from hypothalamic involvement include precocious puberty, diabetes insipidus, emaciation, and vision loss.

Suprasellar germinomas tend to be smooth, round, or lobulated homogeneous midline masses centered on the pituitary stalk, frequently growing from the pituitary gland to the hypothalamus. The lesion can arise in the floor of the third ventricle and invade and/or compress the optic chiasm and infundibulum. The tumor may extend superiorly and infiltrate the walls of the 3rd ventricle. Because this is an intraventricular mass, metastatic spread to the subarachnoid space is common, with involvement of the brain and spinal cord. CT scan or MRI can establish the diagnosis. Nonenhanced CT scan shows a round or lobulated isodense to hyperdense mass that enhances brightly and homogeneously after injection of iodinated contrast material. Occasionally, punctuate calcifications can be seen. On MRI, the lesion is hypointense to isointense on T1-weighted sequences and enhances markedly after injection of gadolinium. Although it may be difficult to distinguish from suprasellar astrocytoma, drop metastasis suggests the diagnosis of germinoma.

Pituitary Adenoma

Pituitary adenomas are rare in children and account for only 1% of pediatric intracranial masses. In contrast, in adults these very lesions constitute nearly 10% of the intracranial neoplasms and are one of the two most common suprasellar masses besides meningiomas. In children, most adenomas are diagnosed in girls between the ages of 9 and 13 years of age. Most of these tumors usually secrete ACTH and PRL. Pituitary adenomas that secrete GH are extremely rare in children. When present, they cause gigantism. In contrast, such GH-producing adenomas are the second most common endocrinologically active tumor in adults and produce acromegaly. Raised PRL does not always indicate the presence of PRL-

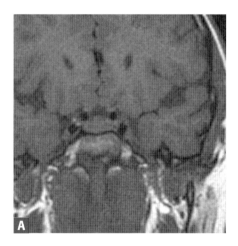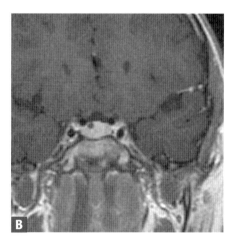

FIGURE 50-5. A to **B.** Pituitary microadenoma (3 mm in diameter) in the right superior lateral aspect of anterior pituitary shown pre (A) and post (B) contrast coronal T1 weighed MRI images. The microadenoma appears as a small black circle on contrast (B).

secreting adenoma, and modest elevation of PRL levels, even up to 200 ng/ml, can occur due to pituitary stalk compression interfering with the delivery of PRL-inhibitory factors. Therefore, any large tumor that compresses the hypothalamus or pituitary stalk can produce this effect, a nonfunctioning pituitary adenoma being the most common. Certain drugs such as phenothiazines can elevate PRL levels modestly, but levels above 200 ng/ml are almost always due to PRL-secreting tumors, the most common of the hormonally active adenomas.

Pituitary microadenomas are less than 10 mm in diameter (Figure 50-5). When they are greater than 10 mm in diameter, they are labeled as macroadenomas. They have a convex upper margin and extend through the diaphragma sellae into the suprasellar cistern. Due to "waisting" at this level, they have a "figure eight" appearance. They can and do extend laterally into the cavernous sinus quite frequently. Necrosis, hemorrhage, and cyst formation are found occasionally. In general, microadenomas are hypodense on contrast-enhanced CT scans and hypointense on MRI images. Macroadenomas are isodense on unenhanced CT scans and in 1% to 8% of cases may show calcification. After intravenous contrast material administration, they may show marked enhancement. These macroadenomas tend to be isointense on T1-weighted sequences and may show heterogeneous enhancement after gadolinium injection.

Langerhans' Cell Histiocytosis (LCH)

Isolated LCH of the central nervous system (CNS) is rare. CNS involvement, however, is found frequently as a part of systemic involvement. The most common endocrine abnormality in LCH is diabetes insipidus (DI), which occurs as a result of deficient secretion of ADH (arginine vasopressin). Although granulomatous infiltration can occur anywhere in the CNS, the hypothalamic nuclei are the most common targets (4). DI is seen in 25% to 33% of children with LCH and is manifest within 2 years of the diagnosis. DI is present in only 5% of patients at the time of diagnosis.

MRI is more effective than CT scanning in the evaluation of children with LCH. Typical findings include thickening of the pituitary stalk and absent hyperintensity of the posterior pituitary on T1-weighted images. A thickened pituitary stalk can be associated with LCH or a hypothalamic mass. With contrast material (Gd) administration, the mass enhances moderately or markedly. Not all patients with LCH have DI. Hence, when LCH is being established as the diagnosis, a skeletal survey, including a skull series and a bone scan, must be obtained to identify or exclude other sites of involvement. Differential diagnostic considerations in children with pituitary stalk thickening include craniopharyngioma, hypothalamic glioma, germinoma, leukemia, lymphoma, metastasis, or sarcoidosis.

Hypopituitary States

Pituitary deficiency results from destruction of the hypothalamic–pituitary axis. Pituitary adenomas, pituitary inflammation (hypophysitis), previous pituitary surgery, and radiation therapy all can produce hypopituitarism. Imaging in these patients may demonstrate an empty or partially empty sella, although there may appear to be a normal amount of pituitary tissue visible within the fossa. Occasionally, parasellar lesions (e.g., meningioma or carotid aneurysm) can involve the pituitary, producing a deficiency state, mostly in adults. The finding of empty sella on MRI simply may be incidental. This may be due to a congenital defect in the diaphragma sella, which allows cerebrospinal fluid (CSF) pulsation to expand the sella and result in compression of pituitary tissue. The so-called empty sella is a very common anatomical variant in which the sella is partially filled with CSF. The infundibular stalk follows its normal course and inserts in the midline of the pituitary gland. The gland itself appears thinned and flattened against the bony floor. On CT scan and MRI, the pituitary gland is flattened to a thin rim along the floor of the sella turcica. The key finding is the fact that the pituitary stalk remains in its normal position and can be traced to the pituitary. This finding diffentiates an empty sella from a cystic tumor in which the stalk is displaced or obliterated. That patients are usually asymptomatic has been attributed to the large functional reserve of the adenohypophysis; if greater than 10% of the gland is functional, the physiology remains undisturbed. When symptomatic, complaints include headache, dizziness, or memory loss and may be due to an elevated intracranial pressure or altered CSF dynamics similar to those seen in pseudotumor cerebri. In some instances, intrasellar herniation of the optic nerve, chiasm, or tract into the empty sella can be seen and visual loss may occur.

THYROID IMAGING

The thyroid gland consists of two lobes of nearly equal size, a bridging isthmus, and occasionally, a pyramidal lobe that is simply a thin extension of thyroid tissue arising off the superior border of the isthmus. The isthmus connects the anteroinferior portions of the lobes (5). The thyroid gland arises from the floor of the embryonic pharynx at the level of the fourth pharyngeal pouch and descends to its normal position anteriorly in the neck, generally below the level of the thyroid cartilage and anterior to trachea. The connection to the base of the tongue is known as the *thyroglossal duct*. The duct usually involutes and disappears after the gland completes its descent in utero. In infants and young children, the thyroid lobes measure 2–3 cm in length, 1–1.5 cm in width, and are approximately 0.2–1.2 cm in thickness. In adolescents, the thyroid lobes reach adult dimensions measuring 5–8 cm in length, 2–4 cm in width, and 1–2.5 cm in thickness (6).

Disorders of the thyroid gland are common. They can be divided into those that are developmental and those that affect function or structure. Ultrasound, CT scanning, MRI, and nuclear medicine imaging techniques are useful in the investigation and management of patients with thyroid disorders. Ultrasonography (US) can differentiate solid from cystic lesions and can detect cysts as small as 2 mm in diameter. It is performed by using a 12- or 15-MHz transducer that is optimal for high-resolution imaging. A 5-MHz transducer frequently is needed for large goiters. Normal thyroid gland is uniformly echogenic and slightly more echogenic than the adjacent muscles. Color-flow or power Doppler techniques are helpful in assessing vascularity. US examinations are invaluable in fine-needle aspiration cytology.

CT scanning helps to characterize large thyroid masses, to assess invasion of adjacent structures, and to identify metastatic lesions in the neck, mediastinum, and lungs. Since iodinated intravenous contrast material is needed for CT examination, TSH levels must be measured prior to CT scanning to assess thyroid function accurately. The normal thyroid gland is of higher attenuation than muscle. MRI is also used to assess large tumors, especially those with mediastinal extension. The normal thyroid has the same or slightly increased signal intensity on T1-weighted images as muscle and slightly lower signal intensity on T2-weighted images. The lack of iodinated contrast material is an advantage, although the specificity of MRI is not different from that of newer multiplanar CT scanning.

Iodine-123 (^{123}I) and technetium-99m are the two commonly used scintigraphic agents. Technetium-99m pertechnetate is trapped like ^{123}I, but its advantage over ^{123}I for routine thyroid imaging is that it is not organified by the thyroid gland. Besides, ^{99}Tc pertechnetate is readily available at a very low cost and has a short physical half-life of 6 hours, gamma energy of 140 keV, and an extremely low radiation dose (a little over 1000 times less than ^{123}I). Pertechnetate is injected intravenously (intramuscularly, if necessary), and the thyroid gland is imaged 15–20 minutes later. ^{123}I is ingested orally either in solution or in capsules. The imaging is performed 24 hours later. When ^{123}I is used for imaging, the percentage of the administered radioactivity accumulating in the thyroid gland is calculated. The normal 4-hour uptake is in the range of 5% to 15% of the ingested dose, whereas 24-hour uptake is 10% to 40%. This can vary from country to country mostly depending on the amount of stable iodine in the diet. ^{123}I has physical half-life of 13 hours and gamma energy of 159 keV.

Developmental Disorders

Neonatal hypothyroidism occurs in approximately 1 per 4000 newborns (7), with thyroid dysgenesis being the most common etiology, accounting for 80% of cases. Aplasia (athyreosis) accounts for 25% thyroid agenesis cases,

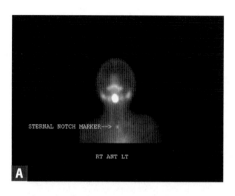
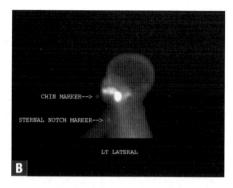

FIGURE 50-6. A to **B.** Elongated lingual thyroid seen in (A) central area of anterior-posterior and (B) lateral views of thyroid scan. Salivary gland activity is seen on both sides.

whereas thyroid ectopia accounts for the remaining 75%. Thyroid ectopia is diagnosed with US and/or scintigraphy. The ectopic thyroid tissue can be located anywhere along the course of the thyroglossal tract, that is, anywhere from the base of the tongue near the foramen cecum to the anterior sublaryngeal level. It appears as a round or an oval-shaped area of uptake in the midline of the upper neck. It is seen most commonly in the lingual or sublingual region (Figure 50-6). On rare occasions, thyroid descent is exaggerated, and it extends down to the substernal region, where it is easily detected on scintigraphy if the area from oropharynx to superior mediastinum is included in the examination. The ectopic thyroid may be present in more than one location in the same patient. The ectopic thyroid tissue typically is dysmorphic, functions poorly, and has a higher incidence of malignant transformation compared with normally placed thyroid.

Hypothyroidism in infants and children results in retarded skeletal maturation that in many cases may be quite pronounced. The ossification of epiphyseal ossification centers is irregular, punctate, and referred as *epiphyseal dysgenesis*. It is best seen involving both the femoral and humeral heads as well as the ossification centers at the knee joint. There is osteoporosis making them more radiolucent. These changes are most pronounced in long bones, ribs, clavicles, and the spine. In the midportion of the vertebral bodies, typical endplate changes cause concave deformities with increased intervertebral disk spaces. There is usually a gibbus deformity, that is, a local prominence at the thoracolumbar junction. There is growth retardation at the base of the skull with large sella turcica. The fontanelles show markedly delayed closure, and multiple intrasutural wormian bones are seen.

Graves Disease

In patients with Graves disease, the iodine turnover is very rapid. As a result iodine-123 uptake at 24 hours may be normal, whereas 4-hour uptake is markedly increased. US shows a diffuse, relatively symmetrical enlargement of the thyroid gland. The homogeneous echo pattern of the normal thyroid gland usually is maintained. Thyroid scintigraphy may not be necessary routinely except where clinical and/or US examination makes one consider other causes of hyperthyroidism, such as toxic adenoma (Plummer disease) or toxic multinodular goiter, hyperfunctioning thyroid carcinoma, and acute suppurative thyroiditis. In Graves disease, the thyroid gland is uniformly enlarged, whereas the various conditions just listed demonstrate focal abnormalities or inhomogeneous appearance of the gland besides high iodine-123 uptake values.

Chronic Lymphocytic Thyroiditis

This is also known as *Hashimoto thyroiditis* and is the most common form of thyroid disease in children (rarely affects children before the age of 5 years) and adolescents, having an estimated incidence of between 1% and 5% of all children. The children present with a diffusely enlarged, firm, and nontender thyroid gland that may have an irregular or lobulated surface. US examination is useful to substantiate the diffuse nature of the thyroid gland abnormality and also to exclude any questionable nodules. The echogenicity of the thyroid gland is diminished, and in some instances, it may appear patchy or irregular. Unfortunately, these findings of chronic lymphocytic thyroiditis are nonspecific and cannot be differentiated from those of other diffuse thyroid disorders such as giant cell or De Quervain's thyroiditis, and thyroiditis after mumps or respiratory viral infections.

On scintigraphy, findings vary depending on the severity and stage of disease. Although scintigraphy is not recommended in every case, it is indicated in severe and longstanding cases of Hashimoto thyroiditis. If there is any questionable nodule in a typical case, scintigraphy is indicated. In most cases, the gland is only mildly enlarged. An irregular and mottled pattern is identified in 50% of cases. Between 15% and 20% of Hashimoto thyroiditis cases show normal homogeneous uptake (early or mild cases). A discrete area of decreased uptake occurs in about 15% to 20% of affected children. Nodules that do not accumulate radiopharmaceutical must be regarded with the same level of suspicion for malignancy as those in patients without the diagnosis of lymphocytic thyroiditis for three reasons: 1) A malignant thyroid nodule may occur in a gland affected by chronic lymphocytic thyroiditis, 2) thyroid malignancy is sometimes associated with elevated serum titers of antibodies to thyroid, which may lead to a mistaken clinical diagnosis of thyroiditis, and 3) lymphocytic infiltration can accompany thyroid malignancy and result in misleading histological evidence of thyroiditis on biopsy (8). Uptake values of iodine-123 and ^{99m}Tc usually are decreased in the patients with hypothyroidism but may be elevated in early phases of the disease when the thyroid is still capable of responding to stimulation by TSH (rarely). The percholate washout test is positive in about half the patients with chronic lymphocytic thyroiditis, indicating that defective organification is a component of the disease process.

Thyroid Neoplasms

Solitary nodules of the thyroid gland are rare in the pediatric population. They are detected in about 1% of asymptomatic children. Most solitary thyroid nodules are produced by benign lesions, although between 20% and 40% of solitary nodules are malignant (9). Follicular adenoma is by far the most common diagnosis. Other benign abnormalities that may produce a solitary, palpable thyroid nodule include thyroglossal duct cyst, colloid cyst, and chronic lymphocytic thyroiditis.

Thyroid malignancies constitute about 5% of head and neck malignancies in children, and these lesions are twice as common in girls. Papillary carcinomas are the most common form (80%) and arise from follicular epithelium. Carcinoma arising from parafollicular cells is termed *medullary carcinoma* and accounts for less than 5% of pediatric cases. The most common clinical presentation of pediatric thyroid neoplasms, whether benign or malignant, is a palpable painless nodule.

US plays an important role in the evaluation of thyroid nodules. It allows for precise localization of the palpable nodule, differentiates cystic from solid lesions, and facilitates identification of any additional nodules that may not be palpable clinically. Presence of multiple nodules indicates a lesser likelihood of malignancy. Cystic thyroid lesions in children almost always indicate a benign process. Most thyroid cysts result from colloid or hemorrhagic necrosis in benign adenomas or multinodular goiter. The cyst walls typically are irregular, but the cyst is free of solid material in the cavity. If the cyst contents do not move easily or layer in different positions, one needs to proceed with needle biopsy even though malignancy in a cyst is extremely rare. Solid thyroid nodules are hyperechoic with respect to normal thyroid and most commonly represent benign adenomas. A hypoechoic halo around the nodule is a sign of benignity. Only rarely is a thyroid carcinoma hyperechoic or mixed echoic. Mixed-echoic pattern in a thyroid nodule usually indicates benign adenoma or a nodular goiter. Most malignant thyroid nodules are hypoechoic compared with normal thyroid tissue, although a benign adenoma also may have such appearance. Approximately 25% of isoechoic thyroid nodules are also malignant. This pattern is most common in follicular adenoma and follicular thyroid carcinoma. These malignant nodules have irregular and infiltrative nodules and may accompany enlarged cervical lymph nodes.

Scintigraphy plays a critical role in evaluation of the solitary palpable thyroid nodule but cannot be used to distinguish benign form malignant lesions. Nodules, depending on the degree of radionuclide accumulation, are classified as cold, warm, or hot. A hot nodule almost always indicates a benign functional adenoma. Only a few rare, well-differentiated thyroid carcinomas may present as hot nodules (1% to 5%). In some nodules, the trapping mechanism is maintained despite failure of organification. These lesions may be visualized as hot nodules on ^{99m}Tc pertechnetate scintigraphy and as cold nodules on ^{123}I scintigraphy. Such discordant nodules need biopsy because malignancy cannot be excluded. A follow-up examination with ^{123}I scintigraphy must be performed in patients with hot nodules on ^{99m}Tc scintigraphy.

Cold nodules must be considered malignant until proven otherwise. Most cold nodules are benign, and only 20% to 30% of cold nodules are malignant (10). In decreasing order of incidence, the differential diagnosis of a solitary cold nodule in children includes follicular adenoma, thyroid carcinoma, chronic lymphocytic thyroiditis, thyroglossal duct cyst, colloid cyst, and abscess (Figure 50-7). Demonstration of tracer uptake in the cervical lymph nodes is a reliable scintigraphic indicator of thyroid carcinoma (11). Warm nodules are equal to or slightly greater in uptake than the adjacent

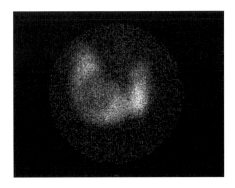

FIGURE 50-7. Thyroid scan showing decrease in 24 hrs uptake (12.6%) and an enlarged right thyroid lobe containing a large cold nodule.

thyroid tissue and are approached clinically with the same level of suspicion for malignancy as cold nodules.

The high iodine content of the thyroid gland provides inherent contrast for separation from adjacent structures on CT scanning. This is also the most sensitive imaging modality for the detection of calcification in a thyroid mass. CT scanning is particularly useful in the evaluation of large thyroid masses and for evaluation of retrotracheal or superior mediastinal extension. Plain chest radiograph and chest CT scan should be performed on anyone suspected of having thyroid carcinoma. Most thyroid nodules appear as low-attenuation lesions on unenhanced CT scans. There are no reliable CT criteria to differentiate benign from malignant thyroid masses unless there is evidence of invasion of adjacent structures or lymphadenopathy. Simple thyroid cysts demonstrate attenuation values approximately equal to those of water, whereas most cystic thyroid masses have higher attenuation value than water because most of them represent degenerated adenomas. With intravenous contrast material administration, the contents of the cyst do not enhance, but the surrounding rim often does. MRI provides information similar to that from CT scanning in the evaluation of the thyroid masses.

PARATHYROID IMAGING

Parathyroid imaging is performed most often for the localization of a parathyroid adenoma in patients with hyperparathyroidism. Primary hyperparathyroidism is rare in children; only 1% to 2% of these patients are younger than 20 years at diagnosis. The condition results from excessive secretion of PTH by hyperplastic glands or by one or more autonomous parathyroid adenomas. Approximately 80% of adult cases are due to a single autonomous parathyroid adenoma, and 20% result from idiopathic parathyroid chief cell hyperplasia that usually affects all four of the glands (12).

Parathyroid glands arise from the 3rd and 4th pharyngeal pouches and usually consist of four glands situated posterior to the thyroid lobes occupying each quadrant. They measure 5 mm × 3 mm × 1 mm and weigh 35–40 mg. Normal parathyroid cannot be imaged reliably by any radiological techniques at the present. Ectopic parathyroids do occur, but they account for less than 5% of cases (6). They are found anywhere from the level of the third pharyngeal pouch structures, just behind the angle of the mandible at the hyoid bone, down to the aortic root. They may lie within or outside the carotid sheath, around the esophagus, or within the thyroid (13). The normal parathyroid glands are small and oval in shape and usually less than 5 mm in diameter. They are frequently difficult to visualize on US due to their small size and also because they have a similar echostructure to that of the thyroid gland itself.

The detection of adenomas or gland hyperplasia on CT scan depends on the size of the tumor. Parathyroids normally are not seen on MRI (12). There are two nuclear medicine techniques to image parathyroid adenomas. Technetium-99m sestamibi and thallium-201 both localize in parathyroid adenomas and normal thyroid gland. Both agents wash out gradually from the thyroid but not from adenomas. Obtaining early and delayed images at 4 hours using one of these agents is usually diagnostic. Sestamibi is preferred because of better imaging characteristics of technetium. The second technique involves administration of sestamibi or thallium followed by pertechnetate, which localizes only in the thyroid gland. The pertechnetate image then is subtracted electronically from sestamibi/thallium image, delineating parathyroid adenoma. Absolute immobilization of the neck is essential during the examination to allow for precise image subtraction and to reach the sensitivity of 80% to 95% reported with this technique (14–16). The chest is also imaged to detect mediastinal disease. A portable radiation detector can be used in the operating room to localize the adenoma. Technetium-99m sestamibi is the single best screening study for parathyroid adenomas, but single photon emission computed tomography (SPECT) is essential, particularly for undescended and deep mediastinal adenomas.

Unlike in the adult age group, where the primary hyperparathyroidism frequently is detected as asymptomatic hypercalcemia on routine blood chemistry screening, the most common initial presentation in children is nephrolithiasis. This occurs in about 37% of patients. Approximately 6% of children with nephrolithiasis have primary hyperparathyroidism. Bony changes in hyperparathyroidism are due to demineralization and have rachitic changes similar to those seen in renal osteodystrophy. The characteristic bone resorption involves subperiosteal cortical bone and is seen mainly on the radial (lateral) aspect of the phalanges of the hands, most pronounced along the middle phalanges of the 2nd and 3rd digits. Other sites of resorption are the tufts of the digits; along the medial aspect of the proximal metaphyseal regions of humerus, femur, and tibia; and along the margins of the rib and lamina dura of the teeth. Brown tumors, also known as *osteoclastomas*, are localized collections of fibrous tissue and giant cells that replace bone and cause expansion. These lesions can degenerate and undergo necrotic liquefaction, producing cystic changes. Osteoclastomas have radiolucent "soap bubble–like" appearance and are seen most frequently in the metaphyseal regions of the long bones, facial bones, ribs, and bony pelvis.

ADRENAL IMAGING

The adrenal glands are situated in the perirenal fascia and are surrounded by adipose tissue. The right adrenal gland is located lateral to the right diaphragmatic crus, medial to the right lobe of the liver, anterior and superior to the upper pole of the right kidney, and posterior to the inferior vena cava. The left adrenal gland is located lateral to the aorta and the left diaphragmatic crus, medial to the spleen, anterior and medial to the upper pole of the left kidney, and posterior to body and tail of the pancreas and the splenic vessels. The left adrenal gland extends down to the level of the renal hilum in 10% of individuals (28). The adrenal cortex arises from the coelomic mesoderm, whereas the medullary portion of the adrenal gland develops from neuroectodermal tissue. During the fetal and neonatal period, the adrenal gland consists of two cortical layers. A thick inner cortex involutes over the first year of life, and a thin outer cortex becomes the adult cortex. Serial US examinations have shown a 40% to 50% decrease in size in the first 6 weeks of life (29). Each limb of the newborn adrenal gland measures 0.9–3.6 cm. in length and 0.2–0.5 cm in thickness, whereas in older children and adults, it measures 4–6 cm in length and 1 cm in thickness.

Adrenal Cortex Tumors

The adrenal cortex produces glucocorticoids, mineralocorticoids, and sex hormones and is controlled by the pituitary through corticotropin (ACTH). Functioning adrenal adenomas have been reported with Gardner syndrome or in patients with multiple endocrine neoplasia type 1 syndrome. Autonomous aldosterone-secreting adenoma is the most frequent cause of primary hyperaldosteronism, with adrenal carcinoma being a rare cause. These adenomas, called *aldosteronomas*, are small, usually less than 3 cm in diameter (30). Their US appearance is identical to that of the adenomas causing Cushing syndrome. On CT scan without contrast material, they classically appear hypodense (31).

Abdominal US shows that adrenal adenomas and carcinomas are moderately echogenic, solid masses ranging between 2 and 5 cm in diameter. Large tumors often exhibit radiating or stellate-type of linear echoes due to fibrous tissue. Sometimes an echogenic capsule-like rim is seen. Echogenic foci secondary to calcifications occur more commonly with carcinoma than with adenoma. Adrenal carcinomas may be bilateral and, in the absence of metastatic disease or gross infiltration of adjacent structures, are indistinguishable from adenomas. In addition, both these lesions cannot be differentiated from neuroblastoma on US examination alone.

On CT scan, small adrenal adenomas and carcinomas appear as well-defined, round homogeneous masses of low attenuation. The tissue density ranges between 0 and 30 Hounsfield units due to the high lipid content (30). Larger adrenal carcinomas frequently have a heterogeneous appearance or may contain central low-attenuation areas due to hemorrhage or necrosis. On MRI, adrenal adenomas larger than 1.5 cm are well visualized, and the signal intensity is usually similar to that of normal adrenal tissue. When there is central necrosis and ill-defined borders, the mass tends to be an adrenal carcinoma.

Enzymatic Defects and Metabolic Diseases of the Adrenal

Congenital Adrenal Hyperplasia Congenital adrenal hyperplasia (CAH) is an autosomal recessive disorder caused by an inborn error in the enzymatic production of cortisol or aldosterone. More than 90% of cases are due to 21-hydroxylase deficiency, whereas most of the remaining cases are due to 11β-hydroxylase and 3β-hydroxysteroid dehydrogenase deficiency.

Microscopically, the adrenal glands show diffuse cortical hyperplasia, most impressively in the zona reticularis. US examination shows that the adrenal glands maintain corticomedullary differentiation but are slightly enlarged or at least are at the upper limit of normal in size. In a neonate with ambiguous genitalia, a mean adrenal length of 20 mm or greater and a mean width of 4 mm or greater while maintaining normal pyramidal configuration is considered consistent with the diagnosis of CAH and helps to differentiate CAH from other causes of ambiguous genitalia in the neonatal period. Al-Allwan reported on 52 children with ambiguous genitalia or salt loss in whom US had a sensivity of 92% and a specificity of 100% for the diagnosis of CAH (32). Overall size, surface characteristics, and internal echo pattern of the adrenal on US examination were used to make the diagnosis. Presence of two or more of the following three signs was considered diagnostic of CAH: 1) measurements of the width of the adrenal limbs over 4 mm are considered abnormal, but some neonates with no clinical signs of CAH may have large adrenals as well; in addition, 28% of neonates with confirmed CAH may not show an absolute enlargement but may have adrenal size in the upper range of normal; 2) the surface of the adrenal glands with CAH is much more undulating than normal; in 25 cases of CAH, 23 had this appearance; 3) the central hyperechoic stripe may be replaced by a diffuse, thickened band of echogenicity.

A rare form of CAH is lipoid adrenal hyperplasia, which leads to markedly enlarged adrenals and defective synthesis of glucocorticoids, mineralocorticoids, and sex steroids (33). On CT examination, massively enlarged adrenal glands show remarkably diminished attenuation values similar to that of fat (34).

Wolman Disease Wolman disease, or familial xanthomatosis, is an autosomal recessive inborn error of lipid metabolism, characterized by massive accumulation of cholesterol esters and triglycerides in all tissues of the body, such as liver, spleen, intestines, kidneys, thymus, adrenals, and blood cells (35). Failure to thrive, anemia, vomiting, diarrhea, steatorrhea and abdominal distension, and hepatosplenomegaly are noted in early infancy. Microscopically, the adrenal cortex contains lipid-laden cells and large areas of necrosis and calcification. The adrenal medulla is not involved. Most patients do not survive beyond their first birthday.

Plain radiographs of the abdomen may show densely calcified enlarged adrenal glands. US examination of the abdomen will confim these findings with hyperechoic enlarged adrenal glands leading to distinct acoustic shadowing in addition to massive hepatosplenomegaly. The adrenal glands show dense cortical calcifications without displacement of the kidneys or distortion of the pelvicaliceal systems. Also noted is a remarkable paucity of subcutaneous fat. The thickened bowel walls secondary to fat deposition within the lamina propria appear highly echogenic. CT scan of the abdomen will show an enlarged liver with a decreased attenuation value that may be less than that of the spleen. CT examination of the thorax shows involuted thymus.

Adrenal Medulla

The adrenal medulla is the site of origin of nearly 90% of all pheochromocytomas, which are catecholamine-secreting tumors arising from chromaffin cells of the sympathetic nervous system. When such a tumor arises in an extra-adrenal location, it is termed as a *paraganglioma*. These tumors can arise from any site along the course of the sympathetic chain, the organ of Zuckerkandl located at the level of bifurcation of abdominal aorta into two common iliac arteries, urinary bladder wall, and periureteral regions. Only 5% of pheochromocytomas are seen in children. There is an increased incidence in patients with multiple endocrine neoplasia (MEN) syndromes, usually MEN types 2A and 2B, and in patients with von Hippel Lindau disease and neurofibromatosis I and II. Multiple or bilateral tumors appear more likely in these syndromes. Pheochromocytomas usually are benign, and only 13% show malignant change (30). Common sites of metastasis are liver, lungs, lymph nodes, and bone.

Clinical features are paroxysmal hypertensive episodes, headaches, tachycardia, and palpitations. US examination of pheochromocytoma is nonspecific, and differentiation from other adrenal tumors requires biochemical studies. Only because many of these tumors are bilateral and multiple can US examination identify a fairly large homogeneous solid mass or masses with sharp margins, measuring more than 2 cm in diameter. Larger lesions show a heterogeneous solid echo pattern. CT scanning, MRI, and scintigraphy are the preferred imaging modalities in patients with clinical and biochemical evidence of pheochromocytoma. CT scanning without intravenous contrast material is the safer and preferred diagnostic imaging modality. Intravenous contrast material should be used only if the patient is premedicated with blocking agents to avoid the risk of a hypertensive crisis. On unenhanced CT scan, the tumor is seen as a low-density mass due to the presence of hemosiderin. Larger tumors may show areas of hemorrhage and necrosis and intense enhancement after intravenous contrast material administration. This enhancement may be mottled or peripheral. Only 10% to 15% of the tumors show punctuate calcifications. On T1-weighted MRI, the mass is isointense to the adjacent renal parenchyma. On T2-weighted imaging, the mass shows increased signal intensity. The presence and the extent of hemorrhage in the tumor can result in variable nonhomogeneity.

Neuroblastomas are common solid malignant tumors of children between the ages of 1 and 5 years. The most common location is the adrenal gland, but they can occur along the entire course of the sympathetic ganglia from the base of the skull down to the floor of the pelvis. US examination shows a large heterogeneous mass of ill-defined margins located in one or both suprarenal areas. Sonolucent areas may be seen in the mass if there is hemorrhage or necrosis. They frequently show small echogenic foci secondary to punctuate calcifications. CT examination shows a large, irregularly shaped mass in the suprarenal area with focal areas of calcifications and with variable contrast enhancement. CT scan helps to evaluate the local extent of the disease and also distant metastasis. MRI is best for detection of bone marrow involvement. On T1-weighted images, the bone marrow metastases have low signal. Congenital neuroblastoma and adrenal hemorrhage can have a similar appearance in the neonatal period. Adrenal hemorrhage usually tends to resolve over the first few weeks or months of life, on occassion leaving behind a few areas of residual calcification. Cystic congenital neuroblastoma may remain unchanged or may enlarge.

Meta-iodo-benzyl-guanidine (MIBG) is a norepinephrine analogue that localizes in both neuroblastomas and pheochromocytomas. It is labeled with iodine-123 (^{123}I). Whole-body scintigraphy is performed 24 and 48 hours after the intravenous injection of the scintigraphic agent. Tomographic images of the areas of interest are obtained. MIBG–^{123}I is a tumor-specific agent rather than being an organ-specific agent and hence localizes to the sites of primary as well as all the metastatic lesions. Standard bone scintigraphy is useful to distinguish bone cortical metastases from bone marrow metastases. Frequently, the primary lesion also may show the radionuclide uptake.

PANCREATIC IMAGING

Pancreatic Neoplasms

Pancreatic tumors are rare in children. They can be classified into nonfunctioning tumors that usually arise from the exocrine portion of the pancreas and functioning or islet cell tumors. Most nonfunctioning pancreatic tumors are adenocarcinomas and are aggressive malignant lesions. They frequently arise from the head of the pancreas or the uncinate process and manifest a propensity for local invasion, obstruction of the pancreatic and common bile ducts, and metastatic disease to adjacent lymph nodes or the liver. Pancreatoblastoma is a well-encapsulated pancreatic carcinoma that is almost always found in the head of the pancreas. It has a very distinctive histopathological appearance resembling the fetal pancreas at about the eighth week of development. Other nonfunctioning pancreatic tumors include hemangioendothelioma, lymphangioma, sarcoma, and lymphoma. The present discussion will be limited only to the functioning pancreatic tumors.

Islet Cell Tumors

The islet cell tumors are endocrine tumors of the pancreas. They arise from neural crest tissue that gives rise to cells of the islets of Langerhans. Most of these tumors are hormonally active and produce increased amounts of polypeptide hormones such as insulin, gastrin, glucagon, vasoactive intestinal peptide, and somatostatin. These islet cell tumors may secrete more than one hormone but usually are labeled after the hormone that is most responsible for the clinical signs and symptoms. Approximately 50% of these tumors are malignant. Lesions less than 3 cm in diameter tend to be benign, and those more than 3 cm in diameter tend to be malignant. Islet cell tumors are seen in children with multiple endocrine neoplasia type 1 (MEN-1 syndrome), von Hippel–Lindau disease, and other phacomatoses (36) and can be found anywhere in the gland; however, the majority of them (52%) are located in the head and the uncinate process of the pancreas.

Insulinomas are the most common type of islet cell tumor. Most insulinomas are benign, solitary, and usually smaller than 2 cm in size. Their US findings are nonspecific and are very much similar to those of other types of islet cell tumors. The tumors are hypoechoic compared with the adjacent pancreas but may have an echogenic capsule. Cystic changes and central necrosis are seen rarely. Color Doppler US shows the tumor to be hypervascular. Intraoperative US examination can be very useful in localizing these small lesions. CT scanning should be done with and without intravenous contrast material. On CT scan, before intravenous contrast administration, the tumor may have slightly lower attenuation than the adjacent pancreatic tissue, but it enhances following administration of contrast material. On MRI, the signal intensity of the normal pancreas is similar to that of the liver parenchyma with both T1- and T2-weighted imaging. The tumors, however, have low signal intensity on T1-weighted imaging and high signal intensity on T2-weighted images. If the tumor has high signal intensity on both T1- and T2-weighted imaging, hemorrhage is likely (37). The tumors tend to enhance with contrast on MRI.

Gastrinomas are the second most common type of islet cell tumor and usually present with peptic ulcer disease and diarrhea. Gastrinomas, unlike the insulinomas, are frequently malignant and tend to have liver metastasis at the time of diagnosis. They tend to be larger, measuring 4–7 cm in diameter. They also tend to have cystic changes secondary to central necrosis, calcifications, local soft tissue or vascular invasion, and distant metastasis. US examination may show cystic changes and calcifications, and their CT scan and MRI appearance is similar to the insulinomas, with the exception of the size, calcifications, and central necrosis and distant metastasis. All types of islet cell tumors with the exception of somatostatinoma can occur in MEN-1 syndrome; however, 75% are gastrinomas and lead to Zollinger–Ellison syndrome, and the majority of the remaining neoplasms are insulinomas.

Glucagonomas, VIPomas (vasoactive intestinal peptide–secreting tumors), and somatostatinomas are extremely rare types of islet cell tumors. If they are smaller than 2 cm in diameter, their imaging characteristics are similar to those of insulinomas, whereas if they are larger than 3 cm in diameter, their imaging pattern more often resembles that of a gastrinoma.

There are a few islet cell tumors that are hormonally inactive, but they are large, with an average size of 8 cm, and usually are detected because they cause pain or symptoms related to metastases. They tend to show necrosis, central cystic changes, dystrophic calcifications, and malignant transformation. Their imaging characteristics are identical to those of many other large pancreatic masses.

GONADAL IMAGING

Radiological Evaluation of Children with Ambiguous Genitalia

The term *ambiguous genitalia* is used when the phenotypic sex of an infant is indeterminate. Various imaging modalities are useful in providing anatomical details of the genital and urinary tracts. These anatomical findings, along with careful clinical, chromosomal, and hormonal evaluation, are critical in determining the sex in infants with ambiguous genitalia.

US of the pelvis should include examination of the scrotal/labial and inguinal regions. Male or female gonadal structures are identified and their morphology carefully analyzed. The examination is performed through a distended urinary bladder for an adequate examination of the pelvic structures. Newborn female infant's ovaries often will contain hypoechoic follicles secondary to stimulation from the maternal estrogen in utero and also through breastfeeding. Undescended testes may be seen in the inguinal regions. Testes have a solid, homogeneous echogenic structure. US appearance of the ectopically located gonadal tissue is often atypical. Fluid-filled structures posterior to the urinary bladder may represent a dilated vagina in a girl but could represent a distended prostatic utricle in a boy. Presence or absence of the uterus is noted. The endometrial canal usually is collapsed and appears as a thin stripe. The presence of fluid/menstrual products can cause prominence and increased echogenicity.

Fluoroscopic genitography is performed by serially injecting water-soluble contrast agents into the catheterized orifices in the perineum. The appearance of the vagina, uterine cervical impression on the cephalic portion of the vagina, urinary bladder, and urethra is studied carefully for any congenital anomalies, including duplications and fistulous communications.

MRI is very useful in demonstrating the presence, absence, or any abnormalities of genital structures, including uterus, vagina, and gonads (Figure 50-8). Undescended intrapelvic testes are better visualized on MRI than on US examination. US examination frequently will detect undescended testis situated in the inguinal canal, but MRI is needed in every other instance of undescended testis. The undescended testis and its epididymis have a normal US appearance. They demonstrate high signal intensity on T2-weighted images.

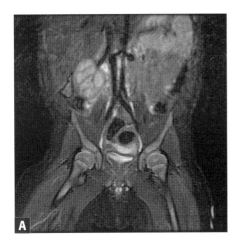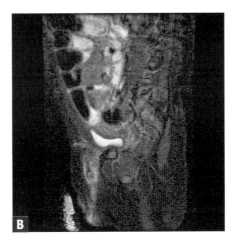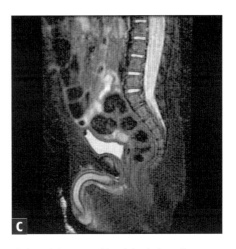

FIGURE 50-8. A to **C.** Persistent Mullerian Duct Syndrome: Coronal and sagittal images showing presence of a phallus, presence of a intrapelvic uterus and intraabdominal gonad. (A) Oblong shape testis to the right of the uterus in coronal image. (B) The bladder appears white with the uterus the oblong structure on top of it. (C) The gonad is on top of the bladder. This gonad has no follicles and its characteristics are consistent with testes (confirmed by microscopic study).

OVARIAN IMAGING

Typically, at least one ovary can be seen by US examination in about 80% of girls younger than 5 years and 90% in girls older than 5 years of age. Both ovaries can be seen in about 65% and 80%, respectively (19). A normal US examination of a menstruating female will show multiple small ovarian follicles (5–7 mm in size) and, depending on the time of the cycle, a dominant follicle (Figure 50-9).

US examination is critical in girls with primary amenorrhea to evaluate presence or absence of the ovaries and the uterus. US assessment of uterine size, shape, and maturity and ovarian developmental status can provide guidance to the etiology of amenorrhea. A small or absent uterus may indicate gonadal dysgenesis, decreased hormonal states, testicular feminization, or isolated uterine hypoplasia or agenesis. Girls with Turner syndrome and pure 45,XO karyotypes have a prepubertal uterus and ovaries that are not visualized; patients with the 45,XO/46,XX karyotype have uterine size ranging from prepubertal to an intermediate length (less than normal adult) and ovaries with variable appearance ranging from absent to streak ovaries to even normal adult-sized ovaries. In Noonan syndrome, there are phenotypic changes of Turner syndrome but normal-appearing and -functioning ovaries. Patients with the 46,XY karyotype and complete androgen receptor defects of testosterone deficiency are phenotypic females and do not have a uterus or ovaries.

When an ovarian follicle continues to grow after failed ovulation, or when it does not collapse after ovulation, ovarian cysts may result. The difference between frequently seen functional cysts and pathological cysts and the physiological follicle in postmenarchal girls is based on size alone, with cysts larger than 3 cm in diameter considered pathological. Simple cysts less than 4 cm in diameter can be followed with serial US until resolution (Figure 50-10). Most of these resolve in 3–4 months. Ovarian cysts can be associated with congenital juvenile hypothyroidism and McCune–Albright syndrome.

In polycystic ovarian disease, the ovaries are enlarged, with mean ovarian volume of 14 mL in 70% of patients. On US examination, there are increased follicles at least 5–8 mm in diameter throughout the ovaries in approximately 40% of patients, although maturing follicles are rare. MRI is more accurate in demonstrating the characteristic peripheral cysts or follicles.

Ovarian neoplasms account for approximately 1% of all childhood neoplasms and are classified according to the cell of origin. In children, 60% of primary ovarian tumors are of germ cell origin. Approximately 75% to 95% of germ cell tumors in childhood are benign teratomas (Figure 50-11). Approximately 10% of teratomas are bilateral. Teratomas may contain hair, teeth, bone and very rarely more complex organs such as eyeball, torso, and hand. Calcification, ossification and teeth are not well seen on MRI and they may cause susceptibility artifact; CT, and to a lesser extent, x-ray and ultrasound show these findings directly. However, in girls younger than 10 years of age, 84% of ovarian germ cell tumors are malignant, and dysgerminoma is the most common malignant germ cell tumor. It occurs frequently before puberty, and 10% are bilateral. The tumor usually is a large, solid, encapsulated, rapidly growing mass containing hypoechoic areas secondary to hemorrhage, necrosis, and cystic degeneration. Retroperitoneal lymphadenopathy is present frequently. Embryonal carcinoma and endometrial sinus tumor are other pediatric malignant germ cell tumors but are less common, and choriocarcinoma is extremely rare.

Approximately 20% are epithelial in origin but rarely occur before puberty. These include serous and mucinous cystadenoma or

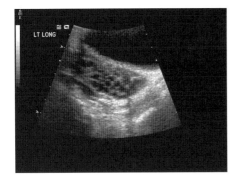

FIGURE 50-9. Normal ovary showing multiple small ovarian follicles on the sixth day of the menstrual cycle. The follicles are between 5-7 mm in size and the dominant follicle has yet to be formed.

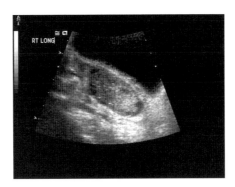

FIGURE 50-10. Ovary with hemorrhagic cyst: Ovary showing normal follicles in the upper half and showing area of hemorrhage in the lower half as an area of increased brightness and echogenicity.

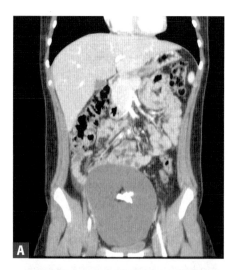

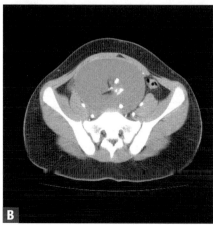

FIGURE 50-11. A to **B.** Ovarian teratoma: Coronal (A) and axial (B) contrast enhanced CT scan showing large ovarian mass (11 × 8 cm) containing multiple areas of calcification. Areas of low attenuation adjacent to these calcifications represent adipose tissue.

cystadenocarcinoma. On US examination, they are predominantly cystic, with septa of variable thickness. About 20% of ovarian tumors in childhood are of stromal cell origin. Of these, granulosa cell tumor is the most common. It is often associated with feminizing effects and precocious puberty as a result of estrogen production. These tumors are bilateral in 10%, and only 3% are malignant. They tend to be predominantly solid in appearance on US examination. Other primary stromal ovarian tumors include the rare Sertoli–Leydig cell tumor (arrhenoblastoma), which may lead to virilization and gonadoblastoma. Gonadoblastoma is a rare ovarian tumor that contains both germ cell and stromal elements and has an increased incidence in patients with Turner syndrome and a karyotype with Y chromosome mosaicism or individuals with the 46,XY karyotype and dysgenetic gonads. They are bilateral in a third of cases, and in 50%, dysgerminoma elements are present (18).

The signs and symptoms of ovarian tumor depend on its size, as well as on whether it is benign or malignant, produces hormone, causes internal hemorrhage, ruptures or undergoes spontaneous torsion, or has any effects on adjacent structures. Hormonally active tumors can produce precocious puberty, vaginal bleeding, or virilization. The most common presentation is asymptomatic abdominal enlargement, palpable pelvic mass, or abdominal pain.

US examination is an invaluable imaging technique. It accurately localizes the mass in the adnexal region and recognizes whether the lesion is cystic, solid, or a combination of both. It detects lymphadenopathy, obstructive uropathy, ascites, and solid-organ metastasis. In the absence of such metastatic disease or frank invasion of adjacent structures, differentiation between benign and malignant lesions is not possible. CT scanning is of greater value than US in evaluation of large ovarian neoplasms. The CT scan is more accurate than US in evaluating any invasion of the adjacent structures. Other US findings are easily confirmed on CT examination. The presence of calcification, ossification, tooth, or fat, characteristic findings seen in teratoma, can be recognized easily on US, CT scan, MRI, or plain radiographic examination.

TESTICULAR IMAGING

The US examination and MRI are the two best imaging modalities for testes. Intrascrotal testicular masses can identified on US examination in nearly 100% of cases, but the accurate differentiation between intra- and extratesticular neoplasms cannot be accomplished in all cases. This differentiation is critical because most intratesticular tumors are malignant (80%), whereas extratesticular lesions tend to be benign.

Cryptorchidism

Testicular descent occurs between 25 and 32 weeks' gestation in 97% of fetuses. At birth, undescended testes are found in about 33% of premature male infants weighing less than 2500 g and 4% of full-term infants. The testicular descent continues in the postnatal period so that by the end of the 1st year in life, only 0.7% to 0.8% of infants have true cryptorchidism (20). Undescended testis tends to be bilateral in 10% to 25%. The testicular migration can be arrested anywhere along the course of descent from the retroperitoneum into the scrotum. Only 20% of undescended testes are not palpable on clinical examination. They can be detected by US examination because about 80% to 90% of these clinically not palpable testes are located in the inguinal

canal. Testes located well above the inguinal ring are identified on MRI. Localization of the undescended testis is important because there is a higher incidence of malignancy, torsion, and infertility. The incidence of malignancy in an abdominal undescended testis is increased by a factor of 30–50.

On US examination, an undescended testis appears as an elliptical-shaped mass with homogeneous echogenicity. The undescended testis tends to be hypoechoic and smaller than the normally descended contralateral testis (Figure 50-12). Gubernaculum testis (i.e., a mesenchymal column of tissue that connects the fetal testis to the developing scrotum and is involved in testicular descent) generally atrophies when the testicular descent is complete and tends to be present as a round or ovoid-shaped hypoechoic fibrous remnant. It can be differentiated from the undescended testis by the presence of a mediastinum testis (i.e., a mass of connective tissue at the back of the testis that encloses the rete testis) (see Figure 50-12A). Even after surgery, the undescended testis tends to stay hypoechoic in appearance.

Testicular Tumors

Testicular tumors account for about 1% of childhood neoplasms and 2% solid malignant tumors in boys (21). Between 70% and 90% of primary testicular tumors are of germ cell

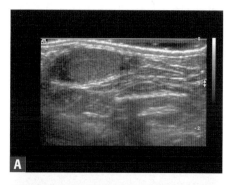

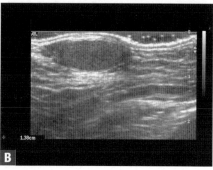

FIGURE 50-12. A to **B.** Normal testis: two longitudinal scans of a testis. Testis is ovoid shaped and has homogeneous medium level echostructure. (A) Central echogenic stripe represents mediastinum testes. (B) The triangular structure proximal to the testes on the second image represents epididymis.

origin, and 66% to 82% of these are endodermal sinus tumors, which are also known as *yolk sac carcinomas*. The remaining germ cell tumors are benign tereatomas, embryonal carcinomas, teratocarcinomas, and choriocarcinomas. Yolk sac carcinomas tend to occur in prepubescent boys (median age 2 years), whereas the other malignancies occur in adolescents or young adults. Teratomas, which are the major benign germ cell tumor, usually are found in boys younger than 4 years of age. Nearly 85% of these have well-differentiated elements from all three germ layers. The other 15%, despite poor differentiation and immature elements, follow a benign course. Teratomas in pubertal boys tend to behave more aggressively and are often malignant. Seminoma, which is the most common testicular tumor in adults, is rare in children. When it does occur in this population, it is usually found during adolescence. Despite it being uncommon in the pediatric age group, it is the neoplasm associated most commonly with an undescended testis. Stromal tumors account for approximately 10% of testicular neoplasms and often present with gynecomastia or premature virilization. Nearly 60% of non–germ cell tumors are Leydig cell tumors, whereas the other 40% are Sertoli cell tumors. Sertoli cell tumors, although commonly hormonally inactive, can produce estrogens, which can lead to gynecomastia. They commonly occur in the first year of life. On the other hand, Leydig cell tumors typically are found in patients between 3 and 6 years of age and produce testosterone with resulting precocious virilization. Both these tumors are benign in prepubertal patients. Another rare tumor is gonadoblastoma, which is found in phenotypic females with streak gonads and in patients with a male karyotype and testes. These lesions are usually small, well circumscribed, and hypoechoic. They become enlarged if there are areas of hemorrhage or necrosis and show large cystic areas. Typically, gonadoblastomas are benign, solid, and hypoechoic masses that usually are found at the time of surgery to remove intra-abdominal dysgenetic gonads.

US examination shows nonspecific findings that are useful in tissue diagnosis in most testicular tumors (Figure 50-13). The lesion may appear as a well-defined testicular mass that is easily distinguishable from the surrounding normal tissue, or there could be diffuse testicular enlargement. In some instances, testicular tumors show a variable echogenicity, ranging from hypoechoic to hyperechoic. In other instances, the tumors may appear homogeneous or may have a heterogeneous appearance. There may be areas of increased echogenicity, representing calcifications, or areas of decreased echogenicity,

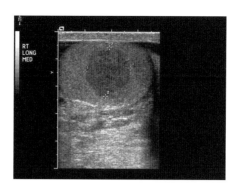

FIGURE 50-13. Leukemic testicular infiltration: Large hypoecoic area in the right testes showing leukemic infiltration. Both testes were enlarged and were affected. Such infiltrations on a much smaller scale are present in 25% of boys at the time of diagnosis. It is seen in 15% of boys while in bone marrow remission but is present in nearly 80% at autopsy.

indicating areas of necrosis and/or hemorrhage. Leydig cell and Sertoli cell tumors typically are small, well-circumscribed, hypoechoic lesions. Cystic spaces resulting from hemorrhage or necrosis may be seen in larger lesions (22).

EVALUATION OF SKELETAL MATURATION

Bone Age

The Greulich and Pyle atlas method (23), developed from films taken in the 1930s and 1940s, is still the most frequently used standard for evaluation of skeletal maturation for children older than 2 years of age. The atlas calls for comprehensive analysis of all bones of the hand and wrist compared with a standard set from the median of a range evaluated for each chronological age. For children under the age of 2 years, the method described by Sontag, Snell, and Anderson in 1939 (24) is preferred because only a very limited number of secondary and primary ossification centers for carpals appear on the radiograph of the hand and wrist before that age.

The advantage of using the hand and wrist area after the age of 2 years is that a single radiograph covers as many as 30 different ossification centers. Osteogenesis is a process of calcification and ossification of cartilage tissue, and chondroplasia is the process of cartilage differentiation and growth. Radiographs of an infant show no secondary ossification centers, and this reflects sheer osteogenesis. Only when the secondary ossification centers of the phalanges and metacarpals appear and the growth plate becomes visible can we have a glimpse at the chondroplasia. In later childhood and adolescence, the appearance of these secondary ossification centers and their maturation and subsequent fusion with the

diaphyses reflect a combination of osteogenesis and chondroplasia. Maturity of the phalanges and metacarpals corresponds with the growth and maturity of the long bones such as the femur and tibia. Maturity of the carpals seems to correspond with growth and maturation of the vertebral column.

GH is a major stimulus of osteogenesis and, to lesser extent, also of chondroplasia. GH deficiency impairs these processes in that order of severity. Thus carpals are much more retarded than other bones. Normal thyroid hormone function is a prerequisite for any growth or bone maturation. Hypothyroidism has a drastic effect on osteogenesis and less severe effect on chondroplasia. Thus, in cretinism, in addition to severely retarded maturation, the epiphyseal ossification centers show stippled appearance and simulate epiphyseal dysplasia.

Gonadal and adrenal steroids (sex steroids) are essential for the growth spurt and bone maturation at puberty, as well as for bone mineral homeostasis. The role of adrenal androgens is less well defined. Some of their effects may be indirect, through estrogen action on the GH–IGF-1 axis, but others have direct effects in cartilage and bone. Estrogen and progesterone receptors are abundant in proliferating and hypertrophic chondrocytes, as well as in osteoclasts, where estrogens inhibit bone resorption and osteoblast activity (26). The fundamental role of sex steroids in bone maturation becomes obvious from the marked delay in skeletal maturity of children with delayed puberty (Figure 50-14) and its

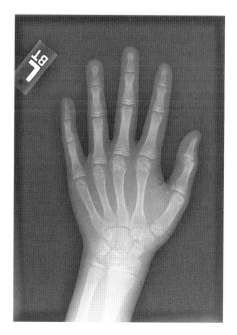

FIGURE 50-14. Retarded Skeletal Maturation: GHD secondary to cranial pharyngioma. This 14 year old boy had a skeletal maturation of a boy of 11 years 6 months of age and is 2.5 SD below mean.

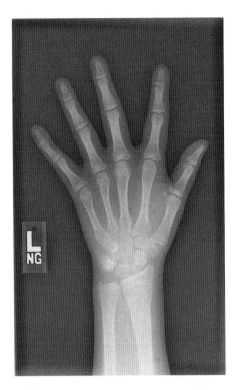

FIGURE 50-15. Advanced Skeletal Maturation: This 9 year and 9 month old girl with precocious puberty has a skeletal maturation of 13 years and 6 months of age, an advance skeletal maturation of 4 SD.

advancement in precocious puberty (Figure 50-15). Bone maturation in precocious puberty is characterized by advanced maturity of both chondroplasia and osteogenesis. Chondroplasia, however, is much more profoundly affected than osteogenesis. Sex steroids affect the maturation process of phalanges and metacarpals to a far greater extent than they affect carpals, radii, or ulnae.

Sex steroids do not affect bone development in utero or during the first 6 months of life. The skeletal maturation of newborns with CAH is normal at birth and for several months later. If untreated, the skeletal maturation of the phalanges and metacarpals progresses very rapidly until such time that the glucocorticoid-replacement therapy can result in complete arrest of bone maturation for several years until catch-down growth is achieved. The same is true for patients with central precocious puberty after they are treated with gonadotropin-suppressing GnRH analogue. At the other extreme, when the patients with delayed puberty are treated with sex steroids, rapid bone maturation proceeds with catch-up growth.

Skeletal maturation is a good predictor of the age of menarche in girls and the age of peak growth velocity in boys.

The mechanism of growth retardation in Turner syndrome has not been resolved. Delay in bone maturation is seen in both pre- and postpubertal Turner patients. Metacarpals and phalanges are shorter, with increasing growth deficiency from distal to proximal and from lateral to medial bones. Metacarpals and phalanges show the most impressive retardation of growth, carpals show moderate retardation, and the least delay in maturation is seen in radius and ulna. The unique profile of bone maturation in Turner syndrome suggests an insult to chondroplasia, which may be related to estrogen deficiency or to an as yet undetermined endocrine or paracrine derangement (25,27).

Radiological Signs Characteristic of Turner Syndrome

Metacarpal Sign A line drawn tangentially to the distal end of the heads of the 4th and 5th metacarpals normally extends distal to the head of the 3rd metacarpal. When it runs tangential, it is considered borderline for Turner syndrome. When the line passes the head of the 3rd metacarpal, it is considered a positive accessory sign of Turner syndrome.

Phalangeal Sign The length of the 4th metacarpal usually is the same as the total of the lengths of the proximal and distal phalanges. It rarely exceeds more than 2 mm. When the total exceeds the length of the metacarpal by 3 mm or more, it is a positive accessory sign of Turner syndrome.

Practical Approach

Bones mature in an orderly fashion. Deviation from such an orderly sequence can be useful in dating a severe systemic insult, malnutrition, or an endocrine pathology. One must recognize that there is a great deal of inter- and intraobserver variability.

For a child older than 2 years of age

- Identify the secondary ossification centers of the phalanges and metacarpals. See how many and which one are present.

- If all the secondary centers have appeared (boys 4–4.5 years; girls 2.5–3 years), note the extent of their maturation by noting their size in comparison with the adjacent metaphysis and their shape at the adjacent articulation. Note the width of the adjacent growth plate and see if is partially or totally fused with the diaphysis. Secondary ossifications usually appear from proximal to distal and fuse from distal to proximal.

- Check as to how many carpals have ossified. Capitate and hamate appear at 3 months in both boys and girls. The pisiform is the last to ossify (boys 10.5 years; girls 8.5–9 years).

- Check if the sesamoid of the thumb has appeared (boys 13 years; girls 11 years).

- Note the sex of the child, and match the collected data with the closest matching standard radiographical plate from the Greulich and Pyle atlas. Make sure to open the correct half of the atlas that is appropriate for the sex of the patient. Note the maturation of the carpals as well as the phalanges and metacarpals separately if the disparity is significant.

- Double check with the next and previous plate to confirm your evaluation. You may give intermediate scores with experience.

- Calculate the difference between skeletal maturation and the chronological age in months.

- Use the given standard deviations to evaluate maturation.

- Look for disease-specific pathology, hypoplastic phalanges or metacarpals, growth arrest lines, irregular epiphysis, and metabolic changes such as rickets or skeletal dysplasia.

- Compare with the previous studies.

For a child younger than 2 years of age, obtain radiographs of the left hemiskeleton. A separate radiograph of the left foot is required frequently. A separate view of the left hand is required only if the radiograph of the upper extremity does not include the entire anteroposterior view of the hand. Count the number of the secondary ossification centers that have appeared, and add that number to that the number of primary ossification centers of the carpals. Primary ossification centers of all tarsals, with the exception of talus and calcaneus, are counted. Now one should refer to the tables and the standard deviations provided by Sontag and colleagues (24) and calculate the skeletal maturation.

Skeletal Dysplasias, Dysostoses, and Metabolic Disorders

Skeletal dysplasias are intrinsic disorders of growth of cartilage or bone. Dysostoses are bone malformations due to disturbance or defect in the development of ectodermal or mesenchymal tissue. There are so far more than 200 well-defined skeletal dysplasias. At least 70% of these are often lethal in the perinatal period. The purpose of this text will be to instruct young physicians on how to identify the key elements of the skeletal malformations. In most instances, by learning the basic principles discussed here and applying them in daily practice, one would be able to make a reasonable assessment of the most likely diagnosis. Later, by referring to more exhaustive texts on this subject, the astute clinician would confirm the initial diagnosis and also gain additional knowledge about other subtle findings associated with the disease.

Dysostoses are malformations secondary to transient signaling defects during organogenesis. Because this defective process is transient, only specific malformations are observed, such as isolated polydactyly or short first metacarpal, as in Holt–Oram syndrome. These signaling defects may occur singly, in combination, or as part of pleiotropic disorders if the controlling gene is expressed in many organ systems. Dysostotic lesions may be distributed asymmetrically. Dwarfism usually is not a primary manifestation.

Dysplasias result if the defects of the prenatally expressing genes continue to express those defects in the postnatal period. Mutated genes expressed in chondro-osseous tissues lead to primary skeletal dysplasias. When extraosseous factors such as errors of metabolism affect the skeleton, secondary dysplasias such as hypophosphatemic rickets are observed.

Most of the bone dysplasias result in clinically disproportionate short stature individuals. Symmetrical shortening simply may represent constitutional delay or familial short stature. However, if an infant or a child were to be dysmorphic on clinical evaluation and/or have multiple congenital anomalies, one needs to obtain a skeletal survey. Although the radiographical findings play a major role in the diagnosis of dysplasia or dysostoses, only by putting together the clinical findings, family history, and laboratory data can one make a tentative diagnosis. Sometimes follow-up skeletal surveys and skeletal surveys of other members of the family lead to an accurate diagnosis.

The very first step in the diagnosis of skeletal dysplasias is to assess if there is any disproportional growth of the skeleton in the first place and, if present, where. Shortening of the extremity may be "rhizomelic", "mesomelic" or "acromelic". In rhizomelic shortening the most impressive shortening involves the proximal third of the limbs closest to the trunk. This means short humeri/upper arms and short femora/thighs. In mesomelic shortening there is disproportionate shortening of radii and ulnae/forearms and shortening of tibiae and fibulae/legs. In acromelic shortening the most impressive shortening involves the distal thirds of the limbs. The hands and feet are small because the bones in hands and feet are short. *Micromelia* refers to severe shortening of bones of all four extremities.

Clinically, the first step would be to assess if the shortening is generalized and symmetrical or instead there is a disproportionate shortening in any particular region, such as trunk, arms/thighs or forearms/legs, or hands/feet. This clinical rhizomelia/mesomelia/acromelia must be confirmed by the radiographic examinations. This is so because the clinical evaluations frequently are guided by the skin creases and folds and not by the true length of the underlying bone. At this stage, it is important to note if there are any vertebral anomalies, such as platyspondyly, to help explain the truncal shortening, if present.

There are several syndromes such as achondroplasia, hypochondroplasia, and metaphyseal dysplasias that manifest rhizomelic shortening on a consistent basis. There are many dysplasias with predominant mesomelic involvement. There are well-defined skeletal anomalies such as Madelung deformity, as noted in dyschondrosteosis. There are various permutations and combinations of this mesomelic shortening with or without acromelic involvement that lead to a variety of other dysplasias. Acromelic dysplasia/dysostosis is secondary to abnormal formation of phalanges or metacarpals and metatarsals. Such brachydactyly occurs in many syndromes as part of a generalized bone dysplasia, as can be observed in patients with achondroplasia or diastrophic dysplasia. The isolated brachydactylies are dysostoses rather than dysplasias. However, they can be a part of a dysplasia noted in brachydactyly B, brachydactyly C, or heterogeneous expression of the Robinow or Grebe dysplasia gene.

Once the presence of skeletal disproportion is confirmed, one must identify whether the abnormal growth pertains primarily or disproprtionately to the epiphyses, metaphyses, or diaphyses of the long bones and/or the vertebral column. If the ossified epiphyses are very small and/or irregular for age, then the diagnosis is epiphyseal dysplasia. If the metaphyses are widened, flared, and/or irregular, the diagnosis is metaphyseal dysplasia. If the diaphyses show widening, marrow space expansion, or cortical thinning or thickening, the diagnosis is diaphyseal dysplasia. If, in addition, there are abnormalities of the vertebrae, such as platyspondyly, the dysplasias get labeled as spondyloepiphyseal or spondylometaphyseal.

If there is abnormality of the epiphyses, one must check to see if there are any punctate calcifications in the cartilaginous epiphyses or around the spine. One also must check to see if there are any dislocations of major joints. Evaluate whether the abnormal-appearing bones have increased or diminished bone density. Identification of the predominant characteristic of the skeletal dysplasias allows one to consult any of the major texts on this subject (38–40). Then the clinician can refer to that specific category of predominant characteristic of skeletal dysplasias and make the appropriate diagnosis. One must ascertain that abnormal or unusual appearance of the bones is not a normal variant. The clinician, once convinced of the abnormal radiographical findings, should refer to the brilliantly presented gamut pages and discussions in the phenomenal textbook written by Drs. Hooshang Taybi and Ralph Lachman (38). Later, one should refer to scholarly textbooks entirely dedicated to the skeletal dysplasias and syndromes written by Drs. Robert Gorlin, M. Cohen, Jr., and L. Stephan Levin (39) and Drs. Jurgen Spranger, Paula Brill, and Andrew Poznanski (40) to confirm the diagnosis and learn more details about the course of the disease process and its prognosis.

Dysostosis Multiplex

The skeletal manifestations seen in children with abnormalities of complex carbohydrate degradation or lysosomal transport are fairly uniform and are summarized under the term *dysostosis multiplex*. The intralysosomal accumulation of partially degraded complex carbohydrates results in a variety of disorders that, depending on the type of stored material, have been classified as mucopolysaccharidoses, oligosaccharidoses, and glycoproteinoses.

The major radiographic findings of dysostosis multiplex are (Figure 50-16) as follows:

- *Skull and facial bones:* J-shaped sella, thick calvarium, macrocephaly, sclerotic facial bones, small or absent paranasal sinuses

- *Thorax:* Bucket handle or oar-shaped ribs, wide sclerotic clavicles, and sclerotic and plump scapulae

- *Abdomen:* Frequent hepatosplenomegaly

- *Vertebral column:* Small, oval-shaped, immature, or hook-shaped vertebral bodies

- *Pelvis and hip joints:* Flared upper iliac bones, overconstricted lower iliac bones, dysplastic capital femoral epiphyses, coxa valga deformity

- *Long bones:* Irregular diaphyseal modeling, submetaphyseal overconstriction, shortening, metaphyseal cloaking in infants with G_{M1}-gangliosidosis type I and mucolipidosis II

- *Short tubular bones:* Shortening; proximal tapering of second to fifth metatarcarpals and metatarsals, eiphyseal dysplasia

- *Overall skeleton:* Generalized osteoporosis with coarse, bony trabecular pattern

These characteristic findings can be seen in many other disorders, and hence the specific diagnosis requires clinical information, such as mental and/or developmental retardation as well as molecular and enzymatic studies. Although the severity of these changes is very useful in the differential diagnosis, one must be aware that there can be a significant phenotypic variability within any specific dysplasia.

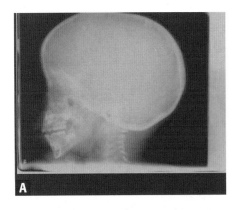

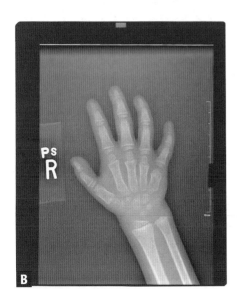

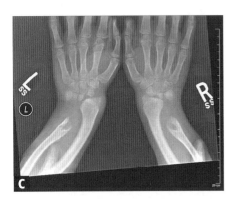

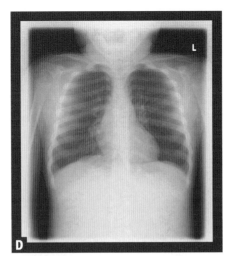

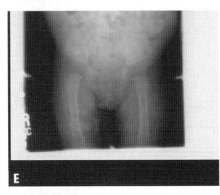

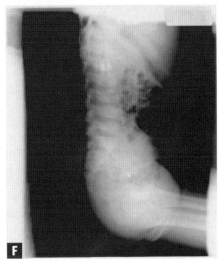

increased tendency for fractures. Osteoporosis could be primary or secondary. Primary osteoporosis is seen in children with osteogenesis imperfecta or in idiopathic forms of osteoporosis. Diseases such as chronic malnutrition, various metabolic disorders in which protein matrix formation is disturbed, or gastrointestinal disorders associated with diarrhea or malabsorption can lead to secondary osteoporosis in children.

Osteomalacia in children is associated with rickets (for details see Chapter 39). Irregular fraying and rarefaction of the provisional zones of calcification leading to metaphyseal widening and cupping are the characteristic radiographic findings (Figure 50-17). These changes are best seen in the metaphyses of the fast-growing bones in the extremities and are seen most impressively at the knees or the wrist joints.

Even though the signs and symptoms of rickets were described some 2000 years ago, it was

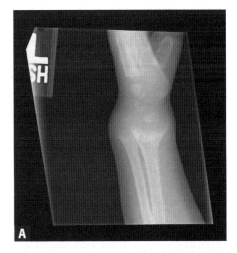

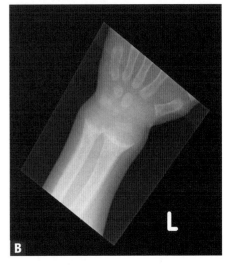

FIGURE 50-16. A to **F.** "Dysostosis Multiplex" (A) shows the lateral view of the skull with the classic "J" shaped sella. (B) shows proximal metacarpal pointing and distal articular surfaces of the radius and ulna slanted toward each other. (C) in addition to the characteristic changes of MPS, also shows Madelung deformity of the wrist. (D) shows short, thick clavicles, paddle-oar shaped ribs and hypoplastic glinoid. (E) shows steep, acetabular angles and narrow base of the ilium. (F) shows gibbus as the result of hypoplastic L1 vertebral body; contrast in the kidneys superimposed over the hypoplastic vertebral body of L1.

Osteoporosis
Osteomalacia–Rickets

Decrease in the bone density is termed as *osteopenia*. This could be secondary to osteoporosis or osteomalacia. Decreased bone mass with relatively normal mineral content is called *osteoporosis*, whereas softening of the bone from a relatively excess amount of uncalcified osteoid tissue is called *osteomalacia*.

Radiographically, in osteoporosis, there is thinning of the bony cortex and loss of bony trabecular matrix but a well preserved provisional zone of calcification. Osteoporosis is a systemic bone disease that shows altered bone architecture with reduced bone mass and an

FIGURE 50-17. A to **B.** "Osteomalacia" Metaphyseal widening, rarefaction, fraying and cupping before treatment (A). Provisional zone of calcification, which was missing, has appeared following the start of treatment (B). While metaphyseal fraying has resolved, cupping is still present.

not until the Industrial Revolution and the rapid movement of rural communities into heavily air-polluted, overcrowded, and dingy dwellings in the cities of Europe that the disease became a public health problem. Following the discovery of vitamin D, the fortification of milk and other foods and the provision of vitamin D eradicated the problem in the industrialized and civilized world. Over the past 30 years, however, there has been a resurgence of the disease, and there has been a realization that the disease has not been uncommon in several developing countries for a long time, where sunlight exposure should not be a problem.

REFERENCES

1. Elster AD, et al. Pituitary gland: MR imaging of physiologic hypertrophy of adolescence. *Radiology.* 1990;174:681–685.
2. Walmsley D, et al. Pituitary size in hypothyroidism as determined by computerized tomography. *Br J Radiol.* 1987;60:935–936.
3. Zimmerman RA. Imaging of intrasellar, suprasellar and parasellar tumors. *Semin Roentgenol.* 1990;25:174–197.
4. O'Sullivan RM, et al. Langerhans' cell histiocytosis of hypothalamus and optic chiasm: CT and MR studies. *J Comput Assist Tomogr.* 1991;15:52.
5. Pansky B. *Review of Gross Anatomy,* 3rd ed. New York: Macmillan; 1984:60–61.
6. Seigel MJ. *Pediatric Imaging,* 3rd ed. Philadelphia: Lippincott Williams & Wilkins; 2002:123–166.
7. Fort P, Brown R. *Pediatric Endocrinology: A Clinical Guide.* New York: Marcel Decker; 1966:369.
8. Sty J, et al. *Diagnostic Imaging of Infants and Children,* Vol. II. Aspen; 1992:300–301.
9. Scott MD, Crawford JO. Solitary thyroid nodules in childhood: Is incidence of thyroid carcinoma declining? *Pediatrics.* 1978;58:521–525.
10. Hung W, et al. Solitary thyroid nodules in children and adolescents. *J Pedatr Surg.* 1982;17:225–229.
11. Vieras F. Preoperative scintigraphic detection of cervical metastasis from thyroid carcinoma with technicium-99m pertechnetate *Clin Nucl Med.* 1985;10:567–569.
12. Stratakis CA, Chrousos GP. Endocrine tumors. In: Pizzo PA, Poplack DG, eds. *Principles and Practices of Pediatric Oncology,* 3rd ed. NewYork: Lippincott-Raven; 1997: 947–976.
13. McIntyre RC Jr, et al. Intrathyroid parathyroid glands can be cause of failed cervical exploration for hyperparathyroidism. *Am J. Surg.* 1997;174:750–753.
14. Picard D, et al. Localization of abnormal parathyroid gland(s) using thallium/iodine-123 subtraction scintigraphy in patients with hyperparathyroidism. *Clin Nucl Med.* 1987;12:60–64.
15. Winzelberg GG, et al. Parathyroid adenomas evaluated with thallium-201/technicium-99m pertechnetate subtraction scintigraphy and high resolution ultrasonography. *Radiology.*1985;155:231–235.
16. Pattou F, et al. Radionuclide scanning in parathyroid diseases. *Br J Surg.* 1998;85: 1605–1616.
17. Norris HJ, et al. Relative frequency of ovarian neoplasms in children and adolescents. *Cancer* 1972;30:713–719.
18. Rosenberg HK. Pediatric pelvic sonography. In: *Diagnostic Ultrasound.* New York: Elsevier–Mosby; 2005:713–719.
19. Orsini LF, et al. Pelvic organs in premenarchal girls by real time ultrasonography *Radiology* 1984;153:113–116.
20. Kogan S, et al. Pediatric andrology. In: Gillenwater JY, et al., eds. *Adult and Pediatric Urology,* 3rd ed. St. Louis: Mosby; 1996: 2623–2674.
21. Skoog SJ. Benign and malignant pediatric scrotal masses. *Pediatr Clin North Am.* 1997;44:1229–1250.
22. Coly BD, Siegel M. *Male Genital Tract in Pediatric Sonography,* 3rd ed. Philadelphia: Lippincott Williams & Wilkins; 2002:586–589.
23. Greulich WW, Pyle JS. *Radiographic Atlas of Skeletal Development of Hand and Wrist,* 2nd ed. Stanford, CA: Stanford University Press; 1959.
24. Sontag LW, et al. Rate of ossification centers from birth to the age of 5 years. *Am J Dis Child.* 1939;58:949–956.
25. Ganey TM, et al. Development of vasculature in chondroepiphysis of rabbit. *J Orthop Res.* 1992;10:496–510.
26. Braidman IP, et al. Preliminary in situ identification of estrogen target cells in bone. *J Bone Miner Res.* 1995;10:74–80.
27. Even L, et al. Bone maturation in girls with Turner syndrome. *Eur J Endocrinol.* 1998;138:59–62.
28. Mitty HA. Embryology, anatomy and anomalies of the adrenal gland. *Semin Roentgenol.* 1988;23:271–279.
29. Scott EM, et al. Serial ultrasonography in normal neonates. *J Ultrasound Med.* 1990;9:279–283.
30. Dunnick NR. Adrenal imaging: Current status. *Am J Roentgenol.* 1990;154:927–936.
31. Doppman JL, et al. Distinction between hyperaldosteronism due to bilateral hyperplasia and unilateral aldosteronoma: Reliability of CT. *Radiology.* 1992;184:677–682.
32. Al-Allwan I, Navarro O, Daneman D, et al. Clinical utility of adrenal ultrasonography in the diagnosis of congenital adrenal hyperplasia. *J Pediatr.* 1999;135:71–75.
33. New MI, et al. Adrenal hyperplasia In: Scriver CR, et al., eds. *The Metabolic Bases of Inherited Disease,* 6th ed. New York: McGraw-Hill; 1989:1881–1917.
34. Ogata T, et al. Computed tomography in the early detection of congenital lipoid adrenal hyperplasia. *Pediatr Radiol.* 1988;18:360–361.
35. Ozmen MN, et al. Wolman's disease: Ultrasonographic and computed tomographic findings. *Pediatr Radiol.* 1992;22:541–542.
36. Davies RP, et al, Ultrasonography of the pancreas in patients with multiple endocrine neoplasia type 1. *J Ultrasound Med.* 1993;12: 67–72.
37. Stark DD, BradleyWG Jr. *Magnetic Resonance Imaging,* 3rd ed. St. Louis: Mosby; 1999:471–501,
38. Taybi and Lachman's Radiology of Syndromes, Metabolic Disorders and Skeletal Dysplasias. Ed. Lachman, RS. 6th Ed. St. Louis, Mosby, 2006.
39. Gorlin RJ, Cohen MM, Levin LS. *Syndromes of the Head & Neck,* 3rd ed. Oxford, England: Oxford University Press; 1990.
40. Spranger JW, Brill PW, Poznanski A. *Dysplasias.* 2nd ed. Oxford, England: Oxford University Press; 2002.

INDEX

Note: Page numbers followed by f indicate figures; page numbers followed by t indicate tables.

A

AADC deficiency. *See* Aromatic L-amino acid decarboxylase (AADC) deficiency
Abetalipoproteinemia, 305
^{131}Ablation, for thyroid cancer, 826–827
ABS. *See* Antley—Bixler syndrome (ABS)
Abuse
  alcohol, male hypogonadism due to, 591
  drug, male hypogonadism due to, 591
Acanthosis nigrans, 282
ACC. *See* Adrenocortical cancer (ACC)
Aceruloplasminemia, 667, 671, 671f
Acetoacetate, laboratory investigations of, in mitochondrial disorders, 864, 864t
N-Acetyl glutamate synthetase (NAGS) deficiency, 142–144, 145f
  clinical presentation of, 142, 144–145
  findings in, 142
N-Acetylaspartic aciduria, 110f, 113–114, 114f
  causes of, 113–114
  clinical presentation of, 110f, 114
  diagnosis of, 114, 114t
  pathophysiology of, 113–114
  treatment and outcome of, 114
N-Acetylglucosamine-β-1,2-galactosyltransferase 1 (CDG-IId) deficiency, 339f, 340, 342, 344f, 350–351, 351t
Acid maltase deficiency, 728, 750–751, 751t
Acid-labile subunit, in GH sufficiency determination, 887t, 890
Acidosis(es)
  lactic, in IBEM, 5
  metabolic
    DKA and, 12, 12t
    normal anion gap and, 699, 699t
    renal tubular, proximal, 694, 698–700, 698f, 699f, 699t
Acrodermatitis acidemia, 88, 88f
Acrodermatitis enteropathica, 668, 672
ACTH concentrations, in adrenal insufficiency, 879
ACTH deficiency
  in cancer survivors, 844, 848–849
  isolated, 420, 422, 432
ACTH measurement, in Cushing syndrome diagnosis, 414–415, 878
ACTH-dependent Cushing syndrome, 411
  diagnosis of, 414–415
ACTH-independent Cushing syndrome, 411
Acute insulin response tests, in recessive K_{ATP} hyperinsulism, 42, 42f

Acylation-stimulating hormone (ASP), in insulin sensitivity, 278
Acylcarnitine profile, laboratory investigations of, 863–864, 863t, 864t
Acyl-CoA oxidase deficiency, 324–325, 326f, 333
Addison disease
  in endocrine testing, 879
  hyperpigmentation associated with, 419, 419f
Adenine phosphoribosyltransferase (APRT) deficiency, 758, 759, 769, 770f
Adenosine deaminase deficiency, 758, 759, 769, 771f, 772
Adenosylcobalamin deficiency cblA cblB, 196–197, 209–210, 209f
S-Adenosyl-homocysteine (SAH), 185
S-Adenosyl-homocysteine hydrolase (SAHH) deficiency, 185f, 186, 188–189, 189f, 189t
  causes of, 188–189
  clinical information related to, 189
  clinical presentation of, 186, 189
  diagnosis of, 189, 189t
  pathophysiology of, 188–189, 189f
  treatment of, 189
S-Adenosylmethionine (SAM), 185
  for MAT I/III deficiency, 188
Adenylosuccinate lyase deficiency, 758, 759, 766, 768f, 769
ADHAPS. *See* Alkyldihydroxyacetonephosphate synthase (ADHAPS)
ADHR. *See* Autosomal dominant hypophosphatemic rickets (ADHR)
Adipocyte factors, in insulin sensitivity, 278
Adipocyte-derived hormones, 277–278, 277t
Adiponectin, 278
Adiposity, measurement of, in overweight evaluation, 284–285, 285t
Adolescent menstrual disorders, 601–616
  amenorrhea, 602–604, 609–615. *See also* Amenorrhea
  dysfunctional uterine bleeding (DUB), 602, 603, 606
  dysmenorrhea, 602, 603, 607–609
  exogenous androgens, 603, 604, 615
  glucocorticoid excess, 603, 604, 613
  hyperprolactinemia, 602, 604, 611–612, 611f
  intermenstrual bleeding, 602, 603, 607
  menometrorrhagia, 602, 603, 607, 608t
  menorrhagia, 602, 603, 606–607
  metrorrhagia, 602, 603, 607
  nonclassic CAH due to 21OHD, 603, 604, 614–615

PCOS, 603, 604, 613–614
  thyroid diseases, 603, 604, 612–613
  tumor-related androgen excess, 603, 604, 615
Adoption studies, obesity related to, 279
Adrenal cortex tumors, imaging of, 901, 908
Adrenal crisis
  acute, emergency assessment and management of, 10–11, 11t
  not associated with salt wasting, 11
  severe, signs and symptoms of, 11t
  treatment of, 11, 11t, 396
Adrenal glands
  anatomy of, 385
  disorders of, 383–437
  embryology of, 385
  function of, tests of, 876, 876t
  imaging of, 901, 908–910
    adrenal cortex tumors, 901, 908
    adrenal medulla, 901, 909–910
    CAH, 901, 908–909
    enzymatic defects, 901, 908–909
    metabolic diseases, 901, 908–909
Adrenal hemorrhage, 420, 432
Adrenal hyperplasia
  congenital, 383–410, 507–508. *See also* Congenital adrenal hyperplasia (CAH)
Adrenal hypoplasia, congenital, 420, 421, 425–426. *See also* Congenital adrenal hypoplasia (AHC)
Adrenal insufficiency, 419–437. *See also specific types and disorders*
  acute, emergency assessment and management of, 10–11, 11t
  aldosterone deficiency, 433–434
  in cancer survivors, 844, 848–849
  candidiasis and, 430–431
  corticosterone methyloxidase deficiency types 1 and 2, 433–434
  described, 419
  familial hyperreninemic hypoaldosteronism type 2, 420, 422, 434
  infectious, 431–432
  newborn screening in, 424
  pseudohypoaldosteronism, 420, 422, 434–435
  prenatal diagnosis of, 424, 424f
  primary, 425–432, 430t
    adrenal hemorrhage, 420, 432
    AHC, 420, 421, 425–426
    adrenal leukodystrophy (ALD), 420, 421, 427
    autoimmune polyglandular syndrome (APS) and, 420–422, 430–431, 430t